ADVANCED
CLINICAL
NATUROPATHIC
MEDICINE

ADVANCED CLINICAL NATUROPATHIC MEDICINE

Leah Hechtman

MSci Med(RHHG), BHSc(Nat), ND, FNHAA

Director, The Natural Health and Fertility Centre
Sydney, Australia

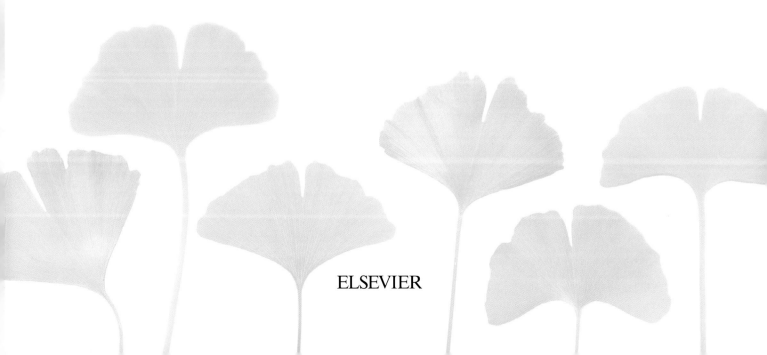

ELSEVIER

ELSEVIER

Elsevier Australia. ACN 001 002 357
(a division of Reed International Books Australia Pty Ltd)
Tower 1, 475 Victoria Avenue, Chatswood, NSW 2067

ISBN: 978-0-7295-4265-4

National Library of Australia Cataloguing-in-Publication Data

 A catalogue record for this book is available from the National Library of Australia

Content Strategist: Larissa Norrie
Content Project Manager: Shruti Raj
Edited by Katie Millar
Proofread by Tim Learner
Permissions Editing and Photo Research: Sarah Thomas and Praveen Kumar
Cover and internal design by Georgette Hall
Index by SPi Global
Typeset by Toppan Best-set Premedia Limited
Printed by Markono Print Media Pte Ltd

Reprinted 2021

Last digit is the print number: 9 8 7 6 5 4 3 2

Acknowledgments

It is with much gratitude that we birth *Advanced Clinical Naturopathic Medicine* (ACNM). ACNM was developed from a yearning to contribute more deeply to the naturopathic body of work, to support the development of the evolving profession and to guide clinicians and students through complicated areas of expertise and specialisation. ACNM brings together a team of true experts to achieve this vision.

As with CNM, a book of this depth requires the commitment and dedication of a number of individuals, and I am again deeply grateful to and humbled by those I have been privileged to work with to achieve this collaborative goal.

In order of their contribution, my appreciation to Natalie Cook, Nicole Bijlsma, Dr Joseph Pizzorno, Dr John Nowicki, Dr Kate Broderick, Dr Jason Hawrelak, Dr Joanna Harnett, Annalies Corse, Dr Rhona Creegan, Dr Margaret Smith, Dr Brad Lichtenstein, Kira Sutherland, Angela Hywood, Jane Hutchens, Dawn Whitten, Tabitha McIntosh, Helen Padarin, Belinda Robson, Justin Sinclair, Dr Janet Schloss, Manuela Boyle, Teresa Mitchell-Patterson and Dr Nicola McFadzean Ducharme. A special note of gratitude goes to Liesl Blott for her contribution of each of the interaction tables for each chapter; as well as Lisa Costa Bir for the dietary plans for each condition. It has been an honour to include your contributions, learn from you and understand your knowledge and expertise more deeply.

Additionally, my heartfelt thanks to Dr Sue Evans for writing the Foreword of this text. For this volume, I was intent on ensuring a balance of the sexes and ideally wanted someone Australian who I perceive as a wise elder, firmly rooted in the history and tradition of our treatments and philosophies and connected to and practising our evolving practice. Sue, you embody all of these admirable attributes and your humble wisdom shines through as always. Thank you.

My sincere appreciation to the wonderful team at Elsevier. The integrity of those involved was highly evident and I am most appreciative of their respective kindness, commitment and dedication to producing the best possible text. Much gratitude to Larissa Norrie, Vanessa Ridehalgh, Shruti Raj, Katie Millar and others.

Thank you to Cheryl le Roux for your dedication and commitment to the project as my research assistant. Your ongoing enthusiasm, kindness and ethical core strove to ensure we produced the most accurate and thorough work. I am blessed to be able to work with you. Many thanks for putting up with my perpetual enquiring mind.

To my colleagues at UNSW, it is from my connections with you all that I am able to critically assess and contribute meaningfully in an academic context. You have supported me to seek and find answers to my enquiries which consistently provide foundational platforms with which to expand as a clinician and educator. Learning, growth and contribution are some of my core values, and my gratitude for these opportunities that you bestow on me are heartfelt and celebrated. Thank you.

To my fellow colleagues clinically and academically, lecturers past and present, mentors and friends, I am blessed to have connected with incredible people who challenge, inspire and guide me so that we can all contribute more meaningfully and help others.

A special thank you to my family, friends and spiritual family. Your love, compassion and kindness enrich and support me to be of greater service and contribution.

Finally, my gratitude to my patients – past, present and future. It is the relationships I share with my patients, their stories, journeys and experiences that drive me to seek out answers to understand and to provide help and support. Without these heartfelt experiences, I would not be as moved or determined to push, to search, to seek and to find how I can help. When your heart is touched and a connection felt, it is the humility of the experience that opens up the universe to you to find answers. I am deeply grateful for each person I am privileged to treat.

Preface

The release of *Advanced Clinical Naturopathic Medicine* (ACNM) is a hallmark achievement supporting the evolving practice of the profession. No longer limited to merely general practice, clinicians have broadened and expanded into specialty practices. This shift in our treatment has seen more specific courses and sub-practices develop, with clinicians narrowing their focus to key areas of expertise.

That the contributors in ACNM are experts in their fields is evident. All have completed advanced training and have years of clinical experience and a deep love of their specialty areas. The chapters showcase the many diverse pathways within the profession and highlight both the opportunities for aspiring clinicians as well as the depth of practice required to truly excel in these specialty areas of expertise.

Each contributor elevates their knowledge. All aspects of their careers aptly highlight the commitment and dedication required to perfect and hone their craft.

ACNM offers both new and experienced clinicians, educators and researchers an opportunity to dive into the hearts and minds of these leaders. It showcases how truly transformative and effective naturopathy is and offers insight into the depth of our practice.

As with *Clinical Naturopathic Medicine*, the publishing of this text is an opportunity for the profession to reclaim and celebrate our vital role in the healthcare system. Our system of healing is unique and relevant; our treatments efficacious and therapeutic; our methodology and outcomes logical and supportive.

I hope this text provides assurance for clinicians and gives them confidence to take on more responsibility and be more active in the welfare of their patients' wellbeing; certainty to be more forthright and transparent with treatment strategies, methodologies and approaches; and determination to consistently strive for excellence and have the patient's best interests at heart.

Naturopathic core principles guide our intentions, with patient-centred care as the primary principle. Our elders always focused on the importance of the inter-relationship between clinician, patient and nature.

My hope is that ACNM provides the platform with which to seek answers and formulate the best care possible.

Leah Hechtman
March 2020

About the Author

MSciMed(RHHG), BHSc(Naturopathy), ND, FNHAA

Leah is an experienced and respected clinician and has been in private practice for over 20 years. She specialises in fertility, pregnancy and reproductive healthcare for men and women and holds fellowships and memberships with a number of International organisations.

She has completed extensive advanced training and is currently completing her PhD through the School of Women's and Children's Health (Faculty of Medicine [UNSW]).

Leah is the Director of The Natural Health and Fertility Centre in Sydney, Australia, where she maintains her clinical practice.

She is a keynote speaker at conferences locally and internationally to both the functional and the complementary medicine communities as well as the wider fertility and gynaecological areas of medicine. She is the author of multiple seminal naturopathic textbooks and is a contributor to journals and other texts within the naturopathic and functional medicine areas, as well as general gynaecology, fertility and infertility.

Most importantly, she is a mother to two gorgeous boys who keep her grounded, humbled and consciously aware. They have helped and continue to help her be a better version of herself and provide insight and direction for her spiritual practice.

Contents

List of Contributors

Nicole Bijlsma
ND, BHScAc(HONS), Grad Dip OHS,
    Adv Dip Building Biology
RMIT researcher
Vice President of Australasian Society
    of Building Biologists, Australia

Liesl Blott
PGradDip(MM), BPharm,
    BHSc(Herbal Med), AdvDip(Nat),
    Cert IV Assessment & Workplace
    Training
Adjunct Senior Lecturer, School of
    Pharmacy and Biomedical
    Sciences, Curtin University, Perth,
    Western Australia, Australia

Kate Broderick
BSc, JD, DNM, DipAcu
Lecturer, Naturopathic Medicine,
    Endeavour College of Natural
    Health, Adelaide, South Australia,
    Australia
Anam Chara Natural Health, Adelaide,
    South Australia, Australia

Manuela Malaguti Boyle
MPH, MHSc, BHSc(Complementary
    Medicine), BA(Journalism), Adv
    Dip Naturopathy. Certified
    Functional Medicine Practitioner
Institute of Functional Medicine,
    Washington, United States
Fellow of Integrative Oncology
    University of Arizona, USA
Clinician
Author
Public speaker
Expert Advisor SDG 3 WHIS, United
    Kingdom, NHAA Australia, AIMA
    Australia

Natalie Cook
MPH, BHSc(Nat), BCom(Mkt)
Director of Innovation, Industry &
    Employability, Health, Torrens
    University Australia (Southern
    School of Natural Therapies and
    Australasian College of Natural
    Therapies), Fitzroy, Victoria,
    Australia
Fellow and Past President of the
    Naturopaths and Herbalists
    Association of Australia
Committee member, World
    Naturopathic Federation

Annalies Corse
BMedSc, BHSc
Senior Lecturer, Health and Medical
    Sciences, Laureate Universities,
    Sydney, New South Wales,
    Australia
Naturopathic Practitioner, Private
    Clinical Practice, Sydney, New
    South Wales, Australia
Academic Writer, Postgrad Lecturer,
    Presenter, Medical and Health
    Sciences, New South Wales,
    Australia

Lisa Costa Bir
BAppSc(Nat), GradDip(Nat), MATMS
Lecturer and Supervisor, Nutrition
    and Naturopathy, Endeavour
    College of Natural Health, Sydney,
    New South Wales, Australia

Rhona Creegan
PhD, MSc Clinical Biochemistry, MSc
    Nutrition Medicine, BSc
    Biomedical Sciences
Owner Omega Nutrition Health,
    Perth, Western Australia,
    Australia

Nicola Ducharme
ND, BHSc(Naturopathy), BA,
    Doctorate of Naturopathic
    Medicine, Bastyr University,
    Seattle, WA, USA
Owner and Medical Director of
    RestorMedicine, San Diego, CA,
    USA
Creator of Lyme-Ed Online Programs
    For Patients and Practitioners
Author of The Lyme Diet, The
    Beginners Guide to Lyme Disease,
    Lyme Disease in Australia, Lyme
    Brain

Joanna Harnett
PhD, MHSc, BHSc(Complementary
    Medicine), Grad Dip Clin
    Nutrition, Grad Cert Educational
    Studies, Adv Dip Naturopathy
Lecturer Complementary Medicines,
    The University of Sydney School
    of Pharmacy, Faculty of Medicine
    and Health, New South Wales,
    Australia
Fellow of the Australian Research
    Centre in Complementary and
    Integrative Medicine, Ultimo,
    New South Wales, Australia

Jason Hawrelak
ND, BNat(Hons), PhD, FNHAA,
    MASN, FACN
Senior Lecturer in Complementary
    and Alternative Medicines,
    College of Health & Medicine,
    University of Tasmania
Visiting Research Fellow, Australian
    Research Centre for
    Complementary & Integrative
    Medicine, University of
    Technology Sydney
Clinical Director, Goulds Natural
    Medicine, Hobart, Tasmania,
    Australia

Leah Hechtman
MSciMed(RHHG), BHSc(Nat), ND, FNHAA
Director, The Natural Health and Fertility Centre, Sydney, New South Wales, Australia

Jane Hutchens
MScMed(RH&HG), BHealthSc, AdvDipNat, BA, RN
Research Assistant, Australian Centre for Public and Population Health Research, The University of Technology, Sydney, New South Wales, Australia
Lecturer, Torrens University, Pyrmont, New South Wales, Australia
Private Practitioner, Minerva Natural Health & Fertility, Blaxland, NSW, Australia

Angela Hywood
BHSc(Complementary Medicine), AdvDipCN, AdvDipNat, AdvDipMH, DipNFM

Brad S. Lichtenstein
ND, BCB, BCB-HRV
Associate and Clinical Professor, Bastyr University, Kenmore, WA

Tabitha McIntosh
BMedSci, AdvDipNat, DipNut, PostGradCert Nutritional and Environmental Science
Director Awaken Your Health, NSW, Australia

Teresa Mitchell-Paterson
AdvDip(Nat), BHSc(CompMed), MHSc(HumNut)
Senior Lecturer, Nutritional Medicine, Torrens University, Sydney, New South Wales, Australia

John Nowicki
BS(Biology), ND
Independent Medical Researcher/ Writer/Editor, Seattle, USA

Helen Padarin
BHSc(Nat), ND, DN, DBM, DRM
Clinical Naturopath, Nutritionist and Herbalist, Sydney, New South Wales, Australia

Joseph Pizzorno
BS(Chemistry), ND
Founding President, Bastyr University, Washington, United States
Co-editor, *Textbook of Natural Medicine*
Editor-in-Chief, *Integrative Medicine, A Clinician's Journal*
Chair, Board of Directors, Institute for Functional Medicine
Member, Board of Directors, Institute for Naturopathic Medicine, Seattle, USA

Belinda Robson
MHlthSc(DD), BNat, AssocDegAppSc
Member of the Naturopaths and Herbalist Association of Australia
Goulds Natural Medicine, Hobart, Tasmania, Australia

Janet Schloss
PhD(medicine), PGC-Clin Nut, AdvDip-HS(Nat), DipNut, Dip HM, BARM
Endeavour College of Natural Health, 269 Wickham St, Fortitude Valley Qld 4006
Fellow at ARCCIM University of Technology Sydney, Ultimo NSW

Justin Sinclair
MHerbMed(USyd), BHSc(Nat)
Research Fellow, NICM Health Research Institute, Western Sydney University, New South Wales, Australia
Coordinator, Australian Medicinal Cannabis Research & Education Collaboration, New South Wales, Australia
Principal Consultant, Traditional Medicine Consultancy, Sydney, New South Wales, Australia
Scientific Advisory Board, United in Compassion (Registered Charity)

Dr Margaret Smith
NZCS, FNZIMLS, MHGSA, BSc(Hons), PhD
Molecular Geneticist, smartDNA Pty Ltd, MHTP Translational Research Facility, Level H04 27-31 Wright Street, Clayton, Victoria 3168, Australia

Kira Sutherland
PostGradDip(Sports Nutrition/IOC), BHSc, AdvDipNat, AdvDipNut, AdvDipHM, DipHom
Lecturer Naturopathy and Nutritional Medicine, Endeavour College of Natural Health, Sydney, New South Wales, Australia
Lecturer Naturopathy and Nutritional Medicine, Torrens University, Sydney, New South Wales, Australia
Member of the Australian Traditional Medicine Society

Dawn Whitten
BNat(Hons), IBCLC
Unit Coordinator, College of Health and Medicine, University of Tasmania, Australia
Clinical Director, Goulds Natural Medicine, Hobart, Tasmania, Australia
Researcher and Educator, ProbioticAdvisor.com

Global naturopathic medicine

Natalie Cook

Naturopathic medicine draws on a rich history of practice that extends many thousands of years. Humans have long needed to rely on the resources of nature for health and healing, and the use of plants as therapeutic agents is well documented through the history of human civilisation. Using plants as a source of medicine as well as for their nutritional value has consistently been observed in cultures over time. Other therapies, including the use of water, heat and cold, and other therapeutic regimens have also variously been used to harness the healing power of nature or *vis medicatrix naturae*. Naturopathy grew from these traditions around the turn of the 20th century and is today practised in over 80 countries around the world. Modern naturopathy combines the best of traditional medicine with contemporary science as a practice that is steeped in tradition while incorporating modern clinical advances. The manner in which the profession is recognised and regulated varies around the world; however, consistency in core beliefs as well as commitment to high standards in education, practice and codes of conduct bind the profession together as a system of medicine that makes a positive contribution to global health.

GLOBAL SCOPE OF NATUROPATHIC MEDICINE

If we could look at a time-lapse image of naturopathy as it has spread around the world from its beginnings until today, we would commence viewing in the 1800s in Europe, specifically in Germany and Austria. The early work of Vincent Priessnitz (1847–1884) and Johann Schroth (1798–1856) from Austria together with Sebastian Kneipp (1821–1897) and Louis Kuhne (1835–1901) from Germany brought together a number of modalities including herbal medicine, hydrotherapy and nutrition, and their 'Nature Cure' movement laid the foundation for modern naturopathy. Benedict Lust (1872–1945), an American who became a student of Kneipp after being cured by his treatments, moved back to the United States in the 1890s and popularised the term 'naturopathy' that was coined by John Scheel around 1900. Prior to this, the term 'naturheilkunde' was first documented by German physician Lorenz Geich (1798–1835), while 'naturheilkuner'

was used by Kneipp. John Scheel translated these terms into English as 'naturopathy' and Lust bought the right to use this term in 1901. Lust went on to found the American School of Naturopathy in New York City as well as the Naturopathic Society of America, which later became the American Naturopathic Association, and thus is regarded as the father of modern naturopathy for the English-speaking world.[1]

The practice of naturopathy spread from these two epicentres in Germanic Europe and north eastern America as students of those forefathers migrated throughout the US and Europe, and swiftly extended as far as Australia by 1904. Today, naturopathy is practised in over 80 countries – over one-third of the countries around the world – by an estimated 75 000–100 000 practitioners.[2,3] The greatest concentrations are found in Germany and Spain, with a reported 20 000 practitioners in each country, and generally it holds true that the longer naturopathy has been practised in a country, the more naturopaths are found to practise there.[2]

The scale of naturopathic medicine can be better appreciated by considering this summary of key figures, which are likely conservative estimates as the global profession continues to be better understood[3]:

- Countries that practise naturopathic medicine = 80+
- National professional associations = 80+
- Naturopathic educational institutions = 90+
- Naturopathic research centres = 20+

Naturopathic practice by world region

TERMINOLOGY

The most common term for those practising naturopathy used in nearly 80% of the world is 'naturopath'. Some countries refer to practitioners as a naturopathic doctor or naturopathic physician, and approximately 10% refer to practitioners as a 'natural medicine doctor' or 'heilpraktiker'. Other terms that may be used around the world to represent naturopathy include: Nature Cure, Natural Medicine, Naturopathía, Naturopathie, Praticien de santé – Naturopathe, Terapêuticas Não Convencionais, Medicina Naturista, Naturopatia ou Medicina Natural, Naturheilkunde.[2]

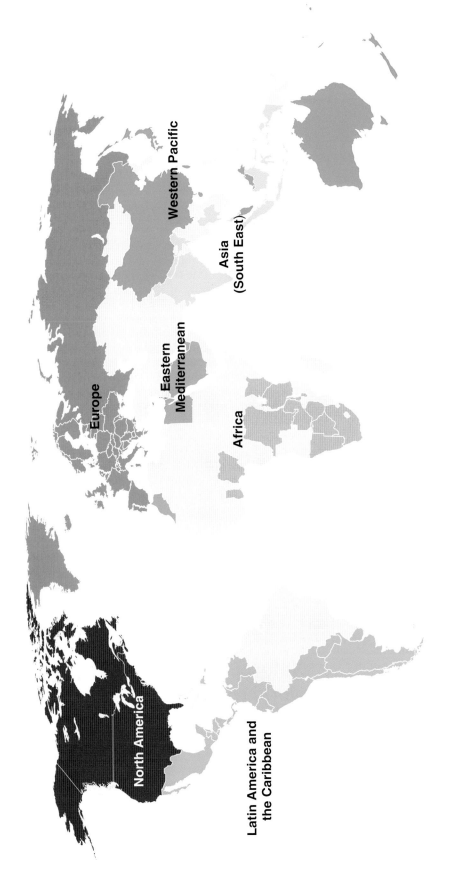

*Note, the world regions are based on the six WHO world regions with the addition of representing the 'Region of the Americas' as 'North America' and 'Latin America and the Caribbean' due to quite different models of practice between the two regions.

Africa: Botswana, Democratic Republic of Congo, Ghana, Kenya, Mauritius, Namibia, Nigeria, South Africa, United Republic of Tanzania, Zambia and Zimbabwe

Asia (South East): India, Indonesia, Nepal and Thailand

Eastern Mediterranean: Bahrain, Egypt, Kuwait, Morocco, Qatar, Saudi Arabia and United Arab Emirates

Europe: Austria, Belgium, Bosnia and Herzegovina, Cyprus, Czech Republic, Denmark, Finland, France, Germany, Greece, Hungary, Iceland, Ireland, Israel, Italy, Luxembourg, Netherlands, Norway, Portugal, Romania, Russia, Slovenia, Spain, Sweden, Switzerland, Ukraine and United Kingdom.

Latin America and the Caribbean: Argentina, Bahamas, Barbados, Bermuda, Chile, Colombia, Costa Rica, Ecuador, El Salvador, Guatemala, Honduras, Mexico, Nicaragua, Panama, Paraguay, Peru, Puerto Rico, Saint Lucia, Uruguay, Venezuela and Virgin Islands (US).

North America: Canada and the US.

Western Pacific: Australia, China, Hong Kong (China), Japan, Malaysia, New Zealand, Singapore and Vanuatu.

FIGURE 1.1 Countries that practise naturopathic medicine, by world region*[3]

The terms 'naturopath' and 'naturopathic doctor' are prevalent in English and non-English-speaking countries alike and although similar, the terms tend not to be interchangeable. History, culture, education and the regulatory environment of the countries in which they practise shape the different terms used to describe practitioners of naturopathy. Naturopaths and naturopathic doctors in particular tend to be differentiated by levels of education and regulation. While there is a great deal of alignment with the fundamental principles and philosophy taught in both cases, the term naturopathic doctor is used in countries where the education standards require more hours and with a greater emphasis on medical assessment in addition to holistic understanding. This often then corresponds to increased scope of practice, as more physically invasive examinations (such as taking blood) and laboratory testing may be included. The regulatory environment supporting naturopathic doctors may include government accreditation of institutions as well as uniform board exams to gain entry to the profession as a registered practitioner. Countries such as the US, Canada and South Africa register their naturopathic practitioners as naturopathic doctors and follow this model. Other countries, such as Australia, may be well recognised for their high standards of education yet are not regulated by national or regional government accreditation processes for either practitioners or institutions. The profession is not subject to statutory regulation and the education required of a naturopath, while based on a strong health science foundation, tends to have some limitations in terms of scope of practice (for more detail, refer to the section 'A global profession – similarities and differences', which discusses the similarities and differences around the world).

Global impact

It is difficult to quantify the impact of naturopathy globally. Arguably, a focus on preventive health and a reduction in reliance on mainstream health systems would suggest that naturopathy could play a significant role in global health goals. Indicators that can be measured in support of this notion include the degree to which traditional medicine is used, particularly in developing countries. The economic value of the herbal and supplement industries is also relevant in considering impact, as naturopathy is a system of health that often prescribes the use of herbal and nutritional supplements. Additionally, as naturopathic practice takes a proactive stance in relation to disease prevention and patient education, it aligns naturally with local and global public health goals.[4]

In a number of countries (such as some African nations), traditional medicine practitioners outnumber medical doctors by a factor of 80 : 1. In these circumstances, traditional medicine is the only viable medical choice for many people.[5] Additionally, where traditional medicine has a strong historical basis and cultural influence, such as in developed countries including Singapore or Korea, it is often preferred even when contemporary medicine services are available.[5]

Herbal medicine sales may be difficult to measure, as regulations differ around the world and definitions of plants as foods or medicines may also vary. As an indication of scale, Chinese herbal medicine sales were worth an estimated US$83.1 billion globally in 2012.[5] In the US, expenditure on natural products was US$14.8 billion in 2008.[5] Market research analysing the worldwide market for herbal supplements estimates this to grow to US$115 billion by 2020.[6]

GLOBAL HEALTH GOVERNANCE: THE WORLD HEALTH ORGANISATION

The World Health Organization (WHO) recognises the important role traditional and complementary medicine (T&CM) plays as part of a global healthcare solution. The following statement made in a speech at the International Conference on Traditional Medicine for South-East Asian Countries (February 2013) reaffirms this value:

> Traditional medicines, of proven quality, safety, and efficacy, contribute to the goal of ensuring that all people have access to care. For many millions of people, herbal medicines, traditional treatments, and traditional practitioners are the main source of health care, and sometimes the only source of care. This is care that is close to homes, accessible and affordable. It is also culturally acceptable and trusted by large numbers of people. The affordability of most traditional medicines makes them all the more attractive at a time of soaring health-care costs and nearly universal austerity. Traditional medicine also stands out as a way of coping with the relentless rise of chronic non-communicable diseases.
>
> **WHO Director-General (2013), Dr Margaret Chan[5] p. 16**

It is important to context naturopathy within WHO policy. Traditional medicine is differentiated from Complementary and Alternative Medicine (CAM), with the former term applied to health systems indigenous to different cultures 'used in the maintenance of health as well as in the prevention, diagnosis, improvement or treatment of physical and mental illness.'[5] While in many cases the terms are used interchangeably, the WHO defines CAM as 'a broad set of health care practices that are not part of that country's own tradition and are not integrated into the dominant health care system'.[5] Given this distinction, and for the purposes of considering global recognition, naturopathy is considered as CAM, although much of the WHO guidelines and policy relate to both without differentiation.

WHO Traditional Medicine Strategy 2014–2023

This strategy document outlines the goals, objectives and actions of the WHO in supporting use of T&CM in a safe, respectful, cost-efficient and effective manner.[5] This applies to all modalities that may be considered T&CM, including naturopathy, and builds on previous WHO reports including the *International Meeting on Global Atlas of Traditional Medicine* and the *WHO Traditional Medicine Strategy 2002-2005*. The goals and objectives of the strategy revolve around the quality and affordable provision of healthcare, which supports the United Nations resolution for universal health coverage, which is considered an essential component of the United Nations sustainable development goals for health.[7] A brief summary of the key elements of the strategy follows:

WHO traditional and complementary medicine goals

Whether as a continuing part of traditional cultural behaviour or as a growing practice in Western countries, T&CM plays a recognised role in global health, and the WHO seeks to harness this contribution in line with the broader mission of ensuring the fundamental right to health for all people of the globe via universal health coverage. The strategy articulates two goals in achieving this[4]:

1   harnessing the potential contribution of T&CM to health, wellness and people-centred healthcare
2   promoting the safe and effective use of T&CM by regulating, researching and integrating TM products, practitioners and practice into health systems, where appropriate.

WHO traditional and complementary medicine objectives

T&CM represents many different health professions globally. Some are steeped in long history of use, while others such as naturopathy have a more recent history. Recognising this diversity both across countries and within countries, yet across modalities, the WHO strives for consistency in policy, safety access and usage:

1   **Policy** – integrate T&CM within national healthcare systems, where feasible, by developing and implementing national T&CM policies and programs.
2   **Safety, efficacy and quality** – promote the safety, efficacy and quality of T&CM by expanding the knowledge base, and providing guidance on regulatory and quality assurance standards.
3   **Access** – increase the availability and affordability of T&CM, with an emphasis on access for poor populations.
4   **Rational use** – promote therapeutically sound use of appropriate T&CM by practitioners and consumers.

Actions at a country level

The WHO recognises challenges associated with achieving these objectives. Challenges include appropriate education and training, professional regulation, research and assurance of product quality, safety and efficacy. The strategy focuses on three key actions member states are encouraged to take:

1   **build the knowledge base** that will allow T&CM to be managed actively through appropriate national policies

that understand and recognise the role and potential of T&CM.
2   **strengthen the quality assurance, safety, proper use and effectiveness** of T&CM by regulating products, practices and practitioners through T&CM education and training, skills development, services and therapies.
3   **promote universal health coverage by integrating T&CM** services into health service delivery and self-healthcare by capitalising on their potential contribution to improve health services and health outcomes, and by ensuring users are able to make informed choices about self-healthcare.

WHO benchmarks for training

The WHO has developed benchmarks for training for a number of T&CM practices including traditional Chinese medicine, chiropractic, osteopathy and naturopathy. The benchmarks for naturopathy are broad, and it should be noted that a number of the consultants involved in creating the naturopathic document were from Ayurvedic medicine and Chinese medicine rather than naturopathic representatives. Areas of study deemed as a requirement include: (1) basic sciences, including anatomy, physiology and pathology; (2) clinical sciences including physical examination and clinical assessment; (3) naturopathic sciences, modalities and principles, including naturopathic history and philosophy, botanical medicine and nutrition; and (4) clinical training and supervised practice.[8]

Regulatory systems

Countries are responsible for establishing their own medicines regulatory authorities (MRAs), and the WHO stipulates these should have a 'solid legal basis ... sustainable financing, access to up-to-date evidence based information (and) capacity to exert effective market control'.[8] In Australia, this agency is the Therapeutic Goods Authority (TGA); in the United States, it is the US Food and Drug Administration (FDA). Often, however, these agencies do not have sufficient knowledge of T&CM. One area of confusion is due to the fact that a plant may be considered as a food, a supplement or a herbal medicine in different countries. The WHO recommendations only extend to the therapeutic substances, not the practice of T&CM.[9]

World health assembly

Every year the WHO convenes a World Health Assembly (WHA) in Geneva, Switzerland. This is the decision-making function of the WHO where all member countries across the six world regions are represented. It is the largest, most important health assembly in the world, and at the 68th World Health Assembly in 2015, representatives from the World Naturopathic Federation (WNF) were in attendance to begin formalising relations with the WHO. In 2016 at the 69th World Health Assembly, resolution WHA69.24 'Strengthening integrated people-centred health services' urged WHO member states to 'integrate, where appropriate, T&CM into health services, based on national context and knowledge-based policies, while assuring the safety, quality and effectiveness of health services and taking into account a holistic approach to health'.[10]

GLOBAL REPRESENTATION: THE WORLD NATUROPATHIC FEDERATION

It is in the best interests of health professions that are practised around the world to have national bodies that support and promote their system of medicine, and to address issues that affect the profession globally. These bodies also provide a vehicle to consult with international organisations such as the WHO and the United Nations on key initiatives. To do so, a federation of national associations must be formed according to WHO guidelines; until recently, while other global professions such as chiropractic and traditional Chinese medicine had been represented at this level, naturopathy had not. To meet WHO guidelines, federations must have member countries from all WHO world regions who are able to vote, and the governing board must also demonstrate global representation. The formation of the WNF in 2015 ensured that naturopathy too has a voice on the world stage. A world federation such as this is able to address issues that affect the profession at large and support standards of education, accreditation and regulation for the profession globally.[11]

History

The WNF was officially incorporated as a not-for-profit organisation in Canada in November 2014. This followed a number of years of work by a small group of dedicated naturopathic practitioners to ensure the naturopathic profession was represented in a way that befits the significant numbers of practitioners positively contributing to healthcare around the world. This was preceded by several key events including the 1st International Congress on Naturopathic Medicine (ICNM) held in Paris in 2013, at which discussions were held about forming a formal world naturopathic organisation. At the 2nd ICNM conference in Paris in July 2014, a meeting of over 30 naturopaths/ naturopathic doctors from 20 countries agreed that the WNF would be established. An interim committee was formed consisting of representatives from Australia, Belgium, Canada, France, India, New Zealand, Spain and the US. The inaugural meeting of the WNF was hosted at the Canadian Association of Naturopathic Doctors (CAND) Health Fusion conference in Calgary in June 2015. The initial executive of the WNF was formed by four practitioners from around the world who had been involved in various aspects of the formation of the WNF: Dr Iva Lloyd, ND from Canada (President of the WNF), Dr Tina Hausser, HP, ND from Spain (Vice President of the WNF), Ysu Umbalo, ND from DR Congo (Secretary of the WNF) and Michael Cronin from the US (Treasurer of the WNF). Additionally, Dr Jon Wardle, PhD from Australia, and Dr Tabatha Parker, ND from the US, who founded Naturopathic Doctors International, were appointed Co-Secretaries General.[2,12]

Membership of the WNF

The primary voting members of the WNF are national naturopathic organisations from countries that practise naturopathy. The largest national professional association in a country that represents naturopathy (as its primary focus) can join as a full member to represent its country. In some instances, a country-based federation of several associations may perform this role, although each country still has only one vote. Full members all share a common commitment to high standards of education, training and professionalism within their country. Associate members are regional naturopathic professional associations that likewise share goals and objectives that are consistent with those of the WNF. Education providers that focus on the education of naturopaths and naturopathic doctors are also able to join the WNF as educational members; like associate members, they are not able to vote, but they are able to observe meetings and participate in working groups. Additionally, as a not-for-profit organisation, the WNF receives financial support from corporate, private and non-profit sponsors. All WHO world regions are represented through membership of the WNF, which is governed by an Executive Council composed of 11 full members, four of which are the WNF Officers.[12]

What the WNF does

The vision of the WNF is to provide a global voice for naturopathy. The mission is to support the growth and diversity of naturopathic medicine worldwide including the appropriate regulation and recognition of naturopathic medicine. In accordance with this, championing accreditation and the highest educational standards for the naturopathic profession is a key focus, as is encouraging naturopathic research. Additionally, the WNF maintains a database of naturopathic organisations, regulation, accreditation, conferences and research activities.[11]

In practical terms, this has generated information that has previously not been available, including surveys to understand and map the naturopathic profession around the world; without this work, much of the detail found in the remainder of this chapter would not be possible. The WNF produced three key documents within the first two years of formation: the *World Naturopathic Profession Report* in 2015,[2] the *Naturopathic Roots Report* in 2016[13] and the 2016 *Naturopathic Numbers Report*.[3] The information in these reports is based on surveying naturopathic associations and education providers around the world. The reports are intended to 'assess the status of the naturopathic profession worldwide'[2] and to 'codify the foundational knowledge of naturopathy including naturopathic history, definitions, principles and theories from around the world'.[13]

Additionally, the WNF collaborates with the WHO to update naturopathic benchmarks as part of the WHO Definitions Project. Professional Mapping Initiatives include examining regulatory and educational infrastructure and policy frameworks that impact on the development of naturopathic medicine within each country around the world. Research Initiatives collect and support ongoing quality naturopathic research. An important milestone for the WNF was the 2016 World Health Assembly attended by WNF Officers (Iva Lloyd, President and Tina Hausser, Vice President) and Co-Secretaries General (Tabatha Parker and Jon Wardle). Meetings with Dr Zhang Qi, who is responsible for T&CM, commenced the process towards official collaboration between the WNF and the WHO, further securing the voice for naturopathic medicine on the world health stage.

A GLOBAL PROFESSION – SIMILARITIES AND DIFFERENCES

The practice of naturopathy is defined by guiding principles and a holistic approach to health and wellbeing – characteristics that are common to the practice around the world. This essential core is flanked by regional differences, and it is through exploring these similarities and differences that we can better understand the factors that define and differentiate the practice of naturopathy and the environment in which this occurs, starting with the foundation of naturopathic principles and then considering the education systems that reinforce these through each generation of graduates. The subsequent practice of naturopathy is where more variation is observed around the world through a range of modalities that are influenced by history, culture, education and regulation. Regulation of the profession is perhaps the area of greatest divergence as recognition, registration and regulation models all differ country by country.

The following sections summarise the similarities and differences between naturopathy around the world and are predominantly based on the results of surveys conducted by the WNF and reported in the *World Naturopathic Profession Report* in 2015[2] and the *Naturopathic Roots Report* in 2016.[14] Although in some instances the response numbers are low, this is the first systematic examination of the profession globally and provides good insight and a foundation upon which further knowledge and understanding can be developed.

Naturopathic principles

Naturopathy is a traditional system of medicine practised in many countries. A system of medicine is defined by integrated principles, philosophies, theories and practice of health and disease,[14] and although naturopathic practitioners use an eclectic array of treatment disciplines, there is a consistent core of philosophy and practice around the world.

The philosophical approach to naturopathy is reflected in six key principles that, although based on traditional values, were formalised in relatively recent times (1989) by the two North American national naturopathic associations (the American Association of Naturopathic Physicians [AANP] and the Canadian Association of Naturopathic Doctors [CAND]).[15]

The six naturopathic principles are:
1 First, Do No Harm (*primum non nocere*)
2 Healing Power of Nature (*vis medicatrix naturae*)
3 Treat the Cause (*tolle causam*)
4 Treat The Whole Person (*tolle totum*)
5 Doctor as Teacher (*docere*)
6 Disease Prevention and Health Promotion

There is a high degree of agreement around the world that these principles reflect the basis of naturopathic practice, indicating that despite other differences in education, specific modes of practice or regulation, the profession is based on strong common principles.[2]

This alignment of principles not only informs educational curriculum but is also influenced by the prevailing theories that are taught. The role of education institutions in maintaining naturopathic principles and high standards of education is paramount in the ongoing sustainability of the profession.

Naturopathic education and training

While there are over 90 institutions teaching naturopathy around the world, these are concentrated in several key geographical regions, with approximately half found in Europe.[3] Given the important role of this region in naturopathic history, this is not surprising; however, it does highlight the reality that over half of the countries where naturopathy is practised do not have locally based educational institutions. Table 1.1 shows the number of naturopathic education institutions by world region.

The genesis of naturopathic teaching institutions starts in 1902 with the formation of the American School of Naturopathy in New York by Benedict Lust. A number of European naturopathic schools also started in the 1920s, such as the Heilpraktiker-Fachschule founded by Josef Angerer (1907–1987) in Munich, Germany, which remains in operation today as the Joseph Angerer Schule. A number of students from Lust's American School of Naturopathy transferred their knowledge and skills to other parts of the world including Spain, by José Castro Blanco (1890–1981), and South America, by Professor Juan Estève Dulin in Argentina, Rosendo Arguello Ramirez in Nicaragua and Juan Antigas y Escobar in Cuba.[1,13] This

TABLE 1.1 Number of naturopathic education institutions by world region	
	Total number of naturopathic educational institutions by world region
Africa	2
Asia	22
Eastern Mediterranean	1
Europe	42
Latin America	12
North America	9
Western Pacific	6
Total	94

process of migration from a central point over the past 100 years helps explain the relatively high degree of alignment between naturopathic educational institutions as to what is taught.

EDUCATION STANDARDS

The WHO describes type I training programs as a minimum standard for naturopathic training, 'aimed at those who have no prior medical or other health-care training or experience. They are designed to produce naturopathic practitioners who are qualified to practise as primary-contact and primary-care practitioners'.[8] A minimum of 1500 hours of study is required with at least 400 hours of supervised clinical training over a two-year full time study period (or longer as equivalent). In practice, there is quite a degree of variation in naturopathic training around the world. A 2015 WNF survey of 85 naturopathic education institutions from 49 different countries identified course duration variation from as low as 1200 hours to some courses requiring over 4000 hours of study. Those at the higher end of the scale tend to align with those courses where the resultant qualification is one of naturopathic doctor such as in North America. The majority of naturopathic courses around the world comprise 3000 hours of study for the course.[2,13] There also tends to be a correlation between the level of course accreditation and the length of the course as shown in Fig. 1.2.

Fig. 1.2 categorises courses as government-accredited, self- or voluntary-accredited, and non-accredited programs. In some instances, the same body accredits education providers as well as course content, which is the situation in the US and Canada. In other regions, such as Australia, separate bodies regulate training providers and professional course content requirements. In some countries, courses may not be subject to either government or voluntary accreditation at all.[2,13]

Entry requirements to study naturopathy vary around the world, mostly in direct relation to the level of government accreditation requirements of the education institutions; that is, those in jurisdictions where the professional and education standards are government accredited tend to have more stringent requirements. In countries such as the US and Canada, where this is the case, an undergraduate degree is required to enrol in naturopathy and standardised exit exams are also part of attaining a qualification in these countries. The US, Canada and South Africa all also have government-approved independent accreditation agencies to maintain these standards of education and graduation. Elsewhere in the world, such as in Australia, where the qualification for all enrolments after 2016 is a bachelor's degree, previous undergraduate qualifications are not required and exit exams vary between education providers.[2,13]

AREAS OF STUDY

Naturopathy courses tend to focus on health sciences, with the sciences forming the core or backbone of the course and naturopathic areas of study built around these foundational requirements. The areas of study common to naturopathic education programs are as follows[2,8]:

1 basic sciences – including anatomy and physiology, biochemistry and pathology
2 clinical sciences – including clinical assessment and diagnosis
3 naturopathic sciences, modalities and principles – including naturopathic history and philosophy, nutrition and botanical medicine
4 clinical training and application – including observation and supervised practice.

While these areas of study are ubiquitous, the time spent within a course on a given study area varies according to where educational institutions are located. For example, those in Europe spend the most time on naturopathic history and philosophy, while Asian schools on average spend a greater percentage of time on the sciences.[2,13]

The high level of agreement internationally in regards to the naturopathic principles is reflected in the

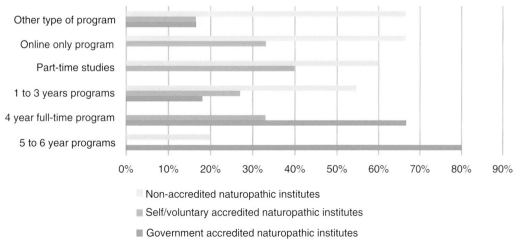

Non-accredited naturopathic institutes

Self/voluntary accredited naturopathic institutes

Government accredited naturopathic institutes

FIGURE 1.2 Type of naturopathic programs based on length

consistency with which these areas are incorporated into naturopathic education. A common element of naturopathic courses is teaching students to treat the whole person as well as a focus on disease prevention and health promotion. The remaining four principles likewise are incorporated into virtually all curricula – First, Do No Harm; Healing Power of Nature; Treat the Cause; and Doctor as Teacher.[13] The importance of naturopathic philosophies and theories in course content may be summarised in the following quote:

> *Naturopathic medicine is a philosophical system of medicine defined by its principles and theories and supported by research. Ensuring that naturopathic programs have a strong focus on naturopathic principles and theories is key to maintaining the essence of naturopathy from generation to generation.*[3]

Naturopathic philosophies, theories and modalities are subject to cultural and historical influences and show variability as to what is taught around the world in naturopathic courses. The philosophy of vitalism, or vital force, for instance, is taught universally, as are naturopathic cures. The treatment modalities that may be taught under the umbrella of naturopathic cures, however, are quite variable, as evidenced by the range of modalities practised (see the section 'Naturopathic practice'). Naturopathic philosophies and theories taught at the majority (over 70%) of naturopathic institutions globally in order of prevalence include[13]:

1 Vital Force*
2 Integration of the Individual*
3 Naturopathic Cures*
4 Value of Fever
5 Therapeutic Order
6 Triad of Health
7 Unity of Disease
8 Hering's Law of Cure
9 Theory of Toxaemia
10 Humoral Theory
   *These are taught nearly universally (96%).

CONTINUING PROFESSIONAL DEVELOPMENT/EDUCATION (CPD OR CPE)

Continuing education is generally required as part of mandatory or voluntary regulation of the profession where stipulated hours of additional study or professional development must be demonstrated to maintain professional membership and/or registration. Continuing education may be formal by way of further study, or through attending seminars most commonly provided by naturopathic associations. Seminars may also be offered by industry such as by complementary medicine companies. In some regions, requirements exist to ensure this education differs from marketing or promotion activity to be eligible as a professional development activity. More informal professional development is also achieved though peer and mentor support arrangements and self-study and research.[2,13]

Naturopathic practice

There is no 'one size fits all' for naturopaths. The range of treatment modalities that may be considered 'naturopathic' and how prevalent these are in practice is influenced by history, culture, professional regulation and any type of practice employed by the practitioner. The following lists the most common naturopathic modalities around the world[13]:

- Clinical Nutrition
- Botanical Medicine (Herbalism)
- Physical Medicine
- Homeopathic Medicine
- Hydrotherapy – Water Cure
- Prevention and Lifestyle Counselling
- Hygiene Therapy
- Nature Cure.

Additionally, practitioners may be trained in other areas, some of which are clearly influenced by history and culture. For example, naturopaths practising in India incorporate Ayurvedic medicine, commonly as part of a qualification that also includes yoga training Bachelor of Naturopathy and Yogic Sciences (BNYS). In other jurisdictions, such as North America, education and practice regulations allow for naturopathic doctors to administer intravenous treatments and perform minor surgery as part of their scope of practice. Other areas that may be included in training and practice additionally include: acupuncture, prescription rights, chelation therapy and colon therapy.[2,13]

The environment in which a practitioner completed their naturopathic education and training also varies and may influence not only the modalities practised, but also the application of them. The majority of naturopaths work in private practice, either as a solo practitioner or as part of a multi-practitioner clinic. Additionally, an estimated 10% of naturopaths are engaged in research and education or work in the complementary medicine industry.[3] It is possible for naturopaths or naturopathic doctors to work in hospital settings, depending on the jurisdiction, but this is not common, except in India, where it is much more prevalent due to a more traditional focus on nature care in an in-clinic setting.[2,13]

Private practice consultations tend to be, on average, significantly longer than those of medical doctors. They tend to be consumed with detailed case taking and clinical assessment of the patient as well as generating prescriptions that may include diet and lifestyle recommendations and herbal and nutritional supplements that may be pre-formulated, extemporaneously formulated or compounded and dispensed on a case-by-case basis. The majority of initial consultations are at least an hour and follow-up visits are commonly 45 minutes in duration.[2,13]

Naturopathic regulation

Professional recognition and systems of regulation are perhaps the areas of greatest difference in naturopathic practice around the world. In some regions, the profession is subject to a national regulatory environment and registration; in others this may vary within a country on a state by state basis, while in other parts of the world various models of self regulation exist. At the minimum, regulation of a health profession provides codes of professional conduct that must be adhered to. Scope of practice and protection of title may also form part of the regulatory process. What is consistent is that where statutory regulation through registration does not exist, there is a strong current of sentiment within the profession to be better recognised and endorsed as part of the primary healthcare system.

REGULATORY MODELS

Naturopathic medicine is regulated in approximately 50% of the world. A third of practising countries are unregulated; however, it is not illegal to practise naturopathy in those areas. Regulation takes a number of forms; for example, in the US and Canada practitioners must study at a government-accredited institution and sit a board exam to gain 'licensure' to practise as a naturopathic doctor in the states and territories where licensing laws exist. Other non-accredited education institutions exist and practitioners who graduate from these may practise as naturopaths.[2]

In Australia, the profession of naturopathy lacks government regulation through a centralised registration body, and instead operates under a less formal third-party regulation of the profession. The professional associations maintain their own codes of conduct, and professional indemnity (malpractice) insurance is only available for practitioners who meet the associations' membership requirements. This includes an appropriate level of education as well as maintaining annual professional development requirements and first aid certification. Additionally, private health insurers will only provide rebates for consultations with practitioners who are verified members of a professional association.[2]

SCOPE OF PRACTICE

The acts that a naturopathic practitioner can perform are generally limited by the scope of education received, which in turn tends to inform professional insurance coverage. Some acts may be frankly prohibited. The regions with the highest levels of recognition tend to have the greatest access to a range of practice options including internal gynaecological examinations, intravenous therapies, minor surgery and laboratory testing. The most common modalities practised as part of naturopathy can be seen in Table 1.2.

Prescribing nutritional supplements and herbal formulations is a common tool of trade in naturopathic practice, and maintaining an in-practice dispensary is usual in Africa, South East Asia, North America and the Western Pacific. In other world regions, this is less usual and is prohibited in some European and Latin American countries where direct dispensing to patients is not possible.[2]

The ability to order laboratory tests also varies around the globe with some practitioners able to not only order laboratory testing but also to take the sample in some

TABLE 1.2 Common naturopathic therapies used in practice	
Therapy	Prevalence allowed in practice
Hydrotherapy	93%
Massage techniques	88%
Botanical medicine	87%
Physical medicine practices	85%
Energetic therapies	85%
Lifestyle counselling	80%
Clinical nutrition	80%
TCM practices	79%
Homeopathy	77%
Colonics	75%

instances, such as naturopathic doctors taking blood tests. Where licensed as primary care practitioners, this generally also extends to the ability to order diagnostic imaging such as x-rays. Others may be limited to the ability to order functional pathology tests such as hair, saliva and stool testing, while some are prohibited from ordering or accessing such testing at all.[2]

USE OF TITLE

Protection of title allows for use of certain professional titles to be protected for use by appropriately qualified practitioners. The level of protection is generally tied to regulatory models and may additionally be covered under regional or national legislation. For example, in the US only graduates of accredited naturopathic medicine courses who have additionally passed a board examination may be licensed to practise as naturopathic doctors. In Germany, the title Heilpraktiker may be used only upon passing a state examination process. In countries such as Spain and Australia, which also have a long history and large numbers of naturopaths, the title of naturopath is not protected, meaning that anyone can call themselves a naturopath and practise even if not appropriately trained.[2]

PROFESSIONAL REPRESENTATION

Some countries have only one national association, while others have multiple professional associations. These may have differing geographical jurisdictions, represent different education standards or have other more philosophical differences within the same geographical areas. As a general rule, those countries more recently establishing associations establish one national body, as is the case in many African nations. In countries with longer histories of practice in an unregulated professional environment such as in Australia and New Zealand, there are multiple associations, some of which represent a variety of 'natural health' modalities.[2]

The core foundations of naturopathic principles temper the rich diversity in the nuances of naturopathic practice.

As a result, what is seen is a global span of practice that has more similarities than differences and that forms a global profession. While naturopathy is relatively young compared to some traditional medicines, its historical roots in botanical medicines and other nature-based cures provides practitioners with strong links to tradition. Combined with contemporary science, naturopathic medicine provides an important element in healthcare provision that is recognised for its value by the WHO. The future of global naturopathic medicine must be shaped by a commitment to high standards of education and practice and a united voice for the profession.

Naturopathy by world region

This final section briefly outlines the history and current practice of naturopathy around the world. The regions are those used by the WHO and WNF.

African region (countries where naturopathy is practised): Botswana, Democratic Republic of Congo, Ghana, Kenya, Mauritius, Namibia, Nigeria, South Africa, United Republic of Tanzania, Zambia and Zimbabwe.

T&CM is practised, taught and regulated variously throughout Africa. With tens of thousands of years of human habitation, long-standing traditional medicine systems have developed throughout the continent. In many parts of Sub-Saharan Africa, reliance on traditional medicine still prevails, as the accessibility to modern medicine practitioners and facilities can be limited. In countries where malaria may afflict children (such as Ghana, Mali, Nigeria and Zambia), home herbal medicine use is the primary treatment for malarial fever in 60% of children.[5] The WHO estimates that 60–80% of people in the African region rely on traditional medicine for their primary healthcare. Traditional medicine is commonly used to treat non-serious, acute illnesses, but also extends to those living with chronic illness such as HIV/AIDS due to limited access to appropriate medication. Practitioners employ herbal medicines, but may also practise bone setting and manage more complex psychiatric conditions as part of traditional practices.[16]

Against this backdrop, naturopathy is clearly a relative newcomer. It was introduced to South Africa after World War II and Zambia in the 1960s by an American, Dr Foster, who was both a medical and a naturopathic doctor.[2] Nonetheless, there are several educational institutions including the University of Western Cape in South Africa and the Zambia Institute of Natural Medicine and Research (also known as the Zinare Centre for Complementary Medicine Studies), both of which offer courses spanning 4200 hours.[13] The University of Western Cape offers a five-year double degree which allows graduates to register as a doctor within the studied discipline.[2,17] The profession is regulated by the Allied Health Professions Council of South Africa (AHPCSA), which was established by the Allied Health Professions Act, 63 of 1982.[18]

See Table 1.3 for information regarding naturopathy in Africa.

South East Asia region (countries where naturopathy is practised): India, Indonesia, Nepal and Thailand.

TABLE 1.3 Naturopathy in Africa: regional snapshot	
Countries practising naturopathy	**11 (representing 23% of countries in this region)**
Number of national naturopathic organisations	5
Number of regional naturopathic organisations	–
Number of other naturopathic organisations	–
Number of educational institutions	2
Estimated number of naturopaths	100–1000

[2,3]

Traditional medicine practices in South East Asia are represented strongly by Ayurvedic, Unani and Siddha philosophies, with Ayurveda arguably the best known in Western cultures. These systems of medicine are known by regionally specific names including Jamu in Indonesia, Dhivelhibeys in the Maldives and Koryo medicine in the Democratic People's Republic of Korea. Several countries, including Bhutan, Myanmar, Nepal and Bangladesh, recognise traditional medicines as valuable contributors to population healthcare and protect these values under Acts of Parliament.[19]

Countries both large and small in the region have rich histories of traditional medicine. Although small, Bhutan is known as Menjong Gyalkhab, meaning 'land of medicinal plants', alluding to its rich abundance of herbal medicines used as part of the traditional medicine system known as Sowa Rigpa. This system evolved from Tibetan medicine and developed after the arrival of Shabdrung Rinpoche from Tibet Region of China in the 16th century.[20]

Ayurvedic, meaning 'science of life', medicine was first documented somewhere between 2500 and 500 BC in India and, as such, is one of the longest continually practised systems of medicine in the world. India's massive population requires significant healthcare resources and it is estimated that 70% of the poorer, rural populations rely on Ayurvedic medicine for their healthcare needs.[21] Homeopathy is a comparatively recent addition and was introduced to India in the 1830s during homeopathy founder Samuel Hahnemann's lifetime. The relative cost effectiveness of this modality has seen its popularity flourish and there are now many homeopathic as well as naturopathic training institutions, practitioners and specialised hospitals throughout the country.[22] Acharya Puccha Venkata Ramaiah originally brought the practice of naturopathy to India around 1885 after having trained under the German naturopath Louis Kuhne. Naturopathic practice was then revived in the 1940s thanks to support from Mahatma Gandhi. In Nepal, naturopathy started in 1968.[2]

In India naturopathic education courses are combined with yoga and known as a Bachelor of Naturopathy and Yogic Sciences (BNYS). This is a five-and-a-half-year

Chapter 1: Global naturopathic medicine

TABLE 1.4 Naturopathy in South East Asia: regional snapshot	
Countries practising naturopathy	4 (representing 36% of countries in this region)
Number of national naturopathic organisations	2
Number of regional naturopathic organisations	11
Number of other naturopathic organisations	3
Number of educational institutions	22
Estimated number of naturopaths	?

[2,3]

TABLE 1.5 Naturopathy in Eastern Mediterranean: regional snapshot	
Countries practising naturopathy	7 (representing 32% of countries in this region)
Number of national naturopathic organisations	2
Number of regional naturopathic organisations	—
Number of other naturopathic organisations	—
Number of educational institutions	1
Estimated number of naturopaths	<100

[2,3]

full-time medical degree that is recognised by the Indian government under the Ministry of AYUSH (Ayurveda, Yoga and Naturopathy, Unani, Siddha, Homoeopathy).[2]

See Table 1.4 for information regarding naturopathy in South East Asia.

Eastern Mediterranean region (countries where naturopathy is practised): Bahrain, Egypt, Kuwait, Morocco, Qatar, Saudi Arabia and United Arab Emirates.

Traditional Arabic and Islamic medicine developed in the eastern Mediterranean region with its generous natural repository of herbal medicines. The medical system developed in the Middle Ages as Arab herbalists, pharmacologists, chemists and physicians built on the ancient medicinal practices of Mesopotamia, Greece, Rome, Persia and India. This legacy is considered an important foundation for contemporary medicine as it developed in Europe. Most famously, the work of Ibn Sina (Avicena in the West), known as Al-Qanun-fil-Tib (*Canon of Medicine*), plays an important role in the history of medicine. This book remained relevant for over 600 years and was published more than 35 times during the 15th and 16th centuries alone.[23] While the medieval Islamic world was spread broadly, wars, including those with the Ottoman Empire, caused the Islamic civilisation into decline by the end of the 1400s.[24]

Traditional medicine remains important in the region, with 88% of the WHO member states of the region acknowledging its continued use. Approximately 40% had established a national policy on T&CM as of 2010.[5] As for regulation, the WHO[5] declared that 'Five Member States reported that they already had regulations for practitioners, with explicit regulations for different disciplines such as acupuncture, ayurveda, homeopathy and herbal medicine in four of them' (p. 64).

The WNF understands that the first legally practising naturopathic doctor in Saudi Arabia was a graduate from the National College of Natural Medicine (NCNM) in the US who began practice in 2005.[2]

See Table 1.5 for information regarding naturopathy in the Eastern Mediterranean.

European region (countries where naturopathy is practised): Austria, Belgium, Bosnia and Herzegovina, Cyprus, Czech Republic, Denmark, Finland, France, Germany, Greece, Hungary, Iceland, Ireland, Israel, Italy, Luxembourg, Netherlands, Norway, Portugal, Romania, Russia, Slovenia, Spain, Sweden, Switzerland, Ukraine and United Kingdom.

Contemporary Western herbal medicine is based on the herbal medicine traditions of Europe, and early European medical advances form the basis of contemporary medical healthcare systems. Germany, in particular, was home to several key practitioners who contributed to the evolution of contemporary naturopathy (as discussed earlier in this chapter). As may be expected, contemporary Germany has recognised naturopathic practitioners for some time under the 'Heilpraktikergesetz' law of 1939 and there is a high degree of utilisation of natural remedies in the population. The first college was established in 1936, and although naturopathic education was prohibited during World War II, the Josef Angerer Schule reopened in 1950 and continues to operate today.[2]

The German situation is, however, not replicated throughout all of Europe. In some countries, such as Spain, naturopathy has been practised virtually since its inception, with the first naturopathic centre opened in Barcelona in 1925 by José Castro Blanco and Nicolas Capo. Today the profession is recognised but yet not government regulated, although the national association OCN-FENACO is actively lobbying for this to occur.[2] In nearby Portugal, naturopathy did not appear until the 1970s. This was followed by naturopathic schools and professional associations and, subsequently, laws in 2004 that regulated a number of natural therapies including naturopathy. Naturopathy arrived in France in the 1940s, with Pierre Valentin Marchesseau considered the father of naturopathy in that country.[2] The European Union of Naturopathy (Union Européenne de Naturopathie – UEN) was formed in 2002 with 17 countries listed as members on its website.[25]

See Table 1.6 for information regarding naturopathy in Europe.

TABLE 1.6 Naturopathy in Europe: regional snapshot	
Countries practising naturopathy	27 (representing 50% of countries in this region)
Number of national naturopathic organisations	43
Number of regional naturopathic organisations	19
Number of other naturopathic organisations	2
Number of educational institutions	42 (nearly half the naturopathic education institutions in the world)
Estimated number of naturopaths	7500+ (however, Germany and Spain are estimated to have in excess of 20 000)

[2,3]

TABLE 1.7 Naturopathy in Latin America and the Caribbean: regional snapshot	
Countries practising naturopathy	22 (representing 43% of countries in this region)
Number of national naturopathic organisations	17
Number of regional naturopathic organisations	5
Number of other naturopathic organisations	–
Number of educational institutions	12
Estimated number of naturopaths	1000–2500

[2,3]

Latin America and the Caribbean region (countries where naturopathy is practised): Argentina, Bahamas, Barbados, Bermuda, Chile, Colombia, Costa Rica, Ecuador, El Salvador, Guatemala, Honduras, Mexico, Nicaragua, Panama, Paraguay, Peru, Puerto Rico, Saint Lucia, Uruguay, Venezuela and Virgin Islands (US).

Traditional medicine in South and Central America has been maintained largely through use by indigenous tribal groups, rural and lower-income urban people. Traditional medicine practice includes herbalists, bone-setters and midwives as well as spiritual healers. Several countries have mixed historical relationships with their traditional healers or 'curandero'. In Peru, a high proportion of people, particularly in more remote regions, use curanderos even though the practice was outlawed for a period of time in 1969. Guatemala, Ecuador and Cuba too have had mixed histories of acceptance since the mid 20th century, yet use prevails, in particular with traditional midwives attending births.[19] Alternatively, in Brazil a national policy on 'Integrative and Complementary Practices' has been implemented in recognition of the economical and cultural benefits of integrating traditional medicines into healthcare systems.[5]

The predominant trend in the region is that in populations under-served by modern medicine – whether due to remote location, indigenous populations or lower socioeconomic status – traditional medicine systems, where they exist, invariably fill the gap. This aligns with the WHO goals to better utilise T&CM to reduce inequities in population health outcomes.[5]

Naturopathy migrated south from the New York-based American School of Naturopathy. Notable students by country include: Carlos Rosendo Arguello Ramirez (Nicaragua), Juan Antigas y Escobar (Cuba) and Juan Esteve Dulin (Argentina). Today there are several higher-education institutions teaching naturopathy in the region. Some of the oldest include HOVINAT, formed in 1986, and Asoeducalt University, formed in 1996, both in Venezuela. Some of the most recent include UPAV, which introduced a degree course after it was formally incorporated in Mexico

in 2012, and the Autonomous University of Tlaxcala, also in Mexico, which launched a course in late 2013.[2]

See Table 1.7 for information regarding naturopathy in Latin America and the Caribbean.

North American region (countries where naturopathy is practised): Canada and the United States.

While based in European traditions, naturopathy as a contemporary system of medicine was born in the US. The practice grew from its beginnings in New York in 1901 with a number of additional schools opening in the US and Canada over the next 20 to 30 years. During this time, the number of naturopathic doctors grew, conferences and professional journals flourished and the profession was regulated in a number of US states and Canadian provinces. While popularity persisted into the 1930s, the profession experienced a downturn from this time to the 1970s 'due to the growing political and social dominance of Western medicine and other economic factors … including (the) impact of wars, the Great Depression, the shifting of funding and support to allopathic-based medical schools and the birth of pharmaceutical medicine and the promise of "miracle cures"' (p. 47).[2] When considering the evolution of naturopathy, the influence of the Native American people and the herbal medicines they introduced to the European settlers can be seen in a number of herbal medicines widely utilised today.

The Council on Naturopathic Medical Education (CNME) accredits naturopathic educational institutions in the US and there are currently five such institutions across the country, including the National University of Natural Medicine (NUNM) in Portland, Oregon, established in 1956, which is the oldest, and also Bastyr University in Seattle, which opened in 1978. These colleges together with two Canadian schools are also recognised by the American Association of Naturopathic Medical Colleges (AANMC), an educational consortium. Graduates from these accredited schools are eligible to sit the Naturopathic Physicians Licensing Examinations (NPLEX), which allows for registration in the states and provinces that have legislation regulating naturopathic doctors. Most states in the US have state naturopathic associations, while the association representing naturopathic doctors nationally is the American Association of Naturopathic Physicians (AANP), founded in 1984.[2] Additionally, the American Naturopathic Medical Association (ANMA) founded in 1981 represents a range of practitioners that practise naturopathy in addition to licensed naturopathic doctors. In some states, it is not legal to practise as a naturopath.[26]

While the majority of Canadian provinces and territories have local naturopathic associations, one national association was established in 1950. The Canadian Association of Naturopathic Doctors (CAND) represents practitioners who have graduated from an accredited naturopathic school. Scope of practice, regulation and protection of title may also vary from province to province, as is the case in the US. The naturopathic profession in both countries developed largely in tandem and, as a result, they are quite closely aligned.[2,15]

See Table 1.8 for information regarding naturopathy in North America.

Western Pacific region (countries where naturopathy is practised): Australia, China, Hong Kong (China), Japan, Malaysia, New Zealand, Singapore and Vanuatu.

Many parts of the Western Pacific region have not only a history of traditional medicine, but maintain a connection to that tradition today. The practice of traditional Chinese medicine in China as well as a number of other countries is an active exemplar of this. This is no doubt related to the strong level of support for traditional medicine by the Chinese government. The Chinese constitution embeds traditional medicine in the healthcare system, and modern and traditional Chinese medicine are often practised side by side. Likewise, in countries including Japan, Mongolia, The Philippines, Singapore and the Republic of Korea (South Korea), government policy actively recognises the contribution and value of traditional medicine systems.[19]

Australia and New Zealand are differentiated by a more recent Western presence influencing their traditional medicine practices, and while New Zealand regulates standards for traditional Māori medicine, this is less apparent when considering Indigenous Australian healing practices.[19] Rongoā is the traditional Māori medicine and is still practised today. It influenced the early western settlers, including Scottish doctor James Neil, who incorporated a mix of native and European herbal remedies in his book *The New Zealand Family Herb Doctor* in 1889.[2]

The presence of naturopathy in the Western Pacific stems from early adoption of the profession in Australia, where records indicate naturopathic practitioners in Queensland and Victoria as early as 1904. Early practice was strongly influenced by the UK and US until Alfred Jacka opened the first formal, four-year training college, the Southern School of Natural Therapies (SSNT) in Melbourne in 1961. In 1995, the college went on to introduce the first government-accredited degree program in naturopathic medicine. Southern Cross University then followed suit with the world's first public university naturopathic program in 1996.[2] Education standards in Australia and New Zealand currently allow both undergraduate degree and diploma level programs in naturopathic medicine. However, in Australia the degree program became the minimum education standard for new graduates at the end of 2018. In Australia and New Zealand, there are a number of national professional associations, and in lieu of government regulation via statutory registration, the associations perform a pseudo-regulatory function. There have been a number of enquiries into regulatory requirements and while naturopathy has been assessed against the Australian National Registration and Accreditation Scheme criteria and meets the criteria for statutory registration, this has not been yet been implemented.[27]

See Table 1.9 for information regarding naturopathy in Western Pacific.

CAN I PRACTISE IN ANOTHER COUNTRY?

Given the widespread nature of naturopathy around the world together with the general similarities in education and naturopathic philosophy, this question is a common one, yet it is not so simple to answer! This chapter outlines the similarities and differences not only in practice, but also in relation to the legal and regulatory environment in which practitioners operate. The bottom line is that local laws and requirements will always need to be met and the onus is on the individual practitioner to demonstrate they have the appropriate education, qualification, experience and credentials to practise in that jurisdiction. There is no 'one size fits all' and transferring from one country to another invariably involves some research into local requirements. Joining a local professional association will generally be your gateway to practise, insurance and other local requirements. You will likely be required to have authenticated/certified copies of all relevant documents as well as course outlines relating to your studies so that equivalence to local requirements can be

TABLE 1.8 Naturopathy in North America: regional snapshot	
Countries practising naturopathy	**2 (representing 67% of countries in this region)**
Number of national naturopathic organisations	2
Number of regional naturopathic organisations	50
Number of other naturopathic organisations	16
Number of educational institutions	9
Estimated number of naturopaths	7500+

[2,3]

TABLE 1.9 Naturopathy in Western Pacific: regional snapshot	
Countries practising naturopathy	8 (representing 22% of countries in this region)
Number of national naturopathic organisations	9
Number of regional naturopathic organisations	2
Number of other naturopathic organisations	1
Number of educational institutions	6
Estimated number of naturopaths	2500–8500

[2,3]

established, so getting paperwork in order is important. You may find there is more than one national association or multiple layers of national and regional associations for you to navigate, so be aware of this and do not assume that the first association you locate from your internet searches is the only one. A useful starting point is the WNF website (worldnaturopathicfederation.org) which lists the membership of national naturopathic organisations.

REFERENCES

[1] Cody GW, Hascall H. The history of naturopathic medicine. In: Pizzorno J, Murray M, editors. Textbook of natural medicine. 4th ed. E-book. Churchill Livingstone; 2013.

[2] World Naturopathic Federation. World Federation Report; 2015. [Internet]. Available from http://worldnaturopathicfederation.org/wp-content/uploads/2015/12/World-Federation-Report_June2015.pdf.

[3] World Naturopathic Federation. 2016 Naturopathic Numbers Report; 2016. [Internet]. Available from http://worldnaturopathicfederation.org/wp-content/uploads/2015/12/2016-Naturopathic-Numbers-Report.pdf.

[4] Wardle J, Oberg EB. The intersecting paradigms of naturopathic medicine and public health: opportunities for naturopathic medicine. J Altern Complement Med 2011;17(11):1079–84.

[5] World Health Organization. WHO Traditional Medicine Strategy: 2014-2023; 2013. [Internet]. Available from http://www.who.int/medicines/publications/traditional/trm_strategy14_23/en/.

[6] Global Industry Analysts, Inc. The global herbal supplements and remedies market trends, drivers and projections; 2015. Available from http://www.strategyr.com/MarketResearch/Herbal_Supplements_and_Remedies_Market_Trends.asp.

[7] United Nations. Sustainable Development Goals. 2015. Available from http://www.un.org/sustainabledevelopment/health/.

[8] World Health Organization. Benchmarks for Training in Naturopathy. [Internet]. 2010. Available from http://apps.who.int/medicinedocs/en/d/Js17553en/.

[9] World Health Organization. Essential medicines and health products. Nd. Available from http://www.who.int/medicines/areas/quality_safety/regulation_legislation/assesment/en/.

[10] WHO. Resolution WHA69.24 'Strengthening integrated people-centred health services'. 2016. Available from http://apps.who.int/gb/ebwha/pdf_files/WHA69/A69_R24-en.pdf.

[11] Wardle J, Cook N, Steel A, et al. The World Naturopathic Federation: global opportunities for the Australian profession. Aust J Herb Med 2016;28(1):3.

[12] World Naturopathic Federation. About WNF. [Internet]. Available from http://worldnaturopathicfederation.org/about-wnf/.

[13] World Naturopathic Federation. Naturopathic Roots Report; 2016. [Internet]. Available from http://worldnaturopathicfederation.org/wp-content/uploads/2015/12/Naturopathic-Roots_final-1.pdf.

[14] Rosenzweig S. Whole medical systems. In: The Merck Manual, consumer edition. 2016. Available from: http://www.merckmanuals.com/home/special-subjects/complementary-and-alternative-medicine-cam/whole-medical-systems. Internet.

[15] Lloyd I. The history of naturopathic medicine, a Canadian perspective. Toronto, Canada: McArthur & Company; 2009.

[16] Mhame PP, Busia K, Kasilo OM. Clinical practices of African traditional medicine. African Health Monitor. 2010 [Internet]. Available from: https://www.aho.afro.who.int/en/ahm/issue/13/reports/clinical-practices-african-traditional-medicine.

[17] University of Western Cape. About us. [Internet]. Available from https://www.uwc.ac.za/Faculties/CHS/SoNM/Pages/About-Us.aspx.

[18] The Allied Health Professions Council of South Africa. [Internet]. Available from http://ahpcsa.co.za/.

[19] Bodeker G, Ong CK, Grundy C, et al. WHO global atlas of traditional, complementary and alternative medicine. World Health Organization. Kobe, Japan: World Health Organization; 2005.

[20] World Health Organization. Review of traditional medicine in the South-East Asia region; 2004. [Internet]. Available from http://apps.searo.who.int/PDS_DOCS/B0514.pdf?ua=1.

[21] Pandey MM, Rastogi S, Rawat AKS. Indian traditional Ayurvedic system of medicine and nutritional supplementation. Evid Based Complement Alternat Med 2013;2013:e376327.

[22] Ministry of AYUSH. Summary of infrastructure facilities under Department of Ayurveda, Yoga and Naturopathy, Unani, Siddha and Homoeopathy. [Internet]. Available from http://ayush.gov.in/infrastructure/summary-infrastructure-facilities-under-ayush.

[23] Azaizeh H, Saad B, Cooper E, et al. Traditional Arabic and Islamic medicine, a re-emerging health aid. Evid Based Complement Alternat Med 2010;7(4):419–24.

[24] Majeed A. How Islam changed medicine. BMJ 2005;331(7531):1486–7.

[25] Union Européenne de Naturopathie – European Union of Naturopathy. Historical. [Internet]. Available from http://www.naturopathy-union.eu/en/presentation-eun/historical/.

[26] American Naturopathic Medical Association. [Internet]. Available from http://www.anma.org/home.html.

[27] Wardle J. The National Registration and Accreditation Scheme: what would inclusion mean for naturopathy and Western herbal medicine? Part I – the Legislation. Aust J Med Herb 2010;22(4):113.

Environmental medicine

2

Nicole Bijlsma

Environmental medicine is the evaluation, management and study of detectable human disease or adverse health outcomes arising from exposure to external physical, chemical and biological factors in the general environment.[1,2] Environmental medicine is a speciality field that has been adopted by occupational and environmental doctors, but largely ignored in patient-centred general practice despite the fact that toxicants alone have been implicated in many chronic diseases typically seen in routine medical practice.[3] There are several reasons why this may be so:

- Most chronic diseases arise from a complex interaction between genes and the environment and, until recently, this relationship has been hampered by limited knowledge of the human genome and the inclination of scientists to study disease using models that consider exposure to single agents at high doses[4]
- Very little of the vast amount of literature on environmental exposure is published in general medical journals[5]
- It takes years to translate scientific discovery to clinical practice[6]
- Clinicians do not undertake house and workplace visits to identify obvious triggers
- There is competition from other disciplines in crowded medical curricula
- There are limitations in adopting a reductionist approach to compartmentalise the body into separate systems
- The need to provide evidence-based medicine that is conclusive and leaves no room for doubt has delayed action on environmental toxicants.

Widespread exposure to toxicants occurs in the human population from the womb to the tomb at levels known to cause adverse health effects.[7–10] This is largely because the burden of proof is not on industry to prove that its products or technologies are safe, and the inadequacies of chemical risk assessment fail to consider multiple routes of exposure, mixture effects, transgenerational epigenetic effects, the impact of endocrine-disrupting chemicals (EDCs) during critical windows of human development and individual susceptibility,[5] although some countries are attempting to address this (for example, the REACH directive in Europe and the Toxic Substance Control Act in the US). Consequently the history of medicine is littered with numerous examples of missed opportunities, wasted resources and counterproductive policies due to an inability to act on available evidence.[11] In 1857, the father of epidemiology, Dr John Snow, was able to demonstrate that 'contagions' in water were responsible for a cholera epidemic[12]; in 1950 Dr Richard Doll published his findings correlating smoking with lung cancer[14]; and in 1956 Dr Alice Stewart was able to prove that one fetal x-ray doubled the incidence of childhood leukaemia.[13] These clinicians were ostracised from their peers and the medical establishment at the time of their findings and it took decades for their work to be validated. There are many environmental hazards that have had devastating consequences on human health, such as lead, mercury, asbestos, benzene, organochlorine pesticides and polychlorinated biphenyls (PCBs).[15] The question we as clinicians need to ask ourselves is, 'When is there sufficient evidence to act?'[5]

Despite calls from numerous organisations[16–19] to provide clinicians with more training and awareness in environmental health, there are multiple barriers to the clinical assessment of toxic environmental exposure. Clinicians are limited in their capacity to test for environmental exposure as many of the tests available have not been validated (e.g. provocation testing, lymphocyte sensitivity tests, DNA-adduct and mitochondrial testing, visual contrast sensitivity tests), are inconsistent or controversial (hair mineral analysis, detoxification profiles), only assess short-term exposure (blood, stool and urine), may not be predictive of adverse health outcomes (genomic profiling), are costly or are not available. In addition, there may be no reliable biomarkers, such as those involved with electromagnetic field exposure. While emerging technologies in the field of metabolomics are predicted to have a profound impact on medical practice in years to come,[20] in the interim clinicians can do many things to address environmental exposure. This starts with taking a thorough history of the patient's health symptoms and environmental exposure, establishing the patient's inherent susceptibility to environmental toxicants and educating the patient on how they can reduce their exposure to toxicants: these topics are the focus of this chapter.

HISTORY-TAKING

According to Bijlsma and Cohen,[5] history-taking should encompass the following:

- A detailed symptom history that includes a timeline from the prenatal period

- A family history that includes previous generations
- An obstetric, paediatric, dietary, environmental and occupational exposure history (links to questionnaires developed for chemical, electromagnetic field and mould exposure are provided in this chapter)
- A history of pharmaceutical and recreational drug use
- A detailed place history that includes places of residence, school and work across the lifespan including primary modes of transportation, with a focus on proximity to toxicants (mining, industry, traffic and other sources of air and water pollution), allergens and electromagnetic fields
- Use of external data sources, geographical information systems and apps to assess exposure to electromagnetic fields (real time) and exposure maps (mining, radon, traffic, pollen), as well as government or non-government environmental pollution reporting regarding ambient air monitoring and drinking water quality
- A physical examination to look for physical signs of metabolic, neurological, reproductive or other disease and comorbidities
- Assessing current toxic load by performing various biomonitoring tests including assessment of biomarkers in various body tissues to evaluate long-term accumulation of toxicants
- Networking with other professionals who can assess the patient's home and/or workplace to establish sources of exposure.

WHO IS SUSCEPTIBLE?

Why is it that a person may work in a department store spraying perfumes day by day, year by year, and be completely unaffected by the environment while a person walking past the same area develops a headache that makes them unwell for the rest of the day? Why do people react differently to pharmaceutical drugs? Why can one person smoke heavily all of their life with no apparent symptoms, while another dies from smoking-related disease in middle age? Establishing a patient's inherent susceptibility to environmental toxicants requires an assessment of their genetic predisposition, age and timing of exposure, gender, gut microbiome, nutrition, drug use and disease states.

Genetic predisposition

> *Genetics loads the gun, but the environment pulls the trigger. Professor Judith Stern*

Environmental exposure and individual susceptibility go hand-in-hand. Simply put, you cannot address one without the other. Until recently, clinicians were limited in their scope to assess individual susceptibility to eliciting the patient's race/ethnicity status and taking a thorough family and personal history, as alterations in highly penetrant genes (mutations) explain only a small fraction of complex diseases. Completion of the human genome in 2003,

however, shifted attention to explore the impact of gene variants or SNPs (single-nucleotide polymorphisms) in the aetiology of chronic disease as the direction and magnitude of the exposure-response effect can vary with different genetic polymorphisms.[4,21,22] For example, there is a higher incidence of asbestos-induced respiratory disease in carpenters with a homozygous deletion of the *glutathione-S-transferase Mu 1* (*GSTM-1*) gene, which plays an important role in phase II liver detoxification.[23] Human variability in phase I and II detoxification can vary more than ten-fold depending on genetic polymorphisms in metabolic enzymes.[24,25]

Studies that explore polymorphisms in the aetiology of chronic disease are frequently inconsistent, inconclusive and contradictory. They often fail to demonstrate cause and effect because multiple genes are involved, polymorphisms in some genes may be compensated by other genes and few studies consider these SNPs within the context of the patient's lifestyle and/or environment. Taking breast cancer as an example, although well-established risk factors have been identified for breast cancer (including age, menarche/parity/menopause, family history, being overweight, drug use, smoking, high penetrance gene mutations [*BRCA1*, *BRCA2*, *TP53* and *PTEN*] and gene variants in detoxification and DNA repair pathways), individually they confer only a small or negligible risk.[3,26] When polymorphisms are combined or considered within the context of relevant environmental and lifestyle exposure, such as being overweight, smoking, using alcohol or drugs, or following toxicant exposure, especially during the prenatal and pubertal periods, the statistical power becomes significant in some[27–31] but not all studies,[32,33] depending on which polymorphisms and environmental factors are investigated. This gene–environment interaction may explain why US-born Asian women have an almost two-fold higher incidence of invasive breast cancer than native Asian women.[34] Like most complex chronic diseases, determining the aetiology and pathogenesis of breast cancer requires big data resources[32] involving large-scale multicentre studies that include detailed individual data, environmental background and gene–gene and gene–environment interactions.[35] The synergistic relationship between genes and the environment in the aetiology of chronic diseases like autoimmune diseases, metabolic disorders, neurodevelopmental disorders such as autism, neurodegenerative disorders such as Parkinson's disease and various cancers has been confirmed by numerous studies.[26,36–39]

While the cost of gene testing has become more affordable, few clinicians implement it because of the time involved, a lack of training, ethical considerations and the fact that very few of the one million-plus SNPs have clear functional implications and actionable outcomes that are relevant to mechanisms of disease.[3,40] Furthermore, current attempts to predict a person's reaction to drugs and toxicants based on their genetic predisposition alone have not met the anticipated success.[41] In addition, the implications for clinical practice have been limited[42] because other compounding factors such as age, gender, gut microbiome, nutrition and lifestyle factors have been shown to influence the way in which toxicants are metabolised in the body.

Age and timing of exposure

Age is an important risk factor for susceptibility, as exposure to toxicants during critical windows of development (prenatal, childhood and prepubescent) has been correlated with a range of adverse health effects. The first association of transgenerational inheritance of disease was documented in the Dutch famine of 1944–1945, when nutritional deprivation in utero was associated with increased risk of obesity later in life.[43] Since then, poor nutrition and chemical exposure in utero have been widely reported.[44–47] However, it wasn't until a series of events beginning in the 1960s – diethylstilboestrol and adverse reproductive outcomes, thalidomide-induced limb defects, tobacco smoke and low birth weight, Minamata disease and mercury, and fetal alcohol syndrome – that our understanding of the placenta as a protective barrier was deemed unfounded.[48]

Early life exposure to toxicants in air, water, food, soil and consumer products can increase the risk of cognitive, behavioural or social impairment, as well as specific neurodevelopmental disorders such as autism and attention deficit hyperactivity disorder.[49] There is convincing evidence that industrial chemicals such as lead, mercury, arsenic, pesticides, fluoride, flame retardants, plastic derivatives, combustion-related air pollutants, PCBs and various solvents like toluene are contributing to a global pandemic of neurodevelopmental disorders.[49–51] Toxicants that persist in the fat and bones of the mother over a life time may expose the fetus to heavy metals such as lead[52] and persistent organic pollutants such as organochlorine pesticides. The fetal and infant brain are vulnerable to lipophilic toxicants as the central nervous system is the dominant repository of fetal fat.[3] Furthermore, concerns about the impact of early life exposure to EDCs have grown following the publication of Rachel Carson's book *Silent Spring* in 1962,[53] Theo Colburn and Pete Myer's text *Our Stolen Future* in 1996,[54] the World Health Organization's report in 2013,[55] the International Federation of Gynecology and Obstetrics' statement in 2015[56] and the TENDR consensus statement in 2016.[49] Since then, there has been a flood of research correlating in utero and early childhood exposure to EDCs with the rising incidence of testicular dysgenesis syndrome, cancers, infertility, metabolic diseases and neurobehavioural disorders.[55] The fetal origins of health and disease proposed by Barker[57] have subsequently morphed into the developmental origins of health and disease (DoHAD), which focuses on the role of early life exposure in chronic disease aetiology.[58]

Breast-fed infants accumulate higher toxicant burden being at the top of the food chain.[59] Compared with adults, neonates are more vulnerable to toxicants because they have fewer binding proteins in the blood,[60] and infants have a higher hand-to-mouth ratio and therefore ingest up to eight times more dirt than adults. Infants also consume more food and drink per unit of body weight to meet their growth and developmental needs, extract more nutrients and toxicants from ingested food, breathe twice as much air, have a breathing zone closer to the ground where most toxicants are found (in household dust), are more susceptible to EDCs, have a longer life expectancy, do not recognise danger, have an undeveloped blood–brain barrier and underdeveloped and immature body systems (e.g. immune, respiratory, renal).[60–62] Apart from immature detoxification pathways, the biodiversity and abundance of a child's gut microbiome (in particular, those that metabolise xenobiotics) is significantly less when compared to an adult's.[63] Consequently the health impact of chemical exposure is most evident in paediatric medicine, where chronic disease has overtaken infectious disease as the major burden of paediatric illness.[64] A well-known example of child–adult differences in metabolic processing is caffeine. Caffeine's half-life in newborns is 14-fold higher than in adults, which is probably the result of the immaturity of the enzyme CYP1A2.[65,66]

Children are also uniquely susceptible to the radiofrequency electromagnetic energy (RF EME) used in wireless technologies because, unlike adults, their skulls are thinner,[67] they absorb twice as much microwave radiation,[68] they are physically smaller in size, they have a longer lifetime exposure and their cells undergo rapid cell division. This is likely to have serious implications for the developing brain, where neurons are being formed at a rate of 250 000 per minute on average in an unborn child over the course of a pregnancy[69] and the proliferation of radial glia and neurons continues to develop until almost 3 years of age.[70]

Gender

Gender differences in toxicant exposure are well documented. For example, women have higher peak blood alcohol levels than men when given the same dose because they metabolise alcohol more slowly than men,[71] have a smaller volume of distribution for alcohol and a higher percentage of body fat.[72] Similarly, multiple chemical sensitivity is significantly higher in women than in men,[73,74] which is suspected to be due to women's higher body fat-to-muscle ratio resulting in a higher body burden of toxicants and because women are often the primary consumers of personal care and cleaning products that contain solvents and EDCs.[7,75] In contrast, autism is four to five times more common in males than in females[76] and has been correlated with exposure to EDCs such as pesticides, phthalates, PCBs, solvents, toxic waste sites, air pollutants and heavy metals.[38] Most of these toxicants are anti-androgens and xeno-oestrogens, which have been shown in animal models to affect both brain and genital development in male progeny[77] and coincides with the sharp rise in the number of male reproductive abnormalities over the past 50 years.[78]

Gut microbiome

The metabolic activity of the gut microbiome is comparable to that of the liver,[79] with 850 bacterial genera involved in the metabolism of xenobiotics[63] and drugs.[79] A study conducted by the Pfizer pharmaceutical group discovered 'accidentally' individual variances in drug metabolism arising from the patient's gut microbiome.[80]

The metabolic profile of a patient's urine was tested before and after ingestion of paracetamol and it was found that the presence of *p*-cresol sulfate (a metabolite from *Clostridium difficile* bacteria found in the gut) significantly altered the ratio of paracetamol-sulfate and paracetamol-glucuronide metabolites in the urine. It was deduced that in patients with a gut microbiome excreting large amounts of *p*-cresol, the *p*-cresol competes for the same enzyme-binding sites and takes up a large part of the rate-limiting phase II sulfation pathway, such that paracetamol is forced to undergo phase II glucuronidation instead of sulfation.[80] In these patients, paracetamol-induced hepatotoxicity is increased, because depletion of glutathione levels causes the reactive metabolites to bind to macromolecules in hepatocytes.[81] Competitive inhibition (between toxicants and metabolites originating from the gut microbiome), resulting in higher blood levels of each chemical, is a phenomenon observed with increasing mixture complexity.[82]

This may explain why many mould-affected patients with associated gut dysbiosis appear to become chemically sensitive. *Why is this significant?* Many drugs, environmental toxicants and their metabolites, catecholamine neurotransmitters such as dopamine, adrenaline and noradrenaline, and hormones undergo phase II sulfation, so this has wide-reaching ramifications for human health. Interestingly, autistic children have been shown to have higher levels of *Clostridia*[83] and low sulfation capacity, which could cause a cerebral increase of catecholamines and subsequent changes in behaviour, especially when they eat foods high in phenolic amines (chocolate, wheat, corn sugar, apples and bananas).[84] Furthermore, *Clostridia* are present in higher numbers in many chronic illnesses such as Alzheimer's, Parkinson's disease and type 2 diabetes,[85] which coincidentally are also diseases commonly associated with various toxicant exposure to pesticides and heavy metals – both of which have been shown to alter gut flora. Depletion of glutathione stores may result in increased oxidative stress levels, especially in neurons and glial cells,[86] as well as many other downstream effects because of glutathione's involvement in iron metabolism, phase II glutathione conjugation, DNA synthesis and repair, protein synthesis, prostaglandin synthesis, amino acid transport and enzyme activation.

The gut microbiome is a major player in the pathogenesis of chronic metabolic and central nervous system diseases.[85,87] Gut microbes can influence the fate of neurons in various regions of the brain,[88] as well as the development and maturation of the microglia; produce neurotransmitters like GABA,[89,90] nitric oxide,[91] serotonin, noradrenaline and dopamine[92]; and influence anxiety and depression,[93] autism spectrum disorder,[88,94] Parkinson's disease[95] and psychiatric disorders in patients with intestinal dysbiosis.[96] Gut microbes produce short-chain fatty acids (SCFAs) from non-digestible carbohydrates, which have many biological actions including: being an important energy source for colonic epithelial cells[97]; regulating gene expression by binding to G-protein-coupled receptors found in a wide variety of tissues and cells (adipocytes, immune and endocrine cells)[98,99]; modulating intestinal gluconeogenesis and appetite[100]; regulating

inflammation by acting on T regulatory cells[101,102]; and regulating the production of leptin.[103–105] This host–microbial relationship is bidirectional and is the end product of a billion years of permanent interaction with our environment.[106] Gut microbial diversity and composition are profoundly influenced by host diet, lifestyle, drugs, disease, the presence of pathogens, genetic background and environmental factors.[100,107–109]

Nutrition

Nutrition plays an important role in both the onset and the prevention of many chronic diseases associated with toxicant exposure. Complex interactions of multiple polymorphisms play a key role in how individuals respond to dietary interventions (*nutrigenetics*) and how some nutrients may affect gene expression (*nutrigenomics*),[110] which may inadvertently affect the way individuals deal with environmental toxicants. About 25 tonnes of food passes through a person's gut in their lifetime, making food the primary source of exposure to microbes and toxicants. The past 20 years have shown that diet and nutrients not only contribute to shaping the gut microbiota composition, but they also affect many genes related to inflammation and oxidative stress and provide key nutrients for a large number of biological processes vital for detoxification, the immune response (including gene expression), protein synthesis, modification and degradation, metabolism, signal transduction, and cellular proliferation and survival.[111,112] Numerous constituents in nutraceuticals (foods that provide health benefits) have been identified, including antioxidant flavonoids, proanthocyanidins, carotenoids, dietary fibre, phyto-oestrogens, glucosinolates, catechins, saponins and lignans,[113] which may explain the effectiveness of health-promoting diets like the traditional Mediterranean diet in lowering the risk of chronic diseases.[114,115]

Recent longitudinal studies investigating dietary intake in human centenarians have shown that micronutrients (zinc, copper, selenium) and polyphenolic antioxidants in fruits and vegetables play a pivotal role in maintaining and reinforcing the performance of the immune and antioxidant systems, as well as in affecting the complex network of genes.[112,116] Similarly, many foods have been implicated in the development of disease. A high-fat diet has been shown to disrupt Gram-negative intestinal populations of animals, liberating lipopolysaccharide and resulting in low-grade chronic inflammation.[79] Alcohol induces CYP2E1 enzyme (which is involved in phase I detoxification, activates various carcinogens and is responsible for metabolising many volatile organic compounds) and simultaneously depletes glutathione levels in the liver, thereby reducing the ability to detoxify other chemicals.[82] It is well established that a Western diet produces chronic inflammation due to excessive levels of omega-6 oils, saturated fat, sugars and starches, as well as a deficiency in micronutrients and antioxidants.[117,118]

Ethnicity

Ethnicity is an important marker for susceptibility to environmental toxicants and is the outcome of the interaction between genetics, diet and geography, as family members who share a family history of heart disease are also more likely to share other risk factors such as diet, activity and place history.[119] Polymorphisms in key detoxification pathways and gut microbiota with distinct xenobiotic metabolising capacities also vary with ethnicity.[63]

ENVIRONMENTAL TRIGGERS OF DISEASE

Chronic non-communicable diseases share a common cluster of environmental and genetic risk factors that ultimately affect the individual's resilience and capacity to cope within their environment. The exposome of the individual, which is the totality of all human environmental exposure from conception to death, will vary depending on the dose, timing, duration, frequency and route of exposure to toxicants, as well as the individual's susceptibility. The increase in allostatic load brought on by environmental exposure results in an increase in the steady-state reactive oxygen species (ROS) known as oxidative stress at the cellular level, and low-grade systemic inflammation, which paradoxically are also the hallmarks of ageing and chronic disease.[86] While nutrition and xenobiotic metabolising enzymes derived from the gut and within the body (detoxification) can modify the risk of exposure to toxicants, in the absence of exposure, the presence or absence of gene polymorphisms becomes irrelevant. Consequently, the focus of clinical practice should be on educating the patient on how to reduce their exposure to harmful toxicants (see Fig. 2.1).[120]

TOXICANTS

The chemicals humans are exposed to, through their diet, home, workplace or environment, can have a profound effect on their health[121]: 27% of global chronic disease mortality is attributed to exposure to radon, ozone, lead,

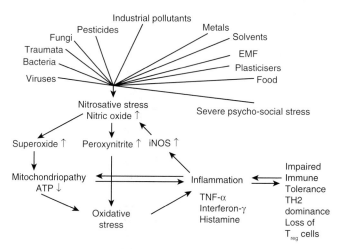

FIGURE 2.1 Pathogenesis of inflammation, mitochondriopathy and nitrosative stress as a result of exposure to environmental triggers.

Von Baehr V. Rationelle labordiagnostik bei chronisch entzündlichen systemerkrankungen. Umwelt Medizin Gesellschaft 2012;25(4):244–247.

workplace chemicals, cigarette smoke, wood smoke (from cooking fires) and air pollution.[122] There are more than 124 million chemicals registered for use on the world's largest database, the Chemical Abstract Service,[123] and most of the artificial portions of these chemicals have never been tested for their impact on human health. Large population biomonitoring studies have revealed widespread exposure to toxicants at levels in humans known to cause adverse health effects.[7–10] While chemical exposure is ubiquitous in the general population, environmental hazards are inequitably distributed according to class, race, location and lifestyle factors.

Diseases associated with toxicant exposure

The list of diseases that have been implicated with toxicant exposure is extensive and growing and includes allergies,[124–127] diabetes,[128,129] infertility,[130–132] testicular dysgenesis syndrome[78,133] (which encompasses hypospadias,[134,135] cryptorchidism,[136,137] testicular cancer[138] and poor semen quality[139–141]), ovarian dysgenesis syndrome,[142] neurodegenerative diseases such as Alzheimer's[143] and Parkinson's disease,[144–146] respiratory disorders such as asthma[147] and chronic obstructive pulmonary disease,[148] autoimmune diseases,[149] obesity,[150–152] cardiovascular disease[153–157] and neurodevelopmental disorders.[50,158]

The environment is likely to play the principal role in most types of cancers as genetic factors have been shown to contribute only a minor role.[159] There is a growing body of evidence associating toxicants with various cancers, including air pollutants such as asbestos, radon, hexavalent chromium, tobacco smoke and benzo(a)pyrene with lung cancer[160–163]; EDCs such as pesticides, dioxins, furans and PCBs with an increased risk of breast cancer,[164] endometrial cancer, testicular cancer and prostate cancer[55,165–167]; arsenic and disinfection by-products with bladder cancer[168,169]; vinyl chloride with liver cancer[170]; benzene with leukaemia[171]; and pesticides with childhood leukaemia.[171–174]

Toxicants have also been linked to the rise in idiopathic environmental intolerance characterised by a chronic, complex multisystem disease that frequently and dramatically limits the activities of sufferers. These sensitivity-related illnesses (SRIs) have no clear aetiology or pathogenesis and attract various diagnoses from multiple chemical sensitivity to chronic fatigue syndrome, myalgic encephalomyelitis, biotoxin illness, sick building syndrome, Gulf War syndrome, fibromyalgia, electromagnetic hypersensitivity and systemic exertion intolerance disease. Clinical similarities and frequent comorbidities between these unexplained multisystem conditions of environmental origin have induced many authors to hypothesise that they may share common genetic and/or metabolic molecular determinants connected with polymorphisms in oxidative stress,[175] antioxidant and detoxification genes[176–178] with subsequent impaired capability to detoxify xenobiotics,[179] and mitochondrial dysfunction,[175,176] along with low-grade systemic inflammation in multiple organ systems.[176,180–182]

Sources of toxicant exposure

Taking an exposure history is essential to detect, treat and prevent toxicant exposure – see the ATSDR case studies.[183] Excluding occupational exposure to toxicants and pharmaceutical drugs, the primary sources of environmental toxicants are air, food and water. Rather than describing the numerous classes of chemicals (pesticides, heavy metals, flame retardants, food additives, preservatives, solvents etc.), this section focuses on the source of exposure.

AIR

Sources of air pollutants

- Natural sources: bushfires, storms, seaspray and volcanic activity
- Industrial emissions: living near industrial areas, mining areas, coal seam gas exploration, shipping ports, airports, military bases, municipal or waste sites and other 'sacrifice zones'
- Vehicle emissions: living, working or exercising in built-up areas close to heavy traffic, bus/truck/taxi depots, flight paths, mining areas, military bases; use of lawn mowers, boat motors
- Agricultural chemicals: living or working in close proximity to farming communities, timber plantations, market gardens, schools, parks, golf courses, bowling clubs and so on; applying pesticides and herbicides for pest management, veterinary and/or gardening purposes
- Volatile organic compounds: environmental tobacco smoke, new clothes, bedding, air fresheners, incense, perfumes, moth balls, dry-cleaning solvents, personal care and cleaning products, new building materials and furnishings, paints, thinners, solvents (spot removers, dry cleaning products)
- Particulates: asbestos and lead dust, as well as particulates generated from vehicle exhaust, mining and industry
- Radon gas: from the radioactive decay of uranium in soil, rock and water – levels in a home depend on the local geology and soil type (it is more commonly found in phosphate and granite deposits), house type, construction, materials and ventilation
- Noxious gases arising from unflued gas appliances, the incomplete combustion of solid fuels (wood/coal/dung/crop waste) for cooking or heating (open fireplace), ground-level ozone and photochemical smog in built-up areas.

Tips to reduce exposure to air pollutants

- Homes, workplaces and schools should be located away from known sources of air pollutants such as industrial zones, shipping ports, mining areas, flight paths, military bases, sewage sites, municipal tips and waste sites, bus/truck/taxi depots, carparks and heavy traffic
- New buildings and renovations should consider the microclimate and topography of the site to maximise the use of natural light, promote passive ventilation and good drainage, and reduce the need for artificial heating and cooling. They should also use natural, unadulterated, sustainable and hygroscopic building materials that are low in volatile organic compounds, are not radioactive and do not adversely impact the electroclimate of the space or the health of the occupants
- Homes located near known sources of air pollutants should be sealed and retrofitted with a whole house filtration system that includes HEPA and carbon filters
- Homes built prior to the 1980s should be tested for lead paint and asbestos by a licensed professional prior to conducting any renovations
- Air-conditioning and heating systems and natural gas appliances should be well maintained and serviced in accordance with the manufacturer's guidelines. The air intake for an air-conditioning system should not be located near food outlets or vehicle exhaust (i.e. garage, carpark)
- Heating and cooking sources that use wood, coal or dung as a fuel source (e.g. open fireplace, wood combustion stove) should be avoided
- Cars should not be left to idle in enclosed garages
- Exhaust fans in the kitchen, bathroom and laundry should be regularly cleaned and vented to the outside
- Environmental tobacco smoke, air fresheners, scented candles, incense, and perfume and fragrances in cleaning and personal care products should be avoided
- Furnishings should be made from natural fibres and materials (timber, glass, metal, bamboo, wool, organic cotton) that have been sourced and made locally
- An integrated pest management plan that avoids the use of chemical pesticides should be implemented
- Occupational exposure should implement the *hierarchy of control* in accordance with legislative requirements.

Lifestyle tips to reduce exposure to air pollutants

- Air the house on dry sunny days
- Avoid exercising in industrial and high-traffic areas
- Remove shoes before entering the home, as most pollutants are tracked into the house
- Expose new furnishings, pillows and mattresses to full sun (outside) to allow volatile organic compounds to outgas
- Wash new clothes, soft toys and bedding before use and air-dry them in the sun
- Limit use of personal care products and cosmetics and use products derived from certified organic plant-based ingredients, or still in their natural state, such as cold-pressed seed, nut or vegetable oils (jojoba oil, camellia nut oil, macadamia nut oil, rosehip oil, argan oil, moringa oil, sweet almond oil, coconut oil, tamanu oil, monoi oil)
- Cover up (hat, sunglasses, UV-resistant clothes) to reduce exposure to midday sun and reduce the need for chemical-based sunscreens
- Use slightly damp microfibre cloths to dust and clean the home and use cleaning products made from food-grade (not industrial-grade) ingredients that are fragrance-free
- Use a vacuum cleaner fitted with HEPA and carbon filters to reduce exposure to airborne pollutants.

FOOD

Sources of toxicants in food

- Pesticides, fungicides and herbicides used on fruits, vegetables, legumes, grains and nuts
- Food additives in processed foods such as food colouring, flavours, preservatives, acidity regulators, antioxidants, emulsifiers, stabilisers, thickeners, anticaking agents and sweeteners
- Eating top predators (fish) that are likely to contain heavy metals and persistent organic pollutants
- Antibiotics, agrochemicals and antiparasitic drugs used in livestock
- Radioactive nuclides occurring naturally in soil and water or arising from nuclear accidents
- Heavy metals in plants and animals (arising from artificial and natural sources)
- Food packaging made from plastic (phthalates, bisphenol-A) and tins (BPA lining, lead solder)
- Cooking utensils: copper or aluminium pots and pans, eroding non-stick cookware, plastic bakeware
- Plastic wraps and containers (numbers 1, 3, 6 and 7), lead- or cadmium-containing glazed ceramics or containers with leaded crystal or radioactive glazes
- Freezing or heating food in plastic.

Tips to reduce exposure to toxicants in food

- Eat food that is:
  Seasonal (has adapted to the microclimate of the region)
  Local (low in embodied energy)
  Organic (free from pesticides)
  Whole (still in its natural state)
- Consume less processed (packaged) food and make meals from scratch using ingredients based on the SLOW principles
- Follow a plant-based diet, which is low on the food chain and less likely to accumulate persistent organic pollutants commonly found in top predators
- Store, freeze and cook food in oven/freezer-proof glass, stainless steel, cast iron, ceramics or Corning Ware
- While non-stick cookware should be avoided, ceramic-lined non-stick cookware is available that does not use perfluorinated chemicals.

WATER

Sources of drinking water pollutants

- Contamination of ground and surface water arising from natural sources: bushfires, storms, seaspray, volcanic activity, high mineral content in rocks (arsenic); and from human sources: industrial emissions, vehicle exhaust, fertilisers, pesticides, mining, effluent (animals and humans), municipal tips and proximity to 'sacrifice zones'
- Disinfectant by-products (fluoride, chlorine, alum) used to purify water
- Radioactive nuclides such as radon gas
- Contaminants arising from the mains distribution and domestic pipes such as asbestos, heavy metals (copper, lead, silver), biofilm and phthalates in plastics
- Contaminants arising from the catchment areas used for tank water such as PVC downpipes, asbestos, lead flashing, microbes, solvents, pesticide drift and sealants on roof and solar panels, animal droppings
- Storage vessels made from plastic (polyvinyl chlorine, polystyrene, polycarbonate), acrylonitrile butadiene styrene (ABS), lead-glazed or radioactive ceramics and heavy metals in older pigments.

Tips to reduce exposure to water pollutants

- Use storage vessels made of glass, food-grade stainless steel, unglazed ceramics or Corning Ware
- While there is no ideal water filter system, the type of water filter used depends on the source of drinking water (tap, tank, bore/well or bottled water), which contaminants you want to remove, water pressure, bench space and how much you are prepared to spend to buy and maintain the unit
- Pre-sediment filters filter out larger particles such as sediment and prolong the life of carbon filters
- Carbon filters filter out chlorine and its by-products, pesticides, petrochemicals and other organic contaminants but not heavy metals or fluoride
- Deioniser filters remove fluoride and heavy metals but not organic contaminants such as pesticides and may leave resin fragments in the water
- Ceramic filters reduce bacteria, chlorine, sediment and rust, but are not effective in removing heavy metals or pesticides, and require weekly maintenance to remove the biofilm
- Ozone oxidises organic contaminants such as pesticides and microorganisms, but is an irritant gas that can be lethal at high doses, which is why it shouldn't be used for domestic water filtration. UV filters are used to kill bacteria, algae and parasites and reduce cysts, but they are ineffective in hard or turbid water and their efficiency dramatically declines when dirt accumulates on the lamp. Reverse osmosis removes most contaminants including fluoride (providing the flow rate is not too high), but it is costly, needs to be plumbed in to remove waste water, needs a lot of space (bench or under the sink) for the storage tank and is slow to filter. Consequently, combination filters are often used for domestic purposes. Water filters should be certified with the National Sanitation Foundation (NSF) to confirm the effectiveness of the filter.

ELECTROMAGNETIC FIELDS

Life on earth has evolved within an exquisite and dynamic array of natural electromagnetic energy sources arising from the earth's magnetic field (geomagnetic field), radioactivity (cosmic and x-rays from the galaxy and radioactivity within the earth's crust), the sun, gravity and the Schumann resonances. The geomagnetic field influences both the magnetic alignment and the migration and homing of various animal species from bees, ants, termites and fruit flies to birds, fish, cows and deer.[184] In the human body, terrestrial radiation provides remarkably low-intensity yet critical frequencies that play an important role in our circadian rhythms, sleep and wake cycles, brainwave activity, neural synchrony, immune function, behaviour and onset of puberty, as well as gene expression, cell communication and metabolism.[185]

In the past 20 years, we have progressively added an enormous amount of artificial frequencies to the planet's natural electromagnetic background to the extent that there is practically nowhere remaining that is not being influenced by it in some way. The rapid uptake of mobile phones (more than 6 billion users worldwide) and deployment of wireless technologies in our homes, schools and workplaces reflects our voracious appetite for technology and has given rise to a plethora of new terms like Google, Facebook, Twitter, Snapchat and digital dementia.[186]

There are four electromagnetic fields that impact the built environment: AC electric fields (voltage), AC magnetic fields (current), radiofrequencies used in wireless technologies, and dirty power (high-frequency spikes and harmonics on electrical wiring). The frequencies that consistently appear in the scientific literature and for which health concerns have been raised are AC magnetic fields and radiofrequencies, and these are the focus of this section.

Mechanism of action

Electromagnetic fields are used in medicine for both diagnostic purposes (magnetic resonance imaging, electrocardiograms, electroencephalograms [EEGs]) and in the treatment of a range of disorders from neonatal jaundice to depression, pain-related disorders, osteoporosis, degenerative affections of peripheral joints, wound healing, rheumatoid arthritis and ankylosing spondylitis.[187–191] Epidemiology and EEG studies provide compelling evidence for the existence of non-thermal effects (low-level exposure effects) arising from the regular use of mobile phones, which use radiofrequency electromagnetic energy.[192] When cells are exposed to low-intensity radiofrequency radiation they produce ROS for several minutes or even hours after irradiation, which can increase the cells' expression of antioxidants.[193,194] Similarly, the health-promoting benefits of magnetic fields are attributed to their ability to alter intracellular concentrations of sodium and potassium ions, resulting in vasodilation, angiogenesis, anticoagulation activity, intensification of the processes of repair and regeneration of soft tissues, and anti-oedematic properties, as well as analgesic activity.[187,190,195] These events may contribute to the activation of protective or damaging processes and are suspected to play a key role in the induction of the radioadaptive response.[196–198] Among 100 currently available peer-reviewed studies dealing with oxidative effects of low-intensity radiofrequency radiation (RFR) used in wireless technologies, 93 confirmed that RFR induces oxidative effects in biological systems.[199]

Paradoxically, the mechanism by which electromagnetic fields may induce protective effects is similar to the way in which they may cause harm. The cell membrane is hydrophobic, consisting of ion pumps to prevent the free movement of ions across the cellular membrane. Electromagnetic fields may cause biological effects by activating L-type voltage-gated calcium channels (VGCCs) in the cell membrane, enabling calcium ions to flow into the cell with subsequent multiple downstream effects.[200,201] This mechanism of action has been confirmed by the observation that these downstream effects can be completely negated with the use of calcium channel blocker drugs.[200,201]

The Russian physicist Igor Lednev demonstrated that when the frequency of the alternating magnetic field is equal to the harmonics, subharmonics or cyclotron frequency of ions (like calcium) bonded to proteins, a resonant response of the biosystem to the magnetic field results that may disrupt or enhance cellular function.[202–204] The subsequent increased intracellular calcium activates nitric oxide synthase enzymes, resulting in the production of nitric oxide, which can lead to one of two pathways: nitric oxide signalling (therapeutic effect) or, after reaction with superoxide, the formation of the very reactive peroxynitrite free radical (harmful effect).[205,206] Low levels of these ROS free radicals activate antioxidant enzymes (superoxide dismutase, catalase and various peroxidases), while high levels inactivate them, resulting in an increase in the steady-state ROS known as oxidative stress.[194,201,207,208]

This may result in mitochondrial dysfunction, DNA strand breaks,[194,201,209,210] inhibition of DNA repair in stem cells[211] and apoptosis (cell death) and cause oxidative damage to proteins, membranes and genes.[116] Furthermore, ROS may contribute to the down regulation of tight junctions and therefore induce the matrix metalloproteinases (MMPs), thereby enhancing the permeability of the blood–brain barrier.[212] Disturbance of this redox balance, uncontrolled activation of free radical processes, overproduction of ROS and/or suppression of antioxidant defence in the cell brought on by radiofrequency exposure[213] at non-thermal effects are often the important signals of some hazardous changes in cell metabolism. Other documented effects include an increase in histamine, which is a major cause of systemic inflammation,[214] and suppression of the 'anticancer' hormone melatonin, which is the body's most potent weapon against cellular and DNA damage.[215,216] The 'dose window theory' in non-ionising radiation-induced adaptive responses[217] is suspected to be nonlinear[193,218] and explains why the impact of low-frequency fields on biological systems appears to induce both protective (within a narrow window) and damaging effects, which makes this field of study both highly controversial and contradictory.

Several authorities (International Commission for Non-Ionising Radiation Protection, US National Cancer Institute, World Health Organization, UK Health Protection Agency, Australian Radiation Protection and Nuclear Safety Authority, Health Canada, New Zealand Ministry for the Environment and the Swedish Radiation Protection Authority) adhere to the concept that non-ionising radiation cannot cause cancer because, unlike ionising radiation, it does not have enough energy to dislodge electrons and harmful effects arising from RF EME occur only due to heating.[219] Applying the ionisation model to non-ionising radiation is inappropriate because peer-reviewed research has shown that RF EME may indirectly induce cancer by generating ROS, which damages DNA and interferes with antioxidant repair mechanisms.[199,219–222] Electromagnetic fields may potentiate the effects of metals and toxicants. In one study, exposure to magnetic resonance imaging and mobile phones significantly accelerated mercury vapour released from dental amalgams.[223]

Health effects attributed to electromagnetic field exposure

Concerns about electromagnetic fields were first brought to light in military personnel on radar bases during World War II and later in electrical workers involved in the telecommunications industry. However, it wasn't until Wertheimer and Leeper published their research on high-voltage power lines and childhood leukaemia in 1979 that concerns about electromagnetic fields on public health came to the fore.[224] While it is recognised that non-ionising electromagnetic fields typically found in the built environment cannot cause gene mutations, cancers that consistently appear in the scientific literature are childhood leukaemia, breast cancer and brain tumours (acoustic neuromas and gliomas). There is a significant body of evidence showing a link between AC magnetic fields in excess of 3 mG and childhood leukaemia,[224–228] with documented exposure zones up to 600 m from high-voltage transmission lines.[229,230] It is estimated that AC magnetic fields above 3 mG are responsible for up to 2% of all cases of childhood leukaemia annually.[227,231] This exposure level can easily be exceeded in a home if individuals spend prolonged periods of time – such as when sleeping, working or relaxing – within 1 m of a smart meter, meter panel, inverter, oven (while it is heating), fridge (while it is cooling) or any other appliance that draws a high level of current. Two pooled analyses on high-voltage transmission lines and childhood leukaemia in the year 2000[225,232] were sufficient to convince the World Health Organization's International Agency for Research on Cancer (IARC) to classify AC magnetic fields as a possible human carcinogen.[233] Using a mobile phone for more than 25 minutes per day reduces production of the body's most potent antioxidant free radical scavenger, melatonin.[234]

The annual incidence of head tumours coincides with the increased rate of mobile phone subscriptions,[235] although there are significant disparities about the rate even among researchers from the same country.[236,237] Part of the problem lies in when the data were collected. Many studies, including the Danish Cancer Registry, analysed data well before mobile phones were adopted by the general public.[238–244] A significant increase in glioma incidence in the Australian population was identified after 2006,[236] which coincides with the time period when mobile phones were widely adopted.[245] However, these findings contradict the Australian government's findings because the cancer registries were not updated. 'Late ascertainment' is common among cancer registries and is

associated with a data lag of between 3 and 5 years.[246] Another issue is that the frequency of brain tumour diagnosis on autopsy has declined substantially due to a general decline in the number of autopsies being performed, rendering some cancer registries unreliable for use in epidemiological studies.[247]

There have been several studies[248–252] and numerous reports[253–256] correlating an increased risk of glioma and acoustic neuroma with mobile phone use. The three most influential case-control studies to date are INTERPHONE (European), CERENAT (French) and Hardell's (Swedish) study, which identified an increased risk of gliomas and acoustic neuromas in people who used their phone for at least 30 minutes per day on one side of the head for a minimum of 10 years. The largest study, the INTERPHONE study involving more than 5000 people, identified a 40% increased risk of glioma,[249] while the CERENAT study calculated a 100% increased risk of glioma,[248] and Hardell's research team identified a 170% increased risk of glioma[251] in addition to increases in other brain tumours (acoustic neuromas and meningiomas).[250,251,257,258] Similar results were obtained in a meta-analysis, which showed an increased risk of gliomas and acoustic neuromas with long-term use of over 10 years.[259] Some have argued that the CERENAT and INTERPHONE studies underestimated the risk because they ignored the radiation emitted from DECT phones.[258,260]

In contrast, there have been many studies for which a correlation has not been observed.[237,243,261–264] Several of these studies analysed brain tumour incidence in patients well before mobile phones were widely adopted by the general public. The INTERPHONE study is an interesting case in point: three groups of researchers came up with completely different conclusions analysing the same data.[263,265,266] The CEFALO multicentre case-control study focused on the possible association between mobile phone use and brain tumours among adolescents and showed no correlation.[267] The authors acknowledged several (major) flaws with their own study, including the fact that mobile phone use was based on the memory of the child or their parents to recall their use (i.e. it didn't measure the dose), the latency period was short as the children had used their phone for less than 4 years and most of the children rarely actually used a mobile phone!

It remains unclear whether the correlation between brain tumours and mobile phone use is coincidental or whether use of mobile phones may cause the development, promotion or progression of specific cancers.[268] There are several reasons why there are discrepancies in mobile phone research:

- The tendency to adjust the research to fit the needs of the industry providing the funding[253]
- Differences in study design – frequency, intensity and duration of exposure – which makes it impossible to compare studies
- The long latency period associated with primary brain tumours
- The time period that the data were analysed
- No exposure data because of reliance on self-reported mobile phone use or data obtained from service providers

- The age of first exposure (higher risks are observed in people who began mobile phone use before the age of 15)[250]
- The use of provocation 'feeling' studies popular among psychologists, which do not allow for the 2–3 days acclimatisation or immune washout typically observed in animal studies.[269–271]

Swedish professor Lennart Hardell, a world expert on mobile phone research, has consistently observed a statistically significant higher risk of developing glioma types of brain tumours in people who use mobile phones using digital frequencies, namely the 3G network, before the age of 20.[250,257] As wide-band microwave signals (3G onwards) were only launched in the early 2000s and it wasn't until 2005 when mobile phones became popular among children,[245] the increased incidence of brain tumours (gliomas and acoustic neuromas) with latency periods of up to 25 years would not be expected until the latter half of the 2020s. Despite this, many existing large-scale population-based studies, including the COSMOS study[272] and the MOBI-Kids study,[273] have failed to gather exposure data, even though apps exist to accurately estimate radiofrequency emissions from mobile devices.[274]

Collecting reliable data on complex and rapidly changing patterns of exposure, while minimising recall bias and errors, will be a significant challenge for ongoing large-scale population-based studies in mobile phone research. Despite this, on 31 May 2011 following an analysis of 900 publications by 30 scientists, the IARC classified radiofrequency electromagnetic energy as a possible human carcinogen.[275] On this basis alone, the precautionary principle should be enacted and the public should be informed about current scientific uncertainty and advised to limit their exposure by adopting the inverse square law (distance).

Electromagnetic fields have also been correlated to other chronic diseases. Two recent reviews concluded an increased risk of female breast cancer following AC magnetic field exposure,[276,277] with some quantifying exposure in excess of 12 mG as being significant[278,279]; however, there are many studies for which an association was not found. Similarly, neurodegenerative diseases like Lou Gehrig's disease (motor neurone disease), Parkinson's disease and Alzheimer's have also been reported following exposure to radiofrequency electromagnetic energy, with inconsistent results.[212,255,280–282]

Electromagnetic hypersensitivity (EHS), or idiopathic environmental intolerance to electromagnetic fields (IEI-EMF), is a syndrome arising from exposure to electromagnetic fields with a broad spectrum of nonspecific symptoms involving multiple organ systems. The wide variation in symptoms experienced by sufferers may be attributed to the local effects that electromagnetic fields may have on voltage-gated calcium channels. EHS is estimated to affect 2–6% of the population (primarily women), with the highest incidence of 13% observed in the Taiwanese population.[283] EHS was first acknowledged as a disability in Sweden when it was documented in computer workers in the 1980s and pressure is mounting on the World Health Organization to recognise it as a

medical disease. According to Bevington,[284] the European Academy for Environmental Medicine,[285] the Austrian Medical Association[286] and the British Society of Ecological Medicine,[287] symptoms of EHS may include the following:

- General: long-term fatigue, headache, sleep disturbance, flu-like symptoms
- Heart and circulation: chest pain, increased heart rate, blood pressure changes, arrhythmias, shortness of breath, nosebleeds, cold extremities
- Brain: brain fog (anomia, poor short-term memory, difficulty concentrating), dizziness, confusion, dyslexia, difficulty learning, mood swings
- Ears: earache, tinnitus (ringing in the ears), problems with balance
- Eyes: dry and gritty, eyelid tics, irritation, pressure behind eyes
- Skin: itchy, prickling and biting sensation on the skin like 'electric shocks', rash, lumps, brown 'sun spots', a sensation of warmth or burning likened to sunburn
- Muscles: body aches and joint pains, jaw and teeth pain, numbness or tingling sensations, muscle spasms/tremors, weakness, restless legs
- Sensitivities: chemical, light, noise and/or smell.

Sufferers can often pinpoint which building and/or rooms make them unwell: the symptoms significantly improve when they are away from the electromagnetic field and they are relieved with avoidance, bathing and shielding.

Testing for electromagnetic fields

- *Clinical testing.* The lack of available clinical biomarkers to test for EHS has been part of the problem in gaining recognition for the syndrome. The Austrian Medical Association in 2012[288] and the European Academy for Environmental Medicine in 2016[285] developed guidelines for doctors on how to diagnose and treat electromagnetic field-related health problems as a duty of care, including a detailed questionnaire, the scope of which is beyond this chapter
- *Exposure data.* Collecting individual exposure data for radiofrequency electromagnetic field exposure is freely available through apps such as Quanta Monitor by Cellraid
- *Home testing* for AC magnetic fields and radiofrequency electromagnetic energy fields in the patient's home and workplace by a qualified building biologist is recommended to identify and reduce exposure to potential sources. While AC magnetic fields can easily be measured using a three-axis digital gauss meter, radiofrequency electromagnetic energy fields require specialist equipment such as a spectrum analyser or high-frequency meter (with a wide range from 27 MHz to 10 GHz). In addition, it requires a thorough knowledge of the various frequencies used by wireless devices, an understanding of the way in which radiofrequencies are influenced by metal building materials such as sarking, reflective foil insulation and metal roofs, knowledge of exposure standards that encompass the precautionary principle and the

limitations involved in spot and short-term measurements. AC magnetic fields above 3 mG can easily be exceeded if you sleep against a wall adjacent to a meter panel, smart meter, inverter, fridge, electric hot water system or oven (when it is heating) or have a digital clock radio within 20 cm of the bed.

Sources of AC magnetic fields

- Outside sources: high-voltage transmission lines, transformers, substations, power lines, tram lines, electricity meters (analogue, digital and smart meters) and inverters (from solar panels)
- Inside sources: all operating appliances that are connected to the building wiring. Higher fields (that draw more current) occur in appliances with a built-in transformer, electronic ballast or motor, including freestanding lamps, halogen desk lamps, energy-saving compact fluorescent lamps and bulbs, older style fluorescent lights, digital clock radios, mobile phone chargers, electronic beds, water beds, fridges, ovens, fish tanks and pool/water feature pumps. High AC magnetic fields also arise when the active and neutral wires are separated, such as in meter panels, switches, some types of electric blankets and electric underfloor heating (hydronic heating is not a high source). Visual display units/monitors are not a high source of AC magnetic fields because they comply with TCO certification (a type of sustainability certification)
- Transient exposure to high AC magnetic fields above 3 mG (such as walking past a meter panel or under powerlines) is unlikely to create a health issue. However, long-term exposure to low levels should be avoided where occupants spend the greatest amount of time, such as in bed, at a desk while studying or working, lying on a favourite sofa or while at the kitchen sink and benchtop where food is prepared. High AC magnetic field readings on the ground floor of older homes may arise if the metal water pipes carry a charge as the earthing system is connected to the power mains neutral conductor.

Tips to reduce exposure to AC magnetic fields

- AC magnetic fields penetrate most materials including concrete, brick and steel and there are few shielding materials (apart from Mu metal) that contain these fields. The most effective method to reduce exposure is distance (inverse square law). Depending on the source of exposure, a distance of at least 1 m from appliances should apply in areas where the occupant spends long periods of time, such as in bed
- When building or rewiring a home, exposure to the AC magnetic field from the wires can be reduced by bundling the cables together and keeping appliances and power boards away from the walls where people spend time, such as walls against a bedhead, sofa or workstation
- Battery-operated and wind-up devices are also recommended.[186]

Sources of RF EME

- Outside sources: mobile phone towers/base stations, radar (military, airport, sea port, traffic and weather control), TETRA (emergency services), digital television and radio towers
- Inside sources: mobile phones, cordless phones, smart meters and wireless devices (routers, computers, laptops, printers, photocopiers, fax machines, iPads, iPods, fitness trackers, Bluetooth, baby monitors, security systems), hearing devices and communication systems such as wireless paging systems used in hospitals and restaurants. Many new appliances coming onto the market will be fitted with ZigBees to enable them to connect wirelessly to a smart meter. This enables the power company to remotely switch off appliances in the home like air conditioners to conserve power. The adverse health effects arising from exposure to these radiofrequencies has not been studied. It is important to avoid using a mobile phone in a car because (apart from causing accidents) the radiofrequency electromagnetic energy will reflect off the metal carriage thereby multiplying the exposure in the same way these frequencies bounce inside a microwave oven.

Tips to reduce exposure to external sources of RF EME

- RF EME reflects off metal and penetrates glass (windows), timber and bricks. As such, metal roofs and foil insulation in the walls will reduce exposure to external sources but will reflect internal sources back into the home. Shielded fabrics, paints and window films can reduce exposure to external sources. Metal blinds that are closed at night also reduce exposure to external sources coming in through a window.[186] The most effective way to reduce exposure to electromagnetic fields is distance. As you double the distance away from an RF source, you will reduce your exposure by 75%.

TIPS WHEN USING CORDLESS AND MOBILE PHONES

- Use a hardwired corded phone whenever possible to make or receive a call
- Keep cordless and mobile phones away from the head by texting or using the loudspeaker function or using an ear piece when making or receiving calls
- Keep calls short
- Do not carry the phone on your body (in your bra or pocket). Carry it in a handbag or place it in a shielded pouch
- If you must use a cordless phone, purchase an analogue model as they emit radiation only when a call is made, and keep the base unit at least two rooms away from bedrooms
- Avoid using a mobile phone in a moving vehicle (tram, train, bus, car) as it emits higher power to maintain a signal with the nearest mobile tower
- Do not charge mobile phones in bedrooms and do not use them as an alarm clock placed under the pillow

- Avoid making calls in areas with poor signal strength: use the phone when the maximum number of bars are on the screen (with fewer bars, the phone emits higher power to maintain the signal)
- Children under the age of 15 should avoid using mobile phones except in an emergency. Texting is preferred as it keeps the phone away from the head. If children play games on a mobile phone, set it to flight mode in order to turn off the wireless connection.[186]

TIPS WHEN USING PORTABLE WIRELESS DEVICES

- Use appliances that use hardwired cable options that don't connect wirelessly
- When in use, place the device on a table or desk away from your body
- Once you have downloaded the information/app from the internet, turn off the wireless connectivity by putting the device in flight mode.[186]

TIPS WHEN USING A ROUTER (MODEM)

- Use a hard-wired cable connection (ADSL) for desktop computers; however, it will restrict internet connectivity to one area of the home. For multiple users, install an ethernet home network which uses a powerline ethernet adapter (such as a TP-Link) plugged into the power socket using the existing electrical wires in your home. This requires a dual modem (with the wi-fi switched off) with an ethernet plug so that it can connect to the TP Link
- Check with the manufacturer to determine how to disable the modem's wireless function. Be mindful that some new modems do not have a cable option
- Keep the router away from areas where people spend time, such as the bedroom, office and living areas. Instead, install it in the garage or a spare room or formal living room that is rarely used
- Power the router down by 95% so that the RF EME fields don't bathe the entire house. For instructions on how to do this, see the manufacturer's website
- Unplug the router when it is not in use, especially at night
- Avoid using extenders (repeaters). Instead, dedicate a specific area of the house to access the internet
- If you live in a multilevel apartment or if your home is attached to another, encourage the neighbours to switch off their wireless devices at night
- In schools, wireless laptops and work stations should be avoided and replaced with standard or fibre-optic cables connected to a rooftop antenna.[186]

ALLERGENS

The interactions between allergens, the immune response, sensitisation and airways disease are highly complex and not yet completely understood.[289] Current thinking suggests a multifactorial model for allergy, in which an initial trigger (viral or environment) stimulates the innate immune response to effect prolonged chronic inflammation, which might – in those with a genetic susceptibility – interact with exposure to an allergen-facilitating allergy.[289] Where pollen sensitisation is strongly associated with the development of allergic rhinitis, indoor allergen sensitisation is associated with asthma.[290] This section focuses on aeroallergens (not allergies arising from exposure to pharmaceutical drugs or food).

In the past two decades, the incidence of allergies such as asthma, atopic eczema, allergic rhinitis and food allergies has steadily increased in Western countries, with strikingly different time courses observed in various locations.[291–295] Australia is leading the allergy epidemic: 25% of the population have been diagnosed with an allergy,[296] 20% of adults have allergic rhinitis, 10% of adults and up to 25% of children have asthma and 10% of children have food allergies and atopic eczema.[297] The increase in respiratory allergic disease since the 1990s has coincided with a 10% increase in food allergies (to cow's milk, egg, nuts, wheat) and a 30% increase in atopic eczema worldwide.[291,298] During this period, hospital admissions for anaphylaxis has more than doubled in the US[299] and increased four-fold in Australia[297] and six-fold in England and Wales,[300] reflecting similar trends in other Western countries.[301,302]

The introduction of allergenic food to infants has been met with much controversy, as delayed introduction has been shown to increase the incidence of developing food allergies.[303] New guidelines recommend breastfeeding for at least 6 months, introducing a variety of solids at around 6 months of age (but not before 4 months of age), and introducing allergenic solid foods including peanut butter, cooked egg, dairy and wheat products in the first year of life.[304] While most childhood food allergies tend to decline with age (except wheat, shrimp and nuts), around 50% of affected children go on to develop inhalant allergies to house dust mites, grass pollens or cat dander (the most prevalent environmental allergens), resulting in allergic rhinitis and asthma later in life. This is known as the 'Atopic (Allergic) March'. With the exception of allergic rhinitis, which appeared in the latter half of the 19th century when changes in farming practices introduced foreign grass pollens following the repeal of the Corn Laws in the UK in 1846,[305] the increase in allergic disease to perennial indoor allergens did not start until post–World War II, when there were significant changes in farming practices, hygiene, housing and lifestyle factors.

The hygiene hypothesis proposes that a lack of infections early in life predisposes children to allergies later in life.[306] The introduction of television in the 1960s and the push to use chemical cleaning products to 'sterilise' the home resulted in children adopting an indoor lifestyle, which significantly reduced their exposure to 'germs'. Furthermore, the move to create airtight and energy-efficient homes that are warmer and more humid, in conjunction with the use of wall-to-wall carpets and an indoor-centric lifestyle, have resulted in an increased exposure to indoor allergens such as house dust mites and mould.[186] It is an interesting coincidence that childhood asthma began to increase from 1960, and by 1990 had increased to epidemic proportions in all countries where children had adopted this lifestyle.[294] Consequently, the immune system (wanting to be busy all the time) turns its attention to otherwise harmless antigens. While the validity of the hygiene hypothesis is still being debated among experts,[307] it is interesting to note that the progressive shift to a Western lifestyle in the Middle East and Asia has correlated with a rise in the prevalence of allergic respiratory diseases.[295,308]

The microflora hypothesis has recently emerged as another theory to explain the rise of allergies in Western countries. There is a significant body of evidence to suggest that the gut microbiome plays an important role in the prevention of allergic disease because of its capacity to 'program' immune responses early in life. The rapid evolution of gut microbiota occurs early in life, arising initially from exposure to the mother's vaginal flora during birth. Babies delivered by caesarean section (which occurs more commonly in Western countries) harbour gut bacterial communities that resemble those found on the skin, which is significantly less diverse compared with gut bacterial communities of babies delivered vaginally.[309] Apart from the mode of birth, other risk factors have been identified to explain how the Western lifestyle limits microbial exposure. Breastfeeding rates continue to decline in Western countries, despite breastfeeding being shown to provide a protective role because it is high in oligosaccharides (prebiotics), which are essential for infant gut health and inhibit the binding of pathogens and toxins.[310,311] The overuse of antibiotic drugs in Western countries has been shown to have dramatic and devastating consequences on the infant's gut microbiome.[312] Increased financial pressures, birth control and delaying motherhood have all resulted in a significant decline in the birth rate in Western countries, which may increase the risk of allergies because not only are humans an important source of microbial diversity in the built environment, but they also contribute to resuspension of microbes in the air.[313] Each person contributes 14–37 million bacterial genome copies per hour in the air, and it is interesting to observe that the presence of older siblings appears to induce a protective role against the development of allergies.[314,315] The ubiquitous and indiscriminate use of chemicals such as pesticides, antibacterial chemicals, disinfectants, preservatives and solvents in household cleaning and personal care products and fungicides in building materials have reduced the microbial biodiversity in household dust.[186] The combination of bacterial exposure in dust and higher allergen levels in the first year of life has been shown to be protective against the development of atopic asthma.[316]

Numerous epidemiological studies have shown that children who grow up on traditional farms with livestock and fodder are protected from asthma, hay fever and allergic sensitisation,[317] especially if exposure occurs in the womb and the first year of life.[318] A recent and important study compared the immune profiles and microbiomes of indoor dust levels of Amish versus Hutterite farm children whose genetic ancestry and lifestyles are similar, but whose prevalence of asthma and allergies are strikingly dissimilar.[319] They discovered that Amish homes have very high endotoxin levels in their household dust, which provides intense and sustained exposure to microbes, triggering a healthy innate immune response – which may explain why Amish children have very low rates of asthma and allergies compared with Hutterite farm children. The idea that microbial exposure in household dust may

influence the composition of an infant's gut microbiome is quite plausible given that an infant's breathing zone is close to the floor and that infants have a very high hand-to-mouth ratio (they can swallow up to eight times more dirt than adults). The primary difference between the Amish and Hutterite communities lies with their farming practices: the Amish use traditional methods, while the Hutterites use industrialised farming practices that include the use of pesticides. It is interesting to note that the 1950s and 1960s experienced significant changes in farming practices with the introduction and ubiquitous use of pesticides in air, food and water – and this period coincides with the time that asthma incidence began to rise. The first 3 years of life are critical in the formation of future allergies,[320] and coincidently this is also the time when the phylogenetic composition of the bacterial communities found within the gut of most children closely mirrors that of the adult.[321] The state of the gut microbiome in the first 3 years of life may therefore provide important clues to the trajectory of allergenic diseases later in life. Children brought up on farms are less likely to develop asthma and allergies.[322,323]

There is a significant body of evidence correlating air pollution with allergic diseases such as eczema, asthma and allergic rhinitis.[125–127,324–326] Part of the problem lies with the fact that many air pollutants are associated with allergic sensitisation, damage the nasal mucosa, impair mucociliary clearance and potentiate the allergic immune response.[126,327,328] Furthermore, individuals with allergic diseases are generally more responsive to airborne irritants.[316] Air pollutants that have been shown to increase asthma and indoor allergen potency include environmental tobacco smoke, ground-level ozone, nitrogen dioxide and traffic-related air pollutants such as diesel particulate matter.[329–331] Atopic individuals living within 200 metres of a major road have an increased risk of asthma and allergic outcomes.[126]

House dust mites

House dust mites (HDMs) affect up to 21% of the population, making it one of the most common allergies in the world.[332,333] HDMs are the leading cause of hay fever and allergic asthma worldwide[333,334] and up to 85% of asthmatics are allergic to them.[335] Atopic individuals react to the combination of allergenic proteins (Der p 1 and Der p 2) and microbial by-products in dust mite faeces (frass).[336] House dust mite ratios are significantly higher in a bed (1884 mites/g of dust) as opposed to a carpet (601 mites/g of dust).[337]

SOURCES OF HOUSE DUST MITES

HDMs require moisture, warmth (above 25°C) and food (human and pet dander, cellulose from textile fibres, pollens and microbes). High levels of mites are typically found in bedding, carpets, soft furnishings, fabric window dressings and soft toys. Levels greater than 10 micrograms/g (equivalent to 500 mites/g of dust) are deemed capable of causing acute asthma in sensitised people.[335] HDM allergies peak in spring and late autumn, 2 months after a spike in mite numbers during late summer when humidity is highest and average monthly temperatures exceed 23°C.[334-338] These conditions occur in beds (where we sweat and shed skin cells), which is why HDMs are most prevalent in bedding. HDM allergens in Australian homes are among the highest recorded worldwide and often well above the 10 micrograms/g (500 mites/g of dust) deemed capable of causing acute asthma in sensitised people.[338, 339]

HEALTH CONCERNS ASSOCIATED WITH HOUSE DUST MITES

Unlike pollens which occur seasonally, HDM allergies occur all year round, so the symptoms are generally always present to some extent, although their intensity varies over time depending on humidity and temperature and the prevalence of mites in the indoor environment. Typical symptoms include itchy and watery eyes; sneezing; an itchy, runny or blocked nose; a dry persistent cough; wheezing; and dermatitis.[289,334,340] Symptoms are worse at night and upon waking and generally improve when sufferers are away from the source. People with an HDM allergy are often diagnosed with asthma, hay fever, perennial sinusitis or eczema. Non-allergic individuals may experience an exacerbation of asthma, and continual exposure to dust mite allergen may be a contributing cause of chronic bronchial hyperreactivity.[341]

TESTING FOR HOUSE DUST MITES

- Allergies can be confirmed by an allergy specialist or clinical immunologist who may perform skin prick tests (used for food and inhaled allergens such as pollen, dander and dust mites) or blood (RAST) tests
- The use of in-home test kits to measure HDMs along with education may beneficially influence behaviours and attitudes towards dust mite reduction strategies and help reduce residential dust mite allergen levels.[342] Safe levels are regarded as less than 2 micrograms of Der p 1/g of dust (100 mites/g of dust).[343]

TIPS FOR REDUCING LEVELS OF HOUSE DUST MITES

As there is no cure for HDM allergy, it is essential to reduce HDM levels as far as is practicable in the home. The best place to start is the bedroom.

- Reduce dust levels in the bedroom: this is important as carpeted floors have been shown to have twice the amount of dust mite allergen.[344] Replace carpets with hard flooring such as timber, linoleum, bamboo or tiles (hot climates) and washable rugs. Avoid using heavy draped curtains, soft furnishings such as decorative pillows and blankets (that aren't used for sleeping), soft toys, books and all forms of clutter (especially under the bed). Use window coverings such as timber or metal blinds that can be wiped with a slightly damp microfibre cloth
- Discard old mattresses, bedding, carpets and soft furnishings. Discard pillows more than 2 years old, and mattresses, wool and feather-filled doonas more than 10 years old. New mattresses and carpets are associated with significantly lower levels of HDM[345]

- Wash bed sheets and pyjamas in hot water on a weekly basis. Washing textiles regularly with a detergent at high temperatures will remove most HDMs.[346] While bed sheets, pillow cases and pyjamas should be washed weekly in hot water (55°C), items such as pillows, soft toys and bedding (blankets, doonas) should be washed at least every 2 months and air-dried in the sun. Only washable toys should be given to a child with HDM allergies. Rugs, blankets, cushions and bedding such as doonas, pillows and mattresses should be aired outside on hot dry days as often as possible. Pull back doonas/blankets daily to allow the mattress to dry
- Use HDM-resistant covers and bedding. HDM-resistant covers are available for mattresses, pillows, doonas and quilts and are an effective way to reduce exposure to dust mites.[347] Breathable covers made from natural fibres such as cotton, silk or eucalyptus are preferred over synthetic materials like nylon, acrylic and polycotton blends with a PVC backing. Dust mite covers should be washed at least every 2 months. Pillow, mattress and doona covers/encasements should be made from natural fibres such as linen, bamboo, organic cotton, hemp or silk. Avoid underlays and blankets made from wool
- Reduce humidity levels. Humidity is a critical factor for mite prevalence, as higher concentrations of mites are found in damp homes[345] and in microclimates where the relative humidity regularly exceeds 60%. A dehumidifier or refrigerated air-conditioning unit (which cools the air by removing water) should be used continuously when the relative humidity exceeds 60%. Optimal relative humidity levels to prevent dust mite and mould growth are between 40% and 55%. Maximise ventilation in wet areas of the home to prevent the build-up of humidity and condensation. Vacuum daily. Vacuum cleaners that are not fitted with a HEPA filter will temporarily increase the amount of HDM allergen in the air (for around 20 minutes)[348] because the mite allergens are attached to large particles.[341] Once you have vacuumed, replace the bag (even though it won't be full) as dust mites thrive in them. Vacuum mattresses daily[349]
- Use space bags: store linen, cushions, blankets and clothes that will not be used for a season or more in a space bag (a bag from which the air has been sucked out) to kill the dust mites.[186] Children who are raised in a house with two or more dogs or cats during the first year of life are less likely to develop allergies.[350]

Pet allergens

Pets that commonly trigger allergic responses include cats, dogs, horses, birds, rabbits, hamsters, guinea pigs, rats and mice. Pets also contribute significant amounts of dust, dander, pesticides and microorganisms into a home. Paradoxically, early life exposure (in the prenatal period and during the first 12 months) to furry pets and their microbial genre appears to be associated with a substantial reduction of allergy and asthma in childhood. This is suspected to be mediated through exposure to a more diverse microbial community in the home,[350] which is in line with the Amish study discussed previously. Individuals with pet allergies are not born with this condition; rather, it takes about 2 years to develop. Contrary to popular belief, it is not pet fur that is the problem, but skin flakes (dander), saliva and urine, which means that there are no 'low allergy' breeds when it comes to dogs and cats.[351] Even after removing a pet from the home, the dander can remain on dust, carpets and furnishings and may take several months of good housekeeping to remove. While the highest concentrations of cat and dog allergens are generally found in the homes of pet owners, the settled dust and air in schools and the cars of pet owners may also be important sites of exposure.[352] Cat and dog allergens remain airborne for much longer than dust mites and the potential for exposure to these pet allergens outside of the home is markedly greater.[353]

SOURCES OF PET ALLERGENS

- Cats produce a protein called Fel d1 in their sweat glands, which they spread when they lick themselves and which can trigger an allergic response in susceptible individuals and exacerbate asthma.[341,351] The allergen is so pervasive that it can be measured in the homes of non-pet owners, in school classrooms and on the clothing of workers who don't have pets. It is thought to be transferred and deposited indoors when attached on the clothes or hair of cat owners.[353,354] Therefore, sensitisation to cat allergens can occur in individuals who do not keep a cat
- The main source of dog allergen (a protein called Can f 1) is in the saliva, which dogs spread to their hair and skin when they lick themselves. This protein may trigger an allergic response in susceptible individuals and exacerbate asthma[341]
- There is limited evidence of an association between exposure to birds and exacerbation of asthma, which may in fact be triggered by the mites harboured by birds.[341] Bedding that contains feathers may be protective for lung problems because it is generally lower in dust mites levels; however, down pillows are suspected to be a risk for asthma because of their higher dust mite content.[341] There are a variety of diseases that birds can pass on to people as a result of microorganisms in their droppings. Psittacosis is one such disease; it causes flu-like symptoms and can progress to pneumonia and death
- Allergies to horses, mice, rats, rabbits and guinea pigs are not as common as cat and dog allergies.

HEALTH CONCERNS ASSOCIATED WITH PET ALLERGENS

Hay fever and asthma are the most common diagnoses attributed to pet allergies. Symptoms range from sneezing, a runny or stuffy nose, itchy and watery eyes, asthma, cough, eczema and hives to an anaphylactic reaction requiring immediate hospital attention. Up to 50% of people with pet allergies will not experience immediate symptoms.[351]

TIPS FOR REDUCING PET ALLERGIES

Individuals with established pet allergies need to implement avoidance strategies to prevent or reduce their symptoms.

- If possible, do not allow pets inside. Indoor pets should be kept away from bedrooms, carpeted areas, furnishings, slippers and stuffed toys. They should be confined to a dedicated mat, which is shaken outside daily as well as washed and air-dried in the sun at least twice a month
- Remove carpets, especially in the bedroom. Alternative types of flooring are timber, bamboo, cork, natural linoleum, slate, marble and ceramic tiles (although the latter may be too cold in a cool temperate climate). To clean these floors, mop with a damp microfibre cloth. Rugs are a better option than carpets, as they can be beaten outside and exposed to the sun
- Brush and wash the pet weekly to remove loose hair and allergens (a non-allergic person should carry out this task). Alternatively, wrap a damp cloth around a brush and brush the pet down rather than bathing them (do this outdoors)
- Wash hands after touching the pet
- Keep pet birds in an outside aviary
- Use air filters fitted with a HEPA filter, as they have been shown to be effective in reducing airborne concentration of pet allergens[316,355-357]
- Use a vacuum cleaner fitted with a HEPA filter and motorised head at least twice weekly.[186]

Pest allergens

Pest allergens such as cockroaches and rodents are present in higher concentrations in urban housing and have repeatedly been linked to asthma morbidity in sensitised children.[329] Pests are generally found in buildings that have a means of ingress, are warm and provide a source of water, food and shelter.

Sources of, and health concerns associated with, pest allergens

- There are more than 4500 species of cockroach, four of which are pests that can exacerbate asthma, hay fever and eczema in allergic individuals.[341,358] Some 30–40% of children with asthma are sensitised to cockroaches and are more likely to miss more school days.[359] Inner-city children who are exposed to high traffic related air pollutants have an increased likelihood of sensitisation to cockroach allergen.[360] Cockroaches have a lifespan of 1–2 years and prefer warm, moist and enclosed habitats. They have a taste for sugar and fat, although they have been known to consume soap, glue and rubbish,[358] and quickly become cannibalistic when food becomes scarce. Cockroaches that are visible in a home are evidence of an active infestation of live cockroaches, which increases the level of exposure to cockroach allergen (Bla g 1/2). In one study cockroach allergen was detected in almost half of all homes tested, even though the occupants reported no signs of cockroaches in the previous 12 months.[344] Individuals who have asthma, hay fever or eczema, or a strong family history of allergies, should be assessed for cockroach sensitivity
- Rodents (mice and rats) carry various infectious diseases such as Salmonella and can enter a hole as

narrow as a pencil to gain access to a building. Mice can mate when they are 1 month old, so it is important to take action as soon as you see one. Wherever they go they leave a trail of urine which contains a protein that can trigger allergic reactions in susceptible individuals. Rodents are more frequent in inner-city homes and have been linked with an increased risk of asthma, rhinitis and eczema in inner-city children[361–363]

• Insect allergies may arise when an individual is stung by a bee, wasp, mosquito, midge, March fly, bedbug, caterpillar, tick or ant. Whereas some individuals experience a localised itch and swelling that settles within a few days after being stung, others may experience hives or develop a potentially life-threatening anaphylactic reaction. The latter generally occurs after a susceptible individual is stung by a honey bee, wasp or Australian Jack Jumper ant[364]

• Ticks attach to the tips of grass blades and bushes and from there transfer themselves to passing animals and humans. Tick bites may result in local irritation and swelling at the site of the bite that can last for several days. Anaphylaxis may occur when the tick is disturbed, so ticks should be killed first (freeze-dried) before they are removed, otherwise the tick may inject more allergen-containing saliva.[365]

Testing for pest allergies

• Allergies can be confirmed by an allergy specialist or clinical immunologist who may perform skin prick tests or blood (RAST) tests. However, there is no reliable skin or blood allergy test to confirm a diagnosis of tick allergy

• Sticky traps strategically placed around the affected area can be used to identify the severity of a cockroach infestation by determining the number of different stages of development in the captured cockroaches. Household dust samples can be used to quantify the allergen load: cockroach antigen Bla g 1 levels should be below 1 unit/g of dust and Bla g 2 should be below 0.02 micrograms/g of dust. An important question to ask is 'Have you seen cockroaches daily, weekly, monthly or never in the recent past?'[358]

Tips for avoiding pest allergies

Allergen avoidance is considered the first line of treatment for patients with indoor allergen sensitivities. Thus the focus should be on creating an environment that doesn't attract pests.

• Food and water will attract pests, so good housekeeping is the key. Don't leave food (including pet food) around the home and clean up after every meal. Ensure all foods are properly stored in sealed containers. Waste and compost bins should be emptied daily and kept away from the house. Ensure the stove exhaust fan is clean and working and that the exhaust air is ducted to the exterior and not the roof cavity, to avoid distributing cooking odours to other parts of the home. Promptly repair water leaks, spills and dampness. Place plugs in all drains

• Avoid clutter in, under (crawl space) and immediately around the house including wood piles and rubbish bins as it provides the ideal home for pests. Keep gutters clean and well maintained

• Inspect the perimeter of the home and crawl space (if you have one) and caulk and seal cracks and holes. Install door sweeps and weatherproofing seals on exterior doors. Install fly screens on windows and doors and attic vents. Remove excess vegetation from around the home and prune branches near the building. Mosquito nets around beds are a cheap and effective physical barrier

• To remove frass (faeces, insect parts), clean carpets with a HEPA vacuum cleaner that is fitted with a motorised head to dig into the carpet pile. Discard the bag after each use

• Discard cockroach-infested mattresses and carpets

• To avoid insect allergies and tick bites cover up with light-coloured clothing (no florals) and wear shoes at all times, wear gloves when gardening, avoid perfumes and fragrances, keep grass areas mowed and get a professional to remove insect mounds and nests[364]

• Consider integrated pest management involving the use of sticky traps, baits, gels, boric acid and food-grade diatomaceous earth. Use chemical-based solutions only as a last resort and use a licensed pest controller. For more information on integrated pest management, refer to www.beyondpesticides.org.

Plant allergens

Pollens are a common cause of seasonal allergies. It is the wind-pollinated plants, however, which account for 10% of all flowering plants, that people with allergies such as asthma and hay fever are likely to react to because they are smaller and lighter (reaching the small airways of the lungs) and produced in large quantities that can be carried over long distances from their source (hundreds of kilometres in some cases). Plants with bright showy flowers are generally pollinated by insects and birds, while plants with small inconspicuous flowers are generally wind-pollinated. Grass pollens also rely on the wind to distribute their pollen over long distances.

SOURCES OF PLANT ALLERGENS

Susceptible individuals may be allergic to one or several types of pollen. With regard to allergic rhinitis and asthma, tree, weed, grass and crop pollinating plants are often the culprits. Grass pollens are the most frequent cause of allergic rhinitis: they are generally released in the early morning in summer and descend in the evening. As such, symptoms that occur in the evening may be indicative of allergies to grass pollen. Pollen maps and apps that provide daily pollen counts are available in many countries. Also contact the local asthma authority for a list of grass, weed and tree pollens in your area.

HEALTH CONCERNS ASSOCIATED WITH PLANT ALLERGENS

Pollens may trigger allergic rhinitis (sneezing, congestion, itchy and watery eyes, and runny nose), asthma, sinus headaches and, less commonly, contact dermatitis, eczema and joint pain, which typically occur seasonally and generally improve after it rains. Symptoms may be immediate upon exposure, or can be delayed by a few days. Thunderstorms and weather changes may trigger asthma attacks in some individuals, as the pollen grains absorb moisture and burst, releasing hundreds of small allergenic particles into the air.[366]

TESTING FOR PLANT ALLERGENS

Allergies can be confirmed by an allergy specialist or clinical immunologist who may perform skin prick tests or blood (RAST) tests.

TIPS FOR AVOIDING PLANT ALLERGENS

- During the allergy season, remain indoors on hot, dry windy days and after thunderstorms when pollen counts are likely to be high
- Use an air conditioner (in the car and/or at home) or air filter that is fitted with a HEPA filter when the outdoor pollen count is high
- To reduce pollens in the home, shower after outdoor activities, damp-brush pets prior to entering the home and avoid hanging clothes on the line on high pollen count days (dry clothes inside instead)
- If allergic to grass pollen, do not mow the lawn or exercise in the early morning in spring and summer. Pollen allergy in tropical climates is more common during the dry season
- Wear glasses that wrap around the eyes during allergy season
- Avoid having flowering plants, including cut flowers, inside the home or office.

Mould

Fungi are nature's greatest decomposers and consequently they are found everywhere on the planet, including in our homes. Approximately 120 fungi are associated with poor indoor air quality and 400 are related to diseases relevant to people, animals or plants. Despite fungi being present for millions of years, their impact on human health has recently gained more attention in the scientific community. Why? The recent push to build airtight and energy-efficient homes with compromised passive ventilation has resulted in an increasing number of new homes experiencing condensation and mould-related complaints. It is estimated that 1 in 4 homes in Nordic countries and New Zealand, 1 in 3 homes in Australia and Canada, and 1 in 2 homes in the US are water-damaged.[367–369] Between one-quarter and one-third of the respiratory health outcomes observed in New Zealand can be explained by indoor dampness[370] attributable to cold, draughty and poorly insulated buildings.[369] The introduction of fungicides into building materials and paints in the 1970s created pathogenic strains of fungi that are more dangerous to human health than those seen previously. The introduction and use of cheap artificial timbers like MDF, plywood, oriented strand board and particle board (chipboard) containing chemicals like formaldehyde have changed the pH, and the type of nutrients (substrate) and therefore the genre of fungi likely to grow in a water-damaged environment. In contrast, solid hard timbers, traditionally used in years gone by, contain resins that are naturally resistant to fungal growth.

SOURCES OF MOULD

Buildings should reflect a Mediterranean type of environment: dry and stable. When we add moisture, we transform a dry stable environment into a living thriving ecosystem where microbes will kill other competing organisms by secreting chemicals to enhance their survival. As mould spores can remain dormant for many years, they will thrive when they are given food and water. As most conventional building materials and furnishings are the ideal 'fast' food for fungi, the key to addressing mould-related problems is to get to the source of the moisture. Within 48 hours of moisture being present, the spores – which are already sitting on all surfaces – will begin to germinate.

Moisture-related problems can occur during building construction, or arise from external or internal sources. Moisture often occurs during building construction with concrete floor slabs, masonry and walls because they contain a large amount of unbound water that needs to cure prior to erecting the frame. Mortar, grout filling and rain can also add moisture to concrete during the construction process. Poor building practices resulting in absent or inadequate water proofing of wet areas (bathrooms, laundry and kitchen) or insufficient drainage in the subfloor or immediately around the home may also cause moisture problems. Timber-framed homes are often exposed to rain or dew during construction, which is why the timbers are commonly contaminated with Trichoderma species. Inadequate insulation and/or single-paned windows commonly result in condensation issues on the walls, around the window frames or behind the curtains.

External sources of moisture that can penetrate the building envelope include: a climate that regularly exceeds 70% relative humidity; natural events such as storms and floods; water damage after a fire; and leaks through the building envelope from blocked and/or damaged gutters, missing or damaged flashing around exits on the roof, cracks in cladding and deteriorating building materials. Buildings that lack eaves or don't have facings around windows are at the mercy of the weather, and enclosed balconies and internal or box gutters are notorious for moisture problems.

Subfloor moisture may occur: due to building on a flood-prone site, swamp or above an aquifer; with blocked, a limited number of or missing subfloor vents; due to landscaping issues where garden beds cover subfloor vents and/or butt up against the house (with no water proofing); from garden sprinklers aimed at the house; with renovations that block off existing subfloor vents; due to the topography of the land (house built on or into a hill), where the surrounding ground level is higher than the ground level under the home; with poor groundwater drainage immediately around the home; from blocked storm water drains or gully traps; or from leaking stormwater, waste or water pipes under the house.

Internal sources of moisture typically occur from: high humidity and condensation generated from bathing, showering, laundering and cooking activities combined with inadequate passive ventilation; unflued gas appliances; indoor spas, pools and saunas; indoor plants, open fish tanks and indoor water features; humidifiers; accidental floods such as an overflowing bath, kitchen sink or laundry sink; steam cleaning of carpets or furnishings that did not dry within 48 hours; leaking plumbing pipes, dripping taps and leaking appliances; and water-damaged furnishings bought from antique or second-hand stores or brought in from a previous water-damaged home. Heating, ventilation and air conditioning (HVAC) systems can also be a source of mould if they are not regularly serviced and maintained.[186]

HEALTH CONCERNS ASSOCIATED WITH MOULD

It has long been established that exposure to mould and dampness results in lung problems like asthma, bronchitis, cold and flu-like symptoms, hay fever and, less commonly, pneumonia and eczema.[371–373] In New Zealand up to one-third of respiratory diseases (in particular, asthma) are attributable to indoor dampness.[370] Traditionally this was thought to be an IgE-mediated response; however, it is now known that fungal products can activate both innate and adaptive immune responses resulting in chronic inflammation.[374]

Water-damaged buildings contain a 'chemical stew' of: airborne bioaerosols from actinomycetes, lipopolysaccharides, bacteria, fungi and their by-products (endotoxins, mycotoxins); ultrafine particles; microbial volatile organic compounds; cell fragments; and inflammagens such as beta glucans, mannans, haemolysins and proteinases.[375–378] In healthy individuals, these microbes are identified by the body's immune system (pattern recognition receptors), which induces downstream events (phagocytosis, cytokine and chemokine release) that in turn polarise a Th17 adaptive immune response designed to eliminate the pathogen from the host.[379] However, advances in gene screening have identified that 24% of the population do not have the immune response genes (*HLA-DR*) required to form antibodies to biotoxins,[380] which means every time these individuals walk into a water-damaged building, a persistent innate immune inflammatory illness ensues, which can affect virtually any organ system of the body.

Chronic inflammatory response syndrome (CIRS) is a chronic, progressive, multisystem, multisymptom syndrome characterised by HLA genetic predisposition, exposure to biotoxins, altered innate and adaptive immunity, peripheral hypoperfusion at multiple sites and multiple hypothalamic-pituitary-end organ dysregulations.[381] Symptoms include fatigue and headache, brain fog (difficulty with recent memory and concentration, and anomia),[382] vertigo, metallic taste, aches and pain in the joints, numbness and tingling, and sleep disturbances. In addition, around half of sufferers experience excessive urination and thirst and increased electric shocks because of alterations to antidiuretic hormone. Remarkably, most of these symptoms disappear during pregnancy, because the anti-inflammatory neuropeptide (melanocyte-stimulating hormone) in the brain increases during pregnancy.

TESTING FOR MOULD

A symptom-based assessment of risk for CIRS following exposure to a water-damaged building is available in a consensus paper in *Surviving Mold*.[383]

Clinical testing

IgE-mediated allergies to fungi can be confirmed by an allergy specialist or clinical immunologist who may perform skin prick tests or blood (RAST) tests. According to McMahon and colleagues[381] and Shoemaker and colleagues,[382] a diagnosis of CIRS requires:

- Exposure to a water-damaged building
- The presence of a multisystem, multisymptom illness
- Laboratory abnormalities in five of the following eight blood protein biomarkers: vasoactive intestinal polypeptide, alpha-melanocyte stimulating hormone, complement component C4a, metallomatrix proteinase-9 (MMP9), vascular endothelial growth factor (VEGF), transforming growth factor beta-1 (TGF β-1), osmolality/antidiuretic hormone balance and cortisol/ACTH balance.

Other useful tests

- A nasal swab can be used to detect multiple antibiotic resistant coagulase negative staphylococcus (MARCoNS)
- Brain scans have identified gliotic areas on MRI scans[382]; elevated lactate and depressed ratios of glutamate to glutamine in MR spectroscopy; atrophy of the caudate nucleus; and bilateral enlargement of the pallidum, forebrain parenchyma and cortical grey using the MRI volumetric software NeuroQuant® [381,382] suggesting inflammation in the brain
- Genetic susceptibility (HLA DR DQ)
- Visual contrast sensitivity (VCS) is a simple, non-invasive eye test that measures the ability to distinguish between finer and finer increments of light versus dark lines, which can affect visual function even with 20/20 vision.[384] Transient deficits in visual contrast have been observed in patients in water-damaged buildings,[385] while permanent deficits have been documented in patients with neurodegenerative and inflammatory diseases affecting the optic nerve such as multiple sclerosis[386] and Alzheimer's disease,[387] ophthalmological disease (glaucoma, cataracts, diabetic retinopathy and macular degeneration) and occupational exposure to solvents, heavy metals and petroleum products.[385]

House testing

House testing should be instigated following a history of water damage that correlates to the development of the above symptoms or the presence of dampness as determined by visible water damage or stains, visible mould and odour from microbial growth.[373,388] Refer to the recent article by Chew and colleagues.[388] There are several reports that document how to test and remediate water-damaged buildings, but the most detailed is ANSI/IICRC S520-2015 on mould remediation.[389] An inspection should be carried out by a qualified building biologist, indoor environmental professional or IICRC-accredited mould remediator and should involve an exterior and interior site inspection of the property including the heating, ventilation and air-conditioning (HVAC) system for evidence of visible mould, damp smells and signs of dampness. It should also involve the use of indoor air quality meters (to compare outdoor and indoor relative and specific humidity levels and temperature), thermal imaging cameras to identify temperature variances with any anomalies verified by a moisture meter, borescopes to identify hidden mould and moisture meters to identify the source and extent of moisture intrusion in building materials. In addition, the inspector should conduct air, dust (ERMI or HERTSMI-2) and/or surface sampling to quantify the genre and prevalence of various fungi and their mycotoxins.

Solutions for water-damaged buildings

The first phase of therapy includes eliminating offending toxin exposure (see below), short-term use of a bile acid sequestrant such as cholestyramine (CSM), and eradicating nasal MARCoNS if present.[381] The second phase includes the correction of antigliadin antibodies, dysregulated androgens, dysregulated ADH (antidiuretic hormone) and osmolality; elevated MMP-9, VEGF (vascular endothelial growth factor; bimodal dysregulation) and complement components C3a, C4a and TGF β-1.[381]

The key to addressing a water-damaged building is to locate and eliminate the source of moisture. Most of the time this will be obvious, such as clogged gutters, inadequate ventilation, broken roof tiles or a history of flooding. If the source of the moisture cannot be identified, a licensed plumber, drainage specialist, building biologist, indoor environmental professional or IICRC-accredited mould remediator may be required to find the source. If the moisture is simply due to living in a hot, humid climate, having the air conditioner or dehumidifier on continuously will keep humidity levels below 70%. Patients with suspected sensitivities to mould should avoid working with garden compost or mulch or mowing the lawn.

For non-porous surfaces, mould can be removed with a microfibre cloth soaked in a solution of dishwashing liquid and water to remove the biofilm. For porous surfaces such as plaster, insulation, particleboard or soft timbers, an alcoholic solution (70% alcohol to 30% water) is effective. If the mould has infiltrated the material, abrasive methods such as wire brushing, sanding or media blasting may need to be employed by an accredited mould remediator.

Non-porous water-damaged contents (metal, laminate, plastic, glass, sealed timber, ceramic and porcelain) and semi-porous items (plasterboard, concrete, plywood, masonry, unsealed timber, oriented strand board and brick) should be vacuumed using a HEPA vacuum cleaner, then wiped with a slightly damp microfibre cloth and vacuumed again. Porous items such as clothing, soft furnishings, carpet, underlay, plasterboard, ceiling tiles, leather, paper (books), taxidermy, fine art, insulation, particle board and medium-density fibreboard that didn't dry within 48 hours

of water damage should be discarded. Clothes that don't have visible mould on them can be washed in a hot cycle and dried in the sun. To save expensive items like fine art and books, specialised laundering companies should be consulted. Note: appropriate personal protective equipment such as a P3 particulate respirator and protective clothing may be warranted during mould remediation.

The HVAC system should be cleaned according to the National Air Duct Cleaners Association 2013 standard and contaminated flex ducting (typically used in residential homes) should be replaced as it is impossible to clean.[186]

REFERENCES

[1] Pope AM, Rall DP. Institute of Medicine. Environmental medicine: integrating a missing element into medical education. Washington, DC: National Academies Press; 1995.

[2] Ducatman AM. Occupational physicians and environmental medicine. J Occup Environ Med 1993;35(3):251–9.

[3] Bijlsma N, Cohen M. Environmental chemical assessment in clinical practice: unveiling the elephant in the room. Int J Environ Res Public Health 2016;13(2):181.

[4] Ramos RG, Olden K. Gene–environment interactions in the development of complex disease phenotypes. Int J Environ Res Public Health 2008;5(1):4–11.

[5] Bijlsma N, Cohen MM. Environmental chemical assessment in clinical practice: unveiling the elephant in the room. Int J Environ Res Public Health 2016;13(2):181.

[6] Institute of Medicine. Crossing the quality chasm: a new health system for the 21st century. Washington, DC: National Academies Press; 2001.

[7] Calafat AM. The US National Health and Nutrition Examination Survey and human exposure to environmental chemicals. Int J Hyg Environ Health 2012;215(2):99–101.

[8] Schindler BK, Esteban M, Koch HM, et al. The European COPHES/DEMOCOPHES project: towards transnational comparability and reliability of human biomonitoring results. Int J Hyg Environ Health 2014;217(6):653–61.

[9] Vandentorren S, Bois C, Pirus C, et al. Rationales, design and recruitment for the Elfe longitudinal study. BMC Pediatr 2009; 9:58.

[10] Magnus P, Irgens LM, Haug K, et al. Cohort profile: the Norwegian Mother and Child Cohort Study (MoBa). Int J Epidemiol 2006;35(5):1146–50.

[11] Whaley P. Systematic review and the future of evidence in chemicals policy. The Policy from Science Project, Réseau Environnement Santé (RES), 2013.

[12] Snow J. On the origin of the recent outbreak of cholera at West Ham. BMJ 1857;1(45):934–5.

[13] Stewart A. Malignant disease in childhood and diagnostic irradiation in utero. Lancet 1956;271(6940):447–8.

[14] Doll R, Hill AB. Smoking and carcinoma of the lung. BMJ 1950;2(4682):739.

[15] Harremoës P, Gee D, MacGarvin M, et al. Late lessons from early warnings: the precautionary principle 1896–2000. Office for Official Publications of the European Communities; 2001.

[16] The role of the internist in occupational medicine: a position paper of the American College of Physicians (September 14, 1984). Am J Ind Med 1985;8(2):95–9.

[17] ACP. Occupational and environmental medicine: the internist's role. Ann Intern Med 1990;113(12):974–82.

[18] Institute of Medicine. Role of the primary care physician in occupational and environmental medicine. Washington, DC: National Academies Press; 1988.

[19] World Health Organization (WHO). Environmental health and the role of medical professionals: report on a WHO consultation. Geneva: WHO; 1996.

[20] National Academies of Sciences, Engineering, and Medicine. Use of metabolomics to advance research on environmental exposures and the human exposome. Washington, DC: The National Academies Press.

[21] Bernstein DI, Kissling GE, Khurana Hershey G, et al. Hexamethylene diisocyanate asthma is associated with genetic polymorphisms of CD14, IL-13, and IL-4 receptor alpha. J Allergy Clin Immunol 2011;128(2):418–20.

[22] Knudsen LE, Loft SH, Autrup H. Risk assessment: the importance of genetic polymorphisms in man. Mutat Res 2001;482(1–2):83–8.

[23] Smith CM, Kelsey KT, Wiencke JK, et al. Inherited glutathione-S-transferase deficiency is a risk factor for pulmonary asbestosis. Cancer Epidemiol Biomarkers Prev 1994;3(6):471–7.

[24] Mizoi Y, Yamamoto K, Ueno Y, et al. Involvement of genetic polymorphism of alcohol and aldehyde dehydrogenases in individual variation of alcohol metabolism. Alcohol Alcohol 1994;29(6):707–10.

[25] Sanderson S, Emery J, Higgins J. CYP2C9 gene variants, drug dose, and bleeding risk in warfarin-treated patients: a HuGEnet systematic review and meta-analysis. Genet Med 2005;7(2):97–104.

[26] Karahalil B, Bohr VA, Wilson DM. Impact of DNA polymorphisms in key DNA base excision repair proteins on cancer risk. Hum Exp Toxicol 2012;31(10):981–1005.

[27] Cerne JZ, Pohar-Perme M, Novakovic S, et al. Combined effect of CYP1B1, COMT, GSTP1, and MnSOD genotypes and risk of postmenopausal breast cancer. J Gynecol Oncol 2011;22(2):110.

[28] Liu G, Sun G, Wang Y, et al. Association between manganese superoxide dismutase gene polymorphism and breast cancer risk: a meta-analysis of 17 842 subjects. Mol Med Rep 2012;6(4):797–804.

[29] Chen Y, Fu F, Lin Y, et al. The precision relationships between eight GWAS-identified genetic variants and breast cancer in a Chinese population. Oncotarget 2016.

[30] Nickels S, Truong T, Hein R, et al. Evidence of gene–environment interactions between common breast cancer susceptibility loci and established environmental risk factors. PLoS Genet 2013;9(3):e1003284.

[31] Nate Seltenrich. Institutes in the lead: identifying environmental factors in breast cancer. Environ Health Perspect 2016;124:A199–205.

[32] Rudolph A, Chang-Claude J, Schmidt MK. Gene–environment interaction and risk of breast cancer. Br J Cancer 2016;114(2):125–33.

[33] Travis RC, Reeves GK, Green J, et al. Gene–environment interactions in 7610 women with breast cancer: prospective evidence from the Million Women Study. Lancet 2010;375(9732):2143–51.

[34] Gomez SL, Quach T, Horn-Ross PL, et al. Hidden breast cancer disparities in Asian women: disaggregating incidence rates by ethnicity and migrant status. Am J Public Health 2010; 100(Suppl. 1):S125–31.

[35] Yan W, Zhang Y, Zhao E, et al. Association between the MTHFR C677T polymorphism and Breast cancer risk: a meta-analysis of 23 case-control studies. Breast J 2016;22(5):593–4.

[36] Thorsby E, Lie BA. HLA associated genetic predisposition to autoimmune diseases: genes involved and possible mechanisms. Transpl Immunol 2005;14(3):175–82.

[37] Hawa MI, Beyan H, Buckley LR, et al. Impact of genetic and non-genetic factors in type 1 diabetes. Am J Med Genet 2002;115(1):8–17.

[38] Rossignol DA, Genuis SJ, Frye RE. Environmental toxicants and autism spectrum disorders: a systematic review. Transl Psychiatry 2014;4(2):e360.

[39] Polito L, Greco A, Seripa D. Genetic profile, environmental exposure, and their interaction in Parkinson's disease. Parkinsons Dis 2016;6465793.

[40] Bland J (ed). Functional medicine & 'omics': a match made in heaven. The 'omics' revolution: nature and nurture. Institute for Functional Medicine Annual International Conference, Austin, TX, 28–30 May 2015.

[41] Cardon LR, Harris T. Precision medicine, genomics and drug discovery. Hum Mol Genet 2016;25(R2):R166–72.

[42] Urban TJ, Goldstein DB. Pharmacogenetics at 50: genomic personalization comes of age. Sci Transl Med 2014;6(220):220ps1.

[43] Ravelli GP, Stein ZA, Susser MW. Obesity in young men after famine exposure in utero and early infancy. N Engl J Med 1976;295(7):349–53.

[44] Barker DJ, Bagby SP, Hanson MA. Mechanisms of disease: in utero programming in the pathogenesis of hypertension. Nat Clin Pract Nephrol 2006;2(12):700–7.

[45] Delisle H. Foetal programming of nutrition-related chronic diseases. Sante 2002;12(1):56–63.

[46] Fernandez-Twinn DS, Constancia M, Ozanne SE. Intergenerational epigenetic inheritance in models of developmental programming of adult disease. Semin Cell Dev Biol 2015.

[47] Rice D, Barone S Jr. Critical periods of vulnerability for the developing nervous system: evidence from humans and animal models. Environ Health Perspect 2000;108(Suppl. 3):511–33.

[48] Fox MA, Aoki Y. Environmental contaminants and exposure. Environmental Impacts on Reproductive Health and Fertility 2010;8–22.

[49] Bennett D, Bellinger DC, Birnbaum LS, et al. Project TENDR: targeting environmental neuro-developmental risks. The TENDR consensus statement. Environ Health Perspect 2016;124(7): A118–22.

[50] Grandjean P, Landrigan PJ. Neurobehavioural effects of developmental toxicity. Lancet Neurol 2014;13(3):330–8.

[51] Grandjean P, Barouki R, Bellinger DC, et al. Life-long implications of developmental exposure to environmental stressors: new perspectives. Endocrinology 2015;156(10):3408–15.

[52] Goyer RA. Lead toxicity: current concerns. Environ Health Perspect 1993;100:177.

[53] Carson R. Silent spring. Houghton Mifflin; 2002.

[54] Colborn T, Dumanoski D, Myers JP. Our stolen future: are we threatening our fertility, intelligence and survival? A scientific detective story. New York: Dutton; 1996.

[55] World Health Organization (WHO). State of the science of endocrine disrupting chemicals, 2012. An assessment of the state of the science of endocrine disruptors prepared by a group of experts for the United Nations Environment Programme (UNEP) and WHO. Geneva: WHO; 2013.

[56] Di Renzo GC, Conry JA, Blake J, et al. International Federation of Gynecology and Obstetrics opinion on reproductive health impacts of exposure to toxic environmental chemicals. Int J Gynaecol Obstet 2015.

[57] Barker DJP, Gluckman PD, Robinson JS. Conference report: fetal origins of adult disease—report of the first international study group, Sydney, 29–30 October 1994. Placenta 1995;16(3):317–20.

[58] Heindel JJ, Balbus J, Birnbaum L, et al. Developmental origins of health and disease: integrating environmental influences. Endocrinology 2015;156(10):3416–21.

[59] Rebelo FM, Caldas ED. Arsenic, lead, mercury and cadmium: toxicity, levels in breast milk and the risks for breastfed infants. Environ Res 2016;151:671–88.

[60] Saadeh R, Klaunig J. Children's inter-individual variability and asthma development. Int J Health Sci 2015;9(4):456–67.

[61] World Health Organization (WHO). Children are not little adults. Children's health and the environment. WHO Training Package for the Health Sector, 2008. Available from www.who.int/ceh/capacity/ Children_are_not_little_adults.pdf?ua=1.

[62] Sly PD, Flack F. Susceptibility of children to environmental pollutants. Ann N Y Acad Sci 2008;1140:163–83.

[63] Das A, Srinivasan M, Ghosh TS, et al. Xenobiotic metabolism and gut microbiomes. PLoS ONE 2016;11(10):e0163099.

[64] Genuis SJ. Evolution in pediatric health care. Pediatr Int 2010;52(4):640–3.

[65] Ginsberg G, Slikker W, Bruckner J, et al. Incorporating children's toxicokinetics into a risk framework. Environ Health Perspect 2004;112(2):272–83.

[66] Dorne J, Walton K, Renwick A. Uncertainty factors for chemical risk assessment: human variability in the pharmacokinetics of CYP1A2 probe substrates. Food Chem Toxicol 2001;39(7):681–96.

[67] Wiart J, Hadjem A, Wong M, et al. Analysis of RF exposure in the head tissues of children and adults. Phys Med Biol 2008;53(13): 3681.

[68] Christ A, Gosselin M-C, Christopoulou M, et al. Age-dependent tissue-specific exposure of cell phone users. Phys Med Biol 2010;55(7):1767.

[69] Abbasi J. Call to action on neurotoxin exposure in pregnant women and children. JAMA 2016;316(14):1436–7.

[70] Rice D, Barone S Jr. Critical periods of vulnerability for the developing nervous system: evidence from humans and animal models. Environ Health Perspect 2000;108(Suppl. 3):511.

[71] Cole-Harding S, Wilson JR. Ethanol metabolism in men and women. J Stud Alcohol 1987;48(4):380–7.

[72] Cederbaum AI. Alcohol metabolism. Clin Liver Dis 2012;16(4): 667–85.

[73] Lavergne MR, Cole DC, Kerr K, et al. Functional impairment in chronic fatigue syndrome, fibromyalgia, and multiple chemical sensitivity. Can Fam Physician 2010;56(2):e57–65.

[74] Sears ME. The medical perspective on environmental sensitivities. Ottawa: Canadian Human Rights Commission; 2007.

[75] Lipson JG, Doiron N. Environmental issues and work: women with multiple chemical sensitivities. Health Care Women Int 2006;27(7): 571–84.

[76] Fombonne E. Epidemiology of pervasive developmental disorders. Pediatr Res 2009;65(6):591–8.

[77] Baskin LS. Hypospadias and genital development. Springer; 2012.

[78] Skakkebaek NE, Rajpert-De Meyts E, Main KM. Testicular dysgenesis syndrome: an increasingly common developmental disorder with environmental aspects. Hum Reprod 2001;16(5):972–8.

[79] Li H, Jia W. Cometabolism of microbes and host: implications for drug metabolism and drug-induced toxicity. Clin Pharmacol Ther 2013;94(5):574–81.

[80] Clayton TA, Baker D, Lindon JC, et al. Pharmacometabonomic identification of a significant host–microbiome metabolic interaction affecting human drug metabolism. Proc Natl Acad Sci USA 2009;106(34):14728–33.

[81] Klaassen CD, Cui JY. Review: mechanisms of how the intestinal microbiota alters the effects of drugs and bile acids. Drug Metab Dispos 2015;43(10):1505–21.

[82] Pohl HR, Scinicariello F. The impact of CYP2E1 genetic variability on risk assessment of VOC mixtures. Regul Toxicol Pharmacol 2011;59(3):364–74.

[83] Song Y, Liu C, Finegold SM. Real-time PCR quantitation of clostridia in feces of autistic children. Appl Environ Microbiol 2004;70(11):6459–65.

[84] Alberti A, Pirrone P, Elia M, et al. Sulphation deficit in 'low-functioning' autistic children: a pilot study. Biol Psychiatry 1999;46(3):420–4.

[85] Ghaisas S, Maher J, Kanthasamy A. Gut microbiome in health and disease: linking the microbiome-gut-brain axis and environmental factors in the pathogenesis of systemic and neurodegenerative diseases. Pharmacol Ther 2016;158:52–62.

[86] Saeidnia S, Abdollahi M. Toxicological and pharmacological concerns on oxidative stress and related diseases. Toxicol Appl Pharmacol 2013;273(3):442–55.

[87] Zhang Y, Zhang H. Microbiota associated with type 2 diabetes and its related complications. Food Science and Human Wellness 2013;2(3):167–72.

[88] Sharon G, Sampson TR, Geschwind DH, et al. The central nervous system and the gut microbiome. Cell 2016;167(4):915–32.

[89] Frost G, Sleeth ML, Sahuri-Arisoylu M, et al. The short-chain fatty acid acetate reduces appetite via a central homeostatic mechanism. Nat Commun 2014;5.

[90] Barrett E, Ross R, O'Toole P, et al. γ-aminobutyric acid production by culturable bacteria from the human intestine. J Appl Microbiol 2012;113(2):411–17.

[91] Ji X-B, Hollocher TC. Reduction of nitrite to nitric oxide by enteric bacteria. Biochem Biophys Res Commun 1988;157(1):106–8.

[92] Clarke G, Stilling RM, Kennedy PJ, et al. Minireview: gut microbiota, the neglected endocrine organ. Mol Endocrinol 2014;28(8):1221–38.

[93] Foster JA, McVey Neufeld KA. Gut-brain axis: how the microbiome influences anxiety and depression. Trends Neurosci 2013;36(5): 305–12.

[94] Krajmalnik-Brown R, Lozupone C, Kang DW, et al. Gut bacteria in children with autism spectrum disorders: challenges and promise of studying how a complex community influences a complex disease. Microb Ecol Health Dis 2015;26:26914.

[95] Sampson TR, Debelius JW, Thron T, et al. Gut microbiota regulate motor deficits and neuroinflammation in a model of Parkinson's disease. Cell 2016;167(6):1469–80.

[96] Bercik P, Denou E, Collins J, et al. The intestinal microbiota affect central levels of brain-derived neurotropic factor and behavior in mice. Gastroenterology 2011;141(2):599–609.

[97] Sa'ad H, Peppelenbosch MP, Roelofsen H, et al. Biological effects of propionic acid in humans; metabolism, potential applications and underlying mechanisms. Biochim Biophys Acta 2010;1801(11): 1175–83.

[98] Le Poul E, Loison C, Struyf S, et al. Functional characterization of human receptors for short chain fatty acids and their role in polymorphonuclear cell activation. J Biol Chem 2003;278(28): 25481–9.

[99] Kimura I, Inoue D, Hirano K, et al. The SCFA receptor GPR43 and energy metabolism. Front Endocrinol (Lausanne) 2014;5:85.

[100] Sanduzzi Zamparelli M, Compare D, Coccoli P, et al. The metabolic role of gut microbiota in the development of nonalcoholic fatty liver disease and cardiovascular disease. Int J Mol Sci 2016;17(8):1225.

[101] Maslowski KM, Vieira AT, Ng A, et al. Regulation of inflammatory responses by gut microbiota and chemoattractant receptor GPR43. Nature 2009;461(7268):1282–6.

[102] Furusawa Y, Obata Y, Fukuda S, et al. Commensal microbe-derived butyrate induces the differentiation of colonic regulatory T cells. Nature 2013;504(7480):446–50.

[103] Schéle E, Grahnemo L, Anesten F, et al. The gut microbiota reduces leptin sensitivity and the expression of the obesity-suppressing neuropeptides proglucagon (Gcg) and brain-derived neurotrophic factor (Bdnf) in the central nervous system. Endocrinology 2013;154(10):3643–51.

[104] Zaibi MS, Stocker CJ, O'Dowd J, et al. Roles of GPR41 and GPR43 in leptin secretory responses of murine adipocytes to short chain fatty acids. FEBS Lett 2010;584(11):2381–6.

[105] Xiong Y, Miyamoto N, Shibata K, et al. Short-chain fatty acids stimulate leptin production in adipocytes through the G protein-coupled receptor GPR41. Proc Natl Acad Sci USA 2004;101(4):1045–50.

[106] Cani PD, Knauf C. How gut microbes talk to organs: the role of endocrine and nervous routes. Mol Metab 2016;5(9):743–52.

[107] Graf D, Di Cagno R, Fak F, et al. Contribution of diet to the composition of the human gut microbiota. Microb Ecol Health Dis 2015;26:26164.

[108] Maslowski KM, Mackay CR. Diet, gut microbiota and immune responses. Nat Immunol 2011;12(1):5–9.

[109] Conlon MA, Bird AR. The impact of diet and lifestyle on gut microbiota and human health. Nutrients 2014;7(1):17–44.

[110] Darnton-Hill I, Margetts B, Deckelbaum R. Public health nutrition and genetics: implications for nutrition policy and promotion. Proc Nutr Soc 2004;63(01):173–85.

[111] Afacan NJ, Fjell CD, Hancock RE. A systems biology approach to nutritional immunology: focus on innate immunity. Mol Aspects Med 2012;33(1):14–25.

[112] Mocchegiani E, Costarelli L, Giacconi R, et al. Micronutrient–gene interactions related to inflammatory/immune response and antioxidant activity in ageing and inflammation. A systematic review. Mech Ageing Dev 2014;136–137:29–49.

[113] Rana S, Kumar S, Rathore N, et al. Nutrigenomics and its Impact on life style associated metabolic diseases. Curr Genomics 2016;17(3):261–78.

[114] Kontogiorgis C, Bompou E-M, Ntella M, et al. Natural products from Mediterranean diet: from anti-inflammatory agents to dietary epigenetic modulators. Anti-Inflammatory & Anti-Allergy Agents in Medicinal Chemistry 2010;9(2):101–24.

[115] Parletta N, Milte CM, Meyer BJ. Nutritional modulation of cognitive function and mental health. J Nutr Biochem 2013;24(5):725–43.

[116] Rahal A, Kumar A, Singh V, et al. Oxidative stress, prooxidants, and antioxidants: the interplay. Biomed Res Int 2014;761264.

[117] Popkin BM, Gordon-Larsen P. The nutrition transition: worldwide obesity dynamics and their determinants. Int J Obes Relat Metab Disord 2004;28(Suppl. 3):S2–9.

[118] Simopoulos AP. Omega-3 fatty acids in wild plants, nuts and seeds. Asia Pac J Clin Nutr 2002;11(s6):S163–73.

[119] Hunt SC, Gwinn M, Adams TD. Family history assessment: strategies for prevention of cardiovascular disease. Am J Prev Med 2003;24(2):136–42.

[120] Von Baehr V. Rationelle labordiagnostik bei chronisch entzündlichen systemerkrankungen. Umwelt Medizin Gesellschaft 2012;25(4):244–7.

[121] Wishart D, Arndt D, Pon A, et al. T3DB: the toxic exposome database. Nucleic Acids Res 2015;43(Database issue):D928–34.

[122] Lim SS, Vos T, Flaxman AD, et al. A comparative risk assessment of burden of disease and injury attributable to 67 risk factors and risk factor clusters in 21 regions, 1990–2010: a systematic analysis for the Global Burden of Disease Study 2010. Lancet 2012;380(9859):2224–60.

[123] American Chemical Society (ACS). CAS REGISTRY: the gold standard for chemical substance information. Available from www.cas.org/content/chemical-substances.

[124] Kim HH, Lee CS, Yu SD, et al. Near-road exposure and impact of air pollution on allergic diseases in elementary school children: a cross-sectional study. Yonsei Med J 2016;57(3):698–713.

[125] Carlsten C, Blomberg A, Pui M, et al. Diesel exhaust augments allergen-induced lower airway inflammation in allergic individuals: a controlled human exposure study. Thorax 2016;71(1):35–44.

[126] Bowatte G, Lodge CJ, Knibbs LD, et al. Traffic-related air pollution exposure is associated with allergic sensitization, asthma, and poor lung function in middle age. J Allergy Clin Immunol 2016.

[127] Brandt EB, Myers JM, Ryan PH, et al. Air pollution and allergic diseases. Curr Opin Pediatr 2015;27(6):724–35.

[128] Chevalier N, Fénichel P. Endocrine disruptors: new players in the pathophysiology of type 2 diabetes? Diabetes Metab 2015;41(2):107–15.

[129] Turyk M, Fantuzzi G, Persky V, et al. Persistent organic pollutants and biomarkers of diabetes risk in a cohort of Great Lakes sport caught fish consumers. Environ Res 2015;140(0):335–44.

[130] Zama AM, Uzumcu M. Epigenetic effects of endocrine-disrupting chemicals on female reproduction: an ovarian perspective. Front Neuroendocrinol 2010;31(4):420–39.

[131] Zeliger HI. Toxic infertility. In: Zeliger HI, editor. Human toxicology of chemical mixtures. 4th ed. Oxford: William Andrew Publishing; 2011. p. 323–40.

[132] Buck Louis GM, Sundaram R, Schisterman EF, et al. Persistent environmental pollutants and couple fecundity: the LIFE study. Environ Health Perspect 2013;121(2):231–6.

[133] Nordkap L, Joensen UN, Blomberg Jensen M, et al. Regional differences and temporal trends in male reproductive health disorders: semen quality may be a sensitive marker of environmental exposures. Mol Cell Endocrinol 2012;355(2):221–30.

[134] Kalfa N, Paris F, Philibert P, et al. Is hypospadias associated with prenatal exposure to endocrine disruptors? A French collaborative controlled study of a cohort of 300 consecutive children without genetic defect. Eur Urol 2015;68(6):1023–30.

[135] Michalakis M, Tzatzarakis MN, Kovatsi L, et al. Hypospadias in offspring is associated with chronic exposure of parents to organophosphate and organochlorine pesticides. Toxicol Lett 2014;230(2):139–45.

[136] Virtanen HE, Adamsson A. Cryptorchidism and endocrine disrupting chemicals. Mol Cell Endocrinol 2012;355(2):208–20.

[137] Voigt K, Brueggemann R, Scherb H, et al. Evaluating the relationship between chemical exposure and cryptorchidism. Environmental Modelling & Software 2010;25(12):1801–12.

[138] Meeks JJ, Sheinfeld J, Eggener SE. Environmental toxicology of testicular cancer. Urol Oncol 2012;30(2):212–15.

[139] Carlsen E, Giwercman A, Keiding N, et al. Evidence for decreasing quality of semen during past 50 years. International Journal of Gynecology & Obstetrics 1993;41(1):112–13.

[140] Fathi Najafi T, Latifnejad Roudsari R, Namvar F, et al. Air pollution and quality of sperm: a meta-analysis. Iran Red Crescent Med J 2015;17(4):e26930.

[141] Vrooman LA, Oatley JM, Griswold JE, et al. Estrogenic exposure alters the spermatogonial stem cells in the developing testis, permanently reducing crossover levels in the adult. PLoS Genet 2015;11(1):e1004949.

[142] Fowler PA, Bellingham M, Sinclair KD, et al. Impact of endocrine-disrupting compounds (EDCs) on female reproductive health. Mol Cell Endocrinol 2012;355(2):231–9.

[143] Genuis SJ, Kelln KL. Toxicant exposure and bioaccumulation: a common and potentially reversible cause of cognitive dysfunction and dementia. Behav Neurol 2015;620143.

[144] Breckenridge CB, Berry C, Chang ET, et al. Association between Parkinson's disease and cigarette smoking, rural living, well-water consumption, farming and pesticide use: systematic review and meta-analysis. PLoS ONE 2016;11(4):e0151841.

[145] Goldman SM, Kamel F, Ross GW, et al. Genetic modification of the association of paraquat and Parkinson's disease. Mov Disord 2012;27(13):1652–8.

[146] Singh NK, Banerjee BD, Bala K, et al. Gene–gene and gene–environment interaction on the risk of Parkinson's disease. Curr Aging Sci 2014;7(2):101–9.

[147] McGwin G, Lienert J, Kennedy JI. Formaldehyde exposure and asthma in children: a systematic review. Environ Health Perspect 2010;118(3):313–17.

[148] Miller MD, Marty MA. Impact of environmental chemicals on lung development. Environ Health Perspect 2010;118(8):1155–64.

[149] Rosenthal GJ. Toxicological assessment of the immune system. Toxicological testing handbook: principles, applications, and data implementation. Boca Raton, FL: CRC Press; 2000. p. 291.

[150] Heindel JJ, vom Saal FS. Role of nutrition and environmental endocrine disrupting chemicals during the perinatal period on the aetiology of obesity. Mol Cell Endocrinol 2009;304(1–2):90–6.

[151] Newbold RR, Padilla-Banks E, Jefferson WN. Environmental estrogens and obesity. Mol Cell Endocrinol 2009;304(1–2):84–9.

[152] Grün F, Blumberg B. Endocrine disrupters as obesogens. Mol Cell Endocrinol 2009;304(1–2):19–29.

[153] Xu X, Freeman NC, Dailey AB, et al. Association between exposure to alkylbenzenes and cardiovascular disease among National Health and Nutrition Examination Survey (NHANES) participants. Int J Occup Environ Health 2009;15(4):385–91.

[154] Hoek G, Krishnan RM, Beelen R, et al. Long-term air pollution exposure and cardiorespiratory mortality: a review. Environ Health 2013;12(1):43.

[155] Zeliger HI. Lipophilic chemical exposure as a cause of cardiovascular disease. Interdiscip Toxicol 2013;6(2):55.

[156] Kaufman JD, Adar SD, Barr RG, et al. Association between air pollution and coronary artery calcification within six metropolitan areas in the USA (the Multi-Ethnic Study of Atherosclerosis and Air Pollution): a longitudinal cohort study. Lancet 2016.

[157] DeJarnett N, Yeager R, Conklin DJ, et al. Residential proximity to major roadways is associated with increased levels of AC133+ circulating angiogenic cells. Arterioscler Thromb Vasc Biol 2015;35(11):2468–77.

[158] Fujiwara T, Morisaki N, Honda Y, et al. Chemicals, Nutrition, and autism spectrum disorder: a mini-review. Front Neurosci 2016;10:174.

[159] Lichtenstein P, Holm NV, Verkasalo PK, et al. Environmental and heritable factors in the causation of cancer: analyses of cohorts of twins from Sweden, Denmark, and Finland. N Engl J Med 2000;343:78–84.

[160] Kim K-H, Jahan SA, Kabir E, et al. A review of airborne polycyclic aromatic hydrocarbons (PAHs) and their human health effects. Environ Int 2013;60:71–80.

[161] Cao J, Yang C, Li J, et al. Association between long-term exposure to outdoor air pollution and mortality in China: a cohort study. J Hazard Mater 2011;186(2–3):1594–600.

[162] Yang WS, Zhao H, Wang X, et al. An evidence-based assessment for the association between long-term exposure to outdoor air pollution and the risk of lung cancer. Eur J Cancer Prev 2015.

[163] Halasova E, Matakova T, Kavcova E, et al. Human lung cancer and hexavalent chromium exposure. Neuro Endocrinol Lett 2009;30(Suppl. 1):182–5.

[164] Teitelbaum SL, Belpoggi F, Reinlib L. Advancing research on endocrine disrupting chemicals in breast cancer: expert panel recommendations. Reprod Toxicol 2015;54(0):141–7.

[165] Kim HS, Lee BM. Endocrine disrupting chemicals and human cancer. In: Nriagu JO, editor. Encyclopedia of environmental health. Burlington: Elsevier; 2011. p. 296–305.

[166] Darbre PD, Williams G. Endocrine disruption and cancer of reproductive tissues. In: Darbre PD, editor. Endocrine disruption and human health. Boston: Academic Press; 2015. p. 177–200.

[167] Le Moal J, Sharpe RM, Jvarphirgensen N, et al. Toward a multi-country monitoring system of reproductive health in the context of endocrine disrupting chemical exposure. Eur J Public Health 2015.

[168] Villanueva CM, Fernandez F, Malats N, et al. Meta-analysis of studies on individual consumption of chlorinated drinking water and bladder cancer. J Epidemiol Community Health 2003;57(3):166–73.

[169] Bhattacharjee P, Chatterjee D, Singh KK, et al. Systems biology approaches to evaluate arsenic toxicity and carcinogenicity: an overview. Int J Hyg Environ Health 2013;216(5):574–86.

[170] Dogliotti E. Molecular mechanisms of carcinogenesis by vinyl chloride. Ann Ist Super Sanita 2006;42(2):163.

[171] Andreoli R, Spatari G, Pigini D, et al. Urinary biomarkers of exposure and of oxidative damage in children exposed to low airborne concentrations of benzene. Environ Res 2015;142:264–72.

[172] Chen M, Chang CH, Tao L, et al. Residential exposure to pesticide during childhood and childhood cancers: a meta-analysis. Pediatrics 2015.

[173] Turner MC, Wigle DT, Krewski D. Residential pesticides and childhood leukemia: a systematic review and meta-analysis. Environ Health Perspect 2010;118(1):33–41.

[174] Van Maele-Fabry G, Lantin A-C, Hoet P, et al. Residential exposure to pesticides and childhood leukaemia: a systematic review and meta-analysis. Environ Int 2011;37(1):280–91.

[175] De Luca C, Gugliandolo A, Calabro C, et al. Role of polymorphisms of inducible nitric oxide synthase and endothelial nitric oxide synthase in idiopathic environmental intolerances. Mediators Inflamm 2015;245308.

[176] De Luca C, Raskovic D, Pacifico V, et al. The search for reliable biomarkers of disease in multiple chemical sensitivity and other environmental intolerances. Int J Environ Res Public Health 2011;8(7):2770–97.

[177] Gugliandolo A, Gangemi C, Calabrò C, et al. Assessment of glutathione peroxidase-1 polymorphisms, oxidative stress and DNA damage in sensitivity-related illnesses. Life Sci 2016;145:27–33.

[178] Korkina L, Scordo MG, Deeva I, et al. The chemical defensive system in the pathobiology of idiopathic environment-associated diseases. Curr Drug Metab 2009;10(8):914–31.

[179] De Luca C, Scordo G, Cesareo E, et al. Idiopathic environmental intolerances (IEI): from molecular epidemiology to molecular medicine. Indian J Exp Biol 2010;48(7):625–35.

[180] Dantoft TM, Elberling J, Brix S, et al. An elevated pro-inflammatory cytokine profile in multiple chemical sensitivity. Psychoneuroendocrinology 2014;40:140–50.

[181] De Luca C, Scordo MG, Cesareo E, et al. Biological definition of multiple chemical sensitivity from redox state and cytokine profiling and not from polymorphisms of xenobiotic-metabolizing enzymes. Toxicol Appl Pharmacol 2010;248(3):285–92.

[182] Palmquist E, Claeson AS, Neely G, et al. Overlap in prevalence between various types of environmental intolerance. Int J Hyg Environ Health 2014;217(4–5):427–34.

[183] Agency for Toxic Substances and Disease Registry. ATSDR case studies in environmental medicine: taking an exposure history. Available from www.atsdr.cdc.gov/csem/exphistory/docs/exposure_history.pdf.

[184] Belova NA, Acosta-Avalos D. The effect of extremely low frequency alternating magnetic field on the behavior of animals in the presence of the geomagnetic field. J Biophys 2015;423838.

[185] Sage C. The implications of non-linear biological oscillations on human electrophysiology for electrohypersensitivity (EHS) and multiple chemical sensitivity (MCS). Rev Environ Health 2015;30(4):293–303.

[186] Bijlsma N. Healthy home, healthy family. 3rd ed. Melbourne: ACES; 2017.

[187] Pasek J, Pasek T, Sieroń-Stołtny K, et al. Electromagnetic fields in medicine: the state of art. Electromagn Biol Med 2016;35(2):170–5.

[188] Tucker JJ, Cirone JM, Morris TR, et al. Pulsed electromagnetic field therapy improves tendon-to-bone healing in a rat rotator cuff repair model. J Orthop Res 2016.

[189] Jauregui JJ, Ventimiglia AV, Grieco PW, et al. Regenerate bone stimulation following limb lengthening: a meta-analysis. BMC Musculoskelet Disord 2016;17(1):407.

[190] Wang R, Wu H, Yang Y, et al. Effects of electromagnetic fields on osteoporosis: a systematic literature review. Electromagn Biol Med 2016;35(4):384–90.

[191] Shreder K, Cucu A, Deloch L, et al. A7.20 low-dose ionising radiation inhibits adipokine induced inflammation in rheumatoid arthritis. Ann Rheum Dis 2016;75(Suppl. 1):A64.

[192] Leszczsynski. Health effects of wireless radiation: possible or probable? Available from https://betweenrockandhardplace .files.wordpress.com/2016/11/leszczynski-arpansa-lecture-nov-2016 .pdf.

[193] Mortazavi SM, Mortazavi SA. Oxidative mechanisms of biological activity of low-intensity radiofrequency radiation. Electromagn Biol Med 2016;35(4):303–4.

[194] Khadra KMA, Khalil AM, Samak MA, et al. Antioxidant profile of saliva among young men using mobile phones. Jordan Journal of Biological Sciences 2014;7(4):275–80.

[195] Pasek J, Mucha R, Sieron A. Magnetostimulation: the modern form therapy in medicine and rehabilitation. Fizjoterapia 2006;14(4):3.

[196] Cao Y, Scarfi MR. Adaptive response in mammalian cells exposed to non-ionizing radiofrequency fields: a review and gaps in knowledge. Mutat Res Rev Mutat Res 2014.

[197] Spitz DR, Azzam EI, Li JJ, et al. Metabolic oxidation/reduction reactions and cellular responses to ionizing radiation: a unifying concept in stress response biology. Cancer Metastasis Rev 2004;23(3–4):311–22.

[198] Sannino A, Sarti M, Reddy SB, et al. Induction of adaptive response in human blood lymphocytes exposed to radiofrequency radiation. Radiat Res 2009;171(6):735–42.

[199] Yakymenko I, Tsybulin O, Sidorik E, et al. Oxidative mechanisms of biological activity of low-intensity radiofrequency radiation. Electromagn Biol Med 2016;35(2):186–202.

[200] Walleczek J. Electromagnetic field effects on cells of the immune system: the role of calcium signaling. FASEB J 1992;6(13):3177–85.

[201] Pall ML. Electromagnetic fields act via activation of voltage-gated calcium channels to produce beneficial or adverse effects. J Cell Mol Med 2013;17(8):958–65.

[202] Lednev VV. Possible mechanism for the influence of weak magnetic fields on biological systems. Bioelectromagnetics 1991;12(2):71–5.

[203] Lednev V, Blank M. Possible mechanism for the effect of weak magnetic fields on biological systems: correction of the basic expression and its consequences. In: Blank M, editor. Electricity and magnetism in biology and medicine. San Francisco: San Francisco Press; 1993. p. 550–2.

[204] Lednev V. Bioeffects of weak combined, constant and variable magnetic fields. Biophysics (Oxf) 1996;1(41):241–52.

[205] Akyol O, Zoroglu SS, Armutcu F, et al. Nitric oxide as a physiopathological factor in neuropsychiatric disorders. In Vivo 2004;18(3):377–90.

[206] Knott AB, Bossy-Wetzel E. Nitric oxide in health and disease of the nervous system. Antioxid Redox Signal 2009;11(3):541–54.

[207] Pilla AA. Electromagnetic fields instantaneously modulate nitric oxide signaling in challenged biological systems. Biochem Biophys Res Commun 2012;426(3):330–3.

[208] Lushchak VI. Free radicals, reactive oxygen species, oxidative stress and its classification. Chem Biol Interact 2014;224:164–75.

[209] Desai NR, Kesari KK, Agarwal A. Pathophysiology of cell phone radiation: oxidative stress and carcinogenesis with focus on male reproductive system. Reprod Biol Endocrinol 2009;7:114.

[210] Cig B, Naziroglu M. Investigation of the effects of distance from sources on apoptosis, oxidative stress and cytosolic calcium accumulation via TRPV1 channels induced by mobile phones and wi-fi in breast cancer cells. Biochim Biophys Acta 2015;1848(10 Pt B):2756–65.

[211] Markova E, Malmgren LO, Belyaev IY. Microwaves from mobile phones inhibit 53BP1 focus formation in human stem cells more strongly than in differentiated cells: possible mechanistic link to cancer risk. Environ Health Perspect 2010;118(3):394–9.

[212] Terzi M, Ozberk B, Deniz OG, et al. The role of electromagnetic fields in neurological disorders. J Chem Neuroanat 2016;75(Pt B):77–84.

[213] Burlaka A, Tsybulin O, Sidorik E, et al. Overproduction of free radical species in embryonal cells exposed to low intensity radiofrequency radiation. Exp Oncol 2013;35(3):219–25.

[214] Belpomme D, Campagnac C, Irigaray P. Reliable disease biomarkers characterizing and identifying electrohypersensitivity and multiple chemical sensitivity as two etiopathogenic aspects of a unique pathological disorder. Rev Environ Health 2015;30(4):251–71.

[215] Lewczuk B, Redlarski G, Żak A, et al. Influence of electric, magnetic, and electromagnetic fields on the circadian system: current stage of knowledge. Biomed Res Int 2014;169459.

[216] European Cancer and Environmental Research Institute (ECERI). Idiopathic environmental intolerance: what role for electromagnetic fields and chemicals? 5th Paris Appeal Congress, 18 May 2015, Paris, France.

[217] Mortazavi SM. Window theory in non-ionizing radiation-induced adaptive responses. Dose Response 2013;11(2):293–4.

[218] Mortazavi SM, Motamedifar M, Namdari G, et al. Non-linear adaptive phenomena which decrease the risk of infection after pre-exposure to radiofrequency radiation. Dose Response 2014;12(2):233–45.

[219] Havas M. When theory and observation collide: can non-ionizing radiation cause cancer? Environ Pollut 2016;219.

[220] Lai H. Neurological effects of non-ionizing electromagnetic fields, Section 9, March 2014, Supplement, BioInitiative Working Group.

[221] Pacher P, Beckman JS, Liaudet L. Nitric oxide and peroxynitrite in health and disease. Physiol Rev 2007;87(1):315–424.

[222] Pall ML. Scientific evidence contradicts findings and assumptions of Canadian Safety Panel 6: microwaves act through voltage-gated calcium channel activation to induce biological impacts at non-thermal levels, supporting a paradigm shift for microwave/lower frequency electromagnetic field action. Rev Environ Health 2015;30(2):99–116.

[223] Mortazavi S, Daiee E, Yazdi A, et al. Mercury release from dental amalgam restorations after magnetic resonance imaging and following mobile phone use. Pak J Biol Sci 2008;11(8):1142–6.

[224] Wertheimer N, Leeper E. Electrical wiring configurations and childhood cancer. Am J Epidemiol 1979;109(3):273–84.

[225] Ahlbom A, Day N, Feychting M, et al. A pooled analysis of magnetic fields and childhood leukaemia. Br J Cancer 2000;83(5):692.

[226] Greenland S, Sheppard AR, Kaune WT, et al. A pooled analysis of magnetic fields, wire codes, and childhood leukemia. Childhood Leukemia-EMF Study Group. Epidemiology 2000;11(6):624–34.

[227] Grellier J, Ravazzani P, Cardis E. Potential health impacts of residential exposures to extremely low frequency magnetic fields in Europe. Environ Int 2014;62:55–63.

[228] Teepen JC, van Dijck JA. Impact of high electromagnetic field levels on childhood leukemia incidence. Int J Cancer 2012;131(4):769–78.

[229] Draper G, Vincent T, Kroll ME, et al. Childhood cancer in relation to distance from high voltage power lines in England and Wales: a case-control study. BMJ 2005;330(7503):1290.

[230] Bunch KJ, Keegan TJ, Swanson J, et al. Residential distance at birth from overhead high-voltage powerlines: childhood cancer risk in Britain 1962–2008. Br J Cancer 2014;110(5):1402–8.

[231] Salvan A, Ranucci A, Lagorio S, et al; on behalf of the SRG. Childhood leukemia and 50 Hz magnetic fields: findings from the Italian SETIL case-control study. Int J Environ Res Public Health 2015;12(2):2184–204.

[232] Greenland S, Sheppard AR, Kaune WT, et al. A pooled analysis of magnetic fields, wire codes, and childhood leukemia. Epidemiology 2000;11(6):624–34.

[233] International Agency for Research on Cancer. IARC monographs on the evaluation of carcinogenic risks to humans. Non-ionizing radiation, Part 1: static and extremely low-frequency (ELF) electric and magnetic fields. Lyon, France: WHO, IARC; 2002.

[234] Burch JB, Reif JS, Noonan CW, et al. Melatonin metabolite excretion among cellular telephone users. Int J Radiat Biol 2002;78(11):1029–36.

[235] de Vocht F, Hannam K, Buchan I. Environmental risk factors for cancers of the brain and nervous system: the use of ecological data to generate hypotheses. Occup Environ Med 2013;70(5):349–56.

[236] Dobes M, Khurana VG, Shadbolt B, et al. Increasing incidence of glioblastoma multiforme and meningioma, and decreasing incidence of Schwannoma (2000–2008): findings of a multicenter Australian study. Surg Neurol Int 2011;2:176.

[237] Chapman S, Azizi L, Luo Q, et al. Has the incidence of brain cancer risen in Australia since the introduction of mobile phones 29 years ago? Cancer Epidemiol 2016;42:199–205.

[238] Christensen HC, Kosteljanetz M, Johansen C. Incidences of gliomas and meningiomas in Denmark, 1943 to 1997. Neurosurgery 2003;52(6):1327–33, discussion 1333–34.

[239] Johannesen TB, Angell-Andersen E, Tretli S, et al. Trends in incidence of brain and central nervous system tumors in Norway, 1970–1999. Neuroepidemiology 2004;23(3):101–9.

[240] Hoffman S, Propp JM, McCarthy BJ. Temporal trends in incidence of primary brain tumors in the United States, 1985–1999. Neuro Oncol 2006;8(1):27–37.

[241] Lonn S, Klaeboe L, Hall P, et al. Incidence trends of adult primary intracerebral tumors in four Nordic countries. Int J Cancer 2004;108(3):450–5.

[242] Cordera S, Bottacchi E, D'Alessandro G, et al. Epidemiology of primary intracranial tumours in NW Italy, a population based study: stable incidence in the last two decades. J Neurol 2002;249(3):281–4.

[243] Inskip PD, Hoover RN, Devesa SS. Brain cancer incidence trends in relation to cellular telephone use in the United States. Neuro Oncol 2010;12(11):1147–51.

[244] Caldarella A, Crocetti E, Paci E. Is the incidence of brain tumors really increasing? A population-based analysis from a cancer registry. J Neurooncol 2011;104(2):589–94.

[245] Soderqvist F, Hardell L, Carlberg M, et al. Ownership and use of wireless telephones: a population-based study of Swedish children aged 7–14 years. BMC Public Health 2007;7:105.

[246] Clegg LX, Feuer EJ, Midthune DN, et al. Impact of reporting delay and reporting error on cancer incidence rates and trends. J Natl Cancer Inst 2002;94(20):1537–45.

[247] Hardell L, Carlberg M. Increasing rates of brain tumours in the Swedish national inpatient register and the causes of death register. Int J Environ Res Public Health 2015;12(4):3793–813.

[248] Coureau G, Bouvier G, Lebailly P, et al. Mobile phone use and brain tumours in the CERENAT case-control study. Occup Environ Med 2014;71(7):514–22.

[249] Group IS. Brain tumour risk in relation to mobile telephone use: results of the Interphone international case–control study. Int J Epidemiol 2010;dyq079.

[250] Hardell L, Carlberg M. Mobile phone and cordless phone use and the risk for glioma: analysis of pooled case-control studies in Sweden, 1997–2003 and 2007–2009. Pathophysiology 2015;22(1):1–13.

[251] Hardell L, Carlberg M, Mild KH. Use of mobile phones and cordless phones is associated with increased risk for glioma and acoustic neuroma. Pathophysiology 2013;20(2):85–110.

[252] Wyde M, Cesta M, Blystone C, et al. Report of partial findings from the National Toxicology Program Carcinogenesis Studies of Cell Phone Radiofrequency Radiation in Hsd: Sprague Dawley® SD rats (Whole Body Exposure). bioRxiv 2016.

[253] CSIRO. Biological effects and safety of electromagnetic radiation (Barnett Report). CSIRO; 1994.

[254] Stewart W. Mobile phones and health: the report of the Independent Expert Group on Mobile Phones. Independent Expert Group on Mobile Phones; 2000.

[255] BioInitiative Report 2012. A rationale for biologically-based exposure standards for low-intensity electromagnetic radiation. Geneva: WHO; 2012.

[256] Russian National Committee on Non-Ionizing Radiation Protection. Children and mobile phones: the health of the following generations is in danger. Moscow: Russian National Committee on Non-Ionizing Radiation Protection; 2008.

[257] Hardell L, Carlberg M, Hansson Mild K. Pooled analysis of case-control studies on malignant brain tumours and the use of mobile and cordless phones including living and deceased subjects. Int J Oncol 2011;38(5):1465–74.

[258] Hardell L, Carlberg M, Soderqvist F, et al. Pooled analysis of case-control studies on acoustic neuroma diagnosed 1997–2003 and 2007–2009 and use of mobile and cordless phones. Int J Oncol 2013;43(4):1036–44.

[259] Khurana VG, Teo C, Kundi M, et al. Cell phones and brain tumors: a review including the long-term epidemiologic data. Surg Neurol 2009;72(3):205–14.

[260] Morgan LL, Miller AB, Sasco A, et al. Mobile phone radiation causes brain tumors and should be classified as a probable human carcinogen (2A) (review). Int J Oncol 2015;46(5):1865–71.

[261] Pettersson D, Mathiesen T, Prochazka M, et al. Long-term mobile phone use and acoustic neuroma risk. Epidemiology 2014;25(2):233–41.

[262] Deltour I, Johansen C, Auvinen A, et al. Time trends in brain tumor incidence rates in Denmark, Finland, Norway, and Sweden, 1974–2003. J Natl Cancer Inst 2009;101(24):1721–4.

[263] Larjavaara S, Schüz J, Swerdlow A, et al. Location of gliomas in relation to mobile telephone use: a case-case and case-specular analysis. Am J Epidemiol 2011;174(1):2–11.

[264] Benson VS, Pirie K, Schuz J, et al. Mobile phone use and risk of brain neoplasms and other cancers: prospective study. Int J Epidemiol 2013;42(3):792–802.

[265] Cardis E, Armstrong B, Bowman J, et al. Risk of brain tumours in relation to estimated RF dose from mobile phones: results from five Interphone countries. Occup Environ Med 2011;68(9):631–40.

[266] Grell K, Frederiksen K, Schüz J, et al. The intracranial distribution of gliomas in relation to exposure from mobile phones: analyses from the Interphone study. Am J Epidemiol 2016.

[267] Aydin D, Feychting M, Schuz J, et al. Mobile phone use and brain tumors in children and adolescents: a multicenter case-control study. J Natl Cancer Inst 2011;103(16):1264–76.

[268] de Vocht F. Inferring the 1985–2014 impact of mobile phone use on selected brain cancer subtypes using Bayesian structural time series and synthetic controls. Environ Int 2016;97:100–7.

[269] Marshall TG, Heil TJ. Electrosmog and autoimmune disease. Immunol Res 2016.

[270] Rubin GJ, Munshi JD, Wessely S. Electromagnetic hypersensitivity: a systematic review of provocation studies. Psychosom Med 2005;67(2):224–32.

[271] Rubin GJ, Nieto-Hernandez R, Wessely S. Idiopathic environmental intolerance attributed to electromagnetic fields (formerly 'electromagnetic hypersensitivity'): an updated systematic review of provocation studies. Bioelectromagnetics 2010;31(1):1–11.

[272] Schuz J, Elliott P, Auvinen A, et al. An international prospective cohort study of mobile phone users and health (Cosmos): design considerations and enrolment. Cancer Epidemiol 2011;35(1):37–43.

[273] Sadetzki S, Langer CE, Bruchim R, et al. The MOBI-Kids Study Protocol: challenges in assessing childhood and adolescent exposure to electromagnetic fields from wireless telecommunication technologies and possible association with brain tumor risk. Front Public Health 2014;2:124.

[274] Quanta Monitor. Available from www.appbrain.com/app/quanta-monitor/com.cellraid.app.play.

[275] International Agency for Research on Cancer. IARC classifies radiofrequency electromagnetic fields as possibly carcinogenic to humans. Press release, 31 May 2011.

[276] Chen Q, Lang L, Wu W, et al. A meta-analysis on the relationship between exposure to ELF-EMFs and the risk of female breast cancer. PLoS ONE 2013;8(7):e69272.

[277] Zhao G, Lin X, Zhou M, et al. Relationship between exposure to extremely low-frequency electromagnetic fields and breast cancer risk: a meta-analysis. Eur J Gynaecol Oncol 2014;35(3):264–9.

[278] Harland JD, Liburdy RP. Environmental magnetic fields inhibit the antiproliferative action of tamoxifen and melatonin in a human breast cancer cell line. Bioelectromagnetics 1997;18(8):555–62.

[279] Blackman C, Benane S, House D. The influence of 1.2 μT, 60 Hz magnetic fields on melatonin-and tamoxifen-induced inhibition of MCF-7 cell growth. Bioelectromagnetics 2001;22(2):122–8.

[280] Haynal A, Regli F. Zusammenhang der amyotrophischen lateralsklerose mit gehäuften elektrotraumata. Stereotact Funct Neurosurg 1964;24(3–4):189–98.

[281] Zhou H, Chen G, Chen C, et al. Association between extremely low-frequency electromagnetic field occupations and amyotrophic lateral sclerosis: a meta-analysis. PLoS ONE 2012;7(11):e48354.

[282] Maes A, Verschaeve L. Can cytogenetics explain the possible association between exposure to extreme low-frequency magnetic fields and Alzheimer's disease? J Appl Toxicol 2012;32(2):81–7.

[283] Kaszuba-Zwolinska J, Gremba J, Galdzinska-Calik B, et al. Electromagnetic field induced biological effects in humans. Przegl Lek 2015;72(11):636–41.

[284] Bevington M. Electromagnetic sensitivity and electromagnetic hypersensitivity: a summary. UK: Capability Books; 2013.

[285] Belyaev I, Dean A, Eger H, et al. EUROPEAN EMF Guideline 2016 for the prevention, diagnosis and treatment of EMF-related health problems and illnesses. Rev Environ Health 2016;31(3):363–97.

[286] Austrian Medical Association. Guideline of the Austrian Medical Association for the diagnosis and treatment of EMF-related health problems and illnesses (EMF syndrome). Group AMAsEW, 3 March 2012.

[287] British Society of Ecological Medicine. Diagnosis and management of electromagnetic hypersensitivity (EHS): rapid overview for a mixed audience. UK: British Society of Ecological Medicine; 2014.

[288] Austrian Medical Association. Guideline of the Austrian Medical Association for the diagnosis and treatment of EMF-related health problems and illnesses (EMF syndrome): consensus paper of the Austrian Medical Association's EMF Working Group. Meeting of environmental medicine officers of the Regional Medical Associations and the Austrian Medical Association, 2012.

[289] Calderon MA, Linneberg A, Kleine-Tebbe J, et al. Respiratory allergy caused by house dust mites: what do we really know? J Allergy Clin Immunol 2015;136(1):38–48.

[290] Bjerg A, Ekerljung L, Eriksson J, et al. Increase in pollen sensitization in Swedish adults and protective effect of keeping animals in childhood. Clin Exp Allergy 2016;46(10):1328–36.

[291] Prescott S, Allen KJ. Food allergy: riding the second wave of the allergy epidemic. Pediatr Allergy Immunol 2011;22(2):155–60.

[292] Asher MI, Montefort S, Bjorksten B, et al. Worldwide time trends in the prevalence of symptoms of asthma, allergic rhinoconjunctivitis, and eczema in childhood: ISAAC Phases One and Three repeat multicountry cross-sectional surveys. Lancet 2006;368(9537):733–43.

[293] Verlato G, Corsico A, Villani S, et al. Is the prevalence of adult asthma and allergic rhinitis still increasing? Results of an Italian study. J Allergy Clin Immunol 2003;111(6):1232–8.

[294] Platts-Mills TA. The allergy epidemics, 1870–2010. J Allergy Clin Immunol 2015;136(1):3–13.

[295] Wang XD, Zheng M, Lou HF, et al. An increased prevalence of self-reported allergic rhinitis in major Chinese cities from 2005 to 2011. Allergy 2016;71(8):1170–80.

[296] Australasian Society of Clinical Immunology and Allergy (ASCIA). Allergy in Australia (AIDA) report 2013: ASCIA; 2013.

[297] Australasian Society of Clinical Immunology and Allergy (ASCIA). Allergy in Australia 2014: a submission for allergic diseases to be recognised as a National Health Priority Area. ASCIA; 2014.

[298] Archer CB. Atopic eczema. Medicine (Baltimore) 2013;41(6):341–4.

[299] Rudders SA, Arias SA, Camargo CA Jr. Trends in hospitalizations for food-induced anaphylaxis in US children, 2000–2009. J Allergy Clin Immunol 2014;134(4):960–2.

[300] Turner PJ, Gowland MH, Sharma V, et al. Increase in anaphylaxis-related hospitalizations but no increase in fatalities: an analysis of United Kingdom national anaphylaxis data, 1992–2012. J Allergy Clin Immunol 2015;135(4):956–63.

[301] Simons FE, Ebisawa M, Sanchez-Borges M, et al. 2015 update of the evidence base: World Allergy Organization anaphylaxis guidelines. World Allergy Organ J 2015;8(1):32.

[302] Panesar SS, Javad S, de Silva D, et al. The epidemiology of anaphylaxis in Europe: a systematic review. Allergy 2013;68(11):1353–61.

[303] Du Toit G, Roberts G, Sayre PH, et al. Randomized trial of peanut consumption in infants at risk for peanut allergy. N Engl J Med 2015;372(9):803–13.

[304] ASCIA. Guidelines. Infant feeding and allergy prevention Australia, 2016. Available from www.allergy.org.au/images/pcc/ASCIA_Guidelines_infant_feeding_and_allergy_prevention.pdf.

[305] Briggs A. The making of modern England, 1783–1867. UK: Harper & Row; 1965.

[306] Strachan DP. Family size, infection and atopy: the first decade of the 'hygiene hypothesis'. Thorax 2000;55(Suppl. 1):S2.

[307] di Mauro G, Bernardini R, Barberi S, et al. Prevention of food and airway allergy: consensus of the Italian Society of Preventive and Social Paediatrics, the Italian Society of Paediatric Allergy and Immunology, and Italian Society of Pediatrics. World Allergy Organ J 2016;9:28.

[308] Goronfolah L. Aeroallergens, atopy and allergic rhinitis in the Middle East. Eur Ann Allergy Clin Immunol 2016;48(1):5–21.

[309] Dominguez-Bello MG, Costello EK, Contreras M, et al. Delivery mode shapes the acquisition and structure of the initial microbiota across multiple body habitats in newborns. Proc Natl Acad Sci USA 2010;107(26):11971–5.

[310] Musilova S, Rada V, Vlkova E, et al. Beneficial effects of human milk oligosaccharides on gut microbiota. Benef Microbes 2014;5(3):273–83.

[311] Pacheco AR, Barile D, Underwood MA, et al. The impact of the milk glycobiome on the neonate gut microbiota. Annu Rev Anim Biosci 2015;3:419.

[312] Lee S-Y, Yu J, Ahn K-M, et al. Additive effect between IL-13 polymorphism and cesarean section delivery/prenatal antibiotics use on atopic dermatitis: a birth cohort study (COCOA). PLoS ONE 2014;9(5):e96603.

[313] Hospodsky D, Yamamoto N, Nazaroff WW, et al. Characterizing airborne fungal and bacterial concentrations and emission rates in six occupied children's classrooms. Indoor Air 2015;25(6):641–52.

[314] Laursen MF, Zachariassen G, Bahl MI, et al. Having older siblings is associated with gut microbiota development during early childhood. BMC Microbiol 2015;15(1):154.

[315] Strachan DP, Aït-Khaled N, Foliaki S, et al. Siblings, asthma, rhinoconjunctivitis and eczema: a worldwide perspective from the International Study of Asthma and Allergies in Childhood. Clin Exp Allergy 2015;45(1):126–36.

[316] Dunlop J, Matsui E, Sharma HP. Allergic rhinitis: environmental determinants. Immunol Allergy Clin North Am 2016;36(2):367–77.

[317] von Mutius E, Vercelli D. Farm living: effects on childhood asthma and allergy. Nat Rev Immunol 2010;10(12):861–8.

[318] Wegienka G, Zoratti E, Johnson CC. The role of the early-life environment in the development of allergic disease. Immunol Allergy Clin North Am 2015;35(1):1–17.

[319] Stein MM, Hrusch CL, Gozdz J, et al. Innate immunity and asthma risk in Amish and Hutterite farm children. N Engl J Med 2016;375(5):411–21.

[320] Illi S, von Mutius E, Lau S, et al. Perennial allergen sensitisation early in life and chronic asthma in children: a birth cohort study. Lancet 2006;368(9537):763–70.

[321] Yatsunenko T, Rey FE, Manary MJ, et al. Human gut microbiome viewed across age and geography. Nature 2012;486(7402):222–7.

[322] Campbell B, Lodge C, Lowe A, et al. Exposure to 'farming' and objective markers of atopy: a systematic review and meta-analysis. Clin Exp Allergy 2015;45(4):744–57.

[323] Ege MJ, Mayer M, Normand AC, et al. Exposure to environmental microorganisms and childhood asthma. N Engl J Med 2011;364(8):701–9.

[324] D'Amato G, Holgate ST, Pawankar R, et al. Meteorological conditions, climate change, new emerging factors, and asthma and related allergic disorders. A statement of the World Allergy Organization. World Allergy Organ J 2015;8(1):25.

[325] Kim BJ, Lee SY, Kim HB, et al. Environmental changes, microbiota, and allergic diseases. Allergy Asthma Immunol Res 2014;6(5):389–400.

[326] Kim HH, Lee CS, Yu SD, et al. Near-road exposure and impact of air pollution on allergic diseases in elementary school children: a cross-sectional study. Yonsei Med J 2016;57(3):698–713.

[327] Diaz-Sanchez D. Pollution and the immune response: atopic diseases — are we too dirty or too clean? Immunology 2000;101(1):11–18.

[328] D'Amato G, Liccardi G, D'Amato M, et al. The role of outdoor air pollution and climatic changes on the rising trends in respiratory allergy. Respir Med 2001;95(7):606–11.

[329] Matsui EC. Environmental exposures and asthma morbidity in children living in urban neighborhoods. Allergy 2014;69(5):553–8.

[330] Kim B-J, Kwon J-W, Seo J-H, et al. Association of ozone exposure with asthma, allergic rhinitis, and allergic sensitization. Ann Allergy Asthma Immunol 2011;107(3):214–19.

[331] Feleszko W, Ruszczynski M, Jaworska J, et al. Environmental tobacco smoke exposure and risk of allergic sensitisation in children: a systematic review and meta-analysis. Arch Dis Child 2014;99(11):985–92.

[332] Bousquet PJ, Chinn S, Janson C, et al. Geographical variation in the prevalence of positive skin tests to environmental aeroallergens in the European Community Respiratory Health Survey I. Allergy 2007;62(3):301–9.

[333] Rao B, Bhat S. Prevalence of IgE mediated airborne allergies in children. Journal of Drug Delivery and Therapeutics 2015;5(3):76–9.

[334] Demoly P, Matucci A, Rossi O, et al. A year-long, fortnightly, observational survey in three European countries of patients with respiratory allergies induced by house dust mites: methodology, demographics and clinical characteristics. BMC Pulm Med 2016;16(1):85.

[335] Platts-Mills TA, de Weck A, Aalberse RC, et al. Dust mite allergens and asthma: a worldwide problem. J Allergy Clin Immunol 1989;83(2 Pt 1):416–27.

[336] Jacquet A. Innate immune responses in house dust mite allergy. ISRN Allergy 2013;735031.

[337] Colloff MJ. Dust mites. Melbourne: CSIRO Publishing and Springer Science; 2009.

[338] Crisafulli D, Almqvist C, Marks G, et al. Seasonal trends in house dust mite allergen in children's beds over a 7-year period. Allergy 2007;62(12):1394–400.

[339] Di Mauro G, Bernardini R, Barberi S, et al. Prevention of food and airway allergy: consensus of the Italian Society of Preventive and Social Paediatrics, the Italian Society of Paediatric Allergy and Immunology, and Italian Society of Pediatrics. World Allergy Organ J 2016;9:28. http://doi.org/10.1186/s40413-016-0111-6.

[340] Poza Guedes P, Sánchez Machín I, Matheu V, et al. Role of predatory mites in persistent nonoccupational allergic rhinitis. Can Respir J 2016;5782317.

[341] Kanchongkittiphon W, Mendell MJ, Gaffin JM, et al. Indoor environmental exposures and exacerbation of asthma: an update to the 2000 review by the Institute of Medicine. Environ Health Perspect 2015;123(1):6–20.

[342] Winn AK, Salo PM, Klein C, et al. Efficacy of an in-home test kit in reducing dust mite allergen levels: results of a randomized controlled pilot study. J Asthma 2016;53(2):133–8.

[343] Kuehr J, Frischer T, Meinert R, et al. Mite allergen exposure is a risk for the incidence of specific sensitization. J Allergy Clin Immunol 1994;94(1):44–52.

[344] Chew GL, Burge HA, Dockery DW, et al. Limitations of a home characteristics questionnaire as a predictor of indoor allergen levels. Am J Respir Crit Care Med 1998;157(5 Pt 1):1536–41.

[345] Simpson A, Simpson B, Custovic A, et al. Household characteristics and mite allergen levels in Manchester, UK. Clin Exp Allergy 2002;32(10):1413–19.

[346] Arlian LG, Vyszenski-Moher DL, Morgan MS. Mite and mite allergen removal during machine washing of laundry. J Allergy Clin Immunol 2003;111(6):1269–73.

[347] Gehring U, de Jongste J, Kerkhof M, et al. The 8-year follow-up of the PIAMA intervention study assessing the effect of mite-impermeable mattress covers. Allergy 2012;67(2):248–56.

[348] Luczynska C, Sterne J, Bond J, et al. Indoor factors associated with concentrations of house dust mite allergen, Der p 1, in a random sample of houses in Norwich, UK. Clin Exp Allergy 1998;28:1201–9.

[349] Wu FF, Wu MW, Pierse N, et al. Daily vacuuming of mattresses significantly reduces house dust mite allergens, bacterial endotoxin, and fungal beta-glucan. J Asthma 2012;49(2):139–43.

[350] Ownby D, Johnson CC. Recent Understandings of pet allergies. F1000Res 2016;5.

[351] Australasian Society of Clinical Immunology and Allergy (ASCIA). Pet allergy. Available from www.allergy.org.au/images/pcc/ASCIA_PCC_Pet_allergy_2015.pdf.

[352] Niesler A, Scigala G, Ludzen-Izbinska B. Cat (Fel d 1) and dog (Can f 1) allergen levels in cars, dwellings and schools. Aerobiologia (Bologna) 2016;32(3):571–80.

[353] Johnston R. Clearing the air: asthma and indoor air exposures. Washington, DC: National Academies Press; 2000.

[354] Karlsson AS, Renstrom A. Human hair is a potential source of cat allergen contamination of ambient air. Allergy 2005;60(7):961–4.

[355] Gore RB, Bishop S, Durrell B, et al. Air filtration units in homes with cats: can they reduce personal exposure to cat allergen? Clin Exp Allergy 2003;33(6):765–9.

[356] van der Heide S, van Aalderen WM, Kauffman HF, et al. Clinical effects of air cleaners in homes of asthmatic children sensitized to pet allergens. J Allergy Clin Immunol 1999;104(2 Pt 1):447–51.

[357] Nishikawa K, Fujimura T, Ota Y, et al. Exposure to positively- and negatively-charged plasma cluster ions impairs IgE-binding capacity of indoor cat and fungal allergens. World Allergy Organ J 2016;9(1):27.

[358] Portnoy J, Chew GL, Phipatanakul W, et al. Environmental assessment and exposure reduction of cockroaches: a practice parameter. J Allergy Clin Immunol 2013;132(4):10.

[359] Gruchalla RS, Pongracic J, Plaut M, et al. Inner city asthma study: relationships among sensitivity, allergen exposure, and asthma morbidity. J Allergy Clin Immunol 2005;115(3):478–85.

[360] Jung KH, Lovinsky-Desir S, Perzanowski M, et al. Repeatedly high polycyclic aromatic hydrocarbon exposure and cockroach sensitization among inner-city children. Environ Res 2015;140:649–56.

[361] Donohue KM, Al-Alem U, Perzanowski MS, et al. Anti-cockroach and anti-mouse IgE are associated with early wheeze and atopy in

an inner-city birth cohort. J Allergy Clin Immunol 2008;122(5): 914–20.

[362] Ahluwalia SK, Peng RD, Breysse PN, et al. Mouse allergen is the major allergen of public health relevance in Baltimore City. J Allergy Clin Immunol 2013;132(4):830–5.

[363] Sedaghat AR, Matsui EC, Baxi SN, et al. Mouse sensitivity is an independent risk factor for rhinitis in children with asthma. J Allergy Clin Immunol Pract 2016;4(1):82–8.

[364] Australasian Society of Clinical Immunology and Allergy (ASCIA). Allergic reactions to bites and stings. Available from www.allergy.org.au/images/pcc/ASCIA_PCC_Allergic_reactions_bites_stings_2015.pdf.

[365] Australasian Society of Clinical Immunology and Allergy (ASCIA). Tick allergy. Available from www.allergy.org.au/images/pcc/ASCIA_PCC_Tick_allergy_2016.pdf.

[366] Australasian Society of Clinical Immunology and Allergy (ASCIA). Thunderstorm asthma. Available from www.allergy.org.au/patients/asthma-and-allergy/thunderstorm-asthma.

[367] Gunnbjörnsdóttir MI, Franklin KA, Norbäck D, et al. Prevalence and incidence of respiratory symptoms in relation to indoor dampness: the RHINE study. Thorax 2006;61(3):221–5.

[368] Mudarri D, Fisk WJ. Public health and economic impact of dampness and mold. Indoor Air 2007;17(3):226–35.

[369] Elkink A. Building basics: internal moisture. New Zealand: Building Research Association of New Zealand; 2012.

[370] Prezant D. Calculating the burden of disease attributable to indoor dampness in NZ: improvements to net benefit model health assessments. Centre for Public Health Research New Zealand: report commissioned by the Energy Efficiency and Conservation Agency, Government of New Zealand; 2011.

[371] Antova T, Pattenden S, Brunekreef B, et al. Exposure to indoor mould and children's respiratory health in the PATY study. J Epidemiol Community Health 2008;62(8):708–14.

[372] Fisk WJ, Eliseeva EA, Mendell MJ. Association of residential dampness and mold with respiratory tract infections and bronchitis: a meta-analysis. Environ Health 2010;9(1):1.

[373] Mendell MJ, Mirer AG, Cheung K, et al. Respiratory and allergic health effects of dampness, mold, and dampness-related agents: a review of the epidemiologic evidence. Environ Health Perspect 2011;119(6):748.

[374] Portnoy JM, Williams PB, Barnes CS. Innate immune responses to fungal allergens. Curr Allergy Asthma Rep 2016;16(9):62.

[375] Shoemaker RC, House D, Ryan JC. Vasoactive intestinal polypeptide (VIP) corrects chronic inflammatory response syndrome (CIRS) acquired following exposure to water-damaged buildings. Health 2013;5(3):396.

[376] Shoemaker RC, House DE. Sick building syndrome (SBS) and exposure to water-damaged buildings: time series study, clinical trial and mechanisms. Neurotoxicol Teratol 2006;28(5):573–88.

[377] Thrasher JD, Crawley S. The biocontaminants and complexity of damp indoor spaces: more than what meets the eyes. Toxicol Ind Health 2009;25(9–10):583–615.

[378] Tang D, Kang R, Coyne CB, et al. PAMPs and DAMPs: signal 0s that spur autophagy and immunity. Immunol Rev 2012;249(1):158–75.

[379] Plato A, Hardison SE, Brown GD. Pattern recognition receptors in antifungal immunity. Semin Immunopathol 2015;37(2):97–106.

[380] Shoemaker R. Differential association of HLA DR by PCR genotypes with susceptibility to chronic, neurotoxin-mediated illnesses. Denver, CO: Poster presentation, American Society for Tropical Medicine and Hygiene; 2002.

[381] McMahon S, Shoemaker R, Ryan J. Reduction in forebrain parenchymal and cortical grey matter swelling across treatment groups in patients with inflammatory illness acquired following exposure to water-damaged buildings. J Neurosci Clin Res 1 2016;1(2).

[382] Shoemaker RC, House D, Ryan JC. Structural brain abnormalities in patients with inflammatory illness acquired following exposure to water-damaged buildings: a volumetric MRI study using NeuroQuant(R). Neurotoxicol Teratol 2014;45:18–26.

[383] Berndtson K, McMahon SW, Ackerley M, et al. Medically sound investigation and remediation of water-damaged buildings in cases of chronic inflammatory response syndrome. Surviving Mold 2016.

[384] Hashemi H, Khabazkhoob M, Jafarzadehpur E, et al. Contrast sensitivity evaluation in a population-based study in Shahroud, Iran. Ophthalmology 2012;119(3):541–6.

[385] Shoemaker RC (ed.). Use of visual contrast sensitivity and cholestyramine in diagnosis and treatment of indoor air acquired, chronic, neurotoxin-mediated illness. Surviving Mold 2003.

[386] Regan D, Silver R, Murray TJ. Visual acuity and contrast sensitivity in multiple sclerosis: hidden visual loss — an auxiliary diagnostic test. Brain 1977;100(3):563–79.

[387] Risacher SL, Wudunn D, Pepin SM, et al. Visual contrast sensitivity in Alzheimer's disease, mild cognitive impairment, and older adults with cognitive complaints. Neurobiol Aging 2013;34(4):1133–44.

[388] Chew GL, Horner WE, Kennedy K, et al. Procedures to assist health care providers to determine when home assessments for potential mold exposure are warranted. J Allergy Clin Immunol Pract 2016;4(3):417–22.

[389] ANSI/IICRC S520 mold remediation. Available from www.iicrc.org/standards/iicrc-s520.

3

Chelation

Joseph Pizzorno, John Nowicki

DESCRIPTION

Toxic metals are considered major environmental pollutants and are a common underlying factor in most cases of toxicant overload. Metals are used in a variety of industrial processes, and as a result, human exposure has dramatically increased during the past 50 years. The general population is exposed to metals at trace concentrations either voluntarily, through supplementation, or involuntarily, through intake of contaminated food and water or contact with contaminated soil, dust or air.

Normal healthy physiology requires biologically based metals and minerals for optimal health, but when in excess or deficient, serious adverse manifestations may result.[1] For example, manganese, iron and chromium are essential for good health, but may be toxic above certain levels.[2] The most prevalent toxic metals in humans are lead, mercury, cadmium and arsenic. These metals are non-essential xenobiotics, and exposure is harmful to human health, primarily damaging the renal, hepatobiliary, neurological, cardiovascular and immune systems. In some individuals, metals are the primary toxins present. Recently the safety of gadolinium has come into question as a result of gadolinium-containing contrast agents used in diagnostic imaging (MRI).[3] Breakdown of metal–ion homeostasis can result in the metal binding to protein sites different from those designed for that purpose or replacement of other metals from their natural binding sites. Toxic metals cause damage in a variety of ways including: increasing free radical production, enzyme poisoning, direct DNA damage, endocrine disruption and mitochondrial or cell wall damage.[4,5]

Chelation therapy involves pharmaceutically derived compounds that form bonds with charged metal ions through a chemical equilibrium reaction. Pharmaceutical chelators are small organic molecules that typically form coordination complexes involving sulfur (e.g. 2,3-dimercaptosuccinic acid [DMSA], 2,3-dimercapto-1-propanesulfonic acid [DMPS]), oxygen and/or nitrogen atoms (e.g. ethylenediaminetetraacetic acid [EDTA]). The intent is to counteract the detrimental effects of the toxic element or to sequester it in a less toxic form. The complexing agent is the chelator, and the involved metal is said to be chelated. Chelators are injected into the blood or muscle, or used orally to bind metals that are present in toxic concentrations so they can be excreted from the body, most frequently in urine.[6] Antidotal treatments range from highly specific (e.g. deferoxamine for iron) to significantly less specific (e.g. EDTA for most divalent cations).

HISTORY

The word chelation is derived from the Greek *chele*, which means pincher and refers to grabbing by the claws of a crab. In the late 19th and early 20th centuries, European and American chemical discoveries recognised that certain chemicals could grab and bind metals and minerals, which led to the development of the word chelation.[7] This understanding led to therapeutic applications as early as World War II when chelation was introduced as an antidote for arsenic-based poisonous gas exposure.[8,9] Chelation is the mainstay in conventional toxicology as a resource for documented acute toxic metal poisoning.[10,11]

CHELATING AGENTS

There are numerous chelating drugs used as antidotes to metal toxicity including: dimercaprol (i.e. British anti-Lewisite, abbreviated BAL), succimer (meso-DMSA), 2,3-dimercapto-1-propanesulfonic acid (i.e. unithiol and abbreviated DMPS), D-penicillamine, N-acetyl-D penicillamine (NAPA), calcium disodium ethylenediaminetetraacetate ($CaNa_2EDTA$), calcium trisodium or zinc trisodium diethylenetriaminepentaacetate ($CaNa_3DTPA$, $ZnNa_3DTPA$), deferoxamine (DFO), deferiprone (L1), triethylenetetramine (trientine), N-acetylcysteine (NAC), and Prussian blue (PB). In addition, several synthetic homologues of these agents have been designed and tested including polyaminopolycarboxylic acids (EDTA and DTPA), derivatives of BAL (DMPS, DMSA and mono- and dialkylesters of DMSA) and carbodithioates. The therapeutic selection of an effective chelating agent is based on the toxicokinetics and chemical considerations of the metal involved and the chelating agent. The most commonly used chelating agents in humans intoxicated with metals are summarised in Table 3.1 and further reviewed below.

TABLE 3.1 Overview of chelation drugs[12]			
Chemical name (common names, abbreviations)	**Activation metabolism**	**Coordination (binding) groups**	**Elements chelated**
2,3-bis(sulfanyl)butanedioic acid (dimercaptosuccinic acid; succimer; DMSA; chemet)	Excretion via urine >90% as DMSA-cysteine disulfide conjugates	Oxygen and sulfhydryl	Lead Arsenic Mercury Cadmium Silver Tin Copper
Sodium 2,3-bis(sulfanyl)propane-1-sulfonate (sodium dimercaptopropanesulfonate; DMPS; unithiol)	84% of IV dose excreted through urine	Oxygen and sulfhydryl	Mercury Arsenic Lead Cadmium Tin Silver Copper, selenium, zinc, magnesium
2-[2-[bis(carboxymethyl)amino]ethyl-(carboxymethyl)amino]acetic acid (ethylenediaminetetraacetic acid; edetic acid; EDTA; endrate; sequestrol; endathamil)	Not metabolised. Excreted unchanged, generally bound with a different cation	Oxygen	Lead Cadmium Zinc
(2S)-2-amino-3-methyl-3-sulfanylbutanoic acid (3-sulfanyl-D-valine; penicillamine; mercaptyl; D-penicillamine; cuprimine)	Rarely excreted unchanged; excreted mainly as disulfides	Oxygen, hydroxyl, sulfhydryl and amine	Copper Arsenic Zinc Mercury Lead
2,3-bis(sulfanyl)propan-1-ol (dimercaprol; British anti-Lewisite; BAL; 2,3-dimercaptopropanol; dicaptol)	Excreted unchanged in urine	Sulfhydryl and hydroxyl	Arsenic Gold Mercury Lead (BAL in combination with $CaNa_2EDTA$)

Desferrioxamine or deferoxamine (DFO)

DFO is a high molecular weight, highly hydrophilic chelator that was first introduced in the 1960s in short-term studies of iron-loaded patients.[13] It is a naturally occurring iron chelator produced by *Streptomyces pilosus*, and was the first iron chelator approved for human use.[14] Deferoxamine prevents iron-catalysed free radical reactions and is used in the treatment of acute iron poisoning and in iron storage disease such as beta-thalassaemia. DFO is poorly absorbed orally and rapidly metabolised in plasma,[15,16] and therefore requires prolonged parenteral infusions (12 hours) to reach plateau plasma concentrations.[17] The usual regimen is 25 to 50 mg/kg/day as a continuous subcutaneous infusion given over 8 to 12 hours. DFO is effective at lowering serum ferritin and hepatic iron levels[18,19] and preventing endocrine complications,[20] and is associated with a reduction in cardiac complications.[21]

DFO has also been used in aluminium toxicity because of its high affinity for aluminium and the high stability of the DFO-Al complex.[22] In animal studies, DFO reduced tissue aluminium concentrations,[23] reversed aluminium-induced LPO[24] and partially reversed aluminium-induced neurofibrillary degeneration.[25]

The burden of prolonged subcutaneous infusions, adverse reactions (primarily pain) and high cost are limiting factors, and as a result, poor compliance remains a significant problem with administration of DFO. Preventable, premature deaths related to iron overload continue to occur.[26]

Dimercaprol (BAL)

Dimercaprol or British anti-Lewisite (BAL) was originally developed to counteract arsenic-containing war gases,[27] but it is now used for the treatment of poisoning with toxic metals such as arsenic, gold, lead and mercury. Dimercaprol is not absorbed orally and must be administered by deep intramuscular injection. BAL is given in a dose of 2.5-5.0 mg/kg intramuscularly (IM) every 4 hours for 48 hours and then 2.5 mg/kg intramuscularly every 12 hours for 1–2 weeks, as necessary. Blood concentrations peak about 30 minutes after IM administration. Dimercaprol has two sulfhydryl groups and forms a stable dimercaptide ring with arsenic. It is metabolised predominantly by glucuronic conjugation, and the metabolites are then excreted in the urine.

BAL has several drawbacks including: its low therapeutic index, its tendency to redistribute metals (e.g. arsenic) to other organs, the need for intramuscular injection and its unpleasant odour.[28] Dimercaprol is contraindicated in patients with glucose-6-phosphate dehydrogenase deficiency because of the risk of haemolysis.[29] BAL is formulated with peanut oil, which increases the adverse effects and is absolutely contraindicated in individuals with peanut allergy.

2,3-dimercaptopropane-1-sulfonate (DMPS)

DMPS was developed in 1951 and patented under the name Dimaval by Heyl Chem-Fabrik GmbH (Berlin) for the treatment of mercury overload. DMPS is not currently approved by the US Food and Drug Administration for metal treatment, although it has been used to treat acute arsenic poisoning.[30] DMPS is a water-soluble dithiol, with an oral bioavailability of the parent drug of approximately 39%. After intravenous administration, DMPS is rapidly transformed to disulfide forms, and the metabolites (acyclical and cyclical disulfide chelates) are excreted in the urine. The elimination half-life of total DMPS is 20 hours.[31] DMPS increases urinary excretion of arsenic, cadmium, lead and mercury and has been shown to increase excretion of essential trace metals (copper, selenium, zinc, magnesium), necessitating supplementation before and after treatment.[32]

Standard oral dosing of DMPS is 10 mg/kg, 5 days on and 9 days off. IV DMPS (3 mg/kg) is dosed once or twice monthly. Transdermal application of DMPS has shown no evidence of absorption into the blood or enhanced mercury excretion.[33]

2,3-dimercaptosuccinic acid (DMSA)

DMSA is a sulfhydryl-containing, water soluble, chelating agent developed in the 1950s as an alternative to more toxic chelating agents. After oral administration, DMSA is absorbed quite rapidly. It has a half-life of 2–3 hours in the blood and is equally excreted through urine and bile.[34] DMSA accumulates in the kidney where it is extensively metabolised in humans to mixed disulfides of cysteine.[35] Approximately 10–25% of an orally administered dose of DMSA is excreted in urine, the majority (>90%) as DMSA-cysteine disulfide conjugates. Urinary excretion of the unaltered (not metabolised) drug peaks at about 2 hours and is essentially complete by 9 hours, whereas urinary excretion of altered DMSA peaks at about 4 hours and is not complete for 24–48 hours.[36] In up to 60% of patients treated at full dosages with DMSA, there is a transient modest rise (typically 14%) in transaminase activity during treatment. Skin reactions occur in approximately 6% of treated patients. It is worth noting that in patients with intestinal dysbiosis, DMSA may have decreased intestinal absorption.[37]

The sulfhydryl group binds tightly to metals located on kidney tissue surfaces and carries them out of the body. Hundreds of articles have been published showing the effectiveness of DMSA in the binding and excretion of toxic metals. DMSA increases urinary excretion of arsenic, cadmium, lead and mercury. DMSA is FDA approved for the treatment of lead, and although it has demonstrated the ability to reduce mercury levels, it is not FDA approved for mercury toxicity.[38]

The full body-weight dose for DMSA is 30 mg/kg/day given in three divided doses of 10 mg/kg each. Dividing the daily dose into three considers the DMSA peak in both the blood and urine that occurs 4 hours post consumption.[39] DMSA is typically given for 5 days, followed by a 9-day rest period, with follow-up metal mobilisation testing done every five cycles. When used with lead-burdened individuals, the blood lead level rebounds close to pre-DMSA levels within 2 weeks of DMSA cessation.[40] If one of the therapeutic goals is reduction of blood lead levels (BLLs), then a rest of less than 14 days between cycles is recommended. There is no single established protocol for DMSA in the treatment of lead that is universally accepted and followed. The dosing is based on either body weight or body surface area. The use of body-weight doses of DMSA has been shown to be safe in children as young as 12 months of age.[41] No harm was observed even after a DMSA overdose (185 mg/kg) in a 3-year-old child.[42] The following protocols have all been utilised:

- 10 mg/kg every 8 hours for a total of 30 mg/kg/day for 5 days, followed by 10 mg/kg twice daily for another 14 days.
- 1050 mg/M²(body size)/day for 7 days, then 700 mg/M²/day for 19 days.
- 10 mg/kg every second day for a month
- 30 mg/kg divided into three daily doses (during waking hours) for 5 days, wait 9 days and then repeat.
- 30 mg/kg divided into three daily doses (during waking hours) for 2 days, wait 5 days and then repeat. This protocol is used in people who begin to experience increased symptoms from mercury mobilisation on day three of DMSA.

Using one of the above protocols, a study of Chinese children with BLLs between 10 and 25 micrograms/dL examined the efficacy of DMSA at the 10 mg/kg level every second day for a month.[43] One of the treatment groups received concurrent daily doses of 1250 mg of calcium and 200 mg of ascorbic acid in addition to the DMSA. The combination of DMSA and nutrients proved to be more efficacious in reducing BLLs, rebalancing ALAD levels and reducing bone lead levels.

DMSA was shown to be safe and effective in removing toxic metals (especially lead) and dramatically effective at normalising red blood cell (RBC) glutathione (GSH) in children with autism.[44] A randomised, double-blind controlled trial of children with autism showed reductions in measures of the severity of autism associated with the difference in urinary excretion of toxic metals before and following treatment with DMSA.[45] Regression analysis found that the body burden of toxic metals was significantly related to the variations in the severity of autism. The metals of greatest influence were lead, antimony, mercury, tin and aluminium.

2-amino-3-mercapto-3 methylbutyric acid (D-penicillamine)

Penicillamine is a sulfur-containing amino acid and is a degradation product of penicillin. Because the levorotatory isomer is toxic, D-penicillamine is used for medicinal purposes. Acetylpenicillamine is a weaker chelating agent than penicillamine and has been used in the treatment of mercury poisoning.[46] Approximately 50–70% of D-penicillamine is absorbed after oral administration and reaches peak plasma concentrations 1.5–4 hours after ingestion.[47] Penicillamine has a half-life of less than 1 hour and is rapidly cleared in the urine, primarily as low-molecular weight disulfides.[48]

Penicillamine can form chelates with many metal ions. The stability of complexes of metals with penicillamine varies in ascending order (i.e. from highest to lowest): mercury, lead, nickel, copper, zinc, cadmium, cobalt, iron and manganese.[49] Penicillamine is used for the treatment of lead poisoning as a chelating agent and is used for the elimination of copper in Wilson's disease. In cases of human poisoning, D-penicillamine has been shown to increase the excretion of lead,[50] arsenic[51] and mercury.[52] However, chelating metals does not necessarily ameliorate toxicity, and, as observed in lead poisoning, relocation of metals may aggravate toxicity and may account for transient worsening upon commencement of penicillamine therapy.[53]

2-[2-[bis(carboxymethyl)amino]ethyl-(carboxymethyl)amino] acetic acid (EDTA)

EDTA is often used to chelate metals because it has high formation constants with several of them.[54] Table 3.2 provides a list of the logarithm values of formation constants of deprotonated EDTA with some metal ions. The formation constant for mercury (Hg^{2+}) is more than 10 orders of magnitude greater than that for calcium (Ca^{2+}), and the formation constant for lead (Pb^{2+}) is about 10 orders of magnitude greater than magnesium (Mg^{2+}). The fact that the formation constants are generally greater for toxic metals than for essential minerals lends a significant safety factor to long-term EDTA use. However, when used in humans and animals, EDTA does not appreciably mobilise mercury. Close monitoring for adverse effects and mineral imbalances is necessary, and oral supplementation with trace minerals (Cu, Zn, Ca, Mg) is appropriate to avoid deficiencies.

$CaNa_2EDTA$ is not metabolised, and EDTA chelates are excreted rapidly in the urine. EDTA binds lead and cadmium strongly and may bind to mercury if other minerals are depleted. The typical dose of intravenous CaEDTA is 50 mg/kg with saline to proper osmolarity delivered over 20 minutes. In animal studies, the lowest dose of EDTA reported to cause toxicity was 750 mg/kg/day, which is equivalent to 45 g/day for a 60-kg person.[55]

N-acetylcysteine (NAC)

NAC is a non-toxic N-acetyl derivative of cysteine containing a thiol group. NAC is widely available, relatively inexpensive, easily administered and well tolerated by patients. It is distributed mainly to extracellular water and is rapidly eliminated in urine, with approximately one-third excreted during the first 12 hours after administration.[56] In humans, the half-life of NAC in blood plasma is approximately 2 hours. In urine, NAC is excreted as the symmetrical disulfide, the mixed disulfide with cysteine and as the free thiol.[57]

NAC is a potent antioxidant/detoxicant that does not alter tissue distribution of essential trace metals (Ca, Mg, Fe, Zn and Cu).[58] NAC produces a transient, dose-dependent increase in urinary excretion of methylmercury (MeHg) that is proportional to the body burden and can decrease brain and fetal levels of methylmercury.[59] Typical oral dose of NAC is 30 mg/kg daily.

Other

Studies show that supplementation of antioxidants along with a chelating agent proves to be a better treatment regimen than monotherapy with chelating agents. Several nutrients including alpha-lipoic-acid,[60] probiotics, vitamin E, melatonin and fibre used concurrently with DMSA not only provide greater reversal of lead-induced biochemical and physiological damage, but significantly increase the excretion of lead itself.[61] Co-administration of NAC with DMSA provided greater lead excretion, likely because cysteine-conjugated DMSA carries the greatest amount of lead from the body.[62] Alpha-lipoic acid has also been shown to prevent neuronal damage from mercury, as well as increase its excretion. Unfortunately, most of the data are from animal studies where the antioxidant substances were injected into the animals, and therefore, little to no

Ion	Formation constant (log₁₀ Kf)
Fe³⁺	25.10
Hg²⁺	21.70
Cu²⁺	18.80
Pb²⁺	18.04
Zn²⁺	16.50
Cd²⁺	16.40
Al³⁺	16.30
Fe²⁺	14.32
Ca²⁺	10.69
Mg²⁺	8.79
Na⁺	1.66
K⁺	0.80

TABLE 3.2 Metal ion formation constants for EDTA[55] — 20°C, 0.1M ion

data exists on the most beneficial doses of these agents for humans.

Spirulina platensis has been found to protect against toxic metal-induced organ damage as well as to prevent anaemia, leukopenia and the deposition of metals in the brain. Forty-one patients with chronic arsenic poisoning were randomly treated orally by either placebo or spirulina extract (250 mg) plus zinc (2 mg) twice daily for 16 weeks.[63] There was a sharp increase in urinary excretion of arsenic (138 micrograms/L) at 4 weeks following spirulina plus zinc administration, and the effect was continued for another 2 weeks. Spirulina extract plus zinc removed 47.1% of arsenic from scalp hair.

Products containing modified citrus pectin plus alginate have been reported to reduce lead and mercury (74% average decrease) in case studies.[64] However, virtually all the data has been from one group of researchers and does not hold up under closer scrutiny.[65]

CHELATABLE TOXICANTS
Aluminium
PRINCIPLES OF TOXICITY

Aluminium is a toxic metal with no known physiological role. Acute toxicity is rare. Aluminium binds to phospholipids, stimulates iron-initiated LPO and it reacts with oxygen to form $Al\text{-}O_2^-$ that increases oxidation of amino acids, leading to generation of protein carbonyls.[66] These reactions reduce the activity of glutathione peroxidase, superoxide dismutase and catalase.[67] The facilitation of superoxide-driven biological oxidation by aluminium has been shown to result from an interaction between the metal and the superoxide radical anion.[68,69] Aluminium may cause impairments in mitochondrial bioenergetics, leading to the generation of oxidative stress and the gradual accumulation of oxidatively modified cellular proteins.[70]

SOURCES

Aluminium is the most widely distributed metal in the environment and exposure occurs through air, food and water. Aluminium sulfate is used as a flocculating agent in the treatment of drinking water and aluminium hydroxide is used therapeutically as a phosphate-binding agent and an antacid. Chronic aluminium toxicity may occur as a result of chronic exposure to extremely high levels of aluminium-containing compounds (e.g. antacids) or direct inoculation of aluminium via dialysates, parenteral nutrition or implanted foreign materials.[71,72]

Aluminium levels in water supplies can be a potential hazard to renal dialysis patients, entering the body across the dialysis membrane and bypassing intestinal absorption. However, acute aluminium toxicity is now quite rare because the water used in dialysis is treated to remove contaminated metals.

Occupational exposure to aluminium compounds primarily occurs through inhalation of airborne particles in dusts and fumes. The air inside aluminium smelters, foundries and remelting plants can contain significant concentrations of aluminium.[73]

BODY LOAD

In general, inhaled soluble particles (e.g. aluminium sulfate, hydrated aluminium chloride and aluminium nitrate) are rapidly absorbed from the lungs, while the less soluble particles (e.g. aluminium metal, aluminium oxide, aluminium hydroxide, aluminium phosphate and aluminium silicate) are retained in the lungs and then slowly released into the systemic circulation.[74] Aluminium is poorly absorbed from the gastrointestinal tract. The usual daily dietary intake of aluminium is 5 to 10 mg. However, most aluminium-containing compounds are relatively insoluble at physiological pH, limiting absorption of aluminium through ingestion.[75] The majority of aluminium is excreted in urine, accomplished by filtration from the blood by the glomerulus of the kidney.[76] If not filtered by the kidneys, aluminium binds to proteins such as transferrin and is distributed throughout the body. Most healthy adults tolerate comparatively large repeated daily oral aluminium exposures (up to 3500–7200 mg/day) without any adverse effect, but other individuals (e.g. pre-term infants, young children, those with reduced kidney function) can be at serious risk for systemic aluminium intoxication even at lower doses.[77] Aluminium has been shown to accumulate in several mammalian tissues including the brain, bones, liver and kidneys.[78,79]

CLINICAL MANIFESTATIONS

The brain appears to be the most vulnerable to the toxic effects of aluminium, and a potential link has been observed between aluminium and Alzheimer's disease, amyotrophic lateral sclerosis (ALS; motor neurone disease [MND]) and autism spectrum disorders.[80] Additional neurological consequences of toxic aluminium exposure include encephalopathy, seizures, parkinsonism and death.[81,82] Aluminium is certainly a potential contributor to the onset, progression and aggressiveness of neurological disease.[83] In workers exposed to aluminium for several years, concerns exist surrounding reduced attention span, impaired cognition and deficits in fine motor skills.[84] Although a causal link has not been proven, several studies have positive outcomes using chelation in the treatment of conditions associated with aluminium overload.

Aluminium toxicity in patients with renal dysfunction causes osteodystrophy and gradual dementia.[85] Pulmonary fibrosis has been reported in relation to aluminium exposure.[86] Higher concentrations of aluminium have been found in tissue bioptates along with elevated serum aluminium levels in patients with laryngeal papilloma and laryngeal cancer.[87]

DIAGNOSTIC TESTING

Acute aluminium toxicity is diagnosed using plasma concentration levels. When performing biological monitoring of aluminium, measurement of urinary levels is recommended due to the higher sensitivity compared to the measurement of aluminium in plasma.[88,89] Preclinical neurotoxic effects have been observed when serum aluminium levels exceed 10 micrograms/L[90] and serum aluminium levels of 6.8–9.5 micrograms/L, and urinary aluminium levels of 4–6 micromols/L appear to represent a threshold for observed neurological effects.[91]

MANAGEMENT/THERAPY

DFO is a trivalent ion chelator that can remove excess aluminium from the body. A small cohort, 2-year, single-blind study of patients with Alzheimer's disease treated with DFO (125 mg intramuscularly twice daily, 5 days per week, for 24 months) demonstrated a significant reduction in the rate of decline of daily living skills in the DFO-treated group compared to the placebo or no-treatment groups.[92] Among haemodialysis patients with aluminium overload, treatment with DFO at both the standard dose (5 mg/kg/week) and the low dose (2.5 mg/kg/week) offered similar therapeutic effects and successful treatment response rates.[93]

Arsenic
PRINCIPLES OF TOXICITY

After exposure to arsine gas, absorbed arsine enters RBCs and is oxidised to arsenic dihydride and elemental arsenic. These derivatives combine with red cell sulfhydryl groups, which results in cell membrane instability and haemolysis. The main mechanism by which monomethylarsonous acid (MMA) and inorganic arsenicals cause cellular and tissue damage is through oxidative stress.[94] Oxidative damage to the DNA results in increased urinary excretion of 8-hydroxy-2′-deoxyguanosine (8-OHdG), which is a valuable marker for both oxidative stress and chronic disease risk.[95] Increases in urinary 8-OHdG levels have been found in those drinking groundwater high in arsenic as well as those occupationally exposed to arsenic.[96] Under physiological conditions, arsenic may also induce toxic effects through the formation of hydrogen peroxide.[97] Higher levels of MMA have also been linked to the presence of elevated homocysteine levels, possibly due to overall methylation defects.[98] Mechanisms of arsenic carcinogenesis include oxidative damage,[99] epigenetic effects[100] and interference with DNA repair.[101]

SOURCES

Arsenic is a ubiquitous metalloid in our food, air and water and is found in both inorganic forms (as trivalent or pentavalent states) and organic forms. Water and dietary sources of arsenic remain the bulk of exposure sources.[102] Groundwater provides a continuous source of inorganic arsenic and its metabolites, while foods provide more of the organic arsenicals (e.g. arsenobetaine, arsenocholine, arsenosugars and arsenolipids), which have very short half-lives and are considered virtually non-toxic. Seafood, rice, mushrooms and poultry are the main food sources of arsenic.[103] Arsenobetaine is primarily found in seafood. Organically grown rice has also been found to have elevated levels of arsenic.[104]

Groundwater is the most common source of arsenic exposure. Arsenic levels up to 3100 micrograms/L have been found in well water samples in regions of the United States.[105] Bangladesh, Taiwan Province of China, Chile, Argentina, China and India have groundwater arsenic levels that are typically >300 micrograms/L (ranging up to 7550 micrograms/L in Argentina). Chronic arsenic poisoning is found in these areas in people drinking an average of 3.3 L of water daily, while those consuming ≤1.9 L have not exhibited poisoning.[106] Arsenic is present in cigarette smoke, and is found in higher levels in smokers.[107,108] Arsenic is a component of certain pigments used in glass making, thereby increasing exposure in individuals working with those colours in glass blowing.[109,110]

BODY LOAD

Elemental arsenic is insoluble in water and bodily fluids, is insignificantly absorbed and is non-toxic. Arsine gas is the most toxic form of arsenic. Both the gastrointestinal and the respiratory tracts absorb arsenic and then widely distribute it through the body, where it is reduced to arsenite (III) and then methylated.[111] A single pass through this methylation pathway produces monomethylarsonous acid (+3) (MMA). MMA can then be passed through the pathway a second time to produce dimethylarsonous acid (+3) (DMA). Methylation primarily occurs enzymatically through the action of arsenic (+3 oxidation) methyltransferases (AS3MT), but can also occur non-enzymatically in the presence of either methylcobalamin or GSH.[112] Ninety-five per cent of methylated inorganic arsenic is excreted in the urine, and 5% is excreted in the bile. Most of the arsenic is eliminated in the first few days, but over time, arsenic can accumulate in hair, nails and skin.

CLINICAL MANIFESTATIONS

Acute and chronic arsenic exposure causes a variety of health effects including dermal changes (e.g. pigmentation, hyperkeratosis and ulceration), respiratory, pulmonary, cardiovascular, gastrointestinal, haematological, hepatic, renal, neurological, developmental, reproductive, immunological, genotoxic, mutagenic and carcinogenic effects.[113] Arsenic ingestion produces violent gastrointestinal pain, haemorrhagic gastroenteritis and vomiting with shock developing. After a latent period of 2–24 hours, exposed individuals experience massive haemolysis, malaise, headache, weakness, dyspnoea, hepatomegaly, jaundice, haemoglobinuria and renal failure. Persistent diarrhoea, dermatitis, haematuria, proteinuria, acute tubular necrosis and polyneuropathy are evidence of chronic ingestion.[114] Lethal doses of arsenates are 5–50 mg/kg, and lethal doses of arsenites are <5 mg/kg.

Inorganic arsenic in drinking water is classified as a Group 1 carcinogen, and observations in highly exposed populations (≥ 100 micrograms/L) reveal that arsenic is an established cause of bladder cancer.[115] A Chilean population of adults (aged 30–49 years) who were in utero or ≤18 years of age when exposed to high concentrations of arsenic had an increased mortality rate (SMR = 8.1; 95% CI: 3.5–16.0) from laryngeal cancer.[116] After adjusting for all appropriate confounders, people consuming groundwater arsenic at levels above 20 micrograms/L (PPM) had an 83% increased risk of lung cancer, while those consuming water with arsenic levels just above 10 micrograms/L had a 47% increased risk.[117] A 2008 study using estimated arsenic levels of participants of the Strong Heart Study from 1989 to 1991 found a corresponding hazard ratio of 2.46 (95% CI: 1.09–5.58) for pancreatic cancer after multivariate adjustment (region, age, sex, education, smoking status, alcohol and BMI).[118] The association of arsenic with pancreatic cancer might be biologically meaningful considering arsenic is reported to induce type 2 diabetes mellitus,[119] and diabetes is thought to be a risk factor for pancreatic cancer.[120] A dose–response relation was observed between arsenic levels in well water and prostate cancer.[121] A study in New Hampshire (US) reported an increased risk for squamous cell carcinoma (SCC) with exposure to arsenic levels common in US groundwater.[122]

Chronic upper and respiratory problems, including dyspnoea, asthma and cough, were noted in a study from India with people consuming groundwater with arsenic levels between 11 and 50 ppm.[123]

Low-level arsenic exposure has been clearly linked in other studies to increasing risks for cardiovascular disease, including hypertension.[124]

Both current and long-term exposure to groundwater arsenic have been significantly related to poorer scores in language, visuospatial skills and executive functioning. Long-term exposure (but not current exposure) to low-level groundwater arsenic is also associated with poorer scores in global cognition, processing speeds and immediate memory.[125]

Low-level arsenic exposure may be associated with hyperuricaemia and gout. In men, the adjusted odds ratio (OR) for hyperuricaemia comparing highest to lowest quartiles of total arsenic was 1.84 (95% CI: 1.26–2.68), and in women, the OR was 1.26 (95% CI: 0.77–2.07).[126]

Arsenic has been shown to increase diabetes risk in a dose-dependent fashion.[127] Comparing participants at the 80th and 20th percentiles, the ORs for type II diabetes were 3.58 for the total level of arsenic, 1.57 for dimethylarsenate and 0.69 for arsenobetaine.[128] Fig. 3.1 demonstrates that there is a direct correlation between the amount of arsenic in a person's body (toenail arsenic is the best measure of body load) and risk of diabetes. In this case, the primary mechanism appears to be the result of damaging pancreatic beta cells with resultant decreased production of insulin.[129]

DIAGNOSTIC TESTING

Random or first-morning urine arsenic levels can be submitted to various laboratories for measurement. To get an accurate reading free of arsenobetaine, it is recommended that seafood be avoided for 48 hours prior to sample collection. Levels <7 micrograms As/g creatinine would be considered optimal. Levels >12 micrograms As/g creatinine would be considered higher risk for cardiovascular disease, diabetes, respiratory problems, cancers and neurological dysfunction. Total arsenic levels >30 micrograms/g creatinine indicate the likelihood that MMA is present in levels high enough to cause genotoxicity.

MANAGEMENT/THERAPY

Chelation for acute arsenic poisoning is most effective when administered as soon as possible after the exposure. For arsenic chelation, DMSA is quite useful for acute exposure, but it is unlikely to remove intracellular levels. In animal studies, the DMSA derivative monoisoamyl dimercaptosuccinic acid (MiADMSA) has been shown to remove arsenic from blood and soft tissue when given with DMSA.[131] Chelation should be continued until 24-hour urinary arsenic levels return to normal (<50 micrograms/L), the patient is symptom free or the remaining toxic effects are believed to be irreversible. Since arsenic does not bioaccumulate, the need for long-term chelation is small.

In rare cases of severe gastrointestinal toxicity secondary to acute arsenic poisoning, BAL is the chelator of choice until the patient can tolerate oral DMSA. The recommended regimen is 2.5 mg/kg IM every 6 hours for the first 2 days, 2.5 mg/kg IM every 12 hours on the third day and then 2.5 mg/kg/day IM for 10 days. The BAL-metal complex is then excreted in urine and bile.

Resveratrol has been shown in cell cultures to protect against arsenic-induced oxidative damage.[132] B vitamins have been shown to increase urinary excretion of arsenic in humans.[133] Curcumin has multiple beneficial effects including enhancing both the methylation and the excretion of inorganic arsenic and reversing arsenic-induced cellular damage.[134,135]

Cadmium

PRINCIPLES OF TOXICITY

Cadmium causes increased oxidative damage to any cell or tissue it encounters. Enhanced oxidative stress and mitochondrial dysfunction from cadmium exposure has been documented along with an increased level of urinary 8-hydroxy-2′-deoxyguanosine. Cadmium also alters DNA methylation[136] and has demonstrated oestrogenic activity.[137] Cadmium is classified as a category 1 human carcinogen by the International Agency for Research on Cancer.[138] The toxic mechanisms of cadmium are not

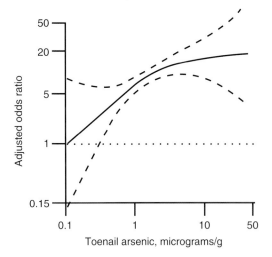

FIGURE 3.1 Arsenic levels correlate with diabetes[130]

completely understood, but it is known to act intracellularly, mainly via free-radical-induced damage, particularly to the lungs, kidneys, bones, central nervous system, reproductive organs and heart.[139]

SOURCES

Cadmium is a toxic heavy metal that is widely distributed throughout the world. Environmental and human contamination by industry has occurred primarily through metal smelting, and more recently in battery manufacturing. It is also used industrially in the manufacturing of pigments, coating, plastic manufacturing and metal plating processes. The main sources of cadmium are tobacco smoking and conventionally grown soybeans. These crops are grown with high phosphate fertilisers that are contaminated with cadmium. Fertilisers produced from industrial waste are then applied to agricultural land where the cadmium content increases in both soil and crops.[140,141] People living in reclaimed industrial areas proximal to former smelting facilities or close to municipal waste incinerators, as well as those downwind of coal-burning facilities, are also exposed. Non-occupational exposure occurs mainly through exposure to tobacco smoke.

BODY LOAD

Cadmium is found ubiquitously in all human studies in all parts of the world. It is readily absorbed through the respiratory tract and, to a far lower extent, in the gastrointestinal tract. Cadmium is absorbed in the intestines via divalent metal transporter 1 (DMT-1) that transports Fe, Cd, Ni, Pb, Co, Mn, Zn and Cu into the bloodstream.[142] This accounts for its increased absorption in those who are iron deficient.[143] Moderate dietary deficiencies of iron, zinc and calcium also enhance the absorption of cadmium, while abundance of these minerals in the body reduces absorption.[144] Men absorb about 5% of dietary cadmium, whereas women absorb twice that amount. Cadmium binds to serum albumin and accumulates in the liver, where it is complexed with metallothionein-1.[145] These compounds are cleared through the glomeruli but are then reabsorbed by the tubules, where they then are trapped. Once cadmium enters the body, much of it binds to metallothioneins. The blood then carries the Cd-metallothionein complex to the kidneys, where it is absorbed in the proximal tubules and then stored in the renal cortex.[146] As the metallothioneins slowly degrade, highly toxic free cadmium is constantly released. While it passively migrates into the urine, it also causes oxidative stress to the tubules.

The blood half-life of cadmium is 3–4 months and represents a combination of body burden and current exposure. Close to 50% of the total body cadmium burden resides in the kidney, where it has a much longer half-life of 10–40 years.

CLINICAL MANIFESTATIONS

Diseases associated with non-occupational, low-level cadmium exposure include osteoporosis, kidney damage, hypertension, insulin resistance, diabetes and cancers. Increased rates of miscarriage are also seen.

Cadmium is a significant kidney toxicant. The concentration of cadmium in the renal tissue of smokers is twice that of non-smokers (40 micrograms/g vs 20 micrograms/g).[147] Cadmium damages the renal cortex and proximal tubules, resulting in increased urinary excretion of proteins and tubular enzymes. Swedish women with a mean urinary cadmium of 0.80 micrograms/g creatinine showed significant elevation of markers for renal damage.[148] Renal damage at urinary cadmium levels as low as 0.6 micrograms/g was found in Japanese men.[149]

The combination of osteoporosis, osteomalacia and kidney damage was first noted in Japan in areas of high cadmium contamination from mining waste leading to cross-contamination of rice fields.[150,151] In a non-exposed population with relatively low kidney levels of cadmium, simply having cadmium tissue levels above the mean significantly increased urinary calcium excretion.[152] An increase in urinary calcium is positively associated with cadmium burden, and hypercalciuria occurs even at relatively subtle levels of cadmium-induced tubular dysfunction.[153] This may be related to a reduced activation of $1,25 (OH)_2$-vitamin D_3 by kidneys damaged by cadmium and increases in parathyroid hormone, leading to decreased calcium absorption and impaired bone mineralisation.[154] A doubling of urinary cadmium increases the risk of bone fractures in women by 73% and loss of height in men by 60%, even at a low degree of environmental exposure.[155] In children, a doubling of urinary cadmium increases risk of bone resorption by 1.72 times.[156]

When people with urinary cadmium levels >0.57 micrograms/g (the 80th percentile for this group) were compared with those with levels <0.14 micrograms/g, the hazard ratio (HR) for all-cause mortality was 1.54, cardiovascular disease mortality was 1.74 and coronary heart disease mortality ratio was 2.09.[157] Other studies have reported both increasing blood pressure[158] and increasing stroke risk linked to elevations in cadmium measurements.[159] Cadmium exposure, especially in adults with hypertension or diabetes, is a significant risk factor in the development of chronic kidney disease.[160]

An experimental study demonstrated that cadmium can malignantly transform human urothelial cells,[161] and these epithelial transformations are consistent with those of a classic transitional-cell carcinoma of the bladder.[162] A case-control study of 172 patients with bladder cancer and 359 population controls found an OR of 8.3 (95% CI 5.0–13.8) for cadmium, comparing the highest to the lowest tertile.[163] A study of people living in Louisiana (US) specifically focused on pancreatic cancer risk in relation to cadmium burden.[164] In this study, urinary cadmium levels were presented in four different quartiles with the following ranges: <0.5 micrograms/g, 0.5 to <1 microgram/g, 1 to <1.5 micrograms/g, and 1.5+ micrograms/g creatinine. People with urinary cadmium levels in the second quartile (0.5 to <1.0 micrograms/g) had a 3.34 increased risk for pancreatic cancer, while those in the third quartile had an OR of 5.58, and those in the fourth quartile had a 7.70 increase in risk.

Women with a history of miscarriage, uterine fibroids and hirsutism have demonstrated evidence of higher kidney cadmium burden.[165] Higher cadmium levels in girls have been associated with delayed puberty,[166] and in pregnant women with the delivery of lower-birth-weight infants.[167] Higher cadmium levels have also been associated with high follicle-stimulating hormone levels and infertility in men.[168]

Low-level cadmium is associated with non-alcoholic fatty liver disease (OR 2.21) and non-alcoholic steatohepatitis (OR 1.30), with urinary cadmium levels of 0.65–0.83,[169] hypomethylation of DNA in Argentinian women (whose urinary cadmium averaged only 0.230)[170] and a reduction in pulmonary function (FEV_1 and FVC).[171]

DIAGNOSTIC TESTING

First morning non-challenged urine cadmium has been shown to be directly related to the kidney burden and is considered to be the best measurement of total body cadmium burden.[172] Approximately 0.007% of the total body burden of cadmium is excreted daily in the urine, with an additional 0.009% excreted faecally.

MANAGEMENT/THERAPY

The most effective agent for the removal of cadmium from the tissues is the polyamino-polycarboxylate compound agent DPTA,[173] which is currently unavailable for use. Intravenous ethylenediaminetetraacetic acid (EDTA), which is readily available, has also demonstrated effectiveness at reducing the kidney burden of cadmium.[174] Similarly, the DMSA derivatives monomethyl DMSA (MmDMSA) and monocyclohexyl DMSA (MchDMSA) have been shown to reduce total body cadmium with no redistribution of brain cadmium.[175] The use of 50 mg/kg of reduced GSH in conjunction with the intravenous CaEDTA increased the post-chelation urinary release of cadmium almost four-fold.[176]

Meso-2,3-dimercaptosuccinic acid (DMSA) has also shown the ability to increase urinary excretion of cadmium, but not to the extent of EDTA.[177] While DMSA has a higher affinity for cadmium compared to other metals, the pH of the urine impacts the strength of the bond. At a pH of 5.5, which is commonly found in the proximal tubules, much of the cadmium is released from its DMSA binding, whereas at a urinary pH of 7.4, the cadmium is completely DMSA-bound and carried out of the body.[178] This may account for the relatively small increases in urinary cadmium noted on post-DMSA urine catches, and may further explain its failure to alleviate cadmium burden in children treated with DMSA.[179]

2,3-dimercaptopropane-1-sulfonate (DMPS) also has an affinity to bind cadmium, but DMPS does not move a significant amount of cadmium.[180] The addition of L-methionine to DMPS significantly enhances both the renal and the faecal clearance of cadmium and reverses cadmium-induced oxidative stress.[181]

Interestingly, the iron-chelating agents deferasirox and deferiprone have both been shown to enhance cadmium clearance from rat tissues,[182] but no human studies have been published. In mice, the use of magnesium at 20 mg/kg prior to cadmium exposure resulted in a significant reduction in renal cadmium burden.[183] In a small human study of cadmium-burdened individuals in China, the daily use of 150 micrograms of selenium resulted in a significant reduction in red blood cell cadmium levels by enhancing faecal cadmium excretion.[184]

NAC plays a dual role of protecting tissues from cadmium-induced oxidative damage and reducing hepatic and renal levels of cadmium.[185,186] The use of NAC was shown to reverse the cadmium-induced reduction of GSH, blood catalase and superoxide dismutase (SOD), and its combination with MiADMS successfully reduced blood and tissue cadmium levels.[187]

Iron
PRINCIPLES OF TOXICITY

Acute iron toxicity most often occurs in small children who have inadvertently swallowed iron tablets. It used to be the leading cause of poisoning death in children. Absorbed iron is initially bound to transferrin, but in large overdoses the iron binding capacity of transferrin can be exceeded, leading to an increase of free iron circulating in the plasma. Unbound iron is directly toxic to target organs. Iron can permeate the gastrointestinal mucosa, initially causing vomiting, diarrhoea and abdominal pain, and later can progress to ulceration and haemorrhage. Free iron is also taken up by the reticuloendothelial system, impairing cellular metabolism and causing cell death, primarily in the heart, liver and central nervous system.[188] Cell membranes are damaged by free-radical-mediated lipid peroxidation. Circulating unbound iron is a potent vasodilator, resulting in hypotension, and in severe cases can cause shock.

Chronic iron overload is associated with several red cell disorders such as sickle cell anaemia, thalassaemia and myelodysplastic syndromes, as well as conditions such as hereditary haemochromatosis. In patients requiring multiple transfusions, iron accumulates and is deposited into multiple organ systems including the heart and liver. Iron chelation may be necessary in these cases to prevent organ failure and decrease mortality.

SOURCES

Iron is commonly found in aqueous oxidation states as ferrous iron (Fe^{2+}) and ferric iron (Fe^{3+}) and is essential to the function of haemoglobin, myoglobin, cytochromes involved in oxygen transport or mitochondrial electron transfer, and several enzyme processes. Iron is found in a variety of foods including eggs, fish, liver, meat and blackstrap molasses. However, dietary sources are not the primary cause of iron toxicity. Numerous iron preparations are available as prescription and over-the-counter supplements, and acute toxicity most commonly results from over-ingestion of these products. The wide availability of iron supplements and iron-containing multivitamins provide easy accessibility for both adults and children. In an iron overdose, it is important to distinguish the amount of elemental iron ingested rather than the amount of iron salt as the cellular toxicity is based on the effects of elemental iron. Toxicity is unlikely to occur unless >60 mg/kg of elemental iron is ingested. Although the LD_{50} of elemental iron is 200 to 250 mg/kg, doses as small as 130 mg have been fatal in children.[189,190]

BODY LOAD

The absorption of iron occurs primarily in the duodenum and is dependent on the form of the mineral as well as total body stores. As little as 10% or as much as 95% of ingested iron is taken into the cell, where it is bound to ferritin, transferred to the serum where it is bound to transferrin or excreted from exfoliated mucosal cells, exuded red blood cells, bile and/or urine and faeces.[191] Iron is tightly regulated physiologically, although the body has no mechanism to excrete excess iron. Approximately two-thirds of the body's iron is concentrated in haemoglobin, with the remaining one-third stored in the liver, bone marrow and spleen.

CLINICAL MANIFESTATIONS

The course of acute iron poisoning is often divided into phases, but not every patient experiences each stage in the same time frame or with the same severity. Table 3.3 describes the time course and the clinical manifestations of acute iron intoxication.

DIAGNOSTIC TESTING

Serum iron concentration is the most useful laboratory test to evaluate the severity of an iron overdose. However,

interpretation can be difficult as haemolysis may interfere with the assay and sustained-release or enteric-coated preparations may have erratic absorption, leading to variable results. In addition, iron is rapidly cleared from the serum and stored in the liver. It is therefore necessary to not only measure serum iron within the first few hours of ingestion, but also to repeat serum concentration levels at 6 to 8 hours after ingestion. It has been recommended that if a patient has clinical features suggesting significant iron toxicity and an initial serum iron concentration of ≥5000 micrograms/L then treatment with deferoxamine is indicated.[192]

Ferritin is an iron storage protein accounting for 20% of the total body iron in normal adults. Serum ferritin levels are the laboratory parameter most often used to assess body iron burden and response to therapy. Most chelation regimens attempt to achieve the goal of lowering serum ferritin below 2500 micrograms/L. Serum ferritin levels are, however, not completely reliable as they may be inappropriately elevated in several medical conditions including cancer, infections, inflammation and acute and chronic liver disease.

MANAGEMENT/THERAPY

The specific antidote for acute iron toxicity is deferoxamine (desferrioxamine). Patients with an iron level above 500 micrograms/dL and those who have signs/symptoms of severe iron poisoning (e.g. shock, acidosis, hypotension, lethargy) require chelation therapy. Continuous subcutaneous infusion of deferoxamine should be administered at a rate of 15 mg/kg/hour and can be stopped when clinical improvement occurs. An intermittent subcutaneous injection schedule has been shown to be as effective in promoting iron excretion as a continuous 12-hour subcutaneous injection.[193] Iron bound to deferoxamine (DFO) is excreted in urine and faeces. When administering chelation to children younger than 5 years old, lower doses of chelation are usually used to avoid toxicity.[194]

Following the introduction of DFO, survival rates for thalassaemia patients increase substantially within a decade.[195] Thalassaemia patients treated with 12-hour subcutaneous DFO infusions have estimated 10-year survival of 100% without cardiac disease.[196] Trials in children with thalassaemia demonstrated intermittent DFO infusions were effective in decreasing liver iron stores and preventing progression of hepatic fibrosis,[197] and intensive chelation significantly reduced liver iron stores in children within 52–83 months of DFO initiation.[198] DFO has also shown significant reductions in mortality and incidence of heart failure in thalassaemia patients.[199]

Two oral agents, deferiprone and deferasirox, have shown some effectiveness in reducing iron levels and complications associated with iron overload, and may contribute to improved compliance, especially among paediatric patients. Newer oral agents are currently under development. However, these agents are typically used in chronic iron overload, and the research available regarding the use of these agents in acute iron poisoning has shown limited to no benefit.

TABLE 3.3 Phases of iron toxicity following an acute overdose		
Phase	Time after ingestion	Clinical features
1 (Gastrointestinal)	<6 hours	• Abdominal pain • Vomiting • Diarrhoea • Haematemesis • Haematochezia
2 (Latent)	6 to 12 hours	• Resolution of gastrointestinal symptoms • Tachycardia • Acidosis • Depressed mental status
3 (Systemic/Hepatic)	12 hours to 5 days	• Return of gastrointestinal symptoms • Shock • Acidosis • Leukocytosis • Coagulopathy • Renal failure • Liver failure with haemorrhage • Lethargy or coma • Cardiovascular collapse
4 (Obstructive)	2 to 6 weeks	• Gastric stricture • Pyloric stenosis • Obstruction

Lead

PRINCIPLES OF TOXICITY

Lead is a powerful pro-oxidant compound causing a tremendous amount of damage to cells and tissues.[200,201,202] Lead not only generates reactive oxygen species (ROS), but also causes a reduction in the activity of ROS-quenching enzymes such as superoxide dismutase, catalase and glutathione peroxidase, resulting in diminished antioxidant defence. Cellular levels of reduced GSH are also seen to drop secondary to lead exposure. In adults, lead-associated oxidative stress is associated with an increase in urinary 8-OHdG levels,[203] but such an increase has not been seen in children with similar blood lead levels (BLLs).[204] Lead also appears to inactivate paraoxonase-1, a potent antioxidant enzyme that protects against organophosphate-pesticide-induced neurotoxicity as well as against cardiovascular disorders.[205]

SOURCES

Once in the indoor air, lead becomes bound to house dust and to fabrics in the home.[206] Household dust lead levels are positively correlated with BLLs in children.[207] Lead is also present in cigarette smoke and is found in higher levels in smokers and those exposed to second-hand smoke. Children who are raised in a smoking household are found to have higher blood lead levels.[208]

The two greatest sources of non-occupational environmental lead contamination came from the addition of tetraethyl lead to commercial petrol (from 1920 until the mid 1980s) and its use as a colour-enhancing additive to paint (until the 1970s). Bone broth made from chicken bones has been found to contain up to 9.5 micrograms/L of lead, equivalent to groundwater lead levels associated with adverse health problems.[209] Dinnerware has been repeatedly found to be contaminated with lead, which is readily leached into acidic foods.[210,211] The migration of lead into such acidic foods can be greatly increased when the food is then microwaved on the contaminated dishware.[212] Ayurvedic and patented Chinese medicines can be sources of lead exposure.[213,214] Lead is used in the manufacturing of polyvinyl chloride (PVC) and has been found in a number of PVC-containing consumer products in the home, including vinyl miniblinds, electrical power cords, artificial Christmas trees, lunchboxes and toys.[215,216,217] Individuals who melt lead to make bullets, fishing weights or toy soldiers, as well as those firing lead bullets in an indoor shooting range, also have greater lead exposure.[218] In addition, people using lead to glaze pottery and utilise lead-glazed pottery for culinary purposes are at risk.[219]

BODY LOAD

Lead is found ubiquitously in populations throughout the world. It is readily absorbed through both the respiratory and the gastrointestinal tracts. Gastrointestinal absorption of lead in children can be up to five times greater than in adults who are exposed to the same sources.[220] Once absorbed, lead is bound to the red blood cells and moved into soft tissue and bones with some excretion via the urine. Up to 70% of lead in the blood comes from the trabecular bone, with the rest coming from current external exposures. Over 90% of the adult total body lead burden is stored in bones, where it is held for decades. Lead crosses both the blood–brain and the placenta barriers in adults, and once in the placenta can easily enter the fetal brain. In children, over 80% of total body lead is found in the bones. The half-life of blood and soft tissue lead averages 35 days. In trabecular bone with greater bone turnover, the lead half-life averages 8 years, while the half-life in cortical bone is up to 40 years.[221]

BLLs in adults >30 micrograms/dL or two readings of >20 micrograms/dL over a period of 4 weeks are the current maximum allowable levels for industrial settings. Pregnant women are advised to have BLLs <5 micrograms/dL, and all adults are advised to have BLLs <10 micrograms/dL in order to prevent long-term health problems.[222]

CLINICAL MANIFESTATIONS

Chronic low-level lead exposure is associated with several adverse health conditions. No threshold for safety exists. Cumulative lead burden in adults, via bone lead assessment, has been associated with the risk of developing parkinsonism,[223,224] Alzheimer's disease[225] and decreased cognition.[226] Several studies have found that EDTA-chelatable lead correlated with renal dysfunction,[227,228] neurobehavioural dysfunction[229] or declines in function of the peripheral nervous system.[230]

Several studies link childhood learning disorders and neurodevelopmental damage to low-level lead exposure, with some evidence showing decreased IQ in children with supposedly safe (<5 micrograms/dL) blood concentrations of lead.[231,232,233]

In vivo animal studies have demonstrated significant alterations in bone mineralisation, resulting in decreased bone density and increased bone turnover associated with lead exposure.[234,235] Lead has complex effects on bone cell function including altering the plasma levels of calcitropic hormones, perturbing calcium-mediated and other sensitive signal transduction pathways, uncoupling osteoblasts and osteoclasts from normal paracrine control by interfering with hormone processes and biochemically inhibiting enzymes resulting in altered cellular energetics.[236] In lead-intoxicated children, blood levels of 1,25-dihydroxyvitamin D_3 are reduced to levels comparable to those of patients with metabolic bone disease.[237]

Positive associations have been demonstrated between lead exposure and risk of meningioma. A Finnish study found an increased risk of brain and nervous system cancer (standardised incidence ratio [SIR] 1.27; 95% CI: 0.81–2.01) in women with occupational exposure to lead.[238]

A significant increase in blood lead level has been detected after menopause secondary to increased bone resorption from decreasing oestrogen levels.[239] The increase was higher in white women compared to Black women, which is consistent with prevalence rates and supports the possibility of lead playing a significant role in postmenopausal osteoporosis.

Among patients in the highest BLL quartile (mean 3.95 micrograms/dL), the prevalence of gout was 6.05% (95% CI: 4.49–7.62%) compared with 1.76% (CI: 1.10–2.42%) among those in the lowest quartile (mean 0.89 micrograms/dL).[240] Each doubling of BLL was associated with an unadjusted OR of 1.74 (CI: 1.47–2.05) for gout and 1.25 (CI: 1.12–1.40) for hyperuricaemia.

Low-level environmental lead exposure has been associated with decreased IQ in children. Around the globe, children with BLLs <10 micrograms/dL have demonstrated significant IQ loss,[241,242,243] and studies have shown that for each 0.19 micrograms/dL increase in BLL, one IQ point was lost.[244] Lead-associated decline of cognitive function in children has been shown to persist into adulthood.[245] BLLs above 1.6 micrograms/dL in children have also been strongly linked to increase risk in attention deficit hyperactivity disorder (ADHD), oppositional defiant disorder (ODD) and conduct disorder (CD).[246]

Studies utilising both bone and blood lead levels have shown correlation with cardiovascular disease. Lead is a potent inactivator of nitric oxide and is therefore associated with increased blood pressure.[247] Increased levels of tibial bone lead also correlate with increased risk for hypertension.[248,249] Higher bone lead levels have also been positively correlated with greater ECG abnormalities and other markers consistent with cardiac disease.[250,251] Lead levels have also been positively correlated with serum levels of homocysteine.[252]

DIAGNOSTIC TESTING

The only method available to clinicians to assess the cumulative lead burden in patients is the lead mobilisation test.[253,254,255] The CaEDTA mobilisation test typically uses a 1 g dose of intravenous sodium CaEDTA (35 mg/kg with saline for proper osmolarity) followed by either an 8- or a 24-hour urine collection. Since 75% of the intravenous dose of CaEDTA is known to be excreted into the urine within 2.5 hours, a 4-hour collection may be sufficient. Children with a pre-challenge lead spill ≥1 microgram/mL are considered to be predictive of a high lead burden.[256] In ongoing trials with adult non-diabetic renal patients, a post-CaEDTA lead spill totalling >80 micrograms/mL was used as the cut-off value for initiation of CaEDTA chelation.[257]

The use of DMSA for the lead mobilisation test only requires a 4-hour urinary collection.[258] The bladder is emptied to provide the pre-provoked sample, then a 1-gram challenge dose of DMSA (approximately half the standard body-weight dose for a 70-kg adult) is used to mobilise soft tissue lead stores. Total lead spills are measured in both the pre-DMSA urine and the 4-hour post-DMSA urine. Published studies have used this basic method to identify 'DMSA-chelatable lead' stores in lead workers.[259,260] Researchers have concluded that, 'DMSA-chelatable lead was found to be the best predictor of lead-related symptoms, particularly of both total symptoms scores and neuromuscular symptoms, than were the other lead biomarkers'.[261]

MANAGEMENT/THERAPY

Oral DMSA and oral and parenteral CaEDTA are both effective chelators of lead, and blood levels of lead drop with the use of either CaEDTA or DMSA. CaEDTA and DMSA have been shown to mobilise lead from different compartments, with EDTA primarily mobilising lead from the trabecular bone and DMSA primarily mobilising lead from soft tissue (primarily the kidneys).[262] Studies utilising DMSA have repeatedly shown that the BLLs rise within 2 weeks of DMSA cessation.[263] The regular release of bone lead into the bloodstream from normal bone turnover daily restores both blood and soft tissue lead levels. For this reason, short-term intermittent use of DMSA is ineffective at reversing neurological dysfunction.[264] Based on this homeostatic balance, the most effective means of achieving long-term reduction of both blood and soft tissue lead levels may be ongoing, rather than intermittent, DMSA therapy.

Based on efficacy and safety, DMSA may be the most appropriate oral chelator as a treatment for lead toxicity in children and adults.[265] In a case series of 17 lead-poisoned adults, DMSA therapy increased lead excretion on average by a factor of 12.[266] Although DMSA may not have a significant effect on lead in bone, it has been shown to reduce hippocampal lead, which may be more directly relevant to changes in health over time.[267] A combination of both EDTA and DMSA may be more effective than either alone. After controlling for blood lead and weight, lead-exposed workers who received EDTA before DMSA excreted, on average, 1068 micrograms more lead after DMSA than did workers who did not receive EDTA before the DMSA ($p = 0.0002$).[268]

EDTA chelates lead by displacement of the central Ca^{2+} ion with Pb^{2+}. Repeated chelation therapy (CaEDTA weekly for 24 months) improved renal function and slowed the progression of renal insufficiency in patients with non-diabetic chronic renal disease and high-normal body lead burdens (at least 80 micrograms but less than 600 micrograms).[269] Subjects in this study were included or excluded based on the lead mobilisation test. Although chelation with EDTA and DMSA both lowered BLLs, children with acute lead intoxication treated with EDTA appeared, on average, to have 6.47 mg/dL (p <0.05: 95% CI: 0.821–12.12) lower BLLs than those treated with DMSA.[270] The use of vitamins E and C, melatonin, alpha-lipoic acid and NAC concurrently with DMSA not only provide greater reversal of lead-induced biochemical and physiological damage, but significantly increase the excretion of lead itself.[271,272]

CaEDTA has been associated with increased gastrointestinal absorption of lead and increased brain lead concentrations. CaEDTA primarily pulls lead from the trabecular bone and secondarily from the kidneys, but while doing so may temporarily increase soft-tissue stores of lead in people with a very high lead burden.[273] Tissue analysis of rats exposed to lead acetate in drinking water for 3–4 months and then injected with CaEDTA indicated that lead was mobilised from bone and redistributed to both brain and liver.[274]

Non-diabetic individuals with renal disease who had a high body lead burden (at least 80 micrograms but less than 600 micrograms) received either intravenous CaEDTA or a placebo weekly for up to 48 months.[275] After the first 3 months of weekly CaEDTA treatment, it was noted that both the BLLs and the total body lead levels dropped dramatically. As the body lead burden levels dropped, the renal function improved as evidenced by reduced serum creatinine and improved glomerular filtration rate. It was estimated that ongoing chelation therapy could delay the need for dialysis by several years.

In addition to the benefit of reducing the total body lead burden, CaEDTA therapy has also been shown to reverse the pro-oxidant effects of lead.[276] These effects included a restoration of SOD and catalase levels, a reduction of malondialdehyde levels, improved PON1 function and a reversal of the depression of acetylcholinesterase activity.

Turmeric contains the flavonoid curcumin which has demonstrated the ability to bind lead and other heavy metals,[277] reduce lead levels in animals and reverse the lead-induced oxidative stress.[278] The lead reduction activity of curcumin appears to be dose related, with more bioavailable forms of curcumin providing greater reduction of lead tissue burden.[279]

Mercury
PRINCIPLES OF TOXICITY

Mercury is a powerful pro-oxidant promoting the formation of hydrogen peroxide, lipid peroxides and hydroxyl radicals.[280] Mercury binds irreversibly with reduced GSH, causing the loss up to two GSH molecules through the bile into the faeces. Compounding this loss is the mercury-induced inhibition of glutathione reductase, preventing the recycling of oxidised glutathione (GSSG) back to GSH.[281] At the same time, mercury also inhibits GSH synthetase reducing the level of GSH production. Not only is mercury known to reduce the functioning of glutathione transferases, but it can also lead to the development of anti-glutathione transferase antibodies.[282] In addition, exposure to mercury reduces the activity of catalase, superoxide dismutase, glutathione peroxidase and paraoxonase 1 (PON1), all of which are necessary to prevent oxidative stress.[283]

MeHg causes a dramatic dissolution of microtubules in platelets, red blood cells, neurons and many other cells.[284] Mercury-induced dissolution of microtubules typically leads to apoptosis of neuronal and/or non-neuronal cells.[285,286] Mercury decreases the phagocytic activity of white blood cells and leads to apoptosis of both monocytes and lymphocytes.[287,288] Apoptosis of these and other cells appears to be secondary to the mercury-induced glutathione depletion in the mitochondrial inner membrane. Regardless of the form of mercury, the percentage of cells undergoing apoptosis is dependent upon the mercury concentration that is present. Mercury (as well as cadmium and lead) also causes a decrease in DNA content and an increase in collagenase-resistant protein formation in synovial joint tissue.[289]

SOURCES

Mercury is a ubiquitous environmental pollutant and potent neurotoxin. Concerns regarding mercury exposure have increased as sources impacting on the general population have also increased. Elemental or metallic mercury is released as a vapour into the environment through combustion of mercury-containing compounds and is also found in older thermometers and thermostats. Dental amalgams, fish, air, water and vaccinations all contain various levels of mercury. Considering mercury is toxic at any level, the cumulative effect of these sources increases the potential for mercury toxicity.

Mercury is present in the environment as a result of natural environmental events (e.g. volcanic eruptions) and/or pollution sources (e.g. burning of coal and oil). Older chlor-alkali plants still use mercury, resulting in end-product mercury contamination (e.g. high-fructose corn syrup), along with higher mercury levels in those living proximal to the facilities.[290,291] Incineration of medical waste and cremations also contribute to the environmental load of mercury.[292] A single crematorium facility releases an average of 5453 kg of mercury per year due primarily to the presence of amalgams in cadavers.[293]

The single greatest source of mercury for humans is the consumption of fish with high MeHg content. It has been shown that women who consume at least nine fish meals per month have blood mercury levels seven times higher than women who do not eat fish.[294] Due to the increased production of coal-fired powerplants in Asia releasing mercury into the air, the mercury level in the Pacific Ocean is expected to increase another 50% by 2050, with an equivalent MeHg increase in fish from those waters.[295] MeHg levels for most fish range from less than 0.01 ppm to 0.5 ppm, with an average of >0.3 ppm.[296]

People with amalgams on their occlusal surfaces have demonstrated nine times higher non-stimulated levels of mercury vapour in their oral cavity than people without amalgams, and chewing stimulation produces an additional six-fold increase in elemental mercury levels.[297] Mercury concentrations remain elevated during 30 minutes of continuous chewing and decline slowly over 90 minutes following chewing cessation.[298] Similar increases in oral mercury levels have also been found in those with amalgams who have bruxism, and during gum chewing, tooth brushing or the consumption of hot drinks.[299,300] Blood mercury concentrations have been positively correlated with both the number and the surface area of amalgam restorations and are significantly higher in those with amalgams than those without.[301]

BODY LOAD

Mercury is found globally in all populations that have been tested. Blood and urine mercury concentrations are commonly used as biomarkers of exposure to mercury, while hair is used to measure MeHg exposure. Recent exposure to mercury is reflected in both blood and urine, with urine giving a greater representation of metallic mercury while blood favours MeHg.

The primary form of mercury in both hair and blood is MeHg with over 90% coming from the consumption of ocean fish and shellfish. Total blood mercury levels are directly associated with fish intake. MeHg present in the circulating blood during hair formation is incorporated into the follicles. Total blood mercury and blood MeHg levels are linearly related to total mercury in the hair. With 80% of the total hair mercury being MeHg, hair mercury levels are an excellent marker of MeHg exposure during the time of hair growth (typically 1–1.5 cm/month). Hair mercury levels have been significantly correlated with mercury levels in the cerebrum, cerebellum, heart, spleen, liver and kidneys.[302]

Elemental mercury vapour is highly absorbed (70–80%) in the lungs and moved into the blood. Once in the circulation, mercury can easily cross both the blood–brain and the placental barriers due to its fat-soluble nature. Elemental mercury is oxidised by catalase-hydrogen peroxide, forming divalent Hg^{2+}, a reactive species. This combines covalently with nearby sulfhydryl groups including haemoglobin, reduced GSH, cysteine and cysteine-containing proteins such as albumin. Once MeHg is complexed with L-cysteine, it can be transported into the brain via methionine-uptake mechanisms.[303] In the brain, MeHg undergoes slow dealkylation to become inorganic mercury.[304]

Elemental mercury has a biphasic biological half-life (t ½), beginning with a rapid 1–3 day half-life, followed by a slower second phase half-life of 1–3 weeks.[305,306] MeHg blood levels peak between 4 and 14 hours after fish consumption, with a blood t ½ of 45–70 days.[307] Approximately two-thirds of MeHg is eliminated in the faeces (complexed with GSH), while the remaining third is rendered inorganic and cleared through the urine. Over 70% of the MeHg dumped into the intestines is reabsorbed via enterohepatic recirculation, accounting for this long t ½.[308] Mercury is moved from the blood into the urine through membrane-bound efflux pumps in the kidneys, primarily through the GSH-dependent multidrug-resistant proteins 2 (MRP2).[309] Transport of both organic and inorganic mercury into the bile for excretion is also dependent upon hepatic GSH stores. Each molecule of mercury binds to two molecules of GSH,[310] thereby reducing GSH stores in the body.[311] A depletion of GSH reduces the hepatic uptake of MeHg by 40% and reduces MeHg uptake by the kidney, thus inhibiting the two major pathways for mercury excretion.[312]

CLINICAL MANIFESTATIONS

Mercury readily moves into the brain in both elemental and organic forms. In the brain, MeHg affects the mitochondria, endoplasmic reticulum, Golgi complex, nuclear envelopes and lysosomes. In nerve fibres, MeHg is localised primarily in myelin sheaths, where it leads to demyelination.[313] A group in New Zealand used a set of mercury-related symptoms that appears to identify people with 'chronic mercury toxicity' (see Box 3.1).[314]

Prenatal exposure to MeHg has resulted in ongoing neurobehavioural and neurocognitive defects in children.[315,316] Children with a cord blood mercury ≥7.5 micrograms/L were four times more likely to have an IQ

BOX 3.1 Mercury toxicity symptom picture used to identify mercury-burdened patients[314]

Chronic mercury toxicity

Gross:
- Ataxia, intention tremor, incoordination, dysarthria
- Psychomotor retardation

Subtle:
- Fine tremor of tongue, lips or outstretched fingers
- Hypersalivation with pooling of saliva
- Cold and erythematous hands and feet
- Labile mood
- Irritability, anxiety, depression, restlessness
- Cognitive problems (memory, concentration, cognition)

<80.[317] Children with higher cord blood mercury levels were also more likely to have ADHD in later years.[318]

Dentists also perform significantly worse on neurobehavioural tests measuring motor speed (finger tapping), visual scanning (trail making), visuomotor coordination and concentration (digit symbol), verbal memory, visual memory and visuomotor coordination speed.[319] Dentists with a mean blood mercury of 3.32 micrograms/L (versus 2.29 micrograms/L) and dental assistants with a mean blood mercury of 1.98 micrograms/L (versus 1.03 micrograms/L) exhibited statistically significant declines on multiple tests.[320]

The kidneys have a high affinity for mercury. Within a few hours of exposure, much of the mercury that gets into the blood ends up in the kidneys. Mercury damages both the glomeruli and the tubules. Proximal tubular necrosis, especially along the straight renal segments in the inner cortex and outer stripe of the outer medulla, is a prominent feature of inorganic mercury nephrotoxicity.[321] Much of the tissue damage appears to result from poisoning of the kidney mitochondria so there is not enough ATP for the cells to protect themselves from the toxicants they are excreting.[322]

Increasing blood mercury levels are associated with increases in aspartate aminotransferase, alanine aminotransferase and elevated gamma-glutamyl transferase (>56 IU/L).[323,324] The primary mechanism of mercury hepatotoxicity may be related to poisoning of cysteine-containing proteins and GSH depletion.[325]

Both short- and long-term increases in blood pressure have been documented among those poisoned in the Minimata Bay area in Japan.[326,327] Two studies utilising hair mercury levels also found positive associations between mercury levels and blood pressure increases.[328,329] Hair mercury levels are associated with atherosclerotic disease resulting in increased carotid intima-media thickness (CIMT).[330] Heart tissue mercury levels in people with cardiomyopathy were found to be 22 000 times higher than in non-CHD controls.[331] A study of Finnish and Swedish men revealed that hair mercury values were significantly associated with myocardial infarction, and that high hair mercury counteracted the benefit of fish oils in preventing heart disease.[332]

Mercury accumulates in the thyroid and reduces the uptake of iodine by binding to the sodium/iodite transporting molecule.[333] Mercury also inhibits deiodinase function in the peripheral tissues preventing the production of triiodothyronine (T3) from thyroxine (T4).[334] Inorganic mercury causes pancreatic beta-cell dysfunction and apoptosis, which can fortunately be prevented with NAC.[335] Data from the 2010-12 KNHANES revealed that when compared with people with the lowest quartile of mercury, those with the highest blood mercury were 62% more likely to have metabolic syndrome.[336] Adults in the CARDIA study with the highest toenail mercury levels were 65% more likely to develop type 2 diabetes than those with lower levels of mercury.[337]

DIAGNOSTIC TESTING

Current mercury exposure can be assessed with blood and urine, while hair gives an indication of exposure over the preceding 30–45 days.[338] As mentioned above, both blood and hair mercury levels provide the clearest indication of methylmercury levels.[339] Urine mercury levels also reflect current exposure but contain far more inorganic than organic mercury.[340]

Both 2,3-dimercaptosuccinic acid (DMSA) and 2,3-dimercaptopropane-1-sulfonate (DMPS) have been utilised as mercury mobilising agents to assess body stores of inorganic mercury.[341,342] Urinary coproporphyrin levels were predictive of a positive mercury mobilisation test indicating a high body burden of mercury in people working in a dental office.[343] DMPS mobilisation resulted in a 10-fold increase in urinary mercury for mercury workers, a 5.9-fold increase for dentists and a 3.8-fold increase in people without amalgams.[344] Another study found 35- to 88-fold increases in urinary mercury in mercury workers after an oral challenge with 300 mg of DMPS.[345] With over 90% of DMPS-bound mercury being released in the urine within the first 6 hours, the use of a 48-hour catch is unnecessary.

MANAGEMENT/THERAPY

Mercury is often chelated with either DMSA or DMPS. DMSA and DMPS contain two sulfhydryl groups each and possess the critical ability to bind mercury tighter than it is bound to extra and intracellular thiols. DMSA is the typical agent of choice because it is less toxic and can be given orally. DMSA primarily moves mercury from the kidneys, which contain the highest mercury concentration in the body,[346] but does not mobilise mercury from amalgams.[347]

DMPS, DMSA and NAC are similar in their mercury mobilising effects. When given separately, DMSA increases urinary mercury excretion by 163%, DMPS by 135% and NAC by 131%.[348] Neither DMSA nor DMPS directly removes CNS mercury, and both chelate several trace minerals, although deficiencies have not been noted.[349]

Several studies have shown DMSA to be effective at increasing mercury excretion. One study looked at urinary excretion of mercury at various lengths of time after cessation of occupational exposure to mercury vapour.[350] Researchers found a clear correlation between exposure currency and mercury levels before and after DMSA. A small study looked at blood and urinary mercury levels associated with fish consumption.[351] An increase in blood mercury was observed in proportion to the amount of fish eaten, but no difference in baseline was found between those who did not eat fish, those who ate 1–2 servings a week and those who ate three or more servings per week. However, significant differences were seen after introduction of DMSA at 30 mg/kg in all groups, with a significantly larger increase in proportion to fish consumption (see Fig. 3.2).[352]

DMPS increases the urinary excretion of mercury and reduces mercury concentrations in the kidneys, blood and brain.[353] DMPS has also shown benefit at reversing mercury-associated symptoms including tremors, memory loss, insomnia and metallic taste in the mouth, and demonstrated objective improvements in neurocognitive testing and in rombergism.[352,354]

Animal studies have shown that DMSA, DMPS and NAC significantly decrease the mercury levels in placental and fetal tissues of pregnant rats and increase urinary excretion of mercury.[355,356] Renal clearance of DMPS, DMSA and NAC-mercury conjugates are all mediated through MRP2 export proteins in the proximal tubules,[357] and elimination of mercury is dependent upon adequate thiol stores.[358]

NAC used in conjunction with haemodialysis of methylmercury-contaminated human blood was quite effective at enhancing MeHg clearance from blood.[359] By itself, NAC supplementation exhibited a 5- to 10-fold increase in urinary methylmercury excretion compared to controls.[360] Studies demonstrate that NAC is effective at attenuating the oxidative damage caused by mercury to the kidneys by increasing the activities of superoxide dismutase (SOD), catalase (CAT) and glutathione-s-transferase (GST), and by decreasing GSH depletion and MDA levels.[361,362]

One case report described a patient who manifested neurological symptoms 10 years after he was administered mercurials for the treatment of syphilis and demonstrated complete resolution of symptoms after long-term EDTA treatment.[363]

Other

THALLIUM

Thallium is highly toxic, and in the past, poisoning often resulted in death.[364] Most human exposure today is associated with contaminated food or drinking water from rodenticide use, and high thallium concentrations have been found in green vegetables such as cabbage.[365] The toxicity of thallium-based compounds is mainly caused by the similarity between thallium ions and potassium ions. Common symptoms in non-fatal cases include fatigue, gastroenteritis, extremely painful sensory neuropathy and alopecia. Prussian blue has been used as a treatment for thallium toxicity as the exchange of potassium ions in the crystal lattice with thallium ions leads to the binding of thallium in the intestine for extraction and elimination.[366]

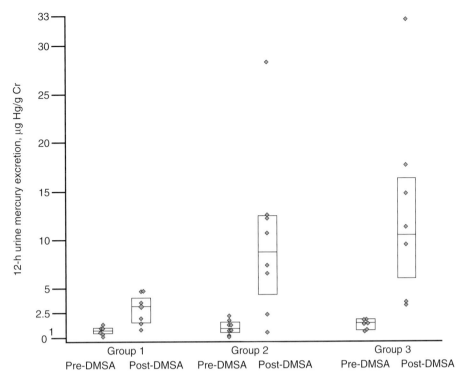

FIGURE 3.2 Results of challenge testing according to amount of fish eaten[352]

Prussian blue is administered in a dose of 10 g orally twice daily and should be continued until urine thallium excretion is 0.5 mg/day.[367] Interestingly, animal studies have found that DL-penicillamine, when given in combination with Prussian blue, had an additive effect in the treatment of acute thallotoxicosis.[368]

COBALT

Although cobalt exposure has generally decreased over the years, there has been a recent upsurge with the use of metal-on-metal (MoM) joint prostheses. Cobalt–chromium alloy is used for most MoM implants, and elevated levels of cobalt and chromium are toxic. The release of cobalt from MoM prostheses is due to the mechanical and oxidative stresses placed on the prosthetic joint, and cobalt exerts its pathological effects through direct cellular toxicity.[369]

Elevated metal ions, such as cobalt, have carcinogenic and biological concerns, as well as concerns regarding hypersensitivity, chromosomal mutation and fetal exposure to high ion levels.[370,371] Several studies show that severe cobalt intoxication leads to hypothyroidism, peripheral neuropathy and cardiomyopathy.[372,373] A relatively common complication associated with MoM total hip arthroplasty is hypersensitivity to the metal. Metal sensitivity should be considered in individuals presenting with persistent pain, marked joint effusion and the development of early osteolysis in the absence of infection. Reactivity to the metal appears to involve the adaptive (macrophage-recruiting) immune system, with elevated proliferation and production of IFN-gamma indicating a

Th1 type response.[374] Asthma, pneumonia, wheezing, respiratory irritation and fibrosis have all been reported as occupational health hazards, especially in workers exposed to cobalt metal powder, cobalt salts and cobalt-containing dusts.[375-378] Peri-articular soft-tissue masses or pseudotumours have been discovered after MoM resurfacing of the hip and total hip replacement. It is estimated that 1% of patients who have a MoM hip resurfacing will develop a pseudotumour within 5 years.[379]

Clinical management of elevated cobalt levels associated with MoM hip prosthesis, particularly surrounding chelation therapy, is greatly debated. Current medical literature provides no consensus on chelation regarding the levels of cobalt in which chelation should be initiated, which agents to use, the timing of administration, the mode of administration and the efficacy of treatment.[380,381] However, animal studies as well as human case studies have shown some benefit.

NAC, GSH, EDTA, DMSA and diethylenetriaminepentaacetic acid (DTPA) have shown the most benefit as chelating agents in acute cobalt toxicity.[382] NAC (liver and spleen) and GSH (spleen) have also been shown to be the most effective at reducing the concentration of cobalt in various tissues.[383] Few human studies exist demonstrating the use of chelating agents in the treatment of MoM cobalt toxicity. Two promising case studies demonstrated the use of NAC to reduce elevated blood metal levels in MoM patients.[384] Considering the safety of NAC, this may be an effective option for treatment at any elevated blood cobalt level. At this time, the use of NAC as a chelating agent, even when cobalt levels appear below the threshold level of 7.0 micrograms/L, appears a safe and effective preventive measure.

ASSESSMENT OF TOXIC METALS

Toxic load is an increasing clinical problem, and accurate assessment is essential, not only for recognition of exposure, but also for tracking efficacy of intervention. Toxins can be directly measured in urine, blood, breath, toenails and adipose tissue. There are several accepted tests for metal toxicity which rely mostly on blood and urine. It is generally recommended that a non-chelator-challenged collection of urine or blood be obtained as a baseline assessment to help determine if there is an ongoing acute exposure that needs to be removed. The limitation of blood or urine tests is that they largely reflect only the level of ongoing exposure to the metal and may bear little relationship to body load. The typical standards for toxin load are population based (i.e. unless a patient is in the top 5% of blood levels, they are usually not considered toxic). While the top 5% is the standard to be considered toxic for most pollutants, there is sufficient reason to question its validity. The assumption that those with lower levels are healthy and are not being damaged by their toxic load is problematic. In addition, since the population has very high levels of ill health and diagnosed disease, normal is not actually healthy.

No single perfect test exists for the diagnosis of chronic metal toxicity. Test results must be interpreted in conjunction with a thorough review of a patient's history, physical findings and symptoms.

With a few interesting exceptions, the standard of assessment for metal 'poisoning' is whole blood levels with reference ranges based on workplace health and safety standards. The blood metal compartment has the shortest biological half-life. Metals leave the blood by excretion and transfer to tissues, where toxic metals have much longer biological half-lives.[385] The analysis of whole blood, plasma and red blood cells can provide valuable information about exposure to specific forms of some metals. However, as previously mentioned, this method is problematic because blood levels can fluctuate with intermittent exposure, primarily indicate current exposure, do not at all consider total body load of these metals and do not consider the huge variation in individual susceptibility to specific toxicants.

Unprovoked urine, representing acute exposure, has reference ranges established for the population for various toxicants. Provocative urine testing is a multi-step process intended to evaluate total body burden of toxic metals (see Challenge Testing below). Urine testing may be beneficial in examining the long-term, low-dose, chronic exposure to toxic compounds, and qualitatively reflect excretion of an unknown fraction of the total body pools of assimilated metals. Assessment of urinary biomarkers of renal damage (e.g. β_2-microglobulin, retinal-binding protein and N-acetyl-β-$_D$-glucosaminidase [NAG]) may be useful in the diagnosis of toxicity in cases of very high exposure.[386] But again, urine testing may not be reliable in assessing total body load.

Hair tissue analysis measures the levels and ratios of minerals and heavy metals in hair. Several studies have been published confirming the efficacy and accuracy of hair testing, especially for toxic metals.[387,388] The concentration of metals in hair is usually far greater than that in blood or urine because there is no back exchange into the body. The test requires a 0.5 g hair sample and reflects the body's exposure for the past 2–3 months. Hair analysis is inexpensive, non-invasive and biologically stable, and may be the most reliable screening test for chronic metal exposure (lead, mercury, cadmium and arsenic). Many variables can affect the results including: gender, hair colour, improper sample collection, hair products (e.g. shampoos, bleaches, hair spray) and inconsistent lab analysis. In addition, reliable results depend on a properly cleaned, collected and prepared sample. Significant controversy exists regarding the use of hair analysis as an indicator of nutritional status and in the diagnosis of disease. A positive hair analysis may suggest an individual has been exposed to metals. However, the clinical significance of that exposure as well as its use to diagnose the presence or absence of disease is limited. The precision of hair analysis in determining long-standing body burdens of most metals is probably too low to base clinical decisions on and may be limited to population screening.[389]

Nail clippings can also be used to identify exposure to a variety of toxicants. Depending on the rate of nail growth, toenail measurements represent exposures that occurred 1–12 months before sample collection.

More detailed information regarding assessment of specific toxic metals can be found under the Diagnostic Testing section for each metal.

CHALLENGE TESTING

There remains significant scientific debate regarding metal mobilisation testing, and the decision to treat subacute levels of metal poisoning requires careful assessment of patient risk versus benefit. There is no scientific disagreement about the use of chelating agents to increase the excretion of toxic metals. Indeed, the removal of toxic metals from the human body can be a useful tool in avoiding the onset or progression of many diseases associated with metal intoxication. The primary way to remove accumulated toxic metals from human organs is to bind these metals to chelating agents with the goal of forming complexes that can be excreted in the urine. Chelation therapy is considered the best treatment against metal poisoning. Before initiating chelation therapy or metal mobilisation testing, it is prudent for the physician to ensure the patient is not allergic or chemically intolerant to the agent, and that the patient has sufficient creatinine clearance to handle the toxic metal flushing.

Initially, a pre-challenge urine sample is collected to determine acute exposure. A chelating agent is then administered to the patient via oral or intravenous means. The chelator forms a complex with the metal and is excreted in the urine. After a set amount of time (e.g. 2 h, 4 h, 24 h), a second urine sample is collected and post-challenge levels are calculated. Comparing pre-challenge urinary metal levels to post-challenge levels may help with the diagnosis, treatment and management of chronic low-level metal toxicity.

There are several limitations to this procedure. Most chelating agents do not extract metals from all tissues and thus do not necessarily represent total body burden. For example, the brain is one of the main target organs for both elemental and organic mercury, yet no chelating agents can extract mercury from the brain.[390] There are no clear reference ranges for provoked urine, and neither DMSA nor DMPS have an optimal dosage for diagnosis or treatment. There is also no standard for safe versus toxic levels. In addition, there are serious confounding factors (e.g. age, gender, BMI) in determining body load of metals and clinical significance.

SIDE EFFECTS

The use of D-penicillamine is associated with significant leukopenia, thrombocytopenia and proteinuria.

In patients with chronic lead intoxication undergoing DMSA chelation therapy, haemolytic anaemia has been observed.[391] However, after termination of therapy, haematological values returned to normal.

Reported risks associated with IV EDTA chelation include renal failure, arrhythmia, tetany, hypocalcaemia, hypotension and prolongation of bleeding time.[392]

Dimercaprol is the most toxic of all chelating agents and is associated with a high incidence of adverse effects at therapeutic doses. Adverse effects of BAL include nausea; vomiting; a burning sensation in the mouth, throat, eyes and sometimes limbs; muscle pain and spasms; lacrimation; rhinorrhoea and hypersalivation. In addition, hypertension, tachycardia, fever and pain in the head, teeth or abdomen can occur. The adverse symptoms develop soon after injection and subside within about 2 hours. Injections can also be painful, and abscesses may develop. BAL may cause haemolysis in glucose-6-phosphate dehydrogenase-deficient individuals.

CASE STUDY

MERCURY

'Doctor, I am afraid I am losing my mind'

CASE SUMMARY

Distraught 67-year-old white woman with progressive early stage dementia. Past history of 2 years of IV DMPS chelation therapy for mercury toxicity. Despite intervention, neurodegeneration symptoms continued to worsen. 18 months of intervention with oral DMSA, fibre and NAC resulted in total reversal of symptoms.

INVESTIGATIONS AND FINDINGS

Presenting symptoms: 'I had the odd feeling that I was living in a fog, that things were very fuzzy and that my memory was very sporadic. I was having trouble sleeping and had a lot of muscle aches during the night. I always had a metal taste in my mouth and felt that my breath lacked

CASE STUDY CONTINUED

freshness other than the first few minutes after brushing my teeth. My skin and scalp were always sore and especially dry.'

Physical examination: within normal limits.

Laboratory findings: IV DMPS challenge test (250 mg DMPS followed by 6-hour urine collection) revealed a very high mercury of 50.0 micrograms/g creatinine (normal <5.0).

Assessment: mercury toxicity likely due to release from bone.

RX

Since the patient no longer had amalgam fillings (typically 55% mercury) and was careful about not eating high-mercury fish, there was no apparent need for exposure reduction.

Treatment:
- 250 mg DMSA every 3rd night
- 2.5 g PGX fibre twice a day
- 500 mg NAC (N-acetylcysteine) twice a day
- Good quality multivitamin and mineral supplement

FOLLOW-UP REVIEW/PROGRESS

6 months. Modest improvement in symptoms and cautiously optimistic patient. Mercury challenge test showed substantial drop in mercury to 12.0 micrograms/g creatinine.

12 months. Substantial decrease in symptoms and feeling more normal. Mercury challenge test down to 7.3.

18 months. Total resolution of all symptoms. Mercury challenge test was now 3.5.

The message, in patient's own words: 'I would caution people to remember that clearing mercury out of one's system is a long process but it is worth the effort even if it takes many years.'

REFERENCES

[1] Bertini I, Cavallaro G. Metals in the 'omics' world: copper homeostasis and cytochrome c oxidase assembly in a new light. J Biol Inorg Chem 2008;13:3–14.

[2] Trumbo P, Yates AA, Schlicker S, et al. Dietary reference intakes: vitamin A, vitamin K, arsenic, boron, chromium, copper, iodine, iron, manganese, molybdenum, nickel, silicon, vanadium, and zinc. J Am Diet Assoc 2001;101(3):294–301.

[3] McDonald RJ, McDonald JS, Kallmes DF, et al. Intracranial gadolinium deposition after contrast-enhanced MR Imaging. Radiology 2015;275:772–82.

[4] Flora SJ, Mittal M, Mehta A. Heavy metal induced oxidative stress & its possible reversal by chelation therapy. Indian J Med Res 2008;128(4):501–23.

[5] Mates JM, Segura JA, Alonso FJ, et al. Intracellular redox status and oxidative stress: implications for cell proliferation, apoptosis, and carcinogenesis. Arch Toxicol 2008;82:273–99.

[6] Rogan WJ, Dietrich KN, Ware JH, et al. The effect of chelation therapy with succimer on neuropsychological development in children exposed to lead. N Engl J Med 2001;344:1421–6.

[7] Rozema T. The protocol for the safe and effective administration of EDTA and other chelating agents for vascular disease, degenerative disease, and metal toxicity. J Adv Med 1997;10:5–100.

[8] Aposhian HV, Maiorino RM, Gonzalez-Ramirez D, et al. Mobilization of heavy metals by newer, therapeutically useful chelating agents. Toxicology 1995;97:23–38.

[9] Flora SJS, Pachauri V. Chelation in metal intoxication. Int J Environ Res Public Health 2010;7:2745–88.

[10] Andersen O. Principles and recent developments in chelation treatment of metal intoxication. Chem Rev 1999;99:2683–710.

[11] Kosnett MJ. The role of chelation in the treatment of arsenic and mercury poisoning. J Med Toxicol 2013;9:347–54.

[12] Sears ME. Chelation: harnessing and enhancing heavy metal detoxification – a review. Sci World J 2013;2013:219840.

[13] Olivieri NF, Brittenham GM. Iron-chelating therapy and the treatment of thalassemia. Blood 1997;89(7):2621.

[14] Brittenham GM, Griffith PM, Nienhuis AW, et al. Efficacy of deferoxamine in preventing complications of iron overload in patients with thalassemia major. N Engl J Med 1994;331(9):567–73.

[15] Callender ST, Weatherall DJ. Iron chelation with oral desferrioxamine. Lancet 1980;2(8196):689.

[16] Summers MR, Jacobs A, Tudway D, et al. Studies in desferrioxamine and ferrioxamine metabolism in normal and iron-loaded subjects. Br J Haematol 1979;42(4):547–55.

[17] Hershko C, Weatherall DJ. Iron-chelating therapy. Crit Rev Clin Lab Sci 1988;26(4):303–45.

[18] Cappellini MD, Cohen A, Piga A, et al. A phase 3 study of deferasirox (ICL670), a once-daily oral iron chelator, in patients with beta-thalassemia. Blood 2006;107(9):3455–62.

[19] Cohen A, Martin M, Schwartz E. Depletion of excessive liver iron stores with desferrioxamine. Br J Haematol 1984;58(2):369–73.

[20] Brittenham GM, Griffith PM, Nienhuis AW, et al. Efficacy of deferoxamine in preventing complications of iron overload in patients with thalassemia major. N Engl J Med 1994;331(9):567–73.

[21] Borgna-Pignatti C, Rugolotto S, De Stephano P, et al. Survival and complications in patients with thalassemia major treated with transfusion and deferoxamine. Haematologica 2004;89(10):1187–93.

[22] Ackrill P, Day JP. Desferrioxamine in the treatment of aluminum overload. Clin Nephrol 1985;24(Suppl. 1):S94–7.

[23] Melograna JM, Yokel RA. Effects of subchronic desferrioxamine infusion on aluminum toxicity in rabbits. Res Commun Chem Pathol Pharmacol 1984;44(3):411–22.

[24] Julka D, Gill KD. Effect of aluminum on regional brain antioxidant defense status in Wistar rats. Res Exp Med (Berl) 1996;196(3):187–94.

[25] Savory J, Herman MM, Erasmus RT, et al. Partial reversal of aluminum-induced neurofibrillary degeneration by desferrioxamine in adult male rabbits. Neuropathol Appl Neurobiol 1994;20(1):31–7.

[26] Ceci A, Bajardi P, Catapano M, et al. Risk factors for death in patients with beta-thalassemia major: results of a case-control study. Haematologica 2006;91(10):1420–1.

[27] Vilensky JA, Redman K. British Anti-Lewisite (dimercaprol): an amazing history. Ann Emerg Med 2003;41(3):378–83.

[28] Muckter H, Liebl B, Reichi FX, et al. Are we ready to replace dimercaprol (BAL) as an arsenic antidote? Hum Exp Toxicol 1997;16(8):460–5.

[29] Janakiraman N, Seeler RA, Royal JE, et al. Hemolysis during BAL chelation therapy for high blood lead levels in two G6PD deficient children. Clin Pediatr (Phila) 1978;17(6):485–7.

[30] Wax PM, Thornton CA. Recovery from severe arsenic-induced peripheral neuropathy with 2,3-dimercapto-1-propanesulphonic acid. J Toxicol Clin Toxicol 2000;38(7):777–80.

[31] Hurlbut KM, Maiorino RM, Mayersohn M, et al. Determination and metabolism of dithiol chelating agents XVI: pharmacokinetics of 2,3-dimercapto-1-propanesulfonate after intravenous administration to human volunteers. J Pharmacol Exp Ther 1994;268(2):662–8. PubMed PMID: 8113976.

[32] Torres-Alanis O, Garza-Ocanas L, et al. Urinary excretion of trace elements in humans after sodium 2,3-dimercaptopropane-1-sulfonate challenge test. J Toxicol Clin Toxicol 2000;38(7):697–700.

[33] Cohen JP, Ruha AM, Curry SC, et al. Plasma and urine dimercaptopropanesulfonate concentrations after dermal application of transdermal DMPS (TD-DMPS). J Med Toxicol 2013;9(1):9–15.

[34] Aposhian HV, Maiorino RM, Rivera M, et al. Human studies with the chelating agents, DMPS and DMSA. J Toxicol Clin Toxicol 1992;30(4):505–28.

[35] Bradberry S, Vale A. Dimercaptosuccinic acid (succimer; DMSA) in inorganic lead poisoning. Clin Toxicol (Phila) 2009;47(7):617–31.

[36] Aposhian HV, Maiorino RM, Dart RC, et al. Urinary excretion of meso-2,3-dimercaptosuccinic acid in human subjects. Clin Pharmacol Ther 1989;45(5):520–6.

[37] Sears ME. Chelation: harnessing and enhancing heavy metal detoxification – a review. Sci World J 2013;2013:219840.

[38] Graziano JH. Role of 2,3-dimercaptosuccinic acid in the treatment of heavy metal poisoning. Med Toxicol 1986;1:155–62.

[39] Aposhian HV, Maiorino RM, Rivera M, et al. Human studies with the chelating agents DMPS and DMSA. Clin Toxicol 1992;30(4):505–28.

[40] Chisolm JJ Jr. Safety and efficacy of meso-2,3-dimercaptosuccinic acid (DMSA) in children with elevated blood lead concentrations. J Toxicol Clin Toxicol 2000;38(4):365–75.

[41] Forman J, Moline J, Cernichiari E, et al. A cluster of pediatric metallic mercury exposure cases treated with meso-2,3-dimercaptosuccinic acid (DMSA). Environ Health Perspect 2000;108(6):575–7.

[42] Sigg T, Burda A, Leikin JB, et al. A report of pediatric succimer overdose. Vet Hum Toxicol 1998;40(2):90–1.

[43] Jin Y, Yu F, Liao Y, et al. Therapeutic efficiency of succimer used with calcium and ascorbic acid in the treatment of mild lead-poisoning. Environ Toxicol Pharmacol 2011;31(1):137–42.

[44] Adams JB, Baral M, Geis E, et al. Safety and efficacy of oral DMSA therapy for children with autism spectrum disorders: part A – medical results. BMC Clin Pharmacol 2009;9:16.

[45] Adams JB, Baral M, Geis E, et al. The severity of autism is associated with toxic metal body burden and red blood cell glutathione levels. J Toxicol 2009;2009:532640.

[46] Florentine MJ, Sanfilippo DJ. Elemental mercury poisoning. Clin Pharm 1991;10:213–21.

[47] Joyce DA. D-penicillamine pharmacokinetics and pharmacodynamics in man. Pharmacol Ther 1989;42:405–27.

[48] Bergstrom RF, Kay DR, Harkcom TM, et al. Penicillamine kinetics in normal subjects. Clin Pharmacol Ther 1981;30:404–13.

[49] Kuchinskas EJ, Rosen Y. Metal chelates of penicillamine. Arch Biochem Biophys 1962;97:370–2.

[50] Lyle WH. Penicillamine in metal poisoning. J Rheumatol 1981;8(Suppl. 7):96–9.

[51] Murphy MJ, Lyon LW, Taylor JW. Subacute arsenic neuropathy: clinical and electrophysiological observations. J Neurol Neurosurg Psychiatry 1981;44:896–900.

[52] Clarkson TW, Magos L, Cox C, et al. Tests of efficacy of antidotes for removal of methylmercury in human poisoning during the Iraq outbreak. J Pharmacol Exp Ther 1981;218:74–83.

[53] Hammond PB. The effects of d-penicillamine on the tissue distribution and excretion of lead. Toxic Appl Pharmac 1973;26:241–6.

[54] Martin BL. Development of a scale for the comparison of metals in enzyme action. J Inorg Biochem 1999;75(4):245–54.

[55] Lanigan RS, Yamarik TA. Final report on the safety assessment of EDTA, calcium disodium EDTA, diammonium EDTA, dipotassium EDTA, disodium EDTA, TEA-EDTA, tetrasodium EDTA, tripotassium EDTA, trisodium EDTA, HEDTA, and trisodium HEDTA. Int J Toxicol 2002;21(Suppl. 2):95–142.

[56] Borgstrom L, Kagedal B, Paulsen O. Pharmakokinetics of N-acetylcysteine in man. Eur J Clin Pharmacol 1986;31(2):217–22.

[57] Hannestad U, Sorbo B. Determination of 3-mercaptolactate, mercaptoacetate and N-acetylcysteine in urine by gas chromatography. Clin Chim Acta 1979;95(2):189–200.

[58] Hjortso E, Fomsgaard JS, Fogh-Andersen N. Does N-acetylcysteine increase the excretion of trace metals (calcium, magnesium, iron, zinc, and copper) when given orally? Eur J Clin Pharmacol 1990;39(1):29–31.

[59] Aremu DA, Madejczyk MS, Ballatori N. N-acetylcysteine as a potential antidote and biomonitoring agent of methylmercury exposure. Environ Health Perspect 2008;116(1):26–31.

[60] Sivaprasad R, Nagaraj M, Varalakshmi P. Combined efficacies of lipoic acid and 2,3-dimercaptosuccinic acid against lead-induced lipid peroxidation in rat liver. J Nutr Biochem 2004;15(1):18–23.

[61] Flora SJ, Pande M, Mehta A. Beneficial effect of combined administration of some naturally occurring antioxidants (vitamins) and thiol chelators in the treatment of chronic lead intoxication. Chem Biol Interact 2003;145(3):267–80.

[62] Flora SJ, Pande M, Kannan GM, et al. Lead induced oxidative stress and its recovery following co-administration of melatonin or N-acetylcysteine during chelation with succimer in male rats. Cell Mol Biol (Noisy-Le-Grand) 2004;50.

[63] Misbahuddin M, Islam AZ, Khandker S, et al. Efficacy of spirulina extract plus zinc in patients of chronic arsenic poisoning: a randomized placebo-controlled study. Clin Toxicol (Phila) 2006;44(2):135–41.

[64] Eliaz I, Weil E, Wilk B. Integrative medicine and the role of modified citrus pectin/alginates in heavy metal chelation and detoxification – five case reports. Forsch komplementmed 2007;14(6):358–64.

[65] Crinnion W. Is modified citrus pectin an effective mobilizer of heavy metals in humans? Altern Med Rev 2008;13(4):283–6.

[66] Toda S, Yase Y. Effect of aluminum on iron-induced lipid peroxidation and protein oxidative modification of mouse brain homogenate. Biol Trace Elem Res 1998;61(2):207–17.

[67] Chaitanya TV, Mallipeddi K, Bondili JS, et al. Effect of aluminum exposure on superoxide and peroxide handling capacities by liver, kidney, testis and temporal cortex in rat. Indian J Biochem Biophys 2012;49(5):395–8.

[68] Exley C. The pro-oxidant activity of aluminum. Free Radic Biol Med 2004;36(3):380–7.

[69] Mujika JI, Ruiperez F, Infante I, et al. Pro-oxidant activity of aluminum: stabilization of the aluminum superoxide radical ion. J Phys Chem A 2011;115(24):6717–23.

[70] Kumar V, Gill KD. Aluminum neurotoxicity: neurobehavioral and oxidative aspects. Arch Toxicol 2009;83(11):965–78.

[71] De Wolff FA. Toxicological aspects of aluminum poisoning in clinical nephrology. Clin Nephrol 1985;24(Suppl. 1):S9–14.

[72] De Wolff FA, Berend K, van der Voet GB. Subacute fatal aluminum poisoning in dialyzed patients: postmortem toxicological findings. Forensic Sci Int 2002;128(1–2):41–3.

[73] Westberg HB, Selden AI, Bellander T. Exposure to chemical agents in Swedish aluminum foundries and aluminum remelting plants – a comprehensive survey. Appl Occup Environ Hyg 2001;16:66–77.

[74] Willhite CC, Karyakina NA, Yokel RA, et al. Systematic review of potential health risks posed by pharmaceutical, occupational and consumer exposures to metallic and nanoscale aluminum, aluminum oxides, aluminum hydroxide and its soluble salts. Crit Rev Toxicol 2014;44(Suppl. 4):1–80.

[75] Soni MG, White SM, Flamm WG, et al. Safety evaluation of dietary aluminum. Regul Toxicol Pharmacol 2001;33(1):66–79.

[76] Colomina MT, Peris-Sampedro F. Aluminum and Alzheimer's disease. Adv Neurobiol 2017;18:183–97.

[77] Krewski D, Yokel RA, Nieboer E, et al. Human health risk assessment for aluminum, aluminum oxide and aluminum hydroxide. J Toxicol Environ Health B 2007;10(Suppl. 1):1–269.

[78] Kumar V, Gill KD. Oxidative stress and mitochondrial dysfunction in aluminum neurotoxicity and its amelioration: a review. Neurotoxicology 2014;41:154–66.

[79] Priest ND. The biological behavior and bioavailability of aluminum in man, with special reference to studies employing aluminium-26 as a tracer: review and study update. J Environ Monit 2004;6(5):375–403.

[80] Shaw CA, Tomljenovic L. Aluminum in the central nervous system (CNS): toxicity in humans and animals, vaccine adjuvants, and autoimmunity. Immunol Res 2013;56(2–3):304–16.

[81] Gupta VB, Anitha S, Hegde ML, et al. Aluminum in Alzheimer's disease: are we still at a crossroad? Cell Mol Life Sci 2005;62(2):143–58.

[82] Miu AC, Benga O. Aluminum and Alzheimer's disease: a new look. J Alzheimers Dis 2006;10(2–3):179–201.

[83] Exley C. What is the risk of aluminum as a neurotoxin? Expert Rev Neurother 2014;14(6):589–91.

[84] Riihimaki V, Aitio A. Occupational exposure to aluminum and its biomonitoring in perspective. Crit Rev Toxicol 2012;42(10):827–53.

[85] Dahl E, Nordal KP, Halse J, et al. The early effects of aluminum deposition and dialysis on bone in chronic renal failure: a cross-sectional bone-histomorphometric study. Nephrol Dial Transplant 1990;5(6):449–56.

[86] Al-Masalkhi A, Walton SP. Pulmonary fibrosis and occupational exposure to aluminum. J Ky Med Assoc 1994;92(2):59–61.

[87] Olszewski J, Latusinski J, et al. Comparative assessment of aluminum and lead concentrations in serum and tissue bioptates in patients with laryngeal papilloma or cancer. B-ENT 2006;2(2):47–9.

[88] Rossbach B, Buchta M, Csanady GA, et al. Biological monitoring of welders exposed to aluminum. Toxicol Lett 2006;162(2–3):239–45.

[89] Riihimaki V, Valkonen S, Engstrom B, et al. Behavior of aluminum in aluminum welders and manufacturers of aluminum sulfate – impact on biological monitoring. Scand J Work Environ Health 2008;34(6):451–62.

[90] Polizzi S, Pira E, Ferrara M, et al. Neurotoxic effects of aluminum among foundry workers and Alzheimer's disease. Neurotoxicology 2002;23(6):761–74.

[91] Riihimaki V, Hanninen H, Akila R, et al. Body burden of aluminum in relation to central nervous system function among metal inert-gas welders. Scand J Work Environ Health 2000;26(2):118–30.

[92] Crapper McLachlan DR, Dalton AJ, et al. Intramuscular desferrioxamine in patients with Alzheimer's disease. Lancet 1991;337(8757):1618.

[93] Kan WC, Chien CC, Wu CC, et al. Comparison of low-dose deferoxamine versus standard-dose deferoxamine for treatment of aluminum overload among haemodialysis patients. Nephrol Dial Transplant 2010;25(5):1604–8.

[94] Bernstam L, Nriagu J. Molecular aspects of arsenic stress. J Toxicol Environ Health B Crit Rev 2000;3(4):293–322.

[95] Valavanidis A, Vlachogianni T, Fiotakis C. 8-hydroxy-2′-deoxyguanosine(8-OHdG): a critical biomarker of oxidative stress and carcinogenesis. J Environ Sci Health C Environ Carcinog Ecotoxicol Rev 2009;27(2):120–39.

[96] Fujino Y, Guo X, Liu J, et al. Japan Inner Mongolia Arsenic Pollution Study Group. Chronic arsenic exposure and urinary 8-hydroxy-2′-deoxyguanosine in an arsenic-affected area in Inner Mongolia, China. J Expo Anal Environ Epidemiol 2005;15(2):147–52.

[97] Jomova K, Valko M. Advances in metal-induced oxidative stress and human disease. Toxicology 2011;283(2–3):65–87.

[98] Hall M, Gamble M, Slavkovich V, et al. Determinants of arsenic metabolism: blood arsenic metabolites, plasma folate, cobalamin, and homocysteine concentrations in maternal-newborn pairs. Environ Health Perspect 2007;115(10):1503–9.

[99] Kitchin KT, Ahmad S. Oxidative stress as a possible mode of action for arsenic carcinogenesis. Toxicol Lett 2003;137(1–2):3–13.

[100] Ren X, McHale CM, Skibola CF, et al. An emerging role for epigenetic dysregulation in arsenic toxicity and carcinogenesis. Environ Health Perspect 2011;119(1):11–19.

[101] Zhang A, Feng H, et al. Unventilated indoor coal-fired stoves in Guizhou province, China: cellular and genetic damage in villagers exposed to arsenic in food and air. Environ Health Perspect 2007;115(4):653–8.

[102] Boyce CP, Lewis AS, Sax SN, et al. Probabilistic analysis of human health risks associated with background concentrations of inorganic arsenic: use of a margin of exposure approach. Hum Ecol Risk Assess 2008;14:1159–201.

[103] Jomova K, et al. Arsenic: toxicity, oxidative stress and human disease. J Appl Toxicol 2011;31(2):95–107.

[104] Holtcamp W. Suspect sweetener: arsenic detected in organic brown rice syrup. Environ Health Perspect 2012;120(5):A204.

[105] Nielsen MG, Lombard PJ, Schalk LF. Assessment of arsenic concentrations in domestic well water, by town, in Maine, 2005-2009. US Geological survey Scientific Investigations Report 2010-5199. http://pubs.usgs.gov/sir/2010/5199/. [Accessed 21 August 2016].

[106] Sinha SK, Misbahuddin M, Ahmed AN. Factors involved in the development of chronic arsenic poisoning in Bangladesh. Arch Environ Health 2003;58(11):699–700.

[107] Wu CC, Chen MC, Huang YK, et al. Environmental tobacco smoke and arsenic methylation capacity are associated with urothelial carcinoma. J Formos Med Assoc 2013;112(9):554–60.

[108] Feki-Tounsi M, Olmedo P, Gil F, et al. Low-level arsenic exposure is associated with bladder cancer risk and cigarette smoking: a case-control study among men in Tunisia. Environ Sci Pollut Res Int 2013;20(6):3923–31.

[109] Haz-Map. https://hazmap.nlm.nih.gov/category-details?id=260&table=tblprocesses. [Accessed 17 August 2016].

[110] Lin TS, Wu CC, Wu JD, et al. Oxidative DNA damage estimated by urinary 8-hydroxy-2′-deoxyguanosine and arsenic in glass production workers. Toxicol Ind Health 2012;28(6):513–21.

[111] Arnold LL, Eldan M, Nyska A, et al. Dimethylarsinic acid: results of chronic toxicity/oncogenecity studies in F344 rats and in B6C3F1 mice. Toxicology 2006;223:82–100.

[112] Zahkaryan R, Aposhian V. Arsenite methylation by methylvitamin B12 and glutathione does not require an enzyme. Toxicol Appl Pharmacol 1999;154:287–91.

[113] Mandal BK, Suzuki KT. Arsenic round the world: a review. Talanta 2002;58(1):201–35.

[114] Dani SU, Walter GF. Chronic arsenic intoxication diagnostic score (CAsIDS). J Appl Toxicol 2018;38(1):122–44.

[115] IARC Working Group on the Evaluation of Carcinogenic Risks to Humans. Arsenic, metals, fibres, and dusts. IARC Monogr Eval Carcinog Risks Hum 2012;100(Pt C):11–465.

[116] Smith AH, Marshall G, et al. Mortality in young adults following in utero and childhood exposure to arsenic in drinking water. Environ Health Perspect 2012;120(11):1527–31.

[117] D'Ippoliti D, Santelli E, De Sario M, et al. Arsenic in drinking water and mortality for cancer and chronic diseases in central Italy, 1990-2010. PLoS ONE 2015;10(9):e0138182.

[118] Garcia-Esquinas E, Pollan M, et al. Arsenic exposure and cancer mortality in a US-based prospective cohort: the strong heart study. Cancer Epidemiol Biomarkers Prev 2013;22(11):1944–53.

[119] Diaz-Villasenor A, Burns AL, et al. Arsenic-induced alteration in the expression of genes related to type 2 diabetes mellitus. Toxicol Appl Pharmacol 2007;225(2):123–33.

[120] Lowenfels AB, Maisonneuve P. Epidemiology and risk factors for pancreatic cancer. Best Pract Res Clin Gastroenterol 2006;20(2):197–209.

[121] Yang CY, Chang CC, Chiu HF. Does arsenic exposure increase the risk for prostate cancer? J Toxicol Environ Health A 2008;71(23):1559–63.

[122] Gilbert-Diamond D, Li Z, Perry AE, et al. A population-based case-control study of urinary arsenic species and squamous cell carcinoma in New Hampshire, USA. Environ Health Perspect 2013;121(10):1154–60. Erratum in: Environ Health Perspect 2013;121(10):1159.

[123] Das D, Bindhani B, Mukherjee B, et al. Chronic low-level arsenic exposure reduces lung function in male population without skin lesions. Int J Public Health 2014;59(4):655–63.

[124] Abhyankar LN, Jones MR, Guallar E, et al. Arsenic exposure and hypertension: a systematic review. Environ Health Perspect 2012;120(4):494–500.

[125] O'Bryant SE, Edwards M, Menon CV, et al. Long-term low-level arsenic exposure is associated with poorer neuropsychological functioning: a Project FRONTIER study. Int J Environ Res Public Health 2011;8(3):861–74.

[126] Kuo CC, Weaver V, et al. Arsenic exposure, hyperuricemia, and gout in US adults. Environ Int 2015;76:32–40.

[127] Coronado-Gonzalez JA, Del Razo LM, Garcia-Vargas G, et al. Inorganic arsenic exposure and type 2 diabetes mellitus in Mexico. Environ Res 2007;104(3):383–9.

[128] Navas-Acien A, Silbergeld EK, Pastor-Barriuso R, et al. Arsenic exposure and prevalence of type 2 diabetes in US adults. JAMA 2008;300(7):814–22.

[129] Liu S, Guo X, Wu B, et al. Arsenic induces diabetic effects through beta-cell dysfunction and increased gluconeogenesis in mice. Sci Rep 2014;4:6894.

[130] Pan WC, Seow WJ, Kile ML, et al. Association of low to moderate levels of arsenic exposure with risk of type 2 diabetes in Bangladesh. Am J Epidemiol 2013;178(10):1563–70.

[131] Bhadauria S, Flora SJS. Response of arsenic-induced oxidative stress, DNA damage, and metal imbalance to combined administration of DMSA and monoisoamyl-DMSA during chronic arsenic poisoning in rats. Cell Biol Toxicol 2007;23(2):91–104.

[132] Chen C, Jiang X, Hu Y, et al. The protective role of resveratrol in the sodium arsenite-induced oxidative damage via modulation of intracellular GSH homeostasis. Biol Trace Elem Res 2013;155(1):119–31.

[133] Argos M, Rathouz PJ, Pierce BL, et al. Dietary B vitamin intakes and urinary total arsenic concentration in the Health Effects of Arsenic Longitudinal Study (HEALS) cohort, Bangladesh. Eur J Nutr 2010;49(8):473–81.

[134] Biswas J, Sinha D, Mukherjee S, et al. Curcumin protects DNA damage in a chronically arsenic-exposed population of West Bengal. Hum Exp Toxicol 2010;29(6):513–24.

[135] Gao S, Duan X, Wang X, et al. Curcumin attenuates arsenic-induced hepatic injuries and oxidative stress in experimental mice through activation of Nrf2 pathway, promotion of arsenic methylation and urinary excretion. Food Chem Toxicol 2013;59:739–47.

[136] Jiang G, Xu L, Song S, et al. Effects of long-term low-dose cadmium exposure on genomic DNA methylation in human embryo lung fibroblast cells. Toxicology 2008;244(1):49–55.

[137] Johnson MD, Kenney N, Stoica A, et al. Cadmium mimics the in vivo effects of estrogen in the uterus and mammary gland. Nat Med 2003;9(8):1081–4.

[138] Waalkes MP. Cadmium carcinogenesis. Mutat Res 2003;533(1–2):107–20.

[139] Waalkes MP. Cadmium carcinogenesis in review. J Inorg Biochem 2000;79:241–4.

[140] Brännvall E, Wolters M, Sjöblom R, et al. Elements availability in soil fertilized with pelletized fly ash and biosolids. J Environ Manage 2015;159:27–36.

[141] Abril JM, García-Tenorio R, Enamorado SM, et al. The cumulative effect of three decades of phosphogypsum amendments in reclaimed marsh soils from SW Spain: (226)Ra, (238)U and Cd contents in soils and tomato fruit. Sci Total Environ 2008;403(1–3):80–8.

[142] Garrick MD, Dolan KG, Horbinshy C, et al. DMT1: a mammalian transporter for multiple metals. Biometals 2003;16:41–54.

[143] Kippler M, Ekström EC, Lönnerdal B, et al. Influence of iron and zinc status on cadmium accumulation in Bangladeshi women. Toxicol Appl Pharmacol 2007;222(2):221–6.

[144] Reeves PG, Chaney RL. Bioavailability as an issue in risk assessment and management of food cadmium: a review. Sci Total Environ 2008;398(1–3):13–19.

[145] Ferraro PM, Costanzi S, Naticchia A, et al. Low level exposure to cadmium increases the risk of chronic kidney disease: analysis of the NHANES 1999-2006. BMC Public Health 2010;10:304.

[146] Ohta H, Cherian MG. Gastrointestinal absorption of cadmium and metallothionein. Toxicol Appl Pharmacol 1991;107:63–72.

[147] Järup L, Berglund M, Elinder CG, et al. Health effects of cadmium exposure – a review of the literature and a risk estimate. Scand J Work Environ Health 1998;24(Suppl. 1):1–51.

[148] Akesson A, Lundh T, Vahter M, et al. Tubular and glomerular kidney effects in Swedish women with low environmental cadmium exposure. Environ Health Perspect 2005;113(11):1627–31.

[149] Uno T, Kobayashi E, Suwazono Y, et al. Health effects of cadmium exposure in the general environment in Japan with special reference to the lower limit of the benchmark dose as the threshold level of urinary cadmium. Scand J Work Environ Health 2005;31(4):307–15.

[150] Tsuritani I, Honda R, et al. Impairment of vitamin D metabolism due to environmental cadmium exposure, and possible relevance to sex-related differences in vulnerability to the bone damage. J Toxicol Environ Health 1992;37(4):519–33.

[151] Emmerson BT. 'Ouch-ouch' disease: the osteomalacia of cadmium nephropathy. Ann Intern Med 1970;73(5):854–5.

[152] Wallin M, Sallsten G, Fabricius-Lagging E, et al. Kidney cadmium levels and associations with urinary calcium and bone mineral density: a cross-sectional study in Sweden. Environ Health 2013;12:22.

[153] Buchet JP, Lauwerys R, Roels H, et al. Renal effects of cadmium body burden of the general population. Lancet 1990;336(8717):699–702.

[154] Nogawa K, Tsuritani I, Kido T, et al. Mechanism for bone disease found in inhabitants environmentally exposed to cadmium: decreased serum 1 alpha, 25-dihydroxyvitamin D level. Int Arch Occup Environ Health 1987;59(1):21–30.

[155] Staessen JA, Roels HA, Emelianov D, et al. Environmental exposure to cadmium, forearm bone density, and risk of fractures: prospective population study. Public Health and Environmental Exposure to Cadmium (PheeCad) Study Group. Lancet 1999;353(9159):1140–4.

[156] Sughis M, Penders J, Haufroid V, et al. Bone resorption and environmental exposure to cadmium in children: a cross-sectional study. Environ Health 2011;10:104.

[157] Tellez-Plaza M, Navas-Acien A, Menke A, et al. Cadmium exposure and all-cause and cardiovascular mortality in the US general population. Environ Health Perspect 2012;120(7):1017–22.

[158] Gallagher CM, Meliker JR. Blood and urine cadmium, blood pressure, and hypertension: a systematic review and meta-analysis. Environ Health Perspect 2010;118(12):1676–84.

[159] Peters JL, Perlstein TS, Perry MJ, et al. Cadmium exposure in association with history of stroke and heart failure. Environ Res 2010;110(2):199–206.

[160] Kim NH, Hyun YY, Lee KB, et al. Environmental heavy metal exposure and chronic kidney disease in the general population. J Korean Med Sci 2015;30(3):272–7.

[161] Somji S, Zhou XD, et al. Urothelial cells malignantly transformed by exposure to cadmium (Cd(+2)) and arsenite (As(+3)) have increased resistance to Cd(+2) and As(+3)-induced cell death. Toxicol Sci 2006;94(2):293–301.

[162] Sens DA, Park S, et al. Inorganic cadmium- and arsenite-induced malignant transformation of human bladder urothelial cells. Toxicol Sci 2004;79(1):56–63.

[163] Kellen E, Zeegers MP, et al. Blood cadmium may be associated with bladder carcinogenesis: the Belgian case-control study on bladder cancer. Cancer Detect Prev 2007;31(1):77–82.

[164] Luckett BG, Su LJ, Rood JC, et al. Cadmium exposure and pancreatic cancer in south Louisiana. J Environ Public Health 2012;2012:180186.

[165] Gerhard I, Monga B, Waldbrenner A, et al. Heavy metals and fertility. J Toxicol Environ Health A 1998;54(8):593–611. Erratum in: J Toxicol Environ Health 1999;56(5):371.

[166] Gollenberg AL, Hediger ML, Lee PA, et al. Association between lead and cadmium and reproductive hormones in peripubertal US girls. Environ Health Perspect 2010;118(12):1782–7.

[167] Johnston JE, Valentiner E, Maxson P, et al. Maternal cadmium levels during pregnancy associated with lower birth weight in infants in a North Carolina cohort. PLoS ONE 2014;9(10):e109661.

[168] Akinloye O, Arowojolu AO, Shittu OB, et al. Cadmium toxicity: a possible cause of male infertility in Nigeria. Reprod Biol 2006;6(1):17–30.

[169] Hyder O, Chung M, Cosgrove D, et al. Cadmium exposure and liver disease among US adults. J Gastrointest Surg 2013;17(7):1265–73.

[170] Hossain MB, Vahter M, Concha G, et al. Low-level environmental cadmium exposure is associated with DNA hypomethylation in Argentinean women. Environ Health Perspect 2012;120(6):879–84.

[171] Lampe BJ, Park SK, Robins T, et al. Association between 24-hour urinary cadmium and pulmonary function among community-exposed men: the VA Normative Aging Study. Environ Health Perspect 2008;116(9):1226–30.

[172] Orlowski C, Piotrowski JK, Subdys JK, et al. Urinary cadmium as indicator of renal cadmium in humans: an autopsy study. Hum Exp Toxicol 1998;17(6):302–6.

[173] Andersen O. Chelation of cadmium. Environ Health Perspect 1984;54:249–66.

[174] Waters RS, Bryden NA, Patterson KY, et al. EDTA chelation effects on urinary losses of cadmium, calcium, chromium, cobalt, copper, lead, magnesium, and zinc. Biol Trace Elem Res 2001;83(3):207–21.

[175] Jones MM, Singh PK, Gale GR, et al. Cadmium mobilization in vivo by intraperitoneal or oral administration of mono alkyl esters of meso 2,3-dimercaptosuccinic acid in the mouse. Pharmacol Toxicol 1992;70(5 Pt 1):336–43.

[176] Gil HW, Kang EJ, Lee KH, et al. Effect of glutathione on the cadmium chelation of EDTA in a patient with cadmium intoxication. Hum Exp Toxicol 2011;30(1):79–83.

[177] Andersen O, Nielsen JB. Oral cadmium chloride intoxication in mice: effects of penicillamine, dimercaptosuccinic acid and related compounds. Pharmacol Toxicol 1988;63(5):386–9.

[178] Fang X, Hua F, Fernando Q. Comparison of rac- and meso-2,3-dimercaptosuccinic acids for chelation of mercury and cadmium using chemical speciation models. Chem Res Toxicol 1996;9(1):284–90.

[179] Cao Y, Chen A, Bottai M, et al. The impact of succimer chelation on blood cadmium in children with background exposures: a randomized trial. J Pediatr 2013;163(2):598–600.

[180] Ruprecht J. Dimaval (DMPS) monograph. 6th ed. Germany: HEYL Chem-pharm Fabrik GmbH & Co. Berlin; 1997.

[181] Tandon SK, Singh S, Prasad S. Influence of methionine administration during chelation of cadmium by CaNa(3)DTPA and DMPS in the rat. Environ Toxicol Pharmacol 1997;3(3):159–65.

[182] Fatemi SJ, Saljooghi AS, Balooch FD, et al. Removal of cadmium by combining deferasirox and desferrioxamine chelators in rats. Toxicol Ind Health 2012;28(1):35–41.

[183] Djukić-Cosić D, Ninković M, Malicević Z, et al. Effect of supplemental magnesium on the kidney levels of cadmium, zinc, and copper of mice exposed to toxic levels of cadmium. Biol Trace Elem Res 2006;114(1–3):281–91.

[184] Wei HJ. Influence of selenium supplement on cadmium metabolism in humans. Zhongguo Yi Xue Ke Xue Yuan Xue Bao 1989;11(3):185–9. Chinese.

[185] Khanna S, Mitra S, Lakhera PC, et al. N-acetylcysteine effectively mitigates cadmium-induced oxidative damage and cell death in Leydig cells in vitro. Drug Chem Toxicol 2016;39(1):74–80.

[186] Tandon SK, Prasad S, Singh S. Chelation in metal intoxication: influence of cysteine or N-acetyl cysteine on the efficacy of 2,3-dimercaptopropane-1-sulphonate in the treatment of cadmium toxicity. J Appl Toxicol 2002;22(1):67–71.

[187] Tandon SK, Singh S, Prasad S, et al. Reversal of cadmium induced oxidative stress by chelating agent, antioxidant or their combination in rat. Toxicol Lett 2003;145(3):211–17.

[188] Robertson A, Tenenbein M. Hepatotoxicity in acute iron poisoning. Hum Exp Toxicol 2005;24:559–62.

[189] Madiwale T, Liebelt E. Iron: not a benign therapeutic drug. Curr Opin Pediatr 2008;18:174–9.

[190] Chang TPY, Rangan C. Iron poisoning: a literature-based review of epidemiology, diagnosis, and management. Pediatr Emerg Care 2011;27:978–85.

[191] Ganz T, Nemeth E. Regulation of iron acquisition and iron distribution in mammals. Biochim Biophys Acta Mol Cell Res 2006;1763:690–9.

[192] Chyka PA, Butler AY, Holley JE. Serum iron concentrations and symptoms of acute iron poisoning in children. Pharmacotherapy 1996;16:1053–8.

[193] Borgna-Pignatti C, Cohen A. Evaluation of a new method of administration of the iron chelating agent deferoxamine. J Pediatr 1997;130:86–8.

[194] Vichinsky E. Consensus document for transfusion-related iron overload. Semin Hematol 2001;38(Suppl. 1):2–4.

[195] Zurlo MG, DeStefano P, Borgna-Pignatti C, et al. Survival and causes of death in thalassemia major. Lancet 1989;2:27–30.

[196] Olivieri NF, Nathan DG, MacMillan JH, et al. Survival in medically treated patients with homozygous B-thalassemia. N Engl J Med 1994;331:574–8.

[197] Barry M, Flynn DM, Letsky EA, et al. Long-term chelation therapy in thalassemia major: effect on liver iron concentration, liver histology, and clinical progress. Br Med J 1974;2:16–20.

[198] Cohen A, Martin M, Schwartz E. Depletion of excessive liver iron stores with desferoxamine. Br J Haematol 1984;58:369–74.

[199] Wolfe L, Oliveri N, Sallan D, et al. Prevention of cardiac disease by subcutaneous deferoxamine in patients with thalassemia major. N Engl J Med 1985;312:1600–3.

[200] Lopes AC, Peixe TS, Mesas AE, et al. Lead exposure and oxidative stress: a systematic review. Rev Environ Contam Toxicol 2016;236:193–238.

[201] Kasperczyk A, Dobrakowski M, Czuba ZP, et al. Environmental exposure to lead induces oxidative stress and modulates the function of the antioxidant defense system and the immune system in the semen of males with normal semen profile. Toxicol Appl Pharmacol 2015;284(3):339–44.

[202] Hsu PC, Guo YL. Antioxidant nutrients and lead toxicity. Toxicology 2002;180(1):33–44.

[203] Hong YC, Oh SY, Kwon SO, et al. Blood lead level modifies the association between dietary antioxidants and oxidative stress in an urban adult population. Br J Nutr 2013;109(1):148–54.

[204] Roy A, Queirolo E, Peregalli F, et al. Association of blood lead levels with urinary F2-8α isoprostane and 8-hydroxy-2-deoxy-guanosine concentrations in first-grade Uruguayan children. Environ Res 2015;140:127–35.

[205] Permpongpaiboon T, Nagila A, Pidetcha P, et al. Decreased paraoxonase 1 activity and increased oxidative stress in low lead-exposed workers. Hum Exp Toxicol 2011;30(9):1196–203.

[206] Dewalt FG, Cox DC, O'Haver R, et al. Prevalence of lead hazards and soil arsenic in US housing. J Environ Health 2015;78(5):22–9, quiz 52.

[207] Etchevers A, Le Tertre A, Lucas JP, et al. Environmental determinants of different blood lead levels in children: a quantile analysis from a nationwide survey. Environ Int 2015;74:152–9.

[208] Richter PA, Bishop EE, Wang J, et al. Trends in tobacco smoke exposure and blood lead levels among youths and adults in the United States: the National Health and Nutrition Examination Survey, 1999–2008. Prev Chronic Dis 2013;10:E213.

[209] Monro JA, Leon R, Puri BK. The risk of lead contamination in bone broth diets. Med Hypotheses 2013;80(4):389–90.

[210] Sheets RW. Acid extraction of lead and cadmium from newly-purchased ceramic and melamine dinnerware. Sci Total Environ 1999;234(1–3):233–7.

[211] Sheets RW. Extraction of lead, cadmium and zinc from overglaze decorations on ceramic dinnerware by acidic and basic food substances. Sci Total Environ 1997;197(1–3):167–75.

[212] Sheets RW, Turpen SL, Hill P. Effect of microwave heating on leaching of lead from old ceramic dinnerware. Sci Total Environ 1996;182(1–3):187–91.

[213] Mathee A, Naicker N, Teare J. Retrospective investigation of a lead poisoning outbreak from the consumption of an Ayurvedic medicine: Durban, South Africa. Int J Environ Res Public Health 2015;12(7):7804–13.

[214] Crinnion WJ. EDTA redistribution of lead and cadmium into the soft tissues in a human with a high lead burden – should DMSA always be used to follow EDTA in such cases? Altern Med Rev 2011;16(2):109–12.

[215] Greenway JA, Gerstenberger S. An evaluation of lead contamination in plastic toys collected from day care centers in the Las Vegas Valley, Nevada, USA. Bull Environ Contam Toxicol 2010;85(4):363–6.

[216] Maas RP, Patch SC, Pandolfo TJ. Artificial Christmas trees: how real are the lead exposure risks? J Environ Health 2004;67(5):20–4, 32.

[217] Daluga M, Miller K. Lead in your child's lunch box. Clin Pediatr (Phila) 2007;46(2):151–3.

[218] Svensson BG, Schütz A, Nilsson A, et al. Lead exposure in indoor firing ranges. Int Arch Occup Environ Health 1992;64(4):219–21.

[219] Hughes JT, Horan JJ, Powles CP. Lead poisoning caused by glazed pottery: case report. N Z Med J 1976;84(573):266–8.

[220] Fourth national report on human exposure to environmental chemicals. 2009. CDC. www.cdc.gov/exposurereport.

[221] Hu H, Shih R, Rothenberg S, et al. The epidemiology of lead toxicity in adults: measuring dose and consideration of other methodologic issues. Environ Health Perspect 2007;115(3):455–62.

[222] Kosnett MJ, Wedeen RP, Rothenberg SJ, et al. Recommendations for medical management of adult lead exposure. Environ Health Perspect 2007;115(3):463–71.

[223] Coon S, Stark A, Peterson E, et al. Whole-body lifetime occupational lead exposure and risk of Parkinson's disease. Environ Health Perspect 2006;114(12):1872–6.

[224] Weisskopf MG, Weuve J, Nie H, et al. Association of cumulative lead exposure with Parkinson's disease. Environ Health Perspect 2010;118(11):1609–13.

[225] Bakulski KM, Rozek LS, Dolinoy DC, et al. Alzheimer's disease and environmental exposure to lead: the epidemiologic evidence and potential role of epigenetics. Curr Alzheimer Res 2012;9(5):563–73.

[226] Shih RA, Glass TA, Bandeen-Roche K, et al. Environmental lead exposure and cognitive function in community-dwelling older adults. Neurology 2006;67(9):1556–62.

[227] Wedeen RP, D'Haese P, Van de Vyver FL, et al. Lead nephropathy. Am J Kidney Dis 1986;8(5):380–3.

[228] Craswell PW, Price J, Boyle PD, et al. Chronic lead nephropathy in Queensland: alternative methods of diagnosis. Aust N Z J Med 1986;16(1):11–19.

[229] Yokoyama K, Araki S, Aono H. Reversibility of psychological performance in subclinical lead absorption. Neurotoxicology 1988;9(3):405–10.

[230] Araki S, Murata K, Aono H. Subclinical cervico-spino-bulbar effects of lead: a study of short-latency somatosensory evoked potentials in workers exposed to lead, zinc, and copper. Am J Ind Med 1986;10(2):163–75.

[231] Tuthill R. Hair lead levels related to children's classroom attention deficit behavior. Arch Environ Health 1996;51(3):214–20.

[232] Needleman H, Schell A, Bellinger D, et al. The long-term effects of exposure to low doses of lead in childhood. N Engl J Med 1990;322(2):83–8.

[233] Iqbal S, Muntner P, Batuman V, et al. Estimated burden of blood lead levels 5 μg/dl in 1999-2002 and declines from 1988 to 1994. Environ Res 2008;107(3):305–11.

[234] Lee CM, Terrizzi AR, Bozzini C, et al. Chronic lead poisoning magnifies bone detrimental effects in an ovariectomized rat model of postmenopausal osteoporosis. Exp Toxicol Pathol 2016;68(1):47–53.

[235] Monir AU, Gundberg CM, et al. The effect of lead on bone mineral properties from female adult C57/BL6 mice. Bone 2010;47(5):888–94.

[236] Goyer RA, Epstein S, et al. Environmental risk factors for osteoporosis. Environ Health Perspect 1994;102(4):390–4.

[237] Rosen JF, Chesney RW, et al. Reduction in 1,25-dihydroxyvitamin D in children with increased lead absorption. N Engl J Med 1980;302(20):1128–31.

[238] Wesseling C, Pukkala E, et al. Cancer of the brain and nervous system and occupational exposures in Finnish women. J Occup Environ Med 2002;44(7):663–8.

[239] Silbergeld EK, Schwartz J, Mahaffey K. Lead and osteoporosis: mobilization of lead from bone in postmenopausal women. Environ Res 1988;47(1):79–94.

[240] Krishnan E, Lingala B, Bhalla V. Low-level lead exposure and the prevalence of gout: an observational study. Ann Intern Med 2012;157(4):233–41.

[241] Canfield RL, Henderson CR Jr, Cory-Slechta DA, et al. Intellectual impairment in children with blood lead concentrations below 10 microg per deciliter. N Engl J Med 2003;348(16):1517–26.

[242] Jusko TA, Henderson CR, Lanphear BP, et al. Blood lead concentrations < 10 microg/dL and child intelligence at 6 years of age. Environ Health Perspect 2008;116(2):243–8.

[243] Lanphear BP, Hornung R, Khoury J, et al. Low-level environmental lead exposure and children's intellectual function: an international pooled analysis. Environ Health Perspect 2005;113(7):894–9.

[244] Lucchini RG, Zoni S, Guazzetti S, et al. Inverse association of intellectual function with very low blood lead but not with manganese exposure in Italian adolescents. Environ Res 2012;118:65–71.

[245] Mazumdar M, Bellinger DC, Gregas M, et al. Low-level environmental lead exposure in childhood and adult intellectual function: a follow-up study. Environ Health 2011;10:24.

[246] Boucher O, Jacobson SW, Plusquellec P, et al. Prenatal methylmercury, postnatal lead exposure, and evidence of attention deficit/hyperactivity disorder among Inuit children in Arctic Québec. Environ Health Perspect 2012;120(10):1456–61.

[247] Vaziri ND, Ding Y. Effect of lead on nitric oxide synthase expression in coronary endothelial cells: role of superoxide. Hypertension 2001;37(2):223–6.

[248] Tsaih SW, Korrick S, Schwartz J, et al. Lead, diabetes, hypertension, and renal function: the normative aging study. Environ Health Perspect 2004;112(11):1178–82.

[249] Park SK, Mukherjee B, Xia X, et al. Bone lead level prediction models and their application to examine the relationship of lead exposure and hypertension in the Third National Health and Nutrition Examination Survey. J Occup Environ Med 2009;51(12):1422–36.

[250] Peters JL, Kubzansky LD, Ikeda A, et al. Lead concentrations in relation to multiple biomarkers of cardiovascular disease: the Normative Aging Study. Environ Health Perspect 2012;120(3):361–6.

[251] Eum KD, Nie LH, Schwartz J, et al. Prospective cohort study of lead exposure and electrocardiographic conduction disturbances in the Department of Veterans Affairs Normative Aging Study. Environ Health Perspect 2011;119(7):940–4.

[252] Schafer JH, Glass TA, Bressler J, et al. Blood lead is a predictor of homocysteine levels in a population-based study of older adults. Environ Health Perspect 2005;113(1):31–5.

[253] Wedeen RP, Batuman V, Landy E. The safety of the EDTA lead-mobilization test. Environ Res 1983;30(1):58–62.

[254] Markowitz ME, Rosen JF. Need for the lead mobilization test in children with lead poisoning. J Pediatr 1991;119(2):305–10.

[255] Wedeen RP. Use of the CaNa2 EDTA Pb-mobilization test to detect occult lead nephropathy. Uremia Invest 1985–1986;9(2):127–30.

[256] Shannon M, Grace A, Graef J. Use of urinary lead concentration in interpretation of the EDTA mobilization test. Vet Hum Toxicol 1989;31(2):140–2.

[257] Chen KH, Lin JL, Lin-Tan DT, et al. Effect of chelation therapy on progressive diabetic nephropathy in patients with type 2 diabetes and high-normal body lead burdens. Am J Kidney Dis 2012; 60(4):530–8.

[258] Hoet P, Buchet JP, Decerf L, et al. Clinical evaluation of a lead mobilization test using the chelating agent dimercaptosuccinic acid. Clin Chem 2006;52(1):88–96.

[259] Tassler PL, Schwartz BS, Coresh J, et al. Associations of tibia lead, DMSA-chelatable lead, and blood lead with measures of peripheral nervous system function in former organolead manufacturing workers. Am J Ind Med 2001;39(3):254–61.

[260] Schwartz BS, Lee BK, Lee GS, et al. Associations of blood lead, dimercaptosuccinic acid-chelatable lead, and tibia lead with neurobehavioral test scores in South Korean lead workers. Am J Epidemiol 2001;153(5):453–64.

[261] Lee BK, Ahn KD, Lee SS, et al. A comparison of different lead biomarkers in their associations with lead-related symptoms. Int Arch Occup Environ Health 2000;73(5):298–304.

[262] Bradberry S, Vale A. A comparison of sodium calcium edetate (edetate calcium disodium) and succimer (DMSA) in the treatment of inorganic lead poisoning. Clin Toxicol (Phila) 2009;47(9):841–58.

[263] Chisolm JJ Jr. Safety and efficacy of meso-2,3-dimercaptosuccinic acid (DMSA) in children with elevated blood lead concentrations. J Toxicol Clin Toxicol 2000;38(4):365–75.

[264] Dietrich KN, Ware JH, Salganik M, et al. Treatment of lead-exposed children clinical trial group. Effect of chelation therapy on the neuropsychological and behavioral development of lead-exposed children after school entry. Pediatrics 2004;114(1):19–26.

[265] Fournier L, Thomas G, Garner R, et al. 2, 3-dimercaptosuccinic acid treatment of heavy metal poisoning in humans. Med Toxicol Adverse Drug Exp 1988;3(6):499–504.

[266] Bradberry S, Sheehan T, Vale A. Use of oral dimercaptosuccinic acid (succimer) in adult patients with inorganic lead poisoning. QJM 2009;102(10):721–32.

[267] Zhang J, Wang XF, Lu ZB, et al. The effects of meso-2,3-dimercaptosuccinic acid and oligomeric procyanidins on acute lead neurotoxicity in rat hippocampus. Free Radic Biol Med 2004;37(7):1037–50.

[268] Lee BK, Schwartz BS, Stewart W, et al. Provocative chelation with DMSA and EDTA: evidence for differential access to lead storage sites. Occup Environ Med 1995;52(1):13–19.

[269] Lin JL, Lin-Tan DT, Hsu KH, et al. Environmental lead exposure and progression of chronic renal diseases in patients without diabetes. N Engl J Med 2003;348(4):277–86.

[270] Tantanasrikul S, Chaivisuth B, Siriratanapreuk S, et al. The management of environmental lead exposure in the pediatric population: lessons from Clitty Creek, Thailand. J Med Assoc Thai 2002;85(Suppl. 2):S762–8.

[271] Pande M, Flora SJ. Lead induced oxidative damage and its response to combined administration of alpha-lipoic acid and succimers in rats. Toxicology 2002;177(2–3):187–96.

[272] Sivaprasad R, Nagaraj M, Varalakshmi P. Combined efficacies of lipoic acid and 2,3-dimercaptosuccinic acid against lead-induced lipid peroxidation in rat liver. J Nutr Biochem 2004;15(1):18–23.

[273] Weiss B, Cory-Slechta DA, Cox C. Modification of lead distribution by diethyldithiocarbamate. Fundam Appl Toxicol 1990;15(4): 791–9.

[274] Cory-Slechta DA, Weiss B, Cox C. Mobilization and redistribution of lead over the course of calcium disodium ethylenediamine tetraacetate chelation therapy. J Pharmacol Exp Ther 1987;243(3):804–13.

[275] Lin-Tan DT, Lin JL, Yen TH, et al. Long-term outcome of repeated lead chelation therapy in progressive non-diabetic chronic kidney diseases. Nephrol Dial Transplant 2007;22(10):2924–31.

[276] Čabarkapa A, Borozan S, Živković L, et al. CaNa2EDTA chelation attenuates cell damage in workers exposed to lead – a pilot study. Chem Biol Interact 2015;242:171–8.

[277] Gupta SC, Prasad S, Kim JH, et al. Multitargeting by curcumin as revealed by molecular interaction studies. Nat Prod Rep 2011;28(12):1937–55.

[278] Shukla PK, Khanna VK, Khan MY, et al. Protective effect of curcumin against lead neurotoxicity in rat. Hum Exp Toxicol 2003;22(12):653–8.

[279] Flora G, Gupta D, Tiwari A. Preventive efficacy of bulk and nanocurcumin against lead-induced oxidative stress in mice. Biol Trace Elem Res 2013;152(1):31–40.

[280] Miller OM, Lund BO, Woods JS. Reactivity of Hg(II) with superoxide: evidence for the catalytic dismutation of superoxide by Hg(II). J Biochem Toxicol 1991;6:293–8.

[281] Zalups RK, Lash LH. Interactions between glutathione and mercury in the kidney, liver and blood. In: Chang LW, editor. Toxicology of metals. Boca Raton: CRC Press; 1996. p. 145–63.

[282] Motts JA, Shirley DL, Silbergeld EK, et al. Novel biomarkers of mercury-induced autoimmune dysfunction: a cross-sectional study in Amazonian Brazil. Environ Res 2014;132:12–18.

[283] Pollack AZ, Sjaarda L, Ahrens KA, et al. Association of cadmium, lead and mercury with paraoxonase 1 activity in women. PLoS ONE 2014;9(3):e92152.

[284] Durham HD, Minotti S, Caporicci E. Sensitivity of platelet microtubules to disassembly by methylmercury. J Toxicol Environ Health 1997;48:57–69.

[285] Falconer MM, Vaillant A, Reuhl KR, et al. The molecular basis of microtubule stability in neurons. Neurotoxicology 1994;15: 109–22.

[286] Miura K, Koide N, Himeno S, et al. The involvement of microtubular disruption in methylmercury-induced apoptosis in neuronal and nonneuronal cell lines. Toxicol Appl Phamacol 1999;160:279–88.

[287] InSug O, Datar S, Koch CJ, et al. Mercuric compounds inhibit human monocyte function by inducing apoptosis: evidence for formation of reactive oxygen species, development of mitochondrial membrane permeability transition and loss of reductive reserve. Toxicol 1997;124:211–24.

[288] Shenker BJ, Guo TL, Shapiro IM. Low-level methylmercury exposure causes human T-cells to undergo apoptosis: evidence of mitochondrial dysfunction. Environ Res 1998;77: 149–59.

[289] Goldberg RL, Kaplan SR, Fuller GC. Effect of heavy metals on human rheumatoid synovial cell proliferation and collagen synthesis. Biochem Pharmacol 1983;32(18):2763–6.

[290] Dufault R, LeBlanc B, Schnoll R, et al. Mercury from chlor-alkali plants: measured concentrations in food product sugar. Environ Health 2009;8:2.

[291] Reis AT, Rodrigues SM, Araújo C, et al. Mercury contamination in the vicinity of a chlor-alkali plant and potential risks to local population. Sci Total Environ 2009;407(8):2689–700.

[292] Agency for Toxic Substances and Disease Registry (ATSDR). 1999 toxicological profile for mercury. http://www.atsdr.cdc.gov/substances/toxsubstance.asp?toxid=24. [Accessed 26 September 2016].

[293] Maloney SR, Phillips CA, Mills A. Mercury in the hair of crematoria workers. Lancet 1998;352:1602.

[294] Mahaffey KR, Clickner RP, Bodurow CC. Blood organic mercury and dietary mercury intake: National Health and Nutrition Examination Survey, 1999 and 2000. Environ Health Perspect 2004;112(5):562–70.

[295] Sunderland EM, Krabbenhoft DP, Moreau JW, et al. Mercury sources, distribution, and bioavailability in the North Pacific Ocean: insights from data and models. Global Biogeochem Cycles 2009;2009:23. doi:10.1029/2008GB003425.

[296] Mercury in fish: cause for concern? U.S. Food and Drug Administration, FDA Consumer September 1994, Revised May 1995.

[297] Vimy MJ, Lorsheider FL. Intra-oral air mercury released from dental amalgams. J Dent Res 1985;64(8):1069–71.

[298] Vimy MF, Lorsheider FL. Serial measurements of intra-oral air mercury: estimation of daily dose from dental amalgams. J Dent Res 1985;64(8):1072–5.

[299] Patterson JE, Weissberg B, Dennison PJ. Mercury in human breath from dental amalgam. Bull Environ Contam Toxicol 1985;34:459–68.

[300] Anthony H, Birtwistle S, Eaton K, et al, editors. Environmental medicine in practice. Southhamptom: BSAENM Publications; 1997. p. 204–8.

[301] Abraham JE, Svare CW, Frank CW. The effect of dental amalgam restorations on blood mercury levels. J Dent Res 1984;63(1):71–3.

[302] Suzuki T, Hongo T, Yoshinaga J, et al. The hair-organ relationship in mercury concentration in contemporary Japanese. Arch Environ Health 1993;48(4):221–9.

[303] Kerper LE, Ballatori N, Clarkson TW. Methylmercury transport across the blood-brain barrier by an amino acid carrier. Am J Physiol 1992;262(5 Pt 2):R761–5.

[304] Clarkson TW, Hursh JB, Sager PR, et al. Mercury. In: Clarkson TW, Friber L, Nordberg GF, et al, editors. Biological monitoring of toxic metals. New York: Plenum Press; 1988. p. 199–246.

[305] Barregård L, Sällsten G, Schütz A, et al. Kinetics of mercury in blood and urine after brief occupational exposure. Arch Environ Health 1992;47(3):176–84.

[306] Sandborgh-Englund G, Elinder CG, Johanson G, et al. The absorption, blood levels, and excretion of mercury after a single dose of mercury vapor in humans. Toxicol Appl Pharmacol 1998;150(1):146–53.

[307] Kershaw TG, Clarkson TW, Dhahir PH. The relationship between blood levels and dose of methylmercury in man. Arch Environ Health 1980;35(1):28–36.

[308] Miettinen JK. Absorption and elimination of dietary mercury(2+) ion and methylmercury in man. In: Miller MW, Clarkson TW, editors. Mercury, mercurials, and mercaptans. Proceedings 4th International Conference on Environmental Toxicology. New York: Plenum Press; 1973.

[309] Bridges CC, Joshee L, van den Heuvel JJ, et al. Glutathione status and the renal elimination of inorganic mercury in the Mrp2(-/-) mouse. PLoS ONE 2013;8(9):e73559.

[310] Fuhr BJ, Rabenstein DL. Nuclear magnetic resonance studies of the solution chemistry of metal complexes. IX. The binding of cadmium, zinc, lead, and mercury by glutathione. J Am Chem Soc 1973;95(21):6944–50.

[311] De Souza Queiroz ML, Pena SC, Salles TSI, et al. Abnormal antioxidant system in erythrocytes of mercury exposed workers. Human & Exp. Toxicol 1998;17:225–30.

[312] Alexander J, Aaseth J. Organ distribution and cellular uptake of methyl mercury in the rat as influenced by the intra- and extracellular glutathione concentration. Biochem Pharmacol 1982;31(5):685–90.

[313] Chang LW. Neurotoxic effects of mercury. A review. Environ Res 1977;14:329–73.

[314] Wojcik DP, Godfrey ME, Christie D, et al. Mercury toxicity presenting as chronic fatigue, memory impairment and depression: diagnosis, treatment, susceptibility, and outcomes in a New Zealand general practice setting (1994–2006). Neuro Endocrinol Lett 2006;27(4):415–23.

[315] Lam HS, Kwok KM, Chan PH, et al. Long term neurocognitive impact of low dose prenatal methylmercury exposure in Hong Kong (China). Environ Int 2013;54:59–64.

[316] Wu J, Ying T, Shen Z, et al. Effect of low-level prenatal mercury exposure on neonate neurobehavioral development in China. Pediatr Neurol 2014;51(1):93–9.

[317] Jacobson JL, Muckle G, Ayotte P, et al. Relation of prenatal methylmercury exposure from environmental sources to childhood IQ. Environ Health Perspect 2015;123(8):827–33.

[318] Boucher O, Jacobson SW, Plusquellec P, et al. Prenatal methylmercury, postnatal lead exposure, and evidence of attention deficit/hyperactivity disorder among Inuit children in Arctic Québec. Environ Health Perspect 2012;120(10):1456–61.

[319] Ngim CH, Foo SC, Boey KW, et al. Chronic neurobehavioural effects of elemental mercury in dentists. Br J Ind Med 1992;49:782–90.

[320] Echeverria D, Woods JS, Heyer NJ, et al. The association between a genetic polymorphism of coproporphyrinogen oxidase, dental mercury exposure and neurobehavioral response in humans. Neurotoxicol Teratol 2006;28(1):39–48.

[321] Bridges CC, Joshee L, Zalups RK. Aging and the disposition and toxicity of mercury in rats. Exp Gerontol 2014;53:31–9.

[322] Atchison WD, Hare MF. Mechanisms of methylmercury-induced neurotoxicity. FASEB J 1994;8(9):622–9.

[323] Lee H, Kim Y, Sim CS, et al. Associations between blood mercury levels and subclinical changes in liver enzymes among South Korean general adults: analysis of 2008-2012 Korean national health and nutrition examination survey data. Environ Res 2014;130:14–19.

[324] Seo MS, Lee HR, Shim JY, et al. Relationship between blood mercury concentrations and serum γ-glutamyltranspeptidase level in Korean adults using data from the 2010 Korean National Health and Nutrition Examination Survey. Clin Chim Acta 2014;430:160–3.

[325] Lin TH, Huang YL, Huang SF. Lipid peroxidation in liver of rats administered with methyl mercuric chloride. Biol Trace Elem Res 1996;54(1):33–41.

[326] Inoue S, Yorifuji T, Tsuda T, et al. Short-term effect of severe exposure to methylmercury on atherosclerotic heart disease and hypertension mortality in Minamata. Sci Total Environ 2012;417–18:291–3.

[327] Yorifuji T, Tsuda T, Kashima S, et al. Long-term exposure to methylmercury and its effects on hypertension in Minamata. Environ Res 2010;110(1):40–6.

[328] Goodrich JM, Wang Y, Gillespie B, et al. Methylmercury and elemental mercury differentially associate with blood pressure among dental professionals. Int J Hyg Environ Health 2013;216(2):195–201.

[329] Hong D, Cho SH, Park SJ, et al. Hair mercury level in smokers and its influence on blood pressure and lipid metabolism. Environ Toxicol Pharmacol 2013;36(1):103–7.

[330] Salonen JT, Seppänen K, Lakka TA, et al. Mercury accumulation and accelerated progression of carotid atherosclerosis: a population-based prospective 4-year follow-up study in men in eastern Finland. Atherosclerosis 2000;148(2):265–73.

[331] Frustaci A, Magnavita N, Chimenti C, et al. Marked elevation of myocardial trace elements in idiopathic dilated cardiomyopathy compared with secondary cardiac dysfunction. J Am Coll Cardiol 1999;33(6):1578–83.

[332] Wennberg M, Strömberg U, Bergdahl IA, et al. Myocardial infarction in relation to mercury and fatty acids from fish: a risk-benefit analysis based on pooled Finnish and Swedish data in men. Am J Clin Nutr 2012;96(4):706–13.

[333] Nishida M, Yamamoto T, Yoshimura Y, et al. Subacute toxicity of methylmercuric chloride and mercuric chloride on mouse thyroid. J Pharmacobiodyn 1986;9(4):331–8.

[334] Tan SW, Meiller JC, Mahaffey KR. The endocrine effects of mercury in humans and wildlife. Crit Rev Toxicol 2009;39(3):228–69.

[335] Chen YW, Huang CF, Yang CY, et al. Inorganic mercury causes pancreatic beta-cell death via the oxidative stress-induced apoptotic and necrotic pathways. Toxicol Appl Pharmacol 2010;243(3):323–31.

[336] Chung JY, Seo MS, Shim JY, et al. Sex differences in the relationship between blood mercury concentration and metabolic syndrome risk. J Endocrinol Invest 2015;38(1):65–71.

[337] He K, Xun P, Liu K, et al. Mercury exposure in young adulthood and incidence of diabetes later in life: the CARDIA Trace Element Study. Diabetes Care 2013;36(6):1584–9.

[338] Harada M, Nakanishi J, Kunuma S, et al. The present mercury contents of scalp hair and clinical symptoms in inhabitants of the Minamata area. Environ Res 1998;77:160–4.

[339] Ruha AM, Curry SC, Gerkin RD, et al. Urine mercury excretion following meso-dimercaptosuccinic acid challenge in fish eaters. Arch Pathol Lab Med 2009;133(1):87–92.

[340] Halbach S, Kremers L, Willruth H, et al. Compartmental transfer of mercury released from amalgam. Hum Exp Toxicol 1997;16:667–72.

[341] Aposhian HV, Maiorino RM, Gonzalez-Ramirez D, et al. Mobilization of heavy metals by newer, therapeutically useful chelating agents. Toxicology 1995;97(1–3):23–38.

[342] Maiorino RM, Gonzalez-Ramirez D, Zuniga-Charles M, et al. Sodium 2,3-dimercaptopropane-1-sulfonate challenge test for mercury in humans. III. Urinary mercury after exposure to mercurous chloride. J Pharmacol Exp Ther 1996;277(2):938–44.

[343] Gonzalez-Ramirez D, Maiorino RM, Zuniga-Charles M, et al. Sodium 2,3-dimercaptopropane-1-sulfonate challenge test for mercury in humans: II. Urinary mercury, porphyrins and neurobehavioral changes of dental workers in Monterrey, Mexico. J Pharmacol Exp Ther 1995;272:264–74.

[344] Molin M, Schütz A, Skerfving S, et al. Mobilized mercury in subjects with varying exposure to elemental mercury vapour. Int Arch Occup Environ Health 1991;63(3):187–92.

[345] Aposhian HV. Mobilization of mercury and arsenic in humans by sodium 2,3-dimercapto-1-propane sulfonate (DMPS). Environ Health Perspect 1998;106(Suppl. 4):1017–25.

[346] Roels HA, Boeckx M, Ceulemans E, et al. Urinary excretion of mercury after occupational exposure to mercury vapour and influence of the chelating agent meso-2,3-dimercaptosuccinic acid (DMSA). Br J Ind Med 1991;48(4):247–53.

[347] Aposhian HV, Bruce DC, Alter W, et al. Urinary mercury after administration of 2,3-dimercaptopropane-1-sulfonic acid: correlation with dental amalgam score. FASEB J 1992;6(7):2472–6.

[348] Hibberd AR, Howard MA, Hunnisett AG. Mercury from dental amalgam fillings: studies on oral chelating agents for assessing and reducing mercury burdens in humans. J Nutr Environ Med 1998;8:219–31.

[349] Aposhian HV. DMSA and DMPS-water soluble antidotes for heavy metal poisoning. Annu Rev Pharmacol Toxicol 1983;23:193–215.

[350] Roels HA, Boeckx M, Ceulemans E, et al. Urinary excretion of mercury after occupational exposure to mercury vapour and influence of the chelating agent meso-2,3-dimercaptosuccinic acid (DMSA). Br J Ind Med 1991;48(4):247–53.

[351] Ruha AM, Curry SC, Gerkin RD, et al. Urine mercury excretion following meso-dimercaptosuccinic acid challenge in fish eaters. Arch Pathol Lab Med 2009;133(1):87–92.

[352] Böse-O'Reilly S, Drasch G, Beinhoff C, et al. The Mt. Diwata study on the Philippines 2000-treatment of mercury intoxicated inhabitants of a gold mining area with DMPS (2,3-dimercapto-1-propane-sulfonic acid, Dimaval). Sci Total Environ 2003;307(1–3):71–82.

[353] Pingree SD, Simmonds PL, Woods JS. Effects of 2,3-dimercapto-1-propanesulfonic acid (DMPS) on tissue and urine mercury levels following prolonged methylmercury exposure in rats. Toxicol Sci 2001;61(2):224–33.

[354] Bradberry SM, Sheehan TM, Barraclough CR, et al. DMPS can reverse the features of severe mercury vapor-induced neurological damage. Clin Toxicol (Phila) 2009;47(9):894–8.

[355] Bridges CC, Joshee L, Zalups RK. MRP2 and the DMPS- and DMSA-mediated elimination of mercury in TR(-) and control rats exposed to thiol S-conjugates of inorganic mercury. Toxicol Sci 2008;105(1):211–20.

[356] Bridges CC, Joshee L, Zalups RK. Effect of DMPS and DMSA on the placental and fetal disposition of methylmercury. Placenta 2009;30(9):800–5.

[357] Zalups RK, Bridges CC. MRP2 involvement in renal proximal tubular elimination of methylmercury mediated by DMPS or DMSA. Toxicol Appl Pharmacol 2009;235(1):10–17.

[358] Zalups RK, Bridges CC. Relationships between the renal handling of DMPS and DMSA and the renal handling of mercury. Chem Res Toxicol 2012;25(9):1825–38.

[359] Lund ME, Banner W Jr, Clarkson TW, et al. Treatment of acute methylmercury ingestion by hemodialysis with N-acetylcysteine (Mucomyst) infusion and 2,3-dimercaptopropane sulfonate. J Toxicol Clin Toxicol 1984;22(1):31–49.

[360] Ballatori N, Lieberman MW, Wang W. N-acetylcysteine as an antidote in methylmercury poisoning. Environ Health Perspect 1998;106(5):267–71.

[361] Ekor M, Adesanoye OA, Farombi EO. N-acetylcysteine pretreatment ameliorates mercuric chloride-induced oxidative renal damage in rats. Afr J Med Med Sci 2010;39(Suppl.):153–60.

[362] Kelly GS. Clinical applications of N-acetylcysteine. Altern Med Rev 1998;3(2):114–27.

[363] Corsello S, Fulgenzi A, Vietti D, et al. The usefulness of chelation therapy for the remission of symptoms caused by previous treatment with mercury-containing pharmaceuticals: a case report. Cases J 2009;2:199.

[364] No authors listed. Toxicity of thallium. Br Med J 1972;3(5829):717.

[365] Ning Z, He L, Xiao T, et al. High accumulation and subcellular distribution of thallium in green cabbage (Brassica oleracea L. Var. Capitata L). Int J Phytoremediation 2015;17(11):1097–104.

[366] Paton WD. Toxicity of thallium. Br Med J 1972;4(5831):49.

[367] Hoffman RS. Thallium toxicity and the role of Prussian blue in therapy. Toxicol Rev 2003;22:29–40.

[368] Montes S, Perez-Barron G, Rubio-Osornio M, et al. Additive effect of DL-penicillamine plus Prussian blue for the antidotal treatment of thallotoxicosis in rats. Environ Toxicol Pharmacol 2011;32:349–55.

[369] Cheung AC, Banerjee S, Cherian JJ, et al. Systemic cobalt toxicity from total hip arthroplasties: review of a rare condition Part 1 – history, mechanism, measurements, and pathophysiology. Bone Joint J 2016;98-B(1):6–13.

[370] MacDonald SJ. Metal-on-metal total hip arthroplasty: the concerns. Clin Orthop Relat Res 2004;429:86–93.

[371] Visuri T, Pukkala E, Paavolainen P, et al. Cancer risk after metal-on-metal and polyethylene-on-metal total hip arthroplasty. Clin Orthop 1996;329(Suppl.):280–9.

[372] Oldenburg M, Wegner R, Baur X. Severe cobalt intoxication due to prosthesis wear in repeated total hip arthroplasty. J Arthroplasty 2009;24(5):825.e15–20.

[373] Dijkman MA, de Vries I, Mulder-Spijkerboer H, et al. Cobalt poisoning due to metal-on-metal hip implants. Ned Tijdschr Geneeskd 2012;156(42):A4983.

[374] Hallab NJ, Caicedo M, Finnegan A, et al. Th1 type lymphocyte reactivity to metals in patients with total hip arthroplasty. J Orthop Surg Res 2008;3:6.

[375] Cugell DW. The hard metal diseases. Clin Chest Med 1992;13(2):269–79.

[376] Cugell DW, Morgan WK, Perkins DG, et al. The respiratory effects of cobalt. Arch Intern Med 1990;150(1):177–83.

[377] Migliori M, Mosconi G, Michetti G, et al. Hard metal disease: eight workers with interstitial lung fibrosis due to cobalt exposure. Sci Total Environ 1994;150(1–3):187–96.

[378] Davison AG, Haslam PL, Corrin B, et al. Interstitial lung disease and asthma in hard-metal workers: bronchoalveolar lavage, ultrastructural, and analytical findings and results of bronchial provocation tests. Thorax 1983;38(2):119–28.

[379] Pandit H, Glyn-Jones S, McLardy-Smith P, et al. Pseudotumours associated with metal-on-metal hip resurfacings. J Bone Joint Surg Br 2008;90(7):847–51.

[380] Devlin JJ, Schwartz M, Brent J. Chelation in suspected prosthetic hip-associated cobalt toxicity. Can J Cardiol 2013;29(11):1533.e7.

[381] Hannemann F, Hartmann A, Schmitt J, et al. European multidisciplinary consensus statement on the use an monitoring of metal-on-metal bearings for total hip replacement and hip resurfacing. Orthop Traumatol Surg Res 2013;99(3):263–71.

[382] Llobet JM, Domingo JL, Corbella J. Comparison of antidotal efficacy of chelating agents upon acute toxicity of Co(II) in mice. Res Commun Chem Pathol Pharmacol 1985;50(2):305–8.

[383] Llobet JM, Domingo JL, Corbella J. Comparison of the effectiveness of several chelators after single administration on the toxicity, excretion and distribution of cobalt. Arch Toxicol 1986;58(4):278–81.

[384] Giampreti A, Lonati D, Ragghianti B, et al. N-acetyl-cysteine as effective and safe chelating agent in metal-on-metal hip-implanted patients: two cases. Case Rep Orthop 2016;2016:8682737.

[385] Physicians' desk reference. 54th ed. Montvale, NJ: Medical Economics; 2000.

[386] Verschoor M, Herber R, Van Hemmen J, et al. Renal function of workers with low-level cadmium exposure. Scand J Work Environ Health 1987;13:232–8.

[387] Suzuki T, Yamamoto R. Organic mercury levels in human hair with and without storage for eleven years. Bull Environ Contam Toxicol 1982;28:186–8.

[388] Airey D. Mercury in human hair due to environment and diet. A review. Environ Health Perspect 1983;52:303–16.

[389] Bencko V. Use of human hair as a biomarker in the assessment of exposure to pollutants in occupational and environmental settings. Toxicology 1995;101:29–39.

[390] Rooney JP. The role of thiols, dithiols, nutritional factors and interacting ligands in the toxicology of mercury. Toxicology 2007;234(3):145–56.

[391] Andersen O, Aaseth J. Molecular mechanisms of in vivo metal chelation: implications for clinical treatment of metal intoxications. Environ Health Perspect 2002;110:887–90.

[392] Knudtson ML, Wyse DG, Galbraith PD, et al. Chelation therapy for ischemic heart disease: a randomized controlled trial. JAMA 2002;287:481–6.

4

Detoxification

Joseph Pizzorno, John Nowicki

INTRODUCTION/OVERVIEW

The incidence of chronic disease is increasing. While medical apologists say this is because the population is ageing, the harsh reality is that chronic disease is increasing in all age groups, including young people.[1] Over 50% of the US population now suffers from one diagnosed chronic disease, and 25% of the population has two or more chronic conditions. In addition, at least 16% of the population describe themselves as chronically unwell.

As the concentration and number of toxic compounds in the environment have increased, so has the incidence of ill health and chronic disease. Exposure to these toxins has consequences. A growing body of research indicates that exposure to endogenous and exogenous toxins is causing metabolic damage and physiological adaptation. Table 4.1 shows just a few of the many strong correlations between toxic load and disease burden.[2] Detoxification is a continual process and an individual's health depends upon their ability to detoxify and eliminate toxins.

TOXINS/TOXICANTS

A toxin is technically defined as a poisonous substance produced by living cells or organisms that when introduced into the body can cause disease. A broader definition would include not only biologically produced substances, but any agent that exerts undesirable effects on physiological function. For this chapter, sources of toxins are grouped into one of three categories: exogenous, endogenous and toxins of choice.

Oxidative damage to cells has long been associated with the development of many chronic diseases, including cancer, heart disease and diabetes. Reactive oxygen species (ROS) (e.g. superoxide radicals, hydrogen peroxide and hydroxyl radicals) are produced through normal biochemical processes in the body such as oxidative phosphorylation in the mitochondria during the production of ATP. They are also produced throughout the body by the cytochrome P450 system that is active in the production, metabolism and catabolism of numerous compounds in the body. In addition, ROS are generated by white blood cells that attack bacterial invaders and by peroxisomes that break down fatty acids. These pro-oxidants then attack and damage lipids, nucleic acids and proteins, leading to DNA damage, abnormal protein folding, lipid peroxidation and mitochondrial membrane damage. Environmental toxicants can easily increase the pro-oxidant load and imbalance the system, leading to greater risk of disease.[3] In fact, a twin-study in Denmark revealed that the bulk of oxidative damage is due to environmental factors.[4]

Sources

EXOGENOUS

Exogenous toxins are comprised of toxic agents that arise from external factors. Sources are primarily environmental and include metals, chemicals (inorganic, fluoride, organic, persistent organic pollutants, drugs, etc.), moulds, radiation (e.g. light, medical, mobile phones) and particulate matter. It is estimated that over 60000 different chemicals are now in use, with 6.5 billion pounds of chemicals released into the air per year in the US alone. Considering only 20% of disease is genetically influenced and 80% of disease results from diet, lifestyle and environmental factors, there is mounting evidence that this high level of toxin exposure is responsible for the rising incidence of chronic disease.

Mould

Indoor environments contain a complex mixture of live and dead microorganisms, fragments of dead organisms, toxins, allergens, volatile microbial organic compounds and other chemicals. Damp building materials contribute to the production of undesirable organisms and toxins including: 1) the growth of moulds which release biological agents, toxic chemicals and spores; 2) the growth of bacteria which release biological agents, toxic chemicals and spores; 3) protozoal growth; 4) virus survival; 5) the proliferation of dust mites (arachnids of many different species); 6) the proliferation of rodents and cockroaches which can carry infectious organisms; and 7) the release of chemicals and particles from building materials. The primary mechanisms for damp-building toxicity include: immunological (e.g. stimulation, suppression, autoimmunity), toxic (e.g. neurotoxicity, genotoxicity, reproductive damage) and inflammatory.

TABLE 4.1 Toxin load and disease risk

Toxin	Disease	Risk
Arsenic	Diabetes	3.6
	Lung cancer	3.0–5.0
Cadmium	Myocardial infarction	1.8
	Osteoporosis	1.4
	Obstructive lung disease	2.52 (top decile)
Lead	Gout	3.6
	Obstructive lung disease	2.37 (top decile)
Organochlorine pesticides	Diabetes	9.1
	Rheumatoid arthritis	3.5
	Hyperuricaemia	2.5
Organophosphate pesticides	IQ in children according to OPs in mother	7.1 point decrease in IQ
	ADHD	2.0
PCBs	Rheumatoid arthritis	8.5
	ADHD	>3.0
Bisphenol A	Prediabetes	1.34 (top tertile)
	Metabolic syndrome	1.51
	Obesity (children)	2.55
Polybrominated diphenyl ethers	Diabetes	2.0–3.0
Phthalates	Osteoporosis	14.1 (MCPP)
		5.9 (MCOP)
		5.9 (MBzP)
	Obesity	1.62 (DEHP, adults)
		1.77 (HMW, adults)
		2.84 (LMW, children)
		4.29 (MiBP, male children)

Moulds are fungi that grow best in warm, damp and humid conditions. In general, any area with a relative humidity of greater than 80% in the presence of metabolisable organic materials supports their growth. Research shows that as many as 50% of residential and work environments have water damage, and 10–50% of indoor environments in Europe, North America, Australia, India and Japan have clinically significant mould problems.[5] The primary mechanisms for damp-building toxicity include: immunological (e.g. stimulation, suppression, autoimmunity), toxic (e.g. neurotoxicity, genotoxicity, reproductive damage) and inflammatory. Toxic metabolites have various physiological effects including disrupting mitochondrial function, misbalancing nitric oxide synthesis, inflammatory mediators, neurotoxicity, cytotoxicity, immune suppression, carcinogenesis and mutagenesis.[6] When adding in biochemical individuality, almost any chronic clinical condition could be caused by these toxins.

Toxic metals

Toxic metals are considered major environmental pollutants and are a common underlying factor in most cases of toxicant overload. Metals are used in a variety of industrial processes and, as a result, human exposure has dramatically increased during the past 50 years. The general population is exposed to metals at trace concentrations either voluntarily, through supplementation, or involuntarily, through intake of contaminated food and water or contact with contaminated soil, dust or air. Toxic metals cause damage in a variety of ways including: increasing free radical production, enzyme poisoning, direct DNA damage, endocrine disruption and mitochondrial or cell wall damage.[7] The severity of signs and symptoms resulting from metal toxicity vary based upon several factors including the dose, route of exposure and chemical species, as well as the age, gender, genetics and nutritional status of exposed individuals. Early symptoms can include impaired ability to think or concentrate, fatigue, headache, indigestion, tremors, poor coordination, myalgia, anaemia, asthma, allergies, 'brain fog', infertility and temperature dysregulation.

Mercury is found globally in all populations that have been tested. The primary form of mercury in both hair and blood is MeHg, with over 90% coming from the consumption of ocean fish and shellfish. Total blood mercury levels are directly associated with fish intake. Mercury is a ubiquitous environmental pollutant and is toxic at any level. MeHg is a potent neurotoxin via several mechanisms including demyelination, oxidative stress and autonomic dysfunction.[8] Metallic mercury interrupts the normal uptake and release of neurotransmitters and can result in excitability and irritability. Mercury causes a great deal of oxidative damage throughout the body including to the DNA. Hydroxyl radical damage to the DNA results in elevated levels of 8-OHdG in the urine. In one study, people without occupational exposure to mercury with mean blood and urine mercury levels of 0.91 microgram/L and 0.95 microgram/L had urinary 8-OHdG levels that averaged 2.08 ng/mg cr. (range 0.95–4.7).[9] The primary mechanism of mercury hepatotoxicity may be related to poisoning of cysteine-containing proteins and glutathione (GSH) depletion.[10]

The two greatest sources of non-occupational environmental lead contamination came from the addition of tetraethyl lead to commercial petrol (from 1920 until the mid 1980s) and its use as a colour-enhancing additive to paint (until the 1970s). Lead is found ubiquitously in populations throughout the world. It is readily absorbed through both the respiratory and the gastrointestinal tracts. Gastrointestinal absorption of lead in children can be up to five times greater than in adults who are exposed to the same sources.[11] Lead not only generates ROS, but also causes a reduction in the activity of ROS-quenching enzymes such as superoxide dismutase, catalase and glutathione peroxidase, resulting in diminished antioxidant defence. In adults, lead-associated oxidative stress is associated with an increase in urinary 8-OHdG levels,[12] but such an increase has not been seen in children with similar blood lead levels (BLLs).[13] Chronic low-level lead exposure is associated with several adverse health conditions. No threshold for safety exists. Cumulative lead burden in adults, via bone lead assessment, has been associated with the risk of developing parkinsonism,[14,15] Alzheimer's disease[16] and decreased cognition.[17] Several studies have found that lead correlated with renal dysfunction,[18,19] neurobehavioural dysfunction[20] and declines in function of the peripheral nervous system,[21] and some evidence shows decreased IQ in children with supposedly safe (<5 micrograms/dL) blood concentrations of lead.[22–24]

Aluminium is a metallo-oestrogen, is genotoxic, is bound by DNA, is a pro-oxidant and has been shown to be carcinogenic in animal studies.[25] Aluminium is certainly a potential contributor to the onset, progression and aggressiveness of neurological disease,[26] and a potential link has been observed between aluminium and Alzheimer's disease, amyotrophic lateral sclerosis (ALS; motor neurone disease [MND]) and autism spectrum disorders.[27] Aluminium-caused toxicity is correlated with multifaceted effects, such as inhibiting the DNA repair system, changing the stability of the DNA structure, repressing protein phosphatase 2 (PP2A) activity, affecting the activity of antioxidant enzymes, disturbing cellular metal homeostasis (especially that of iron), enhancing ROS production, interfering with mitochondrial functions and altering NF-κB, p53, JNK pathway to induce apoptosis.[28]

Arsenic is a ubiquitous metalloid in our food, air and water and is found in both inorganic forms (as trivalent or pentavalent states) and organic forms. Water and dietary sources of arsenic remain the bulk of exposure sources.[29] Groundwater provides a continuous source of inorganic arsenic and its metabolites, while foods provide more of the organic arsenicals (e.g. arsenobetaine, arsenocholine, arsenosugars and arsenolipids), which have very short half-lives and are considered virtually nontoxic. The main mechanism by which monomethylarsonous acid (MMA) and inorganic arsenicals cause cellular and tissue damage is through oxidative stress.[30] Increases in urinary 8-OHdG levels have been found in those drinking groundwater high in arsenic, as well as those occupationally exposed to arsenic.[31] Under physiological conditions, arsenic may also induce toxic effects through the formation of hydrogen peroxide.[32] Mechanisms of arsenic carcinogenesis include oxidative damage,[33] epigenetic effects[34] and interference with DNA repair.[35] Acute and chronic arsenic exposure causes a variety of health effects including dermal changes (e.g. pigmentation, hyperkeratosis and ulceration) and respiratory, pulmonary, cardiovascular, gastrointestinal, haematological, hepatic, renal, neurological, developmental, reproductive, immunological, genotoxic, mutagenic and carcinogenic effects.[36]

Persistent organic pollutants (POPs)

Persistent organic pollutants (POPs) are compounds which are designed for specific chemical/physical/biological effects as well as resistance to environmental degradation through chemical, biological and photolytic processes.[37] Examples of these organic pollutants include pesticides, solvents, plasticisers, herbicides and industrial chemicals.

People are exposed to POPs mostly through the diet, with most exposure coming from the ingestion of animal products.[38] Recent studies have also implicated indoor environments as a major source for human exposure via inhalation and ingestion of indoor dust and air.[39] POPs bio-accumulate in human and animal tissue and bio-magnify in food chains, thus increasing their concentration and toxicity in the environment. POPs are lipophilic in nature and can easily cross the biological membranes and accumulate in fatty tissues. Multiple animal studies show exposure to 2,3,7,8-tetrachlorodibenzo-para-dioxin (TCDD) produces toxic manifestations in the liver including lipid accumulation, hepatocellular hypertrophy, inflammatory cell infiltration and hyperplasia,[40] as well as an increase in total hepatic fatty acids, triglycerides and serum ALT levels.[22,41] In addition, POPs interfere with blood sugar regulation, damage DNA and mitochondria, stimulate tumour necrosis factor-α expression and inflammatory cytokines, disrupt methylation pathways and trigger epigenetic dysmodulation (e.g. higher cord blood levels of hexachlorobenzene associated with twice greater risk for obesity in children).[42] A positive correlation has been found between farmers exposed to pesticides and oxidative stress biomarkers.[43] Pyrethroid exposure induces lipid peroxides and protein oxidation and depletes reduced GSH.[44] POPs are eliminated by phase I biotransformation, followed by phase II conjugation with GSH.

Volatile organic compounds

Volatile organic compound (VOC) exposures, such as toluene, benzene, styrene and xylene, have been associated with both normal liver enzymes and abnormal liver enzymes.[45] Seventy-five per cent of household painters with VOC exposures and abnormal liver enzymes had fatty liver on biopsy,[46] and 100% of toluene-exposed printers with persistent mild liver enzyme elevation had hepatic steatosis.[47]

Chloroalkenes

Vinyl chloride (VC) is metabolised by CYP2E1, forming the highly reactive genotoxic epoxide, chloroethylene oxide.[48] Occupational exposure to VC has been associated with steatohepatitis in lean Brazilian petrochemical workers,[49] and ultrasound studies demonstrated hepatomegaly, steatosis and fibrosis in VC workers.[50]

Air particulate matter (PM)

Rapid industrialisation and urbanisation in many parts of the world have exposed more people to air pollutants now than at any point in human history. Exposure to $PM_{0.1}$ activates signalling pathways (e.g. NF-κB, NADPH oxidase) that induce inflammation, generate reactive oxygen species and lead to cell death.[51] Mice exposed to diesel exhaust particles at 50 micrograms/kg bodyweight developed inflammation and oxidative DNA damage in the liver without systemic inflammation.[52] Obese, diabetic mice had increased levels of aspartate aminotransferase (AST), alanine aminotransferase (ALT), enhanced steatosis and elevated markers of oxidative stress after pulmonary exposure to diesel exhaust particles.[53] It is postulated that inhaled fine PM may aggravate liver damage by crossing the alveolar membranes to reach the circulation, where it accumulates in hepatic Kupffer cells, triggering TLR4-dependent activation of cytokine release, leading to inflammation and hepatic stellate cell collagen synthesis.[54]

ENDOGENOUS

Endogenous toxins are those originating from within an organism and are not attributable to any external or environmental factor. These include gut-derived microbial toxins, normal metabolites not properly detoxified and poorly detoxified hormones. Substantial body load arises from these endogenous toxins, causing significant disruption to body functions.

The role of the digestive system in overall health is difficult to overstate. Unhealthy bowels can indeed be a significant source of metabolic toxins from both 'normal' and 'abnormal' gut bacteria. When the microorganisms die, toxins are secreted and released into the surrounding environment. These toxins are known as endotoxins. Technically only bacterial lipopolysaccharides (LPS) are known as endotoxins; however, it is clinically relevant in this context to use a broader definition including anything harmful released by gut bacteria. Endotoxins bind to receptors, initiating an adaptive immune response and a signalling cascade, leading to activation of pro-inflammatory genes.[55] Impaired digestive function along with gut-derived microbial toxins trigger both the onset and the maintenance of chronic low-grade inflammation.[56] This, in turn, enhances intestinal permeability, increasing the translocation of microbiome-derived LPS to the bloodstream, resulting in a two- to three-fold increase in serum LPS concentration, which can reach a threshold named 'metabolic endotoxaemia' (ME). ME may trigger toll-like receptor (TLR) 4-mediated inflammatory activation, eliciting a chronic low-grade pro-inflammatory and pro-oxidative stress.[57,58] It is associated with the development of several chronic conditions including obesity, cardiovascular disease, diabetes/insulin resistance and non-alcoholic fatty liver disease.[59]

Infection, inflammatory cytokines, nutrient transporter activation and noxious environmental toxins all alter intestinal permeability. In addition, the composition of the gut microbiota is a significant factor associated with intestinal permeability. Exposure of the small intestine to bacteria, independent of the virulence of the microorganisms, triggers the release of zonulin, causing disengagement of the protein zonula occludens 1 from the tight junction complex between the mucosal cells.[60] This opens the space between cells in the gastrointestinal mucosa, allowing water to flush into the gut, washing out the microorganisms and toxins. This opening also dramatically increases gut permeability. The zonulin-driven opening of the paracellular pathway may represent a defensive mechanism, aiding the innate immune system against bacterial colonisation of the small intestine. However, increased intestinal permeability also provides an underlying mechanism in the pathogenesis of allergic,

inflammatory and autoimmune diseases (i.e. most chronic diseases). The tight junctions formerly considered static structures are now being shown to be dynamic and adapt to a variety of developmental, physiological, pathological and dietary circumstances.

The composition of the gut microbiota is thought to influence the development and progression of allergic diseases. In the KOALA Birth Cohort Study, it was demonstrated that differences in gut microbiota composition precede the development of atopic sensitisation during infancy. Specifically, infants with greater amounts of pathogenic *Escherichia coli* or *Clostridium difficile* had a greater incidence of eczema, recurrent wheeze or allergic sensitisation.[61] An overgrowth in the gastrointestinal tract of the yeast *Candida albicans* may be a causative factor in allergic conditions such as asthma. In one study, two atopic asthma patients had significant histamine release and high levels of serum IgE antibodies against an acid protease produced by *C. albicans*.[62] Follow-up studies have confirmed that acid protease is a *C. albicans*-specific allergen, causing human mucosal allergic reaction.[63,64]

The release of fatty acids from dysfunctional and insulin-resistant adipocytes results in lipotoxicity caused by the accumulation of triglyceride-derived toxic metabolites in the liver.[65] Excess adiposity is associated with increased proinflammatory cytokines, oxidative stress and an exaggerated inflammatory response to endotoxin administration.[66]

TOXINS OF CHOICE

Alcohol

Alcohol consumption has been shown to facilitate ROS production, release cytokines, reduce antioxidants and promote an in vivo oxidative microenvironment.[67] Hydroxyethyl free radicals, generated during ethanol metabolism by CYP2E1, react with hepatic proteins, stimulating humoral and cellular immune reactions, which may represent the mechanism by which alcohol-induced oxidative stress contributes to the perpetuation of chronic hepatic inflammation.[68] Induction of CYP2E1 also contributes to increased lipid peroxidation associated with alcoholic liver injury and enhances acetaldehyde production, which in turn impairs defence systems against oxidative stress.[69] Alcohol ingestion also increases intestinal permeability to endotoxins and macromolecules, allowing increased toxic and antigenic effects.[70]

High-fructose corn syrup (HFCS)

Several studies have shown HFCS to be a contributing factor to energy overconsumption, weight gain and the rise in the prevalence of obesity.[71–73] Fructose in sugar-sweetened beverages promotes insulin resistance.[74] HFCS also promotes dyslipidaemia,[75] increases visceral fat deposits and increases hepatic de novo lipogenesis.[76] Fructose provokes a hepatic stress response involving activation of c-Jun N-terminal kinases (JNK) and subsequent reduced hepatic insulin signalling.[77] In hyperglycaemic environments, advanced glycation end-products increase cytosolic ROS, facilitating the production of mitochondrial superoxide.[78] It is hypothesised that the excessive generation of mitochondrial superoxide creates a state of redox imbalance and is the primary initiating event that activates all other pathways of tissue damage.[79]

Tobacco

Chronic tobacco smoke inhalation induces an intracellular oxidative environment characterised by decreased concentrations of circulating antioxidants, increased oxidation of GSH and increased levels of DNA damage.[80] Antioxidants such as vitamin C and vitamin E (daily dosages of 500 mg and 400 IU, respectively) have been shown to protect women smokers from DNA damage,[81] and epicatechins have been shown in mucosal cell cultures to protect against cigarette smoke oxidative DNA damage.[82]

Pharmaceutical medications

Drugs are considered foreign substances by the body to be eliminated like any other toxin. Therefore, understanding genetic variations in enzyme activity among patients, along with the impact of drug interactions that change the systemic exposure of medications due to alterations in metabolism and excretion, is essential to safely and effectively use medications while avoiding excessive toxicity.

From 1999–2000 to 2011–2012, the percentage of US adults reporting use of any prescription medication increased from an estimated 51% to 59%, and polypharmacy (≥5 prescriptions) increased from an estimated 8.2% to 15%.[83] Even those not willingly taking doctor-prescribed or over-the-counter medications may still be exposed. A study conducted by the Environmental Working Group released in 2008 found that at least 40 million Americans drink tap water with detectable levels of prescription medications such as antibiotics, hormones and drugs used to treat epilepsy and depression.[84] All pharmaceuticals reported in drinking water supplies are unregulated in treated tap water, and any level is legal.

Idiosyncratic drug-induced liver injury (DILI) is traditionally believed to be unrelated to dose, and may affect individuals with underlying susceptibility or predisposition. Both genetic and environmental factors likely play a role in determining the occurrence of idiosyncratic DILI. For example, individuals with the HLA-I and HLA-II genotypes have an increased susceptibility to DILI when taking amoxicillin-clavulanate.[85] It has been reported that compounds with more than 50% hepatic metabolism given at doses higher than 50 mg/day were at highest risk of hepatotoxicity.[86] Other offending agents include antimicrobials (e.g. antibacterial agents, antiviral agents, antituberculosis agents), central nervous system agents (e.g. antiepileptic agents, antidepressants, antipsychotics), immunomodulatory agents, analgesics (especially those containing acetaminophen [paracetamol]), antineoplastic agents, antihypertensive agents and lipid-lowering agents.[87]

ASSESSMENT OF TOXINS/ TOXICANTS

With toxic load becoming an increasing clinical problem, accurate assessment is essential, not only for recognition of exposure, but also for tracking efficacy of intervention. There are several accepted tests for metal toxicity, which rely mostly on blood and urine. However, these are known to be useful only for acute exposure and are unreliable for body load. The typical standards for toxin load are population based (i.e. unless a patient is in the top 5% of blood levels, they are usually not considered toxic). While the top 5% is the standard to be considered toxic for most pollutants, there is sufficient reason to question its validity. One problem is the assumption that those with lower levels are healthy and are not being damaged by their toxic load. In addition, since the population has very high levels of ill health and diagnosed disease, normal is not actually healthy. Thus, normal ranges of many standard lab tests now include the effects of physiological adaptation as well as actual damage. Several conventional laboratory tests, within the supposed 'normal' range, show changes in proportion to the body load of specific toxins and toxicants.

Conventional laboratory tests

While a detailed medical history and comprehensive physical exam is foundational in the diagnosis of toxicant exposure, conventional laboratory tests can be used to detect those who are suffering damage from toxicants and to monitor treatment. Examples of conventional laboratory tests that change within the 'normal' range in proportion to toxin load include:
- Full blood count (e.g. RBC, WBC, platelet count, haemoglobin, basophilic stippling)
- Liver enzymes (e.g. ALT, GGT)
- Inflammatory markers (e.g. CRP)
- Lipids (e.g. LDL, ox-LDL, triglycerides)
- Thyroid hormones (e.g. T_3, T_4)
- Blood sugar (e.g. insulin, FBS, 2-hour PP)
- Metabolites (e.g. bilirubin, uric acid, 8-OHdG)

Unfortunately, these tests generally do not indicate the specific toxicant, but rather, represent toxicant classes. Nonetheless, examining lab values in conjunction with detailed history and physical exam is useful in the recognition of toxic exposure. 'Normal' is no longer 'healthy'.

FULL BLOOD COUNT

A full blood count is one of the most common laboratory tests ordered. It is not unusual for individuals to have lab values hovering at the low end of the normal reference range. Studies are now indicating that low normal values of platelets and total white blood cell count may be early indicators of toxic exposure. A study of paint workers exposed to a mixture of benzene-toluene-xylene showed a statistically significant macrocytosis, which may demonstrate an early manifestation of toxicant exposure.[88]

White blood cells (WBC)

White blood count decreases in proportion to total body load of polychlorinated biphenyls (PCBs) and organochlorine pesticides (OCPs).[89] In one study, although the values remained within the normal reference range, there was a 14% decrease in WBC with exposure to PCBs and OCPs. It should be noted that while total PCBs and OCPs correlate well, the correlation with specific chemicals in these classes is inconsistent.

Platelets

A study of auto repair workers showed subclinical abnormalities in platelet count with continuous low-level toluene exposure.[90] Even though the workers wore masks and protective gear, chronic low-level exposure to solvents decreased platelet count by 14% (216 000/mL versus 252 000/mL) compared to office workers in the same facility, who were likely to have been exposed as well, though at lower levels. A study of 42 healthy, non-smoker petrol filling workers demonstrated that workers exposed to solvents for long periods of time (>10 years) had a significant decrease in platelet levels compared to controls (see Fig. 4.1).[91]

Basophilic stippling

Basophilic stippling refers to a unique appearance of red blood cells observed under a microscope in which the erythrocytes display small dots at the periphery. Stippling is a classic sign of lead poisoning as well as arsenic poisoning.

LIVER ENZYMES

The liver is one of the primary organs of detoxification. It activates nutrients, detoxifies harmful substances, makes blood clotting proteins and performs many other vital functions. Enzymes located within the cells of the liver drive these chemical reactions and are induced as needed. Aspartate aminotransferase (AST), alanine aminotransferase (ALT) and gamma-glutamyl transpeptidase (GGT) are three of the most common enzymes tested. When liver cells are damaged or destroyed, the enzymes leak out into the blood where they can be measured. Liver enzymes commonly increase proportionally in response to the load of specific classes of toxicants.

Conventional biomarkers of hepatotoxicity include serum ALT, AST, alkaline phosphatase (ALP) and GGT. Research indicates that several liver enzymes increase proportionally in response to the load of specific classes of toxins. For example, in the NHANES 2003–2004 cohort, individuals with blood mercury levels in the second quartile (25–50 percentile) were twice as likely to have elevated ALT,[92] and data collected from the KNHANES showed that increasing blood mercury levels were associated with increases in AST, ALT and elevated GGT (>56 IU/L).[93,94]

ALT is a transaminase enzyme that catalyses the transfer of an amino group from L-alanine to α-ketoglutarate. The products of this transamination reaction are pyruvate and L-glutamate. For men aged 18–20, ALT values >37 IU/L are considered elevated, while the cut-off for men over the age of 21 is >48 IU/L. For women aged 18–20, ALT values >30 IU/L are considered elevated, and ALT values >31 IU/L are considered elevated for women above the age of 21. ALT increases in a dose-dependent manner with body load of blood cadmium, lead, mercury and PCBs within and above the normal range.[95] Exposure to polycyclic aromatic hydrocarbons causes elevations in AST and ALT.[96] When serum log-perfluorooctanic acid (PFOA – a perfluorinated chemical) increases by one unit, serum ALT increases by 1.86 units (95% CI: 1.24–2.48; p=0.005).[97]

ALP is a hydrolase enzyme responsible for dephosphorylation. It is present in higher concentration in the liver, kidney and bone. Chronic exposure of pesticides in agricultural workers was found to be associated with significantly higher activities of ALP compared to controls, and the number of years exposed to pesticides predicted higher activities of ALP.[98]

Perhaps the most useful liver enzyme is GGT, a key enzyme in GSH recycling. GGT is induced to provide more GSH, likely for phase II conjugation, as well as to neutralise oxidative stress. Cellular GGT metabolises extracellular GSH, allowing precursor cysteine to be reutilised for de novo synthesis of intracellular GSH. Elevations of GGT within the 'normal' range are strongly associated with several chronic diseases including diabetes, coronary heart disease, hypertension, stroke, dyslipidaemia, chronic kidney disease and cancer.[99] An increase in GGT concentration, within its physiological range, has been shown to be a sensitive biomarker for the development of diabetes with concentrations >50 U/L correlating with a 26-fold increased risk of developing diabetes.[100] Compared to men with GGT levels below 15 U/L, the relative risk of all-cause mortality was two times greater for those with GGT levels between 30 and 49 U/L (RR = 2.09) and greater than three times (RR = 3.44) for men with GGT levels ≥50 U/L.[101] Elevations of GGT directly correlate with alcohol consumption (see Fig. 4.2)[102] and, as shown in Fig. 4.3, toxic metal load (cadmium and lead).[103] Serum GGT, within its reference range, is also associated with organochlorine pesticides and polycyclic aromatic hydrocarbons.[104]

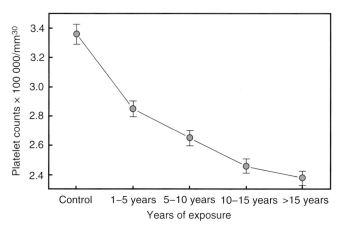

FIGURE 4.1 Platelet count decreases with years of exposure to benzene[91]

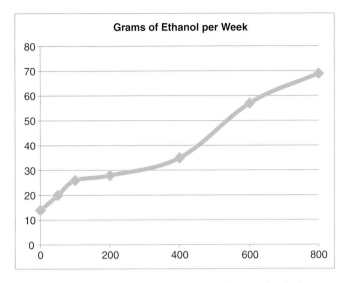

FIGURE 4.2 GGT increases in proportion to alcohol consumption[102]

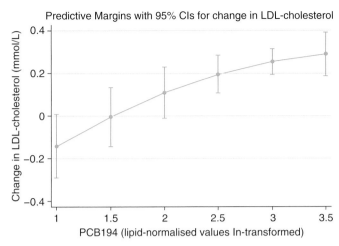

FIGURE 4.4 PCB 194 predictive of LDL-cholesterol elevation[108]

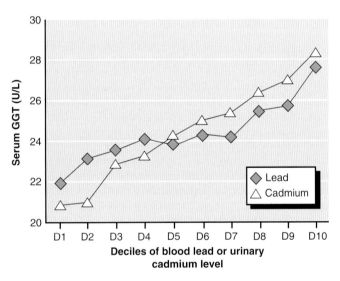

FIGURE 4.3 GGT increases in proportion to toxic metal load[103]

GGT elevates with exposure to other chemicals, especially POPs and several prescription drugs. Workers with a history of sufficient alcohol consumption and high exposure to 2,3,7,8-tetrachlorodibenzo-para-dioxin (TCDD) were found to have a statistically significant elevated risk for out-of-range GGT compared to referents.[105]

INFLAMMATORY MARKERS

C-reactive protein (CRP) is a blood test marker used to detect inflammation. It is produced by the liver and is classified as an acute phase reactant, meaning that levels will rise in response to inflammation. Most environmental toxins are pro-inflammatory and increase oxidative stress in the body. Data from the National Health and Nutrition Examination Survey (NHANES) 2003–2004 shows that exposure to polycyclic aromatic hydrocarbons (specifically

2-hydroxyphenanthrene and 9-hydroxyfluorine) is associated with elevated CRP levels (>3 mg/L).[106] An association has been shown between CRP, body load of PCBs and OC pesticides, and an increased risk of metabolic syndrome.[107]

LIPIDS

An intriguing prospective study evaluated if POP levels could predict future cholesterol levels over time.[108] Results showed a huge variation, with some POPs having little effect while others had a substantial impact. As can be seen in Fig. 4.4, a single POP, PCB 194, showed the best correlation to elevation of LDL-cholesterol over a 5-year period. This is particularly interesting as most reports of POP levels in the blood standardise according to serum lipid levels. In a study of 525 Caucasian and African American residents, total pesticides were more strongly associated with elevations in serum lipids than were total PCBs, and the associations were stronger in African Americans.[109] Individuals in the highest quartile of PFOS exposure had total cholesterol levels that were 13.4 mg/dL (95% CI, 3.8–23.0) higher than those in the lowest quartile.[110] PFC exposure in adolescents is significantly associated with elevated total cholesterol and LDL cholesterol.[111] Considering, in most cases, cholesterol levels increase with age, the research may underestimate actual body load.

Perhaps the most important aspect is that POPs oxidise cholesterol, and oxidised cholesterol is the most artery damaging form. Studies also show a direct correlation between PCBs and the ratio of oxidised glutathione (GSSG) to GSH, a definitive measure of oxidative status. The sum of PCBs shows a strong, significant positive association with ox-LDL, and significant associations with glutathione-related markers (GSSG and GSSG/GSH).[112]

METABOLITES

Bilirubin levels increase in proportion to the level of various PCBs, which is significant as bilirubin is considered the best prognostic measure of chronic liver

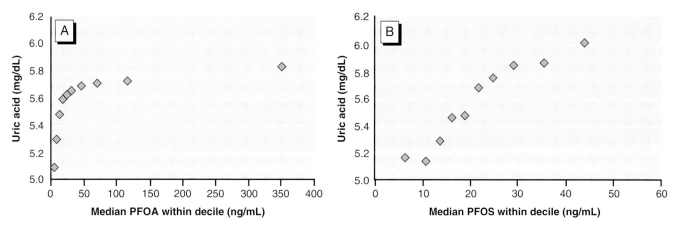

FIGURE 4.5 Serum uric acid increases in proportion to body load of PFOA and PFOS[117]

dysfunction.[113,114] Direct bilirubin is inversely associated with non-alcoholic fatty liver disease, with a significant dose–response relationship ($p = <0.05$), and serves as a protective biomarker which is likely based on the endogenous antioxidant and cytoprotectant properties of bilirubin.[115]

Serum uric acid increases in proportion to body load of perfluorinated hydrocarbons (PFOA and PFOS).[116] Fig. 4.5 demonstrates an interesting threshold effect where low levels of PFOA or PFOS show little effect initially, followed by rapid elevation in uric acid levels with odds ratios (ORs) of hyperuricaemia increasing by quintile of PFOA (ORs = 1.00, 1.33, 1.35, 1.47, and 1.47).[117]

Homocysteine is an endogenous toxin that has been shown to reduce nitric oxide availability, increase levels of reactive oxygen species and induce NF-κB expression.[118,119] Lead levels have been positively correlated with serum levels of homocysteine,[120] a biomarker associated with increased cardiovascular risk. Deficiencies in several B vitamins potentiate the damaging effects of lead on homocysteine. Elevated homocysteine levels have been found among patients with Parkinson's disease, particularly in those taking L-dopa,[121] and the effect is accentuated in those with low folic acid levels.[122]

8-OHdG

Urinary 8-hydroxy-2'-deoxyguanosine (8-OHdG), or urinary 8-oxo-7,8-dihydro-2'-deoxyguanosine (8-oxodG), is an oxidised nucleoside that appears in the urine secondary to DNA damage and is the most common biomarker of oxidative DNA damage. Urinary nucleoside metabolites not only measure DNA damage, but also serve as indirect measures of oxidative stress and toxin load.[123] 8-oxodG is used to estimate exposure to cancer-causing agents, such as tobacco smoke, asbestos fibres, toxic metals and polycyclic aromatic hydrocarbons, and is significantly determined by toxin exposure. 8-OHdG correlates with multiple cancers, mitochondrial damage, mercury levels, rate of ageing and smoking. 8-OHdG is also a fairly accurate predictor of chronic diseases such as atherosclerosis and diabetes.[124] 8-OHdG may be most useful for monitoring toxic load and as a measure of treatment efficacy.

BLOOD SUGAR REGULATION

The incidence of type 2 diabetes has increased almost 10-fold in the past half century. Although sugar consumption has increased, the increase is not consistent with the diabetes epidemic. Considering that most POPs are insulin receptor site poisons, the greatest amount of research on potential disease causation is between toxic load and measures of blood sugar regulation: fasting blood sugar, 2-hour postprandial sugar, HbA$_{1c}$, insulin levels, metabolic syndrome and diabetes. Impaired insulin resistance is the most common mechanism of damage for all POPs, and these chemicals are also implicated in the obesity epidemic.[125–128] Fig. 4.6 shows the results of a 23-year prospective study examining levels of POPs in young adults and changes in glucose-related metabolism.[129] Several critical observations can be made from this study:

- Until the age of 50, there is essentially no difference in blood sugar regulation measurements between those with the lowest and highest PCB levels. This suggests that the increasing toxic load has little impact in younger people.
- In the youngest group, insulin production increases in response to toxin level. This is to be expected since the blocking of insulin receptor sites by PCBs requires more insulin. The ability to adapt decreases with ageing.
- At age 50, all the measures show very strong toxin–dose response, suggesting that the body's adaptive capabilities have become inadequate or are overwhelmed by ever-increasing toxic load.

Non-conventional laboratory tests

HAIR ANALYSIS

Hair tissue analysis measures the levels and ratios of minerals and heavy metals in hair. Several studies have been published confirming the efficacy and accuracy of hair testing, especially for toxic metals.[130,131] Hair analysis is inexpensive, non-invasive and biologically stable, and

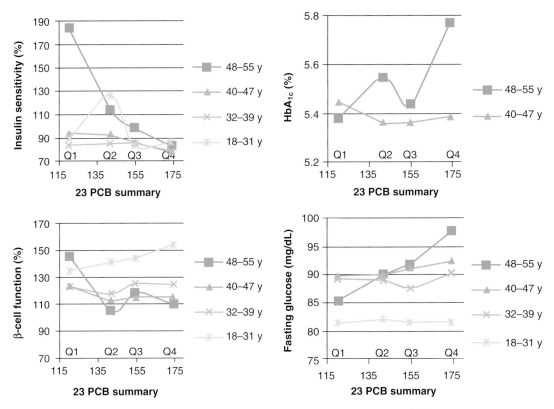

FIGURE 4.6 23-year prospective study on effects of PCBs on blood sugar regulation[129]

may be the most reliable screening test for chronic metal exposure (lead, mercury, cadmium and arsenic). Significant controversy exists regarding the use of hair analysis as an indicator of nutritional status and in the diagnosis of disease. Many variables can affect the results including: gender, hair colour, improper sample collection, hair products (e.g. shampoos, bleaches, hair spray) and inconsistent lab analysis. In addition, reliable results depend on a properly cleaned, collected and prepared sample. A positive hair analysis may suggest an individual has been exposed to metals. However, the clinical significance of that exposure as well as its use to diagnose the presence or absence of disease is limited.

CHALLENGE TESTING

There remains significant scientific debate regarding metal mobilisation testing, and the decision to treat subacute levels of metal poisoning requires careful assessment of patient risk versus benefit. There is no scientific disagreement about the use of chelating agents to increase the excretion of toxic metals. Indeed, the removal of toxic metals from the human body can be a useful tool in avoiding the onset or progression of many diseases associated with metal intoxication.

Provocative urine testing is a multi-step process intended to evaluate total body burden of toxic metals. Initially, a pre-challenge urine sample is collected to determine acute exposure. A chelating agent is then administered to the patient via oral or intravenous means. The chelator forms a complex with the metal and is excreted in the urine. After a set amount of time (e.g. 2 h,

4 h, 24 h), a second urine sample is collected and post-challenge levels are calculated. Comparing pre-challenge urinary metal levels to post-challenge levels may help with the diagnosis, treatment and management of chronic low-level metal toxicity.

There are several limitations to this procedure. Most chelating agents do not extract metals from all tissues and thus do not necessarily represent total body burden. For example, the brain is one of the main target organs for both elemental and organic mercury, yet no chelating agents can extract mercury from the brain.[132] There are no clear reference ranges for provoked urine, and neither DMSA nor DMPS have an optimal dosage for diagnosis or treatment. There is also no standard for safe versus toxic levels. In addition, there are serious confounding factors (e.g. age, gender, BMI) in determining body load of metals and clinical significance.

DIRECT MEASURES OF TOXINS

Toxins can be directly measured in urine, blood, breath, toenails and adipose tissue. Blood levels of metals typically only reflect short term exposure and may not be reliable in assessing total body load. Urine testing may be beneficial in examining the long-term, low-dose, chronic exposure to toxic compounds. But again, urine testing may not be reliable in assessing total body load. Direct measures of some toxicants are available and provide accurate and reliable current exposure levels. However, testing is expensive and is limited to only about 100 of the tens of thousands of toxicants in the environment.

FUNCTIONAL LIVER DETOXIFICATION PROFILE

Phase I and phase II liver detoxification pathways can be measured by exposing the patient to metered doses of three toxins: caffeine, paracetamol and aspirin. Caffeine is primarily absorbed by the intestine and metabolised in the liver by CYP1A2. Paracetamol is metabolised through the phase II pathways GSH conjugation, sulfation and glucoronidation. Aspirin is metabolised through glycine conjugation and glucoronidation. Measuring the presence or absence of the metabolites of these three challenge substances in serum, urine and/or saliva over the next 24 hours can pinpoint imbalances in phase I and phase II detoxification pathways.

ORGANS INVOLVED IN TOXIN ELIMINATION

Toxins and toxicants are expelled from the body through a variety of organ systems. The major systems that work together synchronously to maintain health and balance are discussed below.

Liver

The liver is the main organ for detoxifying lipophilic chemicals and filters about 1 L of blood per minute. The liver metabolises many potentially harmful environmental contaminants and facilitates the excretion of these contaminants from the body. Eighty per cent of the liver is made up of hepatocytes, which play a critical role in the metabolism of amino acids and ammonia, biochemical oxidation reactions and detoxification of a variety of drugs, vitamins, hormones and environmental toxicants. Kupffer cells constitute most of the tissue macrophages present in the body and play a protective role against gut-derived bacterial endotoxins and microbial debris. Upon activation, Kupffer cells release cytokines, prostanoids, nitric oxide and reactive oxygen species which cause inflammation and can influence the noxiousness of environmental toxicants.[133]

The liver protects the body from potential toxic damage via a two-phase detoxification process. During phase I, cytochrome P450 (CYP450) enzymes catalyse the oxidation, reduction, hydrolysis, hydration or dehalogenation of substances, creating more polar and therefore less lipid-soluble intermediary metabolites. The phase I process improves water solubility of the molecule by introducing or exposing functional groups. The cytochrome P450 enzymes are concentrated in the endoplasmic reticulum of the liver and remove accumulated waste from the body. Approximately 50–100 enzymes make up this system, and although each enzyme works best in detoxifying certain types of chemicals, there is considerable overlap in activity among the enzymes. The broad substrate specificity of these enzymes allows for the liver to handle a wide range of chemical exposure. CYP450 enzymes are responsible for the majority of the oxidation of xenobiotic chemicals including drugs, pesticides and

BOX 4.1 Human cytochrome p450 enzymes in xenobiotic metabolism

Xenobiotic P450 enzymes

1A1	2C8	2E1
1A2	2C9	2F1
2A6	2C18	3A4
2A13	2C19	3A5
2B6	2D6	3A7

carcinogens, as well as the metabolism of endobiotics such as steroids, fat soluble vitamins and eicosanoids.[134]

Variations in genetics, dietary factors and nutrient cofactors all impact on an individual's ability to metabolise chemicals effectively and efficiently.[135] Although there are 57 genes for cytochrome enzymes, 10–15 carry out the metabolism for almost all xenobiotics (see Box 4.1).[136] The isoenzymes CYP1A2, CYP2C9, CYP2C19, CYP2D6, CYP2E1 and CYP3A4 are primarily responsible for the metabolism of xenobiotics.[137] CYP3A4 makes up 30% of the total P450 content in the liver and is the predominant cytochrome P450 enzyme expressed in the liver and intestine.

Whenever the mixed function oxidase system (CYP450) is induced, greater levels of ROS will be produced along with increased levels of urinary 8-OHdG.[138] Induction of CYP450 is an epigenetic process that requires constant, regular exposures to an inducer. Cytochrome P450 2E1 (CYP2E1) has emerged as an important cause of ROS overproduction, and higher hepatic CYP2E1 expression and activity may aggravate liver injury from xenobiotic compounds through the generation of harmful reactive metabolites.[139] This is perhaps most recognised in studies examining acetaminophen (APAP, paracetamol) toxicity. CYP2E1 is a very inducible enzyme, particularly by alcohol, with induction resulting in the bioactivation of many toxins and drugs, as well as increased ROS production. Induction combined with exposure to APAP results in the production of the more toxic metabolite N-acetyl-p-benzoquinone imine, which causes an increase in ROS and nitrosamines, mitochondrial poisoning, lipid peroxidation and covalent binding to proteins, with eventual necrosis.[140]

Several other substrates affect CYP450 leading to considerable variations in detoxification capacity. 3-methylcholanthrene and other polycyclic aromatic hydrocarbons (PAHs) from combustion induce the entire 1A series (CYP1A1, 1A2, 1B1), suggesting that all people living in an urban area with vehicular exhaust will be induced. In addition to the 1A series, PAHs, including benzopyrene from vehicular exhaust, and tobacco smoke will induce CYP3A4.

Polymorphic phase I enzymes are responsible for approximately 56% of adverse drug reactions.[141] The drugs hydrocortisone and carbamazepine both produce a dose-dependent increase in CYP3A4 activation.[142] Grapefruit juice, azole antifungals, HIV antivirals and zingiber (ginger) compounds all significantly inhibit CYP3A4,[143] while St John's wort is a well-known inducer of CYP3A4.[144] Steroid hormones such as pregnenalone and DHEA, along with the dioxin 2,3,7,8-TCDD, will all induce CYP1A1. Interestingly, genistein from soy can block the TCDD-elicited induction of CYP1A1.[145] Drinking alcohol and having type 2 diabetes are both associated with an induction of CYP2E1,[146] and the common morning beverage, coffee, is a fantastic inducer of CYP1A2.

Phase II uses conjugation reactions (e.g. sulfation, glucuronidation, acetylation, methylation, amino acid conjugation, GSH conjugation) to convert intermediary metabolites into more water-soluble metabolites, which can then be excreted from the body. Metabolites may be more rapidly eliminated as a result of biotransformation, and their altered specificity may result in increased toxicity.[147] Because most toxins are metabolised through a combination of phase I and phase II activities, the relationship and balance between the phases is important in determining toxicity.

Phase II enzymes are generally much less inducible than phase I. However, a deficit in phase II is often responsible for the accumulation of reactive intermediates. For example, increases in ROS resulting from low levels of GSH and/or glutathione S-transferase (GST) are associated with chronic exposure to chemical toxins and alcohol, cadmium exposure, AIDS/HIV, Parkinson's disease and other neurodegenerative disorders.[148] GSH levels decline as conjugation reactions exceed the cells' ability to regenerate GSH. Chemicals such as PCBs and organochlorine pesticides increase oxidative damage and deplete GSH levels.[149] Depleted GSH has been implicated in several degenerative conditions including: neurodegenerative disorders (Alzheimer's, Parkinson's and Huntington's diseases, ALS (MND), Friedreich's ataxia); pulmonary disease (COPD, asthma and acute respiratory distress syndrome); immune diseases (HIV, autoimmune disease); cardiovascular diseases (hypertension, myocardial infarction, cholesterol oxidation); liver disease; cystic fibrosis; chronic age-related diseases (cataracts, macular degeneration, hearing impairment and glaucoma); and the ageing process itself.[150] There is also an increased risk of cancer and smoking-related heart disease as a result of GSH conjugation polymorphisms in glutathione transferase.[151]

Acetylation (NAT) generally reduces the toxicity of a substrate, but it may also increase toxicity. Conjugation of toxins with acetyl-CoA is the primary method by which the body eliminates sulfa drugs. This is also a good example of the wide individual variability in phase II detoxification activity. The slow acetylator phenotype is found in 52–68% of Caucasians and only 10–15% of Japanese.[152] Clinically, a 40% increase in bladder cancer has been shown for those with the low activity genotype for NAT2, especially when exposed to carcinogens such as cigarette smoke.[153,154]

Methylation of oxygen atoms often inactivates bioactive carboxylates, phenols or alcohols. Inhibition of methylation enzymes (COMT) by S-adenosyl-l-homocysteine leads to a build-up of intermediates and radicals which cause

damage to the cardiovascular and central nervous systems.[155]

Quinone reductase detoxifies quinones produced by phase I enzymes, auto exhaust, cigarette smoke and burned organic materials. Higher enzyme activity resulting from NQO2 gene promoter polymorphisms increases production of ROS and increases the risk of Parkinson's disease.[156]

Gastrointestinal tract

The gastrointestinal (GI) system is the primary gateway by which the external environment interacts with the body.[157] More than 22 tonnes of food will be processed over the course of an individual's lifespan, representing the largest load of antigens and xenobiotics confronting the human body.[158] The GI tract contains an extraordinary number of immune cells that must defend against pathogens, toxins and toxicants while allowing for tolerance to food and commensal bacteria – a balancing act that can have systemic consequences.

The digestive process varies for macronutrients. For example, glucose requires no digestion, while lipid absorption depends on gastric and pancreatic lipases for digestion and bile salts for emulsification and transport of the hydrophobic components. Absorption of these nutrients varies not only by type (monosaccharide versus amino acid) but also by the environment.

Single-sugar carbohydrates (e.g. glucose) do not require digestion to be absorbed. Glucose is absorbed in the small intestine primarily by active transport using the sodium-dependent glucose transporter (SGLT1). However, during sugar-rich meals, this transport becomes saturated and a diffusive process provides a major pathway for absorption. This diffusive absorption is facilitated by glucose transporter type 2 (GLUT2), a receptor normally found in the basolateral membrane which inserts into the apical membrane within minutes in response to a high-sugar meal.[159] As a result of a Western diet high in sugar, there is a constant elevation of GLUT2 in the apical membrane which further increases the absorption of glucose. Artificial sweeteners are likely to have this same effect and may also lead to increased absorption of any natural sugars present in the diet.

Digestive enzymes, such as lactase-phlorizin hydrolase and sucrase isomaltase, are anchored to the mucosal surface of the small intestine where the soluble sugars in the lumen are hydrolysed to free glucose, galactose and fructose, which are absorbed rapidly from the lumen.[160] Damage to the intestinal brush border (such as that due to chronic NSAID use, inflammation, trauma, disease or parasite infection) impairs absorption as a consequence of the loss in enzymatic activity.[161] Altered intestinal barrier function permits increased dietary antigen transport across the intestinal barrier and subsequent exposure of these antigens to the mucosal immune system, leading to the development of antigen-specific responses.

Long-chain triglycerides (TAGs) are the major form of dietary lipids consumed, followed by the phospholipid lecithin. The digestive process converts water-insoluble lipids into absorbable forms that can traverse the aqueous lumen of the GI tract. Digestion and absorption of TAGs begins in the stomach with the initiation of emulsification, creating a stable lipid droplet with a large surface area.[162] Upon entering the small intestine, TAG degradation products cause gall bladder emptying of bile acids, secretion of pancreatic lipase and co-lipase and release of cholecystokinin.[163] The majority of TAG digestion is due to pancreatic lipase. In patients with congenital absence of pancreatic lipase, 50–60% of dietary fats are not absorbed.[164]

Dietary fats and oils are mixed with bile and hydrolysed by pancreatic lipase to be emulsified and absorbed, leading to an increase in the absorption of toxins. Through passive diffusion, fat-soluble toxicants cross the intestinal mucosa to enter lipids. These lipophilic compounds can also be actively transported with bile salts back into the bloodstream.

The best way to eliminate toxic load is to increase the amount of fat excreted in the stool. Orlistat, a potent inhibitor of pancreatic lipase, dramatically increases faecal fat levels and is available as a weight loss product.[165] Both epigallocatechin gallate (EGCG) from green tea and polyphenols from oolong tea inhibit pancreatic lipase activity.[166] This inhibition is different from the inhibition by orlistat, which directly inhibits the production of lipase. Lipase action on lipids can also be inhibited by altering lipid droplet size and surface area (fat emulsion properties) preventing the attachment of lipase. Tea catechins and theaflavins have both demonstrated this ability, which may explain why both green and black teas have been associated with weight loss.[167–169] Tea polyphenols increase faecal fat, and therefore the excretion of persistent pollutants, from 5.5 to 6.9 grams/3 days.[170] By increasing the amount of fat in the stool, the number of fat-soluble toxicants leaving the body automatically increases.

Kidneys

The kidneys play several roles in maintaining health including activation of hormones, maintaining stable levels of key molecules in the blood and excretion of toxins. Most consider the kidneys to be second only to the liver in importance for toxin elimination. However, considering that 20–25% of cardiac output goes through the kidneys, filtering the blood a remarkable 60 times per day, a case could be made that the kidneys are more important than the liver for toxin elimination. The kidneys remove unwanted products of metabolism such as ammonia, urea, uric acid, creatinine, end products of haemoglobin metabolism and hormone metabolites; toxins that have been made water soluble via phase II liver conversion; and direct excretion of industrial toxins such as toxic metals and new-to-nature molecules. They also excrete nutrients or food constituents when consumed in excess, such as salt, vitamin C and B vitamins.

Although the kidneys are good at removing many toxins from the blood, some toxins are difficult to excrete into the urine, allowing them to accumulate in the kidneys. As toxin concentrations increase, a disproportionate amount of damage to the kidneys may result. The key environmental, dietary and endogenous toxins that appear to be the primary causes of the kidney dysfunction epidemic include: heavy metals (cadmium, mercury); persistent organic pollutants (glyphosates and halogenated hydrocarbons – especially those that are fluorinated and released when non-stick pans are heated to typical cooking temperatures); smoking; non-steroidal anti-inflammatory drugs (especially acetaminophen [paracetamol]); lipopolysaccharides from a leaky, toxic gut; and excessive dietary salt and phosphates. These all add up to a damaging load on the kidneys.

The kidneys excrete toxins via three main mechanisms: filtration through the glomeruli; passive diffusion typically from the distal tubules; and active processes where toxins are transported from the blood into the urine. The kidney is exposed to a larger proportion and higher concentration of xenobiotics than other organs through the secretion and reabsorption of toxicants in the renal tubules.[171] This is a normal, controlled process by which the kidneys maintain blood levels of key molecules within a narrow range.

The glomeruli filter out most of the small and medium-sized water-soluble molecules from the blood. Some are then reabsorbed, such as sodium, to ensure stable levels, maintain blood volume, and enable proper physiological body functions. In the proximal tubules are several active, energy-dependent transporters such as organic anion transporters (OATs), organic anion transporting polypeptides (OATPs), organic cation transporters (OCTs), multidrug resistance-associated proteins (MRPs), multidrug-resistant proteins (MDRs), and multidrug and toxin extrusion proteins (MATEs) that transport specific toxins out of the blood and, ideally, into the urine. Finally, there is passive diffusion of the more fat-soluble toxins across the tubules into the urine. These later processes are quite slow, but may be important for some toxins.

Several factors determine how specific toxins are excreted by the kidneys. If the toxin is large or bound to protein, it does not pass through the glomeruli and has to be managed in other ways. As their fat-soluble level increases, toxins that are both water and fat soluble (the octanol/water partition coefficient) are more passively reabsorbed in the distal tubules back into the kidneys and, potentially, into the blood. The active toxin excretion pathways have limited capacity and can be easily saturated. This limitation is used at times to decrease the rate at which an expensive or difficult to obtain drug is excreted so that higher blood levels of the medication can be attained at lower dosages. Finally, as the body uses ATP to actively pump out specific toxins, if the kidney's mitochondria are not working well, these active processes do not work as efficiently. Worse, when the mitochondria are not working adequately, the kidneys cannot protect their own tissue and high concentrations of toxins can accumulate in the kidneys.

Other

The circulatory system mobilises toxins from stored tissues by boosting lymphatic and blood flow, thus increasing toxin elimination. When organs of elimination, such as the kidneys and liver, are overwhelmed and/or failing, the body uses secondary organs (e.g. skin, lungs) to aid the elimination process.

The cardiovascular system and the lymphatic system are intimately related. Lymph is usually a clear fluid, but sometimes may be milky-coloured because of the presence of fats. It is composed of fluids and proteins that move from the bloodstream into the interstitial space, and are then collected by a profusion of microscopic tubules that unite to form larger ducts to collect lymph and carry it to the lymph nodes. The lymphatic system supports a network of defences against microorganisms and plays an essential role in immunological and metabolic processes. Functions of the lymphatic system include maintenance of fluid balance by conserving fluid and plasma that leaks from capillaries; initiation of specific immune responses including the phagocytosis of other cells, bacteria and bits of dead tissue or foreign particles; absorption of lipids and lipid-soluble substances from the intestinal tract; and filtration of fluid by removing harmful substances and microorganisms before they are returned to the bloodstream.

As the largest organ in the body, the integument serves to protect the body from exogenous insults as a physical barrier and also serves as an active metabolic organ regulating the body's interrelation with the environment. The skin contains a variety of cytochrome P450 enzymes, as well as other oxygen and NADP(H)-dependent oxidases that play a fundamental role in the oxidative metabolism of endogenous substances such as steroids, prostaglandins, fatty acids and leukotrienes. Cutaneous CYP enzymes also play a role in the metabolism and detoxification of xenobiotics. Phase II enzyme reactions occur in the skin and constitute an additional detoxification pathway. The skin can eliminate toxic metals and chemical xenobiotics through perspiration. For example, the excretion of trace metals, such as zinc, copper, iron, cadmium and lead, is increased with induced sweating.[172]

Toxins may also be excreted through breast milk and exhaled air. The respiratory system is a site of pollutant ingestion and is also a major pathway for xenobiotic elimination, even when these compounds were absorbed through other routes. The lungs act as a filter for many compounds present in the blood and are the major route of elimination for low-molecular-weight compounds, especially those with low blood solubility and high membrane permeability. Examples of this route of elimination include the smell of garlic in the breath or the measurement of blood alcohol content with a breathalyser. Among the components of breast milk, proteins have a high binding capacity to toxic metals,[173] and lactose and fat may actually enhance and facilitate the absorption of these metals.[174] Routine sampling of breast milk may be worthwhile to provide a better understanding of characterising the levels of elements in breast milk in order to identify and eliminate exposure pathways to toxicants.

DETOXIFICATION STRATEGIES

The body has a number of ways to protect itself from oxidative damage including: enzymes, such as superoxide dismutase, catalase and glutathione peroxidase; antioxidant compounds produced in the body such as ubiquinone, GSH, bilirubin and uric acid; and numerous diet-related antioxidant compounds including the tocopherols, ascorbic acid, polyphenols, carotenoids, N-acetylcysteine and other nutrients. Nutrient deficiencies accentuate the effects of toxins,[175] and the synergy between xenobiotics is often greater than additive effects. The combination of nutrient-depletion, cofactor displacement and high toxicant contamination in the food supply may be some of the main reasons the incidence of all chronic disease is increasing. While the growing sophistication with nutritional biochemistry and toxin elimination is important and of great benefit to patients, these therapies have limited benefit if the basics of health are not ensured: eating organic whole foods rich in nutrients and avoiding toxins as much as possible.

Toxin avoidance

The primary toxic environments are in the individual's control – dietary allergens and toxins/toxicants within the home. Decreasing exposure is primarily accomplished by modifying lifestyle choices. This includes eliminating or significantly reducing consumption of conventionally grown foods (e.g. soybeans), eliminating tobacco smoking, avoiding GMO foods, eliminating or reducing consumption of large fish (e.g. tuna), avoiding non-stick coatings on pots and pans, and avoiding fragrances.

Initial preventive measures include decreasing pollution in the work and home environments, using airway protection during the most-exposed work tasks and cessation of smoking. Eliminating dogs, cats, carpets, rugs and upholstered furniture where allergens can collect is a good first step. Environmental chemicals around the home should be removed. These include: paints, solvents, new furniture, chemical cleaners and scented candles/air fresheners to name a few. Building materials containing formaldehyde (e.g. carpeting, cabinetry) should also be avoided. Perfume, cologne, hair spray, lotions, antiperspirant and scented soaps and shampoos often contain several chemicals that should be avoided. Choosing personal care products that are labelled to be free of phthalates, parabens, triclosan and BP-3 can significantly reduce personal exposure to these harmful toxicants. Use reduction of consumer products has the potential to significantly reduce occupational and residential exposures. Smoking is a modifiable behaviour, and various measures, including nicotine-containing skin patches or chewing gum, acupuncture and hypnosis have all been shown to provide some benefit in helping patients to quit smoking. An air purifier can be used to help improve indoor air quality.

Diet

Increasing hydration is the simplest method of enhancing the elimination of toxins. The consumption of 2–3 L per day of filtered water for an average-sized adult is recommended during a detoxification program.

The nutrient content of conventionally grown foods has decreased precipitously. Modern agricultural methods produce food that is bigger and grows faster, but is lower in nutrients – especially trace minerals.[176] The cause of this mineral loss appears to be the result of three factors: 1) change in cultivars; 2) depletion of soil mineral content after decades of synthetic fertiliser use; and 3) high-phosphate fertilisers that cause foods to grow bigger but dilute their nutrient content.[177] The trace mineral content of US wheat, for example, has decreased 20–33% over the past 122 years, while copper has decreased over 70% in vegetables in the past 50 years. Unfortunately, the foods that the average person consumes are truly depleted of nutrients.[178]

A significant number of toxins come from dietary sources. Organic, mostly plant-based foods should be consumed when possible. Any foods known to cause adverse reactions should also be avoided. Elimination of the offending foods and incorporation of an oligoantigenic diet are primary in reducing inflammation.[179] Fibres, such as pectin, increase excretion of toxins, protect against toxic metal damage and decrease enterohepatic recirculation of toxins.[180] Considering the high prevalence of gluten sensitivities, selecting a gluten-free fibre is necessary to reduce the risk of inflammation in gluten-sensitive individuals. Adequate amounts of water are important to prevent constipation.

Among the most useful interventions to reduce oxidative damage is a diet rich in colourful fruits and vegetables, particularly purple sweet potato leaves and almonds.[181] Greater fruit and vegetable intake is independently associated with reduced 8-OHdG levels.[182] One study found that increasing fruits and vegetables to 12 servings a day decreased urinary 8-oxodG by 57% after only 2 weeks, with those eating the poorest diets beforehand improving the most.[183] A diet high in polyphenols has demonstrated effectiveness at protecting the GSH system.[184] The consumption of brassica family vegetables and flavonoid-containing botanicals, such as *Ginkgo biloba* and green tea, have also demonstrated clear antioxidant benefit.[185,186] Increasing blood flow to the kidneys has a huge impact on improving detoxification as well as decreasing oxidative stress. There is encouraging research evaluating the benefits of foods and nutrients that increase the production of nitrogen oxide in dilating peripheral blood vessels to increase blood flow to the tissues. One study showed an impressive dose-dependent increase in blood flow to the kidneys of up to 26%.[187]

Nutritional factors

NUTRACEUTICALS

Antioxidants protect the liver from damage, support detoxification processes and counteract oxidative stress by reducing the formation of free radicals. Antioxidants such as CoQ10,[188] curcumin,[189] lycopene[190] and green tea have all been shown to significantly reduce oxidative damage.[191]

Vitamin E is a combination of eight different fat-soluble compounds – tocopherols (alpha, beta, gamma and delta) and tocotrienols. Tocopherols tend to be more biologically active, with alpha-tocopherol being the most active of the group. The primary function of vitamin E is

to scavenge free radicals, thereby protecting the body from oxidative damage.[192] Healthy individuals who consumed a balanced diet that supplied adequate (recommended dietary allowance – RDA) vitamin E amounts had decreased oxidative damage when supplemented with vitamin E at 10 times the RDA.[193] Vitamin E functions as an antioxidant, lipoxygenase inhibitor and phospholipase inhibitor.[194]

The importance of GSH in the treatment and prevention of toxicity cannot be overstated. GSH is the major endogenous antioxidant produced by the cells, and participates directly in the neutralisation of free radicals. It is involved in metabolic and biochemical reactions such as DNA synthesis and repair, protein synthesis, prostaglandin synthesis, amino acid transport and enzyme activation. GSH, therefore, affects every system in the body. Nutrients that boost GSH are of critical importance in the treatment and prevention of oxidative damage. If GSH is depleted, de novo synthesis of GSH is up regulated, as is cysteine synthesis.[195] GSH production can be increased using N-acetylcysteine (NAC),[196] whey protein powder,[197] meditation,[198] exercise,[199] alpha-lipoic acid,[200] S-adenosyl L-methionine (SAMe)[201] and/or direct administration of GSH via IV,[202] nebulised or intranasal route.[203] Supplemental selenium may reduce the production of leukotrienes by ensuring optimal activity of glutathione peroxidase in asthmatics.[204,205]

NAC is a precursor to GSH and exhibits direct antioxidant benefits. Studies demonstrate that NAC is effective at attenuating oxidative damage by increasing the activities of superoxide dismutase (SOD), catalase (CAT) and GST and by decreasing GSH depletion and MDA levels.[206,207] Polychlorinated-biphenyl-induced oxidative stress and cytotoxicity in cell lines can be mitigated by NAC.[208]

Curcumin upregulates several phase II enzymes, including GST, and downregulates some phase I enzymes associated with carcinogenic toxicity.[209] In human cells, curcumin protects against DNA damage from PAHs,[210] protects against arsenic toxicity, prevents DNA damage and enhances DNA repair enzymes against arsenic-induced damage.[211]

Quercetin has been shown in animal studies to protect against the oxidative stress induced by dioxins and enhances the protective effects of beta-carotene for DNA from PAHs.[212,213] In human cell lines, EGCG and quercetin protect against CYP1A1 induction and DNA damage from PCBs.[214]

Lipotropic agents such as choline, methionine, betaine, folate and vitamin B_{12} help promote the export of fat from the liver and may be helpful in a variety of liver conditions including chemical-induced liver disease. Supplementation with chlorella decreases toxic metals and metabolites by directly preventing absorption of toxins, increasing stool and urinary excretion of metals and preventing enterohepatic recirculation of toxins.[215]

Commensal bacteria have a very significant impact on intestinal integrity. The probiotic species *Bifidobacterium longum* (BB536) has been found to prevent damage to intestinal cells and to increase production of tight junction cell proteins, improving intestinal integrity. In a trial of patients with ulcerative colitis (UC), BB536 was shown to not only induce remission, but it also upregulated gene expression of tight junction molecules (claudin-1 and ZO-1) known to be key to selective permeability.[216] The combination of prebiotics and probiotics (synbiotic therapy) has been shown to help UC patients achieve greater improvement in quality of life and inflammatory markers than either therapy alone.[217] A double-blind randomised clinical trial demonstrated that the use of probiotics reduced the rate of postoperative septicaemia through reductions in serum zonulin concentration in patients undergoing colectomy for colorectal cancer.[218] *Lactobacillus* spp. are able to breakdown aldehydes in the body through enhancement of the enzyme aldehyde dehydrogenase.[219] In addition, both *Lactobacillus* and *Propionibacterium* are able to bind aflatoxin B1 in the intestine, preventing it from causing damage to the liver and other organs.[220]

Other nutrients have also been shown to stimulate regeneration of intestinal mucosa. L-glutamine, which has long been recognised as the primary amino acid source for intestinal cells, has been shown to regulate intercellular junction integrity.[221] N-acetyl glucosamine (NAG) provides a substrate for the glycosaminoglycans that are normally broken down in a leaky gut and has shown benefit in children with IBD.[222] Zinc deficiency has been shown to disrupt tight junctions, alter membrane permeability, impair immune function and cause intestinal ulceration.[223] Antioxidants, including vitamin C, vitamin E, beta-carotene, grape seed extract and milk thistle extract, protect the GI from oxidant damage and help with hepatic detoxification of compounds associated with intestinal dysfunction. Quercetin appears to be critical to intestinal integrity. In addition to quercetin's antioxidant and anti-inflammatory benefits, it is also involved in the assembly of several tight junction proteins (zonula occludens (ZO)-2, occludin, claudin-1 and claudin-4).[224,225] Quercetin also helps to stabilise mast cells, which are important regulators of intestinal function and tight junction integrity.[226]

BOTANICALS

There is an extensive array of herbal medicines available for the treatment of liver conditions. The most impressive research has been done on *Silybum marianum* (milk thistle) and the extracted flavonoids (e.g. silymarin). These compounds exert a substantial effect on protecting the liver from damage as well as enhancing detoxification processes. Silymarin has been shown to have positive effects in treating liver diseases including cirrhosis, chronic hepatitis, fatty infiltration of the liver (chemical- and alcohol-induced fatty liver) and inflammation of the bile duct.[227–229]

Silymarin prevents damage to the liver by acting as an antioxidant, increasing the synthesis of GSH and increasing the rate of liver tissue regeneration.[230,231] Silymarin not only prevents the depletion of GSH induced by alcohol and other toxic chemicals, but has been shown to increase the level of GSH of the liver by up to 35%.[232] The use of *S. marianum* may provide benefit in the

prevention of drug-induced toxicity.[233] The antioxidant activity of milk thistle has been attributed to its ability to reduce free radical production, reduce lipid peroxidation and support liver detoxification.[234,235]

Bile sequestrants

Bile acid sequestrants (cholestyramine, colestipol and colesevelam) are synthetic resins designed to prevent the reabsorption of cholesterol through the binding of bile acids in the intestines. As a result, the liver is forced to produce more bile to replace the bile that has been lost. Since bile acids are synthesised from cholesterol, interfering with their reabsorption leads to a decrease in circulating levels of cholesterol, specifically low-density lipoproteins.

Ursodeoxycholic acid (UDCA) has choleretic, immunomodulatory and cytoprotective actions. Bile acid therapy with UDCA may be beneficial by reducing bile acid cytotoxicity and protecting hepatocytes against bile acid-induced apoptosis.[236]

Bile acid sequestrants are large particles and are not significantly absorbed leading to the increased excretion of bile acids in the stool. One interesting study showed the potential of bile acid sequestrants (cholestyramine) to bind to ochratoxin-A (OTA), reducing plasma levels and preventing OTA-induced nephrotoxicity.[237] Cholestyramine has also been shown to bind to mycotoxins, such as fumonisin, significantly reducing their toxic effects.[238]

There is significant potential in using bile acid sequestrants to reduce the effects of many toxic agents. However, care should be taken as sequestrants also bind to vitamins, hormones and medications which may alter their effectiveness.

Chelation therapy

Chelation therapy involves pharmaceutically derived compounds that form bonds with charged metal ions through a chemical equilibrium reaction. The complexing agent is the chelator, and the involved metal is said to be chelated. Chelators are injected into the blood or muscle, or used orally to bind metals that are present in toxic concentrations so they can be excreted from the body, most frequently in urine.[239] Chelation is the mainstay in conventional toxicology as a resource for documented acute toxic metal poisoning.[240,241] The therapeutic selection of an effective chelating agent is based on the toxicokinetics and chemical considerations of the metal involved and the chelating agent.

There are numerous chelating drugs used as antidotes to metal toxicity. Deferoxamine is a high-molecular-weight, highly hydrophilic chelator that was first introduced in the 1960s in short-term studies of iron-loaded patients.[242] It is a naturally occurring iron chelator produced by *Streptomyces pilosus* and was the first iron chelator approved for human use.[243] Deferoxamine prevents iron-catalysed free radical reactions and is used in the treatment of acute iron poisoning and in iron storage disease such as beta-thalassaemia. Dimercaprol or British anti-Lewisite (BAL) was originally developed to counteract arsenic-containing war gases,[244] but it is now used for the treatment of poisoning with toxic metals such as arsenic, gold, lead and mercury. DMPS is a water-soluble dithiol that increases urinary excretion of arsenic, cadmium, lead and mercury and has been shown to increase excretion of essential trace metals (copper, selenium, zinc, magnesium), necessitating supplementation before and after treatment.[245] DMSA is a sulfhydryl-containing, water-soluble, chelating agent that increases urinary excretion of arsenic, cadmium, lead and mercury. DMSA is FDA approved for the treatment of lead, and although it has demonstrated the ability to reduce mercury levels, it is not FDA approved for mercury toxicity.[246] Penicillamine is used for the treatment of lead poisoning as a chelating agent and is used for the elimination of copper in Wilson's disease. In cases of human poisoning, d-penicillamine has been shown to increase the excretion of lead,[247] arsenic[248] and mercury.[249] EDTA binds lead and cadmium strongly and may bind to mercury if other minerals are depleted. Considering the formation constants are generally greater for toxic metals compared to essential minerals lends a significant safety factor to long-term EDTA use. Prussian blue has been used as a treatment for thallium toxicity as the exchange of potassium ions in the crystal lattice with thallium ions leads to the binding of thallium in the intestine for extraction and elimination.[250]

NAC is a nontoxic N-acetyl derivative of cysteine containing a thiol group. NAC is widely available, relatively inexpensive, easily administered and well tolerated by patients. NAC produces a transient, dose-dependent increase in urinary excretion of methylmercury that is proportional to the body burden and can decrease brain and fetal levels of methylmercury.[251] Supplementation with chlorella decreases toxic metals and metabolites by directly preventing absorption of toxins, increasing stool and urinary excretion of metals and preventing enterohepatic recirculation of toxins.[252–254] Antioxidants along with a chelating agent have proved to be a better treatment regimen than monotherapy with chelating agents. Several nutrients including alpha-lipoic acid,[255] probiotics, vitamin E, melatonin and fibre used concurrently with DMSA not only provide greater reversal of lead-induced biochemical and physiological damage, but significantly increase the excretion of lead itself.[256]

Sauna therapy

An often-overlooked route of toxicant excretion is via the process of sweating. Induced sweating is a potential method for elimination of many toxic elements from the human body.[257] Sauna therapy is based on the concept that toxins are released through the skin via sweat and has been shown to increase the excretion of toxic metals (arsenic, cadmium, lead, mercury) and chemicals (phthalates, PCBs, PBBs and HCBs).[258–260] Medications including amphetamines (and metabolites),[261] methadone and its metabolites[262] and antiepileptic drugs have been documented to be excreted in sweat.[263] One study measured the antiepileptic drugs phenytoin,

phenobarbitone and carbamazepine after it was noted that several hospitalised patients had lower serum levels of phenytoin during a particularly hot summer.[264] In 80% of patients enrolled in the blood, urine and sweat (BUS) study, BPA was identified in sweat, even in individuals with no BPA detected in their serum or urine samples.[265] The benefit of sweating to reduce the total body load of toxicants is limited by the total millilitres of sweat that can be produced. Regular sauna use is associated with several health benefits including stress reduction, lower blood pressure, detoxification and decreased pain.[266]

Contrast hydrotherapy

An intriguing study evaluated the efficacy of contrast hydrotherapy, the application of hot and/or cold water to the body, in treating lead poisoning.[267] Records for 120 years (3377 patients with lead poisoning) were analysed, with results showing that 45.4% of patients were cured and 93% were improved. Full immersion increased cardiac output by 50% and increased urinary excretion of lead by 250%.

Manual therapy

Manual therapies may be helpful to mobilise and eliminate toxins from the body by mobilising the lymphatic system. Dry skin brushing has traditionally been used to increase lymphatic circulation by gently brushing the skin from the bottom of the feet and the palms of the hands towards the heart. Together with exercise and sauna therapy, massage can enhance the ability of the lymphatic, cardiopulmonary and hepatorenal circulatory systems to eliminate toxins.[268]

Exercise

Exercise stimulates the circulatory and lymphatic systems, helps remove toxins stored in the body tissues and organs, and mobilises stored fat and thus fat-soluble toxins.[269] Acute intense exercise challenges the liver with increased ROS and inflammation, whereas regular exercise training induces hepatic antioxidant and anti-inflammatory improvements.[270]

Exercisers can decrease air pollution exposure by exercising during the early morning hours before pollution accumulates, during periods of increased air movement (i.e. windy days), in less travelled areas or indoors when pollution levels are high.

Mind–body

Treatments that support the mental–emotional–spiritual levels of health should be included when considering a holistic detoxification program. Techniques such as breathing exercises, meditation, tai chi, yoga and/or counselling can be implemented to reduce the impact of stress and negative emotional states.

Adequate sleep supports detoxification and overall wellbeing. This is the body's time for cellular repair and regeneration, with the final 1–2 hours of sleep being the most restorative.[271]

CASE STUDY
Solvents

A VERY SICK BOAT BUILDER

CASE SUMMARY

35-year-old previously healthy white male wooden boat builder becoming progressively debilitated. Problems significantly worse in the winter. Had become so weak, he was having problems getting out of bed in the morning to do his work. Standard assessment by several medical doctors found no apparent cause or identifiable disease. By the time he came to see me, he was very weak, felt like he had the flu all the time and was desperate because he had a wife and young children to support. Assessment was solvent overload caused by working with paints, varnishes and fibreglass with inadequate protection and ventilation.

Intervention with aggressive exposure reduction and liver function/regeneration support resulted in complete remission of all symptoms and return to full functionality.

INVESTIGATIONS AND FINDINGS

Examination revealed an enlarged and very sensitive liver. His hands were discoloured and his complexion appeared waxen. As his family home was next door to his workshop, he was being exposed to toxic chemicals 24/7.

TREATMENT

Eliminated solvent exposure as much as possible: he stopped working for 1 week, moved his family several blocks away from his workshop, added a space heater, opened all doors and windows in the workshop and began using both gloves and a chemical mask whenever he opened a container or could smell solvents.

During the 1 week away from work put on a modified fast, consuming only raw and cooked fruits and vegetables. To this added vitamin C (2 g twice a day) and B complex (50 mg/day). In addition, prescribed two detoxification herbs, *Chionanthus virginicus* (fringe tree) and *Chelidonium majus* (tetterwort).

FOLLOW-UP REVIEW/PROGRESS

As the patient had a good constitution, he responded rapidly to the therapy. Within a few weeks, he was back to his normal energetic self. By improving the ventilation in his workshop and having him rigorously limit contact exposure while strongly supporting his detoxification systems he was able to continue building his beautiful wooden boats.

The message: the chemical solvents in the home and work environments progressively damage health in direct proportion to exposure, genetic susceptibilities and nutritional deficiencies.

REFERENCES

[1] http://www.cdc.gov/nchs/data/databriefs/db100.htm. [Accessed 21 April 2016].

[2] Pizzorno J. Hard to be healthy in North America. Integr Med (Encinitas) 2015;14(3):8–14.

[3] Pilger A, Rüdiger HW. 8-Hydroxy-2'-deoxyguanosine as a marker of oxidative DNA damage related to occupational and environmental exposures. Int Arch Occup Environ Health 2006;80(1):1–15.

[4] Broedbaek K, Ribel-Madsen R, Henriksen T, et al. Genetic and environmental influences on oxidative damage assessed in elderly Danish twins. Free Radic Biol Med 2011;50(11):1488–91.

[5] WHO guidelines for indoor air quality: dampness and mold. World Health Organization; 2009. https://www.who.int/airpollution/guidelines/dampness-mould/en/.

[6] Thrasher JD, Crawley S. The biocontaminants and complexity of damp indoor spaces: more than what meets the eyes. Toxicol Ind Health 2009;25(9–10):583–615.

[7] Flora SJ, Mittal M, Mehta A. Heavy metal induced oxidative stress & its possible reversal by chelation therapy. Indian J Med Res 2008;128(4):501–23.

[8] Farina M, Rocha JB, Aschner M. Mechanisms of methylmercury-induced neurotoxicity: evidence from experimental studies. Life Sci 2011;89(15–16):555–63.

[9] Chen C, Qu L, Li B, et al. Increased oxidative DNA damage, as assessed by urinary 8-hydroxy-2'-deoxyguanosine concentrations, and serum redox status in persons exposed to mercury. Clin Chem 2005;51(4):759–67.

[10] Lin TH, Huang YL, Huang SF. Lipid peroxidation in liver of rats administered with methyl mercuric chloride. Biol Trace Elem Res 1996;54(1):33–41.

[11] Fourth national report on human exposure to environmental chemicals. CDC; 2009. www.cdc.gov/exposurereport.

[12] Hong YC, Oh SY, Kwon SO, et al. Blood lead level modifies the association between dietary antioxidants and oxidative stress in an urban adult population. Br J Nutr 2013;109(1):148–54.

[13] Roy A, Queirolo E, Peregalli F, et al. Association of blood lead levels with urinary F_2-8α isoprostane and 8-hydroxy-2-deoxy-guanosine concentrations in first-grade Uruguayan children. Environ Res 2015;140:127–35.

[14] Coon S, Stark A, Peterson E, et al. Whole-body lifetime occupational lead exposure and risk of Parkinson's disease. Environ Health Perspect 2006;114(12):1872–6.

[15] Weisskopf MG, Weuve J, Nie H, et al. Association of cumulative lead exposure with Parkinson's disease. Environ Health Perspect 2010;118(11):1609–13.

[16] Bakulski KM, Rozek LS, Dolinoy DC, et al. Alzheimer's disease and environmental exposure to lead: the epidemiologic evidence and potential role of epigenetics. Curr Alzheimer Res 2012;9(5):563–73.

[17] Shih RA, Glass TA, Bandeen-Roche K, et al. Environmental lead exposure and cognitive function in community-dwelling older adults. Neurology 2006;67(9):1556–62.

[18] Wedeen RP, D'Haese P, Van de Vyver FL, et al. Lead nephropathy. Am J Kidney Dis 1986;8(5):380–3.

[19] Craswell PW, Price J, Boyle PD, et al. Chronic lead nephropathy in Queensland: alternative methods of diagnosis. Aust N Z J Med 1986;16(1):11–19.

[20] Yokoyama K, Araki S, Aono H. Reversibility of psychological performance in subclinical lead absorption. Neurotoxicology 1988;9(3):405–10.

[21] Araki S, Murata K, Aono H. Subclinical cervico-spino-bulbar effects of lead: a study of short-latency somatosensory evoked potentials in workers exposed to lead, zinc, and copper. Am J Ind Med 1986;10(2):163–75.

[22] Tuthill R. Hair lead levels related to children's classroom attention deficit behavior. Arch Environ Health 1996;51(3):214–20.

[23] Needleman H, Schell A, Bellinger D, et al. The long-term effects of exposure to low doses of lead in childhood. N Engl J Med 1990;322(2):83–8.

[24] Iqbal S, Muntner P, Batuman V, et al. Estimated burden of blood lead levels 5 µg/dl in 1999-2002 and declines from 1988 to 1994. Environ Res 2008;107(3):305–11.

[25] Exley C, Charles CM, et al. Aluminum in human breast tissue. J Inorg Biochem 2007;101(9):1344–6.

[26] Exley C. What is the risk of aluminum as a neurotoxin? Expert Rev Neurother 2014;14(6):589–91.

[27] Shaw CA, Tomljenovic L. Aluminum in the central nervous system (CNS): toxicity in humans and animals, vaccine adjuvants, and autoimmunity. Immunol Res 2013;56(2–3):304–16.

[28] Wu Z, Du Y, Xue H, et al. Aluminum induces neurodegeneration and its toxicity arises from increased iron accumulation and reactive oxygen species (ROS) production. Neurobiol Aging 2012;33:199.e1–12.

[29] Boyce CP, Lewis AS, Sax SN, et al. Probabilistic analysis of human health risks associated with background concentrations of inorganic arsenic: use of a margin of exposure approach. Hum Ecol Risk Assess 2008;14:1159–201.

[30] Bernstam L, Nriagu J. Molecular aspects of arsenic stress. J Toxicol Environ Health B Crit Rev 2000;3(4):293–322.

[31] Fujino Y, Guo X, Liu J, et al. Chronic arsenic exposure and urinary 8-hydroxy-2′-deoxyguanosine in an arsenic-affected area in Inner Mongolia, China. J Expo Anal Environ Epidemiol 2005;15(2):147–52.

[32] Jomova K, Valko M. Advances in metal-induced oxidative stress and human disease. Toxicology 2011;283(2–3):65–87.

[33] Kitchin KT, Ahmad S. Oxidative stress as a possible mode of action for arsenic carcinogenesis. Toxicol Lett 2003;137(1–2):3–13.

[34] Ren X, McHale CM, Skibola CF, et al. An emerging role for epigenetic dysregulation in arsenic toxicity and carcinogenesis. Environ Health Perspect 2011;119(1):11–19.

[35] Zhang A, Feng H, et al. Unventilated indoor coal-fired stoves in Guizhou province, China: cellular and genetic damage in villagers exposed to arsenic in food and air. Environ Health Perspect 2007;115(4):653–8.

[36] Mandal BK, Suzuki KT. Arsenic round the world: a review. Talanta 2002;58(1):201–35.

[37] Ritter L, Solomon KR, Forget J, et al. Persistent organic pollutants. United Nations Environment Program; 1995. https://www.who.int/ipcs/assessment/en/pcs_95_39_2004_05_13.pdf.

[38] Donat-Vargas C, Gea A, Sayon-Orea C, et al. Association between dietary intake of polychlorinated biphenyls and the incidence of hypertension in a Spanish cohort: the Seguimiento Universidad de Navarra project. Hypertension 2015;65(4):714–21.

[39] Cartieaux E, Rzepka MA, Cuny D. Indoor air quality in schools. Arch Pediatr 2011;18(7):789–96.

[40] Kopec AK, D'Souza ML, Mets BD, et al. Non-additive hepatic gene expression elicited by 2,3,7,8-tetrachlorodibenzo-p-dioxin (TCDD) and 2,2′,4,4′,5,5′-hexachlorobiphenyl (PCB153) co-treatment in C57BL/6 mice. Toxicol Appl Pharmacol 2011;256(2):154–67.

[41] Boverhof DR, Burgoon LD, et al. Comparative toxicogenomic analysis of the hepatotoxic effects of TCDD in Sprague Dawley rats and C57BL/6 mice. Toxicol Sci 2006;94(2):398–416.

[42] Smink A, Ribas-Fito N, Garcia R, et al. Exposure to hexachlorobenzene during pregnancy increases the risk of overweight in children aged 6 years. Acta Paediatr 2008;97(10):1465–9.

[43] Lee KM, Park SY, et al. Pesticide metabolite and oxidative stress in male farmers exposed to pesticide. Ann Occup Environ Med 2017;29:5.

[44] Vontas JG, Small GJ, Hemingway J. Glutathione S-transferases as antioxidant defence agents confer pyrethroid resistance in Nilaparvata lugens. Biochem J 2001;357(Pt 1):65–72.

[45] Brautbar N, Williams J. Industrial solvents and liver toxicity: risk assessment, risk factors and mechanisms. Int J Hyg Environ Health 2002;205(6):479–91.

[46] Dossing M, Arlien-Soborg P, et al. Liver damage associated with occupational exposure to organic solvents in house painters. Eur J Clin Invest 1983;13(2):151–7.

[47] Guzelian PS, Mills S, Fallon HJ. Liver structure and function in print workers exposed to toluene. J Occup Med 1988;30(10):791–6.

[48] Huang CY, Huang KL, et al. The GST T1 and CYP2E1 genotypes are possible factors causing vinyl chloride induced abnormal liver function. Arch Toxicol 1997;71(8):482–8.

[49] Cotrim HP, De Freitas LA, et al. Clinical and histopathological features of NASH in workers exposed to chemicals with or without associated metabolic conditions. Liver Int 2004;24(2):131–5.

[50] Hsiao TJ, Wang JD, Yang PM, et al. Liver fibrosis in asymptomatic polyvinyl chloride workers. J Occup Environ Med 2004;46(9):962–6.

[51] Traboulsi H, Guerrina N, Iu M, et al. Inhaled pollutants: the molecular scene behind respiratory and systemic diseases associated with ultrafine particulate matter. Int J Mol Sci 2017;18(2):Pii:E243.

[52] Folkmann JK, Risom L, et al. Oxidatively damaged DNA and inflammation in the liver of dyslipidemic ApoE-/- mice exposed to diesel exhaust particles. Toxicology 2007;237(1–3):134–44.

[53] Tomaru M, Takano H, Inoue K, et al. Pulmonary exposure to diesel exhaust particles enhances fatty change of the liver in obese diabetic mice. Int J Mol Med 2007;19(1):17–22.

[54] Tan HH, Fiel MI, et al. Kupffer cell activation by ambient air particulate matter exposure may exacerbate nonalcoholic fatty liver disease. J Immunotoxicol 2009;6(4):266–75.

[55] Aderem A, Ulevitch RJ. Toll-like receptors in the induction of the innate immune response. Nature 2000;406(6797):782–7.

[56] Laugerette F, Vors C, Peretti N, et al. Complex links between dietary lipids, endogenous endotoxins and metabolic inflammation. Biochimie 2011;93(1):39–45.

[57] Suganami T, Tanimoto-Koyama K, et al. Role of the Toll-like receptor 4/NF-kappaB pathway in saturated fatty acid-induced inflammatory changes in the interaction between adipocytes and macrophages. Arterioscler Thromb Vasc Biol 2007;27(1):84–91.

[58] Cani PD, Amar J, Iglesias MA, et al. Metabolic endotoxemia initiates obesity and insulin resistance. Diabetes 2007;56(7):1761–72.

[59] Everard A, Cani PD. Diabetes, obesity and gut microbiota. Best Pract Res Clin Gastroenterol 2013;27(1):73–83.

[60] El Asmar R, Panigrahi P, Bamford P, et al. Host-dependent zonulin secretion causes the impairment of the small intestine barrier function after bacterial exposure. Gastroenterology 2002;123(5):1607–15.

[61] Penders J, Thijs C, van den Brandt PA, et al. Gut microbiota composition and development of atopic manifestations in infancy: the KOALA Birth Cohort Study. Gut 2007;56(5):661–7.

[62] Akiyama K, Shida T, Yasueda H, et al. Atopic asthma caused by Candida albicans acid protease: case reports. Allergy 1994;49(9):778–81.

[63] Akiyama K. The role of fungal allergy in bronchial asthma. Nippon Ishinkin Gakkai Zasshi 2000;41(3):149–55.

[64] Akiyama K, Shida T, et al. Allergenicity of acid protease secreted by Candida albicans. Allergy 1996;51(12):887–92.

[65] Cusi K. Role of obesity and lipotoxicity in the development of nonalcoholic steatohepatitis: pathophysiology and clinical implications. Gastroenterology 2012;142(4):711–25.

[66] Yang SQ, Lin HZ, Lane MD, et al. Obesity increases sensitivity to endotoxin liver injury: implications for the pathogenesis of steatohepatitis. Proc Natl Acad Sci USA 1997;94(6):2557–62.

[67] Wu D, Cederbaum AI. Alcohol, oxidative stress, and free radical damage. Alcohol Res Health 2003;27(4):277–84.

[68] Albano E. Alcohol, oxidative stress and free radical damage. Proc Nutr Soc 2006;65(3):278–90.

[69] Lieber CS. Role of oxidative stress and antioxidant therapy in alcoholic and nonalcoholic liver diseases. Adv Pharmacol 1997;38:601–28.

[70] Worthington BS, Meserole L, Syrotuck JA. Effect of daily ethanol ingestion on intestinal permeability to macromolecules. Dig Dis 1978;23:23–32.

[71] Ludwig DS, Peterson KE, Gortmaker SL. Relation between consumption of sugar sweetened drinks and childhood obesity: a prospective, observational analysis. Lancet 2001;357:505–8.

[72] Bray GA, Nielsen SJ, Popkin BM. Consumption of high-fructose corn syrup in beverages may play a role in the epidemic of obesity. Am J Clin Nutr 2004;79:537–43.

[73] Elliot SS, Keim NL, Stern JS, et al. Fructose, weight gain, and the insulin resistance syndrome. Am J Clin Nutr 2002;76:911–22.

[74] Stanhope KL. Role of fructose-containing sugars in the epidemics of obesity and metabolic syndrome. Annu Rev Med 2012;63:329–43.

[75] Mock K, Sundus L, Benedito VA, et al. High-fructose corn syrup-55 consumption alters hepatic lipid metabolism and promotes triglyceride accumulation. J Nutr Biochem 2017;39:32–9.

[76] Stanhope KL, Schwarz JM, Keim NL, et al. Consuming fructose-sweetened, not glucose-sweetened, beverages increases visceral adiposity and lipids and decreases insulin sensitivity in overweight/obese humans. J Clin Invest 2009;119(5):1322–34.

[77] Basaranoglu M, Basaranoglu G, Sabunco T, et al. Fructose as a key player in the development of fatty liver disease. World J Gastroenterol 2013;19(8):1166–72.

[78] Coughlan MT, Thorburn DR, et al. RAGE-induced cytosolic ROS promote mitochondrial superoxide generation in diabetes. J Am Soc Nephrol 2009;20(4):742–52.

[79] Nishikawa T, Edelstein D, Du XL, et al. Normalizing mitochondrial superoxide production blocks three pathways of hyperglycaemic damage. Nature 2000;404(6779):787–90.

[80] Mena S, Ortega A, Estrela JM. Oxidative stress in environmental-induced carcinogenesis. Mutat Res 2009;674(1–2):36–44.

[81] Mooney LA, Madsen AM, Tang D, et al. Antioxidant vitamin supplementation reduces benzo(a)pyrene-DNA adducts and potential cancer risk in female smokers. Cancer Epidemiol Biomarkers Prev 2005;14(1):237–42.

[82] Baumeister P, Reiter M, Kleinsasser N, et al. Epigallocatechin-3-gallate reduces DNA damage induced by benzo[a]pyrene diol epoxide and cigarette smoke condensate in human mucosa tissue cultures. Eur J Cancer Prev 2009;18(3):230–5.

[83] Kantor ED, Rehm CD, et al. Trends in prescription drug use among adults in the United States from 1999–2012. JAMA 2015;314(17):1818–31.

[84] Environmental Working Group. 2008. http://www.ewg.org/news/testimony-official-correspondence/ewg-calls-epa-protect-health-americans-and-set-standards (accessed 12 Jun 2017).

[85] Daly AK, Day CP. Genetic association studies in drug-induced liver injury. Semin Liver Dis 2009;29(4):400–11.

[86] Lammert C, Einarsson S, et al. Relationship between daily dose of oral medications and idiosyncratic drug-induced liver injury: search for signals. Hepatology 2008;47(6):2003–9.

[87] Chalasani N, Fontana RJ, et al. Causes, clinical features, and outcomes from a prospective study of drug-induced liver injury in the United States. Gastroenterology 2008;135(6):1924–34.

[88] Haro-Garcia L, Velez-Zamora N, Aguilar-Madrid G, et al. Blood disorders among workers exposed to a mixture of benzene-toluene-xylene (BTX) in a paint factory. Rev Peru Med Exp Salud Publica 2012;29(2):181–7.

[89] Serdar B, LeBlanc WG, Norris JM. Potential effects of polychlorinated biphenyls (PCBs) and selected organochlorine pesticides (OCPs) on immune cells and blood biochemistry measures: a cross-sectional assessment of the NHANES 2003–2004 data. Environ Health 2014;13:114.

[90] Shih HT, Yu CL, Wu MT, et al. Subclinical abnormalities in workers with continuous low-level toluene exposure. Toxicol Ind Health 2011;27(8):691–9.

[91] Uzma N, Salar BM, Kumar BS, et al. Impact of organic solvents and environmental pollutants on the physiological function in petrol filling workers. Int J Environ Res Public Health 2008;5(3):139–46.

[92] Lin YS, Ginsberg G, Caffrey JL, et al. Association of body burden of mercury with liver function test status in the U.S. population. Environ Int 2014;70:88–94.

[93] Lee H, Kim Y, Sim CS, et al. Associations between blood mercury levels and subclinical changes in liver enzymes among South Korean general adults: analysis of 2008-2012 Korean national health and nutrition examination survey data. Environ Res 2014;130:14–19.

[94] Seo MS, Lee HR, Shim JY, et al. Relationship between blood mercury concentrations and serum γ-glutamyltranspeptidase level in Korean adults using data from the 2010 Korean National Health and Nutrition Examination Survey. Clin Chim Acta 2014;430:160–3.

[95] Cave M, et al. Polychlorinated biphenyls, lead, and mercury are associated with liver disease in American adults: NHANES 2003-2004. Environ Health Perspect 2010;118(12):1735–42.

[96] Min YS, Lim HS, Kim H. Biomarkers for polycyclic aromatic hydrocarbons and serum liver enzymes. Am J Ind Med 2015;58(7):764–72.

[97] Lin CY, Lin LY, Chiang CK, et al. Investigation of the associations between low-dose serum perfluorinated chemicals and liver enzymes in US adults. Am J Gastroenterol 2010;105(6):1354–63.

[98] Araoud M, Neffeti F, Douki W, et al. Adverse effects of pesticides on biochemical and haematological parameters in Tunisian agricultural workers. J Expo Sci Environ Epidemiol 2012;22(3):243–7.

[99] Lee DH, Steffes MW, Jacobs DR Jr. Can persistent organic pollutants explain the association between serum gamma-glutamyltransferase and type 2 diabetes? Diabetologia 2008;51(3):402–7.

[100] Lee DH, Ha MH, Kim JH, et al. Gamma-glutamyltransferase and diabetes – a 4 year follow-up study. Diabetologia 2003;46(3):359–64.

[101] Brenner H, Rothenbacher D, Arndt V, et al. Distribution, determinants, and prognostic value of gamma-glutamyltransferase for all-cause mortality in a cohort of construction workers from southern Germany. Prev Med 1997;26(3):305–10.

[102] Nagaya T, Yoshida H, Takahashi H, et al. Dose-response relationships between drinking and serum tests in Japanese men aged 40–59 years. Alcohol 1999;17(2):133–8.

[103] Lee DH, Lim JS, Song K, et al. Graded associations of blood lead and urinary cadmium concentrations with oxidative-stress-related markers in the U.S. population: results from the third National Health and Nutrition Examination Survey. Environ Health Perspect 2006;114(3):350–4.

[104] Lee DH, Jacobs DR. Is serum gamma-glutamyltransferase an exposure marker of xenobiotics? Empirical evidence with polycyclic aromatic hydrocarbon. Clin Chem Lab Med 2009;47(7):860–2.

[105] Calvert GM, Hornung RW, et al. Hepatic and gastrointestinal effects in an occupational cohort exposed to 2,3,7,8-tetrachlorodibenzo-para-dioxin. JAMA 1992;267(16):2209–14.

[106] Everett CJ, King DE, Player MS, et al. Association of urinary polycyclic aromatic hydrocarbons and serum C-reactive protein. Environ Res 2010;110(1):79–82.

[107] Kim KS, Hong NS, Jacobs DR Jr, et al. Interaction between persistent organic pollutants and C-reactive protein in estimating insulin resistance among non-diabetic adults. J Prev Med Public Health 2012;45(2):62–9.

[108] Penell J, Lind L, Salihovic S, et al. Persistent organic pollutants are related to change in circulating lipid levels during a 5 year follow-up. Environ Res 2014;134:190–7.

[109] Aminov Z, Haase R, Olson JR, et al. Racial differences in levels of serum lipids and effects of exposure to persistent organic pollutants on lipid levels in residents of Anniston, Alabama. Environ Int 2014;73:216–23.

[110] Nelsen JW, Hatch EE, Webster TF. Exposure to polyfluoroalkyl chemicals and cholesterol, body weight, and insulin resistance in the general U.S. population. Environ Health Perspect 2010;118(2):197–202.

[111] Geiger SD, Xiao J, Ducatman A, et al. The association between PFOA, PFOS and serum lipid levels in adolescents. Chemosphere 2014;98:78–83.

[112] Kumar J, Monica Lind P, Salihovic S, et al. Influence of persistent organic pollutants on oxidative stress in population-based samples. Chemosphere 2014;114:303–9.

[113] Dufour DR, et al. Diagnosis and monitoring of hepatic injury. II. Recommendations for use of laboratory tests in screening, diagnosis, and monitoring. Clin Chem 2000;46(12):2050–68.

[114] Kumar J, et al. Persistent organic pollutants and liver dysfunction biomarkers in a population-based human sample of men and women. Environ Res 2014;134:251–6.

[115] Tian J, Zhong R, Liu C, et al. Association between bilirubin and risk of nonalcoholic fatty liver disease based on a prospective cohort study. Sci Rep 2016;6:310006.

[116] Geiger SD, Xiao J, Shankar A. Positive association between perfluoroalkyl chemicals and hyperuricemia in children. Am J Epidemiol 2013;177(11):1255–62.

[117] Steenland K, Tinker S, Shankar A, et al. Association of perfluorooctanoic acid (PFOA) and perfluorooctane sulfonate (PFOS) with uric acid among adults with elevated community exposure to PFOA. Environ Health Perspect 2010;118:229–33.

[118] Weiss N. Mechanisms of increased vascular oxidant stress in hyperhomocystenemia and its impact on endothelial function. Curr Drug Metab 2005;6(1):27–36.

[119] Cheung GT, Siow YL, O K. Homocysteine stimulates monocyte chemoattractant protein-1 expression in mesangial cells via NF-kappaB activation. Can J Physiol Pharmacol 2008;86(3):88–96.

[120] Schafer JH, Glass TA, Bressler J, et al. Blood lead is a predictor of homocysteine levels in a population-based study of older adults. Environ Health Perspect 2005;113(1):31–5.

[121] Zesiewicz TA, Wecker L, Sullivan KL, et al. The controversy concerning plasma homocysteine in Parkinson disease patients treated with levodopa alone or with entacapone: effects of vitamin status. Clin Neuropharmacol 2006;29(3): 106–11.

[122] Dos Santos EF, Busanello EN, Miglioranza A, et al. Evidence that folic acid deficiency is a major determinant of hyperhomocysteinemia in Parkinson's disease. Metab Brain Dis 2009;24(2):257–69.

[123] Valavanidis A, Vlachogianni T, Fiotakis C. 8-hydroxy-2'-deoxyguanosine (8-OHdG): a critical biomarker of oxidative stress and carcinogenesis. J Environ Sci Health C Environ Carcinog Ecotoxicol Rev 2009;27(2):120–39.

[124] Wu LL, Chiou CC, Chang PY, et al. Urinary 8-OHdG: a marker of oxidative stress to DNA and a risk factor for cancer, atherosclerosis, and diabetes. Clin Chim Acta 2004;339(1–2):1–9.

[125] Remillard RB, Bunce NJ, et al. Linking dioxins to diabetes: epidemiology and biologic plausibility. Environ Health Perspect 2002;110(9):853–8.

[126] Tang M, Chen K, Yang F, et al. Exposure to organochlorine pollutants and type 2 diabetes: a systematic review and meta-analysis. PLoS ONE 2014;9(10):e85556.

[127] Weinhold B. PCBs and diabetes: pinning down mechanisms. Environ Health Perspect 2013;121(1):A32.

[128] Grün F, Blumberg B. Perturbed nuclear receptor signaling by environmental obesogens as emerging factors in the obesity crisis. Rev Endocr Metab Disord 2007;8(2):161–71.

[129] Suarez-Lopez JR, et al. Persistent organic pollutants in young adults and changes in glucose related metabolism over a 23-year follow-up. Environ Res 2015;137:485–94.

[130] Suzuki T, Yamamoto R. Organic mercury levels in human hair with and without storage for eleven years. Bull Environ Contam Toxicol 1982;28:186–8.

[131] Airey D. Mercury in human hair due to environment and diet. A review. Environ Health Perspect 1983;52:303–16.

[132] Rooney JP. The role of thiols, dithiols, nutritional factors and interacting ligands in the toxicology of mercury. Toxicology 2007;234(3):145–56.

[133] Bilzer M, Roggel F, Gerbes AL. Role of Kupffer cells in host defense and liver disease. Liver Int 2006;26(10):1175–86.

[134] Guengerich FP. Influence of nutrients and other dietary materials on cytochrome P-450 enzymes. Am J Clin Nutr 1995;61(S3): 651S–658S.

[135] Desta Z, Zhao X, et al. Clinical significance of the cytochrome P450 2C19 genetic polymorphism. Clin Pharmacokinet 2002;41(12):913–58.

[136] Guengerich FP. Cytochrome p450 and chemical toxicology. Chem Res Toxicol 2008;21(1):70–83.

[137] Long A, Walker JD. Quantitative structure-activity relationships for predicting metabolism and modeling cytochrome p450 enzyme activities. Environ Toxicol Chem 2003;22(8):1894–9.

[138] Yuan J, Lu WQ, Zou YL, et al. Influence of aroclor 1254 on benzo(a)pyrene-induced DNA breakage, oxidative DNA damage, and cytochrome P4501A activity in human hepatoma cell line. Environ Toxicol 2009;24(4):327–33.

[139] Aubert J, Begriche K, et al. Increased expression of cytochrome P450 2E1 in nonalcoholic fatty liver disease: mechanisms and pathophysiological role. Clin Res Hepatol Gastroenterol 2011;35(10):630–7.

[140] Larson AM. Acetaminophen hepatotoxicity. Clin Liver Dis 2007;11(3):525–48.

[141] Ingelman-Sundberg M. The human genome project and novel aspects of cytochrome P450 research. Toxicol Appl Pharmacol 2005;207(2 Suppl.):52–6.

[142] El-Sankary W, Plant NJ, Gibson GG, et al. Regulation of the CYP3A4 gene by hydrocortisone and xenobiotics: role of the glucocorticoid and pregnane X receptors. Drug Metab Dispos 2000;28(5):493–6.

[143] Pelkonen O, Turpeinen M, et al. Inhibition and induction of human cytochrome P450 enzymes: current status. Arch Toxicol 2008;82(10):667–715.

[144] Di YM, Li CG, Xue CC, et al. Clinical drugs that interact with St. John's Wort and implication in drug development. Curr Pharm Des 2008;14(17):1723–42.

[145] Hukkanen J, Lassila A, Paivarinta K, et al. Induction and regulation of xenobiotic-metabolizing cytochrome P450s in the human A549 lung adenocarcinoma cell line. Am J Respir Cell Mol Biol 2000;22(3):360–6.

[146] Hannon-Fletcher M, O'Kane M, Moles K, et al. Lymphocyte cytochrome P450-CYP2E1 expression in human IDDM subjects. Food Chem Toxicol 2001;39:125–32.

[147] Grant DM. Detoxification pathways in the liver. J Inherit Metab Dis 1991;14:421–30.

[148] Townsend DM, Tew KD, Tapiero H. The importance of glutathione in human disease. Biomed Pharmacother 2003;57(3–4):145–55.

[149] Ludewig G, et al. Mechanisms of toxicity of PCB metabolites: generation of reactive oxygen species and glutathione depletion. Cent Eur J Public Health 2000;8(Suppl.):15–17.

[150] Ballatori N, Krance SM, Notenboom S, et al. Glutathione dysregulation and the etiology and progression of human diseases. Biol Chem 2009;390(3):191–214.

[151] Palma S, Cornetta T, Padua L, et al. Influence of glutathione S-transferase polymorphisms on genotoxic effects induced by tobacco smoke. Mutat Res 2007;633(1):1–12.

[152] Boukouvala S, Fakis G. Arylamine N-acetyltransferases: what we learn from genes and genomes. Drug Metab Rev 2005;37(3):511–64.

[153] Garcia-Closas M, Malats N, Silverman D. NAT2 slow acetylation, GSTM1 null genotype, and risk of bladder cancer: results from the Spanish Bladder Cancer Study and meta-analyses. Lancet 2005;366(9486):649–59.

[154] Zhu Z, Zhang J, Jiang W, et al. Risks on N-acetyltransferase 2 and bladder cancer: a meta-analysis. Onco Targets Ther 2015;8: 3715–20.

[155] Zhu BT. Catechol-o-methyltransferase (COMT)-mediated methylation metabolism of endogenous bioactive catechols and modulation by endobiotics and xenobiotics: importance in pathophysiology and pathogenesis. Curr Drug Metab 2002;3(3):321–49.

[156] Wang W, Le WD, Pan T, et al. Association of NRH:quinone oxidoreductase 2 gene promoter polymorphism with higher gene expression and increased susceptibility to Parkinson's disease. J Gerontol A Biol Sci Med Sci 2008;63(2):127–34.

[157] Jones D. The textbook of functional medicine. Gig Harbor, WA: The Institute for Functional Medicine; 2006.

[158] Liska DJ. The detoxification enzyme systems. Altern Med Rev 1998;3(3):187–98.

[159] Kellett GL, Brot-Laroche E, Mace OJ, et al. Sugar absorption in the intestine: the role of GLUT2. Annu Rev Nutr 2008;28:35–54.

[160] Robayo-Torres CC, Quezada-Calvillo R, Nichols BL. Disaccharide digestion: clinical and molecular aspects. Clin Gastroenterol Hepatol 2006;4(3):276–87.

[161] Basivireddy J, Jacob M, Ramamoorthy P, et al. Indomethacin-induced free radical-mediated changes in the intestinal brush border membranes. Biochem Pharmacol 2003;65(4):683–95.

[162] Tadataka Y. Yamada's textbook of gastroenterology. 4th ed. Philadelphia, PA: Lippincott Williams & Wilkins; 2003.

[163] Mu H, Høy CE. The digestion of dietary triacylglycerols. Prog Lipid Res 2004;43(2):105–33.

[164] Lowe ME. Structure and function of pancreatic lipase and colipase. Annu Rev Nutr 1997;17:141–58.

[165] Ahnen DJ, Guerciolini R, Hauptman J, et al. Effect of orlistat on fecal fat, fecal biliary acids, and colonic cell proliferation in obese subjects. Clin Gastroenterol Hepatol 2007;5(11):1291–9.

[166] Nakai M, Fukui Y, Asami S, et al. Inhibitory effects of oolong tea polyphenols on pancreatic lipase in vitro. J Agric Food Chem 2005;53(11):4593–8.

[167] Glisan SL, Grove KA, Yennawar NH, et al. Inhibition of pancreatic lipase by black tea theaflavins: comparative enzymology and in silico modeling studies. Food Chem 2017;216:296–300.

[168] Shishikura Y, Khokhar S, Murray BS. Effects of tea polyphenols on emulsification of olive oil in a small intestine model system. J Agric Food Chem 2006;54(5):1906–13.

[169] Gilardini L, Pasqualinotto L, Di Pierro F, et al. Effects of Greenselect Phytosome® on weight maintenance after weight loss in obese women: a randomized placebo-controlled study. BMC Complement Altern Med 2016;16:233.

[170] Ashigai H, Taniguchi Y, Suzuki M, et al. Fecal lipid excretion after consumption of a black tea polyphenol containing beverage-randomized, placebo-controlled, double-blind, crossover study. Biol Pharm Bull 2016;39(5):699–704.

[171] Inui KI, Masuda S, Saito H. Cellular and molecular aspects of drug transport in the kidney. Kidney Int 2000;58(3):944–58.

[172] Stauber JL, Florence TM. A comparative study of copper, lead, cadmium, and zinc in human sweat and blood. Sci Total Environ 1988;74:235–47.

[173] Dorea JG. Mercury and lead during breast feeding. Br J Nutr 2004; 92:21–40.

[174] Stephens R, Waldron HA. The influence of milk and related dietary constituents on lead metabolism. Food Cosmet Toxicol 1975;13:555–63.

[175] Lee YM, Lee MK, Bae SG, et al. Association of homocysteine levels with blood lead levels and micronutrients in the US general population. J Prev Med Public Health 2012;45(6):387–93.

[176] Thomas D. A study on the mineral depletion of the foods available to US as a nation over the period 1940 to 1991. Nutr Health 2003;17:85–115.

[177] Hughes M, Chaplin MH, Martin LW. Influence of mycorrhiza on the nutrition of red raspberries. Hort Science 1979;14:521–3.

[178] Garvin DF, Welch RM, Finley JW. Historical shifts in the seed mineral micronutrient concentration of US hard red winter wheat germplasm. J Sci Food Agr 2006;86:2213–20.

[179] Jones VA, Dickinson RJ, Workman E, et al. Crohn's disease: maintenance of remission by diet. Lancet 1985;2(8448):177–80.

[180] Nesterenko VB, Nesterenko AV, Babenko VI, et al. Reducing the 137Cs-load in the organism of 'Chernobyl' children with apple-pectin. Swiss Med Wkly 2004;134(1–2):24–7.

[181] Chen CM, Lin Chen CY, et al. Consumption of sweet potato leaves decreases lipid peroxidation and DNA damage in humans. Asia Pac J Clin Nutr 2008;17(3):408–14.

[182] Cocate PG, Natali AJ, et al. Fruit and vegetable intake and related nutrients are associated with oxidative stress markers in middle-aged men. Nutrition 2014;30(6):660–5.

[183] Thompson HJ, Heimendinger J, Haegele A, et al. Effect of increased vegetable and fruit consumption on markers of oxidative cellular damage. Carcinogenesis 1999;20(12):2261–6.

[184] Pedret A, Valls RM, Fernández-Castillejo S, et al. Polyphenol-rich foods exhibit DNA antioxidative properties and protect the glutathione system in healthy subjects. Mol Nutr Food Res 2012;56(7):1025–33.

[185] Qian G, Xue K, Tang L, et al. Mitigation of oxidative damage by green tea polyphenols and Tai Chi exercise in postmenopausal women with osteopenia. PLoS ONE 2012;7(10):e48090.

[186] He YT, Xing SS, Gao L, et al. Ginkgo biloba attenuates oxidative DNA damage of human umbilical vein endothelial cells induced by intermittent high glucose. Pharmazie 2014;69(3):203–7.

[187] Ferguson SK, Hirai DM, Copp SW, et al. Dose dependent effects of nitrate supplementation on cardiovascular control and microvascular oxygenation dynamics in healthy rats. Nitric Oxide 2014;39:51–8.

[188] Niklowitz P, Sonnenschein A, et al. Enrichment of coenzyme Q10 in plasma and blood cells: defense against oxidative damage. Int J Biol Sci 2007;3(4):257–62.

[189] Kowluru RA, Kanwar M. Effects of curcumin on retinal oxidative stress and inflammation in diabetes. Nutr Metab (Lond) 2007;4:8.

[190] Devaraj S, Mathur S, Basu A, et al. A dose-response study on the effects of purified lycopene supplementation on biomarkers of oxidative stress. J Am Coll Nutr 2008;27(2):267–73.

[191] Hakim IA, Harris RB, Brown S, et al. Effect of increased tea consumption on oxidative DNA damage among smokers: a randomized controlled study. J Nutr 2003;133(10):3303S–3309S.

[192] Burton GW, Ingold KU. Vitamin E as an in vitro and in vivo antioxidant. Ann N Y Acad Sci 1989;570:7–22. In: Diplock AT, Machoin LJ, Parker L, Pryor WA, eds. Vitamin E: biochemistry and health implications.

[193] Horwitt MK. Supplementation with vitamin E. Am J Clin Nutr 1988;47:1088–9.

[194] Panganamala RV, Cornwell DG. The effects of vitamin E on arachidonic acid metabolism. Ann N Y Acad Sci 1982;393:376–91.

[195] Townsend DM, Tew KD, Tapiero H. The importance of glutathione in human disease. Biomed Pharmacother 2003;57(3–4):145–55.

[196] Soltan-Sharifi MS, et al. Improvement by N-acetylcysteine of acute respiratory distress syndrome through increasing intracellular glutathione. Hum Exp Toxicol 2007;26(9):697–703.

[197] Micke P, et al. Oral supplementation with whey proteins increases plasma glutathione levels of HIV-infected patients. Eur J Clin Invest 2001;31(2):171–8.

[198] Sharma H, Datta P, et al. Gene expression profiling in practitioners of Sudarshan Kriya. J Psychosom Res 2008;64(2):213–18.

[199] Rundle AG, Orjuela M, et al. Preliminary studies on the effect of moderate physical activity on blood levels of glutathione. Biomarkers 2005;10(5):390–400.

[200] Jariwalla RJ, et al. Restoration of blood total glutathione status and lymphocyte function following alpha-lipoic acid supplementation in patients with HIV infection. J Altern Complement Med 2008; 14(2):139–46.

[201] Lieber CS, Packer L. S-Adenosylmethionine: molecular, biological, and clinical aspects – an introduction. Am J Clin Nutr 2002;76(5):1148S–50S.

[202] Hauser RA, Lyons KE, et al. Randomized, double-blind, pilot evaluation of intravenous glutathione in Parkinson's disease. Mov Disord 2009;24(7):979–83.

[203] Mischley LK, et al. Safety survey of intranasal glutathione. J Altern Complement Med 2013;19(5):459–63.

[204] Stone J. Reduced selenium status of patients with asthma. Clin Sci 1989;77:495–500.

[205] Kadrabova J, Mad'aric A, Kovacikova Z, et al. Selenium status is decreased in patients with intrinsic asthma. Biol Trace Elem Res 1996;52:241–8.

[206] Ekor M, Adesanoye OA, Farombi EO. N-acetylcysteine pretreatment ameliorates mercuric chloride-induced oxidative renal damage in rats. Afr J Med Med Sci 2010;39(Suppl.):153–60.

[207] Kelly GS. Clinical applications of N-acetylcysteine. Altern Med Rev 1998;3(2):114–27.

[208] Zhu Y, Kalen AL, Li L, et al. Polychlorinated-biphenyl-induced oxidative stress and cytotoxicity can be mitigated by antioxidants after exposure. Free Radic Biol Med 2009;47(12):1762–71.

[209] Garg R, Gupta S, Maru GB. Dietary curcumin modulates transcriptional regulators of phase I and phase II enzymes in benzo[a]pyrene-treated mice: mechanism of its anti-initiating action. Carcinogenesis 2008;29(5):1022–32.

[210] Zhu W, Cromie MM, Cai Q, et al. Curcumin and vitamin E protect against adverse effects of benzo[a]pyrene in lung epithelial cells. PLoS ONE 2014;9(3):e92992.

[211] Mukherjee S, Roy M, et al. A mechanistic approach for modulation of arsenic toxicity in human lymphocytes by curcumin, an active constituent of medicinal herb Curcuma longa Linn. J Clin Biochem Nutr 2007;41(1):32–42.

[212] Ciftci O, Ozdemir I, Tanyildizi S, et al. Antioxidative effects of curcumin, β-myrcene and 1,8-cineole against 2,3,7,8-tetrachlorodibenzo-p-dioxin-induced oxidative stress in rats liver. Toxicol Ind Health 2011;27(5):447–53.

[213] Chang YZ, Lin HC, Chan ST, et al. Effects of quercetin metabolites on the enhancing effect of β-carotene on DNA damage and cytochrome P1A1/2 expression in benzo[a]pyrene-exposed A549 cells. Food Chem 2012;133(2):445–50.

[214] Ramadass P, Meerarani P, Toborek M, et al. Dietary flavonoids modulate PCB-induced oxidative stress, CYP1A1 induction, and AhR-DNA binding activity in vascular endothelial cells. Toxicol Sci 2003;76(1):212–19.

[215] Uchikawa T, Kumamoto Y, et al. Enhanced elimination of tissue methylmercury in Parachlorella beijerinckii-fed mice. J Toxicol Sci 2011;36(1):121–6.

[216] Takeda Y, Nakase H, et al. Upregulation of T-bet and tight junction molecules by Bifidobacterium longum improves colonic inflammation of ulcerative colitis. Inflamm Bowel Dis 2009;15(11):1617–18.

[217] Fujimori S, Gudis K, Mitsui K, et al. A randomized controlled trial on the efficacy of synbiotic versus probiotic or prebiotic treatment to improve the quality of life in patients with ulcerative colitis. Nutrition 2009;25(5):520–5.

[218] Liu ZH, Huang MJ, Zhang XW, et al. The effects of perioperative probiotic treatment on serum zonulin concentration and subsequent postoperative infectious complications after colorectal

cancer surgery: a double-center and double-blind randomized clinical trial. Am J Clin Nutr 2013;97(1):117–26.

[219] Nosova T, Jousimies-Somer H, Jokelainen K, et al. Acetaldehyde production and metabolism by human indigenous and probiotic Lactobacillus and Bifidobacterium strains. Alcohol 2000;35(6):561–8.

[220] Gratz S, Mykkänen H, El-Nezami H. Aflatoxin B1 binding by a mixture of Lactobacillus and Propionibacterium: in vitro versus ex vivo. J Food Prot 2005;68(11):2470–4.

[221] Li N, Neu J. Glutamine deprivation alters intestinal tight junctions via a PI3-K/Akt mediated pathway in Caco-2 cells. J Nutr 2009;139(4):710–14.

[222] Salvatore S, Heuschkel R, Tomlin S, et al. A pilot study of N-acetyl glucosamine, a nutritional substrate for glycosaminoglycan synthesis, in paediatric chronic inflammatory bowel disease. Aliment Pharmacol Ther 2000;14(12):1567–79.

[223] Amasheh M, Andres S, Amasheh S, et al. Barrier effects of nutritional factors. Ann N Y Acad Sci 2009;1165:267–73.

[224] Suzuki T, Hara H. Quercetin enhances intestinal barrier function through the assembly of zonula [corrected] occludens-2, occludin, and claudin-1 and the expression of claudin-4 in Caco-2 cells. J Nutr 2009;139(5):965–74.

[225] Amasheh M, Schlichter S, Amasheh S, et al. Quercetin enhances epithelial barrier function and increases claudin-4 expression in Caco-2 cells. J Nutr 2008;138(6):1067–73.

[226] Bischoff SC, Krämer S. Human mast cells, bacteria, and intestinal immunity. Immunol Rev 2007;217:329–37.

[227] Sarre H. Experience in the treatment of chronic hepatopathies with silymarin. Arzneimittelforschung 1971;21:1209–12.

[228] Salmi HA, Sarna S. Effect of silymarin on chemical, functional, and morphological alteration of the liver. A double-blind controlled study. Scand J Gastroenterol 1982;17:417–21.

[229] Ferenci P, Dragosics H, Frank H, et al. Randomized controlled trial of silymarin treatment in patients with cirrhosis of the liver. J Hepatol 1989;9:105–13.

[230] Hikino H, Kiso Y, Wagner H, et al. Antihepatotoxic actions of flavonolignans from Silybum marianum fruits. Planta Med 1984;50:248–50.

[231] Vogel G, Trost W. Studies on pharmacodynamics, site and mechanism of action of silymarin, the antihepatotoxic principle from Silybum marianum (L.). Gaert Arzneim Forsch 1975;25:179–85.

[232] Valenzuela A, Aspillaga M, Vial S, et al. Selectivity of silymarin on the increase of the glutathione content in different tissues of the rat. Planta Med 1989;55:420–2.

[233] Mooiman KD, Maas-Bakker RF, et al. Milk thistle's active components silybin and isosilybin: novel inhibitors of PXR-mediated CYP3A4 induction. Drug Metab Dispos 2013;41(8):1494–504.

[234] Campos R, Garrido A, Guerra V. Silybin dihemisuccinate protects against glutathione depletion and lipid peroxidation induced by paracetamol on rat liver. Planta Med 1989;55:417–19.

[235] Feher J, Lang I, Nekam KJ, et al. In vivo effect of free radical scavenger hepatoprotective agents on superoxide dismutase (SOD) activity in patients. Tokai J Exp Clin Med 1990;15:129–34.

[236] Paumgartner G, Beuers U. Ursodeoxycholic acid in cholestatic liver disease: mechanisms of action and therapeutic use revisited. Hepatology 2002;36(3):525–31.

[237] Kerkadi A, Barriault C, et al. Cholestyramine protection against ochratoxin A toxicity: role of ochratoxin A sorption by the resin and bile acid enterohepatic circulation. J Food Prot 1999;62(12):1461–5.

[238] Solfrizzo M, Visconti A, et al. In vitro and in vivo studies to assess the effectiveness of cholestyramine as a binding agent for fumonisins. Mycopathologia 2001;151(3):147–53.

[239] Rogan WJ, Dietrich KN, Ware JH, et al. The effect of chelation therapy with succimer on neuropsychological development in children exposed to lead. N Eng J Med 2001;344:1421–6.

[240] Andersen O. Principles and recent developments in chelation treatment of metal intoxication. Chem Rev 1999;99:2683–710.

[241] Kosnett MJ. The role of chelation in the treatment of arsenic and mercury poisoning. J Med Toxicol 2013;9:347–54.

[242] Olivieri NF, Brittenham GM. Iron-chelating therapy and the treatment of thalassemia. Blood 1997;89(7):2621.

[243] Brittenham GM, Griffith PM, Nienhuis AW, et al. Efficacy of deferoxamine in preventing complications of iron overload in patients with thalassemia major. N Engl J Med 1994;331(9):567–73.

[244] Vilensky JA, Redman K. British anti-Lewisite (dimercaprol): an amazing history. Ann Emerg Med 2003;41(3):378–83.

[245] Torres-Alanis O, Garza-Ocanas L, et al. Urinary excretion of trace elements in humans after sodium 2,3-dimercaptopropane-1-sulfonate challenge test. J Toxicol Clin Toxicol 2000;38(7):697–700.

[246] Graziano JH. Role of 2,3-dimercaptosuccininc acid in the treatment of heavy metal poisoning. Med Toxicol 1986;1:155–62.

[247] Lyle WH. Penicillamine in metal poisoning. J Rheumatol 1981;8(Suppl. 7):96–9.

[248] Murphy MJ, Lyon LW, Taylor JW. Subacute arsenic neuropathy: clinical and electrophysiological observations. J Neurol Neurosurg Psychiatry 1981;44:896–900.

[249] Clarkson TW, Magos L, Cox C, et al. Tests of efficacy of antidotes for removal of methylmercury in human poisoning during the Iraq outbreak. J Pharmacol Exp Ther 1981;218:74–83.

[250] Paton WD. Toxicity of thallium. Br Med J 1972;4(5831):49.

[251] Aremu DA, Madejczyk MS, Ballatori N. N-acetylcysteine as a potential antidote and biomonitoring agent of methylmercury exposure. Environ Health Perspect 2008;116(1):26–31.

[252] Uchikawa T, Kumamoto Y, Maruyama I, et al. Enhanced elimination of tissue methylmercury in Parachlorella beijerinckii-fed mice. J Toxicol Sci 2011;36(1):121–6.

[253] Kumar RM, Franklin J, Raj SP. Accumulation of heavy metals (Cu, Cr, Pb and Cd) in freshwater micro algae (Chlorella sp.). J Environ Sci Eng 2013;55(3):371–6.

[254] Lee I, Tran M, Evans-Nguyen T, et al. Detoxification of chlorella supplement on heterocyclic amines in Korean young adults. Environ Toxicol Pharmacol 2015;39(1):441–6.

[255] Sivaprasad R, Nagaraj M, Varalakshmi P. Combined efficacies of lipoic acid and 2,3-dimercaptosuccinic acid against lead-induced lipid peroxidation in rat liver. J Nutr Biochem 2004;15(1):18–23.

[256] Flora SJ, Pande M, Mehta A. Beneficial effect of combined administration of some naturally occurring antioxidants (vitamins) and thiol chelators in the treatment of chronic lead intoxication. Chem Biol Interact 2003;145(3):267–80.

[257] Genuis SJ, Birkholz D, Rodushkin I, et al. Blood, urine, and sweat (BUS) study: monitoring and elimination of bioaccumulated toxic elements. Arch Environ Contam Toxicol 2011;61(2):344–57.

[258] Cohn JR, Emmett EA. The excretion of trace metals in human sweat. Ann Clin Lab Sci 1978;8(4):270–5.

[259] Schnare DW, Ben M, Shields MG. Body burden reductions of PCBs, PBBs, and chlorinated pesticides in human subjects. Ambio 1984;13(5–6):378–80.

[260] Sears ME, Kerr KJ, Bray RI. Arsenic, cadmium, lead, and mercury in sweat: a systematic review. J Environ Public Health 2012;2012:184745.

[261] Vree TB, Muskens JM, Van Rossum JM. Excretion of amphetamines in human sweat. Arch Int Pharmacodyn Ther 1972;199:311–17.

[262] Henderson GL, Wilson KB. Excretion of methadone and metabolites in human sweat. Res Commun Chem Pathol Pharmacol 1973;5(1):1–8.

[263] Johnson HL, Maaibach HI. Drug excretion in human eccrine sweat. J Invest Dermatol 1971;56(3):182–8.

[264] Parnas J, Flachs H, Gram L, et al. Excretion of antiepileptic drugs in sweat. Acta Neurol Scand 1978;58:197–204.

[265] Genuis SJ, Beesoon S, Birkholz D, et al. Human excretion of bisphenol A: blood, urine, and sweat (BUS) study. J Environ Public Health 2012;2012:185731.

[266] Hannuksela ML, Ellahham S. Benefits and risks of sauna bathing. Am J Med 2001;110:118–26.

[267] Heywood A. A trial of bath waters: the treatment of lead poisoning. Med Hist Suppl 1990;10:82–101.

[268] Little L, Porche DJ. Manual lymph drainage (MLD). J Assoc Nurses AIDS Care 1998;9:78–81.

[269] Bulow J. Adipose tissue blood flow during exercise. Dan Med Bull 1983;30:85–100.

[270] Pillon Barcelos R, Freire Royes LF, Gonzalez-Gallego J, et al. Oxidative stress and inflammation: liver responses and adaptations to acute and regular exercise. Free Radic Res 2017;51(2):222–36.

[271] Seigel JM. Why we sleep. Sci Am 2003;89(5):92–7.

5 Naturopathic hydrotherapy

Kate Broderick

INTRODUCTION

Hydrotherapy in the European nature cure tradition historically provided the cornerstone for the formation of naturopathy as a profession. Chapter 1 of *Clinical Naturopathic Medicine* covers a brief history of the contributions of Vincent Priessnitz (1799–1852) and Father Sebastian Kneipp (1821–1897) to the formation of the naturopathic profession in the US, via the migration and teachings of Benedict Lust (1872–1945) and Henry Lindlahr (1852–1925). The history provided here picks up where that chapter left off.

MODERN NATUROPATHIC HYDROTHERAPY

European nature cure, and particularly water cure in the tradition of Father Sebastian Kneipp, has continued to evolve in Europe and remains a robust part of life and culture in Germany to this day. Although today's equipment and facilities are more technologically advanced, and the treatments are administered by highly trained hydrotherapists under medical supervision and prescription, the methods are much the same as Father Kneipp's original water cure: using the thermal and mechanical effects of water, and particularly the targeted application of short cold treatments, to stimulate the nervous and circulatory systems so as to improve the body's capacity to self-regulate, detoxify and heal.[1] Father Kneipp's water cure became the foundation of naturopathy in the late 1800s in the US and that lineage continues to inform the practice of the current generation of US naturopaths.[2]

However, hydrotherapy was already well-established as a natural healing modality in the US decades before the arrival of Benedict Lust and Henry Lindlahr. Starting in the 1840s, non-orthodox practitioners in the Priessnitz tradition began to bring hydrotherapy to the US and set up water cure establishments that attracted a prominent clientele. At the time of the formation of naturopathy as a profession, the most prominent proponent and practitioner of hydrotherapy in the US was an orthodox medical doctor, John Harvey Kellogg (1852–1943). We must return to England in the late 1600s to find the common ancestor of the Kneipp and Kellogg lines. That common ancestor was Dr John Floyer (1649–1734), who in 1697 published his book, *The History of Hot and Cold Bathing*, wherein he espoused the value of cold baths to stimulate health.[3] Dr Floyer was the inspiration for Johann Hahn (1696–1773), who established modern hydrotherapy in Germany to treat acute and chronic diseases successfully, and from whom the line from Priessnitz to Father Kneipp extended. Priessnitz and Kneipp were not doctors – they were both laymen who developed highly effective systems of healing using cold water treatments, raising the ire of the medical establishment of their time, but who, due to their popularity and success in healing, were allowed to practise nonetheless. Lust and Lindlahr both trained with Father Kneipp before migrating to the US and before either had taken up medical training, though both did eventually become licensed doctors.[2]

In contrast, the direct line from John Floyer to John Harvey Kellogg was a line of orthodox US medical doctors who had become disillusioned with the harmful and ineffective treatment methods of the time and had trained in and lent their own expertise to developing Floyer's historical cold water treatments. Kellogg combined hydrotherapy with methods of natural hygiene to form a complete system administered at his well-known Battle Creek Sanitarium in Michigan, which opened in 1903 and focused strongly on the health of the colon and detoxification. He authored the definitive US text, *Rational Hydrotherapy: A Manual of the Physiological and Therapeutic Effects of Hydrotherapy Procedures, and the Technique of Their Application in the Treatment of Disease*, originally published in 1902.[4,5] The influences of Kneipp and Kellogg, through the synthesis of O.G. Carroll (1879–1962) and several of his prominent students, formed the modern practice of naturopathic hydrotherapy in the US, which continues to be taught in the core curriculum in North America's naturopathic colleges and universities, as well as being practised in the teaching clinics of these institutions.[1,6]

The evolution of naturopathic hydrotherapy in Australia charted a somewhat different route than that followed in other countries. Similar to the US, early migration of hydrotherapy to Australia occurred in the 1840s and was evidenced by the publication in 1846 of *Hydropathy; Or the System of Effecting Cures by Means of*

Cold Water by R.T. Claridge. This was 60 years prior to the establishment of naturopathy as a profession. By the 1860s, water cure sanatoriums began to be established, along with recognition of some of the natural sources of mineralised healing springs in Victoria. With the establishment of the profession in the early 1900s, naturopathic journals placed significant focus on hydrotherapy as a treatment modality, indicating it as a core of naturopathic practice. However, a century later, with the establishment of the vocational level National Health Training Package in 2002, the scope of naturopathy was significantly curtailed in Australia, and hydrotherapy was removed from naturopathic education due to perceived complexities involved in training, which has since virtually eliminated its practice by Australian naturopaths.[7]

This chapter aims to weave together current common practice in naturopathic hydrotherapy in the US tradition with current and historical practice in water cure in the Kneipp tradition.

HYDROTHERAPY AND ITS CONNECTION TO MODERN NATUROPATHIC CLINICAL THEORY

A full coverage of modern naturopathic philosophy and clinical theory is provided in *Clinical Naturopathic Medicine*, which may be used as a foundation here. Hydrotherapy is the therapeutic modality in naturopathy that perhaps comes closest to the heart of naturopathic medicine practice when used along with corrections to improper diet and hydration, movement and exposure to the natural elements. Because it relies on the body's natural physiological reactions to temperature change, it is a way to access the *Vis Medicatrix Naturae*, the healing power of nature, in a generalised way. It can be described as a stimulation to the vital force, or as a tonification and training of the body's homeostatic mechanisms. Used in a non-aggressive way, consistently over time, with respect for its power, it comports with the principle of First Do No Harm by gently bringing the body back towards balance to heal and helping maintain that balance for the prevention of future illness.

Used systemically, as opposed to being used for localised injury, the whole person is treated, as the body's homeostatic mechanisms and the balance of the autonomic nervous system impact the entire organism. When the cause of illness is reduced vitality, accumulation of toxins in the system, weakened digestion or even habituated imbalanced patterns of the nervous and circulatory systems created by other disturbing factors, hydrotherapy can be used to address those causes directly. Finally, given that the patient can be taught to engage in many simple hydrotherapy techniques at home as a way to support regaining and maintaining health, hydrotherapy can also be connected to the principle of *Docere*.

Considered in the light of the naturopathic therapeutic order, hydrotherapy is most often noted as falling within

the second level, stimulating the *Vis Medicatrix Naturae*, as explained above. However, it is difficult to find a level in the first four levels of the therapeutic order within which hydrotherapy could *not* be argued to fall. If a patient is taught to do hydrotherapy at home on a regular basis, this can be seen as part of instituting a more healthful regimen at the first level. Considering the impact of hydrotherapy on the nervous and circulatory systems and the digestive and eliminative organs, we must conclude that it is working at level three, tonifying weakened systems. And when the influence of hot and cold water on the body's musculature is considered, as discussed below, it is also possible to argue that hydrotherapy may in some cases be working at level four, influencing the correction of structural integrity.

THE EFFECTS OF WATER ON TISSUES AND SYSTEMS

A detailed review of normal physiology and anatomy is beyond the scope of this text. However, an understanding of how hydrotherapy works requires knowledge of the body's homeostatic control mechanisms, with particular emphasis on the nervous, cardiovascular and lymphatic systems. The overarching aim of naturopathic hydrotherapy is to ensure a normal flow of healthy blood through all body tissues in order to deliver to those tissues what they need to function properly and to prevent metabolic wastes from building up. Following naturally from this is the reasoning that an improved flow of blood to the vital organs of digestion and elimination will also improve the function of those organs and therefore, ultimately, the quality of the blood, by improving digestion and absorption of nutrients and increasing elimination of wastes.[3] These effects are mediated primarily by the autonomic nervous system and the hypothalamus. Lymphatics, as well as metabolic processes and the immune and endocrine systems, are also affected.

Except when using hydrotherapy locally for an acute condition, treatments generally do not directly interact with or intervene in pathogenic processes. Instead, treatments work on the concept of providing a perturbation to the system that, due to the body's compensatory mechanisms, changes the internal environment and thus the terrain in which a disease exists. With consistent serial applications over time, the stimulation of the homeostatic mechanisms has a lasting effect, tonifying the body's self-healing capacities and bringing the system into a more normal balance than the previously imbalanced disease state. This can be particularly useful in the balance of sympathetic and parasympathetic nervous system tone to offset the effects of chronic stress on the system,[8] as well as in the improvement of endothelial function of blood vessels.[9]

Stimulus-reaction-regulation

The various therapeutic properties of water are discussed in the next section. However, for the purposes of elucidating the mechanisms involved in the stimulus-reaction-response strategy of hydrotherapy, it can be noted here that the primary therapeutic property of water as used in naturopathic hydrotherapy is thermal: the capacity to stimulate temperature change on the surface of and within the body. Water of different temperatures is used to therapeutically target the disruption of sensitive temperature regulation systems in the body, which triggers a number of complex nonspecific compensatory mechanisms affecting the systems (discussed in more detail below).

Surface temperature change is perceived via sensors in the skin, which register the change if it exceeds the threshold for the sensor. Depending on the size and intensity of the stimulus, the body's reaction may be localised or general. With a large enough treatment area or an intense stimulus, the body's normal homeostatic mechanisms will react to protect the internal temperature balance, and these mechanisms will then re-establish homeostasis of temperature and other parameters (e.g. blood pressure) that may be disturbed by the temperature change. The body perceives and reacts to hot and cold differently. Cold is often most different from body temperature, so it is perceived as a bigger threat and the body's homeostatic mechanisms react more quickly to it. In contrast, hot is most often closer to body temperature, so it is perceived as less of a threat to homeostasis and the body reacts more slowly to it.[3] Short-term effects and immediate reactions result from single or short-term applications, but with serial applications over longer periods of time there is a possibility of systemic adaptation via consistent 'training' of the systems into new patterns, and thus a return to balance.[8]

Thermal, mechanical and chemical effects of water

As noted above, the primary therapeutic property of water in naturopathic hydrotherapy is thermal. Water has the ability to absorb, give off or carry away large quantities of body heat. Water exists in three states – liquid, solid and gas – which gives it versatility in its application to and therapeutic uses in the body, both externally and internally.

Water above or below body temperature is used in hydrotherapy as a conductor of heat into or out of the body. Generally speaking, the greater the variation from body temperature, the greater the effect, although the patient's vitality level will influence this. Water, a second-class conductor, is about 23 times more thermally conductive than air, making it a much more useful substance for effecting rapid changes of body tissue temperature. Body tissues conduct heat less rapidly than water, so heat from water that is significantly hotter than body temperature will be conducted into the skin and will build up in the local area, as it is conducted into the body at a faster rate than the body can conduct it away from the area.[8] Examples of such treatments include hot baths, hydrocolator packs and hot compresses that are reheated/refreshed before they cool. Heat conduction may be combined with convective action in the case of flowing water to deliver heat to or carry heat away from the body, such as in a rinse.

When local heating of tissues or raising core body temperature is the goal of treatment, longer applications are required to effect the desired change. With local application, skin temperature may typically rise from 32°C to 43°C in 30 minutes, subcutaneous tissue will rise from 34.5°C to 40.8°C in 40 minutes, and intramuscular temperature takes 50 minutes to rise from 34.6°C to 37.6°C using the common temperature range for heating treatments.[10] However, many hydrotherapy applications are aimed not at local tissue effects but at the regulatory effects that result as mediated by the hypothalamus and the autonomic nervous system. To attain lasting effects, serial treatments are required regularly over time, increasing the intensity of hot and cold as the body adapts and becomes inured to larger temperature changes.

Aside from its thermal effects, the mechanical effects of water also play an important role in naturopathic hydrotherapy. For example, with immersion in water or the application of a directed column of water, the hydrostatic pressure that results has the effect of increasing venous return and lymphatic flow, particularly from the extremities, by increasing pressure in the interstitial spaces. This secondarily causes increased kidney filtration and urinary output. The fluidity of water in its liquid state is what enables this effect, as water conforms fully to the surface of the skin. With full-body immersions, increased venous return and lymphatic flow can significantly increase blood pressure by moving blood and interstitial fluid into the arterial side of the system, so caution must be exercised for patients with existing hypertension.[8]

Other mechanical properties of water include its buoyancy effect, which can relieve gravitational tension on the musculoskeletal system, relaxing muscles and allowing ease of mobility. Additionally, the electrical conductivity of water can be used to convey current to or through the body, with potential effects similar to those of electroacupuncture.

Finally, any recounting of the therapeutic effects of water would be remiss in not mentioning its chemical properties. Of course, water taken by mouth has ubiquitous internal effects in the body, but water can also be introduced into a body cavity, such as in enemas or colon hydrotherapy, for its cleansing effects or as a solvent for delivery of medicinal substances, such as with baths or other immersions that use additives.

Physiological responses to thermal stimuli

The response of a local tissue, an organ system or an entire organism to a thermal stimulus will vary depending on factors such as the temperature and length of the application, the surface area covered, the vitality/age/gender of the patient and how the patient was prepared before treatment. Generally, water applications are seen to have both primary and secondary effects. Primary effects are the direct or intrinsic results of the application of a thermal stimulus, while secondary effects are the body's homeostatic reaction and regulation following the primary effects and are thus considered to be indirect. Secondary effects are often the target for therapeutic action.

The direct effects of warm or hot applications are generally sedative and relaxing, including vasodilation and improved general and cutaneous circulation, decreased heart rate, muscle relaxation, loosening of connective tissue, decreased stomach motility and acid production, and analgesia. However, heat secondarily increases heart rate, respiration rate and metabolism, and enhances vagal tone. Very hot applications can be stimulating to the point of being destructive.

The differences in primary and secondary effects of cold applications, particularly on the cardiovascular system, are more pronounced. The primary effects of cold applications are generally tonifying and invigorating, including general and cutaneous vasoconstriction, increased heart rate and blood pressure, increased sympathetic nervous system activity, slowing and deepening of respirations, and increased stomach motility and acid production, as well as local analgesia and decreased inflammation. Secondary effects include general and cutaneous vasodilation and decreased heart rate and blood pressure. The longer the cold application is used, the more intense are the primary effects. In contrast, shorter cold applications give a more effective secondary response, strengthening the whole system and having the strongest medicinal effect of cold water applications. Very cold or prolonged cold applications can be depressive to the point of being destructive; hence, shorter cold applications are preferred in naturopathic hydrotherapy. A summary of the physiological effects of hot and cold applications is shown in Table 5.1.

Through cardiovascular changes that result from hot and cold water as applied to a local pathology, hydrotherapy aims to increase the circulation of nutrient- and oxygen-rich blood to tissues, increase the removal of metabolic wastes and relieve any condition of congestion or ischaemia. In locally heated tissues, vasodilation increases the migration of white blood cells and inflammatory mediators into the tissue space, as well as increasing cellular metabolism and sweating, which can aid in removing metabolic and inflammatory waste products. However, when intense local heat is applied for longer than 7 minutes, it can lead to local congestion caused by blood stasis and oedema.[10] By comparison, local cold applications have the direct effect of reducing

circulation to the area, reducing congestion, pain and inflammation.

For generalised treatments not directed at a local pathology, hydrotherapy aims to use the cardiovascular changes that result from hot and cold applications to stimulate blood flow to the vital organs of digestion and elimination and to train the body's homeostatic mechanisms and balance of sympathetic and parasympathetic nervous system tone. This is generally accomplished by first warming the body and then using a short cold application. Father Kneipp, Vincent Priessnitz and John Harvey Kellogg all believed that repeated prolonged exposure to heat, such as in saunas or hot baths, would weaken a person over time unless they were also engaging in frequent cold water applications.[6] Prolonged heating that is not followed by a cold application will tend to sedate the entire system, having a depressant effect on systemic circulation – particularly circulation to the vital organs of digestion and elimination – and leaving the person with an increased sensitivity to cold. Conversely, a cold application that covers a significant portion of the body, such as a wrap or immersion of the thorax and abdomen, will tend to drive blood towards the internal organs.[10]

With that said, there are instances where a generalised hot application, or whole body hyperthermia, is useful. In cases of chronic or acute infection, hyperthermia can be used to induce or elevate an existing fever; this has stimulating effects on the immune system including increased mobilisation of blood mononuclear cells and increased levels of various stress hormones, which improve the course of the illness.[6]

Principles of blood movement

The combination of nervous and circulatory system reactions to thermal stimuli can be used to create three major effects in the body to impact both pathological local processes and general systemic vitality. Two of these are primary effects that follow on from the discussion in the previous section: derivation and retrostasis (also known as revulsion).

- A derivative effect draws blood or lymph from one part of the body to another. The best example of this is using a hot or warming application on an area that is distant from an area of blood or lymph congestion to draw congestion away from that area and towards the

TABLE 5.1 Effects of thermal stimuli		
Primary effects of heat	**Primary effects of cold**	**Secondary effects of cold**
• Sedation, relaxation • Vasodilation, improved circulation • Decreased, then increased, heart rate • Increased rate of respiration and metabolism • Decreased intestinal motility and secretion • Muscle relaxation • Analgesia	• Stimulation, tonification • Vasoconstriction • Increased heart rate and blood pressure • Decreased and deepened rate of respiration • Increased intestinal motility and secretion • Increased sympathetic nervous system (SNS) tone/activity • Locally decreased pain and inflammation	• Vasodilation • Decreased heart rate and blood pressure

treated area – for example, using a hot foot bath to treat a migraine.

- A retrostatic (or revulsive) effect is the opposite, driving blood or lymph away from a congested part of the body. This is generally achieved through the use of a cold application to the congested area – for example, applying a cold compress to the back of the neck for a congestive headache.[6]

Alternating short hot and cold treatments to an area combines these derivative and retrostatic effects such that each magnifies the effects of the other, alternating between dilation and constriction of blood vessels and toning the endothelium to increase the health of the vascular tissue, thereby stimulating local circulation and metabolism and effectively producing analgesic and decongestant outcomes. This can be done locally, for example alternating hot and cold compresses over the sinuses for a sinus headache or infection, or it can be done to achieve generalised effects on blood flow to vital organs, such as contrast immersions and constitutional hydrotherapy (described later in this chapter). The short cold application need only be long enough to produce vasoconstriction, which can occur in as little as 20 seconds.[10]

The third major effect is the spinal reflex effect, which is an indirect effect as it is a reaction mediated by spinal cord reflex arcs within the nervous system. This reflex effect enables applications of hot or cold to affect organs or areas of the body other than the area directly being treated. There are major patterns of reflex effects: for paired structures such as hands and feet, treating one has a reflex effect on the other, and generally the area of skin over an organ is in a reflex relationship with that organ. In addition to these major patterns, treatments to the hands reflexively affect the brain, lungs and nasal mucosa; treating the feet reflexively affects the brain, pelvic organs, intestines and lungs; and treating the inner thigh reflexively affects the prostate or uterus.[11] Table 5.2 provides a summary of these reflexive relationships.

Reflexive effects tend to be the same as the direct effect at the location of treatment – for example, heat applied to one hand will reflexively cause vasodilation in the contralateral hand. However, an important exception is that heat and cold applied to the skin over the heart have *secondary* effects on the heart – that is, heat increases the heart rate and cold decreases the heart rate. Heat applied to the abdomen decreases gastrointestinal blood flow, motility and gastric secretions, and cold applied to the abdomen has the opposite effect. Reflexive effects are more easily attained with a smaller area of application, as larger areas tend to result in more local direct effects. Higher intensity applications and the proximity of the treatment area to the reflex organ also result in stronger reflexive effects.

GENERAL GUIDELINES FOR ADMINISTERING HYDROTHERAPY

Naturopathic hydrotherapy is an individualised treatment approach that is tailored to the patient's overall condition.

TABLE 5.2 Reflexive treatment areas

Skin area	Organ(s) affected reflexively
Feet and lower legs	Pelvic organs, intestines, brain, lungs
Hands	Brain, lungs and nasal mucosa
Upper inner thigh	Prostate or uterus
Buttocks, groin, front of upper thigh	Genitourinary organs
Lower abdomen just above pubic symphysis, sacrum	Bladder, uterus and ovaries
Central abdomen	Bowels and abdominal viscera in general
Lumbar spine	Bowels and abdominal viscera in general, kidneys
Lower thoracic spine	Stomach
Upper thoracic spine	Lungs and heart
Cervical spine and occiput, lower face	Nasal mucosa
Front and side of lower left ribcage	Spleen and stomach
Front, side and back of lower right ribcage	Liver
Lower sternum	Kidneys
Central sternum	Oesophagus
Suprasternal notch	Larynx and pharynx
Front of chest	Lungs, left side only = heart
Forehead and scalp	Brain

Note: Reflex effects on the distant or deep organs are the same as the direct effects on the skin.
Source: Blake E et al. Naturopathic hydrotherapy. In: Chaitow L, editor. Naturopathic physical medicine. Philadelphia: Churchill Livingstone; 2008.

Regardless of the specific application, there are a number of guidelines and principles that can be adhered to generally to ensure that the patient is properly prepared and cared for, the treatment intensity is appropriate for the patient and their level of vitality, and the outcome is optimal in terms of both patient experience and therapeutic benefits.

The type and intensity of application

The type of application chosen will depend on the condition being treated and the overall treatment aims, as well as other factors discussed below. Although some treatments are generally indicated, with customisation of intensity, for almost anyone (e.g. constitutional hydrotherapy), other treatments are designed for much more specific treatment goals. As discussed above, local treatments are generally aimed at attaining an effect in the location in which the treatment is applied and targeting a specific local pathology – for example, reducing pain and inflammation in a sprained ankle. In contrast, whole body treatments or those covering large areas are aiming for more generalised effects – for example, a full immersion hyperthermia bath to mimic a fever. Reflexive treatments are directed at segmental areas to have a specific reflex effect on a target area or organ – for example, a cold arm bath to reduce the heart rate.

Perhaps some of the most useful generalised or systemic effects that can be attained with hydrotherapy are those that are mediated by the hypothalamus, the immune system and the autonomic nervous system. Daily home hydrotherapy helps general health by reducing stress hormones from the hypothalamus. General or local alternating hot and cold treatments that use higher intensity heating phases can result in generalised or local immunological stimulation. Additionally, alternating hot and cold applications over medium or large portions of the body that are applied serially over time can retrain the balance of tone between the sympathetic and parasympathetic nervous systems.[8]

Beyond customising the type of treatment to the patient's condition, adjusting the intensity of the treatment to the individual's needs is critical. Intensity is generally defined by the temperature, the size of the surface area being treated, the time of day and the duration of the treatment, the frequency of the treatment, and any additives such as herbs. The greater the difference between the patient's body temperature and the temperature of the application, the greater the intensity of the treatment. In treatments that use alternating hot and cold applications, the greater the difference between the hot and the cold, the greater the intensity. At temperatures that are either very hot or very cold, shorter treatments are more intense, as they create a stronger reaction and regulation. However, at temperatures closer to body temperature, longer treatments are more intense due to prolonged effects. Table 5.3 provides guidelines for water temperature selection. Intensity is also affected by the patient's vitality:

in a person whose vitality is relatively strong, repetition of treatment will give a more intense overall effect, but the body's reactive capacities, particularly vasoconstriction, may be exhausted by repetition, so there are diminishing returns with too much repetition. Finally, the more water that is against the skin during the application, the more intense the treatment will be. For example, in a wrap, if the wet layer is wrung loosely before application it will be wetter and provide a more intense effect than if it were wrung tightly to remove more water.

It is interesting to note that while Father Kneipp began his experimentation with hydrotherapy using the very intense stimulus of bathing in the Danube River in winter, over the period of his experience administering treatments he became much more moderate in his approach and finally became a proponent of using the gentlest application possible to gain the desired effect.

Factors influencing appropriate intensity

The individualised nature of hydrotherapy treatment calls for consideration of an array of different factors when determining an appropriate level of intensity for treating a patient. As a priority it is important to consider the patient's current medical condition and medical history, particularly any conditions that could reduce skin sensation of hot or cold, such as diabetes, or conditions that could compromise the cardiovascular system. Additional factors that affect how a patient may respond to treatment include their age, gender, body type, weight, level of vitality, body temperature (noting whether or not they have been exercising just prior to treatment) and general tendency to feel hot or cold, their emotional state and, for women, at what point they are in their menstrual cycle, as well as any medications they are taking, and the season and climate.[6] Less intense treatments are generally used if any factor is indicated that might reduce or compromise the patient's ability to respond physiologically or otherwise to a more intense stimulus. With regard to the patient's emotional state, consideration should be given to their present state of mind and level of resilience, as well as their general psychological tendencies and any stress factors that are present either chronically or acutely in their day or their life.[8]

Conducting treatments

There are a number of basic rules that apply to the practice of hydrotherapy regardless of the type of treatment being administered. These rules are designed not only to achieve the optimum therapeutic effect from treatment, but also to ensure the patient's safety and comfort and to reduce the likelihood of any adverse reactions.

PREPARING THE PATIENT FOR TREATMENT

Treatments are best conducted after the patient has been adequately prepared, in terms of being made aware of (1) what to expect in the treatment so that they won't be surprised, and (2) what behaviours or activities they

TABLE 5.3 Temperature categories for treatment	
Category	**Temperature range**
Very cold	10–15°C
Cold	16–18°C
Moderately cold	19–22°C
Cool	23–27°C
Tepid	28–31°C
Neutral	32–35°C
Warm	36–38°C
Hot	39–41°C
Very hot	42–44°C

Source: Kneipp Schule. Kneipp hydrotherapy [course manual]. Bad Worishofen, Germany; 2016.

should avoid or be attentive to before and after treatment. For the latter, the two most important considerations are to avoid smoking cigarettes before and after treatment, as smoking can negate the effects of treatment due to the effects of nicotine on the nervous and cardiovascular systems, and to avoid eating immediately prior to and after treatment, unless the treatment is specifically aimed at stimulating digestion – in which case eating afterwards is not problematic.[8]

GENERAL TREATMENT RULES[1,6,8]

The following general rules should be widely adhered to during administration of naturopathic hydrotherapy treatments:

1 Hydrotherapy can and should be used in parallel with other naturopathic treatments that are supporting the same treatment goals, such as herbs, nutrition, manual therapies and flower essences or homeopathic remedies.

2 The needs of the patient are paramount; treatment should be modified or stopped and attention given to caring for the patient as appropriate if they are in distress or pronounced discomfort. This requires close monitoring of the patient, particularly when they are undergoing a treatment that they have not had in the past.

3 Cold water should be applied only after warming the body. Warming the body can be done actively, with exercise, or passively with hot water or a sauna. In some circumstances, a cold treatment is possible just after the patient has risen from bed in the morning, in which case warmth can be presumed, but this should be confirmed with the patient.

4 In treatments that alternate between hot and cold applications, the hot application should always be longer than the cold – generally, three to four times longer. In addition, the hot application should always be first and the treatment should always end with a cold application.

5 A short hot application is less than 5 minutes and will have a direct stimulant effect; a long hot application is more than 5 minutes and will have an indirect sedative effect. A short cold application is less than 1 minute and will have an indirect stimulant effect; a long cold application is more than 1 minute and will have a direct sedative effect. Thus, short applications stimulate whether they are hot or cold. With regard to long applications, the implication is that the temperature will be kept relatively constant for the duration of the application.

6 The patient's body temperature, pulse, level of interactivity and emotional state should be monitored during treatment, particularly during intense or long treatments, although some long treatments are quite sedating and the patient may drift off to sleep. If the patient feels faint or loses consciousness during a full-body heating treatment, they must be removed from the heat immediately. In prolonged heat treatments, the pulse of a patient who is relatively vital should be kept below 140 bpm and their body temperature below 40°C – although these thresholds should be adjusted downwards significantly or a

different type of treatment chosen for weaker, young or elderly patients.

7 If the patient becomes chilled during a cold application, the treatment should be stopped and the patient warmed using blankets, warm drinks, heat packs or a hot-water bottle. The patient should never get cold to the point of shivering. Future treatments should be adjusted to a less extreme cold temperature until the patient's vitality has increased.

POST-TREATMENT PATIENT CARE

Patients should be instructed on behaviour and activities after treatment. As treatment almost universally ends with a cold application, care of the body after this phase is important. The patient must be warmed and kept warm, but not through the application of another heating phase, unless the patient is chilled and unable to get warm on their own. Passive warming can be achieved by putting on warm clothes or resting under a warm blanket and avoiding cold weather or being exposed to drafts. The patient should likewise avoid becoming overheated after treatment, either by dressing too warmly, being out in hot weather or exercising. Generally, rest is indicated for about half an hour immediately after treatment, preferably prior to the patient leaving the treatment facility.

After cold applications, the skin should not be dried completely, only wiped off with the hands, so that cooling from evaporation will continue the stimulus for some time. However, there are exceptions to this. For example, the patient should be dried after a full-body treatment before putting on clothing or if they need to go directly out into cold or windy weather or had any dysfunctional reaction to treatment. In addition, body parts covered with hair or areas of skin-to-skin contact, such as intertriginous folds or between the toes, should be dried.[8]

CONTRAINDICATIONS, CAUTIONS AND DYSFUNCTIONAL REACTIONS

There are relatively few absolute contraindications for naturopathic hydrotherapy, particularly when the intensity is well-calibrated to the patient so as to be gentle while still achieving treatment aims. Perhaps the most common contraindication to screen for prior to treatment is the presence of diabetes or any other condition that impairs neurological or cardiovascular function in the treatment area, particularly the extremities. A reduction in the sensation of hot or cold on the skin can make thermal applications dangerous, as the patient cannot feel whether the temperature is too hot or cold. In addition, a compromise in circulation can make thermal applications dangerous: with a hot application heat will build up in the tissue when blood flow is not sufficient to carry the excess heat away, and with a cold application heat will be conducted out of the tissue and if blood flow is not sufficient to keep the tissue somewhat warm, tissue damage can result. However, once any impaired areas have been identified, treatments using reflex effects to influence those impaired areas can still be considered.

Other circumstances in which there may be contraindications to some treatments include concurrent cancer treatment, pregnancy, menstruation or hypertension. In cancer patients receiving radiation treatment, concurrent hyperthermia treatments (local or general) are contraindicated due to the synergy of the treatments. In pregnancy, full-body immersion in water over 40°C is contraindicated and immersion at 40°C should not last more than 10 minutes.[6] For women who are menstruating, cold applications to the pelvic area or lower extremities are contraindicated because they can stop menstrual bleeding through direct or reflexive effects; likewise, hot applications are contraindicated as they can cause excessive bleeding. Finally, caution should be used when considering full-body immersions for hypertensive patients, due to increases in venous return and lymphatic flow moving blood volume into the arterial system, as noted above.[8] While there are two studies that indicate no concern with full immersion at 40°C,[6] perhaps due to the concomitant vasodilation that occurs with such heating, common sense dictates caution in this instance, particularly at other temperatures.

Hydrotherapy may cause a number of possible side effects, particularly when using a treatment that is new to a patient or in the case of a patient who is experiencing unusual stress or acute illness. These include vertigo or light-headedness from transient blood pressure changes, headache or nausea (often a result of a detoxification reaction), nervousness, heart palpitations, increased heart rate, insomnia or hyperventilation (which can result from overstimulation), or feeling chilled or overheated. In the treatment room, these issues can be addressed by placing the patient in a resting situation, lying supine, warming them if indicated, ensuring that they are hydrated and their blood sugar level is stable, and guiding them in breathing exercises.[6] Some effects may occur up to 24 hours after treatment, so patients should be educated about possible side effects and provided with contact details in case they need assistance. Such side effects indicate a need for caution and to moderate the intensity of treatment or change the type of treatment on the next encounter.

There are other dysfunctional reactions that a patient may experience that should be monitored by the practitioner but may be less noticeable to the patient themselves. Arterial dysfunction can result in a mottled red and white appearance on the skin; this is generally caused by too large a difference between the hot and cold applications or a cold application being applied for too long a duration. Venous dysfunction may be evidenced by a blue tinge to the skin and a feeling of tightness, particularly in the lower extremities when the patient is being treated in a standing position; this may be caused by an excessively long hot application resulting in pooling of venous blood. In either circumstance, the next treatment should be moderated to avoid such a reaction.

Finally, a paradoxical reaction may occur any time a patient does not respond as expected for the type of treatment and intensity applied. A paradoxical reaction indicates a need to reassess the patient and treatment plan in the light of that reaction.

COMMONLY PRESCRIBED NATUROPATHIC HYDROTHERAPY TREATMENTS

A full cataloguing of and instruction on naturopathic hydrotherapy treatments would require a book in itself. Thus, this chapter outlines only some of the most commonly prescribed naturopathic hydrotherapy treatments along with general guidance for their administration.

Rinses and douches

A rinse, also known as an affusion or a *guss* (from the German), is the gentle application of water for its thermal effects. A rinse is generally delivered using a stream of water under gentle pressure so that the water forms a plane across the skin's surface and does not splash, stimulating temperature receptors on the treated area without engaging receptors in other areas. A douche, also known as a jet- or flash-rinse, is the application of water in a high-pressure stream to attain both mechanical and thermal effects. Rinses and douches are a line of hydrotherapeutic treatment that come directly from Father Kneipp and his successors.[3,8]

Rinses and douches are applied in a warm room (~24°C) with no drafts, as the patient is either partially or fully disrobed, depending on the area treated. The floor should be non-slip and have a drain so that the patient is not standing in water during the treatment. Natural lighting should be available so as to easily monitor changes in skin colour. Specialised, though inexpensive, equipment is needed in the form of a hose and a regulator that allows independent adjustment of water pressure and temperature, with a thermostat for precise temperature selection, as well as a supportive appliance for the patient to hold onto in some body positions.

For plain rinses, the hose should be 2 cm in diameter and about 2.5 m in length. Water pressure is adjusted such that when the hose is directed vertically, a column of water of about 8 cm high is produced. The hose is held about 10 cm from the skin area being treated, at a 45° angle so that the water forms a sheath around the treatment area. Achieving this without splashing takes considerable practice. Common rinses are generally either cold or alternating hot and cold. Because the temperature changes can be surprising, the patient should be informed beforehand as to how the treatment will proceed. The patient should also be given guidance in breathing, breathing in before water contact and then out as the water contacts them, and repeating this each time there is a change of temperature or treatment area.[8]

As with all hydrotherapeutic treatments, treatment intensity must be individualised to the patient. This may mean moderating the temperature of a cold rinse, or in an alternating rinse, the first cold phase can be moderated and the second one made colder for sensitive patients. Rinses are generally performed until the desired reaction is achieved. The patient should be monitored for skin colour changes due to vasodilation and vasoconstriction, and for breathing and relaxed posture throughout the treatment. For temperature selection, refer to Table 5.3.

KNEE AND THIGH RINSES

Knee and thigh rinses are commonly prescribed for their local, reflexive and systemic tonifying and balancing effects. In the knee rinse, water is applied from the toes to about 5 cm above the knee, while in the thigh rinse, water is applied from the toes to the iliac crest on the back of the leg and to the groin on the front. The thigh rinse is a more intense treatment due to the larger area of water coverage. All areas treated should be unclothed. The right leg is treated first, then the left, and the back of the leg is treated before the front. The treatment is finished by application of cold to the bottoms of both feet. Refer to Table 5.2 to reference areas of the body that are in a reflexive relationship with the skin of the legs and feet.

These rinses can be either cold (assuming the patient is starting warm) or alternating hot and cold, with the patient's condition generally determining selection. The duration of the cold treatment is 70–90 seconds, and it will have more intense effects; the duration of the alternating treatment will be 2–2.5 minutes, remembering that the duration of the hot phase is three to four times longer than the cold phase.

Knee and thigh rinses are contraindicated for women who are menstruating, as the reflexive vasoconstriction in the uterus can stop menstrual flow. They are also contraindicated for patients who are generally cold or feel chilly, for those who have acute conditions of the bladder or kidney and in conditions of diminished arterial function in the legs. In an alternating rinse, caution is needed for patients with hypotension, as dizziness can occur, so patients should be given a stable support to hold onto during treatment of the back of the legs; they can be seated on a stool during treatment of the front of the legs and soles of the feet.[8]

ARM RINSES

Arm rinses are commonly prescribed for their local, reflexive and systemic tonifying and balancing effects. In an arm rinse, water is applied from the fingertips to the shoulder joint without allowing water to contact the thorax. For an extended arm rinse, water is applied to the lower edge of the scapula. Ideally, the entire upper body should be unclothed. The patient is treated in a standing position, bent forwards 90° at the hip and supported by straight arms braced on a stable surface of an appropriate height so that the trunk is parallel to the floor; this allows water to be planed down the arm without running onto the thorax.

The right arm is treated first, then the left, and the back of the arm is treated before the front. The rinse can be either cold or alternating hot and cold, with the patient's condition generally determining selection. The duration of the cold treatment is 60–80 seconds, and it will have more intense effects; the duration of the alternating treatment is 130 to 140 seconds, remembering that the duration of the hot phase is three to four times longer than the cold phase.

Arm rinses are contraindicated for patients who are generally cold or feel chilly, for most heart conditions, for those with Raynaud's syndrome and in conditions of diminished arterial function in the arms.

HYPERTHERMAL RINSES

Two commonly indicated hot rinses are the lumbar rinse and the neck rinse. The hot lumbar rinse is applied to the lower back with the patient in a seated position so that the water does not run down the backs of the legs. Water is applied in a consistent, gentle plane across the unclothed lumbar spine, starting with a neutral temperature and steadily increasing to very hot over a duration of 3–4 minutes. The treated area should become thoroughly warmed and hyperaemic, and the treatment will give both local and reflexive heating effects. The hot lumbar rinse is contraindicated in conditions of acute inflammation or nerve irritation in the lumbar spine, including sciatica.

The hot neck rinse is applied to the back of the neck and the upper back down to the sixth thoracic vertebra. The patient leans forwards bent at 90° at the hip, supported on straight arms to avoid water running down the rest of the back. Other parameters are the same as for the hot lumbar rinse, with an additional contraindication in cases of hyperthyroidism.

BLITZ GUSS

The blitz guss is a type of douche that was a favourite of Father Kneipp and was frequently used in Henry Lindlahr's sanatorium.[3] It is a cold douche to the entire back of the body using water at significant pressure, starting at the feet and moving up to the shoulders in a specific sequence. The blitz guss requires a hose with the capacity to produce a level stream of water spanning about 3 m, resulting in an application of water at a pressure of 0.7–4.2 kg/cm².[1] It is administered to a completely disrobed patient, ideally in the corner of a tiled room or a shower enclosure with handles that the patient can use to steady themselves.

The circuit of water application from the toes to the shoulders is repeated five to ten times according to the patient's vitality and tolerance. It can be done using only cold water, in which case the patient must be warmed first with bath, sauna or exercise; alternatively, it can be done starting with warm water and gradually decreasing the temperature with each repetition until the water is cold. In this instance, the stream of water is moved more slowly when the water is warm, and more quickly when the water reaches colder temperatures. Given the intensity and duration of the treatment, the patient should be dried thoroughly, clothed warmly and left to rest in a warm setting after treatment.

The blitz guss is indicated for most hypotonic, atonic or congestive conditions, although if the patient is of low vitality they will need to be built up to this treatment slowly using less intense treatments over time. This treatment is contraindicated in any acute inflammatory condition or in cases of nervous irritability, heart disease, hypertension, hyperthyroidism, atherosclerosis, skin eruptions or any severe disease. Caution must be observed with water pressure over bony prominences with thin patients.[3]

CONTRAST SHOWERS

A simple and easy to prescribe daily practice for patients at home is the contrast shower. This is essentially a full-body hot rinse followed by a cold rinse, following the general rule that the hot application is three to four times as long as the cold. The patient should allow hot water to tolerance to run on the front and back of the torso and pelvis for 5 minutes, followed by the same with cold water for 1–2 minutes. The cold water does not need to be frigid – the patient can build up slowly to the full cold application, in both temperature and duration.[6] After the round of cold, the patient should turn off the water, dry themselves and get dressed without delay to ensure that they do not become chilled. This daily habit is supportive of the immune system, circulation, digestion, elimination and autonomic nervous system balance.

Wraps

A wrap is an application of water via a wet or damp cotton or linen cloth secured around the body and covered by one or more thermal layers of wool for the purpose of holding in heat. Wraps can be used for acute or chronic conditions or for general tonification and detoxification purposes, depending on the type of wrap applied. There are three basic types of wraps: those that decrease heat or inflammation; those that deliver heat; and those that produce heat and potentially also perspiration.

The effects of the wrap will be determined by the temperature of the water, how tightly the wet layer is wrung out, the duration of the treatment and the size and location of the area treated. Wraps over relatively large areas of the body that are left on for longer and are applied serially over time will have the effect of increasing vagal tone and retraining the balance of the autonomic nervous system by way of an initial increase in sympathetic tone followed by movement into parasympathetic dominance that leaves the patient in a resting state. Even with a single application, wraps over large areas of the body will produce improvements in metabolic processes, circulation and blood pressure. Aside from their thermal effects, wraps can relax tensions in smooth and skeletal muscle, depending on the location of application and the tightness of the wrap.[8]

Wraps have an advantage as a hydrotherapeutic application in that they can be applied in the clinic or at home by the patient or a family member. The most common areas for application are the neck, chest, lumbar region, legs (toes to groin) and calves. Larger areas are wrapped as a short wrap (armpits to just above the knee), three-quarter wrap (armpits to toes) and full wrap (neck to toes).

WARMING COMPRESSES

Warming compresses are also known as heat- or inflammation-reducing wraps or cold double compresses. With a warming compress, the compress itself becomes warmer, not the skin. The warming compress is a cool or cold application that is removed from the skin when the temperature of the damp cloth has risen to that of the skin. The compress can be applied once only or refreshed with a new cool cloth in a serial application, depending on the treatment goals. The compress increases the release of heat from the body by lowering the temperature of the skin or drawing heat from inflamed tissues. A cloth that is wrapped more loosely or that contains more water (i.e. is more gently wrung out) will give a more intense cooling effect.

Warming compresses are indicated in cases of local inflammation (heat, redness, swelling, pain, reduced range of motion) anywhere in the body, as well as in the case of sore throat, bronchitis, influenza or swollen lymph glands.[6] In these instances, application is local to the area of inflammation, and clay can be used as an additive to lengthen the conduction of heat from the body.[8] Warming compresses are also indicated to reduce elevated body temperature from fever, sun exposure or other causes, although they are contraindicated if the patient is shivering or has a cold feeling in their extremities. To reduce elevated body temperature, wraps can be applied serially five to seven times to the legs or calves, including the feet and toes, to draw heat down from the head and away from the core. The first application should be cool, rather than cold, so as not to shock the patient; each successive application can be made cooler. Each time the cloth reaches the temperature of the skin, it should be removed, and after the skin begins to again feel warm and dry, the next application is indicated. If the patient breaks into a sweat during application, it is considered a positive sign, which should be followed by a neutral lavation (described in the next section).

In any use of hydrotherapy to reduce a dangerously high fever, whether using a wrap, a bath or another method, caution should be applied so as not to reduce the fever to a point where it can no longer serve its function of moving the body back to health. Reducing a fever to below 39°C is suppressive and should be avoided; a fever of 40°C or higher should be reduced only to about 39°C – this allows the self-healing action of the fever to proceed, while reducing the danger to the patient.[12] Two studies published in 1997 examined the use of hydrotherapy in the form of cold sponging to reduce fevers in children,[13,14] concluding that sponging is more effective than antipyretic medications for the first 30 minutes, while antipyretic medications are more effective thereafter – the delay being attributed to absorption time for the medication. However, the advantage of hydrotherapy in this instance is that it enables fever reduction to be controlled, mitigating it to reduce the danger to the patient but not suppressing it entirely, as is generally the case with antipyretic medications.[6]

A classic naturopathic variant on the warming compress is the warming sock treatment, which can be used for head or sinus pain or congestion, hot sore throat, otitis media or other conditions of excessive pressure or a sense of fullness or heat in the head. In the warming sock treatment, rather than aiming for a local reduction in heat, the effect is derivative, pulling heat and blood flow from the head to the feet. The patient is first warmed with a bath or shower before bedtime, before putting on a pair of thin cotton socks that have been soaked in very cold water and well-wrung. A pair of thick wool socks is worn over the cotton socks and the patient is sent to bed. The socks are left on overnight; they warm quickly and are generally dry by the morning, with an improvement in the patient's head congestion and pain.

HOT COMPRESSES

Hot compresses, also known as heat-delivering wraps, deliver heat to the body: a hot, damp cloth is quickly applied and covered with wool to minimise loss of heat from the cloth. Hot compresses are indicated for chronic joint pain, intestinal colic or colic of other organs (e.g. gallbladder, urinary tract or uterus), chronic lung and airway diseases, muscle spasms or pain that is not congestive or inflammatory in nature, insomnia and nervous tension.[3,5] Their effects are both local and reflexive to specific organs, but they do not have significant systemic effects. The duration of application can be anywhere 45 minutes to 75 minutes. Hot compresses are contraindicated in acute inflammation or congestive conditions, as they can exacerbate symptoms by increasing local blood flow.

HEAT- AND SWEAT-PRODUCING WRAPS

Wraps that generate internal heat and produce sweating are longer applications that generally consist of three layers: a wet cotton or linen base layer, a second layer of dry thick cotton or other intermediate insulating material, and an outer layer of wool. Sometimes they consist of a wet base layer with two outer layers of wool to ensure the warmth of the patient. They generally cover large areas, are tightly applied and aim for systemic rather than local effects. They tend to influence metabolism and increase the excretion of metabolic wastes through the skin and kidneys, particularly if they are taken into a lengthy sweating phase.

For a heat-producing wrap, the patient must first be warmed using a hot bath, shower or sauna. The wet layer is applied cold to bare skin. During application, the patient must be monitored for temperature and perspiration and to ensure that the wet layer is warming appropriately as the treatment progresses and that the patient does not become chilled. The duration of treatment is generally 45 minutes to 75 minutes, and the wrap should be removed if perspiration begins.[8] If the wet layer is not warm within the first 20 minutes of treatment, the wrap should be removed and the patient dried and warmed – the patient may not have been warm enough at the outset of the application, or the wrap may have been too wet or loose. Some indications for heat-producing wraps are hypertension, metabolic syndrome and autonomic nervous system retraining.

For a sweat-producing wrap, the wet layer is applied either hot or cold; if applied cold, the patient must be warmed first and monitored for appropriate warming during treatment. Generally, the treatment runs for 30 minutes from when sweating starts and is followed by a neutral lavation. An exception to the 30-minute sweating phase is the wet sheet pack, discussed below. Indications for a sweat-producing wrap are excess adiposity, metabolic

disorders, chronic inflammatory disorders of the spine and large joints and fibromyalgia.

The wet sheet pack, an old and reliable treatment, is a specialised sweat-producing wrap credited to Vincent Priessnitz as one of his greatest contributions to modern hydrotherapy. It is a powerful treatment that is useful with a wide array of patients and can be beneficial for almost anyone.[3] The wet sheet pack is a full-body wrap, from the neck to the toes, and is of the longest duration of any treatment covered in this chapter.

The treatment starts with a hydrated patient who has been thoroughly heated in a sauna, bath or shower or with steam and is fully disrobed with an empty bladder. The treatment table is prepared with two wool blankets and a pillow. The treatment starts by laying a cold, damp (well-wrung – which can take two people to achieve) bed sheet on top of the blankets and then having the patient quickly lie supine on the sheet. A twin-sized sheet is adequate for thinner or smaller patients, while a double-sized sheet may be needed for larger patients. The sheet is wrapped around the patient such that there is a layer of sheeting between all areas of normal skin contact (e.g. under the arms and between the legs) and all body surfaces are covered by the sheet. The wool blankets are quickly and tightly wrapped around the patient much like a burrito or mummy, so that only the patient's head is outside the wrap. The wrapping technique takes practice to ensure that the patient's shoulders and neck are well-covered and no outside air can get in. If a patient suffers from claustrophobia or anxiety, one arm can be left out of the first two layers and covered only loosely by the third layer to allow them some movement and sense of control.

The treatment proceeds in four phases, with the length of each stage being dependent on the patient's vitality and constitution:

1 The cooling phase lasts 5–20 minutes. The patient feels cool but gradually warms. This phase is generally tonic and alterative.
2 The neutral phase lasts 15–60 minutes. The patient goes from comfortable to hot. This phase is generally sedative and the patient may drift off to sleep.
3 The heating phase lasts 30–60 minutes. The patient goes from hot to starting to perspire. This phase is generally stimulating and the patient will be more awake.
4 The sweating phase can last from 1–2 hours as indicated by the patient's condition. The patient will sweat continuously until the treatment is terminated. This phase is generally eliminative and detoxifying, as well as working to increase metabolism and decrease general congestion.[3]

All four stages are not indicated for all conditions. If the aim is detoxification, weight loss or addressing acute illness such as cold, influenza or bronchitis, all four phases are used. The patient should be given sips of water every 10 minutes and their oral temperature and pulse monitored, with a cool compress to the head and neck if indicated. If the temperature reaches 40°C or the pulse reaches 140 bpm, the blankets should be loosened or one removed to release some heat. Patients who do not sweat easily can be given diaphoretic herbal teas before and during treatment to encourage sweating. The treatment should be followed by a cool shower or plunge bath, drying the patient and letting them rest comfortably clothed and with water to drink for at least 30 minutes. This is a potent treatment that, particularly when administered serially, can bring on a healing reaction.

The first phase can be used alone for fevers, general weakness or convalescence, anaemia or any conditions that benefit from gentle tonification. For fever, two wet sheets may be needed, or the sheet may be wrung less tightly to leave more water in it. If the goal is to attain calming effects, the first two phases can be used to gain a more sedated psychoemotional state. For most gastrointestinal or congestive conditions, or to prepare a patient for a subsequent cold treatment, the first three phases can be used, stopping at the start of sweating.

Although the wet sheet pack is a good general treatment, it is contraindicated in chilly or extremely devitalised patients, in cases of cold-induced asthma, in skin conditions that are worsened by moisture, in diabetes and circulatory conditions, and in severe colds and flu. The last two phases are contraindicated with anaemia, and caution should be used if the patient is prone to claustrophobia or anxiety, as discussed.

Lavations and simple compresses

A lavation is the application of a thin film of water to the skin using a well-wrung cloth or sponge. A lavation can be applied to specific body parts, such as the extremities or trunk, or to the whole body. A lavation is generally a very gentle and mild treatment, useful in in-patient settings, with very ill or devitalised patients, or in convalescence.

Lavations are generally performed with water that is about 10°C cooler than the patient's skin temperature, in order to achieve a mild stimulation. The ideal time for application is between 5 am and 7 am, when the body tends to be in a parasympathetic state from sleep and is warm, and the nervous system is very receptive to small stimulation. The treatment is applied in the patient's bed, in a warm room with no drafts. The general effects are a reactive relaxation, which can return the person to a deep sleep, increased skin circulation and excretion, increased metabolism and warmth, regulation of blood pressure and improvement of immune function, as well as general balancing of the autonomic nervous system to support healing overall. After treatment, the patient is not dried off, but is kept in bed under covers for at least 30 minutes to warm and dry while resting or sleeping.

In contrast, a neutral lavation is used after sweating treatments, generally given in the nature of a sponge bath. The goal is to cleanse the skin of sweat and toxins, so a neutral water temperature is used in order to not evoke further reaction from the body. The body is also dried after treatment so as not to stimulate evaporative cooling. Other examples of lavations are alternating or hot applications to the extremities for dysfunctional peripheral circulation, alternating or cold applications to pressure points for prevention of bedsores, serial cold applications to the extremities for a fever, and a cool application to the trunk

in the evening to encourage digestion and promote restful sleep.[8]

A simple compress is generally just a single wet cloth applied to the skin, though it may be folded so as to be more than one layer thick. A simple cold compress of a cloth wrung from cold or ice water is used to achieve local and distal vasoconstriction to reduce blood flow and congestion in a local or reflex area. Cold compresses are indicated for acute inflammation or injury, and for reduction of pain, heat and swelling. As the cloth warms, it must be refreshed with cold water, generally every 1–5 minutes. The colder the application, the shorter the duration of treatment. A very cold compress should not be used for more than 20 minutes, as a longer application can impede healing. Cold compresses are contraindicated in patients who are chilly or locally in patients with acute asthma, pleurisy or sinusitis.[6]

Use of simple alternating hot and cold compresses is one of the best ways to achieve a revulsive effect from thermal stimuli to increase blood flow to an area and thus improve the oxygenation and nutrient status of tissues and the removal of inflammation-related metabolic wastes, but without increasing congestion and pain in the area. Alternating compresses are indicated for local subacute inflammation or congestion. Application is made using a hot compress for 3–5 minutes, followed by a cold compress for 30–90 seconds, with this cycle repeated at least three times but always ending on cold to ensure no increase in congestion of blood flow.[6]

Constitutional hydrotherapy

Constitutional hydrotherapy is a naturopathic treatment developed by O.G. Carroll that has been used in North America for more than 80 years.[3] This treatment, like the wet sheet pack, is almost universally applicable to strengthen the vital force, and is particularly useful for increasing blood flow to the organs of digestion, detoxification and elimination, as well as strengthening the immune system and balancing sympathetic and parasympathetic tone. However, it has less effect on detoxification and elimination than a wet sheet pack taken through all four phases. It is a shorter treatment (approximately 45 minutes) and thus perhaps easier to administer when time is an issue, but it requires specialised equipment and the treatment method itself is more complex than other treatments covered in this chapter, requiring hands-on training and practice to master the art and more active participation required from the practitioner during treatment.

The treatment is administered by use of alternating hot and warming (double cold) compresses to the trunk, covering from the clavicles to the anterior superior iliac spine on the front, and from the neck to the sacrum on the back. The patient is disrobed on treated areas. The compresses comprise standard bath towels, folded to create four layers of damp towelling for the hot compresses and two layers of damp towelling for the subsequent cold application. In contrast to other hydrotherapy treatments using alternating hot and cold, the hot is administered for less time than the cold, although the temperature is adjusted to the patient's level of vitality and constitution. The general effect is increased blood flow to all vital organs in the trunk. The patient's entire body is covered with two layers of wool blanket to retain heat during the treatment, and the patient must be monitored to ensure that they do not become chilled.

The treatment effects are increased by using pulsed low-voltage alternating current administered bilaterally to the back at the mid-thoracic level and transabdominally, with the goal of attaining muscular contractions to stimulate lymphatic movement at the thoracic duct/cisterna chyli and in the lymphatics of the gastrointestinal tract. The specialised equipment uses damp sponges as electrodes, rather than needles as in electroacupuncture, though the muscular contraction effects can be similar. All metals – including jewellery, piercings and metal on clothing – should be removed prior to treatment. Due to the use of electrical current, constitutional hydrotherapy is contraindicated in patients who have a pacemaker, metal implant or malignancy in the area of electrical stimulation. Transabdominal electrical stimulation should also not be used during menstruation or pregnancy.

The treatment is particularly indicated for gastrointestinal conditions, respiratory conditions, acute infections, female reproductive conditions, immunodeficiency conditions, nervous system dysregulation and circulatory conditions. It can also be a good treatment to administer late in the day for patients who have trouble sleeping, as the treatment tends to leave the patient in a very relaxed and calm state. Aside from the contraindications and cautions mentioned, the treatment is contraindicated in acute asthma or cold-induced asthma, acute urinary tract infections, high fevers and low body temperatures (less than 36°C). Some patients may not be suitable for this treatment if they have a fear of the electrical stimulation.[3]

Therapeutic baths

The term 'balneotherapy' is used somewhat variably, but traditionally refers to therapeutic bathing in natural, mineralised spring water, which is an integral part of many cultures worldwide. A related practice can be found in thalassotherapy, which refers to the therapeutic use of ocean water for its healing properties. Today, balneotherapy often refers to immersion of part or all of the body in a bath with additives such as minerals, salts, oils, peloids or clays, and herbs. In this section, therapeutic baths are discussed in general from the perspective of clinical naturopathic hydrotherapy, including baths with and without additives, and leaving aside the topic of traditional balneotherapy in mineral springs while acknowledging it as a deep and valuable therapeutic and cultural tradition.

Therapeutic baths have thermal effects that are similar to those of rinses or wraps, with the added benefit of mechanical effects due to hydrostatic pressure on the outside of the body and, when additives are used, the benefit of general or specific chemical effects as well. The effects depend on the size and location of the submerged body part, the temperature and duration of the bath and the nature of any additives. Submersion of a significant portion of the body increases arterial blood volume by increasing venous and lymphatic return and plasma volume; increases kidney filtration, sodium clearance and urine output; decreases plasma concentration of cortisol, adrenaline and other hormones; increases endogenous dopamine and opioid activity; and decreases muscular tension and oxygen consumption.[8]

A full bath is generally considered as submersion to the level of the neck, with a three-quarter bath described as submersion to the chest with the arms in the water, and a half bath described as submersion to the navel with the arms out of the water. For a sitz bath, also known as a hip bath, the patient sits in a specially designed bath with knees and upper body elevated, feet outside the bath, and water covering from the mid-thigh to around the navel. This can be achieved with a regular bath, but it is not as comfortable for the patient and can be challenging for those who have limited mobility, strength or balance. Arm and foot baths are also commonly used, coming from the Kneipp tradition and being valued for their reflexive and homeostatic circulatory and nervous system effects. An arm bath calls for submersion from the fingertips to the middle of the upper arm, and a foot bath calls for submersion from the toes to either the top of the calf or just above the ankle.

Baths can be hot, warm, neutral, cold or contrasting/alternating, depending on the treatment goals. Full-body hot baths result in systemic hyperthermia and are covered in the next section. Additives are generally used only in hot, warm or neutral baths, rather than in cold, due to the short duration of cold baths not allowing adequate time for absorption or direct therapeutic effects on tissues. Most additives fall into the therapeutic categories of anti-inflammatory, anti-rheumatic, circulatory stimulating, astringent, antipruritic, vulnerary, nutritive or nervine.

As with other hydrotherapy techniques, there are general guidelines for clinical therapeutic baths, but these are applicable primarily to immersions in larger baths, rather than to arm and foot baths. Patients need to be supported getting into and out of the bath. When getting out of a full bath, the patient should sit on the side of the bath for a minute before standing to moderate the effects of positional and hydrostatic pressure changes on blood pressure. Once in the bath, the patient's position should be supported so that they do not have to exert effort to hold themselves in place or keep their head above water. This may be easier to achieve with specially designed therapeutic baths, such as a Hubbard tank, but modifications can be made to a home bath to make it suitable for this purpose, assuming it is large enough to submerge the desired portion of the body. While in the bath, the patient must be monitored for reactions, particularly any dysfunctional reactions, and the treatment modified or stopped if necessary. Maintaining consistent interaction with the patient during treatment is an important part of this monitoring; for longer, more relaxing baths in particular, there is an opportunity for use of counselling techniques to achieve additional therapeutic benefits in the bath setting.

Following is an overview of some of the more commonly used therapeutic bath techniques; a more exhaustive coverage is beyond the scope of this book.

FOOT AND ARM BATHS

Foot and arm baths used for their reflexive, circulatory or nervous system effects come directly from the Kneipp tradition, but they are also useful for their local effects, particularly in the case of local injuries or inflammation. Hot, cold or contrasting/alternating applications are most commonly used for foot baths, whereas arm baths tend to be cold or contrasting/alternating. To consider the therapeutic potential for each treatment, refer to Table 5.2.

A hot foot bath is administered at a temperature of 40–43°C for 10–30 minutes,[3] with water either coming to the top of the calf (common in the modern Kneipp tradition) or covering only the feet and ankles (common in modern naturopathic hydrotherapy). Indications for a hot foot bath include congestive headache, nosebleed, chest congestion, pelvic congestion, delayed onset of menstruation, chill or fatigue. The effects are derivative, pulling blood flow and congestion down to the feet. In the case of headache or head congestion, a hot foot bath can be paired with a cold compress to the forehead or the back of the neck to improve treatment outcomes. After the hot foot bath, cold water is poured *briefly* over the patient's feet and ankles, the feet are dried (including between the toes) and covered in socks and the patient rests. As with other similar treatments, the hot foot bath is contraindicated in patients with peripheral circulatory dysfunction or loss of sensation in the feet, such as in diabetes.

Cold foot baths are useful for reduction of swelling or pain in the feet and may be used instead of a cold compress to gain the added effects of water pressure to reduce swelling. This is particularly useful in the acute stage (first 24 hours) after an injury. Otherwise, indications and contraindications for cold arm and foot baths are much the same as for a cold compress or an arm or a knee rinse. Assuming the patient is not chilly, a brief cold footbath can have the effect of drawing blood down towards the feet, similar to a hot foot bath or the wet sock treatment, due to the secondary effect of vasodilation. This is helpful to some in calming the mind before sleep. By comparison, a brief (10–30 seconds) cold arm bath tends to be stimulating and can be useful to increase mental focus and alertness.

Contrasting/alternating hot and cold arm and foot baths used for local effects are indicated in the subacute stage (24–48 hours) after an injury or in chronic arthritis or swelling conditions.[1] A general guideline for these baths is a hot immersion for 3–5 minutes, followed by a cold immersion for 30–90 seconds, with this cycle repeated three times.[6] With hand and foot injuries, baths can give better effects than a compress due to the 100% coverage of the skin, which is often not possible to attain with a compress, and the increased thermal effect from a larger amount of water. That said, the indications and contraindications for contrasting local baths are the same as those for alternating compresses, keeping in mind that these can be used not only for local effects, but also for reflexive and systemic effects.

SITZ BATHS

Sitz baths are indicated for their direct effects in conditions of the pelvic area, including the reproductive organs and genitalia, the rectum and anus, and the lower urinary tract, as well as for their derivative effects in drawing blood or congestion down from the head. As with other baths, sitz baths can be administered hot, neutral or contrasting/alternating, and they very often include additives for therapeutic effects to reduce inflammation, itching, infection, laxity of tissue, or pain. Patients should be disrobed for treatment, but a blanket can be placed around the patient's shoulder or knees, or socks and/or a hot foot bath can be used during longer neutral baths to ensure that the patient does not become chilled.

In a hot sitz bath, the water level should be 1 cm above the patient's navel,[3] and often analgesic or antispasmodic additives are used. Hot sitz baths are indicated for any painful condition caused by or involving muscle tension, spasm or colic in the pelvic area, although they are not indicated in cases of acute inflammation, as the increase of blood flow to the area can further inflame tissues.[6] Other indications include insomnia, delayed onset of menses, congestive headache and painful haemorrhoids. Contraindications include haemorrhage, organ prolapse, menorrhagia, conditions of pelvic congestion such as fibroids, acute infection and during the menses.[3] A hot sitz bath is usually followed by a brief cool sponging of the pelvic area before getting dressed.

In a neutral sitz bath, the water is level with the patient's navel, and often anti-inflammatory, vulnerary or antipruritic additives are used. Neutral sitz baths are indicated for any acute inflammation or pruritus in the pelvic area, including the anal and genital areas. They are particularly useful in acute cystitis and can be used to decrease mental or sexual excitement.[3]

Contrast sitz baths use either hot and cold baths, or a hot bath followed by a cold wet towel applied in the manner of a snug nappy to the entire pelvic area. The water level for the hot sitz bath follows the same guideline as noted above in relation to the navel, while the cold sitz bath uses a water level that is 1 cm below the navel. As with other contrast treatments, the hot application comes first and the treatment ends on a cold application, generally aiming for three to four cycles. Contrast sitz baths have a strongly tonic effect on pelvic organs, so they are indicated for any atonic condition of the pelvic organs or musculature, such as prolapsed organs. Specific indications include chronic urinary tract infections, pelvic congestion, pelvic inflammatory disease, haemorrhoids, fissures, prostatitis, constipation, postpartum discomfort or healing and, via derivative effects, congestive headaches. Contraindications are the same as those listed for hot sitz baths, with the addition of acute inflammation, pain, spasm or colic, as well as acute lung congestion or any heart condition.[3]

CONTRAST FULL BATH

Only the most robust people can take a full-body cold bath without being first warmed, so a contrast full bath is ideal to obtain the beneficial effects of a full cold bath in most people. Regular contrast baths are one of the best overall ways to support vitality, giving both thermal and mechanical effects. As a comparison, full-body contrast showers give outstanding thermal systemic effects, but lack the mechanical effects of baths, although they can be a more efficient regular practice from both a time and water-consumption perspective. Contrast full baths are specifically indicated for systemic or central congestive conditions, such as fibroids, dysmenorrhoea, amenorrhoea, fibromyalgia, haemorrhoids, depression, constipation, water retention or other oedema, benign prostatic hypertrophy and infertility. Like constitutional hydrotherapy they also are very useful generally for increasing blood flow to the vital organs of digestion, detoxification and elimination.[3]

Some sources urge caution in using full-body immersions for hypertension or congestive heart failure.[8] However, two studies have demonstrated the safety and efficacy of warm immersions, either alone or in combination with cold water rinses, in improving some symptoms associated with chronic heart failure.[15,16]

As with other treatments, it is necessary to adjust the hot and cold temperatures for the patient's vitality, age, condition and constitution; the weather and time of day are also valid considerations. Caution should be used in people who are elderly, weak or debilitated, as well as those with cardiovascular concerns. The hot bath will generally be 39–42°C with a duration of 10 minutes or to patient tolerance, while the cold bath will generally be 16–20°C for 30–90 seconds. Patients will have significantly different levels of tolerance for both hot and cold, and it is better to start more moderately on both baths until the patient's response is noted and gradually move towards hotter and colder temperatures as the treatment progresses. Some patients have a very low tolerance to cold at the outset, in which case the bath can be modified from a full immersion to a half or three-quarters immersion until the tolerance is increased.

Patients may be given instructions for a modified form of this treatment to do at home if they have a separate bath and shower and a sufficiently large hot-water tank, with the bath being used for the hot bath and the shower being used for the cold application. Depending on the insulation of the bath and the number of cycles of hot/cold being targeted, it may be necessary to add more hot water to the bath during treatment to maintain the hot temperature. When undertaking a very hot bath at home, the patient should have someone sitting with them to monitor and help them in and out of the bath. If a single cycle is the aim, then a hot bath followed by a cold short wrap can achieve similar treatment effects.

NEUTRAL FULL BATH

The administration of a neutral full bath to achieve the desired effect is a highly individualised endeavour and a bit of an art, but it is also one of the most profound hydrotherapeutic interventions when done properly, particularly for mental and emotional unrest or an excessively excited state of mind or body. The primary effect of a neutral full bath is to sedate, and as a lengthy relaxing treatment, there is opportunity for various counselling techniques while the patient is in a relaxed state, which might enable dialogue that otherwise would not be possible. Neutral baths also have all of the general mechanical benefits of any full-body immersion.

Indications for a neutral full bath include insomnia, anxiety, depression, nervous irritability or mental illness, exhaustion, drug withdrawal and chronic pain, with pain reduction coming from a decrease in nervous system excitation and general relaxation. Neutral full baths may also be used for acute hypertension, pruritus or peripheral oedema. They are contraindicated in cases of cardiovascular weakness or with skin conditions such as eczema that are aggravated by water, and caution should be used with longer baths in patients with kidney conditions.[1,6]

The temperature of a neutral bath is highly dependent on the patient's condition and constitution – they should feel neither warm nor cool while in the bath. The indicated temperature can vary significantly by person and by season, by the temperature of the room and the time of day, as well as by what treatments preceded the bath. Neutral bath temperature is generally considered to be skin temperature, around 32–35°C. Patients who tend to be chilly will not feel this range as neutral and may become chilled, whereas patients who tend to carry excess heat may feel initially cool entering the bath but quickly become equilibrated to it. The patient's sensation is the ultimate key to finding the correct temperature, and in baths longer than 20 minutes, warm water may need to be added periodically to maintain the temperature for the patient. Therapeutic effects on the nervous system will not be achieved if the patient feels warm or chilly.

The duration of a neutral full bath can range from 15 minutes to hours.[6] In colder weather, it may be ideal to heat the patient first in a sauna or hot bath, which will increase the relaxation effects. Due to the calming of the nervous system, the patient may fall asleep, so they need to be properly supported and closely monitored to ensure that their nose and mouth stay above the surface of the water. Because neutral baths tend to gently cool the body, there is a tendency for the patient to become chilled after the bath, so they must be thoroughly dried and left to rest in a warm bed after treatment. If a neutral full bath is undertaken at home, the patient should take it just before bedtime to avoid becoming chilled.

Hyperthermia treatments

Hyperthermia in the therapeutic context aims to increase the core body temperature for therapeutic effect. The most well-known form of hyperthermia treatment is the sauna, although hyperthermia baths are a common naturopathic treatment due to the added mechanical effects of the water and the ability to use additives to achieve therapeutic goals beyond the thermal effects.

The two major therapeutic benefits of whole-body hyperthermia are detoxification[17] and immune system stimulation. Detoxification in this instance is primarily due to increased sweating and excretion of metabolic wastes and toxins through the skin. However, fat tissue may also be mobilised, which mobilises fat-soluble toxins. In addition, volatile compounds may leave the body through the increased rate of breathing, while non-volatile compounds may be processed by the liver and leave the body through the gastrointestinal tract. Immune system stimulation occurs in hyperthermia via mimicking of a 'fever' in the body, which may not only kill heat-labile bacteria and viruses, but also increase circulating white blood cells and cytokines.[18–20] Both of these major effects are useful in preventive and disease treatment settings, assuming that they are not contraindicated for the patient and are not used in a way that is depleting. Other effects of hyperthermia include increasing the metabolic rate, improving vascular endothelial function and, in insulin resistance with serial treatments, significantly reducing elevated blood glucose levels.[10]

The general guidelines for hyperthermia treatments are as follows:

1 Hyperthermia treatment is generally contraindicated in pregnancy and infancy; in those who are the elderly, weak or debilitated; in anaemia; in hypertension or hypotension; during menstruation; if dehydration, hypoglycaemia or electrolyte imbalance is a concern; and in most severe or advanced diseases. Caution should be used for patients with adrenal fatigue or insufficiency, methylation polymorphisms or general heat intolerance. In a dry sauna, caution should be applied for those with dry respiratory conditions.

2 Hyperthermia treatments are attended treatments – the patient must be monitored closely throughout for reactions, either dysfunctional or normal.

3 Treatment should be discontinued immediately if the patient starts to feel dizzy, light-headed or nauseous, has tingling in the hands or feet, has a very rapid heart rate or palpitations, or is otherwise feeling generally unwell. 'Pushing it' is neither advisable nor therapeutically sound or effective.

4 The patient must be kept hydrated. If electrolytes or low blood sugar are a concern, liquids administered during treatment may include diluted fruit or vegetable juices or coconut water. Otherwise, water must be given regularly in small amounts.

5 The patient should be supported when standing up from the sauna or bath and should do so slowly, pausing in a sitting position for a minute to allow the cardiovascular system to respond and prevent pooling of blood in the legs and fainting due to vasodilation.

6 Some patients may hyperventilate during treatment and will require coaching and support in slowing their breathing so as not to cause a respiratory alkalosis.

7 Headaches are a frequent side effect and can be prevented by use of a cold compress to the head, face and ears to keep the head temperature down.

8 The patient should not eat immediately before treatment, but should have had a full meal 3–4 hours beforehand to avoid hypoglycaemia during treatment. The patient should not eat immediately after treatment but rest and wait for their body temperature to return to normal, at which point appetite generally returns as well.

9 Treatments should be partnered with other naturopathic therapeutics to support the treatment goals. For example, if detoxification is the main goal, hyperthermia should be prescribed along with other naturopathic interventions that support the body's detoxification and elimination systems.

10 Resting after treatment is generally advised.

SAUNAS

As with balneotherapy, use of saunas has a widespread cultural history in Russia, Finland, Turkey and other European countries for general health support, as well as having a connection to spiritual practices in traditional cultures such as the Native American sweat lodge. Sauna bathing is well-tolerated by most adults and is well-indicated in moderate hypertension, rheumatic disease and toxic exposure, as well as being generally indicated for health support. For detoxification purposes, extended periods in the sauna at a moderate temperature can be beneficial with proper hydration and electrolyte replacement during treatment. The general contraindications listed above for hyperthermia treatment apply, but specific contraindications include unstable angina pectoris, recent myocardial infarction and severe aortic stenosis.[6]

Procedurally, the aim of the sauna is to attain whole-body sweating and hyperthermia without depleting or weakening the patient. Temperatures should be determined according to the patient's condition and constitution and general tolerance for heat. The sauna is conducted much like a contrast bath, with a heating phase followed by a cool shower or plunge, repeated for several cycles and always ending on cold. After each cold phase, the patient should pat their skin dry before returning to the sauna for another heating/sweating phase. The heating phase should last until the patient is in a full-body sweat; this usually takes longer in the first cycle than in the subsequent cycles. If the patient feels overly hot or has pressure in the head or any other symptoms as discussed in the general guidelines above, at minimum they should have a cold compress applied to the head and the sauna temperature reduced; otherwise, the treatment should be discontinued.

HYPERTHERMIA BATHS

Hyperthermia baths are conducted in-clinic and with close supervision and monitoring. The patient is immersed fully to the neck in a bath with a temperature range of 38–42°C for 20–60 minutes. For longer baths, hot water may need to be added periodically to maintain the temperature. For some conditions and in patients who can tolerate it, higher temperatures can be used for shorter periods. Once a patient's tolerance and reaction have been determined using in-clinic treatment, if the patient has someone at home to supervise and assist with the bath, they can be given instructions for administering hyperthermia baths at home with a maximum temperature of 40°C.

Indications for hyperthermia baths can be extrapolated from the major therapeutic benefits of detoxification and immune stimulation. Additionally, they are indicated for muscle tension and spasms and in some cases of rheumatoid arthritis when the patient reports feeling better from heat.[6] (Note: this is atypical in RA.)

In addition to following the general guidelines for hyperthermia treatment above, during a hyperthermia bath at a temperature of 40°C or higher, the patient's temperature and pulse must be monitored and not allowed to rise above 40°C/140 bpm; if either reaches this level, the patient should carefully get out of the bath. Likewise, if the patient shows signs of dizziness or fainting, the bath should be drained immediately to remove the thermal stimulus; the patient's head should be supported above the water level and the patient removed from the bath as soon as possible. Generally, it is advisable to have two attendants present during hotter hyperthermia baths, as a single attendant will have difficulty handling the necessary procedures if the patient needs to be removed from the bath in a less than fully conscious state.

The treatment process after the bath will vary according to the treatment goals. If extension of the sweating phase of treatment or elevation of body temperature is indicated, the patient may be placed immediately onto a treatment table and wrapped in a dry sheet and wool blankets and allowed to sweat further. The patient must be monitored as if they are still in the bath (i.e. temperature and pulse checked, cold compresses applied to the head, water given to remain hydrated). If detoxification is the primary goal, the bath or extended sweating phase is generally followed by a cool shower with soap, to remove any excreted toxins from the skin surface. However, if an additive was used in the bath, it may be desirable to leave its residue on the skin for some time, so the patient should not shower directly after treatment.

STEAM THERAPIES

The two most commonly prescribed naturopathic hydrotherapy treatments using steam are the Russian steam bath and steam inhalation.

The Russian steam bath is a full-body hyperthermia treatment with the advantage over the classic steam or dry sauna that the patient's head can be easily kept cool and the treatment can be done without any specialised equipment. That said, there are specialised Russian steam cabinets in which the patient sits, leaving only their head outside the top of the cabinet. Inside the cabinet is a heated reservoir of water to produce steam, in which additives can be placed, and the patient is disrobed so as to allow full skin contact with the steam. A towel is wrapped around the patient's neck to prevent steam escaping from the cabinet. The treatment proceeds much like a hyperthermia bath, with similar patient monitoring and post-treatment care.

In the absence of a specialised steam cabinet, the Russian steam bath is still easy to administer in-clinic or to instruct the patient to undertake at home. For the treatment process, the disrobed patient sits on a wooden or plastic chair (metal could get dangerously hot), draped from the neck to the floor with two large wool blankets, front and back, to create a tent around them. The patient's feet are placed into a hot foot bath and under the chair a hotplate with a pan of boiling water or a kettle is placed to produce steam. To avoid burning, the patient should not allow their legs or feet to move under the chair and, if a kettle is used, the spout should be aimed away from the patient's legs. The treatment intensity can be increased by administering diaphoretic herbal teas prior to and during

treatment. Treatment duration is 5–10 minutes for stimulating effects and 15–25 minutes for sedating effects.[3] Cool compresses can be placed on the patient's forehead or back of the neck to keep their head cool, and the treatment ends with a short cold shower.

Indications for the Russian steam bath include colds, influenza, detoxification, hypotension, rheumatoid arthritis, insomnia, nervous agitation, congestive headache, sinus congestion, gout and jaundice, as well as for general health support in a healthy patient. The Russian steam bath is contraindicated in patients with anaemia, diabetes, heart disease, hypertension, peripheral vascular dysfunction, emaciation, weakness or debility.[3]

Stream inhalation is likewise easy to prescribe for patients to undertake at home. It provides a hot, moist air bath for the respiratory tract and is indicated for cough, laryngitis, sinusitis, respiratory congestion or infection,[21] sore throat and allergic rhinitis,[22] and to loosen dry or thick respiratory secretions. It is generally paired with aromatic or essential oils that have therapeutic indications for similar conditions but can be undertaken with plain steam as well. Contraindications include congestive heart failure, cardiac asthma and other severe cardiac conditions, and it is unadvisable in the very young or very old.[3]

The treatment set-up involves a chair and table (often a coffee table works well, as it is lower and the patient can lean forwards over it), on which is placed a large bowl of water just off the boil, with additives as indicated for the patient's condition. The patient sits disrobed from the waist up, with a twin-sized sheet draped over the bowl, the patient's head and upper body. The patient is instructed to breathe deeply through the nose (to the extent possible, if there is nasal congestion) to bring the steam and aromatic compounds into contact with the mucous membranes; the steam will also be in contact with the patient's chest and arms externally. The duration of treatment should be 10 minutes at a minimum, and it can be repeated two to three times daily as needed. In the case of sinus or chest congestion, the treatment can be paired with a hot foot bath to draw congestion down from the head and chest.

Enemas and colonic irrigation

The rectum has reflex relationships throughout the body, so when it is distended or irritated, it can cause widespread symptoms throughout the body.[3] Chronic constipation, with or without other conditions or toxicity concerns, can be a causative or exacerbating factor in a wide range of symptoms and diseases. Enemas and colonic irrigation (also known as colonic hydrotherapy) work to decrease distension and irritation of the colon and rectum by eliminating faecal matter and toxins. Because of the reflexive relationships of the colon and rectum, as well as the generalised effects of detoxification and elimination, the treatment effects tend to be systemic in nature, as well as being beneficial locally to the colon and rectum.

Enemas and colonic irrigation are similar treatments and have a significant overlap in their indications, benefits and contraindications. The salient differences between the two are that enemas can be instructed for patient use at home, they are often used with different additives for specific complaints and water does not reach far into the colon. In contrast, colonic irrigation requires specialised equipment and training, uses water at higher pressures to reach the entire length of the colon and stimulate peristalsis, and generally does not use additives, so is a more generalised treatment.

Colonic irrigation has become popularised outside of the medical sphere by the rising trend for detoxification as a health-supportive regimen in mainstream culture. In many instances this is tied to weight-loss goals and the desire to appear thinner, rather than being directly or solely related to health. Some use the treatment so frequently that it is likely to be detrimental to overall gastrointestinal health. Thus, caution is warranted that enemas and colonic irrigation should not be used other than remedially for addressing illness or frank toxicity concerns; they are not preventive in nature and should not be abused for weight loss or other non-clinical goals.

Enemas are generally indicated for chronic constipation or faecal impaction, or inflammation, congestion and/or pain anywhere in the body when accompanied by the bowels not moving. For these indications, generally plain water is used in treatment. Enemas are also specifically indicated for infant colic, poisoning or other dangerous intoxication, pinworms, ulcerative colitis and chronic diarrhoea. In these instances, additives are used, including herbal infusions, oils and substances such as activated charcoal or clay.[3] The patient should be prepared in advance to be well-hydrated so that the enema solution is not absorbed from the bowel, although it is possible to administer herbs or other medications directly through the rectum, in which case absorption is a goal.

The water temperature should be selected based on the patient's body temperature to avoid cramping and water retention. Generally, a water temperature of 40°C is indicated for a high fever or when the body temperature is only slightly above normal. With a moderate fever, the water temperature should be 38.5–39.5°C, and with a body temperature lower than normal, the water temperature should be gradually increased from 40.5°C to 43°C as the body temperature approaches 35°C, to help warm the patient. Adults require 1–2 L of water for administration of an enema, while children require 250–1000 mL depending on size. Infants only need use of a bulb syringe filled one to three times.[3]

The process calls for the patient to lie supine on a non-absorbent surface with their knees flexed and buttocks elevated by a pillow with a waterproof covering. The nozzle of the apparatus should be lubricated and then inserted gently into the rectum in the direction of the navel; this can be assisted by instructing the patient to bear down as if they are preparing to move their bowels, thus relaxing the sphincters. Water is introduced slowly through the enema apparatus, pausing or stopping if the patient becomes uncomfortable or distended; abdominal massage may ease discomfort. Once the water has been administered, the patient should be instructed to lie still and retain the water for 15–20 minutes, then go quickly to the toilet or nearby receptacle and evacuate completely, before rinsing off if necessary and resting.

Indications for clinical use of colonic irrigation are similar to those for enemas but also include detoxification in cases where toxicity is a true clinical concern and is causing illness or frank pathology. Colonic irrigation is also particularly indicated for chronic constipation or atonic colon, as the water pressure in the colon can assist not only in removing waste matter but also in toning the smooth muscle of the colon and increasing peristalsis. For detoxification, colonic irrigation has greater efficacy in removing toxins when used along with other naturopathic therapeutics that mobilise fat-soluble toxins from the tissues, support the liver and gallbladder, and decrease the reabsorption of toxins from the colon into the bloodstream.

Unlike enemas, colonic irrigation is generally undertaken with plain warm water, with the temperature adjusted to the patient's comfort level. A specialised colonic irrigation unit is used, and modern units generally allow the patient to control the water flow, pressure and temperature. Training for healthcare professionals in the use of a colonic irrigation unit is not complex. Because of the tonifying action of the higher water pressure on the smooth muscle of the colon, colonic irrigation may cause intestinal cramping and other short-term side effects, so patient tolerance of the procedure needs to be monitored to ensure that the treatment is individually appropriate. Colonic irrigation is contraindicated in ulcerative colitis, diverticulitis, inflamed haemorrhoids, intestinal bleeding, pregnancy, colon cancer and hypertension.

EVIDENCE SUPPORTING THERAPEUTIC USES OF WATER

As with other forms of traditional healthcare that have stood the test of time, the therapeutic use of water has been practised for millennia in both formal medicine and folk-healing traditions across many cultures and is still a vital part of culture and healthcare in many countries today. However, like other healing practices that have subtle systemic effects with consistent use over time, such as dietary changes, research demonstrating efficacy at the systemic level or for broader health outcomes can be confounding due to the multitude of factors that must be controlled. Thus, as is generally the case in modern medical research, hydrotherapy studies tend to focus on physiological or biochemical effects in specific pathological conditions with a time-limited course of treatment. This investigates only a fraction of the potential of water therapies, although it does shed light on the power that externally applied water has to effect internal changes, which is not generally recognised in modern conventional medicine.

One of the most studied areas for the therapeutic use of water for its thermal effects is in cardiovascular disease. The mechanical and thermal effects of water, and specifically hyperthermia (including sauna), have been demonstrated to be useful in the treatment of hypertension,[23,24] congestive heart failure[25–27] and vascular endothelial dysfunction in atherosclerosis.[28] The mechanical effects of water in these conditions are primarily through increased venous return, while the thermal effects are primarily through vasodilation and toning of the vascular epithelium. A 2012 study concluded that improvement in exercise tolerance in patients with chronic heart failure resulted from repeated sauna treatment as mediated by improved endothelial function.[29] The use of hyperthermia to tone vascular epithelium has widespread implications, not only for cardiovascular disease, but also for other diseases wherein diminished circulatory function plays a role. For example, a recent study in Finland demonstrated a reduction in risk of dementia as a result of regular sauna usage (four to seven times per week), hypothesised to be mediated by improved endothelial function and reduced inflammation, blood pressure and pulse pressure, all being effects of hyperthermia.[30]

With circulatory compromise being a major concern in diabetes, use of water to improve circulatory function is an area that merits study. Studies of hydrotherapy and diabetes have focused on demonstrating an improvement in insulin resistance in type 2 diabetes through use of hyperthermia treatments as mediated by increased blood flow to skeletal muscles.[31,32] One study showed that a single immersion in the Dead Sea resulted in significantly reduced blood glucose in a group of patients with type 2 diabetes without influencing insulin levels.[33] Heating of local tissues to increase blood flow has also been demonstrated to be effective in healing diabetic ulcers,[34] although this study involved use of dry heat to effect blood flow changes.

Chronic pain and various rheumatic diseases and syndromes have also received attention in the hydrotherapy research. Several studies have examined the effectiveness of balneotherapy for fibromyalgia, finding improvements in a number of tender points as well as the frequency and severity of associated symptoms.[35-37] Evidence is encouraging, if currently scarce, regarding the use of balneotherapy for the treatment of chronic low back pain.[38] Balneotherapy includes not only individual baths with mineral additives, but also therapies such as exercise in water and underwater massage.[39]

Hydrotherapy has demonstrated usefulness in immune stimulation with specific pathologies that create susceptibility to infection. Kneipp hydrotherapy using cold water affusions in patients with chronic obstructive pulmonary disease has indicated potential for improvement in the frequency of respiratory infections via immunomodulation relating to Th-1 cells.[40] A more generalised look at the effects of brief cold exposure on the human immune system demonstrated that whole-body cold exposure subsequent to pre-heating results in increased circulation of leucocytes, granulocytes, natural killer cells and interleukin-6 as mediated by increased noradrenaline.[41] This study used a heated bath followed by a cold air chamber rather than a cold bath, as is commonly practised in hydrotherapy treatments. However, the results of a cold water bath would probably be similar. A study in 2000 using whole-body hyperthermia baths demonstrated an increase in natural killer cell circulation and activity, while total T and B lymphocytes decreased and relative numbers of CD8+ lymphocytes increased.[42] And finally, a small pilot study of naturopathic constitutional hydrotherapy in 2008 with HIV-positive patients demonstrated a statistically significant improvement in energy levels, a trend towards increased physical function, and decreased body fat, pain, systolic blood pressure and C-reactive protein levels.[43]

ACKNOWLEDGMENTS

With gratitude to Father Sebastian Kneipp.

REFERENCES

[1] Kneipp S. My water cure (English language translation). Edinburgh: William Blackwood & Sons; 1893.

[2] Kirchfield F, Boyle W. Nature doctors: pioneers in naturopathic medicine. East Palestine, OH: Buckeye Naturopathic Press; 1994.

[3] Boyle W, Saine A. Lectures in naturopathic hydrotherapy. Sandy, OR: Eclectic Medical Publications; 1988.

[4] Kellogg JH. Rational hydrotherapy: a manual of the physiological and therapeutic effects of hydrotherapy procedures, and the technique of their application in the treatment of disease. 4th ed. Battle Creek, MI: Modern Medicine; 1923.

[5] Cody GW, Hascall H. The history of naturopathic medicine: the emergence and evolution of an American school of healing. In: Pizzorno JE, Murray MT, editors. Textbook of natural medicine. 4th ed. St Louis: Elsevier; 2013.

[6] Huyck A, Broderick K. Hydrotherapy. In: Pizzorno JE, Murray MT, editors. Textbook of natural medicine. 4th ed. St Louis: Elsevier; 2013.

[7] Wardle J. Hydrotherapy: a forgotten Australian therapeutic modality. Aust J of Herbal Med 2013;25(1):12–17.

[8] Kneipp Schule. Kneipp hydrotherapy [course manual]. Bad Worishofen, Germany; 2016.

[9] Imamura M, Biro S, Kihara T, et al. Repeated thermal therapy improves impaired vascular endothelial function in patients with coronary risk factors. J Am Coll Cardiol 2001;38(4):1083–8.

[10] Blake E, et al. Naturopathic hydrotherapy. In: Chaitow L, editor. Naturopathic physical medicine. Philadelphia: Churchill Livingstone; 2008.

[11] Moor FB, Peterson S, Manwell E, et al. Manual of hydrotherapy and massage. Mountain View, CA: Pacific Press; 1964.

[12] Lindlahr H. Nature cure. 20th ed. Holicong, PA: Wildside Press; 1922.

[13] Aksoylar S, Aksit S, Caglayan S, et al. Evaluation of sponging and antipyretic medication to reduce body temperature in febrile children. Acta Paediatr Jpn 1997;39:215–17.

[14] Agbolosu NB, Cuevas LE, Milligan P, et al. Efficacy of tepid sponging versus paracetamol in reducing temperature in febrile children. Ann Trop Paediatr 1997;17:283–8.

[15] Grüner Sveälv B, Cider A, Scharin Täng M, et al. Benefit of warm water immersion on biventricular function in patients with chronic heart failure. Cardiovasc Ultrasound 2009;7:33.

[16] Michalsen A, Lüdtke R, Bühring M, et al. Thermal hydrotherapy improves quality of life and hemodynamic function in patients with chronic heart failure. Am Heart J 2003;146(4):728–33.

[17] Gard ZR, Brown EJ. Literature review and comparison studies of sauna/hyperthermia in detoxification. Townsend Lett 1992;107:470–8.

[18] Kappel M, Stadeager C, Tvede N, et al. Effects of in vivo hyperthermia on natural killer cell activity, in vitro proliferative responses and blood mononuclear cell subpopulations. Clin Exp Immunol 1991;84:175–80.

[19] Kappel M, Barington T, Gyhrs A, et al. Influence of elevated body temperature on circulating immunoglobulin-secreting cells. Int J Hyperthermia 1994;10:653–8.

[20] Zellner M, Hergovics N, Roth E, et al. Human monocyte stimulation by experimental whole body hyperthermia. Wien Klin Wochenschr 2002;114:102–7.

[21] Hendley JO, Abbott RD, Beasley PP, et al. Effect of inhalation of hot humidified air on experimental rhinovirus infection. JAMA 1994;106:1487–92.

[22] Georgitis JW. Local hyperthermia and nasal irrigation for perennial allergic rhinitis; effect on symptoms and nasal airflow. Ann Allergy 1993;71:385–9.

[23] Biro S, Masuda A, Kihara T, et al. Clinical implications of thermal therapy in lifestyle-related diseases. Exp Biol Med 2003;228:1245–9.

[24] Reaven GM, Lithell H, Landsberg L. Hypertension and associated metabolic abnormalities: the role of insulin resistance and the sympathoadrenal system. NEJM 1996;334:374–82.

[25] Kihara T, Biro S, Imamura M, et al. Repeated sauna treatment improves vascular endothelial and cardiac function in patients with chronic heart failure. J Am Coll Cardiol 2002;39(5):754–9.

[26] Cider A, Sveälv B, Täng M, et al. Immersion in warm water induces improvement in cardiac function in patients with chronic heart failure. Eur J Heart Fail 2006;8(3):308–13.

[27] Gabrielsen A, Sorensen V, Pump B, et al. Cardiovascular and neuroendocrine responses to water immersion in compensated heart failure. Am J Physiol Heart Circ Physiol 2000;279(4):H1931–40.

[28] Imamura M, Biro S, Kihara T, et al. Repeated thermal therapy improves impaired vascular endothelial function in patients with coronary risk factors. J Am Coll of Cardiol 2001;38(4):1083–8.

[29] Ohori T, Nozawa T, Ihori H, et al. Effect of repeated sauna treatment on exercise tolerance and endothelial function in patients with chronic heart failure. Am J Cardiol 2012;109(1):100–4.

[30] Laukkanen T, Kunutsor S, Kauhanen J, et al. Sauna bathing is inversely associated with dementia and Alzheimer's disease in middle-aged Finnish men. Age Aging 2016;doi: https://doi.org/10.1093/ageing/afw212.

[31] Baron AD, Steinberg H, Brechtel G, et al. Skeletal muscle blood flow independently modulates insulin-mediated glucose uptake. Am J Physiol 1994;266(2 Pt 1):E248–53.

[32] Hooper PL. Hot tub therapy for type 2 diabetes mellitus. NEJM 1999;341:924–5.

[33] Mizrahi E, Liberty I, Tsedek I, et al. The influence of single immersion in Dead Sea water on glucose, insulin, cortisol and C-peptide levels in type 2 diabetes mellitus patients. Harefuah 2011;150(8):646–9, 688–9.

[34] Petrofsky JS, Besonis C, Rivera D, et al. Does local heating really help diabetic patients increase circulation? J Neurol & Ortho Med Surg 2003;21:40–6.

[35] Buskila D, Abu-Shakra M, Neumann L, et al. Balneotherapy for fibromyalgia at the Dead Sea. Rheum Int 2001;20(3):105–8.

[36] Evcik D, Kizilay B, Gokcen E. The effects of balneotherapy on fibromyalgia patients. Rheum Int 2002;22(2):56–9.

[37] Sukenik S, Baradin R, Codish S, et al. Balneotherapy at the Dead Sea area for patients with psoriatic arthritis and concomitant fibromyalgia. Isr Med Assoc J 2001;3(2):147–50.

[38] Pittler MH, Karagulle MZ, Karagulle M, et al. Spa therapy and balneotherapy for treating low back pain: meta-analysis of randomized trials. Rheumatology 2006;45(7):880–4.

[39] Batsialou I. Balneotherapy in the treatment of subjective symptoms of lumbar syndrome. Med Pregl 2002;55(11–12):495–9.

[40] Goedsche K, Förster M, Kroegel C, et al. Repeated cold water stimulations (hydrotherapy according to Kneipp) in patients with COPD. Forsch Komplementmed 2007;14(3):158–66.

[41] Brenner IKM, Castellani JW, Gabaree C, et al. Immune changes in humans during cold exposure: effects of prior heating and exercise. J Appl Physiol 1999;87(2):699–710.

[42] Blazícková S, Rovenský J, Koska J, et al. Effect of hyperthermic water bath on parameters of cellular immunity. Int J Clin Pharmacol Res 2000;20(1–2):41–6.

[43] Bradley R, Pillsbury C, Huyck A, et al. Clinical pilot of constitutional hydrotherapy in HIV+ adults. Altern Ther Health Med 2009;15:3.

6

The microbiome

Dr Jason Hawrelak, Dr Joanna Harnett

OVERVIEW

Humans, like all animals, coexist in intimate, mutually dependent relationships with microorganisms.[1,2] Animals have had residential microorganisms performing vital metabolic functions for at least 500 million years. Such functions include food digestion and vitamin production, differentiation of host mucosa, metabolism regulation, xenobiotic processing, prevention of the invasion and colonisation of pathogenic microbes and the development and ongoing regulation of the immune system. Given the integral functions of the microbiota, many researchers now consider humans super-organisms or holobionts, composed of both microbe cells and non-microbe cells living in a mutualistic symbiosis.[3–5] The human microbiota is, in fact, a central element of what it means to be human. (See Box 6.1.)

The first observations of the microbiota were made by Antonie van Leeuwenhoek, who in the 1680s, visualised microbes from his own stool, tooth scrapings and skin. Even at that time he could clearly discern differences in the microbes from these habitats.[8] Over the past two decades, the tools used for examining the microbiota have expanded in sophistication, scope and accuracy, giving us a much clearer picture of the microbiota, and its complexity, at different body sites. Anatomical site is one of the most important factors in determining microbiota compositional diversity (see Fig. 6.1).[1] Interestingly, the vast majority of the microbes found on, and in, the human body originate from one of six phylas – Actinobacteria, Bacteroidetes, Firmicutes, Fusobacteria, Proteobacteria and, to a lesser degree, Cyanobacteria.[2] (See Box 6.2.)

Each individual human has a unique microbiota. Composition appears to be influenced by genetics, early microbial exposure, diet, environmental factors and xenobiotic exposures.[9] The differences between individuals are so wide, in fact, that individuals can be accurately identified solely by the microbiota signature left on frequently touched objects such as keyboards and computer mice.[10] Monozygotic twins, while having more similar microbiotas than unrelated individuals, still differ significantly in microbiota composition – demonstrating the overall importance of environmental factors on microbiota development and maintenance.[11] The

ecosystems that have been the subject of the most research to date include the skin, nasal, oral, breastmilk, vagina and gastrointestinal microbiotas.

THE DERMATOLOGICAL MICROBIOTA

The skin is the largest organ of the human body. It provides a protective layer against both microbial infections and physiochemical changes. It is not, however, a static shield, but instead a complex and dynamic organ characterised by indigenous microbial populations and their interplay with the host. The cutaneous microbiome is vital in the enhancement of skin barrier function and colonisation resistance, as well as immune system training and immune homeostasis.[12]

The biogeography of the skin includes several folds, planes and invaginations, creating unique microenvironments and, consequently, specific niches that maintain unique ecologies.[13] These niches can vary in terms of humidity, pH, temperature and the presence of lipids and anti-microbial peptides.[14] All of these factors impact on both the types and the number of microbes present.

The skin has been classified as having four main types of environments – dry, sebaceous, moist and 'other'. Dry areas include the upper buttock and inner forearm areas. Sebaceous areas include the back, retroauricular creases (the skin crease behind the ear), the forehead and the alar creases (side of the nostril). Examples of moist areas are the axilla, inguinal fold and inner elbow. So called 'other' areas refers to the dermal layers, sweat glands and hair follicles.

The cutaneous microbiome is composed of hundreds of species from 19 different phyla, although most species are from the four phyla *Actinobacteria*, *Firmicutes*, *Bacteroidetes* and *Proteobacteria*. Bacterial counts can reach 10^7 bacteria/cm² on the epidermis.[13] Drier sites are colonised predominantly by *Staphylococcus*, *Propionibacterium*, *Micrococcus*, *Corynebacterium* and *Streptococcus* spp. Sebaceous areas provide an anaerobic, lipid-rich environment that is conducive to *Propionibacterium* growth, while moist regions harbour mostly *Staphylococcus* and *Corynebacterium* spp.[15] Fig. 6.2

BOX 6.1 A brief primer on microbiome-related terminology[3,4,6,7]

Dysbiosis

A state in which the microbiota produces harmful effects via: (1) qualitative and quantitative changes in the flora itself; (2) changes in their metabolic activities; and/or (3) changes in their local distribution

Eubiosis

A healthy, balanced ecosystem

Holobiont

A unit of biological organisation composed of a host and its microbiota

Hologenome

The complete genetic content of the host genome, its organelles' genomes and its microbiome

Metagenomics

A method that allows researchers to create catalogues of what bacteria can do based on the genes that they have

Microbiome

A collection of different microbes and their functions or genes

Microbiota

The microbes in or on a host, including bacteria, archaea, viruses, fungi and protists

Mutualism

A relationship benefitting both parties

Pathobiont

A commensal microorganism that is able to promote pathology only when specific genetic or environmental conditions are altered in the host

Symbiosis

Two or more species living closely together in a long-term relationship

BOX 6.2 A primer in taxonomics[3]

Bacteria, like plants and animals, are classified per the Linnaean system, which consists of hierarchies into which an organism is placed.

All life forms are classified into one of three kingdoms – Bacteria, Archaea or Eukaryota.

Humans, for example, are classified at the kingdom level as Eukaryota, phylum Chordata, class Mammalia, order Primates, family *Homininidae*, genus *Homo* and species *sapiens*.

The well-known probiotic species *Lactobacillus acidophilus* is found in the kingdom Bacteria, phylum Firmicutes, class Bacilli, order Lactobacillales, family *Lactobacillaceae*, genus *Lactobacillus* and species *acidophilus*.

The gut commensal *Escherichia coli* is found in the kingdom Bacteria, phylum Proteobacteria, class Gammaproteobacteria, order Enterobacteriales, family *Enterobacteriaceae*, genus *Escherichia* and species *coli*.

Hence, when referring to phyla, or phylum, we are usually describing very large collections of related organisms – some of which will be closely related; others only distantly so.

---

details the main skin environments and the microbes colonising these ecological niches.

Like most microbiomes, a healthy skin ecosystem is characterised by diversity.[15] In addition to intrapersonal biogeographical variations in the skin microbiota, the diversity and abundance of microbes varies due to gender, seasons, age and even ethnicity. Similar to the gastrointestinal tract microbiota, method of birth (vaginal vs caesarean) has a substantial impact on skin microbiota development. Babies born naturally have been found to be colonised by skin bacterial communities very similar to their mothers, while babies born via caesarean had an ecosystem no more similar to their own mother than any other individual.[13] Hence, vertical transmission of the skin microbiota is the biological norm, whereas in

caesarean-born children, incidental exposures provided by hospital staff and environmental surfaces were the greatest contributors to the microbial communities.[13] Whether practices, such as immediate skin-to-skin contact or maternal 'seeding' of the towel or wrap that the newborn will be placed in, help rectify this situation has not yet been investigated. In theory, both practices should help normalise the inoculation of the skin microbiota in these infants.

A lack of diversity, or change in the cutaneous ecosystem composition, can be caused by a number of factors, including frequent washing, application of make-up, cosmetics and moisturisers, ultraviolet radiation, immune deficiencies and even oral antibiotic use.[15–19] Skin dysbiosis has now been implicated in a number of skin conditions such as acne vulgaris, atopic dermatitis, rosacea and psoriasis.[20–23]

THE NASOPHARYNGEAL MICROBIOTA

Microbial composition and dysbiosis

The microbial composition of the nasopharynx is an ecological niche included in The Human Microbiome Project. The top four most abundant genera of the anterior nares of 236 subjects were *Corynebacterium*, *Propionibacterium*, *Staphylococcus* and *Moraxella*.[24] Within the nasopharynx representative genera, species of known potential respiratory tract pathogens such as

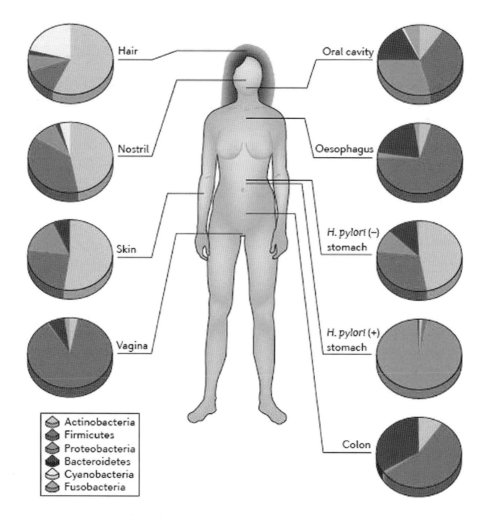

FIGURE 6.1 Compositional differences (phyla) in the microbiome by anatomical site[2]

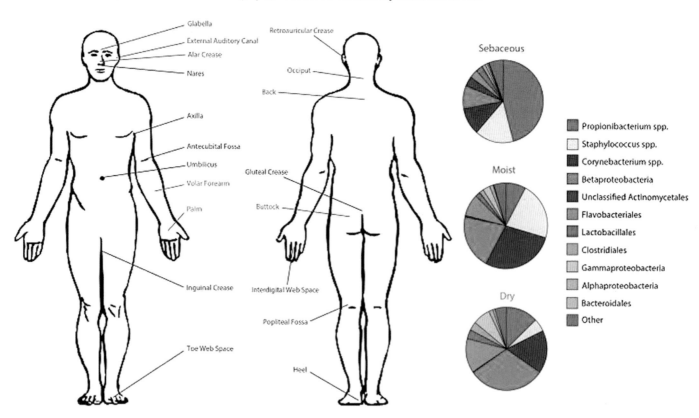

FIGURE 6.2 Regional variation in the skin microbiota[13]
Each pie chart shows the mean bacterial community of a given biogeographical region.

Streptococcus pneumoniae, Haemophilus influenzae, Neisseria meningitides, Moraxella catarrhalis and *Staphylococcus aureus* have been identified in healthy children.[25,26] Disruption that leads to dysbiosis of the nasopharyngeal microbiome may result in these typically asymptomatic bacterial pathogens and viral species causing respiratory tract infections and an increased risk of asthma and severe acute bronchiolitis.[25,27–31]

A core microbiome analysis was conducted on nasal pharyngeal wash specimens collected six months apart from children living with asthma.[30] The five dominant representative genera (95% confidence level) were *Moraxella, Staphylococcus, Streptococcus, Haemophilus* and *Fusobacterium*.[30] In the nasopharyngeal microbiome of children with severe bronchiolitis, *Haemophilus influenzae* and *Moraxella catarrhalis* were associated with respiratory syncytial virus or human rhinovirus infections, and *Moraxella* spp. was associated with acute wheezing.[31] While the findings of these two studies would suggest that dysbiosis of the nasopharyngeal microbiota plays a role in disease predisposition, what causes dysbiosis of this ecological niche is still unfolding.

Factors associated with nasopharyngeal dysbiosis

Breastfed infants have been shown to have characteristics of a more stable nasopharyngeal microbiota community over the first 2 years of life that is positively associated with lower rates of self-reported respiratory infections,[32] suggesting that not breastfeeding may predispose the infant to a less favourable nasopharyngeal tract microbial community. However, this suggestion has been contested.[33]

It is well known that the prevalence of respiratory infections is higher in the colder months of the year. Seasonality has been evaluated as a potential disruptor of the nasopharyngeal microbiome in children.[25] While study results suggested that there was no difference in the diversity of the microbiome between seasons, the abundance of *Lactobacillus* spp. was significantly higher in warmer months, and any differences between abundances were independent of recent antibiotic use or viral infection.[25]

The nasopharyngeal microbiota including *Staphylococcus aureus, Pseudomonas aeruginosa* and other common pathogens (*Streptococcus pneumoniae, Haemophilus influenza, Moraxella catarrhalis* or *Streptococcus pyogenes*) are also implicated in the pathophysiology of chronic rhinosinusitis.[34,35] The longer-term consequences to the sinus microbiota from standard treatment with culture-directed oral antibiotics has been associated with a reduction in the diversity and abundance of nasopharyngeal commensal microbiota[29] and resistance to repeated antibiotic treatments.[36] Of concern is the suggestion that antibiotic treatment may inadvertently allow the growth of *Staphylococcus aureus* due to the suppression of commensal microbiota that would normally play a role in inhibiting growth and colonisation.[25]

Treatment of nasopharyngeal dysbiosis

The efficacy of nasal saline irrigation as a treatment for uncomplicated acute rhinosinusitis in children was compared to the efficacy of amoxicillin.[37] The authors concluded that saline irrigation resulted in the same clinical, bacteriological and cytological cellular changes as 14 days of amoxicillin and had a higher safety profile.[37]

PROBIOTICS

The role of probiotics in altering diversity and abundance of the nasopharyngeal microbiome is still largely unknown. It has been observed that a greater variety of nasopharyngeal microbiota is associated with reduced incidence of upper respiratory tract infections.[38] It is thought that maturation of the host-associated microbial community happens similarly in the nasopharyngeal area and in the gut.[39] Studies exploring the concept that probiotic bacteria may play a role in altering the composition of the nasopharyngeal microbial community have been summarised in a review that reported colonisation of the nasopharyngeal niche by specific probiotic bacteria superior to placebo when administered topically and/or orally.[40] Understanding whether probiotics alter the microbiome of specific niches is an important step in furthering our understanding of studies that report positive or negative clinical outcomes. While a Cochrane review is considered to be of the highest standard and rigour, the approach to the evaluation of the clinical outcomes of probiotic interventions in reducing the risk of upper respiratory tract infections could be considered limited through the inclusion of studies using a range of specified strains and doses in people of all ages.[41] Therefore, only broad conclusions about probiotics in general can be made. Despite this limitation, the authors of a recent review concluded that probiotics were superior to placebo in reducing the prevalence and mean duration of acute upper respiratory tract infections, antibiotic use and cold-related school absence,[41] appropriately noting the quality of the evidence was low or very low.

THE ORAL MICROBIOTA

Composition of the oral microbiome

The oral microbiome, which includes the gingival sulcus, tongue, cheeks, tongue, teeth, soft and hard palates and tonsils, is considered one of the most diverse ecological niches in the human body, comprising bacteria, viruses, fungi, protozoa and archaea.[42,43] The bacterial community of the oral cavity is estimated to be home to ~10 000 bacterial species,[43] placing the oral microbiome second in complexity to the large intestine.[42] The identification of bacterial species and how they interact with the host environment requires a combination of analytical approaches including phylogenetic, metagenomic, transcriptomic, proteomic and metabolomic methodologies.[44] It is thought that a core microbiome exists at a genus level.[42,43,45] However, there are significant inter-individual and intra-individual variations at a bacterial species level which are largely determined by the host[42,45,46] and the specific sites within the oral cavity itself.[47] In addition, further challenges defining the precise composition of oral microbiota relate to the exposure of the oral cavity to exogenous bacteria from food, water, the air and social contact, thus making it difficult to know which bacteria are permanent and which are transient residents.[43,48] Nevertheless, at a phylum level, 96% of species detected belong to the *Firmicutes, Bacteroidetes, Proteobacteria, Actinobacteria, Spirochaetes* and *Fusobacteria* phyla.[43]

Oral dysbiosis and the consequences

The resident commensal bacteria play a critical role in maintaining oral health; paradoxically, some of them play a role in the development of dental caries and periodontal disease.[49] This paradox has been attributed to changes in the abundance and diversity of commensal microbiota, thus 'transforming' their role to pathobionts.[50] Dental and periodontal disease are associated with an accumulation of a biofilm consisting of hundreds of bacteria, salivary glycoproteins and polysaccharides secreted by oral microbes that adhere to teeth and gingiva.[49] Dental caries is considered the most extended infectious disease in the world.[50–52] While the prevalence of dental caries remains uncontested, the term 'infectious disease' has recently been challenged due to our growing knowledge about the composition of the oral microbiome.[49] It was previously thought that *Streptococcus mutans* was the primary ondontopathogen.[53] However, the identification of hundreds of species of oral bacteria has changed our understanding of the aetiology of caries, gingivitis and periodontal disease. Thus, a new definition of dental caries has been proposed (i.e. 'dental caries is a dysbiotic polymicrobial disease caused by pathobionts'[50]). This understanding will require careful consideration of the current and future treatment approaches to dental and periodontal disease.

The prevention and treatment of oral dysbiosis is likely to play a role in the future for chronic disease prevention and treatment. This prediction is based on growing evidence to support a systemic health effect from oral dysbiosis,[54] including a disease association with rheumatoid arthritis,[55] diseases of the head and neck[48,56] and disorders of the respiratory tract,[57] the digestive tract[58,59] and the cardiovascular system.[60–62]

Interventions for oral dysbiosis

Modifiable risks of oral dysbiosis include changes in saliva flow and composition, inflammation of the gingiva, poor oral hygiene, poor dietary choices and smoking.[63]

SMOKING

A large study (n = 1204) exploring the relationship between smoking and the composition of the oral microbiome including 1204 adults identified substantially lower abundance of the phylum *Proteobacteria* and enrichment of *Firmicutes* and *Actinobacteria* in smokers compared to non-smokers. This difference was not observed between former and never smokers, suggesting that any disruption to the oral microbiota caused by smoking may resolve over time,[50] and further supporting that smoking cessation remains the best practice to restore a healthy phenotype.[64]

SALIVA

The saliva and gingival fluid contain constituents with antimicrobial properties and nutrients for microbial growth.[65] In addition to supporting microbial equilibrium, saliva is necessary for normal mastication and swallowing of food, and is a source of enzymes for the initial stage of the digestive process. Studies investigating the microbial composition of saliva have detected 10^8 microorganisms per mL of saliva that are most reflective of the tongue microbiota.[65] Other salivary constituents include anti-microbial peptides including histatins, defensins, lactoferrin[66]; immune modulators including lactoferrin[67]; and protective proteins including secretory IgA and the enzyme lactoperoxidase.[68] The absence of these important constituents that keep microbial balance in check in combination with the presence of dietary risk factors play a role in the origin of oral dysbiois.

DIET

A relationship between the intake of refined sugar, fermentable carbohydrates and a cariogenic microbial ecology has been made.[69,70] In caries, carbohydrates are fermented to organic acids such as lactic acid, which demineralises the tooth enamel.[63] In addition, lactic-acid-loving bacteria proliferate, resulting in dysbiosis of the oral microbiome. Thus, limited intake of refined sugars and fermentable carbohydrates is considered important in the overall prevention and management of recurrent dental caries via modifying the pH and hence the microbial composition of the oral cavity.[70]

PROBIOTICS

The role of probiotic interventions in disorders associated with oral dysbiosis is promising, but larger studies are required before definitive guidelines can be confidently developed.[71] At this point in time, there appear to be no significant differences in outcomes between species or strains of probiotics employed in studies measuring microbial endpoints of dysbiosis.[71]

One randomised controlled trial involving 113 children evaluated the effect of maternal *Lactobacillus reuteri* strain ATCC 55730 supplementation during the last 4 weeks of pregnancy and the infants' first year of life. Specifically, it addressed the prevalence of dental caries at 9 years of age in children following gestational exposure of supplementation during the last 4 weeks of pregnancy and the first 12 months of life.[72] Samples of saliva and plaque were analysed for the presence of *Streptococcus mutans* and lactobacilli in addition to salivary secretory IgA. Significantly fewer children in the group supplemented with *Lactobacillus reuteri* strain ATCC 55730 than those in the placebo group had caries and/or gingivitis. Interestingly, there were no differences in dietary practices, oral hygiene practices, plaque or fluoride supplementation or any of the microbial or immune markers between the groups.[72]

A separate randomised controlled trial evaluated the prevalence of caries and the presence of cariogenic microbiota in 179 9-year-old children who had been supplemented with *Lactobacillus paracasei* F19 during the 4th to 13th months of life.[73] No intergroup variations were observed for dental health or for the presence of *Streptococcus mutans* or lactobacilli. In addition, there was no colonisation of *Lactobacillus paracasei* F19.[73]

In a randomised control trial involving 54 adults with hyposalivation, two different probiotic gums and placebo were evaluated for effects on saliva flow rate, saliva IgA levels and saliva pH. The participants were given either placebo chewing gum, or *Bifidobacterium animalis* ssp. *lactis* Bb12 (ATCC 27536) or *Lactobacillus rhamnosus* LGG (ATCC 53103), *Bifidobacterium longum* 46 (DSM 14583) and *Bifidobacterium longum* 2C (DSM 14579) gum to chew daily for 3 months. All three groups had a positive outcome with increased salivary flow rate and saliva pH and IgA levels.[74]

A group of 29 healthy adults were given a lozenge containing *Lactobacillus rhamnosus* GG and *Bifidobacterium animalis* subsp. *lactis* Bb12 or placebo for 4 weeks, and the effects on salivary mutans streptococci, plaque, gingival inflammation and the oral microbiota were evaluated.[75] The probiotic lozenge decreased both plaque and gingival inflammation, but no changes were found in the specific microbial compositions of saliva in either group.[75]

Summary

The role of the oral microbiome in both regional and systemic health and disease is apparent. The advent of molecular technology in the assessment of the oral microbiome has expanded our knowledge regarding the composition and behaviour of this complex ecosystem. This expansion of knowledge challenges a reductionist approach towards studying the oral microbiome's impact on oral and systemic health in the future. Future research endeavours in this important area require consideration of a systems-based biology approach to enquiry.

THE BREASTMILK MICROBIOTA

The breastmilk microbiota is covered in great depth in Chapter 14.

THE VAGINAL MICROBIOTA

Research conducted over the past few decades has found the vaginal microbiota to provide a first line of defence in the female reproductive tract. It was once believed that a healthy vaginal ecosystem was dominated by *Lactobacillus acidophilus*. However, using modern molecular techniques, this has been found to be incorrect. A healthy vaginal microbiota *is* dominated by lactobacilli, but species other than *L. acidophilus* play a major role. The four most common species found in healthy vaginal ecosystems are *L. crispatus, L. iners, L. jensenii* and *L. gasseri*.[76] They are typically present in concentrations of 10^7 to 10^8 CFU per mL of vaginal fluid.[77]

A healthy vaginal microbiota, unlike the others discussed so far, is characterised by a lack of diversity at a genus level.[78] Lactobacilli typically comprise >70% of a healthy ecosystem. This single genus dominance is unique, not only among human microbiomes, but also among other mammalian vagina ecosystems, where lactobacilli usually comprise <1%. Lactobacilli dominance is maintained in most women by the constant secretion of both glycogen and α-amylase. Interestingly, some vaginal lactobacilli strains lack the capacity to metabolise glycogen.[79] Vaginal epithelial cells appear to release α-amylase into the vagina environment, to break down glycogen into maltose, maltotriose and maltodextrins, which can be used as food sources by vaginal lactobacilli.[80] So it appears the host does its best to nurture its 'garden' of lactobacilli. The important functions of vaginal lactobacilli are highlighted in Box 6.3. The optimal pH of the vaginal environment (pH 3.5–4) is maintained by a lactobacilli-dominated ecosystem. At this pH range, lactic acid works as a potent bactericide and a virucide, inhibiting pathogen growth.[81,82]

BOX 6.3 Properties of vaginal lactobacilli that enhance host health[83–85]

Inhibition of binding of potential pathogens to epithelial cells

Down-regulation of the innate immune response to microbial antigens; thereby preventing inflammation

Production of anti-microbial compounds that inhibit other species of bacteria

Lyse bacteria commonly associated with bacterial vaginosis

Inhibition of histone deacetylases, leading to increased gene transcription and DNA repair

Inhibition of cyclical AMP, leading to induction of autophagy to kill intracellular microorganisms and protect against inflammation

Production of D- and L-lactic acid, which modify the pH of the vagina and protect against pathogen and pathobiont growth

Inhibition of extracellular matrix metalloproteinase inducer production (via D-lactic acid production), which strengthens the vaginal barrier, protects against upper genital tract infections and, consequently, premature birth during pregnancy

Production of hydrogen peroxide, which displays anti-microbial activity, as well as enhancing the activity of the host-produced anti-microbial peptides lactoferrin and muramidase

The vaginal microbiota of reproductive-aged women generally falls into one of five community states – although this is still subject to some debate.[86] Four of these states are lactobacilli dominated, whereas the final one is composed of a diverse collection of anaerobes and strict anaerobes. This last scenario may or may not be associated with vaginal symptoms (e.g. bacterial vaginosis). Community state type one (CST-I) is dominated by *Lactobacillus crispatus* isolates, CST-II dominated by *L. gasseri*, CST-III by *L. iners* and CST-V by *L. jensenii* strains. CST-IV is composed of a polymicrobial mixture of species of the genera *Gardnerella*, *Atopobium*, *Mobiluncus* and *Prevotella*. Lactobacilli are not dominant players in CST-IV and aerobic species, such as group B *Streptococcus*, *Staphylococcus aureus*, *Escherichia coli* and *Enterococcus*, may also be present.

It has been recognised for decades that the healthy vaginal microbiota (i.e. a lack of vaginal symptoms, absence of infections and good pregnancy outcomes) is dominated mainly by *Lactobacillus* species. Lactobacilli are, in fact, the dominant species in ~70% of women.[87] However, there are still many unknowns about what constitutes a 'healthy' ecosystem, as the use of molecular techniques to examine the vaginal ecosystem has given substantial insight, but their use is relatively recent.

Current thinking is that CST-I, CST-III and CST-V are healthy, whereas a *L. iners*-dominated ecosystem (CST-II) may be healthy or may be transitional. Both CST-II and CST-IV (non-lactobacilli dominated) can be seen as layovers on the journey from eubiosis to symptomatic dysbiosis (and vice versa), and both are risk factors for the development of bacterial vaginosis. Strains of *L. iners* appear to have less capacity to protect against potential pathogen growth when compared to the other lactobacilli species. Ethnicity appears to play a role too, in that women from African and Hispanic descent have a far greater incidence of CST-IV (and consequently a higher risk of bacterial vaginosis [BV]) than women of European or Asian descent. Whether this is a result of genetic factors that impact on vaginal immunity and metabolic pathways, or differences in hygiene practices, such as douching, has not yet been explored. The varying percentages of each CST as found in Ravel et al.'s landmark study[81] are also detailed in Fig. 6.2. At the time of publication, few commercial laboratories offer comprehensive vagina microbiota assessment, but this will undoubtedly change over the next few years. (See Fig. 6.3.)

The vaginal ecosystem is considered relatively dynamic in some women, and transitions between CSTs can occur. Research to date suggests that women with *L. crispatus*- or

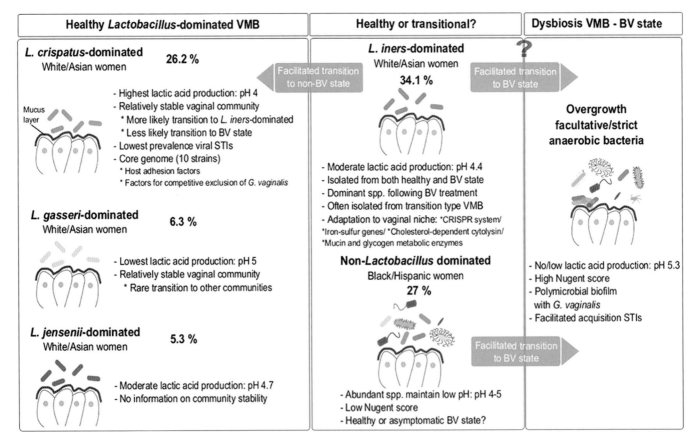

FIGURE 6.3 Composition of the vaginal microbiota during healthy and dysbiotic states

VMB = vaginal microbiota; BV = bacterial vaginosis; STIs = sexually-transmitted infections.

Adapted from Petrova MI, Lievens E, Malik S, et al. Lactobacillus species as biomarkers and agents that can promote various aspects of vaginal health. Front Physiol 2015;6:81.

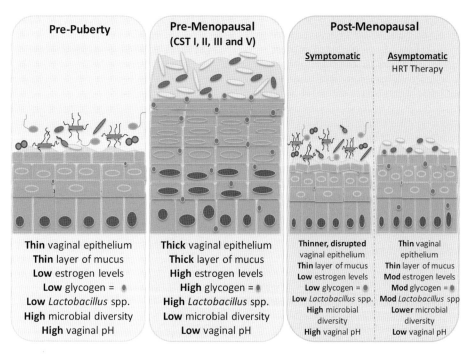

FIGURE 6.4 The vaginal microbiome through the female lifecycle

The vaginal epithelium prior to puberty is thin, composed of stratified squamous epithelium and covered with little mucus. After puberty (but pre-menopause), women are producing high levels of oestrogen resulting in more glycogen deposits in the epithelial cells and significant amounts of free glycogen available for lactobacilli in the vagina, which predominate in a healthy vaginal microbiota (CST I, II, III and V). Community State Type IV, though found in some otherwise healthy women, is not depicted for the sake of simplicity. During this phase, the vaginal epithelium is thick and covered by a thick layer of mucus. After menopause, as serum levels of oestrogen drop, glycogen production and subsequent release into the vagina decrease. In some cases, this leads to depletion of lactobacilli, an increase in diverse microbial species and a change in community state type to CST IV.

CST = community state types.

Modified from Muhleisen AL, Herbst-Kralovetz MM. Menopause and the vaginal microbiome. Maturitas 2016;91:42–50.

L. gasseri-dominated ecosystems are the most stable over time. Even in women with these ecosystems, however, there can be a shift at the time of menses to an alternative ecosystem (often a *L. iners*-type). These tend to revert back to their original CST post menses. Women with CST-II vary widely in terms of both species composition and stability – with some women remaining *L. iners*-dominated over time and others moving into a BV-like composition.[88]

The microbiota also varies dramatically throughout a woman's life stages (see Fig. 6.4).[89] Pre-puberty, when oestrogen levels are low, correlates with low glycogen production. This results in a highly diverse ecosystem, with a relatively high vaginal pH, where lactobacilli play only a minor role. In reproductive-aged women, high oestrogen levels induce greater secretion of glycogen and, consequently, the vagina is dominated by lactobacilli and the vaginal environment has an acidic pH – at least when the ecosystem is healthy. In menopause, however, the lower oestrogen levels result in decreased glycogen production.[90] In many women, this results in a change in the microbiota, with a decrease in lactobacilli concentrations, an increase in microbial diversity (including colonisation by enteric bacteria) and a more neutral pH. These microbiome changes appear to be risk factors for recurrent urinary tract infections and vulvovaginal atrophy, which are both fairly common in this population.[91,92]

The lactobacilli-dominated microbiota

A lactobacilli-dominated microbiota has been found to:

ENHANCE FERTILITY

In infertile women, both bacterial vaginosis and CST-IV are frequently found with a recent study finding 21% of infertile women attending an IVF clinic to have undiagnosed BV and 28% to have CST-IV. IVF-assisted pregnancy rates were significantly reduced among the women with non-lactobacilli-dominated ecosystems – 9% versus 35% ($p = 0.004$).[93] Hence, focusing on restoration of a lactobacilli-dominated ecosystem should be an intervention strategy in women who are having trouble getting pregnant.

REDUCE HIV TRANSMISSION

Research has consistently found increased risk of HIV acquisition in women with non-lactobacilli-dominated vaginal microbiotas.[94–96] One study found a four-times greater risk of HIV in women with high-diversity bacterial communities compared to women with CST-I.[94] This reduced risk of HIV transmission in lactobacilli-dominated ecosystems, and particularly CST-I microbiotas, is most likely related to the high lactic acid production in these ecosystems. In such concentrations, lactic acid is virucidal against HIV. Lactic acid also upregulates the local immune response to viral RNA and downregulates the local inflammatory response, resulting in a more intact epithelium.[96]

REDUCE STI RISK

The transmission of sexually transmitted infections (STIs) is significantly increased in women with a non-lactobacilli-dominated ecosystem.[95] This protective effect is believed to be mediated mostly by the bactericidal and virucidal effects of lactobacilli-produced lactic acid.

PREVENT VULVOVAGINAL ATROPHY

Research has found a strong correlation between post-menopausal vulvovaginal atrophy and a CST-IV microbiota. In fact, women with vaginal atrophy have 26-fold greater odds of being classified as CST-IV than those who are *L. crispatus*-dominated.[92]

PROTECT AGAINST CERVICAL CANCER

Cervical cancer and its pre-malignant precursor, cervical intraepithelial neoplasia (CIN), are caused by strains of the human papillomavirus (HPV). Over 80% of sexually active women will be infected by the virus by the age of 50. The vast majority (~90%) of these infections are transient, however, being cleared within 6–18 months after infection initiation. Persistence of the virus is essential for the development of high-grade CIN and cervical cancer. Emerging evidence has suggested an important role of the cervicovaginal microbiota in the persistence or regression of the viral infection and subsequent disease. Research has consistently shown HPV-positive women have less lactobacilli present and a more diverse microbiota compared to HPV-negative women. Research has also found that increased severity of CIN is associated with higher microbiota diversity and decreased relative abundance of *Lactobacillus* spp. A lactobacilli-dominated microbiota maintains the low vaginal pH that is essential for optimal cervical epithelial barrier function that appears to inhibit entry of HPV to the basal keratinocytes, where the virus thrives.[97]

PROTECT AGAINST URINARY TRACT INFECTIONS

The vagina is a key anatomical site in the pathogenesis of urinary tract infections (UTIs) in women, serving as a potential reservoir for infecting bacteria.[98] The microbiota of UTI-prone women has been characterised by diminished lactobacilli concentrations, a more diverse ecosystem and higher Nugent scores compared to healthy controls.[99] A healthy, acidic vagina cannot be a reservoir for urinary tract pathogens, such as *E. coli*, as the low pH, characteristic of this environment, is inhibitory to their growth.

How to restore a lactobacilli-dominated ecosystem

Given the importance of having a lactobacilli-dominated ecosystem, knowledge of some of the main causes of vaginal dysbiosis is paramount in order to better educate patients and improve treatment outcomes. The main causes of vaginal dysbiosis are highlighted in Box 6.4.

Given the main aim of treatment is to restore a lactobacilli-dominated microbiota, and in light of the current state of research, one dominated by *L. crispatus* isolates agents capable of modifying the microbiota to this end would be valuable. The best way of creating such an ecosystem, however, is still being researched. To date, there has been little investigation done to evaluate techniques to optimise the vaginal ecosystem. Probiotics have been the most investigated intervention category. Prebiotics are currently under-researched interventions, with great potential to create a *Lactobacillus*-dominated ecosystem.

Several probiotic strains and strain combinations have shown efficacy in the treatment of BV in human trials, thus demonstrating their capacity to improve a dysbiotic vaginal ecosystem.[109–111] Currently, however, only a couple of these preparations are commercially available in Australia, Canada and/or the US. *L. rhamnosus* Lcr35 and the combination of *L. rhamnosus* Gr-1 and *L. fermentum* RC-14 have both shown the capacity to normalise the vaginal microbiota. Sadly, supplements containing strains of *L. crispatus* are not currently available in these markets. They are, however, commercially available in many Western European countries.

In a randomised controlled trial (RCT), intra-vaginal application of *L. rhamnosus* Lcr35 (1.0×10^9 CFU/day) in women with BV for 7 days post antibiotic treatment resulted in the restoration of vaginal flora in 83% of subjects compared to 35% in the antibiotics-only group 1 month after antibiotic treatment ($p < 0.001$).[112]

BOX 6.4 Agents and practices that have been shown in human or in in vitro research to negatively impact on vaginal lactobacilli

Cigarette smoking[100]
Diaphragm use[101]
Increased intercourse frequency[102]
Low dietary intake of magnesium, zinc and vitamin E[103]
Multiple sexual partners[104]
Oral antibiotic use[105]
Spermicide[106]
Topical anti-fungals (e.g. miconazole)[107]
Use of bidet toilets[108]
Vaginal antiseptics (e.g. chlorhexidine gluconate)[107]
Vaginal douching (with water or soap and water)[105]

The combination of *L. rhamnosus* GR-1 and *L. fermentum* RC-14 has been evaluated in three BV trials. In the first RCT, intra-vaginal application nightly for 5 days resulted in a 90% cure rate (e.g. normalisation of the ecosystem) by day 30.[113] In the second trial, the probiotic combination was taken orally for 4 weeks after a single dose of tinidazole. Compared to the placebo control group, the BV cure rate was significantly better (88% vs 50%; *p* = 0.01), and the vaginal flora normalised in 75% of women versus 34% of controls (*p* = 0.011).[114] In the final trial, women with BV ingested the probiotic combination for 6 weeks. This resulted in 61.5% restitution to a healthy, balanced vaginal microbiota compared to 26.9% in the placebo group (*p* <0.001). Six weeks after cessation of treatment tests revealed a normal vaginal microbiota was still present in 51.1% of the probiotic group compared to 20.8% of the placebo group (*p* <0.001).[115] Recent research has confirmed that treatment with this probiotic combination results in an increased abundance of indigenous *L. iners* or *L. crispatus* strains, suggesting that these strains work, at least in part, by enhancing endogenous lactobacilli populations, rather than via permanent colonisation.[116]

Prebiotics, selectively fermented ingredients that create specific beneficial changes, both in the composition and/or in the activity of the microbiota, are obvious choices for the task of optimising the vaginal ecosystem.[117] But they are little researched to date, with only glucooligosaccharides and hydrolysed glucomannan oligosaccharides being evaluated in human trials.

Glucooligosaccharides display prebiotic activity in vitro (specifically feeding vaginal lactobacilli isolates)[118] and have been shown to alter the vaginal ecology in a single human trial.[119] Use of a vaginal gel containing a novel glucooligosaccharide (at a daily dose of 300 mg oligosaccharide for 16 days), by women with BV undergoing metronidazole treatment resulted in a significant improvement in vaginal ecosystem normalisation (100% vs 67% in the placebo group; *p* <0.05). At this point in time, the gel used in this trial is not commercially available; nor are the active ingredients – glucooligosaccharides. It does, however, provide proof of concept data that vaginally administered prebiotics can improve the vaginal ecosystem.

Hydrolysed glucomannan oligosaccharides (HGO) have been evaluated in one trial assessing their impact on the vaginal ecosystem. Administration of HGO (200 mg twice weekly for 4 weeks) alongside standard anti-fungal therapy in women with vaginal candidiasis resulted in a quicker recovery of a healthy ecosystem versus controls.[120] In an in vitro study, glucomannan hydrolysates were shown to stimulate the growth of vaginal lactobacilli while simultaneously inhibiting *Candida* growth.[121]

Other prebiotics that have not yet been assessed for vaginal prebiotic activity in human trials include fructooligosaccharides and lactulose. In vitro, fructooligosaccharides (FOS) are utilised as a food source by many lactobacilli strains, including strains of *L. crispatus*.[118,122] Some in vitro research suggests that *L. crispatus* strains may specifically prefer small-chain fructooligosaccharides, such as oligofructose or Actilight,

compared to long-chain FOS such as inulin,[118,123] although inulin was well fermented in another study.[121] In consideration of the previous vaginal research on glucooligosaccharides, dosages of ≥300 mg/day of a small-chain FOS (i.e. oligofructose) or a combination product (such as oligofructose-enriched inulin) locally administered at least twice weekly should have the desired prebiotic effect.

Lactulose has proven prebiotic effects in the human GIT after oral ingestion, including increasing intestinal lactobacilli concentrations.[124] It has also been shown to feed numerous lactobacilli strains in vitro.[125,126] As with FOS above, research has not yet been done on vaginal applications. It should work as an effective vaginal prebiotic when administered locally, however. Dosages of 2 mL made into a pessary or diluted in a little liquid can be used at least twice weekly.

Another intervention with evidence of a vaginal-microbiota-normalising effect is hydrogen peroxide. There have been two human trials using hydrogen peroxide applications in the treatment of BV. In one trial, a single administration of 20 mL 3% hydrogen peroxide resulted in complete clearance of BV in 63% of women.[127] In another trial, application of 30 mL of a 3% solution nightly for 7 days resulted in the restoration of a lactobacilli-dominated ecosystem in all women with BV and normalised the pH in 98% of women.[128] It should be noted that while these applications were well-tolerated in the above two trials, in some women, a 3% solution can sting an irritated vaginal mucosa. Consequently, it can be worth administering a weaker dilution, such as a 1% or 1.5% solution, for the initial applications to ensure tolerability before using the 3% solution.

Topical vitamin C applications have also shown efficacy in the normalisation of the vaginal ecosystem in BV. In one RCT, 250 mg of vitamin C was given intravaginally once daily for 6 days to women with BV. Cure rates were 55.3% in the vitamin C group versus 25.7% in placebo-treated controls (*p* <0.001).[129] In another trial, in women with non-specific vaginitis, topical vitamin C application (250 mg daily for 6 days) resulted in normalisation of vaginal pH in significantly more women than in the placebo group, suggesting a normalising effect on the microbiota.[130]

CASE STUDY 6.1: VAGINAL DYSBIOSIS

PRESENTATION

A 28-year-old female presented with a 6-week history of vaginitis symptoms – thin white discharge, vaginal itching and dyspareunia. She was very recently diagnosed by her GP with bacterial vaginosis (via the Amsel's criteria). In-clinic pH testing revealed a vaginal pH of 5.5.

TREATMENT PROTOCOL

The patient was prescribed a probiotic and vaginal prebiotic douche to address the imbalanced ecosystem. A probiotic product containing a combination of *Lactobacillus rhamnosus* GR-1 and *Lactobacillus reuteri* RC-14 was advised to be taken orally (5×10^9 CFU combined/day) for 30 days. The probiotic was also used intravaginally as part of the prebiotic douche. The vaginal application contained 2 mL lactulose syrup and 5×10^9 CFU of the probiotic combination mixed into ~20 mL water. This was applied via a small syringe nightly for 7 nights and then twice weekly for the following 3 weeks.

OUTCOME

Vaginitis symptoms improved within the first 10 days of treatment, as did the white discharge. In-clinic pH testing after 30 days of treatment revealed a pH of 4.3. Normalisation of the vaginal ecosystem was inferred by the correction of the pH and the cessation of vaginal symptoms.

THE GASTROINTESTINAL MICROBIOTA

The gastrointestinal tract has long been a focus of naturopathic practice. In 400 BCE, Hippocrates stated that, '... death sits in the bowels ...' and '... bad digestion is the root of all evil ...'. This focus on the gut has been maintained throughout the history of naturopathic medicine. Nineteenth-century naturopath Louis Kuhne, for example, proposed that excess food intake, or the intake of the wrong types of food, resulted in increased growth of bacteria within the bowel, the production of intestinal toxins and, subsequently, disease.[131] Therefore, improving gastrointestinal tract function and the health of the GIT ecosystem have long been key treatment approaches in naturopathic medicine.

Over the past 20 years, research examining the role of the GIT ecosystem in human health has expanded exponentially – mostly due to recent advances in technology that have given unprecedented insights into this ecosystem. The GIT microbiota is considered an ecosystem of the highest complexity, composed of bacteria, archaea, fungi, viruses and protozoa. Thus far, research has focused predominantly upon the bacterial components of the microbiota. Over 50 genera of bacteria accounting for over 1000 different species have been found in the human gut.[132] The adult human GIT is estimated to contain 10^{13}–10^{14} viable microorganisms, which means there are more gastrointestinal microbes than eukaryotic cells found within the human body.

Some researchers have labelled this microbial population the 'microbe' organ or the 'forgotten organ' – an organ similar in size and metabolic functionality to the liver. As previously detailed, other researchers consider humans super-organisms. From both perspectives, the GIT microbiota is essential for human health and 'normal' metabolism and physiology.[3–5]

The functions of the GIT microbiota

As a rapidly evolving area of research, each passing year finds additional insights into the functional attributes of the GIT microbiota. Given that over 3 million microbial genes have been isolated and that microbial genes outnumber human genes by ~150 to 1, it is unsurprising that the GIT microbiota plays a number of critical roles in human health.[133]

PRODUCTION OF VITAMINS

Some indigenous bacteria from the gut microbiota possess the ability to synthesise vitamin K (menaquinone), as well as many of the B vitamins. In contrast to dietary vitamins, which are absorbed primarily in the upper small intestine, microbially produced vitamins are predominantly absorbed in the colon and distal small bowel.[134] Vitamin K_2 can be synthesised by a number of intestinal inhabitants, including strains of *Bacteroides fragilis*, *E. coli*, *Eubacterium* spp.,[135] *Veillonella* spp. and *Propionibacterium* spp.[136] Microbially produced K_2 is produced in substantial enough amounts to contribute to meeting the human nutritional requirements for this vitamin.

B group vitamins are also produced by members of the GIT microbiota. Thiamine is synthesised in considerable amounts by as-yet unknown species of intestinal bacteria, as are riboflavin, niacin, pantothenic acid and biotin.[137] Bifidobacteria are known producers of these vitamins (with the exception of riboflavin), but other species are likely to be involved.[138] Thiamine is produced as both free thiamine and in phosphorylated forms, while riboflavin, niacin and biotin appear to be synthesised mainly in their free forms, which are highly bioavailable. Colonic transporters for some B vitamins, such as thiamine and niacin, have only recently been discovered,[139,140] whereas colonic absorption of biotin and pantothenic acid has been known about for a considerable time. In general, colonic production of water-soluble vitamins is enhanced in plant- and fibre-rich diets.[137]

The colonic microbiota synthesise folate in amounts that can approach, or even exceed, the level in the diet.[137] Microbial folate production appears to be upregulated by consuming prebiotics (such as oligofructose) and higher amounts of fibre. This is perhaps not surprising, given many strains of bifidobacteria are capable of producing folate.[141] Microbially produced folate is actively and efficiently absorbed by colonocytes.

Cobalamin (vitamin B_{12}) is produced in considerable amounts by the microbiota. Colonocytes, however, lack the pathways necessary to absorb this vitamin from the colonic lumen. So, humans do not get the benefit of microbially produced B_{12}. On the other hand, microbes within the colonic ecosystem do. It has been estimated that up to 80% of colonic bacterial species have a metabolic need for cobalamin (or closely related corrinoids), where they are used as enzyme cofactors and regulators of gene expression. Some authors have even speculated that supplementation of vitamin B_{12} may be a novel approach to altering the microbiota.[142]

PRODUCTION OF SHORT-CHAIN FATTY ACIDS

The vast majority of intestinal microorganisms are saccharolytic species (i.e. they derive their energy through the fermentation of carbohydrates).[143] Most simple dietary carbohydrates are broken down and/or absorbed in the small intestine, with the exception of some indigestible oligosaccharides (e.g. fructooligosaccharides and galactooligosaccharides) and sugar alcohols (e.g. sorbitol and xylitol). It is these latter carbohydrates, in addition to resistant starch, plant cell wall polysaccharides (dietary fibre) and small amounts of unabsorbed mono- and disaccharides from the upper gut that make up the main food sources of the colonic microbiota. It is estimated that resistant starch constitutes the major fermentation substrate (8–40 g/day), followed by dietary fibre (8–18 g/day), unabsorbed sugars (2–10 g/day), oligosaccharides (2–8 g/day) and endogenous carbohydrates (2–3 g/day) in the typical Western diet.[144] This pattern will obviously vary considerably depending upon a patient's dietary choices. Protein can also be utilised as growth substrates by some members of the microbiota. This fermentable protein can total 25 g/day, but again, dietary choices can have a significant influence on the amount of unabsorbed proteins that reach the colon.[143] Individuals with higher dietary protein intakes will have greater amounts of protein reaching the colon.

As fermentable substrates are utilised by the microbiota, various byproducts are formed. Fermentation of carbohydrates produces short-chain fatty acids (SCFAs) and the gases methane, carbon dioxide and hydrogen. The metabolism of protein, referred to as putrefaction, yields branched-chain fatty acids (isobutyrate and isovalerate) and smaller amounts of SCFAs, hydrogen and methane, ammonia, phenolic compounds, indoles, hydrogen sulphide gas and amines.[143]

SCFA production is one of the most crucial functions of the colonic microbiota. The term SCFAs refers to a group of C_1–C_6 monocarboxylic acids, which are produced in significant amounts in the human colon.[145] There are many factors that determine the proportion and amount of SCFAs derived from fermentation. These include the amount and type of substrate, the extent of substrate breakdown and the predominant species present in the microbiota, as well as the gastrointestinal transit time, mucus secretion and medication use of the host. The predominant SCFAs produced are acetic acid (acetate), propionic acid (propionate) and butyric acid (butyrate), while minor fatty acids include formate, lactate, isobutyrate, valerate, isovalerate and caproic acid. The fermentation of carbohydrates results in the production of mainly acetate, propionate and butyrate, while the putrefaction of amino acids yields branched-chain fatty acids such as isobutyrate, 2-methylbutyrate and isovalerate, in addition to the three major SCFAs.[143]

In general, acetate appears to contribute 50–60% of total SCFAs, and butyrate and propionate 15–20% and 20–25%, respectively.[146] However, the exact amounts depend upon the above-mentioned variables, and in particular, dietary substrates. Table 6.1 outlines the

TABLE 6.1 Examples of differing short-chain fatty acid ratios produced by faecal microorganisms via fermentation of different carbohydrates and foods[147]

Substrate	Production ratios		
	Acetate	Propionate	Butyrate
Starch	62	15	23
Psyllium husks	77	10	12
Pectin (from apples)	82	11	7
Cellulose	62	23	15
Inulin	72	19	8
Oat bran	57	21	22
Glucose	62	16	22
Cabbage	73	15	9
Sugar beet	93	7	1

fermentation end products of a number of carbohydrates and foods. As can be seen, acetate consistently comprises the greatest proportion of total SCFAs, while the proportion of butyrate and propionate varies significantly depending upon the substrate.

Daily production of SCFAs in humans is approximately 300 mmol[148] (again depending upon the quantity and type of dietary substrates). About 95–99% of these SCFAs are rapidly absorbed from the colonic lumen.[149] Through their presence in the lumen, and upon absorption, they produce a range of health benefits to the host. Some of these benefits are detailed in Table 6.2. Microbial production of SCFAs contributes greatly to the health and functioning of the GIT as well as to the overall wellbeing of the body. Major colonic bacterial species and their fatty acid byproducts are highlighted in Table 6.3.

Given the known, and emerging, health benefits of butyrate, dietary or supplemental strategies that enhance colonic production of this SCFA are actively being researched. Foods and supplemental fibres known to enhance colonic butyrate production include: foods rich in resistant starch and supplemental resistant starch,[167] partially hydrolysed guar gum,[168] psyllium seeds[169] (and to a lesser degree husks),[170] oat bran,[171] germinated barley,[172] inulin[173] and legumes and whole grains generally.[174,175]

IMMUNITY

The GIT microbiota plays an essential role in the induction, education and function of the human immune system.[176,177] The human immune system is a complex web of adaptive and innate components endowed with an astonishing capacity to adapt and respond to diverse challenges. Collectively, the immune system acts as a formidable regulator of homeostasis, sustaining and restoring tissue function in the context of continual environmental and microbial encounters. The two arms of the human immune system have evolved to maintain symbiotic relationships with diverse microbial communities. In turn, these microbial communities stimulate and calibrate multiple aspects of immune system functioning. When operating optimally, the microbiota–immune system alliance interweaves the adaptive and innate arms of the system in a highly orchestrated dialogue that selects, adjusts and concludes responses in the most suitable manner. Diseases that are increasingly affecting humans, such as allergies and inflammatory, metabolic and autoimmune disorders, all have at their core a failure to control misdirected immune responses against self, microbiota-derived or environmental antigens. Alterations in the composition and functioning of the microbiota due to antibiotic use, dietary changes, changes in birth and infant feeding practices and the extermination of some constitutive microbial partners have disrupted this highly orchestrated, microbiota–immune system choreography.

Research done over the past 50 years using the gnotobiotic mouse model (i.e. microbiota-free or germ-free mice) has demonstrated the importance of the GIT microbiota for specific components of normal immune system function. Using these models, researchers have shown that numbers of mucosal IgA-plasma cells are significantly decreased in germ-free animals compared to animals with a microbiota. Quantitative studies on both the large and the small bowel have shown that the IgA-plasma cell population in germ-free mice was only 10% the density of that found in their normal counterparts. Similarly, concentrations of IgA in intestinal secretions and serum were very low and did not exceed 10% of the control values.[178] Other research with this model showed microbiota decontamination to result in significant atrophy of the thymus and spleen, decreased lymphocyte function and natural killer cell activity, fewer T-cell types, reduced expression of antimicrobial peptides

TABLE 6.2 Host-associated benefits of microbial SCFA production[143,150–161]		
SCFA	**Specific effect**	**Benefit**
Total SCFA	Decrease colonic pH	Growth inhibition of pH-sensitive pathobionts Protects against colonic carcinogenesis by reducing bioavailability of toxic amines Increased solubility and absorption of major and trace minerals
	Relax colonic blood vessels	Increased colonic and hepatic venous blood flow
	Stimulate colonic epithelial proliferation, causes hypertrophy of the caecal wall and increases crypt column height	Possible increased absorptive capacity, leading to enhanced absorption of major and trace minerals
	Enhance sodium, chloride and water absorption; increased bicarbonate secretion	Diminished faecal loss of ions and fluid; prevention of diarrhoea
	Trophic effect on small intestinal mucosa	Increased absorptive capacity, leading to enhanced absorption of nutrients
	Increase production of enterotrophic hormones	Proliferation of colonocytes
	Relax proximal stomach	Slows down gastric emptying (ileo-colonic brake)
	Stimulate emptying of the distal small bowel	Protects the ileal mucosa against the potentially harmful effects of colonic bacterial reflux
	Enhance expression of the tight junction proteins occludin and claudin-5 in the blood–brain barrier	Maintains integrity of the blood–brain barrier
	Increase glucagon-like peptide-1 secretion by intestinal L cells	Lowers plasma glucose concentrations, improves insulin secretion and sensitivity, and preserves pancreatic beta-cell function
Acetate	Enhances muscular contraction in colon	Improved laxation
	Improves calcium absorption	Diminished faecal loss of calcium
	Utilised in the synthesis of long-chain fatty acids, glutamine, β-hydroxybutyrate and glutamate	Consumed as metabolic fuel in muscle, kidney, heart and brain tissue
	Stimulates proliferation of normal colonic crypt cells	Maintenance of mucosal integrity
	Decreases lipopolysaccharide-stimulated TNF-α release from neutrophils	Local and systemic anti-inflammatory effects
	Used by cross-feeding species as a co-substrate to produce butyrate	Enhances colonic butyrate production and 'feeds' numerous butyrate-producing species
Propionate	Substrate for hepatic gluconeogenesis	Increased glycogen stores
	May inhibit hepatic cholesterol synthesis	Decreased serum cholesterol levels
	Increases production of leptin	Reduction in food intake and improved satiety
	Induces mitochondrial adenine nucleotide transports	Encourages colorectal cancer apoptosis

TABLE 6.2 Host-associated benefits of microbial SCFA production[146,153–164]—cont'd

SCFA	Specific effect	Benefit
Butyrate	Preferred metabolic fuel of colonocytes	Maintenance of colonic mucosa integrity; proliferation of colonocytes
	Increases colonic mucin synthesis	Improved protection of the surface mucosal cells
	Promotes migration of colonic epithelial cells	Enhanced wound closure and maintenance of mucosal integrity
	Suppresses colonic production of urokinase	Improved colonic epithelial barrier function
	Increases colonic transglutaminase activity	Promotes re-epithelisation and increased tensile strength of damaged colonic tissue
	Promotes differentiation of colonic epithelial cells	Diminished risk of colorectal malignancy
	Inhibits histone deacetylase	Alters gene expression; induction of apoptosis, cell cycle arrest, and inhibition of angiogenesis and metastasis in colonocytes
	Improves insulin sensitivity	Prevention and treatment of conditions associated with insulin resistance
	Enhances mitochondrial function	Improved thermogenesis and weight regulation
	Increased expression of peptides involved in appetite regulation, peptide YY and proglucagon	Improved appetite regulation and reduced kilojoule intake
	Improves leptin production and sensitivity	Improved appetite regulation and reduced kilojoule intake
	Increased colonic 5-HT release	Decreases abdominal pain and sensation of faecal urgency in patients with visceral hypersensitivity; enhances colonic motility
	Suppresses the growth of *Methanobrevibacter smithii*	Increasing butyrate production can be used as an interventional strategy to deal with conditions associated with excessive methanogenesis (e.g. methane-dominant SIBO or chronic constipation)
	Downregulates pathogen virulence gene-expression	Protection against gastrointestinal viral and bacterial infections
	Inhibits cholesterol synthesis	Helps maintain healthy cholesterol levels
	Decreases systematic inflammation via suppression of the release of pro-inflammatory mediators (e.g. TNF-α, NFκB, IF-γ IL-6 and IL-12) in the liver, adipose tissue and WBCs	Helps maintain a healthy systemic inflammatory milieu

TNF-α = tumour necrosis factor-alpha; 5-HT = 5-hydroxytryptamine; SIBO = small intestinal bacterial overgrowth; NFκB = nuclear factor kappa-B; IF-γ = interferon gamma; IL-6 = interleukin-6; IL-12 = interleukin-12; WBCs = white blood cells

TABLE 6.3 Summary of fatty acids produced by major groups of fermentative gut microorganisms[143,162–166]

Acetate	Propionate	Butyrate	Lactate
Atopobium	*Bacteroides*	*Anaerostipes*	*Atopobium* (L)
Bacteroides	*Clostridium*	*Anaerotruncus*	*Bacteroides* (D)
Butyrivibrio	*Megasphaera*	*Blautia*	*Bifidobacterium* (L)
Enterococcus	*Porphyromonas*	*Butyrivibrio*	*Clostridium* (L)
Enterobacteria	*Prevotella*	*Clostridium*	*Enterobacteria* (D/L)
Clostridium	*Propionibacterium*	*Coprococcus*	*Enterococcus* (L)
Bacteroides	*Veillonella*	*Eubacterium*	*Escherichia coli* (D/L)
Bifidobacterium		*Faecalibacterium*	*Eubacterium* (L)
Eubacterium		*Fusobacterium*	*Faecalibacterium* (D)
Fusobacterium		*Intestinibacter*	*Fusobacterium* (L)
Lactobacillus		*Peptococcus*	*Klebsiella* (D/L)
Peptococcus		*Peptostreptococcus*	*Lactobacillus* (D/L)
Peptostreptococcus		*Pseudobutyrivibrio*	*Peptococcus* (L)
Propionibacterium		*Roseburia*	*Peptostreptococcus* (L)
Ruminococcus		*Ruminococcus*	*Ruminococcus* (L)
Streptococcus		*Subdoligranulum*	*Streptococcus* (D/L)
Veillonella			

(L) and (D) indicate stereoisomers of lactate.

and increased susceptibility to infection.[179–181] Germ-free mice also fail to develop tolerance to dietary antigens – a situation only reversible when the microbiota is reconstituted in infancy.[182]

A number of microbial metabolites have the capacity to alter immune regulatory responses.[183] Lipoteichoic acids, peptidoglycans, lipopolysaccharides and SCFAs are among the most researched.[184,185] Lipoteichoic acids are found on the surface of Gram-positive bacteria, peptidoglycans are present in both Gram-positive and Gram-negative bacteria, while lipopolysaccharides are expressed only by Gram-negative organisms.

MOOD MANAGEMENT

A growing body of literature has demonstrated bidirectional signalling between the brain and the GIT microbiota, involving multiple immunological, endocrine and neurocrine pathways (see Fig. 6.5). While it has long been known that psychological stress could negatively impact on GIT microbiota composition, recent research suggests that alterations in the composition of the ecosystem modifies both emotional behaviour and brain function.[186]

The microbiota may interact with the gut–brain axis and alter brain function through a number of different mechanisms:[188,189]

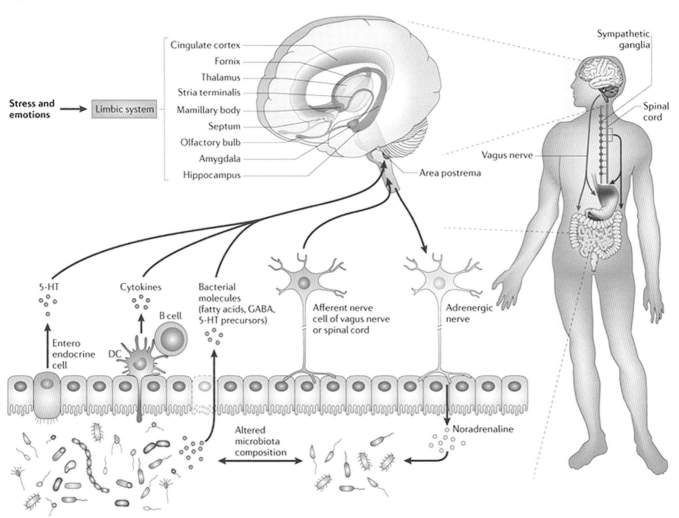

Nature Reviews | Microbiology

FIGURE 6.5 The bidirectional microbiota gut–brain axis[187]

The neural, immunological, endocrine and metabolic pathways by which the microbiota influences the brain and the proposed brain-to-microbiota component of this axis. Putative mechanisms by which bacteria access the brain and influence behaviour include bacterial products that gain access to the brain via the bloodstream and the area postrema, via cytokine release from mucosal immune cells, via the release of gut hormones such as 5-hydroxytryptamine (5-HT) from enteroendocrine cells or via afferent neural pathways, including the vagus nerve. Stress and emotions can influence the microbial composition of the gut through the release of stress hormones or sympathetic neurotransmitters that influence gut physiology and alter the habitat of the microbiota. Alternatively, host stress hormones such as noradrenaline might influence bacterial gene expression or signalling between bacteria, and this might change the microbial composition and activity of the microbiota.

DC = dendritic cell; GABA = γ-aminobutyric acid.

- production of bacterial metabolites such as neurotransmitters and SCFAs
- alterations in the integrity of the intestinal barrier
- modulation of sensory afferent nerve function
- pro-inflammatory bacterial products such as lipopolysaccharides
- impacts on blood sugar regulation and insulin sensitivity
- mucosal immune regulation.

Preclinical studies involving germ-free rodent models have demonstrated the importance of the microbiota in behavioural regulation. Bacterial colonisation in infancy has been found to be central to the development and maturation of both the enteric nervous system (ENS) and the central nervous system (CNS). Significant alterations in the expression and turnover of neurotransmitters in both the ENS and the CNS are observed in germ-free animals. This leads to alterations in gut sensory motor functions, such as delayed gastric and intestinal transit time and reduced migrating motor complex recurrence. Memory dysfunction also occurs, which is believed to be mediated by the lack of brain-derived neurotrophic factor in the hippocampus. Reconstitution of the microbiota has been found to significantly improve most of these observed abnormalities (if performed in the right time window).[187,188]

Human research in this area is, in many respects, still in its infancy. Research has just started to link specific mood disorders to specific dysbioses. For example, patients with major depression disorder have been found to have higher concentrations of Bacteroidetes and Proteobacteria microbes, and more specifically, high levels of *Alistipes* and endotoxin-rich Enterobacteriaceae. On the other hand, a negative correlation was observed between *Faecalibacterium* populations and severity of depressive symptoms.[190] Results like these provide microbiota treatment targets, in that once the imbalance is noted, it can be targeted therapeutically and corrected. Correcting this underlying dysbiosis may result in improved mood – the subject of current research endeavours. Clinical trials assessing the efficacy of specific probiotic strains and prebiotics in altering mood is a booming area of research that has produced very promising results so far.[191–193]

PHYTOCHEMICAL METABOLISM

The microbiota is involved in the metabolism of many xenobiotic substances, including phytochemicals and some pharmaceutical drugs.[194] This metabolism plays an important role in the medicinal action of many botanical medicines. For example, herbs that have polyphenols as their active compounds will often have much of their medicinal activity dependent upon microbiota metabolism.[195] This means that if the microbiota is severely altered, it is possible that metabolism of many of these polyphenols will also be altered or, in some cases, absent, meaning diminished effectiveness of the medicines.

Polyphenols are a broad class of phytochemicals found in many commonly consumed foods, as well as in a significant number of medicinal herbs.[196] Examples of polyphenols include lignans, phenolic acids, anthocyanins, flavonols, flavanols, chalcones, flavonones, flavones, condensed tannins, proanthocyanidins and isoflavones. Only a small percentage of consumed polyphenols appear to be absorbed intact, with approximately 95% of ingested polyphenols reaching the colon, where they interact with the microbiota.[197] This both nourishes members of the microbiota and at the same time modifies the polyphenol to a form that is both active and absorbable.[198] Most polyphenols occur in the form of glycosides, polymers and esters, and many of these rely heavily on microbial activity in the colon to free the medicinally active aglycones for absorption. Bacterial species that have so far been elucidated to play vital roles in polyphenol transformation include bifidobacteria, eubacteria, clostridia, *Butyrivibrio*, *Bacteroides*, enterococci and lactobacilli.[199] Consumption of foods and herbs rich in polyphenols should increase colonic concentrations of species that facilitate polyphenol metabolism over time, as will regular and ongoing consumption of prebiotics such as FOS, inulin, lactulose and partially hydrolysed guar gum. Supplementation with FOS, for example, has been found to increase colonic bifidobacteria populations, enhance colonic β-glucosidase activity[200] and increase serum concentrations of isoflavone aglycones.[201]

An example showing the importance of this polyphenol-modification process is the bark of *Salix alba* (willow), used for its analgesic and anti-inflammatory actions. Willow bark contains the ester glycoside salicortin. After ingestion of an extract of *Salix alba*, the ester linkages of salicortin are hydrolysed in the alkaline intestinal fluid to yield salicin. This glycoside is entirely dependent on the β-glycosidase action of the intestinal biota to be hydrolysed to release the aglycone saligenin. Saligenin is subsequently absorbed and oxidised in the bloodstream and liver to yield salicylic acid, the pharmacologically active agent. Thus, without the aid of the intestinal microbiota, *Salix alba* would be unable to perform its analgesic and anti-inflammatory actions.[202]

The medicinal activities of isoflavones and lignans are also dependent upon the GIT microbiota. Both isoflavones and lignans are modified by the intestinal flora, converting these compounds to their active forms. For example, flaxseeds (*Linum usitatissimum*) are an abundant source of plant lignans. When ingested, these lignans, secoisolariciresinol-diglucoside and matairesinol, are converted to the mammalian lignans enterodiol and enterolactone, respectively. This conversion occurs by hydrolysis, dehydroxylation, demethylation and oxidation reactions catalysed by members of the intestinal microbiota.[203]

COLONISATION RESISTANCE

One of the most important functions performed by the colonic microbiota is acting as a barrier against pathogenic and opportunistic microorganisms. This barrier role has been termed 'colonisation resistance' and has been defined as 'the protection against colonisation of the intestinal tract with potentially pathogenic bacteria afforded by the intestinal flora'.[204] The endogenous flora maintains strong control over the growth of potentially pathogenic microorganisms (PPMs). On entering the colon, any PPM intent on colonisation must compete with the endogenous microbiota, which occupies every available physical, physiological and metabolic niche. Resistance is conferred by the release of antimicrobial substances (e.g. hydrogen peroxide and bacteriocins), enhancement of the gut immune response, competition for adhesion sites and substrates, and metabolic byproducts (e.g. SCFAs), as well as the inactivation of toxins secreted by pathogens.[205]

Colonisation resistance has been confirmed using animal models and the introduction of pathogenic microorganisms. This barrier effect can be demonstrated by decontaminating the GIT with antibiotics (or even just altering microbiota dynamics) and observing how this procedure effects subsequent infection rates when pathogenic organisms are orally administered. Such experiments have shown that significant alterations in the normal intestinal microbiota substantially decreases the number of pathogenic organisms required to cause an infection, lengthens the time of infection and increases faecal levels of the pathogen.[205] This effect has been noted in studies utilising *E.coli, Klebsiella pneumoniae, Pseudomonas aeruginosa,*[206] *Candida albicans,*[207] *Clostridium difficile,*[208] *vancomycin-resistant Enterococcus,*[209] *Shigella flexneri, Vibrio cholerae* and *Salmonella enteriditis.*[210]

WEIGHT AND METABOLISM REGULATION

Over the past decade, the gut microbiota has received considerable attention as a novel factor contributing to the pathobiology of metabolic diseases. This research started from observations on germ-free mice (i.e. mice kept sterile without a GIT microbiota). Researchers observed that germ-free mice had 40% less total body fat than normal mice, while consuming 30% less food.[211] These initial observations were followed by Turnbaugh et al.'s ground-breaking study showing that obesity could be transferred from obese mice to germ-free mice via faecal inoculation. The newly inoculated mice became obese, despite no change in kilojoule input or output.[212]

The microbiota is thought to impact metabolism via a number of different mechanisms. The obese microbiome appears to extract more energy from a given diet compared to a lean microbiome (as demonstrated in Turnbaugh's experiments described above).[213] Initial research focused on the ratio of the two main phyla, Bacteroidetes and Firmicutes,[214] with the observation that obese mice have a lower abundance of Bacteroidetes and proportionally more Firmicutes compared to lean mice – an observation that was also initially corroborated in human research.[214] Considerable research has now been published, however, that has refuted this finding,[215,216] while other research is still supportive.[217,218] So, at this point in time, the clinical significance of the Bacteroidetes:Firmicutes ratio remains unclear. While exactly what constitutes an 'obese microbiome' in humans is still being defined (and debated), it does seem to be characterised by a lack of diversity compared to healthy controls[219,220] and changes at the Genus and species level. Lower concentrations of *Akkermansia muciniphila,*[221]

bifidobacteria[222] and *Faecalibacterium prausnitzii*[220] have been observed fairly consistently in obese individuals.

The GIT microbiota can also effect metabolism through its production of SCFAs. SCFAs modulate energy homeostasis via effects on multiple cellular metabolic pathways and receptor-mediated mechanisms.[223] Acetate, propionate and butyrate are all ligands of G-protein-coupled receptors – free fatty acid receptor-2 (FFAR2) and free fatty acid receptor-3 (FFAR3). These receptors are expressed in enteroendocrine L cells in the colon, ileum, adipocytes and even some immune cells and skeletal muscles. Activation of FFAR2 and FFAR3 by SCFAs in enteroendocrine cells triggers the secretion of peptide YY (PYY), while in adipocytes, stimulation of FFAR2 induces the release of leptin.[224,225] Both compounds are known for their ability to inhibit appetite. Acetate and propionate have also been found to increase the secretion of glucagon-like peptide 1 (GLP-1) by L cells along the colon, as well as leptin secretion from adipocytes. Glucagon-like peptide 1 is known to improve insulin sensitivity, enhance pancreatic insulin production and enhance satiety.[226] Other research has found butyrate capable of enhancing mitochondrial function and energy expenditure in skeletal muscle and biogenesis in brown fat.[227]

Another mechanism through which the microbiota may alter metabolism is through metabolic endotoxaemia. In their seminal paper, Cani et al.[228] showed that a high-fat, low-fibre diet induced dysbiosis, obesity, insulin resistance and, importantly, high serum levels of lipopolysaccharide (LPS). These changes were accompanied by increased pro-inflammatory markers such as TNF-α, IL-6 and IL-1. They termed this condition metabolic endotoxaemia. Lipopolysaccharide (aka endotoxin) is a component of the cell membrane of Gram-negative bacteria (mainly from the phyla Bacteroidetes and Proteobacteria), which are common members of the human GIT microbiota. It is continually produced due to constant breakdown and turnover of intestinal Gram-negative bacteria. Lipopolysaccharide can translocate from the intestine to several tissue sites, cause intestinal permeability and, when bound to toll-like receptor (TLR) 4, triggers a pro-inflammatory response.[229] The consequences of this metabolic endotoxaemia are fasting glycaemia, fasting insulinaemia and insulin resistance, weight gain, increased hepatic triglyceride content and systemic low-grade inflammation (see Fig. 6.6). The specific dysbiosis induced by the high-fat, low-fibre diet was characterised by a decrease in bifidobacteria populations, as well as key butyrate-producing species, and an increase in Gram-negative bacteria. These dysbiotic changes resulted in an enlarged endotoxin pool in the GIT, increased plasma endotoxin concentrations and a reduced capacity of the GI epithelial tissue to heal.[228]

Composition

The human gastrointestinal tract is home to approximately two hundred trillion microbial cells from over 1000 different microbial species, the vast majority of them belonging to the bacterial domain.[231] The GIT of a typical Westerner is a unique and individual ecosystem containing

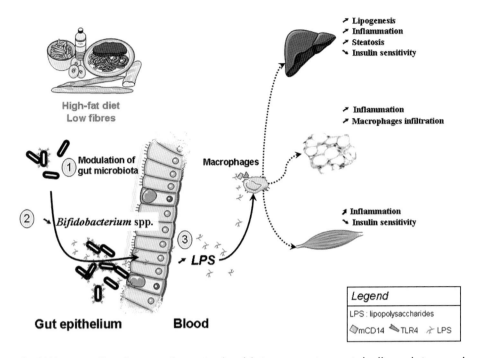

FIGURE 6.6 The typical Western diet changes the gut microbiota, promotes metabolic endotoxaemia and triggers the development of metabolic disorders[230]

1) A diet high in fat and low in fibre modulates the microbiota by 2) selectively decreasing bifidobacteria concentrations and increasing levels of endotoxin-rich, Gram-negative bacteria. This combination of events results in 3) increased LPS absorption and the release of proinflammatory cytokines that cause low-grade inflammation and a range of metabolic abnormalities. LPS = lipopolysaccharide.

an average of 160 species,[133,232] although 30–40 of them dominate the ecosystem (see Fig. 6.7). The vast majority of these species originate from one of five phyla – Firmicutes, Bacteroidetes, Actinobacteria, Proteobacteria and Verrucomicrobia.

Microbial communities in the gut include native (or autochthonous) species that colonise the intestine permanently and a variable number of microbes that are temporary visitors transiting through the GIT (allochthonous microbes).[234] The stomach is kept relatively sterile owing to the low pH of this environment, as well as rapid transit. Organisms in the stomach are generally autochthonous, visitors from the oral cavity, with the exception of *Helicobacter pylori*, the only microbe that could be considered native to the stomach environment. Microbe concentrations in the small intestine vary considerably along its length, with low levels in the duodenum (10^{3-4} per mL) and relatively high levels in the ileum (10^8 per mL). Low numbers in the proximal small bowel are maintained by the pH of the incoming gastric chyme, the propulsive motor activity that impedes stable colonisation, and high concentrations of digestive secretions such as bile and pancreatic secretions.[231] However, the immune system is also thought to play a role through the production of sIgA and antimicrobial compounds, such as defensins and cathelicidins, in part due to the large amount of organised lymphoid structures in the small bowel mucosa. The colon is the most densely populated area of the GIT, with levels of organisms reaching concentrations of 10^{11} CFU/mL. Transit time here

is slow, so microorganisms have plenty of time to proliferate by consuming available substrates from both the diet and endogenous sources (such as mucus and shed cells). Autochthonous microbes far outnumber transients in this environment (see Fig. 6.8).

Development of the GIT microbiota

Our knowledge regarding the development of the human microbiome has grown substantially over the past two decades. It was previously thought that the development of the human microbiome started at birth. However, emerging pre-conceptual factors, including the mother's weight at time of conception, have been identified as shaping the composition of her offspring's microbiota.[235] Infants born vaginally by women who were overweight pre-conceptually had differences in their neonatal acquisition of microbiota compared to infants born to women who were of normal weight.[235] In addition, the placenta is thought to harbour its own microbial community that plays a role in shaping the infant's microbiome.[236]

The succession of the microbial species in the first months and years of life is dynamic and complex.[237] There is constant traffic involving transient microbial species whose colonisation is restricted or allowed by numerous environmental and genetic factors.[237,238] At birth, there is early colonisation of the gastrointestinal tract by facultative anaerobes including *E. coli* and other

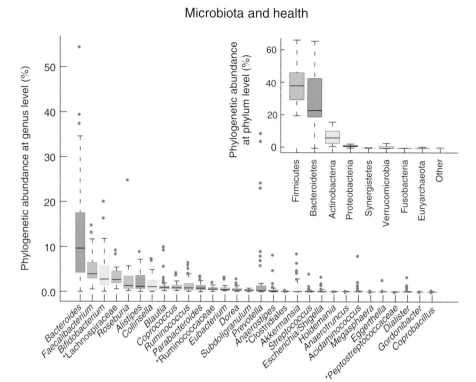

FIGURE 6.7 Genus variation box plot for the thirty most abundant genera of the human gut microbiota[233] Inset (upper right) shows phylum abundance box plot.
*= Bacterial Family (rather than Genus).

Enterobacteriaceae.[237] Over the following days, the anaerobic environment of the gastrointestinal tract dominates with *Bifidobacterium, Clostridium, Bacteroides* and *Ruminococcus* spp.[239] Over the following 3 years of life, the microbial composition of the gastrointestinal tract increases in diversity.[238] By the age of 3 years, it is thought the child's microbiome has a similar composition and metabolic function to that of the adult microbiome.[238]

IN THE BEGINNING: PLACENTA AND UTERINE ENVIRONMENT

The development of microbial programming in utero and during birth shapes the development of the immune system, and the immune system in turn shapes the composition of the microbiota.[240] An association, and in some cases a causal relationship, has emerged between the influence of the maternal microbiome on pregnancy outcomes and an individual's health beyond infancy.[241] It was thought that the development and interactions between the microbiota and the host immune system begin at the time of birth. However, the maternal uterine environment is not as sterile as was previously thought, with a distinctive placental microbiome composition being identified.[236,242,243] The Placenta Microbiome Project has now been added to the list of projects that seek to identify the characteristics and influences of niche microbial ecosystems within the human body. The characterisation of the microbiome obtained from the 320 placentas

suggested the composition was most characteristic of the maternal oral microbiome.[236] In this same study, microbial 'fingerprints' were identified in the placentas of women who had experienced a urinary tract infection during the first trimester of pregnancy.[236] Placental microbiome composition patterns have also been associated with preterm births.[236,244]

MODE OF DELIVERY AND THE INFANT MICROBIOME

The mode of delivery at birth has been shown to result in the development of different microbial compositions in infants and their subsequent health trajectories.[245–247] During a vaginal birth, the infant is inoculated with microbiota from the mother's vaginal, cervix, vulva and faecal microbiota that is principally comprised of members from the order of *Lactobacillaceae, Clostridiales, Bacteroidales* and *Actinomycetales*.[248] A variety of *Lactobacillus* dominates the vaginal microbiota composition.[249]

However, the proportion of individuals being born by caesarean delivery has reached unprecedented levels globally.[250] Data collected from 150 countries indicated that 18.6% of total live births were by caesarean, with the lowest prevalence (6%) being in countries with less resources.[250] The life-saving gift of a caesarean intervention is inarguable; however, the long-term sequelae of caesarean delivery on an individual's health have not

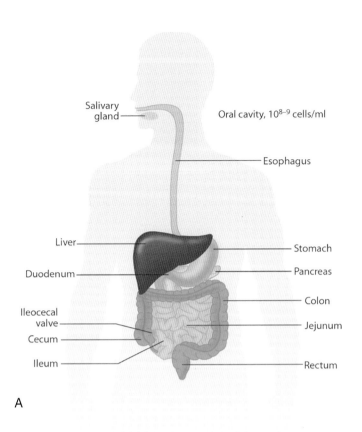

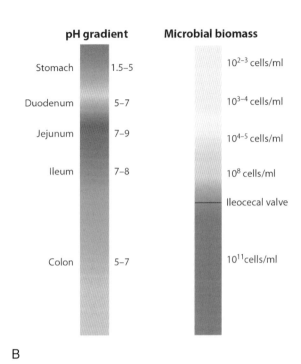

A

B

Bacterial population present

Oral cavity:
Gemella (e.g., *G. haemolysans*), *Granulicatella*,
Streptococcus (e.g., *S. mitis*), *Veillonella*, *Prevotella*,
Porphyromonas, *Rothia*, *Neisseria*, *Fusobacterium*,
Lactobacillus

Allochthonous microbes are generally outnumbered
by autochthonous microbes.

Stomach:
Helicobacter pylori

Allochthonous: *Gemella* (e.g., *G. haemolysans*),
Granulicatella, *Streptococcus* (e.g., *S. mitis*), *Veillonella*,
Prevotella, *Porphyromonas*, *Rothia*, *Neisseria*,
Fusobacterium, *Lactobacillus*

Small intestine:
Escherichia coli, *Klebsiella*, *Enterococcus*, *Bacteroides*,
Ruminococcus, *Dorea*, *Clostridium*, *Coprococcus*,
Weissella, *Lactobacillus* (some species)

Allochthonous: *Granulicatella*, *Streptococcus*
(e.g., *S. mitis*), *Veillonella*, *Lactobacillus*

Large intestine:
Five major phyla: *Firmicutes*, *Bacteroidetes*,
Actionobacteria, *Verrucomicrobia*, and *Proteobacteria*.
Hundreds of species.

Allochthonous microbes are generally outnumbered
by autochthonous microbes.

C

FIGURE 6.8 Characteristics of the major habits of the human gastrointestinal tract and their inhabitants[234]

A) The major sections of the GIT. B) Bars in the centre indicate pH levels moving from stomach to distal gut (*left*) and biomass levels
(*right*). C) Boxes indicate the dominant types of microbes either allochthonous or autochthonous to those habitats.

been fully elucidated. Fundamental differences in
microbiome development, which may in turn contribute to
variations in normal physiology and predisposition to a
number of diseases, have been identified in infants born
by caesarean.[240,245,251] Infants born by caesarean have
been found to have a microbiome that more closely
resembles that of the mother's skin (i.e. *Staphylococcus*,

Corynebacterium and *Propionibacterium*).[252] A prospective
cohort study following 1441 mothers who delivered their
baby vaginally or by caesarean found that compared with
vaginally delivered children, caesarean-delivered children
were at 1.4 greater times greater risk of becoming
overweight or obese in childhood.[253] A longitudinal study
including 10219 children, of whom 926 were delivered by

caesarean, reported significantly lower birth weights and increased adiposity at 6 weeks through to 15 years of age for the caesarean-delivered children.[246] At age 11, caesarean-delivered children had 1.83 times the odds of being overweight or obese.[246]

The quest to identify unifying risk factors in the development of diseases associated with an aberrant response of the immune system prompted a large Danish study to examine hospital records of children born by caesarean delivery over a 35-year period.[245] The authors concluded that caesarean delivery exemplified a shared risk factor in early life with asthma, systemic connective tissue disorders, juvenile arthritis, inflammatory bowel disease, immune deficiencies and leukaemia, but not type 1 diabetes, psoriasis or coeliac disease.[245] However, a meta-analysis conducted in 2008, including 20 studies worldwide, reported that caesareans, independent of maternal age, birth weight and breastfeeding, contributed a 20% increase in the risk of type 1 diabetes.[254] Earlier studies found an increased risk of coeliac disease among children who were born by caesarean.[255,256]

While the mode of delivery is an important foundational step in establishing an individual's microbiome, other influential factors in infancy are known to play an integral role in what appears to be a cohesive progression in establishing a unique microbiome in the first years of life.[257]

BREASTFEEDING AND THE DEVELOPMENT OF THE MICROBIOME

The composition of the infant's microbiome is shaped by feeding practices.[258] Breast milk contains commensal and probiotic bacteria, oligosaccharides and bioactive proteins that support the intestinal colonisation of beneficial bacteria, interplay with the developing immune system and protect the infant from gastrointestinal and respiratory infections.[259–263] The presence of microbiota in human breast milk is thought to possibly originate from the maternal gut via an enteromammary pathway. During lactation, cells from gut-associated lymphoid tissue of the mother travel to the breast via the lymphatics and peripheral blood.[264,265] Sustained long-term mucosal protection after breastfeeding has ceased has also been demonstrated.[266] This adds the composition of the maternal gastrointestinal microbiota to the web of influences on the neonate's microbiome development.

While there are clear limitations with both culture-dependent and culture-independent identification techniques, they both contribute to our understanding of breast milk composition and the factors that are associated with variations to that composition. These studies suggest a predominance of the facultative anaerobes including Staphylococcus and Streptococcus spp. and Propionibacterium, and a sub-dominance of obligate anaerobes Bifidobacteria and Veillonella in human breast milk.[267,268] The advent of molecular identification techniques reveals members common to the gut microbiome in breast milk including Bacteroides, Clostridia, Faecalibacterium and Roseburia.[268] Species from Bifidobacterium, Coprococcus, Faecalibacterium and

Roseburia are all producers of the SCFA butyrate, which plays an important role in maintaining the health of colonic cells.[265] Members of the phylum Firmicutes, including species from the Lactobacillus, Lactococcus and Enteroccus genus, are known to possess probiotic properties.[265]

The composition of human breast milk has been shown to vary depending on the birth delivery method, gestation age and the stage of lactation.[269] Thirty-two healthy mothers representing 19 preterm and 13 term births, and 15 vaginal and 17 caesarean deliveries, had the composition of their colostrum, transitional and mature breast milk analysed for microbiota composition.[269] The total bacteria, Bifidobacterium and Enterococcus spp. counts increased throughout the lactation period. Bifidobacteria was detected more frequently in the milk of mothers who had delivered their babies vaginally. All three milk samples from mothers who carried their babies to full-term contained a significantly higher concentration of Bifidobacterium spp. than those who gave birth prematurely.[269] In a separate study, the composition of breast milk from obese mothers had a less diverse bacterial community compared with milk from normal-weight mothers.[270]

Interestingly, in another study, the genes that facilitate the breakdown of plant-derived polysaccharides were present during the exclusive breastfeeding period.[271] The presence of microbial enzymes in breast milk that degrade non-digestible polysaccharides of plant origin have also been reported by other groups, suggesting a microbial priming in preparation for the introduction of solid foods.[272]

FORMULA FEEDING AND THE DEVELOPMENT OF THE MICROBIOME

Formula feeding plays an important and essential role in the nutrition of many children where breastfeeding is not possible or a preference for the mother. There are ongoing developments in identifying the many components of breast milk, including the microbial composition.[273] There are also extensive reviews focused on the influence of formula feeding versus breastfeeding upon the developing microbiome.[258,273] A study involving 207 3-month-old infants who were exclusively breastfed, partially breastfed or exclusively formula-fed found that Lactobacilli could only be cultured from exclusively and partially breastfed infants' saliva samples.[274] Interestingly, the microbiota of breastfed infants was further differentiated between those who were born vaginally or by caesarean delivery.[274] Furthermore, the presence of Lactobacillus plantarum, L. gasseri and L. vaginalis in one salivary sample inhibited growth of one bacteria associated with tooth decay, S. mutans.[274] The authors concluded that oral microbiota differs between breastfed and formula-fed infants, which is possibly related to cariogenic species suppression by lactobacilli indigenous to breast milk.[274]

ANTIBIOTICS

Antibiotics are known disruptors to the diversity and abundance of the intestinal microbiome.[275] The impact of antibiotic use during the microbiome development period of the first 3 years of life is an area of interest. The results of a longitudinal study involving the molecular evaluation of faecal samples from 39 children, of whom half had ≥9 courses of antibiotics over their first 3 years of life, were recently reported.[276] The children who had received antibiotics had less bacterial and strain diversity and a less stable microbiome.[276] In addition, infants as young as 2 months harboured antibiotic-resistant genes.[276] A separate study evaluated the effect of prematurity and perinatal antibiotic administration in the first 3 months of life in term and preterm infants.[277] Preterm infants had a reduced percentage distribution of the *Bacteroidaceae* family and a temporary peak of *Lactobacillaceae* compared to full-term infants. Infants whose mothers had received antibiotics perinatally had an increased percentage distribution of the *Enterobacteriaceae* family compared to infants whose mother had not received antibiotics.[277] The temporal impact of antibiotics and diet on the composition of the microbiome has also been observed by other groups.[278,279]

LESS TRAVELLED FRONTIERS OF MICROBIOME DEVELOPMENT

As discussed, pre-conceptual maternal weight, the intrauterine environment, delivery method, breastfeeding and antibiotic use are factors that shape the development of the intestinal microbiome. However, less explored factors including infant stress,[239] proton pump inhibitor use,[280] a family's shared microbiome,[281] hygiene practices and having a pet[282] are also being explored as shaping the development of the microbiome. In one study, children who were born vaginally, at home, who had a greater number of siblings and who were breastfed had greater microbial diversity and fewer infections than those born in hospital who were bottle fed and had fewer siblings, suggesting the immunological benefits of greater exposure to a broad range of microbiota.[283]

OLD FRIENDS AND HYGIENE – A HYPOTHESIS

The 'hygiene hypothesis', or 'old friends hypothesis', can be traced back to the 1870s when Charles Harrison Blackley noticed that aristocrats and city dwellers were more likely to have hayfever than were farmers.[284] Similarly, Leibowitz et al.[285] noted that the incidence of multiple sclerosis in Israel was positively related to sanitation. The term 'hygiene hypothesis' was coined and popularised by the media when Strachan et al.[286] noted that hayfever was less frequent in larger families containing many siblings. This directed focus towards allergic disorders, despite the clear evidence that other inflammatory conditions were increasing in parallel in Western societies. Popular media provided a polarised interpretation of these findings, suggesting that all early childhood illness and poor hygiene practices were a prerequisite for the normal development of the immune system.

The 'old friends hypothesis' was presented to provide a Darwinian synthesis and to focus attention on the fact that modern domestic hygiene practices are not the primary issue.[284] The 20th century witnessed an unprecedented rise in the incidence of many chronic inflammatory disorders in wealthy developed countries. These included autoimmune disorders such as coeliac disease, diabetes mellitus and multiple sclerosis.[287] Although genetics and specific triggering mechanisms such as molecular mimicry and viruses are involved, the increase in these diseases has been so rapid that an explanation that omits environmental change is incomplete. These environmental factors, most of them microbial, have led to a decrease in the efficacy of our immunoregulatory mechanisms. This is likely to be attributable to a state of evolved dependence on organisms with which we have co-evolved and which have been tolerated as inducers of immunoregulatory circuits. These organisms have been referred to as 'old friends' whose numbers are depleted in the modern urban environment.[288] Rook[284] cautioned against a reductionist approach when investigating depletion of our 'old friends'.

SUMMARY

There are a number of well-established and emerging factors that influence the development of the microbiome. It is suggested an integrative study model that considers a range of factors that influence microbial fetal and neonatal programming, including the family and social environment, hygiene practices, psychological and physical stressors, medication use and dietary practices are considered when seeking to understand this important area related to human health trajectories.[284]

Clinical assessment techniques

Tools for assessing the microbiota have changed considerably over the past 20 years.[132] Prior to the year 2000, most microbiota assessment studies used technology that, in some respects, was little changed from the late 1800s. This approach, termed culturing, is dependent upon collecting live microorganisms, putting them into a suitable growth medium, creating the appropriate conditions for the growth of that organism and then observing what grows. A considerable number of microbes that we are all familiar with, such as *E. coli*, lactobacilli, bifidobacteria and bacteroides, were first isolated in the early 20th century using very basic microbiology techniques. A breakthrough in anaerobic culturing techniques in the late 1960s substantially increased the number of discoverable GI microbes to give a clearer picture of the GIT microbiota.

Despite these advances, culturing as a technique to evaluate the microbiota has been found to have significant limitations. It is, for example, particularly poor in detecting changes in the microbiota from dietary and pharmaceutical interventions.[6] We now know this is mostly due to the fact that currently cultivable faecal bacteria represent only a fraction of the species actually present in the GIT – perhaps as little as 10%.[289] Using modern culture-independent, molecular methods has revealed a far more diverse ecosystem than previously believed, containing myriad hitherto undiscovered species. Many species that make up significant proportions of a healthy

GIT ecosystem that play vital roles in the ecosystem are not readily cultured, most notably *Faecalibacterium prausnitzii* and *Akkermansia muciniphila*. Trying to assess the health and balance of the GI ecosystem using approaches that cannot detect the majority of species in the GIT, nor evaluate the microbial richness and diversity of the ecosystem, is obviously problematic.

Another issue with commercially available faecal analyses that are dependent upon culturing is whether populations of cultivable microbes accurately represent the fresh state by the time the stool sample arrives at the lab. The journey from anus to lab can take a number of days, with the sample potentially being exposed to a wide range of temperatures along the journey. Bacterial populations can significantly alter during this journey, meaning that concentrations at the commencement of the culturing process are no longer representative of the fresh faecal sample (Hawrelak, unpublished data).

Culturing still has a place in clinical practice in determining the presence of bacterial and fungal pathogens in the stool and in evaluating their sensitivity to anti-microbials, but it should not be used as a tool to assess the balance or diversity of the GIT microbiota. Molecular, culture-independent methods should be used for this purpose.[290]

The switch to culture-independent assessment techniques that occurred from the turn of the century is responsible for the renaissance of interest in, and the explosion of new research about, the GIT microbiota. Molecular techniques overcome the drawbacks of culture-dependent techniques and have completely revolutionised and deepened our understanding of this ecosystem.[290]

Molecular microbiology techniques work by assessing the differences in the sequence of nucleotides of microbial genes. The majority of these techniques consist of the extraction of DNA from a stool sample, followed by amplification and sequencing of a specific component – the 16S ribosomal RNA genes.[233] This gene is present in all bacteria and fungi and has an appropriate balance of variability and conservation, with enough variation to distinguish between different species and enough similarity to identify organisms belonging to closely related groups. Techniques based on 16S rRNA gene sequences have become the standard method to identify and classify different microbial species.[290] Identification is based on sequence similarity analysis of this gene; essentially comparing what is found in a stool sample with reference sequences in a library database. In this way, the 16S rRNA genes provide information about microbial composition and diversity of species in a given sample. The amount of specific genes present in the sample also gives an indication of the amount of that organism in the stool.[233]

Alterations in the microbiota – dysbiosis

Gastrointestinal dysbiosis is now being linked to myriad pathological conditions (see Table 6.4). For some of these conditions, dysbiosis appears to contribute to the onset of

| TABLE 6.4 A list of conditions currently linked to GI dysbiosis[291–311] ||
GI conditions	Non-GI conditions
Alcoholic liver disease	Anxiety
Antibiotic-associated diarrhoea	Asthma
Chemotherapy-associated diarrhoea	Atopic eczema
Clostridium-difficile-associated disease	Autism
Coeliac disease	Chronic fatigue syndrome
Crohn's disease	Depression
Diverticular disease	Kidney stones
Irritable bowel syndrome	Metabolic syndrome
Liver cirrhosis	Multiple sclerosis
Non-alcoholic fatty liver disease	Obesity
Radiotherapy-associated diarrhoea	Parkinson's disease
Ulcerative colitis	Rheumatoid arthritis
	Type I diabetes
	Type II diabetes

the condition, whereas in others there is an association, but causality has not yet been confirmed.

The causes of dysbiosis

A number of factors have been found to negatively impact on the health and balance of the GIT ecosystem. The most researched ones are highlighted, alongside their impact on the microbiota, in Table 6.5.

Interventions to improve the health of the ecosystem

A number of tools can be utilised to improve the balance of the GIT microbiota and to enhance the growth of specific members of the ecosystem:

PROBIOTICS

Probiotics are live microorganisms that when administered in adequate amounts confer a health benefit on the host, are frequently recommended as tools to improve the microbiota.[332] Despite the reputation that probiotics and fermented foods have as being able to restore an imbalanced microbiota, research suggests this is not the case.[333] To date, probiotics have shown only a limited capacity to alter the GI microbial ecosystem. Current generation probiotics (i.e. those based on lactobacilli and bifidobacteria) do not have the capacity to permanently colonise the GIT after oral ingestion either, despite claims in the blogosphere to the contrary.[334] A limited number of probiotic strains have shown some capacity to alter levels of specific indigenous microbes, however:

TABLE 6.5 Factors that have been found to negatively impact on the GIT microbiota

Intervention	Study type	Impact on the microbiota
Pharmaceutical agents		
Antibiotics	Human	Each antibiotic has a unique impact on the microbiota. Antibiotic combinations generally have the strongest and longest-lasting impacts. Changes can vary between minor population alterations in just a few species to massive alterations in dozens of species, with some species even becoming extinct. The impact of some antibiotics is now known to linger for years after their use, in terms of both damage to microbial diversity and alterations in crucial functions of the microbiome[6,312–314]
Chemotherapy	Human	Chemotherapy caused an absolute decrease in faecal bacterial concentrations with specific decreases in populations of bacteroides, bifidobacteria and *Clostridium* clusters IV (including *Faecalibacterium prausnitzii*) and XIVa; *Enterobacterium faecium* populations increased. Some patients became colonised with *Clostridium difficile*[315]
Non-steroidal anti-inflammatory drugs (NSAIDs)	Human	NSAID users had significantly lower faecal lactobacilli and *Collinsella* spp. concentrations[316]
	Rat	Increased abundance of *Bacteroides* spp. and decreased levels of butyrate-producing bacteria; increased bile cytotoxicity[317]
Proton pump inhibitors (PPIs)	Human	Marked decline in microbiota diversity beginning in just 7 days. This loss in diversity was only partly reversed 1 month after cessation of PPI use[318]
	Human	Significantly lower faecal concentrations of *Faecalibacterium prausnitzii*. No impact on diversity[319]
	Human	Significantly lower microbial diversity in PPI users. Higher abundance of *Rothia*, *Steptococcus*, *Enterococcus*, *Staphylococcus* and *E. coli*[320]
	Human	Significantly lower abundance of total gut bacteria and lower microbial diversity in PPI users. Higher abundance of Proteobacteria, *Rothia* and *Streptococcus*[321]
	Rat	PPI administration resulted in significant reductions in small intestinal populations of bifidobacteria[322]
Radiotherapy	Human	Pelvic radiotherapy resulted in significant reductions in microbial diversity[323]
Dietary additives		
Emulsifiers	Mouse	Ingestion of carboxymethylcellulose and polysorbate-80 both significantly decreased overall microbial diversity and both compounds increased levels of inflammation-promoting proteobacteria[324]
Saccharin	Mouse	Increased populations of bacteroides and staphylococci; decreased concentrations of *Lactobacillus reuteri* and *Akkermansia muciniphila*[324]
Sucralose	Rat	Reductions in total anaerobe populations and bifidobacteria, bacteroides and lactobacilli concentrations specifically[325]
Diet		
High-protein, low-carbohydrate diet	Human	50% decline in bifidobacteria concentrations after 4 weeks. Significant decreases in concentrations of butyrate-producing bacteria *Roseburia* spp. and *Eubacterium rectale*, with a corresponding reduction in faecal butyrate levels[326]
Ketogenic diet	Human	A very low-carbohydrate, high-fat diet resulted in a significant reduction in bifidobacteria populations and a decrease in faecal SCFA and butyrate concentrations[327]
	Human	A classic ketogenic diet resulted in a significant increase in *Desulfovibrio* spp. concentrations. There was no significant impact on other microbial species[328]
	Mouse	The ketogenic diet had an 'anti-microbial-like' effect, significantly reducing total bacterial populations. Faecal concentrations of bifidobacteria, lactobacilli and *Roseburia* spp. were all significantly reduced on the ketogenic diet. Faecal bacteroides and enterobacteria concentrations were significantly increased[329]
Low FODMAP diet	Human	Following a low FODMAP diet resulted in a reduction in total bacterial abundance and decreased abundance of *Akkermansia muciniphila*, *Faecalibacterium prausnitzii*, *Ruminococcus* spp., lactobacilli and bifidobacteria[330]
	Human	Four weeks on the low FODMAP diet resulted in significant decreases in faecal bifidobacteria concentrations[331]

TABLE 6.6 The better researched prebiotics and their impact on the GIT ecosystem		
Prebiotic	**Dose**	**Effects on the GIT microbiota**
Fructooligosaccharides	4 g/day	Increase in bifidobacteria; decrease in β-glucuronidase activity[342]
	10 g/day	Increase in bifidobacteria and *Faecalibacterium prausnitzii*[343]
	15 g/day	Increase in bifidobacteria; decrease in faecal bacteroides, clostridia and fusobacteria concentrations[344]
	40 g/day	Increase in bifidobacteria; decrease in faecal concentrations of enterococci and enterobacteria[345]
Galactooligosaccharides	2.5 g/day	Increase in bifidobacteria; decrease in faecal concentrations of protein putrefactive byproducts (indoles and isovaleric acid)[346]
	2.6 g/day	Faecal bifidobacteria counts increased significantly, as did faecal levels of *Lactobacillus-Enterococcus* spp.; concentrations of *Bacteroides* spp., the *Clostridium histolyticum* group, *E. coli* and *Desulfovibrio* spp. decreased compared with placebo treatment[347]
	5 g/day	Increase in bifidobacteria and *Faecalibacterium prausnitzii*; decrease in *Bacteroides* spp.[348]
Lactulose	3 g/day	The faecal concentration of bifidobacteria increased significantly after treatment, whereas the number of Bacteroidaceae and clostridia decreased; faecal concentrations of protein putrefactive byproducts (skatol, indole and phenols) were reduced with lactulose intake; faecal beta-glucuronidase, azoreductase and nitroreductase activities also decreased; mean faecal pH also dropped from 7.0 to 6.4[349]
	5 g twice daily	After ingestion, faecal populations of bifidobacteria increased[350]
	10 g twice daily	After treatment, populations of bifidobacteria and lactobacilli increased by 3.0 and 1.9 log units, respectively; populations of *Bacteroides*, *Clostridium* and coliforms decreased by 4.1, 2.3 and 1.8 log units, respectively; mean faecal pH also dropped from 6.9 to 5.8[124]
Partially-hydrolysed guar gum	6 g/day	Enhanced growth of bifidobacteria, as well as butyrate-producing bacteria in the *Roseburia/Eubacterium rectale* group, *Eubacterium hallii* and the microbe SS2/1

- *Bacillus coagulans* GBI-30 6086 – significant increase in populations of *Faecalibacterium prausnitzii*[335]
- *Bifidobacterium lactis* HN019 – significant increases in faecal concentrations of bifidobacteria, lactobacilli and enterococci compared to baseline, as well as a decrease in coliforms[336]
- *Bifidobacterium longum* BB536 – significant increase in faecal bifidobacteria concentrations[337]; significant decrease in enterotoxigenic *Bacteroides fragilis* populations[338]
- *Lactobacillus acidophilus* NCFM – significant increase in faecal bifidobacteria, lactobacilli and eubacteria[339]
- *Lactobacillus casei* Shirota – significant increase in faecal bifidobacteria concentrations[340]
- *Lactobacillus rhamnosus* GG – significant increases in faecal concentrations of bifidobacteria and lactobacilli, as well as decreases in lecithinase-negative clostridia concentrations[341]

PREBIOTICS

Prebiotics are selectively fermented ingredients that result in specific changes in the composition and/or activity of the gastrointestinal microbiota, thus conferring benefit(s) upon host health.[117] Prebiotics have the greatest capacity to balance and restore a dysbiotic environment. Their use, over the short term, can specifically enhance the growth of key species that have been negatively impacted by dietary or pharmaceutical interventions (see Table 6.6). Over the

long-term, however, they have an amazing capacity to increase microbial diversity. Given the number of dysbiotic factors highlighted in Table 6.5 that negatively impact microbial diversity, agents capable of improving diversity are sorely needed.

The golden rule of prebiotic dosing is to *start low and slow*. The dose of the prebiotic should be slowly increased over a period of weeks to finally achieve the therapeutic or optimal dose. Most individuals will experience only minor digestive discomfort and increased flatulence upon commencement of prebiotic therapy. Others, particularly those patients who are prone to bloating and distension, will experience an exacerbation of those symptoms when commencing prebiotic treatment. In these patients, starting at ¼–½ the typical dose is advisable.

PREBIOTIC-LIKE FOODS

Prebiotic-like foods are foods that when consumed result in specific changes in the composition and/or activity of the gastrointestinal microbiota that improve host health. Prebiotic-like foods and their impact on the microbiota are highlighted in Table 6.7.

RESISTANT STARCH

Resistant starch is defined as the total amount of starch, and the products of starch degradation, that resists digestion in the small intestine.[358] Resistant starches (RS) are thus able to reach the colon, where they can be

TABLE 6.7 The effects of prebiotic-like foods on the microbiota		
Prebiotic-like food	Dose	Effects on the GIT microbiota
Almonds (roasted with skins)	56 g/day = ~ ⅓ cup	Increased faecal concentrations of bifidobacteria and lactobacilli; decreased faecal β-glucuronidase, nitroreductase and azoreductase activities[351]
Apples	2 medium apples/day	Increased faecal concentrations of bifidobacteria; trend for increased concentrations of lactobacilli; decrease in faecal clostridia; decreased faecal sulphide concentrations[352]
Blackcurrants	4 capsules/day black currant powdered extract	Increased faecal concentrations of bifidobacteria and lactobacilli; decreased counts of *Bacteroides* spp. and *Clostridium* spp.; decrease in faecal pH; decreased faecal β-glucuronidase activity; increased β-glucosidase activity[353]
Blueberries (wild)	25 g of powdered wild blueberries per day	Increased faecal concentrations of bifidobacteria[354]
Brown rice	~550 g/day = 4 cups cooked	Increased numbers of bifidobacteria; decreased counts of *Bacteroides* spp., *Escherichia coli* and *Clostridium* spp.[355]
Cocoa powder	~14 g dark cocoa powder/day	Increased faecal concentrations of bifidobacteria and lactobacilli; decrease in faecal clostridia[356]
Green tea	300 mg catechins/day; equivalent to ~5–6 cups/day	Increased faecal concentrations of bifidobacteria and lactobacilli; decreased concentrations of bacteroides, clostridia and enterobacteria; decrease in faecal pH; decrease in faecal concentrations of potentially toxic protein putrefactive byproducts ammonia, sulfide, skatol, indole and cresol; increased production of SCFAs[357]

fermented by members of the microbiota, producing a variety of end-products including SCFAs. There are four different types of RS:[359,360]

1 RS1 – resists digestion due to the starch being trapped within cellulose cell walls; and thus is physically inaccessible. RS1 is found in all grains, seeds and legumes. When cooked as whole kernels or coarsely ground, the thick cell wall of legumes and the protein matrix of cereal grains prevent water penetration into the starch. This means the starch granules do not gelatinise and swell, making them resistant to human digestive enzymes. The more finely milled the grain, seed or legume, the less the RS1 content.

2 RS2 – a type of starch with a high amylose content. Amylose is not easily broken down by human digestive enzymes. Significant amounts of RS2 is found in raw potatoes, legumes, plantains and green (unripe) bananas. However, cooking these foods alters the starch structure to make it digestible, so these foods (or products from these foods) must be consumed in their raw state to get the benefit of the RS2 content. Hi-maize corn is rich in RS2.

3 RS3 – termed retrograde starch. RS3 is formed when starchy foods are cooked and then cooled. The cooling process alters some of the starches to make them indigestible – via a process termed retrogradation. Substantial amounts of RS3 are found in cooked and cooled root vegetables (i.e. potatoes and sweet potatoes) and cooked and cooled grains and legumes.

4 RS4 – includes chemically modified or re-polymerised starches. Includes starches which have been etherised,

esterified or cross-bonded with chemicals in such a manner as to decrease their digestibility.

Research to date suggests that the different forms of RS may have slightly differing effects on the microbiota. For example, RS2 appears to increase concentrations of bifidobacteria, *Ruminococcus bromii* and *Eubacterium rectale*[361,362]; RS3 has been found to increase both *Ruminococcus bromii* and *Eubacterium rectale*[363]; RS4 increases *Bifidobacterium adolescentis* and *Parabacteroides distasonis*, but decreases *Faecalibacterium prausnitzii* and ruminococci.[362] In general, RS appears to be butyrogenic; that is, it feeds butyrate-producing bacteria, thereby enhancing colonic butyrate production (although RS4 appears to be the exception).

To make the area even more complex, however, the impact of RS is also patient-specific, in that some patients will not get the expected microbiota alterations when consuming that RS type. Presumably this is because those species are lacking in their unique microbiota, or the specific strains of those species contained in that individual's ecosystem lack the fermentation pathways specifically needed to utilise that RS type, and so the RS cannot be fermented. Given this, it seems prudent to suggest dietary recommendations that incorporate all three naturally occurring RS forms on a daily basis to ensure the patient has the best chance of benefitting from the potential prebiotic-like actions of RS.

Using a mixture of these interventions, particularly prebiotic supplements and prebiotic-like foods, will provide the greatest benefits in restoring a dysbiotic ecosystem.

CASE STUDY 6.2: GASTROINTESTINAL DYSBIOSIS

PRESENTATION

A 24-year-old female presented with a 9-month history of idiopathic colitis. After working with a number of gastroenterologists, she had decided to proceed down the path of a faecal microbial transplant (FMT) to treat the colitis and wanted guidance on how best to encourage robust populations of beneficial GIT species post transplant. Characteristics of her GIT microbiota (using culture-independent methods) pre-FMT are highlighted in Table 6.8. Her genera richness and diversity were both low. Her comparative diversity score was only 21%, which means that 79% of all the hundreds of thousands of stool samples analysed had a more diverse microbial pattern than hers. Concentrations of the pathobiont *Bacteroides* were well above the healthy range, and levels of key beneficial species such as *Akkermansia* and *Faecalibacterium* were extremely low and sub-optimal, respectively. Additionally, bifidobacteria were either completely absent from her ecosystem or below detectable levels (culture independent methods in general can only detect microbial populations $\geq 10^6$ CFU/mL).

TREATMENT PROTOCOL AND OUTCOMES

During the 6-week FMT process and for the following 4 months, the patient was prescribed two prebiotic supplements and told to consume microbiota-nourishing foods daily (both prebiotic-like foods and foods rich in resistant starch). Partially hydrolysed guar gum (7 g/day) was prescribed to nourish the butyrate-producing organisms in the GIT, while galactooligosaccharides (2.75 g/day) were prescribed to feed her *Faecalibacterium prausnitzii* and bifidobacteria. She was also advised to commence an exercise regimen, significantly increase the diversity of her diet (aiming for 40+ whole, plant foods each week) and implement a daily meditation practice to help reduce stress levels. Stress has been shown to negatively impact the microbiota,[364] while moderate exercise has been shown to improve microbial diversity.[365] A diet rich in food diversity has also been shown to enhance microbiota diversity.[366]

Characteristics of her GIT microbiota immediately following a series of 7 FMTs and 6 weeks of concurrent microbiota support are shown in Table 6.8. As can be seen, microbiota diversity had improved so that her faecal microbial ecosystem was now more diverse than 49% of the samples in the microbiome library and contained an additional 20 genera compared to the pre-FMT sample. Levels of the *Bacteroides* genus decreased, while concentrations of butyrate-producing bacteria, such as *Roseburia*, *Subdoligranulum* and *Blautia* increased markedly. *Akkermansia* populations also increased, as did concentrations of bifidobacteria.

Lactulose was added in at this point at a starting dose of 5 mL/day, with the idea of slowly increasing the dose upwards towards 10 mL b.i.d. over the subsequent 6 weeks. Lactulose was added to further support diversity, and bifidobacteria, *Akkermansia* and *Faecalibacterium* populations.[367,368]

A final microbiota assessment was done 8 weeks after the final FMT (see Table 6.8). Genera richness further increased and diversity score improved markedly to 98%, meaning that only 2% of samples in the microbiome library were more diverse than hers. Concentrations of *Bacteroides* had decreased to healthy levels and concentrations of beneficial bacteria and butyrate-producers had substantially increased compared to both baseline and the 6-week treatment time points.

This case illustrates the benefits of FMT therapy in improving the GIT ecosystem, but even more so, the power of prebiotics and dietary and lifestyle interventions in substantially improving the GIT microbiota – in terms of species balance, genera richness and diversity, and concentrations of key beneficial species.

TABLE 6.8 Culture-independent GIT microbiota characterisation of a 24-year-old patient – pre faecal microbial transplant (FMT), immediately post FMT and 8 weeks after final FMT. Genera richness refers to the number of different genera found in the stool specimen

		Pre FMT	Immediately post FMT	8 weeks post FMT
Microbiota diversity	Genera richness	45	65	72
	Comparative Diversity score	21%	49%	98%
Key beneficial species	*Akkermansia*	0.04%	0.13%	1.25%
	Bifidobacterium	ND	0.32%	1.65%
	Faecalibacterium	6.82%	8.35%	10.32%
Butyrate producers	*Blautia*	2.19%	5.13%	3.39%
	Roseburia	1.32%	9.60%	9.12%
	Subdoligranulum	0.52%	2.08%	5.21%
Key pathobiont	*Bacteroides*	51.03%	42.85%	19.10%

REFERENCES

[1] Relman DA. The human microbiome and the future practice of medicine. JAMA 2015;314(11):1127–8.

[2] Cho I, Blaser MJ. The human microbiome: at the interface of health and disease. Nat Rev Genet 2012;13(4):260–70.

[3] Marchesi JR, Adams DH, Fava F, et al. The gut microbiota and host health: a new clinical frontier. Gut 2016;65(2):330–9.

[4] Bordenstein SR, Theis KR. Host biology in light of the microbiome: ten principles of holobionts and hologenomes. PLoS Biol 2015;13(8):e1002226.

[5] D'Argenio V, Salvatore F. The role of the gut microbiome in the healthy adult status. Clin Chim Acta 2015;451(Pt A):97–102.

[6] Hawrelak JA, Myers SP. Intestinal dysbiosis: a review of the literature. Altern Med Rev 2004;9:180–97.

[7] Chow J, Mazmanian SK. A pathobiont of the microbiota balances host colonization and intestinal inflammation. Cell Host Microbe 2010;7(4):265–76.

[8] Ursell LK, Metcalf JL, Parfrey LW, et al. Defining the human microbiome. Nutr Rev 2012;70(Suppl. 1):S38–44.

[9] Consortium HMP. Structure, function and diversity of the healthy human microbiome. Nature 2012;486(7402):207–14.

[10] Fierer N, Lauber CL, Zhou N, et al. Forensic identification using skin bacterial communities. Proc Natl Acad Sci USA 2010;107(14):6477–81.

[11] Tims S, Derom C, Jonkers DM, et al. Microbiota conservation and BMI signatures in adult monozygotic twins. ISME J 2013;7(4):707–17.

[12] Ferretti P, Farina S, Cristofolini M, et al. Experimental metagenomics and ribosomal profiling of the human skin microbiome. Exp Dermatol 2017;26(3):211–19.

[13] SanMiguel A, Grice EA. Interactions between host factors and the skin microbiome. Cell Mol Life Sci 2015;72(8):1499–515.

[14] Schommer NN, Gallo RL. Structure and function of the human skin microbiome. Trends Microbiol 2013;21(12):660–8.

[15] Dréno B, Araviiskaia E, Berardesca E, et al. Microbiome in healthy skin, update for dermatologists. J Eur Acad Dermatol Venereol 2016;30(12):2038–47.

[16] Zhang M, Jiang Z, Li D, et al. Oral antibiotic treatment induces skin microbiota dysbiosis and influences wound healing. Microb Ecol 2015;69(2):415–21.

[17] Callewaert C, Hutapea P, Van de Wiele T, et al. Deodorants and antiperspirants affect the axillary bacterial community. Arch Dermatol Res 2014;306(8):701–10.

[18] Oh J, Freeman AF, Program NCS, et al. The altered landscape of the human skin microbiome in patients with primary immunodeficiencies. Genome Res 2013;23(12):2103–14.

[19] Staudinger T, Pipal A, Redl B. Molecular analysis of the prevalent microbiota of human male and female forehead skin compared to forearm skin and the influence of make-up. J Appl Microbiol 2011;110(6):1381–9.

[20] Salava A, Lauerma A. Role of the skin microbiome in atopic dermatitis. Clin Transl Allergy 2014;4:33.

[21] Fry L, Baker BS, Powles AV, et al. Is chronic plaque psoriasis triggered by microbiota in the skin? Br J Dermatol 2013;169(1):47–52.

[22] Picardo M, Ottaviani M. Skin microbiome and skin disease: the example of rosacea. J Clin Gastroenterol 2014;48(Suppl. 1):S85–6.

[23] Szabo K, Erdei L, Bolla BS, et al. Factors shaping the composition of the cutaneous microbiota. Br J Dermatol 2016;176(2):344–51.

[24] Zhou Y, Mihindukulasuriya KA, Gao H, et al. Exploration of bacterial community classes in major human habitats. Genome Biol 2014;15(5):R66.

[25] Bogaert D, Keijser B, Huse S, et al. Variability and diversity of nasopharyngeal microbiota in children: a metagenomic analysis. PLoS ONE 2011;6(2):e17035.

[26] Allen EK, Koeppel AF, Hendley JO, et al. Characterization of the nasopharyngeal microbiota in health and during rhinovirus challenge. Microbiome 2014;2(1):22.

[27] Rosas-Salazar C, Shilts MH, Tovchigrechko A, et al. Differences in the nasopharyngeal microbiome during acute respiratory tract infection with human rhinovirus and respiratory syncytial virus in infancy. J Infect Dis 2016;214(12):1924–8.

[28] Alamri L, Crandall KA, Freishtat RJ. Nasopharyngeal microbiome diversity changes over time in children with asthma. PLoS ONE 2016;12(1):e0170543.

[29] Teo SM, Mok D, Pham K, et al. The infant nasopharyngeal microbiome impacts severity of lower respiratory infection and risk of asthma development. Cell Host Microbe 2015;17(5):704–15.

[30] Pérez-Losada M, Alamri L, Crandall KA, et al. Nasopharyngeal microbiome diversity changes over time in children with asthma. PLoS ONE 2017;12(1):e0170543.

[31] Hyde ER, Petrosino JF, Piedra PA, et al. Nasopharyngeal Proteobacteria are associated with viral etiology and acute wheezing in children with severe bronchiolitis. J Allergy Clin Immunol 2014;133(4):1220–2.

[32] Biesbroek G, Tsivtsivadze E, Snaders EA, et al. Early respiratory microbiota composition determines bacterial succession patterns and respiratory health in children. Am J Respir Crit Care Med 2014;190(11):1283–92.

[33] Berrington JE, Cummings SP, Embleton ND. The nasopharyngeal microbiota: an important window of opportunity. Am J Respir Crit Care Med 2014;190(3):246–8.

[34] Liu CM, Soldanova K, Nordstrom L, et al. Medical therapy reduces microbiota diversity and evenness in surgically recalcitrant chronic rhinosinusitis. Int Forum Allergy Rhinol 2013;3(10):775–81.

[35] Thanasumpun T, Batra PS. Endoscopically-derived bacterial cultures in chronic rhinosinusitis: a systematic review. Am J Otolaryngol 2015;36(5):686–91.

[36] Bhattacharyya N, Kepnes LJ. Assessment of trends in antimicrobial resistance in chronic rhinosinusitis. Ann Otol Rhinol Laryngol 2008;117(6):448–52.

[37] Ragab A, Farahat T, Al-Hendawy G, et al. Nasal saline irrigation with or without systemic antibiotics in treatment of children with acute rhinosinusitis. Int J Pediatr Otorhinolaryngol 2015;79(12):2178–86.

[38] Stearns JC, Davidson CJ, McKeon S, et al. Culture and molecular-based profiles show shifts in bacterial communities of the upper respiratory tract that occur with age. ISME J 2015;9(5):1246–59.

[39] Adlerberth I, Wold AE. Establishment of the gut microbiota in Western infants. Acta Paediatr 2009;98(2):229–38.

[40] Tapiovaara L, Pitkaranta A, Korpela R. Probiotics and the upper respiratory tract – a review. Pediatric Infectious Diseases 2016;1:19.

[41] Hao Q, Dong BR, Wu T. Probiotics for preventing acute upper respiratory tract infections. Cochrane Database Syst Rev 2015;(2):CD006895, https://doi.org//10.1002/14651858.CD006895.pub3.

[42] Consortium THM. Structure, function and diversity of the healthy human microbiome. Nature 2012;486(7402):207–14.

[43] Dewhirst FE, Chen T, Izard J, et al. The human oral microbiome. J Bacteriol 2010;192:5002–17.

[44] Wade WG. The oral microbiome in health and disease. Pharmacol Res 2013;69(1):137–43.

[45] Zaura E, Keijser BJF, Huse SM, et al. Defining the healthy 'core microbiome' of oral microbial communities. BMC Microbiol 2009;9(1):259.

[46] Lazarevic V, Whiteson K, Hernandez D, et al. Study of inter- and intra-individual variations in the salivary microbiota. BMC Genomics 2010;11(1):523.

[47] Segata N, Haake SK, Mannon P, et al. Composition of the adult digestive tract bacterial microbiome based on seven mouth surfaces, tonsils, throat and stool samples. Genome Biol 2012;13:R42.

[48] Wade WG. The oral microbiome in health and disease. Pharmacol Res 2013;69:137–43.

[49] Belda-Ferre P, Alcaraz LD, Cabrera-Rubio R, et al. The oral metagenome in health and disease. ISME J 2012;6(1):46–56.

[50] Simón-Soro A, Mira A. Solving the etiology of dental caries. Trends Microbiol 2015;23(2):76–82.

[51] Dye BA, Thornton-Evans G, Li X, et al. Dental caries and sealant prevalence in children and adolescents in the United States, 2011–2012. 2015. US Department of Health and Human Services, Centers for Disease Control and Prevention, National Center for Health Statistics.

[52] Kassebaum NJ, Bernabé E, Dahiya M, et al. Global burden of untreated caries. J Dent Res 2015;94(5):650–8.

[53] Loesche WJ. Role of Streptococcus mutans in human dental decay. Microbiol Rev 1986;50(4):353–80.

[54] Wu J, Peters BA, Dominianni C, et al. Cigarette smoking and the oral microbiome in a large study of American adults. ISME J 2016;10(10):2435–46.

[55] Mikuls TR, Payne JB, Reinhardt RA, et al. Antibody responses to Porphyromonas gingivalis (P. gingivalis) in subjects with rheumatoid arthritis and periodontitis. Int Immunopharmacol 2009;9(1):38–42.

[56] He J, Li Y, Cao Y, et al. The oral microbiome diversity and its relation to human diseases. Folia Microbiol 2015;60:69–80.

[57] Beck JM, Young VB, Huffnagle GB. The microbiome of the lung. Transl Res 2012;160:258–66.

[58] Ahn J, Chen CY, Hayes RB. Oral microbiome and oral and gastrointestinal cancer risk. Cancer Causes Control 2012;23:399–404.

[59] Fan X, Alekseyenko AV, Wu J, et al. Human oral microbiome and prospective risk for pancreatic cancer: a population-based nested case-control study. Gut 2018;67(1):120–7.

[60] Koren O, Spor A, Felin J, et al. Human oral, gut, and plaque microbiota in patients with atherosclerosis. Proc Natl Acad Sci USA 2011;108:4592–8.

[61] Slocum C, Kramer C, Genco C. Immune dysregulation mediated by the oral microbiome: potential link to chronic inflammation and atherosclerosis. J Intern Med 2016;280(1):114–28.

[62] Kholy KE, Genco RJ, Van Dyke TE. Oral infections and cardiovascular disease. Trends Endocrinol Metab 2015;26(6):315–21.

[63] Kilian M, Chapple IL, Hannig M, et al. The oral microbiome – an update for oral healthcare professionals. Br Dent J 2016;221(10):657–66.

[64] Godtfredsen NS, Prescott E. Benefits of smoking cessation with focus on cardiovascular and respiratory comorbidities. Clin Respir J 2011;5:187–94.

[65] Marsh PD, Do T, Beighton D, et al. Influence of saliva on the oral microbiota. Periodontol 2000 2016;70(1):80–92.

[66] Khurshid Z, Naseem M, Sheikh Z, et al. Oral antimicrobial peptides: types and role in the oral cavity. Saudi Pharm J 2016;24(5):515–24.

[67] Legrand D. Overview of lactoferrin as a natural immune modulator. J Pediatr 2016;173(Suppl.):S10–15.

[68] Gornowicz A, Tokajuk G, Bielawska A, et al. The assessment of sIgA, histatin-5, and lactoperoxidase levels in saliva of adolescents with dental caries. Med Sci Monit 2014;20:1095–100.

[69] Yang F, Zeng X, Ning K, et al. Saliva microbiomes distinguish caries-active from healthy human populations. ISME J 2012;6(1):1–10.

[70] Bradshaw DJ, Lynch RJ. Diet and the microbial aetiology of dental caries: new paradigms. Int Dent J 2013;63(Suppl. 2):64–72.

[71] Jørgensen MR, Keller MK. Use of probiotics in future prevention and treatment of oral infections, in oral infections and general health: from molecule to chairside. In: Pedersen AML, editor. Oral infections and general health. Cham. Switzerland: Springer International Publishing; 2016. p. 125–36.

[72] Stensson M, Koch G, Coric S, et al. Oral administration of Lactobacillus reuteri during the first year of life reduces caries prevalence in the primary dentition at 9 years of age. Caries Res 2014;48(2):111–17.

[73] Hasslof P, West CE, Videhult FK, et al. Early intervention with probiotic Lactobacillus paracasei F19 has no long-term effect on caries experience. Caries Res 2013;47(6):559–65.

[74] Gueimonde L, Vesterlund S, García-Pola MJ, et al. Supplementation of xylitol-containing chewing gum with probiotics: a double blind, randomised pilot study focusing on saliva flow and saliva properties. Food Funct 2016;7(3):1601–9.

[75] Toiviainen A, Jalasvuori H, Lahti E, et al. Impact of orally administered lozenges with Lactobacillus rhamnosus GG and Bifidobacterium animalis subsp. lactis BB-12 on the number of salivary mutans streptococci, amount of plaque, gingival inflammation and the oral microbiome in healthy adults. Clin Oral Investig 2015;19(1):77–83.

[76] van de Wijgert JH, Borgdorff H, Verhelst R, et al. The vaginal microbiota: what have we learned after a decade of molecular characterization? PLoS ONE 2014;9(8):e105998.

[77] Boris S. Barbés C. Role played by lactobacilli in controlling the population of vaginal pathogens. Microbes Infect 2000;2(5):543–6.

[78] Miller EA, Beasley DE, Dunn RR, et al. Lactobacilli dominance and vaginal pH: why is the human vaginal microbiome unique? Front Microbiol 2016;7:1936.

[79] Martin R, Soberon N, Vaneechoutte M, et al. Characterization of indigenous vaginal lactobacilli from healthy women as probiotic candidates. Int Microbiol 2008;11(4):261–6.

[80] Spear GT, French AL, Gilbert D, et al. Human alpha-amylase present in lower-genital-tract mucosal fluid processes glycogen to support vaginal colonization by Lactobacillus. J Infect Dis 2014;210(7):1019–28.

[81] Ravel J, Brotman RM. Translating the vaginal microbiome: gaps and challenges. Genome Med 2016;8(1):35.

[82] O'Hanlon DE, Moench TR, Cone RA. Vaginal pH and microbicidal lactic acid when lactobacilli dominate the microbiota. PLoS ONE 2013;8(11):e80074.

[83] Ravel J, Gajer P, Abdo Z, et al. Vaginal microbiome of reproductive-age women. Proc Natl Acad Sci USA 2011; 108(Suppl. 1):4680–7.

[84] Witkin SS, Linhares IM. Why do lactobacilli dominate the human vaginal microbiota? BJOG 2016;124(4):606–11.

[85] Sgibnev AV, Kremleva EA. Vaginal protection by H2O2-producing lactobacilli. Jundishapur J Microbiol 2015;8(10):e22913.

[86] Smith SB, Ravel J. The vaginal microbiota, host defence and reproductive physiology. J Physiol 2016;595(2):451–63.

[87] Petrova MI, Lievens E, Malik S, et al. Lactobacillus species as biomarkers and agents that can promote various aspects of vaginal health. Front Physiol 2015;6:81.

[88] Gajer P, Brotman RM, Bai G, et al. Temporal dynamics of the human vaginal microbiota. Sci Transl Med 2012;4(132):132ra52.

[89] Muhleisen AL, Herbst-Kralovetz MM. Menopause and the vaginal microbiome. Maturitas 2016;91:42–50.

[90] Mirmonsef P, Modur S, Burgad D, et al. Exploratory comparison of vaginal glycogen and Lactobacillus levels in premenopausal and postmenopausal women. Menopause 2015;22(7):702–9.

[91] Farage MA, Miller KW, Song Y, et al. The vaginal microbiota in menopause. In: Farage MA, Miller KW, Maibach HI, editors. Textbook of aging skin. Heidelberg: Springer Berlin Heidelberg; 2017. p. 1417–31.

[92] Brotman RM, Shardell MD, Gajer P, et al. Association between the vaginal microbiota, menopause status, and signs of vulvovaginal atrophy. Menopause 2014;21(5):450–8.

[93] Haahr T, Jensen JS, Thomsen L, et al. Abnormal vaginal microbiota may be associated with poor reproductive outcomes: a prospective study in IVF patients. Hum Reprod 2016;31(4):795–803.

[94] Gosmann C, Anahtar MN, Handley SA, et al. Lactobacillus-deficient cervicovaginal bacterial communities are associated with increased HIV acquisition in young South African women. Immunity 2017;46(1):29–37.

[95] Borgdorff H, Tsivtsivadze E, Verhelst R, et al. Lactobacillus-dominated cervicovaginal microbiota associated with reduced HIV/STI prevalence and genital HIV viral load in African women. ISME J 2014;8(9):1781–93.

[96] Buvé A, Jespers V, Crucitti T, et al. The vaginal microbiota and susceptibility to HIV. AIDS 2014;28(16):2333–44.

[97] Mitra A, MacIntyre DA, Marchesi JR, et al. The vaginal microbiota, human papillomavirus infection and cervical intraepithelial neoplasia: what do we know and where are we going next? Microbiome 2016;4(1):58.

[98] Stapleton AE. The vaginal microbiota and urinary tract infection. Microbiol Spectr 2016;4(6).

[99] Kirjavainen PV, Pautler S, Baroja ML, et al. Abnormal immunological profile and vaginal microbiota in women prone to urinary tract infections. Clin Vaccine Immunol 2009;16(1):29–36.

[100] Brotman RM, He X, Gajer P, et al. Association between cigarette smoking and the vaginal microbiota: a pilot study. BMC Infect Dis 2014;14:471.

[101] Hooton TM, Fihn SD, Johnson C, et al. Association between bacterial vaginosis and acute cystitis in women using diaphragms. Arch Intern Med 1989;149(9):1932–6.

[102] Vallor AC, Antonio MA, Hawes SE, et al. Factors associated with acquisition of, or persistent colonization by, vaginal lactobacilli:

role of hydrogen peroxide production. J Infect Dis 2001;184(11):1431–6.

[103] Tuddenham S, Rovner A, Ma B, et al. Association between dietary intake and dysbiotic vaginal microbiota. Sex Transm Infect 2015;91(Suppl. 2):A54–5.

[104] Beigi RH, Wiesenfeld HC, Hillier SL, et al. Factors associated with absence of H2O2-producing Lactobacillus among women with bacterial vaginosis. J Infect Dis 2005;191(6):924–9.

[105] Baeten JM, Hassan WM, Chohan V, et al. Prospective study of correlates of vaginal Lactobacillus colonisation among high-risk HIV-1 seronegative women. Sex Transm Infect 2009;85(5):348–53.

[106] Gupta K, Hillier SL, Hooton TM, et al. Effects of contraceptive method on the vaginal microbial flora: a prospective evaluation. J Infect Dis 2000;181(2):595–601.

[107] Neut C, Verrière F, Nelis HJ, et al. Topical treatment of infectious vaginitis: effects of antibiotic, antifungal and antiseptic drugs on the growth of normal vaginal Lactobacillus strains. Open J Obstet Gynecol 2015;5:173–80.

[108] Ogino M, Iino K, Minoura S. Habitual use of warm-water cleaning toilets is related to the aggravation of vaginal microflora. J Obstet Gynaecol Res 2010;36(5):1071–4.

[109] Heczko PB, Tomusiak A, Adamski P, et al. Supplementation of standard antibiotic therapy with oral probiotics for bacterial vaginosis and aerobic vaginitis: a randomised, double-blind, placebo-controlled trial. BMC Womens Health 2015;15:115.

[110] Pendharkar S, Brandsborg E, Hammarstrom L, et al. Vaginal colonisation by probiotic lactobacilli and clinical outcome in women conventionally treated for bacterial vaginosis and yeast infection. BMC Infect Dis 2015;15:255.

[111] Vicariotto F, Mogna L, Del Piano M. Effectiveness of the two microorganisms Lactobacillus fermentum LF15 and Lactobacillus plantarum LP01, formulated in slow-release vaginal tablets, in women affected by bacterial vaginosis: a pilot study. J Clin Gastroenterol 2014;48(Suppl. 1):S106–12.

[112] Petricevic L, Unger FM, Viernstein H, et al. Randomized, double-blind, placebo-controlled study of oral lactobacilli to improve the vaginal flora of postmenopausal women. Eur J Obstet Gynecol Reprod Biol 2008;141:54–7.

[113] Anukam KC, Osazuwa EO, Ahonkhai I, et al. Lactobacillus vaginal microbiota of women attending a reproductive health care service in Benin City, Nigeria. Sex Transm Dis 2006;39:59–62.

[114] Martinez RC, Franceschini SA, Patta MC, et al. Improved cure of bacterial vaginosis with single dose of tinidazole (2 g), Lactobacillus rhamnosus GR-1, and Lactobacillus reuteri RC-14: a randomized, double-blind, placebo-controlled trial. Can J Microbiol 2009;55:133–8.

[115] Vujic G, Jajac Knez A, Despot Stefanovic V, et al. Efficacy of orally applied probiotic capsules for bacterial vaginosis and other vaginal infections: a double-blind, randomized, placebo-controlled study. Eur J Obstet Gynecol Reprod Biol 2013;168(1):75–9.

[116] Macklaim JM, Clemente JC, Knight R, et al. Changes in vaginal microbiota following antimicrobial and probiotic therapy. Microb Ecol Health Dis 2015;26:27799.

[117] Gibson GR, Scott KP, Rastall R, et al. Dietary prebiotics: current status and new definition. Food Science and Technology Bulletin: Functional Foods 2010;7(1):1–19.

[118] Rousseau V, Lepargneur JP, Roques C, et al. Prebiotic effects of oligosaccharides on selected vaginal lactobacilli and pathogenic microorganisms. Anaerobe 2005;11(3):145–53.

[119] Coste I, Judlin P, Lepargneur J-P, et al. Safety and efficacy of an intravaginal prebiotic gel in the prevention of recurrent bacterial vaginosis: a randomized double-blind study. Obstet Gynecol Int 2012;2012:7.

[120] Tester R, Al-Ghazzewi F, Shen N, et al. The use of konjac glucomannan hydrolysates to recover healthy microbiota in infected vaginas treated with an antifungal agent. Benef Microbes 2012;3(1):61–6.

[121] Sutherland A, Tester R, Al-Ghazzewi F, et al. Glucomannan hydrolysate (GMH) inhibition of Candida albicans growth in the presence of Lactobacillus and Lactococcus species. Microbial Ecology in Health and Disease 2011;20(3).

[122] Vongsa RA, Minerath RA, Busch MA, et al. In vitro evaluation of nutrients that selectively confer a competitive advantage to lactobacilli. Benef Microbes 2016;7(2):299–304.

[123] Ganzle MG, Follador R. Metabolism of oligosaccharides and starch in lactobacilli: a review. Front Microbiol 2012;3:340.

[124] Ballongue J, Schumann C, Quignon P. Effects of lactulose and lactitol on colonic microflora and enzymatic activity. Scand J Gastroenterol 1997;1997(Suppl. 222):41–4.

[125] Pham TT, Shah NP. Effect of Lactulose on biotransformation of isoflavone glycosides to aglycones in soymilk by Lactobacilli. J Food Sci 2008;73(3):M158–65.

[126] De Souza Oliveira RP, Rodrigues Florence AC, Perego P, et al. Use of lactulose as prebiotic and its influence on the growth, acidification profile and viable counts of different probiotics in fermented skim milk. Int J Food Microbiol 2011;145(1):22–7.

[127] Chaithongwongwatthana S, Limpongsanurak S, Sitthi-Amorn C. Single hydrogen peroxide vaginal douching versus single-dose oral metronidazole for the treatment of bacterial vaginosis: a randomized controlled trial. J Med Assoc Thai 2003;86(Suppl. 2): S379–84.

[128] Cardone A, Zarcone R, Borrelli A, et al. Utilisation of hydrogen peroxide in the treatment of recurrent bacterial vaginosis. Minerva Ginecol 2003;55(6):483–92.

[129] Petersen EE, Genet M, Caserini M, et al. Efficacy of vitamin C vaginal tablets in the treatment of bacterial vaginosis: a randomised, double blind, placebo controlled clinical trial. Arzneimittelforschung 2011;61(4):260–5.

[130] Petersen EE, Magnani P. Efficacy and safety of vitamin C vaginal tablets in the treatment of non-specific vaginitis. A randomised, double blind, placebo-controlled study. Eur J Obstet Gynecol Reprod Biol 2004;117(1):70–5.

[131] Kuhne L. The new science of healing. London: Williams & Norgate; 1892.

[132] Rajilic-Stojanovic M, de Vos WM. The first 1000 cultured species of the human gastrointestinal microbiota. FEMS Microbiol Rev 2014;38(5):996–1047.

[133] Qin J, Li R, Raes J, et al. A human gut microbial gene catalogue established by metagenomic sequencing. Nature 2010;464(7285):59–65.

[134] LeBlanc JG, Milani C, de Giori GS, et al. Bacteria as vitamin suppliers to their host: a gut microbiota perspective. Curr Opin Biotechnol 2013;24(2):160–8.

[135] Ramotar K, Conly JM, Chubb H, et al. Production of menaquinones by intestinal anaerobes. J Infect Dis 1984; 150(2):213–18.

[136] Fernandez F, Collins MD. Vitamin K composition of anaerobic gut bacteria. FEMS Microbiol Lett 1987;41(2):175–80.

[137] Said HM. Recent advances in transport of water-soluble vitamins in organs of the digestive system: a focus on the colon and the pancreas. Am J Physiol Gastrointest Liver Physiol 2013;305(9):G601–10.

[138] Deguchi Y, Morishita T, Mutai M. Comparative studies on synthesis of water-soluble vitamins among human species of bifidobacteria. Agric Biol Chem 1985;49(1):13–19.

[139] Nabokina SM, Inoue K, Subramanian VS, et al. Molecular identification and functional characterization of the human colonic thiamine pyrophosphate transporter. J Biol Chem 2014;289(7):4405–16.

[140] Kumar JS, Subramanian VS, Kapadia R, et al. Mammalian colonocytes possess a carrier-mediated mechanism for uptake of vitamin B3 (niacin): studies utilizing human and mouse colonic preparations. Am J Physiol Gastrointest Liver Physiol 2013;305(3):G207–13.

[141] Pompei A, Cordisco L, Amaretti A, et al. Folate production by bifidobacteria as a potential probiotic property. Appl Environ Microbiol 2007;73(1):179–85.

[142] Degnan PH, Taga ME, Goodman AL. Vitamin B12 as a modulator of gut microbial ecology. Cell Metab 2014;20(5):769–78.

[143] Macfarlane GT, Macfarlane S. Bacteria, colonic fermentation, and gastrointestinal health. J AOAC Int 2012;95(1):50–60.

[144] Gibson GR. Dietary modulation of the human gut microflora using prebiotics. Br J Nutr 1998;80(Suppl. 2):S209–12.

[145] Cherbut C, Aube AC, Blottiere HM, et al. Effects of short-chain fatty acids on gastrointestinal motility. Scand J Gastroenterol 1997;32(Suppl. 222):58–61.

[146] Topping DL. Short-chain fatty acids produced by intestinal bacteria. Asia Pac J Clin Nutr 1996;5(Suppl.):15–19.

[147] Cummings JH. Short chain fatty acids. In: Gibson GR, Macfarlane GT, editors. Human colonic bacteria: role in nutrition, physiology and pathology. Boca Raton: CRC Press; 1995. p. 101–30.

[148] Latella G. Effects of SCFA on human colonocytes. Gastroenterology International 1998;11(Suppl. 1):76–9.

[149] Scheppach W. Effects of short chain fatty acids on gut morphology and function. Gut 1994;35(Suppl. 1):S35–8.

[150] Tedelind S, Westberg F, Kjerrulf M, et al. Anti-inflammatory properties of the short-chain fatty acids acetate and propionate: a study with relevance to inflammatory bowel disease. World J Gastroenterol 2007;13(20):2826–32.

[151] Braniste V, Al-Asmakh M, Kowal C, et al. The gut microbiota influences blood-brain barrier permeability in mice. Sci Transl Med 2014;6(263):263ra158.

[152] Gao Z, Yin J, Zhang J, et al. Butyrate improves insulin sensitivity and increases energy expenditure in mice. Diabetes 2009;58(7):1509–17.

[153] Puddu A, Sanguineti R, Montecucco F, et al. Evidence for the gut microbiota short-chain fatty acids as key pathophysiological molecules improving diabetes. Mediators Inflamm 2014;2014:9.

[154] Berni Canani R, Di Costanzo M, Leone L. The epigenetic effects of butyrate: potential therapeutic implications for clinical practice. Clin Epigenetics 2012;4(1):4.

[155] Berni Canani R, Di Costanzo M, Leone L, et al. Potential beneficial effects of butyrate in intestinal and extraintestinal diseases. World J Gastroenterol 2011;17.

[156] Soliman MM, Ahmed MM, Salah-Eldin AE, et al. Butyrate regulates leptin expression through different signaling pathways in adipocytes. J Vet Sci 2011;12(4):319–23.

[157] Abell GCJ, Conlon MA, McOrist AL. Methanogenic archaea in adult human faecal samples are inversely related to butyrate concentration. Microbial Ecology in Health and Disease 2011;18(3–4).

[158] D'Argenio G, Mazzacca G. Short-chain fatty acid in the human colon. In: Zappia V, Ragione F, Barbarisi A, et al, editors. Advances in nutrition and cancer 2. Advances in experimental medicine and biology. US: Springer US; 1999. p. 149–58.

[159] Gibson PR, Rosella O, Rosella G, et al. Butyrate is a potent inhibitor of urokinase secretion by normal colonic epithelium in vitro. Gastroenterology 1994;107(2):410–19.

[160] Hatayama H, Iwashita J, Kuwajima A, et al. The short chain fatty acid, butyrate, stimulates MUC2 mucin production in the human colon cancer cell line, LS174T. Biochem Biophys Res Commun 2007;356(3):599–603.

[161] Riviere A, Selak M, Lantin D, et al. Bifidobacteria and butyrate-producing colon bacteria: importance and strategies for their stimulation in the human gut. Front Microbiol 2016;7:979.

[162] Chang D-E, Jung H-C, Rhee J-S, et al. Homofermentative production of d-or-lactate in metabolically engineered escherichia coli RR1. Appl Environ Microbiol 1999;65(4):1384–9.

[163] Smith SM, Eng RHK, Buccini F. Use of D-lactic acid measurements in the diagnosis of bacterial infections. J Infect Dis 1986;154(4):658–64.

[164] Louis P, Flint HJ. Diversity, metabolism and microbial ecology of butyrate-producing bacteria from the human large intestine. FEMS Microbiol Lett 2009;294(1):1–8.

[165] Pryde SE, Duncan SH, Hold GL, et al. The microbiology of butyrate formation in the human colon. FEMS Microbiol Lett 2002;217(2):133–9.

[166] Wrzosek L, Miquel S, Noordine ML, et al. Bacteroides thetaiotaomicron and Faecalibacterium prausnitzii influence the production of mucus glycans and the development of goblet cells in the colonic epithelium of a gnotobiotic model rodent. BMC Biol 2013;11:61.

[167] Kelly J, Ryan S, McKinnon H, et al. Dietary supplementation with a type 3 resistant starch induces butyrate producing bacteria within the gut microbiota of human volunteers. Appetite 2015;91(Complete):438.

[168] Noack J, Timm D, Hospattankar A, et al. Fermentation profiles of wheat dextrin, inulin and partially hydrolyzed guar gum using an in vitro digestion pretreatment and in vitro batch fermentation system model. Nutrients 2013;5(5):1500–10.

[169] Fernandez-Banares F, Hinojosa J, Sanchez-Lombrana JL, et al. Randomized clinical trial of Plantago ovata seeds (dietary fiber) as compared with mesalamine in maintaining remission in ulcerative colitis. Am J Gastroenterol 1999;94(2):427–33.

[170] Campbell JM, Fahey GC. Psyllium and methylcellulose fermentation properties in relation to insoluble and soluble fiber standards. Nutr Res 1997;17(4):619–29.

[171] Hallert C, Bjorck I, Nyman M, et al. Increasing fecal butyrate in ulcerative colitis patients by diet: controlled pilot study. Inflamm Bowel Dis 2003;9(2):116–21.

[172] Kanauchi O, Iwanaga T, Mitsuyama K, et al. Butyrate from bacterial fermentation of germinated barley foodstuff preserves intestinal barrier function in experimental colitis in the rat model. J Gastroenterol Hepatol 1999;14(9):880–8.

[173] Jung TH, Jeon WM, Han KS. In vitro effects of dietary inulin on human fecal microbiota and butyrate production. J Microbiol Biotechnol 2015;25(9):1555–8.

[174] Higgins JA. Whole grains, legumes, and the subsequent meal effect: implications for blood glucose control and the role of fermentation. J Nutr Metab 2012;2012:7.

[175] Mallillin AC, Trinidad TP, Raterta R, et al. Dietary fibre and fermentability characteristics of root crops and legumes. Br J Nutr 2008;100(3):485–8.

[176] Belkaid Y, Hand Timothy W. Role of the microbiota in immunity and inflammation. Cell 2014;157(1):121–41.

[177] Lathrop SK, Bloom SM, Rao SM, et al. Peripheral education of the immune system by colonic commensal microbiota. Nature 2011;478(7368):250–4.

[178] Crabbe PA, Bazin H, Eyssen A, et al. The normal microbial flora as a major stimulus for proliferation of plasma cells synthesising IgA in the gut. The germ-free intestinal tract. Int Arch Allergy Appl Immunol 1968;34:362–75.

[179] Pulverer G, Ko HL, Roszkowski W, et al. Digestive tract microflora liberates low molecular weight peptides with immunotriggering activity. Zentralbl Bakteriol 1990;227:318–27.

[180] Roszkowski K, Roszkowski W, Ko HL, et al. Intestinal microflora of BALB/c mice and function of local immune cells. Zentralbl Bakteriol Mikrobiol Hyg A 1988;270:270–9.

[181] Tomkovich S, Jobin C. Microbiota and host immune responses: a love–hate relationship. Immunology 2016;147(1):1–10.

[182] Guarner F. Functions of the gut microbiota. In: Guarner F, editor. World gastroenterology organisation handbook on gut microbes. Milwaukee, USA: World Gastroenterology Organisation; 2014. p. 9–11.

[183] Arnolds KL, Lozupone CA. Striking a balance with help from our little friends – how the gut microbiota contributes to immune homeostasis. Yale J Biol Med 2016;89(3):389–95.

[184] Correa-Oliveira R, Fachi JL, Vieira A, et al. Regulation of immune cell function by short-chain fatty acids. Clin Transl Immunology 2016;5(4):e73.

[185] Turroni F, Ventura M, Buttó LF, et al. Molecular dialogue between the human gut microbiota and the host: a Lactobacillus and Bifidobacterium perspective. Cell Mol Life Sci 2014;71(2):183–203.

[186] Mayer EA, Knight R, Mazmanian SK, et al. Gut microbes and the brain: paradigm shift in neuroscience. J Neurosci 2014;34(46):15490–6.

[187] Collins SM, Surette M, Bercik P. The interplay between the intestinal microbiota and the brain. Nat Rev Microbiol 2012;10(11):735–42.

[188] Carabotti M, Scirocco A, Maselli MA, et al. The gut-brain axis: interactions between enteric microbiota, central and enteric nervous systems. Ann Gastroenterol 2015;28(2):203–9.

[189] Biesmans S, Meert TF, Bouwknecht JA, et al. Systemic immune activation leads to neuroinflammation and sickness behavior in mice. Mediators Inflamm 2013;2013:14.

[190] Jiang H, Ling Z, Zhang Y, et al. Altered fecal microbiota composition in patients with major depressive disorder. Brain Behav Immun 2015;48:186–94.

[191] Wallace CJ, Milev R. The effects of probiotics on depressive symptoms in humans: a systematic review. Ann Gen Psychiatry 2017;16:14.

[192] Schmidt K, Cowen PJ, Harmer CJ, et al. Prebiotic intake reduces the waking cortisol response and alters emotional bias in healthy volunteers. Psychopharmacology (Berl) 2015;232(10):1793–801.

[193] Azpiroz F, Dubray C, Bernalier-Donadille A, et al. Effects of scFOS on the composition of fecal microbiota and anxiety in patients

with irritable bowel syndrome: a randomized, double blind, placebo controlled study. Neurogastroenterol Motil 2017;29(2):e12911.

[194] Spanogiannopoulos P, Bess EN, Carmody RN, et al. The microbial pharmacists within us: a metagenomic view of xenobiotic metabolism. Nat Rev Microbiol 2016;14(5):273–87.

[195] Li H, Zhou M, Zhao A, et al. Traditional Chinese medicine: balancing the gut ecosystem. Phytother Res 2009;23(9):1332–5.

[196] Tsao R. Chemistry and biochemistry of dietary polyphenols. Nutrients 2010;2(12):1231–46.

[197] Clifford MN. Diet-derived phenols in plasma and tissues and their implications for health. Planta Med 2004;70(12):1103–14.

[198] Ozdal T, Sela DA, Xiao J, et al. The reciprocal interactions between polyphenols and gut microbiota and effects on bioaccessibility. Nutrients 2016;8(2):78.

[199] Marin L, Miguelez EM, Villar CJ, et al. Bioavailability of dietary polyphenols and gut microbiota metabolism: antimicrobial properties. Biomed Res Int 2015;2015:905215.

[200] Rowland IR, Rumney CJ, Coutts JT, et al. Effect of Bifidobacterium longum and inulin on gut bacterial metabolism and carcinogen-induced aberrant crypt foci in rats. Carcinogenesis 1998;19(2):281–5.

[201] Teekachunhatean S, Techatoei S, Rojanasthein N, et al. Influence of fructooligosaccharide on pharmacokinetics of isoflavones in postmenopausal women. Evid Based Complement Alternat Med 2012;2012:9.

[202] Wohlmuth H. Pharmacognosy and medicinal plant pharmacology. Lismore: Southern Cross University Press; 1998. p. 72–3.

[203] Landete JM, Arques J, Medina M, et al. Bioactivation of phytoestrogens: intestinal bacteria and health. Crit Rev Food Sci Nutr 2016;56(11):1826–43.

[204] Hentges DJ. Role of the intestinal microflora in host defense against infection. In: Hentges DJ, editor. Human intestinal microflora in health and disease. New York: Academic Press; 1983. p. 311–32.

[205] Buffie CG, Pamer EG. Microbiota-mediated colonization resistance against intestinal pathogens. Nat Rev Immunol 2013;13(11):790–801.

[206] Van der Waaij D, Berghuis-de Vries JM, Lekkerkerk V. Colonization resistance of the digestive tract in conventional and antibiotic-treated mice. J Hyg (Lond) 1971;69(3):405–11.

[207] Kennedy MJ, Volz PA. Ecology of Candida albicans gut colonization: inhibition of Candida adhesion, colonization, and dissemination from the gastrointestinal tract by bacterial antagonism. Infect Immun 1985;49(3):654–63.

[208] Britton RA, Young VB. Role of the intestinal microbiota in resistance to colonization by Clostridium difficile. Gastroenterology 2014;146(6):1547–53.

[209] Ubeda C, Taur Y, Jenq RR, et al. Vancomycin-resistant Enterococcus domination of intestinal microbiota is enabled by antibiotic treatment in mice and precedes bloodstream invasion in humans. J Clin Invest 2010;120(12):4332–41.

[210] Hentges DJ. Intestinal flora in defence against infection. In: Hentges DJ, editor. Human intestinal microflora in health and disease. London: Academic Press; 1983. p. 311–31.

[211] Backhed F, Ding H, Wang T, et al. The gut microbiota as an environmental factor that regulates fat storage. Proc Natl Acad Sci USA 2004;101(44):15718–23.

[212] Turnbaugh PJ, Ley RE, Mahowald MA, et al. An obesity-associated gut microbiome with increased capacity for energy harvest. Nature 2006;444(7122):1027–31.

[213] Goffredo M, Mass K, Parks EJ, et al. Role of gut microbiota and short chain fatty acids in modulating energy harvest and fat partitioning in youth. J Clin Endocrinol Metab 2016;101(11):4367–76.

[214] Ley RE, Backhed F, Turnbaugh P, et al. Obesity alters gut microbial ecology. Proc Natl Acad Sci USA 2005;102(31):11070–5.

[215] Schwiertz A, Taras D, Schäfer K, et al. Microbiota and SCFA in lean and overweight healthy subjects. Obesity (Silver Spring) 2010;18(1):190–5.

[216] Duncan SH, Lobley GE, Holtrop G, et al. Human colonic microbiota associated with diet, obesity and weight loss. Int J Obes (Lond) 2008;32(11):1720–4.

[217] Verdam FJ, Fuentes S, de Jonge C, et al. Human intestinal microbiota composition is associated with local and systemic inflammation in obesity. Obesity (Silver Spring) 2013;21(12):E607–15.

[218] Jumpertz R, Le DS, Turnbaugh PJ, et al. Energy-balance studies reveal associations between gut microbes, caloric load, and nutrient absorption in humans. Am J Clin Nutr 2011;94(1):58–65.

[219] Turnbaugh PJ, Gordon JI. The core gut microbiome, energy balance and obesity. J Physiol 2009;587(Pt 17):4153–8.

[220] Andoh A, Nishida A, Takahashi K, et al. Comparison of the gut microbial community between obese and lean peoples using 16S gene sequencing in a Japanese population. J Clin Biochem Nutr 2016;59(1):65–70.

[221] Yassour M, Lim MY, Yun HS, et al. Sub-clinical detection of gut microbial biomarkers of obesity and type 2 diabetes. Genome Med 2016;8(1):1–14.

[222] Kalliomaki M, Collado MC, Salminen S, et al. Early differences in fecal microbiota composition in children may predict overweight. Am J Clin Nutr 2008;87(3):534–8.

[223] Chambers ES, Morrison DJ, Frost G. Control of appetite and energy intake by SCFA: what are the potential underlying mechanisms? Proc Nutr Soc 2015;74(3):328–36.

[224] Blaut M. Gut microbiota and energy balance: role in obesity. Proc Nutr Soc 2015;74(3):227–34.

[225] Kasubuchi M, Hasegawa S, Hiramatsu T, et al. Dietary gut microbial metabolites, short-chain fatty acids, and host metabolic regulation. Nutrients 2015;7(4):2839–49.

[226] Chambers ES, Morrison DJ, Frost G. Control of appetite and energy intake by SCFA: what are the potential underlying mechanisms? Proc Nutr Soc 2015;74(3):328–36.

[227] Gao Z, Yin J, Zhang J, et al. Butyrate improves insulin sensitivity and increases energy expenditure in mice. Diabetes 2009;58(7):1509–17.

[228] Cani PD, Amar J, Iglesias MA, et al. Metabolic endotoxemia initiates obesity and insulin resistance. Diabetes 2007;56(12):e20.

[229] Scheithauer TP, Dallinga-Thie GM, de Vos WM, et al. Causality of small and large intestinal microbiota in weight regulation and insulin resistance. Mol Metab 2016;5(9):759–70.

[230] Cani PD, Delzenne NM. The role of the gut microbiota in energy metabolism and metabolic disease. Curr Pharm Des 2009;15(13):1546–58.

[231] Herrera C, Guarner F. Microbial communities. In: Guarner F, editor. World gastroenterology organisation handbook on gut microbes. Milwaukee, US: World Gastroenterology Organisation; 2014.

[232] Lozupone CA, Stombaugh JI, Gordon JI, et al. Diversity, stability and resilience of the human gut microbiota. Nature 2012;489(7415):220–30.

[233] Robles Alonso V, Guarner F. Linking the gut microbiota to human health. Br J Nutr 2013;109(S2):S21–6.

[234] Walter J, Ley R. The human gut microbiome: ecology and recent evolutionary changes. Annu Rev Microbiol 2011;65:411–29.

[235] Mueller NT, Shin H, Pizoni A, et al. Birth mode-dependent association between pre-pregnancy maternal weight status and the neonatal intestinal microbiome. Sci Rep 2016;6:23133.

[236] Aagaard K, Ma J, Antony KM, et al. The placenta harbors a unique microbiome. Sci Transl Med 2014;6(237):237ra65.

[237] Koenig JE, Spor A, Scalfone N, et al. Succession of microbial consortia in the developing infant gut microbiome. Proc Natl Acad Sci USA 2011;108(Suppl. 1):4578–85.

[238] Nicholson J. Host-gut microbiota metabolic interactions. Science 2012;336(6086):1262–7.

[239] Matamoros S, Gras-Leguen C, Le Vacon F, et al. Development of intestinal microbiota in infants and its impact on health. Trends Microbiol 2013;21(4):167–73.

[240] Mueller NT, Bakacs E, Combellick J, et al. The infant microbiome development: mom matters. Trends Mol Med 2015;21(2):109–17.

[241] Fox C, Eichelberger K. Maternal microbiome and pregnancy outcomes. Fertil Steril 2015;104(6):1358–63.

[242] Stout MJ, Conlon B, Landeau M, et al. Identification of intracellular bacteria in the basal plate of the human placenta in term and preterm gestations. Am J Obstet Gynecol 2013;208(3):e1–7.

[243] Antony KM, Ma J, Mitchell KB, et al. The preterm placental microbiome varies in association with excess maternal gestational weight gain. Am J Obstet Gynecol 2015;212(5):653.e1–16.

[244] Prince AL, Ma J, Kannan PS, et al. The placental membrane microbiome is altered among subjects with spontaneous preterm birth with and without chorioamnionitis. Am J Obstet Gynecol 2016;214(5):627.

[245] Sevelsted A, Stokholm J, Bønnelykke K, et al. Cesarean section and chronic immune disorders. Pediatrics 2015;135(1):e92–8.

[246] Blustein J, Attina T, Liu M, et al. Association of caesarean delivery with child adiposity from age 6 weeks to 15 years. Int J Obes (Lond) 2013;37(7):900–6.

[247] Chu DM, Ma J, Prince AL, et al. Maturation of the infant microbiome community structure and function across multiple body sites and in relation to mode of delivery. Nat Med 2017;23(3):314–26.

[248] Aagaard K, Riehle K, Ma J, et al. A metagenomic approach to characterization of the vaginal microbiome signature in pregnancy. PLoS ONE 2012;7(6):e36466.

[249] Petrova MI, Lievens E, Malik S, et al. Lactobacillus species as biomarkers and agents that can promote various aspects of vaginal health. Front Physiol 2015;6:81.

[250] Betrán AP, Ye J, Moller AB, et al. The increasing trend in caesarean section rates: global, regional and national estimates: 1990–2014. PLoS ONE 2016;11(2):e0148343.

[251] Pflughoeft KJ, Versalovic J. Human microbiome in health and disease. Annu Rev Pathol 2012;7:99–122.

[252] Dominguez-Bello MG, Costello EK, Contreras M, et al. Delivery mode shapes the acquisition and structure of the initial microbiota across multiple body habitats in newborns. Proc Natl Acad Sci USA 2010;107(26):11971–5.

[253] Mueller NT, Mao G, Bennet WL, et al. Does vaginal delivery mitigate or strengthen the intergenerational association of overweight and obesity? Findings from the Boston Birth Cohort. Int J Obes (Lond) 2017;41(4):497–501.

[254] Cardwell C, Stene LC, Joner G, et al. Caesarean section is associated with an increased risk of childhood-onset type 1 diabetes mellitus: a meta-analysis of observational studies. Diabetologia 2008;51(5):726–35.

[255] Decker E, Engelmann G, Findeisen A, et al. Cesarean delivery is associated with celiac disease but not inflammatory bowel disease in children. Pediatrics 2010;125(6):e1433–40.

[256] Mårild K, Stephansson O, Montgomery S, et al. Pregnancy outcome and risk of celiac disease in offspring: a nationwide case-control study. Gastroenterology 2012;142(1):39–45.e3.

[257] Penders J, Thijs C, Vink C, et al. Factors influencing the composition of the intestinal microbiota in early infancy. Pediatrics 2006;118(2):511–21.

[258] Guaraldi F, Salvatori G. Effect of breast and formula feeding on gut microbiota shaping in newborns. Front Cell Infect Microbiol 2012;2:94.

[259] Walker A. Breast milk as the gold standard for protective nutrients. J Pediatr 2010;156(2, Suppl.):S3–7.

[260] Victora CG, Bahlr R, Barros AJD, et al. Breastfeeding in the 21st century: epidemiology, mechanisms, and lifelong effect. Lancet 2016;387(10017):475–90.

[261] Walker WA, Iyengar RS. Breast milk, microbiota, and intestinal immune homeostasis. Pediatr Res 2015;77(1–2):220–8.

[262] Lönnerdal B. Bioactive proteins in human milk: mechanisms of action. J Pediatr 2010;156(2, Suppl.):S26–30.

[263] Rogier EW, Frantz AL, Bruno ME, et al. Secretory antibodies in breast milk promote long-term intestinal homeostasis by regulating the gut microbiota and host gene expression. Proc Natl Acad Sci USA 2014;111(8):3074–9.

[264] Rigon G, Vallone C, Lucantoni V, et al. Maternal factors pre-and during delivery contribute to gut microbiota shaping in newborns. Front Cell Infect Microbiol 2012;2:93.

[265] Jost T, Lacroix C, Braegger C, et al. Impact of human milk bacteria and oligosaccharides on neonatal gut microbiota establishment and gut health. Nutr Rev 2015;73(7):426–37.

[266] Eidelman AI, Schanler RJ, Johnston M, et al. Breastfeeding and the use of human milk. Pediatrics 2012;129(3):e827–41.

[267] Hunt KM, Foster JA, Forney LJ, et al. Characterization of the diversity and temporal stability of bacterial communities in human milk. PLoS ONE 2011;6(6):e21313.

[268] Jost T, Lacroix C, Braegger C, et al. Assessment of bacterial diversity in breast milk using culture-dependent and culture-independent approaches. Br J Nutr 2013;110(7):1253–62.

[269] Khodayar-Pardo P, Mira-Pascual L, Collado MC, et al. Impact of lactation stage, gestational age and mode of delivery on breast milk microbiota. J Perinatol 2014;34(8):599–605.

[270] Cabrera-Rubio R, Collado MC, Laitinen K, et al. The human milk microbiome changes over lactation and is shaped by maternal weight and mode of delivery. Am J Clin Nutr 2012;96(3):544–51.

[271] Vaishampayan PA, Kuehl JV, Froula JL, et al. Comparative metagenomics and population dynamics of the gut microbiota in mother and infant. Genome Biol Evol 2010;2:53–66.

[272] Kurokawa K, Itoh T, Kuwahara T, et al. Comparative metagenomics revealed commonly enriched gene sets in human gut microbiomes. DNA Res 2007;14(4):169–81.

[273] Fernández L, Langa S, Martin V, et al. The human milk microbiota: origin and potential roles in health and disease. Pharmacol Res 2013;69(1):1–10.

[274] Holgerson PL, Vestman NR, Claesson R, et al. Oral microbial profile discriminates breastfed from formula-fed infants. J Pediatr Gastroenterol Nutr 2013;56(2):127–36.

[275] Theriot CM, Koenigsknecht MJ, Carlson PE Jr, et al. Antibiotic-induced shifts in the mouse gut microbiome and metabolome increase susceptibility to Clostridium difficile infection. Nat Commun 2014;5:3114.

[276] Yassour M, Vatanen T, Siljander H, et al. Natural history of the infant gut microbiome and impact of antibiotic treatment on bacterial strain diversity and stability. Sci Transl Med 2016;8(343):343ra81.

[277] Arboleya S, Sanchez B, Milani C, et al. Intestinal microbiota development in preterm neonates and effect of perinatal antibiotics. J Pediatr 2015;166(3):538–44.

[278] Beaugerie L, Petit J-C. Antibiotic-associated diarrhoea. Best Pract Res Clin Gastroenterol 2004;18(2):337–52.

[279] Dethlefsen L, Huse S, Sogin ML, et al. The pervasive effects of an antibiotic on the human gut microbiota, as revealed by deep 16S rRNA sequencing. PLoS Biol 2008;6(11):e280.

[280] Freedberg DE, Lamousé-Smith ES, Lightdale JR, et al. Use of acid suppression medication is associated with risk for C. difficile infection in infants and children: a population-based study. Clin Infect Dis 2015;61:432.

[281] Schloss PD, Iverson KD, Petrosino JF, et al. The dynamics of a family's gut microbiota reveal variations on a theme. Microbiome 2014;2(1):25.

[282] Azad MB, Konya T, Maughan H, et al. Infant gut microbiota and the hygiene hypothesis of allergic disease: impact of household pets and siblings on microbiota composition and diversity. Allergy Asthma Clin Immunol 2013;9(1):15.

[283] Adlerberth I. Factors influencing the establishment of the intestinal microbiota in pregnancy. J Paediatr Child Health 2008;62:13–29.

[284] Rook GA. 99th Dahlem conference on infection, inflammation and chronic inflammatory disorders: darwinian medicine and the 'hygiene' or 'old friends' hypothesis. Clin Exp Immunol 2010;160(1):70–9.

[285] Leibowitz U, Antonovsky A, Medalie JM, et al. Epidemiological study of multiple sclerosis in Israel. II. Multiple sclerosis and level of sanitation. J Neurol Neurosurg Psychiatry 1966;29(1):60–8.

[286] Strachan DP. Hay fever, hygiene, and household size. BMJ 1989;299(6710):1259–60.

[287] Ponsonby A-L, Hughes AM, Lucas RM. The 'hygiene hypothesis' and the development of multiple sclerosis. Neurodegenerative Disease Management 2011;1(4):285–94.

[288] Janoff EN, Gustafson C, Frank DN. The world within: living with our microbial guests and guides. Transl Res 2012;160(4):239–45.

[289] Blaut M, Clavel T. Metabolic diversity of the intestinal microbiota: implications for health and disease. J Nutr 2007;137(3):751S–5S.

[290] Gong J, Yang C. Advances in the methods for studying gut microbiota and their relevance to the research of dietary fiber functions. Food Res Int 2012;48(2):916–29.

[291] Mulle JG, Sharp WG, Cubells JF. The gut microbiome: a new frontier in autism research. Curr Psychiatry Rep 2013;15(2):337.

[292] Zhang Y, Zhang H. Microbiota associated with type 2 diabetes and its related complications. Food Science and Human Wellness 2013;2(3–4):167–72.

[293] Knip M, Siljander H. The role of the intestinal microbiota in type 1 diabetes mellitus. Nat Rev Endocrinol 2016;12(3):154–67.

[294] Young VB, Schmidt TM. Antibiotic-associated diarrhea accompanied by large-scale alterations in the composition of the fecal microbiota. J Clin Microbiol 2004;42(3):1203–6.

[295] Chang JY, Antonopoulos DA, Kalra A, et al. Decreased diversity of the fecal microbiome in recurrent Clostridium difficile-associated diarrhea. J Infect Dis 2008;197(3):435–8.

[296] Touchefeu Y, Montassier E, Nieman K, et al. Systematic review: the role of the gut microbiota in chemotherapy- or radiation-induced gastrointestinal mucositis – current evidence and potential clinical applications. Aliment Pharmacol Ther 2014;40(5):409–21.

[297] Sartor RB, Mazmanian SK. Intestinal microbes in inflammatory bowel diseases. Am J Gastroenterol Suppl 2012;1(1):15–21.

[298] Barbara G, Scaioli E, Barbaro MR, et al. Gut microbiota, metabolome and immune signatures in patients with uncomplicated diverticular disease. Gut 2016;66(7):1252–61.

[299] Usami M, Miyoshi M, Yamashita H. Gut microbiota and host metabolism in liver cirrhosis. World J Gastroenterol 2015;21(41):11597–608.

[300] Distrutti E, Monaldi L, Ricci P, et al. Gut microbiota role in irritable bowel syndrome: new therapeutic strategies. World J Gastroenterol 2016;22(7):2219–41.

[301] Evrensel A, Ceylan ME. The gut-brain axis: the missing link in depression. Clin Psychopharmacol Neurosci 2015;13(3):239–44.

[302] Neufeld KA, Kang N, Bienenstock J, et al. Effects of intestinal microbiota on anxiety-like behavior. Commun Integr Biol 2011;4(4):492–4.

[303] Fujimura KE, Lynch SV. Microbiota in allergy and asthma and the emerging relationship with the gut microbiome. Cell Host Microbe 2015;17(5):592–602.

[304] Abrahamsson TR, Jakobsson HE, Andersson AF, et al. Low diversity of the gut microbiota in infants with atopic eczema. J Allergy Clin Immunol 2012;129(2):434–40.e2.

[305] Giloteaux L, Goodrich JK, Walters WA, et al. Reduced diversity and altered composition of the gut microbiome in individuals with myalgic encephalomyelitis/chronic fatigue syndrome. Microbiome 2016;4(1):30.

[306] Kaufman DW, Kelly JP, Curhan GC, et al. Oxalobacter formigenes may reduce the risk of calcium oxalate kidney stones. J Am Soc Nephrol 2008;19(6):1197–203.

[307] Boulangé CL, Neves AL, Chilloux J, et al. Impact of the gut microbiota on inflammation, obesity, and metabolic disease. Genome Med 2016;8(1):42.

[308] Wu X, He B, Liu J, et al. Molecular insight into gut microbiota and rheumatoid arthritis. Int J Mol Sci 2016;17(3):431.

[309] Chen J, Chia N, Kalari KR, et al. Multiple sclerosis patients have a distinct gut microbiota compared to healthy controls. Sci Rep 2016;6:28484.

[310] Felice VD, Quigley EM, Sullivan AM, et al. Microbiota-gut-brain signalling in Parkinson's disease: implications for non-motor symptoms. Parkinsonism Relat Disord 2016;27:1–8.

[311] Cenit MC, Olivares M, Codoner-Franch P, et al. Intestinal microbiota and celiac disease: cause, consequence or co-evolution? Nutrients 2015;7(8):6900–23.

[312] Langdon A, Crook N, Dantas G. The effects of antibiotics on the microbiome throughout development and alternative approaches for therapeutic modulation. Genome Med 2016;8(1):39.

[313] Francino MP. Antibiotics and the human gut microbiome: dysbioses and accumulation of resistances. Front Microbiol 2015;6:1543.

[314] Ferrer M, Méndez-García C, Rojo D, et al. Antibiotic use and microbiome function. Biochem Pharmacol 2017;134:114–26.

[315] Zwielehner J, Lassl C, Hippe B, et al. Changes in human fecal microbiota due to chemotherapy analyzed by TaqMan-PCR, 454 sequencing and PCR-DGGE fingerprinting. PLoS ONE 2011;6(12):e28654.

[316] Makivuokko H, Tiihonen K, Tynkkynen S, et al. The effect of age and non-steroidal anti-inflammatory drugs on human intestinal microbiota composition. Br J Nutr 2010;103(2):227–34.

[317] Blackler RW, De Palma G, Manko A, et al. Deciphering the pathogenesis of NSAID enteropathy using proton pump inhibitors and a hydrogen sulfide-releasing NSAID. Am J Physiol Gastrointest Liver Physiol 2015;308(12):G994–1003.

[318] Seto C, Jeraldo P, Orenstein R, et al. Prolonged use of a proton pump inhibitor reduces microbial diversity: implications for Clostridium difficile susceptibility. Microbiome 2014;2(1):42.

[319] Tsuda A, Suda W, Morita H, et al. Influence of proton-pump inhibitors on the luminal microbiota in the gastrointestinal tract. Clin Transl Gastroenterol 2015;6:e89.

[320] Imhann F, Bonder MJ, Vich Vila A, et al. Proton pump inhibitors affect the gut microbiome. Gut 2016;65(5):740–8.

[321] Jackson MA, Goodrich JK, Maxan M-E, et al. Proton pump inhibitors alter the composition of the gut microbiota. Gut 2016;65(5):749–56.

[322] Wallace J, Syer S, Denou E, et al. Proton pump inhibitors exacerbate NSAID-induced small intestinal injury by inducing dysbiosis. Gastroenterology 2011;141:1314–22.

[323] Nam YD, Kim HJ, Seo JG, et al. Impact of pelvic radiotherapy on gut microbiota of gynecological cancer patients revealed by massive pyrosequencing. PLoS ONE 2013;8(12):e82659.

[324] Suez J, Korem T, Zeevi D, et al. Artificial sweeteners induce glucose intolerance by altering the gut microbiota. Nature 2014;514(7521):181–6.

[325] Abou-Donia MB, El-Masry EM, Abdel-Rahman AA, et al. Splenda alters gut microflora and increases intestinal p-glycoprotein and cytochrome p-450 in male rats. J Toxicol Environ Health A 2008;71(21):1415–29.

[326] Duncan SH, Belenguer A, Holtrop G, et al. Reduced dietary intake of carbohydrates by obese subjects results in decreased concentrations of butyrate and butyrate-producing bacteria in feces. Appl Environ Microbiol 2007;73(4):1073–8.

[327] Brinkworth GD, Noakes M, Clifton PM, et al. Comparative effects of very low-carbohydrate, high-fat and high-carbohydrate, low-fat weight-loss diets on bowel habit and faecal short-chain fatty acids and bacterial populations. Br J Nutr 2009;101(10):1493–502.

[328] Tagliabue A, Ferraris C, Uggeri F, et al. Short-term impact of a classical ketogenic diet on gut microbiota in GLUT1 Deficiency Syndrome: a 3-month prospective observational study. Clin Nutr ESPEN 2017;17:33–7.

[329] Newell C, Bomhof MR, Reimer RA, et al. Ketogenic diet modifies the gut microbiota in a murine model of autism spectrum disorder. Mol Autism 2016;7(1):37.

[330] Halmos EP, Christophersen CT, Bird AR, et al. Diets that differ in their FODMAP content alter the colonic luminal microenvironment. Gut 2015;64(1):93–100.

[331] Staudacher HM, Lomer MC, Anderson JL, et al. Fermentable carbohydrate restriction reduces luminal bifidobacteria and gastrointestinal symptoms in patients with irritable bowel syndrome. J Nutr 2012;142(8):1510–18.

[332] Sanders ME. Probiotics: definition, sources, selection, and uses. Clin Infect Dis 2008;46(Suppl. 2):S58–61.

[333] Kristensen NB, Bryrup T, Allin KH, et al. Alterations in fecal microbiota composition by probiotic supplementation in healthy adults: a systematic review of randomized controlled trials. Genome Med 2016;8(1):52.

[334] Hawrelak J. Probiotics. In: Braun LA, Cohen M, editors. Herbs & natural supplements: an evidence-based guide 2. Sydney: Elsevier; 2015. p. 771–95.

[335] Nyangale EP, Farmer S, Cash HA, et al. Bacillus coagulans GBI-30, 6086 modulates Faecalibacterium prausnitzii in older men and women. J Nutr 2015;145(7):1446–52.

[336] Ahmed M, Prasad J, Gill H, et al. Impact of consumption of different levels of Bifidobacterium lactis HN019 on the intestinal microflora of elderly human subjects. J Nutr Health Aging 2007;11(1):26–31.

[337] Kondo J, Xiao JZ, Shirahata A, et al. Modulatory effects of Bifidobacterium longum BB536 on defecation in elderly patients receiving enteral feeding. World J Gastroenterol 2013;19(14):2162–70.

[338] Odamaki T, Sugahara H, Yonezawa S, et al. Effect of the oral intake of yogurt containing Bifidobacterium longum BB536 on the cell numbers of enterotoxigenic Bacteroides fragilis in microbiota. Anaerobe 2012;18(1):14–18.

[339] van Zanten GC, Krych L, Roytio H, et al. Synbiotic Lactobacillus acidophilus NCFM and cellobiose does not affect human gut bacterial diversity but increases abundance of lactobacilli, bifidobacteria and branched-chain fatty acids: a randomized,

double-blinded cross-over trial. FEMS Microbiol Ecol 2014;90(1):225–36.

[340] Spanhaak S, Havenaar R, Schaafsma G. The effect of consumption of milk fermented by Lactobacillus casei strain Shirota on the intestinal microflora and immune parameters in humans. Eur J Clin Nutr 1998;52:899–907.

[341] Benno Y, He F, Hosoda M, et al. Effects of Lactobacillus GG yoghurt on human intestinal microecology in Japanese subjects. Nutr Today 1996;31:9S–12S.

[342] Buddington RK, Williams CH, Chen S, et al. Dietary supplement of neosugar alters the fecal flora and decreases activities of some reductive enzymes in human subjects. Am J Clin Nutr 1996;63:709–16.

[343] Ramirez-Farias C, Slezak K, Fuller Z, et al. Effect of inulin on the human gut microbiota: stimulation of Bifidobacterium adolescentis and Faecalibacterium prausnitzii. Br J Nutr 2009;101(4):541–50.

[344] Gibson GR, Beatty ER, Wang X, et al. Selective stimulation of bifidobacteria in the human colon by oligofructose and inulin. Gastroenterology 1995;108:975–82.

[345] Kleesen B, Sykura B, Zunft HJ, et al. Effects of inulin and lactose on fecal microflora, microbial activity, and bowel habit in elderly constipated persons. Am J Clin Nutr 1997;65:1397–402.

[346] Ito M, Deguchi Y, Matsumoto K, et al. Influence of galactooligosaccharides on the human fecal microflora. J Nutr Sci Vitaminol 1993;39:635–40.

[347] Vulevic J, Drakoularakou A, Yaqoob P, et al. Modulation of the fecal microflora profile and immune function by a novel trans-galactooligosaccharide mixture (B-GOS) in healthy elderly volunteers. Am J Clin Nutr 2008;88(5):1438–46.

[348] Davis LMG, Martinez I, Walter J, et al. Barcoded pyrosequencing reveals that consumption of galactooligosaccharides results in a highly specific bifidogenic response in humans. PLoS ONE 2011;6(9):e25200.

[349] Terada A, Hara H, Kataoka M, et al. Effect of lactulose on the composition and metabolic activity of the human faecal flora. Microbial Ecology in Health and Disease 1992;5:43–50.

[350] Bouhnik Y, Attar A, Joly FA, et al. Lactulose ingestion increases faecal bifidobacterial counts: a randomised double-blind study in healthy humans. Eur J Clin Nutr 2004;58(3):462–6.

[351] Liu Z, Lin X, Huang G, et al. Prebiotic effects of almonds and almond skins on intestinal microbiota in healthy adult humans. Anaerobe 2014;26:1–6.

[352] Shinohara K, Ohashi Y, Kawasumi K, et al. Effect of apple intake on fecal microbiota and metabolites in humans. Anaerobe 2010;16(5):510–15.

[353] Molan A-L, Liu Z, Plimmer G. Evaluation of the effect of blackcurrant products on gut microbiota and on markers of risk for colon cancer in humans. Phytother Res 2014;28(3):416–22.

[354] Vendrame S, Guglielmetti S, Riso P, et al. Six-week consumption of a wild blueberry powder drink increases bifidobacteria in the human gut. J Agric Food Chem 2011;59(24):12815–20.

[355] Benno Y, Endo K, Miyoshi H, et al. Effect of rice fiber on human fecal microflora. Microbiol Immunol 1989;33(5):435–40.

[356] Tzounis X, Rodriguez-Mateos A, Vulevic J, et al. Prebiotic evaluation of cocoa-derived flavanols in healthy humans by using a randomized, controlled, double-blind, crossover intervention study. Am J Clin Nutr 2011;93(1):62–72.

[357] Goto K, Kanaya S, Nishikawa T, et al. The influence of tea catechins on fecal flora of elderly residents in long-term care facilities. Ann Long-Term Care 1998;6:43–8.

[358] Zaman SA. Sarbini SR. The potential of resistant starch as a prebiotic. Crit Rev Biotechnol 2016;36(3):578–84.

[359] Fuentes-Zaragoza E, Sánchez-Zapata E, Sendra E, et al. Resistant starch as prebiotic: a review. Starch – Stärke 2011;63(7):406–15.

[360] Birt DF, Boylston T, Hendrich S, et al. Resistant starch: promise for improving human health. Adv Nutr 2013;4(6):587–601.

[361] Venkataraman A, Sieber JR, Schmidt AW, et al. Variable responses of human microbiomes to dietary supplementation with resistant starch. Microbiome 2016;4(1):33.

[362] Martínez I, Kim J, Duffy PR, et al. J. Resistant starches types 2 and 4 have differential effects on the composition of the fecal microbiota in human subjects. PLoS ONE 2010;5(11):e15046.

[363] Walker AW, Ince J, Duncan SH, et al. Dominant and diet-responsive groups of bacteria within the human colonic microbiota. ISME J 2011;5(2):220–30.

[364] Rea K, Dinan TG, Cryan JF. The microbiome: a key regulator of stress and neuroinflammation. Neurobiol Stress 2016;4:23–33.

[365] Mach N, Fuster-Botella D. Endurance exercise and gut microbiota: a review. J Sport Health Sci 2017;6(2):179–97.

[366] Heiman ML, Greenway FL. A healthy gastrointestinal microbiome is dependent on dietary diversity. Mol Metab 2016;5(5):317–20.

[367] Bajaj JS, Heuman DM, Hylemon PB, et al. Altered profile of human gut microbiome is associated with cirrhosis and its complications. J Hepatol 2014;60(5):940–7.

[368] Mao B, Li D, Ai C, et al. Lactulose differently modulates the composition of luminal and mucosal microbiota in C57BL/6J mice. J Agric Food Chem 2016;64(31):6240–7.

7

Methylation

Annalies Jane Corse

INTRODUCTION

Methylation is very much a contemporary subject in naturopathic education and practice. In our profession today, it is essential to have an understanding of biochemistry, genetics, physiology and nutritional biochemistry in order to comprehend the enormity of what the successful treatment of methylation disorders means for the individual and for human health in the future. Every year, a myriad of research is published in the scientific literature regarding methylation disorders. Naturopathic practitioners are incredibly well positioned to safely and effectively manage methylation disorders, but this requires a commitment to understanding the scientific evidence that underpins methylation research. The study of methylation is deeply embedded in the subspecialisations of molecular biology and biochemistry, both of which require continual learning. The clinical application of nutritional and lifestyle interventions can then follow, supported further by science, novel therapeutics research and the clinical insights of experienced practitioners.

Practitioners of naturopathic and orthodox medicine find themselves at what may be described as a clinical impasse: merging our knowledge and treatment approaches represents the best way forward in managing methylation issues for long-term patient health. The capability of medical science to determine the exact mechanisms linking methylation disorders with disease is remarkable and will continue. The naturopathic approaches of nutritional, environmental and lifestyle medicine offer a means of treating and managing these conditions from an evidence-based perspective.

Molecular biology is a scientific specialisation that studies nucleic acids, genes and their protein products. Molecular biology has revolutionised modern science, having a particularly profound impact on medicine and health with respect to pathophysiology, diagnostics and epigenetics. The mapping of the human genome during the 1990s and early 21st century was only a momentary culmination of what molecular biology has to offer medical science. The Human Genome Project provided a scientific springboard from which the exploration of epigenetics, the emergence of our knowledge regarding single nucleotide polymorphisms (SNPs) and the potential of gene therapy can shape the future of modern healthcare, in both naturopathic and conventional medical practice. The process of methylation is inextricably linked to all three of these burgeoning areas of medical science.

The essential nature of methylation to life is irrefutable: it is one of the most important and commonly occurring biochemical processes in the human body and in other living organisms. As a biochemical process, methylation occurs every second of life in every cell, from the moment of conception until death. Molecular biology has also demonstrated that epigenetic methylation is activated post mortem. Thousands of biochemical reactions rely on correct methylation. There is no subspecialty of medicine unaffected by methylation: genetics, oncology, neurology, cardiology, immunology, biochemistry, physiology, pathophysiology, endocrinology, embryology, obstetrics and gynaecology, andrology, hepatology, toxicology and metabolism are some of the more common areas of clinical application.

The importance of methylation to human health often focuses on its role in epigenetics. However, methylation is a ubiquitous biochemical process, reaching far beyond molecular biology. The scope of this chapter encompasses the biochemical, genetic and metabolic features of methylation, and the clinical relevance of methylation to the individual and the wider implications of aberrant methylation to human health. The relationship between methylation, metabolic pathways and their enzyme catalysts is exemplified beyond simple diagrams, highlighting the importance of methylation to fundamental biochemical and physiological processes.

As clinicians, we frequently see cases of erroneous methylation in our clinics – although this may not be immediately evident. In clinical practice and methylation education, there can be a heavy focus on supratherapeutic dosing of key nutrients known to support methylation biochemistry. For some patients, such a strategy may be essential for the long term, or a short time. For other patients, robust dosage regimens are unnecessary. Many dietary and environmental obstacles place excessive burden on methylation metabolic pathways, or diminish the cache of methyl groups required for well-balanced biochemistry. This can occur without the usual presence of genetic polymorphisms associated with methylation disorders. In clinic, it is important to remember that methylation problems have both genetic *and* lifestyle causes. Some people require robust nutraceutical prescriptions, while others respond better to nutritional, lifestyle and phytochemical therapies addressing the microbiome, stress, sleep and lifestyle.

There is no one clinical protocol for the treatment of methylation disorders. Although methylation disorders arise from common genetic polymorphisms, they frequently evolve from the intricate biochemical results of toxin overexposure, poor sleep hygiene, disordered stress response, medication use, diet, exercise patterns and physical fitness. The clinical sections of this chapter focus on both paediatric and adult presentations of disordered methylation, including a discussion of conditions correlating with methylation concerns. Molecular diagnostic testing and the therapeutic interventions necessary to safely and effectively support patients are also presented.

DEVELOPMENTAL AND EVOLUTIONARY ORIGINS

Methylation is commonly referred to as one-carbon metabolism, or 1C metabolism.[1] It is a vital biochemical process in all living organisms, from both a genetic and a metabolic perspective. Methyl groups are transferred and chemically bonded to thousands of biological compounds in every cell, every day: life for any organism would not exist without methylation.

Methylation is also significant from a developmental and an embryological perspective. The deoxyribonucleic acid (DNA) of the early embryo is hypomethylated. Via environmental cues within the embryo-fetal-maternal milieu, DNA methylation progressively increases. This facilitates organogenesis and tissue differentiation.[1] In this regard, methylation is crucial to healthy embryogenesis and the formation of a living organism from the very first stages of life. During embryogenesis and early postnatal life, the DNA methylation patterns of the fetus and the infant are established. These patterns are heavily affected by environmental signals, including nutrient supply and maternal and fetal stress, and the patterns established in utero and in early infancy are imperative to the future health of the individual. Silencing imprinted genes (genes that will not be expressed) and the emergence of transgenerational diseases not linked to gene mutations reflect the methylation process.[2] These topics are discussed later in the chapter.

From an evolutionary perspective, the role of methylation is only beginning to be explored. The concept of developmental plasticity examines how methylation is involved when an individual's genotype responds to the environment by modifying its phenotype to suit the environment.[2] In evolutionary terms, this may describe why certain phenotypic traits (both favourable and unfavourable) present in the population. Species-specific adaptations and variable phenotypes were linked with methylation four decades ago, but the exact mechanisms have only been investigated solidly in the past decade.[3] Different mammalian species have very similar genomes, but it is the pattern of DNA methylation that possibly makes us different, or has favoured the retaining or emergence of favourable evolutionary traits. This emerging aspect of genetics is known as the methylome as opposed to the genome.[4] Optimising the parental–fetal environment towards one promoting a healthy methylome represents a huge opportunity in the practice of preventive healthcare.

CHEMISTRY AND BIOCHEMISTRY OF THE METHYL GROUP

Before delving into the intricacies of epigenetic and metabolic methylation, it is important to understand the basic chemical foundations that underpin these processes. Doing so helps practitioners to understand exactly why certain prescriptions are made for the treatment of methylation disorders. Revising biochemistry and genetics helps us to explain the evidence base behind naturopathic interventions. Revisiting the simple chemistry and biochemistry of the methyl group is necessary to facilitate a deeper understanding of how such a diminutive chemical entity influences human health in profound ways. The dictum *structure equals function* is, regrettably, overlooked by many when studying biology and physiology. Many processes can be explained by relating the actions of a chemical back to its molecular structure. Analysing chemical structures reveals a wealth of information regarding their eventual functions.

- The methyl group is an example of an organic molecule, as its structure is based on carbon to hydrogen bonds. A methyl group contains only carbon (C) and hydrogen (H) atoms and is considered a simple organic molecule for this reason; no other elements are present.
- Other organic molecules include the alkanes, alkenes and alkynes (carbon-to-carbon single, double and triple bonds, respectively). More complex organic molecules retain the carbon-to-hydrogen base structure, but also include elements such as oxygen (O), nitrogen (N), phosphorus (P) and sulfur (S).
- All molecules pertaining to living organisms (e.g. hormones, enzymes, carbohydrates, proteins, lipids, nucleic acids, vitamins, neurotransmitters) are organic molecules based on carbon to hydrogen bonding. Many contain significant structures such as benzene rings, a steroid nucleus or other functional groups. Functional groups are additions, bonded to the 'parent' carbon to hydrogen structure. The methyl group is an example of a functional group. Functional groups are also referred to as alkyl groups. In biochemistry, most chemical reactions occur between the functional groups on separate biological molecules. Functional groups are quite reactive, while the 'parent' hydrocarbon structure is comparatively inert.
- These structural modifications, and the sheer variety of structural combinations occurring in nature, give rise to the infinite variety of chemical compounds observed in the living world. Arguably, the methyl group is the smallest of them all.

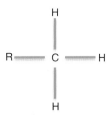

FIGURE 7.1 One carbon atom: the basic structural formula of the methyl group. The 'R' group represents the various organic substrates to which methyl groups can bond (e.g. nucleic acids, proteins, peptides, lipids).

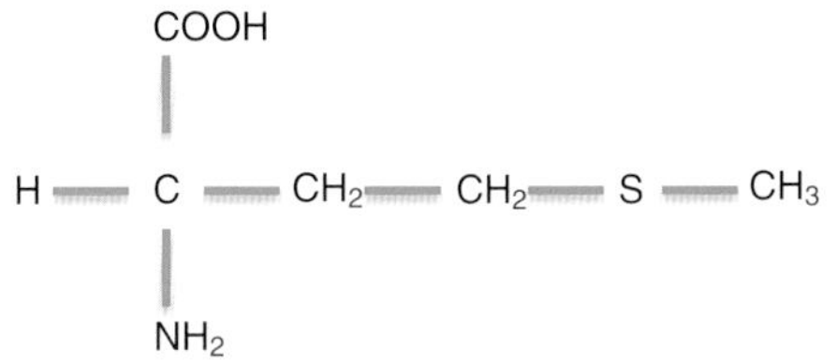

$$H - C - CH_2 - CH_2 - S - CH_3$$

with COOH above C and NH₂ below C

FIGURE 7.2 The basic structural formula of methionine. In methionine, the methyl group is bonded directly to the sulfur atom.

A closer look at the methyl group reveals the following:

- Molecular formula: CH_3. One carbon atom is bonded to three hydrogen atoms, all via single bonds (see Fig. 7.1). A carbon atom always forms four bonds with other atoms; with a methyl group, the remaining bond attaches the methyl group to the parent carbon chain. Such carbon chains may be proteins, nucleic acids and other complex biological molecules.
- Bonding within the methyl group involves covalent bonding (i.e. between non-metallic elements). Covalent bonds within the methyl group display a non-polar arrangement, making the methyl group hydrophobic. This property prevents the methyl group from reacting with nearby water molecules, an important quality for many biological molecules.
- Due to the single bonds present, methyl groups are chemically quite stable and unreactive; the reactivity of any methyl group is usually dictated by the properties of adjacent alkyl groups to which the methyl group is attached.
- Methyl groups are synthesised endogenously via reduction (addition of one hydrogen atom) to a methylene (CH_2) group. This can be observed as part of the folate cycle.
- Exogenous methyl groups can be obtained via the diet, starting with the essential amino acid, methionine (see Fig. 7.2). Our biochemistry has the ability to recover methionine once the methyl group has been removed. This can be observed as part of the methionine cycle.
- Demethylation involves the removal of a methyl group from a compound. The addition of a methyl group to a compound describes methylation. The removal or addition of methyl groups changes the chemical structure of a molecule, thus changing its shape and altering its function. Methylation, demethylation and remethylation are all common processes in living organisms.

REVISION OF KEY BIOCHEMICAL STRUCTURES

Rapid advances in our understanding of molecular genetics and methylation are providing new approaches to clinical problems. For naturopathic medicine, this focus is largely based on nutritional biochemistry and lifestyle medicine, while orthodox medicine focuses on genomics.[5] Regardless of the focus, revisiting some key concepts of molecular genetics is required to understand and appreciate the role of methylation in the health of the genome. This section provides a brief overview only; readers are encouraged to supplement the detail provided here with further revision of basic molecular biology.

Nucleic acid structure

The nitrogenous bases found in DNA and RNA are named due to their alkaline pH; this property is a direct result of their chemical structure. All bases are examples of heterocyclic aromatic amines: all are based on cyclic structures containing nitrogen, with additional attachment of other structures and functional groups. All contain amine groups (N atoms bonded to C atoms). The amine group is alkaline.[4] There are five bases important to the structure of DNA and RNA, and each can be classified further based on its chemical structure:

- Adenine (A) is a purine base. It is found in both DNA and RNA. From the structure, there is an amine functional group located at position 6 of the ring structure.
- Guanine (G) is a purine base. It is found in both DNA and RNA. From the structure, there is a ketone functional group at position 6 and amine groups at positions 1 and 2.
- Cytosine (C) is a pyrimidine base. It is found in both DNA and RNA. From the structure, there is an amine group at position 1. All pyrimidines contain ketone groups on position 2. The cytosine nucleotide is significant to the process of methylation, as methyl groups are known to attach to cytosine bases. Methylation occurs in DNA in locations where cytosine is followed by guanosine (the CpG dinucleotide).[3]
- Thymine (T) is a pyrimidine base. It is found in DNA only. From the structure, there is an amine group at position 3 and a methyl group at position 5.
- Uracil (U) is a pyrimidine base. It is found in RNA only, present instead of T bases in RNA. From the structure, an amine group is present at position 3.

Fig. 7.3 presents the five principal bases of DNA and RNA. Purines are bicyclic, containing two nitrogenous rings fused together. Pyrimidines are smaller and monocyclic, containing only one nitrogenous ring. The hydrogen atoms (shaded) are removed when a base bonds with either deoxyribose or ribose.[4]

The bases are complementary: during all chemical interactions between bases in DNA structure and processes such as transcription and translation, a base will match

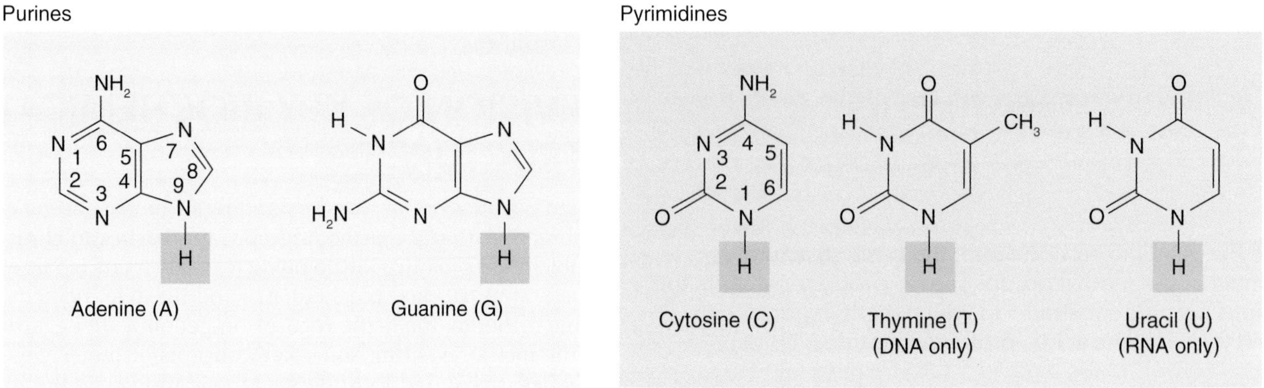

Purines

Adenine (A)　　　　　Guanine (G)

Pyrimidines

Cytosine (C)　　　Thymine (T)　　　Uracil (U)
　　　　　　　　　(DNA only)　　　(RNA only)

FIGURE 7.3 Purine and pyrimidine bases of DNA and RNA.

Bettelheim F, Brown W, Campbell M, et al. Nucleotides, nucleic acids, and heredity. In: Introduction to general, organic and biochemistry. 10th edn. Belmont: Brooks/Cole, Cengage Learning; 2013, p. 689.

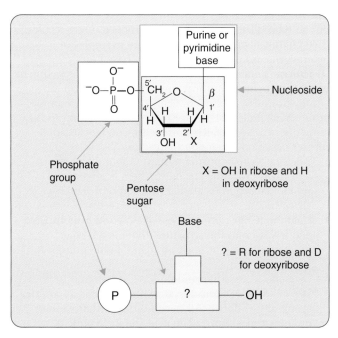

FIGURE 7.4 The general structure of a nucleotide.

Batmanian L, Ridge J, Worrall S. Nucleic acids: biological molecules for information storage, retrieval and usage. In: Biochemistry for health professionals. Sydney: Elsevier; 2011, pp. 101–109.

only to its complementary base. A large purine will match with a small pyrimidine. In DNA, this facilitates an even and uniform structure for the eventual double helix conformation.

DNA

DNA molecules are large and consist of smaller subunits called deoxyribonucleotides. Each subunit consists of one base (A, G, C or T) bonded to deoxyribose (a pentose sugar), bonded to a phosphate group (PO_4^-).

Fig. 7.4 presents the structure of a deoxyribonucleotide. A nucleoside refers to a base attached to a sugar

(deoxyribose in this case). Once the nucleoside attaches to a phosphate group, it is known as a nucleotide. When multiple nucleotides join together, a molecule of DNA begins to form.[5] DNA is a double helix consisting of two strands. Recall that these strands are chemically bonded via complementary base pairs. The helical shape allows for considerable compaction of huge amounts of DNA to produce chromosomes. The chromosomes are located in the nucleus of eukaryotes (multicellular organisms).

RNA

Ribonucleic acid (RNA) structure is also based on nucleotides, known as ribonucleotides. Another pentose sugar, ribose, is present instead of deoxyribose. Thymine is replaced by uracil in RNA. RNA is a single-stranded molecule but with various forms based on its function.

mRNA

Messenger RNA (mRNA) is a mobile molecule.[5] mRNA is significant in the process of transcription, where information encoded in DNA must be copied and transported out of the nucleus to the site of protein synthesis, the ribosomes.

tRNA

The transfer RNA (tRNA) family consists of multiple small RNA molecules.[5] tRNA molecules transfer specific amino acids to ribosomes during the process of protein synthesis.

rRNA

Ribosomal RNA (rRNA) accounts for approximately 80% of all the RNA in a cell and is a major component of the structure of ribosomes.[5] rRNA helps decode information presented by mRNA and facilitates the correct insertion of amino acids into a growing peptide chain.[5]

REVISION OF BASIC MOLECULAR BIOLOGY

Chromatin

For conceptual reasons, the genome is often represented in a linear fashion. In reality, the genome is a far more dynamic three-dimensional landscape.[6] As long segments of DNA begin to condense, the material becomes more visible under microscopy. This condensed DNA within the nucleus is known as chromatin. Chromatin is not bare DNA double helices, but rather is DNA in complex with several classes of specialised proteins known as histones.[7]

Histones

There are five major protein histones crucial to the correct packaging of chromatin in the nucleus.[6] Not only do histones provide a scaffold for the spooling of DNA for compaction, but the various types are also highly specialised. Histone structure can be modified via chemical changes, leading to a structure and function pattern that varies from cell type to cell type. This possibly dictates how accessible DNA is to methylation and other regulatory processes involved in gene expression.[7] As more and more chromatin is in complex with histones, chromosomes begin to form. In addition to DNA, histones are known to undergo methylation, representing another point for epigenetic gene regulation.

Fig. 7.5 illustrates the levels of chromatin packaging in human chromosomes.

Chromosomes

In humans, there are normally 46 chromosomes, ordered in 23 pairs. The first 22 pairs are known as autosomes, with the final pair consisting of the sex chromosomes (XX in a female and XY in a male). One chromosome from each pair is inherited from the mother and the other is inherited from the father.[8] Alterations to the number of chromosomes result in specific genetic conditions. For the purposes of locating genes or their mutation, this is often done by naming their exact location on a specific chromosome.

Cell division

Many cell populations in adult tissues are quiescent: they are biochemically active and functional, yet they do not undergo frequent or rapid cell division.[9] Some populations including haematopoietic cells, integumentary tissue and gastrointestinal mucosal cells replicate frequently, but the control of cell division in other tissue types is tightly regulated.[9] Cell proliferation is also highly regulated, influenced by factors such as nutrients, growth factors and inhibitory factors.[10] Disruption of the cell cycle and cell division control is a distinctive trait of malignant growth. Methylation changes in genes related to cell cycle control are just one of the molecular mechanisms involved in malignant transformation.[11]

As a cell prepares to divide, it must first enter the cell cycle, where every gene on every chromosome must be replicated with high fidelity. Somatic cells divide once via mitosis, resulting in two daughter cells with the full

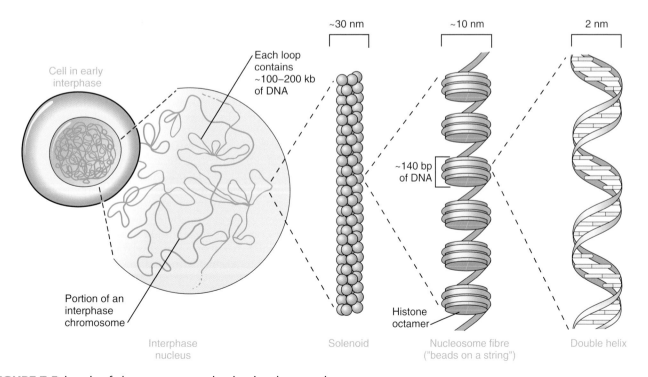

FIGURE 7.5 Levels of chromosome packaging in a human chromosome.

Nussbaum R, McInnes C, Willard H. The human genome: structure and function. In: Thomson and Thomson genetics in medicine. 8th edn. Philadelphia: Elsevier; 2016.

complement of 23 chromosome pairs. Gametes (ova and spermatozoa) divide twice via meiosis, resulting in four daughter cells, each with one single chromosome from the 23 pairs.

Gene structure and function

As methylation is intricately involved in epigenetics and gene expression, it is important to briefly review gene structure and function. Genes are the basic unit of inheritance, transmitted from parents to offspring, passing on countless physical and possibly emotional traits. Certain diseases can be passed on via genetic inheritance; methylation may be involved in whether or not these diseases are physically expressed. Genes ultimately influence every aspect of body structure and function.[12]

INTRONS

The term 'intron' refers to DNA sequences within a gene and their corresponding sequences in RNA after DNA transcription. Introns form the major portion of most eukaryotic genes.[12] Intron derives from the term 'intragenic region' (a region inside a gene).[13] Introns do not code for proteins, though they are pivotal for the regulation of gene expression.[13]

EXONS

Exons are regions of a gene containing the sequence ultimately transcribed to mRNA. Exons appear to have a higher level of methylation compared to flanking introns. This is most likely a transcriptional control provided by methylation.[14]

CODONS

The term 'codon' refers to triplets of three base nucleotides in either DNA or RNA. Each codon of the genetic code translates to or encodes an amino acid in the 'language' of proteins.[15]

THE GENETIC CODE

Functional proteins of living organisms range from small peptides through to large polypeptides consisting of several individual peptide chains. Regardless of their size and length, all proteins are composed of sequences of amino acids.[12] The actual sequence of amino acids is unique for every protein. The genetic code simply refers to the language of genes and how it is translated into the language of amino acids.

There are 20 different amino acids necessary for protein structure and only 4 or 5 (depending on DNA or RNA structure) base nucleotides, thus a single base does not translate to a single amino acid. To reach the required number of 20, bases are translated by codons. Each codon translates to an amino acid; this is known as the genetic code. Arranging the 4 bases into codons gives us 64 possible codon combinations: 3 signify the end of a gene (stop codons), the other 61 specify amino acids, thus most amino acids are specified by more than one codon.[12]

As a chemical process, methylation can take place on the minute chemical structures of base nucleotides, through to complex and physiologically active histones and functional proteins. This encompasses the fundamental role of methylation in epigenetics or gene expression, a facet of health that medical and clinical research is hastening to understand.

METHYLATION AND MITOCHONDRIA

Questioning a potential role for methylation in mitochondrial function is natural, as mitochondria are known to possess their own genes and DNA, known as mitochondrial DNA (mtDNA). mtDNA contains the genes governing many of the vital functions of mitochondria, including regeneration of adenosine triphosphate (ATP) via the electron transport chain (ETC) and oxidative phosphorylation. Mitochondria are also responsible for beta-oxidation of fatty acids. While mtDNA methylation is attracting increasing attention as a potential biomarker for certain diseases, this interest remains controversial.[16]

Each mitochondrion contains multiple copies of DNA molecules, and the arrangement of mtDNA is distinct from nuclear DNA (nDNA). mtDNA exists as a closed circular, double-stranded molecule.[17] Coding regions contain 13 protein-coding genes responsible for the ETC and the genes required for mitochondrial RNA (required for protein synthesis).[17] Unlike nDNA, mtDNA is not protected by chromatin, thus the mutation rate of mtDNA is relatively high.[17] These mutations give rise to a large and diverse cluster of diseases known as the mitochondrial disorders. Mitochondrial disorders are genetic, inherited diseases of maternal lineage; all mtDNA in an individual is derived from the ovum at fertilisation. Spermatozoa contribute no mitochondria to the zygote.[17] On the other hand, some genes for mitochondrial function are located in nDNA, thus some mitochondrial disorders follow the usual Mendelian inheritance patterns.[18]

The epigenome of mtDNA does appear to involve methylation. Methyltransferase enzymes are present and active in mitochondria, but the isolation of these enzymes from mitochondria has been successful only from certain tissues.[19] Additionally, epigenetic changes in the nuclear genome may be due to altered methylation in mDNA, but the exact links remain unknown.[19] Some studies are showing that aberrant methylation of mtDNA might be influenced by ageing, chronic disease and stress, specific environmental toxin exposure and certain medications, particularly those that deplete B complex vitamins.[16]

Mitochondria are known to alter methylation patterns in nDNA. This occurs via a mitochondrial influence on folate metabolism and the cytoplasmic folate cycle, resulting in the production of S-adenosylmethionine (SAMe). SAMe is a critical chemical entity for the donation of methyl groups (discussed later). mtDNA alterations are also known to influence both hyper- and hypomethylation in numerous nuclear genes.[20]

TRANSCRIPTION AND TRANSLATION

In order for a gene to be expressed and to offer an organism the physical protein product encoded within its sequence of base nucleotides, several subcellular mechanisms must be initiated. These include DNA transcription to mRNA, transport of this mRNA transcript from the nucleus to the cytoplasm, translation of the transcript into a protein and post-translational processing of the protein.[21] Each step is highly regulated, and each step provides options for a cell to progress to the next phase or to mitigate or terminate the process. The significance of this is that faulty mRNA transcripts are not transported out of the nucleus and the production of faulty proteins is eliminated. Ultimately, each phase represents a point in time when the expression of a gene can be regulated. For brevity, transcription and translation are reviewed here.

Transcription

Essentially, transcription means to transcribe: information held in protein-coding genes is copied onto a transcript, a molecule of mRNA. mRNA is not pre-existing; it forms when expression of a gene is initiated. The base nucleotide sequence of DNA is read and a corresponding sequence of mRNA is generated, according to complementary base pairing. The formation of mRNA is catalysed by the enzyme RNA polymerase II (RNAPol II).[21] mRNA then exits the nucleus and is transported to cytoplasmic ribosomes in preparation for protein synthesis.

Methylation is more often associated with regions of DNA that are less active in transcription. In order for DNA to be transcribed, it must be in a hypomethylated state, thus demethylation of coding sequences of a gene is required for efficient transcription.[20] Methylation is involved in blocking regions of a gene not to be transcribed, representing an important epigenetic control mechanism. DNA demethylation exposes DNA to transcriptional activators; however, the enzymes responsible for DNA demethylation during normal gene transcription remain elusive.[22] The emerging science of nutrigenomics examines the role of nutritional factors in regulating methylation and other epigenetic controls of gene expression, such as histone acetylation and phosphorylation.[21]

Translation

Once a molecule of mRNA makes contact with a ribosome, it travels through the ribosome. mRNA enters via its chain-initiating codon, with its chain-terminating codon signalling the end of the gene transcript.[23] During this process, both tRNA and rRNA are working to translate the nucleotide sequence of mRNA, codon by codon, to a sequence of amino acids. A growing peptide or polypeptide chain begins to form within the ribosome, under the influence of numerous chemical reactions.

Methylation is critical to protein translation in two key areas:

1   Many protein products undergo post-translation modifications, methylation being one of them.[24] Methylation confers subtle changes to the primary structure of a peptide chain, ultimately influencing its three-dimensional structure and physiological function. Depending on the biological role of the methylated protein, different results are produced. For example, methylated proteins are often involved in DNA repair, control of transcription and protein translocation (the transport of proteins across cellular compartments).[25]

2   Proteins involved in translation, such as ribosomal proteins and translation proteins (both part of the ribosomal milieu), are significantly methylated.[24]

PROTEIN SYNTHESIS

It is estimated that a typical human cell is required to synthesise approximately 10000 different proteins.[26] As described, this occurs according to the instructions encoded in mRNA molecules during transcription and translation. Protein synthesis is a dynamic collection of reactions involving many enzymes, multiple ribosomes, translation factors and every form of RNA. Orchestrating a process such as protein synthesis is a monumental task for a cell, yet in most cases it unfolds without fault. Protein synthesis is often divided into three phases: initiation, elongation and termination.[26] All must proceed correctly for a functional protein to be synthesised correctly.

Several biochemical guardians are critical during the three stages of protein biosynthesis, methylation being one of these. Structurally, all ribosomes and many translation factors are proteins: their structure alone makes them susceptible to the effects of protein methylation.[27] The biological significance of ribosomal and translation factor methylation is an ongoing question in research. However, it appears that methylation modulates the affinity of ribosomes and translation factors for their RNA at the molecular level. This would probably influence the regulation of transcription (an epigenetic control) and the accuracy of translation.[27]

A newly synthesised protein is not functional until it acquires its unique three-dimensional structure. Once the termination point of the protein's amino acid sequence has been identified by a ribosome, structural refining commences. This is known as post-translational modification.[24]

PROTEIN METHYLATION AND POST-TRANSLATIONAL MODIFICATION

For a protein to completely 'mature', numerous modifications to protein architecture are required. Recall from protein biochemistry that protein structure consists of a primary structure (correct and unique amino acid sequence), followed by a secondary structure (the presence and arrangement of alpha helices and beta-pleated sheets) and a tertiary structure. Only some proteins (usually those with several subunits) develop a further quaternary structure. The tertiary structure is commonly modified in several important ways, one of these being the addition of functional groups of molecular appendages along the protein chain.[28] Examples of post-translational modifications include methylation, phosphorylation, glycosylation, ubiquitylation (also referred to as ubiquitination), acetylation and lipidation.[28]

Post-translational modifications occur at precise locations on the amino acid chain, at any phase of protein chain assemblage and growth. These modifications are mediated by enzyme activity. During post-translational modification via methylation, a family of enzymes known as the methyltransferases attach methyl groups to arginine or lysine residues.[28] During protein methylation, a methyl group donor known as SAMe provides the supply of methyl groups.[29]

Methylation is an important mechanism of epigenetic regulation. For example, changes in the methylation status of protein-based histones influence the availability of DNA for transcription.[28] Many methylating enzymes are specific for histones (thus they are essential for modulating DNA transcription and are an important epigenetic control mechanism), but many modify non-histone protein substrates such as ribosomes and RNA.[30] As research accumulates, it is believed that evidence for methyltransferase activity beyond genomic activities will increase, revealing a greater impact for this enzyme family on specific aspects of mammalian cellular physiology and possible disease states.[30] The essentiality of methyltransferases to the post-translational modification of proteins involved in lipid biosynthesis, protein repair, hormone inactivation and tissue differentiation has been known for several decades.[31] Non-epigenetic roles for the methyltransferase enzyme family are featured later in the chapter.

EPIGENETICS, METHYLATION AND GENE EXPRESSION

For the past few decades, we have observed enormous progress in genetics and molecular biology, yet the nucleotide sequence–gene–amino acid sequence–protein product aspect of genetics does not adequately explain certain facets of human biology.[32] There is far more to a gene than its sequence of base nucleotides. The human genome project revealed that our genome possesses only one-third of the predicted number of genes, thus other factors are involved in the functionality of our genome. The development and evolution of the human species have required differentiation of cells to create not only functional organs, but also various cell types within the same organ. This highly specialised development relies on epigenetics, the science of what occurs 'on the top of' genes.[33]

> Epigenetics refers to modifications to DNA and its associated proteins that define the distinct gene-expression profiles for individual cell types at specific developmental stages.[32]

Some phenotypical traits are epigenetic as opposed to genetic traits. During cell differentiation, genes interact with their environment to produce a certain 'physical' phenotype. Subject to the environment encountered, a gene's activity can be upregulated or downregulated.[33] Depending on the gene involved, this activity may be inconsequential, advantageous, mildly problematic or potentially lethal to the organism. Epigenetic traits are sometimes stable enough to be inherited and result from changes to a chromosome, without any alteration to the DNA base sequence.[33] Epigenetic changes occur far more rapidly than gene mutations, thus providing a mechanism for a swift cellular response to environmental change.[34] This is often referred to as the plasticity of the epigenome.[33] In a dynamic sense, it is important for an organism to change to suit its environment. This becomes problematic when the resulting phenotype is not suitable for future environmental changes – for example, a reduced nutrient supply in utero versus a lifetime diet of high-energy food, leading to the metabolic syndrome.

Various biochemical processes are collectively responsible for epigenetic changes. Methylation is a critical epigenetic mechanism; it can take place at various points within the superstructure of chromosomes and create a methylation pattern in the wider genome. Depending on the pattern of these modifications, certain epigenetic traits may be maintained, activated or silenced.[32] Methylation is known to repress gene activity.[34] Again, subject to the gene implicated, methylation may be favourable or unfavourable (e.g. a methylated versus an unmethylated tumour suppressor gene). Methylation is fundamental to gene regulation; further epigenetic processes are known to maintain methylation across cell division, while others lead to de novo DNA methylation events.[32] Methylation exerts its control over genes at restricted sites, specifically where a cytosine nucleotide is followed by a guanine nucleotide in a gene sequence (CpG). These are usually referred to as CpG islands.[34] Fig. 7.6 outlines the fundamentals of epigenetics.

The disruption of epigenetic control mechanisms is associated with a variety of diseases (see Fig. 7.7). These have been known in medical research for some time; what has been lacking is the significance of epigenetics to clinical health and medicine, although this is now becoming more established.[32]

The significance of methylation to the gene–protein product aspect of our genetics is clear: methylation is a critical biochemical component of DNA replication, mRNA transcription, translation and post-translational protein modification. The fact that subcellular methylation reactions are occurring in every cell of the body, on every chromosome, thousands of times per day may seem astounding in itself, yet the critical importance of methylation to human health is well beyond the genetic processes already discussed. Methylation is also critical to metabolism; immune regulation; endocrine, cardiovascular and neurological physiology; hepatic detoxification; and mitochondrial function. Methylation relies on the body's proficient and constant biosynthesis of methyl groups, which must be produced endogenously via specific macro- and micronutrients ingested in the diet. As with all biosynthetic processes, specific genes, biochemical pathways, enzymes and nutrient cofactors must all operate correctly for this to be achieved.

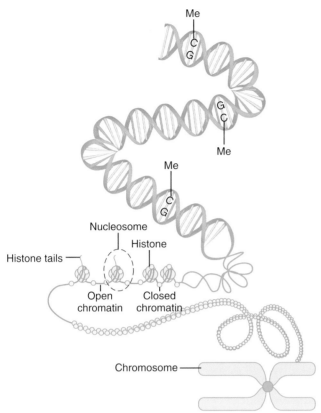

DNA methylation
- Methyl marks repress gene activity (usually at a cytosine residue)

Histone modification
- Different chemical groups in combination bind to the tails of the histones and alter DNA activity
- There are more than 200 post-translational modifications

3D structure
- DNA is tightly compacted around histones into chromatin
- Chromatin can be in an open (active) or closed (inactive) conformation
- Chromatin packaging necessitates inter- and intra-chromosome contacts that are dynamic and non-random
- Connections work to repress or activate certain regions of the genome

FIGURE 7.6 Fundamentals of epigenetics
Schierding W et al. Foetal and neonatal physiology. 5th edn. Elsevier; 2017.

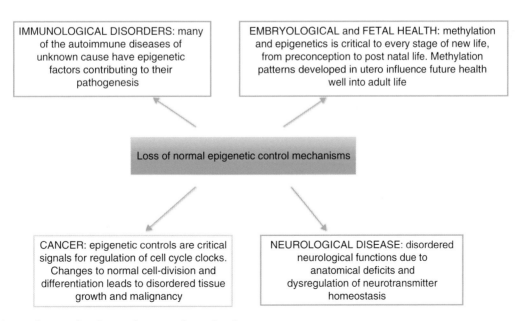

FIGURE 7.7 Loss of normal epigenetic control mechanisms

METABOLIC PATHWAYS

The methionine or methylation cycle is one of the most fundamentally important metabolic pathways of human biochemistry. Commencing with dietary methionine (the essential sulfur-containing amino acid), a series of amino acids is synthesised before methionine is ultimately regenerated in the final step of the pathway. This regeneration of methionine facilitates the continuation of the cycle. Most tissues and cell types express the genes for enzymes of the methionine cycle, but hepatic tissue appears to be a major location.[35]

Simply examining amino acid or protein biochemistry alone reveals the critical importance of methionine in the human diet: it is the only essential amino acid containing sulfur and is the precursor amino acid for other endogenously synthesised amino acids including cysteine, taurine and homocysteine. In addition to sulfur atoms, methionine has another aspect to its molecular structure making it vital to human health: the presence of a methyl group attached to its sulfur group. Methionine is the body's major source of methyl groups for the infinite methylation reactions that must be sustained throughout life. A constant supply of methyl groups and continual

regeneration of methionine are imperative to life. Methionine regeneration in itself occurs via remethylation, relying on other methyl donor chemical entities. Herein lies the complexity of methylation biochemistry, where several related metabolic pathways intersect and operate in tandem to achieve homeostasis. A single problem in one pathway may have minor or disastrous effects on the entire methylation network, depending on the exact biochemical error. See Fig. 7.8.

Methionine cycle

- In order for methionine to serve as a methyl donor, it must first be activated. This occurs in two steps that enable methionine to be converted into S-adenosylmethionine (SAMe). Steps 1 and 2 require adenosine triphosphate (ATP) to donate adenosine.
  - Step 1 requires magnesium (Mg) as a nutrient cofactor (which stabilises ATP)
  - Step 2 is the rate-limiting step of the whole methionine cycle (i.e. the slowest step, determining the reaction rate of the entire pathway)
- SAMe donates its methyl group via the action of methyltransferase enzymes. This donation is accepted

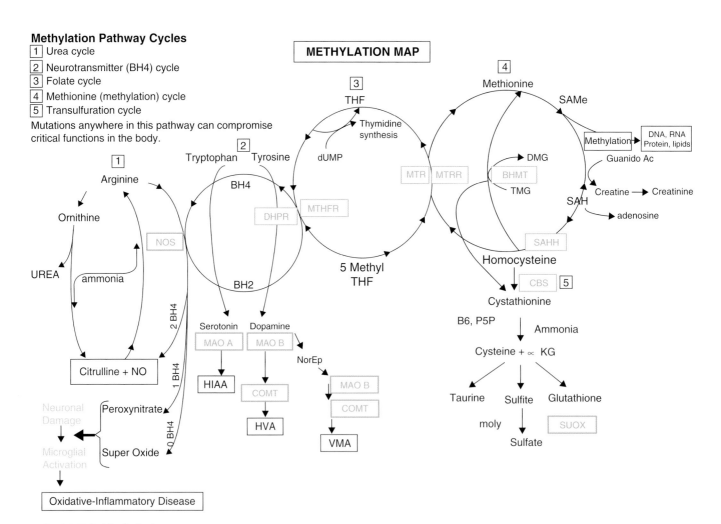

Methylation Pathway Cycles
1 Urea cycle
2 Neurotransmitter (BH4) cycle
3 Folate cycle
4 Methionine (methylation) cycle
5 Transulfuration cycle

Mutations anywhere in this pathway can compromise critical functions in the body.

FIGURE 7.8 Methylation map

by nucleic acids, proteins, lipids, carbohydrates and other small molecules via transmethylation reactions. This is the step of the pathway on which our epigenetic and metabolic transmethylation reactions rely.

- Upon demethylation, SAMe is converted to S-adenosylhomocysteine (SAH). SAH has an inhibitory effect on transmethylation.[36] SAH elevations can inhibit the previous step to ensure continual SAH elevations do not occur. In a reversible step, SAH is hydrolysed to homocysteine (Hcy). In homeostasis, the reaction direction favouring SAH synthesis is favoured; the rapid removal or 'drain' of Hcy products (including methionine, cysteine and its downstream products) favours the Hcy direction. This point represents the biochemical junction where the methionine cycle, folate cycle, neurotransmitter cycle and transsulfuration pathway all intersect.[36]

- Hcy can be methylated back to methionine via one of two ways: the first (predominant in most tissues) requires methylcobalamin and 5-methyltetrahydrofolate (5-MTHF). These are obtained via an intersection between the methionine and the folate cycles. The second (predominant in hepatic tissue) uses betaine as a methyl donor and requires Zn as a cofactor. If not converted to methionine, Hcy can enter the transsulfuration pathway, an important pathway during times of high oxidative stress.

- Elevated SAMe levels have inhibitory effects on the folate-dependent remethylation of Hcy to methionine. SAMe has stimulatory effects on the first enzyme of the transsulfuration pathway. Therefore, when SAMe/methionine levels are low, Hcy undergoes remethylation. The methionine cycle continues and Hcy can form again. When SAMe/methionine levels are elevated, Hcy is directed towards transsulfuration, where it is ultimately degraded.[36]

- SAMe can also enter another cyclic pathway known as the methionine salvage pathway. This salvage pathway leads to the biosynthesis of polyamines, which appear to have several important roles in cancer prevention.[36]

Folate cycle

- Tetrahydrofolate (THF, which occurs in several forms) is the activated form of vitamin B_9. THFs are crucial biochemical entities for the remethylation of homocysteine to methionine. In addition to their role in the methionine/methylation cycle network, THFs are essential for the biosynthesis of the purine base nucleotides (adenine and guanine) and thymidine, critical for the synthesis of DNA and RNA.[37]

- Being an essential micronutrient vitamin, B_9 must be obtained via the diet or supplementation. Folates ingested in the diet require activation before they can service their support functions in the methionine cycle. The various biochemical reactions of folate uptake, activation and interconversion collectively establish the metabolic pathway known as the folate cycle.[37]

- Dietary folates exist in a form known as the polyglutamate. This is preferred by folate-dependent enzymes and by cells for optimal folate retention. In

contrast, the uptake and transport of folates requires them to be in a monoglutamate form, tetrahydrofolate (THF).[37]

- Dietary folates in polyglutamate form are absorbed in the duodenum and jejunum. Once taken up by the cells, folates are converted to the monoglutamate form, THF. If a supplement or fortified food contains folic acid, it is reduced (twice) to dihydrofolate (DHF) before further conversion to THF. This conversion occurs in hepatic tissue, but appears to be low or at least variable in the human liver.[37]

- Once activated, THF is largely concerted to 5,10-methylene-THF. Serine (as a methyl donor) and P-5-P are required at this step, and the reaction is reversible.

- 5,10-methylene-THF is metabolised via a number of pathways, but for its purpose in servicing the methionine cycle, it is reduced to 5-MTHF via an irreversible reaction. This step requires vitamins B_2 and B_3 (as components of FAD and NAD, respectively).[37] 5-MTHF serves as a methyl donor for the remethylation of homocysteine to methionine in the methionine cycle. The enzyme at this point (methionine synthase) requires cobalamin (B_{12}). The methyl group from 5-MTHF is donated to cobalamin, generating methylcobalamin (the cofactor for methionine synthase). This step regenerates THF, which re-enters the folate cycle. Methylcobalamin donates its methyl group to homocysteine, methionine is recovered and the methionine cycle continues.[37]

- Methionine synthase does become inactive, as cobalamin is progressively oxidised in these reactions. Methionine synthase reductase (B_3-dependent) restores the function of methionine synthase via reductive methylation.[37]

Transsulfuration pathway

- The transsulfuration pathway is one of several routes of metabolism for Hcy. SAMe is an activator of the first step of the transsulfuration pathway. As previously stated, this serves as a means of methionine/SAMe reduction when levels become too high.

- Hcy entry into the transsulfuration pathway is very important during times of high oxidative stress. This is the pathway for the biosynthesis of glutathione, one of the most effective endogenous antioxidant molecules in the human body.[38]

- The first step of transsulfuration involves conversion of Hcy to cystathionine: this requires both serine and P-5-P. The second step involves the conversion of cystathione to cysteine. This also requires P-5-P.[38] The first step is irreversible, thus Hcy is committed to this pathway.

- When SAMe production is low, Hcy may be spared from entering the transsulfuration pathway. This relies on the effective recycling of glutathione via glutathione reductase activity and the cofactors FADH and NADH (containing B_2 and B_3, respectively).[38]

- Cysteine is the rate-limiting precursor for the potent endogenously synthesised anti-oxidant, glutathione. If SAMe/methionine levels are low, the transsulfuration pathway is inhibited, potentially reducing glutathione biosynthesis.[38]

- In addition to glutathione biosynthesis, cysteine can be metabolised via an oxidative pathway for taurine biosynthesis, or a non-oxidative pathway for the control of sulfur metabolism.[38]

Tetrahydrobiopterin cycle

In addition to the above three metabolic pathways, a fourth cycle, known as the tetrahydrobiopterin (BH4) cycle, is linked to the methionine cycle at two points: via a direct interaction with the folate cycle, and from an interaction delivered via SAMe generated in the methionine cycle. The BH4 cycle is the major pathway for the synthesis of several neurotransmitters. Methylation errors arising in either the folate or the methionine cycles can have a negative impact on neurotransmitters synthesised in the BH4 cycle.

- The amino acids phenylalanine, tyrosine and tryptophan are converted to tyrosine, dopamine and serotonin, respectively. Each of these three conversion pathways requires BH4 (synthesised endogenously) as a cofactor.
- BH4 is oxidised to dihydrobiopterin (BH2) and must be regenerated. Activated folates converted in the folate cycle serve in the regeneration of BH4 from BH2. MTHFR mutations and SNPs are both implicated in compromised regeneration of BH4 and the negative downstream effects on both monoamine and catecholamine metabolism.
- A second cofactor, P-5-P (B$_6$), is also required for the synthesis of both dopamine and serotonin.[39]
- In itself, dopamine is a critical neurotransmitter in the human body, but it is also the precursor substrate for the biosynthesis of the catecholamines, noradrenaline (norepinephrine) and adrenaline (epinephrine).
- Neurotransmitters synthesised via the BH4 cycle can enter the urea cycle (in the liver). Briefly, this cycle serves as a means of nitrogenous waste removal via urea and ammonia.
- SAMe generated in the methionine cycle has links to the BH4 cycle. SAMe (as a methyl donor) is involved in the methylation of noradrenaline (norepinephrine) to adrenaline (epinephrine).[39]

MAJOR METHYL DONORS

For clinical and dietary considerations, the major methyl donors of these biochemical networks include:

- Methionine
- SAMe
- 5-MTHF
- Methylcobalamin
- Serine
- Betaine
- Choline.

The major micronutrient cofactors for these same networks are:

- FAD (requires vitamin B$_2$)
- NAD (requires vitamin B$_3$)
- P-5-P (activated B$_6$)
- Methyl-THF (activated B$_9$)
- Methylcobalamin (activated B$_{12}$)
- Magnesium
- Zinc.

A deficiency in any one of these nutrients can potentially disrupt the metabolic homeostasis these pathways are designed to maintain. In the clinical setting, it is essential to remember that deficiencies arise not only from poor dietary intake, but also from malabsorption at the various anatomical locations of micronutrient absorption (may be related to disease), increased nutrient excretion (may also be related to disease), the presence of competing pharmacological agents or increased nutrient need (e.g. phase of life cycle, presence of disease state).

Correction of flawed methylation biochemistry does not simply involve the prescription of supplement formulations based on these methyl donor/nutrient cofactors. Correction must be based on careful consideration of a patient's diet, lifestyle, gender and phase of life. The presence of further complicating factors such as nutrient-depleting medications, chronic disease states and genetic aberrations may require further management to fully address methylation issues.

ALTERED METHYLATION PATTERNS: HYPOMETHYLATION AND HYPERMETHYLATION

As previously described, transcription of DNA occurs only when the chromatin structure of DNA unravels to a much looser arrangement and histones are displaced from DNA. Eukaryotic genes (such as those in humans and all higher-order living organisms) are 'silent' unless histones are removed from DNA.[39] Methylation of histone lysine residues facilitates the tight condensation of chromatin, thus reducing transcription.[39] Under conditions of 'normal' methylation (i.e. the absence of extensive hyper- or hypomethylation to induce pathology), this epigenetic control mechanism is critical to the cellular processes discussed in Table 7.1.[39,40,41,42]

Hypomethylation

DNA hypomethylation, demethylation and undermethylation all refer to the loss of the methyl group from the CG nucleotide. The terms usually apply to unmethylated CG sites in the genome that, under normal circumstances, should be methylated. Hypomethylation may also be a general feature affecting the bulk of the genome.[43] In cancer, global hypomethylation is present within specific gene bodies, within mobile elements, at areas of repetitive sequences.[41]

Many genome-wide studies have confirmed that DNA hypomethylation is the 'almost constant companion' of hypermethylation of the genome in cancer.[44] DNA hypomethylation is not limited to cancer, but is also implicated in atherosclerosis and certain autoimmune diseases such as multiple sclerosis (MS), systemic lupus erythematosus (SLE), Alzheimer's disease and psychiatric disorders.[45,46] The reasons why demethylation occurs remain the question of extensive research to elucidate both the causes and the mechanisms of hypomethylation.[45]

TABLE 7.1 Functions and genetic significance of methylation	
Functions of DNA methylation	**Physiological and pathological significance**
Gene regulation	Approx. 60% of human genes contain CG islands at promoter regions (i.e. the area initiating gene transcription). This reflects a genome highly reliant on methylation for normal and healthy expression of genes. The methylation state of CG promoter regions varies across different tissue types, reflecting the crucial role of methylation in normal and healthy tissue differentiation. Impaired CG methylation is linked with many forms of cancer.
Suppression of mobile elements	CG sequences at mobile elements are kept methylated to prevent their transcription. Mobile elements shape an organism's genome via mutations, base pair rearrangements and sequence duplications. Mobile elements have a variety of functions depending on the organism; in humans, they are often linked with disease, thus their inactivation via methylation is crucial.
X inactivation	This is observed in females, as the XX karyotype necessitates the silencing/inactivation of the second X chromosome. Widespread DNA methylation of the inactive X chromosome is observed; this structure is known as the Barr body. X inactivation occurs in both paternally and maternally derived X chromosomes, resulting in a mosaic pattern of inactivation. Without X inactivation, females would exhibit gene expression of both copies of a gene, and extra copies of genes or chromosomes affect normal development. X inactivation, via methylation, is a compensatory mechanism for the extra X chromosome.
Imprinting	In oocytes and spermatozoa, some genes are selectively methylated. These methylated genes are silent, a phenomenon known as imprinting. If a gene of either maternal or paternal origin is imprinted, the same gene from the corresponding maternal or paternal genome is expressed. Most imprinted genes appear to be involved in control of embryonic growth. Some conditions linked to imprinted genetic disorders include the inherited Prader-Willi and Angelman syndromes, and some forms of breast and ovarian cancers.

Source: [39,40,41,42]

Hypermethylation

In many disease states, hypermethylation is considered an important 'epigenetic lesion'.[47] In cancer, hypermethylation occurs at the normally unmethylated CG promoters of tumour suppressor genes.[41] This is the opposite methylation change observed in the widespread hypomethylation of cancer, but is a constant feature of the cancer genome.[44] Many forms of cellular repair are inactivated by hypermethylation of tumour suppressor genes, including DNA repair cycles, cell cycle controls, apoptosis, cell adherence and cellular detoxification.[47] Immune dysfunction and Trisomy 21 (Down syndrome) are also associated with hypermethylated areas of the genome.[41] DNA hypermethylation has been associated with patients who have a deficiency of methyl donors as well as patients undergoing methyl donor supplementation. The clinical results of supratherapeutic dosing for methylation issues are largely unknown, as research in this area is still underway. Proceeding with caution to avoid hypermethylation may be a very real clinical goal.

Key enzymes of methylation

The key enzymes involved in methylation are the large methyltransferase superfamily. Several enzyme categories belong to this group, all of which are defined by various structural (thus, functional) features. Methyltransferase enzymes catalyse the transfer of a methyl group from the cofactor SAMe to a variety of organic substrates, including:

- Proteins (including histones and transcription factors)
- DNA (for epigenetic control)
- RNA (for epigenetic control)
- Lipids (including phosphatidylethanolamine for phosphatidylcholine synthesis)
- Noradrenaline (norepinephrine) (for synthesis of adrenaline)
- Dopamine
- Histamine (for deactivation)
- Arginine (for creatine synthesis)
- Oestrogens (for deactivation and detoxification).[48,49]

It has become clear that methyltransferases can target proteins beyond those involved in genetics and transcription. This represents a greater impact on normal physiology and pathophysiology.[48] Some 208 proteins in the human genome have been identified as methyltransferase enzymes, with approximately 30% linked to disease conditions, most notably cancer and neurological disorders.[49] Methyltransferases have varied roles in diverse biological pathways; there are hundreds of known substrates to which the methyltransferase enzymes can bind. These methyltransferase + substrate interactions are essential for epigenetic control, but also for lipid biosynthesis, protein repair, hormone inactivation and tissue differentiation.[49]

- *Seven-beta-strand superfamily:* the most abundant of the classes. These enzymes methylate a wide variety of substrates, including small metabolites, nucleic acids, lipids and proteins.[50]
- *SPOUT methyltransferase superfamily.* Catalyses methylation of RNA substrates.[48] The potential substrate appears to be guanine and uracil.[49]
- *SET methyltransferase superfamily.* Methylation of lysine residues in histones and ribosomes is predominant here.[49]

Smaller super families have been identified and include the precorrin-like homocysteine and radical SAMe methyltransferases, the MetH activation domain, the TYW3 protein and the membrane-bound family.[49]

In the clinical setting, several factors may influence the function of methyltransferase enzymes, including:

- Mutations in any of the genes encoding the structure of a methyltransferase enzyme. Types and severity of consequent diseases arising from such mutations are incredibly vast, depending on the precise biological role of the faulty methyltransferase gene.
- SNPs are also responsible for many aspects of disordered methylation. Several genes encoding proteins of the methylation cycle are known to contain SNPs in some individuals. Some SNPs play a very direct role in disordered methylation and a host of disease states.
- The absence or deficiency of essential micronutrient cofactors required by methyltransferase enzymes. With so many methyltransferase enzymes now identified and sequenced, their list of required micronutrient cofactors grows as more research accumulates. In general, the minerals (inorganic cofactors) and vitamins (organic cofactors) involved in the metabolic pathways for endogenous synthesis of methyl groups are critical to many methyltransferase enzymes. These micronutrients include the minerals copper (Cu), manganese (Mn), magnesium (Mg), selenium (Se) and zinc (Zn) and vitamins B_1, B_2, B_3, B_6, B_9, B_{12} and C. The amino acids cysteine, glycine, methionine (essential) and serine are also necessary for the normal functioning of some enzymes in the methylation cycle.
- Exposure to any substance known to act as an enzyme inhibitor for methyltransferase enzymes. For example, methyltransferase inhibitors are under the lens of pharmacological research as inhibitors of hypermethylation for some cancers, particularly through the potential restoration of tumour suppressor gene function. The clinical efficacy of these agents remains under investigation.[51]

BEYOND GENETICS: METHYLATION AND OUR BROADER PHYSIOLOGY

Nervous system physiology

Methylation is essential in supporting nervous system physiology via a number of biological pathways. Methylation reactions support the correct function of the hypothalamic-pituitary-adrenal (HPA) endocrine axis.[52] Methylation is involved in the biosynthesis of all monoamine neurotransmitters (including serotonin, dopamine, noradrenaline [norepinephrine] and adrenaline [epinephrine]) and acetylcholine.[52] The conversion of noradrenaline (norepinephrine) to adrenalin (epinephrine) is based on methylation and is catalysed by the enzyme phenylethanolamine N-methyltransferase (PNMT), which relies on SAMe supplied by methylation cycles.[53] Any stress response that increases stress hormones can upregulate PNMT activity. Consequently, more noradrenaline (norepinephrine) is converted to adrenaline (epinephrine). The catecholamine response to stress is potentiated; sympathetic nervous system responses increase via positive feedback on the HPA axis.[53]

In the clinical setting, the effects of insufficient methylation on the nervous system may present as patients with apathy/low mood, depression, anxiety, chronic and generalised fatigue, poor cognitive health, insomnia or poor sleep maintenance. It is likely that these are linked with reduced neurotransmitter synthesis. Alzheimer's disease has shown some links with reduced PNMT activity.[53] SAMe is essential for phosphatidylcholine production, which in turn is present in all cell membranes and is the precursor substrate for acetylcholine. Low levels of SAMe have been implicated in demyelination.[52] Additionally, the early embryonic development of the central nervous system is dependent on folates to prevent a host of neurological deficits including neural tube defects. While folate deficiency is an established contributing factor, methylation deficits may also be implicated here.[53]

Biosynthesis and recycling of glutathione

Endogenous glutathione (GSH) is well-established as the most abundant and one of the most important defences against oxidative stress. Glutathione is vital in redox reaction signalling and the detoxification of xenobiotics.[54] This antioxidant species is also a powerful regulator of cell proliferation, apoptosis, immune function, fibrogenesis and some transcription factors.[54]

GSH is ubiquitous and is synthesised in the cytoplasm of all mammalian cells in a highly regulated manner.[55] The major biochemical precursor for GSH synthesis is the availability of cysteine.[55] Cysteine (being a non-essential amino acid) can be synthesised endogenously, but only if the biochemical pathways leading to cysteine biosynthesis function properly (this includes precursor substrate availability and correct enzyme function). This is where GSH synthesis conjoins with the methylation cycle. A situation of glutathione depletion–methylation cycle block has been hypothesised as a possible contributing factor in glutathione depletion. This may be due to ineffective enzyme function (including nutrient cofactors) or restriction of key precursors of the methylation cycle.[56]

In clinical practice, reduced GSH availability has been associated with many diverse chronic disease pathologies including cancer, Parkinson's disease, Alzheimer's disease, chronic fatigue syndrome, fibromyalgia, autism, multiple sclerosis, hypertension and atherosclerosis.[57] In all cases, pathogenesis is linked to oxidative stress, with glutathione depletion regarded as an indicator of such stress.[57] Studies have shown that depletion of GSH results in a cascade of biochemical events known to cause cellular injury and cell death.[57] Due to the ubiquitous production of GSH as a major intracellular antioxidant, deficiency links with many diseases across multiple tissue types are not unexpected.

Methylation and the immune response

A host of immune effects including the inflammatory response, swift reaction to infection and regulation of the immune system are reliant upon and influenced by healthy patterns of genomic methylation. DNA methylation plays an eminent role in guiding diverse immune processes such as growth and differentiation of the haematopoietic cell line, immune competence, the antigen receptor pool, antigenic reactivity, autoimmunity, viral life cycle, tumour surveillance, haematopoietic neoplasia and changes in immune status due to age.[58] Natural killer (NK) cell and T-cell maturation (particularly T2 cytokine regulation) rely on methylation. Histamine (which is both a pro-inflammatory mediator and a neurotransmitter) is normally metabolised and deactivated via methylation, with SAMe as the methyl donor. Reduced SAMe levels are linked to the accumulation of histamine and its consequent pro-inflammatory clinical picture.[58]

With regard to bacterial infections, recent research has uncovered the induction of thousands of changes in DNA methylation. This appears to occur only hours after pathogen invasion and in cells and genes of the innate immune response.[59] The immunosurveillance of cancer theory suggests that cellular escape mechanisms contribute to tumour growth; methylation appears to regulate molecules of the tumour immune response.[60]

In clinical practice, pathogenic methylation changes in the immune genome manifest across the entire immune disease landscape, including atopy, asthma, rheumatoid arthritis (RA), ICF syndrome, scleroderma, Sjögren's syndrome, lupus, complications of Epstein-Barr virus (EBV) infection, and immune and non-immune malignancies.[60,61] A vast number of factors contribute to immune disorders besides methylation issues, so pinpointing aberrant methylation as the cause of disease can be problematic. Screening patients for potential methylation issues beyond the immune system is required; this is achieved via thorough medical and health history taking, and possibly with the assistance of specific functional and pathology laboratory investigations.

Support for all mitochondrial functions

As previously described, research strongly suggests that mtDNA is subject to the same epigenetic modifications as nDNA. These modifications to mtDNA methylation patterns are implicated in the development of specific diseases, potentially meaning that altered mtDNA methylation can be used as a detection and diagnostic biomarker.[16,62]

The mitochondria's most renowned biological role is the biochemical production of energy. Additionally, the mitochondria have a pivotal role in the detection of foreign substances as they entr the body, potentising the resulting inflammasome of the immune response.[62] Recent evidence has demonstrated that virally infected cells can be eliminated via mitochondria-driven apoptosis.[62] Mitochondrial function also contributes to both the regeneration and the structural integrity of all organ tissues, particularly via stem cells.[62] Any change to the 'healthy state' epigenetic landscape of mtDNA towards one that alters the correct expression of mitochondrial genes is potentially deleterious to human health. Additionally, transmethylation reactions occur during the biosynthesis of coenzyme Q10 (CoQ10), carnitine and ATP. All are fundamental biomolecules for mitochondrial cellular respiration and energy production.[62]

The implications of disordered mitochondrial methylation patterns on the wider general population are enormous; bioenergetics, immune potency and tissue repair are fundamental to the anatomy and physiology of every body system. Considering the public health concerns of an ageing population, addressing methylation problems to prevent defective mitochondrial gene expression is likely to be a necessity for naturopathic and integrative medicine. Without doubt, patients enduring conditions associated with premature ageing and general ageing will require mitochondrial support, with methylation support being a natural clinical query to investigate further in such patients.

Biosynthesis of lipids

Methylation reactions feature in several enzyme catalysed reactions in phospholipid biosynthesis, such as the synthesis of phosphatidylcholine. Endogenous production of phosphatidylcholine occurs in hepatic tissue via two pathways, one of which relies on the methyltransferase enzyme, phosphoethanolamine methyltransferase (PEMT).[63] Methylation reactions occur at three points in this pathway, with SAMe being the major donor of methyl groups for these reactions (see Fig. 7.9).

Phosphatidylcholine is the major cell membrane phospholipid in mammals and is a component of lipoproteins, pulmonary surfactant and bile.[63] It is also used as substrate for potent eicosanoids, including leukotrienes, prostaglandins and lipoxins.[64] Clinical conditions such as

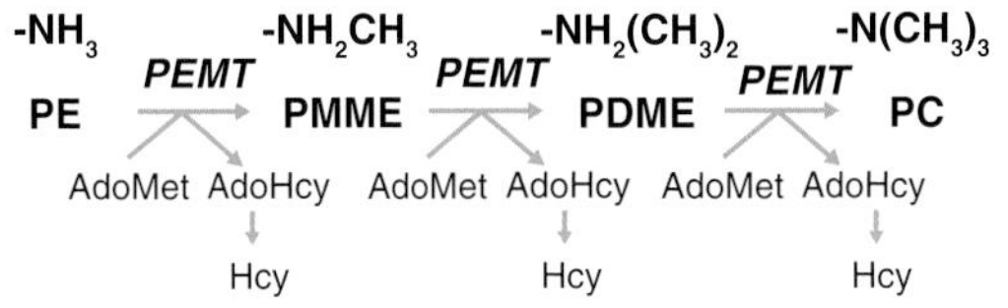

FIGURE 7.9   Phosphatidylcholine synthesis
PEMT, phosphoethanolamine methyltransferase; PC, phosphatidylcholine; PE, phosphatidylethanolamine; PMME, phosphatidylmonomethylethanolamine; PDME, phosphatidyldimethylethanolamine.

non-alcoholic fatty liver disease (NAFLD), steatosis, lipid peroxidation and generalised oxidative stress are linked to inadequate phosphatidylcholine production.[65] The requirement of a methyltransferase enzyme such as PEMT as the catalyst for this pathway confirms a biochemical link with the methionine cycle, as methyl groups are obtained via the donation from SAMe.[63] Phosphatidylcholine biosynthesis would be diminished without the adequate and continued supply of SAMe.

Detoxification of xenobiotics and hormones

Hepatic glucuronidation, sulfuration, acetylation and methylation are all significant pathways for phase II biotransformation and detoxification.[66] A patient's methylation status is also a factor in the regulation, biotransformation and clearance of oestrogens, which is important to consider in patients (female or male) with oestrogen-dominant conditions or oestrogen-receptor positive tumours.[66] Methylation of oestrogens can occur via the COMT pathway.[67]

Other transmethylation reactions

In addition to the methylated products of transmethylation described above (namely, noradrenaline [norepinephrine] to adrenaline [epinephrine] and phosphatidylethanolamine to phosphatidylcholine), a variety of important biomolecules undergo transmethylation reactions. These biomolecules are only physiologically and biochemically active once they are methylated. They are summarised in Table 7.2.[65,68–72]

KEY NUTRIENTS

Folate

While folate refers to a group of 1-carbon derivatives of folic acid, methylation is reliant upon the activation of folate via the folate cycle.[73] As depicted by the cycle, folate is first reduced to tetrahydrofolate (THF) and further to methylenetetrahydrofolate (MeTHF); this occurs in the liver and/or intestine.[74] MeTHF function then intercedes in the methionine cycle, serving in the replenishment of

methionine from homocysteine (along with vitamin B_{12} and betaine). Several SNPs are associated with variations in the 5,10-methylenetetrahydrofolate reductase gene (MeTHFR), which codes for the key enzyme in folate metabolism.[73] The negative consequences of impaired folate activation are pervasive; the resulting biochemical inefficiency of the methionine cycle places stress on homocysteine recycling, regeneration of methionine, DNA/RNA/protein methylation and lipid synthesis.

Pyridoxal-5-phosphate

There are a number of points in the methionine, folate and transsulfuration pathways where B_6 is essential. In the folate cycle, once folic acid or dietary folate has been converted to the THF coenzyme, it is further converted to 5,10-methylene-THF by serine hydroxymethyltransferase. This is a B_6-dependent enzyme.[75] B_6 is also required in the transsulfuration pathway in the conversion of homocysteine to cystathione and cysteine, by the enzymes cystathione beta synthase and cystathionine lyase.[76]

Cobalamin

The methylation of homocysteine to methionine (methionine recycling or replenishment) requires methylcobalamin, the activated form of B_{12}.[77] The B_{12}-dependent enzyme at this point of the methionine cycle is methionine synthase.[78] This reaction is another example of the intricate links between the methionine and folate cycles: methyl-THF (activated in the folate cycle) donates its methyl group to cobalamin, producing methylcobalamin (activated B_{12}). Methylcobalamin donates this methyl group to homocysteine, thus producing methionine to continue the methionine cycle.[77] Without B_{12}, homocysteine accumulates and the amount of methionine regenerated is reduced, weakening the entire methylation biochemical network.

Riboflavin

Vitamin B_2 is an essential component of the coenzymes flavin adenine dinucleotide (FAD) and flavin mononucleotide (FMN). FAD is required as a cofactor for the MTHFR enzyme, the key enzyme of the folate cycle for

TABLE 7.2 Transmethylation reactions in human biochemistry			
Methyl group acceptor	Methylated product	Tissue type	Major functions
Methionine	Carnitine	Highest in kidneys, liver, skeletal muscle, cardiac muscle and brain	Transport of fatty acids to mitochondria for catabolism via β-oxidation
Guanidinoacetate	Creatine	Liver and kidneys	Buffer for ATP in conjunction with creatine phosphate
Methionine and serine	Cysteine and cystine	Ubiquitous tissue synthesis	3D protein shaping and modifications via disulphide bonds
Acetyl serotonin	Melatonin	Pineal organ	Regulation of day/night circadian rhythms
Serine	Choline	Liver	Major cell membrane phospholipid
Uracil	Thymine	Ubiquitous tissue synthesis	Pyrimidine base nucleotide of DNA; energy carrier

Source: [65,68,69,70,71,72]

activation of methyl TH4.[79] B_2 is also required by methionine synthase reductase, the enzyme responsible for reactivating methionine synthase when it becomes inactive, allowing the conversion of homocysteine to methionine to continue.[80]

Magnesium

The activation of methionine to SAMe requires catalysation by the methionine adenosyltransferase (MAT) enzyme. This is an 'energy expensive' reaction: MAT cleaves a molecule of ATP in order to harvest a molecule of adenosine. Methionine is hence activated by this chemical attachment of adenosine.[81] ATP exists as a chelate with magnesium, thus this reaction is not only ATP- dependent, but also magnesium-dependent.[82] This reaction also requires potassium ions. The biochemistry suggests that magnesium deficiency may prevent the activation of methionine.

Selenium

Selenium has important interactions with methionine. Selenium is required by the methionine sulfoxide reduction system, which functions as a potent antioxidant system.[83] It is also an essential nutrient cofactor for the antioxidant glutathione peroxidase enzymes; this occurs via the incorporation of selenium into selenocysteine, the precursor for glutathione peroxidases (which are generated from homocysteine via the transsulfuration pathway).[84]

Zinc

Methionine synthase and betaine homocysteine methyltransferase (BHMT) are both zinc-dependent methyltransferases.[85] Methionine synthase has been discussed previously. Betaine is an important methyl group donor for transmethylation reactions and is synthesised endogenously (mostly in the liver and kidneys) via choline.[36] BHMT participates in the transfer of a methyl group from trimethylglycine (TMG) to form dimethylglycine; this methyl group is then used to methylate homocysteine to regenerate methionine.[86] Researchers are investigating the implications of zinc deficiency on the activity of BHMT and methionine synthase and the consequences for elevated homocysteine and its abundant negative health effects.[85,86] Zinc deficiency also has broader implications for genome health beyond methylation.

Sulfur

The importance of sulfur in the transsulfuration pathway is clear: via homocysteine, sulfur-containing compounds such as cystathione, cysteine, sulfite, sulfate, taurine and glutathione are produced. These compounds have a widespread impact on malignant growth, immune health, cardiovascular health and antioxidant and detoxification systems.[87] The requirement for sulfur is significant and continual and it must be supplied by methionine via homocysteine and cysteine. Being the only sulfur-containing essential amino acid, methionine must be ingested in the diet in optimal amounts every day.

L-ascorbic acid

In addition to zinc and selenium, specific vitamins are important to the methylation of DNA, RNA and histones from an epigenetic standpoint. While not related specifically to methylation cycles, these vitamins are essential when methyl groups from methylation cycles become available for epigenetic functions. L-ascorbic acid (vitamin C) appears to maintain imprinted DNA methylation patterns in some areas of mammalian genomes.[88] Vitamin C is also required by specific dioxygenase enzymes for regulating histone and DNA methylation.[88]

1,25-dihydroxycholecalciferol

1,25-dihydroxycholecalciferol (active vitamin D) has a well-established role in regulating gene expression via the vitamin D receptor (which functions as a transcription factor).[89] A possible bidirectional relationship exists between vitamin D metabolism and DNA methylation: genes encoding enzymes of the vitamin D metabolism pathway are possibly regulated by methylation, while vitamin D appears to influence the methylation status of genes involved in cell cycle regulation.[89]

SAMe

SAMe is synthesised endogenously in the cytoplasm of every cell of the body. Hepatic tissue is the most significant site for the biosynthesis and degradation of SAMe. After ATP, SAMe is the second most used cofactor in cellular biochemistry. It is estimated that over 100 methyltransferase enzymes require SAMe for the donation of methyl groups.[90] Approximately half of our ingested dietary methionine enters the methionine cycle for conversion to SAMe.[91] As signified by the methionine cycle, SAMe biosynthesis is entirely dependent on the presence of other nutrients, namely the methyl donation from activated B_9, activated B_{12} and choline.[91] The critical importance of this nutrient to cell membrane structural integrity, cholinergic neurotransmission, lipid biosynthesis, neurotransmitter synthesis, DNA/RNA/protein stabilisation, anti-oxidant capacity, detoxification and cell signalling via epigenetic cues cannot be overstated.

Dimethylglycine and trimethylglycine

Both dimethylglycine (DMG) and trimethylglycine (TMG) are methylated derivatives of the amino acid glycine. They contain two or three methyl groups, respectively.[92] DMG is produced via the methylation of TMG (betaine) from homocysteine in the methionine cycle. While the methyl group removed from TMG is donated to regenerate methionine, the resulting DMG molecule can donate electrons to the electron transport chain (ETC) of mitochondria to possibly support cellular respiration. Research is examining the effects of DMG deficiencies on mitochondrial health.[93] DMG synthesis may be impaired in cases of elevated homocysteine levels with low regeneration of methionine.

N-acetyl cysteine

Cysteine is the antioxidant precursor of glutathione; its endogenous biosynthesis occurs via conversion of homocysteine to cysteine via the transsulfuration pathway of glutathione synthesis, which also requires vitamin B₆.[94] Cysteine deficiency is linked to inefficient transsulfuration of homocysteine; the resulting glutathione deficiency is associated with a myriad of clinical conditions, including cognitive decline and cardiovascular disease.[94] N-acetyl cysteine has been used clinically as a nutrient and prodrug for more than three decades, replenishing glutathione levels in paracetamol toxicity, genetic defects, metabolic disorders

of the folate and methionine cycles, homocysteinuria and combatting the oxidative stress associated with human immunodeficiency virus (HIV) infection and chronic obstructive pulmonary disease (COPD).[95] While not directly involved in the folate or methionine cycles, cysteine is synthesised when the genetic, nutritional and environmental requirements for these cycles are primed; cysteine and glutathione deficiency are indirect sequelae of disordered methylation cycles.

Refer to Table 7.7 and the dietary and lifestyle modification sections later in this chapter for further discussion of the key nutrients for methylation support.

METHYLATION DEFICITS AND ASSOCIATED CONDITIONS

See Fig. 7.10 for more discussion of conditions correlated with methylation deficits.

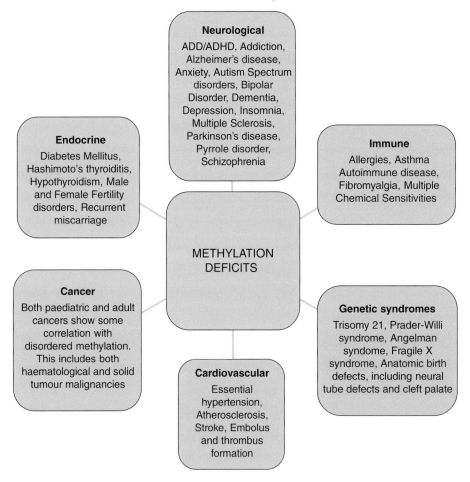

FIGURE 7.10 Conditions associated with methylation deficits
[96,97,98,99,100]

SPECIAL TOPICS

Embryogenesis and pregnancy

Well before the moment of conception, the health of potential embryos, fetuses and infants is being moulded in the primordial cells from which mature ova and

spermatozoa differentiate. The months (potentially years) of preconception time that elapses before a successful fertilisation takes place is a critical time of genetic plasticity, where environmental factors, lifestyle choices and the nutrient status of both parents shapes many health outcomes in their future offspring. These outcomes are experienced in all phases of life: embryonic, fetal,

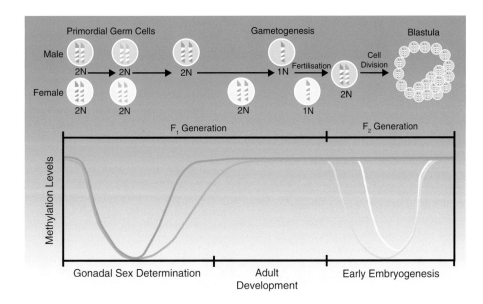

FIGURE 7.11 Epigenetic mechanisms including methylation are implicated in fetal programming

infancy, childhood, adolescence and adulthood. This is a well-established genetic concept known as fetal programming.[101] All epigenetic mechanisms including methylation are implicated in fetal programing (see Fig. 7.11).

Fetal programming is crucial in cementing the correct genetic expression of imprinted genes. Genetic imprinting is an important epigenetic mechanism, where certain genes are silenced (imprinted) via methylation. Epigenetic 'imprints' are established in germ cells (ova and spermatozoa); thus, they are inherited. If an imprinted gene is present in an allele of maternal or paternal origin, it is not expressed. The corresponding non-imprinted allele is expressed instead. Genetic imprints are preserved in the somatic genome of offspring, with some evidence that they are maintained across familial generations.[101] Imprinting has been implicated in developmental disorders, autism, some gynaecological cancers and the genetic disorders Prader-Willi syndrome and Angelman syndrome.[101,102]

Research examining the in utero environment has demonstrated that the fetal epigenome and imprinted genes are very sensitive to environmental stimuli. Epigenetic modifications including DNA methylation and histone methylation control the expression of genes during embryonic and fetal development.[102] This serves an evolutionary role, whereby specific epigenetic changes ensure fetal survival. However, some modifications may be required for only a small window of time; if maintained into adulthood, some changes can elicit various clinical diseases.[102] Certain endocrine-disrupting compounds (EDCs) have been found to cause not only congenital birth defects, but also changes to epigenetic fetal programming. These include:

- Bisphosphenol A (BPA)
- Phthalates
- Methoxychlor (a pesticide)
- Vinclozolin (a fungicide)

- Polychlorinated biphenyls (PCBs)
- Polybrominated diphenyl ethers (PBDEs)
- Polycyclic aromatic hydrocarbons (PAHs).[102]

Environmental pollutants (including cigarette smoke, heavy metals and indoor allergens), certain hormones (e.g. oestrogens), specific viral pathogens (e.g. *H. pylori*, EBV, HPV, HBV), some medications, disordered eating and maternal hyponutrition states have been defined as environmental inducers of epigenetic change. The length and level of exposure are both significant in determining the epigenetic outcome. Diseases states in later life believed to result from these altered epigenetic landscapes include:

- Malignant cancers
- Pulmonary diseases, including asthma
- Cardiovascular diseases
- Autoimmune diseases
- Neurobehavioural disorders
- Neurodegenerative disorders
- Obesity and metabolic syndromes.[101,102]

In the clinical setting, males and females of reproductive age must be educated on and screened for harmful exposure to EDCs. This is critically important for those planning a family, ideally well before conception. The hypomethylating effects of EDCs demonstrate widespread activity not restricted to patients with methylation polymorphisms.[103] The methylome appears to have a great degree of plasticity, and parental supplementation or dietary intervention with key methylation nutrients is important for healthy methylation patterns during embryogenesis and pregnancy. Screening for and rectifying nutrient deficiencies linked to methylation is important in all aspects of preconception and antenatal naturopathic healthcare.

Other negative pregnancy outcomes associated with methylation disorders include neural tube defects, congenital birth defects such as cleft palate, atrial or ventricular septal defects, placental abruption and spontaneous abortion.[103]

Autoimmune diseases

Various epigenetic mechanisms are implicated in the pathogenesis of several autoimmune diseases. This most likely originates from the epigenetic malfunctions of genes expressed in immune cells and tissues. These genes are often involved in both the activation and the controlled proliferation of specific immune cells.[104] Examples of autoimmune diseases linked to methylation problems include:

- Autoimmune pancreatitis: genes involved in immune cell trafficking and the control of autoimmunity appear incorrectly methylated in this condition. The same gene (*MST1*) is implicated in some cases of rheumatoid arthritis.[105]
- Systemic sclerosis (scleroderma): the exact pathogenesis of scleroderma remains multifactorial, yet largely unknown. The characteristic immune abnormalities and sclerotic/fibrotic changes may be the result of epigenetic changes.[104] Anti-fibrotic genes (*Fli-1*, *BMPRII*) may be silenced via hypermethylation in some patients. Hypomethylation (thus, activation) of specific pro-inflammatory CD immune cells (CD11a, CD40L and CD70) results in their overexpression.[104,106]

Other autoimmune diseases that display specific epigenetic marks include autoimmune thyroid disease, rheumatoid arthritis, type 2 diabetes, systemic lupus erythematosus, Sjögren's syndrome and multiple sclerosis.[106]

Cancer

It is well-known that cancer is not a single disease, but a term grouping many diseases of abnormal and uncontrolled cellular differentiation and proliferation together. Currently, more than 100 different cancer subtypes have been established, and much of the evidence for this is a result of the molecular biology revolution experienced over the past several decades.[107] In its genetic aspects, cancer is not simply a disease of disordered methylation. Cell cycle deregulation, mutations, uncontrolled growth inhibition, insensitivity to extracellular growth controls and failure of cell growth checkpoints all contribute to malignant transformation.[107] While methylation is only one molecular aspect of carcinogenesis, it can play a role in any one of these mechanisms. Many, if not most, of these processes are under the control of genes. Hypomethylation of oncogenes and hypermethylation of tumour suppressor genes are hallmarks of cancer. Both genome-wide and lesion-localised patterns of DNA methylation are examples of the earliest and most numerous events to occur in human cancers.[107] Two fundamental changes in methylation status occur during carcinogenesis: regional hypermethylation of gene promoter regions and genome-wide hypomethylation.[108] Some well-established clinical examples of the links between abnormal methylation patterns and human cancers include:

- Prostate cancer: aberrant methylation of glutathione-S-transferase genes is expressed in more than 90% of prostatic carcinomas. Hypermethylation of RAS tumour suppressor genes is also implicated.[107]
- Bladder cancer: mutations of the *p53* gene may be silenced via methylation, though demethylation of this mutagen is frequent in both early and invasive forms of bladder cancer. Hypermethylation of RAS and global hypomethylation are also observed.[107,108]
- Colon cancer: hypermethylation in the SFRP gene family is often present. This gene family is normally involved in extracellular signals controlling abnormal cell proliferation and is silenced by hypermethylation.[109]

While most cancers have established molecular links to abnormal methylation activities, other examples with strong evidence include haematological malignancies, small-cell lung cancer, breast cancer and ovarian cancer.[109] Methylation issues may be suspected in families with a high incidence of specific cancers or a combination of various cancers. They may also occur over different generations. Diet, lifestyle, SNPs and mutations may all be implicated to some degree.

Cardiovascular disease

The relationship between methylation cycles, homocysteine and cardiovascular disease emerged approximately four decades ago.[110] This was established when paediatric patients with the very rare genetic condition homocysteinuria (autosomal recessive inheritance) displayed the clinical signs of advanced atherosclerosis, despite the absence of lipids within the plaques.[111] Elevated levels of homocysteine in both blood plasma (hyperhomocysteinaemia) and urine (homocysteinuria) have been implicated in many other conditions of disordered methylation discussed in this chapter, including diabetes mellitus, neurological disorders and inflammatory and autoimmune conditions.

Elevated homocysteine levels are now viewed as an independent risk factor for a host of cardiovascular disease presentations, including atherosclerosis, stroke, myocardial infarction and coronary artery disease.[110,111] The pathogenic mechanisms leading to cardiovascular damage from homocysteine remain somewhat unclear; however, damage to the endothelial intima, reduced blood vessel flexibility and atypical haemostasis are possible contributing factors.[112] As viewed in the metabolic pathways, homocysteine is normally metabolised via two routes:

- Continuation of the methionine cycle, where the methionine synthase enzyme catalyses a transmethylation reaction of homocysteine to produce methionine. Methionine is thus regenerated. Methyl donors for this reaction include betaine, MTHF and methylcobalamin.
- If not converted to methionine, homocysteine can enter the transsulfuration pathway and is converted to cysteine over two steps. This pathway requires P-5-P.

While elevated levels of homocysteine can arise from genetic defects and SNPs related to a variety of methylation cycle enzymes, they can also result from deficiencies of vitamins B$_6$, B$_9$ and B$_{12}$, or any medications that interfere with their metabolism (particularly folate antagonists).[112] The majority of clinical trials and evidence supporting the use of micronutrient therapies for homocysteine reduction include a combination of oral B_6, B_9 and B_{12} therapy.[112]

LABORATORY ASSESSMENT OF METHYLATION

Health practitioners have access to a great variety of functional and pathology testing methods for the clinical evaluation of methylation status. This includes genetic profiling and key nutrient assessments, as well as direct measurements of neurotransmitters (including their metabolites), specific amino acids, hormones (including their metabolites), detoxification markers and indicators of oxidative load. Methylation is incredibly intricate, involving genetics, environment, diet and lifestyle. No laboratory assessment should be interpreted in isolation, nor should results be interpreted without the clinical context provided through medical, health, diet and lifestyle histories. No single assessment is diagnostic; all results must be interpreted with care by practitioners and patients alike.

Genetic testing

As observed in the folate cycle, the 5,10-methylene THF reductase enzyme catalyses the conversion of 5,10-methylene THF (5-MeTHF) to 5-MTHF (the major and most active form of folate). It is clear that this conversion is required for the remethylation of homocysteine to methionine and the further conversion to SAMe as the major methyl donor of the human body. Problems may arise at this point, as there are several genetic polymorphisms associated with the MTHFR gene.[113] The two most common variants are:

- The thermolabile variant, c.665C>T (p.Ala222Val), more commonly referred to as C677T. The inheritance of two copies of the gene polymorphism (i.e. one from each parent) confers a *homozygous* status; the inheritance of only one copy (i.e. from either parent) confers *heterozygous* status.
- The c.1298A>C (p.Glu429Ala) variant, commonly known as the A1298C polymorphism. Again, individuals may have either *homozygous* or *heterozygous* status for this polymorphism.

An inheritance pattern of *heterozygosity* for both gene variants is known as *compound heterozygosity in trans.* Homozygosity for one variant in combination with heterozygosity for the other variant is rare.[113] While the C677T variant is the most common variant associated with hyperhomocysteinaemia, a total of 34 rare deleterious mutations and nine common SNPs are associated with the MTHFR gene. Only the 677CT and 1298AC variants appear to reduce MTHFR enzyme activity.[114] See Table 7.3 for a summary of common MTHFR gene variants.

These occur commonly in the general population, possibly reducing an individual's ability to metabolise and activate folate. Reduced MTHFR activity is a genetic risk factor for elevated homocysteine levels in blood and urine, particularly when coupled with low folate levels.[113]

The MTHFR gene acts in association with a number of other genes, thus abnormalities are considered as threshold risk factors.[117] As an individual abnormality, its significance remains contentious. In isolation, genetic testing for MTHFR polymorphisms is not diagnostic and should be considered as investigational only. As described, other nutrient cofactors such as vitamins B_6, B_9 and B_{12} are involved intimately with homocysteine levels, with B_2, zinc, magnesium, selenium, choline, methionine and betaine having a less direct, yet important, biochemical role. Wider clinical investigation of the patient, including medical and diet histories, lifestyle factors and other pathology testing, help to strengthen the investigation of methylation disorders.

In Australia, MTHFR testing is covered by Medicare only in specific situations, such as a diagnosed deep vein thrombosis, diagnosed pulmonary embolism or a known MTHFR mutation in a first-degree relative.[113] MTHFR testing is often requested when investigating infertility,

TABLE 7.3 Biochemical impact of selected MTHFR polymorphisms		
MTHFR polymorphism	**Population genetics**	**Functional impact**
677CT	Homozygosity is most common in Asian, Mediterranean and Caucasian ancestral genetics, and is rare in black African ancestral genetics	Residual enzyme activity reduced to 45% of wild-type enzyme Homozygosity: 70% loss of function Heterozygosity: 40% loss of function
1298AC	Similar to 677CT variant	Residual enzyme activity reduced to 68% of wild-type enzyme Homozygosity: 40% loss of function Heterozygosity: unknown
677CT + 1298AC compound heterozygosity	Mixed ancestral genetic origins	Biochemical profile is similar to 677CT homozygosity; significantly elevated plasma homocysteine levels
1793GA	Homozygosity appears only in Caucasians	Unknown
1068TC	Silent allele	Appears to be unexpressed with insignificant impact

Source: [114,115,116]

| TABLE 7.4 Other genetic SNPs associated with methylation genetic profiling ||
Gene	Function
AHCY (adenosylhomocysteinase)	Conversion of SAH to adenosine and homocysteine in the methionine cycle. Altered activity can lead to hypermethioninaemia and impaired methylation. Mutations (leading to severe myopathies and developmental delay) and SNPs (less severe clinical presentation) are both associated with this gene.
COMT (catechol-O-methyltransferase)	COMT catalyses the transfer of a methyl group from SAMe to catecholamines, a major degradative pathway for dopamine, noradrenaline (norepinephrine) and adrenaline (epinephrine). Impaired COMT is associated with impaired inactivation of catecholamines and is linked with a range of mental health disorders. COMT is also involved in the deactivation and clearance of oestrogens. The COMT gene is associated with several clinically relevant SNPs.
MTRR (methionine synthase reductase)	Methionine synthase becomes inactive over time due to oxidation of its B_{12} cofactor. It is regenerated by methionine synthase reductase via methylation. This enzyme is encoded by the MTRR gene, which is associated with several SNPs and possibly linked to hypomethylation.
CBS (cystathionine-B-synthase)	Irreversible synthesis of cystathionine from homocysteine in the transsulfuration pathway. Depending on severity, homocysteine elevations and glutathione/taurine/sulfate depletion may result.
BHMT (betaine-homocysteine methyltransferase)	Involved in the alternative pathway of homocysteine to methionine conversion in hepatic tissue. Possibly implicated in elevated homocysteine levels.
MAT1A (methionine adenosyltransferase I alpha)	Conversion of methionine to SAMe in first reaction of the methionine cycle. Enzyme appears inhibited by ethanol. Reduced SAMe, increased homocysteine and poor methylation in general may result.
MAO-A and MAO-B (monoamine oxidase A and B)	MAO-A (catabolism of serotonin, dopamine and noradrenaline [norepinephrine]). MAO-B (catabolism of dopamine and histamine). SNPs may be implicated in conditions associated with poor clearance of biogenic amines, catecholamines and histamine.

Source: [121,122,123]

cancer, autism, cardiovascular diseases, thrombophilia and congenital birth defects, though these do not currently attract a Medicare rebate. Some companies offer direct-to-consumer MTHFR genetic testing for a cost, though the validity of the methods must be scrutinised first. In many cases, direct-to-consumer testing may not involve a health practitioner for clinical interpretation and efficacious treatment, undermining the clinical significance of MTHFR testing.

Other genetic polymorphisms do occur in other genes governing the folate cycle, though they are far less common in the population and are not tested for as frequently. These include the methionine synthase (MTR) A2756G polymorphism and the three-functional enzyme, methylenetetrahydrofolate dehydrogenase/ methylenetetrahydrofolate cyclohydrolase/ formyltetrahydrofolate synthetase (MTHFD1) G1958A polymorphism.[118,119] Both appear to increase circulating homocysteine levels, but only if the individual has a homozygous status for these more rare polymorphisms.[118] Research is accumulating to confirm that various inheritance patterns of the above polymorphisms are linked with elevated homocysteine levels. The severity of the clinical end points associated with these polymorphisms is a contentious issue in orthodox, integrative and naturopathic medicine and remains a prevalent topic in medical research. The varied inheritance patterns, with multiple clinical presentations over several physiological systems, make methylation disorders difficult conditions to both accept clinically and diagnose in areas of health and medicine not yet cognisant of methylation research.

Current statistics estimate that 60–70% of the general population will have inherited at least one polymorphism. Approximately 8.5% are homozygous for thermolabile C677T or A1298C, with 2.25% having compound heterozygosity. An estimated 10% of the population are homozygous or compound heterozygous for these two main polymorphisms.[120] Other SNPs in genes beyond the MTHFR gene are implicated in methylation disorders and these are summarised in Table 7.4.

Biomarkers

Effective laboratory biomarkers of methylation status are presented in Table 7.5.

Additional parameters besides those present in blood are useful biomarkers for specific nutrient deficiencies associated with methylation. Measurements of specific organic acids excreted in urine are indirect measurements of methylated B_{12} and methylated folate in tissues.[127] These include formiminoglutamic acid (FIGLU) and methylmalonic acid (MMA). In the catabolism of the amino acid histidine, FIGLU is an intermediate preceding the production of glutamic acid (the final product).[128] FIGLU is normally removed from tissues in complex with THF, thus elevated levels in urine represent the extent of folate deficiency. Elevated urinary FIGLU may also be linked to B_{12} deficiency.[128] The body normally converts MMA to succinyl coenzyme A. This is a B_{12}-dependent reaction, thus deficiencies of B_{12} can lead to elevated levels of MMA in blood and urine.[127] Urinary MMA is possibly a better biomarker than serum homocysteine levels for the clinical assessment of B_{12} deficiency, with

TABLE 7.5 Laboratory biomarkers of methylation status

Analyte	Clinical interpretation
Plasma homocysteine	Elevated due to increased need for folate, B_6 and/or B_{12}. Reductions follow improved methylation activity, but also during times of high oxidative stress (glutathione need).
Plasma SAMe	Low values indicate diminished methylation capacity.
Plasma SAH	Product of SAMe methylation. Elevated levels indicate high homocysteine, as SAH is not converted to homocysteine when homocysteine levels are high.
Plasma SAMe:SAH ratio	The important methylation index. The normal ratio is 2:1. Generally, low or high levels of both indicate low or high dietary intake of methionine, respectively. A low SAMe/high SAH is a sensitive marker of poor methylation and oxidative stress. A high SAMe/low SAH may indicate overmethylation as a result of methionine intake. SAH is well-known as a potent inhibitor of methylation reactions. To prevent SAH accumulation, Hcy levels must remain normal via correct operation of the methionine cycle with MTHF, B_{12} and betaine as major methyl donors. Novel research suggests that the ratio may be a superior predictor of cardiovascular risk over plasma Hcy levels.
Plasma glutathione (oxidised and reduced)	Reduced glutathione is of more diagnostic value than total glutathione and is more indicative of antioxidant capacity. Oxidised glutathione is normally converted back to reduced glutathione, thus elevated oxidised glutathione indicates high oxidative stress. Glutathione is also required to keep B_{12} from oxidising to support the methionine synthase enzyme.
Plasma histamine	Plasma histamine concentration is usually very low. Elevations are often noted in cases of severe allergic reaction. However, in the absence of or coinciding with allergic reaction, investigation of methylation disorders (clinically and lab based) is required. Plasma histamine may be elevated in conjunction with MAO SNPs or general methylation defects. Elevated histamine is associated with undermethylation (note any concurrent low homocysteine, low zinc, low copper, poor response to B complex vitamins). Low histamine is possible and is linked to overmethylation (also look for reduced zinc or elevated Cu).
Plasma methionine	Both low and high levels are associated with disordered methylation and low B_6/B_9/B_{12}. Elevated and reduced levels are also associated with dietary intake. Patients are advised to fast before testing to limit falsely elevated results.
Plasma folic acid/folinic acid	Elevations are most often due to poor conversion of supplemental folic acid to active folates.
5-MTHF	Levels are often reduced with MTHFR SNPs, B_{12} deficiency, SAMe deficiency or other methionine cycle deficits (nutrient- or SNP-based).
THF	Level is indicative of the metabolically active form of folate.

Source: [124,125,126]

some clinicians finding urinary testing to be superior to serum testing.[129]

Additional urinary markers include vanilmandelate (VMA) and homovanillate (HVA) levels. These are often tested or interpreted in conjunction with COMT SNP testing, as low levels may be linked to poor clearance of catecholamines.[128] COMT SNP testing may also prompt the analysis of the oestrogen methylation ratio in urine. This measures the capacity to methylate oestrogen for detoxification and clearance. Problems in this pathway may be linked to gynaecological cancers.[128]

Routine pathology

The routine pathology tests shown in Table 7.6 may be considered before, during or after functional testing. They must be interpreted with the individual's full medical and health case history in mind. Omitting thorough physical examination in favour of extensive laboratory testing is a clinical oversight to be avoided. Valuable clinical data can be captured on physical examination, including obvious nutrient deficiencies and criteria for disease diagnosis.

CASE 7.1 ADULT PRESENTATION OF METHYLATION DISORDER DUE TO SNPS

A 42-year-old male presented with a recent history of emboli formation (femoral and splenic) and a long-term history of anxiety and panic disorder since his early teens. Genetic profiling revealed a homozygous status for MTHFR and heterozygous status for COMT SNPs. Other biomarkers included elevated plasma homocysteine, reduced plasma SAMe and reduced plasma THF, indicating aberrant methionine and folate cycles. Urinary organic acid screening specifically looking at VMA and HVA was normal, indicating the COMT SNP was not significantly impeding catecholamine clearance. Peripheral blood films revealed moderate macrocytosis (possible B_9/B_{12} deficiencies) and neutrophilic leucocytosis (coinciding with a concurrent surgical wound infection). Fasting BGL was normal. Lipid and biochemistry profiles showed no major abnormalities.

Family history revealed maternal Alzheimer's disease (mother living) and paternal bladder cancer (father deceased). He has one son and one daughter, with his daughter experiencing a similar anxiety and panic disorder. Lifestyle revealed high workplace stress and long hours (legal profession), high ethanol ingestion (at least two standard drinks every day), past history of elite contact sport (representative rugby union), past history of social smoking and regular self-prescription of OTC antacids (calcium salts) for acid reflux. Diet analysis revealed an overconsumption of processed food, very little fresh fruit/vegetables and a liking for sweet carbonated beverages. Physical examination revealed excess central adiposity and mild angular stomatitis. Other physical complaints included arthritic pain in both knees, likely due to high-level sport.

Supplementation was not immediately initiated due to recent surgery and current high-level anxiety. Dietary intervention included immediate reduction of alcohol to two standard drinks per week and a transition to a wholefood diet for his entire family. A broad-spectrum probiotic was prescribed for recent antibiotic therapy, to be continued for 6 weeks minimum. The patient displayed excellent diet compliance and experienced improved sleep and less intense anxiety in the first month post dietary intervention. Bowels were regular and 3 kg weight loss was noted. Light exercise (swimming) commenced at 3x/week.

Supplementation with B-complex vitamins commenced, along with a methyl donor (SAMe) plus magnesium and zinc compound. The patient experienced some nausea and increased inflammatory knee pain on this regimen, indicating

a degree of methyl donor intolerance. SAMe was then prescribed at the same dose, but only as a single morning dose every second day. After 3 months of therapy and a complete dietary overhaul, anxiety attacks diminished and appeared linked to the now rare occasions of poor sleep. SAMe supplementation was discontinued, but the B-complex regimen remained in place in conjunction with zinc and magnesium. Knee pain remained an issue, but was less acute (knee replacement likely). Follow-up scans for emboli formation all clear at the 6-month mark, with B vitamins, lifelong diet and lifestyle changes all directed at preventing their recurrence and minimising adverse cardiovascular events. Homocysteine levels currently at high end of normal range.

THERAPEUTICS AND PRESCRIPTIONS

A variety of intrinsic factors (mutations, SNPs, imprinting, disease states, life cycle phase) and extrinsic factors (response to stressors, nutritional deficiencies, pharmaceuticals) contribute to methylation issues. The role of the clinician is to identify the contributing factors and formulate a holistic prescription that does not simply involve high-dose supplementation. 'Methyl donor intolerance' is a term applied to patients who experience an aggravation of their symptoms, or experience new symptoms in response to supplementation.[131] Methylation substrates and cofactors can be supplied via a nutritious

TABLE 7.6 Methylation correlates from routine pathology	
Analyte	**Clinical interpretation**
Serum vitamin B_6	If reduced, consider further testing for B_9, B_{12} or comprehensive methylation panels with integrative pathology testing.
Serum vitamin B_{12}	If reduced, consider further testing for B_6, B_9 or urinary organic acid screening (MMA specifically). Look for B_9/B_{12} abnormalities on peripheral blood film.
Red cell folate	If reduced, consider further testing for B_6, B_{12} or urinary organic acid screening (FIGLU specifically). Look for B_9/B_{12} abnormalities on peripheral blood film.
Serum ammonia	Elevated levels indicate urea cycle defects or other upstream pathway defects in the folate or methionine cycle. Useful for screening only and not for interpretation in isolation.
Serum copper	Elevated levels indicate possible copper toxicity, a metal known to inhibit specific enzymes of methylation pathways. The source of copper toxicity should be determined and eliminated for effective treatment. Urinary copper or blood caeruloplasmin is often more reliable. Note: levels are increased during the acute phase response and by oestrogens (physiological and therapeutic). Both situations may mask a deficiency state.
Plasma zinc	Reduced levels may be seen with copper toxicity, with consequences for methylation cycles. May also indicate dietary deficiency and increased physiological requirement for zinc. Plasma zinc is not an accurate assessment of zinc stores. Hair analysis preferred if zinc assessment is a priority.
Red cell and serum magnesium	Deficiency is rarely noted on blood; urine analysis is an alternative. Physical exam correlates are important, including muscle spasm and cardiac arrhythmias.
Peripheral blood film	Clinical B_9/B_{12} deficiency causes megaloblastic anaemia. This is observed on the peripheral blood film as hypersegmented neutrophils, hypochromasia of red blood cells, macrocytosis of red blood cells and red cell fragments. Macrocytosis is also noted as a high MCV on red cell indices (part of full blood count).

Source: [130]

diet, while lifestyle modifications can support changes in physiology less diminishing on methylation reserves.

Dietary modifications

In addition to the specific food recommendations presented in Table 7.7, individuals with suspected methylation issues respond well to broader anti-inflammatory health interventions:

- Blood glucose regulation and healthy weight maintenance: central adiposity and elevated general adiposity are both linked with the production of pro-inflammatory cytokines and disordered DNA methylation.
- Anti-inflammatory dietary practices, i.e. a high phytonutrient, high organic-based foods, low refined sugar, low processed food, low refined vegetable oil, low hydrogenated fat-based diet.
- While dietary changes can be overwhelming for patients, most of the goals can be achieved with a patient-led, practitioner-supervised conversion to a wholefood diet.
- Regarding folates specifically, evidence suggests that folate receptors can be blocked by folate autoantibodies. What elicits folate autoantibody production remains unclear. Several immune-based links are currently the subject of research, including a possible link between folate autoantibody production and consumption of dairy products in the diet.[131–134]

Supplementation

A number of treatment protocols for methylation issues are described in clinical scientific literature, passed forth by educators and clinicians and published by nutraceutical manufacturers. As with all facets of naturopathic medicine, the clinical reality is that no one protocol is entirely suitable (or safe) for patients with a suspected or laboratory-confirmed methylation disorder. One piece of advice serves as a ubiquitous clinical platform for all patient prescriptions: *proceed with caution*. Aggressive supplementation with methyl donors is often unnecessary and can be detrimental (particularly in the long term). For many patients, the role of the practitioner is to provide clinical tools and patient education to promote the body's inherent biochemical mechanisms for methylation, returning them to a state of efficiency. Attempting to countermand aberrant biochemistry with high-dose supplementation may be clinically indicated, but only for a small portion of patients or for a brief period of time.

- Initial phase: thorough case history taking, including a screening health history of the patient's first-degree relatives (parents, siblings and children). Any possible or recurring conditions related to disordered methylation should be noted. Environmental and diet history should follow. Depending on the information gleaned, routine and/or functional pathology and/or genetic profiling can be considered. Dietary and lifestyle changes can be initiated, as they can address

TABLE 7.7 Food-based sources of key methylation nutrients	
Methylation nutrient	**Rich food sources**
Betaine (TMG)	Beets, liver, amaranth, red meat, quinoa, spinach, kamut, rye, sunflower seeds
Cobalamin	Eggs, liver, molluscs, red meat, poultry, fish, crustaceans
Choline	Eggs, poultry, red meat, whey, soy beans, chick peas, mung beans, peas, legumes, cauliflower, flaxseeds
Cysteine	Eggs, liver, poultry, red meat, soy beans, seaweeds, spirulina, oats, pumpkin seeds, clams, walnuts
Folate	Dark-green leafy vegetables, mung beans, beans and legumes, Daikon radish, poultry, liver, lentils, chard, kale, cress, bok choy, turnip greens, mushrooms, okra, artichokes
Magnesium	Legumes, Daikon radish, dark-green leafy vegetables, rice bran, molasses, seeds and seed kernels, beans, brazil nuts, teff, amaranth, almonds, cocoa, hazel nuts, bulgur
Methionine	Eggs, poultry, red meat, nuts, seeds, seaweed, spirulina, fish, cheeses
Potassium	Legumes, dark-green leafy vegetables, radishes, potatoes, beans, molasses, seeds, dried apricots, dried herbs
P-5-P	Daikon radish, liver, turkey, rice bran, garlic, pistachio nuts, nuts, seeds, amaranth, walnuts, paprika, chervil, soft cheeses, rosemary, prunes, chickpeas, dried apricots
Riboflavin	Daikon radish, eggs, liver, seaweed, spirulina, red meat, almonds, soy beans, blueberries
Sulfur compounds	Eggs, legumes, alliums, nuts, seeds, soy beans, red meat, poultry, beans, cabbage, brassicas, horseradish, oats, barley, red meat, poultry
Selenium	Brazil nuts, nuts, poultry, eggs, fish, crustaceans, sunflower seeds
Taurine	Animal and fish proteins, eggs, yeast, fish roe
Zinc	Molluscs, red meat, beans, sesame seeds, poultry, pumpkin seeds, teff, peas, lentils, basil, cashew nuts, parsley, peanuts, crustaceans, thyme, dark rye

Source: [131,132,133]

general health issues such as inflammation, gut health, detoxification, nutritional deficits and contributing environmental factors.

- Supplementation phase: depending on the clinical situation and the results of investigations, a variety of nutraceuticals may be prescribed (see Table 7.8).

Every practitioner well versed in the management of methylation disorders advises to prescribe low and initiate dosage increases or prescription additions *slowly*. It is often necessary to titrate supplement dosages to lower levels in response to any negative health exacerbations. This is very important when managing patients with mental health issues. Every patient is uniquely different, with some experiencing more intense clinical signs/symptoms (or novel signs/symptoms) before improvements are noted.

As noted above, methylation is exceptionally complex, influencing the metabolic activities of several body systems

TABLE 7.8 Precursor and supportive nutrients for disordered methylation		
Precursor nutrients	**Clinical considerations**	**Formulation**
Methyl donors: Methionine Betaine SAMe Serine	Initiate treatment with lower dosages to avoid overmethylation. Monitor closely for exacerbation of symptoms, particularly those associated with inflammation and mental health imbalances. These nutrients are usually necessary to reduce homocysteine levels.	If using betaine, zinc is a necessary cofactor. Often necessary to prescribe methyl donors with B_6/B_9/B_{12}. Consider protein and B vitamin malabsorption issues.
Choline	Easily obtained through dietary intervention alone.	Lecithin (both animal and plant derived) is an easily obtained supplemental form of choline. Consider lipid malabsorption issues.
Cofactor nutrients	**Clinical considerations**	**Formulation**
L-5-MTHF and folinic acid	Both need to be prescribed with methyl B_{12} (each nutrient requires the other). Avoid folic acid-fortified foods. L-5-MTHF is the active form of B_9, requiring no conversion. It enters cells directly, thus its usefulness for supporting methylation cycle defects directly. It may exacerbate symptoms of inflammation, thus addressing these issues before supplementation is often necessary. The folinic acid vitamer (L-5-formyltetrahydrofolate) is readily converted to THF independent of dihydrofolate reductase (DHFR). It also enters cells directly, but this form is able to directly enter the pathway of nucleotide biosynthesis, making it a preferred form for supporting DNA repair as opposed to methylation defects. The general therapeutic indication for either form is patients with *known* mutations or SNPs of the MTHFR gene, though L-5-MTHF is preferable for these patients, particularly those with homozygous status. These forms are also preferred for patients prescribed medications known to block DHFR activity (e.g. oral contraceptives, aspirin and cholesterol-lowering medications).	Either L-5-MTHF or folinic acid is the preferred biochemical form of B_9 for supplementation. Folic acid is synthetic and may not be activated in hepatic tissue to L-5-MTHF. Oral supplementation generally works well. Prescription with other activated B-complex vitamins, especially methylcobalamin, is usually required. Folinic acid has the same biochemical activity and profile as L-5-MTHF. It displays rapid conversion to L-5-MTHF. The most common form in supplements is calcium folinate. Folinic acid also has a long history of use as a bone-marrow and GIT mucosa-sparing agent following methotrexate treatment and other pharmacological therapies involving DHFR inhibition. Both forms only require very small dosing regimens to be clinically effective. Caution does exist for folinic acid and L-5-MTHF supplementation. Without viewing the patient's entire methylation cycle, overmethylation can rapidly occur, often within days of supplementation commencing (signs include musculoskeletal pain, anxiety, nausea, migraines, increased atopy, low mood). The excess levels of methyl groups may precipitate increased levels of neurotransmitters further downstream of the primary methylation pathway.
Methylcobalamin	Often required in conjunction with other B vitamins. An important nutrient to consider in patients who follow a vegetarian or vegan diet.	Transdermal, sublingual or intramuscular administration is best, as absorption is notoriously reduced via the oral route.
P-5-P	Required for 5-MTHF synthesis. Required for glutathione synthesis.	Usually prescribed in conjunction with other B vitamins and not in isolation.
Magnesium	Required for ATP stabilisation and necessary for methionine conversion to SAMe.	Usually present as a cofactor in methyl donor preparations. Supplement separately if clinically indicated.

TABLE 7.8 Precursor and supportive nutrients for disordered methylation—cont'd		
Cofactor nutrients	**Clinical considerations**	**Formulation**
Selenium	May be prescribed as adjunct therapy for cases of oxidative stress.	Supplement separately only if clinically indicated.
Zinc	Enzyme cofactor for betaine-dependent conversion of homocysteine to methionine in the liver.	Usually present as a cofactor in methyl donor preparations. Supplement separately if clinically indicated.
Supportive nutrients	**Clinical considerations**	**Formulation**
Glutathione	Generally only supplemented when reduced or total glutathione is low or oxidised glutathione is very high. Supporting other pathways can correct glutathione status, as can assessing medication use (particularly acetaminophen [paracetamol]).	N-acetyl cysteine is often prescribed as a precursor for glutathione synthesis, along with zinc and magnesium as nutrient cofactors.
N-acetyl cysteine	Associated with a long history of prescription. Used to treat glutathione deficiency.	Often prescribed with its cofactors, zinc and magnesium.
Mitochondrial support: CoQ10 Acetyl-l-carnitine D-ribose	Generally only supplemented in specific situations of chronic fatigue, known mitochondrial disorders, cardiovascular complications, ageing and high oxidative stress.	Ubiquinone is the preferred form for maximal absorption of CoQ10.
Microbial producers of folates: *Lactobacillus plantarum* *Bifidobacterium bifidum* *Bifidobacterium infantis* *Bifidobacterium breve* *Bifidobacterium longum* *Bifidobacterium adolescentis* *Bifidobacterium pseudocatenulatum*	Prebiotic foods support the growth and metabolism of microbial folate producers.	Multi-strain probiotic preparations are easily obtained. It is important to consider any impediment to folate absorption, such as intestinal inflammation. Medical history for antibiotic therapy is important when screening for a possible altered microbiome.

Source: [125,131,133,135]

and the entire landscape of our epigenome. Genetics, environment, diet and lifestyle contribute to the individual's unique metabolism and epigenetics – supplementation alone cannot accomplish the entirety of clinical treatment goals.

Lifestyle modifications

- *Smoking cessation:* the carbon monoxide produced by cigarettes is known to deactivate several vitamins, including B6.
- *Stress management and sleep hygiene:* assess and manage situations leading to psychological and/or physical stress. Methyl donors are required for both the production and the deactivation of catecholamines, which are in high demand during chronic stress responses. Methyl donor supplies may become depleted during extended periods of stress. Herbal medicine prescriptions for an appropriate adaptogen, sedative hypnotic or nervine may be required.
- *Exercise habits:* excessive high-intensity cardiovascular exercise can induce a stress response. B vitamins can be quickly depleted if not replaced by the diet. Protein and lipid stores (for methionine, betaine, choline) can also be catabolised for energy and depleted if not

replaced by the diet. Sedentary lifestyles are considered to be pro-inflammatory, which is possibly causative of or negatively influential to abnormal methylation.[133]
- *Caffeine intake:* excess caffeine consumption is linked to the depletion of several B vitamins, most likely via its diuretic effect. All sources of caffeine must be considered: coffee (brewed, instant, iced), tea (black, green, white, iced), soft drinks, energy drinks and coffee-containing desserts.
- *Ethanol intake:* ethanol (drinking alcohol) is known to deplete water-soluble vitamins when consumed in excess. All forms of alcoholic beverages need to be included in the assessment of ethanol intake, paying particular attention to any single serving higher than a standard drink (i.e. size of wine or beer glass, nips of spirits, cocktails).
- *Cooking methods:* several cooking methods are known to destroy B vitamins including frying, high heat and microwave radiation. Include low-heat methods of cooking, slow cooking and fresh/raw no cooking methods of appropriate foods to minimise B vitamin loss.
- *Digestive physiology:* many people do not assimilate the micronutrients in food due to poor digestion. Assess and address any issues linked to malabsorption

including dental issues, fast and non-mindful eating, drinking excess liquids with meals, inflammatory digestive conditions, disordered eating, poor diet, chronic digestive diseases, GIT infections and dysbiosis. Herbal medicine prescriptions for mucous membrane trophorestoratives, GIT anti-inflammatories, carminatives, bitter principles and cholagogues/choleretics may be necessary.

- *Toxin exposure through employment or hobbies:* pesticides, fertilisers, phthalates, persistent organic pollutants (POPs), heavy metals and vehicle exhaust have been linked to altered methylation of DNA. Individuals are advised to assess their level of exposure via work, hobbies and the home, minimising exposure or protecting their body as far as possible. Dietary changes to support methylation are essential if exposure is high. Herbal medicine prescriptions for botanical antioxidants can be useful.

Medications

- *Prescription medications:* a variety of prescribed medications are known to deplete the body of certain B vitamins. These include methotrexate (prescribed for certain autoimmune diseases, specific cancers and some forms of arthritis), oral contraceptives, phenytoin, metformin, some antibiotics and proton-pump inhibitors (PPIs). Patients who require a medication known to deplete B-complex vitamins need follow-up for possible deficiencies, particularly if their therapy is long term. Some drugs need regular review from the prescribing medical practitioner (for dose, type and clinical necessity).
- *OTC medications:* OTC antacids are known to block nutrient absorption, particularly for B vitamins. Regular and long-term reliance on OTC antacids may interfere with B vitamin status, particularly for patients with low B-complex vitamin intake or medical conditions such as pernicious anaemia, malabsorption or inflammatory conditions of the GIT and thyroid conditions. Pregnant women have an increased need for B vitamins, but regular use of OTC antacids may block their absorption. The elderly often have issues with malabsorption; any frequent use of OTC antacids can compound this problem.

REFERENCES

[1] Ross M, Desai M. Developmental origins of adult health. In: Gabbe S, Niebyl J, Simpson J, et al, editors. Obstetrics: normal and problem pregnancies. 7th ed. Philadelphia: Elsevier; 2017. p. 83–99.
[2] Schierding W, Vickers M, O'Sullivan J, et al. Epigenetics. In: Polin R, Abman S, Rowtich D, et al, editors. Foetal and neonatal physiology. 5th ed. Philadelphia: Elsevier; 2017. p. 89–100.
[3] Hernando-Herraez I, Garcia-Perez R, Sharp A, et al. DNA methylation: insights into human evolution. PLoS Genet 2015;11(12):e1005661.
[4] Bettelheim F, Brown W, Campbell M, et al. Nucleotides, nucleic acids, and heredity. In: Introduction to general, organic and biochemistry. 10th ed. Belmont: Brooks/Cole, Cengage Learning; 2013. p. 687–9.
[5] Batmanian L, Ridge J, Worrall S. Nucleic acids: biological molecules for information storage, retrieval and usage. In: Biochemistry for health professionals. Sydney: Elsevier; 2011. p. 101–9.
[6] Nussbaum R, McInnes C, Willard H. The human genome: structure and function. In: Thomson and Thomson genetics in medicine. 8th ed. Philadelphia: Elsevier; 2016. p. 21–42.
[7] Nussbaum R, McInnes C, Willard H. Introduction to the human genome. In: Thomson and Thomson genetics in medicine. 8th ed. Philadelphia: Elsevier; 2016. p. 3–20.
[8] Stein C. Applications of cytogenetics in modern pathology. In: McPherson R, Pincus M, editors. Henry's clinical diagnosis and management by laboratory methods. 23rd ed. St Louis: Elsevier; 2017. p. 1337–59.
[9] Malumbres M, Barbacid M. To cycle or not to cycle: a critical decision in cancer. Nat Rev Cancer 2001;1:222–31.
[10] Malumbres M. Control of the cell cycle. In: Niederhuber J, Armitage J, Doroshow J, et al, editors. Abeloff's clinical oncology. 5th ed. Philadelphia: Saunders; 2014. p. 52–68.
[11] Vandiver A, Idrizi A, Rizzardi L, et al. DNA methylation is stable during replication and cell cycle arrest. Sci Rep 2015;5:17911.
[12] Jorde L, Carey J, Bamshad M. Basic cell biology. In: Jorde L, Carey J, Bamshad M, editors. Medical genetics. 5th ed. Philadelphia: Mosby; 2016. p. 6–27.
[13] Wagner A, Berliner N, Benz E. Anatomy and physiology of the gene. In: Hoffman R, Benz E, Silberstein L, et al, editors. Haematology: basic principles and practice. 6th ed. Philadelphia: Saunders; 2013. p. 2–15.
[14] Maor G, Yearim A, Ast G. The alternative role of DNA methylation in splicing regulation. Trends Genet 2015;31(5):274–80.
[15] Scott D, Lee B. The human genome. In: Kliegman R, Stanton B, St Geme J, et al, editors. Nelson's textbook of paediatrics. 20th ed. Philadelphia: Elsevier; 2016. p. 588–93.
[16] Iacobazzi V, Castegna A, Infantino V, et al. Mitochondrial DNA methylation as a next-generation biomarker and diagnostic tool. Mol Genet Metab 2013;110(1–2):25–34.
[17] FitzPatrick D, Seckl J. Molecular and genetic factors in disease. In: Walker B, Colledge N, Ralston S, et al, editors. Davidson's principles and practice of medicine. 22nd ed. Philadelphia: Churchill-Livingstone; 2014. p. 41–70.
[18] Wallace D, Lott M, Procaccio V. Mitochondrial medicine. In: Rimoin D, editor. Emery and Rimoin's principles and practice of medical genetics. 6th ed. Philadelphia: Elsevier; 2013. p. 1–153.
[19] Shock L, Thakkar P, Peterson E, et al. DNA methyltransferase 1, cytosine methylation and cytosine hydroxymethylation in mammalian mitochondria. Proc Natl Acad Sci USA 2011;108(9):3630–5.
[20] Smiraglia D, Kulawiec M, Bistulfi G, et al. A novel role for mitochondria in regulating epigenetic modifications in the nucleus. Cancer Biol Ther 2014;7(8):1182–90.
[21] Patton J, Hunt M, Jamieson A. Regulation of gene expression. In: Baynes J, Dominiczak M, editors. Medical biochemistry. 4th ed. Philadelphia: Saunders; 2014. p. 453–65.
[22] Roldan-Arjona T, Ariza R. DNA demethylation. In: Madame Curie Bioscience Database 2009. Available from: www.ncbi.nlm.nih.gov/books/NBK6365.
[23] Hall J. Genetic control of protein synthesis, cell function, and cell reproduction. In: Guyton and Hall's textbook of medical physiology. 13th ed. Philadelphia: Elsevier; 2016. p. 27–43.
[24] Polevoda B, Sherman F. Methylation of proteins involved in translation. Mol Microbiol 2007;65(3):590–606.
[25] Bedford M, Clarke S. Protein arginine methylation in mammals: who, what and why. Mol Cell 2009;33(1):1–13.
[26] Meisenberg G, Simmons W. DNA, RNA and protein synthesis. In: Meisenberg G, Simmons W, editors. Principles of medical biochemistry. 3rd ed. Philadelphia: Elsevier; 2012. p. 64–92.
[27] Patton J, Bannon G. Protein synthesis and turnover. In: Baynes J, Dominiczak M, editors. Medical biochemistry. 4th ed. Saunders Elsevier; 2014. p. 441–52.
[28] Wang J, Toms A, Zhou M, et al. Protein architecture. In: Hoffman R, Benz E, Silberstein LE, et al, editors. Haematology: basic principles and practice. 6th ed. Philadelphia: Saunders; 2013. p. 48–54.
[29] Walsh C. Post-translational modification of proteins: expanding nature's inventory. Englewood, CO: Roberts & Co.; 2006.

[30] Clarke S. Protein methylation at the surface and buried deep: thinking outside the histone box. Trends Biochem Sci 2013;38(5):243–52.

[31] Petrossian T, Clarke S. Uncovering the human methyltransferasome. Mol Cell Proteomics 2011;10(1):M110.000976.

[32] Weksberg R, Butcher D, Grafodatskaya D, et al. Epigenetics. In: Emery and Rimoin's principles and practice of medical genetics. 6th ed. Philadelphia: Elsevier; 2013. p. 1–31.

[33] Berger S, Kouzarides T, Shiekhattar R, et al. An operational definition of epigenetics. Genes Dev 2009;23:781–3.

[34] Bennett-Baker P, Wilkowski J, Burke D. Age-associated activation of epigenetically repressed genes in the mouse. Genetics 2003;165:2055–62.

[35] Ji Y, Nordgren K, Chai Y, et al. Human liver methionine cycle: MAT1A and GNMT gene resequencing, functional genomics and hepatic genotype-phenotype correlation. Drug Metab Dispos 2012;40(10):1984–92.

[36] The Rat Genome Database 2015. Methionine cycle/metabolic pathway. Bioinformatics Program, HMGC. Medical College of Wisconsin, Milwaukee. Available from: http://rgd.mcw.edu/rgdweb/pathway/pathwayRecord.html?acc_id=PW:0000048. [Accessed 11 October 2016].

[37] The Rat Genome Database 2015. Folate cycle metabolic pathway. Bioinformatics Program, HMGC. Medical College of Wisconsin, Milwaukee. Available from: http://rgd.mcw.edu/rgdweb/pathway/pathwayRecord.html?acc_id=PW:0001207. [Accessed 11 October 2016].

[38] The Rat Genome Database 2015. Transsulfuration pathway of homocysteine metabolism. Bioinformatics Program, HMGC. Medical College of Wisconsin, Milwaukee. Available from: http://rgd.mcw.edu/rgdweb/pathway/pathwayRecord.html?acc_id=PW:0000400. [Accessed 11 October 2016].

[39] Hyland K. Inherited disorders affecting dopamine and serotonin: critical neurotransmitters derived from aromatic amino acids. J Nutr 2007;137(6):1568S–72S.

[40] Singh P, Bourque G, Craig N, et al. Mobile genetic elements and genome evolution. Mob DNA 2014;5:26.

[41] Vinson C, Chatterjee R. CG methylation. Epigenomics 2012;4(6):655–63.

[42] Uno E, Berry D. X inactivation and epigenetics. Walter + Eliza Hall Institute of Medical Research. Sydney; 2012. Available from: www.wehi.edu.au/wehi-tv/x-inactivation-and-epigenetics.

[43] Peinado M. Hypomethylation of DNA. In: Schwab M, editor. Encyclopaedia of cancer. 3rd ed. Berlin: Springer-Verlag; 2012. p. 1791–2.

[44] Ehrlich M. DNA hypomethylation in cancer cells. Epigenomics 2009;1(2):239–59.

[45] Wilson A, Power B, Molloy P. DNA hypomethylation and human diseases. Biochim Biophys Acta 2007;138–62.

[46] Pogribny I, Beland F. DNA hypomethylation in the origin and pathogenesis of human diseases. Cell Mol Life Sci 2009;66(14):2249–61.

[47] Estellar M. CpG island hypermethylation and tumour suppressor genes: a booming present, a brighter future. Oncogene 2002;21(35):5427–40.

[48] Boriack-Sjodin A, Swinger K. Protein methyltransferases: a distinct, diverse and dynamic family of enzymes. Biochemistry 2016;55(11):1557–69.

[49] Petrossian T, Clarke S. Uncovering the human methyltransferosome. Mol Cell Proteomics 2011;10:M110.000976.

[50] Falnes P, Jakobsson M, Davydova E, et al. Protein lysine methylation by seven-beta-strand methyltransferases. Biochem J 2016;473(14):1995–2009.

[51] Goffin J, Eisenhauer E. DNA methyltransferase inhibitors: state of the art. Ann Oncol 2002;13:1699–716.

[52] Bottiglieri T. S-adenosyl-L-methionine (SAMe): from the bench to the bedside — molecular basis of a pleiotrophic molecule. Am J Clin Nutr 2002;76:1151S–7S.

[53] Levkovitz Y, Alpert J, Brintz C, et al. Effects of S-adenosylmethionine augmentation on serotonin-reuptake inhibitor antidepressants on cognitive symptoms of major depressive disorders. Eur Psychiatry 2011;136(3):1174–8.

[54] Lu S. Glutathione synthesis. Biochim Biophys Acta 2013;1830(5):3143–53.

[55] Lu S. Regulation of glutathione synthesis. Mol Aspects Med 2009;30(1–2):42–59.

[56] Van Konynenburg R. Is glutathione depletion an important part of the pathogenesis of chronic fatigue syndrome? Presented at AACFS Seventh International Conference Madison, Wisconsin, 8–10 October 2004. Available from: http://phoenixrising.me/research-2/glutathione-depletionmethylation-blockades-in-chronic-fatigue-syndrome/is-glutathione-depletion-an-important-part-of-the-pathogenesis-of-chronic-fatigue-syndrome-by-richard-van-konynenburg-independent-researcher.

[57] Mytilineou C, Kramer B, Yabut J. Glutathione depletion and oxidative stress. Parkinsonism Relat Disord 2002;8(6):385–7.

[58] Teitell M, Richardson B. DNA methylation in the immune system. Clin Immunol 2003;109:2–5.

[59] Pacis A, Tailleux L, Morin A, et al. Bacterial infection remodels the DNA methylation landscape of human dendritic cells. Genome Res 2015;doi:10.1101/gr.192005.115.

[60] Serrano A, Castro-Vega I, Redondo M. Role of gene methylation in anti-tumour immune response: implication for tumour progression. Cancers (Basel) 2011;3(2):1672–90.

[61] Jeffries M, Sawalha A. Autoimmune disease in the epigenetic era: how has epigenetics changed our understanding of disease and how can we expect the field to evolve? Expert Rev Clin Immunol 2015;11(1):45–58.

[62] Cherry C, Thompson B, Saptarshi N, et al. 2106: a 'mitochondria' odyssey. Trends Mol Med 2016;22(5):391–403.

[63] Vance D. Phospholipid methylation in mammals: from biochemistry to physiological function. Biochim Biophys Acta 2014;1838(6):1477–87.

[64] Kanno K, Wu M, Scapa E, et al. Structure and function of the phosphatidylcholine transfer protein (PC-TP)/StarD2. Biochim Biophys Acta 2007;1771(6):654–62.

[65] Linus Pauling Institute. Choline. Micronutrient Information Center, Oregon State University. Available from: http://lpi.oregonstate.edu/mic/other-nutrients/choline. [Accessed 17 October 2016].

[66] Guo Y, Yu S, Zhang C, et al. Epigenetic regulation of Keap1-Nrf2 signaling. Free Radic Biol Med 2015;88(Pt B):337–49.

[67] Yager J. Mechanisms of oestrogen carcinogenesis: the role of E2/E1-quinone metabolites suggests new approaches to preventive intervention — a review. Steroids 2015;99(Pt A):56–60.

[68] Vaz F, Wanders J. Carnitine biosynthesis in mammals. J Biochem 2002;361:417–29.

[69] Da Silva R, Nissim I, Brosnan M, et al. Creatine synthesis: hepatic metabolism of guanidinoacetate and creatine in the rat in vitro and in vivo. Am J Physiol Endocrinol Metab 2009;296(2):E256–61.

[70] UniProt. Cysteine biosynthesis. UniProt Consortium. Available from: www.uniprot.org/keywords/KW-0198. [Accessed 18 October 2016].

[71] Schomerus C, Korf H. Mechanisms regulating melatonin synthesis in the mammalian pineal organ. Ann N Y Acad Sci 2005;1057:372–83.

[72] Berg J, Tymoczko J, Stryer L. Section 25.1: In de novo synthesis, the pyrimidine ring is assembled from bicarbonate, aspartate, and glutamine. Biochemistry. 5th ed. New York: W.H. Freeman & Company; 2002.

[73] Dominiczak M, Broom J. Vitamins and minerals. In: Baynes J, Dominiczak M, editors. Medical biochemistry. 4th ed. Philadelphia: Saunders; 2014. p. 126–41.

[74] Locasale J. Serine, glycine and one-carbon units: cancer metabolism in full circle. Nat Rev Cancer 2013;13:572–83.

[75] Crider K, Yang T, Berry R, et al. Folate and DNA methylation: a review of molecular mechanisms and the evidence for folate's role. Adv Nutr 2012;3:21–38.

[76] Aitkin S, Lodha P, Morneau D. The enzymes of the transsulfuration pathways: active site characterisations. Biochim Biophys Acta 2011;1814(11):1511–17.

[77] Meisenberg G, Simmons W. Amino acid metabolism. In: Meisenberg G, Simmons W, editors. Principles of medical biochemistry. 3rd ed. Philadelphia: Saunders; 2012. p. 441–62.

[78] Banks E, Doughty S, Toms S, et al. Inhibition of cobalamin-dependent methionine synthase by substituted benzofused heterocycles. FEBS J 2007;274(1):287–99.

[79] Linus Pauling Institute. Riboflavin. Micronutrient Information Center, Oregon State University. Available from: http://lpi

.oregonstate.edu/mic/vitamins/riboflavin. [Accessed 21 October 2016].

[80] National Institutes of Health. MTRR gene. In: US National Library of Medicine. Available from: https://ghr.nlm.nih.gov/gene/MTRR. [Accessed 21 October 2016].

[81] Shafqat N, Muniz J, Pilka E, et al. Insight into the S-adenosylmethionine biosynthesis from the crystal structures of the human methionine adenosyltransferase catalytic and regulatory subunits. Biochem J 2013;452(1):27–36.

[82] Williams N. Magnesium ion catalyzed ATP hydrolysis. J Am Chem Soc 2000;122(48):12023–4.

[83] Hy K. The methionine sulfoxide reduction system: selenium utilization and methionine sulfoxide reductase enzymes and their functions. Antioxid Redox Signal 2013;19(9):958–69.

[84] Joseph J. Selenistasis: epistatic effects of selenium on cardiovascular phenotype. Nutrients 2013;5(2):340–58.

[85] Jing M, Rech L, Goltz D, et al. Effects of zinc deficiency and zinc supplementation on homocysteine levels and related enzyme expression in rats. J Trace Elem Med Biol 2015;30:77–82.

[86] Craig S. Betaine in human nutrition. Am J Clin Nutr 2004;80(3):539–49.

[87] Belalcazar A, Ball J, Frost L, et al. Transsulfuration is a significant source of sulfur for glutathione production in human mammary epithelial cells. ISRN Biochem 2013; doi:10.1155/2013/637897. 637897.

[88] Monfort A, Wutz A. Breathing-in epigenetic change with vitamin C. EMBO Rep 2013;14(4):337–46.

[89] Beckett E, Duesing K, Martin C, et al. Relationship between methylation status of vitamin D-related genes, vitamin D levels, and methyl-donor biochemistry. J Nutr Intermed Metab 2016;6:8–15.

[90] Imbard A. Plasma choline and betaine correlate with serum folate, plasma. Clin Chem Lab Med 2013;51:683–92.

[91] Braun L, Cohen M. S-adenosyl-L-methionine (SAMe). In: Braun L, Cohen M, editors. Herbs and natural supplements, vol. 2. 4th ed. Sydney: Elsevier; 2015. p. 856–64.

[92] Avula S, Parikh S, Demarest S, et al. Treatment of mitochondrial disorders. Curr Treat Options Neurol 2014;16(6):292.

[93] Yang M, Vousden H. Serine and one-carbon metabolism in cancer. Nat Rev Cancer 2016;16:650–62.

[94] Miller A. The methionine-homocysteine cycle and its effects on cognitive diseases. Altern Med Rev 2003;8(1):7–19.

[95] Atkuri K, Mantovani J, Herzenberg L, et al. N-acetylcysteine: a safe antidote for cysteine/glutathione deficiency. Curr Opin Pharmacol 2007;7(4):355–9.

[96] Oakes C, Claus R, Gu L, et al. Evolution of DNA methylation is linked to genetic aberrations in chronic lymphocytic leukemia. Cancer Discov 2014;4(3):348–61.

[97] Lv J, Lui H, Su J, et al. DiseaseMeth: a human disease methylation database. Nucleic Acids Res 2012;40(database issue): D1030–5.

[98] Kumar V, Abbas A, Aster J. Genetic disorders. In: Kumar V, Abbas A, Aster J, editors. Robbins and Cotran pathologic basis of disease. 9th ed. Philadelphia: Elsevier; 2014. p. 137–83.

[99] Conerly M, Grady W. Insights into the role of DNA methylation in disease through the use of mouse models. Dis Model Mech 2010;3(5–6):290–7.

[100] Lord R, Bralley A. Genomics. In: Lord R, Bralley A, editors. Laboratory evaluations for integrative and functional medicine. 2nd ed. Georgia: Metametrix Institute. 2008. p. 589–98.

[101] Ho S, Johnson A, Tarapore P, et al. Environmental epigenetics and its implications, disease risk and health outcomes. ILAR J 2012;53(3–4):289–305.

[102] Bernal A, Jirtle R. Epigenomic disruption: the effects of early developmental exposures. Birth Defects Res A Clin Mol Teratol 2010;88(10):938–44.

[103] Geraty A, Lindsay K, Alberdi G, et al. Nutrition during pregnancy impacts offspring's epigenetic status: evidence from human and animal studies. Nutr Metab Insights 2015;8(Suppl. 1):41–7.

[104] Luo Y, Wang Y, Shu Y, et al. Epigenetic mechanisms: an emerging role in pathogenesis and its therapeutic potential in systemic sclerosis. Int J Biochem Cell Biol 2015;67:92–100.

[105] Meda F, Folci M, Baccarelli A, et al. The epigenetics of autoimmunity. Cell Mol Immunol 2011;8(3):226–36.

[106] Zhao M, Wang Z, Yung S, et al. Epigenetic dynamics in immunity and autoimmunity. Int J Biochem Cell Biol 2015;67:65–74.

[107] Gonzalgo M, Sfanos K, Meeker A. Molecular genetics and cancer biology. In: Wein A, Kavoussi L, Partin A, et al, editors. Campbell-Walsh urology. 11th ed. Philadelphia: Elsevier; 2016. p. 459–81.

[108] Yang B. Epigenetics: DNA hypermethylation in cancer. In: Tubbs R, Stoler M, editors. Cell and tissue-based molecular pathology: a volume in the foundations in diagnostic pathology series. Philadelphia: Elsevier; 2009.

[109] Baylin S. Epigenetics and cancer. In: Mendelsohn J, Gray J, Howley P, et al, editors. The molecular basis of cancer. 4th ed. Philadelphia: Elsevier; 2015. p. 67–78.

[110] Bope E, Kellerman R. The cardiovascular system. In: Bope E, Kellerman R, editors. Conn's current therapy. Philadelphia: Elsevier; 2016. p. 439–518.

[111] Miller A, Kelly G, Tran J. Homocysteine metabolism. In: Pizzorno J, Murray M, editors. Textbook of natural medicine. 4th ed. St Louis: Churchill Livingstone; 2013. p. 488–504.

[112] Bleie O, Refsum H, Ueland P. Changes in basal and post methionine load concentrations of total homocysteine and cystathione after B vitamin intervention. Am J Clin Nutr 2004;80: 641–8.

[113] Hickey S, Curry C, Toriello H. ACMG practice guideline: lack of evidence for MTHFR polymorphism testing. Genet Med 2013;15(2): 153–6.

[114] Leclerc D, Sibani S, Rozen R. Molecular biology of methylenetetrahydrofolate reductase (MTHFR) and overview of mutations/polymorphisms. Madame Curie Bioscience Database. Available from: www.ncbi.nlm.nih.gov/books/NBK6561. [Accessed 17 October 2016].

[115] Nazki F, Sameer A, Ganaie B. Folate: metabolism, genes, polymorphisms and the associated diseases. Gene 2014;533(1): 11–20.

[116] Fisher M, Cronstein B. Meta-analysis of methylenetetrahydrofolate reductase (MTHFR) polymorphisms affecting methotrexate toxicity. J Rheumatol 2009;36(3):539–45.

[117] NSW Health. About MTHFR: information for GPs. Centre for Genetics Education, NSW Government. Available from: www. genetics.edu.au/Professionals/mthfr-dna-test. [Accessed 22 October 2016].

[118] Sniezawska A, Dorszewska J, Rozycka A, et al. MTHFR, MTR, and MTHFD1 gene polymorphisms compared to homocysteine and asymmetric dimethylarginine concentrations and their metabolites in epileptic patients treated with antiepileptic drugs. Seizure 2011;20(7):533–40.

[119] Ho V, Massey T, King W. Effects of methionine synthase and methylenetetrahydrofolate reductase gene polymorphisms on markers of one-carbon metabolism. Genes Nutr 2013;8(6): 571–80.

[120] Wilcken B, Bamforth F, Li Z. Geographical and ethnic variation of the 677C>T allele of 5,10 methylenetetrahydrofolate reductase (MTHFR): findings from over 7000 newborns from 16 areas worldwide. J Med Genet 2003;40(8):619–25.

[121] Feng Q, Pelleymounter L, Moon I, et al. Human S-adenosylhomocysteine hydrolase: common gene sequence variation and functional genomic characterization. J Neurochem 2009;110(6):1806–17.

[122] Hoth K, Paul R, Williams L, et al. Associations between the COMT Val/Met polymorphism, early life stress, and personality among healthy adults. Neuropsychiatr Dis Treat 2006;2(2):219–25.

[123] Rai V, Yadav U, Kumar P, et al. Analysis of methionine synthase reductase polymorphism (A66G) in Indian Muslim population. Indian J Hum Genet 2013;19(2):183–7.

[124] Richie J, Nichenametla S, Neidig W, et al. Randomised controlled trial of oral glutathione supplementation on body stores of glutathione. Eur J Nutr 2015;54(2):251–63.

[125] NutriPATH Integrative Pathology Services. Methylation and MTHFR. Practitioner Manual. Available from: http://nutripath .com.au/wp-content/uploads/2015/11/NPATH-METHYLATIO N-MTHFR-Practitioner-Manual-v3.1.pdf. [Accessed 22 October 2016].

[126] Costello J, Plass C. Methylation matters. J Med Genet 2001;38:285–303.

[127] American Association of Clinical Chemistry. Methylmalonic acid. Available from: https://labtestsonline.org/understanding/analytes/mma/tab/sample. [Accessed 22 October 2016].

[128] NCBI. FIGLU Test. MeSH Database. Available from: www.ncbi.nlm.nih.gov/mesh?Db=mesh&term=FIGLU+Test. [Accessed 22 October 2016].

[129] Norman E. Urinary methylmalonic acid test may have greater value than the total homocysteine assay for screening elderly individuals for cobalamin deficiency. Clin Chem 2004;50(8):1482–3.

[130] Royal College of Pathologists of Australasia (RCPA). Manual of use and interpretation of pathology tests. 7th ed. Surry Hills: RCPA; 2015. Available from: www.rcpa.edu.au/Library/Practising-Pathology/RCPA-Manual/Home. [Accessed 11 September 2016].

[131] Fitzgerald K, Hodges R. The methylation diet and MTHFR. BioIndividual Nutrition Institute. Available from: http://bioindividualnutrition.com/methylation-diet-mthfr. [Accessed 23 October 2016].

[132] USDA. UDSA food composition databases. Agricultural Research Service, United States Department of Agriculture. Available from: https://ndb.nal.usda.gov/ndb. [Accessed 23 October 2016].

[133] Fitzgerald K, Hodges R. Food-based nutrients. In: Fitzgerald K, Hodges R, editors. Methylation diet and lifestyle. 2016. p. 47. Available from: www.drkarafitzgerald.com/product/methylation-diet-lifestyle-ebook.

[134] Frye R, Sequeira J, Quadros E, et al. Cerebral folate receptor autoantibodies in autism spectrum disorder. Mol Psychiatry 2013;18:369–81.

[135] Jadavji N, Wieske F, Dirnagl U, et al. Methylenetetrahydrofolate reductase deficiency alters levels of glutamate and γ-aminobutyric acid in brain tissue. Mol Genet Metab Rep 2015;3:1–4.

8 Genetics and epigenetics

Rhona Creegan and Margaret Smith

Terminology

- Copy number variant: sections of the genome are repeated or deleted and the number of repeats varies between individuals
- Epigenetics: modification of gene expression rather than alteration of the genetic code itself, which occurs in response to environment and metabolic cues
- Germline mutation: inherited genetic alterations that occur in sperm and oocytes and are present in all cells of offspring (e.g. cystic fibrosis, haemoglobinopathies, haemophilia)
- Nutrigenetics: the effect of genetic variation on dietary response (e.g. APOE and fat intake)
- Nutrigenomics: the effect of nutrients and other compounds on gene expression (e.g. resveratrol, curcumin and sulforaphanes on SIRT1, COX and GSTM, respectively)
- SNP (single nucleotide polymorphism): a variation in a single nucleotide at a specific position in the genome; occurs in >1% of the population
- Somatic mutation: genetic alteration acquired by the cell that can be passed onto the progeny cells during cell division. These acquired alterations are frequently caused by environmental factors such as exposure to UV light or chemicals. Typically, somatic mutations give rise to various diseases such as cancer
- Wild type: the gene sequence that prevails and produces the typical phenotype occurring in nature as distinct from an atypical mutant type.

THE 'OMICS' REVOLUTION

The 'omics' revolution has changed the way that practitioners view the human body in relation to preventive health and disease states. The omics suffix refers to various technologies that are used to characterise and measure biological molecules, or biomolecules, present in cells. Biomolecules include the larger macromolecules such as lipids, proteins, carbohydrates, nucleic acids, hormones, neurotransmitters and RNA molecules (transcriptomics) as well as smaller molecules such as natural products and primary and secondary metabolites (metabolomics) in cells, and genomes. Omics-based medicine is now part of the preventive health landscape allowing us to explore roles, relationships and actions in human cells.

Genomics, the study of our genes, and nutrigenomics, the study of gene–nutrient interactions, have hit centre stage in the preventive health arena. Practitioners globally are now being presented with a plethora of seemingly complicated information that they are required to decipher. Companies are using omic-based data to connect genomic information with biochemical assays to provide greater insights into human health.

It is common practice to use both genomic and metabolomics information, since both are equally important. Each data set validates the other and provides more in-depth knowledge. For example, a biochemical result is useful, but if we do not understand the genomic contribution or the dysregulated pathway, we are only seeing an output without understanding the causation. While single nucleotide polymorphisms (SNPs) may not be our genetic destiny, they are molecular beacons that provide greater insight into the interplay between genes, lifestyle and environment.

Importantly for practitioners, this burgeoning area requires education and ongoing practitioner support delivered by appropriately qualified geneticists and nutritional biochemists. Companies that offer support and more importantly provide evidence-based information will remain at the forefront of preventive health.

REGULATION OF GENETIC SCREENING

Many companies provide genetic information, either directly to consumers or to practitioners only. A global consensus regarding privacy of information has not been reached since each country has its own regulatory bodies that provide the framework for laboratories providing human genetic analysis. This is largely because genomic technologies are moving so quickly that regulatory bodies cannot keep up with the ethical and clinical issues associated with genetic analysis.

Laboratories providing genetic information fall into either clinically relevant genetic assessment or non-clinical risk assessment analysis. For example, testing for genes associated with familial breast cancer, *BRCA1* and *BRCA2*, is considered genetically relevant and operates under strict accreditation guidelines. In contrast, the risk assessment genotypes obtained from direct-to-consumer companies and genomic companies providing a service to practitioners fall under other regulatory standards. The regulatory standard for non-clinical risk assessment limits the release of genetic information as raw data. There are several companies that for a fee upload the raw data providing information relating to the individual's genotype.

Within this testing and consultation construct, practitioners have an obligation in the first instance to understand how a genetic test result will be obtained and how accurate the data are. The most affordable test is often ordered without due consideration for the differences in how the result will be obtained and the accuracy of the data. Selecting a test without understanding the technology means that a more informative test may be overlooked. Importantly, practitioners must ask several questions before selecting a genetic test:

- What will the test tell me and what are the limitations of the technology?
- How can I use this information to create a treatment plan for my client?
- Does this result fit the clinical picture for this client? Functional pathology and pathology testing should be queried if a result is not as expected: do not assume that a result is correct.

Identifying SNPs in DNA is performed using various types of technologies, each of which has its own unique set of limitations. The gold standard test, Sanger sequencing, is too expensive for routine genetic testing. Traditionally, medical genetic testing used Sanger sequencing to confirm a mutation detected by another, usually more cost-effective, method. In contrast, non-clinical risk assessment using array-based technologies, providing genetic information on millions of DNA changes, remains unvalidated. There are simply too many DNA changes to validate and it would be a costly exercise to compare with data sets from Sanger sequencing.

While information on genetic variants provides molecular beacons to altered activity of various enzymes in biochemical pathways, epigenetics also needs to be considered.

INTRODUCTION TO DNA AND GENE EXPRESSION

Epigenetics

Certain classical inherited diseases result from DNA sequence changes of germline cells that markedly alter the function of the coded protein, such as occurs in Huntington's disease, cystic fibrosis, haemophilia and some familial cancers. Advances in technology and the availability of testing have resulted in many practitioners delving into the complex area of genetics without a clear understanding of what an inherited disease is and what a genetic variant means.

What is the difference between a genetic variant and a mutation? Generally, the term 'variant' should be used to describe a change in DNA sequence that is present in a percentage of the population but does not result in disease, whereas the term 'mutation' (germline or somatic) should be used to describe a change in DNA sequence that results in disease.[1] This is very relevant for interpretation of results

and communication of any genetic information to patients.

In addition to understanding the implications of genetic variants in terms of disease risk, we now know that alterations in the expression of genes (i.e. whether a gene is switched on or off) can have a major influence on how the body adapts to its environment and can impact overall health. This relates to the concept of genetic plasticity: major advances in the past few decades have shown that our genes are not always our destiny or a prescription for disease; rather, they respond to both the external and the internal environment and metabolic cues to alter transcription of genes that influence cellular biochemistry.[2] This is epigenetics – a change in phenotype without a change in genotype – and results from the dynamic alteration of genetic transcription to adapt and influence cellular processes without any change in the DNA sequence. Abnormal gene transcription can therefore have the same effect in terms of contributing to disease risk even in the absence of DNA sequence variants. This is an important concept in terms of understanding disease risk and using targeted interventions in the field of personalised medicine. It is important to realise that the gene sequence alone, whether a variant or wild type, does not provide the whole picture and should rarely be used in isolation for therapeutic intervention.

Epigenetic control of gene expression is required for both development and survival. An obvious epigenetic modification is the terminal differentiation of cells. All cells start out the same but go on to become specific tissue cells. At the developmental stage 'imprinting' is the expression of certain genes, the pattern of which is inherited from a parent and usually acts to silence genes.[3,4] The imprinted genes discovered to date are involved in embryonic growth, development of the placenta and, in the postnatal period, suckling and metabolism.[5,6]

Epidemiological studies have shown that prenatal and postnatal environmental factors influence the risk of developing chronic disease and behavioural problems in adulthood.[7] For example, children born during the Dutch famine of 1944–1945 have a higher incidence of cardiovascular disease and obesity if their mothers were exposed to famine in the prenatal period compared to children born to mothers who were not exposed to famine.[8] This may provide some rationale for the passing down of unhealthy lifestyle habits or adversity and the influence of metabolic disease in subsequent generations, regardless of any true genetic variants predisposing to disease. From a mechanistic point of view, the association described in the Dutch famine study appears to be caused by hypomethylation or activation of the insulin-like growth factor II gene (*IGF2*).[9] Further studies have reported a link between prenatal exposure to famine and schizophrenia.[10,11]

Throughout life, changes in gene expression or epigenetic modifications are necessary as all nucleated cells contain a complete set of all the genes required by the body. Clearly, selective expression of specific genes will depend on the tissue and requirements for the cell's activity at a given time. Different cellular conditions require flexibility in biochemical pathways to support

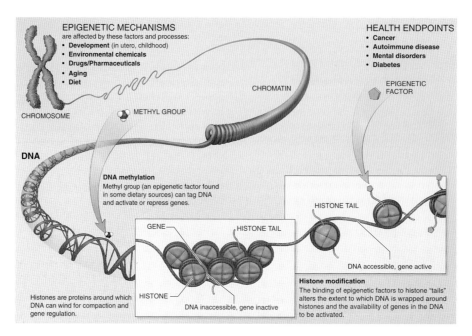

FIGURE 8.1 Epigenetic mechanisms[14]

unique bioenergetic demands and dynamic balance between anabolic and catabolic pathways. Epigenetic modifications are also therefore influenced by age, environment, diet, lifestyle and the presence of disease. Research in the field of epigenetics has shown associations between altered gene expression and various chronic disorders including cancer, mental retardation, immune dysfunction and neuropsychiatric conditions.

Several mechanisms have been identified to date that produce changes in gene expression.[12,13] These are covalent modifications of DNA directly, remodelling of chromatin with histone modification and the use of non-coding RNA transcripts. Typically, acetylation of histones enhances transcription whereas methylation suppresses transcription. It is likely that all of these mechanisms work in concert to regulate gene expression (see Fig. 8.1).

DNA methylation

Direct methylation of DNA is a common means of controlling gene transcription that is distinct from methylation of histone proteins described later in the chapter. Methylation of DNA occurs at the cytosine residues where DNA methyltransferase enzymes convert cytosine to 5-methylcytosine (5-MC), which usually results in gene silencing as the methyl group projects into the major groove of DNA and prevents binding of transcription factors.[12] In the promotor regions of genes, the cytosine bases are usually adjacent to a guanine base (CpG sites), resulting in two methylated cytosines sitting on diagonally opposing DNA strands. When proteins bind to these methylated CpG sites, they form complexes with other proteins involved in deacetylation of histones, which results in 'closing' of the chromatin (see following section). The addition of methyl groups to the cytosine bases is carried out by a group of DNA methyltransferases (DNMT).

There are three main enzymes involved in the establishment and maintenance of DNA methylation patterns. DNMT3a and DNMT3b are mainly involved with *de novo* methylation that occurs post-implantation. This methylation pattern triggers a 'gene silencing' cascade involving deacetylation and then methylation of histones, resulting in the formation of heterochromatin or 'closed' chromatin. After DNA replication, the newly synthesised DNA strand is unmethylated and is referred to as hemi-methylated. DNMT1 then rapidly scans the unmethylated strand and adds methyl groups complementary to the original strand, resulting in replication of methylation patterns.[12,15]

DNA methylation is also a crucial part of DNA repair. DNA damage occurs frequently, occurring on average around 60 000 times per day in each cell.[16] A double strand break is repaired in a precise manner and after repair a series of methyl groups is left at the repair site to mark genes and so they are packed and silenced. This is probably an adaptive response by the cell to protect the genome, as packed chromatin DNA is more resistant to damage and gene silencing prevents expression of a damaged gene (see Fig. 8.2).

While methylation acts to silence gene transcription, demethylation or removal of the methyl group is also required to initiate gene expression and for epigenetic reprogramming of genes. The removal of the methyl group can occur passively or actively, or a combination of both. Passive demethylation occurs during DNA replication via reduced activity or inhibition of DNMT1. Although the exact mechanisms for the active process are unclear, it is thought to occur by removal of 5-methylcytosine by a series of modifications to the cytosine bases that have been oxidised by TET enzymes (ten-eleven translocases). These enzymes bind to CpG-rich regions to prevent overactivity of DNMT and to convert 5-MC to 5-hydroxymethylcytosine,

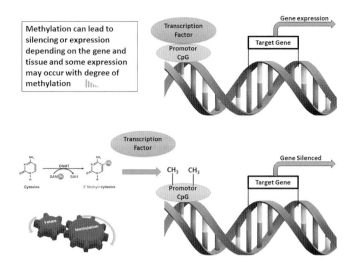

Methylation can lead to silencing or expression depending on the gene and tissue and some expression may occur with degree of methylation

FIGURE 8.2 Epigenetic modification by DNA methylation
The binding of a transcription factor to the promotor region of a gene usually results in gene expression. If the CpG island on the promotor region is methylated, the transcription factor cannot bind due to steric hindrance. The gene is therefore silenced. CpG: cytosine-guanine island (C and G base on same DNA strand); CH₃: methyl group; DNMT: DNA methyl-transferase; SAMe: S-adenosyl methionine; SAH: S-adenosyl-homocysteine.

© Reproduced by kind permission of Dr Rhona Creegan (Omega Nutrition Health).

5-formylmethylcytosine and then to 5-carboxylcytosine via hydroxylase activity. These TET enzymes influence gene expression and repression, tumour suppression and epigenetic reprogramming processes.[17,18]

Chromatin remodelling

If the DNA in each cell was stretched out it would measure several metres – therefore, it must be coiled and kinked to fit into the nucleus. To achieve this, the DNA winds itself around proteins called histones, forming a condensed complex known as chromatin.[19] The basic unit of chromatin is called a nucleosome, which consists of 147 base pairs of DNA wrapped around a core of eight histone proteins. When this structure is tightly bound or 'closed' it is referred to as heterochromatin.

The structure of chromatin itself provides complex levels of control over gene expression. If the way the DNA is wound around the histones is modified or the histones are themselves modified, the chromatin can be 'opened' (referred to as euchromatin), which gives access to specific transcription factors that bind to target sequences of selected genes to recruit RNA polymerases and initiate gene expression.[20] Enzymes known as writer, reader and eraser complexes remodel nucleosomes and reversible epigenetic modifications of histone proteins include methylation, acetylation, phosphorylation, biotinylation and the addition of ubiquitin and SUMO (small ubiquitin-like modifier) proteins or ADP-ribose.[21,22] The N-terminus of histone proteins forms a tail that protrudes from the complex and enables modification typically by acetylation and methylation of lysine residues,[23] but many other

modifications have been described which have been called the histone code.[24] Histone acetylation is balanced by the action of histone acetyl-transferases (HAT) and histone deacetylases (HDAC). Histone methylation is maintained by histone methyltransferases and histone demethylases.

The effect of nutrients on epigenetic modification

It is well known that diet can influence epigenetic modification and will therefore impact physiological and pathological processes. Various nutrients and bioactive food components can influence epigenetic processes by directly modifying enzymes that catalyse DNA methylation or histone modification or by altering the availability of substrates and cofactors required for enzyme activity. Folate, vitamins B₂ and B₁₂, methionine, choline and betaine can alter one-carbon metabolism, which directly affects DNA and histone methylation. S-adenosyl methionine (SAMe) is the primary methyl donor for these reactions.[25] When SAMe donates its methyl group S-adenosyl homocysteine is formed, which is a potent inhibitor of methyltransferase reactions.[26] Therefore, any nutrient, bioactive food component or condition that can impair the methionine/methylation cycle has the potential to alter DNA or histone methylation. Methylation is covered in more detail in Chapter 7. Other vitamins such as biotin, niacin (B₃) and pantothenic acid (B₅) also have roles in histone modification.

Certain nutrients and food components such as polyphenols have been shown to increase levels of DNA repair enzymes such as MGMT (O⁶-methylguanine DNA methyltransferase), MLH1 (MutL homologue 1) and p53.[27] Other food components such as isothiocyanates (broccoli), epigallocatechin gallate (green tea), curcumin (turmeric), genistein (soybeans), quercetin (apples), anacardic acid (cashews), resveratrol (red grapes), cinnamic acid (cinnamon), lycopene (tomatoes) and diallyl disulphide (garlic) have been shown to influence epigenetic changes in cell line studies.[28,29]

Dietary antioxidants are important for preventing the formation of oxidised DNA lesions where 8-hydroxy-2-deoxyguanosine (8-OHdG) replaces guanine and diminishes the binding of DNA methyltransferases and other proteins.[30] Demethylation of DNA can also occur as a result of TET-mediated hydroxymethylation.[31] In vitro studies have shown that depletion of glutathione by oxidative stress leads to global DNA hypomethylation, possibly through the depletion of SAMe.[32]

THE ROLE OF GENETIC TESTING IN HEALTHCARE

Genetic testing in healthcare can be separated into two distinct categories. First, there is its use in a diagnostic/predictive setting where single gene mutations are known to cause disease, such as *CFTR* in cystic fibrosis and *APC*, *BRCA1*, *BRCA2*, *MLH1* and *MSH6* in familial cancers. However, most common conditions, such as cardiovascular disease, type 2 diabetes and mental health disorders, are multifactorial in aetiology with no single gene being identified as causative. Multifactorial conditions are likely to be a result of an interaction between genes and environment. These conditions have multiple components involving nutrient status, inflammation, oxidation, detoxification, impaired methylation and glycation.

As these conditions are considered lifestyle disorders that take many years to develop, there are opportunities for appropriate intervention if we can identify an individual's biochemical vulnerabilities. This is where identification of genetic variants in specific pathways can help tailor personalised nutrition and lifestyle programs that may reduce an individual's risk of developing certain conditions. It is important to select variants that have been shown in the research literature to be associated with specific outcomes and to realise that identification of a variant is not the whole story – treatment and interventions should not be based on genetic information alone. However, the identification of genetic variants does underpin faulty biochemical processes and they can be used not only in preventive health strategies but also in interventions.

APOE (apolipoprotein E) genotyping is not performed for cardiovascular disease assessment because carriers of the *ApoE4* allele are also at increased risk of developing Alzheimer's disease. However, the APOE genotype is not diagnostic of either disease. APOE genotyping has poor predictive value since not everyone with an *ApoE4* allele will develop Alzheimer's, while some who develop Alzheimer's will not have the *ApoE4* allele. The *APOE* gene dual-disease risk has created a public health issue in relation to treatment and drug efficacy: since APOE testing has been actively discouraged by the genetics community, this has hampered nutritional-based approaches in the treatment of cardiovascular disease.

The clinical utility of screening the *APOE* gene is as an adjunct test when an individual has symptoms of progressive dementia including decreasing intellectual ability such as language and speech skills, memory loss and personality and behavioural changes that are interfering with daily living. However, historically genetic testing of the *APOE* gene was not performed routinely because of potential psychological and social harms. If APOE genotyping was performed, the results were delivered by a team including a clinical geneticist, a genetic counsellor or another specialist. However, we now live in an era where many thousands of individuals have learned about their genetic risk factors for common complex disorders, including their APOE genotype, through consumer genomics companies. Such testing provides personal autonomy and the current restrictions on genetic risk assessment testing are often viewed as paternalistic, hindering an individual's inherent right to their decoded genome. Arguably there is a personal utility beyond that which the medical genetics community has defined. One clinical trial reported that individuals who received genetic test results for Alzheimer's disease risk were more likely to improve their diet, increase their exercise frequency and take vitamin supplements.[33] It has also been reported that individuals who discuss their genetic test results with their healthcare practitioner are likely to reduce their dietary fat intake and exercise more frequently.[34]

Second, whether genetic testing is ordered as a direct-to-consumer test or performed in a medical setting, we need certainty in relation to the accuracy of the test being performed. In the context of genetic testing in healthcare, cardiovascular and metabolic disease can be used to illustrate the integration of genetic information and functional testing.

Cardiovascular health assessment protocol

The protocol for personalised assessment of cardiovascular health begins with lipoprotein profiling for dyslipidaemia (see Fig. 8.3). An abnormal cholesterol profile is indicative of dyslipidaemia. Dyslipidaemia interventions can be enhanced by using targeted genomic analysis followed by other complementary testing including fatty acid profiling, LDL sub-fractions and oxidised LDL, homocysteine, methylene tetrahydrofolate reductase (MTHFR) genotyping, markers of inflammation and apolipoproteins A and B, lipoprotein (a) and fibrinogen. A CT angiogram with calcium score may also be recommended if atherosclerosis is suspected. A test that measures all the lipoprotein classes and subclasses would be superior to the current lipid profile as part of a treatment protocol.

OVERVIEW OF LIPOPROTEIN METABOLISM

As lipids are non-soluble in water they are transported in blood in lipoproteins, which are particles consisting of various amounts of lipid (triglycerides, phospholipids and cholesterol and their associated fatty acids), apolipoproteins and other proteins and fat-soluble compounds such as vitamins. Lipoprotein metabolism is complex and involves the transfer of lipids between the lipoproteins and the delivery of several components to tissues via interaction with various receptors and transfer proteins. Numerous genetic variants have been identified in several key genes involved in lipoprotein and lipid metabolism and this information can be used to identify and modify cardiovascular disease risk. Fig. 8.4 summarises lipoprotein metabolism and illustrates some of the polymorphic genes that can influence disease risk.

FATTY ACID PROFILING

Fatty acids are components of all lipids (triglycerides, phospholipids, sphingolipids and cholesteryl esters); the fatty acid composition of lipids can have a marked impact on health. Fatty acid profiling is very useful in determining the levels and impact of fatty acids. Each fatty acid affects plasma cholesterol levels differently due to its impact on the LDL (low-density lipoprotein) receptor, the activity of which is regulated by the sterol content of the cell via the master transcription factor sterol regulatory element binding protein (SREBP).[35] When the sterol content of the cell is low, a fragment of SREBP is cleaved by a protease that acts as a transcription factor to activate the LDL receptor gene. Dietary fatty acids and cholesterol can increase the sterol regulatory pool by their effects on the enzyme acylCoA-cholesterol acyl transferase (ACAT).[36,37] The activity of this enzyme is determined in part by the

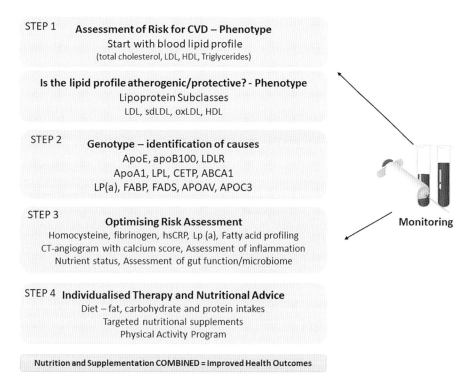

FIGURE 8.3 Protocol for assessment of cardiovascular health

© Reproduced by kind permission of Dr Margaret Smith (SmartDNA) and Dr Rhona Creegan (Omega Nutrition Health).

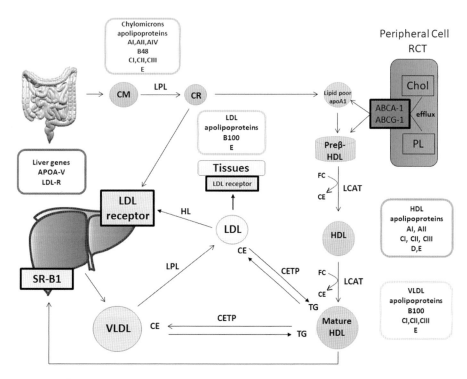

FIGURE 8.4 Lipoprotein metabolism and associated genes

CM: chylomicrons; LPL: lipoprotein lipase; CR: chylomicron remnants; RCT: reverse cholesterol transport; Chol: cholesterol; PL: phospholipid; ABCA, ABCG: ATP-binding cassette transporters; LDL: low-density lipoprotein; LDL-R: LDL receptor; HDL: high-density lipoprotein; VLDL: very-low-density lipoprotein; HL: hepatic lipase; FC: free cholesterol; CE: cholesteryl ester; LCAT: lecithin-cholesterol acyl transferase; CETP: cholesteryl ester transfer protein; SR-B1: scavenger receptor B1.

© Reproduced by kind permission of Dr Rhona Creegan (Omega Nutrition Health).

amount and type of dietary fatty acid, which therefore affects plasma cholesterol levels.[35] The saturated fatty acid, palmitic acid, partially inhibits cholesteryl ester (CE) formation by ACAT, therefore increasing the amount of free cholesterol. As the sterol regulatory pool increases, SREBP cleavage is inhibited, leading to the reduced expression and activity of the LDL receptor. In contrast, if the liver cells are enriched with monounsaturated fatty acids (MUFAs) and polyunsaturated fatty acids (PUFAs), ACAT activity is increased as it is a preferred substrate and CE formation is promoted.[38]

A fatty acid profile can give important information:

- Dietary intake
- Interconversions between the different fatty acid types
- Requirement for cofactors for normal action of the fatty acid desaturase (coded for by FADS genes)
- Requirement for elongase enzymes required to synthesise the longer chain fatty acids from the 18-carbon essential fatty acids of the omega-6 and omega-3 series.

Ultimately, the fatty acid profile will influence cholesterol levels via the effect on other signalling molecules, inflammation and membrane fluidity.

Specifically, fatty acid profiling measures the plasma levels of the following:

- *Saturated fatty acids* which, apart from the effect on ACAT and the LDL receptor, if present in excess may contribute to increased risk of arteriosclerosis and metabolic disease. One mechanism by which this may occur is the association between insulin resistance and the accumulation of toxic ceramides (a type of sphingolipid). These ceramides may be the intermediary that links excess dietary saturated fatty acids (particularly palmitic acid) and inflammatory cytokines, a major contributor to cardiovascular disease[39,40]
- *Monounsaturated fatty acids*, such as found in olive oil, which may help lower total cholesterol and LDL levels by the effect on ACAT as described above. Insulin resistance also impairs action of stearoyl CoA desaturase, the enzyme required to add a double bond to stearic acid to form MUFA[41]
- *Polyunsaturated fatty acids*, which measure plasma omega-3 and omega-6 levels, influence lipid pathways and inflammation and can alter cellular membranes, which influence the risk of cardiovascular disease. The omega-3s DHA (docosahexaenoic acid) and EPA (eicosapentaenoic acid) are important in reducing plasma triglyceride levels as they regulate the activity of various nuclear receptors, resulting in a repartitioning of fatty acids away from storage as triglycerides and towards oxidation. These receptors include LXR (liver X receptor), hepatocyte nuclear factor 4α, farnesoid X-activated receptor (FXR) and peroxisome proliferator-activated receptors (PPARs). Each of these receptors is in turn regulated by SREBP-1c.[42] EPA and DHA reduce SREBP-1c, which is the main genetic switch controlling lipogenesis. This reduces the amount of free fatty acids available for VLDL (very-low-density lipoprotein) synthesis. EPA and DHA are highly unsaturated and prone to peroxidation, which stimulates the degradation

of apolipoprotein B (ApoB), required for VLDL synthesis. Their presence in lipoproteins may also enhance postprandial chylomicron clearance by stimulating lipoprotein lipase activity[42]

- *Trans fatty acids*, which are known to increase LDL cholesterol and decrease HDL (high-density lipoprotein) cholesterol in the blood. Dietary trans fatty acids are known to contribute to dyslipidaemia and associated increased disease risk.[43] Most naturally occurring fatty acids have double bonds in a cis configuration, which allows the chain to bend. The trans bond imparts a rigid structure, which is similar to saturated fatty acids, and increased consumption from processed and fast foods can lead to dyslipidaemia.[43,44] Trans fatty acids alter membrane fluidity and responses of various membrane receptors through their incorporation into membrane phospholipids. As fatty acids are ligands for nuclear receptors, such as PPARs, LXR and SREBP, regulation of gene transcription can be altered,[45–47] directly modulating metabolic and inflammatory responses in an adverse way. The effects on lipid metabolism are due to several mechanisms. Trans fatty acids alter the secretion, composition and size of apolipoprotein B-100 produced in the liver. This decreases the rate of LDL catabolism. The catabolism of ApoA-I is increased, which reduces plasma HDL cholesterol. Trans fatty acids increase the cellular accumulation and secretion of free cholesterol and cholesterol esters by the liver.[48] The effects on reducing HDL are thought to be due to an increase in cholesteryl ester transfer protein (CETP), which transfers cholesterol esters from HDL to LDL and VLDL.[49] Additionally, the fluidity, determined by the fatty acid at the sn-2 position of phosphatidylcholine, is a major regulator of lecithin-cholesterol acyltransferase (LCAT), which is required for the formation of mature HDL. Trans fatty acids reduce fluidity and can therefore reduce the activity of LCAT.[50]

BLOOD LIPID PROFILES AND LIPOPROTEIN SUBCLASS PHENOTYPING

Lipoprotein sub-fractionation measures cholesterol concentration in all 12 lipoprotein fractions and subfractions:

- VLDL – associated with hypertriglyceridaemia
- IDL (intermediate-density lipoprotein) and VLDL remnants associated with increased cardiovascular disease risk
- The large buoyant LDL subtypes 1 and 2 associated with average coronary heart disease risk
- The small dense LDL3 to LDL7 associated with a three times increased risk of cardiovascular disease
- The levels of HDL cholesterol associated with additional risk factors or reduced risk.[51,52]

Generally, if low-density lipoprotein cholesterol (LDL-C) is raised, measuring the sub-fraction gives an indication of the atherogenicity of the LDL particles.[53] The small dense particles LDL 3 to LDL 7 and oxidised LDL are much more damaging to the endothelium than the larger particles[51,54,55] (see Fig. 8.5).

(a)

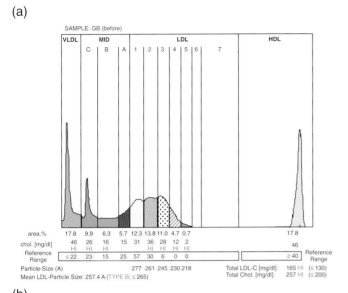

(b)

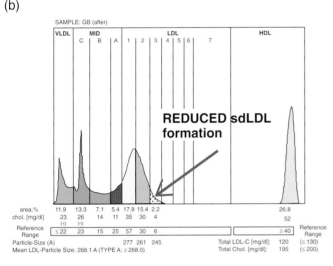

REDUCED sdLDL formation

FIGURE 8.5 Examples of an LDL lipoprotein sub-class profile

(a) Increased small dense LDL and an abnormal type pattern (atherogenic profile). (b) The small dense LDL have reduced to a more normal pattern.

IMUNPRO Australia (www.imupro.com.au).

Lipoprotein profiling and elevated VLDL

VLDL cholesterol is produced in the liver and released into the bloodstream to supply body tissues with triglycerides. The VLDL level is not normally provided during routine cholesterol screening. Triglycerides comprise 50% of a VLDL particle. High levels of VLDL cholesterol are associated with the development of plaque deposits on artery walls, which narrow the passage and restrict blood flow. The best way to lower VLDL cholesterol is to lower triglycerides. Losing weight and exercising regularly are important in addition to avoiding sugary food and alcohol.

HDL sub-fractions

The value of using HDL sub-fractions for cardiovascular disease risk assessment is not so clear cut as with LDL sub-fractions. The role of HDL in reverse cholesterol transport and contribution to cardiovascular disease is complex (see Fig. 8.6). It may be that the level of circulating HDL is misleading in terms of cardio-protection and that HDL function is more important.[56] Although high-density lipoprotein cholesterol (HDL-C) and the CETP variants are considered protective, this is only relevant if blood levels of C-reactive protein (CRP) are normal and the HDL sub-fraction results indicate highly lipidated forms or mature forms of HDL.[57,58] When HDL is separated into sub-fractions there are three groups: large, intermediate and small. The large and intermediate sizes are considered anti-atherogenic, but this also depends on the LDL subclass and whether the LDL is oxidised.[59] HDL particles, by their interaction with ATP binding cassette (ABC) transporters and exchange of cholesteryl esters between other lipoproteins, promote reverse cholesterol transport – the removal of cholesterol from tissues for delivery to the liver for excretion in bile or to be used by steroidogenic tissues. However, it is now clear that HDL, due to the presence of ApoA-1, also modulates inflammation and itself is subject to post-translational modification by oxidation.[60] If ABC transporters and ApoA-1 are dysfunctional, HDL particles will not mature and small HDL particles will increase. A functional assay for HDL in conjunction with genetic variants remains the goal for determining whether HDL is anti-atherogenic or not.[56]

Lipoprotein sub-fraction cholesterol measurements are used as an aid in evaluating lipid metabolism disorders in conjunction with other lipid tests, genetics, patient risk assessment and clinical evaluation. This assessment protocol provides individualised therapy and nutritional advice and ongoing lipoprotein assessment.

Lipid metabolism genotyping

WHY DOES GENETIC ANALYSIS MAKE SENSE IN DYSLIPIDAEMIAS?

It is known that 90% of the disorders of lipid metabolism are caused by genes that are involved in fat absorption, fat transport, conversions of lipoproteins and degradation of fat. Dyslipidaemias have various genetic causes that can be influenced by environmental factors such as nutrition, alcohol, smoking and sex-specific differences, all of which can induce metabolic dysfunction and problems with insulin signalling. In general, a Mediterranean-style diet is considered beneficial for the prevention of coronary heart disease (i.e. a large quantity of fresh fruit, vegetables and olive oil, as well as red wine, which is said to have an antioxidant effect).[61]

WHY ARE NUTRITIONAL INTERVENTIONS BASED ON PERSONALISED GENOMICS SO IMPORTANT?

Based on current knowledge, 50% of patients don't respond to a Mediterranean diet because the standard recommendation of energy sources, alcohol and medication are at genetic odds with 50% of those with cardiovascular disease. Personalised genomics identifies the causes of the dyslipidaemia and the individual's metabolism specificities, enabling individualised therapies and nutritional advice.

(a)

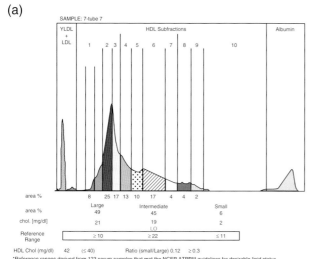

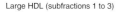

Large HDL (subfractions 1 to 3)

(b)

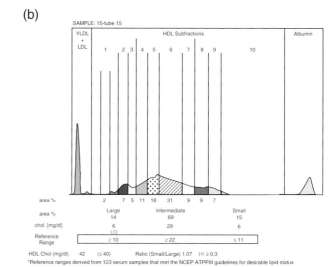

Intermediate HDL (subfractions 4 to 7)

(c)

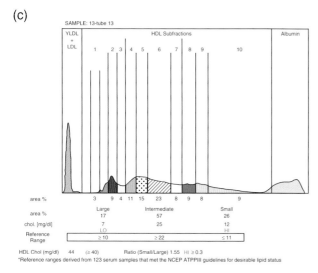

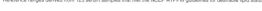

Small HDL (subfractions 8 to 10)

FIGURE 8.6 HDL sub-fractions

(a) A normal profile with high large HDL and low small HDL. (b) An intermediate pattern with a predominance of intermediate size. (c) A low large and a high small HDL.

IMUNPRO Australia (www.imupro.com.au).

APOE ASSESSMENT AND NUTRITIONAL MANAGEMENT OF DYSLIPIDAEMIA

Genetic assessment for cardiovascular disease risk is a good example of how genetics can be used to underpin dietary interventions and cholesterol biochemistry. Several genetic variants have been identified in genes associated with heart health that involve lipid metabolism, inflammation, metabolic function and nutrient status – abnormalities that contribute to cardiovascular disease. A major contributor to cardiovascular health is the *APOE* gene. The *APOE* gene is considered the main dietary hub for nutritional interventions. Two polymorphisms, denoted as rs7412 and rs429358, determine three common variants of APOE: E2, E3 and E4. Since we inherit one half of our genome from each parent, this results in six APOE constellations: E2/E2, E2/E3, E2/E4, E3/E3, E3/E4 and E4/E4.[62,63] The most common genotype (50–65% of the population) is E3/E3, which is associated with normal cholesterol metabolism. The distribution of E2, E3 and E4 is variable, with Asians, Mexican Americans and American Indians having the highest frequency of the E3 genotype, African Americans and Caucasians having the highest frequency of the E2 genotype and African Americans and Africans having the highest frequency of the E4 genotype.[64]

The six *APOE* constellations are associated with gene dose-dependent risk profiles. Genotypes E2/E2 and E4/E4 represent two opposing enzymatic activities, while E2/E4 and E3/E3 have similar enzymatic activities. E3/E3 has 'normal' lipid metabolism; however, other genes may contribute to altered cholesterol profiles and dyslipidaemia. Carriers of the E2 and E4 genotypes should not smoke tobacco since it is a major contributor to cardiovascular disease in these groups.[65]

The *APOE* gene encodes the apolipoprotein E protein, which is involved in the production, delivery and use of cholesterol in the body. It is the structural differences of the ApoE2, ApoE3 and ApoE4 proteins that determine protein domain-to-domain interaction, binding affinity and protein stability. Each genotype therefore has a structural difference that affects the function of the Apo E protein and the metabolism of lipoproteins:[66]

- ApoE2 and ApoE4 have opposing effects on plasma lipids
- ApoE2 is an intermediate coronary heart disease risk, expressing less efficient VLDL and chylomicron formation and transfer from the blood to the liver, leading to slower clearance of dietary fat. Slow conversion has markedly decreased LDL receptor binding compared to the other genotypes
- ApoE2 preferentially binds to HDL-C
- The ApoE4 genotype is associated with a limitation on HDL-C affinity with preferential binding of VLDL
- ApoE4 rapidly converts IDL to LDL. Overall this leads to increased total cholesterol, LDL-C, small dense LDL (sdLDL) and triglyceride
- The ApoE2 constellation produces a protein that is associated with slower cholesterol metabolism, which results in lower total cholesterol, lower LDL and higher triglyceride concentrations
- The structural confirmation of the ApoE4 constellation produces a protein that is characterised by faster cholesterol metabolism, which results in higher total cholesterol, elevated LDL and suppressed HDL.

A form of dyslipidaemia identified by Addison and Gull in 1851 is an ApoE2 carrier disease risk associated with increased blood chylomicrons remnants and IDL levels and premature vascular disease, including both coronary heart disease and peripheral artery disease.

The well-studied and recommended Mediterranean diet, if applied to all individuals regardless of APOE genotype, may result in deleterious cholesterol profiles. The standard Mediterranean diet recommends intakes of fat, protein and carbohydrate with the addition of one or two glasses of red wine, but is not suitable for all *APOE* constellations. The Framingham Heart Study demonstrated that alcohol increased LDL cholesterol in males with an ApoE4 genotype more than any other APOE constellation. In contrast, males with an ApoE2 genotype who consumed alcohol had reduced LDL cholesterol when compared with males with an ApoE2 genotype who didn't consume alcohol.[67] Generally, *ApoE3* carriers respond well to a standard Mediterranean diet. The modified dietary recommendations for *ApoE4* carriers is a low fat, high-carbohydrate diet, while lower carbohydrate and higher fat diets are recommended for *ApoE2* carriers.

OTHER GENETIC POLYMORPHISMS ASSOCIATED WITH COMMON DYSLIPIDAEMIAS

Common forms of dyslipidaemia are polygenic, meaning that multiple genetic variations contribute and,

importantly, the genetic contribution is variable from person to person. This translates into personalised approaches for prevention and if dyslipidaemia is detected, a targeted intervention can be used.[68]

Genetic polymorphisms contributing to dyslipidaemia may be associated with elevated triglycerides, the formation of small dense LDL particles, total cholesterol or non-protective HDL cholesterol. These common forms of dyslipidaemia are often found in association with obesity, metabolic syndrome, type 2 diabetes, hypothyroidism and kidney disease. The most effective approach is targeted diet, exercise and supplementation of specific nutrients. Other contributing factors are smoking tobacco, and some pharmaceutical drugs – oestrogens and progestins, anabolic steroids, glucocorticoids and immunosuppressants – also increase the risk of dyslipidaemia.

ELEVATED TRIGLYCERIDES AND RISK REDUCTION WITH TARGETED NUTRITION AND LIFESTYLE CHOICES

Individuals carrying risk polymorphisms in the *LPL*, *ApoC3* and *ApoA-5* (apolipoprotein A-V) genes often develop elevated blood triglycerides due to the reduced ability to transport triglycerides from blood plasma to the liver and muscles where it can be used to produce energy. The *nitric oxide synthase 3* (*NOS3*) gene variant rs1799983 nutrient response is associated with elevated triglyceride levels and low omega-3 intake. This gene–nutrient interaction determines the individual's response to omega-3 fatty acids by modulation of triglyceride levels.

The *ApoC3* gene plays a crucial role in lipid metabolism, slowing the breakdown of triacylglycerol, which results in higher blood levels of triglycerides. The variant rs5182 is associated with a four-fold increase in risk for hypertriglyceridaemia, as well as increased risk of heart attack, cardiovascular disease and the formation of sdLDLs.

ApoA-5 plays a key role in influencing fasting lipids and in determining plasma triglyceride levels. Variants in this gene have been reported to be associated with increased likelihood of developing coronary artery disease. The *ApoA-5* variant rs662799 has an increased effect when the supply of omega-6 fatty acids exceeds 6% of the total energy supply. Cardiovascular risk is increased because more aggressive sdLDL particles are formed under these circumstances. Women and men are equally affected.

The genetic variant rs1260326 in the glucokinase regulatory protein (GCKR) has been shown to drive the production of triglycerides for storage, thereby increasing the risk of elevated blood triglycerides and fatty liver disease. This is due to the poor regulation of glucose uptake by the liver, which results in more glucose being metabolised and ultimately the production of triglycerides and large VLDL.[69]

Individuals carrying these risk variants can reduce their risk of developing elevated triglyceride levels by avoiding excessive intake of processed carbohydrates and simple refined sugars, reducing total dietary fats (in particular, saturated fats), increasing omega-3 intake and reducing omega-6 intake to improve their blood lipid profile.

ELEVATED LDL AND THE *ApoB, ApoB-100* AND *LDL-R* GENES

In addition to APOE, several other variants contribute to elevated LDL levels. Genetic polymorphisms in the *ApoB* (*apolipoprotein* B), *ApoB-100* (*apolipoprotein B-100*) and *LDL-R* (*low-density lipoprotein receptor*) genes are associated with elevated LDL-C level in response to dietary saturated fat intake. The *ApoB* gene product is the main apolipoprotein of chylomicrons and LDLs. ApoB occurs in plasma as two main isoforms: ApoB-48 and ApoB-100 – the former is synthesised exclusively in the gut and the latter is synthesised in the liver. ApoB-100 is a key component of LDL-C with an important role in the binding of LDL to LDL receptors. LDL-R plays a crucial role in lipid metabolism, being responsible for the uptake of lipoproteins into the cells. The genetic LDL-R variant rs688 exerts its effect by shortening the length of the LDL receptor. It was reported that the effect on splicing may be physiologically relevant because the presence of the rs688 minor allele was associated with increased total and LDL-C in female members of the Framingham Offspring Study. The largest rs688-associated cholesterol differences were observed in premenopausal women. The risk allele is present in approximately 60% of Caucasians and is associated with a significant 10% increase in total and LDL-C in premenopausal women.

A high LDL-C level indicates that while cholesterol is circulating it can adhere to vascular walls, particularly if the sdLDL is elevated. As previously described, there are subclasses of LDL that differ in size: smaller LDL particle size and oxidised LDL are related to increased atherogenic potential and can form part of extended testing for cardiovascular disease risk.

Genetic risk variants in these LDL-associated genes are associated with higher blood cholesterol levels due to the reduced clearance of plasma LDL particles. A high-fat and cholesterol-rich diet exaggerates this effect. Reducing the intake of refined carbohydrates and cholesterol-rich foods such as egg yolks, pastries, fatty meats and dairy products, coupled with increasing fibre intake, can help.

NUTRITIONAL MODULATION OF HDL

In the Framingham study, it was reported that the nutrigenomic modulation of HDL showed that the ApoA-1 risk genotype is associated with lower HDL-C level when PUFA intake is greater than 4% of calories. Conversely, ApoA-1 non-risk genotypes are associated with higher HDL-C blood levels when PUFA is greater than 6–8% of calories. No recommendation can be made in relation to modulating HDL levels unless HDL is reported to be non-protective as part of a standard or advanced lipoprotein analysis. Just as with LDL particle size, HDL particle size is also relevant. As previously mentioned, a subgroup of patients with 'protective' HDL levels has been shown to be at increased risk of cardiovascular disease if inflammation is present, as indicated by high CRP levels and altered CETP activity.[58]

Lipoprotein lipase (LPL) hydrolyses triglycerides in lipoproteins (mainly chylomicrons and VLDL) into glycerol and free fatty acids by recognition of the ApoC-II apolipoprotein.[70] The free fatty acids can then be used by various tissues. As LPL is also involved in promoting cellular uptake of chylomicron remnants and cholesterol-rich lipoproteins, LPL genetic variants are associated with higher triglyceride and lower HDL levels in the blood. A diet low in saturated fat and calorie restriction can help improve these levels for variant carriers, thereby reducing risk of cardiovascular disease. Two common variants of the *LPL* gene (S477X and Hind II) mildly affect LPL activity. Each is associated with increased triglyceride and decreased HDL-C levels in response to a high-fat diet.

The ATP-binding cassette transporter ABCA1 (member 1 of the human transporter subfamily ABCA) is also known as the cholesterol efflux regulatory protein. ABCA1 is a major regulator of cellular cholesterol and phospholipid homeostasis. With cholesterol as its substrate, this protein functions as a cholesterol efflux pump in the cellular lipid removal pathway. A genetic variant resulting in a single amino acid change called R219K SNP results in a single amino acid change at codon 219 from an arginine (R) to a lysine (K) residue and is associated with higher HDL-C, especially in the Asian population, and a lower risk of coronary artery disease in the Asian and Caucasian populations.

CETP genetic variants are associated with elevated blood HDL-C levels. It has been reported that individuals with the CETP rs5882 *GG* genotype have increased lipoprotein sizes and lower serum CETP concentrations. The findings suggest that lipoprotein particle sizes are heritable and promote a healthy ageing phenotype.[58,71]

APOLIPOPROTEIN (A) AND CARDIOVASCULAR DISEASE RISK

Apolipoprotein (a) or Lp(a) is a specific heterogeneous class of lipoprotein particles found in human plasma consisting of an apolipoprotein (a) molecule attached to an ApoB-100 and lipid-rich LDL-like core. However, Lp(a) is metabolically distinct from LDL. The protein has two components: a single copy of ApoB-100 linked to a single copy of apolipoprotein (a).

Numerous studies have documented the relationship of high plasma Lp(a) concentrations with a variety of cardiovascular disorders, including peripheral vascular disease, cerebrovascular disease and premature coronary disease. However, the exact mechanism is as yet unknown. It is assumed that Lp(a) contributes to the atherosclerotic process as it is found at sites of vascular injury. Lp(a) has been linked to the promotion of both early and advanced-stage atherosclerosis. Elevated Lp(a) is associated with increased coagulation and a three- to five-fold increased incidence of cardiovascular disease. An elevated level of Lp(a) is an independent risk factor for cardiovascular disease. In combination with other abnormal disease markers, the risk increases further. Lp(a) is inherited in a dominant fashion. *LPA*-Intron 25 carriers may have an increased risk of coronary heart disease. *LPA*-Intron 25 is a one-time genetic test. The test results may help healthcare providers to characterise and reduce other risk factors that can contribute to the initiation or progression of heart disease and to increase patients' adherence to treatment recommendations. Lp(a) levels may vary depending on physiological status, so practitioners may choose to monitor this risk factor over time.

A 2009 meta-analysis of 36 cohort and case-control studies, with data from 126 334 patients, concluded that Lp(a) is continuously, independently and modestly associated with risk of coronary heart disease and stroke. The review found a 13% greater risk of coronary heart disease per 3.5-fold higher than usual Lp(a) concentration, after adjusting for other risk factors. This preceded an endorsement of widespread screening for Lp(a) by the European Atherosclerosis Society, which has sparked dialogue and debate across the world. Although Lp(a) has now been identified definitively as an independent risk factor for cardiovascular disease, we still know relatively little about what its purpose is, how to lower it effectively and safely and whether attempts to do so will translate into positive clinical outcomes.

FAT ABSORPTION

The fatty acid-binding protein 2 (FABP2) is a protein encoded by the *FABP2* gene. Intestinal FABP2 is an abundant cytosolic protein in small intestine epithelial cells. The analysed genetic variant rs1799883 provides information on the absorption of fat in the small intestine. Since fat has a high energy value (9 kCal/g) and polymorphism is associated with increased fat absorption in the intestine, it is important to ensure that the individual does not gain weight. A high-fibre diet may help reduce this impact.

FADS GENE AND OMEGA-3 AND OMEGA FATTY ACID METABOLISM

An individual's ability to convert the plant-based essential fatty acids alpha linolenic acid (ALA) and linoleic acid (LA) to the longer chain omega-3 eicosapentaenoic acid (EPA) and the omega-6 arachidonic acid (AA), is determined by the variant rs174450 located in the *fatty acid desaturase (FADS)* gene, which codes for the delta desaturase enzymes involved in adding double bonds to fatty acids in PUFA metabolism. Carriers of the variant are at risk of fat accumulation and elevated blood triglycerides due to reduced utilisation of plant-based oils and the role of the longer chain fatty acids as transcription factors influencing peroxisome activity and fatty acid oxidation. A variant in the *FADS1* gene, rs147547, is associated with decreased blood levels of AA and EPA. Since both AA and EPA are precursors of the biologically important eicosanoids (prostaglandins, leukotrienes and thromboxanes) involved with inflammation, blood clotting and vascular tone, individuals carrying the variant should increase their intake of omega-3 fatty acids and monitor their intake of omega-6 fatty acids to optimise these pathways and reduce their cardiovascular disease risk.

As described previously, fatty acid profiling is an important adjunct test to determine the impact of any genetic variants in the *FADS* gene. Red cell fatty acid profiles, including measurement of AA and EPA, can

---

Next steps: Lipid metabolism genetics and future treatment directions

If variants in any of these genes or other genes associated with lipid metabolism and cardiovascular risk factors are identified, the following tests should also be considered:

- LDL sub-fractions
- Oxidised LDL
- HDL sub-fractions
- hsCRP
- Homocysteine
- Apolipoproteins A and B
- Lipoprotein (a)
- Fibrinogen
- Asymmetrical dimethylarginine (ADMA) – inhibits NO synthesis[72]
- CT-angiogram with calcium score
- Fatty acid profiling
- Assessment of inflammation, oxidation, nutrient and methylation status
- Urine organic acid testing (OAT) for markers of gut dysbiosis, mitochondrial function and functional nutrient status
- Gut function and microbiome testing (link between gut bacteria, lipopolysaccharide (LPS) and metabolic syndrome).[73]

---

determine impairment of this enzyme and the need to supplement with omega-3 fatty acids or provide additional support with cofactors such as zinc and magnesium.

Metabolic function genotyping

Metabolic dysfunction is a key contributor to chronic disease and ageing, including cardiovascular disease, and therefore genes associated with metabolic function impact many aspects of health. The genes discussed below come from three main sources: evidence gathered from large studies, known effects in pathways and a demonstrated increased vulnerability to develop metabolic syndrome if these variants have been inherited.

Practitioners will benefit from this information as to how these genetic variants exert their effects in relation to the processing of dietary fats, dietary modification based on the genetic variants detected and incorporating this information into a weight management program. The patient should be engaged in the process and will better understand how important this information is if they have a family history of type 2 diabetes.

The *acetyl-CoA carboxylase β* (ACC2) gene plays a key role in fatty acid synthesis and oxidation pathways. Disturbance of these pathways is associated with impaired insulin responsiveness and metabolic syndrome. Studies have determined a gene–nutrient interaction between ACC2 rs4766587 and metabolic syndrome risk: minor A allele carriers of rs4766587 have increased metabolic syndrome risk compared with GG homozygotes. Risk was modulated by dietary fat intake, where risk conferred by the A allele was exacerbated among individuals with a high-fat intake (>35% energy), particularly a high intake (>5.5% energy) of omega-6 polyunsaturated fat (PUFA). Saturated and monounsaturated fat intake did not modulate risk. These findings were replicated in an independent cohort. The authors concluded that the ACC2 rs4766587 polymorphism influences metabolic syndrome risk, which is modulated by dietary fat, suggesting novel gene–nutrient interactions.[74]

LONG-CHAIN *ACSL1* GENE

Acyl CoA synthetase 1 (ACSL1) plays an important role in fatty acid metabolism and triglyceride synthesis. Disturbance of these pathways may result in dyslipidaemia and insulin resistance, hallmarks of the metabolic syndrome. Dietary fat is a key environmental factor that may interact with genetic determinants of lipid metabolism to affect metabolic syndrome risk. Researchers investigated the relationship between ACSL1 polymorphisms (rs4862417, rs6552828, rs13120078, rs9997745 and rs12503643) and metabolic syndrome risk and determined potential interactions with dietary fat. *GG* homozygotes for rs9997745 had increased metabolic syndrome risk, displayed elevated fasting glucose and insulin concentrations and increased insulin resistance relative to the A allele carriers. However, metabolic syndrome risk was modulated by dietary fat: the risk conferred by *GG* homozygosity was abolished among individuals consuming either a low-fat (<35% energy) or a high-PUFA (>5.5% energy) diet. The researchers concluded that the ACSL1 polymorphism rs9997745 influences metabolic syndrome risk, most likely via disturbances in fatty acid metabolism, which is modulated by dietary fat consumption, particularly PUFA intake, suggesting novel gene–nutrient interactions.[75]

G6PG2 GENE

The *glucose-6-phosphatase catalytic 2* (G6PG2) gene encodes an enzyme that enables the release of glucose into the bloodstream. Polymorphisms in this gene are associated with significant reductions in two main areas: fasting plasma glucose level and glycated haemoglobin A1C (HbA_{1c}). Scientific evidence suggests that for individuals with the rs560887 polymorphism, small changes in blood glucose can affect morbidity and mortality as the non-enzymatic addition of glucose (glycation) to proteins can affect function and contribute to the ageing process.[76]

SLC30A8 GENE

Research shows that the *solute carrier family 30 (zinc transporter) member 8* (SLC30A8) gene has a key role in pancreatic beta cell function and insulin secretion. Polymorphisms in this gene have been shown to be associated with an increased likelihood of developing type 2 diabetes. The polymorphism rs13266634 is associated with decreased beta cell function and impaired insulin secretion.[77]

TCF7L2 GENE AND *WFS1* GENE

Research shows that the *transcription factor 7-like 2* (TCF7L2) gene and the *Wolfram syndrome 1* (WFS1) gene are involved in insulin secretion, and polymorphisms in

these genes have been shown to be associated with an increased likelihood of developing type 2 diabetes. This can affect the individual's ability to remove glucose from the blood, which may result in elevated blood glucose levels.[78,79]

FTO GENE

The exact function of the *fat mass and obesity-associated* (FTO) gene is unknown; however, research suggests that it has a role in the control of food intake and food choice, with some polymorphisms leading to preference for energy-dense foods.[80,81] The rs9939609 polymorphism is also thought to modify energy expenditure depending on fat intake.[82] Some polymorphisms have been associated with an increased likelihood of developing type 2 diabetes. Individuals carrying this genetic variant may benefit from eating protein with every meal, as well as increasing exercise and fibre intake.[83]

PEROXISOME PROLIFERATOR-ACTIVATED RECEPTOR GAMMA GENE

Peroxisome proliferator-activated receptors (PPARs) are 'lipid sensing' ligand/metabolite-activated transcription factors that alter gene expression in a tissue-specific but overlapping manner. They form heterodimers with retinoid-x-receptors (RXR), which when complexed bind to the PPARs of various genes. In the absence of ligand, the heterodimers are bound to DNA with co-repressors such as histone deacetylases (e.g. SIRT1) to repress/activate target genes.[84,85] Three PPARs have been identified to date (PPARα, PPARγ and PPARδ) that have specific patterns of distribution and often opposing functionality designed to maintain coordinated glucose and lipid homeostasis.[86] For example, PPARα and PPARδ promote fatty acid oxidation in liver and muscle, respectively. PPARγ promotes adipocyte differentiation and lipogenesis in adipose tissue, which helps store fat appropriately and prevent the accumulation of harmful ectopic fat in tissues such as muscle and liver not designed to store fat, thereby improving insulin sensitivity.[87] Endogenous ligands of PPARs are unsaturated fatty acids, oxidised PUFAs, eicosanoids and oxidised components of lipoproteins (LDL and VLDL).[88] In addition, the pharmacological ligands for PPARα (fibrates) and PPARγ (thiazolidinediones) are used extensively for their triglyceride and insulin sensitising actions, respectively.[89,90]

The *peroxisome proliferator-activated receptor gamma* (PPARG) gene codes for PPARγ. The rs1801282 polymorphism in this gene appears to be associated with greater BMI and lower insulin sensitivity in some populations including Caucasians and obese individuals,[91] and may also be gender-dependent.[92] This polymorphism does not appear to have a significant effect on diabetes-related traits in non-diabetic individuals.[93]

Inflammation markers

Although inflammation is an important and necessary protective response by the body, chronic inflammation is linked to many disease states. Low-grade chronic inflammation is characterised by a two- to three-fold increase in systemic concentrations of cytokines such as

Next steps: Metabolic function genetics and future treatment directions

If variants in any of these genes or other metabolic function genes are identified, the following tests should also be considered:

- Assessment for cardiovascular disease risk, including lipids
- Fasting blood glucose and insulin
- Glycated haemoglobin and other advanced glycation end-product proteins such as carbonyl AGE proteins
- Cytokines such as IL-6
- Assessment of inflammation, oxidation, nutrient and methylation status
- Urine organic acid testing (OAT) for markers of gut dysbiosis, mitochondrial function and functional nutrient status
- Gut function and microbiome testing (link between gut bacteria, LPS and metabolic syndrome).[73]

tumour necrosis factor alpha (TNF-α), interleukin-6 (IL-6) and C-reactive protein (CRP). The circulating levels of these cytokines can be influenced by variations in the *TNF-α*, *IL-6* and *CRP* genes. Low-grade inflammation is a major contributor to chronic disease and is connected to risk factors for metabolic and cardiovascular disease by many mechanisms including modification of ApoA-1 and adipose tissue dysfunction with excess production of ceramides as previously described when saturated fat intake is high. These inflammatory cytokines also interfere with insulin signalling cascades.[39,40]

Research shows that genetics can influence the blood levels of inflammatory markers or cytokines such as IL-6, TNF-α and CRP.[94–96] Genetic variations that predispose individuals to inflammation may interact with environmental factors, for example diet, which may increase the individual's susceptibility to developing inflammatory-related problems.[97]

IL-6 GENE

The IL-6 polymorphism −174 SNP (rs1800795) was first described in 1998,[94] when it was shown that the rs1800795 *C* allele produces less IL-6 than the *G* allele, which supported the hypothesis that a protective genotype against systemic-onset juvenile rheumatoid arthritis would be rs1800795 *CC* – and indeed, few juvenile rheumatoid arthritis patients had that genotype.[98] Position '−174' is located in the promoter of the *IL-6* gene affecting levels of this cytokine. Carriers of this *IL-6* gene polymorphism may benefit from a Mediterranean diet containing virgin olive oil, nuts and anti-inflammatory plant compounds, especially if they are at increased risk of coronary artery disease.[97]

TNF-α GENE

The -308G>A SNP in the *TNF-α* gene, rs1800629, is also known as TNF-308 SNP. Occasionally, the rs1800629 *A* allele is referred to as 308.2 or TNF2, with the more common *G* allele being 308.1 or TNF1. The TNF-α *A* allele is associated with higher levels of TNF expression.[95] This SNP has been linked to a wide variety of conditions, including asthma.[99] The TNF-α -308 *A* allele has been shown to be associated with higher TNF-α levels in the blood. Some research suggests that the anti-inflammatory effect of fish oil may benefit those genetically predisposed to increased inflammation. As such, those with the *TNF-α A* allele may benefit from consuming deep-sea fish or by taking fish oil supplements. Practitioners should consider the mercury content of deep-sea fish, especially in those with heavy metal toxicity and genetic variants in detoxification and glutathione genes. Fish that contain higher levels of mercury include shark, ray, swordfish, barramundi, gemfish, orange roughy, ling and southern bluefin tuna.

CRP GENE

The *CRP* gene variant has been reported to have significant correlation with increasing BMI and waist circumference in males and has also been reported to be associated with cardiovascular disease and type 2 diabetes.[96] Another study of the rs1205 SNP showed increases in CRP levels in both males and females with this genotype. Research has shown that high blood levels of CRP, a marker of inflammation, are associated with increased risk of cardiovascular disease.[100] But what isn't clear is whether CRP actually *causes* heart disease or just indicates the presence of artery-blocking atherosclerosis.[101]

Researchers from Imperial College London set out to answer this question using a genetic approach. They reasoned that if high CRP levels really do *cause* heart disease, genetic variants associated with increased CRP should also be associated with increased heart disease risk. Using a sample of 28 000 heart disease patients and 10 000 controls, they examined several SNPs in the *CRP* gene. They found a significant association between the SNPs and CRP levels, and between CRP levels and heart disease. However, no association was detected between the genetic variations and heart disease.

The rs1205 *TT* genotype is associated with a 20% lower circulating CRP blood level when compared to individuals with the *CT* and *CC* genotypes. Conversely, the *TC* and *CC* genotypes are associated with higher circulating CRP levels when compared to individuals harbouring the T allele. Based on previous studies of CRP, this should have translated to 6% lower odds of heart disease. There was no association between rs1205 and heart disease.[102]

The association between measures of adiposity and CRP levels was reported to be dependent on variation in the rs1205 SNP of the *CRP* gene. A correlation was reported between higher CRP levels and adiposity by the presence of the C allele in males. Another study of the rs1205 SNP reported increases in CRP levels in both males and females with this genotype.[103]

Food sensitivities

SODIUM SENSITIVITY GENETICS

Results from testing sodium sensitivity genetics will indicate whether the patient has one or more genetic variations associated with a sodium-sensitive genotype

---

Next steps: Inflammation genetics and future treatment directions

If variants in any of these genes or other genes associated with inflammation are identified, the following tests should also be considered:

- hsCRP
- Cytokine panel (interleukins, TNF-α, interferon γ, GM-CSF)
- AA:EPA ratio (see section on fatty acid profiling)
- Urinary 17-keto-steroids, which are derived from androgen and glucocorticoid metabolism and can provide information on the balance between anabolic and catabolic processes. Elevated cortisol metabolites can indicate high levels of stress and inflammation.

---

or a predisposition to hypertension. If they do, the practitioner may recommend that the patient reduce their dietary sodium intake and ensure that their potassium intake meets the Australian recommended daily intake (RDI). This genetic information may be useful as a preventive approach or for those patients who have developed hypertension or type 2 diabetes, are overweight or have kidney disease. For some individuals, a higher dietary salt intake is associated with a significant increase in blood pressure; these individuals are considered to be 'salt sensitive'. A reduction in salt intake has been reported to significantly lower their blood pressure.

Several genetic variations have been found in genes that encode for important enzymes involved in blood pressure regulation. Two genes in particular – *ACE* (*angiotensin-converting enzyme*) and *AGT* (*angiotensinogen*) – have an important role in the renin-angiotensin-aldosterone system and have been linked with salt sensitivity.[104–106] The *ACE* gene encodes for ACE, which converts angiotensin I to blood pressure boosting angiotensin II in the lungs. The *AGT* gene encodes for AGT (the precursor to angiotensin I), which is converted to angiotensin I by renin when blood pressure is low.

Carriers of the ACE rs4343 *AA* and *AG* genotypes and the AGT rs699 *CC* and *CT* genotypes are associated with increased risk of sodium sensitivity based on the Australian recommended upper level of intake for adults. Individuals with these genotypes are more likely to have significantly greater blood pressure response associated with higher salt intake. This is referred to as 'salt sensitive' hypertension when compared with individuals carrying the 'GG' genotype. Individuals who lower their salt intake are more likely to have a reduction in blood pressure if their salt intake is currently high.[107–109]

COELIAC DISEASE

The field of application for coeliac disease testing is patients with a family history of coeliac disease, those with a negative serology result and a strong family history, patients who have started a gluten-free diet but have not had a confirmed diagnosis of coeliac disease, patients who feel ill after eating gluten and patients who present with the following symptoms: diarrhoea and/or abdominal pain, fatigue, weight loss, nausea and vomiting.[110,111] Genetic testing for coeliac HLA is a screening tool, thereby ruling out true coeliac disease, which is the local autoimmune destruction of intestinal mucosa by immune cross-reactivity to gluten.[112]

The advantage of genetic testing is that it prevents the need for further invasive tests if the patient is negative, assists when a serology test is negative and can be performed without the need to consume gluten. The main contributor to coeliac disease is the HLA markers DQ2.2, DQ2.5 and DQ8.[113,114] The presence of HLA markers does not mean that a patient may not be sensitive to gluten and wheat. An acquired sensitivity/reaction to the protein component of wheat (gluten) or the sugar component (fructans) may develop if there are digestive system or microbiome abnormalities.

LACTOSE INTOLERANCE

The field of application for lactose intolerance testing is patients presenting with abdominal discomfort after consuming dairy products and having a family history of lactose intolerance or with an Asian, Australian Aboriginal, Torres Strait Islander, South American, Southern European or African background, and anyone taking IBS supplements. Carriers of the *MCM6* gene polymorphism rs4988235 *CC* genotype are at high risk of being lactose intolerant.[115] This polymorphism does not exclude the possibility of developing a secondary lactose intolerance due to small intestinal bacterial overgrowth or dysbiosis.

CAFFEINE METABOLISM

CYP1A2 caffeine metabolism gene

Caffeine is one of the most popular and widely used stimulant drugs in the world. Research has shown that daily intake of caffeine over 300 mg is unhealthy and can be damaging to the brain, putting significant strain on the heart, liver and kidneys. Individuals who are slow metabolisers of caffeine are at higher risk of organ damage. The field of application for caffeine metabolism genetics is women who want to conceive, patients with a history of heart disease, patients with risk factors for heart disease or high blood pressure, patients who consume high quantities of caffeine, patients with difficulty sleeping or insomnia, anyone who feels over-stimulated or anxious after consuming caffeine, and sports and exercise enthusiasts. The clinical benefit of dietary caffeine removal is a reduction in cardiovascular disease risk, a reduction in hypertension risk, reducing fertility issues in women who are slow metabolisers of caffeine, assisting individuals with stress or anxiety to understand how caffeine may be affecting them, and helping sports enthusiasts to understand the implications of their caffeine intake.[116] Slow metabolisers of caffeine who drink 2–3 cups of coffee per day have an increased risk of heart attack of 67%, while an intake of more than 4 cups per day increases the risk to >133%.

Carriers of the *CYP1A2* gene rs762551 *C* allele are slow metabolisers.[117]

Oxidative stress

Oxidation is a normal part of metabolism and cellular signalling but when the generation of oxidation overwhelms the endogenous and exogenous antioxidant systems, cellular damage can occur. Genetic variants in several genes that code for cellular antioxidant enzyme systems can influence enzyme function and knowing whether they have such variants can be useful for patients who want to understand their need for antioxidant support, patients interested in anti-ageing strategies, disease prevention and preconception care for males to ensure good sperm quality. The clinical benefit is multifactorial, providing information in relation to antioxidant support and as part of an anti-ageing strategy with the main areas of influence being weight management, cardiovascular health, blood sugar levels, respiratory function, joint mobility, immune response, brain health and preconception care.

Manganese superoxide dismutase MnSOD (rs4880) is a mitochondrial biomarker for oxidative stress that neutralises superoxide, a toxic type of free radical. Glutathione peroxidase (rs1050450) is a selenium-dependent

glutathione.[118,119] Dietary sources of selenium are Brazil nuts, shell fish, meat, eggs, mushrooms and grains. Catalase (rs1001179) reduces oxidative stress by converting hydrogen peroxide into water and oxygen.[120,121]

Methylation

The process of methylation can be thought of as an on/off switch and involves the addition of a methyl group (CH_3). This process is involved in hundreds of reactions involving DNA synthesis and repair, immune function, mitochondrial energy generation, detoxification and antioxidant pathways, hormone metabolism and neurotransmitter and catecholamine pathways. Abnormalities in the methylation cycle/pathways can have far-reaching consequences for health (see Table 8.1).

The methyl group is supplied by the integrated function of the methionine, folate and biopterin pathways. There are many genetic variants in the numerous genes involved in these pathways. Genetic variants in the *MTHFR* gene can reduce the methylfolate available for the methylation of cobalamin, which is required for the conversion of homocysteine to methionine and subsequently the production of SAMe, the major methyl donor in the body. This variant sometimes leads to elevated homocysteine[122] and s-adenosyl-homocysteine, which are risk factors for cardiovascular disease.[123] S-adenosyl-homocysteine is a potent inhibitor of methyltransferase enzymes[124] required for numerous methylation reactions such as catechol-O-methyltransferase (COMT) involved in neurotransmitter and oestrogen metabolism and phosphatidylethanolamine-

TABLE 8.1 Biochemical processes involving methylation and adverse consequences

Biochemical process	Adverse consequence
DNA and RNA	Turn on/off genetic expression and enzymes
Neurotransmitters	Depression, anxiety, cognition (adrenaline, noradrenaline, dopamine, serotonin)
Cell membranes	Neuro-degeneration, membrane receptors and fluidity, lipid abnormalities
Hormones	Thyroid abnormalities, stress response, poor sleep, oestrogen metabolism
Immune function	Poor wound healing, infection, autoimmunity, cancer, food allergies
Detoxification	Degenerative disease, cancer, food sensitivities, increased oxidation and inflammation, antioxidants (glutathione)
Energy generation	Chronic fatigue, mitochondrial abnormalities (carnitine, CoQ10)

Source: © Reproduced by kind permission of Dr Rhona Creegan and Dr Margaret Smith.

TABLE 8.2 MTHFR enzyme activity for the combined SNP contributions of C677T and A1298C polymorphisms

MTHFR genotype	677CC homozygous normal	677CT heterozygous one T allele	677TT homozygous two TT alleles
1298AA homozygous normal	100% normal enzyme activity	65% normal enzyme activity	25% normal enzyme activity
1298AC heterozygous one C allele	83% normal enzyme activity	48% normal enzyme activity	Not known
1298CC homozygous two C alleles	61% normal enzyme activity	Not known	Not known

Source: © Reproduced by kind permission of Dr Margaret Smith (SmartDNA).

TABLE 8.3 MTHFR enzyme activity and homocysteine level

MTHFR genotype	677CC homozygous normal	677CT heterozygous one T allele	677TT homozygous two TT alleles
1298AA homozygous normal	No impact on homocysteine metabolism	No impact on homocysteine metabolism	Associated with elevated homocysteine level
1298AC heterozygous one C allele	No impact on homocysteine metabolism	Associated with elevated homocysteine level	Associated with elevated homocysteine level*
1298CC homozygous two C alleles	No impact on homocysteine metabolism	Associated with elevated homocysteine level*	Associated with elevated homocysteine level*

*Rare MTHFR gene SNP pairing. Refer to hwww.omim.org/entry/607093
Source: © Reproduced by kind permission of Dr Margaret Smith (SmartDNA).

methyltransferase (PEMT) required for the production of phosphatidylcholine for membrane function and synthesis of choline and acetylcholine. Variants in the *MTHFR* gene are often tested for to assess the function of methylation and research has focused on two SNPs: C677T and A1298C. Tables 8.2 and 8.3 highlight the effects of these two common genetic variants on enzyme activity and homocysteine levels.[123,125]

Because the methylation cycle involves complex interactions of integrated pathways, genetic variants in other genes should be considered when making therapeutic decisions. Some of these include *MTR, MTRR, TCN2, SLC19A1, CBS, MTHFD1* involved with methionine synthesis, remethylation of vitamin B_{12}, transport of B_{12}, folate and choline, interconversion of folates and the transsulfuration pathway for producing cysteine and glutathione. Variants in these genes can also influence methylation pathways and affect plasma levels of homocysteine.[126,127] If therapeutic decisions are based solely on MTHFR variants and plasma homocysteine levels, the wrong therapeutic strategies may be used. For example, certain variants in the transsulfuration pathway (CBS rs234706 699C>T) may upregulate the cystationine-β-synthase enzyme, which converts homocysteine to cystathionine and can lower homocysteine levels. However, the activity of this enzyme is upregulated in the presence of oxidative stress, even when the wild-type gene is present, as it acts as a redox sensor to increase production of glutathionine in times of need.[128,129]

Most identified variants in genes involved in the methylation cycle lead to elevated homocysteine and S-adenosyl-homocysteine (SAH). The impact of these variants on methylation status varies depending on factors such as nutrient availability, overall requirement for methylation reactions at a given time, oxidative stress and overall toxin load. Homocysteine can be measured in the blood and elevated levels are a risk factor for cardiovascular disease. If homocysteine is elevated, support nutrients such as folate, vitamin B_{12}, vitamin B_2, vitamin B_6, choline and trimethylglycine (betaine) can be used to lower levels. The form of the nutrients used will depend on the genetic variants identified and needs to be individualised. Nutrient status can be assessed by various methods including urine organic acid and amino acid testing. Urine organic acid testing provides a functional assessment of the nutrients by measuring the nutrient sensitive pathways and whether the reactions are proceeding (e.g. methylmalonic acid for vitamin B_{12} and foriminoglutamic acid [FIGLU] or pyrimidine metabolites for folate status).

The form of folate may be important, depending on the SNPs; individuals appear to react differently to the various activated forms (methylfolate vs folinic vs folic acid). There is considerable confusion among practitioners about the various forms of folate. One report showed that unmetabolised folic acid reduced the activity of natural killer cells[130] but this has not been verified in subsequent studies and any role for unmetabolised folic acid as a contributor to disease is disputed.[131] It is likely that the enzyme dihydrofolate reductase (DHFR, which reduces dietary folic acid into active folates) becomes saturated when folic acid intake is high and that the unmetabolised folic acid is a transient phenomenon. As folic acid is not a cofactor for any biochemical reactions, it is unlikely to adversely affect pathways, although this is still an active area of research. The active forms of folate supplements may be beneficial if the DHFR activity is reduced, such as with genetic variants, excess alcohol consumption and certain medications.

If homocysteine levels are normal or low, methylation may still be impaired, as an upregulated cystathionine B synthase (CBS) enzyme in the transsulfuration pathway may be diverting the homocysteine away from regenerating methionine. A plasma methylation profile can be used to functionally assess the methylation cycle. The ratio between SAMe and SAH is important. SAH is a potent inhibitor of methyltransferase enzymes, including DNMT (epigenetic regulation), HNMT (histamine metabolism) and COMT (neurotransmitter and oestrogen metabolism). This test will also measure cystathionine levels. An important cause of abnormal methylation is inhibition of many of the enzymes by accumulation of toxins regardless of genetic status, although this is exacerbated by genetic variants and subsequent reduced enzyme function. It is a perpetuating cycle where toxins inhibit the enzymes and methylation is required for detoxification pathways. Methylation pathways provide the methyl and glycine groups directly in phase II liver pathways and support the transsulfuration pathway to produce glutathione for the glutathione transferase enzymes in phase II conjugation. Many of these enzymes (CBS) and phase I cytochrome

p450 detoxification enzymes are dependent on the synthesis of haem and therefore overall toxin burden can be assessed by measuring urinary porphyrins, heavy metals or environmental pollutants.

Detoxification

Detoxification of exogenous and endogenous compounds is vital for health in order to prevent the accumulation of potentially harmful substances including products of metabolism, hormones, heavy metals, pharmaceuticals and pollutants. Detoxification occurs mainly in the liver by phase I and phase II reactions. Phase I activates compounds by the action of the cytochrome P450 enzymes, followed by conjugation of these reactive intermediates in phase II. Phase II conjugates are more water-soluble and can be excreted from the body via the bile and kidneys in phase III. There is substrate competition between the detoxification enzymes which, when combined with the polymorphic nature of the genes that encode for these enzymes, can slow down or speed up removal of compounds, resulting in excess accumulation of unwanted substances (such as environmental chemicals and hormones), and altered elimination of pharmaceutical compounds, resulting in reduced efficacy or enhanced toxicity. This is the basis of pharmacogenetics which is applied to several areas of medicine, including oncology, psychiatry, cardiology and pain management.

The genes encoding CYP2D6, CYP2C19, CYP2C9, CYP3A4 and CYP3A5 account for the metabolism of 80–90% of all prescription drugs and testing for genetic variants in these genes may help reduce adverse drug reactions, especially in the modern era of polypharmacy.[132,133]

Oestrone (E1) and oestradiol (E2) are metabolised to 2-, 4- and 16-hydroxy metabolites. These metabolites are further metabolised into methylated products. Variants in the CYP450s and methylating enzymes involved can therefore lead to abnormal amounts of the metabolites, which differ in their oestrogenicity and effect on disease risk.

CYP1A1 catalyses the 2-hydroxylation of E1 (oestrone) and E2 (oestradiol) to form the catechols 2-hydroxy-E1 (2-OHE1) and 2-hydroxy-E2 (2-OHE2). These are considered more anti-oestrogenic than the 4-OH and 16-OH metabolites and are therefore considered more protective in terms of breast cancer risk.[134] The CYP1A1 rs4646903 variant has been shown to increase enzyme activity.[135] Additionally, CYP1A1 activates pro-carcinogens such as polycyclic aromatic hydrocarbons (PAH) and heterocyclic aromatic amines (HA) found in tobacco smoke and chargrilled meat, which have been reported to play a role in the development of some cancers such as lung and breast. Females with CYP1B1 rs1056836 *CG* or *GG* who smoke have been shown to have a 2.3-fold increased risk of developing breast cancer.[136]

CYP1B1 hydroxylates E1 and E2 into the 4-OH metabolites, which are mutagenic.[137] It also produces toxic intermediates from xeno-oestrogens that mimic oestrogens by binding to oestrogen receptors. The CYP1B1 rs1056836 variant is upregulated by xeno-oestrogens, which increases production of the 4-OH metabolites and has been shown to increase risk of uterine fibroids and breast and prostate

Methylation genetics and future treatment directions

If variants in any of these genes or other genes associated with methylation are identified, the following tests should also be considered:
- Plasma methylation profile (SAMe, SAH, SAMe:SAH ratio, homocysteine, cystathionine, methionine)
- Folate metabolism profile (5-MTHF, folinic acid, THF)
- Urinary porphyrins (intermediates in haem pathways)
- Hepatic detoxification profiles
- Heavy metals (hair, urine or blood)
- Urine organic acids (nutrient status, mitochondrial function, neurotransmitter metabolism, ammonia)
- Urine amino acids
- Urine pyrroles (for zinc and vitamin B$_6$ status)
- Urine hormone metabolites, including oestrogen and cortisol
- Histamine (take caution with this assessment as a significant amount may be produced in gut).

cancer.[134,138,139] Once the 2- and 4-hydroxylated metabolites are produced, they are methylated (inactivated) by COMT, which relies on adequate enzyme activity and which can be slowed by various SNPs in both MTHFR and COMT (rs4680). Accumulated fat-soluble 4-hydroxy oestrone can be further oxidised to produce catechol quinones, which can damage DNA and activate oncogenes.[140] If variants in phase I and oestrogen metabolism genes are present as described, exposure, PAHs, PCBs and xeno-oestrogens should be reduced. Activity of COMT may also be impaired with being overweight, excessive alcohol consumption and stress.

Glutathione-S-transferase enzymes detoxify many water-soluble environmental toxins including solvents, PAHs, steroids, herbicides, pesticides, lipid peroxidases and heavy metals (mercury, cadmium and lead) by conjugating glutathione with phase I derived products. Decreased glutathione conjugation capacity can therefore overwhelm detoxification capacity, leading to toxin accumulation and increased oxidative stress. Copy number variations in the GSTT1 and GSTM1 enzymes are associated with less effective detoxification of potential carcinogens and an increased susceptibility to heavy metal accumulation and some types of cancer.[141] When looking at the copy number of a gene, the variant is assigned as being either present or absent (null). The GSTP1 gene encodes for the glutathione-S-transferase P1 enzyme located in the brain, skin and lungs and is involved in detoxification of carcinogens, xenobiotics, steroids, heavy metals and oxidative stress. The rs1695 variant produces an enzyme with lower activity and less detoxification capacity.

The association between certain dietary components (e.g. isothiocyanates in cruciferous vegetables) and reduced cancer risk is thought to be due to the effect on the detoxification genes/enzymes including CYP1A1, GSTT1 and GSTM1.[142,143] Analysis of genetic variants in the detoxification genes is important therefore for identification of risk of the damaging effects of both endogenous and exogenous toxin exposure and the implementation of dietary and lifestyle strategies to assist with the detoxification capacity.

PUTTING IT ALL TOGETHER

If genetic variants are identified in any genes, additional testing may be required to determine whether the variants are affecting biochemical pathways at a functional level. As many modern chronic health concerns are multifactorial in aetiology, it is likely that abnormalities in metabolic function, detoxification, oxidation, inflammation and methylation are present, which can be made worse when biochemical weaknesses are exposed by underlying genetic variability. The genetic polymorphisms do not indicate the presence of disease, but when used in combination with the individual's clinical presentation, information on their diet, lifestyle, environment and specific biochemical testing, powerful personalised interventions can be employed.

The best time to assess genetic variability is when the person is well, because ultimately the goal is to prevent the development of chronic conditions by focusing on where any weaknesses in their biochemistry lie. However, many practitioners see patients who are trying to regain lost health and genomic profiling will assist in revealing possible dysfunctional pathways. Our health is a complex interaction of diet, lifestyle and environment with our genome and microbiome, involving numerous signalling molecules to provide metabolic and survival cues that instruct our genes to express or repress (epigenetics), so that appropriate biochemical pathways are activated/deactivated to ensure survival. When imbalances in metabolism, detoxification, inflammation, methylation, glycation and oxidation occur, there will also be abnormalities with hormones, neurotransmitters, gut function and energy generation. Knowing our biochemical vulnerabilities is a key piece of the complex health puzzle. With certain genotypes, general diet and lifestyle recommendations can be made, but specific recommendations should not usually be made based on genotype alone – this needs to be based on phenotype.

Detoxification genetics and future treatment directions

If variants in any of these genes or other genes associated with detoxification are identified, the following tests should also be considered:
- Phase I liver detoxification profile – caffeine clearance.
- Phase II liver detoxification profile – measures of glucuronidation, glycination, glutathionation and sulfation.
- Urine mercapturic acid.
- Profiles looking at toxic exposure to volatile solvents, chlorinated pesticides, polychlorinated biphenyls, organophosphates, bisphenol A, phthalates and parabens.
- Urine organic acids.
- Urinary oestrogen metabolites.
- Heavy metal analysis.
- Oxidative stress markers (as described).
- Methylation assessment (as described).

REFERENCES

[1] Karki R, Pandya D, Elston RC, et al. Defining 'mutation' and 'polymorphism' in the era of personal genomics. BMC Med Genomics 2015;8:37.
[2] Burdge GC, Lillycrop KA. Nutrition, epigenetics, and developmental plasticity: implications for understanding human disease. Annu Rev Nutr 2010;30:315–39.
[3] Feil R, Berger F. Convergent evolution of genomic imprinting in plants and mammals. Trends Genet 2007;23(4):192–9.
[4] Court F, Tayama C, Romanelli V, et al. Genome-wide parent-of-origin DNA methylation analysis reveals the intricacies of human imprinting and suggests a germline methylation-independent mechanism of establishment. Genome Res 2014;24(4):554–69.
[5] Tycko B, Morison IM. Physiological functions of imprinted genes. J Cell Physiol 2002;192(3):245–58.
[6] Isles AR, Holland AJ. Imprinted genes and mother–offspring interactions. Early Hum Dev 2005;81(1):73–7.
[7] Jirtle RL, Skinner MK. Environmental epigenomics and disease susceptibility. Nat Rev Genet 2007;8(4):253–62.

[8] Painter RC, Roseboom TJ, Bossuyt PM, et al. Adult mortality at age 57 after prenatal exposure to the Dutch famine. Eur J Epidemiol 2005;20(8):673–6.

[9] Heijmans BT, Tobi EW, Stein AD, et al. Persistent epigenetic differences associated with prenatal exposure to famine in humans. Proc Natl Acad Sci USA 2008;105(44):17046–9.

[10] van Os J, Selten JP. Prenatal exposure to maternal stress and subsequent schizophrenia. The May 1940 invasion of The Netherlands. Br J Psychiatry 1998;172:324–6.

[11] St Clair D, Xu M, Wang P, et al. Rates of adult schizophrenia following prenatal exposure to the Chinese famine of 1959–1961. JAMA 2005;294(5):557–62.

[12] Egger G, Liang G, Aparicio A, et al. Epigenetics in human disease and prospects for epigenetic therapy. Nature 2004;429(6990):457–63.

[13] Saha A, Wittmeyer J, Cairns BR. Chromatin remodelling: the industrial revolution of DNA around histones. Nat Rev Mol Cell Biol 2006;7(6):437–47.

[14] https://en.wikipedia.org/wiki/Epigenetics.

[15] Issa JP. CpG island methylator phenotype in cancer. Nat Rev Cancer 2004;4(12):988–93.

[16] Cuozzo C, Porcellini A, Angrisano T, et al. DNA damage, homology-directed repair, and DNA methylation. PLoS Genet 2007;3(7):e110.

[17] Pfeifer GP, Kadam S, Jin SG. 5-hydroxymethylcytosine and its potential roles in development and cancer. Epigenetics Chromatin 2013;6(1):10.

[18] Kohli RM, Zhang Y. TET enzymes, TDG and the dynamics of DNA demethylation. Nature 2013;502(7472):472–9.

[19] Holliday R. Epigenetics: a historical overview. Epigenetics 2006; 1(2):76–80.

[20] Clapier CR, Cairns BR. The biology of chromatin remodeling complexes. Annu Rev Biochem 2009;78:273–304.

[21] Ernst J, Kellis M. Discovery and characterization of chromatin states for systematic annotation of the human genome. Nat Biotechnol 2010;28(8):817–25.

[22] Chi P, Allis CD, Wang GG. Covalent histone modifications: miswritten, misinterpreted and mis-erased in human cancers. Nat Rev Cancer 2010;10(7):457–69.

[23] Turner BM. Reading signals on the nucleosome with a new nomenclature for modified histones. Nat Struct Mol Biol 2005;12(2):110–12.

[24] Cosgrove MS, Boeke JD, Wolberger C. Regulated nucleosome mobility and the histone code. Nat Struct Mol Biol 2004;11(11):1037–43.

[25] Selhub J. Homocysteine metabolism. Annu Rev Nutr 1999;19:217–46.

[26] Chen NC, Yang F, Capecci LM, et al. Regulation of homocysteine metabolism and methylation in human and mouse tissues. FASEB J 2010;24(8):2804–17.

[27] Fang M, Chen D, Yang CS. Dietary polyphenols may affect DNA methylation. J Nutr 2007;137(1 Suppl.):223S–8S.

[28] Gerhauser C. Epigenetic impact of dietary isothiocyanates in cancer chemoprevention. Curr Opin Clin Nutr Metab Care 2013;16(4):405–10.

[29] Gerhauser C. Cancer chemoprevention and nutriepigenetics: state of the art and future challenges. Top Curr Chem 2013;329:73–132.

[30] Valinluck V, Tsai HH, Rogstad DK, et al. Oxidative damage to methyl-CpG sequences inhibits the binding of the methyl-CpG binding domain (MBD) of methyl-CpG binding protein 2 (MeCP2). Nucleic Acids Res 2004;32(14):4100–8.

[31] Chia N, Wang L, Lu X, et al. Hypothesis: environmental regulation of 5-hydroxymethylcytosine by oxidative stress. Epigenetics 2011;6(7):853–6.

[32] Niedzwiecki MM, Hall MN, Liu X, et al. Blood glutathione redox status and global methylation of peripheral blood mononuclear cell DNA in Bangladeshi adults. Epigenetics 2013;8(7):730–8.

[33] Chao S, Roberts JS, Marteau TM, et al. Health behavior changes after genetic risk assessment for Alzheimer disease: the REVEAL Study. Alzheimer Dis Assoc Disord 2008;22(1):94–7.

[34] Bloss CS, Schork NJ, Topol EJ. Effect of direct-to-consumer genomewide profiling to assess disease risk. N Engl J Med 2011;364(6):524–34.

[35] Gropper SS, Groff J. Advanced nutrition and human metabolism. 4th ed. Belmont, CA: Thomson Wadsworth; 2004.

[36] Puglielli L, Tanzi RE, Kovacs DM. Alzheimer's disease: the cholesterol connection. Nat Neurosci 2003;6(4):345–51.

[37] Woollett LA, Spady DK, Dietschy JM. Saturated and unsaturated fatty acids independently regulate low density lipoprotein receptor activity and production rate. J Lipid Res 1992;33(1):77–88.

[38] Spady DK, Woollett LA, Dietschy JM. Regulation of plasma LDL-cholesterol levels by dietary cholesterol and fatty acids. Annu Rev Nutr 1993;13:355–81.

[39] Summers SA. Ceramides in insulin resistance and lipotoxicity. Prog Lipid Res 2006;45(1):42–72.

[40] Chavez JA, Summers SA. A ceramide-centric view of insulin resistance. Cell Metab 2012;15(5):585–94.

[41] Dobrzyn P, Jazurek M, Dobrzyn A. Stearoyl-CoA desaturase and insulin signaling: what is the molecular switch? Biochim Biophys Acta 2010;1797(6–7):1189–94.

[42] Davidson MH. Mechanisms for the hypotriglyceridemic effect of marine omega-3 fatty acids. Am J Cardiol 2006;98(4A):27i–33i.

[43] Ascherio A, Katan MB, Zock PL, et al. Trans fatty acids and coronary heart disease. N Engl J Med 1999;340(25):1994–8.

[44] Mauger JF, Lichtenstein AH, Ausman LM, et al. Effect of different forms of dietary hydrogenated fats on LDL particle size. Am J Clin Nutr 2003;78(3):370–5.

[45] Khan SA, Vanden Heuvel JP. Role of nuclear receptors in the regulation of gene expression by dietary fatty acids (review). J Nutr Biochem 2003;14(10):554–67.

[46] Vanden Heuvel JP. Cardiovascular disease-related genes and regulation by diet. Curr Atheroscler Rep 2009;11(6):448–55.

[47] Vanden Heuvel JP. Diet, fatty acids, and regulation of genes important for heart disease. Curr Atheroscler Rep 2004;6(6):432–40.

[48] Matthan NR, Welty FK, Barrett PH, et al. Dietary hydrogenated fat increases high-density lipoprotein apoA-I catabolism and decreases low-density lipoprotein apoB-100 catabolism in hypercholesterolemic women. Arterioscler Thromb Vasc Biol 2004;24(6):1092–7.

[49] van Tol A, Zock PL, van Gent T, et al. Dietary trans fatty acids increase serum cholesterylester transfer protein activity in man. Atherosclerosis 1995;115(1):129–34.

[50] Parks JS, Huggins KW, Gebre AK, et al. Phosphatidylcholine fluidity and structure affect lecithin:cholesterol acyltransferase activity. J Lipid Res 2000;41(4):546–53.

[51] Duncan D, Morais J, Muniz N, et al. Lipoprotein subfraction testing with the lipoprint R system: easy, accurate and comprehensive. Presented at CLAS, Northbrook, IL, May 2004.

[52] Lamarche B, Tchernof A, Moorjani S, et al. Small, dense low-density lipoprotein particles as a predictor of the risk of ischemic heart disease in men. Prospective results from the Quebec Cardiovascular Study. Circulation 1997;95(1):69–75.

[53] Mack WJ, Krauss RM, Hodis HN. Lipoprotein subclasses in the Monitored Atherosclerosis Regression Study (MARS). Treatment effects and relation to coronary angiographic progression. Arterioscler Thromb Vasc Biol 1996;16(5):697–704.

[54] Rajman I, Maxwell S, Cramb R, et al. Particle size: the key to the atherogenic lipoprotein? QJM 1994;87(12):709–20.

[55] Kholodova YD, Harris WS. Identification and characteristic of LDL-subfractions in human plasma. Ukr Biokhim Zh 1995;67(6):60–5.

[56] Fisher EA, Feig JE, Hewing B, et al. High-density lipoprotein function, dysfunction, and reverse cholesterol transport. Arterioscler Thromb Vasc Biol 2012;32(12):2813–20.

[57] Kontush A, Chapman MJ. Functionally defective high-density lipoprotein: a new therapeutic target at the crossroads of dyslipidemia, inflammation, and atherosclerosis. Pharmacol Rev 2006;58(3):342–74.

[58] Dullaart RP. Increased coronary heart disease risk determined by high high-density lipoprotein cholesterol and C-reactive protein: modulation by variation in the CETP gene. Arterioscler Thromb Vasc Biol 2010;30(8):1502–3.

[59] Navab M, Reddy ST, Van Lenten BJ, et al. HDL and cardiovascular disease: atherogenic and atheroprotective mechanisms. Nat Rev Cardiol 2011;8(4):222–32.

[60] Oravec S, Dostal E, Dukat A, et al. HDL subfractions analysis: a new laboratory diagnostic assay for patients with cardiovascular diseases and dyslipoproteinemia. Neuro Endocrinol Lett 2011;32(4):502–9.

[61] Estruch R, Ros E, Salas-Salvado J, et al. Primary prevention of cardiovascular disease with a Mediterranean diet. N Engl J Med 2013;368(14):1279–90.

[62] Rall SC Jr, Weisgraber KH, Mahley RW. Human apolipoprotein E. The complete amino acid sequence. J Biol Chem 1982;257(8):4171–8.

[63] Weisgraber KH, Innerarity TL, Mahley RW. Abnormal lipoprotein receptor-binding activity of the human E apoprotein due to cysteine–arginine interchange at a single site. J Biol Chem 1982; 257(5):2518–21.

[64] Eisenberg DT, Kuzawa CW, Hayes MG. Worldwide allele frequencies of the human apolipoprotein E gene: climate, local adaptations, and evolutionary history. Am J Phys Anthropol 2010;143(1):100–11.

[65] Grammer TB, Hoffmann MM, Scharnagl H, et al. Smoking, apolipoprotein E genotypes, and mortality (the Ludwigshafen Risk and Cardiovascular Health study). Eur Heart J 2013;34(17):1298–305.

[66] Mahley RW, Weisgraber KH, Huang Y. Apolipoprotein E: structure determines function, from atherosclerosis to Alzheimer's disease to AIDS. J Lipid Res 2009;50(Suppl.):S183–8.

[67] Corella D, Tucker K, Lahoz C, et al. Alcohol drinking determines the effect of the APOE locus on LDL-cholesterol concentrations in men: the Framingham Offspring Study. Am J Clin Nutr 2001;73(4): 736–45.

[68] Kathiresan S, Willer CJ, Peloso GM, et al. Common variants at 30 loci contribute to polygenic dyslipidemia. Nat Genet 2009;41(1):56–65.

[69] Santoro N, Zhang CK, Zhao H, et al. Variant in the glucokinase regulatory protein (GCKR) gene is associated with fatty liver in obese children and adolescents. Hepatology 2012;55(3):781–9.

[70] Kinnunen PK, Jackson RL, Smith LC, et al. Activation of lipoprotein lipase by native and synthetic fragments of human plasma apolipoprotein C-II. Proc Natl Acad Sci USA 1977;74(11): 4848–51.

[71] Barzilai N, Atzmon G, Schechter C, et al. Unique lipoprotein phenotype and genotype associated with exceptional longevity. JAMA 2003;290(15):2030–40.

[72] Schulze F, Lenzen H, Hanefeld C, et al. Asymmetric dimethylarginine is an independent risk factor for coronary heart disease: results from the multicenter Coronary Artery Risk Determination investigating the Influence of ADMA Concentration (CARDIAC) study. Am Heart J 2006;152(3):493.e1–e8.

[73] Mazidi M, Rezaie P, Kengne AP, et al. Gut microbiome and metabolic syndrome. Diabetes Metab Syndr 2016;10(2 Suppl. 1): S150–7.

[74] Phillips CM, Goumidi L, Bertrais S, et al. ACC2 gene polymorphisms, metabolic syndrome, and gene–nutrient interactions with dietary fat. J Lipid Res 2010;51(12):3500–7.

[75] Phillips CM, Goumidi L, Bertrais S, et al. Gene–nutrient interactions with dietary fat modulate the association between genetic variation of the ACSL1 gene and metabolic syndrome. J Lipid Res 2010; 51(7):1793–800.

[76] Renström F, Shungin D, Johansson I, et al. Genetic predisposition to long-term nondiabetic deteriorations in glucose homeostasis: ten-year follow-up of the GLACIER study. Diabetes 2011;60(1):345–54.

[77] Zeggini E, Weedon MN, Lindgren CM, et al. Replication of genome-wide association signals in UK samples reveals risk loci for type 2 diabetes. Science 2007;316(5829):1336–41.

[78] Scott LJ, Mohlke KL, Bonnycastle LL, et al. A genome-wide association study of type 2 diabetes in Finns detects multiple susceptibility variants. Science 2007;316(5829):1341–5.

[79] Dupuis J, Langenberg C, Prokopenko I, et al. New genetic loci implicated in fasting glucose homeostasis and their impact on type 2 diabetes risk. Nat Genet 2010;42(2):105–16.

[80] Speakman JR, Rance KA, Johnstone AM. Polymorphisms of the FTO gene are associated with variation in energy intake, but not energy expenditure. Obesity (Silver Spring) 2008;16(8):1961–5.

[81] Frayling TM, Timpson NJ, Weedon MN, et al. A common variant in the FTO gene is associated with body mass index and predisposes to childhood and adult obesity. Science 2007;316(5826):889–94.

[82] Sonestedt E, Roos C, Gullberg B, et al. Fat and carbohydrate intake modify the association between genetic variation in the FTO genotype and obesity. Am J Clin Nutr 2009;90(5):1418–25.

[83] Kilpelainen TO, Qi L, Brage S, et al. Physical activity attenuates the influence of FTO variants on obesity risk: a meta-analysis of 218,166 adults and 19,268 children. PLoS Med 2011;8(11):e1001116.

[84] Glass CK, Rosenfeld MG. The coregulator exchange in transcriptional functions of nuclear receptors. Genes Dev 2000;14(2):121–41.

[85] Berger J, Moller DE. The mechanisms of action of PPARs. Annu Rev Med 2002;53:409–35.

[86] Evans RM, Barish GD, Wang YX. PPARs and the complex journey to obesity. Nat Med 2004;10(4):355–61.

[87] Yamauchi T, Kamon J, Waki H, et al. The mechanisms by which both heterozygous peroxisome proliferator-activated receptor gamma (PPARgamma) deficiency and PPARgamma agonist improve insulin resistance. J Biol Chem 2001;276(44):41245–54.

[88] Bensinger SJ, Tontonoz P. Integration of metabolism and inflammation by lipid-activated nuclear receptors. Nature 2008;454(7203):470–7.

[89] Staels B, Dallongeville J, Auwerx J, et al. Mechanism of action of fibrates on lipid and lipoprotein metabolism. Circulation 1998;98(19):2088–93.

[90] Lehmann JM, Moore LB, Smith-Oliver TA, et al. An antidiabetic thiazolidinedione is a high affinity ligand for peroxisome proliferator-activated receptor gamma (PPAR gamma). J Biol Chem 1995;270(22):12953–6.

[91] Kilpelainen TO, Lakka TA, Laaksonen DE, et al. SNPs in PPARG associate with type 2 diabetes and interact with physical activity. Med Sci Sports Exerc 2008;40(1):25–33.

[92] Hsiao TJ, Lin E. The Pro12Ala polymorphism in the peroxisome proliferator-activated receptor gamma (PPARG) gene in relation to obesity and metabolic phenotypes in a Taiwanese population. Endocrine 2015;48(3):786–93.

[93] Rocha RM, Barra GB, Rosa EC, et al. Prevalence of the rs1801282 single nucleotide polymorphism of the PPARG gene in patients with metabolic syndrome. Arch Endocrinol Metab 2015;59(4):297–302.

[94] Fishman D, Faulds G, Jeffery R, et al. The effect of novel polymorphisms in the interleukin-6 (IL-6) gene on IL-6 transcription and plasma IL-6 levels, and an association with systemic-onset juvenile chronic arthritis. J Clin Invest 1998;102(7):1369–76.

[95] Louis E, Franchimont D, Piron A, et al. Tumour necrosis factor (TNF) gene polymorphism influences TNF-alpha production in lipopolysaccharide (LPS)-stimulated whole blood cell culture in healthy humans. Clin Exp Immunol 1998;113(3):401–6.

[96] Benjamin EJ, Dupuis J, Larson MG, et al. Genome-wide association with select biomarker traits in the Framingham Heart Study. BMC Med Genet 2007;8(Suppl. 1):S11.

[97] Urpi-Sarda M, Casas R, Chiva-Blanch G, et al. Virgin olive oil and nuts as key foods of the Mediterranean diet effects on inflammatory biomakers related to atherosclerosis. Pharmacol Res 2012;65(6):577–83.

[98] Pascual M, Nieto A, Mataran L, et al. IL-6 promoter polymorphisms in rheumatoid arthritis. Genes Immun 2000;1(5):338–40.

[99] Elahi MM, Asotra K, Matata BM, et al. Tumor necrosis factor alpha-308 gene locus promoter polymorphism: an analysis of association with health and disease. Biochim Biophys Acta 2009;1792(3):163–72.

[100] Hage FG, Szalai AJ. C-reactive protein gene polymorphisms, C-reactive protein blood levels, and cardiovascular disease risk. J Am Coll Cardiol 2007;50(12):1115–22.

[101] Wypasek E, Potaczek DP, Undas A. Association of the C-reactive protein gene (CRP) rs1205 C>T polymorphism with aortic valve calcification in patients with aortic stenosis. Int J Mol Sci 2015;16(10):23745–59.

[102] Elliott P, Chambers JC, Zhang W, et al. Genetic loci associated with C-reactive protein levels and risk of coronary heart disease. JAMA 2009;302(1):37–48.

[103] Eiriksdottir G, Smith AV, Aspelund T, et al. The interaction of adiposity with the CRP gene affects CRP levels: age, gene/ environment susceptibility – Reykjavik study. Int J Obes (Lond) 2009;33(2):267–72.

[104] Yamagishi K, Tanigawa T, Cui R, et al. High sodium intake strengthens the association of ACE I/D polymorphism with blood pressure in a community. Am J Hypertens 2007;20(7):751–7.

[105] Zhang L, Miyaki K, Araki J, et al. Interaction of angiotensin I-converting enzyme insertion-deletion polymorphism and daily salt intake influences hypertension in Japanese men. Hypertens Res 2006;29(10):751–8.

[106] Norat T, Bowman R, Luben R, et al. Blood pressure and interactions between the angiotensin polymorphism AGT M235T and sodium intake: a cross-sectional population study. Am J Clin Nutr 2008;88(2):392–7.

[107] Giner V, Poch E, Bragulat E, et al. Renin-angiotensin system genetic polymorphisms and salt sensitivity in essential hypertension. Hypertension 2000;35(1 Pt 2):512–17.

[108] Poch E, Gonzalez D, Giner V, et al. Molecular basis of salt sensitivity in human hypertension. Evaluation of renin-angiotensin-aldosterone system gene polymorphisms. Hypertension 2001;38(5):1204–9.

[109] Hunt SC, Cook NR, Oberman A, et al. Angiotensinogen genotype, sodium reduction, weight loss, and prevention of hypertension: trials of hypertension prevention, phase II. Hypertension 1998;32(3):393–401.

[110] Anderson RP. Coeliac disease is on the rise. Med J Aust 2011; 194(6):278–9.

[111] Anderson RP. Coeliac disease. Aust Fam Physician 2005;34(4): 239–42.

[112] Pietzak MM, Schofield TC, McGinniss MJ, et al. Stratifying risk for celiac disease in a large at-risk United States population by using HLA alleles. Clin Gastroenterol Hepatol 2009;7(9):966–71.

[113] Monsuur AJ, de Bakker PI, Zhernakova A, et al. Effective detection of human leukocyte antigen risk alleles in celiac disease using tag single nucleotide polymorphisms. PLoS ONE 2008;3(5):e2270.

[114] Koskinen L, Romanos J, Kaukinen K, et al. Cost-effective HLA typing with tagging SNPs predicts celiac disease risk haplotypes in the Finnish, Hungarian, and Italian populations. Immunogenetics 2009;61(4):247–56.

[115] Enattah NS, Sahi T, Savilahti E, et al. Identification of a variant associated with adult-type hypolactasia. Nat Genet 2002;30(2): 233–7.

[116] Yang A, Palmer AA, de Wit H. Genetics of caffeine consumption and responses to caffeine. Psychopharmacology (Berl) 2010;211(3): 245–57.

[117] Josse AR, Da Costa LA, Campos H, et al. Associations between polymorphisms in the AHR and CYP1A1-CYP1A2 gene regions and habitual caffeine consumption. Am J Clin Nutr 2012;96(3): 665–71.

[118] Pourvali K, Abbasi M, Mottaghi A. Role of superoxide dismutase 2 gene ala16val polymorphism and total antioxidant capacity in diabetes and its complications. Avicenna J Med Biotechnol 2016;8(2):48–56.

[119] Soerensen M, Christensen K, Stevnsner T, et al. The Mn-superoxide dismutase single nucleotide polymorphism rs4880 and the glutathione peroxidase 1 single nucleotide polymorphism rs1050450 are associated with aging and longevity in the oldest old. Mech Ageing Dev 2009;130(5):308–14.

[120] Goth L, Nagy T, Kosa Z, et al. Effects of rs769217 and rs1001179 polymorphisms of catalase gene on blood catalase, carbohydrate and lipid biomarkers in diabetes mellitus. Free Radic Res 2012; 46(10):1249–57.

[121] Wenten M, Gauderman WJ, Berhane K, et al. Functional variants in the catalase and myeloperoxidase genes, ambient air pollution, and respiratory-related school absences: an example of epistasis in gene–environment interactions. Am J Epidemiol 2009;170(12): 1494–501.

[122] Hustad S, Midttun O, Schneede J, et al. The methylenetetrahydrofolate reductase 677C→T polymorphism as a modulator of a B vitamin network with major effects on homocysteine metabolism. Am J Hum Genet 2007;80(5):846–55.

[123] Frosst P, Blom HJ, Milos R, et al. A candidate genetic risk factor for vascular disease: a common mutation in methylenetetrahydrofolate reductase. Nat Genet 1995;10(1):111–13.

[124] Kennedy BP, Bottiglieri T, Arning E, et al. Elevated S-adenosylhomocysteine in Alzheimer brain: influence on methyltransferases and cognitive function. J Neural Transm (Vienna) 2004;111(4):547–67.

[125] Weisberg I, Tran P, Christensen B, et al. A second genetic polymorphism in methylenetetrahydrofolate reductase (MTHFR) associated with decreased enzyme activity. Mol Genet Metab 1998;64(3):169–72.

[126] Fredriksen A, Meyer K, Ueland PM, et al. Large-scale population-based metabolic phenotyping of thirteen genetic polymorphisms related to one-carbon metabolism. Hum Mutat 2007;28(9):856–65.

[127] Lord RFK. Significance of low plasma homocysteine. Metametrix Clinical Laboratories; 2006. Available from: www.metametrix.com.

[128] Jhee KH, Kruger WD. The role of cystathionine beta-synthase in homocysteine metabolism. Antioxid Redox Signal 2005;7(5–6): 813–22.

[129] Banerjee R, Zou CG. Redox regulation and reaction mechanism of human cystathionine-beta-synthase: a PLP-dependent hemesensor protein. Arch Biochem Biophys 2005;433(1):144–56.

[130] Troen AM, Mitchell B, Sorensen B, et al. Unmetabolized folic acid in plasma is associated with reduced natural killer cell cytotoxicity among postmenopausal women. J Nutr 2006;136(1):189–94.

[131] Obeid R, Herrmann W. The emerging role of unmetabolized folic acid in human diseases: myth or reality? Curr Drug Metab 2012; 13(8):1184–95.

[132] Gomes AM, Winter S, Klein K, et al. Pharmacogenomics of human liver cytochrome P450 oxidoreductase: multifactorial analysis and impact on microsomal drug oxidation. Pharmacogenomics 2009;10(4):579–99.

[133] Hart SN, Wang S, Nakamoto K, et al. Genetic polymorphisms in cytochrome P450 oxidoreductase influence microsomal P450-catalyzed drug metabolism. Pharmacogenet Genomics 2008;18(1):11–24.

[134] Meilahn EN, De Stavola B, Allen DS, et al. Do urinary oestrogen metabolites predict breast cancer? Guernsey III cohort follow-up. Br J Cancer 1998;78(9):1250–5.

[135] Oliveira CB, Cardoso-Filho C, Bossi LS, et al. Association of CYP1A1 A4889G and T6235C polymorphisms with the risk of sporadic breast cancer in Brazilian women. Clinics (Sao Paulo) 2015;70(10):680–5.

[136] Feldman DN, Feldman JG, Greenblatt R, et al. CYP1A1 genotype modifies the impact of smoking on effectiveness of HAART among women. AIDS Educ Prev 2009;21(3 Suppl.):81–93.

[137] Mauras N, Santen RJ, Colon-Otero G, et al. Estrogens and their genotoxic metabolites are increased in obese prepubertal girls. J Clin Endocrinol Metab 2015;100(6):2322–8.

[138] Reddy EK, Mansfield CM, Hartman GV, et al. Carcinoma of the uterine cervix: review of experience at University of Kansas Medical Center. Cancer 1981;47(7):1916–19.

[139] Tang YM, Green BL, Chen GF, et al. Human CYP1B1 Leu432Val gene polymorphism: ethnic distribution in African-Americans, Caucasians and Chinese; oestradiol hydroxylase activity; and distribution in prostate cancer cases and controls. Pharmacogenetics 2000;10(9):761–6.

[140] Parl FF, Dawling S, Roodi N, et al. Estrogen metabolism and breast cancer: a risk model. Ann N Y Acad Sci 2009;1155:68–75.

[141] Norskov MS, Frikke-Schmidt R, Bojesen SE, et al. Copy number variation in glutathione-S-transferase T1 and M1 predicts incidence and 5-year survival from prostate and bladder cancer, and incidence of corpus uteri cancer in the general population. Pharmacogenomics J 2011;11(4):292–9.

[142] Brennan P, Hsu CC, Moullan N, et al. Effect of cruciferous vegetables on lung cancer in patients stratified by genetic status: a mendelian randomisation approach. Lancet 2005;366(9496):1558–60.

[143] Palli D, Masala G, Peluso M, et al. The effects of diet on DNA bulky adduct levels are strongly modified by GSTM1 genotype: a study on 634 subjects. Carcinogenesis 2004;25(4):577–84.

9

Mind–body medicine

Brad S Lichtenstein

INTRODUCTION

Western medicine has been steeped in a dichotomous split between mind and body for centuries. Traditional and indigenous healing methods do not suffer from this same bipolar relationship when either classifying illness or addressing methods of healing.[1–4] The conventional Western paradigm fails to integrate these two worlds, segregating conditions into either psychological or physiological constructs. At its very foundation, naturopathic medicine is an integrated, person-centred approach, whose practice is based on a codified system of theories and principles.[5,6] In relation to conventional biomedical care, naturopathic medicine embraces a holistic paradigm where body and mind are inseparable and a single provider treats all aspects of the person rather than distinct components. Mind–body medicine, a subdiscipline of behavioural medicine, is an approach to care that seeks to create and restore health, rather than eradicate disease, through the interplay of mind and its capacity to affect bodily function and symptoms. Thus, mind–body medicine aligns well with the principles of naturopathic medicine.

BIOMEDICINE

In his article, 'Role of behavioral medicine in primary care', Feldman defines behavioural medicine 'as an interdisciplinary field that aims to integrate the biological and psychosocial perspective on human behavior and apply them to the practice of medicine'.[7] He makes a point of using the word 'medicine' since it implies actively providing care, which includes the treatment of illness and disease, as well as prevention. The definition put forth by the Society of Behavioral Medicine (SBM), a not-for-profit organisation comprised of practitioners from a wide array of professions, does not differ significantly from that of Feldman. The SBM defines behavioural medicine as an 'interdisciplinary field concerned with the development and integration of behavioral, psychosocial, and biomedical science knowledge and techniques relevant to the understanding of health and illness, and the application of this knowledge and these techniques to prevention, diagnosis, treatment, and rehabilitation'.[8] These definitions also describe naturopathic medicine, as the core principles are the same.

The biomedical approach

The emergence of behavioural medicine in the 1970s was a reaction to the reductionist biomedical approach to disease. Throughout much of the 20th century, the prevailing healthcare paradigm was biomedical. According to the biomedical approach:

- The cause of disease is some force or entity outside the individual, such as a pathogen or trauma
- Responsibility for care falls upon another, such as a doctor, nurse or other practitioner, who administers a treatment to target the specific disease entity
- Health does not exist on a continuum but is stated in absolute terms – an individual is either healthy or ill
- The interaction between mind and body is irrelevant, since thoughts and emotions do not contribute to the individual's state of health.

The biopsychosocial model

In 1977, Engel[9,10] argued for a *biopsychosocial model* in healthcare, recognising that the biomedical approach works well for the treatment of acute pathology, yet fails to successfully treat the majority of chronic diseases, to which Engel believed lifestyle and behavioural factors directly contributed. These factors are not only psycho-emotional, such as how emotional states affect disease (e.g. the impact of anger and anxiety on cardiovascular disease), or the relationship of emotions to disease (e.g. the increased prevalence of depression in those with cancer). Additional factors are socioeconomic, political and cultural: issues such as equality, diversity, social justice and socioeconomic status are inseparable and intrinsic to behavioural medicine and the biopsychosocial paradigm. Complete healing cannot take place if these factors are ignored.

According to Kroenke and Mangelsdorff,[11] 80% of patients who present to primary care providers have no diagnosable organic aetiology, and only 10% present with psychological disorders without any physiological symptomology as cofactors. Gatchel and Oordt[12] estimated that up to 70% of medical visits to primary care providers are for problems related to psychosocial issues. Since primary care providers treat patients throughout their entire lifespan, they tend to see a wide array of conditions. While these may include specific psychological or psychiatric conditions (e.g. anxiety, depression, posttraumatic stress disorder [PTSD]), the majority of complaints – up to 85% in one estimate – are considered somatic with no organic aetiology by conventional medical standards. For these conditions (e.g. tension headaches, insomnia, chronic pain, irritable bowel syndrome [IBS]), medication is often unwarranted or unnecessary, although patients continue to seek treatment from biomedical primary care providers.

Integrated science model

Sahler and Carr[13] have presented an integrated science model for healthcare that identifies five domains covering all aspects of the biopsychosocial model. The patient is viewed as a complex system with all of these variables influencing their life and behaviours. Comprehensive care must include a full evaluation and assessment of each of these domains:

- Biological
- Environmental
- Cognitive
- Behavioural
- Sociocultural.

For some, this list remains incomplete. Depending on definition, emotional and spiritual domains are distinct from the others and warrant attention since they hold tremendous influence on health and wellness, as will be discussed later in this chapter.

The idea of viewing the patient in a comprehensive, multidimensional manner is far from revolutionary to the naturopathic doctor. The formal definition adopted by the house of delegates of the American Association of Naturopathic Physicians states that:[14]

> *Naturopathic medicine is a distinct system of primary health care – an art, science, philosophy and practice of diagnosis, treatment and prevention of illness. Naturopathic medicine is distinguished by the principles upon which its practice is based. These principles are continually reexamined in the light of scientific advances. The techniques of naturopathic medicine include modern and traditional, scientific and empirical methods. The following principles are the foundation of naturopathic medical practice:*
> - *The Healing Power of Nature (Vis Medicatrix Naturae): Naturopathic medicine recognizes an inherent self-healing process in the person which is ordered and intelligent. Naturopathic physicians act to identify and remove obstacles to healing and recovery, and to facilitate and augment this inherent self-healing process.*
> - *Identify and Treat the Causes (Tolle Causam): The naturopathic physician seeks to identify and remove the underlying causes of illness, rather than to merely eliminate or suppress symptoms.*
> - *First Do No Harm (Primum Non Nocere): Naturopathic physicians follow three guidelines to avoid harming the patient:*
>   - *Utilize methods and medicinal substances which minimize the risk of harmful side effects, using the least force necessary to diagnose and treat;*
>   - *Avoid when possible the harmful suppression of symptoms;*

> - *Acknowledge, respect, and work with the individual's self-healing process.*
> - *Doctor as Teacher (Docere): Naturopathic physicians educate their patients and encourage self-responsibility for health. They also recognize and employ the therapeutic potential of the doctor–patient relationship.*
> - *Treat the Whole Person (Tolle Totum): Naturopathic physicians treat each patient by taking into account individual physical, mental, emotional, genetic, environmental, social, and other factors. Since total health also includes spiritual health, naturopathic physicians encourage individuals to pursue their personal spiritual development.*
> - *Prevention (Preventare): Naturopathic physicians emphasize the prevention of disease – assessing risk factors, heredity, and susceptibility to disease and making appropriate interventions in partnership with their patients to prevent illness. Naturopathic medicine is committed to the creation of a healthy world in which humanity may thrive.*

We could argue, then, that behavioural medicine is an alternative expression of the principles and theory of naturopathic medicine developed for conventional mainstream medical culture. When naturopaths claim to treat the whole person (*Tolle Totum*) and address the cause or causes (*Tolle Causam*) of suffering, naturopathic medicine is a biopsychosocial model that examines the multifactorial determinants of health. When treatment is not hurried and is carefully considered, naturopathic medicine maintains the principle of First Do No Harm (*Primum Non Nocere*). Furthermore, a significant amount of behavioural medicine research has been conducted around the prevention of disease in conventional care (*Preventare*). Finally, the naturopathic model of healing states that illness occurs when a disturbance disrupts the vital force. While conventional biomedicine seeks to treat a pathogen or physical trauma as sole disturbance, an integrated naturopathic model attempts to examine all domains, including the biological, but also the environmental, cognitive, emotional, behavioural, socio-political and spiritual disturbances that impact on health and wellbeing.

MIND–BODY MEDICINE

Mind–body medicine, as a modality, falls under the heading of behavioural medicine. The National Institutes of Health (NIH) define mind–body therapies as 'interventions that use a variety of techniques designed to facilitate the mind's capacity to affect bodily function and symptoms'.[15] A broader and more inclusive definition from the National Center for Complementary and Alternative Medicine (NCCAM) defines mind–body medicine as any approach that enhances the 'interactions among the brain, mind, body and behavior, and on the powerful ways in which emotional, mental, social, spiritual, and behavioral factors can directly affect health'. The techniques and practices that fall into this category are any 'intervention strategies believed to promote health; [such as] relaxation, hypnosis, visual imagery, meditation, yoga, biofeedback, tai chi, qi gong, cognitive-behavioral therapies, group support, autogenic training, and spirituality'.[16] Some authors also include other practices such as automatic writing, humour, music, dance and exercise.

Regardless of the type of practice, several key factors are important:

- Mind–body medicine emphasises the individual's innate capacity for growth and healing
- Mind–body medicine focuses on quality of life, self-awareness, self-knowledge and self-empowerment
- Mind–body medicine views disease as a means of transformation rather than something to be cured and eradicated
- Mind–body medicine practitioners consider themselves to be trainers and catalysts, and see the individuals with whom they work as empowered partners, rather than sick or diseased patients.

An increasing number of patients are using both traditional healing practices (such as Ayurveda, yoga, qi gong, Sufi healing and shamanic, faith and psychic healing) and integrative practices (such as naturopathic medicine, traditional Chinese medicine and Western herbalism) concurrently with conventional medical approaches.[3] According to the 2015 US National Health Statistics Report[17] reviewing trends from 2002 to 2012, the use of mind–body approaches has increased over time:

- Yoga, tai chi and qi gong practice has increased linearly over time. Yoga was the most commonly used of these three at all time points
  - While all age groups showed increased use of yoga over the 10-year period, use decreased with age. The highest prevalence was in adults aged 18–44. No significant differences were observed in yoga use among adults aged 45–64 and those aged 65 and over between 2002 and 2007; however, an increase was seen between 2007 and 2012 for both age groups
  - Use of yoga among Hispanic and non-Hispanic black adults doubled between 2007 and 2012. Non-Hispanic white adults showed a consistent increase in yoga use across time. Use of yoga among non-Hispanic other adults increased by approximately 30% from 2002 to 2012
- Deep-breathing exercises were the second most commonly used mind–body medicine approach, used independently or as a part of other approaches
- Meditation was among the top five most commonly used approaches
- Biofeedback, guided imagery and hypnosis had consistently low prevalence and had no significant changes across time.

Mechanisms of action

Identifying specific mechanisms of action in regards to mind–body medicine is challenging. This can negatively influence consensus among disciplines.[18] A few considerations include outcome measures and techniques used (many and varied within the field). Despite these challenges, research continues. As the name implies, mind–body medicine has a bidirectional mechanism of action, involving both top-down (brain down to peripheral tissues) and bottom-up (peripheral tissues up to the brain) feedback loop systems. Telles and colleagues[19] state that mind–body medicine practices have numerous mechanisms of action at multiple levels with bidirectional feedback loops. Not only have mind–body medicine practices demonstrated efficacy in improving acute and chronic pain, anxiety, depression, posttraumatic stress, insomnia, hypertension and irritable bowel syndrome, but studies have also identified physiological changes due to these practices including decreased inflammatory response, improved immune parameters, enhanced glucose tolerance and increased cardiac-vagal tone and cardiovascular function. These changes support the concept of creating or maintaining psychophysiological balance. Pioneers in the field of mind–body medicine, such as Edmund Jacobson, developer of progressive muscle relaxation, and Johannes Heinrich Schultz, developer of autogenic training, emphasised relaxation versus treating particular pathology, despite the fact that both techniques have demonstrated improvement for a multitude of illnesses and symptoms.[20,21]

Stress, stressors and the stress response

The Oxford English Dictionary defines stress as 'hardship, adversity or affliction', yet the word 'stress' first appeared around the 14th century in Middle French from the word *destresse* ('distress'), which had its roots in the Latin word *strictus,* meaning 'to compress'. Initially, the word 'stress' involved a physical force, but by the 16th century it had entered the common vernacular connoting overwork or fatigue as a result of subjecting an entity to force or strain. Thus stress occurs whenever an individual feels a disruption in normal function, equilibrium or homeostasis. The agent of that change, that which causes the disruption, is referred to as the stressor, and can exist on all levels including environmental (e.g. excessive temperature, pollution, natural disasters), social (e.g. crowding, traffic, war), physiological (e.g. disease, broken bones, allergens) and psychological (e.g. guilt, shame, humiliation, worry, rumination).

In the naturopathic model of healing, the stressor is the stimulus that disturbs the vital force, which can be acute or short term, chronic or long term, or episodic, coming and going. This way of classifying stressors reflects the five domains of the integrated science model, and understanding the nature of each can inform treatment. The process that the mind and body undergo to restore balance after exposure to a stressor is considered the *stress response* and it too can be acute, chronic or episodic. The stress response is a constellation of events, which involve a stimulus (stressor – a force), that causes some sort of reaction in the brain that activates a physiological reaction in the body.

Homeostasis is the state of physical balance, thought of as an ideal set point reached through local regulatory mechanisms. Claude Bernard first used this term in the mid-19th century, believing that the body needs to maintain a constant state of internal balance, or the *le milieu interieur.* Body temperature, blood pH and oxygen concentrations are all examples of systems that operate and function in a very narrow band and must be kept very consistent. Not all physiological systems need to stay constant. *Allostasis* refers to constancy through change, where the ideal depends on the conditions and stability is maintained through change. This form of stability can be achieved through physiological or behavioural change, such as alterations in hormones and cytokines. In the short term, these changes can be adaptive, bringing about stability. Processes like respiration and heart rate require constancy through change in order to maintain overall health. Running to catch a bus that is pulling away from the bus stop is one example. Muscles contract, the heart pounds faster and breathing quickens and deepens. Once the bus is boarded and a seat is found, these systems settle down: they changed to match the physiological and metabolic demands of the moment. Heart rate, breathing rate and muscle tension should not stay constant, but adjust to demand.

Allostasis can go awry, as in chronic stress, where the mind and body perpetually respond without rest. The term 'allostatic load' was coined by McEwan and Stellar[22] to describe the damaging consequences of continual and chronic exposure to stress. Neural and neuroendocrine responses designed to keep the body balanced through change continually fluctuate, causing the systems to break down and function improperly. This wear and tear results from repeated and continued cycles of allostasis.

According to the cognitive appraisal theory of stress, the stressor itself does not induce the stress response, rather the individual's *perception* determines:
- The likelihood of a response
- The type of response
- The degree of response.

Individual assessment of an event, positive or negative, affects outcomes. Therefore, psychotherapy often views stress as a *response* rather than a *stimulus*. Much of mind–body medicine involves shifting perspective, reframing or reappraising expectations.

Not all stress is bad, and not all stressors induce a negative response. Stress is simply a force exerted on a system, such as gravity. In a weightless environment, muscles atrophy without the force of gravity to act on them. Such types of stress can be called *eustress*, or good stress, as opposed to *dys-stress*. Keller and colleagues[23] demonstrated that people who appraised their physical experiences as bad, negative or detrimental had poorer physical and mental health, with a 43% increased risk of dying prematurely. When participants interpreted any observed changes in their pulse or breathing rate as negative, such as indicating some physiological pathology, increased blood pressure was observed in these individuals. On the other hand, participants who appraised the same physiological changes more positively, such as indications of excitement or engagement, felt more alive and energised, had greater confidence and vitality and suffered from less anxiety and depression. Furthermore, the positive group maintained relaxed blood vessels despite an elevated heart rate.

Emotional resilience

Some people tend to be more inclined towards emotional resiliency than others. In her research, Kobassa[24] found that resilient individuals, including some survivors of cancer and other diseases, demonstrated hardiness, consisting of:
- Commitment
- Challenge
- Control.

Commitment involves appraising life more broadly than one singular domain, such as an individual thinking that they are more than their diagnosis or career. Commitment is the state of actively participating in life. The individual is committed to their health, and views themselves as an integral part of their own healthcare team. Rather than blindly following every suggestion made by their provider, those with commitment remain active and engaged with a sense of agency and purpose. Furthermore, they continue to participate in all aspects of their life and engage in meaningful relationships and activities like family, spiritual and religious groups, exercise and hobbies.

Regarding the *control* parameter, the individual realises that while they may not be able to control the events around them, such as whether or not they get a particular disease, they can control their appraisal of the events and can choose to adapt to the situation at hand. Those able to do this have more emotional resiliency.

The *challenge* parameter involves appraisal of the actual event or issue itself. Those with this characteristic frame all information received, from diagnosis to prognosis, as a challenge with which to work and an opportunity for growth rather than a threat. People who exhibit the challenge parameter do not spend much time asking, *Why me?* but ask rather *What now?*

Mind–body medicine approaches focus on strengthening resiliency, and hence hardiness, through reappraising stressors as challenges and helping patients find inner strength.

Stress response

Once a stressor has been perceived and appraised negatively, the stress response begins. All perceptions of stress involve safety in one way or another. When a threat to our safety is perceived, whether immediate and physical, such as a car speeding through a red light, or more existential, such as a mortgage payment due, the nervous system, and particularly the amygdala of the limbic system, activates. One of the main functions of the amygdala is to assess for safety. Whenever a situation is deemed unsafe, the amygdala stimulates the nervous system.

Walter Cannon, a medical doctor and physiologist, coined the phrase the 'fight or flight response' in 1915 after he conducted experiments on laboratory animals by exposing them to extremes in temperature or lack of food and water. His subjects activated the same physiological responses as if fleeing or fighting a predator. Cannon believed this to be an evolutionarily adaptive survival mechanism. He was one of the first doctors to recognise that mental–emotional stressors in humans can incite the same mechanisms and to urge doctors to discuss psychological wellbeing with their patients as well. Considering the prevailing biomedical paradigm of the times, this was revolutionary.

Hans Selye elaborated on Cannon's model almost by accident. A young endocrinologist at McGill University in the 1930s, Selye was studying the effects of ovarian extract in rats. On autopsy at the end of the study, Selye found that his rats had peptic and duodenal ulcers, enlarged adrenal glands and atrophied thymus and other lymphatic tissues. At first he was excited, believing that he had found a new hormone; however, his enthusiasm quickly waned when he realised that his control subjects, rats injected with pure saline alone, experienced the same physiological changes. Selye went on to repeat the experiment with other injections, such as formalin, and other types of stressors, such as exposure to different temperatures, exercise, pain, etc. No matter what the stressor, Selye observed similar physiological findings, leading him to outline his general adaptation syndrome of stress. The reactions listed are not solely physiological, but cover all domains of behavioural health.

The phases of his general adaptation syndrome are as follows:

1   *Alarm phase:* similar to Cannon's fight or flight response, this occurs on first exposure to the stressor and disruption of homeostasis.
2   *Resistance phase:* the body begins to adapt to continued exposure to stress. The body returns to the prior state of arousal only as long as the necessary material for energy expenditure is available.
3   *Exhaustion and burnout phase:* energy stores have been completely depleted and the body is no longer able to mount a resistance. Permanent damage and illness or death result. A great example of this is salmon: after their evolutionary drive to swim upstream and spawn, salmon die of exhaustion and burnout.

Two adaptive response systems are engaged during the general adaptation syndrome: the sympathetic adrenal medullary (SAM) axis and the hypothalamic pituitary adrenal (HPA) axis. Activation of the SAM axis is swift, occurring within seconds of a perceived threat, stimulating the locus coeruleus, located in the pons of the brainstem, to signal the preganglionic nerve fibres of the spinal cord to release acetylcholine, causing the adrenal medulla to secrete noradrenaline and adrenaline directly into the bloodstream through postganglionic nerve fibres. These catecholamines stimulate the liver to convert glycogen to glucose to release into the bloodstream for fuel, to allow for an increase in metabolic activity, heart rate, respiration, blood pressure, blood flow to the muscles, pupil size and platelet aggregation. Simultaneously, less vital systems, including urinary output and digestive function, decrease.

The HPA axis is often considered the long-term system. Most modern stressors are not short in duration. In long-term situations, the HPA axis kicks in several minutes later and is longer acting. When a threat is detected, the hypothalamus releases corticotropin-releasing hormone (CRH) within 15 seconds, which then signals the anterior pituitary to release adrenocorticotropic hormone (ACTH).

ACTH stimulates the adrenal cortex to release mineralocorticoids and glucocorticoids. Mineralocorticoids directly impact the kidneys by causing the retention of sodium and water, thus increasing blood pressure and volume. Glucocorticoids enable fats and proteins to be converted to glucose for immediate energy, thereby increasing blood glucose, energy levels and pain threshold. Immunologically, glucocorticoids induce a shift from Th1-directed (cell mediated) immunity to Th2-directed (antibody) immunity. This decreases a host of cytokines involved in immunity, such as IL-1, IL-2, TNF-α and IFN gamma and alpha, while increasing the pro-inflammatory cytokines, such as IL-4, IL-10, IL-13 and cAMP. As a result, NK cell cytotoxicity decreases and CD4:CD8 ratios fall, limiting the ability to fight microbes.

In the acute phase, both the SAM and the HPA axes are activated. As a stressor continues, the resistance phase begins and SAM activity declines as the HPA axis takes over. Should the stressor resolve, the entire system returns to homeostasis. However, often this is not the case. Dickerson and Kemeny[25] note that the types of stressors that lead to the greatest release of glucocorticoids and ACTH are those that are uncontrollable or performance tasks that involve evaluation by others. Most individuals reporting chronic ongoing stress seem to have a stressor in these categories, which only maintains the cycle. If the stress continues for too long, exhaustion occurs and SAM activity re-emerges. At this point, organ and tissue damage ensue until inevitable collapse.

Polyvagal theory and the vagus nerve

While these models have been used to describe stress for quite some time, Stephen Porges[26–30] has outlined a phylogenetically ordered, adaptive neuroregulation of the autonomic nervous system, expanding on the work of Cannon and Selye. Porges suggests that the nervous system is ordered along a continuum from threat to safety, initiating distinct involuntary subsystems that are linked to behaviour. According to Porges' polyvagal theory, during periods of perceived threat the first subsystem activated for all mammals is the ancient and oldest branch of the vagus nerve (the 10th cranial nerve), which is unmyelinated and arises from the dorsal motor nucleus. Activation of this subsystem results in immobilisation of the entire mind/body, with commonly expressed behaviours of vasovagal syncope, feigning death, dissociation, withdrawal and shutdown. This strategy can be life-sustaining if predators deem such immobilisation as death and therefore an unappetising meal. The second subsystem, activation of the sympathetic nervous system, is the traditional fight-or-flight reaction with the strategy of mobilisation to escape danger. The third subsystem is engaged only in times of perceived safety. Here, the newer and myelinated branch of the ventral vagal complex, only seen in mammals, arises from the nucleus ambiguus. Activation of this vagal system leads to social engagement, with such overt behavioural changes as slower and deeper breathing, softening of the facial muscles, and increased intonation and prosody of the voice.

TABLE 9.1 Phylogenetic stages of Porges' polyvagal theory

Phase	ANS component	Lower motor neuron	Neurobiological adaptive function
1st	Unmyelinated vagus (dorsal vagal complex)	Dorsal motor nucleus of the vagus	Immobilisation (feigning death, fainting, passive avoidance)
2nd	Sympathetic adrenal system	Spinal cord	Mobilisation (fight-or-flight, active avoidance)
3rd	Myelinated vagus (ventral vagal complex)	Nucleus ambiguus	Social engagement, social communication, self-soothing and calming, inhibiting arousal

Source: Modified from Porges, SW. The polyvagal perspective. Biological Psychology 2007;74:120.

The first and third subsystems (immobilisation and social engagement) are innervated by the parasympathetic nervous system. Thus the belief that all stress responses result from sympathetic activation is unsubstantiated. The vagal nerve is bidirectional, providing enervation to organs and viscera, as well as afferent communication about the state of such tissues back to the brain. Approximately 80% of all vagal fibres are sensory, and only 15% of the total motor fibres (20%) are myelinated.

When activated in times of safety rather than threat, the dorsal motor vagus functions in growth and regeneration by regulating the activity of sub-diaphragmatic organs. In contrast, the ventral vagus regulates supra-diaphragmatic organs such as the heart and lungs. The newer subsystem has an inhibitory impact on the first and second subsystems. Thus social engagement and communication in a safe environment can 'turn off' the immobilisation and mobilisation systems by slowing down the heart and breathing rate. The ventral vagal complex comprises neurophysiologically connected nerves that innervate muscles of the head and neck necessary for social engagement, namely larynx and facial muscles, allowing the individual to regulate the tone, pitch and prosody of the voice and demonstrate facial expressions that signal listening, caring and attentiveness. Thus activating the social engagement system can dampen the SAM and HPA axes, alter the immunological response and create a sense of calm, peace and relaxation.[30]

Table 9.1 outlines the phylogenetic stages of the polyvagal theory as outline by Porges.

Trauma research grounded in the polyvagal theory posits that individuals can become neurobiologically conditioned for a predominance in one subsystem over another. Perpetual activation of either the immobilisation or the mobilisation subsystem will have psychological and physiological consequences downstream. Regardless of theory, perpetual activation of the stress response has been associated with a wide array of symptoms and diseases including cardiovascular disease, recurrent colds and flu, poor wound healing and tissue destruction, weight gain, insomnia, chronic fatigue and disruption of memory. On the other hand, use of mind–body medicine techniques has been correlated with improvement of the immune system, as well as a 43% reduction in healthcare use.[31] The approach of mind–body medicine is not eradication of any particular disease, but cultivation of resilience, balance and social engagement. Researchers resist the claim that stress is a causative factor for any particular disease, yet understanding the proposed stress response systems outlined above, chronic immobilisation or mobilisation fails to improve health. Rather than validate any particular mind–body technique for treatment of a specific disease, shifting the neurobiological adaptive response towards social engagement and ventral vagal activation may be the more appropriate approach.

Self-stressing theory

Determining which of the numerous mind–body approaches to use can be confusing. Researchers and clinicians typically focus on one particular method, failing to address variations in individual stress response patterns. To address this issue, Smith[32,33] has proposed a self-stress theory, recognising that individuals maintain and perpetuate heightened nervous system arousal by responding to stressors in one of six particular psychological or physiological patterns (outlined below). Interestingly, each pattern corresponds to a family or group of mind–body techniques. To obtain optimal results, providers and patients need to select the strategy that matches the self-stress target. However, Smith does not imply that only one mind–body approach be reserved for a particular target. Rather, the patterns should be considered as a guide to navigate the field of mind–body practices.

When their safety is called into question, people respond in one of the following six ways:

- *Stressed posture and position:* the individual reacts to stressors by adopting a physical posture to create a sense of safety. For instance, the person could collapse and curl up, or stand more erect and thrust the chest forwards. If a stress posture becomes habituated and maintained over time, the person's health declines due to restriction and lack of movement. Blood flow decreases and muscle tension increases, leading to exhaustion and fatigue
- *Stressed skeletal muscles:* various emotions are associated with overt muscular patterns.[34] Muscle tension and bracing is often seen in anxiety disorder, for instance. An individual who responds to stress by contracting skeletal muscles is chronically ready to fight or flee. This pattern is commonly demonstrated by those with a chronic mobilisation subsystem
- *Stressed breathing:* activation of immobilisation and mobilisation subsystems alters breathing, leading to erratic, uneven, shallow breathing, potentially punctuated with sighs, breath holding, gasps and

yawns. Breathing volume may grow deeper. All of these changes alters blood pH mediated by CO_2 and O_2 levels, and hence lead to a variety of health complications

- *Stressed body focus:* the individual experiences an intensification of somatic complaints, such as rapid heart rate, increased breathing or digestive discomfort, simply by directing their attention to the symptoms. Consider an individual in the midst of a panic attack who is focusing on their breathing: they begin to hyperventilate, worrying that they are not getting enough oxygen. Not only is this untrue, but an intense focus on the symptom aggravates their condition and perpetuates the over-breathing, creating more anxiety
- *Stressed emotion:* in order to manage stress, the individual compensates by engaging in scenarios or self-talk that intensify and perpetuate the already distressing effect
- *Stressed attention:* this strategy is exemplified by a ruminating mind, intent on solving the problem of safety. Thoughts and cognitions end up shifting away from the experience of the present moment towards multi-tasking.

Individuals may demonstrate more than one of these strategies when confronted with triggers and a threat to safety, but identifying the predominant pattern can aid in selecting the most beneficial corresponding mind–body intervention. Table 9.2 lists the mind–body practices associated with each stress response pattern. These practices include the following:

- *Stretching exercises:* any mind–body approach that incorporates stretching of the muscles with postural awareness would fit into this category. This includes the movement and postural portion of yoga as well as approaches that increase awareness of posture and position such as Pilates, the Feldenkrais method, the Alexander technique and somatics
- *Progressive muscle relaxation:* in order to release chronically constricted skeletal muscles, the individual must be aware of the tension. Progressive muscle relaxation involves systematically tensing then releasing specific muscles groups in order to bring about a state of relaxation
- *Breathing exercises:* any modality that involves awareness and alteration of the breath would be classified as breathing exercises – such as any yoga technique that focuses on the breath, as well as spiritual practices and religious practices that involve chanting or recitation of prayers which impact the breathing rate
- *Autogenic training:* developed by Johannes Schultz in the 1920s, this involves silent and self-generated repetition of specific phrases about particular physical sensations, such as heaviness and warmth. Directing attention to a particular body part, the individual repeats to themselves, for example, 'My arm is heavy'. This shifts attention away from worrying about distressing physical sensations and induces a state of calm and relaxation
- *Imagery, self-talk:* rather than rehearsing negative affect-arousing narratives, this approach employs positive imagery and affirmations. It includes mind–body therapies such as hypnosis and some spiritual or religious practices such as loving kindness or compassion meditation
- *Meditation and mindfulness:* mindfulness can be defined as attention to the present moment without judgment. It involves focusing the mind away from distraction or rumination, such as the physical postures in yoga when attention is completely directed to the experience of the physical sensation within the pose
- Smith distinguishes three types of relaxation methods: self-relaxation, assisted relaxation and casual relaxation
  - In self-relaxation, the individual doesn't rely on anything or anyone in order to engage in the process. Listening to a recorded guided meditation may be considered self-relaxation if afterwards the individual can recall the instructions and practise on their own
  - Assisted-relaxation techniques require someone or something in the process, such as computer screens and hardware, massage practitioners, music or animals for 'pet therapy'
  - Casual relaxation comprises those daily activities that induce a relaxation response without that being the intention, such as reading, exercising, listening to music (when not used therapeutically) and stroking a pet.

Placebo

While an in-depth review is beyond the scope of this book, any discussion of mind–body medicine demands, at the very least, a brief mention of placebo, since a few critics of mind–body medicine have claimed that the benefits seen are no more than a placebo response. Any treatment – whether substance, procedure or device – that is deemed pharmacologically and physiologically inert and incapable of producing a physiological change is considered a placebo. Placebo effects are responses that ensue from administration of the placebo.

However, as Finniss and colleagues explain,[35] these definitions are problematic for clinicians and researchers based on their inherent contradiction. Despite reports of positive outcomes, how can placebos produce a physiological effect if they are inert? Finniss and

TABLE 9.2 Self-stressing theory	
Stress response pattern	**Associated mind–body practice**
Stressed posture and position	Stretching exercises, yoga, Pilates and movement
Stressed skeletal muscles	Progressive muscle relaxation
Stressed breathing	Breathing exercises
Stressed body focus	Autogenic training
Stressed emotion	Guided imagery/visualisation/ self-talk, hypnotherapy
Stressed attention	Meditation and mindfulness

TABLE 9.3 External biopsychosocial contexts and the placebo effect	
External context	**Example**
Location	Emergency room Community clinic Doctor's office
Treatment type	Pharmacological – oral, IV, injection, surgical Physical involving touch Verbal – talk therapy Device administered
Treatment duration/ frequency	Single incident Single or multiple daily treatment
Verbal	'This will make you feel better quickly' 'You'll feel a quick jab but then it will be brief' 'This will take the pain away'
Social	Communication style and empathy Eye contact Body language Prosody and intonation of voice White coat, gloves, stethoscope

Source: Adapted from Wager TD, Atlas LY. The neuroscience of placebo effects: connecting context, learning and health. Nat Rev Neurosci 2015;16:403–18.

TABLE 9.4 Internal biopsychosocial contexts and the placebo effect	
Internal context	**Example**
Expectations (of future responses)	'Pain will go away' 'Medication will help' 'My doctor cares'
Past experience	Relief of symptoms following treatment Improved performance after treatment
Memory	Past witnessing of another person responding positively to a treatment
Meaning	'My doctor cares about me' 'I am safe now'
Emotions	'This feels calming' 'I am less anxious'

Source: Adapted from Wager TD, Atlas LY. The neuroscience of placebo effects: connecting context, learning and health. Nat Rev Neurosci 2015;16:403–18.

colleagues suggest shifting the focus away from the placebo itself, instead emphasising the mechanisms through which observed responses occur. Taking a biopsychosocial perspective to treatment, or the patient–practitioner relationship, the placebo responses can then be attributed to the 'context' of the therapeutic delivery.[35,36] Just as orienting strategy (immobilisation, mobilisation, social engagement) results in activation of various neurological subsystems, researchers have begun outlining the neurological and neurochemical mediators induced by placebo effects, which are witnessed in all therapeutic encounters whether the specific therapeutics are active or inert. External and internal biopsychosocial cues are perceived and interpreted by the patient, which colour the treatment context and induce brain–mind responses and neurochemical changes. Tables 9.3 and 9.4 provide examples of several external and internal biopsychosocial contexts that surround the treatment encounter, potentially generating placebo effects.

Based on what has been presented thus far about orientation strategy and the goal of the naturopathic doctor steeped in mind–body medicine, rather than speaking of placebo effects, the changes witnessed – both the subjective report of the patient, and neurological and neurohormonal mediators – are merely results of shifting orientation towards safety. Only when patients feel safe can they begin to assign new meaning to their symptoms, healthcare providers, treatment regimen and the world. Once they are able to socially engage with their care, neurological changes take place that decrease stress hormones, shift the neuro-endocrine-immune systems and impact health.

MIND–BODY THERAPEUTICS

The following discussion introduces various mind–body medicine therapeutics in more detail. Using Smith's categorisation as a frame of reference, the techniques are discussed in reverse order, starting with meditation and mindfulness, as they are the basis of all other modalities.

Meditation and mindfulness

MEDITATION

Throughout the literature, consensual agreement about the definition of meditation is difficult to find and this speaks to the issues regarding evaluation of meditation-based therapies. Smith recognises that several therapies overlap in implementation. Most researchers agree that the process of meditation involves some level of mental focus and concentration. The word 'meditation' itself is derived from the Latin, *meditari*, meaning 'to participate in contemplation or deliberation'. Shapiro and colleagues[37] describe meditation as a family of self-regulation practices that aim to bring mental processes under voluntary control through focusing attention, resulting in psychological and spiritual wellbeing and maturity. While historically used for spiritual and religious pursuits, meditation may or may not have any connection with religious contemplation or introspection.

Cardoso and colleagues[38] have outlined the distinct components found in the multitude of meditation practices reviewed – any mind–body approach incorporating these components can therefore be considered meditation:

- The techniques are specific and clearly defined
- Physical (and muscular) relaxation occurs at some point during the process
- Cognitive (mental or logical) relaxation occurs during the process, which involves releasing expectations for a

particular outcome, along with analytical and judgmental thought
- The process is a self-induced state and can be practised without requiring any support (this supports Smith's self-relaxation category)
- 'Self-focus skill' describes the direction and focus of attention; it is also known as the anchor.

Broadly speaking, meditation is an intentional self-regulatory process of directing and focusing one's attention for the purpose of self-inquiry. Depending on the form of meditation, the object of focus, also known as the anchor, may vary. The anchor is used to direct attention away from unwanted cognitive processes, such as rumination, judgment, analysis, sleepiness, lethargy and boredom. Meditation practices can be categorised into two groups based on their anchor:[39]

- Concentration meditation practices use a single point of focus to give the mind an object on which to grasp in an attempt to still the mind. The use of a word or phrase, or mantra, is at the root of transcendental meditation created by Maharishi Mahesh Yogi. Through silent repetition, one directs the mind back to the anchor to prevent its wandering
- Mindfulness is a broader approach that is reviewed more fully below. Briefly, during mindfulness, the entire spectrum of experiences that arise moment to moment, thoughts, sensations and emotions, are observed and noted without judgment or reactivity.

Whenever distractions arise, the distraction is acknowledged before attention is redirected back to the anchor. Although not universal, breathing work is a common factor in several forms of meditation. Sustaining focus on a specific object of attention has been described as executive attention or conflict monitoring, and several studies have reported that meditating for even short periods of time can improve scores on attention regulation measurements.[40]

Many people struggle with meditation, believing that their mind should be blank without thoughts, yet this is not necessarily the goal. Through daily practice, meditation trains the mind to develop a capacity for attention and focus. Emphasising the neurological changes of meditation practice, Ott and colleagues note: '[f]rom a scientific perspective, the effects of these traditional exercises are based on the plasticity of the brain. Sustained efforts to focus attention and to cultivate emotional balance leave traces in the underlying neural substrate and circuitry. Over time, these changes in brain structure in turn support the intended changes in mental faculties and personality'.[41] However, the goal is not a calm and relaxed state of being, but remaining present to momentary experiences without the need to dissociate or distract away from them.

Hussain and Bhushan[39] highlight their review of 813 meditation studies by the University of Alberta Evidence-Based Practice Center, which categorises meditation practices into five groups (again we see overlap based on self-stressing theory):
- *Mantra meditation* (comprising transcendental meditation (TM), relaxation response and clinically standardised meditation)

- *Mindfulness meditation* (comprising Vipassana, Zen Buddhist meditation, mindfulness based on stress reduction and mindfulness-based cognitive therapy)
- *Yoga* (based on Indian Yogic tradition developed by Patanjali, incorporating a variety of techniques like body postures, breath control and meditation)
- *Tai chi* (based on Chinese martial arts that incorporate various slow rhythmic movements to emphasise force and complete relaxation)
- *Qi gong* (based on Chinese practice that combines breathing patterns with various physical postures, bodily movements and meditation).

MINDFULNESS

As a mind–body medicine approach, mindfulness is considered the technique best suited for those with stressed attention. The term 'mindful' can be found in the English language as early as the 14th century and denoted attention, being cautious, careful and paying heed. In the 16th century, the word 'mindfulness' became synonymous with 'attention', 'awareness' and 'memory'. The first use of the English word 'mindfulness' can be attributed to the British civil servant, Thomas William Rhys Davids (1843–1922), who translated original Buddhist Pali texts into English. Struggling to encapsulate the essence of the Buddhist term *sati*, Davids initially used words such as 'recollect' and 'remember', and this perpetual remembering focused on the present moment. Slowly the term 'mindfulness' became synonymous with this process.[42] Modern definitions elaborate on this process of remembering. Bishop and colleagues[43] define mindfulness as 'non-elaborative, non-judgmental, present-centered awareness in which each thought, feeling, or sensation that arises in the attentional field is acknowledged and accepted as it is'. Kabat-Zinn,[44] creator of Mindfulness-Based Stress Reduction, describes mindfulness as the 'awareness that emerges through paying attention on purpose, in the present moment, and non-judgmentally to the unfolding of experience moment by moment'.

Mindfulness can be conceptualised as a state rather than a trait,[45] which requires continual practice to train cognitive capacity for sustained focus and concentration. The anchor is the experience of the arising present moment, which can focus on internal or external objects. Originating from within, internal objects of focus pertain to bodily sensations (heat, cold, vibration, pain, pressure) or cognitions (this is boring, my body aches, how long do I have to sit here?). External objects are experienced as arising from outside the person (visual objects, scents, sounds). For either type of object, should the focus drift from the anchor, the individual gently remembers to turn their attention back to the experience of the phenomenon or the arising present moment sensations and thoughts.

Two concepts are fundamental to the practice of mindfulness: non-elaboration and non-judgment. Whenever thoughts arise that describe, evaluate or analyse the experienced phenomenon, elaboration and judgment occur. This may take the form of thoughts about sensations or thoughts about thoughts. Rather than becoming stuck in cycles of ceaseless ruminations, mindfulness practice reminds us to return our attention to the present experience. Distress and suffering increase when the ruminations involve cognitive appraisal of the currently arising phenomenon. When mind and body, thoughts and sensations are deemed 'good' or 'bad', stress response subsystems activate, since these experiences are perceived through the lens of safety. Cravings, desires, aversions and rejections all arise, and subsequently attempts are made to avoid or distract from the potential threat of the undesired experience. Mindfulness offers freedom from suffering through the practice of sustaining attention on unpleasant or painful sensations and cognitions without judgment or elaboration, thereby reducing emotional reactivity, building tolerance and cultivating a new way of orienting our experiences.

Regardless of the desire or aversion for the phenomenon, in order to approach a mindful state, the individual must orient to every phenomenon with openness, curiosity and acceptance.[43] The Five Facet Mindfulness Questionnaire was developed by Baer and colleagues[46] to identify mindfulness behaviours. These include:

- Observing (sustaining attention on the internal or external anchor or phenomenon)
- Describing (providing a cognitive label of the anchor)
- Acting with awareness (remaining present to the momentary experience without acting habitually without awareness)
- Non-judging of inner experience (suspending judgment of experienced phenomenon)
- Non-reactivity to inner experience (suspending elaboration of the experienced phenomenon to refrain from emotionally reacting to the experience).

The definition of mindfulness poses an interesting conundrum for researchers. Since mindfulness is about process not outcome, studying mindfulness as a treatment of particular conditions appears incongruous. Simply put, mindfulness *is* the goal of mindfulness. Clinging to any desired outcome is antithetical to its basic tenets. However, the association between mindlessness and health has been reported. Chronic rumination and perseveration have been associated with poorer overall outcomes, such as elevated heart rate, decreased heart rate volume (HRV), increased risk of cardiovascular disease and poor sleep.[47] Conversely, mindfulness training has been reported to improve health parameters. Davidson and colleagues[48] noted how 25 healthy subjects showed increased antibody production in response to flu vaccination after 8 weeks of training, while Carlson and colleagues[49] found a decrease in cortisol levels and systolic blood pressure in participants with breast and prostate cancer after training, with a continual reduction in Th1 (pro-inflammatory) cytokines one-year post follow-up. Women recently diagnosed with breast cancer who participated in an 8-week mindfulness-based stress reduction (MBSR) intervention demonstrated reduced levels of stress hormones, better immune system biomarkers, improved coping skills and better quality of life.[50] Paul and colleagues[51] found a reduction in susceptibility to depression and other psychological states from a decrease in rumination through mindfulness training.

Numerous studies have examined the connection between mindfulness and meditation and changes in morphological and neurological brain structure. As Fox and colleagues[52] point out in their meta-analysis and review of 21 neuroimaging studies, determining a causative relationship between meditation and alterations in brain structure remains suspect. However, after reviewing these studies with more than 300 meditation practitioners, they found approximately 123 morphological brain differences. Of most interest are studies comparing meditation-naïve and meditation-experienced practitioners, where significant changes in morphology were seen. This begs the question: were such changes pre-existing, predisposing practitioners to meditation? Or were these changes enhanced by practice? Though unanswered, most surprising was the evidence that minimal time was required practising meditation before structural changes were observed. Fox identified the most consistently altered areas of the brain as follows:

- Left rostrolateral prefrontal cortex (involved in introspection and metacognition, abstract information processing and integration of cognitive process as relates to higher order behavioural goals)
- Anterior/midcingulate cortex (crucial for executive attention, self-control and emotional regulation, focused-problem solving, orienting, alerting and diminished attentional blink effect)
- Primary and secondary somatosensory cortices (involved with tactile information processing, pressure, temperature, pain, proprioception)
- Anterior insula (involved in enhanced body awareness)
- Orbitofrontal cortex (involved in discerning relationship between stimuli and motivational outcome; connected to primary sensory areas, as well as limbic structures such as amygdala, striatum and hypothalamus)
- Left inferior temporal gyrus (involved in high-level visual processing, potentially related to visual imagery arising during meditation versus visual perception)
- Hippocampus (involved in memory processing and emotional learning, associated with appropriateness of expression of stress response).

Brewer[53] found reduced activation in the default mode network, an area of the brain that includes the posterior cingulate cortex, the precuneus and temporoparietal junction, and the angular gyrus. This decreased functional connectivity may potentially explain how experienced meditators demonstrate less rumination and an increased ability to focus on a single anchor. Hölzel[40] found a decrease in right basolateral amygdala grey matter density in participants after an 8-week mindfulness training program, and correlated this with decreased perceived stress. Zeidan and colleagues[54] found reduction in pain correlating to pain-related activation of the contralateral primary somatosensory cortex in those trained in mindfulness for only 4 days.

What can be concluded from all of this? Meditation and mindfulness are orientation strategies that affect the stress response, which in turn impacts the neurological, immunological and endocrine systems. Mindfulness can reduce rumination and negative thinking, which is linked to improved overall health. Even within a short period of time, structural changes can be seen on fMRI in individuals trained in meditation and mindfulness.

Spirituality, religion and prayer

If the word 'meditation' has its roots in contemplation, it stands to reason that spirituality – a contemplation on the sacred and the transcendent – fits under the heading of mind–body medicine. As mentioned earlier, mind–body, behavioural and naturopathic medicine emphasise integration of all parts of the individual, but trends in conventional care are also moving in this direction. The Joint Commission on Accreditation of Healthcare Organizations (JCAHO)[55] has stated that 'patients deserve care, treatment, and services that safeguard their personal dignity and respect their cultural, psychosocial, and spiritual values. These values often influence the patient's perceptions and needs. By understanding and respecting these values, providers can meet care, treatment, and service needs and preferences.'

Spirituality is commonly defined as a subjective human experience of the sacred in life connected with a search for understanding and meaning.[56–58] Elkins and colleagues[59] describe spirituality as a multidimensional way of experiencing and being in the world that arises from an awareness of a transcendent dimension. Spirituality is characterised by certain specific values about life (self, others, world, nature and the sense of ultimate) and consists of nine major components. According to Elkins and colleagues, all people with a sense of spirituality share these common components, despite individual variations in each component:

1 *Transcendent dimension:* the acceptance in and belief of a transcendent dimension consisting of something beyond the self and what is seen.
2 *Meaning and purpose in life:* an authentic belief that all life and personal existence has significance, importance, meaning and purpose.
3 *Mission in life:* the recognition that in order to fulfil our purpose, we must pursue our particular life 'vocation'.
4 *Sacredness of life:* a sense that all life, not just certain events or aspects, are 'holy' and worthy of awe, wonder and reverence; the ability to separate mundane and sacred, as all life is valued and appreciated.
5 *Material value:* the understanding that money and material possessions are useful tools for daily living, yet are unable to provide a life of meaning and purpose.
6 *Altruism:* the recognition of interconnectedness of all life and all people, with a deeply held belief that as one person suffers, all people suffer, leading to a sense of social justice.
7 *Idealism:* holding high values and ideals for the betterment of the world and each person, including oneself.
8 *Awareness of the tragic:* the insight and acknowledgment that joy, value and meaning are all inextricably linked to pain, loss and suffering.
9 *Fruits of spirituality:* the experience that engaging in spirituality enriches and benefits life in the present moment through improved relationships with the self, others, nature, life and the world.

Based on these components, an individual can be spiritual and live a spiritual existence, yet fail to follow any particular religious tradition. Religion attempts to answer spiritual questions about existence, providing value and purpose through an organised and systematic set of beliefs, teachings and practices. Religion requires a group, collective or community that share a common framework. By providing structure for enquiry, spiritual needs may be met. For the remainder of this chapter, the term 'spirituality' is used to discuss both concepts in mind–body medicine.

The association between spirituality and health is quite strong. First, spiritual beliefs influence how an individual experiences their state of health, since concepts like illness and disease are inseparable from worldview. Any holistic, person-centred paradigm recognises that how a patient responds to a diagnosis is contingent on their appraisal of the diagnosis, which can activate various subsystems of the stress response. If the individual embraces a spiritual orientation, feels a connection with the transcendent, has a sense that all life is sacred, yet recognises and appreciates the tragic events, they may be more inclined to perceive a terminal diagnosis as a step in their path towards connection with the Divine. Without any spiritual belief, a patient may feel adrift and alone, perceiving any ailment as unjustified victimisation.

Second, since spiritual beliefs affect appraisal, they impact medical choices. In interviews with 21 doctors about the relationship between spirituality and health, all practitioners agreed that spiritual beliefs influenced a patient's understanding and meaning of illness.[60] When spirituality supported coping skills, doctors deemed it as a positive association. However, when spiritual beliefs contradicted or conflicted with medical recommendations and advice, doctors considered spirituality as harmful.

Third, mounting evidence shows a positive relationship between spirituality and health outcomes. Regarding the connection between mental health and spirituality, Koenig[61] reports that prior to the year 2000, more than 700 studies examined this relationship, and 'nearly 500 of those studies demonstrated a significant positive association with better mental health, greater well-being, or lower substance abuse'. Furthermore, other significant mental health associations were decreases in anxiety and depression, rates of suicide and rates of substance abuse and increases in sense of wellbeing, marital satisfaction and stability, social support and sense of purpose and meaning in life. If spiritual beliefs improve mental health outcomes, improvements in physical health parameters should be found as well, modulated by a reduction in the stress response. A review of the literature by Clark[62] found that spiritual beliefs were associated with decreases in mortality rates from cancer, cardiovascular disease, blood pressure and cholesterol and increases in immune function, health behaviours (increased exercise and sleep, and reduction in smoking) and longevity.

Finally, patients want their emotional and spiritual needs to be met by their medical providers. Studies show that 77% of patients want to have their spiritual concerns discussed by their providers, yet only 10–20% of practitioners engage in such conversations.[63–65] If they were gravely ill, 66% of patients report that they would want their providers to enquire about their religious beliefs, while up to 40% believe that doctors should ask about spirituality to a greater extent than they do. In order to create a therapeutic alliance, enquiring about a patient's beliefs may be one of the single most important factors in healing, allowing them to relax into the medical visit or procedure with a sense of safety, social engagement and trust.

Many doctors agree with patients on this matter: 77% want patients to share their religious beliefs during the medical encounter, and an even greater percentage, 96%, believe that spiritual wellbeing is important to overall health. However, doctors surveyed felt inadequately trained (59%), unable to determine which patients were interested in such conversations (56%) and reported lack of time (71%) as the biggest challenges to broaching spiritual conversations.[63–67] Other reasons cited included lack of comfort and fear of reaching beyond their level of expertise. However, as Koenig[61] points out, doctors constantly screen for a wide array of health conditions, many of which are beyond their expertise and require consultation with a specialist. If during a conversation about spiritual needs, the doctor deems an expert is warranted, a referral to a chaplain or other spiritual advisor can easily be made.

TAKING A SPIRITUAL HISTORY

Initiating spiritual conversations may appear daunting, yet several authors have outlined clear and concise questions that practitioners can use. For example, Lo and colleagues[68] recommend starting with these questions:

1   Is faith (religion, spirituality) important to you in this illness?
2   Has faith been important to you at other times in your life?
3   Do you have someone to talk to about religious matters?
4   Would you like to explore religious matters with someone?

Anandarajah and Hight[65] propose the following to assist in spiritual assessment:

H: enquire about sources of **H**ope, meaning, comfort, strength, peace, love and connection
O: ask about participating in any particular **O**rganised religion
P: discuss any **P**ersonal spirituality or **P**ractices
E: explore how spiritual issues might have an **E**ffect on medical care and **E**nd-of-life.

Underwood and Teresi[69] created the Daily Spiritual Experience Scale to assist in understanding the link between spirituality and health and wellbeing. The first 15 questions are answered on a Likert scale ranging from 'never experience' a particular item to 'experience many times a day' while the final question is scaled from 'not at all' to 'as close as possible':

1   I feel God's presence.
2   I experience a connection to all of life.
3   During worship, or at other times when connecting with God, I feel joy which lifts me out of my daily concerns.
4   I find strength in my religion or spirituality.
5   I find comfort in my religion or spirituality.
6   I feel deep inner peace and harmony.
7   I ask for God's help in the midst of daily activities.
8   I feel guided by God in the midst of daily activities.
9   I feel God's love for me, directly.
10 I feel God's love for me, through others.
11 I am spiritually touched by beauty of creation.
12 I feel thankful for my blessings.
13 I feel a selfless caring for others.
14 I accept others even when they do things I think are wrong.
15 I desire to be closer to God or in unison with the Divine.
16 In general, how close do you feel to God?

Conversations about spirituality are a mind–body medicine practice. Such discussions in no way necessitate the need to pray within the medical visit. According to Koenig,[61] praying with a patient is appropriate when the patient directly request this, if the patient is highly religious, if the patient and practitioner are of a similar religious background, and when the situation is serious and warrants prayer. However, practitioners should consent only if they feel comfortable doing so. Otherwise, they should consult a chaplain, family member or someone of the same religious and spiritual background to assist, never losing sight of the ultimate goal – to create a sense understanding, support and care, allowing for social engagement and balance of the nervous system.

Guided imagery, hypnosis and autogenic training

For those who engage in mental scenarios or self-talk that perpetuates and intensifies their emotional reactions when stressed, guided imagery and hypnosis are the associated self-relaxation strategies. Forms of imagery and hypnosis have been practised throughout the millennia, yet French pharmacist Émile Coué de la Châtaigneraie has been credited by some as the father of guided imagery. Coué firmly believed that healing is linked to imagination, and that the object of our mental focus impacts both body and mind. In 1922 he wrote *Self Mastery through Autosuggestion*, providing instructions on positive suggestions to manifest health and wellbeing.

Imagery, also known as visualisation, has been defined by Achterberg as 'the thought process that invokes and uses senses: vision, audition, smell, taste', as well as the 'senses of movement, position, and touch'.[70] Since all senses are activated in the process, imagery is the preferred term. These images are internal mental representations of real or imaginary experiences in the absence of any external stimuli. When guided, a practitioner or therapist introduces the images, yet audio recordings may be considered guided as well. The goal, however, is the ability to self-generate images. Initially, imagery may focus on general relaxation combined with techniques like muscle relaxation or breathing. With mastery, the process shifts to addressing a specific issue or health condition. Guided imagery is commonly used for relaxation and stress reduction, pain management, immune system regulation and healing.[71–77]

Imagery may take many forms, according to Naparstek in her influential book on the subject:[78]

- *Feel-state imagery:* recalling an image that induces a positive emotion, like a safe place or peaceful setting
- *End-state imagery:* visualising the desired state or outcome occurring in the present, such as passing a final exam or finishing a race
- *Energetic imagery:* imagining healing waves emitting from the area of pain or discomfort, unblocking the flow of energy
- *Cellular imagery:* imagining healing and repairing of cellular level processes, as in imagining immune cells killing cancer cells
- *Physiological imagery:* picturing the body in a state of healing, such as imagining a painfully contracted muscle softening and relaxing
- *Metaphoric imagery:* using specific symbols or metaphors as images, such as picturing immune cells to be Pac-Men or sharks attacking cancer cells
- *Psychological imagery:* changing an emotional state by imagining adopting a compassionate response, such as imagining the love and compassion your grandmother might express towards you
- *Spiritual imagery:* envisioning connection with a transcendent higher power or Divinity.

Imagery has been suggested as the basis of hypnosis, or at least a subcategory of the modality due to the similarities in techniques.[75,79,80] In Europe, Anton Mesmer was one of the first to popularise a consistent methodology for hypnosis, although it was not until the 1950s that hypnotherapy became more widely embraced as a serious mind–body modality. Hypnosis has been described as a trance-like state in which focus and concentration are increased. Techniques are typically guided at the onset of training. The practitioner (hypnotist) suggests words or phrases for mental repetition along with images to activate the senses, although audio recordings may be used. Hypnosis is indicated for situations where guided imagery is warranted and efficacious, such as relaxation, pain relief (e.g. headaches, chronic low back pain, arthritis, burns, postoperative healing), anxiety, depression and phobias.[81,82]

The first step in hypnosis is called induction, where a series of instructions is provided to assist the person in voluntarily invoking an absorbed attentional state of focus. Inductions are voluntary and can be cognitive instructions – 'Focus on the feeling of your tummy rising and falling as you breathe' – or cognitive strategies (guided imagery) – 'Imagine your mind and body growing more and more relaxed as you descend a flight of stairs.' Although frequently the case, induction need not involve relaxation. Induction is used to prepare the person for suggestions. Suggestions consist of statements describing changes in experience and do not require the participant's volitional engagement – 'Your legs are becoming heavy; you find you are unable to move them.'

What enables a person to become hypnotised? The Stanford Hypnotic Susceptibility Scale was created in 1959 by Weitzenhoffer and Hildgard to assess the degree of responsiveness to hypnotic suggestion while performing a series of 12 activities.[83] A sample task might include the person keeping their arm at shoulder height during the suggestion of holding a heavy object. Should their arm begin to lower, a positive score is given. Research has shown that a person's susceptibility to hypnosis remains fairly stable throughout adult life, regardless of how hard they might try to be hypnotised. Susceptibility doesn't seem to be linked to psychological or personality traits, and identical twins show a greater likelihood than same-sex fraternal twins for susceptibility.[84] In one study, those who were highly hypnotisable had a 32% larger rostrum of the corpus callosum on brain imaging, the area of the brain responsible for attention and inhibition of unwanted stimuli.[85] Furthermore, in another study a 16% increase in blood flow was seen on fMRI during hypnosis, and decreased activation of the default mode network.[86]

Autogenic training, created by Johannes Schultz and expanded on by Wolfgang Luthe, is a structured form of guided imagery. Though often defined as self-hypnosis, autogenic training more accurately translated as self-regulation. Autogenic training was conceived as a means of self-empowerment, where the individual heals themselves without the assistance of a practitioner. As categorised by Smith, autogenic training is appropriate for those with a somaticised stress response where attending to a specific bodily sensation evokes or intensifies it. Initially taught individually or in groups, autogenic training involves silent recitation of self-suggestion phrases, called formulas, using physiological imagery to passively induce a relaxed and calm somatic process.[87,88] The formulas are introduced one at a time, in a consistent order, over an 8-week period, with daily home practice required for mastery. Here is the classic list of six bodily sensations induced with their associated formula to be recited silently:

- Heavy: 'My arms (legs, low back, jaw, etc.) are heavy'
- Warm: 'My arms (legs, low back, jaw, etc.) are warm'
- Cardiac: 'My heart is steady and calm'
- Breath: 'My breath breathes me'
- Solar plexus: 'My abdomen is warm'
- Forehead: 'My forehead is cool'.

Similar to mindfulness, autogenic training is approached with an attitude of passive concentration, a non-judgmental mindset where the individual remains detached from the outcome (non-striving).

The benefits of all three of these techniques (guided imagery, hypnosis and autogenic training) may rest in the shift in subjective experience that interrupts rumination and reframes negative beliefs and appraisals to those that are more pleasant or favourable. With practice and mastery come a sense of internal locus of control, a reduction in anxiety and an increased sense of wellbeing. Decreased rumination reduces sympathetic nervous system and HPA axis activation, and normalises immune function, as seen in appropriate changes in white blood cell counts.[72,75,89] When practised in an environment with reduced sensory stimulation, similar outcomes are seen with all three approaches; namely, a reduction in sympathetic tone, and balance between sympathetic and parasympathetic activity.

Progressive muscle relaxation

For those who respond to stressors by tensing their muscles, progressive muscle relaxation, also known as progressive relaxation or muscle relaxation therapy, is the indicated tool. Progressive muscle relaxation is a classic example of the bottom-up approach to mind–body medicine, which emphasises changing the physical body to influence mental and emotional states, rather than focusing on calming the mind first. In fact, Edmund Jacobson, who developed progressive muscle relaxation, rarely addressed mental relaxation or training, considering the release of muscular tension all that was required. He believed it was inaccurate to assume that thinking was generated solely in the brain. For him, cognition was an entire mind–body event.[90] This worldview took shape for Jacobson in the 1930s after observing minute physical movements in his patients that accompanied stressful and anxious thoughts. His emotionally tense patients demonstrated chronic muscle tension with increased startle reflexes. He proposed that an emotionally calm state was impossible when muscles were physically contracted, and his research was able to demonstrate how cognition slowed down when muscles became more relaxed. His system of progressive muscle relaxation taught patients to regulate skeletal muscle tension in order to reduce unwanted emotional and mental states.[91]

Muscles are the anchor in progressive muscle relaxation. Finding a comfortable and relaxed posture, usually reclining, in a room free from distractions and interruptions, the patient is instructed to remain still and silent throughout, since talking engages facial muscles, which activate the nervous system. The practitioner guides the patient in a series of contractions and relaxations targeting muscles in a systematic way. The key is to keep the other muscles completely still and passive, especially muscles that were just contracted then relaxed. In Jacobson's classic methodology, the dominant arm was used to differentiate between maximum to minimum levels of tension. Contractions are held for approximately 5–7 seconds, then swiftly and completely disengaged in an attempt to drop tension below baseline levels. Once able to detect the presence and degree of tension, the patient practises relaxing muscles at will. Ultimately this will generalise to other areas of the body as the patient masters greater control of physical tension.

Jacobson's basic protocol consisted of many stages and was time-intensive. More than 50 private sessions per year, each lasting upwards of 60 minutes, along with hour-long daily practice at home were required. Bernstein and Borkovec[92] abbreviated Jacobson's protocol and combined it with cognitive-behavioural therapy to teach patients stress reduction. Training can be as brief as 8–12 weekly sessions, with 20 minutes of home practice per day. Initially 16 muscle groups are trained; over time, muscles are combined into groups of seven and four. Finally, relaxation is practised without the need for a tension-release cycle by recalling the muscle(s), recalling and counting backwards, then counting alone.[93] Table 9.5 details one potential training schedule.

Several authors argue that while learning to decrease muscle tension and become more relaxed is important overall, progressive muscle relaxation alone is insufficient to interrupt anxiety or panic reactions. Jacobson's concepts have been modified and combined with other techniques for additional benefit or to address particular conditions. For example, in 1967 Farmer combined tension and release cycles with breathing and silent recitation of relaxing words, while Burrows (1976), Kleinsorge and Klumbies (1964) and Boom and Richardson (1931) combined elements of progressive muscle relaxation with imagery and autogenic-type phrases. Wolpe incorporated muscle relaxation in his process of systematic desensitisation, while the modification by Öst led to applied relaxation, efficacious in the treatment of phobias, panic and generalised anxiety.[94–96]

Lehrer and colleagues[97] outline the typical steps in the abbreviated progressive muscle relaxation protocol as follows:

1   Ask the patient to adopt a comfortable, relaxed, reclined posture and to remain still so as not to engage any muscles.
2   Direct the patient to focus their attention on the specific targeted muscle group.
3   Direct the patient to tense the muscle group for 5–7 seconds, breathing freely while tensing.
4   Direct the patient to relax the muscle group swiftly, completely and instantly.
5   Direct the patient to focus on the sensations of relaxation for 30–40 seconds.
6   Prior to moving to a new muscle group, ask the patient if the muscle group is relaxed. Invite them to respond with a movement of a finger to prevent nervous system activation through speaking. If still tense, repeat the tension-relaxation cycle for 50–60 seconds up to five times.
7   Repeat the process for the specified sequence of muscles.
8   When all muscle groups are relaxed, review each group with the patient.
9   To end the session, instruct the patient to move their feet, arms, head and neck.

In addition to efficacy in reducing anxiety and panic,[95,98,99] progressive muscle relaxation has shown promise in addressing conditions such as depression,[93] attention deficit hyperactivity disorder (by improving attention and decreasing impulsivity),[100] trauma (by improving distress tolerance), cardiovascular disease (by decreasing heart rate and decreasing diastolic and systolic blood pressure),[101] inflammation (by decreasing TNF-α and IL-6)[102] and Parkinson's disease (by increasing dopamine and adrenaline levels).[103]

Stretching and movement: yoga

Stretching and movement is the category of mind–body medicine techniques appropriate for those who respond to stress by changing their posture. Numerous

TABLE 9.5 Sample progressive muscle relaxation training schedule 16 muscle group series

Muscle group	Instructions (Keep all other muscles, especially those previously contracted-released, still, relaxed and unengaged)
1. Dominant hand and forearm	Make a fist with the dominant hand.
2. Dominant upper arm	Press the dominant elbow into the chair.
3. Non-dominant hand and forearm	Make a fist with the non-dominant hand.
4. Non-dominant upper arm	Press the non-dominant elbow into the chair.
5. Forehead	Raise the eyebrows as high as possible.
6. Upper cheeks and nose	Squeeze the eyes together as if squinting, while wrinkling the nose.
7. Lower face	Clench the teeth and pull the corners of the mouth back as if showing the teeth.
8. Neck	If reclining, slightly press the back of the head into the chair. Without head support, neck counterpose (moving antagonist muscles): attempt to raise the chin while simultaneously lowering it.*
9. Chest, shoulders, upper back	Draw the shoulders and shoulder blades back and together while taking a deep breath and holding it.
10. Abdomen	Abdominal counterpose: attempt to draw in the abdomen while simultaneously pushing it out.
11. Dominant upper leg	Simultaneously contract the muscles on the top and bottom of the dominant upper leg.
12. Dominant calf	Point the dominant toes towards the head.*
13. Dominant foot	Point the dominant toes downwards, turn the foot inwards and curl the toes under.*
14. Non-dominant upper leg	Simultaneously contract the muscles on the top and bottom of the non-dominant upper leg.
15. Non-dominant calf	Point the non-dominant toes towards the head.*
16. Non-dominant foot	Point the non-dominant toes downwards, turn the foot inwards and curl the toes under.*

Seven muscle group series

1. Dominant hand, forearm and upper arm
2. Non-dominant hand, forearm and upper arm
3. All facial muscles
4. Neck*
5. Chest, shoulders, upper back and abdomen
6. Dominant upper leg, calf and foot*
7. Non-dominant upper leg, calf and foot*

Four muscle group series

1. Both arms and hands
2. Face and neck*
3. Chest, shoulders, back and abdomen
4. Both legs and feet

*To prevent cramping, avoid contracting muscles as vigorously.

movement-oriented approaches exist, but this chapter concentrates on yoga, the most commonly used mind–body modality according to the 2015 US National Health Statistics Reports.[17] The word 'yoga' comes from the Sanskrit term *yuj*, which means 'to yoke' or 'to join' – yoga is considered the practice of forging a union of mind, body and spirit. Originating around 4000 years ago in India, yoga is a comprehensive philosophical system leading to self-awareness.[104] Although modern-day practice tends to highlight postures, known as *asanas*, yoga is more than a physical discipline. In the *Yoga Sutras*, Patanjali codified eight parts to the practice of yoga in the 2nd century (*asthanga* in Sanskrit means eight limbs). Known

as *Raja*, or royal yoga, this system details the following limbs:[105]

- *Yamas*: moral and ethical code of behaviour
- *Niyamas*: techniques for self-discipline
- *Asanas*: postures for cleansing the physical body to prepare it for higher states of consciousness and meditation
- *Pranayama*: breathing exercises, also used for physical purification and to raise energy
- *Pratyahara*: sensory withdrawal practice to prevent distraction from mundane experiences
- *Dhyana*: concentration practices to expand awareness and direct focus, called *dharana*

- *Meditation*
- *Samadhi:* enlightenment or union with universal consciousness.

All forms of yoga strive to bring mind, body and spirit together in order to achieve the ultimate goal of Samadhi. Some systems of yoga arose between the 6th and 15th centuries, each underscoring a different path to reach transcendence. Hatha Yoga used physical development as the means to obtain divine union, while Jnana (also known as Gnyana) Yoga used introspection, knowledge, contemplation and wisdom to identify ultimate Truth. Intense spiritual devotion, love, compassion and service to God were the way to reach Samadhi in Bhakti Yoga, while Karma Yoga focused on the law of cause and effect to engage practical action and service to others to discover enlightenment.[105]

Since yoga incorporates physical posture with breathing and mental focus, determining the precise form of yoga attributing to the growth change can be a challenge, especially when studies often fail to detail the therapeutic intervention. However, it should come as no surprise that yoga demonstrates improvements in stress, mood and symptoms. According to Khalsa,[106] reduction in the HPA axis and autonomic nervous system activation, along with decreased basal glucocorticoids and catecholamines, reduced metabolic rate and oxygen consumption, and increased parasympathetic activity, may be the mechanisms behind yoga's health benefits. Salmon and colleagues[107] have identified positive changes in chronic low back pain, irritable bowel syndrome, type II diabetes and chronic disease. Physiological changes in body weight, blood pressure, cholesterol and blood glucose levels have also been reported.

Questions about the safety of yoga have been raised on several occasions. In a systematic review and meta-analysis of randomised control trials of yoga, Cramer found that, when compared with standard physical exercise, yoga is a safe intervention with no differences in the frequency of adverse events or dropouts due to adverse events between the comparison groups.[108]

Breathwork

The second most popular mind–body method, breathwork, can be examined through the lens of yoga, as a component to another modality such as meditation, autogenic training or progressive muscle relaxation, or as an isolated practice. In Sanskrit, the term *prana* means 'life force', and in yogic philosophy life force is said to be regulated through breathing. Pranayama, one of the limbs of yoga, involves breathing practices designed to control this vital life force energy in order to purify the mind and body from toxic energies.[109] With the exception of mindfulness training, all breathwork involves manipulation of one or more of the following components:

- *Timing/rate:* number of breaths per minute, the inhalation to exhalation ratio, and pausing or retaining the breath
- *Volume:* the amount of air inhaled, exhaled or retained
- *Location/placement:* nose versus mouth breathing, diaphragmatic versus thoracic/clavicular breathing

- *Effort:* laboured or easy breathing, the smoothness of transitions between the stages of breathing, recruitment of extra muscles
- *Posture:* physical alignment facilitating laboured or effortless breath.

For instance, sudarshan kriya is a cyclic pranayama practice that adjusts the rate and timing of breathing with several longer breaths followed by medium and short breaths.[109] In alternate nostril breathing, known as nadi shodhana, the flow of air is controlled by closing one nostril at various times during the inhalation and exhalation cycle.[110] Buteyko breathing involves holding the breath after a normal exhalation for upwards of 60 seconds to change CO_2 and O_2 levels in the bloodstream.[111] Whole-person breathing teaches slow, diaphragmatic breathing, typically 4–8 breaths per minute, in a smooth, effortless fashion.[112]

Breathing impacts health by improving cardiovascular and neurological functions. Specifically defining the exact mechanism may be easy to grasp yet challenging to outline. Due to the complexity of the process of respiration, discussion on its mechanism of action is beyond the scope of this book. Research suggests that sudarshan kriya results in changes in immune function (decrease in neutrophils, increase in NK cells), mood, such as anxiety and depression (mediated by elevation in oxytocin, decrease in glucocorticoids and ATCH) and blood pressure (reduction in diastolic blood pressure).[113] Breathwork in general has been shown to impact cardiovascular health by increasing vagal tone, improving chemoreflex and baroreflex sensitivity, increasing heart rate variability and decreasing sympathetic excitation. In their review of the literature, Brown and colleagues[114] cite research that demonstrates psychological improvement from breathwork for those with posttraumatic stress disorder, anxiety, panic, stress and depression.

Biofeedback

Biofeedback capitalises on the work of all previously mentioned mind–body approaches. Schwartz[115] defines biofeedback as:

> *a process that enables an individual to learn how to change physiological activity for the purpose of improving health and performance. Precise instruments measure physiological activity such as brainwaves, heart function, breathing, muscle activity, and skin temperature. These instruments rapidly and accurately 'feed back' information to the user. The presentation of this information – often in conjunction with changes in thinking, emotions, and behavior – support desired physiological changes. Over time, these changes can endure without continued use of instrument.*

The common physiological systems measured are:

- Electromyographic activity: measures muscular contraction
- Electrodermal activity: measures skin conduction and resistance based on amount of sweat on the palms of the hands or soles of the feet

- Temperature: measures peripheral temperature, reflects blood vessel dilation or contraction
- Pulse: measures heart rate
- Respiration: measures breathing rate
- Electroencephalography: measures brain waves.

While machinery is typically used, anything can function as a biofeedback sensor – a mirror, a thermometer, a practitioner's hands, even a practitioner's words – as long as information about physiological processes can be fed back then used to modify physical responses. When combined with other techniques, biofeedback allows the individual to 'see' in real time how their body responds to practice. For instance, practising autogenic training while connected to electromyography and temperature sensors, the individual can see whether visualising and reciting the phrase, 'My right arm is heavy and warm', decreases muscle contraction and increases hand temperature.

REFERENCES

[1] Vukic A, Gregory D, Martin-Misener R, et al. Aboriginal and Western conceptions of mental health and illness. Pimatisiwin 2011;9(1):65–86.

[2] So JK. Somatization as cultural idiom of distress: rethinking mind and body in a multicultural society. Couns Psychol Q 2008;21(2):167–74.

[3] Moodley R, Sutherland P, Oulanova O. Traditional healing, the body and mind in psychotherapy. Couns Psychol Q 2008;21(2):153–65.

[4] Benning TB. Should psychiatrists resurrect the body? Adv Mind Body Med 2016;30(1):32–8.

[5] Fleming S, Gutknecht NC. Naturopathy and the primary care office. Prim Care 2010;37:119–36.

[6] Dunn N. Naturopathic medicine: what a patient expects? J Fam Pract 2005;54(12):1067–72.

[7] Feldman MD, Berkowitz SA. Role of behavioral medicine in primary care. Curr Opin Psychiatry 2012;25(2):121–7.

[8] Society for Behavioral Medicine. Behavioral medicine: definition. Available from: www.sbm.org/resources/education/behavioral-medicine.

[9] Engel GL. The need for a new medical model: a challenge for biomedicine. Science 1977;196(4286):129–36.

[10] Engel GL. The clinical application of the biopsychosocial model. Am J Psychiatry 1980;137(5):101–24.

[11] Kroenke K, Mangelsdorff AD. Common symptoms in ambulatory care: incidence, evaluation, therapy, and outcome. Am J Med 1989;86(3):262–6.

[12] Gatchel RJ, Oordt MS. Clinical health psychology and primary care: practical advice and clinical guidance for successful collaboration. Washington, DC: American Psychological Association; 2003.

[13] Sahler OJZ, Carr JE, Frank JB, et al. The behavioral sciences and health care. 3rd ed. Cambridge MA: Hegrefe Publishing; 2012.

[14] Snider P, Zeff J. Report of the Select Committee on the Definition of Naturopathic Medicine. Washington, DC: AANP; 1988.

[15] National Center for Complementary and Integrative Medicine. Mind and body information for researchers. Available from: http://nccam.nih.gov/grants/mindbody.

[16] National Center for Complementary and Alternative Medicine (NCCAM). Mind-body medicine: an overview. NCCAM; 2007.

[17] Clarke TC, Black LI, Stussman BJ, et al. Trends in the use of complementary health approaches among adults: United States, 2002–2012. Natl Health Stat Report 2015;79:1–15.

[18] Wahbeh H, Haywood A, Kaufman K, et al. Mind-body medicine and immune system outcomes: a systematic review. Open Complement Med J 2009;1:25–34.

[19] Telles S, Gerbarg P, Kozasa EH. Physiological effects of mind and body practices. Biomed Res Int 2015;1–2.

[20] Jacobson E. Progressive relaxation. 2nd ed. Chicago: University of Chicago Press; 1938.

[21] Luthe W, Schultz JH. Autogenic therapy: applications in psychotherapy. New York: Gronne Statton; 1969.

[22] McEwan BS, Stellar E. Stress and the individual: mechanisms leading to disease. Arch Intern Med 1993;153(18):2093–101.

[23] Keller A, Litzelman K, Wisk LE, et al. Does perception that stress affects health matter? The association with health and mortality. Health Psychol 2012;32(5):677–84.

[24] Kobassa SC, Puccetti MC. Personality and social resources in stress resistance. J Pers Soc Psychol 1983;45(4):839–50.

[25] Dickerson SS, Kemeny ME. Acute stressors and cortisol responses: a theoretical integration and synthesis of laboratory research. Psychol Bull 2004;130(3):355–91.

[26] Porges SW. Orienting in a defensive world: mammalian modification of our evolutionary heritage – a polyvagal theory. Psychophysiology 1995;32:301–18.

[27] Porges SW. The polyvagal perspective. Biol Psychol 2007;74:116–43.

[28] Porges SW. The polyvagal theory: new insights into adaptive reactions of the autonomic nervous system. Cleve Clin J Med 2009;76(2):S86–90.

[29] Porges SW, Furman SA. The early development of the autonomic nervous system provides a neural platform for social behavior: a polyvagal perspective. Infant Child Dev 2011;20(1):106–18.

[30] Geller SM, Porges SW. Therapeutic presence: neurophysiological mechanism mediating feeling safe in therapeutic relationships. J Psychother Integr 2014;24(3):178–92.

[31] Stahl JE, Dossett ML, LaJoie AS, et al. Relaxation response and resiliency training and its effect on healthcare resource utilization. PLoS ONE 2015;10(10):1–14.

[32] Smith JC. The new psychology of relaxation and renewal. Biofeedback 2007;35(3):85–9.

[33] Smith JC. Relaxation today. In: Schwartz MS, Adrasik F, editors. Biofeedback: a practitioner's guide. 4th ed. New York: Guilford Press; 2015. p. 189–95.

[34] Craske MG, Rauch SL, Ursana R, et al. What is anxiety disorder? Depress Anxiety 2009;26:1066–85.

[35] Finniss DG, Kaptchuk TJ, Miller F, et al. Placebo effects: biological, clinical and ethical advances. Lancet 2010;375(9715):686–95.

[36] Wager TD, Atlas LY. The neuroscience of placebo effects: connecting context, learning and health. Nat Rev Neurosci 2015;16:403–18.

[37] Shapiro SL, Walsh R, Britton WB. An analysis of recent meditation research and suggestions for future directions. J Medit & Medit Res 2003;3:69–90.

[38] Cardoso R, de Souza E, Camano L, et al. Meditation in health: an operational definition. Brain Res Brain Res Protoc 2004;14:58–60.

[39] Hussain D, Bhushan B. Psychology of meditation and health: present status and future directions. Int J Psychol Psychol Ther 2010;10(3):439–51.

[40] Hölzel BK, Lazar SW, Gard T, et al. Does mindfulness meditation work? Proposing mechanisms of action from a conceptual and neural perspective. Perspect Psychol Sci 2011;6:537–59.

[41] Ott U, Vaitl D, Hölzel B. Brain structure and meditation: how spiritual practices shape the brain. In: Walach H, Schmidt S, Jonas WB, editors. Neuroscience, consciousness, and spirituality. New York: Springer; 2011. p. 119–28.

[42] Shonin E, van Gordon W, Singh NN, editors. Buddhist foundations of mindfulness. New York: Springer; 2015. p. 97.

[43] Bishop SR, Lau M, Shapiro S, et al. Mindfulness: a proposed operational definition. Clin Psychol Sci Pract 2004;11(3):230–41.

[44] Kabat-Zinn J. Mindfulness-based interventions in context: past, present, and future. Clin Psychol Sci Pract 2003;10(2):144–56.

[45] Davis D, Hayes J. What are the benefits of mindfulness? A practice review of psychotherapy-related research. Psychotherapy (Chic) 2011;48(2):198–208.

[46] Baer RA, Smith GT, Hopkins J, et al. Using self-report assessment methods to explore facets of mindfulness. Assessment 2006;13:27–45.

[47] Brosschot JF, Gerin W, Thayer JF. The perseverative cognition hypothesis: a review of worry, prolonged stress-related physiological activation, and health. J Psychosom Res 2006;60:113–24.

[48] Davidson RJ, Kabat-Zinn J, Schumacher J, et al. Alterations in brain and immune function produced by mindfulness meditation. Psychosom Med 2003;65:564–70.

[49] Carlson LE, Speca M, Faris P, et al. One year pre-post intervention follow-up of psychological, immune, endocrine and blood pressure outcomes of mindfulness-based stress reduction (MBSR) in breast and prostate cancer outpatients. Brain Behav Immun 2007;21:1038–49.

[50] Witek-Janusek L, Albuquerque K, Chroniak KR, et al. Effect of mindfulness based stress reduction on immune function, quality of life and coping in women newly diagnosed with early stage breast cancer. Brain Behav Immun 2008;22:969–81.

[51] Paul NA, Stanton SJ, Greeson JM, et al. Psychological and neural mechanisms of trait mindfulness in reducing depression vulnerability. Soc Cogn Affect Neurosci 2013;8:56–64.

[52] Fox KCR, Nijeboer S, Dixon ML, et al. Chirstoff K. Is meditation associated with altered brain structure? A systematic review and meta-analysis of morphometric neuroimaging in meditation practitioners. Neurosci Biobehav Rev 2014;43:48–73.

[53] Brewer JA, Worhunsky PD, Grey JR, et al. Meditation experience is associated with differences in default mode network activity and connectivity. Proc Natl Acad Sci USA 2011;108(50):20254–9.

[54] Zeidan F, Martucci KT, Kraft RA, et al. Brain mechanisms supporting modulation of pain by mindfulness meditation. J Neurosci 2011;31(14):5540–8.

[55] Joint Commission Resources. 2007 comprehensive accreditation manual for hospitals: the official handbook. Oakbrook Terrace, IL: Joint Commission on Accreditation of Healthcare Organizations; 2007.

[56] Vaughan F. Spiritual issues in psychotherapy. J Transpers Psychol 1991;23:105–19.

[57] Sheehan MN. Spirituality and the care of people with life-threatening illnesses. Tech Reg Anesth Pain Manag 2005;9(3):109–13.

[58] McDonald C, Wall K, Corwin D, et al. The perceived effects of psycho-spiritual integrative therapy and community support groups on coping with breast cancer: a qualitative analysis. Eur J Pers Cent Healthc 2012;1(2):298–309.

[59] Elkins DN, Hedstrom LJ, Hughes LL, et al. Toward a humanistic-phenomenological spirituality: definition, description, and measurement. J Humanist Psychol 1998;28(4):5–18.

[60] Curlin FA, Roach CJ, Gorawara-Bhat R, et al. How are religion and spirituality related to health? South Med J 2005;98(8):761–6.

[61] Koenig HG. Religion, spirituality, and medicine: research findings and implications for clinical practice. South Med J 2004;97(12):1194–200.

[62] Clark PA, Drain M, Malone MP. Addressing patients' emotional and spiritual needs. Jt Comm J Qual Saf 2003;29(12):659–70.

[63] King DE, Bushwick B. Beliefs and attitudes of hospital inpatients about faith healing and prayer. J Fam Pract 1994;39:349–52.

[64] Maugans TA, Wadland WC. Religion and family medicine: a survey of physicians and patients. J Fam Pract 1991;32:210–13.

[65] Anandarajah G, Hight E. Spirituality and medical practice: using the HOPE questions as a practice tool for spiritual assessment. Am Fam Physician 2001;63(1):81–8.

[66] Oyama O, Koenig HG. Religious beliefs and practices in family medicine. Arch Fam Med 1998;7:431–5.

[67] Ehman JW, Ott BB, Short TH, et al. Do patients want physicians to inquire about their spiritual or religious beliefs if they become gravely ill? Arch Intern Med 1999;159:1803–6.

[68] Lo B, Quill T, Tulsky J. Discussing palliative care with patients. Ann Intern Med 1999;130(9):772–4.

[69] Underwood LG, Teresi J. The Daily Spiritual Experience Scale: development, theoretical description, reliability, exploratory factor analysis, and preliminary construct validity using health related data. Anns Behav Med 2002;24(1):22–33.

[70] Achterberg J. Imagery in healing. Boston, MA: Shambala; 1985.

[71] Lewandowski W, Jacobson A. Bridging the gap between mind and body: a biobehavioral model of the effects of guided imagery on pain, pain disability, and depression. Pain Manag Nurs 2013;14(4):368–78.

[72] Lewandowski W, Jacobson A, Palmieri PA, et al. Biological mechanism related to the effectiveness of guided imagery for chronic pain. Biol Res Nurs 2011;13(4):364–75.

[73] Posadzki P, Lewandowski W, Terry R, et al. Guided imagery for non-musculoskeletal pain: a systematic review of randomized clinical trials. J Pain Symptom Manage 2012;44(1):95–104.

[74] Gozales AE, Ledesma RJA, Perry SM, et al. Effects of guided imagery on postoperative outcomes in patients undergoing same-day surgical procedures: a randomized, single-blind study. AANA J 2010;78(3):185–8.

[75] Trakhtenberg E. The effects of guided imagery on immune system: a critical review. Int J Neurosci 2008;118:839–55.

[76] van Kuiken D. A meta-analysis of the effect of guided imagery practice on outcomes. J Holist Nurs 2004;22(2):164–79.

[77] Halpin LS, Speir AM, CapoBianco P, et al. Guided imagery in cardiac surgery. Outcomes Manag 2002;6(3):132–7.

[78] Naparstek B. Staying well with guided imagery. How to harness the power of your imagination for health and healing. New York: Hachette Book Group; 1994.

[79] Miller GE, Cohen S. Psychological interventions and the immune system: a meta-analytic review and critique. Health Psychol 2001;20(1):47–63.

[80] Rider MS, Achterberg J. Effect of music-assisted imagery on neutrophils and lymphocytes. Biofeedback Self Regul 1989;14:247–57.

[81] Montgomery GH, DuHamel KN, Redd WH. A meta-analysis of hypnotically induced analgesia: how effective is hypnosis? Int J Clin Exp Hypn 2000;48(2):134–49.

[82] Walker WR. Hypnosis as an adjunct in management of pain. South Med J 1980;73(3):362–4.

[83] Benham G, Smith N, Nash MR. Hypnotic susceptibility scales: are the mean scores increasing? Int J Clin Exp Hypn 2002;50(1):5–16.

[84] Lichtenberg P, Bachner-Melman R, Ebstein RP, et al. Hypnotic susceptibility: multidimensional relationship with Cloninger's tridimensional personality questionniare, COMPT polymorphisms, absorption, and attentional characteristics. Int J Clin Exp Hypn 2003;52(1):47–72.

[85] Horton JE, Crawford HJ, Harrington G, et al. Increased anterior corpus callosum size associated positively with hypnotizability and the ability to control pain. Brain 2004;127(Pt 8):1741–7.

[86] Vanhaudenhuyse A, Laureys S, Faymonville ME. Neurophysiology of hypnosis. Clin Neurophysiol 2014;44:343–53.

[87] Stetter F, Kupper S. Autogenic training: a meta-analysis of clinical outcome studies. Appl Psychophysiol Biofeedback 2002;27(1):45–98.

[88] Kanji N, Ernst E. Autogenic training for stress and anxiety: a systematic review. Complement Ther Med 2000;8:106–10.

[89] Serra D, Parris CR, Carper E, et al. Outcomes of guided Imagery in Patients Receiving Radiation Therapy for Breast Cancer. Clin J Oncol Nurs 2012;16(6):617–23.

[90] Elton D, Burrows GD, Stanley GV. Relaxation theory and practice. Aust J Physiother 1978;24(3):143–9.

[91] Jacobson E. Progressive relaxation. Chicago: University of Chicago Press; 1938.

[92] Bernstein DA, Borkovec TD. Progressive relaxation training: a manual for the helping professions. Champaign, IL: Research Press; 1973.

[93] Safi SZ. A fresh look at the potential mechanisms of progressive muscle relaxation therapy on depression in female patients with multiple sclerosis. Iran J Psychiatry Behav Sci 2015;9:340–8.

[94] Elton D, Burrows GD, Stanley GV. Relaxation theory and practice. Aust J Physiother 1978;24(3):143–9.

[95] Conrad A, Roth WT. Muscle relaxation therapy for anxiety disorders: it works but how? J Anxiety Disord 2006;21:243–64.

[96] Hayes-Skelton SA, Roemer L. A contemporary view of applied relaxation for generalized anxiety disorder. Cogn Behav Ther 2014;42(4):1–12.

[97] Lehrer PM, Woolfolk RL, Sime WE. Principles and practice of stress management. 3rd ed. New York, NY: The Guilford Press; 2007.

[98] Lee EJ, Bhattacharya J, Sohn C, et al. Monochord sounds and progressive muscle relaxation reduce anxiety and improve relaxation during chemotherapy: a pilot EEG study. Complement Ther Med 2012;20(6):409–16.

[99] Ranjita L, Sarada N. Progressive muscle relaxation therapy in anxiety: a neurophysiological study. IOSR-JDMS 2014;13(2):25–8.

[100] Chan E. The role of complementary and alternative medicine in attention-deficit hyperactivity disorder. J Dev Behav Pediatr 2002;23(Suppl.).

[101] Sheu S, Irvin BL, Lin H, et al. Effects of progressive muscle relaxation on blood pressure and psychosocial status for clients with essential hypertension in Taiwan Province of China. Holist Nurs Pract 2003;17(1):41–7.

[102] Koh KB, Lee Y, Beyn KM, et al. Counter-stress effects of relaxation on proinflammatory and anti-inflammatory cytokines. Brain Behav Immun 2008;22(8):1130–7.

[103] Hernandez-Reif M, Field T, Largie S, et al. Parkinson's disease symptoms are differentially affected by massage therapy vs. progressive muscle relaxation: a pilot study. J Bodyw Mov Ther 2002;6(3):177–82.

[104] Riley D. Hatha yoga and the treatment of illness. Altern Ther Health Med 2004;10(2):20–1.

[105] da Silva TL, Ravindran LN, Ravindran AV. Yoga in the treatment of mood and anxiety disorders: a review. Asian J Psychiatr 2009;2(2009):6–16.

[106] Khalsa SBS. Yoga as a Therapeutic intervention: a bibliometric analysis of published research studies. Indian J Physiol Pharmacol 2004;48(3):269–85.

[107] Salmon P, Lush E, Jablonski M, et al. Yoga and mindfulness: clinical aspects of an ancient mind/body practice. Cogn Behav Pract 2009;16:59–72.

[108] Cramer H, Ward L, Saper R, et al. The safety of yoga: a systematic review and meta-analysis of randomized controlled trials. Am J Epidemiol 2015;1–13.

[109] Brown RP, Gerbarg PL. Yoga breathing, meditation and longevity. Ann N Y Acad Sci 2009;1172:54–62.

[110] Dhanvijay AD, Bagade AH, Choudhary AK, et al. Alternate nostril breathing and autonomic function in healthy young adults. IOSR-JDMS 2015;14(3):62–5.

[111] Cooper S, Oborne J, Newton S, et al. Effect of two breathing exercises (Buteyko and pranayama) in asthma: a randomised controlled trial. Thorax 2003;58:674–9.

[112] Peper E, Tibbetts V. Effortless diaphragmatic breathing. Phys Ther Prod 1994;6(2):67–71.

[113] Sharma P, Thapliyal A, Chandra T, et al. Rhythmic breathing: immunological, biochemical, and physiological effects on health. Adv Mind Body Med 2015;29(1):18–25.

[114] Brown RP, Gerbarg PL, Muench F. Breathing practices for treatment of psychiatric and stress-related medical conditions. Psychiatr Clin North Am 2013;36:121–40.

[115] Schwartz MS, Adrasik F, editors. Biofeedback. A practitioner's guide. 4th ed. New York, NY: The Guilford Press; 2016.

Sports naturopathy

Kira Sutherland

10

INTRODUCTION

The concept of using foods and fluids to enhance sports performance is not new. As far back as ancient Greece it is known that athletes focused on their diet before competition or sport. As the Olympic motto states, 'Faster, Higher, Stronger' – and this is what athletes and those participating in sport are looking for. Much of what is covered in this chapter pertains to people participating in sports at a medium to high level. Although these principles can be adjusted and applied to anyone participating in physical fitness and recreation, most of the research and clinical suggestions are for those involved in physical activity on a regular basis.

Sports nutrition is the domain of dietitians and sports scientists. It is a heavily researched field of human nutrition and biochemistry. As a naturopath approaching the use of sports nutrition there are many philosophical differences that need to be put aside, as the application of dietetics-style sports nutrition will need to prevail in the idea that fuelling the body for sport may not always follow the food-is-medicine guidelines of naturopathic nutrition. This is not to say that many sports nutrition principles cannot be brought within naturopathic principles, but at times use of glucose, sucrose or large doses of sodium, for example, may be required to keep an athlete moving and safe. As naturopaths learn to apply these principles, it is up to each practitioner and their clients to find their level of food as medicine versus food as fuel during sport.

A complete overview of all sports nutrition principles is beyond the scope of this book, but this chapter aims to teach the basics of fuelling for active people and athletes and to bring an understanding of its application in everyday life.

EXERCISE PHYSIOLOGY

Energy metabolism

A basic understanding of how the body uses macronutrients as fuel during different types of output and exercise is vital to the application of sports nutrition principles. A good understanding of exercise physiology goes a long way to interpreting why certain sports nutrition principles are applied and when. A short summary is provided below; more detail can be found in other publications.[1,2] Many systems must coordinate when a body is in motion. Exercise requires an increase in energy metabolism, while fuel and oxygen must be supplied to the working muscles. The body must attempt to remove heat and waste products while also trying to maintain fluid and electrolyte balance.

Energy systems

A clear understanding of the body's three energy systems is vital. The aerobic (oxidative) and anaerobic (phosphate or glycolytic) systems use different fuels and are available for differing intensities and types of exercise. Knowing the metabolic profile of a sport is imperative to applying accurate sports nutrition principles for supporting optimum training, recovery and competition. Figs 10.1 and 10.2 and Table 10.1 review these three systems.[2–4]

The phosphate system has a high power output but can supply energy for only a very short period of time; however, replenishment of this system is rapid. The glycolytic system has a greater ability for adenosine triphosphate (ATP) generation but has a lower power output and a much slower ability to replenish itself as glycogen (carbohydrate) stores must be replaced.

Oxidative/aerobic metabolism of carbohydrate (CHO) and lipids provides the vast majority of ATP for muscle contraction. Amino acid oxidation occurs to a limited extent. The contribution of carbohydrate or lipids is influenced by the person's exercise intensity, diet prior to exercise, substrate availability and fitness level as well as environmental factors such as hot or cold climates.

No energy system is ever used exclusively, and the systems do not run independently of each other. Many factors come into play as to which system is used and to what extent, including the intensity, type, duration and frequency of training, and the person's overall fitness level, gender and substrate availability (see Table 10.2).

Fuel sources

Muscle glycogen is important for both intense and prolonged forms of exercise (see Fig. 10.3). Its rate of usage is most rapid during the early stages of exercise and is correlated to exercise intensity. As exercise continues and muscle glycogen declines, blood glucose becomes an

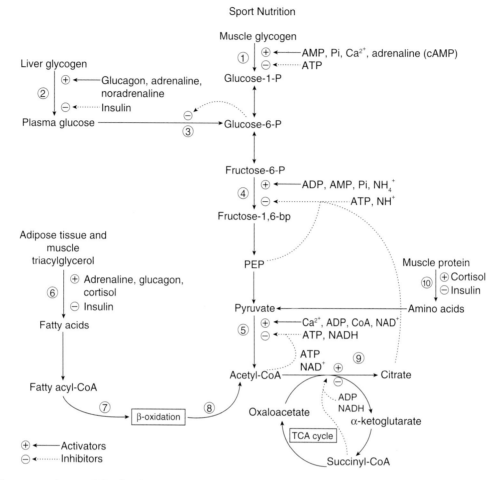

FIGURE 10.1 Energy systems of the body

Jeukendrup AE, Gleeson M. Sports nutrition: an introduction to energy production and performance. 4th edn. Champaign, IL: Human Kinetics Publishers; 2004.

TABLE 10.1 Working energy systems			
	Phosphate (anaerobic)	**Glycolytic (anaerobic)**	**Oxidative metabolism (aerobic)**
Intensity of effort	Very high intensity 95–100% of maximum effort, explosive	High intensity 60–95% of maximum effort	Low intensity Up to 60% of maximum effort
Duration	Approximately 8–10 seconds	Primary system for high-intensity exercise lasting 10–180 seconds	Primary system for exercise lasting longer than 2 minutes
Fuel	Phosphocreatine (PC) and adenosine triphosphate (ATP)	Carbohydrate in the form of muscle glycogen and blood glucose	Carbohydrates Muscle/liver glycogen Fats Intramuscular lipids Adipose triglycerides Amino acids from Muscle Liver Blood Gut Exogenous sources can also be used for energy production in prolonged exercise

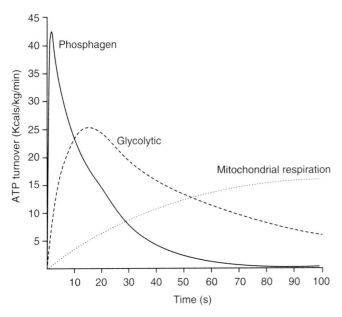

FIGURE 10.2 Interaction of metabolic energy systems

Baker JS, McCormick MC, Robergs RA. Interaction among skeletal muscle metabolic energy systems during intense exercise. Journal of Nutrition and Metabolism 2010:1–13.

TABLE 10.2 Approximate contributions of anaerobic and aerobic energy supply to total energy demand in races over different distances

Distance	Duration (min)	Anaerobic (%)	Aerobic (%)
100 m	0:9.58	90	10
400 m	0:43.18	70	30
800 m	1:40.91	40	60
1500 m	3:26.00	20	80
5000 m	12:37.35	5	95
10 000 m	26:17.53	3	97
42.2 km	122:57	1	99

Note: The times given are for the men's world records for these distances in 2014.
Source: Maughan R, Shirreffs S. Physiology of sport. In Burke L, Deakin V. Clinical sports nutrition. 5th edn. Australia: McGraw-Hill Australia; 2015.

important carbohydrate fuel source. Exogenous carbohydrate eaten at this time can become a major source of fuel during prolonged events.

Muscle also obtains energy from the beta oxidation of plasma free fatty acids (FFAs), from lipolysis of adipose tissue. Its use as a fuel may reduce the reliance on glycogen stores and blood glucose, especially during prolonged exercise such as endurance events.

The body's use of differing substrates is primarily influenced by the intensity of exercise, as well as the style of diet the athlete chooses to follow. Fig. 10.4 illustrates the percentage of different fuels the body uses at increasing

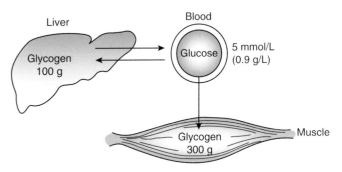

FIGURE 10.3 Glycogen storage in the body

Jeukendrup AE, Gleeson M. Sports nutrition: an introduction to energy production and performance. 4th edn. Champaign, IL: Human Kinetics Publishers; 2004.

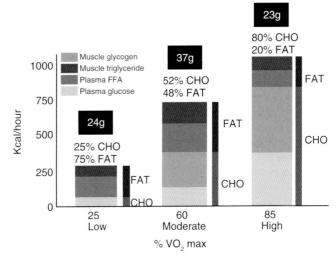

FIGURE 10.4 Fuel usage breakdown

Tucker R. Exercise and weight loss, part 3: fat. The Science of Sport; 2010 [Cited 18 December 2016. Available from http://sportsscientists.com/2010/01/exercise-and-weight-loss-part-3-fat.]

levels of activity.[5] Regarding diet, if an endurance athlete eats a higher carbohydrate diet in the days prior to an event – better known as carbohydrate loading – their body will have a higher volume of muscle glycogen prior to the event, as well as an increased rate of glycolysis at rest and during exercise. If an athlete eats a higher fat diet with lower carbohydrate levels, this will shift metabolism during aerobic exercise in favour of fat oxidation.[4] The idea of eating a high-fat, low-carbohydrate (HFLC) diet is increasing in popularity and its merits and limitations are discussed later in this chapter.

ENERGY REQUIREMENTS

Proper energy intake is the foundation of an athlete's health and ability to perform. There are multiple ways to measure energy and food intake, such as using diet apps, a food frequency questionnaire, 24-hour recall or a simple food diary kept for 3–7 days. Each method has its benefits and limitations but most likely an athlete will underreport their volume of eating no matter which method is used. Although no method is perfect, it is important to obtain and assess an athlete's daily intake of foods, liquids and supplements in order to have an overall understanding of kilojoule intake, food preferences and timing habits of eating around training.

Factors that increase an athlete's energy requirements include increased training and intensity, a hot or cold climate, high altitude, certain injuries, caffeine intake, an increase in the body's fat-free mass and potentially the luteal phase of the female cycle.[6,7] Factors that may decrease energy requirements include decreased training volume and intensity, ageing, a decrease in muscle mass and potentially the follicular phase of the reproductive cycle.[8]

When working with physically active people it is important to match food intake with energy expenditure. The volume of training can change dramatically from pre-season to mid-season or even on a daily basis depending on the training program and rest days. It is vital to take such factors into account when designing food intake and meal plans. What an athlete needs to eat on a double-session training day is very different from their intake on a rest day.

The need for athletes to maintain a healthy body composition and weight is vital for performance as well as their mental state. There is a balancing act that must occur between maintaining muscle mass, decreasing fat mass and fuelling properly for high-level training and performance. Each sport has its own metabolic profile and potential range of optimum body composition: practitioners must be aware of these parameters and consider what is potentially attainable for their patients. In addition, many people engaging in sports will not fit this 'metabolic profile' and care needs to be taken to avoid disordered eating habits, body image issues and so on. Practitioners should be aware of the warning signs for such disorders and refer their patients when needed to other healthcare professionals as appropriate, such as doctors, sports psychologists and dietitians.

CARBOHYDRATES

Carbohydrates are vital to fuel an exercising body: they are the dominant fuel source for anaerobic (glycolytic) activity and are one of the two main sources for aerobic activity. The amount of carbohydrate stored within the body (glycogen) is limited but can be manipulated via training and dietary intake on a daily basis.[8] Low glycogen stores are associated with fatigue, reduced work rate, impaired skill and concentration as well as an increased perception of effort.[6]

The amount of glycogen within the muscle cells plays a role in regulating muscle adaptation to training by altering the physical, metabolic and hormonal environment in which the signalling responses to exercise are exerted.[9] Training and nutrition strategies that use carbohydrate restriction before, during and after training or in an overall diet are referred to as 'training low' and are being recognised as having potential benefit for certain sports or specific training sessions.[10]

The amount of carbohydrate a person needs to consume on a daily basis will vary depending on many factors. No longer are strict 'high-carb' guidelines being given, but rather varying amounts of intake are suggested depending on training goals, the volume of exercise undertaken and proximity to competition or race day. Nutrition strategies are focusing on high performance or training adaptations with the nutrition tailored depending on the desired outcomes.

Carbohydrate intake guidelines

Guidelines for suggested carbohydrate intake are provided according to:
- The athlete's body weight
- The type of exercise undertaken and the training goals
- The timing of carbohydrate intake needed in relation to training or competition
- The volume of carbohydrate needed over the day in relation to training volume
- The athlete's total energy needs and body composition goals.

A higher carbohydrate intake is recommended when undertaking high-quality training, while a lower intake is suggested prior to training to promote stimulus response and prior to adaptive training with lower glycogen stores.[11] See Table 10.4 below for more details on adjusting carbohydrate intake for differing training goals. Most importantly, carbohydrate targets should be individualised for an athlete's specific needs.

Carbohydrate recommendations were previously given as a percentage of daily diet. New guidelines aim to move away from daily percentages as these were found to be too general and hard to apply in real food terms. The most recent recommendations are given in calculations of training volume and grams per kilogram of body weight. The guidelines are not absolute amounts that must be followed: individual variations must be taken into account, as some athletes will perform better at the higher end of the recommendations while others will prefer the lower end.

Table 10.3 is a simplified table of general recommendations by the International Society of Sports Nutrition, while Table 10.4 is part of the 2010 IOC

TABLE 10.3 Carbohydrate intake suggestions for physical activity	
Activity level	**Grams/kg/day**
30–60 minutes/day, 3–4 times/week	3–5
5–7 hours /week	4–6
Moderate to high intensity, 2–3 hours/day, 5–6 times/week	5–8
High-volume intense exercise, 3–6 hours/day, 1–2 sessions day, 5–6 times/week	8–10

Source: Potgieter S. Sport nutrition: a review of the latest guidelines for exercise and sport nutrition from the American College of Sport Nutrition, the International Olympic Committee and the International Society for Sports Nutrition. South African Journal of Clinical Nutrition 2013;26(1):6–16.

TABLE 10.4 Carbohydrate targets

	Situation	Carbohydrate targes	Comments on type and timing of carbohydrate intake
Daily needs for fuel and recovery			
1. The following targets are intended to provide high carbohydrate availability (i.e. to meet the carbohydrate needs of the muscles and central nervous system) for different exercise loads for scenarios where it is important to exercise with high quality and/or at high intensity. These general recommendations should be fine-tuned with individual consideration of total energy needs, specific training needs and feedback from training performance. 2. On occasions when exercise quality or intensity is less important, it may be less important to achieve these carbohydrate targets or to arrange carbohydrate intake over the day to optimise availability for specific sessions. In these cases, carbohydrate intake may be chosen to suit energy goals, food preferences or food availability. 3. In some scenarios, when the focus is on enhancing the training stimulus or adaptive response, low carbohydrate availability may be deliberately achieved by reducing total carbohydrate intake or by manipulating carbohydrate intake related to training sessions (e.g. training in a fasted state, undertaking a second session of exercise without adequate opportunity for refuelling after the first session).			
Light	Low-intensity or skill-based activities	3–5 g/kg of athlete's body weight/day	• Timing carbohydrate intake over the day may be manipulated to promote high carbohydrate availability for a specific session by consuming carbohydrate before or during the session, or in recovery from a previous session. • Otherwise, as long as total fuel needs are provided, the pattern of intake may simply be guided by convenience and individual choice. • Athletes should choose nutrient-rich carbohydrate sources to allow overall nutrient needs to be met.
Moderate	Moderate exercise program (e.g. ~1 h per day)	5–7 g/kg/day	
High	Endurance program (e.g. 1–3 h/day moderate to high-intensity exercise)	6–10 g/kg/day	
Very high	Extreme commitment (e.g. 4–5 h/day moderate to high-intensity exercise	8–12 g/kg/day	
Acute fuelling strategies			
These guidelines promote high carbohydrate availability to promote optimal performance in competition or key training sessions.			
General fuelling up	Preparation for events < 90 min exercise	7–12 g/kg per 24 h as for daily fuel needs	• Athletes may choose carbohydrate-rich sources that are low in • fibre/residue and easily consumed to ensure that fuel targets are met, and to meet goals for gut comfort or lighter 'racing weight'.
Carbohydrate loading	Preparation for events >90 min of sustained/ intermittent exercise	36–48 h of 10–12 g/kg body weight per 24 h	
Speedy refuelling	<8 h recovery between 2 fuel-demanding sessions	1–1.2 g/kg/h for first 4 h then resume daily fuel needs	• There may be benefits in consuming small regular snacks. • Carbohydrate-rich foods and drink may help ensure that fuel targets are met.
Pre-event fuelling	Before exercise >60 min	1–4 g/kg consumed 1–4 h before exercise	• Timing, amount and type of carbohydrate foods and drinks should be chosen to suit the practical needs of the event and individual preferences/experiences. • Choices high in fat/protein/fibre may need to be avoided to reduce risk of gastrointestinal issues during the event. • Low glycaemic index choices may provide a more sustained source of fuel for situations where carbohydrate cannot be consumed during exercise.
During brief exercise	<45 min	Not needed	
During sustained high intensity exercise	45–75 min	Small amounts including mouth rinse	• A range of drinks and sports products can provide easily consumed carbohydrate. • The frequent contact of carbohydrate with the mouth and oral cavity can stimulate parts of the brain and central nervous system to enhance perceptions of wellbeing and increase self-chosen work outputs.

Continued

	Situation	Carbohydrate targes	Comments on type and timing of carbohydrate intake
During endurance exercise including 'stop and start' sports	1–2.5 h	30–60 g/h	• Carbohydrate intake provides a source of fuel for the muscles to supplement endogenous stores. • Opportunities to consume food and drink vary according to the rules and nature of each sport. • A range of everyday dietary choices and specialised sports products ranging in form from liquid to solid may be useful. • Athletes should experiment to find a refuelling plan that suits their individual goals including hydration needs and gut comfort.
During ultra-endurance exercise	> 2.5–3 h	Up to 90 g/h	• As above. • Higher intakes of carbohydrate are associated with better performance. • Products providing multiple transportable carbohydrates (glucose:fructose mixtures) achieve high rates of oxidation of carbohydrate consumed during exercise.

TABLE 10.4 Carbohydrate targets—cont'd

Source: Burke LM, Hawley JA, Wong SHS, Jeukendrup AE. Carbohydrates for training and competition. Journal of Sports Sciences 2011;29(suppl):S17–27.

guidelines for carbohydrate in a training diet.[12,13] It is imperative that the practitioner understands an athlete's sport, its time commitment, energy system usage and general training schedule in order to use these guidelines.

CONSIDERATIONS FOR CARBOHYDRATE CHOICES

The choice of carbohydrate use has become a 'hot' topic of late. There are many differing opinions regarding this choice and it is up to the individual athlete and their practitioner to decide what works best for them. Issues to consider when choosing a carbohydrate source include:

- Personal food preference and willingness to consume foods in the quantities needed
- Food convenience and availability
- How much money the athlete has for a 'food budget'
- Whether the athlete is travelling after training and needs something compact and portable
- Whether refuelling is time-sensitive due to further training on the same day and thus there is a need for quick glycogen recovery
- Whether the athlete is attempting to follow 'train low' or 'sleep low' practices (low-glycogen training – see below)
- Food allergies and sensitivities; digestive comfort
- Whether nutrient-dense foods are needed in order to achieve higher carbohydrate intake targets
- Whether other macronutrients are needed in the same meal for recovery (such as protein)
- Whether the athlete has dietary restrictions such as coeliac, vegetarian or paleo
- Whether the meal needs to be low in fibre, residue, protein or fat due to timing near an event
- Whether the athlete has goals of weight loss or muscle gain.

Another factor to take into consideration is who is doing the cooking for the athlete – are they living with their parents, by themselves or with others who are sharing the meal preparation? Above all, the athlete needs to be motivated to eat the meals that are suggested. It is useless trying to make an athlete, especially a teenager, eat a food or meal they do not like. They will be more likely to skip this meal and thus compromise their glycogen stores and recovery.

Table 10.5 gives examples of carbohydrate sources in approximately 30-g amounts for ease of calculating volumes needed. It includes a range of examples and is not meant to be a list of 'health' foods, as it contains foods that are not within normal naturopathic suggestions but that athletes may use during training or events where high-glycaemic index (GI), low-fibre carbohydrates are needed.

WHOLEFOODS VERSUS FUELLING FOR SPORT

The recent focus on wholefoods and minimal sugar and processed food intake to decrease inflammation is a great move towards improved general health. However, at times athletes will need to ingest more concentrated sugars depending on their chosen sport and fuelling needs. In many endurance sports (lasting longer than 2 hours) it is vital for an athlete to have a portable, non-perishable, fast-digesting carbohydrate for fuel as their glycogen stores become depleted. Sports drinks, gels and chews have been created specifically for this need. There are wholefood options, but these may not be the most realistic choice during a race or hectic training schedule.

Carbohydrates do not always have to come from grains – many people focus on getting the majority of their carbohydrate from fruit and vegetables. Rather, the individual needs to be aware of the volume of carbohydrate in different foods and their individual needs. Each person functions better on differing amounts: athletes should start on the lower end of the guidelines and see how they feel,

TABLE 10.5 What 30 g carbohydrate looks like

General carbohydrates (30 g)

Bread	2 slices	Pasta, cooked	¾ cup
Bread roll	1 roll	Rice, cooked	½ cup
Crumpet	1.5	Hot-cross bun	1 average
Weet-Bix	3	Untoasted muesli	½ cup
Cereal (average)	½ cup	Cooked oats	1 cup
Rice cakes	4	Pancakes	2 average
Yoghurt, plain full-fat	300 g	Fruit-flavoured yoghurt	200 g
Milk	600 mL	Muesli bar	1–2 (read label)
Chocolate muesli bar	2	Crisp bread	6 biscuits

Concentrated forms of carbohydrate (30 g)

Fruit juice	300 mL	Cordial	300 mL
Soft drink	250–300 mL	Sports drink	350–400 mL
Jam	2 tablespoons	Jellybeans	10
Sugar	2 tablespoons	Honey	2 tablespoons
Sports gel	1–1.5 packets	Maple syrup	2 tablespoons

Fruit (30 g)

Fruit salad	1 cup	Orange/apple/pear	2 medium
Banana	1 large	Grapes	1 cup (12–14)
Dried figs	4 medium	Dried apricots	10 halves
Peach	2 large	Watermelon	3 cups
Sultanas/raisins	1/3 cup/45 g	Blueberries	1.5 cups
Dates	6 small	Strawberries	3 cups
Dates	2.5–3 large	Raspberries	2 cups
Kiwi	3	Mango	1 medium
Rock melon	2.2 cups	Avocado	2
Pineapple	1.5 cups	Nectarine	2

Carbohydrate-dense vegetables (30 g)

Taro root	90 g	White potato	140 g
Butternut pumpkin	300 g	Carrots	300 g
Sweet potato	150 g	Beetroot	300 g
Yam	100–110 g	Sweetcorn	120 g

working their way higher if needed, depending on their sport, volume of training and energy levels.

PROTEIN

Protein is of major importance for all athletes as it is involved in recovery, muscle building, supporting the immune system, repair and adaptation post-exercise. Exercise in combination with an adequate protein intake provides the body with the stimulus and fuel for the synthesis of contractile and metabolic proteins.[14,15] The rise in leucine concentrations and supply of exogenous amino acids is suggested to be the stimulus for this activity.[16] Research with resistance exercise has shown an upregulation of muscle protein synthesis (MPS) for at least 24 hours post-exercise and an increased sensitivity to proteins ingested.[17]

Current recommendations and variable needs

Recommendations for protein now focus on the timing of protein intake throughout the day as well as intake post-training[15] rather than just the total daily intake.

Protein intake should be assessed using the following criteria: total daily protein needs, placement for intake throughout the day, post-training needs, quality of protein ingested such as high biological value and leucine content.

Current data suggest that dietary protein intake necessary to support metabolic adaptation, repair and remodelling and for protein turnover generally ranges from 1.2 to 2.0 g/kg/d.[7] Guidelines based on per meal intake suggest 0.25–0.3 g/kg body weight, providing ~10 g essential amino acids in the early recovery phase (0–2 hours) post-exercise to optimise muscle protein synthesis, as well as other meals and snacks.[6,15,18,19] This is approximately 15–25 g of protein post-training for an average-size athlete. More or less may be needed depending on the athlete's body size. Recent research has also shown that whole-body resistance training may benefit from an intake of up to 40 g of protein to enhance muscle protein synthesis.[20] Higher intake of protein can be applied in such situations as short-term high-intensity training or when there is a decreased energy budget in order to lose weight while supporting retention of muscle mass.[14,21]

FATS

Fat is an essential part of an athlete's healthy diet. It is needed to provide fuel for the body, to assist in the absorption of fat-soluble vitamins, as part of cell membranes, for hormone production and for insulation and protection of vital organs. Each athlete will have an individual amount of fat needed in their diet depending on their body weight, body composition goals, training volume, sport of choice and nutrition goals such as fat adaptation strategies. Fat intake of less than 20% is not recommended for athletes unless it occurs in the few days before an endurance event and carbohydrate loading is being undertaken. Typical ranges vary from 20% to 35% of total energy intake for daily training. The goal is to choose healthy fats and to be aware of the overall intake in relation to body composition goals. Healthy fats to focus on are olive oil, linseed (flax) oil, avocados, coconut oil, deep-sea oily fish, raw seeds and nuts.

Fuel source

Fat is used as a major fuel source along with carbohydrate during aerobic exercise. The burning of fat as a fuel plays an important role in sparing glycogen stores during exercise up to moderate intensities. Consuming a higher fat diet while training can potentially increase fat oxidation levels, decrease reliance on glycogen and endogenous carbohydrates, and delay fatigue in endurance events.[22]

Fat adaptation strategies

Training with low glycogen stores is becoming increasingly popular with endurance athletes and those wanting to further use body fat stores for fuel. Recent research has suggested that doing this leads to improvements in increased lipid oxidation, mitochondrial biogenesis and

TABLE 10.6 Strategies used to 'train low'

Strategy	Application
Training in a fasted state	6–10 h after consumption of last meal
Training twice per day	Second session performed with low glycogen stores
Restricting carbohydrate intake during recovery period post-training	Decrease carbohydrate available post-training
Sleep low	Training in the evening, sleeping without carbohydrate replenishment and performing morning training to further decrease glycogen stores

Source: [29–34].

increased fatigue resistance.[23,24] There are multiple ways in which to 'train low' and each needs to be considered in its application, ability for the athlete to adhere to such eating schedules and ability to maintain high performance levels when necessary. The research in this area is expanding and will provide more information in the next few years. Most important for the practitioner is to consider the type of athlete and sport that may benefit from this protocol, rather than applying such ideas to all sports in a generalised manner. In-depth explanation of this topic as well as research and discussion on fat adaptation is available in several articles.[22,25–28]

Table 10.6 outlines some strategies used to 'train low'.[29–34]

The benefits of such applications need to be considered within the whole picture of wellbeing. Previous research has shown that increasing training stress may influence immune function, leading to an increased risk of illness or injury[35] and thus limiting performance gains if the athlete must take time out of training to recover from being unwell. One of the major issues with the use of these new strategies is an awareness of which sports may benefit from such methods and which may be hindered or have a negligible benefit for effort involved. The research to date is equivocal as to performance benefits for many sports and there is the potential for the downregulation of carbohydrate oxidation at higher levels.[36,37] It is of little use for a sprint athlete or swimmer who needs to perform at high intensity to upregulate fat burning when the majority of their performance needs to be well above their anaerobic threshold. The idea of fat adaptation can be applied to many sports in the off-season when lower intensity training may be undertaken for the time it takes to 'adapt'. The use of fat adaptation or low-carbohydrate high-fat diets can be more easily applied to people trying to stay fit, lose weight and not be competitive within their sport, especially in the first few months of its application. Great consideration needs to be given as to which sports and athletes may benefit from such approaches and who may be disadvantaged. The next decade of research in this area will be fascinating to watch.

FUELLING FOR TRAINING AND RECOVERY

Pre-training

Eating before training depends on multiple factors and ultimately needs to suit the athlete and their digestive system. Factors that need to be considered are the length of the session, the time of day the training is occurring, whether there are two training sessions per day or only one, the type of session occurring and the goal of the session, and the person's ability to handle food pre-training.

If the session being performed is 1 hour or less, it can easily be done with no food intake beforehand or a small snack of mainly carbohydrate. If the training is occurring early in the morning, many athletes find they don't like to eat anything then as it can make them feel unwell; if this is the case, training on empty is fine. Others don't feel well training on empty and thus need to consume a small snack. If a high-intensity, weights or strenuous session is planned, most athletes find a small snack helps them to have enough energy through the demanding session. When a session is longer than 1 hour, it is best to have a small snack before training to help sustain energy levels. For training sessions longer than 1.5 hours the athlete will probably need to fuel during the session as well. If the session is occurring later in the day, aim for a meal 2 hours prior to training or a small snack half an hour to an hour beforehand consisting of mainly carbohydrate with a little protein for stable blood sugar levels.

FOOD CHOICES

Food choices for pre-training can be almost anything that suits the athlete and their tastes. Common choices are banana, fresh dates, toast or gluten-free toast with nut butter and honey or avocado, healthy muesli bars, sports bars or homemade date-and-nut bars or a piece of fresh fruit. Approximately 20–30 g of carbohydrate is a volume that's easy to consume pre-training without creating digestive distress. It becomes a trial and error of what works for the individual.

Eating during training and sports

An athlete's training goals must be taken into consideration when deciding whether they should eat during training. Other factors include the length of the session; the goals of the session; whether the session is high intensity, slow and longer endurance, or strength; the time of day; what meals have already been eaten; and whether it is the only session of the day or there are multiple training sessions. Many people become focused on the idea of 'fat burning' within a training session and undertake exercise with prior food and no kilojoule intake during the session. At times this can benefit an athlete, but for a high-intensity session or strength work it may be more advantageous for the athlete to consume a small amount of carbohydrate during the session in order to finish their training strong and well-fuelled. The following sections explain these ideas in more detail.

SESSION LENGTH

A training session <75 minutes needs only a small snack pre-training or a small snack halfway through the session. Toast, a banana, dates, a sports bar, juice or sports drink (containing electrolytes and carbohydrate) are all great options that are easy to digest and give a good amount of carbohydrate to fuel the session.

A training session >75 minutes should be fuelled by fluids and foods consumed during the session. Athletes can eat prior to training if that is their choice but sessions of this length and longer are assisted by ingestion of carbohydrate during sport. Athletes should aim to consume 30–60 g of carbohydrate per hour for sessions of this nature. Fluid intake is also vital for longer sessions (see the hydration section below). The specific amount required depends on the athlete's training intensity, session goals and digestive comfort. Creating a quality sports nutrition plan is vital to get the most out of a training session. It is also important to consume foods or sports gels with an adequate amount of water to facilitate rapid absorption of both foods and fluids across the intestinal lining (approximately 250–300 mL for 20–25 g of carbohydrate). However, combining foods/gels with a sports drink containing carbohydrate will greatly decrease gastrointestinal absorption rates and is more likely to cause gastrointestinal disturbances. Foods and fluids must be absorbed, not just consumed, in order to assist the body.

Suggested food options during training include sports bars, sports drinks, gels and chews, banana, dates, muesli bars, and bread with honey or nut butter. Ultimately, it's about what suits the athlete and their stomach. There are many recipes for homemade sports drinks and gels to keep exposure to sucrose and artificial colourings to a minimum if that is what is desired.

MULTIPLE TRANSPORTABLE CARBOHYDRATES

Fig. 10.5[38] is an easy-to-follow guide to the volume of carbohydrate needed to be ingested depending on the length of exercise session or race. The values are not absolute and intake ultimately needs to be tailored for each individual, their digestive comfort and their training or racing needs.

Research shows that up to 90 g of multiple transportable carbohydrates can be ingested[39] during endurance events but for some athletes this will be far too much for their digestive system to handle, thus the recommendation of upwards of 60 g of carbohydrate per hour rather than a definitive amount. Each person will have to practise their intake, trialling multiple forms of carbohydrate at differing amounts to know where their individual best intake resides. Starting at the lower end of the scale and working upwards is an easier way to trial such a process than starting high and experiencing gut issues until personal comfort is reached.

Glucose can be absorbed at a rate of 60 g per hour through the digestive system, see Fig. 10.6.[40] Research has shown that it is possible to eat upwards of this amount if multiple sources of carbohydrate are ingested, such as a 2:1 glucose/fructose combination. Fructose is absorbed through a different pathway in the gut lining

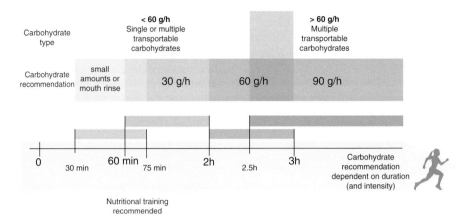

FIGURE 10.5 Recommended carbohydrate intake during exercise

www.mysportscience.com

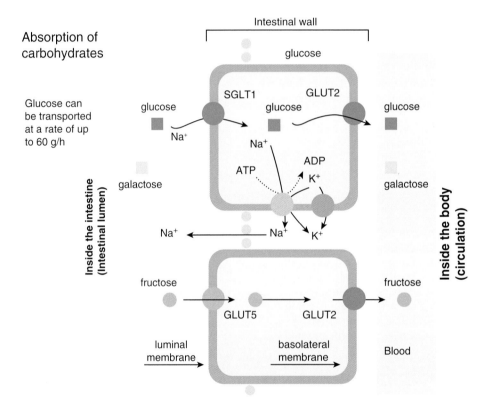

FIGURE 10.6 Absorption of carbohydrates

www.mysportsscience.com

than glucose, thus enabling higher volumes of carbohydrate ingestion when glucose transports are already saturated.[39,41–43]

A NATUROPATHIC PERSPECTIVE

The use of pure sugars, specifically fructose, is a controversial topic within complementary medicine. The general population ingests large volumes of processed foods and sugars and as practitioners there is a move to decrease sugar intake. When applying holistic health principles to sports nutrition research there is a divide regarding how to optimise an athlete's performance while attempting to do as little harm as possible. There is the option to use wholefoods instead of sports products, especially during training, but when an athlete is undertaking an event that lasts 4–6 hours or an entire day they need compact, heat-stable nutrition. Many athletes prefer to use wholefoods but care must be taken not to use high-fibre foods that slow the gastrointestinal emptying rate and potentially cause more issues than benefits. The choice of which sugars to use in training and racing is up to the practitioner and their awareness of current science, as well as ultimately what works for the athlete and their digestive system.

PROTEIN DURING TRAINING

The benefit of eating protein during training is inconclusive. There is some evidence that adding a small amount of protein to carbohydrate in a ratio of 4 : 1 during exercise may have some benefit. There is a potential improvement in endurance performance, increasing muscle glycogen stores, reducing muscle damage and promoting better training adaptations after resistance training.[44] The most recent joint position statement[6] states that 'Protein ingestion pre and during exercise seems to have less of an impact on muscle protein synthesis (MPS) than the post exercise provision but may still enhance muscle reconditioning depending on the type of training that takes place'.

Though not considered necessary for everyone, whether to eat protein during training will depend on the goals of the athlete and the training involved. Those wanting to focus on muscle protein synthesis after resistance exercise and those looking to enhance recovery from ultra-endurance training may benefit from protein intake pre- and during training.[6] Ultra-endurance athletes often choose to intake a small amount of protein and sometimes fat during events for stabilisation of blood sugar levels, for flavour variety as well as for alternative fuel sources and potentially increasing time to exhaustion. Examples are demonstrated in case study 1. For a review of the ingestion of protein during training, see the article by van Loon.[45]

Post-exercise nutrition

GOALS POST-EXERCISE

Athletes may have the following post-exercise goals:
- Change the body from a catabolic state to an anabolic state
- Replace glycogen stores
- Repair damaged tissue and build muscle
- Support immune function
- Replace fluid and electrolyte losses.

Post-training is the most vital time in an athlete's day to get their nutrition correct. The body has been challenged, has used fuels and fluids and is in a catabolic state. Proper nutrition protocols post-training can have far-reaching effects in many areas of health as well as recovery from training. Depending on the type of training the nutrition goals will vary slightly, but there are many similarities no matter the sport.

TIME BETWEEN TRAINING SESSIONS

If there are fewer than 8 hours between training sessions, carbohydrate intake should start as soon as possible post-training in order to facilitate glycogen replacement. Glycogen storage rates are at their highest in the first hour after exercise.[46,47] Glycogen synthase has been activated as well as an increase in insulin sensitivity[48] and muscle cell membrane permeability to glucose[49] post-exercise. Common recommendations are to eat a meal or snack within 30–60 minutes. Many athletes will not feel hungry at this time but encouraging them not to wait to eat will potentially enhance their recovery. A small snack or liquid meal replacement/smoothie is often an easy alternative until a proper meal can be eaten. A small amount of protein (20–25 g) at this time is also beneficial for recovery, as noted above. With an athlete undertaking two training sessions per day the importance of restocking glycogen after the first session is vital for a quality second session. Medium to high GI carbohydrate may be consumed at this time to enhance the speed of glucose delivery to the body.

If there is longer recovery between sessions (i.e. 24 hours), the pattern of meals and snacks is not as important, but it is still wise to eat a meal or snack close to finishing a training session to assist in recovery and glycogen replacement. Suggested volumes for carbohydrate intake are shown in Tables 10.3 and 10.4 and range from 1 g/kg to 1.5 g/kg in the hour post-training. Protein is also beneficial at this time in the suggested amount of 0.25–0.3 g/kg for the meal post-training. Over-restrictive eating in the post-exercise window can lead to suboptimal training, poor recovery, potential immune issues, lack of energy and a decrease in training adaptations.

OTHER CONSIDERATIONS IN EATING POST-TRAINING

Common suggestions for post-training ratios of carbohydrate to protein are 3–4 : 1, depending on the sport and individual needs.[12] See Tables 10.7 and 10.11 below for many foods and their approximate carbohydrate and protein amounts. (It is important to note that these suggestions are for an athlete's needs – as a practitioner working with individuals who want to stay fit and exercise but potentially do not do large volumes of training, these intake levels may be too high.) Trial and error, awareness of training volume and individual variation all need to be taken into account. Start at the lower end of the scale and adjust up or down depending on training volume and the athlete's feedback regarding energy levels, ability to sustain training and overall wellbeing. If an individual undertakes only a light training session, the levels may be adjusted lower to accommodate the decreased urgency for glycogen replacement post-training and consider intake to be consumed with regular meals and snacks.

POST-TRAINING PROTEIN NEEDS

Protein is important for the recovery phase after training to promote muscle hypertrophy, support the immune system and assist the repair and adaptations that occur in the body following exercise. The most recent guidelines recommend 0.25–0.3 g/kg of protein be consumed in the post-training meal.[14] Intact protein or a complete mixture of amino acids is also important.[50] Note that if insufficient volume of carbohydrate is ingested in the 4 hours post-training it can be augmented by the intake of protein (20–25 g) and thus assist in glycogen storage. If sufficient intake of carbohydrate occurs, the added protein will not give a further benefit to glycogen levels.[51]

Protein needs and muscle protein synthesis

Muscle protein synthesis after resistance exercise is an area of great focus in post-training fuelling suggestions. Recent research focuses on a variety of factors including

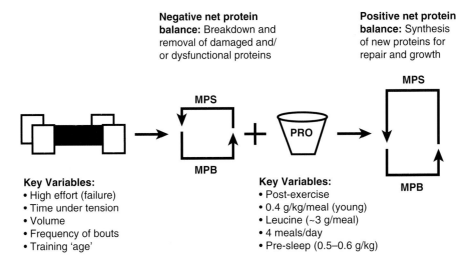

Negative net protein balance: Breakdown and removal of damaged and/or dysfunctional proteins

Positive net protein balance: Synthesis of new proteins for repair and growth

Key Variables:
- High effort (failure)
- Time under tension
- Volume
- Frequency of bouts
- Training 'age'

Key Variables:
- Post-exercise
- 0.4 g/kg/meal (young)
- Leucine (~3 g/meal)
- 4 meals/day
- Pre-sleep (0.5–0.6 g/kg)

FIGURE 10.7 Schematic showing how resistance exercise variables and protein ingestion can impact muscle protein turnover

MPS, muscle protein synthesis; MPB, muscle protein breakdown; PRO, protein.

Morton JP, Croft L, Bartlett JD, et al. Reduced carbohydrate availability does not modulate training-induced heat shock protein adaptations but does upregulate oxidative enzyme activity in human skeletal muscle. Journal of Applied Physiology 2009;106(5):1513–21.

the amount of protein ingested, the source of protein, and the potential distribution and timing of post-exercise protein ingestion.[52] Fig. 10.7 summarises important points when focusing on muscle protein synthesis.

Protein amounts

Table 10.7 lists the amount of protein in common serving sizes. The foods shown are not necessarily high in protein, or healthy; they are given as examples only. All amounts are approximate.

HYDRATION AND DEHYDRATION

Dehydration can be a serious problem for athletes and affect their ability to perform. For every 1% of body weight lost via dehydration, blood volume decreases by 2.5%, muscle water decreases by 1% and the body's core temperature can increase by 0.4–0.5°C. Losses equal to 2% of body mass are sufficient to cause a detectable decrease in performance and a risk of nausea, vomiting, diarrhoea and other gastrointestinal problems.[53]

Table 10.8 outlines the signs and symptoms of dehydration.[54]

Compromises in exercise performance

Many athletes are under the misconception that they can train their body to cope with dehydration. This is not the case and they would do well to prevent dehydration from occurring. When working with athletes it is important to explain the potential loss of performance that occurs when a person becomes dehydrated (see Table 10.9).[55–57] It is also important to enlighten athletes on the dangers of over-hydration and hyponatraemia. Individual fluid intake should be calculated and practised for appropriate

temperatures and climates in order to safely prescribe the required volume of fluid replacement.

Heat risks

The temperature a person exercises in can greatly influence their sweat rate. Climates at or below 20–21°C have insignificant dehydration effects if the exercise is <90 minutes in duration; however, >90 minutes at this temperature can lead to dehydration of more than 2% and impair performance. In a hot climate such as 31°C, exercise >60 minutes in duration can significantly impair performance if fluids are not ingested.[58,59]

Sweat rate

Factors that affect the sweat rate include:
- Genetics
- Body size – larger athletes tend to have increased sweat rates
- Fitness – fitter people sweat earlier and in larger quantities
- Environment – sweat losses are higher in heat and humidity
- Intensity – sweat losses increase the harder a person exercises.

Maintaining adequate fluid intake

Maintaining adequate fluid intake is vital for people undertaking sports, especially in hot environments such as Australia. The goal of drinking during exercise is to address the sweat losses that occur and to assist thermoregulation without drinking in excess of one's sweat rate. Fluid deficits after training need to be replenished: ingestion of fluids with post-exercise meals will aid the retention of fluids due

TABLE 10.7 The amount of protein in common serving sizes

Food	Protein (g)
Almond butter 1 tbsp	2
Almonds 33 g	6.6
Anchovies (5) 20 g	5.8
Bacon 2 slices, thick-style	10–12
Baked beans 220 g, cooked	20
Brown rice 1/2 cup, cooked	2.3
Cashews 25 g, raw	4
Chicken breast 100 g, cooked	20–25
Cottage cheese 100 g	15–18
Egg (1) 50 g, raw	5–6
Egg whites (2) 70 g, raw	7–8
Feta 28 g	4
Fish 120 g, cooked	20
Goats cheese 100 g, soft	18–19
Greek yoghurt 150 g, full-fat	11–12
Haloumi 30 g	6
Kidney beans 175 g, cooked	6.7
Lean beef or lamb 120 g, cooked	25
Milk 250 mL, low-fat 2%	11
Mozzarella 60 g	11–12
Muesli 100 g, not toasted	11
Muesli 100 g, toasted	9
Oysters 50 g, raw	6
Pine nuts 33 g	4.3
Protein powder, 1 serve	20–25
Quinoa 85 g, dry	12
Ricotta cheese 246 g	28
Rolled oats 100 g, raw	11–14
Salmon 100 g, cooked	25
Snapper/swordfish 85 g, cooked	21
Soymilk 250 mL	7
Sunflower seeds 33 g	7.6
Tofu 100 g	12
Tuna 100 g, tinned	25
White rice 1/2 cup, cooked	2.1

TABLE 10.8 Signs and symptoms of dehydration

Mild dehydration

Dry lips and mouth

Thirst

Low urine output

Moderate dehydration

Thirst

Very dry mouth

Sunken eyes

Tenting of skin when pinched with no bounce back

Low or no urine output

Severe dehydration – all signs of 'Moderate' plus

Rapid and weak pulse

Cold hands and feet

Rapid breathing

Blue lips

Lethargic, comatose, seizures

Requires immediate hospitalisation

Source: Meletis C. Dehydration: an imbalance of water and electrolytes. Water International 2002 27(3):456.

TABLE 10.9 How dehydration compromises exercise performance

Dehydration may compromise exercise performance by causing the following:

Increased perception of effort and decreased work capacity

Increased risk of heat illness

In a cold environment, cooling of core and limb temperature may lead to decreased performance

Impaired skill and concentration

Decline in cardiovascular and thermoregulatory function

Reduced rate of fluid absorption from the intestines, making it difficult to rehydrate

Thirst, irritability, dizziness, weakness, headache, chills, cramps, nausea, vomiting

Source: Murray R. Fluid needs in hot and cold environments. International Journal of Sport Nutrition 1995;5(s1):S62–73. Casa DJ, DeMartini JK, Bergeron MF, et al. National Athletic Trainers' Association position statement: Exertional heat illnesses. Journal of Athletic Training 2015;50(9):986–1000.

to the food's sodium content.[60] Athletes should aim to replace 150% of their post-exercise fluid deficit over the next 2–4 hours as fluid losses via urine and sweating will continue during the recovery period.

Athletes can estimate their own fluid requirements[60] by weighing themselves before and after a 1-hour exercise session in different seasons, temperatures, sports, etc.: each kg of weight lost is equivalent to approximately 1 L of fluid loss. There is only a small error (~10%) in this assumption.[58] Athletes cannot train their body to adapt to dehydration. It is important for athletes to practise their fluid intake during training to train their body for the intake of larger volumes.[57,61] An intake of 400–800 mL is a good starting point until the person knows their sweat rate.[59]

Fluid choices

Which fluids should be consumed is an area of great debate within sports nutrition and especially in naturopathic medicine. The inclusion of bright artificial colours and high-fructose corn syrup leaves many athletes and practitioners feeling very negative about sports drinks. However, the market now contains many drinks with more natural sugars as well as no colouring. The aim of sports drinks is to fuel an athlete with carbohydrate, electrolytes and water. There is a time and a place for their use, but unfortunately the general population is choosing them when they are not needed.

SPORTS DRINKS

For increased absorption of fluids via the small intestines, the carbohydrate content of a sports drink should be 8% (8 g per 100 mL of fluid) or lower.[62] Drinks that contain higher than a 10% solution will inhibit absorption rates and decrease the amount of fuel getting to the working muscles, potentially causing gastrointestinal disturbances. Research has shown[39] that glucose and maltodextrin saturate the intestinal transporters at 60 g/h but with the inclusion of fructose up to another 30 g can be consumed if needed (2:1 glucose to fructose ratio). This volume of carbohydrate may not be necessary or even tolerable for an athlete and they must trial the intake of carbohydrate that works for them while exercising.

Sweat losses lead to a loss of electrolytes, with higher losses of sodium and chloride and smaller amounts of potassium, calcium and magnesium.[63] Sodium and other electrolytes are added to drinks and sports drinks to: encourage fluid intake by driving the thirst mechanism, increase fluid absorption and retention and assist with salt replacement for athletes in endurance events. Electrolyte capsules and water-dissolving (effervescent) tablets are available for those looking for electrolyte replacement without the added carbohydrate of sports drinks.

Sports drinks are designed to be used during extended sporting events, when the need for fluids, electrolytes and carbohydrate is high. It is possible to consume other foods or gels and chews with plain water for the same outcome, but there are times when drinks are the easiest, most portable form of fuelling. During endurance events and sports taking place in hot environments, such products can be invaluable. It is up to the practitioner's discretion and ultimately the athlete to choose what works for them and their specific sport's profile. Sodium needs may be quite high when competing in hot environments or endurance sports or when the individual is a high sweater. If an athlete consumes fluid without adequate sodium or consumes more fluid than their sweat rate, the issue of hyponatraemia becomes a real danger. Most sports drinks do not contain sufficient sodium to equal blood sodium levels as the taste would be a deterrent to ad lib ingestion. Caution and care need to be taken in certain endurance events with electrolyte ingestion, and specifically with sodium amounts.

Extracellular sodium levels should remain between 130 and 160 mmol/L or issues of hyponatraemia can occur. This volume of sodium intake can be ingested through fluids, gels, foods and capsules. The sodium level in many sports drinks is 10–25 mmol/L – this is enough to stimulate the thirst mechanism and enhance fluid absorption but is insufficient to meet total sodium needs.[62] Higher sodium sports drinks (30–50 mmol/L) and gels may be of use if the taste can be tolerated.[64] The need for electrolyte or sodium tablets is dependent on the event being undertaken and the choice of food eaten during the event, as well as the sodium losses of the athlete.

What to look for in a sports drink

Look for the following in a sports drink:
- 4–8% carbohydrate (4–8 g carbohydrate per 100 mL) – the amount of carbohydrate will depend on what fuelling strategy is needed
- 10–25 mmol/L sodium – aim for higher sodium levels if exercising in hot/humid environment or if known high sweating athlete
- Broad spectrum of electrolytes
- Affordable and tastes good.

Table 10.10 outlines some ready-made sports drinks currently on the market.

Homemade sports drinks

Homemade sports drinks are becoming popular as people try to avoid high-fructose corn syrup and food colourings. They are not always as scientific in their recipes, especially with sodium content, but they are easy and very inexpensive to make. The internet has hundreds of examples, but the following basic recipe makes a 6% solution (6 g per 100 mL of fluid)

Recipe for homemade sports drink
- 4 tbsp maple syrup
- 1 L warm water
- 450 mg sea salt

Mix the ingredients together until the maple syrup and salt has dissolved. Alternatively, replace the maple syrup with *one* of the following:
- 4 tbsp honey or rice malt syrup
- 60 g pure glucose
- 450 mg sea salt

Drink	TABLE 10.10 Sports drinks Carbohydrate (%)	Sodium (mmol/L)
Gatorade	6	18
PowerAde	8	12
Endura	6	14
Staminade sport	7.5	14
PB	6.8	25
Cola	11	Low
Coconut water	3–4	Low

- 500 mL of fruit juice plus 500 mL of water (although this much fructose could be hard on the stomach to absorb; and it is only 55 g of carbohydrate on average)
- 2.5 tbsp glucose (40 g carbohydrate) plus 240 mL fruit juice (approximately 20 g of carbohydrate), a 2:1 glucose to fructose mix.

ALTERNATIVE FLUIDS

Coconut water has gained in popularity as a sports drink recently. It typically contains less carbohydrate and sodium than a standard sports drink but has no added food colourings. Research so far has not shown it to be more or less effective in rehydration than water or sports drinks, but neither has it been found to be worse.[65–67] If preferred as a drink post-training, there is no problem with using coconut water, although it is potentially an expensive alternative to plain water. Furthermore, in an endurance event lasting a few hours or longer it would be insufficient to supply all the necessary carbohydrate and sodium. Some research has noted gastrointestinal upset with coconut water in certain individuals, as well as decreased intake due to taste, while other studies have found increased intake due to palatability and fewer stomach issues with fresh coconut water compared with commercial sports drinks or bottled coconut water. Many fluids have been assessed for their ability to rehydrate after exercise in comparison to water. Recent research[68] has developed a beverage index for assessing a fluid's ability to rehydrate. Among the top performers are oral rehydration mix, orange juice, full-fat and skim milk and sports drink.

Carbohydrate content of foods and drinks

When working with athletes and giving them macronutrient targets to aim for, it is very useful to get them to do the calculations themselves so that they learn about the volume of food they need to ingest. Smartphone apps are also a fantastic tool to empower patients and enable them to track their intake and energy expenditure. Table 10.11 lists the carbohydrate content of many fruits and vegetables as well as milk, milk alternatives and

TABLE 10.11 Carbohydrate content of foods and drinks		
Vegetables	**Volume**		**Amount of carbohydrate (g)**
Avocado	½ cup	115 g	10
Asparagus	½ cup	90 g	4
Artichoke hearts	½ cup	85 g	10
Brussel sprouts	½ cup	80 g	6
Broccoli	½ cup	80 g	5.5
Beetroot	½ cup	85 g	8
Carrots	½ cup	80 g	5.8
Cauliflower	½ cup	50 g	2.6
Cabbage (raw)	1 cup	70 g	4
Capsicum	½ cup	75 g	3.5
Cherry tomato	5 pieces	85 g	3.3
Cucumber	¼ of	75 g	2.7
Celery	2 stalks	80 g	2.4
Chard (Swiss)	1 cup	36 g	1.6
Corn (sweet)	½ cup	82 g	20
Eggplant (cooked)	½ cup	50 g	4.3
Kale (raw)	1 cup	67 g	6.7
Kimchi	1 cup	150 g	6
Lentils (boiled)	¼ cup	50 g	10
Lettuce	1 cup	55 g	1.5
Mushrooms	1 cup	85 g	2.8
Onions (raw)	½ cup	80 g	7.5
Onions (red)	½ cup	60 g	5.8

Continued

TABLE 10.11 Carbohydrate content of foods and drinks—cont'd		
Vegetables	**Volume**		**Amount of carbohydrate (g)**
Peas (sugar/snap)	½ cup	32 g	2.4
Pumpkin (cooked)	½ cup	125 g	6
Radicchio	1 cup	40 g	1.8
Radish	6 pieces	30 g	1
Sauerkraut	½ cup	118 g	5.1
Seaweed (kelp)	½ cup	40 g	3.8
Seaweed (spirulina)	½ cup	8 g	1.8
Tofu		90 g	2.2
Spinach (raw)	1 cup	30 g	1.1
Squash, butternut (cooked)	½ cup	100 g	11
Sweet potato (cooked)	½ cup	100 g	20
Tomato (raw)	1 piece	125 g	4.8
Zucchini	½ cup	90 g	4
Fruits	**Volume**		**Amount of carbohydrate (g)**
Apple	1 piece	135 g	10
Apricot (dried)	¼ cup	33 g	20
Banana	1 medium	115 g	25
Blackberries	½ cup	75 g	8
Blueberries	½ cup	75 g	9.5
Cherries	½ cup	75 g	10
Cranberries (raw)	½ cup	55 g	6.7
Dates	¼ cup	45 g	33.5
Figs (fresh)	2 pieces	100 g	19
Grapefruit	½ cup	115 g	12.2
Grapes	½ cup	75 g	14
Grapes (raisins)	¼ cup	40 g	32.5
Guava	1 piece	55 g	8
Kiwi fruit	1 piece	75 g	11
Lemon	1 piece	110 g	11
Mandarin orange	1 medium	88 g	11
Mango	½ cup	85 g	14
Melon	½ cup	85 g	6
Melon (water)	½ cup	75 g	5.7
Orange	1 piece	130 g	15
Papaya	½ cup	70 g	7
Passionfruit	1 piece	18 g	4.2
Peach	1 medium	150 g	14.3
Pear	1 piece	150 g	20
Pineapple	½ cup	78 g	10
Plum (large)	1 piece	66 g	7.5
Pomegranate	1 piece	155 g	26
Prunes (dried)	2 pieces	17 g	10.7

| TABLE 10.11 Carbohydrate content of foods and drinks—cont'd |||
Fruits	Volume		Amount of carbohydrate (g)
Raspberries	½ cup	62 g	7.3
Strawberries	½ cup	72 g	5.5
Tangerine	1 piece	88 g	11.7
Seeds and nuts	**Volume**		**Amount of carbohydrate (g)**
Almonds	¼ cup	35 g	6
Almond butter	1 Tbs	16 g	3.5
Brazil nuts	¼ cup	35 g	4.3
Cashews	¼ cup	35 g	11
Cashew butter	1 Tbs	16 g	4.5
Flax/linseed	¼ cup	45 g	12.3
Hazelnuts	¼ cup	30 g	5.2
Macadamias	¼ cup	35 g	4.5
Peanuts	avoid		
Pecans	¼ cup	27 g	3.8
Pine nuts	1 Tbs	9 g	1
Pistachios	¼ cup	30 g	8.5
Pumpkin seeds / pepitas	¼ cup	57 g	7.6
Sesame seeds	3 Tbs	10 g	2.4
Sesame butter / tahini	1 Tbs	15 g	3.2
Sunflower seeds	1 Tbs	8 g	1.8
Sunflower seed butter	1 Tbs	16 g	4.4
Walnuts	¼ cup	30 g	4
Milks	**Volume**		**Amount of carbohydrate (g)**
Cows milk	1 cup	245 mL	12
Lactose-free milk	1 cup	245 mL	12
Rice milk	1 cup	240 mL	25
Soy milk	1 cup	240 mL	14
Coconut milk	1 cup	240 mL	7
Almond milk	1 cup	240 mL	8
Cashew milk	1 cup	240 mL	9

seeds/nuts. It does not contain grain or breads as these are previously covered in Table 10.5 or can be calculated from the back of the packaging.

FUELLING FOR COMPETITIONS AND RACE DAY

The precise nutritional needs of each sport during competitions or race days vary greatly depending on many factors, including the duration of the sport and whether there are multiple heats or games in one day. This chapter introduces the basic principles of eating for exercise, as an in-depth description of competition nutrition is beyond the scope of this textbook. The Australian Institute of Sport (AIS) and Sports Dietitians Australia both have in-depth handouts that focus on individual sports' needs during competitions or race day: see www.ausport.gov.au/ais/nutrition and www.sportsdietitians.com.au/factsheets. The case studies provided at the end of this chapter cover both training nutrition and race day needs in an attempt to demonstrate the use of sports nutrition on competition days. One case covers endurance sport and the other covers a competition day for a competitive swimmer.

DRUGS IN SPORT

Within the sporting arena, whether athletes are competing at a professional or Olympic level, routine drug testing occurs. It is an unfortunate part of sport that some competitors choose to take illegal and banned substances in order to enhance their performance. If an athlete tests positive, they can be banned for 2 years or face up to a life-time ban. Within the banned list are not only drugs but also certain methods of doping, medications and herbal substances.

The World Anti-Doping Agency (WADA) is responsible for the World Anti-Doping Code and publishes a document aiming to harmonise regulations on doping in all sports and countries. Within Australia the Australian Sports Anti-Doping Authority (ASADA) governs sports and regulations regarding such matters. Education and information are available to athletes, with yearly updates on both organisations' websites. It is up to individual athletes to make themselves aware of all the rules and regulations: failure to do so has severe penalties. The volume and variety of supplements available via pharmacies, health-food stores, practitioners and the internet is astounding. The assurance of quality within a product is under the regulation of each country's 'code' of manufacturing and this leaves athletes at risk of an accidental 'positive' result if a product contains banned substances.

Naturopathic practitioners must be aware of these guidelines and regulations. In Australia, manufacturing of supplements falls under the jurisdiction of the Therapeutic Goods Administration (TGA). Australia has very strict rules and testing procedures but this is by no means a guarantee of no prohibited substances. Neither the TGA nor Australian supplement companies can give a guarantee of product. Third-party independent testing companies are available to test batches of product for prohibited substances and an athlete and their practitioner would be advised to only use products that have been through such a process. The assumption that a product is 'clean' because it contains no banned substances is a very dangerous attitude to take. Cross-contamination within manufacturing can occur and lead to an accidental 'positive'. Other companies may knowingly place banned substances into products yet fail to disclose all ingredients. Geyer and colleagues purchased and analysed 634 supplements from 215 suppliers in 13 countries and found that 94 supplements (15%) contained banned substances.[69]

The AIS and ASADA have lists of banned substances on their websites. The AIS has created the AIS Sports Supplement Framework to educate athletes regarding the ranking of sports foods and supplements for scientific evidence, safety, legality and potential for improving sports performance. The AIS' ABCD classification system outlined in Table 10.12 is for sports foods and individual ingredients rather than specific supplements and brands.[70]

EVIDENCE-BASED SUPPLEMENTS

The American College of Sports Medicine's joint position statement on nutrition and athletic performance contains a table of dietary supplements and sports foods with evidence-based uses in sports nutrition (see Table 10.13). This table is not exhaustive: many nutrients that are not on the list may have benefit but research is not significant

TABLE 10.12 The AIS ABCD classification system for sports foods and supplement ingredients

Group A

Overview of category	Sub-categories	Examples
Evidence level Supported for use in specific situations in sport using evidence-based protocols. **Use within supplement programs** Provided or permitted for use by some athletes according to best practice protocols.	**Sports foods** – specialised products used to provide a practical source of nutrients when it is impractical to consume everyday foods.	Sports drink Sports gel Sports confectionery Liquid meal Whey protein Sports bar Electrolyte replacement Iron supplement Calcium supplement Multivitamin/mineral Vitamin D Probiotics (gut/immune) Caffeine B-alanine Bicarbonate Beetroot juice Creatine
	Medical supplements – used to treat clinical issues, including diagnosed nutrient deficiencies. Requires individual dispensing and supervision by appropriate sports medicine/science practitioner	
	Performance supplements – used to directly contribute to optimal performance. Should be used in individualised protocols under the direction of an appropriate sports medicine/science practitioner. While there may be a general evidence base for these products, additional research may often be required to fine-tune protocols for individualised and event-specific use.	

TABLE 10.12 The AIS ABCD classification system for sports foods and supplement ingredients—cont'd

Group B

Overview of category	Sub-categories	Examples
Evidence level Deserving of further research and could be considered for provision to athletes under a research protocol or case-managed monitoring situation. **Use within supplement programs** Provided to athletes within research or clinical monitoring situations.	**Food polyphenols** – food chemicals that have purported bioactivity, including antioxidant and anti-inflammatory activity. May be consumed in food form or as isolated chemical. **Other**	Quercetin Tart cherry juice Exotic berries (acai, goji etc.) Curcumin Antioxidants C and E Carnitine HMB Glutamine Fish oils Glucosamine

Group C

Overview of category	Sub-categories	Examples
Evidence level Have little meaningful proof of beneficial effects. **Use within supplement programs** Not provided to athletes within supplement programs. May be permitted for individualised use by an athlete where there is specific approval from (or reporting to) a sports supplement panel.	Category A and B products used outside approved protocols. The rest – if you can't find an ingredient or product in Groups A, B or D, it probably deserves to be here. Note that the Framework will no longer name Group C supplements or supplement ingredients in this top-line layer of information. This will avoid the perception that these supplements are special.	See list for Category A and B products. Fact sheets and research summaries on some supplements of interest that belong in Group C may be found on the 'A–Z of Supplements' page in the AIS Sports Nutrition section of the ASC website.

Group D

Overview of category use within AIS system	Sub-categories	Examples
Evidence level Banned or at high risk of contamination with substances that could lead to a positive drug test. **Use within supplement programs** Should not be used by athletes.	**Stimulants** http://list.wada-ama.org	Ephedrine Strychnine Sibutramine Methylhexanamine (DMAA) Other herbal stimulants
	Prohormones and hormone boosters http://list.wada-ama.org	DHEA Androstenedione 19-norandrostenione/ol Other prohormones Tribulus terrestris and other testosterone boosters Maca root powder
	GH releasers and 'peptides' http://list.wada-ama.org Technically, while these are sometimes sold as supplements (or have been described as such) they are usually unapproved pharmaceutical products.	
	Other http://list.wada-ama.org	Glycerol used for re/hyperhydration strategies – banned as a plasma expander Colostrum – not recommended by WADA due to the inclusion of growth factors in its composition

Source: Australian Sports Commission. ABCD Classification; 2016 [Cited 19 December 2016. Available from www.ausport.gov.au/ais/nutrition/supplements/classification.]

TABLE 10.13 Dietary supplements and sports foods with evidence-based uses in sports nutrition

Category	Example	Use	Concern	Evidence
Sports food	Sports drinks Sports confectionery Sports gels Electrolyte supplements Protein supplements Liquid meal supplements	Practical choice to meet sports nutritional goals especially when access to food, opportunities to consume nutrients or gastrointestinal concerns make it difficult to consume traditional food and beverages	Cost is greater than whole foods May be used unnecessarily or in inappropriate protocols	Burke & Cato (2015)
Medical supplements	Iron supplements Calcium supplements Vitamin D supplements Multi-vitamin/mineral Omega-3 fatty acids	Prevention or treatment of nutrient deficiency under the supervision of appropriate medical/nutritional expert	May be self-prescribed unnecessarily without appropriate supervision or monitoring	Burke & Cato (2015)

Specific performance	Ergogenic effects	Physiological effects/ mechanism of ergogenic effect	Concerns regarding	Evidence
Creatine	Improves performance of repeated bouts of high-intensity exercise with short recovery periods - Direct effect on competition performance - Enhanced capacity for training	Increases Creatine and Phosphocreatine concentrations May also have other effects such as enhancement of glycogen storage and direct effect on muscle protein	Associated with acute weight gain (0.6–1 kg) which may be in weight sensitive sports May cause gastrointestinal problems Some products may not contain appropriate amounts of creatine	Tarnopolsky (2010)
Caffeine	Reduces perception of fatigue Allows exercise to be sustained at optimal intensity/output for longer	Adenosine antagonist with effects on many body targets including central nervous system Promotes Ca^{2+} release from sarcoplasmic reticulum	Causes side effects (tremor, anxiety, increased heart rate, etc.) when consumed in very high doses Rules of National Collegiate Athletic Association competition prohibit the intake of large doses that produce urinary caffeine levels exceeding 15 micrograms/mL Some products do not disclose caffeine dose or may contain other stimulants	Astorino & Roberson (2010) Tarnopolsky (2010) Burke et al. (2013)
Sodium bicarbonate	Improves performance of events that would otherwise be limited by acid–base disturbances associated with high rates of anaerobic glycolysis - High intensity events of 1–7 minutes - Repeated high-intensity sprints - Capacity for high-intensity 'sprint' during endurance exercise	When taken as an acute dose pre-exercise, increases extracellular buffering capacity	May cause gastrointestinal side effects which cause performance impairment rather than benefit	Carr et al. (2011)
Beta-alanine	Improves performance of events that would otherwise be limited by acid–base disturbances associated with high rates of anaerobic glycolysis - Mostly targeted at high-intensity exercise lasting 60–240 seconds - May enhance training capacity	When taken in a chronic protocol, achieves increase in muscle carnosine (intracellular buffer)	Some products with rapid absorption may cause paraesthesia (tingling sensation)	Quesnele et al. (2014)

TABLE 10.13 Dietary supplements and sports foods with evidence-based uses in sports nutrition—cont'd

Specific performance	Ergogenic effects	Physiological effects/ mechanism of ergogenic effect	Concerns regarding	Evidence
Nitrate	Improves exercise tolerance and economy Improves performance in endurance exercise at least in non-elite athletes	Increases plasma nitrite concentrations to increase production of nitric oxide with various vascular and metabolic effects that reduces O_2 cost of exercise	Consumption in concentrated food sources (e.g. beetroot juice) may cause gut discomfort and discolouration of urine Efficacy seems less clear cut in high-calibre athletes	Jones (2014)

Source: [108–115]

TABLE 10.14 Evidence-based functional foods

Functional food	Justification/action	Evidence
Tart cherry juice	Facilitates recovery by modulating inflammation and/or oxidative stress; reduces some markers of muscle damage including muscle pain and soreness	[73–79]
Turmeric/curcumin	Antioxidant, anti-inflammatory, decreases pain, decreases oedema, increases nitric oxide	[80,81]
Probiotics	Immune and digestive system support, decreased incidence of illness (URTI) and decreased illness duration	[82–84]
Other foods of interest: berries, blueberries, green tea, pomegranate, spirulina, mushrooms (beta-glucans) and bromelain (pineapple), pickle juice, ginger and bitter tonics	For a review of some of these foods in relation to exercise-induced muscle damage, see the article by Sousa and colleagues.[72] Comprehensive reviews on many foods and supplements can be found at www.examine.com.[85]	

enough or may show both negative and positive effects and thus is not included. An example is vitamins C and E being nutrients that in high doses have been found to reduce indices of oxidative damage but have also been shown to have detrimental effects on the adaptive and recovery processes of exercise as they can interfere with the signalling functions of reactive oxygen species.[71] Sousa and colleagues[72] have written a comprehensive review on dietary strategies for reducing exercise-induced muscle damage looking at both wholefoods and specific nutrients. The evidence behind certain complementary medicines may be strong but it is not specific for sports performance. Thus practitioners need to use their knowledge and understanding of human physiology and biochemistry to assist athletes and those undertaking sports to enhance their health in a holistic manner.

Evidence-based, non-sports specific supplements

The information in Table 10.14 is specifically for those athletes competing at the higher levels of sport: the use of nutritional supplements and herbal medicine for non-drug tested athletes is not an issue. The use of complementary medicine to enhance general wellbeing, support the body while under stress, correct nutritional deficiencies and support the immune and musculoskeletal system are areas that naturopaths are well educated in.

However, the application of naturopathic principles to the domain of sports nutrition is a newer concept. The ability of naturopaths to look at athletes from a holistic perspective gives athletes a further area of support beyond macronutrient-based sports nutrition guidelines. The ability to go beyond dietary interventions and support the body's systems with herbal medicine and nutrients enables a more holistic treatment of athletes and their needs.

Nutrients and foods

Proper nutrition is vital for sports performance. As training loads increase, so too do the demands on the body for many nutrients. There is a growing body of evidence for the use of functional foods and nutritional supplements for athletes. Funding for research in this area is on the increase as science looks to natural foods and nutrients to support energy demands and overall health. Table 10.15 contains a general list of nutrients that may benefit individuals undertaking exercise; this is not an evidence-based list specific to athletes (that can be found in Table 10.14 above). It also contains the RDI (recommended dietary intake) for each nutrient.[86] Athletes' needs may be higher, especially during times of large-volume training, but foods should always be the focus first, with supplements used when there is a dietary shortfall or when an injury or illness potentially increases needs.

TABLE 10.15 Nutrients			
Nutrient	**Justification**	**RDI**	**Dietary source**
Alpha lipoic acid	Blood sugar regulation	No RDI available	Red meat, liver, heart, kidney
Bioflavonoids	Enhances the absorption of vitamin C; helps maintain the health of small blood vessel walls	No RDI available	Citrus fruits, buckwheat, vegetables
Calcium	Bone health; muscle contraction; nerve impulse transmission	1000–1300 mg/day	Almonds, dairy, figs, small fish with edible bones, tahini, sesame seeds, molasses, tofu, green leafy vegetables
Chromium	Component of glucose tolerance factor, required for blood sugar regulation, glucose and fat metabolism	25–35 micrograms/day	Apples, asparagus, oysters, prunes, cheese, meat, broccoli, apples, bananas
Coenzyme Q10	Minimises oxidative damage; necessary for cellular metabolic processes and ATP production	No RDI available	Almonds, broccoli, mackerel, sardines, salmon, sesame seeds
Glutamine	The most prevalent amino acid in muscles, important in maintaining immune function; a key nutrient for the health of the intestines and digestive tract integrity	No RDI available	Beans, legumes, cottage cheese, ham, most protein sources, ricotta cheese, rolled oats, whey protein and products
Iodine	Healthy thyroid function	150 micrograms/day	Iodised salt, seaweed, seafood
Iron	Involved in transportation and storage of oxygen in the body and in the creation of energy; involved in general growth, reproduction, healing and the immune system; indicated in anaemia	8–18 mg/day	Red meat, apricots, oysters, sunflower seeds, pumpkin seeds, pine nuts, spinach, molasses, kidney beans
Magnesium	Essential for hundreds of enzymatic reactions in the body, the burning of glucose for fuel and for muscle contractions; assists in carbohydrate and fat metabolism, DNA and protein synthesis, active transport of ions across cell membranes	310–420 mg/day	Green leafy vegetables, cocoa, almonds, brewer's yeast, cashews, kelp, wheat bran, wheatgerm, buckwheat, nuts and seeds
N-acetyl-cysteine (NAC)	Antioxidant (reactive scavenging species)	No RDI available	Supplement only
Omega-3 fatty acids	Precursor to eicosanoids; anti-inflammatory and cell wall integrity	90–160 mg/day (DHA + EPA + DPA)	Salmon, sardines, trout, herring, mackerel
Potassium	Maintains fluid balance; principal cation of intracellular fluid; involved with nerve impulse transmission	2800–3800 mg/day adequate intake (AI) as no RDI available	Vegetables, sardines, avocados, bananas, dates, citrus fruits, yams, squash, Swiss chard, artichokes, spinach, tomatoes
Probiotics	Help strengthen digestive tract health and support immune system, potentially reducing the incidence of some illnesses	Strain dependent; multi-strains are advisable	Yoghurt, miso soup, sauerkraut, kefir, kombucha, pickles, tempeh, kimchi
Quercetin and other plant polyphenols	Antioxidant, anti-inflammatory, antipathogenic	No RDI available	Cocoa, apples, pears, pomegranates, citrus fruits, red grapes, green leafy vegetables, red wine, green tea
Silica	Repair of scar tissue; reduction of adhesion formation	No RDI available	Barley, oats, wholegrain cereals, root vegetables, horsetail tea
Sodium	Assists in absorption of glucose, amino acids and water; regulator of extracellular fluid status; involved with electrochemical gradient; important for nerve cell transition, muscle contraction and heart function	460–920 mg/day Western diet likely ample, may need supplementation in some endurance and ultra-endurance events (see case study 1)	Table salt, wholegrains, vegetables, meats, legumes, nuts and seeds, sports drinks, many packaged foods
Vitamin A	Involved in supporting normal immune system function; antioxidant; involved in synthesis of proteins and red blood cell development	700–900 micrograms/day	Kohlrabi; egg yolk; carrots; apricots; cod and salmon liver oil; green leafy vegetables; red, yellow and orange fruits and vegetables

Nutrient	Justification	RDI	Dietary source
TABLE 10.15 Nutrients—cont'd			
Vitamin B₁ (thiamine)	Co-enzyme in the body with essential roles in metabolism and ATP production; synthesis in DNA and RNA	1.1–1.2 mg/day	Legumes, wheatgerm, wholegrains, nuts, asparagus, lettuce, mushrooms, lentils
Vitamin B₂ (riboflavin)	Co-factor within numerous enzyme systems within the body; red blood cell production; part of the electron transporter FAD	1.1–1.3 mg/day	Avocados, beans, sprouts, broccoli, eggs, milk, mushrooms, asparagus, green leafy vegetables
Vitamin B₃ (niacin)	Required for energy production (part of electron transporter NAD); involved in the synthesis of certain hormones (e.g. oestrogen, progesterone and testosterone); assists in DNA repair	14–16 mg/day	Almonds, chicken, eggs, legumes, salmon, sardines, tuna, asparagus, mushrooms, halibut, sea vegetables such as kelp and wakame, lentils and lima beans
Vitamin B₅ (pantothenic acid)	Required for steroid hormone, cholesterol and neurotransmitter production, formation of acetyl-CoA	4–6 mg/day	Avocados, egg yolk, sweet potato, green vegetables, cauliflower, broccoli, mushrooms
Vitamin B₆ (pyridoxine)	Helps in the creation of neurotransmitters and steroid hormones; supports nervous and immune systems	1.3–1.5 mg/day	Chicken, egg yolk, legumes, salmon, tuna, walnuts, beans, oats, potato, bananas, hazelnuts
Vitamin B₉ (folic acid)	Co-enzyme in the metabolism of amino and nucleic acids; assists in red blood cell creation	400 micrograms/day	Leafy green vegetables, lentils, eggs, beans, citrus and wholegrains
Vitamin B₁₂	Enzyme co-factor in creating and maintaining nerve and red blood cells and DNA synthesis	2.4 micrograms/day	Salmon, sardines, egg yolk, oysters, trout, beef, yoghurt, tuna, fermented foods
Vitamin C	Antioxidant, immune stimulant	45 mg/day	Blackcurrants, kiwi fruits, mangoes, guava, rosehips, strawberries, parsley, citrus fruits
Vitamin D₃	Key role in immunity and bone health	5–10.0 micrograms/day	Fish liver oils, egg yolk, sprouted seeds, milk
Vitamin E	Antioxidant; helps support the immune system; aids to protect cells from damage	7–10 mg/day (natural mixed forms)	Almonds, wheatgerm, safflower, egg yolks, corn, beef, nuts
Zinc	Involved in muscle growth; vital for the immune system and hormone creation; role in the structure of proteins and cell walls (membranes), regulation of gene expression, cell signalling and nerve impulse transmission	8–14 mg/day	Beef, baked beans, wholegrains, oysters, pumpkin seeds, cashews, sunflower seeds, sesame seeds, wild game, poultry

Source: ww.nrv.gov.au/nutrients

Herbal medicines

An array of herbal medicines can be used to support the body while undertaking large volumes of exercise. Their application should follow traditional naturopathic concepts of treating and supporting the whole person. Many classes of herbs shown in Table 10.16 are given for general support or are indicated in acute situations where athletes undertake high volumes of training that are exhausting, leading to overtraining and immune suppression.[87] When applying support with herbal medicine, practitioners should view each athlete, their sport, training volume, previous medical history, current medications, stress levels, and so on.

SPECIFIC HERBAL MEDICINES AND SPORTS PERFORMANCE

The term 'adaptogen' is applied to a classification of herbs containing phytonutrients that assist in the regulation of metabolism when the body is under physical or mental stress. They help the body adapt by (a) normalising system functions, (b) developing resistance to future such stress and (c) elevating the body's functioning to a higher level of performance.[88,89] The use of adaptogens to support the wellbeing of athletes is an area where naturopathic practitioners can greatly assist their patients. Supporting the body in times of stress, from both daily life and

TABLE 10.16 Herbal medicine classes			
Specific herbal medicine classes	**Action**	**Potential holistic application to sport**	**Examples**
Adaptogen	Increases resistance to physical, environmental, emotional or biological stress; assists the body in adapting at heightened times of stress	High-volume training, overtraining and exhaustion	• *Panax ginseng* (Korean ginseng) • *Eleutherococcus senticosus* (Siberian ginseng) • *Panax quinquefolius* (American ginseng) • *Astragalus membranaceus* (Astragalus) • *Rhodiola rosea* (Rhodiola) • *Schisandra chinensis* (Schisandra) • *Withania somnifera* (Ashwagandha) • *Codonopsis pilosula* (Codonopsis) • *Bacopa monnieri* (Bacopa/Brahmi) • *Lentinula edodes* (Shiitake)
Adrenal tonic	Aids in nourishing and renewing the adrenal gland, where there has been stress leading to exhaustion and debility	High-volume training; adrenal support	• *Glycyrrhiza glabra* (Liquorice) • *Withania somnifera* (Ashwagandha) • *Rehmannia glutinosa* (Rehmannia)
Anodyne/analgesic	Used to relieve pain	Assists in pain relief from training and delayed-onset muscle soreness	• *Corydalis ambigua* (Corydalis) • *Curcuma longa* (Turmeric)
Antibacterial/ antiviral/ antimicrobial	Destroys or inhibits bacterial or viral growth	Athletes with immunity issues; increased incidence of upper respiratory tract infections; supports the immune system while under heavy training load	• *Echinacea* spp. (Echinacea) • *Sambucus nigra* (Elder) • *Hydrastis canadensis* (Golden seal) • *Glycyrrhiza glabra* (Liquorice) • *Berberis vulgaris* (Barberry) • *Allium sativum* (Garlic) • *Astragalus membranaceus* (Astragalus) • *Hypericum perforatum* (St John's wort)
Anti-inflammatory (musculoskeletal)	Reduces the response to injury, infection or irritation	Assists the body during inflammation caused by injury and training	• *Curcuma longa* (Turmeric) • *Zingiber officinale* (Ginger) • *Rehmannia glutinosa* (Rehmannia) • *Centella asiatica* (Gotu kola) • *Salix alba* (White willow)
Antioxidant	Protects the body from oxidative damage and is a potential free radical scavenger	Oxidative damage due to training load	• *Schisandra chinensis* (Schisandra) • *Rhodiola rosea* (Rhodiola) • *Curcuma longa* (Turmeric) • *Rosmarinus officinalis* (Rosemary) • *Olea Europa* (Olive leaf)
Antispasmodic (muscles)	Reduces muscular cramping, spasm or tension	Injury and spasm due to training and racing	• *Chamomilla recutita* (Chamomile) • *Coleus forskohlii* (Coleus) • *Glycyrrhiza glabra* (Liquorice) • *Viburnum opulus* (Cramp bark) • *Mentha x piperita* (Peppermint) • *Corydalis ambigua* (Corydalis)
Bitter tonic	Promotes appetite, digestion and absorption of nutrients	Increases appetite when suppressed due to heavy training load and exhaustion	• *Gentiana lutea* (Gentian) • *Andrographis paniculata* (Andrographis) • *Cynara scolymus* (Globe artichoke) • *Picrorhiza kurroa* (Picrorhiza)
Blood sugar modulator/regulator	Assists to regulate the concentration of blood glucose	Assists in general health and blood sugar regulation, weight maintenance	• *Codonopsis pilosula* (Codonopsis) • *Gymnema sylvestre* (Gymnema) • *Cinnamomum zeylanicum* (Cinnamon) • *Glycyrrhiza glabra* (Liquorice)
Connective tissue regenerator	Assists to regenerate tissues that provide support and structure in the body	Assists in healing and injury from sport	• *Centella Asiatica* (Gotu kola)
Energy production	Assists in energy production	Assists in energy production and wellbeing	• *Eleutherococcus senticosus* (Siberian ginseng) • *Panax ginseng* (Korean ginseng) • *Rhodiola rosea* (Rhodiola)

	TABLE 10.16 Herbal medicine classes—cont'd		
Specific herbal medicine classes	**Action**	**Potential holistic application to sport**	**Examples**
Immunomodulator/ stimulant	Assists, enhances or modifies immune functions and regulation	Supports immune system under heavy training load	• *Echinacea* spp. (Echinacea) • *Astragalus membranaceus* (Astragalus) • *Cordyceps militaris* (Cordyceps)
Lymphatic	Improves the flow of lymphatic fluid or drainage	Supports immune system and recovery with increased lymphatic flow	• *Galium aparine* (Cleavers) • *Phytolacca decandra* (Poke root) • *Calendula officinalis* (Calendula)
Nervine tonic	Nourishes and strengthens the nervous system and its function; can have a relaxant effect on the body	Supports holistically for exhausted and stressed athletes; increases relaxation to assist in sleep and recovery	• *Melissa officinalis* (Lemon balm) • *Scutellaria lateriflora* (Skullcap) • *Verbena officinalis* (Vervain) • *Leonurus cardiaca* (Motherwort) • *Avena sativa* (Oats) • *Bacopa monnieri* (Bacopa/Brahmi) • *Hypericum perforatum* (St John's wort) • *Zizyphus spinosa* (Zizyphus) • *Passiflora incarnata* (Passionflower) • *Withania somnifera* (Ashwagandha)
Sleep enhancement, hypnotic/sedative	Assists the body and nervous system in relaxing and higher quality sleep	Assists the body in recovery from training; supports healthy immune system and weight management via enhancing sleep; potentially decreases stress levels	• *Chamomilla recutita* (Chamomile) • *Scutellaria lateriflora* (Skullcap) • *Eschscholzia californica* (California poppy) • *Lavandula angustifolia* (Lavender) • *Passiflora incarnata* (Passionflower) • *Piscidia erythrina* (Jamaican dogwood) • *Valeriana officinalis* (Valerian) • *Zizyphus spinosa* (Zizyphus)

training, can have a large impact on an individual's health and wellbeing. There is varied research as to the use of the following adaptogens with athletes and this is an area of future investigation that should be undertaken with well-designed trials to bring these ancient herbs into the 21st century of evidence-based complementary medicine.

Korean ginseng

Korean ginseng has been investigated for its adaptogenic and stress-attenuating activity. It has been shown to enhance cognitive performance in healthy young adults[90,91] but review of data by Bucci[92] showed the effect of ginseng on human exercise performance to be dose- and duration-of-supplementation-sensitive. In chronic use it is believed to improve cardiorespiratory function and lower lactate concentrations in the blood, as well as improving physical performance. Its effects were more noted for those in a poor physical condition.[93] Chen and colleagues[94] suggest future studies take into consideration number of participants, longer length of trial and dosage to better substantiate the ergogenic effects of Korean ginseng on humans and exercise performance.

Siberian ginseng

Siberian ginseng is a herb with long traditional use as an adaptogen and to combat fatigue and exhaustion. Recent research that examined the impact of an 8-week intake of the herb found that it enhances endurance capacity,

elevates cardiovascular function and has a metabolic glycogen-sparing effect in recreationally trained athletes.[95] Much of the research on Siberian ginseng is from Russia and is either unavailable or dated, although substantial in its claims and participant numbers. Goulet and Dionne[96] reviewed the literature on Siberian ginseng and found the methodology in many trials to be weak. Eschback and colleagues[97] produced no significant results from their trial but supplementation was only administered for one week prior to testing. Traditional use of Siberian ginseng is much longer in its administration and it is typically used at times of debility, exhaustion and convalescence. Further research would be of interest with well-controlled methodology, traditional dosages and length of administration.

Rhodiola

Rhodiola has robust traditional and pharmacological evidence of use in fatigue and potential emerging evidence for cognition and mood enhancement.[98] Research has demonstrated a decrease in fatigue and an increased perception of wellbeing as related to life stress.[99] Further studies have shown a decrease in C-reactive protein and creatine kinase levels in exhaustive exercise,[100,101] thus having potential application in decreasing muscle damage from physical activity. Rhodiola appears to be able to reduce the effects of physical exhaustion and fatigue experienced from life stress and low-intensity exercise.[102]

Ashwagandha

Traditionally ashwagandha has been used as a tonic and adaptogen in Ayurvedic medicine for supporting those with general debility, nervous exhaustion, muscular fatigue and memory and sleep issues. It has been shown to relieve insomnia and stress-induced depression,[103] which could potentially aid athletes if they fall into overtraining issues where stress and sleeplessness become a concern. It has also been shown to reduce cortisol levels and thus assist in the immunosuppression that occurs with high stress.[104] It can assist both sedentary and athletic populations by improving physical performance and memory.[105] Wankhede[106] recently found that supplementation is associated with significant increases in muscle mass and strength, and suggests it has potential to be used alongside strength training.

WORKING WITH SPORTS CLIENTS

Sportspeople are some of the most positive patients to work with. Their attitude, motivation and willingness to take on large-scale changes to diet and lifestyle are impressive. It is common to be working with such people to reach optimum health rather than dealing with chronic disease and long-term poor health habits. They can be fast to adopt changes suggested and at times may even need to be slowed down in their optimism for overhauling their entire food intake. Practitioners working with athletes who already have a good standard of health with no underlying issues may only need two or three appointments as the practitioner takes on more of an education role regarding sports nutrition principles and practices.

The harder aspects of working with sportspeople comes in the form of a singular focus leaning towards obsessiveness around food choices, weight, body fat and training schedules. They can be motivated but at the same time want results very quickly, and at times the human body doesn't heal as quickly as they want it to. Teaching moderation and passive recovery in the form of good sleep hygiene, rest days when unwell and relaxing their eating regimen at times can be difficult. The media and internet are great sources of information for many athletes and practitioners may have to 'retrain' patients into a more evidence-based approach to food and health that may be contradictory to what they have read on the internet or learned from their training partners.

One of the largest hurdles in working with athletes and those undertaking high volumes of training is to teach them to rest and take time off from their training when they are unwell. Many athletes have a fear of losing fitness or muscle mass or not being ready for an upcoming race or event. Practitioners need to explain the dangers of further immune stress and that taking a few days off to let the body recover may be far less intrusive to a training schedule than trying to train through an illness and prolonging ultimate recovery. The idea of nourishing the body and supporting its inherent needs is a concept that many hyper-focused athletes find hard to incorporate into their fitness and health regimens.

Application of scientific and naturopathic principles

Understanding the science and principles of sports nutrition is one thing, but learning how to apply them with patients is another. What needs to be taken into consideration and how should research be used? What is the evidence-based science and on whom was research done? Is the research applicable to the patient and their level of sport participation and fitness? After using the applicable research, what individual things need to be considered with the specific person? Practitioners must be aware of and educated in differentiating between clearly evidence-based research and media hype and testimonials by elite athletes or well-written marketing hype by companies. Athlete endorsements are not proof that a certain diet or supplement works: the latest 'fad diet' can be just that, a fad and not an evidence-based nutritional approach. Evidence-based sports nutrition should always be the foundation for patient treatment protocols, and then individual variation and the application of naturopathic principles can be brought in to complement the case in hand. Athletes are not just their sport – the rest of their stress and lifestyle will have a dynamic influence on their health and this needs to be assessed and treated.

Case taking

Things to consider about a sports patient that may be different from a non-athlete patient include the following:
- Are they an elite/professional athlete who will be drug tested and thus giving anything more than food and diet suggestions takes on a much larger consideration?
- Are they a serious competitor, trying to qualify for Masters or world championships within their age group, or are they a weekend warrior just out having fun?
- What is their general fitness routine, training schedule, racing schedule or competition season?
- Is there a clear understanding by both practitioner and patient of the metabolic profile and demands of the sport being undertaken?
- Is there a need for training nutrition and a separate protocol for race day nutrition?

These questions do not form part of the regular case history and questions asked in a naturopathic consultation. Understanding the individual and their sport is of utmost importance before an evidence-based protocol of sports nutrition can be suggested.

Food diary

A seven-day food, fluid and training diary undertaken by the patient before the first appointment can be vital in helping the practitioner to understand the patient's needs. However, not all people are motivated to keep a food diary and there are multiple ways to assess a person's intake of food and fluids. Nutrition apps for smartphones, taking photos of foods eaten and simply keeping a paper journal diary can all be used.

A food, fluid and training diary gives great insight into the patient's general habits, snacking routine, food likes and dislikes, and intake of supplements, powders, gels and bars, as well as presenting the practitioner with a foundation of food intake to build on rather than suggesting a completely different diet from what the person normally eats. The less change the practitioner suggests, the more likely the person will be able to follow the new protocol. The diary also provides information on the person's training schedule, length of training sessions, types of exercise undertaken and hydration habits (or lack thereof). In addition, a well-planned diary can be constructed to chart the person's digestive function, bowel movements, emotional state at the time of eating and stress levels. The following should be considered when undertaking a food, fluid and training diary:

- It is important to record the exact time of food and fluid intake for the entire day (e.g. 7.30 am, not 'breakfast'), as there is a need to understand what foods and fluids are consumed before, during and after training
- The length of the training session, the time of day it occurred and the type of exercise need to be considered in order to construct a meal plan that fits into the patient's lifestyle and habits
- The food and fluids taken during training sessions will give a clear understanding of the patient's habits in fuelling, over-fuelling or under-fuelling their training sessions
- Single or double training sessions per day will make a big difference to kilojoule and carbohydrate needs, and post-training fuelling will become more important in order to replenish glycogen stores for the second session of the day unless 'training low' is being implemented.

Issues to consider when assessing a food diary include the following:

- Is there adequate protein at each meal and snacks for the training volume undertaken?
- Is the patient eating at the appropriate time post-training and with the right volume of carbohydrates and protein for their individual needs?
- Is the patient hitting their carbohydrate targets each day or eating their carbohydrates at the appropriate meals if they are 'training low'?
- Is the patient over-focusing on the little things and missing the big picture of food intake and general health?
- How is the patient's hydration intake? Is it adequate and at the correct time for training?
- When the patient is craving or eating sweets, is it a mental or a physical craving? Are they eating at appropriate times in order to avoid blood sugar lows that may trigger sweet cravings?
- Is the patient taking too many supplements in order to enhance performance and not focusing on the basics of good sports nutrition? Where do they need supplement support and what can be done using a food first protocol?
- Does the patient follow good meal preparation and planning or are they short of time, defaulting to unhealthy choices because of lack of availability? If so, what can be done about this, such as weekly meal planning, shopping and preparation, or home delivery of groceries or pre-made meals?
- Does the patient know what healthy snacks can be found at supermarkets and convenience stores if they get caught short rather than skipping meals or making poor choices?

Systems review

Sports patients may arrive at the naturopathic consultation as healthy individuals. The case history may be shortened, depending on the person. Many athletes want only a food and fuelling focus and are not aware or overly concerned with other body systems and their workings. Practitioners need to consider their holistic training as well as the patient's wants in order to support what the individual is seeking from the appointment. Areas of greater concern for many athletes seeking a holistic focus to their health include a medical history, blood tests, previous injuries, sporting background, weight concerns, ability to recover quickly, energy levels, immune system issues, musculoskeletal problems, digestion and bowel health, kilojoule intake adjustment, sleep, work–life balance and stress management.

Note with athletes that it is best to take bloods at least 24 hours after the person's last training session. Exercise can create false results for many blood tests, especially iron studies. Ask the person to abstain from exercise as they will not know this. The morning after a full rest day is best as the person will have had more than 30–35 hours without training.

Considerations with athletes

As noted previously, athletes have different needs to regular naturopathic patients dealing with chronic health issues. Many of the general wellness suggestions given will be the same, as all individuals need certain volumes of sleep, fluids, etc. However, the questions a practitioner may also need to cover when working with athletes include:

- What sport is being undertaken (power, endurance etc.)?
- How long is the sports season and where is the person currently in the season?
- In what environment does the sport occur? Is it a summer or winter sport? Does it occur outdoors or indoors?
- How often does the person train? Daily, twice per day or a few times per week?
- What time of day does training or racing occur and for how long?
- What foods does the person consume pre-, during and post-training or racing?
- What is the food availability at the training venue?
- Who does the person live with and who is involved in meal preparation and shopping? If they live in a dormitory or on campus at an institution, what foods are available for them there? What is the person's ability and desire to cook their own food? What is their general attitude to cooking and money spent on food?

There are many more things to consider for the individual athlete, but the above questions are a great starting point in understanding an individual's nutritional needs and habits.

RACE DAY/COMPETITION CONSIDERATIONS

Considerations for racing and competition include:
- What are the person's food needs in the week or days leading up to a race?
- Does the person need to change their diet to increase carbohydrates and so on?
- What is the food availability if the person is flying to another country or town? What are they allowed to take with them across international borders?
- What does the person need to consume during a race? Has this been planned appropriately?

Special needs of certain athletic populations

This chapter covers many of the basics of working with athletes and gives general guidelines and recommendations. Each sport has its own metabolic profile and this must always be considered, along with the individual sitting in front of the practitioner. There are also 'special populations' that partake in sport and need more specific assistance and guidelines. This includes injured athletes, children, teens, vegetarians, vegans,

diabetics and those with food allergies, eating disorders, compromised immune systems, digestive or female reproductive disorders, bone density issues or needing a change in body composition and fat loss. The special needs of these groups is beyond the scope of this textbook but more information can be found in research papers such as the ACSM position statement[6] or textbooks such as *Clinical Sports Nutrition.*[107]

Knowing your limits as a practitioner

It is vital that naturopathic practitioners know their limits and abilities in treating individuals. When these limits of expertise are reached it is vital that practitioners refer on or ask for assistance from professionals whose scope of knowledge or practice can assist the patient. Professionals who may need to be called on when working with the sporting population include:
- General practitioners
- Sports doctors
- Sports psychologists
- Exercise physiologists
- Sports dietitians
- Coaches/trainers
- Physiotherapists/massage therapists
- Chiropractors, osteopaths, acupuncturists.

CASE STUDY 1: GENERAL AND RACE NUTRITION FOR A FEMALE TRIATHLETE

A healthy triathlete is looking to increase her energy, support her immune system and learn the basics of healthy naturopathic sports nutrition.

OVERVIEW

KW, a 35-year-old female athlete, presented with minimal health concerns and no longstanding health issues. She was seeking education around diet and sport as she was aiming to race a long-distance triathlon within 3 months. She is an age group triathlete, which means she competes within a 5-year age bracket against other women, and is undertaking the sport for fun.

GENERAL INFORMATION

- Female
- Age 35
- Height 173 cm
- Weight 60 kg (healthy range for height)
- Average sweat rate 600–800 mL per hour
- Racing Ironman triathlon in 3 months' time
- Estimated finish time 11.5–13 hours
- Works full-time in an office with flexible schedule.

SYSTEMS REVIEW

- Digestion, gastrointestinal tract and bowels: no issues
- Female cycle: 26–28 days, 5-day bleed with nothing remarkable, mild sugar cravings

- Immune system slightly compromised from high training load, urinary tract infections (URTIs) every 2–3 months lasting 3–5 days, with only 3 days taken off training
- Cramping in legs and feet, especially with swimming or long training sessions, 2–3 times per week
- Work stress 7/10, life stress 6/10
- Sleeps 7 hours per night due to early training
- Complains of tiredness and inability to stay awake at work
- Happy with current weight
- No known food allergies or sensitivities.

TRAINING SCHEDULE (VARIABLE AND FLEXIBLE AS PER WORKLOAD AND TIREDNESS)

	AM	PM
Monday	Rest day	Yoga or Pilates
Tuesday	Bike 1–2 hours	Run 1–1.5 hours
Wednesday	Swim 1–1.5 hours	
Thursday	Bike 1–2 hours	Swim 1–1.5 hours
Friday	Run 1 hour	
Saturday	Bike 4–7 hours, run 30 minutes	Swim 1 hour
Sunday	Run 1–2.5 hours	Rest

RACE

- Start at 7.00 am
- 3.8-km swim in open water (1 hour to 1 hour 10)
- 180-km bike ride (aiming for 6 hours)
- 42.2-marathon run (aiming for 4–4.5 hours).

FOOD, FLUID AND SUPPLEMENT DIARY

- 7-day food training diary completed
- Forgets to eat after training as rushing to work
- Generally healthy choices: organic fruit and vegetables and meats
- Low fish intake
- Poor snack choices when tired from training
- No food allergies or sensitivities, limits gluten by choice, fine with dairy
- Good amount of carbohydrate; protein intake slightly low
- Fluid intake of 1–1.5 L plus training fluid though can be forgetful
- 2 black coffees per day with a dash of milk, or a cappuccino
- 2–3 glasses of wine per week, dropping to zero closer to race
- Takes no supplements unless unwell.

INVESTIGATIONS REFERRAL

The following investigations were ordered:
- FBC (full blood count)
- Iron studies
- Vitamin D
- TSH (thyroid-stimulating hormone) test.

KW had very few health complaints and thus the investigations requested were minimal. Many athletes need little blood work as they are healthy eaters who get more than adequate exercise and are seeing the practitioner for optimum health rather than chronic disease. KW's fatigue was not low enough to request further testing, as a change in diet and supplementation of nutritionals and herbal medicine was the first line of treatment.

INVESTIGATION RESULTS

Investigation	Result	Treatment
FBC	Within range	None given
Iron studies	Ferritin low, 15 micrograms/L	Supplementation given
Vitamin D	45 nmol/L, mild deficiency	Supplementation given
TSH	1.8 mU/L	None given, within range

TREATMENT PROTOCOL

KW is a typical endurance athlete who is pushing her body at work as well as through sports. Education focused on general eating for sports and recovery to support her heavy training load.

Initial treatment

- Increase protein intake to match training needs. Started with 1.5 g/kg of body weight = 90 g of protein spread throughout the day with 20–25 g in the post-training meal.
- Post-training carbohydrate targets to be met for optimum glycogen synthesis and recovery, especially on double training days. Started with 1 g/kg of body weight post-training = 60 g and will assess results at next appointment.
- Eat within 30 minutes of finishing all training sessions in correct carbohydrate to protein ratios.
- Increase sleep to 8 hours per night and nap when possible.
- Focus on protein at each meal and snack.
- Red meat 2–3 times per week for increased iron needs, eaten with vitamin C foods for increased absorption.
- Suggested increase in fish intake inclusive of sardines and herring for vitamin D needs.
- Suggested healthier snacks and preparing foods on Sunday to be ready for the week ahead.

Suggested meal ideas			
Breakfast	**Lunch and dinner**	**Snacks**	**Other**
150 g plain full-fat yoghurt with 1 piece of fruit and 25 g raw seeds/nuts; can add protein powder if necessary, honey if need more carbs	120 g meat (20–25 g protein) such as red meat, chicken, fish plus vegetable stir fry and rice or sweet potato	120 g plain yoghurt and ½ punnet of berries or 20 g seeds and nuts on top	Fluids: best is water, mineral water and herbal tea Need 1.5 L per day plus training fluids
Smoothie: 20 g protein powder, liquid of choice, 1 frozen banana, ½ cup frozen berries, honey to taste, yoghurt if desired	120 g meat (20–25 g protein) such as red meat, chicken, fish plus unlimited veggie salad and starchy vegetables if post-training	2–3 tbsp hummus or tzatziki with veggie sticks (carrot, zucchini, cucumber, capsicum)	2 coffees per day, try to limit milk (black is best), no sugar; substitute with green tea
Porridge with LSA (linseeds, sunflower seeds and almonds) or 20 g raw seeds/nuts or protein powder and a few sultanas or berries	Frittata (eggs and veggies) plus unlimited salad	Miso soup and 1 boiled egg	Limit alcohol, best none in 6 weeks before race
2 eggs scrambled with stir fry of veggies (onions, capsicum, zucchini, mushrooms) and 2 pieces wholemeal or gluten-free toast	Steamed or baked veggies plus 120–150 g meat/fish/beans/tofu (20–25 g protein)	Healthy sports bar or homemade protein ball	1 meal per day should be free of grains/potato/sweet potato/bread/corn/rice, best *not* the meal post-training

Continued

Suggested meal ideas—cont'd

Breakfast	Lunch and dinner	Snacks	Other
2 eggs with spinach, fetta and mushroom sauté and 2 pieces of toast	Meat lasagne with veggies or salad or thin-crust pizza with healthy toppings (protein and veggies)	45 g raw seeds/nuts plus 1 piece fresh fruit or 3 fresh dates	Starchy carbohydrate is best consumed in a meal post-training (within 30 minutes)
Recovery drink with correct carb:protein ratio if after training	Homemade slow-cook stew/soup with protein and veggies, add quinoa, potato, sweet potato or rice	½ cup cottage cheese plus veggie sticks	Any breakfast can be eaten for lunch or dinner, and vice versa
120–150 g cottage cheese plus 1 piece of fruit and 25 g seeds and nuts	Vegetarian protein source that = 20–25 g protein (beans, tofu, tempeh) plus salad or stir fry and rice/quinoa if need to add carbohydrate	Small smoothie or 1 piece of fruit, coconut water and 20 g protein powder	Post-training 4:1 or 3:1 ratio of carb:protein is best recovery ratio Within 30 minutes Do not skip meals, especially post-training
2 eggs plus tomato, bacon, spinach, avocado and sweet potato mash or 2 pieces of toast	Wrap or sandwich with 100 g protein of choice (20 g of pure protein) and plenty of veggies/salad; use a salad leaf to wrap if wanting no grain	Turmeric tea, 45 g seeds and nuts	Continue to keep a food and training diary Treats happen, try for 2 squares of dark chocolate
Buckwheat pancakes with maple syrup, plain yoghurt and fruit (Saturday or Sunday after long training session)	Recovery drink if short of time and post-training (4:1 ratio)	Small beetroot and fetta salad	Meals post-training need to hit carbohydrate and protein goals Meals not around training are great to have a small amount of protein and salad

Suggested nutrient requirements

Nutrient	Dosage	Rationale
Magnesium	350 mg/day	Energy production, muscle cramping, stress, assists sleep
Probiotic (multi-strain)	1 capsule/day	Supports immune system and digestive function
B complex	2 capsules/day	Supports energy production, stress support
High-strength fish oil (omega 3 fatty acids)	2000 mg/day	Low fish intake in diet, cell membrane support, assists with fat-soluble vitamin absorption
Vitamin D$_3$	1000–2000 IU/day	Mild deficiency, immune support
Iron	30–40 mg/day	Borderline ferritin levels, oxygenation of blood, endurance sport increasing demand, immune support
Vitamin C with bioflavonoids	2000 mg/day (or more)	Immune support, antioxidant; given when acute URTI, not given all the time as can potentially inhibit training adaptations

Suggested herbal medicines

Herbal medicine	Quantity	Rationale
Withania somnifera (Ashwagandha)	40 mL	Stress, exhaustion, sleep
Rehmannia glutinosa (Rehmannia)	40 mL	Immune support, adrenal restorative, anti-inflammatory
Echinacea spp. (Echinacea)	40 mL	Immune support and modulation, lymphatic, increased incidence of URTI
Astragalus membranaceus (Astragalus)	40 mL	Immune support, tonic
Glycyrrhiza glabra (Liquorice)	40 mL	Immune support, adrenal support
Phytolacca decandra (Poke root)	5 mL	Lymphatic, general support

Dosage: 7 mL BD in a small amount of water or juice.
Source: Thomsen M, Gennat H. Phytotherapy: a clinical handbook. 4th edn. Hobart: Global Natural Medicine; 2009

At the time of presentation KW did not have an URTI but had previously had one the month before and was prone to infections. She was complaining of tiredness and is undergoing a large volume of training (upwards of 10–15 hours per week depending on her schedule). The herbal tonic was designed to support the immune system and the lymphatics: KW was in need of a general adaptogen tonic and immune support. This combination of herbs is a common recipe used with athletes, although with long-term use it is advisable to supply other adaptogens.

Herbal teas recommended as coffee alternatives and for general health and wellbeing	
Herbal tea	**Justification**
Ayurvedic Vata tea (combination of digestive, nervine and aromatic herbs)	Assists digestion and relaxes the nervous system before bed
Matricaria recutita (Chamomile)	Digestive, nervine before bed
Camellia sinensis (Green tea)	Antioxidant, coffee substitute
Taraxacum officinalis (Dandelion)	Liver support, coffee alternative

Follow-up

KW returned 3 weeks later to review protocols, assess energy levels and report on dietary changes. Her assessment of her health is as follows:

- Energy fantastic, now 8/10, and hoping it will go higher as iron levels increase
- Sleeping 8 hours per night with much less sleepiness during the day, except on really hard training days
- Eating after training is a big focus and she has noticed a substantial difference in her energy levels, ability to train hard and, most helpfully, she has fewer cravings for sugar and bad snacks
- Eating plan is great, loving the ideas and implementing most of the suggestions
- Has not had an URTI since her first visit
- Periods normal
- Seeking assistance with her race nutrition plan at this appointment
- Sweat rate for the bike is 800 mL/hour
- Sweat rate for run is 600–700 mL/hour.

Treatment plan

KW is doing so well that the treatment plan will stay the same up to and including her race in 2 months' time. Supplements and herbal medicine will stay the same unless she has an URTI or is unwell and then a specific immune mix will be used. Adaptogens in her mix will be varied with substitution of Rhodiola and Siberian or Korean ginseng

likely for Glycyrrhiza and Rehmannia as race time approaches.

The largest part of the treatment plan is to teach KW about race nutrition for an endurance event. Specific protocols need to be followed for the few days before the race as she will benefit from an adapted carbohydrate loading protocol since her race will take her more than 11 hours. In addition, there is the actual protocol for during the race. Endurance events that last for more than 2 hours need specific guidelines so that athletes fuel themselves properly every hour while trying to minimise fatigue, gastric discomfort, dehydration and glycogen depletion.

KW is given the following guidelines for adapted carbohydrate loading and foods to be eaten in the 2–3 days before the race as well as on the day itself.

NUTRITION PROTOCOL FOR THE 3 DAYS PRIOR TO THE RACE/ADJUSTED CARB LOADING

- Increase carbohydrate intake to 65–75% of total daily intake
- Suggestion: intake 8–12 g of carbohydrate per kg of body weight (KW is 60 kg so 480–720 g of carbohydrate per day)
- Since KW has not carb loaded before and is not an elite athlete, her chosen level will be at the lower end of this range. It is up to KW to trial how she feels on different amounts and then move forward with the plan
- KW is aiming for 480–500 g of carbohydrate per day, which is a large volume for most people. This will increase her glycogen stores above normal, giving her more fuel reserves for race day
- For every gram of glycogen, the body holds approximately 2.5 g water – thus KW will be holding extra water in her body, which will be of benefit come race day. This can amount to an extra 2 kg in body weight
- As KW's carbohydrate increases she will need to decrease her fibre, protein and fat volumes, as this is not about kilojoule loading but carb loading
- Many athletes feel much better on race day by minimising high-fibre foods so their gut is lighter and they are less likely to have gastrointestinal problems
- Carb loading has been shown to enhance endurance and postpone fatigue in endurance athletes competing at a steady state. It does not help them go faster. Carb loading is where naturopathic nutrition sometimes has to take a back seat. KW will need to consume large volumes of carbohydrate and thus may need to eat dense forms such as white rice, fruit juice, honey, jam, dates, flavoured yoghurt and sports drinks. Some athletes also eat gummy bears and other lollies. It is up to the athlete and how they want to roll with their nutrition.

The following meal suggestions are provided to KW as examples of higher carbohydrate, lower fibre meals for the few days before the race. KW will calculate the exact volume of meals using her specific target goals from the carbohydrate tables.

Eating with increased carbohydrate intake pre-race			
Breakfast	**Lunch and dinner**	**Snacks**	**Other**
Yoghurt with 1–2 pieces of fruit and a sprinkle of seeds and nuts	120–150 g protein such as red meat, chicken, fish plus vegetable stir fry (unlimited veggies) and white rice	Yoghurt with a piece of fruit and 1 tbsp honey (berries, banana, fresh dates etc.)	Fluids: best is water, mineral water and herbal tea to keep fluid levels topped up for race day
Smoothie: 20 g protein powder, yoghurt, fluid of choice (juice, milk, coconut water etc.), 1 banana, ½ cup berries and honey	120–150 g protein plus unlimited veggie salad and 1 of the following: toast, pasta, potato, sweet potato or rice	Hummus or guacamole and rice crackers or crumpets with honey	If you are short on carbohydrate it is okay to add a few jelly snakes, honey or sports drink to get to your carbohydrate goals
Porridge (oats, quinoa or rice) with a few sultanas or strawberries and some honey (not race morning as high fibre (too much fibre))	Frittata (eggs and veggies with a lot of potato and sweet potato) plus salad	Fresh fruit, dried fruit or dates and small amount of raw nuts	Best to avoid alcohol in the week before the race: beer is not good for carbohydrate loading
2 eggs cooked as preferred, 1/3 avocado and 2–3 pieces of low-fibre or gluten-free toast plus fruit or juice	Baked veggies plus 120–150 g meat/fish/other protein source	Muesli bar, gluten-free muesli bar, hot-cross bun or high-carb sports bar	Add a little extra salt to food in the few days before the race
2 eggs with spinach, fetta and mushroom sauté and 2–3 pieces toast or potato/sweet potato mash	Lasagne made with a lot of veggies or served with a salad	Jelly snakes or jelly beans	Do not over-hydrate, but be sure not to be dehydrated
150 g of low-fibre cereal (2 cups) plus milk, 1 banana and berries/dates	Homemade slow-cook stew/goulash with protein and many veggies; add potato, sweet potato or rice for increased carbohydrate	Chocolate milk, fruit juice, sports drink, 4:1 recovery drink are great high carbohydrate snacks	Any breakfast can be eaten for lunch or dinner, and vice versa
Pancakes with maple syrup, yoghurt and fresh fruit	Wrap or sandwich with 120 g protein and plentiful veggies/salad or baked potato	Small smoothie: see breakfast recipe	Post-training 4:1 carb:protein is your best recovery ratio Within 30 minutes
2–3 crumpets with honey or jam and a nut butter	Recovery drink in a 4:1 (carb:protein) ratio	Rice pudding or sushi rolls with rice	If in doubt use a food diary app such as mynetdiary or myfitnesspal

The following meal plan suggestions equate to approximately 480 g of carbohydrate:

Breakfast
- 200 g vanilla yoghurt (45 g carbohydrate)
- 1 large banana (30 g carbohydrate) or 3 large dates
- 2 tbsp honey (30 g)
- Sprinkle of seeds/nuts (minimal carbs).

Snack
- Sports bar (45 g carbohydrate)
- Fruit juice 250 mL (30 g).

Lunch
- 2 pieces of bread (30 g)
- Salad for sandwich such as tomatoes, lettuce, etc. (10 g carbohydrate)
- Protein for sandwich such as chicken or turkey
- 1 cup of grapes (30 g carbohydrate).

Snack
- 3 tbsp hummus (6–7 g carbohydrate)
- 15 rice crackers (30 g)
- Chocolate milk 350 mL (35 g carbohydrate) or fruit juice 300 mL (33 g carbohydrate).

Dinner
- Protein of choice (beef, lamb, chicken, fish)
- 1.5 cups white rice (65 g)
- Tamari sauce to add extra sodium
- Stir fry veggies (approx. 20–30 g).

After-dinner snack
- 15 jelly beans (45 g) or
- 1.5 hot-cross buns (45 g) or
- 120 g vanilla yoghurt plus 2 large dates (45 g).

RACE MORNING NUTRITION

- Discussed with KW that race morning can be very nervous time: stomach and digestion can feel poor and nerves can make you feel like you don't want to eat
- The golden rule is to never eat or drink anything new on race morning
- The entire race day nutrition plan should have been trialled at least twice on long training days to know it works and feels great
- Timing of pre-race meal depends on what time KW wants to get up

- Race start is 7 am and KW needs to be there 1–1.5 hours before this to check in and get ready
- KW will wake around 4.30 am; she needs to eat a meal that has time to digest before the race start
- Aim on race morning is to eat a meal that contains 1–4 g of carbohydrate per kg of body weight to replenish liver glycogen stores and be ready for race start. KW has trialled a 2 g/kg of body weight breakfast and feels comfortable with this (at 60 kg of body weight = 120 g of carbohydrate; if her nerves get really bad, she will drop this to 100 g). The meal needs to be high in low-fibre, easy-to-digest carbohydrate with only a small portion of protein or fat
- Many athletes love oats on race morning but if they tend to have gastrointestinal issues during races they should have a less fibrous breakfast like creamed rice.

Breakfast options

- Recovery drink 4 : 1 ratio (carb:protein)
- Bread with jam or honey and a nut butter
- Crumpets and honey
- Banana and dates
- Smoothie or sports bars
- Top-up fluid.

RACE NUTRITION PLAN
Pre-race/swim

- Water only in the last hour before race start and then 15 minutes out have either a gel with 300 mL water or a 300 mL sports drink. This will provide carbohydrate during the swim when KW is unable to eat anything.

Bike

- Once out of the water and onto the bike, intake water only for 15–20 minutes to flush the system and let heart rate settle down, find your rhythm
- Aiming for 60 g of carbohydrate per hour
- Fluid rate: 800 mL/hour – adjust up or down depending on temperature and weather
- Salt tablets: 500 mg every hour or 1 g every second hour to keep levels topped up; continue with this on the run
- KW's gel choice has 30 g of carbohydrate, so intake a gel every 30 minutes with 350 mL of water
- Plus sip extra water during the hour to get intake to 800 mL/hour
- Solid food eaten 2–3 times on the ride for fullness and flavour change, often in hours 2 and 4 for an estimated 6-hour ride
- KW's choice is a sports bar high in carbohydrate and low in protein, fibre and fat, cut into portions of 30 g of carbohydrate each so that she replaces a gel with the bar
- Food options to eat on the ride: bars, banana, dates, Vegemite sandwich with white bread, gels, carbohydrate chew, gummy bears, pretzels or just about anything that dense in carbohydrate that can be digested
- No food or gel with sports drink – only water to dilute contents in stomach for fast absorption
- Have plenty of water with solid food and remember to chew
- Set watch to beep every 30 minutes as a reminder to eat

- If get really uncomfortable in the stomach and feel like nothing is digesting, sip water and skip one eating session, allowing digestion to ride/rest for a while.

Examples of how and when food and fluid will be ingested on the bike ride		
Time ingested	**Food: 30 g carbohydrate**	**Fluid**
0–15 minutes	—	Water only
15–30 minutes	Gel	350 mL water
30–60 minutes	Gel	350–400 mL water
60 minutes	Gel	350–400 mL water
1 hour 30 minutes	Gel	350–400 mL water
2 hours	Bar/food	350–400 mL water
2 hours 30 minutes	Gel	350–400 mL water
And so on		

Run

- On the run KW's digestion is more temperamental so she will consume only 50 g per hour of carbohydrate
- Fluid intake needs be about around 600 mL/hour
- Swap to a different carbohydrate gel that has only 25 g of carbohydrate to make calculations easier
- Have 1 gel every 30 minutes with 250–300 mL water
- Have 1 gel that contains caffeine every 3 gels to assist in delaying fatigue
- Continue with salt/electrolyte tablets
- Have just gels, water and salt tablets on the run
- If need solid food, drop a gel and have a banana or 3 dates or approximately 400 mL sports drink.
  Race plans can include sports drinks but for simplicity's sake KW has chosen not to. In long-distance events water, sports drinks and degassed cola will be available for athletes at drink stations. Food is often available as well in the form of fruit, gummy lollies and cookies. Lists are available pre-race of what is being offered.

OTHER IMPORTANT INFORMATION
FLAVOUR FATIGUE

- If you hit flavour fatigue with the gels, you may like to move to cola
- Aim to consume about 400–450 mL cola per hour to get enough carbs
- Consume some water to dilute the cola as it's 11%: at a drink station aim for 150–200 mL cola and a few sips of water
- Practise what 100 mL and 200 mL of fluid looks like.

STOMACH ISSUES AND HOW YOU 'FEEL'

- If your stomach feels too full, burping or sloshing, let it ride, only sipping water and slow down slightly to increase digestion function
- Always check in with yourself and 'feel' how you are going, especially with your digestion
- Don't force food/fluids down
- Best of all, enjoy the race!

CASE STUDY 2: AN ELITE MALE SWIMMER

A swimmer competing at a high level needs a nutrition focus on both training days and carnival days where he is competing in multiple heats. The information from this case study can easily be applied to other sports with multiple races or games per day.

OVERVIEW

TD, an 18-year-old male swimmer, has a high training load. He is mid-season and is looking to maintain his weight and muscle mass while increasing his energy for training and racing. He has been a competitive swimmer since the age of 10. He is not currently drug tested, although if he goes further this will be the case.

GENERAL INFORMATION

- Male
- Age 18
- Height 187 cm
- Weight 80 kg.

SYSTEMS REVIEW

- Digestion, gastrointestinal tract and bowels: normal, no issues
- Immune system: strong, only 1–2 infections per year, recovers quickly
- Musculoskeletal: no issues
- Skin: mild facial acne since puberty and at times on upper back but not recently

- Sleeps 9 hours per night, would like more but gets to the pool at 5 am
- Stress 7–8/10 due to final year of high school and exams
- Happy with current weight and muscle mass
- No known food allergies or sensitivities.

TRAINING SCHEDULE (VARIABLE)

	AM	PM
Monday	Swim 5–6.30	Pilates 1 hour
Tuesday	Swim 5–7.00 endurance session	Weights 1 hour
Wednesday	Swim 5–6.30	Weights or Pilates 1 hour
Thursday	Swim 5–6.30	Run 1 hour
Friday	Swim 5–6.30	Rest
Saturday	Race (all-day carnival)	
Sunday	Day off or further racing	

RACE DAY

Competes in 2–3 events over the course of the day
Sometimes heats and finals occur on the same day, other times the final is on the next day
Races last <3 minutes

FOOD, FLUID AND SUPPLEMENT DIARY (SAMPLE OF HANDOUT GIVEN TO ATHLETE)

Time/date	Food	Carb/protein calculations	Fluid	Feelings/ energy	Supplements	Sleep	Stress

INVESTIGATIONS

None: TD had minimal complaints so no blood tests were needed. Often in athletes under the age of 20 there is a preference for no blood tests unless warranted. If health issues arise, this will be reassessed.

TREATMENT PROTOCOL

Initial appointment

TD is an average 18-year-old with not a lot of variety in his food choices. After looking over his food and training diary, as well as an uneventful systems review, the appointment focused on education of basic sports nutrition principles to assist recovery and increase energy levels. As with many teenagers who do not want to listen to their parents about

good nutrition, TD was more than willing to learn from someone else. He also enquired about creatine usage and whether this would help in his sport and in maintaining muscle mass.

Initial treatment
PROTEIN

- Increase protein levels to match required intake. At 80 kg TD's intake is estimated to be around 130–150 g per day, with a focus on protein in the meal post-training of 0.3 g/kg = 25 g minimum and up to 35 g after larger volume training sessions
- Each meal to have 25–35 g of protein and each snack to have 15–20 g; if short on intake, a protein snack could be consumed just before bed

- Bedtime snack can be plain full-fat yoghurt plus seeds and nuts (30 g) or a homemade protein ball if aiming for dairy-free choice.

CARBOHYDRATE

- As an 18-year-old male there were no issues with volume of carbohydrate consumed. Often meals were carbohydrate heavy and protein short. Discussion centred on amounts needed and how to focus carbohydrates strategically around training sessions
- At times TD does not eat before morning training and the suggested carbohydrate intake during training will assist to fuel the session when no food is ingested prior
- Add a small snack pre-morning sessions if TD has time: 20–30 minutes before training have 15–20 g of high GI (fast digesting) carbohydrate. Suggested foods: banana, dates, toast plus honey or 200 mL juice (fruit and vegetable combination)
- Suggested carbohydrate intake 5–7 g/kg/day, aiming for lower end on lower training days and higher end on double training days
- Keep track of energy levels and 'feel' during training so carbohydrate can be adjusted further
- Fill out a food diary over next 2 weeks.

FLUID INTAKE

- Fluid intake low considering the volume of training undertaken: often has only 300 mL water during a 1.5-hour swim session. States that he doesn't feel thirsty
- Take 2 water bottles to training in the morning, one filled with water and the other with a sports drink containing approximately 50 g of carbohydrate (regular sports drink, homemade drink or diluted fruit juice)
- Discussed how consuming carbohydrate during the session will help with finishing his swim session strong and fuelled as well as sparing glycogen, which is especially important for recovering on days when there are two training sessions
- Total fluid intake needs to be a focus: TD is sweating in the pool, he just don't notice it as much as with a run. Needs to consume about 800 mL/hour for training plus regular fluid intake for the day. Advised how to do a personal fluid test.

EATING POST-TRAINING

- Dietary suggestions focused on the importance of post-training eating. TD often had long periods of time between finishing swim squad and arriving at school and eating. Discussed that energy levels and refuelling need to happen faster than 1.5 hours post-training
- Take a smoothie to consume post-training on the bus to school. Suggested 1–1.2 g/kg in carbohydrate after morning squad = 82–90 g of carbohydrate plus 25–30 g of protein. TD very happy with smoothie idea and will try to take to all morning sessions
- TD very responsive to being given carbohydrate and protein sheets that lists foods and amounts of carbohydrate and protein. TD happy to try to calculate amounts from diet to see if he is hitting targets.

Post-training smoothie recipe

Smoothie (post-training)	Carbohydrate or protein (approximate)
1 banana	25 g carbohydrate
3 mejool dates	35 g carbohydrate
1 cup strawberries	10 g carbohydrate
Protein powder	20 g protein
1.5 cups cow's milk	18 g carbohydrate, 16 g protein
2 cups almond milk if wanting a milk alternative	16 g carbohydrate, 2–3 g protein (add in more protein to hit goals)
Total: 88 g of carbohydrate and 36 g of protein (calculation with cow's milk not almond milk), hitting very close to target meal suggestion.	

DAILY GOALS

- Carbohydrate: 5–7 g/kg/day at 80 kg = 400–560 g per day (may need to adjust later)
- Protein: 0.3 g/kg per meal and 0.25 g/kg per snack = 25 g on average per meal and 20 g per snack, plus 35 g in post-training meal. Total of 3 meals and 2 snacks = 130–150 g
- May need to add a night-time snack to get total up to 140–150 g per day.

Suggested supplements

Nutrient	Dosage	Rationale
Probiotic (multi-strain)	1 capsule/day	Supports immune system, decreases incidence of URTIs in athletes
Zinc citrate 25 mg	1 capsule/day with food	Acne/skin health, immune and hormone production support
B complex	2 capsules/day	Energy production, general health and stress support
Creatine monohydrate	5 g/day for 4–8 weeks during heavy strength work training schedule	Increased energy for weights sessions, muscle growth

Suggested herbal medicines

Herbal medicine	Quantity	Rationale
Schisandra chinensis (Schisandra)	40 mL	Stress, energy support with high-volume training, exhaustion; nerve tonic, adaptogen and antioxidant
Glycyrrhiza glabra (Liquorice)	40 mL	Adaptogen, anti-inflammatory and taste
Rhodiola rosea (Rhodiola)	40 mL	Adaptogen, energy, stress support, immune modulator, anti-inflammatory

Suggested herbal medicines—cont'd		
Herbal medicine	**Quantity**	**Rationale**
Withania somnifera (Ashwagandha)	40 mL	Adaptogen, stress support, nervine tonic, exhaustion
Scutellaria lateriflora (Skullcap)	40 mL	Nervous system support, stress support

Dosage: 5 mL BD with food in a small amount of water or juice.

TD is only 18 years old and has never taken herbal medicine. The dose chosen is low but will potentially be increased as he weighs 80 kg – being cautious at first and waiting for feedback on how his energy and stress levels feel. The herbs chosen are for support of energy and stress levels due to his high training volume and school exams. Herbs with both adaptogenic and immune modulation have been chosen, even though he is not immunocompromised, as his volume of training and stress both put him at greater risk of immune issues.

TD's change in diet and proper fuelling after sport should have a great impact on his energy and concentration. TD is asking a lot of his body and between the dietary changes, supplements and herbal medicine there should be a good amount of support for his overall health and wellbeing. He was asked to keep track of his stress and energy levels on a scale of 1 to 10.

Follow-up

TD returned 3 weeks later to assess his food diary and discuss his energy levels, race day nutrition and acne. His assessment of changes is as follows:

- Energy levels much better, especially mid-morning – consistently rating 8 or 9/10. Doesn't look for sugar as much to bolster energy levels
- Working on his fluid intake; still not great drinking during the day, but hitting fluid targets for training

- Loves the smoothie for breakfast post-training. He pre-packs all dry ingredients into a Ziploc and places them in the freezer so that he has 5 prepared for the week. Bought a new thermos and thinks it is the easiest thing ever
- Calculating carbohydrate and protein has been a great learning process and he feels much more in control over food choices that are smart rather than convenient. He lives at home and his mum is assisting in the meal preparation. Bulk meals being made and frozen so that there are easy and correct choices to hit targets
- Not feeling low-energy slumps mid-morning or low with training, so sticking to carbohydrate and protein targets set at last appointment
- Skin is a little clearer; unsure if much has changed as it's only been 3 weeks
- Sleeping really well, especially with protein snack before bed
- Herbs and supplements are fine, when he remembers.

FOOD DIARY ASSESSMENT AND DISCUSSION
- Eating is heavy on wheat and dairy products
- Very repetitive food choices
- Low on fluids still
- Sometimes looking for sugar in the afternoon for an energy hit before training
- Compliant with carbohydrate and protein suggestions, just needs more variety
- Vegetable intake could be higher
- Needs better snack options, especially pre-afternoon training; meals appear to be consistently good.

TREATMENT PLAN
- Continue with all supplements at same dosage
- Stick with smoothie post-training
- Bigger focus on taking right snack when running around to training sessions in the afternoon
- Meal plan provided: keep to calculations of carbohydrate and protein targets
- If needed, use smartphone app to track food diary and intake of macronutrients.

Meal plan suggestions			
Breakfast	**Lunch and dinner**	**Snacks**	**Other**
Plain full-fat yoghurt with 1 piece fruit and 25–30 g raw seeds/nuts or added protein powder	Protein of choice plus vegetables/salad and sweet potato or potato	Plain full-fat yoghurt with added protein powder to hit target of 25–30 g protein plus a piece of fruit or a cup of berries	Protein: aim for 20–30 g of pure protein in meals to hit suggested targets
Smoothie: milk or milk substitute, protein powder, berries, banana, honey or dates	Sushi, sashimi being aware to intake enough protein	Hummus with veggie sticks (carrot, zucchini, cucumber, capsicum) or rice crackers	Choose a variety of protein from meats, fish, eggs and vegetable sources such as tofu, beans, seeds and nuts
Porridge or healthy muesli with a few raw seeds/nuts or protein powder and topped with berries or fruit of choice	Frittata, quiche or omelette with salad	Miso soup and 2 boiled eggs or sushi; if hungry and pre-training carbohydrate hit needed in the afternoon	Eat in the correct ratios post-training and try to eat within 30 minutes of finishing all training sessions

Meal plan suggestions—cont'd			
Breakfast	**Lunch and dinner**	**Snacks**	**Other**
2–3 eggs scrambled with a stir fry of veggies (onions, capsicum, zucchini, mushrooms) and 2 pieces of wholemeal or gluten-free toast	Lasagne or pasta (gluten-free or regular) with protein and vegetables	Sports bar with a 4 : 1 ratio or a homemade protein ball of the same ratio	Any breakfast can be eaten for lunch or dinner, and vice versa
2–3 eggs with spinach, fetta, avocado and mushroom sauté and 2 pieces of toast	Goulash/stew with enough protein (meat or legumes) and plenty of root vegetables	45 g raw seeds/nuts plus 1 piece fresh fruit or 3 fresh dates	Post-training 4 : 1 or 3 : 1 ratio of carb:protein is your best recovery ratio Within 30 minutes
Recovery drink: if short on time use pre-mixed recovery drink specific for sport in 3–4 : 1 ratio of carbs:protein	Protein source with stir fry vegetables and rice or rice noodles	Chocolate milk (cow's milk or milk substitute) (homemade is best)	Fluids: best is water, mineral water and herbal tea Need 1.5 L/day plus training fluids
Buckwheat pancakes or French toast with maple syrup, plain yoghurt and fruit (great on the morning of a swim meet) for topping up carbohydrate stores	Wrap or sandwich with protein (meat, cheese, etc.) and salad	Small smoothie or 1 piece fruit, coconut water and 20 g protein powder	Limit alcohol and caffeine intake where possible
2–3 eggs plus tomato, bacon, spinach, avocado and sweet potato mash or toast	Thin-crust pizza (regular or gluten-free) with cheese/protein and healthy vegetable toppings and salad	Smoothie (see previous recipe)	Contact me if there are any questions

SWIM MEET: THINGS TO CONSIDER

- Eat a good breakfast 2–3 hours before first race, if possible
- To replace glycogen stores, have 1–2 g/kg of easily digestible carbohydrate (low-fibre may feel better for race morning) and a small amount of protein and fat as breakfast – for an 80 kg athlete = 80–160 g of carbohydrate
- If very nervous and having trouble eating, try a smoothie for digestive ease
- Top up fluid levels so arrive well-hydrated for the start of the day
- Be aware of what food is available at the pool facilities. Best to take your own food in a small cool bag or thermos
- Probably will not be able to eat regular meals depending on heats/races. Plan for small meals or larger snacks to be eaten when you know there is ample time for digestion (1–2 hours). If less than 1 hour between heats, have a small mainly carbohydrate snack and some water to top up fluid levels
- Remember to stay hydrated throughout the day without over-drinking
- Freezing water or sports drink so it remains cool during the day can be an added bonus on a hot day
- Pack a variety of foods so you have choices during the day
- Be sensible with food choices and do not eat sugary snacks unless you are about to have a high-energy demand period and need the added fuel, otherwise you can end up on a blood sugar low and feel tired at the start of a race

- Aim for 3–4 : 1 carb:protein ratio with most snacks/meals to keep carbohydrate levels high but with the added protein
- Many people find having salty, savoury and sweet options is important so they don't experience flavour fatigue
- The smoothie recipe for post-training is a great drink between races. There are also pre-mixed recovery drinks in a 4 : 1 or 6 : 1 ratio of carb:protein if you run short on time. These can be adjusted with added protein or carbohydrate to change the ratio if needed for easier digestion
- Never try anything new on race day! Only have what you find easy to digest. The stress of competing can make it hard on your digestion.

Suggested foods to take

- Toast with nut butters and honey
- Pasta (regular or gluten-free) with bolognaise sauce
- Chicken and rice
- Smoothie
- Homemade fruit and protein balls/bars
- Healthy muesli/cereal bars/sports bars
- Boiled eggs and bread or gluten-free bread
- Wraps and sandwiches with protein
- Banana, dates and seeds/nuts (if allowed at school)
- Yoghurt and fruit
- Homemade hot chocolate or chocolate milk
- Pumpkin soup
- Whatever you are comfortable with and have trialled in training or at previous swim meets.

REFERENCES

[1] Maughan RJ, Gleeson M, Maughlan RJ. The biochemical basis of sports performance. 2nd ed. New York: Oxford University Press; 2010.

[2] Jeukendrup AE, Gleeson M. Sports nutrition: an introduction to energy production and performance. 4th ed. Champaign, IL: Human Kinetics Publishers; 2004.

[3] Burke L, Deakin V. Clinical sports nutrition. 5th ed. Australia: McGraw-Hill Australia; 2015.

[4] Baker JS, McCormick MC, Robergs RA. Interaction among skeletal muscle metabolic energy systems during intense exercise. J Nutr Metab 2010;1–13.

[5] Tucker R. Exercise and weight loss, part 3: fat. The Science of Sport; 2010. Available from: http://sportsscientists.com/2010/01/exercise-and-weight-loss-part-3-fat. [Accessed 18 December 2016].

[6] Kira S. Überhealth. Available from: www.kirasutherland.com.au. [Accessed 18 December 2016].

[7] Thomas DT, Erdman KA, Burke LM. Position of the Academy of Nutrition and Dietetics, Dietitians of Canada, and the American College of Sports Medicine: nutrition and athletic performance. J Acad Nutr Diet 2016;116(3):501–28.

[8] Spriet LL. New insights into the interaction of carbohydrate and fat metabolism during exercise. Sports Med 2014;44(S1): 87–96.

[9] Philp A, Hargreaves M, Baar K. More than a store: regulatory roles for glycogen in skeletal muscle adaptation to exercise. Am J Physiol Endocrinol Metab 2012;302(11):E1343–51.

[10] Stellingwerff T. Contemporary nutrition approaches to optimize elite marathon performance. Int J Sports Physiol Perform 2013;8(5):573–8.

[11] Burke LM, Hawley JA, Wong SHS, et al. Carbohydrates for training and competition. J Sports Sci 2011;29(Suppl. 1):S17–27.

[12] Potgieter S. Sport nutrition: a review of the latest guidelines for exercise and sport nutrition from the American College of Sport Nutrition, the International Olympic Committee and the International Society for Sports Nutrition. South Afr J Clin Nutr 2013;26(1):6–16.

[13] Burke LM, Hawley JA, Wong SHS, et al. Carbohydrates for training and competition. J Sports Sci 2011;29(Suppl. 1):S17–27.

[14] Phillips SM, Van Loon LJC. Dietary protein for athletes: from requirements to optimum adaptation. J Sports Sci 2011;29(Suppl. 1):S29–38.

[15] Phillips SM. Dietary protein requirements and adaptive advantages in athletes. Br J Nutr 2012;108(S2):S158–67.

[16] Churchward-Venne TA, Burd NA, Mitchell CJ, et al. Supplementation of a suboptimal protein dose with leucine or essential amino acids: effects on myofibrillar protein synthesis at rest and following resistance exercise in men. J Physiol 2012;590(11):2751–65.

[17] Burd NA, West DWD, Moore DR, et al. Enhanced amino acid sensitivity of myofibrillar protein synthesis persists for up to 24 h after resistance exercise in young men. J Nutr 2011;141(4): 568–73.

[18] Beelen M, Burke LM, Gibala MJ, et al. Nutritional strategies to promote postexercise recovery. Int J Sport Nutr Exerc Metab 2010;20(6):515–32.

[19] Moore DR, Robinson MJ, Fry JL, et al. Ingested protein dose response of muscle and albumin protein synthesis after resistance exercise in young men. Am J Clin Nutr 2008;89(1):161–8.

[20] Macnaughton LS, Wardle SL, Witard OC, et al. The response of muscle protein synthesis following whole-body resistance exercise is greater following 40 g than 20 g of ingested whey protein. Physiol Rep 2016;4(15):e12893.

[21] Mettler S, Mitchell N, Tipton KD. Increased protein intake reduces lean body mass loss during weight loss in athletes. Med Sci Sports Exerc 2010;42(2):326–37.

[22] Hawley JA, Burke LM, Phillips SM, et al. Nutritional modulation of training-induced skeletal muscle adaptations. J Appl Physiol 2010;110(3):834–45.

[23] Bartlett JD, Hawley JA, Morton JP. Carbohydrate availability and exercise training adaptation: too much of a good thing? Eur J Sport Sci 2014;15(1):3–12.

[24] Impey SG, Hammond KM, Shepherd SO, et al. Fuel for the work required: a practical approach to amalgamating train-low paradigms for endurance athletes. Physiol Rep 2016;4(10):e12803.

[25] Close G, Hamilton L, Philp A, et al. New strategies in sport nutrition to increase exercise performance. Free Radic Biol Med 2016;98:144–58.

[26] Volek JS, Noakes T, Phinney SD. Rethinking fat as a fuel for endurance exercise. Eur J Sport Sci 2014;15(1):13–20.

[27] Burke LM. Re-examining high-fat diets for sports performance: did we call the 'nail in the coffin' too soon? Sports Med 2015;45(S1):33–49.

[28] Phinney SD, Bistrian BR, Evans WJ, et al. The human metabolic response to chronic ketosis without caloric restriction: preservation of submaximal exercise capability with reduced carbohydrate oxidation. Metabolism 1983;32(8):769–76.

[29] Hansen AK, Fischer C, Plomgaard P, et al. Skeletal muscle adaptation: training twice every second day versus training once daily. Scand J Med Sci Sports 2005;15(1):65–6.

[30] Morton JP, Croft L, Bartlett JD, et al. Reduced carbohydrate availability does not modulate training-induced heat shock protein adaptations but does upregulate oxidative enzyme activity in human skeletal muscle. J Appl Physiol 2009;106(5):1513–21.

[31] Van Proeyen K, Szlufcik K, Nielens H, et al. Beneficial metabolic adaptations due to endurance exercise training in the fasted state. J Appl Physiol 2010;110(1):236–45.

[32] Yeo WK, Paton CD, Garnham AP, et al. Skeletal muscle adaptation and performance responses to once a day versus twice every second day endurance training regimens. J Appl Physiol 2008;105(5):1462–70.

[33] Marquet LA, Hausswirth C, Molle O, et al. Periodization of carbohydrate intake: short-term effect on performance. Nutrients 2016;8(12):755.

[34] Lane SC, Camera DM, Lassiter DG, et al. Effects of sleeping with reduced carbohydrate availability on acute training responses. J Appl Physiol 2015;119(6):643–55.

[35] Gleeson M. Immune function in sport and exercise. J Appl Physiol 2007;103(2):693–9.

[36] Stellingwerff T. Decreased PDH activation and glycogenolysis during exercise following fat adaptation with carbohydrate restoration. Am J Physiol Endocrinol Metab 2005;290(2):E380–8.

[37] Havemann L. Fat adaptation followed by carbohydrate loading compromises high-intensity sprint performance. J Appl Physiol 2006;100(1):194–202.

[38] Jeukendrup A. Trusted sports nutrition advice & exercise science news. My Sport Science. Available from: www.mysportscience.com.

[39] Currell K, Jeukendrup A. Superior endurance performance with ingestion of multiple transportable Carbohydrates. Med Sci Sports Exerc 2008;40(2):275–81.

[40] Available from www.mysportsscience/shopify.

[41] Jentjens RLPG. Exogenous carbohydrate oxidation rates are elevated after combined ingestion of glucose and fructose during exercise in the heat. J Appl Physiol 2005;100(3):807–16.

[42] Jentjens R, Underwood K, Achten J, et al. High exogenous carbohydrate oxidation rates following glucose and fructose ingestion during exercise in the heat. Med Sci Sports Exerc 2005;37(Suppl.):S307–8.

[43] Jentjens RLPG, Achten J, Jeukendrup AE. High oxidation rates from combined carbohydrates ingested during exercise. Med Sci Sports Exerc 2004;36(9):1551–8.

[44] Kerksick C, Harvey T, Stout J, et al. International Society of Sports Nutrition position stand: nutrient timing. J Int Soc Sports Nutr 2008;5(1):17.

[45] van Loon LJC. Is there a need for protein ingestion during exercise? Sports Med 2014;44(S1):105–11.

[46] Ivy J, Katz A, Cutler C, et al. Muscle glycogen synthesis after exercise: effect of timing of carbohydrate ingestion. J Appl Physiol 1988;64:1480–5.

[47] Ivy JL. Muscle glycogen synthesis before and after exercise. Sports Med 1991;11(1):6–19.

[48] Prats C, Helge JW, Nordby P, et al. Dual regulation of muscle glycogen synthase during exercise by activation and compartmentalization. J Biol Chem 2009;284(23):15692–700.

[49] Burke L, Deakin V. Clinical sports nutrition. 5th ed. Australia: McGraw-Hill Australia; 2015.

[50] Tipton KD, Elliott TA, Cree MG, et al. Ingestion of casein and whey proteins result in muscle anabolism after resistance exercise. Med Sci Sports Exerc 2004;36(12):2073–81.

[51] Betts JA, Williams C. Short-term recovery from prolonged exercise. Sports Med 2010;40(11):941–59.

[52] Morton RW, McGlory C, Phillips SM. Nutritional interventions to augment resistance training-induced skeletal muscle hypertrophy. Front Physiol 2015;6.

[53] Wilmore JH, Costill DL, Gleim GW. Physiology of sport and exercise. Med Sci Sports Exerc 1995;27(5):792.

[54] Meletis C. Dehydration: an imbalance of water and electrolytes. Water Int 2002;27(3):456.

[55] Murray R. Fluid needs in hot and cold environments. Int J Sport Nutr 1995;5(s1):S62–73.

[56] Casa DJ, DeMartini JK, Bergeron MF, et al. National Athletic Trainers' Association position statement: exertional heat illnesses. J Athl Train 2015;50(9):986–1000.

[57] Rehrer NJ, van Kemenade M, Meester W, et al. Gastrointestinal complaints in relation to dietary intake in triathletes. Int J Sport Nutr 1992;2(1):48–59.

[58] Cheuvront SN, Haymes EM, Sawka MN. Comparison of sweat loss estimates for women during prolonged high-intensity running. Med Sci Sports Exerc 2002;34(8):1344–50.

[59] Coyle EF. Fluid and fuel intake during exercise. J Sports Sci 2004;22(1):39–55.

[60] Maughan RJ, Shirreffs SM. Development of individual hydration strategies for athletes. Int J Sport Nutr Exerc Metab 2008;18(5):457–72.

[61] Kreider RB. Physiological considerations of ultraendurance performance. Int J Sport Nutr 1991;1(1):3–27.

[62] Casa D, Armstrong L, Hillman S, et al. National Athletic Trainers Association position statement: fluid replacement for athletes. J Athl Train 2000;35:212–24.

[63] Maughan RJ, Shirreffs SM. Dehydration and rehydration in competitive sport. Scand J Med Sci Sports 2010;20:40–7.

[64] van Kemenade MC, Meesler TA, Saris WHM, et al. Nutrition in relation to GI complaints among triathletes. Med Sci Sports Exerc 1990;22(2):S107.

[65] Kalman DS, Feldman S, Krieger DR, et al. Comparison of coconut water and a carbohydrate-electrolyte sport drink on measures of hydration and physical performance in exercise-trained men. J Int Soc Sports Nutr 2012;9(1):1.

[66] Saat M, Singh R, Sirisinghe RG, et al. Rehydration after exercise with fresh young coconut water, carbohydrate-electrolyte beverage and plain water. J Physiol Anthropol Appl Human Sci 2002;21(2):93–104.

[67] Ismail I, Singh R. Percentage of volume intake for rehydration after exercise-induced dehydration. Br J Sports Med 2010;44(Suppl. 1):i41.

[68] Maughan RJ, Watson P, Cordery PA, et al. A randomized trial to assess the potential of different beverages to affect hydration status: development of a beverage hydration index. Am J Clin Nutr 2015;103(3):717–23.

[69] Geyer H, Parr M, Mareck U, et al. Analysis of non-hormonal nutritional supplements for anabolic-androgenic steroids: results of an international study. Int J Sports Med 2004;25(2):124–9.

[70] Australian Sports Commission. ABCD Classification; 2016. Available from: www.ausport.gov.au/ais/nutrition/supplements/classification. [Accessed 19 December 2016].

[71] McGinley C, Shafat A, Donnelly AE. Does antioxidant vitamin supplementation protect against muscle damage? Sports Med 2009;39(12):1011–32.

[72] Sousa M, Teixeira VH, Soares J. Dietary strategies to recover from exercise-induced muscle damage. Int J Food Sci Nutr 2014;65(2):151–63.

[73] Levers K, Dalton R, Galvan E, et al. Effects of powdered Montmorency tart cherry supplementation on acute endurance exercise performance in aerobically trained individuals. J Int Soc Sports Nutr 2016;13(1).

[74] Bell P, Stevenson E, Davison G, et al. The effects of Montmorency tart cherry concentrate supplementation on recovery following prolonged, intermittent exercise. Nutrients 2016;8(8):441.

[75] Dimitriou L, Hill JA, Jehnali A, et al. Influence of a Montmorency cherry juice blend on indices of exercise-induced stress and upper respiratory tract symptoms following marathon running—a pilot investigation. J Int Soc Sports Nutr 2015;12(1).

[76] Connolly DAJ. Efficacy of a tart cherry juice blend in preventing the symptoms of muscle damage. Br J Sports Med 2006;40(8):679–83.

[77] Bell P, Walshe I, Davison G, et al. Montmorency cherries reduce the oxidative stress and inflammatory responses to repeated days high-intensity stochastic cycling. Nutrients 2014;6(2):829–43.

[78] Howatson G, McHugh MP, Hill JA, et al. Influence of tart cherry juice on indices of recovery following marathon running. Scand J Med Sci Sports 2009;20(6):843–52.

[79] Cote K, Connolly DA, McHugh MP, et al. The efficacy of cherry juice supplementation in preventing the symptoms of exercise-induced muscle damage. Med Sci Sports Exerc 2006;38(Suppl.):S404.

[80] Belcaro G, Hosoi M, Pellegrini L, et al. A controlled study of a lecithinized delivery system of curcumin (Meriva®) to alleviate the adverse effects of cancer treatment. Phytother Res 2013;28(3):444–50.

[81] Epstein J, Sanderson IR, MacDonald TT. Curcumin as a therapeutic agent: the evidence from in vitro, animal and human studies. Br J Nutr 2010;103(11):1545–57.

[82] Pyne DB, West NP, Cox AJ, et al. Probiotics supplementation for athletes: clinical and physiological effects. Eur J Sport Sci 2014;15(1):63–72.

[83] Santesso N. A summary of a Cochrane review: probiotics to prevent acute upper respiratory tract infections. Glob Adv Health Med 2015;4(6):18–19.

[84] Gleeson M, Bishop NC, Struszczak L. Effects of Lactobacillus casei Shirota ingestion on common cold infection and herpes virus antibodies in endurance athletes: a placebo-controlled, randomized trial. Eur J Appl Physiol 2016;116(8):1555–63.

[85] Available from https://examine.com/supplements.

[86] National Health and Medical Research Council. Nutrient reference values for Australia and New Zealand. Available from: www.nrv.gov.au/nutrients. [Accessed 19 December 2016].

[87] Thomsen M, Gennat H. Phytotherapy: a clinical handbook. 4th ed. Hobart: Global Natural Medicine; 2009.

[88] Abascal K, Yarnell E. Increasing vitality with adaptogens: multifaceted herbs for treating physical and mental stress. Altern Complement Ther 2003;9(2):54–60.

[89] Wankhede S, Langade D, Joshi K, et al. Examining the effect of Withania somnifera supplementation on muscle strength and recovery: a randomized controlled trial. J Int Soc Sports Nutr 2015;12(1).

[90] Kennedy DO, Scholey AB. Ginseng: potential for the enhancement of cognitive performance and mood. Pharmacol Biochem Behav 2003;75(3):687–700.

[91] Kennedy DO, Scholey AB, Wesnes KA. Modulation of cognition and mood following administration of single doses of ginkgo biloba, ginseng, and a ginkgo/ginseng combination to healthy young adults. Physiol Behav 2002;75(5):739–51.

[92] Bucci L. Selected herbals and human exercise performance. Am J Clin Nutr 2000;72(2):624S–636S.

[93] Kim S, Park K, Chang M, et al. Effects of panax ginseng extract on exercise-induced oxidative stress. J Sports Med Phys Fitness 2005;45(2):178–82.

[94] Chen C, Muhamad A, Ooi F. Herbs in exercise and sports. J Physiol Anthropol 2012;31(1):4.

[95] Kuo J. The effect of eight weeks of supplementation with Eleutherococcus senticosus on endurance capacity and metabolism in human. Chin J Physiol 2010;53(2):105–11.

[96] Goulet EDB, Dionne IJ. Assessment of the effects of Eleutherococcus senticosus on endurance performance. Int J Sport Nutr Exerc Metab 2005;15(1):75–83.

[97] Eschbach LC, Webster MJ, Boyd JC, et al. The effect of Siberian ginseng (Eleutherococcus senticosus) on substrate utilization and performance during prolonged cycling. Int J Sport Nutr Exerc Metab 2000;10(4):444–51.

[98] Panossian A, Wikman G, Sarris J. Rosenroot (Rhodiola rosea): traditional use, chemical composition, pharmacology and clinical efficacy. Phytomedicine 2010;17(7):481–93.

[99] Ishaque S, Shamseer L, Bukutu C, et al. *Rhodiola rosea* for physical and mental fatigue: a systematic review. BMC Complement Altern Med 2012;12(1).

[100] Abidov M, Grachev S, Seifulla RD, et al. Extract of *Rhodiola rosea* radix reduces the level of C-reactive protein and creatinine kinase in the blood. Bull Exp Biol Med 2004;138(7):63–4.

[101] Parisis A, Tranchita E, Duranti G, et al. Effects of chronic *Rhodiola rosea* supplementation on sports performance and antioxidant capacity in trained males: preliminary results. J Sports Med Phys Fitness 2010;50(1):57–63.

[102] Hung SK, Perry R, Ernst E. The effectiveness and efficacy of *Rhodiola rosea*: a systematic review of randomized clinical trials. Phytomedicine 2011;18(4):235–44.

[103] Andrade C, Aswath A, Chaturvedi S, et al. A double-blind, placebo-controlled evaluation of the anxiolytic efficacy of an ethanolic extract of *Withania somnifera*. Indian J Psychiatry 2000;42(3):295–301.

[104] Chandrasekhar K, Kapoor J, Anishetty S. A prospective, randomized double-blind, placebo-controlled study of safety and efficacy of a high-concentration full-spectrum extract of ashwagandha root in reducing stress and anxiety in adults. Indian J Psychol Med 2012;34(3):255.

[105] Pratte MA, Nanavati KB, Young V, et al. An alternative treatment for anxiety: a systematic review of human trial results reported for the Ayurvedic herb ashwagandha (*Withania somnifera*). J Altern Complement Med 2014;20(12):901–8.

[106] Wankhede S, Langade D, Joshi K, et al. Examining the effect of *Withania somnifera* supplementation on muscle strength and recovery: a randomized controlled trial. J Int Soc Sports Nutr 2015;12(1).

[107] Burke L, Deakin V. Clinical sports nutrition. 5th ed. Australia: McGraw-Hill Australia; 2015.

[108] Thomas DT, Erdman KA, Burke LM. Position of the Academy of Nutrition and Dietetics, Dietitians of Canada, and the American College of Sports Medicine: nutrition and athletic performance. Med Sci Sports Exerc 2016;48:543–68.

[109] Burke LM, Cato L. Supplements and sports foods. In: Burke LM, Deakin V, editors. Clinical sports nutrition. 5th ed. Sydney: McGraw-Hill; 2015. p. 493–591.

[110] Tarnopolsky MA. Caffeine and creatine use in sport. Ann Nutr Metab 2010;57(Suppl. 2):1–8.

[111] Astorino TA, Roberson DW. Efficacy of acute caffeine ingestion for short-term high-intensity exercise performance: a systematic review. J Strength Cond Res 2010;24(1):257–65.

[112] Burke L, Desbrow B, Spriet L. Caffeine for sports performance. Champaign, IL: Human Kinetics; 2013.

[113] Carr AJ, Hopkins WG, Gore CJ. Effects of acute alkalosis and acidosis on performance: a meta-analysis. Sports Med 2011;41(10):801–14.

[114] Quesnele JJ, Laframboise MA, Wong JJ, et al. The effects of beta-alanine supplementation on performance: a systematic review of the literature. Int J Sport Nutr Exerc Metab 2014;24(1):14–27.

[115] Jones AM. Influence of dietary nitrate on the physiological determinants of exercise performance: a critical review. Appl Physiol Nutr Metab 2014;39(9):1019–28.

Fertility – Female and male

Leah Hechtman

11

EPIDEMIOLOGY

Fertility rate

The fertility rate is defined as the average number of children that women produce during their lifetimes. At the end of World War II, the rate was low in Australia, at 2.7, but still above the replacement rate of 2.3. During the late 1950s and early 1960s, the fertility rate increased, reaching a maximum of 3.6 in 1961. Since then there was a persistent decline until 2003. The zero population growth rate was passed in 1974, and in 2003 the lowest rate of 1.7 was reached. This was then followed by the Australian government initiative to offer a financial 'baby bonus' and to increase the Medicare safety net for funding fertility procedures. In addition, there has been the baby boom echo, which refers to women deferring childbearing because of their careers, and giving birth in their thirties. These factors have led to an increase in fertility rate, with recent statistics from the Australian Bureau of Statistics[1] indicating the following information.

In 2011, Australia's total fertility rate (TFR) was 1.88 babies per woman, down very slightly from the 2010 TFR of 1.89 babies per woman. Since 1976, the TFR for Australia has been below replacement level; that is, the average number of babies born to a woman throughout her reproductive life (measured by the TFR) has been insufficient to replace herself and her partner. The TFR required for replacement is currently considered to be around 2.1 babies per woman. The TFR reached a low of 1.73 babies per woman in 2001 before increasing to a 30-year high of 1.96 babies per woman in 2008.

Fertility rates decreased slightly for women aged 20–24 years, 30–34 years and 35–39 years between 2010 and 2011, and increased for all other age groups. Fertility rates remained highest for women aged 30–34 years, recording 122 babies per 1000 women, which was a very slight decrease from 123 babies per 1000 women in the previous year. At the national level, the teenage fertility rate was 16 babies per 1000 women aged 15–19 years in 2011.

Infertility

Infertility is a prevalent problem in Australia. Infertility is defined as the inability to conceive after 12 months or more of regular unprotected intercourse with the same partner. After 12 months, intervention and treatment is recommended. The Fertility Society of Australia estimates that one in six couples (15%) of reproductive age suffer from fertility problems,[2] accounting for over 3 million Australians. It is advisable to initiate earlier intervention and treatment for women over the age of 35 years, the recommendation being to treat after 6 months of unsuccessful attempts at conception.

Infertility is not only a female issue. In approximately 40% of infertile couples, the problem is a male factor; in about 40%, it is a female factor; in 10%, it is a joint problem; and in the remaining 10%, the cause is unknown.[2] However, other research has suggested that female causes contribute to 30%, male causes to 30%, joint causes to 30% and unknown causes to 10% of infertility cases.[3]

Stillbirth

The incidence of stillbirth is difficult to ascertain, as methods of data collection and reporting vary. Data suggest that the overall incidence of stillbirth may be slightly lower, the estimated rate being 5.3 per 1000 deliveries for women aged 15–44 years in developing countries.[4]

Pregnancy loss

Recurrent pregnancy loss is a condition distinct from infertility, and is defined as two or more failed pregnancies.[5] When the cause is unknown, each pregnancy loss merits careful review to determine whether specific evaluation may be appropriate. After three or more losses, a thorough evaluation is warranted. For purposes of determining when evaluation and treatment for infertility or for recurrent pregnancy loss is appropriate, pregnancy is defined as a clinical pregnancy documented by ultrasonography or histopathological examination (see Fig. 11.1).

In Australia, miscarriage is defined as a baby who dies before 20 weeks of gestation and/or has a birth weight <400 g. Babies who die after 20 weeks of gestation (or who weigh >400 g) are classified as stillborn. This definition is not applied worldwide. For example, the World Health Organization (WHO) defines miscarriage as loss of a pregnancy up to 23 weeks of gestation or <500 g birth

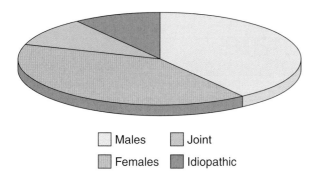

☐ Males	☐ Joint
☐ Females	☐ Idiopathic

FIGURE 11.1 The scope of infertility

weight, and other countries define it as a loss of pregnancy up to 24, 26 or 28 weeks of gestation. The definition of miscarriage is usually divided into early miscarriage (before 13 weeks) and late miscarriage (after 13 weeks and before 20 weeks). Approximately, 80% of miscarriages occur before 12 weeks.[6]

The risk of miscarriage is highest immediately after implantation. It is thought that around 50% of all fertilised eggs do not survive, coming away with a normal (or slightly late) period. This is often referred to as an 'unnoticed miscarriage' because it is usually not formally acknowledged by the woman, who is never aware of her pregnancy.

The normal rate of clinically apparent miscarriage in young women is approximately 12%. The rate rises independently with age, the number of previous pregnancies and, in particular, the number of previous miscarriages. The rate is also higher in many cases of infertility, whether conception occurs with or without treatment. It is estimated that approximately 12–15% of known pregnancies will end in miscarriage, with this figure increasing to 20% for those previously classified as infertile.

Assisted reproduction technologies

The growing trend for women to delay childbearing has a significant impact on their individual fecundity and consequent need for assisted reproductive technology (ART) and other treatments. Chromosomal anomalies and growth defects are the most common causes, and increase with the age of the mother.

Data obtained from the Perinatal and Reproductive Epidemiology Research Unit of the University of New South Wales (UNSW)[7] showed that there were 81 062 ART treatment cycles reported from Australian and New Zealand clinics in 2016 (74 357 and 6705, respectively), representing a 4.0% increase in Australia and 7.4% increase in New Zealand on 2015. This represented 14.8 cycles per 1000 women of reproductive age (15–44 years) in Australia, compared to 7.0 cycles per 1000 women of reproductive age in New Zealand. Women used their own oocytes or embryos (autologous cycles) in 94.1% of treatments. Embryos that had been frozen and thawed were used in 38.1% of autologous cycles.

There were 39 980 women who undertook 76 255 autologous fresh and/or thaw cycles in Australia and New Zealand in 2016. On average, 1.9 fresh and/or thaw cycles per woman were undertaken in 2016, with more cycles per woman in Australia (1.9 cycles per woman) than in New Zealand (1.5 cycles per woman). The number of cycles where embryos were selected using preimplantation genetic testing (PGT) increased from 5773 in 2015 to 7425 in 2016 (28.6% increase).

CLASSIFICATION

Fertility

A person's fertility is a reflection of their general health and wellbeing. As we are genetically constructed to pass on the best information to the next generation, fertility is believed to be optimal at 18–35 years for a woman and 16–40 years for a man.

Delaying having children until later in life contributes considerably to the proportion of couples who are involuntarily childless. Demographic[8] and clinical studies[9] have shown that women experience optimal fertility before the age of 30–31 years. After the age of 31 years, the probability of conception falls rapidly, but this can be partly compensated for by continuing insemination for more cycles. In addition, the probability of an adverse pregnancy outcome starts to increase at about the same age.[9]

Thereafter, fertility gradually decreases, with an acceleration, towards the age of 40 years. In women, fertility remains relatively stable until 30 years of age, generally producing more than 400 pregnancies per 1000 exposed women per year, and then begins to decrease substantially. By 45 years of age, the fertility rate is only 100 pregnancies per 1000 exposed women.[10] Already at an age of 40–41 years, half of women will have completely lost their capacity for reproduction. It is generally accepted that reproductive ageing is in fact ovarian ageing, and is related to the decreasing quantity and quality of the pool of follicles preserved in the ovary.[11]

CONCEPTION REQUIREMENTS

The requirements for normal conception include:
- production of viable sperm with respect to motility, morphology, count and DNA integrity
- transport of sperm through the male genital tract and deposition in the female genital tract, usually near the cervix of the uterus during sexual intercourse
- normal oocyte production (ovulation) by the ovaries
- transport of sperm and the oocyte within the female genital tract to the site of fertilisation in one fallopian tube
- penetration of sperm into the oocyte, fertilisation, development of a pre-embryo and its transport to and implantation in the uterus.

Infertility

Australia is one of a long list of nations experiencing a recent and dramatic decline in fertility rate.[1] The reasons behind this trend are complex and recent, and generally appear to be independent of the socioeconomic status of the country. However, deferred childbearing and improved contraceptive use are undoubtedly major factors. That said, it is intriguing that there is negative population growth in several countries, such as Sri Lanka, Denmark and Spain, where there have been no obvious increases in abortion rates or contraceptive use. This loss of fertility has affected countries such as Denmark to the point where approximately 7% of all babies are now born due to assisted conception.[12] In Australia and New Zealand, the number of babies born as a result of assisted conception procedures has increased three-fold over the past 10 years and, despite recent increases, the birth rate in Australia is still well below that needed to maintain the population at its present level.

'NORMAL' PREGNANCY RATES

Three out of five couples conceive within 6 months of trying, and one in four take between 6 months and a year. For the rest, conception takes more than a year, indicating that there may be a problem.

PRIMARY INFERTILITY

A couple is defined as having primary infertility if pregnancy has not occurred despite regular, unprotected intercourse for a year or more.

The cause of primary infertility involves many and varied factors (see Box 11.1), including:
- the production of gametes (sperm or eggs)
- the structure or function of the male or female reproductive system
- hormone disorders in the man or woman
- antibody (autoimmune) disorders in the man or woman.

SECONDARY INFERTILITY

A couple is defined as having secondary infertility if, despite having achieved a pregnancy in the past (which may or may not have resulted in the birth of a child), they are unable to do so again after a year or more of regular, unprotected intercourse.

Causes of secondary infertility include:
- Sexual function – that is, how often and when in the menstrual cycle a couple is having intercourse.
- Ovulation – that is, whether the woman is producing an egg each month.
- Sperm function – that is, whether the man has enough normal moving sperm per ejaculate. A previous pregnancy does not provide sufficient proof of this.
- Tubal function – that is, whether the egg and sperm can meet normally in the woman's body. Tubal problems are more common in secondary than primary infertility (20% of couples compared to the usual 10% incidence), due to infective or inflammatory complications that can occur after delivery or the end of the pregnancy.

UNEXPLAINED INFERTILITY

Unexplained infertility occurs in approximately 5–10% of couples trying to conceive. Generally, assessments reveal

---

BOX 11.1 Evolution – why does infertility exist?

Reproductive success is defined as successful reproduction in one's offspring. It is important to survive long enough to rear children who grow into fertile adults, to continue the cycle of life. However, if a couple has too many children, the chance that any will survive to adulthood is reduced.

Strategies in nature to provide reproductive fitness include R-selection and K-selection. R-selection is contingent on the rate of reproduction (i.e. how rapidly a species can produce offspring), and features rapid sexual maturity, superabundant production of eggs, low survival rates of offspring and short life span. An example of an R-selection group is butterflies and moths.

Conversely, K-selection strategises competition in the longer term, and involves a longer time to reach sexual maturity, high survival of offspring, usually singleton births and several episodes of gestation in a lifetime. *Homo sapiens* is the most K-selected species, and of all species on earth, human infants are the most dependent at birth, and have the longest childhood dependency and vulnerability. For optimal reproductive fitness, *H. sapiens* requires biological devices for spacing pregnancies. One method – natural contraception – involves lactational amenorrhoea, which provides contraception to delay subsequent conceptions. Some theories consider subfertility to be a highly evolved human condition, whereby multiple miscarriages, low sperm count or other conditions may occur to reduce fecundity scores and thus protect the survival of the species.

Strategy	R-selection	K-selection
Size	Small	Large
Numbers	Huge	Small
Time to maturity	Short	Long
Parity	Semelparity (one big episode)	Iteroparity (repeated)

---

limited information and no apparent cause of the infertility. In a much higher percentage of couples, only minor abnormalities are found that are not severe enough to result in infertility. In these cases, the infertility is referred to as unexplained. Couples with unexplained infertility may have problems with egg quality, tubal function or sperm function that are difficult to diagnose and/or treat. The likelihood of unexplained infertility being a true diagnosis is often a reflection of poor investigation or lack of current assessment strategies to accurately determine the cause. All too often, couples are simply poorly investigated and assessed, and are directed to the easiest solution (ART) without assessing what may actually be causing the problem.

CALCULATING FECUNDITY

Fecundity is defined as the couple's chance of conception in a single menstrual cycle. The normal monthly success

No. of factors	Average monthly fecundity (%)	Pregnant in 2 years (%)	Pregnant in 3 years (%)	Average time needed to pregnancy
0	20	94	97	3 months
1	5	64	76	2 years
2	1	21	29	7 years
3	0.2	5	7	40 years

TABLE 11.1 Calculating fecundity

rate for couples trying to conceive naturally at age 25 years is 25%. This figure decreases with increasing age, particularly after 35 years of age for women. It was once believed that the woman's age was the only major contributing factor, but it is now known that male fertility reduces with age concurrently with abnormalities in semen parameters. For example, 74.6% of couples aged 25 years will conceive in less than 6 months, but by 25–29 years of age the chance of conception in less than 6 months reduces to 25.5%.

A couple's fecundity is calculated to determine the monthly chance that couple has of conceiving a child. It factors in a number of variables and considerations for both the male and the female partners. When presented with an infertile couple, it is important to consider all variables as pieces of their specific jigsaw puzzle of reproductive and fertility health. While not as common, blatant fertility issues can direct the treatment direction definitively. More commonly, patients will present with a number of more minor irregularities or imbalances that combine to produce an infertile presentation.

Each half of a couple may have minor health concerns that alone are insufficient as a cause but when combined have a major influence on successful fertility outcomes. For example:

- the woman may have multiple minor fertility concerns (irregular menstrual cycle, weight gain, sugar imbalance, diagnosis of polycystic ovarian syndrome [PCOS]), digestive disturbances affecting her nutrient absorption, multiple nutrient deficiencies and other general health complaints
- the man may have subnormal semen analysis results, sleep irregularities, a strong family history of cardiovascular disease (presents with pre-cardiovascular disease concerns) and asthma.

The combination of the effect of all these minor abnormalities is summarised in Table 11.1.

Aetiology

Fertility is a reflection of one's general health and wellbeing and can indicate latent or undiagnosed genetic abnormalities or other aetiological considerations. The causes of fertility problems are many and varied, and a comprehensive and holistic review is essential.

The causes of male and female factor infertility are summarised in Boxes 11.2 and 11.3, respectively.

Optimising natural fertility

When presented with a couple who have experienced infertility, it is essential to ascertain their existing fertility strategies and any assessment tools they use to detect ovulation.

CONCEPTION

Humans reproduce by the coming together of two cells (gametes) – an ovum, or egg, which is produced by the woman, and a sperm, which is produced by the man. Each gamete contributes half of the genetic material in the resulting individual. For normal conception to take place, therefore, the man must be able to produce a sufficient number of normal, actively moving sperm, and the woman must be able to produce a healthy egg. In addition, the parts of the woman's body that carry and sustain a fertilised egg must all be fully functional.

The mature egg can survive for only 24–36 hours after ovulation. Sperm can survive in the presence of fertile-quality cervical fluid for 3–5 days. At ejaculation, the sperm swim, guided by the fertile cervical fluid, through the cervix and into the uterus. The uterus contracts in such a way as to help move the sperm up into the fallopian tubes to reach the egg. However, so many sperm are lost along the way that only a few hundred get this far. Around the egg is a shell (the zona pellucida). Once a single sperm has penetrated this shell, it sets up a barrier that further sperm are unable to penetrate. The head of this single sperm releases its contents inside the egg, and the egg is said to have been fertilised.

The egg (a cell) then begins to divide and grow, and becomes an embryo. Over the course of about 3 days, the embryo moves along the fallopian tube, via muscle action and the movement of fine hairs (cilia), into the uterus. After about another 3 days, the embryo implants in the endometrium. Once it has implanted, it starts to produce a hormone called human chorionic gonadotrophin (hCG), and the pregnancy can be detected. All pregnancy tests done on blood or urine test for the presence of hCG.

SPERM PRODUCTION

The male genital system consists of the testes, a system of ducts and some other glands opening into the ducts. The testes produce sperm and testosterone. Sperm are produced by repeated division of cells in small, coiled tubules within the testes at an average rate of approximately 100 million/day in healthy young men.

BOX 11.2 Causes of male factor infertility[13]

- Unknown (40–50%).
- Primary hypogonadism (30–40%):
  - androgen insensitivity
  - congenital or developmental testicular disorder (e.g. Klinefelter syndrome)
  - cryptorchidism
  - medication (e.g. alkylating agents, antiandrogens, cimetidine, ketoconazole, spironolactone).
- Orchitis, including mumps orchitis.
- Radiation.
- Systemic disorder.
- Testicular trauma.
- Varicocele.
- Y chromosome defect: genetic defects, such as microdeletions on the long arm of the male-determining Y chromosome, and other yet to be discovered mutations, are responsible for some of the more severe defects of sperm production or function, and these defects may be transmitted directly to sons or to future generations.
- Altered sperm transport (10–20%):
  - absent vas deferens or obstruction
  - epididymal absence or obstruction
  - erectile dysfunction
  - retrograde ejaculation.
- Secondary hypogonadism (1–2%):
  - androgen excess (e.g. tumour, exogenous administration)
  - congenital idiopathic hypogonadotrophic hypogonadism
  - oestrogen excess (e.g. tumour)
  - infiltrative disorder (e.g. sarcoidosis, tuberculosis)
  - medication
  - multiorgan genetic disorder (e.g. Prader–Willi syndrome)
  - pituitary adenoma
  - trauma.
- Other:
  - infection
  - hormone imbalances
  - hepatic cirrhosis
  - infection
  - excessive heat
  - radiation exposure
  - heavy metal toxicity
  - cigarette smoking
  - xenobiotic exposure
  - pesticide exposure
  - high intake of cottonseed oil.

BOX 11.3 Causes of female factor infertility[13]

- Ovulation disorders (40%):
  - ageing
  - diminished ovarian reserve
  - endocrine disorder (e.g. hypothalamic amenorrhoea, hyperprolactinaemia, thyroid disease, adrenal disease)
  - polycystic ovary syndrome
  - premature ovarian failure
  - tobacco use.
- Tubal factors (30%):
  - obstruction (e.g. history of pelvic inflammatory disease, tubal surgery).
  - Endometriosis (15%).
  - Other (approximately 10%).
- Uterine/cervical factors (>3%):
  - congenital uterine anomaly
  - fibroids
  - endometrial polyps
  - poor cervical mucus quantity/quality (due to smoking, infection); mucus hostility (sperm antibodies)
  - uterine synechiae or adhesions (Asherman's syndrome).

Sperm production is a lengthy process; from the beginning of the division of the stem cell to the appearance of mature sperm in the semen takes 72–76 days. Leading from each testis is a long, highly coiled tube called an epididymis. The sperm spend 2–10 days passing through the epididymis, during which time they mature and become capable of swimming and penetrating oocytes. At the beginning of ejaculation, sperm are transported from the tail of the epididymis via the vas deferens to the urethra. The seminal vesicles, prostate gland and Cowper's glands secrete most of the volume of semen – these secretions help deliver the sperm during ejaculation. The volume of liquid coming from the two epididymides is less than 5% of the total semen volume. Approximately 60% of the semen volume comes from the seminal vesicles, and 30% from the prostate gland. The average semen volume for healthy men ejaculating every 2 days is 3 mL, and the sperm concentration is 85 million/mL (for more detail, see below). During ejaculation, usually the sperm and the prostatic fluid come out first, and the seminal vesicle fluid follows. The seminal vesicle fluid coagulates, giving the semen a lumpy, gel-like appearance. Liquefaction occurs after 20 minutes or so and the gel disappears.

MATURING FERTILITY

Fertility is generally highest in the first months of unprotected sex and declines gradually thereafter in the population as a whole. If no conception occurs within the first 3 months, monthly fecundity decreases substantially among those who continue their efforts to conceive.[14]

FREQUENCY OF INTERCOURSE

In some cases, practitioners may need to explain the basics of the reproductive process. Assessment and discussion is best conducted earlier in the treatment process to avoid misinterpretation and misunderstanding. In the past decade, abstinence intervals have varied greatly. A widely held misinterpretation is that frequent ejaculations decrease male fertility. A retrospective study analysed 9489 men with normal semen quality, sperm concentration and sperm motility, and found that profiles remained normal even with daily ejaculation.[15] Of more importance is the finding that in males with abnormalities such as oligozoospermia, low sperm concentration and low sperm motility, fertility may be higher with more frequent (daily) ejaculation.[15]

Couples should be informed that reproductive efficiency increases with the frequency of intercourse, and is highest when intercourse occurs every 1–2 days. However, optimal frequency is best defined by the couple's own preference within this context.

FERTILE WINDOW

The fertile window is best defined as the 6-day interval ending on the day of ovulation.[16] As oestrogen increases in the woman in the lead up to ovulation, she produces fertile-quality cervical fluid. This fluid then provides a medium to protect the sperm from the acidic pH of the vagina, a medium for the sperm to travel in, and sustenance for the sperm to survive. Sperm are theoretically able to survive for up to 5 days in the presence of this fluid.

MAKING BABIES

There are a number of recommendations available. However, some are simply ridiculous, and others unnecessary. Ultimately, conception simply requires one sperm to meet one oocyte. A number of general recommendations can be followed to increase the chances of natural conception.

During intercourse, the woman's position should encourage a slight pelvis tilt (pillow under hips) and positions where the sperm cannot leak from the vagina. Experts therefore recommend that a couple avoids having sex in positions that defy gravity (as this lessens the likelihood of the man's sperm reaching the cervix) and chooses positions that encourage deeper penetration in order to place sperm as close as possible to the cervix. Sperm can be found in the cervical canal seconds after ejaculation, regardless of coital position, but increasing the quantity of sperm that can pass through the cervical opening is advisable. The use of lubricants should be discouraged as most act as mild contraceptives (see the discussion later in this chapter).

It is required that the sperm travel time through the cervix is minimal. However, a lack of movement and activity after ejaculation is advisable. Women do not need to literally have their legs raised in the air, but they should be encouraged to avoid urinating for a minimum of 10 minutes after intercourse.

In addition, some research suggests that the female orgasm is important in promoting sperm transport. Research suggests that orgasm should be encouraged after ejaculation, as the contractions that accompany the female orgasm may help carry sperm further into the cervix. However, there is no known relationship between orgasm and fertility outcome.

Ultimately, the focus should be on love making and not baby making, as this can cause unnecessary stress and pressure on the couple.

AGE ON FERTILITY

Age is rapidly becoming the biggest preventable cause of failure to conceive. Approximately 20% of women wait until after age 35 years to begin their families. Several factors have contributed to this trend:

- contraception is readily available
- more women are in the workforce and furthering their careers
- women are marrying at an older age
- the divorce rate remains high
- married couples are delaying pregnancy until they are more financially secure
- many women do not realise that their fertility begins to decline in their late twenties or early thirties.

After 35 years of age, a woman's fertility declines rapidly in conjunction with deteriorating egg quality. She may enter oopause in her thirties, depending on her genetic make-up, and this will further reduce her fertility. Even though women today are healthier and taking better care of themselves than ever before, improved health in later life does not offset the natural age-related decline in fertility.

While at the age of 35 years over 95% of healthy couples will conceive within 3 years of trying, by age 38 years, this figure has dropped to 77%. By the age of 41 years, less than half of healthy couples will conceive after 3 years of trying (see Table 11.2).

The effects of ageing

A number of considerations regarding the effects of age on fertility should be considered, and these are described below (see Table 11.3).

TABLE 11.2 Age and fertility in partnered women[13]		
Age group (years)	Infertile (%)	Chance of remaining childless (%)
20–24	7	6
25–29	9	9
30–34	15	15
35–39	22	30
40–44	29	64

TABLE 11.3 The effects of ageing	
Ovarian function	As women age, fertility declines due to normal age-related changes that occur in the ovaries. Women are born with all the eggs they will ever have, with approximately 300 000 follicles remaining at menarche. She then will lose between 20 and 30 follicles each cycle. Of the eggs remaining at puberty, it is believed that approximately 360–400 of these follicles, over 30 years, will mature and be released by the body, with the remainder being lost from each cycle. The rest will undergo atresia – a degenerative process that occurs regardless of whether a woman is pregnant, has normal menstrual cycles, uses birth control or is undergoing infertility treatment. Smoking appears to accelerate atresia and is linked to earlier menopause.
Ovarian reserve	Ovarian reserve declines with each cycle. Diminished ovarian reserve is usually age related and occurs due to the natural loss of eggs and decrease in the average quality of the eggs that remain. The remaining eggs become 'poor responders' to follicle-stimulating hormone (FSH) and luteinising hormone (LH), thus shortening menstrual cycles. Young women may also have reduced ovarian reserve due to smoking, family history of premature menopause and prior ovarian surgery. Premature ovarian failure is unfortunately common, and comprehensive investigations are required.
Genetic abnormalities	Ageing affects oocyte quality and increases the chance of neonatal genetic abnormalities. (See Table 11.4 for elaboration.)
Miscarriage risk	Older oocytes increase the risk of miscarriage. (See Table 11.5 for elaboration.)
Ageing male	While men can father children when they are older, as men age their testes reduce in size and get softer, sperm morphology and motility tend to decline and there is a slightly higher risk of gene defects in their sperm. Ageing men may develop medical illnesses that adversely affect their sexual and reproductive function.

TABLE 11.4 Maternal age and risk of chromosomal abnormality in newborns[13]

Maternal age (years)	Risk of Down syndrome	Total risk of chromosomal abnormalities
20	1/1667	1/526
25	1/1250	1/476
30	1/952	1/385
35	1/378	1/192
40	1/106	1/66
41	1/82	1/53
42	1/63	1/42
43	1/49	1/33
44	1/38	1/26
45	1/30	1/21
46	1/23	1/16
47	1/18	1/13
48	1/14	1/10
49	1/11	1/8

TABLE 11.5 Maternal age and miscarriage risk[13]

Maternal age (years)	Spontaneous abortion (%)
15–19	10
20–24	10
25–29	10
30–34	12
35–39	18
40–44	34
≥45	53

WEIGHT BALANCE

Obesity

Obesity has an impact on reproduction in women in a number of ways (see Table 11.6).[17]

BMI classification

The BMI classification uses the definitions outlined in Table 11.7.[20]

Anorexia

Women with a BMI <19 and who have irregular or absent menstruation should be advised to increase body weight to improve their chance of conception.

IMMUNOLOGICAL CONSIDERATIONS

As optimal production of gametes requires a healthy immune response, any deviation from 'normal' can significantly affect the outcome. In males, this is commonly experienced as sperm antibodies, while in women, any immunological requirement, including general health, conception, implantation and sustaining a pregnancy, can cause problems. A thorough discussion of immunological considerations is provided in Chapter 12.

HORMONAL CONSIDERATIONS

The intricate balance between the hormone pathways is a complex interrelationship. Any irregularity can have significant effects on specific reproductive pathways and subsequent gamete production, sustenance of a successful

TABLE 11.6 Impact of obesity on fertility[17]	
Ovulation potential	Ovulation returns with a relatively modest degree of weight loss from diet and exercise. Approximately 90% of obese women will resume ovulation if they lose >5% of their pre-treatment weight, and 30% will conceive. In very obese women, this is a higher pregnancy rate than can be expected from a single IVF cycle, so this is incredibly encouraging for obese women wishing to have children.
IVF outcome	The success rate of assisted reproductive techniques is reduced in obese women. IVF success rates may be reduced by as much as 25% in obese patients, and 50% in very obese patients. IVF centres are very reluctant to perform fertility treatment on women with a BMI greater than 35 kg/m^2, and generally recommend a target BMI of 30 kg/m^2 before starting the treatment.[18]
Semen analysis	Obese men are also at risk. The effect of weight loss on male fertility is less well understood, but weight loss does seem to lead to an improvement in testosterone levels and sexual dysfunction. Obese men generally have lower sperm counts (up to 50%), reduced spermatogenesis, increased DNA fragmentation of sperm and increased levels of erectile dysfunction. Hormonal changes are primarily responsible for the changes in obese men. The level of total and free testosterone is reduced in obese men in proportion to the level of obesity. Oestrogen is increased due to the peripheral aromatisation of androgens in adipose tissue. The oestrogens produced have a negative feedback effect on gonadotrophin production, reducing FSH. A reduction in the level of FSH in obese men reduces testosterone production and spermatogenesis. Increased body fat and a sedentary lifestyle are also associated with raised testicular temperature, which further adversely affects spermatogenesis.[18] Heat stress modifies gene expression in the testes, causing impaired spermatogenesis. Sperm cells are extremely vulnerable and respond by apoptosis and DNA damage.[19]
Miscarriage	The risk of miscarriage in the first trimester increases from 12 to 15% in normal-weight women (under 37 years old) to 31% for BMI > 35 kg/m^2. The rate of recurrent miscarriage increases four-fold in obese women.
Birth defects	Maternal obesity has a detrimental impact on fetal development (e.g. three times the risk of neural tube defects, structural heart defects). Folic acid supplementation is less effective in preventing neural tube defects, so high-dose supplementation is required for obese women (always beneficial to calculate nutrient requirements based on patient's presenting weight).
Pregnancy complications	Pregnancy complications are more common in obese women (gestational diabetes is six times more common); pregnancy-induced hypertensive diseases are more common (gestational hypertension and preeclampsia). Complications increase the risk of premature delivery/caesarean section. Babies born to obese women have heavier birthweights (fetal macrosomia) which increases the risk of traumatic vaginal delivery. There is a higher complication rate for caesarean and vaginal deliveries in obese women (e.g. excessive blood loss, thromboembolic disease and post-operative infection).
Pregnancy outcomes	Increasing BMI increases risk of stillbirth (two times the risk vs normal-weight women).
The newborn	Maternal obesity carries long-term risks for the newborn infant (e.g. increased risk of being overweight as adults and having weight-related diseases in adulthood).

TABLE 11.7 BMI classification	
BMI (kg/m^2)	**Classification**
Less than 18.5	Underweight
18.5–24.9	Healthy weight range
25–29.9	Overweight
30-40	Obese
>40	Morbidly obese

pregnancy and delivery of a healthy child. Additional information on the various hormone relationships is given throughout this chapter. However, readers are encouraged to review the endocrine system, and the female and male reproductive system chapters in *Clinical Naturopathic Medicine* (CNM).

GENETIC FACTORS

There are numerous genetic disorders that affect fertility. A simple karyotyping is often performed by reproductive specialists. However, additional assessments may be conducted, depending on the presentation of either parent. For example, cystic fibrosis is a common autosomal recessive disease, and may present with normal pH and low semen volume. Alternatively, a woman may present with amenorrhoea and have undiagnosed Turner's syndrome.

There are a number of recessive genetic inheritance patterns that may eventuate due to the coupling of the parents. Table 11.8 summarises some of these patterns and gives examples of genetic diseases. In addition, various ethnic groups have increased frequencies of disease carriers, as shown in Table 11.9.

There are also a number of genetic factors that can influence the health of either parent and the subsequent success of pregnancy and health of the future child. These include markers such as coeliac gene markers, methylenetetrahydrofolate reductase (MTHFR) mutations

TABLE 11.8 Genetic inheritance patterns and examples of genetic diseases[21]

Inheritance pattern	Explanation	Examples
Autosomal recessive	A mutation in the same gene is inherited from each parent. Each parent is a healthy carrier as they have a second unaffected copy of the gene. If both parents are carriers of an autosomal recessive condition, there is 1 : 4 (25%) chance that each child will be affected. It is estimated that all people carry 5–10 autosomal recessive mutations	Cystic fibrosis* Spinal muscular atrophy* Haemochromatosis Alpha-thalassaemia* Beta-thalassaemia* Sickle-cell disease* Tay Sachs disease*
Autosomal	Having a mutation in one of a pair of a particular gene is sufficient to result in the disease. The child of a person with a dominant condition has a 1 : 2 (50%) chance of inheriting the condition	Neurofibromatosis type 1 Huntington's disease
X linked	Because females have two X chromosomes, mutation in the X chromosome gene cause mild or no manifestations in females but fully manifest in males, who only have one X chromosome. If a woman carries a mutation in a gene on one of her X chromosomes, there is a 1 : 2 (50%) chance that any son she has will be affected by the particular condition.	

*Condition for which community screening for carrier status may be offered.

TABLE 11.9 Frequency of carriers and disease in ethnic groups for conditions for which carrier screening is commonly offered[21]

Disease	Ethnic group	Carrier frequency	Incidence in newborns
Cystic fibrosis	Caucasians	1 : 25	1 : 2500
Tay Sachs disease	Ashkenazi Jews	1 : 28	1 : 3100
Sickle-cell disease	Black Africans	Up to 1 : 5	Up to 1 : 100
Beta-thalassaemia	Mediterranean	Up to 1 : 5	Up to 1 : 100
Alpha-thalassaemia	South-East Asians and Chinese	1 : 10	1 : 400

TABLE 11.10 Percentage of embryos that will be affected, normal and carriers of single gene mutations having different patterns of inheritance[22]

Mutation	Affected	Normal	Carrier	Example
Autosomal dominant	50%	50%	–	Marfan syndrome
Autosomal recessive	25%	25%	50%	Cystic fibrosis
X-linked (female carrier)	25% (male)	50%	25% (female)	Haemophilia A

For each type of mutation, the sum of normal and carrier embryos equals the total percentage of all embryos potentially available for transfer.

and prothrombin genes. Further discussion of these markers is given later in this chapter.

In instances of known or presumed chromosomal irregularities, patients should be referred for preimplantation genetic diagnosis (PGD) to determine whether a specific mutation or an unbalanced chromosomal complement has been transmitted to the oocyte or embryo (see Table 11.10).

ENVIRONMENTAL FACTORS

Although it has long been acknowledged that both male and female partners contribute to human infertility, the past 20 years have witnessed a growing awareness of the importance of the male factor in the aetiology of this condition. In one paper, it was asserted that defective sperm function is the largest single, defined cause of human infertility.[23] Current estimates suggest that one in 20 Australian men suffer some degree of infertility.[24]

Human semen quality is notoriously poor compared to that of other mammalian species, and in some major capital cities, such as Paris and Copenhagen, there is evidence that it is getting poorer over time.[12] Leading researchers in this area have found that, whatever factors are responsible for this deterioration in semen quality, they do not appear to be universal, because in other areas, such as Finland[25] and the US,[26,27] similar changes have not been found. The same researchers have found that, at present, 30% of young Danish men seem to have sperm counts that are in the subnormal range according to WHO guidelines, and in 10% of this population, the semen parameters are indicative of substantially reduced fertility prospects.[12] Furthermore, they have found that declining semen parameters correlate with increased rates of testicular cancer, leading to the suggestion that testicular dysgenesis syndrome (TDS) is environmentally triggered, and warranting concern for population survival.

The particularly low sperm counts recorded in Denmark are linked with other male reproductive pathologies, including one of the highest rates of testicular cancer in the world and an increasing occurrence of other male genital tract abnormalities such as cryptorchidism and hypospadias.[28] It has been proposed that environmental factors are involved in the aetiology of TDS, and that these factors have their effect during early fetal life when the male genital tract is attempting to differentiate from the default female condition.[15] Whether the outcome of TDS is impaired spermatogenesis or testicular cancer may depend on the timing and nature of the xenobiotic attack and the genetic background on which these factors are acting. Therefore, the outcome will be determined by the man's polymorphism profile for proteins involved in detoxification, such as the cytochrome P450s and glutathione-S-transferases.

The environmental impact cannot be underestimated. Industrial growth since the end of World War II has introduced many complex chemicals into the environment that are novel to biological detoxification systems. Some of these molecules are reproductive toxins, capable of impairing fertility and inducing developmental abnormalities in the embryo, including errors in normal sexual differentiation.

One example of such an effect is the ability of environmental endocrine disruptors (including certain insecticides and detergent-derived products) to impair male sexual development in aquatic species, including oysters, alligators and fish.[29] Another example is the ability of vinclozolin, a fungicide used in the wine industry, to disrupt the fertility of male rats.[30] Alarmingly, just one exposure of a pregnant female rat to this fungicide was found to disrupt spermatogenesis in more than 90% of the male offspring for at least four generations via an effect that was exclusively transmitted through the male germ line.

This epigenetic phenomenon cannot be underestimated. The power of reproductive toxins that target the germ line lies in their capacity to generate damage that can be passed down the generations via genetic or epigenetic means.

In humans, a prime example is the effect of paternal smoking. Men who smoke heavily generate spermatozoa that suffer from high levels of DNA damage, largely as a result of oxidative stress. One of the consequences of this DNA damage is that the children of such men exhibit an increased incidence of childhood cancer.[31] While we have traditionally focused on the ability of cigarette smoke to induce lung cancer, a far more sinister effect of this activity is its ability to induce DNA damage in the germ line, and thereby influence the health and wellbeing of future generations.

In view of these findings, research on reproductive toxins is accelerating rapidly. Groups of toxins that might be involved in the aetiology of male infertility and possibly TDS include phenols (including oestrogen-like compounds) and phthalate esters, both of which are heavily represented in the environment (including dietary sources) of industrialised countries.

Exposure route

Toxic compounds may exert their genetic or epigenetic effects on the germ line via several potential routes of exposure:

- Women may be exposed to xenobiotics during pregnancy, thereby disrupting the normal differentiation of the germ line in the fetus.
- Women exposed to toxins may transmit xenobiotics to their offspring via breast milk.
- Paternally mediated toxicity through effects on DNA integrity in the male germ line. Toxicological studies in animal models reporting infertility, abortion and birth defects as a result of male exposure to xenobiotics demonstrate that such associations are possible.[32] Epidemiological studies suggest that these associations are clinically significant.[12,28]

Although there are no data to suggest that semen quality in Australia is deteriorating with time, testicular cancer rates are rising in every state, and this may suggest an environmental effect on germ cell development. That exposure to environmental chemicals can impair semen quality is clearly plausible and, in some heavily polluted environments in Europe, such effects are clearly evident.[12,33] Other countries, including in Europe and the US, are implementing various strategies to monitor the effects of toxins on reproductive processes. As such, it is prudent that Australian authorities establish whether environmental factors are to blame for the significant rates of testicular cancer and infertility seen in Australian men.[34]

Environmental toxins

PESTICIDES, SOLVENTS AND HEAVY METALS

Pesticides and solvents have been shown to disrupt neurological function, are immunotoxic, endocrinologically toxic (disrupt cascades and integration between subsystems) and can also cause various dermatological, gastrointestinal, genitourinary, respiratory, musculoskeletal and cardiological problems. Heavy metals are classed as poisons, with a diverse range of enzyme functions affecting virtually every system of the body.

Since 1976, the Environmental Protection Agency has organised a National Human Adipose Tissue Survey (NHATS) that measures the toxin levels in samples of adipose tissue from cadavers and elective surgeries from all regions of US.[35] It expanded investigation in 1982 to include an additional 54 environmental toxins. The results are alarming, indicating that it is not a question of if we are exposed to toxic xenobiotic compounds, but rather how much we are exposed and what the effects are on public health and the health of the next generations.

Overall, 20 toxic compounds were found in more than 76% of individuals in the NHATS. The following toxins were found in the percentages of individuals listed below:

- 100%: octachlorodibenzo-p-dioxin (OCDD), styrene, 1,4-dichlorobenzene, xylene, ethylphenol

Parameter	Phone use			
	None (n = 40)	<2 h/day (n = 107)	2–4 h/day (n = 100)	>4 h/day (n = 114)
Volume (mL)	2.86 ± 1.67	3.16 ± 1.62	2.83 ± 1.40	3.37 ± 1.80
Liquefaction time (minutes)	20.00 ± 3.58	20.04 ± 3.18	20.85 ± 3.56	20.39 ± 4.11
pH	7.67 ± 0.20	7.67 ± 0.18	7.76 ± 0.19	7.78 ± 0.16
Viscosity	3.00 ± 1.01	2.98 ± 1.03	3.11 ± 1.21	2.95 ± 1.14
Sperm count ($\times 10^6$/mL)	85.89 ± 35.56	69.03 ± 40.25	58.87 ± 51.92	50.30 ± 41.92
Motility (%)	67.80 ± 6.16	64.57 ± 8.47	54.72 ± 10.97	44.81 ± 16.30
Viability (%)	71.77 ± 6.75	68.21 ± 8.65	57.95 ± 11.28	47.61 ± 16.67
WHO morphology (% normal)	40.32 ± 13.06	31.24 ± 12.24	21.36 ± 10.12	18.40 ± 10.38

TABLE 11.11 Semen analysis results (mean ± SD)* in four mobile phone use groups[40]

*Means and SD were based on data on the original scale; all analyses were done with appropriately transformed data.

- 91–98%: benzene, toluene, chlorobenzene, ethylbenzene, dichlorodiphenyldichloroethylene (DDE), three dioxins, one furan
- 87%: β-benzene hexachloride (BHC)
- 83%: polychlorinated biphenyl (PCB)
- 31–69%: phthalates
  - diethyl phthalate (42%), di-n-butyl phthalate (44%), butylbenzyl phthalate (69%), di-n-octyl phthalate (31%).

Recommendation – assessment

The recommendation is to thoroughly review all presenting patients for environmental exposure and assess treatment according to the results. Specific areas to consider include:
- full occupational exposure review
- non-occupational exposure
  - where they live
  - age of structure
  - age of carpet, floor coverings, floorboards
  - renovations – when, what, how?
  - type of heating and air-conditioning
  - indoor or outdoor pesticides
  - attached garage
  - blinds, curtains
  - cleaning products
  - pool/spa/sauna
  - pets – type, medicines, foods
  - food sources
  - water source
  - others.

Recommendation – treatment

It is best to recommend avoidance of other exposure to items such as paints, solvents, fumes, chemical products, perfumes, hair spray, new furniture, new carpets or cabinets, plastics, gas, chemical gases and many others. Organic, environmentally sound and sustainable practices are generally the best recommendations.

RADIATION

Mobile phones operate at frequencies of 400–2000 MHz and emit radiofrequency electromagnetic waves (EMWs). Analogue phones operate at 450–900 MHz, digital phones (global system for mobile communications [GSM]) at 850–1900 MHz, and third-generation phones at approximately 2000 MHz.[36] Potential adverse effects of radiofrequency EMWs on the brain, heart, endocrine system and DNA of humans and animals are widely reported in the literature. Specifically from a fertility context, they have been also implicated in DNA strand breaks.[37] However, the concern that mobile phone use might have adverse impacts on semen quality has not been extensively addressed. The relationship between mobile phone use and male infertility remains unclear. Harmful EMWs emitted from mobile phones may interfere with normal spermatogenesis and result in a significant decrease in sperm quality. Specific findings pertaining to effects of mobile phones on sperm motility in humans have been noted.[38,39] When considering these factors, it is also important to acknowledge the additional impact of cordless household phones.

In one observational study,[40] the use of mobile phones decreased the semen quality in men by decreasing sperm count, motility and viability, and inducing changes in normal morphology (Table 11.11). The decrease in sperm parameters was dependent on the duration of daily exposure to mobile phones, but independent of the initial semen quality. Of greatest importance was that sperm count, viability and morphology reduced as mobile phone use increased. Specifically, using the phone for more than 4 hours/day led to a 25% drop in the number of sperm produced, and only 20% of these had normal morphology.

This study was a specialised population, as all study participants were attending an infertility clinic. Therefore, until more studies have been completed it is advisable to recommend reduction in or avoidance of mobile phone usage for all men and to review further research as it becomes available.

SMOKING

Both active and passive cigarette smoking are known to have a significant effect on both pregnancy rates and long-term ovarian function. Smokers are more likely to have a premature menopause, and smoking is thus an important preventable cause of difficulty in conceiving.

Cigarette smoking is known to have a number of detrimental consequences on general health, including noxious effects on both male and female fertility. A Cochrane systematic review in 2010 found that both active and passive smoking is associated with reduced fertility and a decreased chance of a healthy, live birth in both fertile and infertile populations.[41]

In women, cigarette smoking has been shown to contribute to decreased ovarian vascularisation and reduced oocyte maturation,[42] and in women of reproductive age, it has been linked to premature ovarian ageing[43] (thus contributing to premature decline in fertility) and increased risk of miscarriage. Results from an Australian survey involving 14 779 women aged 18–23 years showed that current smokers and ex-smokers had an increased risk of menstrual symptoms and miscarriages compared to women who had never smoked.[44] Women who smoked 20 or more cigarettes were most at risk, the odds ratio generally increasing with younger age of starting to smoke. In women, smoking has also been shown to compromise IVF[45] and ART[46] outcomes.

The negative impacts of smoking are not limited to women. In men, cigarette smoking has been observed to impair sperm respiration, affecting their mitochondrial function,[47] and to decrease sperm motility and semen quality.[48] The male partner smoking has also been found to be associated with increased risk of the female miscarrying.[49] Furthermore, smoking is likely to further contribute to oxidative damage of sperm, increasing sperm DNA damage. The DNA damage that smoking induces in sperm and its abhorrent repair in the fertilised egg can result in embryo mutations that induce miscarriage or impair the health and fertility of the child.[50]

In view of the above findings, it is thus widely accepted that prior to conception both prospective parents should cease smoking and minimise their exposure to secondary cigarette smoke.

RECREATIONAL DRUGS

No association has been demonstrated between excessive female alcohol intake (considered as more than one to two drinks per day) and infertility, although excessive alcohol consumption is known to have adverse effects on the fetus. In contrast, excessive alcohol consumption in men is associated with diminished sperm function.

After cigarettes and alcohol, marijuana is the most commonly used recreational drug.[51] Although considered by many to be a 'soft' drug, marijuana is a known fertility toxicant. Marijuana contains constituents known as cannabinoids, which have been shown to impair signalling pathways, alter hormone regulation and lead to incorrect timing during embryo implantation.[52] Specifically, in men, cannabinoids have been found to inhibit the mitochondrial respiration of human sperm,[53] reduce testosterone production[52] and decrease sperm motility, morphology and function, including capacitation and acrosome reaction.[54] In women, smoking marijuana has been associated with an elevated risk of infertility due to ovulatory abnormality/disrupted ovarian function.[55] Clearly, acknowledging the adverse effects of marijuana on

both male and female fertility, its use must be excluded in all patients undergoing preconception care.

Complications

IMPLANTATION ERRORS AND MISCARRIAGE

To begin to understand the prevention, investigation and treatment of miscarriage, it is important to understand implantation and how the placenta forms through the first trimester.

Implantation of the developing embryo into the receptive endometrium is a critical key event in the establishment of early pregnancy in the human. The unique process of cell adhesion of the trophoblast to the endometrium at the time of implantation and its subsequent invasion into the maternal tissue is dynamically balanced through the expression of specific cell adhesion molecules and endocrine, paracrine and autocrine signals. The process can be viewed as a series of distinct events, many of which are similar to those of an inflammatory reaction, and it is greatly influenced by the factors present in the uterine microenvironment, which include hormones, growth factors and inflammatory and proinflammatory cytokines.[56] The secretion of a number of factors achieves modulation of the immunological response of the trophoblast. Cytokines produced at the fetal–maternal interface play a key role in regulating maternal tolerance to the fetus and successful pregnancy.

A brief summary of the process of implantation and placenta formation is given in Table 11.12.

Investigations

FEMALE INVESTIGATIONS

The following is a summary of recommended assessments. A naturopath may conduct some of these assessments, but some will require referral to a fertility centre, general practitioner or reproductive specialist. Thorough questioning should be conducted by the naturopath to elucidate a full history and assess causative or contributing factors.

Physical examination (by general practitioner)

- Breast formation.
- Galactorrhoea.
- Genitalia (e.g. patency, development, masses, tenderness, discharge).
- Signs of hyperandrogenism (e.g. hirsutism, acne, clitoromegaly).

Stage one investigations

The investigations carried out in the first stage are summarised in Tables 11.13 and 11.14, and a description of the assessment of ovarian reserve is given in Box 11.4. In addition to the investigations listed in Table 11.15, the general investigations and treatments shown in Tables 11.16 and 11.17 are carried out in stage one.

TABLE 11.12 Implantation, placental formation and miscarriage (adapted from Jansen[57])

Step		Explanation
1	Embryo cleavage, blastulation and hatching	Requires significant cell turnover and optimal nutritional environment
2	Penetration	The mother needs to 'switch down' her immune response to allow the embryo to penetrate the endometrium
3	Avoiding rejection: fetal HLA-G and maternal uterine CD56+ NK cells	Early pregnancy failure (subclinical miscarriage or biochemical pregnancy) can alter these maternal mechanisms
4	Coagulation cascade and placental construction	Embryonic miscarriage or 'blighted ovum' are often due to conditions that cause thrombophilia, which increases the likelihood of miscarriage at this stage
5	Conversion of maternal placental arterioles	Antiphospholipid antibodies in either late or early pregnancy can initiate miscarriage due to prevention of maternal blood flow into the intervillous space, contributing to poor vascularisation of the mature placenta. This can result in preeclampsia if the pregnancy proceeds to the second or third trimester
6	Allograft survival and cytokine balance	Between weeks 6 and 11, maternal white blood cells enter the placental site, causing a rush of cytotoxic T cells and aggressive intrauterine disturbance, which can lead to miscarriage without a specific immune reaction
7	Make or break with syncytiotrophoblast turnover	The syncytiotrophoblast has functions in filtration, facilitated diffusion for nutrients and excretion and is in immediate contact with maternal blood without HLA antigen. It influences maternal metabolic pathways, blood coagulation, the immune response and synthesises progesterone. Importantly, it must grow with the pregnancy. Any condition from hyperthyroidism to coagulation disorders or nutritional deficiencies can affect this development and cause miscarriage – even later miscarriages once a heartbeat has been detected – as growth can be interrupted, delayed or halted at any stage of this delicate interrelationship between the embryo and placental growth
8	Final pathways to miscarriage	When the syncytiotrophoblast and progesterone production fail, Th1 cytokines are produced and fibrin forms at the imminent cleavage between the placenta and the mother. Late miscarriages can be triggered by infection, cervical incompetence or inflammation

HLA = human leucocyte antigen; HLA-G = human leucocyte antigen G; NK = natural killer; Th1 = T helper 1.

Stage two investigations

The investigations and treatments carried out in stage two are summarised in Tables 11.18 and 11.19.

Miscarriage screen (female)

A summary of the assessments included in this screen, and the normal reference ranges for each, are given in Table 11.20. Interpretation and treatments are given in Table 11.21.

MALE INVESTIGATIONS

A summary of recommended assessments is shown in Tables 11.22–11.27. A naturopath may conduct some of

Text continued on p. 275

TABLE 11.13 Key elements of infertility evaluation in women

Female investigation[58]

History	Coital practices Medical history (e.g. genetic disorders, endocrine disorders, history of pelvic inflammatory disease) Medications (e.g. hormone therapy, psychotropics, NSAIDs) Menstrual history Potential sexually transmitted disease exposure, symptoms of genital inflammation (e.g. vaginal discharge, dysuria, abdominal pain, fever) Previous fertility Substance use, including caffeine Surgical history (previous genitourinary surgery) Toxin exposure
Physical examination	Breast formation Galactorrhoea Genitalia (e.g. patency, development, masses, tenderness, discharge) Signs of hyperandrogenism (e.g. hirsutism, acne, clitoromegaly)

TABLE 11.14 Stage one investigations: female		
Assessment	**Time in menstrual cycle**	**Justification for assessment**
Follicle-stimulating hormone (FSH)	Days 2–3	FSH stimulates follicle development. High levels can indicate menopause or declining fertility (possible primary ovarian failure). It is useful to assess the FSH:LH ratio to ensure that the hormone status is optimal. Day 3 is essential.
Luteinising hormone (LH)	Days 2–3	LH triggers ovulation when it surges. Excessive levels may indicate polycystic ovarian syndrome (PCOS). It is useful to assess the FSH:LH ratio to ensure that hormone status is optimal. Day 3 is essential.
Progesterone (P4)	Day 21 (7 days post ovulation)	To evaluate adequacy of progesterone and to confirm ovulation. Eliminates luteal phase defect. 7 days post-ovulation is the most important and will vary with women.
Prolactin (PRL)	Any day	Inhibits ovarian production of oestrogen, inhibitory role with progesterone if high, stimulates production of breast milk
Oestradiol (E$_2$)	Day 3	E$_2$ stimulates egg maturation and endometrial maturation for implantation; responsible for fertile-quality cervical fluid
Testosterone, free androgen index, androstenedione	Any day	To eliminate PCOS or testosterone dominance
Specific hormone binding globulin (SHBG)	Any day	To evaluate if the concentration of SHBG is affecting the amount of testosterone available to body tissues
Transvaginal and transabdominal ultrasound scan	Days 6–11	To evaluate follicle maturation, antral follicle count, ovulation and endometrial thickness and appearance. General assessment of pelvic organs to diagnose abnormalities of the uterus and ovaries. To assess the thickness and appearance of the endometrium and to count antral follicles
Beta-human chorionic gonadotrophin (β-hCG)	Any day	To eliminate pregnancy or tumour
Anti-Müllerian hormone (AMH)	Days 2–3	To assess ovarian reserve (best done combined with an antral follicle count using ultrasound scan)

BOX 11.4 Assessing ovarian reserve: anti-Müllerian hormone (AMH)

There is growing awareness that in some women, even quite young women, an important factor in the difficulty in conceiving is that the number of oocytes available have reduced prematurely. In this circumstance, more rapid referral with earlier intervention is important, with assessment of the ovarian oocyte reserve therefore forming an important part of the initial assessment in all women, regardless of age. This was formerly done by checking the FSH concentration on day 2 or 3 of the menstrual cycle. However, apart from the timing challenge, a raised day 2 or day 3 FSH concentration is not a particularly sensitive marker of ovarian reserve, only being elevated in cases of severe depletion. There is also considerable intercycle variation and, as a consequence of early follicle recruitment, oestradiol secretion may occasionally falsely inhibit the FSH concentration, giving a misleading impression of normality.

Measurement of AMH is an important tool for assessing ovarian reserve. It is a protein hormone secreted by the granulosa cells of immature (pre-antral) ovarian follicles due to the stimulatory effects of FSH. As a consequence, the concentration of AMH in serum is a more useful reflection of the large number of small, growing follicles left in the ovary, rather than the small number of more mature antral follicles nearing dominance.

Another useful option for assessing ovarian reserve is to count the more mature antral follicles using transvaginal ultrasound. However, while very useful, this technique requires considerable skill and sophisticated equipment, and is best performed by an experienced sonologist/sonographer.

The developing sophistication of these approaches means that an AMH level should now be a routine part of assessing even young women in order to identify the small proportion of women with a reduced ovarian reserve of oocytes, for whom accelerated referral and treatment is indicated.

TABLE 11.15 Interpretation and treatment for stage one investigations (female)

Assessment	Potential treatment*
Follicle-stimulating hormone (FSH)	Reduce increasing FSH levels and improve oocyte sensitivity with oestrogen support and herbal medicines such as *Dioscorea villosa* (wild yam) and *Asparagus racemosus* (shatavari); or nutrients such as vitamin E, coenzyme Q10, zinc and B vitamins
Luteinising hormone (LH)	Regulate the FSH/LH ratio using the protocols recommended in Chapter 13
Progesterone (P4)	Support progesterone levels with *Vitex agnus-castus* (chaste tree), zinc and vitamin B_6 (Note: there is a competitive relationship between prolactin and progesterone)
Prolactin (PRL)	Reduce prolactin levels with *Vitex agnus-castus* (chaste tree), zinc and vitamin B_6 (Note: there is a competitive relationship between prolactin and progesterone)
Oestradiol (E_2)	Support regulated oestrogen pathways with calcium, zinc and B vitamins, and herbal medicines such as *Dioscorea villosa* (wild yam) and *Asparagus racemosus* (shatavari)
Testosterone, free androgen index, androstenedione, specific hormone binding globulin (SHBG)	Reduce androgenisation with specific herbal medicines, such as *Paeonia lactiflora* (peony), or nutrients, including zinc, B vitamins and chromium
Transvaginal and transabdominal ultrasound	Treatment is dependent on the findings. For example, if PCOS is diagnosed, follow the protocols given in Chapter 13
Beta-human chorionic gonadotrophin (β-hCG)	Assess for pregnancy or tumour, and refer as necessary
Anti-Müllerian hormone (AMH)	Assess the reading to determine the ovarian reserve. If the reserve is compromised and waning, referral for ART procedures with supportive treatment is ethically appropriate

*Recommendations are not definitive and individual assessment is essential.

TABLE 11.16 General health investigations: female

Assessment	Justification
General health assessments	
FBC U and E, LFT Homocysteine Iron studies Fasting glucose, insulin, HbA_{1c} Cholesterol profile Thyroid function assessment TSH, anti-TPO, anti-TG, T3, T4, urinary iodine Vitamin D Zinc and copper Pap smear BMI (eliminate disordered eating) Hip:waist ratio	General health assessments to eliminate other abnormalities
General pre-pregnancy assessments	
Blood group and antibody screen General STI screen Infectious disease screening Rubella immunity	General pre-pregnancy assessments (if not already organised)
Cervical swab	
Bacterial culture Ureaplasma Mycoplasma	Assess for infective pathogen compromising fertility
Other	
BBT, cervical fluid changes Ovulation kit (urine)	Assessment of self-directed assessments (if used)
Advanced fertility assessments	
See miscarriage screen	Advanced fertility assessments if previous results show no abnormality or if infertility remains unexplained

TABLE 11.17 Interpretation and treatment for general health investigations (female)

Assessment	Potential treatment
General health assessments	
FBC U and E, LFT Homocysteine Iron studies Fasting glucose, insulin, HbA$_{1c}$ Cholesterol profile Thyroid function assessment: TSH, anti-TPO, anti-TG, T3, T4, Urinary iodine Vitamin D Zinc and copper Pap smear BMI (eliminate disordered eating) Hip:waist ratio	Treatment is specific to findings. For example, a low vitamin D level will require supplementation, and an increased BMI will require weight reduction
General pre-pregnancy assessments	
Blood group and antibody screen General STI screen Infectious disease screen Rubella immunity	Referral likely; however treatment is specific to findings
Cervical swab	
Bacterial culture Ureaplasma Mycoplasma	Assessment of partner is essential. Treatment is specific to isolated infective pathogen and focused on general immune support strategies such as vitamin C, zinc, *Thymus vulgaris* (thyme) and *Echinacea* spp. (echinacea)

TABLE 11.18 Stage two investigations: female

Assessment	Timing in menstrual cycle	Justification for assessment
Sperm antibodies (serum)	Any day	To determine if antibodies are present against partner's sperm. If blood results are positive, cervical mucus may need to be analysed for sperm antibodies
Laparoscopy + hysteroscopy + salpingoscopy	Before ovulation	Inspection of uterotubal junctions. Diagnosis and treatment of pelvic disease (endometriosis) or adhesions. Hysteroscopy complements HSG in revealing pathology that disturbs the shape of the endometrial cavity, especially intrauterine adhesions, submucosal fibroids and endometrial polyps. These can be diagnosed with HSG, but hysteroscopy is required to locate the pathology accurately if found, and to treat accordingly
Hysterosalpingogram (HSG) ± selective salpingogram (if indicated)	Day 7	Vaginal examination and injection of radiographic fluid into the uterus to visualise fallopian tubes on x-ray. Determines whether fallopian tubes are clear and uterine cavity is normal
Clomiphene challenge test	Day 3 – FSH and oestradiol Day 10 – FSH	Determines ovarian reserve and whether pregnancy can occur before ARTs are implemented.
Curettage or endometrial biopsy	Day 26 (just before menses is expected)	Reveals the tissue structure of the endometrium. Estimates normal ovulation due to timing. Not advised regularly due to risk of scarring

TABLE 11.19 Interpretation and treatment for stage two investigations (female)

Assessment	Potential treatment
Sperm antibodies (serum)	If results are positive, cervical mucus sperm antibodies may be required. Abstinence or barrier methods until the immune system has been regulated, and concurrent autoimmune treatment is essential through herbal medicines, dietary modifications, lifestyle modifications and nutritional supplementation
Laparoscopy + hysteroscopy + salpingoscopy	Treatment is dependent on findings. For example, if endometriosis is diagnosed, follow the protocols given in Chapter 18: Female Reproductive System in CNM
Hysterosalpingogram (HSG) ± selective salpingogram (if indicated)	

TABLE 11.20 Miscarriage screen: female	
Assessment	**Reference range**
Immunological assessments	
Lupus anticoagulant	24.0–38.0 s
Immunoglobulin A (IgA)	0.69–3.09 g/L
Anti-gliadin antibodies – IgA	<34 AU/mL
Anti-gliadin antibodies – IgG	<20 AU/mL
Antinuclear antibodies	Negative
Transglutaminase antibody	<7 AU/mL
Endomysial antibodies	Negative
Anti-thyroglobulin antibodies	undetectable
Anti-TPO	undetectable
Anti-cardiolipin antibodies – IgM	<5
Anti-cardiolipin antibodies – IgG	<5
Biochemical assessments	
Serum copper	12–22 micromol/L
Plasma zinc	9–19 micromol/L (diurnal variation occurs)
Caeruloplasmin	0.24–0.58 g/L
CA125	<35
Protein S	60–140%
Protein C	69–140%
Anti-thrombin III	50–150%
APC resistance	1.8–3.6
Fasting insulin	4–10 mU/L
Fasting glucose	3.0–5.4 mmol/L
Fasting homocysteine	5–13 micromol/L
Active B_{12}	180–790 pmol/L
Red cell folate	>650 nmol/L
Genetic tests	
Extended karyotype	46 XX (female)
MTHFR C677T	Does not carry
MTHFR 1298C	Does not carry
Prothrombin G20210A	Does not carry
Factor V Leiden	Does not carry
Ultrasound and procedures	
Pelvic ultrasound	No abnormalities detected
Sonohysterogram	No abnormalities detected
Vaginal swab	No cultures
Cervical swab	No cultures
Endometrial biopsy	Assessment dependent on phase of cycle
Endometrial T-cell subsets	CD56+ (uterine) NK cells and CD57+ NK cells present in endometrial stromal cell density (as a percentage)

Continued

TABLE 11.20 Miscarriage screen: female—cont'd

Assessment	Reference range
Haematological tests	
Blood group	Various
Blood group antibodies	Negative
Syphilis	Not detected
Hepatitis B	Not detected
Hepatitis C+	Not detected
HIV	Not detected
Rubella	Immune (>40 IU/mL)
T-cell subsets	Normal
FBC	Normal
Endocrine tests	
FSH, LH, PRL, SHBG, FAI, TT, β-hCG, 17 OHP, P4, TSH, fT4, fT3	Various
Ovulation tracking over 2 months: E$_2$, LH, P4	Various

TABLE 11.21 Interpretation and treatment for miscarriage screen (female)

Assessment	Potential treatment
Immunological assessments	
Lupus anticoagulant Immunoglobulin A (IgA)	Autoimmune management, with treatment specific to the presentation. Note correlating evidence of compounding autoimmune factors (see Chapter 7)
Anti-gliadin antibodies – IgA Anti-gliadin antibodies – IgG Transglutaminase antibodies Endomysial antibodies	Autoimmune treatment principles, with strict avoidance of gluten. Referral for coeliac gene screen ± biopsy (endoscopy) is essential. Full discussion of the assessment is given in Chapter 9
Antinuclear antibodies	Autoimmune management, with treatment specific to the presentation. Note correlating evidence of compounding autoimmune factors (see Chapter 7)
Anti-thyroglobulin antibodies Anti-TPO	Treat for the autoimmune presentation (see Chapter 17 for a full discussion)
Anti-cardiolipin antibodies – IgM Anti-cardiolipin antibodies – IgG	Autoimmune management, with treatment specific to the presentation. Note correlating evidence of compounding autoimmune factors. Assess for blood coagulation abnormalities or antiphospholipid syndrome. Treat for autoimmune presentation.
Biochemical assessments	
Serum copper	Supplement as required, or address zinc/copper imbalance
Plasma zinc	Supplement as required
Caeruloplasmin	Assess iron metabolism and query copper+zinc status
CA125	Query endometriosis or cancer. Refer for further investigation. See Chapter 13 for more information.
Protein S Protein C Anti-thrombin III APC resistance	Support blood coagulation and cardiovascular function with various prescriptions, including herbal medicines such as *Ginkgo biloba* (ginkgo), *Curcuma longa* (turmeric) or vitamin E, coenzyme Q10 and vitamin K

TABLE 11.21 Interpretation and treatment for miscarriage screen (female)—cont'd	
Assessment	**Potential treatment**
Biochemical assessments	
Fasting insulin	Query hypoglycaemia and diabetes. Treat depending on the fluctuation (see Chapter 17 for a full discussion of blood sugar management)
Fasting glucose	
Fasting homocysteine	Homocysteine-lowering strategies, such as vitamins B_6, B_9 and B_{12}. Query MTHFR polymorphism and cardiovascular health
Active B_{12}	Assess for anaemia. Query intrinsic factor, thalassaemia. Supplement as required
Red cell folate	Assess for anaemia. Query MTHFR polymorphism and thalassaemia. Supplement as required
Genetic tests	
Extended karyotype	Refer
MTHFR C677 T	Query homocysteine and supplement with high-dose or methylated folate or folinic acid
MTHFR 1298C	
Prothrombin G20210A	Support blood coagulation and cardiovascular function with various prescriptions, including herbal medicines such as *Ginkgo biloba* (ginkgo), *Curcuma longa* (turmeric), vitamin E, coenzyme Q10 and vitamin K. The condition is compounded if the male partner is also a carrier
Factor V Leiden	
Ultrasound and procedures	
Pelvic ultrasound	Treatment is dependent on findings
Sonohysterogram	
Vaginal swab	Assessment of the male partner is essential. Treatment is specific to the isolated infective pathogen, and the focus is on general immune supportive strategies
Cervix swab	
Endometrial biopsy	If endometrial proliferation is poor, focus on building endometrial lining with hormone support (progesterone) and key nutrients for tissue growth (protein and B vitamins)
Endometrial T-cell subsets	Address with immune-modulating protocol
Haematological tests	
Blood group + antibodies	Assess and compare with male partner's blood type and antibody screen. Refer if antibodies are found
Syphilis	Treatment is dependent on findings
Hepatitis B	
Hepatitis C+	
HIV	
Rubella	Refer for vaccination if indicated
T-cell subsets	Treatment is dependent on findings; however, immune modulation will generally be required
FBC	Treatment is dependent on finding. For example: blood building and regulation of red blood cell parameters through protein, B vitamins and iron and blood building herbal medicines; regulation of white blood cell parameters through zinc, vitamin C and immune-regulating herbal medicines
Endocrine tests	
FSH, LH, prolactin, SHBG, FAI, TSH, testosterone, β-hCG	Various treatments depending on findings
Ovulation tracking over 2 months: E_2, LH, P4	

these assessments, but some will require referral to a fertility centre, general practitioner or reproductive specialist. Thorough questioning should be conducted by the naturopath to elucidate a full history and assess causative or contributing factors.

A summary of the terminology associated with semen and sperm is given in Box 11.5.

Semen analysis and treatments are shown in Tables 11.28 and 11.29.

Sperm chromatin structure assay (SCSA)

Research indicates that sperm with high levels of DNA fragmentation have a lower probability of producing a successful pregnancy. Samples with a DFI >29% are likely

TABLE 11.22 General assessment: male[58]

Assessment	Elaboration and explanation
Age	What is the age of the couple?
Fertility history	How long have they been trying to conceive, and have they ever conceived previously (together/separately)? Do they have any idea why they have not been able to conceive?
Sexual history	STI screen – potential sexually transmitted disease exposure, symptoms of genital inflammation (e.g. urethral discharge, dysuria)
Medication history	E.g. sulfasalazine, methotrexate, colchicine, cimetidine, spironolactone
Surgical history	E.g. previous genitourinary surgery
Contraception history	When it was ceased, and what was the likely speed of its reversibility?
Fertile times	Does the couple engage in regular intercourse during fertile times?
Lifestyle factors	Diet, exercise, alcohol, smoking cessation, recreational drug usage, environmental toxin screen

TABLE 11.23 Reproductive history: male[58]

Assessment	Elaboration and explanation
Prior paternity	Previous fertility
Psychosexual issues (erectile, ejaculatory)	Interference with conception
Pubertal development	Poor progression suggests underlying reproductive issue
A history of undescended testes	Risk factor for infertility and testis cancer
Previous genital infection (STI) or trauma	Risk for testis damage or obstructive azoospermia
Symptoms of androgen deficiency (AD)	Indicative of hypogonadism
Previous inguinal, genital or pelvic surgery	Testicular vascular impairments, damage to vasa, ejaculatory ducts, ejaculation mechanisms
Medications, drug use	Transient or permanent damage to spermatogenesis
General health (diet, exercise, smoking)	General health screen

TABLE 11.24 Physical examination: male[58]

Assessment	Elaboration and explanation
General examination	Acute/chronic illness, nutritional status
Genital examination (by GP)	Assess for varicocele, testicular size and other genital factors Testes: small testes suggests spermatogenic failure Presence of vas deferens: may be congenitally absent Epididymides: thickening or cysts may suggest previous infection and resultant obstructive problems Varicoceles: detected when standing, coughing or performing Valsalva manoeuvre Penis: assess for abnormalities (e.g. Peyronie's) that may interfere with intercourse
Degree of virilisation	Assess for signs of virility Signs of androgen deficiency (e.g. increased body fat, decreased muscle mass, decreased facial and body hair, small testes, Tanner stage <5)
Prostate examination	Assess if history suggests prostatitis/STI

BOX 11.5 Semen terminology

Aspermia: an absence of semen despite male orgasm
Azoospermia: a complete absence of sperm (spermatozoa) in the semen
Teratozoospermia: sperm with abnormal morphology
Asthenozoospermia: reduced sperm motility
Necrospermia: death of sperm
Oligoasthenoteratozoospermia (OAT): a low count, weak motility and abnormal morphology of sperm
Oligozoospermia: reduced number of normal motile sperm cells (spermatozoa) in the ejaculate (compare with azoospermia, where there is no sperm in the ejaculate). It includes terms such as: asthenozoospermia, teratozoospermia and (OAT)

to have significantly reduced fertility potential, including a significant reduction in term pregnancies and an increase in the miscarriage rate. Sperm that appear to be normal by traditional semen analysis parameters may have extensive DNA fragmentation.

The DFI threshold for humans was first established in the Georgetown Male Factor Infertility Study, which used data from 200 presumed fertile couples attempting to conceive naturally.[60] Fertility data from this study were used to establish the statistical thresholds of DFI >30% for 'significant lack of', DFI 15–30% for 'reasonable' and DFI <15% for 'high' fertility status (see Table 11.30). It is normal for up to 20% of sperm to have some DNA fragmentation. Mature sperm are protected from damage as 85% of the chromosomes are bound by protamines into a condensed, compact structure. If more than 20% of sperm have DNA damage, there is an increased risk of infertility, impaired embryo development, miscarriage and recurrent miscarriage (up to three- to four-fold higher), and genetic disease or childhood cancer in the next generation.

Reasons for testing include unexplained infertility, low fertility rates, poor embryo quality, implantation failure after IVF, recurrent miscarriage, exposure to environmental toxins, abnormal semen analysis and age above 45 years.

TABLE 11.25 Blood assessments: male

Assessment	Justification for assessment
Follicle-stimulating hormone (FSH) Progesterone (P4) Prolactin (PRL) Luteinising hormone (LH)	Assessment to ensure hormonal status is optimal, eliminates hormonal irregularities **FSH** Elevated levels are seen when spermatogenesis is poor (primary testicular failure), in normal men the upper reference value is approximately 8 IU/L. Azoospermic men: 14 IU/L strongly suggests spermatogenic failure, 5 IU/L suggests obstructive azoospermia but a testis biopsy may be required to confirm that diagnosis
Total testosterone, free testosterone	**Testosterone** Testosterone is often normal 8–27 nmol/L, even in men with significant spermatogenic defects. Some men with severe testicular problems display a fall in testosterone levels and rise in serum LH; these men should undergo evaluation for androgen deficiency. The finding of low serum testosterone and low LH suggests a hypothalamic–pituitary problem (e.g. prolactinoma, serum prolactin levels required)
Specific hormone binding globulin (SHBG)	Evaluates if concentration of SHBG is affecting the amount of testosterone available to body tissues
TSH, T3, T4, Thyroid antibodies, reverse T3, urinary iodine	Query thyroid function

TABLE 11.26 Other: male

Assessment	Justification
General health assessments	
FBC, blood type U and E, LFT Homocysteine Vitamin D Fasting glucose and other diabetes screening if indicated (insulin, HbA$_{1c}$, GTT) Cholesterol profile General STI screen	General health assessments to eliminate other abnormalities
Urinalysis	
Urinalysis and swabs	To assess for *Chlamydia trachomatis*, *Ureaplasma urealyticum*, *Mycoplasma hominis*, *Neisseria gonorrhoeae*
Advanced fertility assessments	
Karyotyping and subsequent genetic testing	Advanced fertility assessments if previous results show no abnormality or if infertility remains unexplained
Scrotal (testicular) ultrasonography	History of undescended testes or concern regarding testicular cancer
Transrectal ultrasonography	If ejaculatory duct obstruction is suspected

TABLE 11.27 Andrology assessment

Assessment	Justification
Semen analysis (SA)	General semen analysis including an assessment of motility, morphology, concentration, volume, appearance
Sperm chromatin structural assay (SCSA)	To determine level of DNA damage to sperm
Immunobead test (IBT)	To assess for antibodies present against sperm
Semen culture	To assess for presence of infection
Retrograde ejaculatory testing	Performed if semen analysis has extremely low count to assess for retrograde semen flow
Trial wash	Conducted prior to IVF/ICSI procedures to assess sperm factors and determine if IVF or ICSI is more appropriate
Micro-epididymal sperm aspiration (MESA)/testicular sperm extraction (TESE) and percutaneous epididymal sperm aspiration (PESE)	Specialised sperm extraction from the male genitals when sperm count is low or if ejaculation is not possible

Current research indicates a trend in increased human spontaneous abortions when the DFI ≥30%. A DFI ≥30% is associated with increased miscarriage rates and a higher rate of spontaneous abortion at 12 weeks of gestation (*p* <0.01) in comparison with a DFI <30%. Data suggest that 39% of miscarriages are related to a DFI >30%.[61] In addition, a 31% abortion rate was reported when

spermatozoa from men with cryptozoospermia (<1 million sperm/cm³) or severe oligoasthenoteratozoospermia (OAT) syndrome were used for intracytoplasmic sperm injection (ICSI).[62] The high abortion rate in this study possibly reflects genetically compromised sperm.

Sperm DNA damage

Various methods have been developed to measure sperm DNA strand breaks in situ. Currently, there are four major tests for sperm DNA fragmentation, including the COMET assay, TUNNEL assay, SCSA and the acridine orange test.

TABLE 11.28 Semen analysis (adapted from WHO[59])	
Semen parameter	Lowest reference (reference range)
General parameters	
Abstinence	Parameters are defined based on abstinence of 3 days
Collection method	Optimal collection is via masturbation. However, specialised condoms can be provided for men with religious restrictions in this regard
Specimen	The semen sample must be complete (always check the comments section)
Analysis time	Sample must be analysed within 60 minutes
Appearance	Nil debris Nil clumping or viscosity changes Liquefaction complete
pH	>7.2 (range 7.2–7.8)
Volume	>1.5 mL (range 1.4–1.7 mL)
Concentration	
Sperm concentration	>15 million/mL (12–16 million/mL)
Total sperm count	>39 million per ejaculate (33–46 million per ejaculate)
Motility	
Total motility	40% (range 38–42%) (>25% rapid, >40% progressive, >50% motile)
Progressive rating	>3
Progressive motility	>32% (range 31–34%) with forward movement
Vitality	>58% (range 55–63%) live
Morphology	
Sperm morphology	4% (range 3–4%) normal forms Note: the trial wash can provide specific information about morphological abnormalities (i.e. head, neck, tail)
Teratozoospermia index (TZI)	<1.64
Immune involvement	
Peroxidase-positive leucocytes	<1.0 million/mL
Semen culture	Negative
Mixed anti-globulin reaction (MAR) test (motile sperm with bound particles)	<50%
Immunobead test (motile spermatozoa with bound beads) (refers to assessment for sperm antibodies)	<50% sperm with adherent particles
Growth-associated molecule (GAM) or isotype	>20% positive >50% pathologically significant (except tail tip binding)
Other	
Seminal zinc	>2.4 micromol/ejaculate
Seminal fructose	>13 micromol/ejaculate
Seminal neutral glucosidase	>20 mU/ejaculate

DNA fragmentation can be attributed to various pathological conditions (see Box 11.6), including cryptorchidism, cancer, varicocele, fever, age, infection and leucocytospermia. Many environmental conditions can also affect DNA fragmentation, such as chemotherapy, radiation, prescribed medicines, air pollution, smoking, pesticides, chemicals, heat and ART preparation protocols.

Current thought suggests that DNA fragmentation is due to an apoptotic event or to ROS. Given the clear relationship between high DNA fragmentation and lower pregnancy rates, it seems plausible that DNA damage may be due to reactive oxygen species (ROS). ROS are molecules that are highly disruptive to cell function in general, and have been shown to play a role in male factor

TABLE 11.29 Interpretation and treatment for semen analysis

Semen parameter	Treatment
General parameters	
Specimen	Incomplete samples are frequent and will distort readings. Assessment can only be done by reviewing a full sample due to variations in prostatic secretion versus epididymis involvement
Analysis time	Samples that are assessed after longer than 60 minutes will produce inaccurate findings
Appearance	Debris, clumping, viscosity or liquefaction issues can suggest systemic congestion, poor hydration, poor elimination or immune processes. It can also indicate poor ejaculation frequency
pH	pH control is essential for sperm survival. An abnormally high or low semen pH can kill sperm or affect their ability to move or to penetrate an egg. The pH of the sample will be affected if there is a delay between sample collection and analysis. If the pH is <7.0 and the sample is azoospermic, there may be an obstruction of the ejaculatory ducts or congenital bilateral absence of the vas deferens (CBAVD). pH irregularities can relate to dietary intake and hydration level. Very acidic samples can indicate obstruction and require referral
Volume	Volume can be affected by the period of abstinence (3 days are recommended), incomplete ejaculation, retrograde ejaculation. It generally indicates dehydration, and treatment should consist of hydration calculation based on weight and energy expenditure.

Sperm concentration

Concentration can be affected by a number of factors including:
Incomplete collection of the sample
Health status of the individual
An obstruction
Genetic condition
The WHO guidelines[59] suggest that peripheral blood karyotyping analysis can be diagnostically helpful. Abnormal genotype may be present in up to 12% of azoospermic men and 4% of oligospermic men. Cystic fibrosis screening is recommended for azoospermia if it is due to CBAVD. Optional screening for Y-chromosome microdeletion if sperm count is <5 million/mL.
An individual's semen quality can vary considerably between samples, even in men with normal semen parameters. As a result at least two, and occasionally three, semen analyses are needed, each several weeks apart, in order to get a good idea of an individual's average semen quality. It is well recognised that sperm count can be adversely affected by illness, especially fevers, which may temporarily suppress sperm count in normal men for several months. In this case, the semen analysis should be delayed for several months.
The finding of no sperm in the ejaculate suggests either an absence of sperm production or obstruction to sperm outflow. It is most important that an azoospermic semen sample is spun down to carefully examine whether the ejaculate contains even a few sperm. Naturopathic approach considers defects in internal processes and hormonal pathways as potential hindrances to optimal count. Nutritional deficiencies are essential and interferences with pathways for spermatogenesis require exploration.

Motility and vitality

Sperm must be able to move forward (or 'swim') through cervical mucus to reach an egg. A high percentage of sperm that cannot swim properly may impair a man's ability to father a child.
There are other important conditions which predominantly affect sperm motility, such as sperm autoimmunity, a condition that accounts for about 6% of male infertility. Sperm that show no movement (immotile sperm) may be due to structural problems in the sperm tail or due to death of the sperm.
The percentage of sperm that are alive (sperm vitality) is noted because this declines in association with genital tract infections and disorders of sperm transport through the genital tract.
Proportion of live sperm is assessed if total motility is <50%. Low motility and high vitality could indicate a disturbance of the motility apparatus. If >75% of sperm are dead, immobilising antisperm antibodies might be present and testing is encouraged.
Poor motility can often indicate autoimmune processes, infection, lack of mitochondrial energy to propel the sperm or medication, alcohol or other toxins that affect semen quality.

Morphology

Sperm shape is an important predictive indicator of sperm fertilising ability. Compared to other species, the human has a relatively small percentage of sperm showing a 'normal' morphology (actually defined as being perfectly shaped), with as few as 15% normal forms being regarded as the lower limit of normal. Fertility declines as this percentage falls, particularly in men with ejaculates with less than 5% normal-shaped sperm.
Sperm can be abnormal in several ways and may be unable to move normally or to penetrate an egg. Some abnormal sperm are usually found in every normal semen sample. However, a high percentage of abnormal sperm may impair a man's ability to father a child.
Morphology is performed on Papanicolaou stained sperm using the strict Tygerberg criteria method of assessment. This method has a strong correlation between the presence of abnormalities and clinical pregnancies and only accepts sperm that are clearly completely normal in every way.
The fifth edition of the WHO criteria[59] suggests that morphology should be >4% normal forms and provides stricter criteria for subcategories associated with morphology. (See Appendix 11.6.)
Morphology is often a direct reflection of generalised toxicity in the body as semen is a by-product of the body and is a major eliminatory channel. Detoxification, avoidance of environmental toxins and immaculate dietary practices are essential. Key nutrients in sperm structure must be considered including essential fatty acids, antioxidants especially coenzyme Q10, zinc, selenium and protein.

Continued

TABLE 11.29 Interpretation and treatment for semen analysis—cont'd	
Semen parameter	Treatment
Immune involvement	
Peroxidase-positive leucocytes	The presence of white blood cells or bacteria indicates that an infection is present (genito-urinary). Even in the absence of a relevant history or symptoms, the finding of a high white cell count may prompt investigation of infection and may warrant a course of appropriate antibiotic therapy. Such infections may contribute to sperm damage and are easily treatable. Identification of infection is the primary objective with subsequent targeted treatment to eradicate the infection. It is essential to assess the partner if infection is detected.
MAR test (motile sperm with bound particles) Immunobead test (motile spermatozoa with bound beads) (refers to assessment for sperm antibodies) GAM or isotype	The immune system produces antibodies as part of the normal defence against foreign substances and organisms. Sperm are normally protected from exposure to immune system. However, some men produce sperm antibodies following surgery or trauma to the testicles. In other men, there is no apparent cause for their development. The antibodies attach to the surface of the sperm and reduce their life span, impair sperm motility and ability to penetrate the partner's cervical mucus. Antibodies located on the sperm head may prevent the sperm fertilising the egg. Abstinence or barrier methods until the immune system is regulated and concurrent autoimmune treatment is essential through herbal medicines, dietary modifications, lifestyle modifications and nutritional supplementation.
DNA fragmentation	
Once male germ cells have completed meiosis, they lose their capacity for DNA repair, discard their cytoplasm (containing the defensive enzymes that protect most cell types from oxidative stress) and eventually become separated from the Sertoli cells that have nursed and protected them throughout their differentiation into spermatozoa. In this isolated state, spermatozoa must spend a week or so journeying through the male reproductive tract and, uniquely in our species, a further period (up to 3 or 4 days) in the female tract waiting for an egg. During this period of isolation, sperm DNA is vulnerable to damage by both xenobiotics and electromagnetic radiation. Such DNA damage is associated with male infertility, and its aberrant repair in the fertilised egg may result in mutations in the embryo with the potential to either induce abortion or impair the health and fertility of the offspring.[32,34] Treatment consists of environmental review and modification as well as exceptionally high doses of antioxidant prescription.	
Other	
Seminal zinc	Low levels suggest supplementation is required.
Seminal fructose	Normal levels are 300 mg/100 mL ejaculate. Absence may indicate that the man was born without seminal vesicles or may have a blockage of seminal vesicles. As such, referral is essential for further investigations.

TABLE 11.30 Sperm chromatin structure assay: DNA fragmentation index					
DNA fragmentation index				High green (HG)	
<15%	15–24%	25–29%	>29%	<15%	15–100%
Excellent DNA integrity	Good DNA integrity	Fair DNA integrity	Poor DNA integrity	Normal	Abnormal

BOX 11.6 Causes of DNA fragmentation

Pathologies	Environmental	Other
Protamine deficiencies	Air pollution/chemicals	Age
Cryptorchidism	Smoking	
Cancer	Heat	
Varicocele	Chemotherapy/radiotherapy	
Fever	Prescription/illicit drugs	
Infection	High levels of ROS	
	Stress (mental, physical, emotional, environmental)	

infertility. ROS are free radicals (i.e. contain unpaired electrons), which tend to bind other molecules and alter them. The ROS of primary interest are the superoxide anion, the hydroxyl radical and the hypochlorite radical. These damage cells of all types, and may play a role in as much as 40% of male factor infertility.

Sperm are produced in the testes and spend approximately 10 days in the epididymis, where they undergo important maturation stages. It is in the epididymis that oxidative damage to the sperm may occur. Sperm contain polyunsaturated fatty acids, making up approximately 40% of the lipids in the sperm head, which are important for membrane fluidity, sperm motility, capacitation and sperm binding to the zona pellucida. These polyunsaturated fatty acids are extremely susceptible to oxidative damage.

BOX 11.7 Outcome of elevated sperm DNA fragmentation

- Poor oocyte fertilisation
- Defective embryo development
- Increased probability of implantation failure
- Recurrent miscarriage
  Note: All are independent of other semen parameters.

TABLE 11.31 Miscarriage screen: male	
Assessment	**Reference range**
Semen assessments	
Sperm chromatin structure assay (SCSA)	DFI <15%
Biochemical assessments	
Selenium assay	0.8–1.90
Fasting homocysteine	5–13 micromol/L
Genetic tests	
Extended karyotype	46 XY (male)
MTHFR C677T	Does not carry
MTHFR 1298C	Does not carry
Prothrombin G20210A	Does not carry
Factor V Leiden	Does not carry

The immature sperm cell is highly susceptible to damage by these highly reactive molecules because of its unique structure. The spermatozoon has a unique lipid membrane covering its head. This membrane is involved in the attachment to the zona pellucida as well as important changes that occur in the capacitation reaction. The sperm head also contains important acrosome enzymes as well as the chromosomes that will eventually fuse with the maternal chromosomes. The midpiece of the sperm generates the power to propel the tail by generating energy using its mitochondria. These mitochondria generate reactive oxygen molecules and are the aerobic source of cell energy. Semen also contains white blood cells, a very important source of ROS.

Sperm may naturally produce ROS when they utilise their oxidative metabolism to provide movement. This can occur during hyperactivation, capacitation, acrosome reaction, oocyte penetration and signal transduction (via tyrosine phosphorylase).

The internal sources of sperm ROS are the mitochondria, which generate hydrogen peroxide (H_2O_2) and the sperm plasma membrane NADPH oxidase system. External sources include white blood cells in the semen, and generation by other cells in the male reproductive tract, including endothelial cells, fibroblasts, mesangial cells and vascular smooth muscle cells. Other sources of ROS include infection of the prostate, which is associated with decreased sperm motility, anti-sperm antibodies and oxidative stress. ROS may be increased by certain medications, radiation, pollutants and in patients with spinal cord injury.

The consequences of elevated sperm DNA fragmentation are listed in Box 11.7.

Treatment

Originally, the only effective treatment for reducing the number of damaged sperm and to improve pregnancy rates was ICSI. However, seminal plasma and spermatozoa have several antioxidant mechanisms that help counteract the harsh effects of ROS, and antioxidant supplementation has shown promise in decreasing sperm DNA fragmentation in male infertility factor patients.

The sperm scavengers in seminal plasma include vitamin E (alpha-tocopherol), vitamin C (ascorbic acid), uric acid, glutathione, taurine, hypotaurine and albumin. In addition, a group of enzymes (glutathione peroxidase, catalase, indolamine dioxygenase and superoxide dismutase) helps to scavenge oxygen radicals throughout the male reproductive tract. A number of research papers support antioxidant prescriptions, which are discussed in detail later in this chapter.[63–67]

Another recommendation is to freeze a sperm sample and then defrost it, with the aim of improving the DFI, but this is generally not very successful.

Miscarriage screen (male)

A summary of the assessments included in this screen and the normal reference ranges for each are given in Table 11.31. Treatments are given in Table 11.32.

Specific naturopathic investigations

NUTRIENT AND TOXIC ELEMENT SCREENING

The nutrient and toxic element screen is a useful test to measure levels of toxic elements, including aluminium, arsenic, cadmium, lead and mercury. Excess exposure to heavy metals has detrimental effects on fertility,[68,69] and therefore this needs to be corrected (e.g. with detoxification and chelation therapy) before preconception treatment is commenced to enhance fertility status and to ensure healthy conception and a healthy fetus.

ADRENAL HORMONE PROFILE

The adrenal hormone profile determines adrenal function and may help to determine the presence or extent of acute and/or chronic mental and/or physical stress. Prolonged stress has documented suppressive effects on the fertility of both the man and the woman, and hence, where required, adrenal health needs to be supported in those undergoing fertility treatment.

FEMALE SEX HORMONE PROFILE

The female sex hormone profile measures female hormones and provides valuable information on an individual's hormone status and the potential impact this may have on the subsequent ability to reproduce. The profile obtained

TABLE 11.32 Interpretation and treatment for miscarriage screen (male)

Assessment	Treatment
Semen assessments	
SCSA	High-dose antioxidant therapy with both herbal medicines and nutritional supplementation
Biochemical assessments	
Selenium assay	Selenium supplementation
Fasting homocysteine	Homocysteine-lowering strategies such as vitamins B_6, B_9 and B_{12}. Query MTHFR polymorphism and cardiovascular health
Genetic tests	
Extended karyotype	Referral
MTHFR C677T	Query homocysteine, and supplement with high-dose folate, methylated folate or folinic acid; the dose required will be dependent on whether there is hetero- or homozygosity and which allele is affected
MTHFR 1298C	
Prothrombin G20210A	Support blood coagulation and cardiovascular function with various prescriptions including herbal medicines such as *Ginkgo biloba* (ginkgo), *Curcuma longa* (turmeric), vitamin E, coenzyme Q10 and vitamin K. The condition is compounded if the female partner is also a carrier
Factor V Leiden	

from using a saliva or urine sample is significantly more accurate than that obtained using a blood sample. DUTCH hormone profile should be considered.

MALE SEX HORMONE PROFILE

The male sex hormone profile measures the male hormones and provides valuable information on an individual's hormone status and the potential impact this may have on subsequent reproduction. The profile obtained from using a saliva or urine sample is significantly more accurate than that obtained using a blood sample.

GENITOURINARY INFECTION SCREENING

Urogenital infections (such as with *Neisseria gonorrhoeae*, *Chlamydia trachomatis* or the anaerobic organisms characterising bacterial vaginosis) have been found to play a part in the genesis of miscarriage[70,71] and infertility.[72] However, patients may be unaware of their presence due to the asymptomatic nature of many infections. Screening for a range of genitourinary infections is a necessary part of preconception care to detect possible infection and thus barriers to conception. The most common and essential infections that should be screened for include:
* primary genitourinary infections:
  – *Chlamydia trachomatis*
  – *Ureaplasma urealyticum*
  – *Mycoplasma hominis*
  – *Neisseria gonorrhoeae*.
* secondary genitourinary infections:
  – *Gardnerella vaginalis*
  – group B streptococcus
  – β-haemolytic streptococcus
  – *Staphylococcus aureus*
  – *Staphylococcus milleri*.

FERTILITY CHARTING

Fertility charting incorporates consideration of basal body temperature (BBT; the waking temperature), cervical fluid

changes and cervix position changes. Infertility treatment and assessments can be extremely invasive and disempowering. Fertility charting is a simple, cost effective and empowering screening tool that enables a female patient to intricately understand the inner fertility workings of her body.

Fertility sign 1 – waking temperature

Waking temperature is a hindsight measurement that confirms the occurrence of ovulation. It can only be used to assist in predicting ovulation once a woman is connected to and aware of the changes that occur during her cycle. It is used to confirm the luteal shift to progesterone, and is beneficial to assess the follicular and luteal phase lengths. It is also used to assess progesterone stability in the luteal phase. This is an effective predictor of progesterone stability to support implantation and pregnancy, and can also confirm anovulatory cycles.

Progesterone causes the endometrium to remain conducive to the implantation of a fertilised ovum. It also causes the body temperature to rise perceptibly, typically by 0.2°C. Therefore, it is advisable to document readings on a chart to two decimal places for greater accuracy (see Appendix 11.1). Pregnancy can be detected by a classic triphasic appearance of the chart, often caused by a second surge in progesterone after implantation, and by confirming a luteal phase length of more than 18 days.

It is important to advise women to maintain consistent timing for assessments and to have a minimum of 4 hours of unbroken sleep.

Ideally, the luteal phase lasts for 12–14 days, as this indicates that sufficient progesterone is produced and will enable the woman to maintain pregnancy following implantation. It should be noted that there are many possible appearances of a 'normal' chart, as many cycle lengths are possible. The main criteria for a normal cycle are:
* The follicular phase should ideally be <16 days. This phase can be affected by numerous factors; however,

stress is one of the main causes of an extended follicular phase.

- The luteal phase should ideally be >10 days. Each woman will have a set luteal phase, but the follicular stage can, and will, differ.

Fertility sign 2 – cervical fluid

Fertile-quality cervical fluid is produced 3–5 days prior to ovulation in response to the increasing oestrogen levels that precede the LH surge. Sperm can theoretically survive for 3–5 days in the presence of fertile-quality cervical fluid.

The role of cervical fluid is multifaceted. It:

- buffers the pH of the vagina to provide a hospitable environment for sperm survival
- provides a medium for sperm to swim in on its journey through the cervix
- provides nutritional food for sperm survival
- acts as a lubricant to increase sexual pleasure and increase sexual frequency for greater conception opportunity.

Assessment should be conducted from vaginal assessment (inserting a finger into the vaginal opening and extracting fluid for assessment) rather than relying on toilet paper or underwear changes.

SPINNBARKEIT

Spinnbarkeit (German for 'possible to spin'), also known as spin mucus, is considered the most fertile cervical fluid. It typically occurs 1–2 days before actual ovulation, resembles clear egg whites and has tremendous stretch (usually >6–10 cm). However, not all women will produce spinnbarkeit, but all that is required for conception is fluid that resembles clear egg whites.

Fertility sign 3 – cervical position

The assessment of cervical position is the most controversial of the self-assessments, and reproductive specialists often discredit its value. This is due to the cervix position being affected by numerous variables, including the timing of bowel movement.

The cervical tissue is responsive to oestrogen fluctuations and produces physical and tangible changes when ovulation is approaching. Fertile signs include a softening, opening of the cervical os, increased wetness from cervical fluid and a lengthening of the vaginal canal as the cervix shortens away from the vaginal opening. Infertile signs include a closed os, hardening, shortening and dryness.

This technique can be very beneficial for very nervous patients, as it is the most 'physical' and tangible sign, changing conclusively from fertile to non-fertile times. In addition, it is one sign that both partners can be aware of, specifically with different positions during intercourse.

Therapeutic considerations
CLINICAL DECISION MAKING AND RATIONALE

It is important to incorporate a number of considerations when determining the treatment approach:

- whether either partner has been pregnant before
- duration of infertility
- time left for conception (age of partners)
- severity of pathology
- individual factors.

It is essential that the naturopath acknowledges the presenting couple holistically and rationally. While it is ideal for all couples to experience natural conception in a loving, committed relationship, infertility can modify this ideal significantly. One may be presented with an older couple in whom the female partner presents with declining ovarian reserve, suggesting greater urgency for conception. The woman may simply not have much time left to partake in a lengthy preconception process. Alternatively, one may be presented with a couple who require donor gametes, and in such a case, the practitioner cannot address any health factors associated with the donor.

Naturopathic treatment cannot address all variables, including genetic factors or overt physical impediments. However, it can attenuate various presentations and factors. Above all, the above-mentioned principles should be considered in order to respectfully support and treat each couple individually.

Therapeutic application
ALLOPATHIC PERSPECTIVE

Please see Interactions table for potential interactions. See Fig. 11.2.

Stage 1: ovulation induction

Ovulation induction with controlled ovarian stimulation may be recommended for women who have normal tubes, but who rarely or never ovulate, and whose partners have a normal semen analysis. For women who do ovulate regularly, stimulation can be used to increase the chance of pregnancy by increasing the number of follicles that develop fully and, therefore, increasing the number of eggs that are released during a cycle.

Ovulation induction is achieved by using 3 types of medications, including:

- letrozole, which works by inhibiting aromatase, thereby suppressing oestrogen production
- clomiphene citrate, which blocks oestrogen receptors
- follitropin alfa/beta, synthetic FSH.

The outcome from all three options is that the pituitary gland produces more of the hormones needed to stimulate the ovaries. Patients are generally prescribed a course of five tablets/cycle for three cycles, usually taken on days 2–6 or 5–9 of their cycle.

Stage 2: assisted insemination

Assisted insemination is a technique in which sperm are placed into a woman's cervix or uterus around the time of ovulation via a soft, thin plastic tube. An assisted insemination cycle may or may not include ovarian stimulation. The woman's cycle is monitored by means of blood tests and ultrasound scans so that insemination can be timed precisely. The technique is rarely used

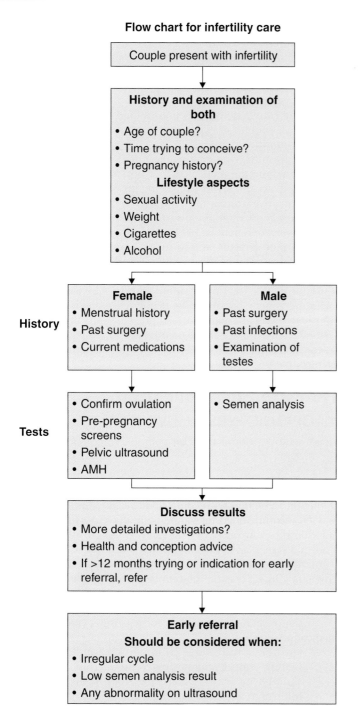

Flow chart for infertility care

Couple present with infertility

History and examination of both
- Age of couple?
- Time trying to conceive?
- Pregnancy history?

Lifestyle aspects
- Sexual activity
- Weight
- Cigarettes
- Alcohol

History

Female
- Menstrual history
- Past surgery
- Current medications

Male
- Past surgery
- Past infections
- Examination of testes

Tests

- Confirm ovulation
- Pre-pregnancy screens
- Pelvic ultrasound
- AMH

- Semen analysis

Discuss results
- More detailed investigations?
- Health and conception advice
- If >12 months trying or indication for early referral, refer

Early referral
Should be considered when:
- Irregular cycle
- Low semen analysis result
- Any abnormality on ultrasound

FIGURE 11.2 Summary of allopathic assessment for infertility care[73]

sequentially, unless requested by patients, and is often only recommended in a few circumstances, including if there is a physical problem with sexual intercourse, scarring of the cervix prevents sperm penetration or if donor sperm are required.

Assisted insemination is not as effective as IVF in cases where there is a low sperm count, or if there is endometriosis. In addition, the fallopian tubes must not be blocked, nor is it recommended when the cause of

infertility is unknown. The success rate of assisted insemination is directly related to a woman's age, and offers no better chance than that of a couple without subfertility who are having regular intercourse. Pregnancy rates are generally 5–10% per month, or 35–40% over a 6-month course of treatment. Assisted insemination is generally trialled for three cycles, and if unsuccessful the couple is referred for IVF procedures.

Stage 3: in vitro fertilisation

IVF is considered when stage 1 (ovulation stimulation) and stage 2 (assisted insemination) interventions have proven unsuccessful. A few factors are considered to accurately determine successful outcome, and ideally these are assessed prior to the procedure:
- tubal status
- endometriosis severity
- uterine factors
- ovarian status
- male factor
- female age.

However, in some instances, IVF is initiated without thorough investigation and consideration of these variables.

IVF is generally safe, with a low incidence of side-effects. Most women undergoing IVF will experience some bloating, particularly close to the site of egg collection. However, there are two serious possible consequences:

1 Ovarian hyperstimulation syndrome (OHSS), which sometimes involves severe ascites and fluid shifts, occurs in about 1% of patients, with young women and women with PCOS being at higher risk. Women developing OHSS were formerly advised to increase their fluid intake. It is now clear that this is not helpful, and can in fact sometimes lead to severe fluid overload. Adequate analgesia and sometimes paracentesis are now the main aspects of management.
2 Pelvic infection after oocyte retrieval (rare).
Other important considerations:
- In the longer term, careful studies of former IVF patients have not found any increased incidence of serious disorders such as breast cancer or ovarian cancer.
- It is clear that the rate of congenital anomaly in children conceived by IVF is slightly higher than the congenital anomaly rate in spontaneously conceived children. Of importance is Beckwith–Wiedemann syndrome, which appears to be higher in IVF parents with MTHFR polymorphism due to derangement in folate metabolism and subsequent effects on cell replication. It is not yet clear whether this is a consequence of the IVF procedures or whether couples who cannot conceive naturally are already at higher risk of there being problems in their offspring.

IVF PROTOCOL

If IVF is considered appropriate for the couple, the IVF cycle will consist of the following steps.

First the couple will undergo a thorough assessment:
- Step 1 – assessment of the woman's ovarian reserve

- Step 2 – male factor assessment
- Step 3 – infectious disease screening
- Step 4 – mock embryo transfer (controversial and rarely performed)
- Step 5 – evaluation of the uterus (transabdominal/ transvaginal ultrasound, hysterosalpingogram, laparoscopy)
- Step 6 – the woman's natural cycle (if preferred and accepted by the IVF specialist)
- Step 7 – a clomiphene-citrate-stimulated cycle (if preferred by the couple).

The standard IVF protocol is implemented after review and consideration of the above-mentioned assessments:
- Step 1 – controlled ovarian stimulation
- Step 2 – egg collection
- Step 3 – sperm collection
- Step 4 – micromanipulation of gametes (if indicated by other assessments)
- Step 5 – IVF fertilisation
- Step 6 – embryo transfer (preferably as a day 5 blastocyst)
- Step 7 – post-implantation luteal (endometrial) support (if the endometrium does not increase in thickness)
- Step 8 – vitrification (freezing) of excess embryos.

For a more thorough discussion of the steps involved in an IVF cycle, see Appendix 11.4.

Stage 4: intracytoplasmic sperm injection (ICSI)

ICSI was an accidental discovery and has revolutionised infertility practice. In this procedure, a single sperm is injected into the cytoplasm of each oocyte by means of a fine glass needle. By means of this procedure, any man with viable sperm found at any point in the genital tract can father his own children. The sperm used in the procedure is often obtained through TESE or a similar method.

ICSI is used for the treatment of infertility due to male factors or selected female factors, including, but not limited to, morphological anomalies of the oocytes, limited quantities of oocytes or anomalies of the zona pellucida. It is often required if polyspermy or poor fertilisation occurred in a prior cycle where insemination alone was used, or if PGD is planned, especially for single defects.[74]

Provided that a live sperm can be found for each oocyte, good results can be obtained, with average normal fertilisation rates being the same as those for normal semen in standard IVF. However, ICSI does not address issues relating to fertilisation or implantation.

Stage 5: donor gametes

Donor gametes (sperm or oocyte) are especially recommended for older women with poor oocyte response (oopause). Australian legislative changes (January 2010) led to significant restriction of oocyte and sperm donation. Genetic heritage rights for the child now stipulate that they must be able to determine who their genetic parents are, which excludes anonymity. Therefore, all individuals must know their donor and provide information for Australian ART procedures. Because of these legal

restrictions in Australia, some individuals may be required to travel overseas to obtain gamete donation.

Stage 6: surrogacy

Surrogacy is required if the woman's assessments indicate that no treatment would be effective and that pregnancy would be impossible. A number of general criteria need to be considered in such cases. As an overview, the commissioning woman and the surrogate are required to meet all the following requirements:
- There is a clear medical indication for surrogacy.
- There is a close and ongoing relationship with the commissioning couple and surrogate (in instances of gestational surrogacy).
- The surrogate must have at least one child and be over 21 years old.

Stage 7: adoption

Adoption may be considered if all other avenues have been exhausted. Each country, state and territory has its own laws and jurisdictions. However, many prevent adoption in instances of increasing age and by unmarried persons, or other unfortunate restrictions.

Historical perspective

Fertility disorders are not a modern phenomenon, and a range of botanicals were identified and documented by the Eclectic physicians as enhancing healthy fertility. While there is a wide array of information pertaining to female fertility problems, including miscarriage and subfertility, male subfertility and infertility remain relatively undocumented, suggesting that this domain was largely undiscovered. The majority of the literature reviewed suggests that when managing fertility the Eclectics concentrated on abnormalities in the structure and function of the reproductive system, and on stress. Modern day factors that have been implicated in the aetiology of impaired fertility, such as nutrition and environmental toxins, enjoy little mention.

Acknowledging the wide range of herbs that have been identified to help prevent miscarriage, this appears to have been a common occurrence during the time of the Eclectics. Ellingwood describes the use of *Caulophyllum thalictroides* (blue cohosh) for its toning effects on the reproductive organs, thus helping to prevent threatened miscarriage:

> *The growth of the fetus has been compared to an apple, which, when fully ripened, falls from the tree. The effect of caulophyllum is to prolong gestation till the fetus is fully developed, labor being a physiological process at full term, and not pathological, therefore less protracted, less painful, and less liable to accidents.*[75]

The nervine sedative and uterine tonic actions of *Viburnum prunifolium* (black haw) led it to be considered one of the best remedies to administer in the prevention of miscarriage due to its action on irritated uterine structures.[75] *Viburnum prunifolium* was found to combine well with *Packera aurea* (life root), although the latter was also known for its beneficial effects in overcoming female sterility,[75] as was *Actaea racemosa* (black cohosh). Another botanical deemed useful for its reversible effects on female sterility was *Serenoa repens* (saw palmetto):

> An exceedingly important use for this remedy that I have not been able to find in the books, is its use for sterility. In simple cases where there is no organic lesion on the part of the patient, this agent has an excellent reputation for restoring the ovarian action properly and assisting in putting the patient into an excellent condition. One conscientious reliable lady physician assures me that in five definite cases, pregnancy has followed the use of this remedy where sterility was pronounced previously, and thought to be incurable.[75]

The Eclectic physician Ellingwood detailed the use of *Aletris farinosa* (true unicorn root), suggesting it to not be reliable for immediate results in the presence of miscarriage, but to be more of a regulator due to its ability to correct the tendency to habitual abortion, improve the function of the ovaries and promote fertility. He also noted the use of the uterine tonic *Chamaelirium luteum* for its anti-abortive action. Ellingwood also details the example of Dr Hemminger of Pennsylvania and his use of *Mitchella repens* (squaw vine) to prevent miscarriage, given as 20-drop doses three times daily throughout the entire period of gestation.

For males, a range of botanicals were identified and documented by the Eclectic physicians as enhancing healthy fertility. While there is a wide array of information pertaining to female fertility problems, including miscarriage and subfertility, male subfertility and infertility remain relatively undocumented, suggesting that this domain was largely undiscovered. This is not surprising, as the known causes of male infertility, such as sperm DNA fragmentation, are modern day discoveries. Given that we now know that the male factor contributes to almost half of all cases of infertility, we are reminded of the enormous growth in modern naturopathy in the last century alone. The majority of the literature reviewed suggests that when managing fertility, the Eclectics concentrated on abnormalities in the structure and function of the reproductive system and on stress. Modern day factors that have been implicated in the aetiology of impaired fertility, such as nutrition and environmental toxins, enjoy little mention.

There is relatively little documented information on specific remedies to increase and enhance fertility in men. Instead, the majority of the literature focuses on increasing the 'sexual power' of men by means of male tonics such as *Turnera diffusa* (damiana) and *Serenoa repens*. Many of the traditional male tonics employed in the modern day treatment of male fertility, such as *Tribulus terrestris* (tribulus), *Panax ginseng* (Korean ginseng) and *Ginkgo biloba* (ginkgo), have been borrowed from the Ayurvedic and traditional Chinese systems of medicine.

Naturopathic perspective
A REVIEW OF THE CURRENT STATUS

The National Fertility Study undertaken in 2006[76] was the first of its kind and gave an interesting insight into the modern day Australian experience and knowledge of fertility issues. The study used the opinions of 2400 Australians (equal numbers of men and women) aged 18 years or over living in various states in Australia.

Although the benefits of preconception care (particularly in those experiencing fertility problems) are obvious to the majority of naturopaths, the same cannot be said for the general public. Of the men and women interviewed who were experiencing fertility problems, 39% of women and 36% of men smoked, 30% of men and 19% of women reported they drank more than two alcoholic drinks a day (≥14 drinks/week), and 42% of men and 52% of women reported being overweight. In sharp contrast to 30 years ago, when 92% of women had their first child before age 30 years, just 27% of Australian women now have their first child before this age. A desire to be in a stable relationship with a positive financial status was the main reason cited by participants for choosing to conceive later in life. As one in three women in their late twenties and thirties have no partner, this poses a problem. Additionally problematic is that 2–3 children was seen as the ideal, desired family size. As a reduced conception window is clearly evident, the question remains how realistic the decision is to delay conception until a later age.

The study findings suggested that there is some misunderstanding with regard to the effect of age on fertility: 51% of childless women aged 39–49 years believed they could conceive whenever they wanted to, despite 95% acknowledging that fertility declined with age. Of significance is the fact that both men and women appeared to underestimate the male contribution to fertility, with only 2% believing that the male factor was a reason for IVF (in fact male factors are actually the most prevalent reason why Australian couples undergo IVF). Furthermore, only 4% of women believed their partner's fertility could affect their chance of conceiving.

Lastly, 59% of participants with fertility problems had never consulted a doctor. Family and friends made up a large percentage of those asked for advice, while 48% of women and 34% of men also sought the help of a natural therapist. This highlights the important role of the naturopathic practitioner and suggests that they may play a key role in educating and informing patients of their fertility options.

As the design of this study was aimed at producing a sample that is representative of the general Australian population, it is clear that there are some major misconceptions about fertility that need to be dispelled. Where appropriate, the topic of fertility is something that may need to be tactfully discussed with patients of reproductive age, so that they are made aware of the relationship between age and optimal fertility.

NATUROPATHIC PRECONCEPTION TREATMENT

Preconception treatment adheres to the philosophy that the final stages of gamete production can be modified and influenced. The final stages of spermatogenesis last for

72–76 days, while the final stages of oocyte development take approximately 100 days. The environment to which each gamete is exposed during this period of development can influence various abnormalities.

In addition, consideration of current nutrient status throughout this developmental stage can also significantly influence the prospective outcome. The concept of nutrient repletion suggests that nutrient prescriptions need to be prescribed for a minimum of 3 months in order to properly correct all defects that the individual nutrient can affect. For example, zinc is involved in numerous pathways within the body, including those that affect reproductive health and function. To rectify all deficiencies, sufficient zinc supplementation at a repletion dosage (typically higher than general prescriptions) for an extended period of time (i.e. at least 3 months) can enable optimal correction. At lower doses or if taken for an insufficient duration, zinc treatment may only address the highest priority requirements (i.e. immune function rather than sperm production).

Finally, it is always important to acknowledge that healthy fertility occurs when the individual's health is optimal. The body is primed to pass on genetic material only when the environment and conditions are at their best. If survival from an evolutionary perspective is compromised, fertility will be hindered. Everything a person eats, drinks, experiences or is exposed to can and will influence their fertility. True naturopathic fertility care supports, acknowledges and considers absolutely all variables for holistic health. Couples should be encouraged to participate in treatment for 3–4 months in order to properly address all nutritional and gamete variables.

Foresight research and preconception healthcare

Foresight, the Association for the Promotion of Preconceptual Care, was established in the UK in 1978. It is a preconception program that incorporates dietary and lifestyle advice to enhance fertility, thereby increasing the chances of a healthy conception. The association is the pioneer of preconception care, and its education of the general public and clinicians has been invaluable.

The association has undertaken two studies, both of which produced promising results. The first study, conducted in 1995, showed an 89% success rate of live births, and a 2003 study showed a conception rate of 78.4%. The combined results of these studies leave no doubt that preconception care can improve fertility and conception outcomes. This is especially evident as the Foresight program covers nutritional status, environmental toxins, genitourinary infections, smoking and other substance abuse.

However, on review of this research, it is evident that it is of poor quality. The majority of the research is unpublished, and one study was published only as a letter to the editor. Therefore, before a rigorous evidence-based opinion can be ascertained, additional research is required. It is recommended that future studies should be scrupulously designed and reported so that they can be appraised accordingly.

ATTENUATING AND ADDRESSING INFLUENCING HEALTH CONDITIONS

The naturopathic approach to attenuating fertility issues is based on a number of parameters, each of which suggests specific processes and irregularities in the body. Therefore, treatment can be specifically targeted for optimal outcome.

Treating the female

NUTRITIONAL MEDICINE (DIETARY)

Therapeutic objectives

1 Provide nutritional sustenance to foster health and wellbeing.
2 Improve fertility parameters.
3 Avoid dietary factors that compound infertility, such as sugar, caffeine, alcohol, trans fatty acids, artificial sweeteners and anything that deviates from a wholefood diet as they are low in essential nutrients and inhibit vitamin and mineral absorption.
4 Address macro- and micronutrient deficiencies, paying particular attention to hydration and protein requirements.

Specific dietary recommendations

Advanced glycation end products (AGEs)

Advanced glycation end products (AGEs) have been shown to have a negative impact on ART outcomes and appear to be related to diminishing ovarian reserve or abnormally functioning folliculogenesis.[77] Dietary AGEs are formed during the cooking process, especially animal-derived foods that are high in fat and protein.[78] Reduce their formation by cooking with moist heat instead of dry, using shorter cooking times, cooking at lower temperatures and using acidic ingredients such as lemon juice or vinegar. Artificial sweeteners have been found to be associated with unfavourable embryo development.[79] Sugared beverages, independent of their caffeine content, are associated with lower oocyte and embryo quality in women undergoing IVF treatment.[80] High-fat diets have been associated with changes in reproductive function, including altered menstrual cycle length, changes in reproductive hormone levels and embryo quality in ART settings. These impacts on reproductive function are present in normal-weight women, and the effect is worsened in obesity.[81]

Fertility diet

The concept of a fertility diet is not new. There is significant research suggesting that dietary modulation improves ovulation, conception and the chances of the birth of a healthy child. A detailed prospective study[82] used the platform of the Nurses' Health Study II. Strengths of this study include its prospective design, where information on dietary and lifestyle characteristics was collected at least 2 years before the report of infertility, making it unlikely that subsequent diagnosis or treatment of infertility influenced the results. The use of previously validated questionnaires to assess ovulatory disorder infertility, as well as diet, physical activity and body weight, add to the strengths of this study.

During 8 years of follow-up, 25 217 pregnancies and pregnancy attempts were accrued among 7544 women. Of these, 3209 were incident reports of infertility (all causes), of which 2032 were of women who reported undergoing diagnosis for infertility, and 416 were of women reporting ovulatory disorder infertility. As expected, a high 'fertility diet' score was characterised by a lower intake of trans fat with a simultaneous greater intake of monounsaturated fat; a lower intake of animal protein with greater vegetable protein intake; a higher intake of high-fibre, low glycaemic index carbohydrates; higher non-haem iron intake; and higher frequency of multivitamin use. In addition, women with a high fertility diet score were more likely to consume coffee and alcohol and to be physically active. They were also less likely to be smokers, have long menstrual cycles and be recent users of hormonal contraception.

The positive dietary modifications as outlined above constitute a positive fertility outcome. As such, the fertility diet pattern may have favourable effects on the fertility of otherwise healthy women, and combining this dietary strategy with body weight control and increased physical activity may help prevent the majority of infertility cases due to problems with ovulation.

Please note, these findings were contradicted in newer research,[83] and lower rates of ovulation were found in groups consuming larger amount of dairy foods (cream, yoghurt).[84]

Similarly, in ART, diet has been found to play an important role. A cohort study found that women undergoing IVF/ICSI treatment had improved chances of success if they adhered to the Netherlands Nutrition Centre guidelines during the preconception period. These guidelines include eating at least four slices of wholemeal bread daily (or comparable servings of cereals), the use of monounsaturated or polyunsaturated oils, ≥200 g of vegetables daily, ≥2 pieces of fruit daily, ≥3 servings of meat or meat replacers weekly and ≥1 serving of fish weekly.[85]

Despite the increasing evidence suggesting that a healthy preconception diet might increase fecundity (or a woman's chances of becoming pregnant), results from the NHS-II cohort found no relationship between preconception adherence to several healthy dietary patterns prior to pregnancy and risk of pregnancy loss.[86]

Dietary inclusions

Oily fish

Adequate intake of omega-3 fatty acids is required to ensure stable cell membrane fluidity and energy production of the oocyte. While oily fish are a known source of omega-3 fatty acids, patients must be educated about the high methylmercury content of some fish. Due to this potential toxicity, current general guidelines advise that women undergoing preconception care refrain from intake of shark, swordfish and king mackerel, and limit their intake of tuna to two 85 g meals per week during the preconception period.[87] The general recommendation by naturopaths is to avoid all high-methylmercury-content fish throughout the preconception window. For a full discussion on the recommendations of mercury and fish, see the discussion of angina in CNM Chapter 20: Cardiovascular System.

Wholefood diet

Similarly to males, a wholefood diet is essential for women to ensure optimal development and maturation of oocytes. An unbalanced diet is associated with low intakes of vitamins and minerals and with subfertility.[88,89] For more information on this topic, please refer below to the Male section.

Protein

As every cell of the body requires protein, it is essential that protein requirements are assessed for all patients. When reviewing protein needs, it is important to consider the future requirements of a woman with regard to expected pregnancy. One study[90] observed that consumption of protein from animal sources, including chicken and red meats, was associated with an increased risk of infertility, whereas consuming protein from vegetable sources appeared to have the opposite effect. Similarly, in women ($n = 269$) attending a fertility clinic, consumption of red meat prior to IVF had a negative influence on embryo development and the likelihood of clinical pregnancy; however, higher fish intake was associated with a higher likelihood of blastocyst formation.[91]

As such, it may be beneficial to assess the protein quality and source when reviewing and recommending for patients.

Mediterranean diet

A study in the Dutch community observed that high adherence in preconception by couples undergoing IVF or ICSI treatment to a diet based on the principles of the Mediterranean diet increased the chance of achieving a successful pregnancy.[92] This type of diet was found to be more effective than a 'low processed diet', which was actually based on very similar principles. The authors suggested the high content of B vitamins, in particular vitamin B_6, combined with a high intake of vegetable oils in the Mediterranean diet may be the mechanism behind the differences observed between these two diets.

These findings are supported by a case control study of 485 Spanish women which showed improved fertility in women who adhered to a Mediterranean diet compared to those who followed a Western dietary pattern.[93] Adequate folic acid intake is associated with female fertility, and a study of three generations of women in Spain showed that a higher adherence to a Mediterranean diet was significantly related to a greater folate intake.[94]

Specialised diet

Where the reason for subfertility is known, such as in PCOS, the patient should follow a modified diet specific for their condition. For example, in PCOS, dietary principles, such as foods with a low glycaemic load, need to be followed strictly (see PCOS in Chapter 18: Female Reproductive System in CNM for more information), while in patients with autoimmune conditions that impact on fertility, such as thyroid disorders, a diet that supports thyroid health is required in addition to a standard preconception diet.

Dietary exclusions

Caffeine

Caffeine consumption is associated with an increased time to conception[95–97] and has been linked with other causes of infertility, including endometriosis and risk of spontaneous abortion.[98] Although the mechanism by which caffeine delays conception is undetermined, alterations in hormone levels, including higher early follicular E_2 levels in females, have been observed.[99] A study analysing serum and follicular fluid samples of women undergoing IVF confirmed that caffeine can reach the follicular fluid. The results showed that caffeine consumption is associated with a decrease in the number of harvested eggs in relation to increase in serum caffeine levels. There was no association found between caffeine intake and pregnancy rate in this study.[100] Excess intake of caffeine is also likely to place stress on the adrenal glands, and its diuretic action will impact on nutritional status, increasing the loss of vital nutrients required to enhance fertility, such as the B vitamins. One study[96] showed that women who consumed less than one cup of coffee a day were twice as likely to become pregnant compared to moderate coffee drinkers, with the risk of failing to become pregnant increasing with higher consumption. Studies have however produced conflicting results, with a New Zealand study of 250 women undergoing ART finding no association between coffee intake and treatment outcomes. In this study, the consumption of caffeinated herbal tea was associated with decreased pregnancy rates.[101] In a prospective cohort study of 3628 women who were planning pregnancy, it was found that caffeine in general does not show a significant negative impact on time to pregnancy in healthy women.[102] A recent prospective cohort study of 2135 women found that there was no significant association between caffeine intake and fecundity. Once again, caffeinated tea was associated with slight reductions in female fecundability.[103] Given the inconclusive nature of the evidence thus far, caffeine should be avoided in those trying to optimise their fertility.

Alcohol

The data on alcohol consumption and its relationship with fertility is mixed. While some have suggested there is no link between alcohol and fertility,[104,105] other studies have suggested a link between alcohol intake and miscarriage,[106] and between alcohol and adverse effects on oocyte retrieval, and therefore a lower chance of subsequent pregnancy, in IVF.[107]

Several theories have been proposed for the detrimental effects of alcohol on female fertility, including negative effects on blastocyst development and implantation, as well as the ability of alcohol to increase oestrogen, which in turn reduces FSH secretion, suppressing folliculogenesis and leading to anovulation and infertility.[108] Acute alcohol consumption can cause increases in oestradiol, testosterone and LH levels,[109] and regular alcohol use leads to overproduction of ROS and is associated with delayed conception. A Danish study demonstrated an increased risk of infertility in women over the age of 30 who consumed seven or more alcohol serves per week, and concluded that alcohol might exacerbate age-related infertility.[110] A prospective cohort study of 2545 couples undergoing IVF found that women drinking four or more drinks per week had 16% lower odds of a live birth compared to those who drank less than four drinks per week.[111] In contrast to these results, consumption of less than 14 servings of alcohol per week was found to have no discernible effect on fertility.[112] However, a recent systematic review and meta-analysis of the literature concluded that female alcohol consumption is associated with reduced fertility, and that the association is dose dependent.[113]

Thus, for these reasons, from a naturopathic perspective it is highly advisable for those wanting to optimise their fertility to exclude all alcohol from their diet.

Trans fatty acids

Trans fats may increase the risk of ovulatory infertility, particularly when consumed instead of carbohydrates or unsaturated fats.[114] They also offer little in the way of nutrition and are associated with adverse health outcomes, and thus they should be excluded from the diet.

Women in the highest trans fatty acid intake had reduced fecundability in a North American cohort.[95] A recent prospective cohort study of 60 women undergoing IVF treatment found a negative correlation between the trans fatty acid index and IVF outcomes.[115]

Sugar

Entering pregnancy with poor glycaemic control increases the risk of gestational diabetes, macrosomia and effects on the fetus. Therefore, it is important to ensure blood sugar levels are under control during the preconception period.

NUTRITIONAL MEDICINE (SUPPLEMENTAL)

Therapeutic objectives

1 Address deficiencies and provide nutrient repletion to restore nutrient pathways.
2 Improve fertility potential and relevant fertility factors.
3 Address attenuating factors such as infection, inflammation, toxicity and stress.
4 Provide antioxidants to reduce oxidation influence on gametes.
5 Support communication between the endocrine and reproductive systems.
6 Support hormone production and delivery to all reproductive tissues.
7 Encourage optimal eliminatory pathways.
8 Support optimal general health.

SAMPLE DAILY DIET

BREAKFAST	Avocado boat filled with curried chickpeas and baby spinach	Avocado and spinach are both excellent sources of folate. Adequate folate is required for DNA methylation and integrity. Elevated levels of homocysteine in follicular fluid as a result of folate insufficiency correlate with immaturity of the oocyte and poor early embryo quality,[116] and may impair female fecundity and compromise implantation, as well as the chance of a live birth.[116] Adequate folate needs to be consumed prior to conception to reduce risk of spina bifida and other neural tube defects because the neural tube closes by the 28th day after conception.[117] Avocado also provides a source of monounsaturated fatty acids, which are required for synthesis of cholesterol, and steroid hormones, such as oestradiol, which are needed for fertility.
LUNCH	Lamb, brown lentil, kale, goat's cheese and roasted vegetable salad (tomatoes, pumpkin, basil, rocket)	A high-quality diet before pregnancy may reduce the risk of gestational hypertension[118] and gestational diabetes.[119] A Mediterranean diet high in vegetable oils, fish, vegetables and legumes is positively associated with a 40% increase in the probability of pregnancy.[120] Red meat provides coenzyme Q10 and zinc. Coenzyme Q10 is able to rejuvenate mitochondrial energy stores in granulosa cells, restoring mitochondrial oocyte function, while zinc is essential for hormone regulation.
DINNER	Wakame, tamari, sesame seed and ginger seaweed salad with marinated tofu	Seaweed provides a source of omega-3, iodine and vitamin B_{12}. Iodine is crucial for maternal thyroid function. Thyroid hormones are involved in fertility, affecting the actions of FSH and LH on steroid biosynthesis by specific triiodothyronine sites on oocytes.[121] Vitamin B_{12} is required to prevent epigenetic alterations in DNA and histone methylation in genes that regulate key developmental processes in the embryo.[122]
SNACK	Sardine pâté made from wild sardines with crudites and walnuts Fresh fruit	Sardines and walnuts provide omega-3 fatty acids. Omega-3 improves embryo morphology.[123] Sardines may also provide a source of vitamin D. Vitamin D is required for decidualisation of the endometrium as well as regulating gene OXA-10 expression for implantation to take place.[124] Provides vitamin C and other antioxidants to the follicular environment to protect from damage and improve oocyte competence.

Specific nutrients required

Amino acids

Arginine

Arginine is an amino acid that may be used to enhance female fertility. Via its role as a precursor to nitric oxide synthesis, arginine is required for angiogenesis, embryogenesis, fertility and hormone secretion.[125]

Supplementation with oral arginine (16 g/day) in 'poor responder' female patients (patients who failed to achieve an adequate number of mature follicles and/or adequate serum oestradiol levels after gonadotrophin stimulation) undergoing assisted fertilisation may improve ovarian response, endometrial receptivity and pregnancy rates. In a small study, females undergoing ovarian stimulation were allocated to one of two groups: 1) flare-up gonadotrophin-releasing hormone analogue (GnRHa) plus elevated pure follicle-stimulating hormone (pFSH) ($n = 17$); or 2) flare-up GnRHa plus elevated pFSH plus oral L-arginine ($n = 17$).[126] Those females receiving L-arginine demonstrated a lower cancellation rate, and an increased number of oocytes collected and embryos transferred, than the control group. Three out of 17 individuals conceived in the arginine group, compared to none in the control group.

Carnitine

Carnitine is a naturally occurring amino acid that plays a vital role in fatty acid metabolism for energy. It is essential to ensure that it is prescribed in the L-form and not the DL-form. It works synergistically with CoQ10, so it is advisable to co-prescribe these two nutrients together.

Supplementation with carnitine is desirable in females trying to optimise their fertility. Aside from its effects on the mitochondria, carnitine has been found to exert a protective effect on the mouse oocyte, reducing oocyte cytoskeleton damage and embryo apoptosis induced by incubation in peritoneal fluid from patients with endometriosis.[127] A review on the role of L-carnitine in fertility suggests that carnitines improve female fertility through their integrated actions in reducing cellular stress, maintaining hormonal balance and enhancing energy production.[128] However, studies in humans are needed to determine whether carnitine supplementation is beneficial for endometriosis in patients with proven oocyte concerns due to peritoneal factors. A small in vitro study of follicular fluid from 22 infertile women with mild endometriosis undergoing IVF treatment found that L-carnitine with N-acetylcysteine prevented oocyte damage.[129]

A double-blinded RCT study in 170 clomiphene-resistant PCOS women found that administering L-carnitine (3 g/day) in conjunction with clomiphene citrate (250 mg/day, days 3–7 of the cycle) significantly improved ovulation and pregnancy rates. The lipid profile and BMI of the women was also improved.[130] A small prospective study (n = 24) of women with stress-induced hypothalamic amenorrhoea found that 16-week supplementation with acetyl-L-carnitine (1 g/day) resulted in a significant increase in LH levels in hypo-LH women, via modulation of the HPG axis. LH response to naloxone was restored in the treatment group.[131] These results were confirmed in a study of women with functional hypothalamic amenorrhoea (n = 27) who were administered L-carnitine (500 mg/day) with acetyl-L-carnitine (250 mg/day) over 12 weeks. Once again, LH plasma levels increased in hypo-LH women, while cortisol and amylase levels decreased significantly.[132]

Antioxidants

Oxidative stress causes alterations in certain protein pathways, the abnormal expression of which could possibly lead to the pathophysiology of infertility.[133] Excessive ROS production (through lifestyle factors such as smoking, alcohol intake, recreational drug use and exposure to environmental pollutants) can overpower the body's natural antioxidant defence system, creating an environment unsuitable for normal female physiological reactions, leading to unexplained infertility.[134] Characteristics such as advanced age and obesity are also associated with increased oxidative stress and decreased fertility.[133,135,136]

It is hypothesised that peritoneal fluid with increased ROS and decreased antioxidant status diffuses into the fallopian tubes and can damage the sperm, which is highly sensitive to oxidative stress. Lower total antioxidant status is observed in the peritoneal fluid of women with idiopathic infertility compared to fertile controls.[136] Oocyte quality is also affected by oxidative stress, limiting successful ovulation and fertilisation. Follicular fluid contains high level of antioxidants which protect oocytes from ROS damage, and a small pilot study has shown that higher levels of melatonin (a powerful antioxidant) in the follicular fluid are associated with both quantity and quality of oocytes, and can predict IVF outcomes.[137] Glutathione is the major non-enzymatic antioxidant found in oocytes and embryos.[134] Selenium and glutathione peroxidase levels have been found to be lowest in follicular fluid in patients with unexplained infertility, and follicular antioxidant capacity levels were higher in those whose oocytes fertilised successfully compared to those whose did not.[138]

It is important to note that physiological levels of ROS are required for healthy oocyte development and better IVF outcomes. They are a prerequisite for the first meiotic phase (meiosis I) and are also required for folliculogenesis; however, if levels are abnormally high, they are negatively associated with oocyte and embryonic development and pregnancy outcomes. Antioxidant intake is important to suppress ROS build-up and maintain physiological levels of free radicals for homeostasis and proper cell functioning.[133]

While is it clear that antioxidant status plays a role in reproduction and infertility, the success of antioxidant supplementation in female subfertility is not so clear. A 2013 Cochrane review found that the quality of the evidence in the studies was low due to poor reporting of outcomes, the size of the studies and reporting bias, and that antioxidant supplementation was not associated with an increased live birth rate or clinical pregnancy rate.[139] This conclusion was supported by a later randomised controlled trial of 218 women with unexplained subfertility undergoing IVF treatment, which showed that daily oral antioxidant supplementation (multivitamins and minerals) did not improve oocyte quality and pregnancy rates.[140]

A data analysis was carried out on women in the fast track and standard treatment (FASTT) trial (n = 503), which consisted of couples with unexplained fertility undergoing IVF treatment. Analysis of the diet and supplement intake was carried out by age and BMI (known factors affecting fertility). Results showed that increased intakes of beta-carotene, vitamin C and vitamin E were associated with decreased time to pregnancy, but the effect of individual antioxidants varies by age and BMI. In women under 35 years of age with BMI ≥25, beta-carotene supplementation was associated with short time to pregnancy. In women under 35 years of age with a BMI <25, vitamin C was associated with a shorter time to pregnancy. In women who were older than 35, vitamin E supplementation was associated with shorter time to pregnancy.[135]

A Cochrane review assessed the use of vitamin supplementation in the prevention of miscarriage and found that multivitamins plus iron and folic acid had reduced risk for stillbirth, but no effect on miscarriage risk.[141]

Alpha-lipoic acid

Alpha-lipoic acid (ALA) is able to scavenge fat-, water- and lipid-soluble free radicals. It is indicated for disease states associated with oxidative stress, and is thus helpful to support fertility.[142,143] Oxidative stress has a detrimental effect on female fertility, including increased time to conception; decreased fertilisation; decreased oocyte penetration, function and viability; decreased implantation; and increased reduction in implantation rates.[144] Due to its potent antioxidant potential, it can be expected that ALA can exert a protective role to assist in the protection from the above-mentioned concerns. However, as yet there are insufficient human clinical trials to confirm these extrapolations.

In addition, it is beneficial to review the role of ALA in the treatment of blood sugar irregularities, glucose metabolism and gestational diabetes. This is especially pertinent in patients presenting with PCOS (for a full discussion of this application see Chapter 18: Female Reproductive System in CNM).

Vitamin A

Vitamin A is an antioxidant required for cell growth and differentiation, which is especially pertinent for the development of the embryo.[145] It is required for gene expression and cell differentiation in organogenesis and embryonic development.[146] It is also required for immunity, regulatory functions and epithelial tissue integrity. It is necessary for the health of the cilia in the fallopian tubes. It has a direct interrelationship with zinc, and vitamin A deficiency has been linked with infertility, miscarriage and cleft palate. These malformation and congenital abnormality risks are aggravated by supplementation during pregnancy. However, toxic doses in pregnancy are believed to be above 25 000 IU/day. Therefore, doses below 10 000 IU/day are recommended, allowing a considerable margin for safety. A full discussion regarding vitamin A and pregnancy is given in Chapter 13: Pregnancy and Labour.

Vitamin A is a cofactor of 3β-dehydrogenase in steroidogenesis. Deficiencies may result in impaired enzyme activity,[147] and thus low oestrogen. Low concentrations of vitamin A are associated with anovulation in females.[148] Plasma levels of antioxidants, including vitamin A, have been observed to be decreased in females suffering from habitual miscarriage, leading to the suggestion that a decrease in antioxidant status may be one factor contributing to miscarriage.[149] However, a Cochrane review has found no evidence to support the use of vitamin A supplementation to reduce the risk of miscarriage.[141]

Carotenoids/beta-carotene

Beta-carotene is a powerful fat-soluble antioxidant that is converted to retinoic acid in the body, which assists the healthy functioning of the immune system and also plays an important role in the development of the baby's limbs, heart, eyes and ears.

In females, beta-carotene has been suggested to have a possible role in ovarian oocyte follicular maturation and function.[150]

Coenzyme Q10

CoQ10 is a fat-soluble antioxidant and free radical scavenger found in every cell in the body. It plays a vital role in all energy-dependent processes, and is also required for the maintenance of healthy cell membrane integrity and cell functioning. As such, it is of specific importance for new cells, including oocytes.

CoQ10 exists in both an oxidised and a reduced form, and thus can take part in oxidation and reduction reactions. It is required for mitochondrial ATP synthesis, and functions as an antioxidant in cell membranes and lipoproteins. It is involved in cell respiration and energy production in all cells of the body, and supports the immune and cardiovascular systems.

The presence of CoQ10 in human follicular fluid indicates its role in reproductive health. Higher follicular fluid CoQ10 levels were found in mature oocytes and good grade embryos compared to immature eggs and poor grade embryos, respectively.[151,152] Therefore, its application to ensure the health of the oocytes is highly desirable. It supports mitochondrial function and has positive applications for maturing oocytes, which are at greater risk of oxidative damage and zona pellucida issues. Receptivity of the zona is strongly correlated with antioxidant status,

specifically CoQ10 levels. This is understandably more important in situations of ART.

CoQ10 supplementation (600 mg/day) in women undergoing IVF resulted in reduced aneuploidy and increased pregnancy rates compared to placebo.[153] In women with clomiphene-resistant PCOS, it was found that CoQ10 supplementation (180 mg/day) in conjunction with clomiphene citrate resulted in significantly improved ovarian response, luteinisation (midluteal progesterone), endometrial thickness, ovulation and pregnancy rate compared to treatment with clomiphene citrate alone.[154]

Vitamin C

Vitamin C is the primary water-soluble antioxidant in the body. In addition to its protective effects against free radicals, vitamin C protects against oxidation of folate and vitamin E, both of which are important for healthy fertility. Vitamin C has been proposed as a highly important vitamin in both male and female reproduction. It is required for collagen production, synthesis of hormones and, acknowledging that oxidative stress has been repeatedly implicated in the pathophysiology of infertility and assisted fertility, as an antioxidant.

The ovary is believed to be the site of ascorbate accumulation. The midcycle change of retention and excretion of ascorbate is one of the main markers of ovulation.

Reviews of vitamin C highlight its structurally important role in female fertility via its effects on collagen biosynthesis, and in particular, its effects on growth and repair of the ovarian follicle as well as the development of the corpus luteum.[155] Ascorbic acid concentrations have been identified in the ovaries, including in the luteal compartment. Changes have been noted in ascorbic acid retention midway in the menstrual cycle, and these have been suggested to assist in luteal steroidogenesis.

Vitamin C is necessary for maturation of the pre-ovulatory follicle and the production of collagen (skin, tissue, bone), and reduces the risk of preeclampsia when prescribed with vitamin E. Deficiency causes increased risk of miscarriage, spontaneous rupture of membranes and brain tumour in offspring. Evidence is still very limited, and a Cochrane review concluded that there is insufficient evidence to support the use of vitamin C supplementation alone, or in combination with other supplements, to help prevent stillbirth, poor fetal growth, preterm birth or preeclampsia.[156]

Bioflavonoids

It is important to mimic nature and always prescribe vitamin C with concurrent bioflavonoids. The function of bioflavonoids is to enhance the absorption of vitamin C, and they have been shown to strengthen capillaries and help prevent miscarriage and breakthrough bleeding.

Vitamin E

Vitamin E is a powerful, lipid-soluble antioxidant that is essential for fertility and reproduction.

Vitamin E maintains the health of the ovaries[157] and regulates hormone balance. A recent study observed vitamin E levels to be low in infertile females compared to controls, suggesting that antioxidant capacity may also subsequently be low, thus increasing the risk of oxidative damage.[158] A clinical study assessing the effect of vitamin E on treatment outcomes in women with unexplained infertility undergoing ART showed that vitamin E (400 IU/day) combined with clomiphene citrate resulted in increased endometrial thickness, but no statistical difference was found in implantation or ongoing pregnancy rates compared to clomiphene citrate treatment without vitamin E.[159] A recent cross-sectional study of women undergoing IVF treatment (*n* = 50) found that higher levels of serum vitamin E (10–15 mL/dL) were associated with higher-quality embryos.[160] A double-blind RCT of 105 infertile women with PCOS undergoing IVF treatment showed that clinical pregnancy and implantation rates were significantly higher in the treatment group compared to placebo. Treatment consisted of 8-week supplementation with vitamin E (400 mg/day) and vitamin D$_3$ (50 000 IU/once every 2 weeks). Antioxidant status was not improved and oxidative stress was not reduced in the treatment group in this study, leading the authors to conclude that the positive results were due to the increase in vitamin D$_3$ levels of the participants.[161] A 2015 Cochrane review found no evidence to support vitamin E supplementation in pregnancy to prevent stillbirth, baby death, preterm birth, preeclampsia or low-birth-weight babies.[156]

Selenium

Selenium is a trace element that displays powerful antioxidant and immune-regulating functions. Selenium is also highly important for thyroid function, and hence will work in concert with iodine for infertility related to hypothyroidism. Selenium deficiency has been linked to female infertility, miscarriage, preeclampsia, gestational diabetes, fetal growth restriction, preterm labour and obstetric cholestasis.[162]

In females, selenium supplementation may help reduce the risk of miscarriage, such as in thyroid autoimmunity, which may be linked to recurrent miscarriage and infertility.[163] In one study,[164] there was an observed decrease in serum selenium in females who suffered miscarriage in the first trimester and in females who suffered recurrent miscarriage. Lowered selenium levels have also been observed in the hair, but not the serum, of females with recurrent miscarriage compared to controls who have undergone successful pregnancy.[163]

Serum and follicular fluid levels of selenium are reduced in women undergoing IVF and this is associated with non-fertilisation of the oocytes picked up for IVF.[165] Serum and follicular fluid levels have been shown to normalise with multivitamin/mineral supplementation.[166] Selenium levels in hair correlate positively with follicle number and oocyte yield after ovarian stimulation, suggesting that selenium has a positive effect on ovarian response to gonadotrophin therapy for IVF.[167] Thus, selenium clearly plays an important role in female fertility, although further studies are required to explore this topic further.

In pregnancy, selenium supplementation (100 micrograms/day) reduces pre-labour membrane rupture and preeclampsia.[168,169] In a preliminary study of healthy women, dietary selenium was significantly associated with lower odds of luteal phase deficiency. A 10 microgram increase in average daily selenium consumption decreased the odds of luteal phase deficiency by 20%. Luteal phase deficiency refers to inadequate progesterone secretion by the corpus luteum, which may render the endometrium less receptive to implantation and result in infertility or early pregnancy loss.[170]

Zinc

Zinc is an essential trace element that is known to play an important role in all human living cells, including the transcription of RNA, the replication of DNA and the synthesis of protein, all of which are crucial for reproduction and fertility. Zinc exerts antioxidant properties to protect against free radicals and ROS that may damage oocyte quality.

Zinc is required for reproduction and ovulation, as well as DNA synthesis for the development of the oocyte in females.[89] Deficiency may result in altered synthesis/secretion of FSH and LH,[171] abnormal ovarian development, risk of miscarriage[172] and teratogenicity[172] due to its role in DNA and RNA, to name but a few complications.

Specific functions of zinc with regard to female fertility are:
- It is the single most important nutrient for the pregnant woman.
- It is disrupted by the use of the oral contraceptive pill, copper intrauterine devices and inorganic iron supplements.
- It is necessary for the formation of elastin chains in connective tissue.
- In pregnancy, an inadequate zinc level leads to common problems such as stretch marks, cracked nipples and prolonged labour.
- Fetal growth retardation and congenital malformations may also result from zinc deficiency.
- There are links with postnatal depression.
- Zinc-deficient babies cry excessively and are difficult to calm.

Women with endometriosis who successfully achieved pregnancy after IVF had higher intra-follicular zinc levels than those women who failed to achieve pregnancy.[173] However, a Cochrane review found that while zinc supplementation in pregnancy leads to a slight reduction in preterm births, it does not prevent other problems such as low birth weight or preeclampsia.[174]

B group vitamins

The B vitamins are a group of water-soluble vitamins that have an indispensable role during preconception due to their multifaceted actions within the body. Deficiencies of B vitamins have been associated with a number of fertility problems, including fetal abnormalities such as neural tube defects,[175] neonatal or perinatal death, low birth weight and miscarriage.[176,177] Therefore, it is important to ensure that the B vitamin requirements of each individual couple are identified and maintained during the preconception period. It is important to consider that alcohol, carbohydrate-rich diets and the oral contraceptive pill increase the body's requirements for B vitamins. As such, any couple that wants to optimise their fertility and has a history involving these variables may require additional B vitamins to prepare their bodies for future conception. Acknowledging that stress also increases requirements for B vitamins and that stress has been identified as playing a major factor in couples who have difficulty conceiving, the importance of adequate B vitamin intake is further emphasised. As always, it is essential to prescribe B complex preparations in stable formulations for optimal outcome.

Vitamin B₁ (thiamine)

Vitamin B_1 is a water-soluble vitamin that participates in numerous enzymatic reactions within the body. One paper[178] details the potentially beneficial effects of thiamine observed in animal studies, in which vitamin B_1 has been shown to stabilise the membranes of newly generated neuronal cells during embryogenesis, while also slowing down cell death. Furthermore, vitamin B_1 has also been shown to be involved in the plasma membrane transformation of uterine epithelial cells during pregnancy.

Vitamin B_1 also plays a key role in female reproductive function. Deficiency is associated with altered cell differentiation and proliferation and altered breakdown of carbohydrates, leading to inadequate energy supply, as well as interference with normal hormone processes that control gestation. Due to these factors, a subsequent increased risk of miscarriage has been hypothesised.[179] To date, the majority of research with regard to female fertility and vitamin B_1 has been largely experimental or undertaken in vivo. However, acknowledging the indispensable role of vitamin B_1 in the body is sure to be of use. Periconceptional intake of vitamin B_1 as well as B_3 and B_6 has also been found to contribute to the prevention of oral facial cleft.[180]

Vitamin B₂ (riboflavin)

Vitamin B_2 is crucial for energy production, antioxidant defence and numerous enzyme systems that are reliant on the presence of B vitamins.

Vitamin B_2 is required for the development of the fetus. It has been shown in animal studies that a deficiency of vitamin B_2 affects embryonic growth and cardiac development, and thus it has been suggested that ensuring adequate intake of riboflavin in humans may prevent these same complications.[181] Low intake of dietary vitamin B_2 has also been linked to low birth weight.[182] One study has shown an increased risk of having a child with congenital heart defects in mothers who consumed a diet high in saturated fat and who did not use vitamin supplements in the periconceptional period.[183]

Vitamin B₅ (pantothenic acid)

Vitamin B_5 is essential for life and is found as part of coenzyme A, an enzyme system required for numerous functions within the body, including the synthesis of steroid hormones such as testosterone.

Female rats deprived of vitamin B_5 become sterile or experience a high percentage of stillbirths. Although it is uncertain whether these same results can be translated to humans, they indicate the significant role of vitamin B_5 on both male and female reproduction.

Vitamin B₆ (pyridoxine)

Vitamin B_6 is required for the metabolism of amino acids, lipids, pathways of gluconeogenesis and synthesis of neurotransmitters during the periconception period.[145]

Vitamin B_6 is required for the synthesis of prostaglandins and also plays a key role in the regulation of homocysteine, which when elevated has been linked to infertility and miscarriage,[184] suggesting that lower plasma concentrations of vitamin B_6 and other B vitamins may precede recurrent spontaneous miscarriage.[185] Elevated homocysteine concentrations in follicular fluid are also associated with poor oocyte and embryo qualities in PCOS patients undergoing assisted reproduction[186]; hence the benefits of supplementing with B vitamins known to lower homocysteine.

In addition, vitamin B_6 is beneficial in reducing elevated prolactin levels, supports the luteal phase by increasing progesterone, increases the influx of magnesium into the myometrium, improves absorption of zinc and prevents preeclampsia, toxaemia and infarction of placenta. Serum levels are often low in hyperemesis gravidarum, and deficiency may be associated with a higher incidence of gestational diabetes.

Vitamin B₉ (folate)

Folate is required for healthy DNA and RNA synthesis, as well as normal protein synthesis[187] and regulation of gene expression. Deficiency is associated with impaired DNA synthesis and repair and the subsequent complications.

Folate has been identified as being important for oocyte quality and maturation.[89] Inadequate folate results in elevated homocysteine and alters DNA methylation, negatively influencing oocyte and early embryo quality.[188] Inadequate B vitamin status and raised concentrations of homocysteine are also associated with early loss of pregnancy, as evidenced by a systematic review which found that folate deficiency and hyperhomocysteinaemia were risk factors for placenta-mediated diseases such as preeclampsia, spontaneous abortion and placental abruption.[189] A recent study found that folate and vitamin B_{12} levels were largely inadequate among women attending an infertility clinic for IVF treatment.[190]

Folate appears to exert a protective effect, with a prospective cohort study involving 18 555 females reporting decreased risk of ovulatory infertility in females regularly taking multivitamins containing folic acid and other B vitamins.[82] The most important variation in folate metabolism in terms of reproduction impact is the MTHFR polymorphism. Impaired folate metabolism disturbs endometrial maturation and results in poor oocyte quality.[191] Live birth rates in women undergoing IVF were found to be 20% higher among women with the highest amount of supplemental folate intake (>800 micrograms/day) compared to women taking the lowest amount (<400 micrograms/day). This study also suggested that folate supplementation was superior to dietary folate.[192] Similarly, higher serum concentrations of folate and vitamin B_{12} before ART treatment were associated with

BOX 11.8 Folate and vitamin B$_{12}$ – a combined therapeutic relationship

The importance of folate cannot be refuted. This poses both positive and negative implications for future childbearing. Folate and vitamin B$_{12}$ work synergistically in the maintenance and regulation of DNA and RNA in every cell in the body. Supplementation of one without the other (or one in excessively high doses) can disrupt this balance, causing subsequent masked anaemias. As such, it is prudent to concurrently prescribe vitamins B$_9$ and B$_{12}$ in combination throughout the preconception and pregnancy periods.

higher live birth rates.[193] Folate intake has been related to a lower frequency of sporadic anovulation in a prospective cohort of young healthy women,[194] and folic acid supplementation was associated with shorter time to pregnancy in healthy women.[195] Contrary to these positive findings, a 2014 study found that neither folic acid supplementation nor folate status had a positive effect on pregnancy outcome following infertility treatment in women with unexplained infertility.[196]

Folate protects against neural tube defects and spina bifida, improving pregnancy outcomes, as confirmed in a 2015 Cochrane review.[197] However, a 2016 Cochrane review found no evidence to support the use of folic acid supplementation for reducing the risk of early or late miscarriage or stillbirth.[141]

In women undergoing IVF treatment, higher urinary bisphenol A (BPA) concentrations were associated with a 66% lower probability of implantation. This effect was ameliorated by higher levels of dietary folate intake (more than 400 micrograms/day). The same protective effect was not seen with supplemental folate.[198]

Prescription recommendations are a minimum of 3 months preconceptually to address the life cycle of a red blood cell (see Box 11.8).

Vitamin B$_{12}$ (hydroxo- or methyl-cobalamin)

Vitamin B$_{12}$ is essential for cell replication, folate and amino acid metabolism, as well as the synthesis of myelin, which forms a protective case around the spinal cord and brain of the fetus.

In terms of maternal health, vitamin B$_{12}$ deficiency has been linked to infertility and recurrent spontaneous miscarriage,[199] as well as to high levels of homocysteine. Pregnancy has also been shown to occur following correction of vitamin B$_{12}$ deficiency.[199]

Vitamin D

Vitamin D is a lipid-soluble vitamin that is required structurally and functionally. It enhances male and female fertility, and facilitates the absorption of calcium. It acts as a potent immunomodulator and can support skeletal health in both the mother and the developing fetus.

The active form of vitamin D, 1-25-dihydroxyvitamin D$_3$, has been shown to regulate the transcription and function of genes associated with placental invasion, normal implantation and angiogenesis.[200] Specifically, its application is best considered in incidences of miscarriage, implantation issues or general infertility. The presence of vitamin D receptor in the ovaries, uterus, placenta and endometrium indicate that vitamin D is involved in female reproduction processes and vitamin D deficiency is a factor influencing female fertility and IVF outcomes.[201]

A number of studies have yielded positive results of the association of vitamin D and fertility outcomes. However, a similar number of studies have found no associations, and one study even observed a negative association.

Positive associations have been found in women undergoing IVF treatment.

In one study, higher serum and follicular fluid levels of 25(OH)D were related to increased pregnancy rates. Each ng/mL increase in follicular fluid 25(OH)D increased the chance of becoming pregnant by 6%.[202] Sufficient levels of serum 25(OH)D have been associated with increased pregnancy and implantation.[203–205] While the effect of vitamin D deficiency is unclear, it is likely that deficiency does not have a detrimental effect on ovarian reserve.[206] A positive association of vitamin D with endometrial thickness has been observed.[207]

These findings were not supported in other studies.[208–211] No association was found between serum or follicular fluid levels of vitamin D and IVF outcomes.[212,213] In women undergoing euploid embryo transfer, vitamin D status was unrelated to pregnancy outcomes.[214] A case control study compared early pregnancy levels of vitamin D between women who took 12–24 months to get pregnant compared to age-matched women conceiving in less than 1 year and found no association.[215] A recent study of 70 infertile women found that 64% of the women were vitamin D deficient, but this did not correlate with anti-Müllerian hormone levels.[216]

A retrospective study on 101 women who underwent IVF showed that higher follicular fluid levels of 25(OH)D negatively affected embryo quality and led to poorer IVF outcome.[217]

A retrospective cohort study found that the relationship between vitamin D status and pregnancy rates differed by race. In non-Hispanic white women, pregnancy rates declined with lower levels of vitamin D, while in Asian women, the reverse association was seen.[218] A study in donor-recipient IVF cycles showed that insufficient vitamin D levels of the recipients (rather than the donors) was associated with lower pregnancy rates, suggesting that the effects of vitamin D may be mediated through the endometrium rather than through the follicle or oocyte.[219] Once again, however, these results were not supported by another study which found no difference in pregnancy rates in egg donation recipients who had differing vitamin D levels (normal, insufficient or deficient).[220]

Maternal vitamin D deficiency has also been suggested to be an independent risk factor for preeclampsia. The optimal dose of vitamin D during the preconception period is unknown, but it is prudent to assess patients thoroughly in the preconception review and supplement as required based on the findings. A recently published meta-analysis found no association between vitamin D insufficiency and risk of spontaneous abortion.[221]

Given the heterogeneity of findings, little can be conclusively stated from the results on vitamin D and fertility. Vitamin D deficiency might be detrimental to fertility, but it is not clear whether higher levels of vitamin D confer additional benefit once sufficiency has been achieved.

A Cochrane review concluded that supplementing with vitamin D during pregnancy may reduce the risk of preeclampsia, low birth weight and preterm birth. However, vitamin D and calcium supplementation combined increases the risk of preterm birth.[222]

Vitamin K

Vitamin K aids blood clotting, and thus helps to protect against haemorrhagic disease of newborns. It is also highly important for bone health.[223] It is also an important consideration for maternal health in females presenting with implantation or miscarriage factors that contribute to poor blood coagulation or clotting factors.

Calcium

Calcium is an essential nutrient for both female and male fertility, where it is required both structurally and functionally.

Calcium signalling is required for oocyte maturation and for fertilisation.[224] In addition, calcium, together with magnesium, is required for bone formation. Mineral fluxes from mother to child during gestation result in the loss of minerals, especially calcium, for the mother. Calcium supplementation has been shown to exert a protective effect against preeclampsia, with a Cochrane review showing that calcium supplementation appears to almost halve the risk of this condition.[225] Females undergoing preconception care may need to be informed about the importance of meeting the recommended daily intake of calcium via diet or through supplementation, and where necessary, calcium supplements should be recommended if dietary sources are inadequate.[226]

Chromium

Chromium may be used to improve glucose tolerance. This is particularly important in patients with disorders such as PCOS, where fertility may be impaired due to insulin resistance.[227] Pregnancy may reduce the ability of insulin to control blood sugar; hence the importance of blood sugar balancing nutrients to prevent the risk of gestational diabetes.[223] By stabilising blood sugar levels, one can hypothesise that cravings for sugar may decrease, leading to weight loss and improved weight management. The growing fetus relies on blood glucose for energy, and therefore in a deficient mother subsequent development issues, including adult obesity and macrosomia, are possible. A pilot study investigation levels of trace elements associated with IVF outcomes found that higher urinary chromium levels were associated with higher number of retrieved oocytes. However, higher follicular fluid levels of chromium were negatively associated with the proportion of mature oocytes. While this is a preliminary investigative study with no clear clinical

implications, it highlights the potential role that chromium plays in reproductive health.[228]

Iodine

Iodine is an essential trace element. Iodine deficiency has re-emerged in Australia, one of the major reasons being the reduction of iodine in milk since the dairy industry replaced iodine-rich cleaning solutions with other cleaning products.[229] More than 30% of non-pregnant women of childbearing age have suboptimal urinary iodine concentrations.[230,231] Adequate dietary intake of iodine during the preconception period is imperative, and can minimise the risk of iodine deficiency during early attempts at conceiving as well as later during the critical period of fetal development. A recent population-based prospective cohort study of 501 women found that moderate to severe iodine deficiency is associated with a 46% decrease in fecundability.[232]

The maturing oocytes are dependent on healthy thyroid hormone levels, and thus any deviation in these levels will affect reproductive function.[233] Thyroid autoimmunity is significantly higher among infertile females than among fertile females, and increases miscarriage rate.[234] Iodine is well known for its effects on the thyroid gland, where it is required for the synthesis of thyroid hormones as well as the development of the fetus, in particular its central nervous system. Adequate intake of iodine is paramount for healthy fertility. However, it is known that many people in Australia are not getting the recommended daily intake, and this is significant given that deficiency of iodine may result in a spectrum of disorders including miscarriage, stillbirth, mental retardation and cretinism (deaf mutism and spasticity).[235,236]

As early as 1939, Kemp[237] acknowledged a link between deficiency of iodine and stillbirth of unknown origin. In the late 1970s, Potter et al.[238] discussed the decline in stillbirth rates in Tasmania (compared to Australia as a whole) following iodine supplementation in the 1950s, this time highlighting the positive relationship that ensued between iodine (when taken at the correct dose) and a reduced incidence of stillbirth.

Now, with iodine deficiency once again recognised as a problem, one could hypothesise that females may be at increased risk of stillbirth due to this deficiency. This certainly seems true when one observes statistics published by the Stillbirth Foundation of Australia in 2006,[239] which show that there are 2000 stillborn babies every year in Australia. In spite of advances in technology, one-third of these deaths are of unknown cause and, sadly for the parents, many of these idiopathic deaths occur at late-term gestation, often after a normal, uneventful pregnancy.

Acknowledging the link between iodine deficiency in pregnancy and increased risk of stillbirth, iodine levels (and thyroid function) should be tested in all females contemplating conception. However, it is recognised that a diagnosis of hypothyroidism based on TSH values in isolation may not be enough to recognise mild to moderate iodine deficiency in a pregnant woman.[240] A 2017 Cochrane review found no conclusive evidence of the benefits or harms of iodine supplementation in women before, during or after pregnancy. Iodine supplementation appears to decrease the likelihood of postnatal hyperthyroidism, and increases the likelihood of digestive intolerance in pregnancy.[241]

Iron

Adequate intake of iron is paramount for healthy fertility due to the multifaceted role of iron in the body, particularly with regard to its blood tonic effects. Iron is required for the formation of red blood cells, subsequent transport of oxygen to the tissues via haemoglobin and nucleic acid metabolism, as well as being involved in numerous enzyme systems within the body.[145] It is important to note, however, that excessive amounts of iron (or any nutrient) may hamper fertility. Therefore, it is prudent to assess a woman's iron levels preconceptually to ensure a proven need for supplementation is evident.

Adequate iron intake during the preconception period is likely to help prevent iron deficiency during the pregnancy, and thus screening for iron deficiency anaemia is crucial.[226] Results from the Nurses' Health Study II suggest that females who consume iron supplements have a significantly lower risk of ovulatory infertility than do females who do not use iron supplements.[138,242] Furthermore, it is beneficial to increase iron stores preconceptually in preparation for the increase in circulating blood volume during pregnancy. Iron is also supportive to ensure the correct formation of fetal blood, brain, eyes and bones and healthy growth rate.

Magnesium

Magnesium is involved in numerous reactions in the body relevant to fertility, including cell signalling and energy production.

Females undergoing spontaneous abortion have been observed to have lower plasma magnesium levels than healthy controls, and the relationship between magnesium deficiency and spontaneous abortion requires further investigation.[243] Magnesium and B vitamins supplementation for both sexes may also be required to address the stress aspect associated with fertility, as infertility and miscarriage are both recognised as being highly stressful. Stress is associated with impaired fertility, including impotence in males and miscarriage and failed pregnancy outcomes in females.[244]

Essential fatty acids

Omega-3 fatty acids are essential polyunsaturated fatty acids that are structurally required to maintain the lipid bilayer in all cell membranes, and as precursors for prostaglandin synthesis.

Females undergoing preconception care are encouraged to consume a diet rich in essential fatty acids.[226] Omega-3 fatty acids have regulatory effects on the cell membrane and effects on oocyte quality and embryo implantation.[245] A prospective study in the Netherlands on women undergoing IVF/ICSI treatment ($n = 235$) showed that omega-3 fatty acid intake has a beneficial effect on fertility. Higher ALA intake was associated with higher baseline oestradiol levels. ALA and DHA intake was associated with improved embryo morphology.[245] A study investigating the associations between serum levels of polyunsaturated

fatty acids and embryo implantation in women undergoing IVF found that an increased omega-6 to omega-3 ratio was more important than individual levels of PUFAs for improving implantation and pregnancy rate.[246] DHA has been associated with a reduced risk of anovulation in healthy, regularly menstruating women.[247] In overweight and obese women undergoing IVF treatment, intake of PUFAs, specifically omega-6 PUFAs and linoleic acid, and possibly omega-3 PUFAs, was associated with improved pregnancy rates. However there were no association with live birth rates.[248] Similarly, in a cohort study of women undergoing IVF treatment in Iran, serum levels of eicosapentaenoic acid (EPA) were significantly higher in women who achieved pregnancy compared to those who did not.[249] In a North America cohort, women with the lowest omega-3 fatty acid intake had lower fecundability compared to women with higher intake.[250]

In the prevention of miscarriage, omega-3 fatty acids 4 g/day (providing 795 mg DHA and 1190 mg EPA) have been found to improve uterine artery blood flow velocity in females with recurrent miscarriage due to impaired uterine perfusion.[251] While aspirin was deemed more effective, many people would be likely to find omega-3 more therapeutically beneficial to address multiple treatment objectives and also to provide a safer treatment margin for both mother and growing fetus. As such, it is prudent to initially supplement and then consider treatment with aspirin as required.

Probiotics

Changes in the microflora of the vagina and subsequent genital and intrauterine infections[252] have been linked to reproductive failure and adverse pregnancy outcomes such as preterm labour, miscarriage and spontaneous preterm birth.[252–254] Bacterial vaginosis is associated with ascending infections which may lead to tubal factor infertility. Selected *Lactobacillus* strains are typically used for treating bacterial vaginosis, as the human vaginal microbiota is a predominantly *Lactobacillus* community.[255] In one study, during the first half of pregnancy, females with altered vaginal flora of bacterial origin evidenced by atypical Gram-positive rods or pronounced vaginal leucocytosis had an adjusted odds ratio of 5.2 for spontaneous preterm birth compared to females with normal lactobacilli-dominated microflora, who were four times less likely to have a spontaneous preterm birth compared to the overall preterm birth rate.[256] Acknowledging that altered vaginal flora may be related to reproductive failure and miscarriage, using probiotics to restore healthy flora may help to improve pregnancy outcomes. Further studies are warranted.

Dosage requirements

The dose requirements listed in Table 11.33 are based on adult doses reported in the literature. Due to the varying range of recommendation, it is essential to review and ascertain the requirements of patients on an individual basis. Furthermore, it is beneficial to calculate the dose according to the patient's body weight, as the recommendations given in the table are for an average adult.

TABLE 11.33 Supplementation dosage requirements in preconception treatment

Nutrient	Women (dose per day)	Nutrient	Women (dose per day)
Vitamins		**Minerals**	
Vitamin A*	10 000–25 000 IU	Calcium	1000–2000 mg
Vitamin B₁ (thiamine)	50–100 mg	Chromium‡	100–400 micrograms
Vitamin B₂ (riboflavin)	50 mg	Copper§	2–4 mg
Vitamin B₃ (niacin)	50–200 mg	Iodine¶	250–400 micrograms
Vitamin B₅ (pantothenic acid)	50–200 mg	Iron**	10–100 mg
Vitamin B₆ (pyridoxine)	50–250 mg	Magnesium	500–1000 mg
Vitamin B₉ (folate)	800–5000 micrograms	Manganese	10–50 mg
Vitamin B₁₂ (hydroxo/methyl cobalamin)	800–2000 micrograms	Potassium	3–8 g
Vitamin C§§	1000–5000 mg	Selenium	150–300 micrograms
Vitamin D†	1000–5000 IU	Silica	20–30 mg
Vitamin E	500–1000 IU	Zinc	40–80 mg
Vitamin K	60–120 micrograms	**Essential fatty acids**	
Beta-carotene	3–6 mg	Total omega-3 essential fatty acids	1000–5000 mg
Bioflavonoids	600–1500 mg	Total omega-6 essential fatty acids	1000–2000 mg
Biotin	500–5000 micrograms	DHA	600–800 mg
Choline	1000–2000 mg	EPA	1000–1200 mg
Inositol	25 mg	Evening primrose oil	1000–1500 mg
PABA	50 mg	**Animo acids**	
Coenzyme Q10	100–600 mg	Arginine	3000–16 000 mg
		Carnitine	900–3000 mg
		Other	
		Probiotics (mixed strains)	$25–50 \times 10^9$

*Retinol equivalents (RE) are now used: 1 microgram RE = 1 microgram retinol = 6 micrograms beta-carotene = 12 micrograms other carotenoids.
†Prescribe based on pathology results.
‡Dose is dependent on blood sugar level (BSL) control and weight requirements.
§Avoid in instances of Wilson's disease (assess prior to prescription) and ensure that prescription is only recommended when the zinc:copper ratio has been considered.
¶Assessment prior to prescription is essential, and should only be conducted when thyroid function values can be reviewed.
**Must have a pathology interpretation prior to recommending a prescription in order to determine the required dosage.
§§In divided doses.

HERBAL MEDICINE – FEMALE

See Table 11.34 for a summary of herbal medicine classes specific to female fertility treatment.

Therapeutic objectives – female

1 Improve fertility potential and relevant fertility factors.
2 Improve oocyte health and receptivity to sperm.
3 Prevent miscarriage and address relevant miscarriage factor(s) if present.
4 Support optimal general health.
5 Encourage optimal eliminatory pathways.
6 Support hormone production and delivery to all reproductive tissues.
7 Support communication between the endocrine and reproductive systems.
8 Address attenuating factors such as infection, inflammation, toxicity and stress.

Specific herbal medicines – female

Alchemilla vulgaris (lady's mantle)

Alchemilla vulgaris is a herbaceous perennial prized for its astringent properties (due to its tannin content), which make it ideal for halting bleeding and healing wounds.[257] It is used for the treatment of female reproductive conditions, including menstrual disorders, prevention of miscarriage and as a preconception aid.[258] As yet, there have been no well-designed human clinical studies assessing the effects of *A. vulgaris* on fertility or miscarriage. However, the traditional application of this herb appears to have stood the test of time, and it is still

TABLE 11.34 Herbal medicine classes – female

Herbal class	Justification
Adaptogens	Infertility causes a great deal of stress; however, stress may also negatively impact on fertility. Adaptogens may be used to help the body adapt to stressors. Useful herbs that display adaptogen action include *Panax ginseng* (Korean ginseng), *Eleutherococcus senticosus* (Siberian ginseng), *Glycyrrhiza glabra* (liquorice), *Rehmannia glutinosa* (rehmannia) and *Withania somnifera* (ashwagandha)
Adrenal tonic	Excessive cortisol has been demonstrated to have a detrimental effect on fertility; hence, adrenal tonics should be employed in patients at risk of adrenal exhaustion. These herbs include *Glycyrrhiza glabra* (liquorice) and *Rehmannia glutinosa* (rehmannia)
Antidepressants	It is recognised that a high percentage of women undergoing fertility experience depression; hence, antidepressant herbs such as *Turnera diffusa* (damiana) or *Hypericum perforatum* (St John's wort) may require consideration
Anti-miscarriage	Traditional anti-miscarriage herbal medicines are recommended where there is risk of miscarriage to tone the uterus and correct uterine displacements. Examples of herbal medicines are *Aletris farinosa* (true unicorn root), *Chamaelirium luteum* (false unicorn root) or *Viburnum prunifolium* (black haw)
Antioxidant	Oxidative stress has been implicated in female infertility as well as miscarriage; hence the importance of antioxidant botanicals such as *Vitis vinifera* (grape seed extract) and *Curcuma longa* (turmeric) to protect the female reproductive structures as well as the oocyte against the effects of free radical damage
Anticoagulants	Blood coagulation is implicated in a number of miscarriage factors and requires specific herbal medicines to normalise blood production and coagulation. Useful herbal medicines include *Curcuma longa* (turmeric) or *Ginkgo biloba* (ginkgo)
Detoxification	Detoxification should be implemented in all individuals contemplating conception to ensure optimal fertility outcomes. A wide array of toxins have been identified as detrimental to female fertility and the oocyte; hence the importance of herbs that support healthy detoxification such as *Silybum marianum* (St Mary's thistle), *Schisandra chinensis* (schisandra), *Curcuma longa* (turmeric) and *Camellia sinensis* (green tea)
Immune modulating	Immune-modulating herbs are highly indicated where autoimmunity is implicated in the cause of infertility; this may be true of conditions such as Hashimoto's disease and rheumatoid arthritis. Botanicals in this class include *Rehmannia glutinosa* (rehmannia), *Echinacea* spp. (echinacea), *Hemidesmus indicus* (hemidesmus) or *Albizia lebbeck* (albizia)
Hormone modulation	HPO modulation: *Vitex agnus-castus* (chaste tree) Androgen modulation: *Glycyrrhiza glabra* (liquorice) or *Paeonia lactiflora* (peony) Prolactin modulation: *Dioscorea villosa* (wild yam) or *Vitex agnus-castus* (chaste tree) Oestrogen modulation: *Asparagus racemosus* (shatavari), *Actaea racemosa* (black cohosh), *Chamaelirium luteum* (false unicorn root) LH modulation: *Actaea racemosa* (black cohosh) FSH modulation: *Tribulus terrestris* (tribulus) Progesterone modulation: *Vitex agnus-castus* (chaste tree) and *Alchemilla vulgaris* (lady's mantle)

favoured and used successfully by modern day herbalists to enhance fertility.

Aletris farinosa (true unicorn root)

Aletris farinosa is another botanical that has a long history of use for female gynaecological conditions. The Eclectic physician Ellingwood detailed its use in correcting sterility due to deficient menstruation, and stated that it is the perfect remedy in situations where there is threat of miscarriage:

> *Aletris farinosa may be given for three, four, five and 6 months, the woman going her full term without any untoward effect, rendering the labor easy and safe.*[75]

With regard to the threat of abortion, Ellingwood states there is no better combination than *A. farinosa* and the *Viburnum* spp. to prevent miscarriage. Grieve[257] also suggests it to be valuable for its effects on the female generative organs, due to its tonic effects, as well as for habitual miscarriage.

Angelica sinensis (dong quai)

Angelica sinensis is a traditional Chinese medicine with a gentle, warming action. It is believed to nourish the blood and restore the body back to its natural balance. In traditional Chinese medicine, it is used as a female tonic and for a number of gynaecological conditions, including amenorrhoea. However, there is a lack of clinical studies to support this use. *A. sinensis* remains a popular botanical in Western herbal medicine for optimising fertility, although further study of its actions is required.

Asparagus racemosus (shatavari)

Asparagus racemosus is an Ayurvedic botanical renowned for its effects on the female reproductive system, and has been used for this purpose since the 16th century. It is believed to function as an aphrodisiac, promoting strength and enhancing sexual appetite, while preventing miscarriage and promoting healthy fertility. In Western herbal medicine, *A. racemosus* is primarily employed as a female reproductive herb, but in Ayurvedic medicine, it may also be employed to enhance male fertility, particularly where there is a low sperm count. The roots of *A. racemosus* were traditionally boiled in milk and consumed with sugar to promote sperm production, cleanse sperm and increase 'ojas' (which can be likened to the naturopathic notion of 'vital force'). In animal studies, *A. racemosus* has been observed to exert oestrogenic effects,[259] but there has been little in the way of well-blinded human clinical studies. In Ayurveda, *A. racemosus* has been used safely over long periods of time, even during pregnancy and lactation.[260]

Chamaelirium luteum (false unicorn root)

The rhizomes of *Chamaelirium luteum* function as a uterine tonic and have been used to correct problems of the female reproductive tract since the time of the Eclectics. *King's American Dispensatory* documents the use of *C. luteum* for treating repeated and successive miscarriage, while Ellingwood[75] highlights its use for uterine displacements, particularly where there is threatened abortion. In the latter situation *C. luteum* should be combined with *Viburnum prunifolium* and given in full doses.

C. luteum is an extremely clinically beneficial prescription. However, as it is threatened due to excessive wildcrafting, practitioners are encouraged to try other steroidal saponin-containing herbal medicines such as *Dioscorea villosa* and prescribe *C. luteum* only if the required clinical outcome is not achieved with the alternative botanical.

Actaea racemosa (black cohosh)

Actaea racemosa has historically been used for disorders affecting the organs of the female reproductive system. It is described by the Eclectics as a utero-ovarian tonic for:

> *pains of a dull aching character; dragging pains in the womb, with sense of soreness; the dull tensive pains incident to reproductive disorders of the female, as well as the annoying pains accompanying pregnancy; false pains; after-pains.*[261]

A. racemosa may be useful for restoring suppressed menses, which otherwise would result in infertility, as well as in situations characterised by a lack of functional power in the uterus resulting in infertility. A primary study of 147 patients showed that in women with unexplained fertility who were undergoing clomiphene induction, supplementation with *A. racemosa* (120 mg/day on days 1–12 of the cycle) resulted in increased LH, progesterone and oestradiol, in addition to increased endometrial thickness and clinical pregnancy rates.[262] A subsequent study of 134 women with unexplained infertility, undergoing clomiphene induction, compared clomiphene citrate cycles with follicular-phase supplementation with *A. racemosa* (120 mg/day on days 1–12 of the cycle) or ethinyl oestradiol. Results showed that *A. racemosa* supplementation improved endometrial thickness,

follicular maturation and oestradiol levels. There was no statistically significant difference in clinical pregnancy rates between the two treatment groups.[263] Similar results were seen in a study of women with PCOS and infertility. Treatment with clomiphene citrate alone or clomiphene citrate combined with *A. racemosa* (120 mg/day) found that the *A. racemosa* group had improved cycle outcomes and pregnancy rates.[264]

Dioscorea villosa (wild yam)

Traditionally, *Dioscorea villosa* was prescribed in instances of ovarian or uterine spasm. It is still used in this application. However, it is also clinically beneficial in regulating and optimising oestrogen levels, and thus in increasing the quality and quantity of cervical fluid.

Glycyrrhiza glabra (liquorice)

Glycyrrhiza glabra is particularly useful for treating suboptimal fertility related to PCOS, where it combines well with *Paeonia lactiflora* (for a full discussion of this combination see Chapter 13: Pregnancy and Labour). *G. glabra* has been found to reduce elevated prolactin,[265] which may further aid fertility. It may also help to support adrenal health, which is extremely important, as stress is known to negatively impact on fertility.

Paeonia lactiflora (white peony)

Paeonia lactiflora has long been used in traditional Chinese medicine for its effects on the female reproductive system. In Chinese medicine, *P. lactiflora* is used as one herb in a formulation known as Dang Gui Shao Yao San, a combination of medicinal herbs used for the treatment of ovulatory disorders, to improve ovulation and thus promote a good fertility outcome. Another formulation, unkei-to (a traditional Japanese herbal medicine consisting of shakuyaku [*P. radix*, *P. lactiflora* Pallas] and keihi [*Cinnamomi cortex*, *Cinnamomum cassia* Blume]), demonstrates stimulatory effects on the ovulatory process and human granulosa cells in vitro.[266] This formulation has been found to promote steroidogenesis, cytokine secretion, 17-β-oestradiol secretion and progesterone secretion in highly luteinised granulosa cells obtained from IVF patients.

Rehmannia glutinosa (rehmannia)

Rehmannia glutinosa is a potent immune regulator, anti-inflammatory, adaptogen and adrenal restorative. It is specifically recommended for patients with threatened miscarriage or autoimmune processes that hinder conception, implantation or carrying a pregnancy to term. It may also be used to prevent the suppressive effects of corticosteroid drugs on endogenous levels, and thus may be used as an adjuvant therapy for females on corticosteroids who are attempting to improve their fertility. Unfortunately, there is a scarcity of well-designed clinical trials in humans. As such, more research is required into this effective herbal medicine.

Tribulus terrestris (tribulus)

Tribulus terrestris is generally thought of as a male tonic. However, it is used extensively in Western herbal medicine for the treatment of female reproductive disorders, including infertility.

Most papers and documentation refer back to a poorly designed study by Tabakova et al.,[267] who conducted a non-randomised trial in 51 females with endocrine sterility to assess the effect of Tribestan (a standardised *T. terrestris* extract) on infertility. Although the results of this study were encouraging, larger studies of better design are needed in order to evaluate the effectiveness of Tribestan in the treatment of female infertility. In the study, subjects took Tribestan 1–2 tablets (250 mg/tablet) t.i.d. by mouth, either on days 5–14 of their cycle (schedule I) or on days 1–12 of their cycle (schedule II) for the first 3 months. After a washout period, 20 out of 36 patients went on to receive a combination treatment. In this phase, patients were treated with Tribestan 1–2 tablets t.i.d. by mouth on days 1–12 of their cycle plus either Stimovul 1–2 tablets daily on days 5–14 of their cycle or Clomifen 1–2 tablets daily on days 5–9 of their cycle. It was found that 67% of patients treated with Tribestan had normalised ovulation with or without pregnancy. When compared to other drugs, Tribestan was inferior to Stimovul alone.

T. terrestris is commonly applied in clinics for its FSH stimulating properties. It is given at the start of the woman's cycle to initiate ovulation and improve conception rates. Most of the substantiating evidence for this claim, while clinically relevant, lacks credibility. In a clinical context, one can expect to see a marked increase in cervical fluid within a few days of taking the prescription. This increase precedes ovulation and markedly supports conception outcome. It is especially beneficial for patients who have delayed ovulation or absent ovulation as it regulates the FSH/LH ratio. Patients are generally aware of increased 'fertile' awareness, libido and cervical fluid release. This has a positive effect on mood and confidence in the patient's fertility potential.

Viburnum prunifolium (black haw)

The roots and stems of *Viburnum prunifolium* have long been employed for miscarriage and infertility. The Eclectic physicians of the 1800s used *V. prunifolium* to treat a range of disorders of the female reproductive organs, although the greatest value of *V. prunifolium* was said to be its ability to protect and prevent against the threat of miscarriage, for which it was deemed extremely useful provided the membranes had not ruptured. *V. prunifolium* was employed in small doses for long periods of time to protect against miscarriage.[268] According to the *King's American Dispensatory*, *V. prunifolium* tones the uterus, and it was well utilised for sterility. *V. prunifolium* has been identified as containing the constituents salicin and scopoletin, which are thought to be responsible for some of its pharmacological effect. Although there have been no clinical trials in humans, *V. prunifolium* is considered safe for long-term use in pregnancy.

Vitex agnus-castus (chaste tree)

There is good evidence to support the use of *Vitex agnus-castus* in combination with other herbs and nutrients to enhance female fertility. As anovulatory cycles, hyperprolactinaemia and hypothalamic dysfunction may all have a detrimental effect on fertility, *V. agnus-castus*, which has demonstrated effects of lowering prolactin as well as regulating the hypothalamic–pituitary–ovarian axis, and promotes a regular menstrual cycle, would appear useful. In one study,[269] 96 females with secondary amenorrhoea, luteal insufficiency or idiopathic infertility received either a preparation containing *V. agnus-castus* together with other botanicals or a placebo over three menstrual cycles. Of these females, 15 went on to conceive (seven with amenorrhoea, four with idiopathic infertility, four with luteal insufficiency).

An uncontrolled study using a blend of *V. agnus-castus* combined with green tea extract and nutrients (L-arginine; vitamins E, B$_6$ and B$_{12}$, folate; iron; magnesium; zinc; and selenium) administered to 30 females who had been unsuccessful in their attempt to conceive despite trying for 6–36 months also showed beneficial results.[270] After 5 months of treatment, five of the 15 females in the treatment group were pregnant (33% versus 0%, *P* <0.01), and four of these went on to have healthy live births.

LIFESTYLE INTERVENTIONS

General recommendations

Recommendations include consideration of all factors associated with infertility (Table 11.35). These include avoidance of the following:

- cigarette smoking – cigarette smoke is composed of many toxic chemicals and pro-oxidants that increase ROS. Smokers, including passive smokers, have a significantly increased odds ratio for infertility and increased time to conception, likely due to the

	TABLE 11.35 Lifestyle factors that may impact fertility[271]	
Factor	**Impact on fertility**	**Study**
Obesity (BMI >35)	Time to conception increased two-fold	Hassan and Killick, 2004
Underweight (BMI <19)	Time to conception increased four-fold	Hassan and Killick, 2004
Smoking	RR of infertility increased 60%	Clark et al., 1998
Alcohol (>2 drinks/day)	RR of infertility increased 60%	Eggert et al., 2004
Caffeine (>250 mg/day)	Fecundability decreased 45%	Wilcox et al., 1988
Illicit drugs	RR of infertility increased 70%	Mueller et al., 1990[55]
Toxins, solvents	RR of infertility increased 40%	Hruska et al., 2000

BMI = body mass index; RR = relative risk

activation of oxidative stress mechanisms.[134] Each stage of reproductive function – folliculogenesis, steroidogenesis, embryo transport, endometrial receptivity, endometrial angiogenesis, uterine blood flow and uterine myometrium – is a target for cigarette smoke components.[272] In women undergoing IVF, smoking has been associated with delayed conception and a significant decrease in the odds for pregnancy and live delivery per cycle. There is also a marked increase in the odds for spontaneous miscarriage and ectopic pregnancy.[134]

- alcohol (see above in dietary section)
- recreational drugs – regular marijuana use results in an elevated risk of primary infertility compared to non-users.[134]
- excessive exposure to radiation, including mobile phone use and Wi-fi exposure.[273]
- exposure to environmental hazards, including pesticides, solvents, heavy metals and other toxins.[134,274] While there have been an increasing number of experimental and clinical studies investigating the effects of exposure to endocrine disrupting chemicals (such as BPA, phthalates, parabens and triclosan) on fertility, a causal relationship has yet to be established.[275–277] A recent study of 32 women undergoing IVF treatment found that ongoing exposure to persistent organic pollutants (POPs) had a negative impact on clinical IVF outcomes.[278]
- excessive body weight – the risk of infertility in obese women is three times that of normal weight women.[279] Obesity affects female reproduction by disturbing the general body metabolism, hormone metabolism and follicular environment. Obesity is associated with suboptimal oocyte quality and development, oocyte fertilisation, embryo development and implantation,[134,280–282] and may adversely affect ovarian reserve.[283,284] Obesity may cause LH surge and corpus luteum dysfunction,[285–287] and promote inflammatory markers which are negatively correlated with pregnancy rates in women undergoing IVF treatment.[288] In women undergoing ART, higher BMI is associated with lower pregnancy rates and a 68% reduction in live births compared to women of normal weight.[289] In women undergoing IVF treatment, the pregnancy rate in women with higher BMI (overweight or obese) was found to be significantly lower than in women with normal BMI. The study authors proposed that altered endometrial gene expression in obese patients may contribute to the lower implantation rates and increased miscarriage rates seen in obese infertile patients.[290] It is noted that in women undergoing ART, obesity has a greater impact on fertility in women under 35 years of age. After age 35, age becomes a more important factor than obesity in regards to chances of conception.[280,291]
- A recent Cochrane review was unable to suggest any evidence-based recommendations on the best interventions for improving pregnancy outcomes for women who are overweight or obese[292]; however, weight loss is crucial. In a retrospective cohort study, meaningful weight loss (10% of their maximum weight) was found to increase conception rates (88% vs 54%) and live birth rates (71% vs 37%) in patients with infertility compared to women who did not lose weight.[293] A systematic review of the literature concluded that weight loss interventions were more likely to result in ovulation improvements and pregnancies. Miscarriage rates were not affected by weight-loss interventions.[294]
- A recent prospective cohort study of 501 couples found that both partners' body composition need to be taken into account. In couples where both partners are obese, a longer time to pregnancy was observed than in leaner couples.[295]
- It is beneficial to avoid douches, vaginal sprays, scented tampons and other feminine products that change the pH of the vagina and disturb the vaginal microecology.

Counselling and emotional impact

The emotional impact of infertility can be very pronounced. In one study, 50% of females rated their infertility as one of the most stressful times in their lives.[296] Other clinical studies have reported feelings of depression and psychological distress, including suicidal thoughts.[297] Women undergoing infertility treatment report higher levels of anxiety, depression and emotional stress compared to those who conceive naturally.[298] A recent Cochrane review of the effects of psychological interventions on mental health in subfertile couples concluded that the quality of the evidence is too low to recommend specific interventions and called for further higher-quality studies.[299] Infertility can be a profound psychological burden to patients, and thus counselling is highly recommended. Counselling provides emotional support, particularly when conception attempts are unsuccessful, and may enable patients to understand better the implications of their treatment choices.

Counselling may also help to foster a better relationship between the couple. Social pressure ('When are you going to have a baby?'), financial stress (e.g. due to the cost of IVF or ICSI) and loss of self-esteem are all factors that may place strain on and test a couple's relationship. Counselling for infertile couples with a desire to conceive should include tactful reference to sexuality and any sexual dysfunction,[300] as the latter is a problem commonly cited by patients undergoing fertility treatment.[301,302]

Stress and fertility

Difficulty conceiving is often a stressful and challenging situation for couples. Unfortunately, stress is a catch-22 situation. Although an individual may say they cannot help but feel stressed due to the perceived enormity of the situation, it is important for individuals to know that stress has a proven negative effect in both male and female fertility.

Stress has been observed to negatively alter semen quality in men,[303] and in females it may be associated with a reduced probability of conceiving in a given cycle or, in more serious cases, with miscarriage.[304] A study on salivary stress biomarkers and their relationship to female fecundity found that salivary alpha-amylase, but not cortisol or adrenalin, was associated with decreased probability of conception. The mechanism of action of alpha amylase on fertility is unknown. It is hypothesised that catecholamine receptors in the reproductive tract might alter blood flow to the fallopian tubes.[305,306] Stressful life events have also been suggested to reduce the chances of a successful outcome following IVF.[307] However, a 2011 meta-analysis of 14 prospective studies concluded that emotional distress (due to fertility problems or other life events) did not compromise the chance of becoming pregnant using ART.[308]

Because of the potentially detrimental effects of stress on fertility, both partners should be screened for potential stressors, and appropriate stress management techniques discussed and implemented where necessary.

Exercise and fertility

Excessive exercise can alter energy balance in the body and negatively affect the reproductive system.[309] A study of 3628 women undergoing IVF treatment found that while physical activity of any type might improve fertility outcomes in overweight or obese women, lean women who engage in vigorous physical activity (5 or more hours per week) had reduced chances of conceiving.[310] These results are supported in a recent systematic review which concluded that extremely heavy exercisers (>60 min/day) increased the risk of anovulation, and vigorous exercise of 30–60 min/day reduced the risk of anovulatory infertility. These effects are probably produced via modulation of the hypothalamic–pituitary–gonadal (HPG) axis due to increased activity of the hypothalamic–pituitary–adrenal (HPA) axis. In overweight and obese women (with or without PCOS), exercise contributed to lower insulin and free androgen levels, leading to the restoration of HPA regulation of ovulation.[311]

Conversely, very low physical activity may increase the risk of menstrual cycle disruptions in healthy women and may have a detrimental effect on reproductive health.[312] An observational study of obese women undergoing ART ($n = 216$) found that women who exercised regularly had an over three-fold higher success rate with IVF compared to those who were sedentary.[313]

Lubricants

Cervical fluid

A number of medications affect the quality of cervical fluid and interfere with conception outcome. These include antihistamines, some cough mixtures, dicyclomine, progesterone (taken prior to or at ovulation), propantheline and tamoxifen.

Effect on sperm

Many studies have found a deleterious effect of personal lubricants on sperm function, such as motility, including a decreased ability of sperm to penetrate cervical mucus after exposure to lubricants. Several studies have shown that commonly used lubricants kill sperm equivalently to contraceptive jellies.[314–326] Some lubricants and gels have been incorrectly labelled as 'non-spermicidal'.[327]

Optimal lubricants

Ideal lubricants are those that are most natural and do not affect the pH of the vagina. The optimal lubricant is egg whites as they have a similar nutritional profile to cervical mucus and an ability to sustain the longevity of sperm.

Treating the male
NUTRITIONAL MEDICINE (DIETARY)
Therapeutic objectives

1 Provide nutritional sustenance to foster health and wellbeing.
2 Improve fertility parameters.
3 Avoid dietary factors that compound infertility, such as sugar, caffeine, alcohol, trans fatty acids and anything that deviates from a wholefood diet.
4 Address macro- and micronutrient deficiencies, paying particular attention to hydration and protein requirements.

Specific dietary treatments

Dietary inclusions
Oily fish

Adequate intake of omega-3 fatty acids is required to ensure stable cell membrane fluidity and energy production of the sperm. Similarly to their female counterparts, patients must be educated about the high methylmercury content of some fish. Acknowledging that the male component makes up half of the genetic material of the future child, the same recommendations of avoidance of high mercury containing fish should apply to men. The general recommendation by naturopaths is to avoid all high methylmercury-content fish throughout the preconception window.

Wholefood diet

A healthy diet provides a wide variety of nutrients required for the development and maturation of healthy sperm. While an unbalanced diet characterised by a low intake of minerals and vitamins has been associated with subfertility,[88,89] a wholefood diet based on a variety of fresh, seasonal foods, organic where possible, will contain a blend of synergistic nutrients required for healthy preconception. A prospective study in the US of 155 male partners in subfertile couples found that total fruit and vegetable consumption was not related to semen quality parameters; however, high-pesticide-residue fruit and vegetable intake was.[328] Foods such as processed meats and smallgoods should always be avoided due to negative impact on sperm parameters.[329]

A study comparing two different dietary patterns found that adhering to a prudent diet (high intake of fish, chicken, fruits, vegetables, legumes and whole grains) was associated with increased sperm motility. Adherence to a Western diet (high intake of red and processed meat, refined grains, pizza, snacks, high-energy drinks and sweets) was not associated with any semen parameter.[330] Similarly, a recent review of observational studies concluded that adherence to a healthy diet (such as the Mediterranean diet pattern and diets characterised by higher intakes of seafood, poultry, whole grains, fruits and vegetables in non-Mediterranean countries) has been consistently associated with better semen parameters in a wide range of studies in North America, Europe, the

Middle East and East Asia.[331–333] It has been shown that following a diet characterised by higher intakes of legumes, vegetables, cereals, fruits and olive oil, and low intakes of dairy, mayonnaise, margarines, sauces, snacks and sweets is associated with semen quality – particularly sperm concentration and progressive motility – among men from couples planning pregnancy.[334] A study in men with asthenozoospermia showed an association between following a dietary nutrient intake pattern comprising mainly antioxidants, vitamin D, fibre and polyunsaturated fatty acids and a significantly lower risk of asthenozoospermia.[335]

A longitudinal study on the effects of dairy on semen parameters found that low-fat dairy intake (particularly low-fat milk) was associated with increased sperm concentrations and motility, whereas cheese intake was associated with lower sperm concentration.[336]

Protein

Please review the discussion on protein and fertility in the Treating the female section for more information.

Antioxidant-rich foods

Acknowledging the role of oxidative stress and its detrimental effects on male fertility, the inclusion of a wide variety of dietary antioxidants is recommended. Antioxidants are well known for their health benefits and have demonstrated significant benefits in improving a wide range of fertility outcomes, including effects on sperm health.

Phyto-oestrogens

There is conflicting information available on the effect of phyto-oestrogens on sperm parameters and fertility. Various studies have found improvements in sperm count and motility with soy consumption; others have found the intake of soy and isoflavones was inversely related to sperm concentration.[337] A 2010 meta-analysis found that neither soy foods nor isoflavone supplement intake has an effect on testosterone levels.[338] A recent prospective cohort study found that soy food intake in men was not related to clinical outcomes among couples attending a fertility clinic.[339]

Dietary exclusions

Caffeine

An in vitro study on the effects of caffeine on Sertoli cell metabolism and oxidative profile found that high dosages of caffeine increased protein oxidative damage in the cells, but moderate doses of caffeine stimulated lactate production, which can promote germ cell survival. Moderate consumption of caffeine appears to be safe in male reproductive health in this study.[340] This is supported by an analysis of a cohort of 4474 semen samples in an epidemiological study which found that semen volumes were higher among caffeine consumers, but concentration was lower. No relationship was observed for motility, morphology or DNA fragmentation.[341] A study of more than 2500 Danish men investigating caffeine intake from various sources, including cola, found that caffeine intake of less than 800 mg/day and cola consumption of less than 14 bottles (500 mL) per week was not associated with reduced semen quality. There was

an apparent threshold with cola consumption of 1 L per day, which was associated with a reduction in sperm quality. The authors concluded that this effect is probably due to constituents in cola other than caffeine, or the effects might be associated with a less healthy diet and lifestyle of high-quantity cola consumers.[342] In summary, a recent systematic review of the relationship between caffeine and parameters of male fertility found that caffeine intake may negatively affect male reproductive function; however, the data to date are inconsistent and inconclusive.[343]

As far as ART outcomes are concerned, an observational study on the effects of caffeine and alcohol on men at a fertility clinic found no association between caffeine or alcohol intake on semen parameters. However, pretreatment caffeine and alcohol intake did affect live birth outcome after ART. Caffeine intake was associated with a lower probability of achieving live birth.[344]

Alcohol

The data on alcohol consumption and its relationship with fertility is mixed. While some have suggested there is no link between alcohol and fertility,[104] others have shown a direct link to decreased male fertility.

Alcohol consumption has been shown to impair gonadal function and is associated with defective sperm morphology, impaired sperm motility and lowered sperm counts.[48,345]

A review of the literature in 2013 suggested that alcohol consumption alters sperm parameters (most commonly morphologically abnormal spermatozoa) and testicular pathology. It is noted that genetic factors as well as nutritional deficiencies may modulate the impact of alcohol on spermatogenesis.[346]

More recently, a cross-sectional study of 8344 healthy men in Europe and the US found that moderate alcohol intake was not associated with a reduction in semen quality. However, this study only looked at alcohol consumed the week prior to the semen testing, which does not account for the long term effects of alcohol consumption.[347] Another study of 347 men investigating the effect of the past 5 days' worth of alcohol intake found that alcohol intake was associated with impairment of most semen characteristics. There was a tendency towards lower semen parameters with higher intake of alcohol, but no statistically significant dose–response association was found.[348]

A recent review of 15 cross-sectional studies has shown a detrimental effect of daily, but not occasional, alcohol consumption on semen volume and morphology. This suggests that a moderate consumption of alcohol should not adversely affect semen quality parameters.[349] Without further rigorous studies, the best available evidence suggests that alcohol intake and fertility are linked only with high levels of consumption (more than eight drinks per week or more than 40 g alcohol per day, depending on the study).[350]

From a naturopathic perspective, however, it is highly advisable for those wanting to optimise their fertility to exclude all alcohol from their diet. A case report of a 6-year follow-up of a male patient showed that stopping alcohol consumption led to a rapid, dramatic improvement in semen characteristics. Normal semen parameters were observed after 3 months.[351]

Dietary fats

A preliminary cross-sectional study of 99 men attending a fertility clinic found that high intake of saturated fat was negatively associated with sperm count and sperm concentration, and a higher intake of omega-3 fats in the diet was positively related to sperm morphology. Nutrient intake was estimated based on food frequency questionnaires. Total energy intake, age, abstinence time, BMI, smoking and intake of alcohol and caffeine were adjusted for in this study.[352] In support of these results, a Danish study of young men (n = 701) and a cross-sectional study of 120 men found that intake of saturated fat was associated with lower sperm count, sperm concentration and sperm volume.[353,354]

The consumption of trans fats compromises male fertility. These fats cannot be endogenously synthesised, and excessive consumption contributes to fat accumulation within the testicular environment.[355] A cross-sectional study of 209 men found that trans fatty acid intake was inversely related to total sperm count.[356] An analysis of the same set of data found that trans fatty acid intake was also inversely related to testicular volume, while the intake of omega-3 polyunsaturated fatty acids was positively related to testicular volume.[357]

High-energy diets and obesity

It has been suggested that the overconsumption of high-energy diets disrupt the male reproductive function at either central (HTP axis) and/or gonadal levels, affecting testicular physiology and disrupting its metabolism and bioenergetics capacity. This might lead to adverse reproductive outcomes such as inefficient energy supply to germ cells, sperm defects or spermatogenesis issues. High-energy intake enhances oxidative stress within the testicular environment. The major decline in fertility seen in high-energy diets might largely be due to the types of fats consumed.[355] High consumption of sugar-sweetened beverages has been associated with lower sperm motility among healthy young men. The association was stronger in lean men and absent in overweight or obese men.[358]

Overconsumption of high-energy diets leads to weight gain and obesity, and reduced fertility is recognised as one of the consequences of obesity promoted by dietary lifestyle. Obesity adversely affects sperm concentration and may affect sperm quality, in particular altering the physical and molecular structure of germ cells in the testes and, ultimately, mature sperm. Obesity is linked to low serum testosterone levels. However, treatment with exogenous testosterone is likely to have a further adverse effect on fertility.[359,360] A meta-analysis of 21 studies demonstrated an increased risk of azoospermia or oligozoospermia in overweight or obese men.[361] Obesity induces a state of inflammation with increased pro-inflammatory cytokines such as tumour necrosis factor alpha (TNF-α) and interleukin-6 in the serum, testicular tissue and seminal plasma. In the testes, pro-inflammatory cytokines can

directly impair the seminiferous epithelium. A pro-inflammatory state can also damage epididymal epithelium function, impeding sperm maturation and fertilisation ability.[362] Obesity also causes damage to DNA and plasma membrane integrity in sperm due to excess ROS and oxidative stress.[363] Obesity has been shown to affect semen parameters, including decreased sperm concentration, decreased sperm motility and vitality and increased abnormal morphology.[363–366]

A 2011 Danish cohort study on the effects of weight reduction in severely obese (BMI >33) males established an association between obesity and poor semen quality. A 15% reduction in weight over 14 weeks led to improvements in total sperm count, semen volume, testosterone, sex-hormone-binding globulin and anti-Müllerian hormone. The study group that lost more weight had a statistically significant increase in total sperm count and normal sperm morphology.[367] Maintaining an adequate or normal body weight is an important factor for male fertility.[368]

Furthermore, epidemiological and animal studies have shown that obese fathers are more likely to father an obese child, with metabolic and reproductive health consequences passed on to the next generation. Animal studies have shown that simple diet and exercise interventions can reverse the damaging effect of obesity on sperm function.[360]

Metabolic syndrome and sperm parameters

In a small case-controlled pilot study, it was shown that men with metabolic syndrome have compromised sperm parameters. It is hypothesised that a systemic inflammatory state with associated oxidative stress may provide an explanation.[369]

NUTRITIONAL MEDICINE (SUPPLEMENTAL)

Therapeutic objectives

1. Address deficiencies and provide nutrient repletion to restore nutrient pathways.
2. Improve fertility potential and relevant fertility factors.
3. Address attenuating factors such as infection, inflammation, toxicity and stress.
4. Provide antioxidants to reduce oxidation influence on gametes.
5. Support communication between the endocrine and reproductive systems.
6. Support hormone production and delivery to all reproductive tissues.
7. Encourage optimal eliminatory pathways.
8. Support optimal general health.

Specific nutrients required

Amino acids

Arginine

Arginine is an amino acid that may be used to enhance male fertility. Via its role as a precursor to nitric oxide synthesis, arginine is required for angiogenesis, spermatogenesis, fertility and hormone secretion.[125]

In males, a combination of antioxidants and arginine appears to be useful for increasing the health of sperm, and thus leading to increased chance of optimal fertility.

SAMPLE DAILY DIET

BREAKFAST	Tomato, grapefruit and carrot juice Omelette served with potato, ample leafy greens and avocado	Regular consumption of tomato juice has been shown to improve sperm motility in infertile men,[370] thus improving chances of conception. The antioxidant action of lycopene, beta-carotene and retinol reduces sperm DNA fragmentation and lipid peroxidation,[371] suggesting wholefoods containing these constituents, such as tomato, grapefruit and carrot, should be consumed regularly in the diet. Uncooked leafy greens and avocado contain optimal quantities of folate. Low folate is associated with reduced sperm density and count[372] as well as increased sperm DNA damage.[373] Animal studies also suggest that paternal folate deficiency increases the risk of birth defects in the offspring, highlighting the importance of folate beyond male fertility.[374]
LUNCH	Walnut-pesto-crusted salmon with buckwheat pasta and marinated roast vegetables: carrot, eggplant, leek, rocket and chives	Sperm are made up of a high proportion of polyunsaturated fatty acids, and the presence of these is required for healthy fertilisation. In particular, the human sperm head contains a higher concentration of DHA and is sensitive to dietary omega-3 PUFA.[375] Walnuts and salmon are both sources of omega-3 fatty acids. Consumption of supplemental DHA is associated with improved seminal antioxidant status and decreased sperm DNA fragmentation[376]; thus, it can be hypothesised that oily fish in the diet would produce similar benefits.
DINNER	Tomato-based bolognaise sauce made with extra virgin olive oil, tomato passata, tomato paste; mixed vegetables served with zucchini noodles (zoodles)	Since oxidative stress increases sperm membrane lipid peroxidation, DNA damage and apoptosis, leading to decreased sperm viability and motility, a diet rich in antioxidants from fruits and vegetables should be emphasised for optimal sperm function. Cooked tomato products contain lycopene. Lycopene concentration is increased from cooked rather than raw foods and in the presence of fats. Favourites such as spaghetti bolognaise can be modified to a healthier version to support sperm health. The lycopene in cooked tomato products increases in bioavailability when consumed with healthy oils (e.g. extra virgin olive oil or avocado).
SNACK	Trail mix: walnuts, sunflower seeds, pumpkin seeds, goji berries, Brazil nuts Salsa and guacamole with rice crackers	Sunflower and pumpkin seeds offer zinc. Zinc is found in sunflower and pumpkin seeds and is required for testosterone production, spermatogenesis and sperm motility, and may protect sperm from chromosomal damage.[377] Brazil nuts contain selenium. Selenium is a powerful antioxidant that may improve sperm morphology and concentration. Salsa is a source of lycopene. Avocado in combination with tomato salsa has been shown to increase lycopene and beta-carotene levels in humans compared to when salsa is consumed alone.[378]

An improvement in semen parameters was observed in a double-blind, randomised, placebo-controlled, cross-over clinical trial examining the effects of Prelox, a combination of 80 mg/day Pycnogenol and 3 g/d L-arginine-L-aspartate.[379] In 50 males with idiopathic infertility, over a treatment period of 4 weeks there was an observed significant increase in ejaculate volume, concentration and number of spermatozoa and percentage of vital spermatozoa compared to placebo. The percentage of spermatozoa with good progressing motility also increased significantly, while the percentage of immotile spermatozoa decreased. This appears to be due to a combination of the antioxidant activity of Pycnogenol and/or the activity of arginine to stimulate the activity of endothelial nitric oxide synthase, leading to enhanced motility of spermatozoa.

L-carnitine
Carnitine is a naturally occurring amino acid that plays a vital role in fatty acid metabolism for energy. It is essential to ensure that it is prescribed in the L-form and not the DL-form. It works synergistically with CoQ10, and it is advisable to co-prescribe these two nutrients together.

Carnitine is found in high concentrations in the seminal fluid, where it functions as an energy substrate for the sperm, assisting in their motility and maturation. Carnitine also functions as an antioxidant, providing protection against ROS. Clinical trials have demonstrated the ability of carnitine, in combination with other nutrients, to improve sperm motility in men.

In a placebo-controlled, double-blind, randomised study, 60 infertile male with a low sperm concentration and poorly motile sperm were administered a combined treatment of L-carnitine (2 g/day) and L-acetylcarnitine (1 g/day) or placebo for 6 months.[380] Increased sperm parameters were observed after combined carnitine treatment. The most significant improvement in sperm motility (both forward and total) was seen in patients who had lower initial absolute values of motile sperm ($<4 \times 10^6$ forward or $<5 \times 10^6$ total motile spermatozoa per ejaculate), suggesting that carnitine is particularly effective in patients with the lowest levels of poorly motile sperm.

In a similar study,[381] 60 infertile male underwent double-blind therapy with L-carnitine 3 g/day, acetyl-L-carnitine 3 g/day, a combination of L-carnitine 2 g/day and acetyl-L-carnitine 1 g/day, or placebo over 6 months. Sperm cell motility (total and forward) increased in patients who received acetyl-L-carnitine, either alone or in combination with L-carnitine. The total oxyradical scavenging capacity of the seminal fluid also improved, highlighting the antioxidant role of carnitine. L-carnitine (145 mg L-carnitine and 64 mg acetyl-L-carnitine) in combination with fructose (250 mg), citric acid (50 mg), selenium (50 micrograms), zinc (10 mg), CoQ10 (20 mg), vitamin B_{12} (1.5 micrograms), folic acid (200 micrograms) and vitamin C (90 mg) improved sperm motility in men with idiopathic asthenozoospermia over a 4-month period.[382] Similarly, a small study of 20 infertile men with asthenoteratozoospermia found that 3 months of supplementation with L-carnitine (1500 mg), in combination with other antioxidants, vitamin C (60 mg), coenzyme Q10 (20 mg), vitamin E (10 mg), zinc (10 mg), vitamin B_9 (200 micrograms), selenium (50 micrograms) and vitamin B_{12} (1 microgram), resulted in a significant reduction in DNA fragmentation and also an increase in sperm concentration, motility, vitality and morphology parameters.[383] These results are supported by another randomised interventional study in which L-carnitine (2 g/day) was administered in conjunction with a multivitamin for 3 months. Improvements were seen in sperm concentration, sperm count and sperm motility in men with idiopathic oligo- and/or asthenozoospermia. The results were more significant in L-carnitine combined with multivitamins than in either of those interventions alone, compared to control.[384] Similarly, a 3-month study of 199 subfertile men showed that supplementation with a combination of L-carnitine (440 mg), L-arginine (250 mg), zinc (40 mg), vitamin E (120 mg), glutathione (80 mg), selenium (60 micrograms), CoQ10 (15 mg) and folic acid (800 micrograms) once per day resulted in a significantly better improvement in sperm density and motility compared to supplementation with L-carnitine alone (500 mg twice a day).[385] In ART, L-carnitine had an enhancing effect on sperm motility and viability after cryopreservation.[386]

Antioxidants

Antioxidant support has been suggested for the preparation of good-quality sperm for ICSI where high levels of ROS have been detected.[387]

Spermatozoa are particularly susceptible to oxidative damage. Their cell membrane contains high levels of unsaturated fatty acids, which are affected by oxidation (lipid peroxidation), and their cytoplasm contains only small concentrations of the enzyme, which can neutralise ROS. Lipid oxidation of the cell membrane leads to loss of membrane integrity, increased permeability, inactivation of cellular enzymes, structural DNA damage and cell apoptosis, resulting in reduced sperm count and activity, decreased motility and abnormal morphology.[388,389] Antioxidants are required to protect sperm against oxidative damage, as well as to instigate cell repair for damage caused by factors such as environmental factors and ageing. In the healthy male, the seminal plasma is naturally rich in antioxidants to protect from this damage, whereas it is estimated that between 25 and 80% of infertile men present elevated levels of ROS in the semen and lower antioxidant capacity of semen.[388,390] Clinical studies carried out on the effects of antioxidant supplementation on sperm parameters have been difficult to compare and draw conclusive results from, due to the lack of uniformity in study designs, target populations, differences in type, dosages and duration of antioxidant therapy, and small sample sizes. A review of 17 carefully selected studies did find that 14 of the 17 trials showed an improvement in sperm quality (predominantly motility, but including concentration and morphology). In six out of 10 trials measuring pregnancy rates, an increase was found.[391] Another review assessing measures of sperm oxidative stress or DNA damage found that 95% of the studies reported significant reductions in oxidative stress or DNA damage after treatment with oral antioxidants.[392] A 2014 Cochrane review on the effect of oral antioxidant supplementation for male partners of subfertile couples undergoing ART cycles concluded that taking oral antioxidants had a statistically significant effect on live birth rate and pregnancy rates.[393]

Apart from oxidative damage affecting the fertility of the male, it has been found that oxidative damage to sperm DNA has consequences for the offspring. Paternal (but not maternal) smoking is associated with a significant increase in the risk of childhood cancer in the offspring – a clinical consequence of the relationship between oxidative DNA damage in the paternal germ line and long-term health consequences in future generations.[394]

In terms of reproductive health in older men (>44 years), a study found that men with greater intakes of vitamin C, vitamin E and zinc had lower levels of DNA fragmentation, similar to levels in younger men.[395]

A study of 169 men with oligoasthenozoospermia found that antioxidant therapy consisting of vitamin C (80 mg/day), vitamin E (40 mg/day) and CoQ10 (120 mg/day) for a period of 6 months resulted in significant improvements in sperm concentration and motility.[396] Similarly, combination therapy with L-carnitine (440 mg), CoQ10 (ubiquinol 30 mg), vitamin E (75 IU) and vitamin C (12 mg), two or three times per day for 3–6 months improved sperm concentration in infertile men.[397]

In a study of 120 men with idiopathic infertility, supplementation with N-acetylcysteine (600 mg/day) for 3 months resulted in improvements in semen volume, motility and viscosity. Serum antioxidant capacity was increased and the total peroxide and oxidative stress index were lower.[398]

A 10-week trial found that curcumin supplementation (80 mg/day) resulted in statistically significant improvements in semen parameters and total antioxidant capacity compared to placebo in infertile men.[399]

Alpha-lipoic acid

Alpha-lipoic acid (ALA) is an antioxidant found in virtually all cells of the body. It is particularly unique as it is soluble in water as well as lipids. Therefore, it is able to scavenge both fat- and water-soluble free radicals. Due to this free radical scavenging ability, it is indicated for disease states associated with oxidative stress. For example, it has been proven that optimal fertility is hampered by oxidative stress.[142,143] ALA also aids the removal of metals from the body via chelation, thus minimising the risk of cellular damage. For this reason, ALA should be considered during preconception care for any patient that presents with heavy metal toxicity. Another useful feature of ALA is its ability to regenerate other antioxidants, including vitamins C and E as well as CoQ10 and glutathione.[400] This action is highly important, given the role of these nutrients in male fertility.

ALA exhibits marked antioxidant activity on sperm in animal studies.[401–403] On review of research, it appears that ALA acts as a shield for the sperm, forming a protective barrier surrounding the midpiece (aqueous layer) of the sperm and within the structure itself (lipid layer). This protection is crucial, as this area has been identified as one of the first places where free radicals attack.[403] It is therefore useful to consider ALA in patients with high free radical damage, especially elevated DNA fragmentation levels. By exerting this protective armour, ALA helps prevent damage via cracks and the formation of deep pores that would otherwise disable the structural integrity of the sperm.

In addition, animal studies have revealed the ability of ALA to improve sperm motility and viability, minimise DNA damage,[403] protect against bacterial lipopolysaccharides (which can induce acute inflammation)[404] and possibly assist with energy supply to the sperm.[403] Finally, ALA has been found to enter the Krebs cycle, and can therefore be used for ATP production, which is required for healthy, viable sperm.[403]

In a small ($n = 44$) randomised, triple-blind, placebo-controlled clinical trial, ALA supplementation (600 mg/day) for 12 weeks improved sperm count, concentration and motility and seminal levels of total antioxidant capacity in infertile men.[405]

Vitamin A

Vitamin A is an antioxidant and is necessary for the health of the testes and sperm production. Low concentrations of vitamin A are associated with abnormal semen parameters in males.[148] In addition, deprivation of vitamin A in animals has been shown to lead to loss of spermatogenesis due to degeneration of the germ cells,[406] which is restored once vitamin A is reintroduced.[407] Studies on vitamin A in combination with other nutrients have demonstrated positive effects on sperm motility and sperm count. However, studies are lacking in investigating the effect of Vitamin A alone.[408]

Carotenoids/beta-carotene

Beta-carotene is a powerful fat-soluble antioxidant that is converted to retinoic acid in the body. Levels of beta-carotene are significantly reduced in immunoinfertile males. Beta-carotene intake is positively associated with a higher sperm concentration, as well as a higher quantity of motile sperm,[409] which is likely to be due to synergy of antioxidant supplementation in the prevention of free radical damage. A study of 189 young healthy men showed that higher beta-carotene and lutein intake from food sources was associated with better sperm motility, while higher lycopene intake was associated with better morphology. A moderate intake of beta-carotene and vitamin C was associated with higher sperm concentration and sperm count.[410]

Coenzyme Q10

CoQ10 is a fat-soluble antioxidant and free radical scavenger. It is found in the seminal fluid and the sperm,[411] where its role in the mitochondrial respiration chain is likely to be well utilised, particularly with regard to sperm motility. Furthermore, the antioxidant role of CoQ10 is also likely to be useful as free radical damage has been associated with defective functioning of the sperm. Decreased levels of CoQ10 have also been found in the seminal plasma and sperm cells of male with idiopathic and varicocele-associated asthenospermia.[412] A 6-month, double-blind, randomised, placebo-controlled trial in which male patients with idiopathic infertility were administered CoQ10 200 mg/day found an increase in sperm motility. Interestingly, although pregnancy was not a primary outcome measure, six pregnancies occurred in the CoQ10 treatment group.[413] This confirms earlier work,[414] which showed similarly beneficial effects in an open, uncontrolled pilot study of CoQ10 supplementation (200 mg/day) in infertile males with idiopathic asthenozoospermia. In this study, supplementation resulted in increased CoQ10 in the seminal plasma and increased sperm motility over a 6-month period. A 2009 RCT of 212 infertile men with idiopathic oligoasthenoteratospermia found that supplementation with 300 mg CoQ10 daily over 26 weeks resulted in statistically significant improvement in sperm count, sperm motility and sperm morphology.[415] A later RCT confirmed these findings. Supplementation with CoQ10 (200 mg/day) for 3 months resulted in a significant improvement in sperm morphology in men with idiopathic OAT. The treatment group also had higher catalase and superoxide dismutase activity, indicating improved oxidative stress in seminal plasma.[416] Similarly, in men with varicocele, supplementation with CoQ10 (100 mg/day) for 3 months resulted in improved seminal plasma antioxidant status (40% increase) and a small improvement in semen parameters.[417] In a study of 187 infertile men with idiopathic OAT, treatment with 300 mg CoQ10 daily for 12 months resulted in significant improvements in sperm motility and sperm morphology. There was also a beneficial effect on pregnancy rate in the group.[418] Administration of 200 mg/day of ubiquinol over 26 weeks in a group of 228 men with unexplained infertility resulted in significant improvements in sperm density, motility and morphology.[419] These results were supported in a 6-month trial of 60 men, in which ubiquinol (150 mg daily) was found to increase sperm count and motility.[420] While CoQ10 supplementation has been shown to be of benefit in improving various parameters of male infertility, CoQ10 intake from food was not related to semen parameters (sperm concentration, total and progressive motility and morphology) among subfertile men. A study of 211 participants showed that these men had a mean dietary CoQ10 intake of 19.2 mg/day (ranging from 2 mg/day to 247 mg/day). Intake estimate varied greatly and was based on a validated food frequency questionnaire.[421]

Vitamin C

Vitamin C is the primary water-soluble antioxidant in the body and improves all semen parameters. A marginal deficiency causes oxidative damage to sperm, resulting in reduced sperm motility and viability. Supplementation leads to improvement in both viability and motility, reduced numbers of abnormal sperm and reduced sperm agglutination.

The generation of ROS and associated links with infertility have been established and studied extensively. In particular, work has focused on the effects of increased ROS in the serum, semen and testicular tissues of patients. Changes in the testicular microenvironment and haemodynamics can increase the production of ROS and/or decrease local antioxidant capacity, resulting in the generation of excessive oxygen species.

Vitamin C (ascorbic acid), a major antioxidant present in extracellular fluid, is present at a high concentration in seminal fluid compared to blood plasma (364 mM vs 40 mM), and is present in detectable amounts in sperm,[422] where it prevents sperm agglutination and oxidative damage. In infertile men, vitamin C has been found in reduced quantity in the seminal plasma.[423,424] Males with inadequate seminal vitamin C have also been observed to suffer from sperm DNA damage,[423] suggesting that a defect or inadequate intake of vitamin C may initiate ROS to cause breakage and oxidation of sperm DNA. A small open study involving 13 oligospermic, infertile males revealed that vitamin C supplementation (1000 mg/day b.i.d. for 2 months) may improve sperm count, sperm motility and sperm morphology, thus theoretically improving chances of conception.[425] A study undertaken in Iranian males observed that sperm count, motility and normal morphology in fertile males were associated with significantly higher vitamin C intakes than those in idiopathically infertile males.[426]

Antioxidant treatment appears particularly beneficial for patients undergoing ICSI. In a study of 38 males with DNA-fragmented spermatozoa given 1 g/day vitamin C and 1 g/day vitamin E for 2 months after one failed ICSI attempt, 76% of males taking antioxidants showed a decrease in the percentage of DNA-fragmented spermatozoa, and a second ICSI attempt was performed.[65] While there were no differences in fertilisation rates or embryo morphology before and after antioxidant supplementation, there was a significant increase in pregnancy (48.2% vs 6.9%) and implantation (19.6% vs 2.2%) compared to the pretreatment ICSI

outcomes, suggesting that antioxidant treatment with vitamins C and E may help to repair DNA damage, thus increasing fertility and chances of a successful conception.

A study (n = 115) showed that 3 months of daily vitamin C supplementation (500 mg/day) as an adjunt therapy resulted in a significant improvement in sperm motility and morphology compared to placebo in men after undergoing varicocelectomy.[427] Supplementation with 1000 mg vitamin C per day for 6 months resulted in improvements in sperm concentration and motility, but no change in semen volume or percentage of normal sperm morphology.[428]

A full review of the literature shows that interventional studies have produced promising but inconsistent results, and have often provided incomplete reporting of study outcomes. Changes to semen parameters are frequently noted. However, there is little or no information documenting successful pregnancies or characteristics of the study population, thereby hindering accurate interpretation of results. As such, further research is required to evaluate better the effects of vitamin C in male fertility.

Vitamin E

Vitamin E is a powerful, lipid-soluble antioxidant that is essential for fertility and reproduction.

Like vitamin C, vitamin E is an important antioxidant that protects the health of the sperm. Serum and seminal vitamin E concentrations (along with total antioxidant capacity) have been found to be significantly lower in infertile men than in fertile subjects.[429] Free radicals, if left alone, lead to peroxidation of phospholipids in the mitochondria of the sperm, making the sperm immotile. Treatment of patients with immotile sperm with vitamin E (100 IU t.i.d.) improved sperm motility, resulting in 21% of males impregnating their spouses,[430] compared to no pregnancies reported in the spouses of the placebo-treated patients. Following the completion of the study, 26 of the placebo patients were switched to vitamin E and, during its course, four were then able to successfully impregnate their spouses. Combined therapy of vitamin E (400 IU/day) and selenium (200 micrograms/day) administered over 6 months resulted in a significant increase in sperm motility and a reduced percentage of defective spermatozoa in 690 infertile men.[431] A prospective randomised study comparing the effectiveness of vitamin E alone, clomiphene citrate alone or a combination of both treatments on semen parameters in 90 patients with idiopathic OAT showed a significant improvement in sperm concentration and sperm motility in the combined treatment group.[432]

Supplementation with vitamin E may also be useful for couples undergoing IVF. Vitamin E (200 mg/day for at least 3 months) was found to improve the IVF rate of fertile normospermic males with low fertilisation rates after 1 month of treatment, possibly by reducing the lipid peroxidation potential.[433] Beneficial results have also been observed in patients undergoing ICSI, where vitamin E helps to prevent DNA fragmentation and thus improves ICSI outcomes.[66]

Selenium

Selenium is a potent antioxidant that is essential for male fertility due to its role in testosterone synthesis, normal sperm maturation and motility.[434,435]

Diets that are excessive or deficient in selenium affect the gross as well as histological morphology of the testis. A supply of selenium for the selenoproteins in the testis is critical to spermatogenesis, and deficiency or excess of dietary selenium may impair spermatogenesis, resulting in poor semen characteristics and quality and infertility.[436]

Clinical trials reveal the ability of selenium to increase sperm motility and promote healthy spermatozoa.[437] Aside from its functional roles, selenium is also required structurally; the sperm capsular selenoprotein is involved in the stability and motility of the mature sperm and also forms part of the glutathione peroxidase antioxidant system, which is paramount for spermatogenesis and protects the sperm against the effects of ROS.[164]

Lack of selenium leads to atrophy of the seminiferous epithelium, testis volume reduction and disorders of spermatogenesis and maturation of spermatozoa in the epididymis. Selenium in seminal plasma correlates with good spermatozoa concentrations, motility and morphology.[438]

In animal studies, depletion of mitochondrial glutathione peroxidase has been found to cause impaired sperm quality and severe structural abnormalities in the midpiece of spermatozoa, leading to infertility.[439]

The effects of selenium on sperm motility were highlighted in a study involving a subgroup of individuals with poorly motile sperm and subsequent subfertility.[440] Over a 3-month period, males administered selenium (either on it its own or as part of a combination of antioxidants including vitamins A, C and E) showed increased sperm motility compared to males receiving placebo. Five males (11%) achieved paternity in the treatment group, in contrast to none in the placebo group. This small study highlights the efficacy of selenium supplementation in subfertile men, and suggests that improving selenium status can in turn improve sperm motility and the chance of successful conception. Although some may consider this number of subjects to be small, in terms of the outcome for those who were successful in conceiving the outcome is highly significant, and more so when one compares the cost and convenience of supplementation with that of IVF or ICSI.

More recently, selenium 200 micrograms/day in combination with the antioxidant N-acetylcysteine 600 mg/day was found to improve semen parameters in males with idiopathic OAT in a double-blind, placebo-controlled, randomised study undertaken over 6.5 months.[441] Increases in sperm count, motility and normal morphology were all observed. However, once supplementation was stopped, the parameters reverted back to their baseline values in two spermatogenesis cycles. This study did not include data on pregnancy rate.

Zinc

Zinc exerts antioxidant properties specific to the reproductive system, and thus its presence is likely to protect against free radicals and ROS that may impair sperm.[442]

Zinc is highly important for male reproductive function and is found in high concentrations in the reproductive organs of the healthy male, including in the prostate and testes. Particularly high amounts of zinc are found in the semen. Approximately 2.5 mg of zinc is lost per ejaculate. Zinc is required for the development of the testicles and for spermatogenesis and sperm motility.[443] Deficiency of zinc in males may lead to gonadal dysfunction,[443] and has been associated with idiopathic male infertility[442] and impotence. Synthesis of testosterone by the Leydig cells is dependent on zinc, and hence a lack of zinc results in a lack of testosterone. Zinc is also required for the conversion of testosterone into its active form via its role in the 5-reductase enzyme.

The role of zinc with regard to sperm health is as follows:

1 Zinc is found in the maturing spermatozoa.
2 Zinc in seminal plasma influences the oxygen consumption of the spermatozoa, nuclear chromatin decondensation and acrosin activity.
3 Zinc is important in the stabilisation of cell membranes and sperm chromatin.[444]
4 Zinc influences the motility and head–neck connection of the sperm.[445]
5 Zinc may increase sperm count and morphology,[446] and the number and motility of sperm are strongly correlated with zinc status.[438]
6 Zinc has been shown in vitro to improve seminal antioxidant states in infertile men, but it does not prevent sperm lipid peroxidation.[447]
7 Zinc exerts an antimicrobial effect in the seminal plasma.[448,449]
8 Zinc deficiency can cause chromosomal aberrations and lowered testosterone levels.

In a study of 45 asthenozoospermic men, it was found that supplementing with zinc (zinc sulphate 200 mg b.i.d.) alone, or in combination with vitamin E (10 mg b.i.d.), or in combination with both vitamins E (10 mg b.i.d.) and C (5 mg b.i.d.) over 3 months was associated with improved sperm parameters, less oxidative stress, sperm apoptosis and sperm DNA fragmentation index compared to placebo. There was no difference in effect between the three treatment groups.[450] Two other studies have shown that zinc sulphate supplementation (24 mg elemental zinc for 45–50 days and 89 mg zinc for 4 months) significantly increased testosterone, seminal zinc levels and sperm count.[451] Supplementation with zinc sulphate (220 mg/day) for 3 months resulted in increased semen volume, sperm motility and normal sperm count, and improved antioxidant status in spermatozoa and seminal plasma.[452] Oral zinc supplementation (440 mg zinc sulphate per day) successfully restored seminal catalase-like activity and improved sperm concentration and progressive motility in a group of asthenozoospermic men.[453]

A recent systematic review and meta-analysis of 22 studies including 2600 cases and 867 controls concluded that seminal plasma zinc concentrations in infertile males were significantly lower than those in fertile males, and zinc supplementation could significantly increase the sperm quality of infertile males.[454]

Lycopene

Lycopene is a fat-soluble nutrient with antioxidant activity. It is found in high concentrations in the testes and seminal plasma. Decreased levels have been demonstrated in males suffering from infertility.[455] Levels of lycopene in the semen can be significantly increased with dietary intake of natural sources of lycopene.[456] A randomly controlled study found that regular consumption of tomato juice (one can per day, 30 mg lycopene) significantly increased seminal plasma lycopene levels and increased sperm motility in 44 infertile men in a 12-week period. Improved results were seen after 6 weeks of the trial.[457] Thirty males with idiopathic non-obstructive OAT were given lycopene 2 mg b.i.d. for 3 months.[458] Twenty patients (66%) showed an improvement in sperm concentration, 16 (53%) had improved motility and 14 (46%) showed improvement in sperm morphology.

B group vitamins

The B vitamins are a group of water-soluble vitamins that have an indispensable role during preconception due to their multifaceted actions within the body.

Vitamin B_1 (thiamine)

Vitamin B_1 is a water-soluble vitamin that participates in numerous enzymatic reactions within the body.

The effect of vitamin B_1 deficiency on spermatogenesis in humans has not been reported. However, in mice deprived of vitamin B_1, decreased testicular mass and absence of sperm have been observed, and this is thought to occur as a result of germ cell apoptosis, leading to subsequent infertility.[459,460]

Vitamin B_5 (pantothenic acid)

Vitamin B_5 is essential for life and is found as part of coenzyme A, an enzyme system required for numerous functions within the body, including the synthesis of steroid hormones such as testosterone.

In male rats, vitamin B_5 has been shown to be essential for testicular endocrinology, including testosterone production and normal sperm motility.[461] Male rats fed a vitamin-B_5-deficient diet demonstrated damaged germinal epithelium and impaired spermiogenesis.

Vitamin B_6 (pyridoxine)

Vitamin B_6 is required for the metabolism of amino acids, lipids, pathways of gluconeogenesis and synthesis of neurotransmitters during the periconception period.[145] It is required for the regulation of homocysteine and also promotes the absorption of zinc.

Vitamin B_9 (folate)

Folate is required for healthy DNA and RNA synthesis, as well as normal protein synthesis[187] and regulation of gene expression. Deficiency is associated with impaired DNA synthesis and repair and the subsequent complications.

Spermatogenesis is reliant on DNA synthesis; hence the importance of adequate folate,[187] in particular for germ cell growth and rapid division of cells. Low vitamin B_9 in seminal plasma is associated with increased sperm DNA damage.[462] Infertile men have been found to have lower concentrations of serum folate compared to fertile men; however, serum folate concentration was not correlated with any semen parameters.[463] A recent study of 269 men found that seminal plasma folate level was significantly lower among men with azoospermia than those with normozoospermia. In men with normozoospermia, low seminal plasma folate level was significantly correlated with low sperm concentration.[464] Folic acid 5 mg/day together with zinc sulfate 66 mg/day has been shown to be efficacious in enhancing male fertility in both subfertile and healthy males. In a double-blind, randomised, placebo-controlled trial conducted over 6.5 weeks, subfertile male patients administered with the latter supplements revealed a significant 74% increase in total normal sperm count and a minor increase of 4% in abnormal spermatozoa. Similar beneficial results were also seen in the fertile males.[187] These results were not supported by a later 16-week RCT of 83 subfertile men. Daily treatment with folic acid (5 mg/day) and zinc sulphate (220 mg/day) did not improve sperm quality in the men in any of the folic acid only, zinc sulphate only or combination treatment groups.[465] Another study did find that co-administration of folic acid (5 mg/day) and zinc sulphate (66 mg/day) for 6 months significantly improved sperm parameters post surgical repair of varicocele.[466] A recent study investigating high-dosage folic acid supplementation (5 mg/day) for 6 months found that methylation of promoter regions in several genes involved in cancer and neurobehavioural disorders was altered. Folic acids supplementation must be done carefully in order to avoid causing overdose problems, particularly in patients who are homozygous for the MTHFR C677T polymorphism.[467]

Vitamin B_{12} (hydroxo- or methyl-cobalamin)

Vitamin B_{12} is essential for cell replication, folate and amino acid metabolism, as well as the synthesis of myelin, which forms a protective case around the spinal cord and brain of the fetus.

Vitamin B_{12} is required for DNA and RNA synthesis, and thus plays a key role in healthy fertility and reproduction. Vitamin B_{12} is involved in spermatogenesis,[468] and deficiency has been associated with reduced sperm motility and count. There have been a number of studies[451,469] in which supplementation with vitamin B_{12} (1000–6000 micrograms/day) has produced beneficial effects on sperm parameters in infertile males and males with low sperm counts. Increases in sperm count, sperm motility and sperm concentration and a reduction in sperm DNA damage were all observed between 4 and 60 weeks. The beneficial effects of vitamin B_{12} on semen quality may be due to increased functionality of reproductive organs, decreased homocysteine toxicity, reduced amounts of generated nitric oxide, decreased levels of oxidative damage to sperm, reduced amount of energy produced by spermatozoa, decreased inflammation-induced semen impairment and control of nuclear factor-κB activation.[470] A recent small study showed that in infertile men with varicocele, supplementation with a multivitamin including vitamin

B_{12} at 1 microgram/day for 3 months resulted in approximately 22.1% lower sperm DNA fragmentation.[471] In men with the MTHFR gene polymorphisms, vitamin B_9 and vitamin B_{12} dietary intake was associated with a decrease in homocysteine and improvement of sperm concentration, motility and morphology. The greatest benefits were seen in men with the T allele of MTHFR C677T polymorphism.[472]

Vitamin D

Vitamin D is a lipid-soluble vitamin that is required structurally and functionally. It enhances male and female fertility, and facilitates the absorption of calcium. It acts as a potent immunomodulator and can support skeletal health in both the mother and the developing fetus.

The vitamin D receptor and enzymes that metabolise vitamin D are found in human sperm (in particular the sperm head and midpiece), the testes and male reproductive tract of rats, and have been suggested to play an important role in the production and transport of sperm.[473] Expression levels of vitamin D receptor in CYP24A1 in spermatozoa are positive markers for semen quality.[474] Men with vitamin D sufficiency have a higher percentage of motile spermatozoa compared to those with vitamin D deficiency.[475,476] A cross-sectional study of 170 healthy men found that serum vitamin D levels at both low and high levels are associated with a decline in semen parameters.[477] This association is supported by another study investigating the association between vitamin D status and semen quality in 307 young healthy men. High vitamin D levels were associated with lower total sperm count and percentage of normal morphology sperm.[478]

A study of 54 men showed that vitamin D supplementation increases testosterone levels. All men in the study were vitamin D deficient at the start of the study and had testosterone levels at the lower end of the reference range.[479] This is in contrast to other studies that found that vitamin D supplementation did not affect testosterone levels.[476,480] A cross-sectional study of 1362 men did find that plasma 25(OH)D levels were positively associated with total and free testosterone levels.[481] Given the level of evidence available, supplementation with vitamin D might improve semen quality in at least some of the idiopathic cases of male infertility in a safe and non-invasive manner. Data from small intervention studies and a recent prospective study of more than 1000 men indicate that vitamin D supplementation may only be beneficial for men with vitamin D deficiency.[482,483] Vitamin D supplementation (5000 IU/day for 2 months) was found to improve sperm motility in a small study of idiopathic infertility patients ($n = 117$) who had low vitamin D levels.[484] Similarly in a prospective pilot study of infertile men, the incidence of low vitamin D was 76.9% (mean serum vitamin D level 23.6 ng/mL). After treatment with vitamin D supplements, the rate of low sperm motility (<40%) improved.[485]

Calcium

Calcium is essential for sperm function via its role in calcium signalling, which plays a pivotal role in sperm physiology and function, being involved in the regulation of acrosome reaction, chemotaxis and sperm motility and metabolism.[486] Inadequate calcium results in the inability of the sperm to partake in chemotaxis and acrosome reactions. Calcium is also highly important for a special style in which the sperm swim known as 'hyperactivation', a process that is paramount in fertilisation.[486] Hyperactivation is characterised by asymmetrical flagellar beating and the development of high-amplitude flagellar waves.

Iodine

Hypothyroidism is less common in males than females, but still does occur and may affect fertility. Hypothyroidism in males is associated with altered sperm morphology and motility,[487] and iodine supplementation may be considered appropriate to rectify thyroid function and improve sperm quality. A recent study of 96 couples undergoing fertility treatment found that an increase in serum iodine is associated with a lower total motile sperm count and with more years without successfully achieving pregnancy.[488]

Iron

Small amounts of transferrin are produced in the Sertoli cells of the testes, signifying a relationship between iron metabolism and fertility status in males.[489] Increased secretion of transferrin in the male testis has also been linked to impaired spermatogenic function,[490] further highlighting the involvement of iron in fertility. In men, iron overload due to haemochromatosis has been linked to impaired gonadotrophin secretion and hypogonadism.[489] Taking this into account, iron status (excess and deficiency) needs to be investigated in all males presenting with infertility.

Magnesium

Magnesium is found in the seminal fluid and is involved in numerous enzyme systems within the body, including the synthesis of nucleic acids and its functions as an energy substrate. Although magnesium is known to be involved in spermatogenesis, its specific role is unclear.[491]

Essential fatty acids

Omega-3 fatty acids are essential polyunsaturated fatty acids that are structurally required to maintain the lipid bilayer in all cell membranes, and as precursors for prostaglandin synthesis.

The presence of omega-3 fatty acids in sperm ensures that they are kept fluid and flexible.[492] This fluidity regulates acrosome reaction, sperm oocyte fusion and sperm oocyte fertilisation. By improving the sperm membrane and these functions, fertility is likely to be increased.[493] Of the omega-3 fatty acids, docosahexaenoic acid (DHA) in particular appears to be most important, with studies showing that sperm motility is strongly correlated with sperm membrane DHA levels.[494] DHA is also important for cryogenic tolerance.[495] Safarinejad et al.[493] observed that deficiency of omega-3 fatty acids was associated with poor sperm quality, and that infertile males had a high proportion of omega-6 fatty acids in their spermatozoa and a higher seminal plasma omega-6 to omega-3 fatty acid ratio. This suggests that an excess or an imbalance of omega-6 fatty acids is associated with decreased sperm concentration, sperm motility and sperm morphology in males with idiopathic OAT. A double-blinded, placebo-controlled RCT with 238 men with idiopathic oligoasthenoteratospermia receiving 1.84 g of omega-3 fatty acids (DHA and EPA) or placebo daily for 32 weeks resulted in a significant improvement of sperm cell total count and sperm cell concentration in the omega-3 groups compared to placebo.[496] Supplementation with DHA-enriched oil (990 mg of DHA and 135 mg of EPA per day) over 10 weeks in a randomised controlled trial ($n = 57$) resulted in a significant decrease in sperm DNA fragmentation compared to placebo. There was an insignificant effect on semen parameters.[497]

Another study found that 75 g of walnuts per day over 12 weeks improved sperm vitality, motility and morphology in a group of healthy men consuming a Western-style diet.[498] Walnuts contain not only essential fatty acids, but are also a good source of antioxidants in the diet.

Probiotics

Two small preliminary studies into the use of probiotics for improving male fertility have been carried out recently. In the first 6-week study, men with asthenozoospermia ($n = 9$) were administered two different antioxidant probiotic strains (*L. rhamnosus* CECT8361 and *B. longum* CECT7347). Each capsule contained an equal amount of each strain corresponding to 10^9 CFU/day. Results showed a significant improvement in sperm motility and a decrease in DNA fragmentation and intracellular ROS. Cell viability was not affected by the treatment. The authors concluded that the results were due to the antioxidant activity of the probiotic strains.[499]

In the second randomised trial, men with idiopathic oligoasthenoteratospermia ($n = 41$) were administered a proprietary probiotic/prebiotic therapy (Flortec) over 6 months. The treatment consists of *L. paracasei* B21060 5×10^9 cells, arabinogalactan 1243 mg, oligo-fructosaccharides 700 mg and L-glutamine 500 mg. The probiotic/prebiotic treatment group had improved volume of ejaculate, sperm concentration, number of ejaculated spermatozoa, motility and percentage of typical forms compared to placebo. FSH, LH and testosterone levels were also improved. The mechanism of action is unknown, but the authors hypothesised that these improvements may be mediated by normalisation of subtle alterations in hypothalamic–pituitary function, an antioxidant effect and/or possible improvements in the prostatic microenvironment.[500] An alternative hypothesis regarding the improvements seen in this study has been proposed.[501] Improvement in gut bacteria leads to improvement in intestinal mucosa barrier function, thereby resolving 'leaky gut' and reducing endotoxin-containing gut bacteria from migrating into the systemic circulation. Endotoxin is a powerful immune stimulant, and recent data has linked endotoxin activation of the immune system with impaired Leydig and Sertoli cell function via systemic inflammation and hypogonadism. *Lactobacillus* probiotic has been shown to exert a beneficial effect on testicular function in mice via modulation of the immune system.[501] While these small

studies are preliminary pilot studies, they show promise for a new avenue of treatment in male infertility. Hopefully larger trials will be forthcoming.

Dosage requirements

The dose requirements listed in Table 11.36 are based on adult doses reported in the literature. Due to the varying range of recommendation, it is essential to review and ascertain the requirements of patients on an individual basis. Furthermore, it is beneficial to calculate the dose according to the patient's body weight, as the recommendations given in the table are for an average adult.

HERBAL MEDICINE – MALE

See Table 11.37 for a summary of herbal medicine classes specific to male fertility treatment.

Therapeutic objectives – male

1　Improve fertility potential and relevant fertility factors.
2　Support optimal general health.
3　Encourage optimal eliminatory pathways.
4　Support hormone production and delivery to all reproductive tissues.
5　Support communication between the endocrine and reproductive systems.
6　Address attenuating factors such as infection, inflammation, toxicity and stress.
7　Provide antioxidants to reduce the influence of oxidation on sperm parameters.

Specific herbal medicines – male

Avena sativa seed (oat seed)

Avena sativa traditionally has been used for its tonifying action on the male reproductive system. The Eclectics favoured *A. sativa* to normalise sperm production where there was nervous debility, exhaustion and convalescence, particularly in spermatorrhoea (seminal emission) or in simple spermatorrhoea when not due to self-abuse.[268] Due to its gentle and restorative action on the body, *A. sativa* may be considered as an adjuvant and supportive botanical for males contemplating fertility treatment, as well as males wanting to support normal healthy physiology and function.

Centella asiatica (Gotu kola)

Centella asiatica is widely used to treat venous insufficiency, where it has been used to improve venous distension[503] and correct impairment of the microcirculation, thus reducing inflammation and strengthen and healing connective tissue.[504,505] *C. asiatica* is best known for its effects in treating venous insufficiency of the lower extremities such as the legs.[503] However, it may also be used to improve the microcirculation of the male reproductive system, thus enhancing male fertility. Although no studies have been undertaken in this area, the application of *C. asiatica* is particularly relevant if varicocele, a common cause of infertility in men, is suspected, due to the ability of this botanical to enhance the connective tissue of varicosities via a regulatory effect on the metabolism in the connective tissue of the vascular wall.[506]

TABLE 11.36 Supplementation dosage requirements in preconception treatment				
Nutrient	Men (dose per day)		Nutrient	Men (dose per day)
Vitamins			Minerals	
Vitamin A*	10 000–25 000 IU		Calcium	1000–1500 mg
Vitamin B$_1$ (thiamine)	50–100 mg		Chromium‡	100–400 micrograms
Vitamin B$_2$ (riboflavin)	50 mg		Copper§	2–4 mg
Vitamin B$_3$ (niacin)	50–200 mg		Iodine¶	250–400 micrograms
Vitamin B$_5$ (pantothenic acid)	50–200 mg		Iron**	10–80 mg
Vitamin B$_6$ (pyridoxine)	50–150 mg		Magnesium	500–1000 mg
Vitamin B$_9$ (folate)	800–5000 micrograms		Manganese	10–50 mg
Vitamin B$_{12}$ (hydroxo- or methyl-cobalamin)	800–5000 micrograms		Potassium	3–8 g
Vitamin C	1000–5000 mg§§		Selenium	200–300 micrograms
Vitamin D†	1000–5000 IU		Silica	20–30 mg
Vitamin E	500–1000 IU		Zinc	40–80 mg
Vitamin K	60–120 micrograms		Essential fatty acids	
Beta-carotene	3–6 mg		Total omega-3 essential fatty acids	1000–5000 mg
Bioflavonoids	600–1500 mg		Total omega-6 essential fatty acids	1000–2000 mg
Biotin	500–5000 micrograms		DHA	400–700 mg
Choline	1000–2000 mg		EPA	800–1000 mg
Inositol	25 mg		Evening primrose oil	1000–1500 mg
PABA	50 mg		Animo acids	
Coenzyme Q10	100–600 mg		Arginine	3000–4000 mg
			Carnitine	900–3000 mg
			Other	
			Probiotics (mixed strains)	25–50 × 10^9

*Retinol equivalents (RE) are now used: 1 microgram RE = 1 microgram retinol = 6 microgram beta-carotene = 12 microgram other carotenoids.
†Prescribe based on pathology results.
‡Dose is dependent on blood sugar level (BSL) control and weight requirements.
§Avoid in instances of Wilson's disease (assess prior to prescription) and ensure that prescription is only recommended when the zinc/copper ratio has been considered.
¶Assessment prior to prescription is essential, and should only be conducted when thyroid function values can be reviewed.
**Must have a pathology interpretation prior to recommending a prescription, in order to determine the required dosage.
§§In divided doses.

Ginkgo biloba (ginkgo)

Ginkgo biloba is an antioxidant that improves circulation and increases peripheral blood flow to the reproductive organs, helping to maintain healthy blood vessel tone. *G. biloba* has been hypothesised to increase nitric oxide bioavailability,[507] and animal studies have shown a smooth muscle relaxant action on the penis. Clinical studies have demonstrated the effects of *G. biloba* in individuals with antidepressant sexual dysfunction. However, there are no studies assessing the effects of *G. biloba* in male fertility, although it is widely used by naturopaths in clinical practice for this purpose due to the actions described above.

Panax ginseng (Korean ginseng)

Panax ginseng is one of the most widely researched botanicals for male reproductive health and has been used for centuries in traditional Chinese medicine as a male tonic to support virility and healthy fertility. *P. ginseng* is an energy tonic indicated where there is lowered vitality and where physical performance and sexual function require enhancement. It appears to work by enhancing nitric oxide production[508] and by affecting different levels of the hypothalamus–pituitary–testis axis.[509]

In vitro studies have demonstrated the ability of *P. ginseng* to enhance male physiology. The active constituents in *P. ginseng*, the ginsenosides, have been found to enhance intracellular nitric oxide production (nitric oxide plays a key role in modulating sperm functions). Acknowledging this, it is no surprise that ginsenoside Re has been shown to be useful in regulating the capacitating process of spermatozoa, thus improving fertilisation,[508] and in improving sperm motility.[502] Semen samples were obtained from 10 fertile volunteers and 10

TABLE 11.37 Herbal medicine classes – male

Herbal class	Justification
Adaptogen	Adaptogens may be used to increase resistance to stress and are especially important for patients undergoing fertility treatment because of the known detrimental effects of stress on fertility and libido. Positive example adaptogens include *Panax ginseng* (Korean ginseng), *Eleutherococcus senticosus* (Siberian ginseng), *Rhodiola rosea* (rhodiola) and *Withania somnifera* (ashwagandha).
Alterative/depurative	Acknowledging that the semen pass through the urinary structures, alteratives/depuratives such as *Sarsaparilla officinalis* (smilax), *Galium aparine* (cleavers) and *Arctium lappa* (burdock) are required for their cleansing and detoxifying action within the body.
Anti-infective	Infection is implicated in the pathogenesis of some male infertility; hence the importance of anti-infective botanicals. Choice of botanical will be dependent upon the infective organism; e.g. *Arctostaphylos uva-ursi* (uva ursi) for *Mycoplasma* and *Artemesia annua* (wormwood) for toxoplasmosis.
Anti-inflammatory	Botanicals with a specific anti-inflammatory action on the male reproductive structures such as *Serenoa repens* (saw palmetto) may be well utilised to modulate inflammation and DNA damage to the sperm.
Antioxidant	Antioxidant botanicals such as *Vitis vinifera* (grape seed extract), *Curcuma longa* (turmeric), *Silybum marianum* (St Mary's thistle) and *Camellia sinensis* (green tea) may be used to protect the cells of the male reproductive system and reduce DNA damage to the sperm from free radicals and radiation (e.g. laptops and mobile phones), and environmental-induced damage (e.g. heavy metals, pesticides).
Aphrodisiac	Aphrodisiacs such as *Turnera diffusa* (damiana) and *Serenoa repens* (saw palmetto) may be used to increase sexual desire and libido. This may be particularly relevant for patients experiencing sexual dysfunction and loss of desire due to such factors as timed intercourse, loss of sexual spontaneity etc. In these instances it may also be useful to use a botanical with a secondary function as a nervine.
Hepatoprotective and detoxicant	Optimal detoxification and elimination mechanisms within the body are imperative in acknowledging the hazardous role of toxicity in male infertility; hence, a detoxification protocol needs to be implemented by the male prior to conception. Build-up of toxins such as xeno-oestrogens, pesticides, heavy metals and the like, combined with improper breakdown and clearance from the body, has a detrimental effect on sperm and subsequent fertility; hence the importance of applying botanicals that work on detoxification and elimination such as *Silybum marianum* (St Mary's thistle), *Schisandra chinensis* (schisandra), *Curcuma longa* (turmeric) and *Camellia sinensis* (green tea).
Male tonic	Male tonics such as *Serenoa repens* (saw palmetto), *Panax ginseng* (Korean ginseng) and *Turnera diffusa* (damiana) have an affinity for the male sex and improve the tone of the male reproductive organs.
Testosterone stimulant	As their name suggests, testosterone stimulants enhance testosterone in the body. These herbal medicines include *Panax ginseng* (Korean ginseng), *Sarsaparilla officinalis* (smilax), *Avena sativa* (oats), *Turnera diffusa* (damiana) and *Tribulus terrestris* (tribulus).
Nervines	The nervine class of herbs is particularly important for patients undergoing fertility treatment due to their ability to support the nervous system and include *Avena sativa* (oats), *Passiflora incarnata* (passionflower), *Scutellaria lateriflora* (skullcap) and *Melissa officinalis* (lemon balm).
Venous structural health	Herbs that aid in the repair of connective tissue and have a supportive/strengthening action on the venous structures on the male reproductive structures are well utilised for the management of conditions such as varicocele; e.g. *Centella asiatica* (Gotu kola).
Increase sperm count	Botanicals with the ability to increase sperm count may be used to enhance fertility and chances of conception in males with low sperm count. *Panax ginseng* (Korean ginseng) has been clinically proven to increase sperm count, thus enhancing fertility and chances of conception.
Improve sperm motility	Botanicals that exhibit an ability to improve sperm motility are highly indicated for patients who present with altered sperm motility, including such herbs as *Panax ginseng* (Korean ginseng) and Astragalus *membranaceus* (astragalus). Ginsenoside Re, a constituent within *Panax ginseng*, has been shown to enhance both fertile and infertile sperm motility, nitrous oxide systems activity and nitric oxide production.[502]
Improve sperm morphology	Botanicals such as *Schisandra chinensis* (schisandra) and *Ginkgo biloba* (ginkgo) may be used to improve sperm morphology by improving detoxification and peripheral and general circulation.
Peripheral vascular tonics	Peripheral vascular tonics support the vascular components of the male reproductive system, increasing blood flow, circulation and nutrition to the male reproductive structures, leading to healthier sperm. These include *Ginkgo biloba* (ginkgo) and *Vitis vinifera* (grape seed extract).

asthenozoospermic infertile patients, and spermatozoa were incubated with ginsenoside Re.[502] Ginsenoside Re was shown to enhance fertile and infertile sperm motility, nitric oxide synthetase activity and nitric oxide production, highlighting the beneficial effect of this compound on sperm motility. An RCT of 80 male infertile patients with varicocele showed that treatment with Korean red ginseng root powder (500 mg t.i.d.) resulted in significant improvement in sperm concentration, viability, motility and morphology. Participants were divided into four groups: non-varicocelectomy with placebo or treatment; varicocelectomy with placebo or treatment. Improved sperm parameter results were similar in all groups at the end of the study except for the non-varicocelectomy with placebo group.[510]

Serenoa serrulata (saw palmetto)

Serenoa serrulata is another botanical traditionally renowned for its effects as a male tonic. The Eclectics stated that *Serenoa serrulata* could 'relieve any undue irritation, due to excess and exhaustion that may be present in any part of the genitourinary apparatus'.[75] The National Standards monographs make mention of the use of *S. serrulata* for low sperm count, but concede that there is no scientific evidence to support this use. *S. serrulata* has also been found to reduce the androgen dihydrotestosterone. While dihydrotestosterone is essential for the maturation of spermatozoa,[511] increased levels are associated with problems with sperm.

Tribulus terrestris (tribulus)

Tribulus terrestris is a popular herb that has been traditionally used all over the world – in Ayurvedic medicine as a tonic and aphrodisiac, and in European folk medicine to increase sexual potency. Different parts of the *T. terrestris* plant contain active constituents in varying ratios. Studies have shown that the constituents known as the saponins are the most important with regard to the biological activities displayed by *T. terrestris*. The steroidal saponin protodioscin is considered the chief constituent responsible for the herb's effects on libido and sexual function. In animal studies, *T. terrestris* has been shown to increase certain sex hormones, including testosterone as well as nitric oxide synthesis.[512] However, such results have not been observed in some human studies.[513] These differences in the results obtained may possibly be due to the use of different extracts or plant parts, as well as the fact that many of the studies were done in healthy males with normal testosterone levels rather than males with testosterone abnormalities.

T. terrestris appears to be useful in enhancing male fertility due to its ability to increase sperm count, viability and libido. A recent in vitro study found that the addition of *T. terrestris* to human sperm enhanced sperm motility, number of progressive motile spermatozoa and curvilinear velocity. Sperm viability was also significantly enhanced.[514] *T. terrestris* also had an enhancing effect on sperm motility and viability after cryopreservation.[515] However, due to the lack of well-designed studies, a definitive opinion regarding its efficacy cannot be drawn. A case series in patients with idiopathic oligoasthenozoospermia given Tribestan 250 mg t.i.d. for

2 months showed an increase in ejaculate volume, sperm concentration and motile sperm.[516] Similarly, in a case series of 20 patients aged 14–43 years diagnosed with primary or secondary hypogonadism,[517] individuals were given Tribestan 500 mg t.i.d. for 4–8 weeks. Two patients with Noonan syndrome reported improved libido, erections, a genital pelage and improved confidence, while three patients out of nine (33%) with Klinefelter syndrome experienced increased libido: erections occurred in one patient, and two patients had an increase in coital and masturbatory activity, although azoospermia and aspermia still persisted. The effects of Tribestan in patients with idiopathic oligoasthenozoospermia have been assessed in unpublished trials.[518] In one double-blind, placebo-controlled multicentre study in 48 subfertile couples with husbands, 39 subfertile males were treated with Tribestan 500 mg/day for 3 months, while nine subfertile males were given placebo. Eight (22%) pregnancies were noted after 4 months.[518]

More recent studies have produced conflicting results. In a recent prospective, randomised, double-blind, placebo-controlled trial, Tribestan (500 mg three times per day for 12 weeks) was found to successfully improve sexual function in men with mild to moderate erectile dysfunction ($n = 180$).[519] These results are in contrast to an earlier study using 400 mg of *T. terrestris* twice per day for 30 days. The treatment was found to be no better than placebo at improving erectile dysfunction, possibly due to suboptimal dosing and/or too short a study period.[520] A randomised trial of 30 male patients with idiopathic infertility found no significant improvement in levels of testosterone or semen parameters after 3 months of treatment with *T. terrestris* (750 mg/day).[521] However, a trial of 65 men with abnormal semen evaluation found that administering Androsten (250 mg dried extract per capsule, including 37.5 mg protodioscin) three times per day over 12 weeks resulted in significant enhancement in sperm count and motility, but not morphology.[522] In conclusion, the exact role of *T. terrestris* in male infertility is still inconclusive and controversial, and there may be a need to determine different mechanisms of action other than the current hypothesis that its desirable effects are due to androgen-enhancing properties.[523] Acknowledging that *T. terrestris* has not yet been the subject of extensive scientific study, and that the majority of studies undertaken have been of poor design, it is clear that more good quality studies are needed.

Turnera diffusa (damiana)

Turnera diffusa is another herb that has been used traditionally by the Eclectics as a male tonic. It is mentioned in *King's American Dispensatory* for its positive aphrodisiac effects, acting energetically on the genitourinary organs of both sexes, and is strongly indicated for sexual weakness and debility.[268] It is also mentioned by the Eclectic physician Ellingwood[75] as a stimulant tonic of the sexual apparatus and as a general tonic, especially if there is enfeeblement of the central nervous system. *T. diffusa* has been shown to facilitate sexual behaviour in male rats with sexual dysfunction, reducing ejaculation latency.[524] Another study undertaken in rats demonstrated *T. diffusa* to have a restorative effect in sexually exhausted male rats, hastening their recovery.[525] *T. diffusa* has been observed to suppress aromatase activity, leading to the hypothesis that it may increase testosterone in the body.[526] However, to date there have been few studies on the effects of *T. diffusa* in human male fertility. The traditional application of *T. diffusa* as a male tonic and the effects demonstrated in animals suggest that it would be useful particularly in the subfertile male who requires nervous system support due to debility, fatigue and mild depression.

Astragalus membranaceus (astragalus)

Poor sperm motility is an important cause of male infertility, and *Astragalus membranaceus* has been observed in experimental studies to increase the motility of sperm in semen.[527] However, further studies in humans are required to confirm these effects.

Mucuna pruriens (velvet bean)

In the ancient Indian Ayurvedic and Unani medicine systems, numerous plants and their products have been recommended for endurance against stress, general resistance against infection, retardation of the ageing process and eventual improvement of male sexual function, alleviating disorders such as psychogenic impotence and unexplained infertility.[528] One study[529] has provided evidence that *Mucuna pruriens* seed powder helps fight stress-mediated poor semen quality, and acts as a restorative and invigorator tonic or aphrodisiac in infertile subjects. A follow-up study[530] was aimed at determining how *M. pruriens* achieved this dramatic improvement (success for 70% of study participants). It was found that treatment with *M. pruriens* regulated steroidogenesis and improved semen quality in infertile males. What was most interesting was the finding that treatment with *M. pruriens* significantly improved testosterone, LH, dopamine, adrenaline and noradrenaline levels in infertile men, and reduced levels of FSH and prolactin. Sperm count and motility were also significantly recovered in infertile males after treatment. A summary of the findings of this study is given in Tables 11.38 and 11.39. In a study of *M. pruriens* seed powder administered to 180 infertile men over 3 months, nuclear magnetic resonance analysis showed a significant improvement in seminal plasma metabolic profile. Improvements were seen in alanine, citrate, glycerophosphocholine, histidine and phenylalanine concentrations in seminal plasma.[531]

Withania somnifera (ashwagandha)

Countless practitioners acknowledge the importance of addressing the effects of stress on fecundity scores. An interesting paper[532] supports the prescription of *Withania somnifera* for more than its adaptogenic properties, and highlights the importance of holistic prescription. In the study, treatment with *W. somnifera* effectively reduced oxidative stress, as assessed by decreased levels of various oxidants, and improved the level of diverse antioxidants (see Table 11.40). As antioxidant requirements are significant for the health of semen parameters, this finding is especially clinically relevant. Moreover, the levels of testosterone, LH, FSH and prolactin (PRL), which are good indicators of semen quality, were also reversed in infertile subjects after treatment with *W. somnifera* (Table 11.41). Therefore, the prescription of *W. somnifera* should be considered specifically for infertile men, especially those presenting with depletion, emotional stress and fatigue. A pilot study of 46 men with oligospermia found that daily supplementation with *W. somnifera* (675 mg/d of high-concentration, full-spectrum root extract) over 90 days resulted in a 167% increase in sperm count, 53% in semen volume and 57% increase in sperm motility compared to placebo. Improvement and regulation of serum hormone levels (testosterone and LH) was also observed in the treatment group as compared to placebo.[533]

W. somnifera acts on semen quality by repairing disturbed concentrates of lactate, alanine, citrate, glycerophosphocholine, histidine and phenylalanine in

TABLE 11.38 Clinical parameters of patients before and after treatment with *Mucuna pruriens*[530]							
Physiological parameters	**Control**	**Normozoospermic**		**Oligozoospermic**		**Asthenozoospermic**	
		Pre treatment	Post treatment	Pre treatment	Post treatment	Pre treatment	Post treatment
Semen volume (mL)	2.70 ± 0.32	2.56 ± 0.47 (−5)	2.78 ± 0.61 (+8)	2.65 ± 0.35 (−2)	2.72 ± 0.43 (+3)	2.18 ± 0.40 (−19)	2.29 ± 0.19 (+5)
Liquefaction time (min)	20.85 ± 2.22	25.10 ± 2.92[a] (+20)	19.40 ± 2.16[b] (−23)	24.15 ± 1.79 (+16)	18.75 ± 2.49[b] (−22)	58.10 ± 6.38[c] (+179)	35.80 ± 4.96[b] (−38)
Motility (%)	56.75 ± 5.05	62.50 ± 6.44[d] (+10)	67.15 ± 6.27 (+7)	68.00 ± 9.60 (+20)	70.80 ± 15.45 (+4)	12.85 ± 2.39[c] (−77)	18.10 ± 2.86[b] (+41)
Sperm comcentration (× 10^8/mL)	58.07 ± 7.61	56.10 ± 7.31[d] (−3)	70.65 ± 7.17[b] (+26)	8.31 ± 2.82[c] (−86)	56.20 ± 6.69[b] (+576)	54.55 ± 6.37 (−6)	57.70 ± 9.16 (+6)

Note: Results are expressed as mean ± SD. Values in parentheses indicate percentage change (pretreatment groups vs control and posttreatment groups vs respective pretreatment groups).
[a] $P<0.05$ vs control group.
[b] $P<0.001$ vs pretreatment group.
[c] $P<0.001$ vs control group.
[d] $P<0.01$; vs control group.

TABLE 11.39 Hormone parameters of patients before and after treatment with *Mucuna pruriens*[530]

Hormonal parameters	Control	Normozoospermic		Oligozoospermic		Asthenozoospermic	
		Pre treatment	Post treatment	Pre treatment	Post treatment	Pre treatment	Post treatment
LH (mIU/mL)	7.35 ± 0.52	6.08 ± 0.93[a] (−17)	7.50 ± 0.96[b] (+23)	5.15 ± 0.97[c] (−30)	7.28 ± 0.92[b] (+41)	4.14 ± 1.35[c] (−43)	5.79 ± 0.97[b] (+40)
FSH (mIU/mL)	6.22 ± 1.71	7.11 ± 1.30[a] (+14)	6.28 ± 1.94[b] (−11)	8.30 ± 1.06[c] (+33)	6.32 ± 1.46[b] (−24)	7.28 ± 2.05[c] (+17)	6.67 ± 1.29[b] (−8)
Testosterone (ng/mL)	5.63 ± 0.81	4.49 ± 0.53[a] (−20)	5.72 ± 0.36[b] (+27)	3.89 ± 0.95[c] (−30)	5.40 ± 0.48[b] (+39)	2.65 ± 0.73[c] (−52)	3.66 ± 0.39[b] (+17)
PRL (ng/mL)	6.68 ± 2.03	6.75 ± 1.13[a] (+1)	5.45 ± 0.66[b] (−19)	10.76 ± 2.94[c] (+61)	7.28 ± 1.66[b] (−32)	6.92 ± 1.53[c] (+4)	6.16 ± 1.74[b] (−11)

Note: Results are expressed as mean ± SD. Values in parentheses indicate percentage change (pre-treatment groups vs control and post-treatment groups vs respective pre-treatment groups).
[a]P <0.05 vs control group.
[b]P <0.05 vs pretreatment group.
[c]P <0.05 vs control group.

TABLE 11.40 Effect of *Withania somnifera* on the seminal plasma levels of antioxidant vitamins and corrected fructose in infertile men[532]

Group	Treatment	Vitamin A (microgram/dL)	Vitamin E (mg/dL)	Vitamin C (mg/dL)	Corrected fructose (mg/dL)
Control (n = 75)		28.61 ± 4.43	0.143 ± 0.012	5.64 ± 0.71	3.63 ± 0.34
Normozoospermic (n = 25)	Pre treatment[a]	17.86 ± 3.02	0.109 ± 0.013	4.18 ± 0.42	2.49 ± 0.30
	Post treatment	21.73 ± 4.05[b]	0.129 ± 0.019[b]	5.12 ± 0.49[b]	2.77 ± 0.52*
Oligozoospermic (n = 25)	Pre treatment[a]	16.86 ± 3.66	0.089 ± 0.016	4.95 ± 0.77	2.18 ± 0.29
	Post treatment	19.50 ± 3.41[b]	0.123 ± 0.026[b]	6.03 ± 0.91[b]	2.51 ± 0.29*
Asthenozoospermic (n = 25)	Pre treatment[a]	15.23 ± 2.39	0.078 ± 0.020	5.05 ± 0.88	2.32 ± 0.40
	Post treatment	17.91 ± 3.06[b]	0.108 ± 0.031[b]	6.13 ± 0.90[b]	2.55 ± 0.41*

[a]P <0.01 compared to control (Dunnett test).
[b]P <0.01 compared to pretreatment (paired t test)
*P <0.01 compared to pretreatment (paired t test)

TABLE 11.41 Effect of *Withania somnifera* on the hormone profile in the serum of infertile men[532]

Group	Treatment	LH (mIU/mL)	T (ng/mL)	FSH (mIU/mL)	PRL (ng/mL)
Control (n = 75)		7.94 ± 1.00	7.09 ± 0.63	5.67 ± 0.91	7.10 ± 0.67
Normozoospermic (n = 25)	Pre treatment	6.87 ± 0.60[a]	5.80 ± 0.88[a]	6.07 ± 0.69[NS]	7.21 ± 0.72[NS]
	Post treatment	7.85 ± 0.53[b]	6.65 ± 0.78[b]	5.75 ± 0.60**	6.93 ± 0.67[NS]
Oligozoospermic (n = 25)	Pre treatment	4.02 ± 0.57[a]	3.51 ± 0.56[a]	7.78 ± 0.77[a]	10.57 ± 1.42[a]
	Post treatment	5.98 ± 0.80[b]	4.94 ± 0.54[b]	6.27 ± 0.76[b]	8.75 ± 1.28[b]
Asthenozoospermic (n = 25)	Pre treatment	3.82 ± 0.59[a]	4.32 ± 0.89[a]	6.49 ± 0.85[a]	7.78 ± 0.82*
	Post treatment	5.37 ± 0.61[b]	5.23 ± 0.80[b]	5.95 ± 0.96**	7.19 ± 0.82[b]

[a]P <0.01 compared to control.
[b]P <0.01 compared to pretreatment.
*P <0.05 compared to control.
**P <0.05 compared to pretreatment.
[NS]Not significant

seminal plasma, thereby normalising seminal plasma metabolites. In addition, *W. somnifera* acts on regulating reproductive hormones, fatty acid metabolism and enzymatic activity of the tricarboxylic acid cycle (Krebs cycle).[534] A study into the effect of *W. somnifera* on stress-related male fertility found that treatment with *W. somnifera* powder (5 g/day dried root powder for 3 months) resulted in a decrease in stress, improved antioxidant levels and improvement in sperm concentration and motility and sperm liquefaction time. The study was conducted on 60 infertile men (with 60 control subjects), categorised into heavy smokers, those under psychological stress and infertility with unknown aetiology. Seminal lipid peroxides were elevated in the infertile group at baseline compared to the control group, but were decreased after the treatment period. Treatment with *W. somnifera* also resulted in significantly decreased cortisol levels and increased serum testosterone and LH levels.[535] A 3-month treatment of normozoospermic, oligozoospermic and asthenozoospermic men ($n = 75$) with *W. somnifera* (5 g/day root powder) found improved semen quality by restoring the altered levels of intracellular ROS in spermatozoa and cell death and improving essential metal ion (Cu^{2+}, Zn^{2+}, Fe^{2+} and Au^{2+}) concentrations.[536]

Nigella sativa (black cumin)

Nigella sativa is a herb displaying antioxidant properties. Thymoquinone and unsaturated fatty acids (linoleic and oleic acid) are the main antioxidant components. In a study of 68 infertile men with abnormal semen parameters, treatment with *N. sativa* seed oil (2.5 mL b.i.d.) over 2 months improved sperm count, motility, morphology and semen volume compared to placebo.[537] This study follows on from previous animal studies which showed that *N. sativa* improves sperm parameters, semen Leydig cells, reproductive organs and reproductive hormones.[538]

LIFESTYLE INTERVENTIONS

General recommendations

Recommendations include consideration of all factors associated with infertility (Table 11.35). These include avoidance of the following:

- Cigarette smoking – tobacco smoking leads to reduced semen quality including semen volume, sperm density, motility, viability, DNA fragmentation, seminal zinc levels and normal morphology. Furthermore, reproductive hormone system disorders, dysfunction of spermatogenesis, sperm maturation process and impaired spermatozoa function have been observed in smokers. The effects are directly correlated with cigarette quantity and duration of smoking.[539,540] Tobacco smoke contains high levels of ROS which cause DNA damage. Cadmium, lead and nicotine in cigarettes also cause DNA strand breaks.[541] Stopping smoking for 3 months allows sperm quality to improve.[542] A systematic review and meta-analysis ($n = 5865$) on the effects of cigarette smoking suggested an overall negative effect on semen parameters. An association was seen with reduced sperm count and motility, and the effect is greater in moderate and heavy smokers.[543]

- Alcohol.

- Recreational drugs – the illicit drugs that have been found to have an adverse effect on male fertility are marijuana, opioid narcotics, methamphetamines, cocaine and anabolic–androgenic steroids.[544,545] Consuming cannabis several times per week for 5 years results in a reduction in the volume and number of spermatozoa and changes their morphology and motility, reducing their fertilisation capacity.[546] In vivo and in vitro studies have shown that cannabis may disrupt the hypothalamus–pituitary–gonadal axis, spermatogenesis and sperm function (motility, capacitation, acrosome reaction).[547]

- Excessive exposure to radiation, including mobile phone use – the literature suggests that mobile phone use alters sperm parameters, particularly motility and morphology, and increases oxidative stress.[548] A longitudinal cohort study of men attending a fertility clinic ($n = 153$) found inconsistent results between different patterns of mobile phone usage, and overall, no evidence was found for a relationship between mobile phone use and semen quality.[549] In contrast, a retrospective analysis of men attending a fertility clinic ($n = 468$) showed that mobile phone storage in trouser pockets had an effect on sperm morphology and LH levels, and was significantly associated with increased varicocele, which in turn have an effect on sperm concentration and testosterone levels.[550] A 2014 meta-analysis reported a statistically significant decrease in sperm motility with mobile phone use, but no relationship with sperm concentration.[551] A second meta-analysis reported that mobile phone use in epidemiological studies was not related to semen volume, motility, sperm concentration or normal morphology. However, mobile phone EMF was related to significant decreases in sperm motility in in vitro studies as well as decreases in motility and concentration in animal studies.[552] Both of these meta-analyses, despite inconsistent results from a small number of studies, concluded that mobile phone use may negatively affect semen quality. Studies have also shown a negative correlation between wireless internet usage duration and the total sperm count, and Wi-Fi was shown to have a more destructive effect than mobile phone use.[553] A recent in vitro study found that the effects of EMFs emitted from 3G+ Wi-Fi modems cause a significant decrease in sperm motility and velocity.[554]

- Exposure to environmental hazards, including pesticides, solvents, heavy metals and other toxins – cadmium and BPA compromise testis function directly by affecting Sertoli–Sertoli and Sertoli–germ cell junctions. They can also affect testis function indirectly via their effect on other tissues and organs (e.g. adipose tissue), thereby leading to subfertility and infertility. A recent meta-analysis of 20 case control studies concluded that men with lower fertility have higher semen levels of lead and cadmium and lower semen zinc levels. Lead and cadmium have a direct toxic effect on the testis, which leads to a decline in the quality and quantity of semen by inhibiting the formation of sperm and inducing sperm morphology changes.[555] Persistent organic pollutants, phthalates and polychlorinated biphenyls (PCBs) serum levels in males are associated with up to 30% reduction in fecundity in couples trying to conceive.[556] One source of phthalate exposure that is relatively easier to control and remove is via prescription medications. Phthalates and polymers are used as excipients to enable timed release of active ingredients. A recent case control study of participants in the Danish IVF register over a period of 10 years included over 18 500 males with poor semen quality and over 31 000 controls. Exposure to medicinal products containing orthophthalates and/or polymers within 90 days of testing was associated with a 30% and 71% increased risk of poor semen quality, respectively. The highest association was found in exposure to polymers from alimentary tract and metabolism drugs (bisacodyl and sulfasalazine).[557]

- Sedentary lifestyle – a study of 189 young men found that sperm concentration and total sperm count were directly related to physical activity. TV watching was inversely associated with sperm concentration and sperm count. Measurement of physical and leisure time activities was not related to sperm motility and morphology in this study.[558] In a study of 31 healthy males, it was found that physically active men have a more anabolic hormonal environment and healthier semen production compared to their sedentary counterparts.[559] Physical activity also helps to maintain a healthy weight: BMI and waist circumference are associated with a decrease in total sperm count and ejaculate volume.[560] Regular physical activity has beneficial impacts on sperm parameters, as demonstrated in a cross-sectional study of 32 men which found significant enhancement in semen volume, viability, motility and morphology in the physically active men compared to sedentary men.[561]

- A study of 419 sedentary men attending a fertility clinic found that moderate aerobic exercise training for 24 weeks favourably improved seminal markers of inflammation and oxidative stress and enhanced the antioxidant defence system. This correlated with improvements in semen parameters, sperm DNA integrity and pregnancy rate. Improvements were seen after 12 weeks of the trial.[562] These results are supported by an additional study showing that in healthy men, moderate intensity aerobic exercise training can induce significant improvements in semen parameters and sperm DNA integrity, mainly through adaptations in the seminal antioxidant defence system and attenuating seminal markers of inflammation.[563] Further studies have demonstrated the beneficial effects of aerobic exercise on sperm parameters and recommend that it is included as a lifestyle approach in treating male infertility.[564–566] It should be noted that prolonged intensive exercise and training may lead to alterations in reproductive hormone levels, atrophy of the testicular germinal epithelium and adverse effects on spermatogenesis, and changes in semen parameters including abnormal sperm morphology and reduced sperm motility.[567] It is advisable to avoid hot tubs, saunas, bike riding, tight clothing or anything that causes overheating to the testicles and the subsequent effects on sperm parameters.

REFERENCES

[1] Australian Bureau of Statistics. 3301.0 – Births, Australia, 2011. Available from: http://www.abs.gov.au/ausstats/abs@.nsf/Products/3301.0~2011~Main+Features~Fertility+rates. [Accessed 9 September 2018].

[2] The Fertility Society of Australia. 2018. Available from: http://www.fertilitysociety.com.au. [Accessed 9 September 2018].

[3] Hughes G, Steigrad S, Persson J, et al. Fertility in the over-35-year-old. In: Australian doctor. How to treat yearbook. Chatswood, NSW: Australian Doctor; 2006.

[4] Stanton C, Lawn J, Rahman H, et al. Stillbirth rates: delivering estimates in 190 countries. Lancet 2006;367:1487–94.

[5] American Society for Reproductive Medicine. Definitions of infertility and recurrent pregnancy loss. Fertil Steril 2008;3.

[6] Villar J, Gulmezoglu AM, Khanna J, et al. Evidence-based reproductive health in developing countries. The WHO Reproductive Health Library, No. 5. Geneva: World Health Organization; WHO/RHR/02.1.

[7] Australia's mothers and babies. Perinatal and Reproductive Epidemiology Research Unit. Sydney: University of New South Wales; 2018. Available from: https://npesu.unsw.edu.au/surveillance/assisted-reproductive-technology-australia-and-new-zealand-2016. [Accessed 9 September 2018].

[8] Wood JW. Fecundity and natural fertility in humans. Oxf Rev Reprod Biol 1989;11:61–109.

[9] Noord-Zaadstra BM, Looman CW, Alsbach H, et al. Delaying childbearing: effect of age on fecundity and outcome of pregnancy. BMJ 1991;302:1361–5.

[10] Heffner LJ. Advanced maternal age – how old is too old? N Engl J Med 2004;351:1927–9.

[11] te Velde ER, Pearson PL. The variability of female reproduction ageing. Hum Reprod Update 2002;8:141–54.

[12] Skakkebaek NE, Jørgensen N, Main NE, et al. Is human fecundity declining? Int J Androl 2006;29:2–12.

[13] American Society for Reproductive Medicine. 2003.

[14] Gnoth C, Godehardt E, Frank-Hermann P, et al. Time to pregnancy: results of the German prospective study and impact on the management of infertility. Hum Reprod 2003;18:1959–66.

[15] Levitas E, Lunenefeld E, Weiss N, et al. Relationship between the duration of sexual abstinence and semen quality: analysis of 9,489 semen samples. Fertil Steril 2005;83:1680–6.

[16] Wilcox AJ, Weinberg CR, Baird DD. Timing of sexual intercourse in relation to ovulation – effects on the probability of conception, survival of the pregnancy and sex of the baby. N Engl J Med 1995;333:1517–21.

[17] ESHRE Capri Workshop Group. Nutrition and reproduction in female. Hum Reprod Update 2006;12(3):193–207.

[18] Lighten A. A weighty issue: managing reproductive problems in the obese. Conceptions, Sydney: IVF; 2009. p. 9.

[19] Durairajanayagam D, Agarwal A, Ong C. Causes, effects and molecular mechanisms of testicular heat stress. Reprod Biomed Online 2015;30(1):14–27.

[20] National Health and Medical Research Council. Clinical practice guidelines for the management of overweight and obesity in adults, adolescents and children in Australia. Melbourne: NHMRC; 2013.

[21] Antenatal and pre-pregnancy screening for genetic conditions. In: Australian doctor. Chatswood, NSW: Australian Doctor; 2005.

[22] American Society for Reproductive Medicine. Preimplantation genetic testing: a Practice Committee opinion. Fertil Steril 2008;90:S136–43.

[23] Hull MGR, Glazener CMA, Kelly NJ, et al. Population study of causes, treatment and outcome of infertility. BMJ 1985;291:1693–7.

[24] McLachlan RI, deKretser DM. Male infertility: the case for continued research. Med J Aust 2001;174:116–17.

[25] Vierula M, Niemi M, Keiski A, et al. High and unchanged sperm counts of Finnish male. Int J Androl 1996;19:11–17.

[26] Saidi JA, Chang DT, Goluboff ET, et al. Declining sperm counts in the United States? A critical review. J Urol 1999;161:460–2.

[27] Handelsman DJ. Estrogens and falling sperm counts. Reprod Fertil Dev 2001;13:317–24.

[28] Boisen K, Chellakooty M, Schmidt IM, et al. Hypospadias in a cohort of 1072 Danish newborn boys: prevalence and relationship to placental weight, anthropometrical measurements at birth, and reproductive hormone levels at 3 months of age. J Clin Endocrinol Metab 2005;90:4041–6.

[29] Porte C, Janer G, Lorusso LC, et al. Endocrine disruptors in marine organisms: approaches and perspectives. Comp Biochem Physiol C Toxicol Pharmacol 2006;143:303–15.

[30] Anway MD, Cupp AS, Uzumcu M, et al. Epigenetic transgenerational actions of endocrine disruptors and male fertility. Science 2005;308:1466–9.

[31] Ji BT, Shu XO, Linet MS, et al. Paternal cigarette smoking and the risk of childhood cancer among offspring of nonsmoking mothers. J Natl Cancer Inst 1997;89:238–44.

[32] Lewis SE, Aitken RJ. DNA damage to spermatozoa has impacts on fertilization and pregnancy. Cell Tissue Res 2005;322:33–41.

[33] Rubes J, Selevan SG, Evenson DP, et al. Episodic air pollution is associated with increased DNA fragmentation in human sperm without other changes in semen quality. Hum Reprod 2005;20:2776–83.

[34] Aitken RJ, Koopman P, Lewis SE. Seeds of concern. Nature 2004;432:48–52.

[35] Environmental Protection Agency. Office of Toxic Substances. EPA-560/5-86-035 Broad scan analysis of the FY82 National Human Adipose Tissue Survey specimens. Washington, DC: EPA; 1986.

[36] British Medical Association Board of Science and Education. Mobile phones and health: an interim report. BMA Policy Report. London: BMA; 2001. p. 115.

[37] Lai H, Singh NP. Single- and double-strand DNA breaks in rat brain cells after acute exposure to radiofrequency electromagnetic radiation. Int J Radiat Biol 1996;69:513–21.

[38] Fejes I, Zavaczki Z, Szollosi J, et al. Is there a relationship between cell phone use and semen quality? Arch Androl 2005;51:385–93.

[39] Davoudi M, Brossner C, Kuber W. The influence of electromagnetic waves on sperm motility. Urol Urogynaecol 2002;18–22.

[40] Agarwal A, Deepinder F, Sahrma RK, et al. Effect of cell phone usage on semen analysis in male attending infertility clinic: an observational study. Fertil Steril 2008;1(89):124–8.

[41] Anderson K, Norman RJ, Middleton P. Preconception lifestyle advice for people with subfertility. Cochrane Database Syst Rev 2010;(4):CD008189.

[42] Motejlek K, Palluch F, Neulen J, et al. Smoking impairs angiogenesis during maturation of human oocytes. Fertil Steril 2006;86(1):186–91.

[43] Waylen AL, Jones GL, Ledger WL. Effect of cigarette smoking upon reproductive hormones in female of reproductive age: a retrospective analysis. Reprod Biomed Online 2010;20(6):861–5.

[44] Mishra GD, Dobson AJ, Schofield MJ. Cigarette smoking, menstrual symptoms and miscarriage among young female. Aust N Z J Public Health 2000;24(4):413–20.

[45] Feichtinger W, Papalambrou K, Poehl M, et al. Smoking and in vitro fertilization: a meta-analysis. J Assist Reprod Genet 1997;14(10):596–9.

[46] Waylen AL, Metwally M, Jones GL, et al. Effects of cigarette smoking upon clinical outcomes of assisted reproduction: a meta-analysis. Hum Reprod Update 2009;15(1):31–44.

[47] Chohan KR, Badawy SZ. Cigarette smoking impairs sperm bioenergetics. Int Braz J Urol 2010;36(1):60–5.

[48] Gaur DS, Talekar MS, Pathak VP. Alcohol intake and cigarette smoking: impact of two major lifestyle factors on male fertility. Indian J Pathol Microbiol 2010;53(1):35–40.

[49] Fuentes A, Muñoz A, Barnhart K, et al. Recent cigarette smoking and assisted reproductive technologies outcome. Fertil Steril 2010;93(1):89–95.

[50] Aitken RJ, Skakkebaek NE, Roman SD. Male reproductive health and the environment (editorial). Med J Aust 2006;185(8):414–15.

[51] Day NL, Richardson GA. Prenatal marijuana use: epidemiology, methodologic issues, and infant outcomes. Clin Perinatol 1991;18(1):77–91.

[52] Battista N, Pasquariello N, Di Tommaso M, et al. Interplay between endocannabinoids, steroids and cytokines in the control of human reproduction. J Neuroendocrinol 2008;20(Suppl. 1):82–9.

[53] Badawy ZS, Chohan KR, Whyte DA, et al. Cannabinoids inhibit the respiration of human sperm. Fertil Steril 2009;91(6):2471–6.

[54] Rossato M. Endocannabinoids, sperm functions and energy metabolism. Mol Cell Endocrinol 2008;16:286. (1–2 Suppl. 1): S315.

[55] Mueller BA, Daling JR, Weiss NS, et al. Recreational drug use and the risk of primary infertility. Epidemiology 1990;1(3):195–200.

[56] Das C, Senthil Kumar V, Gupta S, et al. Network of cytokines, integrins and hormones in human trophoblast cells. J Reprod Immunol 2002;53:257–68.

[57] Jansen R. Miscarriage. In: Australian doctor. How to treat yearbook. Chatswood, NSW: Australian Doctor; 2004.

[58] Andrology Australia. Male infertility – diagnosis and management. GP Summary Guide. Clayton, Victoria: Andrology Australia; 2007.

[59] World Health Organization. WHO laboratory manual for the examination and processing of human semen. 5th ed. Geneva: WHO; 2010.

[60] Evenson DP, Jost LK, Marshall D, et al. Utility of the sperm chromatin structure assay as a diagnostic and prognostic tool in the human fertility clinic. Hum Reprod 1999;14(4):1039–49. doi:10.1093/humrep/14.4.1039.

[61] Evenson DP, Larson KL, Jost LK. Sperm chromatin structure assay: its clinical use for detecting sperm DNA fragmentation in male infertility and comparisons with other techniques. J Androl 2002;23:25–43.

[62] Sanchez R, Stalf T, Khanaga O, et al. Sperm selection methods for intracytoplasmic sperm injection (ICSI) and andrological patients. J Assist Reprod Genet 1996;13:228–33.

[63] Strzezek J, Fraser L, Kuklinska M, et al. Effects of dietary supplementation with polyunsaturated fatty acids and antioxidants on biochemical characteristics of boar semen. Reprod Biol 2004;4(3):271–87.

[64] Silver EW, Eskenazi B, Evanson DP, et al. Effect of antioxidant intake on sperm chromatin stability in healthy nonsmoking male. J Androl 2005;26(4):550–6.

[65] Greco E, Romano S, Iacobelli M, et al. ICSI in cases of sperm DNA damage: beneficial effect of oral antioxidant treatment. Hum Reprod 2005;20(9):2590–4.

[66] Greco E, Iacobelli M, Rienzi L, et al. Reduction of the incidence of sperm DNA fragmentation by oral antioxidant treatment. J Androl 2005;26(3):349–53.

[67] Rolf C, Cooper TG, Yeung CH, et al. Antioxidant treatment of patients with asthenozoospermia or moderate oligoasthenozoospermia with high-dose vitamin C and vitamin E: a randomized, placebo-controlled, double-blind study. Hum Reprod 1999;14(4):1028–33.

[68] Kasperczyk A, Kasperczyk S, Horak S, et al. Assessment of semen function and lipid peroxidation among lead exposed male. Toxicol Appl Pharmacol 2008;228(3):378–84.

[69] Wu HM, Lin-Tan DT, Wang ML, et al. Cadmium level in seminal plasma may affect the pregnancy rate for patients undergoing infertility evaluation and treatment. Reprod Toxicol 2008;25(4):481–4.

[70] Penney GC. Preventing infective sequelae of abortion. Hum Reprod 1997;12(Suppl. 11):107–12.

[71] Hay PE, Lamont RF, Taylor-Robinson D, et al. Abnormal bacterial colonisation of the genital tract and subsequent preterm delivery and late miscarriage. BMJ 1994;308(6924):295–8.

[72] Gaudoin M, Rekha P, Morris A, et al. Bacterial vaginosis and past chlamydial infection are strongly and independently associated with tubal infertility but do not affect in vitro fertilization success rates. Fertil Steril 1999;72(4):730–2.

[73] Illingworth P. Infertility. How to treat. Australian Doctor 2010;May:7.

[74] ASRM. Intracytoplasmic sperm injection. Fertil Steril 2008;90:3.

[75] Ellingwood F. The American materia medica, therapeutics and pharmacognosy. Portland, OR: Eclectic Materia Medica Publications; 1919.

[76] Fertility Society of Australia. National Fertility Survey 2006. Available from: http://www.fertilitysociety.com.au/2008/11/10/national-fertility-study-2006/.

[77] Merhi Z. Advanced glycation end products and their relevance in female reproduction. Hum Reprod 2014;29(1):135–45.

[78] Uribarri J, Woodruff S, Goodman S, et al. Advanced glycation end products in foods and a practical guide to their reduction in the diet. J Am Diet Assoc 2010;110(6):911–16.

[79] Setti AS, Braga DP, Halpern G, et al. Is there an association between artificial sweetener consumption and assisted reproduction outcomes? Reprod Biomed Online 2018;36(2): 145–53.

[80] Machtinger R, Gaskins AJ, Mansur A, et al. Association between preconception maternal beverage intake and in vitro fertilization outcomes. Fertil Steril 2017;108(6):1026–33.

[81] Hohos NM, Skaznik-Wikiel ME. High-fat diet and female fertility. Endocrinology 2017;158(8):2407–19.

[82] Chavarro JE, Rich-Edwards JW, Rosner BA, et al. Diet and lifestyle in the prevention of ovulatory disorder infertility. Obstet Gynecol 2007;110:1050–8.

[83] Wise LA, Wesselink AK, Mikkelsen EM, et al. Dairy intake and fecundability in 2 preconception cohort studies. Am J Clin Nutr 2016;105(1):100–10.

[84] Kim K, Wactawski-Wende J, Michels KA, et al. Dairy food intake is associated with reproductive hormones and sporadic anovulation among healthy premenopausal women–3. J Nutr 2016;147(2):218–26.

[85] Twigt JM, Bolhuis ME, Steegers EA, et al. The preconception diet is associated with the chance of ongoing pregnancy in women undergoing IVF/ICSI treatment. Hum Reprod 2012;27(8):2526–31.

[86] Gaskins AJ, Rich-Edwards JW, Hauser R, et al. Prepregnancy dietary patterns and risk of pregnancy loss. Am J Clin Nutr 2014;100(4):1166–72.

[87] McDiarmid MA, Gardiner PM, Jack BW. The clinical content of preconception care: environmental exposures. Am J Obstet Gynecol 2008;199(Suppl. 6):357–61.

[88] Homan GF, Davies M, Norman R. The impact of lifestyle factors on reproductive performance in the general population and those undergoing infertility treatment: a review. Hum Reprod Update 2007;13:209–23.

[89] Ebisch IM, Thomas CM, Peters WH, et al. The importance of folate, zinc and antioxidants in the pathogenesis and prevention of subfertility. Hum Reprod Update 2007;13:163–74.

[90] Chavarro JE, Rich-Edwards JW, Rosner BA, et al. Protein intake and ovulatory infertility. Am J Obstet Gynecol 2008;198(2):210.e1–e7.

[91] Braga DP, Halpern G, Setti AS, et al. The impact of food intake and social habits on embryo quality and the likelihood of blastocyst formation. Reprod Biomed Online 2015;31(1):30–8.

[92] Vujkovic M, deVries JH, Lindemans J, et al. The preconception Mediterranean dietary pattern in couples undergoing in vitro fertilization/intracytoplasmic sperm injection treatment increases the chance of pregnancy. Fertil Steril 2010;94(6):2096–101.

[93] Toledo E, Lopez-del Burgo C, Ruiz-Zambrana A, et al. Dietary patterns and difficulty conceiving: a nested case–control study. Fertil Steril 2011;96(5):1149–53.

[94] Monteagudo C, Mariscal-Arcas M, Palacin A, et al. Estimation of dietary folic acid intake in three generations of females in Southern Spain. Appetite 2013;67:114–18.

[95] Bolumar F, Olsen J, Rebagliato M, et al. Caffeine intake and delayed conception: a European multicenter study on infertility and subfecundity. Am J Epidemiol 1997;145:324–34.

[96] Wilcox AJ, Weinberg C, Baird DD. Caffeinated beverages and decreased fertility. Lancet 1988;2(8626–7):1453–6.

[97] Stanton CK, Gray RH. Effects of caffeine consumption on delayed conception. Am J Epidemiol 1995;142(12):1322–9.

[98] Fernandes O, Sabharwal M, Smiley T, et al. Moderate to heavy caffeine consumption during pregnancy and relationship to spontaneous abortion and abnormal foetal growth: a meta-analysis. Reprod Toxicol 1998;12:435–44.

[99] Lucero J, Harlow BL, Barbieri RL, et al. Early follicular phase hormone levels in relation to patterns of alcohol, tobacco, and coffee use. Fertil Steril 2001;76:723–9.

[100] Al-Saleh I, El-Doush I, Grisellhi B, et al. The effect of caffeine consumption on the success rate of pregnancy as well various performance parameters of in-vitro fertilization treatment. Med Sci Monit 2010;16(12):CR598–605.

[101] Gormack AA, Peek JC, Derraik JG, et al. Many women undergoing fertility treatment make poor lifestyle choices that may affect treatment outcome. Hum Reprod 2015;30(7):1617–24.

[102] Hatch EE, Wise LA, Mikkelsen EM, et al. Caffeinated beverage and soda consumption and time to pregnancy. Epidemiology 2012;23(3):393.

[103] Wesselink AK, Wise LA, Rothman KJ, et al. Caffeine and caffeinated beverage consumption and fecundability in a preconception cohort. Reprod Toxicol 2016;62:39–45.

[104] Practice Committee of American Society. Optimising natural fertility. Fertil Steril 2008;90(Suppl. 5):S1–6.

[105] Hansen KR, He AL, Styer AK, et al. Predictors of pregnancy and live-birth in couples with unexplained infertility after ovarian stimulation–intrauterine insemination. Fertil Steril 2016;105(6):1575–83.

[106] Windham GC, Fenster L, Swan SH. Moderate maternal and paternal alcohol consumption and the risk of spontaneous abortion. Epidemiology 1992;3:364–70.

[107] ESHRE Task Force on Ethics and Law. Lifestyle-related factors and access to medically assisted reproduction. Hum Reprod 2010;25(3):578–83.

[108] Gill J. The effects of moderate alcohol consumption on female hormone levels and reproductive function. Alcohol 2000;35(5):417–23.

[109] Schliep KC, Zarek SM, Schisterman EF, et al. Alcohol intake, reproductive hormones, and menstrual cycle function: a prospective cohort study, 2. Am J Clin Nutr 2015;102(4): 933–42.

[110] Tolstrup JS, Kjær SK, Holst C, et al. Alcohol use as predictor for infertility in a representative population of Danish women. Acta Obstet Gynecol Scand 2003;82(8):744–9.

[111] Rossi BV, Berry KF, Hornstein MD, et al. Effect of alcohol consumption on in vitro fertilization. Obstet Gynecol 2011; 117(1):136.

[112] Mikkelsen EM, Riis AH, Wise LA, et al. Alcohol consumption and fecundability: prospective Danish cohort study. BMJ 2016;354:i4262.

[113] Fan D, Liu L, Xia Q, et al. Female alcohol consumption and fecundability: a systematic review and dose-response meta-analysis. Sci Rep 2017;7(1):13815.

[114] Chavarro JE, Rich-Edwards JW, Rosner BA, et al. Dietary fatty acid intakes and the risk of ovulatory infertility. Am J Clin Nutr 2007;85(1):231–7.

[115] Eskew AM, Wormer KC, Matthews ML, et al. The association between fatty acid index and in vitro fertilization outcomes. J Assist Reprod Genet 2017;34(12):1627–32.

[116] Laanpere M, Altmäe S, Stavreus-Evers A, et al. Folate-mediated one-carbon metabolism and its effect on female fertility and pregnancy viability. Nutr Rev 2010;68(2):99–113.

[117] Mills JL. Strategies for preventing folate-related neural tube defects: supplements, fortified foods, or both? JAMA 2017;317(2):144–5.

[118] Gresham E, Collins CE, Mishra GD, et al. Diet quality before or during pregnancy and the relationship with pregnancy and birth outcomes: the Australian Longitudinal Study on Women's Health. Public Health Nutr 2016;19(16):2975–83.

[119] Abell SK, Nankervis A, Khan KS, et al. Type 1 and type 2 diabetes preconception and in pregnancy: health impacts, influence of obesity and lifestyle, and principles of management. Semin Reprod Med 2016;34(2):110–20.

[120] Vujkovic M, de Vries JH, Lindemans J, et al. The preconception Mediterranean dietary pattern in couples undergoing in vitro fertilisation/intracytoplasmic sperm injection treatment increases the chance of pregnancy. Fertil Steril 2010;94(6):2096–101.

[121] Medenica S, Nedeljkovic O, Radojevic N, et al. Thyroid dysfunction and thyroid autoimmunity in euthyroid women in achieving fertility. Eur Rev Med Pharmacol Sci 2015;19(6):977–87.

[122] Xu J, Sinclair KD. One-carbon metabolism and epigenetic regulation of embryo development. Reprod Fertil Dev 2015;27(4):667–76.

[123] Hammiche F, Vujkovic M, Wijburg W, et al. Increased preconception omega-3 polyunsaturated fatty acid intake improves embryo morphology. Fertil Steril 2011;95(5):1820–3.

[124] Mmbaga N, Luk J. The impact of preconceptual diet on the outcome of reproductive treatments. Curr Opin Obstet Gynecol 2012;24(3):127–31.

[125] Wu G. Amino acids: metabolism, functions, and nutrition. Amino Acids 2009;37(1):1–17.

[126] Battaglia C, Salvatori M, Maxia N, et al. Adjuvant L-arginine treatment for in-vitro fertilization in poor responder patients. Hum Reprod 1999;14(7):1690–7.

[127] Mansour G, Abdelrazik H, Sharma RK, et al. L-Carnitine supplementation reduces oocyte cytoskeleton damage and embryo apoptosis induced by incubation in peritoneal fluid from patients with endometriosis. Fertil Steril 2009;91(Suppl. 5):2079–86.

[128] Agarwal A, Sengupta P, Durairajanayagam D. Role of L-carnitine in female infertility. Reprod Biol Endocrinol 2018;16(1):5.

[129] Giorgi VS, Da Broi MG, Paz CC, et al. N-acetyl-cysteine and L-carnitine prevent meiotic oocyte damage induced by follicular fluid from infertile women with mild endometriosis. Reprod Sci 2016;23(3):342–51.

[130] Ismail AM, Hamed AH, Saso S, et al. Adding L-carnitine to clomiphene resistant PCOS women improves the quality of ovulation and the pregnancy rate. A randomized clinical trial. Eur J Obstet Gynecol Reprod Biol 2014;180:148–52.

[131] Genazzani AD, Lanzoni C, Ricchieri F, et al. Acetyl-L-carnitine (ALC) administration positively affects reproductive axis in hypogonadotropic women with functional hypothalamic amenorrhea. J Endocrinol Invest 2011;34(4):287–91.

[132] Genazzani AD, Despini G, Czyzyk A, et al. Modulatory effects of l-carnitine plus l-acetyl-carnitine on neuroendocrine control of hypothalamic functions in functional hypothalamic amenorrhea (FHA). Gynecol Endocrinol 2017;33(12):963–7.

[133] Gupta S, Ghulmiyyah J, Sharma R, et al. Power of proteomics in linking oxidative stress and female infertility. Biomed Res Int 2014;2014:916212.

[134] Agarwal A, Aponte-Mellado A, Premkumar BJ, et al. The effects of oxidative stress on female reproduction: a review. Reprod Biol Endocrinol 2012;10(1):49.

[135] Ruder EH, Hartman TJ, Reindollar RH, et al. Female dietary antioxidant intake and time to pregnancy among couples treated for unexplained infertility. Fertil Steril 2014;101(3):759–66.

[136] Pereira AC, Martel F. Oxidative stress in pregnancy and fertility pathologies. Cell Biol Toxicol 2014;30(5):301–12.

[137] Tong J, Sheng S, Sun Y, et al. Melatonin levels in follicular fluid as markers for IVF outcomes and predicting ovarian reserve. Reproduction 2017;153(4):443–51.

[138] Tvrdá E, Kňazická Z, Lukáčová J, et al. Antioxidants, nutrition and fertility. Potravinárstvo 2011;5:407–16.

[139] Showell MG, Brown J, Clarke J, et al. Antioxidants for female subfertility. Cochrane Database Syst Rev 2013;(8):CD007807.

[140] Youssef MA, Abdelmoty HI, Elashmwi HA, et al. Oral antioxidants supplementation for women with unexplained infertility undergoing ICSI/IVF: randomized controlled trial. Hum Fertil 2015;18(1):38–42.

[141] Balogun OO, da Silva Lopes K, Ota E, et al. Vitamin supplementation for preventing miscarriage. Cochrane Database Syst Rev 2016;(5):CD004073.

[142] Agarwal A, Gupta S, Sharma RK. Role of oxidative stress in female reproduction. Reprod Biol Endocrinol 2005;3:28.

[143] Agarwal A, Saleh RA, Bedaiwy MA. Role of reactive oxygen species in the pathophysiology of human reproduction. Fertil Steril 2003;79(4):829–43.

[144] Ruder EH, Hartman TJ, Blumberg J, et al. Oxidative stress and antioxidants: exposure and impact on female fertility. Hum Reprod Update 2008;14(4):345–57.

[145] Cetin I, Berti C, Calabrese S. Role of micronutrients in the periconceptional period. Hum Reprod Update 2010;16(1):80–95.

[146] Morriss-Kay GM, Sokolova N. Embryonic development and pattern formation. FASEB J 1996;10(9):961–8.

[147] Lithgow DM, Politzer WM. Vitamin A in the treatment of menorrhagia. S Afr Med J 1977;51(7):191–3.

[148] Al-Azemi MK, Omu AE, Fatinikun T, et al. Factors contributing to gender differences in serum retinol and alpha-tocopherol in infertile couples. Reprod Biomed Online 2009;19(4):583–90.

[149] Simşek M, Nazıroğlu M, Simşek H, et al. Blood plasma levels of lipoperoxides, glutathione peroxidase, beta carotene, vitamin A and E in female with habitual abortion. Cell Biochem Funct 1998;16(4):227–31.

[150] Palan PR, Cohen BL, Barad DH, et al. Effects of smoking on the levels of antioxidant beta carotene, alpha tocopherol and retinol in human ovarian follicular fluid. Gynecol Obstet Invest 1995;39(1):43–6.

[151] Turi A, Giannubilo SR, Brugè F, et al. Coenzyme Q10 content in follicular fluid and its relationship with oocyte fertilization and embryo grading. Arch Gynecol Obstet 2012;285(4):1173–6.

[152] Akarsu S, Gode F, Isik AZ, et al. The association between coenzyme Q10 concentrations in follicular fluid with embryo morphokinetics and pregnancy rate in assisted reproductive techniques. J Assist Reprod Genet 2017;34(5):599–605.

[153] Bentov Y, Hannam T, Jurisicova A, et al. Coenzyme Q10 supplementation and oocyte aneuploidy in women undergoing IVF-ICSI treatment. Clinical Medicine Insights. Reprod Health 2014;8:31–6.

[154] El Refaeey A, Selem A, Badawy A. Combined coenzyme Q10 and clomiphene citrate for ovulation induction in clomiphene-citrate-resistant polycystic ovary syndrome. Reprod Biomed Online 2014;29(1):119–24.

[155] Luck MR, Jeyaseelan I, Scholes RA. Ascorbic acid and fertility. Biol Reprod 1995;52(2):262–6.

[156] Rumbold A, Ota E, Nagata C, et al. Vitamin C supplementation in pregnancy. Cochrane Database Syst Rev 2015;(9):CD004072.

[157] Osiecki H. The nutrient bible. 6th ed. Eagle Farm, Qld: Bio Concepts Publishing; 2004.

[158] Mehendale SS, Kilari Bams AS, Deshmukh CS, et al. Oxidative stress-mediated essential polyunsaturated fatty acid alterations in female infertility. Hum Fertil 2009;12(1):28–33.

[159] Cicek N, Eryilmaz OG, Sarikaya E, et al. Vitamin E effect on controlled ovarian stimulation of unexplained infertile women. J Assist Reprod Genet 2012;29(4):325–8.

[160] Bahadori MH, Sharami SH, Fakor F, et al. Level of Vitamin E in follicular fluid and serum and oocyte morphology and embryo quality in patients undergoing IVF treatment. J Family Reprod Health 2017;11(2):74.

[161] Fatemi F, Mohammadzadeh A, Sadeghi MR, et al. Role of vitamin E and D3 supplementation in Intra-Cytoplasmic Sperm Injection outcomes of women with polycystic ovarian syndrome: a double blinded randomized placebo-controlled trial. Clin Nutr ESPEN 2017;18:23–30.

[162] Mistry HD, Pipkin FB, Redman CW, et al. Selenium in reproductive health. Am J Obstet Gynecol 2012;206(1):21–30.

[163] Al-Kunani AS, Knight R, Haswell SJ, et al. The selenium status of female with a history of recurrent miscarriage. Br J Obstet Gynaecol 2001;108(10):1094–7.

[164] Rayman MP, Rayman MP. The argument for increasing selenium intake. Proc Nutr Soc 2002;61:203–15.

[165] Mirone M, Giannetta E, Isidori AM. Selenium and reproductive function. A systematic review. J Endocrinol Invest 2013;36(10 Suppl.):28–36.

[166] Özkaya MO, Nazıroğlu M, Barak C, et al. Effects of multivitamin/mineral supplementation on trace element levels in serum and follicular fluid of women undergoing in vitro fertilization (IVF). Biol Trace Elem Res 2011;139(1):1–9.

[167] Dickerson EH, Sathyapalan T, Knight R, et al. Endocrine disruptor & nutritional effects of heavy metals in ovarian hyperstimulation. J Assist Reprod Genet 2011;28(12):1223–8.

[168] Tara F, Rayman MP, Boskabadi H, et al. Selenium supplementation and premature (pre-labour) rupture of membranes: a randomised double-blind placebo-controlled trial. J Obstet Gynaecol 2010;30(1):30–4.

[169] Tara F, Maamouri G, Rayman MP, et al. Selenium supplementation and the incidence of preeclampsia in pregnant Iranian women: a randomized, double-blind, placebo-controlled pilot trial. Taiwan Province of China J Obstet Gynecol 2010;49(2):181–7.

[170] Andrews MA, Schliep KC, Wactawski-Wende J, et al. Dietary factors and luteal phase deficiency in healthy eumenorrheic women. Hum Reprod 2015;30(8):1942–51.

[171] Bedwal RS, Bahuguna A. Zinc, copper and selenium in reproduction. Experientia 1994;50(7):626–40.

[172] Breskin MW, Worthington-Roberts BS, Knopp RH, et al. First trimester serum zinc concentrations in human pregnancy. Am J Clin Nutr 1983;38(6):943–53.

[173] Singh AK, Chattopadhyay R, Chakravarty B, et al. Markers of oxidative stress in follicular fluid of women with endometriosis and tubal infertility undergoing IVF. Reprod Toxicol 2013;42: 116–24.

[174] Ota E, Mori R, Middleton P, et al. Zinc supplementation for improving pregnancy and infant outcome. Cochrane Database Syst Rev 2015;(2):CD000230.

[175] Kondo A, Kamihira O, Ozawa H. Neural tube defects: prevalence, etiology and prevention. Int J Urol 2009;16(1):49–57.

[176] George L, Mills JL, Johansson AL, et al. Plasma folate levels and risk of spontaneous abortion. JAMA 2008;288(15): 1867–73.

[177] Hübner U, Alwan A, Jouma M, et al. Low serum vitamin B12 is associated with recurrent pregnancy loss in Syrian women. Clin Chem Lab Med 2008;46(9):1265–9.

[178] Bâ A. Metabolic and structural role of thiamine in nervous tissues. Cell Mol Neurobiol 2008;28(7):923–31.

[179] Bâ A. Alcohol and B1 vitamin deficiency-related stillbirths. J Matern Fetal Neonatal Med 2009;22(5):452–7.

[180] Krapels IP, vanRooij IA, Ocké MC, et al. Maternal dietary B vitamin intake, other than folate, and the association with orofacial cleft in the offspring. Eur J Nutr 2004;43(1):7–14.

[181] Chan J, Deng L, Mikael LG, et al. Low dietary choline and low dietary riboflavin during pregnancy influence reproductive outcomes and heart development in mice. Am J Clin Nutr 2010;91(4):1035–43.

[182] Haggarty P, Campbell DM, Duthie S, et al. Diet and deprivation in pregnancy. Br J Nutr 2009;102(10):1487–97.

[183] Smedts HP, Rakhshandehroo M, Verkleij-Hagoort AC, et al. Maternal intake of fat, riboflavin and nicotinamide and the risk of having offspring with congenital heart defects. Eur J Nutr 2008;47(7):357–65.

[184] Wouters MGAJ, Boers GHJ, Blom HJ, et al. Hyperhomocysteinemia: a risk factor in female with unexplained recurrent early pregnancy loss. Fertil Steril 1993;60:820–82.

[185] Ronnenberg AG, Venners SA, Xu X, et al. Preconception B-vitamin and homocysteine status, conception, and early pregnancy loss. Am J Epidemiol 2007;166(3):304–12.

[186] Berker B, Kaya C, Aytac R, et al. Homocysteine concentrations in follicular fluid are associated with poor oocyte and embryo qualities in polycystic ovary syndrome patients undergoing assisted reproduction. Hum Reprod 2009;24(9):2293–302.

[187] Wong WY, Merkus HM, Thomas CM, et al. Effects of folic acid and zinc sulfate on male factor subfertility: a double-blind, randomized, placebo-controlled trial. Fertil Steril 2002;77:491–8.

[188] Laanpere M, Altmäe S, Stavreus-Evers A, et al. Folate-mediated one-carbon metabolism and its effect on female fertility and pregnancy viability. Nutr Rev 2010;68(2):99–113.

[189] Ray JG, Laskin CA. Folic acid and homocyst(e)ine metabolic defects and the risk of placental abruption, pre-eclampsia and spontaneous pregnancy loss: a systematic review. Placenta 1999;20:519–52.

[190] La Vecchia I, Paffoni A, Castiglioni M, et al. Folate, homocysteine and selected vitamins and minerals status in infertile women. Eur J Contracept Reprod Health Care 2017;22(1):70–5.

[191] Altmäe S, Stavreus-Evers A, Ruiz JR, et al. Variations in folate pathway genes are associated with unexplained female infertility. Fertil Steril 2010;94(1):130–7.

[192] Gaskins AJ, Afeiche M, Wright DL, et al. Dietary folate and reproductive success among women undergoing assisted reproduction. Obstet Gynecol 2014;124(4):801.

[193] Gaskins AJ, Chiu YH, Williams PL, et al. Association between serum folate and vitamin B-12 and outcomes of assisted reproductive technologies. Am J Clin Nutr 2015;102(4): 943–50.

[194] Gaskins AJ, Mumford SL, Chavarro JE, et al. The impact of dietary folate intake on reproductive function in premenopausal women: a prospective cohort study. PLoS ONE 2012;7(9):e46276.

[195] Cueto HT, Riis AH, Hatch EE, et al. Folic acid supplementation and fecundability: a Danish prospective cohort study. Eur J Clin Nutr 2016;70(1):66.

[196] Murto T, Svanberg AS, Yngve A, et al. Folic acid supplementation and IVF pregnancy outcome in women with unexplained infertility. Reprod Biomed Online 2014;28(6):766–72.

[197] De-Regil LM, Peña-Rosas JP, Fernández-Gaxiola AC, et al. Effects and safety of periconceptional oral folate supplementation for preventing birth defects. Cochrane Database Syst Rev 2015;(12):CD007950.

[198] Mínguez-Alarcón L, Gaskins AJ, Chiu YH, et al. Dietary folate intake and modification of the association of urinary bisphenol A concentrations with in vitro fertilization outcomes among women from a fertility clinic. Reprod Toxicol 2016;65:104–12.

[199] Reznikoff-Etiévant MF, Zittoun J, Vaylet C, et al. Low vitamin B12 level as a risk factor for very early recurrent abortion. Eur J Obstet Gynecol Reprod Biol 2002;104(2):156–9.

[200] Bodnar M, Catov JM, Simhan HN, et al. Maternal vitamin D deficiency increases the risk of preeclampsia. J Clin Endocrinol Metab 2007;92:3517–22.

[201] Shahrokhi SZ, Ghaffari F, Kazerouni F. Role of vitamin D in female Reproduction. Clin Chim Acta 2016;455:33–8.

[202] Ozkan S, Jindal S, Greenseid K, et al. Replete vitamin D stores predict reproductive success following in vitro fertilization. Fertil Steril 2010;94(4):1314–19.

[203] Garbedian K, Boggild M, Moody J, et al. Effect of vitamin D status on clinical pregnancy rates following in vitro fertilization. CMAJ Open 2013;1(2):E77–82.

[204] Paffoni A, Ferrari S, Viganò P, et al. Vitamin D deficiency and infertility: insights from in vitro fertilization cycles. J Clin Endocrinol Metab 2014;99(11):E2372–6.

[205] Polyzos NP, Anckaert E, Guzman L, et al. Vitamin D deficiency and pregnancy rates in women undergoing single embryo, blastocyst stage, transfer (SET) for IVF/ICSI. Hum Reprod 2014;29(9):2032–40.

[206] Drakopoulos P, van de Vijver A, Schutyser V, et al. The effect of serum vitamin D levels on ovarian reserve markers: a prospective cross-sectional study. Hum Reprod 2016;32(1):208–14.

[207] Abdullah UH, Lalani S, Syed F, et al. Association of Vitamin D with outcome after intra cytoplasmic sperm injection. J Matern Fetal Neonatal Med 2017;30(1):117–20.

[208] Abadia L, Gaskins AJ, Yu-Han C, et al. Serum 25-hydroxyvitamin D concentrations and treatment outcomes of women undergoing assisted reproduction, 2. Am J Clin Nutr 2016;104(3): 729–35.

[209] Neville G, Martyn F, Kilbane M, et al. Vitamin D status and fertility outcomes during winter among couples undergoing in vitro fertilization/intracytoplasmic sperm injection. Int J Gynaecol Obstet 2016;135(2):172–6.

[210] Aflatoonian A, Arabjahvani F, Eftekhar M, et al. Effect of vitamin D insufficiency treatment on fertility outcomes in frozen-thawed embryo transfer cycles: a randomized clinical trial. Iran J Reprod Med 2014;12(9):595.

[211] Asadi M, Matin N, Frootan M, et al. Vitamin D improves endometrial thickness in PCOS women who need intrauterine insemination: a randomized double-blind placebo-controlled trial. Arch Gynecol Obstet 2014;289(4):865–70.

[212] Aleyasin A, Hosseini MA, Mahdavi A, et al. Predictive value of the level of vitamin D in follicular fluid on the outcome of assisted reproductive technology. Eur J Obstet Gynecol Reprod Biol 2011;159(1):132–7.

[213] Firouzabadi RD, Rahmani E, Rahsepar M, et al. Value of follicular fluid vitamin D in predicting the pregnancy rate in an IVF program. Arch Gynecol Obstet 2014;289(1):201–6.

[214] Franasiak JM, Molinaro TA, Dubell EK, et al. Vitamin D levels do not affect IVF outcomes following the transfer of euploid blastocysts. Am J Obstet Gynecol 2015;212(3):315.

[215] Somigliana E, Paffoni A, Lattuada D, et al. Serum levels of 25-hydroxyvitamin D and time to natural pregnancy. Gynecol Obstet Invest 2016;81(5):468–71.

[216] Lata I, Tiwari S, Gupta A, et al. To study the vitamin D levels in infertile females and correlation of Vitamin D deficiency with AMH levels in comparison to fertile females. J Hum Reprod Sci 2017;10(2):86.

[217] Anifandis GM, Dafopoulos K, Messini CI, et al. Prognostic value of follicular fluid 25-OH vitamin D and glucose levels in the IVF outcome. Reprod Biol Endocrinol 2010;8(1):91.

[218] Rudick B, Ingles S, Chung K, et al. Characterizing the influence of vitamin D levels on IVF outcomes. Hum Reprod 2012;27(11):3321–7.

[219] Rudick BJ, Ingles SA, Chung K, et al. Influence of vitamin D levels on in vitro fertilization outcomes in donor-recipient cycles. Fertil Steril 2014;101(2):447–52.

[220] Fabris A, Pacheco A, Cruz M, et al. Impact of circulating levels of total and bioavailable serum vitamin D on pregnancy rate in egg donation recipients. Fertil Steril 2014;102(6):1608–12.

[221] Amegah AK, Klevor MK, Wagner CL. Maternal vitamin D insufficiency and risk of adverse pregnancy and birth outcomes: a systematic review and meta-analysis of longitudinal studies. PLoS ONE 2017;12(3):e0173605.

[222] De-Regil LM, Palacios C, Lombardo LK, et al. Vitamin D supplementation for women during pregnancy. Cochrane Database Syst Rev 2016;(2):CD008873.

[223] Zimmermann MD. Burgerstein's handbook of nutrition micronutrients in the prevention of disease. New York: Thieme; 2001.

[224] Martín-Romero FJ, Ortíz de Galisteo JR, Lara-Laranjeira J, et al. Store-operated calcium entry in human oocytes and sensitivity to oxidative stress. Biol Reprod 2008;78(2):307–15.

[225] Hofmeyr GJ, Atallah AN, Duley L. Calcium supplementation during pregnancy for preventing hypertensive disorders and related problems. Cochrane Database Syst Rev 2006;(3):CD001059.

[226] Gardiner PM, Nelson L, Shellhaas CS, et al. The clinical content of preconception care: nutrition and dietary supplements. Am J Obstet Gynecol 2008;2:S345–56.

[227] Lucidi R, Thyer A, Easton C, et al. Effect of chromium supplementation on insulin resistance and ovarian and menstrual cyclicity in female with polycystic ovary syndrome. Fertil Steril 2005;84(6):1755–7.

[228] Ingle ME, Bloom MS, Parsons PJ, et al. Associations between IVF outcomes and essential trace elements measured in follicular fluid and urine: a pilot study. J Assist Reprod Genet 2017;34(2):253–61.

[229] Li M, Ma G, Boyages SC, et al. Re-emergence of iodine deficiency in Australia. Asia Pac J Clin Nutr 2001;10(3):200–3.

[230] Pan Y, Caldwell KL, Li Y, et al. Smoothed urinary iodine percentiles for the US population and pregnant women: National Health and Nutrition Examination Survey, 2001–2010. Eur Thyroid J 2013;2(2):127–34.

[231] Stagnaro-Green A, Dogo-Isonaige E, Pearce EN, et al. Marginal iodine status and high rate of subclinical hypothyroidism in Washington DC women planning conception. Thyroid 2015; 25(10):1151–4.

[232] Mills JL, Buck Louis GM, et al. Delayed conception in women with low-urinary iodine concentrations: a population-based prospective cohort study. Hum Reprod 2018;33(3):426–33.

[233] Poppe K, Velkeniers B, Glinoer D. The role of thyroid autoimmunity in fertility and pregnancy. Nat Clin Pract Endocrinol Metab 2008;4(7):394–405.

[234] Redmond GP. Thyroid dysfunction and female's reproductive health. Thyroid 2004;14(Suppl. 1):S5–15.

[235] Australian Government, Department of Health & Ageing. Nutrient reference values for Australia and New Zealand. 2005. Available from: http://www.nhmrc.gov.au/_files_nhmrc/file/publications/synopses/n35.pdf. [Accessed 16 September 2010].

[236] Picciano MF. Pregnancy and lactation: physiological adjustments, nutritional requirements and the role of dietary supplements. J Nutr 2003;133(6):S1997–2002.

[237] Kemp MD. Iodine deficiency in relation to the stillbirth problem. Can Med Assoc J 1939;41(4):356–61.

[238] Potter JD, McMichael AJ, Hetzel BS. Iodization and thyroid status in relation to stillbirths and congenital anomalies. Int J Epidemiol 1979;8(2):137–44.

[239] Robinson J. Perinatal Society of Australia and New Zealand (PSANZ) Perinatal Mortality Group. Media release. Available from: http://www.stillbirthfoundation.org.au/research. [Accessed 17 September 2010].

[240] Melse-Boonstra A, Jaiswal N. Iodine deficiency in pregnancy, infancy and childhood and its consequences for brain development. Best Pract Res Clin Endocrinol Metab 2010;24:29–38.

[241] Harding KB, Peña Rosas JP, Webster AC, et al. Iodine supplementation for women during the preconception, pregnancy and postpartum period. Cochrane Database Syst Rev 2017;(3):CD011761.

[242] Chavarro JE, Rich-Edwards JW, Rosner BA, et al. Iron intake and risk of ovulatory infertility. Obstet Gynecol 2006;108:1145–52.

[243] Borella P, Szilagyi A, Than G, et al. Maternal plasma concentrations of magnesium, calcium, zinc and copper in normal and pathological pregnancies. Sci Total Environ 1990;99(1–2):67–76.

[244] Anderson K, Nisenblat V, Norman R. Lifestyle factors in people seeking infertility treatment – a review. Aust N Z J Obstet Gynaecol 2010;50(1):8–20.

[245] Hammiche F, Vujkovic M, Wijburg W, et al. Increased preconception omega-3 polyunsaturated fatty acid intake improves embryo morphology. Fertil Steril 2011;95(5):1820–3.

[246] Jungheim ES, Frolova AI, Jiang H, et al. Relationship between serum polyunsaturated fatty acids and pregnancy in women undergoing in vitro fertilization. J Clin Endocrinol Metab 2013;98(8):E1364–8.

[247] Mumford SL, Chavarro JE, Zhang C, et al. Dietary fat intake and reproductive hormone concentrations and ovulation in regularly menstruating women, 2. Am J Clin Nutr 2016;103(3):86–7.

[248] Moran LJ, Tsagareli V, Noakes M, et al. Altered preconception fatty acid intake is associated with improved pregnancy rates in overweight and obese women undertaking in vitro fertilisation. Nutrients 2016;8(1):10.

[249] Mirabi P, Chaichi MJ, Esmaeilzadeh S, et al. The role of fatty acids on ICSI outcomes: a prospective cohort study. Lipids Health Dis 2017;16(1):18.

[250] Wise LA, Wesselink AK, Tucker KL, et al. Dietary fat intake and fecundability in 2 preconception cohort studies. Am J Epidemiol 2017;187(1):60–74.

[251] Lazzarin N, Vaquero E, Exacoustos C, et al. Low-dose aspirin and omega-3 fatty acids improve uterine artery blood flow velocity in female with recurrent miscarriage due to impaired uterine perfusion. Fertil Steril 2009;92(1):296–300.

[252] Goldenberg RL, Hauth JC, Andrews WW. Intrauterine infection and preterm delivery. N Engl J Med 2000;342:1500–7.

[253] Simhan HN, Caritis SN, Krohn MA, et al. Elevated vaginal pH and neutrophils are associated strongly with early spontaneous preterm birth. Am J Obstet Gynecol 2003;189:1150–4.

[254] Slattery MM, Morrison JJ. Preterm delivery. Lancet 2002;360:1489–97.

[255] Mastromarino P, Hemalatha R, Barbonetti A, et al. Biological control of vaginosis to improve reproductive health. Indian J Med Res 2014;140(Suppl. 1):S91.

[256] Verstraelen H, Verhelst R, Roelens K, et al. Modified classification of Gram-stained vaginal smears to predict spontaneous preterm birth: a prospective cohort study. Am J Obstet Gynecol 2007;196(6):528.e1–6.

[257] Grieve M. A modern herbal. Lady's mantle. Available from: http://botanical.com/botanical/mgmh/l/ladman05.html. [Accessed 19 September 2010].

[258] Natural Standard. Professional monograph: lady's mantle (Alchemilla vulgaris). Available from: http://www.naturalstandard.com. [Accessed on 19 September 2010].

[259] Pandey SK, Sahay A, Pandey RS, et al. Effect of Asparagus racemosus rhizome (shatavari) on mammary gland and genital organs of pregnant rat. Phytother Res 2005;19(8):721–4.

[260] Goyal RK, Singh J, Lal H. Asparagus racemosus – an update. Indian J Med Sci 2003;57:408.

[261] Felter HW. The Eclectic materia medica, pharmacology and therapeutics. Portland, OR: J.K. Scudder; 1922.

[262] Shahin AY, Ismail AM, Zahran KM, et al. Adding phytoestrogens to clomiphene induction in unexplained infertility patients – a randomized trial. Reprod Biomed Online 2008;16(4):580–8.

[263] Shahin AY, Ismail AM, Shaaban OM. Supplementation of clomiphene citrate cycles with Cimicifuga racemosa or ethinyl oestradiol – a randomized trial. Reprod Biomed Online 2009; 19(4):501–7.

[264] Shahin AY, Mohammed SA. Adding the phytoestrogen Cimicifugae Racemosae to clomiphene induction cycles with timed intercourse in polycystic ovary syndrome improves cycle outcomes and pregnancy rates – a randomized trial. Gynecol Endocrinol 2014; 30(7):505–10.

[265] Werner S, Brismar K, Olsson S. Hyperprolactinaemia and liquorice. Lancet 1979;1(8111):319.

[266] Sun WS, Imai A, Tagami K, et al. In vitro stimulation of granulosa cells by a combination of different active ingredients of unkei-to. Am J Chin Med 2004;32(4):569–78.

[267] Tabakova P, Dimitrov M, Ognyanov K, et al. Clinical study of Tribestan in females with endocrine sterility. Documentation for Registration (unpublished); 1999.

[268] Felter HW, Lloyd JU. King's American dispensatory. Portland, OR: Eclectic Materia Medica Publications; 1905.

[269] Dennehy C. The use of herbs and dietary supplements in gynecology: an evidence-based review. J Midwifery Womens Health 2006;51(6):402–9.

[270] Westphal LM, Polan ML, Trant AS, et al. A nutritional supplement for improving fertility in female: a pilot study. J Reprod Med 2004;49(4):289–93.

[271] ASRM. Optimising natural fertility. Fertil Steril 2008;90:S1–6.

[272] Dechanet C, Anahory T, Daude JM, et al. Effects of cigarette smoking on reproduction. Hum Reprod Update 2011;17(1):76–95.

[273] Nazıroğlu M, Yüksel M, Köse SA, et al. Recent reports of Wi-Fi and mobile phone-induced radiation on oxidative stress and reproductive signaling pathways in females and males. J Membr Biol 2013;246(12):869–75.

[274] Chalupka S, Chalupka AN. The impact of environmental and occupational exposures on reproductive health. J Obstet Gynecol Neonatal Nurs 2010;39(1):84–102.

[275] Mínguez-Alarcón L, Gaskins AJ. Female exposure to endocrine disrupting chemicals and fecundity: a review. Curr Opin Obstet Gynecol 2017;29(4):202–11.

[276] Sifakis S, Androutsopoulos VP, Tsatsakis AM, et al. Human exposure to endocrine disrupting chemicals: effects on the male and female reproductive systems. Environ Toxicol Pharmacol 2017;51:56–70.

[277] Scsukova S, Rollerova E, Mlynarcikova AB. Impact of endocrine disrupting chemicals on onset and development of female reproductive disorders and hormone-related cancer. Reprod Biol 2016;16(4):243–54.

[278] Bloom MS, Fujimoto VY, Storm R, et al. Persistent organic pollutants (POPs) in human follicular fluid and in vitro fertilization outcomes, a pilot study. Reprod Toxicol 2017;67:165–73.

[279] Skrzypek M, Wdowiak A, Marzec A. Application of dietetics in reproductive medicine. Ann Agric Environ Med 2017;24(4):559–65.

[280] Jungheim ES, Travieso JL, Hopeman MM. Weighing the impact of obesity on female reproductive function and fertility. Nutr Rev 2013;71(Suppl. 1):S3–8.

[281] Broughton DE, Moley KH. Obesity and female infertility: potential mediators of obesity's impact. Fertil Steril 2017;107(4):840–7.

[282] Pantasri T, Norman RJ. The effects of being overweight and obese on female reproduction: a review. Gynecol Endocrinol 2014;30(2):90–4.

[283] Bernardi LA, Carnethon MR, de Chavez PJ, et al. Relationship between obesity and anti-Müllerian hormone in reproductive-aged African American women. Obesity (Silver Spring) 2017;25(1):229–35.

[284] Kiranmayee D, Talla Praveena YH, Sriharibabu M, et al. The effect of moderate physical activity on ovarian reserve markers in reproductive age women below and above 30 years. J Hum Reprod Sci 2017;10(1):44.

[285] Chosich J, Bradford AP, Allshouse AA, et al. Acute recapitulation of the hyperinsulinemia and hyperlipidemia characteristic of metabolic syndrome suppresses gonadotropins. Obesity (Silver Spring) 2017;25(3):553–60.

[286] Kuokkanen S, Polotsky AJ, Chosich J, et al. Corpus luteum as a novel target of weight changes that contribute to impaired female reproductive physiology and function. Syst Biol Reprod Med 2016;62(4):227–42.

[287] Roth LW, Allshouse AA, Bradshaw-Pierce EL, et al. Luteal phase dynamics of follicle-stimulating and luteinizing hormones in obese and normal weight women. Clin Endocrinol (Oxf) 2014;81(3):418–25.

[288] Buyuk E, Asemota OA, Merhi Z, et al. Serum and follicular fluid monocyte chemotactic protein-1 levels are elevated in obese women and are associated with poorer clinical pregnancy rate after in vitro fertilization: a pilot study. Fertil Steril 2017;107(3):632–40.

[289] Moragianni VA, Jones SM, Ryley DA. The effect of body mass index on the outcomes of first assisted reproductive technology cycles. Fertil Steril 2012;98(1):102–8.

[290] Comstock IA, Diaz-Gimeno P, Cabanillas S, et al. Does an increased body mass index affect endometrial gene expression patterns in infertile patients? A functional genomics analysis. Fertil Steril 2017;107(3):740–8.

[291] Luke B, Brown MB, Stern JE, et al. Female obesity adversely affects assisted reproductive technology (ART) pregnancy and live birth rates. Hum Reprod 2011;26(1):245–52.

[292] Opray N, Grivell RM, Deussen AR, et al. Directed preconception health programs and interventions for improving pregnancy outcomes for women who are overweight or obese. Cochrane Database Syst Rev 2015;(7):CD010932.

[293] Kort JD, Winget C, Kim SH, et al. A retrospective cohort study to evaluate the impact of meaningful weight loss on fertility outcomes in an overweight population with infertility. Fertil Steril 2014;101(5):1400–3.

[294] Best D, Avenell A, Bhattacharya S. How effective are weight-loss interventions for improving fertility in women and men who are overweight or obese? A systematic review and meta-analysis of the evidence. Hum Reprod Update 2017;23(6):681–705.

[295] Sundaram R, Mumford SL, Buck Louis GM. Couples' body composition and time-to-pregnancy. Hum Reprod 2017;32(3):662–8.

[296] Freeman EW, Boxer AS, Rickels K, et al. Psychological evaluation and support in a program of in vitro fertilization and embryo transfer. Fertil Steril 1985;43:48–53.

[297] Baram D, Tourtelot E, Muechler E, et al. Psychosocial adjustment following unsuccessful in vitro fertilization. J Psychosom Obstet Gynaecol 1988;9(3):181–90.

[298] Vahratian A, Smith YR, Dorman M, et al. Longitudinal depressive symptoms and state anxiety among women using assisted reproductive technology. Fertil Steril 2011;95(3):1192–4.

[299] Verkuijlen J, Verhaak C, Nelen WL, et al. Psychological and educational interventions for subfertile men and women. Cochrane Database Syst Rev 2016;(3):CD011034.

[300] Wischmann TH. Sexual disorders in infertile couples. J Sex Med 2010;7:1868–76.

[301] Nelson CJ, Shindel AW, Naughton CK, et al. Prevalence and predictors of sexual problems, relationship stress, and depression in female partners of infertile couples. J Sex Med 2008;5:1907–14.

[302] Shindel A, Nelson CJ, Naughton CK, et al. Sexual function and quality of life in the male partner of infertile couples: prevalence and correlates of dysfunction. J Urol 2008;179:1056–9.

[303] Gollenburg A, Liu F, Brazil C, et al. Semen quality in fertile men in relation to psychosocial stress. Fertil Steril 2010;93(4):1104–11.

[304] Bashour H, Abdul Salam A. Psychological stress and spontaneous abortion. Int J Gynaecol Obstet 2001;73(2):179–81.

[305] Louis GM, Lum KJ, Sundaram R, et al. Stress reduces conception probabilities across the fertile window: evidence in support of relaxation. Fertil Steril 2011;95(7):2184–9.

[306] Lynch CD, Sundaram R, Maisog JM, et al. Preconception stress increases the risk of infertility: results from a couple-based prospective cohort study – the LIFE study. Hum Reprod 2014;29(5):1067–75.

[307] Ebbesen S, Zachariae R, Mehlsen MY, et al. Stressful life events are associated with a poor in-vitro fertilization (IVF) outcome: a prospective study. Hum Reprod 2009;24(9):2173–82.

[308] Boivin J, Griffiths E, Venetis CA. Emotional distress in infertile women and failure of assisted reproductive technologies: meta-analysis of prospective psychosocial studies. BMJ 2011;342:d223.

[309] Ösz BE, Tero-Vescan A, Imre S, et al. Reproductive function and a menstrual cycle linked diet in sportswomen. Palestrica of the Third Millennium Civilization & Sport 2017;18(1).

[310] Wise LA, Rothman KJ, Mikkelsen EM, et al. A prospective cohort study of physical activity and time to pregnancy. Fertil Steril 2012;97(5):1136–42.

[311] Hakimi O, Cameron LC. Effect of exercise on ovulation: a systematic review. Sports Med 2017;47(8):1555–67.

[312] Gudmundsdottir SL, Flanders WD, Augestad LB. Menstrual cycle abnormalities in healthy women with low physical activity: the North-Trøndelag population-based health study. J Phys Act Health 2014;11(6):1133–40.

[313] Palomba S, Falbo A, Valli B, et al. Physical activity before IVF and ICSI cycles in infertile obese women: an observational cohort study. Reprod Biomed Online 2014;29(1):72–9.

[314] Anderson L, Lewis SE, McClure N. The effects of coital lubricants on sperm motility in vitro. Hum Reprod 1998;13:3351–6.

[315] Frishman GN, Luciano AA, Maier DB. Evaluation of Astroglide, a new vaginal lubricant: effects of length of exposure and concentration on sperm motility. Fertil Steril 1992;58:630–2.

[316] Kutteh WH, Choe CH, Ritter JO, et al. Vaginal lubricants for the infertile couple: effect on sperm activity. Int J Fertil Menopausal Stud 1996;41:400–4.

[317] Miller B, Klein TA, Opsahl MS. The effect of surgical lubricant on in vivo sperm penetration of cervical mucus. Fertil Steril 1994;6:1171–3.

[318] Tagatz GE, Okagake T, Sciarra JJ. The effect of vaginal lubricants on sperm motility and viability in vitro. Am J Obstet Gynecol 1972;113:88–90.

[319] Tulandi T, Plouffe L Jr, McInnes RA. Effect of saliva on sperm motility and activity. Fertil Steril 1982;38:721–3.

[320] Tulandi T, McInnes RA. Vaginal lubricants: effect of glycerin and egg white on sperm motility and progression in vitro. Fertil Steril 1984;41:151–3.

[321] Ozgur K, Franken DR, Kaskar K, et al. The influence of a mineral oil overlay on the zona pellucida binding potential of human spermatozoa. Andrologia 1995;27:155–9.

[322] Wright RW, Ellington JE. Effects of personal lubricants on in vitro fertilisation and embryo development. Phoenix, AZ: American Society of Andrology; 2003.

[323] Ellington JE, Short RA, Schimmels J. Effect of new intimate moisturizer on sperm motility. Phoenix, AZ: American Society of Andrology; 2003.

[324] Ellington JE, Short RA. Prevalence of vaginal dryness in trying to conceive couples. Rancho Mirage, CA: Pacific Coast Reproductive Society Meeting; 2003.

[325] Ellington JE, Schimmels J. The effects of vaginal lubricants on computer assisted sperm analysis parameters associated with cervical mucus penetration. Birmingham, AL: ASRM; 2004.

[326] Agarwal TM, Said K, Seifarth DP, et al. Changes in sperm motility and chromatin integrity following contact with vaginal lubricants. Submitted to American Society of Reproductive Medicine 2005.

[327] Vargas J, Crausaz M, Senn A, et al. Sperm toxicity of 'nonspermicidal' lubricant and ultrasound gels used in reproductive medicine. Fertil Steril 2011;95(2):835–6.

[328] Chiu YH, Afeiche MC, Gaskins AJ, et al. Fruit and vegetable intake and their pesticide residues in relation to semen quality among men from a fertility clinic. Hum Reprod 2015;30(6):1342–51.

[329] Afeiche MC, Gaskins AJ, Williams PL, et al. Processed meat intake is unfavorably and fish intake favorably associated with semen quality indicators among men attending a fertility clinic. J Nutr 2014;144(7):1091–8.

[330] Gaskins AJ, Colaci DS, Mendiola J, et al. Dietary patterns and semen quality in young men. Hum Reprod 2012;27(10):2899–907.

[331] Salas-Huetos A, Bulló M, Salas-Salvadó J. Dietary patterns, foods and nutrients in male fertility parameters and fecundability: a systematic review of observational studies. Hum Reprod Update 2017;23(4):371–89.

[332] Liu CY, Chou YC, Chao JC, et al. The association between dietary patterns and semen quality in a general Asian population of 7282 males. PLoS ONE 2015;10(7):e0134224.

[333] Karayiannis D, Kontogianni MD, Mendorou C, et al. Association between adherence to the Mediterranean diet and semen quality parameters in male partners of couples attempting fertility. Hum Reprod 2016;32(1):215–22.

[334] Oostingh EC, Steegers-Theunissen RP, de Vries JH, et al. Strong adherence to a healthy dietary pattern is associated with better semen quality, especially in men with poor semen quality. Fertil Steril 2017;107(4):916–23.

[335] Eslamian G, Amirjannati N, Rashidkhani B, et al. Nutrient patterns and asthenozoospermia: a case-control study. Andrologia 2017;49(3).

[336] Afeiche MC, Bridges ND, Williams PL, et al. Dairy intake and semen quality among men attending a fertility clinic. Fertil Steril 2014;101(5):1280–7.

[337] Ko EY, Sabanegh ES. The role of nutraceuticals in male fertility. Urol Clin North Am 2014;41(1):181–93.

[338] Hamilton-Reeves JM, Vazquez G, Duval SJ, et al. Clinical studies show no effects of soy protein or isoflavones on reproductive hormones in men: results of a meta-analysis. Fertil Steril 2010;94(3):997–1007.

[339] Mínguez-Alarcón L, Afeiche MC, Chiu YH, et al. Male soy food intake was not associated with in vitro fertilization outcomes among couples attending a fertility center. Andrology 2015;3(4):702–8.

[340] Dias TR, Alves MG, Bernardino RL, et al. Dose-dependent effects of caffeine in human Sertoli cells metabolism and oxidative profile: relevance for male fertility. Toxicology 2015;328:12–20.

[341] Belloc S, Cohen-Bacrie M, Dalleac A, et al. Caffeine intake and sperm parameters. Analysis of a cohort of 4474 consecutive semen samples. Fertil Steril 2013;100(3):S212.

[342] Jensen TK, Swan SH, Skakkebæk NE, et al. Caffeine intake and semen quality in a population of 2,554 young Danish men. Am J Epidemiol 2010;171(8):883–91.

[343] Ricci E, Viganò P, Cipriani S, et al. Coffee and caffeine intake and male infertility: a systematic review. Nutr J 2017;16(1):37.

[344] Karmon AE, Toth TL, Chiu YH, et al. Male caffeine and alcohol intake in relation to semen parameters and in vitro fertilization outcomes among fertility patients. Andrology 2017;5(2):354–61.

[345] Donnelly GP, McClure N, Kennedy MS, et al. Direct effect of alcohol on the motility and morphology of human spermatozoa. Andrologia 1999;31(1):43–7.

[346] La Vignera S, Condorelli RA, Balercia G, et al. Does alcohol have any effect on male reproductive function? A review of literature. Asian J Androl 2013;15(2):221.

[347] Jensen TK, Swan S, Jørgensen N, et al. Alcohol and male reproductive health: a cross-sectional study of 8344 healthy men from Europe and the USA. Hum Reprod 2014;29(8):1801–9.

[348] Hansen ML, Thulstrup AM, Bonde JP, et al. Does last week's alcohol intake affect semen quality or reproductive hormones? A cross-sectional study among healthy young Danish men. Reprod Toxicol 2012;34(3):457–62.

[349] Ricci E, Al Beitawi S, Cipriani S, et al. Semen quality and alcohol intake: a systematic review and meta-analysis. Reprod Biomed Online 2017;34(1):38–47.

[350] Barazani Y, Katz BF, Nagler HM, et al. Lifestyle, environment, and male reproductive health. Urol Clin North Am 2014;41(1):55–66.

[351] Sermondade N, Elloumi H, Berthaut I, et al. Progressive alcohol-induced sperm alterations leading to spermatogenic arrest, which was reversed after alcohol withdrawal. Reprod Biomed Online 2010;20(3):324–7.

[352] Attaman JA, Toth TL, Furtado J, et al. Dietary fat and semen quality among men attending a fertility clinic. Hum Reprod 2012;27(5):1466–74.

[353] Jensen TK, Heitmann BL, Jensen MB, et al. High dietary intake of saturated fat is associated with reduced semen quality among 701 young Danish men from the general population. Am J Clin Nutr 2013;97(2):411–18.

[354] Dadkhah H, Kazemi A, Nasr-Isfahani MH, et al. The relationship between the amount of saturated fat intake and semen quality in men. Iran J Nurs Midwifery Res 2017;22(1):46.

[355] Rato L, Alves MG, Cavaco JE, et al. High-energy diets: a threat for male fertility? Obes Rev 2014;15(12):996–1007.

[356] Chavarro JE, Mínguez-Alarcón L, Mendiola J, et al. Trans fatty acid intake is inversely related to total sperm count in young healthy men. Hum Reprod 2014;29(3):429–40.

[357] Mínguez-Alarcón L, Chavarro JE, Mendiola J, et al. Fatty acid intake in relation to reproductive hormones and testicular volume among young healthy men. Asian J Androl 2017;19(2):184.

[358] Chiu YH, Afeiche MC, Gaskins AJ, et al. Sugar-sweetened beverage intake in relation to semen quality and reproductive hormone levels in young men. Hum Reprod 2014;29(7):1575–84.

[359] Stokes VJ, Anderson RA, George JT. How does obesity affect fertility in men – and what are the treatment options? Clin Endocrinol (Oxf) 2015;82(5):633–8.

[360] Palmer NO, Bakos HW, Fullston T, et al. Impact of obesity on male fertility, sperm function and molecular composition. Spermatogenesis 2012;2(4):253–63.

[361] Sermondade N, Faure C, Fezeu L, et al. BMI in relation to sperm count: an updated systematic review and collaborative meta-analysis. Hum Reprod Update 2012;19(3):221–31.

[362] Liu Y, Ding Z. Obesity, a serious etiologic factor for male subfertility in modern society. Reproduction 2017;154(4):R123–31.

[363] Shukla KK, Chambial S, Dwivedi S, et al. Recent scenario of obesity and male fertility. Andrology 2014;2(6):809–18.

[364] Guo D, Wu W, Tang Q, et al. The impact of BMI on sperm parameters and the metabolite changes of seminal plasma concomitantly. Oncotarget 2017;8(30):48619.

[365] Wang EY, Huang Y, Du QY, et al. Body mass index effects sperm quality: a retrospective study in Northern China. Asian J Androl 2017;19(2):234.

[366] Oliveira JB, Petersen CG, Mauri AL, et al. Association between body mass index and sperm quality and sperm DNA integrity. A large population study. Andrologia 2017;50(3).

[367] Håkonsen LB, Thulstrup AM, Aggerholm AS, et al. Does weight loss improve semen quality and reproductive hormones? Results from a cohort of severely obese men. Reprod Health 2011;8(1):24.

[368] Luque EM, Tissera A, Gaggino MP, et al. Body mass index and human sperm quality: neither one extreme nor the other. Reprod Fertil Dev 2017;29(4):731–9.

[369] Leisegang K, Udodong A, Bouic PJ, et al. Effect of the metabolic syndrome on male reproductive function: a case-controlled pilot study. Andrologia 2014;46(2):167–76.

[370] Yamamoto Y, Aizawa K, Mieno M, et al. The effects of tomato juice on male infertility. Asia Pac J Clin Nutr 2017;26(1):65–71.

[371] Ghyasvand T, Goodarzi MT, Amiri I, et al. Serum levels of lycopene, beta-carotene, and retinol and their correlation with sperm DNA damage in normospermic and infertile men. Int J Reprod Biomed (Yazd) 2015;13(12):787–92.

[372] Wallock LM, Tamura T, Mayr CA, et al. Low seminal plasma folate concentrations are associated with low sperm density and count in male smokers and nonsmokers. Fertil Steril 2001;75(2):252–9.

[373] Boxmeer JC, Smit M, Utomo E, et al. Low folate in seminal plasma is associated with increased sperm DNA damage. Fertil Steril 2009;92(2):548–56.

[374] Lambrot R, Xu C, Saint-Phar S, et al. Low paternal dietary folate alters the mouse sperm epigenome and is associated with negative pregnancy outcomes. Nat Commun 2013;4:2889.

[375] Esmaeili V, Shahverdi AH, Moghadasian MH, et al. Dietary fatty acids affect semen quality: a review. Andrology 2015;3(3):450–61.

[376] Martínez-Soto JC, Domingo JC, Cordobilla B, et al. Dietary supplementation with docosahexaenoic acid (DHA) improves seminal antioxidant status and decreases sperm DNA fragmentation. Syst Biol Reprod Med 2016;62(6):387–95.

[377] Kothari RP, Chaudhari AR. Zinc levels in seminal fluid in infertile males and its relation with serum free testosterone. J Clin Diagn Res 2016;10(5):CC5–8.

[378] Unlu NZ, Bohn T, Clinton SK, et al. Carotenoid absorption from salad and salsa by humans is enhanced by the addition of avocado or avocado oil. J Nutr 2005;135(3):431–6.

[379] Stanislavov R, Nikolova V, Rohdewald P. Improvement of seminal parameters with Prelox: a randomized, double-blind, placebo-controlled, cross-over trial. Phytother Res 2009;23(3):297–302.

[380] Lenzi A, Sgrò P, Salacone P, et al. A placebo-controlled double-blind randomized trial of the use of combined L-carnitine and L-acetylcarnitine treatment in male with asthenozoospermia. Fertil Steril 2004;81:1578–84.

[381] Balercia G, Regoli F, Armeni T, et al. Placebo-controlled, double-blind, randomized trial on the use of L-carnitine, L-acetylcarnitine, or combined L-carnitine and L-acetylcarnitine in male with idiopathic asthenozoospermia. Fertil Steril 2005;84:662–71.

[382] Busetto GM, Koverech A, Messano M, et al. Prospective open-label study on the efficacy and tolerability of a combination of nutritional supplements in primary infertile patients with idiopathic astenoteratozoospermia. Arch Ital Urol Androl 2012;84(3):137–40.

[383] Abad C, Amengual MJ, Gosálvez J, et al. Effects of oral antioxidant treatment upon the dynamics of human sperm DNA fragmentation and subpopulations of sperm with highly degraded DNA. Andrologia 2013;45(3):211–16.

[384] Aram JJ, Al-Shamma KJ, Al-Hassani AN. Effect of L-carnitine, multivitamins and their combination in the treatment of idiopathic male infertility. Iraqi J Pharm Sci 2017;21(1):14–20.

[385] Lipovac M, Bodner F, Imhof M, et al. Comparison of the effect of a combination of eight micronutrients versus a standard mono preparation on sperm parameters. Reprod Biol Endocrinol 2016;14(1):84.

[386] Banihani S, Agarwal A, Sharma R, et al. Cryoprotective effect of l-carnitine on motility, vitality and DNA oxidation of human spermatozoa. Andrologia 2014;46(6):637–41.

[387] Donnelly E, McClure N, Lewis S. The effect of ascorbate and α-tocopherol supplementation in vitro on DNA integrity and hydrogen peroxide-induced DNA damage in human spermatozoa. Mutagenesis 1999;14(5):505–11.

[388] Walczak-Jedrzejowska R, Wolski JK, Slowikowska-Hilczer J. The role of oxidative stress and antioxidants in male fertility. Cent European J Urol 2013;66(1):60–7.

[389] Atig F, Kerkeni A, Saad A, et al. Effects of reduced seminal enzymatic antioxidants on sperm DNA fragmentation and semen quality of Tunisian infertile men. J Assist Reprod Genet 2013;34(3):373–81.

[390] Ko EY, Sabanegh ES, Agarwal A. Male infertility testing: reactive oxygen species and antioxidant capacity. Fertil Steril 2014;102(6):1518–27.

[391] Ross C, Morriss A, Khairy M, et al. A systematic review of the effect of oral antioxidants on male infertility. Reprod Biomed Online 2010;20(6):711–23.

[392] Gharagozloo P, Aitken RJ. The role of sperm oxidative stress in male infertility and the significance of oral antioxidant therapy. Hum Reprod 2011;26(7):1628–40.

[393] Showell MG, Mackenzie-Proctor R, Brown J, et al. Antioxidants for male subfertility. Cochrane Database Syst Rev 2014;(12):CD007411.

[394] Aitken RJ, Smith TB, Jobling MS, et al. Oxidative stress and male reproductive health. Asian J Androl 2014;16(1):31.

[395] Schmid TE, Eskenazi B, Marchetti F, et al. Micronutrients intake is associated with improved sperm DNA quality in older men. Fertil Steril 2012;98(5):1130–7.

[396] Kobori Y, Ota S, Sato R, et al. Antioxidant cosupplementation therapy with vitamin C, vitamin E, and coenzyme Q10 in patients with oligoasthenozoospermia. Arch Ital Urol Androl 2014;86(1):1–4.

[397] Gvozdjáková A, Kucharská J, Dubravicky J, et al. Coenzyme Q10, α-tocopherol, and oxidative stress could be important metabolic biomarkers of male infertility. Dis Markers 2015;2015.

[398] Ciftci H, Verit A, Savas M, et al. Effects of N-acetylcysteine on semen parameters and oxidative/antioxidant status. Urology 2009;74(1):73–6.

[399] Alizadeh F, Javadi M, Karami AA, et al. Curcumin nanomicelle improves semen parameters, oxidative stress, inflammatory biomarkers, and reproductive hormones in infertile men: a randomized clinical trial. Phytother Res 2017;32(3):514–21.

[400] Bilska A, Wlodek L. Lipoic acid – the drug of the future? Pharmacol Rep 2005;57(5):570–7.

[401] Selvakumar E, Prahalathan C, Sudharsan PT, et al. Chemoprotective effect of lipoic acid against cyclophosphamide-induced changes in the rat sperm. Toxicology 2006;217(1):71–8.

[402] Prahalathan C, Selvakumar E, Varalakshmi P. Modulatory role of lipoic acid on adriamycin-induced testicular injury. Chem Biol Interact 2006;160(2):108–14.

[403] Ibrahim SF, Osman K, Das S, et al. A study of the antioxidant effect of alpha lipoic acids on sperm quality. Clinics 2008;63(4):545–50.

[404] Aly HA, Lightfoot DA, El-Shemy HA. Modulatory role of lipoic acid on lipopolysaccharide-induced oxidative stress in adult rat Sertoli cells in vitro. Chem Biol Interact 2009;182(2–3):112–18.

[405] Haghighian HK, Haidari F, Mohammadi-asl J, et al. Randomized, triple-blind, placebo-controlled clinical trial examining the effects

of alpha-lipoic acid supplement on the spermatogram and seminal oxidative stress in infertile men. Fertil Steril 2015;104(2):318–24.

[406] Kim KH, Wang ZQ. Action of vitamin A on the testis: role of the Sertoli cell. In: Russel LD, Grisworld MD, editors. The sertoli cell. Clearwater, FL: Cache River Press; 1993.

[407] Morales A, Cavicchia JC. Spermatogenesis and blood–testis barrier in rats after long-term vitamin A deprivation. Tissue Cell 2002;34(5):349–55.

[408] Eslamian G, Amirjannati N, Rashidkhani B, et al. Intake of food groups and idiopathic asthenozoospermia: a case-control study. Hum Reprod 2012;27(11):3328–36.

[409] Eskenazi B, Kidd SA, Marhs AR, et al. Antioxidant intake is associated with semen quality in healthy male. Hum Reprod 2005;20(4):1006–12.

[410] Zareba P, Colaci DS, Afeiche M, et al. Semen quality in relation to antioxidant intake in a healthy male population. Fertil Steril 2013;100(6):1572–9.

[411] Mancini A, De Marinis L, Oradei A, et al. Coenzyme Q10 concentration in normal and pathological human seminal fluid. J Androl 1994;15:59159.

[412] Balercia G, Arnaldi G, Fazioli F, et al. Coenzyme Q10 levels in idiopathic and varicocele-associated asthenozoospermia. Andrologia 2002;34:107–11.

[413] Balercia G, Buldreghini E, Vignini A, et al. Coenzyme Q10 treatment in infertile male with idiopathic asthenozoospermia: a placebo-controlled, double-blind randomized trial. Fertil Steril 2009;91(5):1785–92.

[414] Balercia G, Mosca F, Mantero F, et al. Coenzyme Q10 supplementation in infertile male with idiopathic asthenozoospermia: an open, uncontrolled pilot study. Fertil Steril 2004;81:93–8.

[415] Safarinejad MR. Efficacy of coenzyme Q10 on semen parameters, sperm function and reproductive hormones in infertile men. J Urol 2009;182(1):237–48.

[416] Nadjarzadeh A, Shidfar F, Amirjannati N, et al. Effect of coenzyme Q10 supplementation on antioxidant enzymes activity and oxidative stress of seminal plasma: a double-blind randomised clinical trial. Andrologia 2014;46(2):177–83.

[417] Festa R, Giacchi E, Raimondo SE, et al. Coenzyme Q10 supplementation in infertile men with low-grade varicocele: an open, uncontrolled pilot study. Andrologia 2014;46(7):805–7.

[418] Safarinejad MR. The effect of coenzyme Q10 supplementation on partner pregnancy rate in infertile men with idiopathic oligoasthenoteratozoospermia: an open-label prospective study. Int Urol Nephrol 2012;44(3):689–700.

[419] Safarinejad MR, Safarinejad S, Shafiei N, et al. Effects of the reduced form of coenzyme Q 10 (ubiquinol) on semen parameters in men with idiopathic infertility: a double-blind, placebo controlled, randomized study. J Urol 2012;188(2):526–31.

[420] Thakur AS, Littarru GP, Funahashi I, et al. Effect of ubiquinol therapy on sperm parameters and serum testosterone levels in oligoasthenozoospermic infertile men. J Clin Diagn Res 2015;9(9):BC01.

[421] Tiseo BC, Gaskins AJ, Hauser R, et al. Coenzyme Q10 intake from food and semen parameters in a subfertile population. Urology 2017;102:100–5.

[422] Patel SR, Sigman M. Antioxidant therapy in male infertility. Urol Clin North Am 2008;35:319–30.

[423] Song GJ, Norkus EP, Lewis V. Relationship between seminal ascorbic acid and sperm DNA integrity in infertile male. Int J Androl 2006;29(6):569–75.

[424] Kao SH, Chao HT, Chen HW, et al. Increase of oxidative stress in human sperm with lower motility. Fertil Steril 2008;89(5):1183–90.

[425] Akmal M, Qadri JQ, Al-Waili NS, et al. Improvement in human semen quality after oral supplementation of vitamin C. J Med Food 2006;9(3):440–2.

[426] Colagar AH, Marzony ET. Ascorbic acid in human seminal plasma: determination and its relationship to sperm quality. J Clin Biochem Nutr 2009;45(2):144–9.

[427] Cyrus A, Kabir A, Goodarzi D, et al. The effect of adjuvant vitamin C after varicocele surgery on sperm quality and quantity in infertile men: a double blind placebo controlled clinical trial. Int Braz J Urol 2015;41(2):230–8.

[428] Rafiee B, Morowvat MH, Rahimi-Ghalati N. Comparing the effectiveness of dietary vitamin C and exercise interventions on fertility parameters in normal obese men. Urol J 2016;13(2):2635–9.

[429] Benedetti S, Tagliamonte MC, Catalani S, et al. Differences in blood and semen oxidative status in fertile and infertile men, and their relationship with sperm quality. Reprod Biomed Online 2012;25(3):300–6.

[430] Suleiman SA, Ali ME, Zaki ZM, et al. Lipid peroxidation and human sperm motility: protective role of vitamin E. J Androl 1996;17(5):530–7.

[431] Moslemi MK, Tavanbakhsh S. Selenium–vitamin E supplementation in infertile men: effects on semen parameters and pregnancy rate. Int J Gen Med 2011;4:99.

[432] El Sheikh MG, Hosny MB, Elshenoufy A, et al. Combination of vitamin E and clomiphene citrate in treating patients with idiopathic oligoasthenozoospermia: a prospective, randomized trial. Andrology 2015;3(5):864–7.

[433] Geva E, Bartoov B, Zabludovsky N, et al. The effect of antioxidant treatment on human spermatozoa and fertilization rate in an in vitro fertilization program. Fertil Steril 1996;66(3):430–4.

[434] Ursini F, Heim S, Kiess M, et al. Dual function of the selenoprotein PHGPx during sperm maturation. Science 1999;285:1393.

[435] Hawkes WC, Turek PJ. Effects of dietary selenium on sperm motility in healthy men. J Androl 2001;22(5):764–72.

[436] Ahsan U, Kamran Z, Raza I, et al. Role of selenium in male reproduction – a review. Anim Reprod Sci 2014;146(1):55–62.

[437] Vézina D, Mauffette F, Roberts KD, et al. Selenium–vitamin E supplementation in infertile male. Effects on semen parameters and micronutrient levels and distribution. Biol Trace Elem Res 1996;53(1–3):65–83.

[438] Camejo MI, Abdala L, Vivas-Acevedo G, et al. Selenium, copper and zinc in seminal plasma of men with varicocele, relationship with seminal parameters. Biol Trace Elem Res 2011;143(3):1247–54.

[439] Schneider M, Förster H, Boersma A, et al. Mitochondrial glutathione peroxidase 4 disruption causes male infertility. FASEB J 2009;23(9):3233–42.

[440] Scott R, MacPherson A, Yates RW, et al. The effect of oral selenium supplementation on human sperm motility. Br J Urol 1998;82(1):76–80.

[441] Safarinejad MR, Safarinejad S. Efficacy of selenium and/or N-acetyl-cysteine for improving semen parameters in infertile men: a double-blind, placebo controlled, randomized study. J Urol 2009;181(2):741–51.

[442] Colagar AH, Marzony ET, Chaichi MJ. Zinc levels in seminal plasma are associated with sperm quality in fertile and infertile male. Nutr Res 2009;29(2):82–8.

[443] Wong WY, Thomas CM, Merkus JM, et al. Male factor subfertility: possible causes and the impact of nutritional factors. Fertil Steril 2000;73:435–42.

[444] Caldamone AA, Freytag MK, Cockett AT. Seminal zinc and male infertility. Urology 1979;13:28028.

[445] Bjorndahl L, Kvist U. Importance of zinc for human sperm head–tail connection. Acta Physiol Scand 1982;126:51–5.

[446] Chia SE, Ong C, Chua L, et al. Comparison of zinc concentration in blood and seminal plasma and various sperm parameters between fertile and infertile male. J Androl 2000;21:53–7.

[447] Ajina T, Sallem A, Haouas Z, et al. Total antioxidant status and lipid peroxidation with and without in vitro zinc supplementation in infertile men. Andrologia 2017;49(7).

[448] Carreras A, Mendosa C. Zinc levels in seminal plasma of infertile and fertile male. Andrologia 1990;22:279–83.

[449] Wong WY, Flik G, Groenen PM, et al. The impact of calcium, magnesium, zinc, and copper in blood and seminal plasma on semen parameters in men. Reprod Toxicol 2001;15(2):131–6.

[450] Omu AE, Al-Azemi MK, Kehinde EO, et al. Indications of the mechanisms involved in improved sperm parameters by zinc therapy. Med Princ Pract 2008;17(2):108–16.

[451] Ghareeb DA, Sarhan EM. Role of oxidative stress in male fertility and idiopathic infertility: causes and treatment. J Diagn Tech Biomed Anal 2014;12:2.

[452] Alsalman AR, Almashhedy LA, Hadwan MH. Zinc supplementation attenuates lipid peroxidation and increases antiperoxidant activity

in seminal plasma of Iraqi asthenospermic men. Life Sci J 2013;10(4):989–97.

[453] Hadwan MH, Almashhedy LA, Alsalman AR. Oral zinc supplementation restores superoxide radical scavengers to normal levels in spermatozoa of Iraqi asthenospermic patients. Int J Vitam Nutr Res 2015;85(3–4):165–73.

[454] Zhao J, Dong X, Hu X, et al. Zinc levels in seminal plasma and their correlation with male infertility: a systematic review and meta-analysis. Sci Rep 2016;6:22386.

[455] Durairajanayagam D, Agarwal A, Ong C, et al. Lycopene and male infertility. Asian J Androl 2014;16(3):420.

[456] Goyal A, Chopra M, Lwaleed BA, et al. The effects of dietary lycopene supplementation on human seminal plasma. BJU Int 2007;99(6):1456–60.

[457] Yamamoto Y, Aizawa K, Mieno M, et al. The effects of tomato juice on male infertility. Asia Pac J Clin Nutr 2017;26(1):65–71.

[458] Gupta NP, Kumar R. Lycopene therapy in idiopathic male infertility – a preliminary report. Int Urol Nephrol 2002;369–72.

[459] Fleming JC, Tartaglini E, Kawatsuji R, et al. Male infertility and thiamine-dependent erythroid hypoplasia in mice lacking thiamine transporter Slc19a2. Mol Genet Metab 2003;80(1–2):234–41.

[460] Oishi K, Barchi M, Au AC, et al. Male infertility due to germ cell apoptosis in mice lacking the thiamin carrier, Tht1. A new insight into the critical role of thiamin in spermatogenesis. Dev Biol 2004;266(2):299–309.

[461] Yamamoto T. Effects of pantothenic acid on testicular function in male rats. J Vet Med Sci 2009;71(11):1427–32.

[462] Boxmeer JC, Smit M, Utomo E, et al. Low folate in seminal plasma is associated with increased sperm DNA damage. Fertil Steril 2009;92(2):548–56.

[463] Murphy LE, Mills JL, Molloy AM, et al. Folate and vitamin B12 in idiopathic male infertility. Asian J Androl 2011;13(6):856.

[464] Yuan HF, Zhao K, Zang Y, et al. Effect of folate deficiency on promoter methylation and gene expression of Esr1, Cav1, and Elavl1, and its influence on spermatogenesis. Oncotarget 2017;8(15):24130.

[465] Raigani M, Yaghmaei B, Amirjannti N, et al. The micronutrient supplements, zinc sulphate and folic acid, did not ameliorate sperm functional parameters in oligoasthenoteratozoospermic men. Andrologia 2014;46(9):956–62.

[466] Azizollahi G, Azizollahi S, Babaei H, et al. Effects of supplement therapy on sperm parameters, protamine content and acrosomal integrity of varicocelectomized subjects. J Assist Reprod Genet 2013;30(4):593–9.

[467] Aarabi M, San Gabriel MC, Chan D, et al. High-dose folic acid supplementation alters the human sperm methylome and is influenced by the MTHFR C677T polymorphism. Hum Mol Genet 2015;24(22):6301–13.

[468] Boxmeer JC, Smit M, Weber RF, et al. Seminal plasma cobalamin significantly correlates with sperm concentration in male undergoing IVF or ICSI procedures. J Androl 2007;28(4):521–7.

[469] Sinclair S. Male infertility: nutritional and environmental considerations. Altern Med Rev 2000;5(1):28–38.

[470] Banihani SA. Vitamin B12 and semen quality. Biomolecules 2017;7(2):42.

[471] Gual-Frau J, Abad C, Amengual MJ, et al. Oral antioxidant treatment partly improves integrity of human sperm DNA in infertile grade I varicocele patients. Hum Fertil 2015;18(3):225–9.

[472] Najafipour R, Moghbelinejad S, Aleyasin A, et al. Effect of B9 and B12 vitamin intake on semen parameters and fertility of men with MTHFR polymorphisms. Andrology 2017;5(4):704–10.

[473] Corbett ST, Hill O, Nangia AK. Vitamin D receptor found in human sperm. Urology 2006;68(6):1345–9.

[474] Jensen MB. Vitamin D and male reproduction. Nat Rev Endocrinol 2014;10(3):175–86.

[475] Jensen MB, Bjerrum PJ, Jessen TE, et al. Vitamin D is positively associated with sperm motility and increases intracellular calcium in human spermatozoa. Hum Reprod 2011;26(6):1307–17.

[476] Tirabassi G, Cutini M, Muscogiuri G, et al. Association between vitamin D and sperm parameters: clinical evidence. Endocrine 2016;58(1):194–8.

[477] Hammoud AO, Meikle AW, Peterson CM, et al. Association of 25-hydroxy-vitamin D levels with semen and hormonal parameters. Asian J Androl 2012;14(6):855.

[478] Ramlau-Hansen CH, Moeller UK, Bonde JP, et al. Are serum levels of vitamin D associated with semen quality? Results from a cross-sectional study in young healthy men. Fertil Steril 2011;95(3):1000–4.

[479] Pilz S, Frisch S, Koertke H, et al. Effect of vitamin D supplementation on testosterone levels in men. Horm Metab Res 2011;43(03):223–5.

[480] Heijboer AC, Oosterwerff M, Schroten NF, et al. Vitamin D supplementation and testosterone concentrations in male human subjects. Clin Endocrinol (Oxf) 2015;83(1):105–10.

[481] Nimptsch K, Platz EA, Willett WC, et al. Association between plasma 25-OH vitamin D and testosterone levels in men. Clin Endocrinol (Oxf) 2012;77(1):106–12.

[482] Boisen IM, Hansen LB, Mortensen LJ, et al. Possible influence of vitamin D on male reproduction. J Steroid Biochem Mol Biol 2016;173:215–22.

[483] Blomberg Jensen M, Gerner Lawaetz J, Andersson AM, et al. Vitamin D deficiency and low ionized calcium are linked with semen quality and sex steroid levels in infertile men. Hum Reprod 2016;31(8):1875–85.

[484] Alzoubi A, Mahdi H, Al Bashir S, et al. Normalization of serum vitamin D improves semen motility parameters in patients with idiopathic male infertility. Acta Endocrinol (Buchar) 2017;13(2):180–7.

[485] Waud K, Bocca S. Role of vitamin D deficiency in male fertility. Fertil Steril 2015;103(2):e39.

[486] Bedu-Addo K, Costello S, Harper C, et al. Mobilisation of stored calcium in the neck region of human sperm – a mechanism for regulation of flagellar activity. Int J Dev Biol 2008;52(5–6):615–26.

[487] Krassas GE, Papadopoulou F, Tziomalos K, et al. Hypothyroidism has an adverse effect on human spermatogenesis: a prospective, controlled study. Thyroid 2008;18(12):1255–9.

[488] Partal-Lorente AB, Maldonado-Ezequiel V, Martinez-Navarro L, et al. Iodine is associated to semen quality in men who undergo consultations for infertility. Reprod Toxicol 2017;73:1–7.

[489] Buretić-Tomljanović A, Vlastelić I, Radojcićbadovinac A, et al. The impact of hemochromatosis mutations and transferrin genotype on gonadotrophin serum levels in infertile male. Fertil Steril 2009;91(5):1793–800.

[490] Anaplitoou ML, Goulandris N, Douvara R. Seminal fibronectin-like antigen and transferrin concentrations in infertile and fertile male. Andrologia 1995;27:137–42.

[491] Wong WY, Flik G, Groenen PM, et al. The impact of calcium, magnesium, zinc, and copper in blood and seminal plasma on semen parameters in male. Reprod Toxicol 2001;15(2):131–6.

[492] Lenzi A, Gandini L, Maresca V, et al. Fatty acid composition of spermatozoa and immature germ cells. Mol Hum Reprod 2000;6(3):226–31.

[493] Safarinejad MR, Hosseini SY, Dadkhah F, et al. Relationship of omega-3 and omega-6 fatty acids with semen characteristics, and anti-oxidant status of seminal plasma: a comparison between fertile and infertile male. Clin Nutr 2010;29(1):100–5.

[494] Gulaya NM, Margitich VM, Govseeva NM, et al. Phospholipid composition of human sperm and seminal plasma in relation to sperm fertility. Arch Androl 2001;46(3):169–75.

[495] Giraud MN, Motta C, Boucher D, et al. Membrane fluidity predicts the outcome of cryopreservation of human spermatozoa. Hum Reprod 2000;15(10):2160–4.

[496] Safarinejad MR. Effect of omega-3 polyunsaturated fatty acid supplementation on semen profile and enzymatic anti-oxidant capacity of seminal plasma in infertile men with idiopathic oligoasthenoteratospermia: a double-blind, placebo-controlled, randomised study. Andrologia 2011;43(1):38–47.

[497] Martinez-Soto JC, Domingo JC, Cordobilla B, et al. Dietary supplementation with docosahexaenoic acid (DHA) improves seminal antioxidant status and decreases sperm DNA fragmentation. Syst Biol Reprod Med 2016;62(6):387–95.

[498] Robbins WA, Xun L, FitzGerald LZ, et al. Walnuts improve semen quality in men consuming a Western-style diet: randomized control dietary intervention trial. Biol Reprod 2012;87(4):101.

[499] Valcarce DG, Genovés S, Riesco MF, et al. Probiotic administration improves sperm quality in asthenozoospermic human donors. Benef Microbes 2017;8(2):193–206.

[500] Maretti C, Cavallini G. The association of a probiotic with a prebiotic (Flortec, Bracco) to improve the quality/quantity of spermatozoa in infertile patients with idiopathic oligoasthenoteratospermia: a pilot study. Andrology 2017;5(3):439–44.

[501] Tremellen K, Pearce K. Probiotics to improve testicular function (Andrology 2017;5:439–444) – a comment on mechanism of action and therapeutic potential of probiotics beyond reproduction. Andrology 2017;5(5):1052–3.

[502] Zhang H, Zhou QM, Li XD, et al. Ginsenoside R(e) increases fertile and asthenozoospermic infertile human sperm motility by induction of nitric oxide synthase. Arch Pharm Res 2006;29(2):145–51.

[503] Pointel JP, Boccalon H, Cloarec M, et al. Titrated extract of Centella asiatica (TECA) in the treatment of venous insufficiency of the lower limbs. Angiology 1987;38:46–50.

[504] Anon. Centella asiatica. Altern Med Rev 2007;12(1):69–72.

[505] Incandela L, Cesarone MR, Cacchio M, et al. Total triterpenic fraction of Centella asiatica in chronic venous insufficiency and in high-perfusion microangiopathy. Angiology 2001;52(Suppl. 2):S9–13.

[506] Arpaia MR, Ferrone R, Amitrano M, et al. Effects of Centella asiatica extract on mucopolysaccharide metabolism in subjects with varicose veins. Int J Clin Pharmacol Res 1990;10(4):229–33.

[507] McKay D. Nutrients and botanicals for erectile dysfunction: examining the evidence. Altern Med Rev 2004;9(1):4–16.

[508] Zhang H, Zhou Q, Li X, et al. Ginsenoside Re promotes human sperm capacitation through nitric oxide-dependent pathway. Mol Reprod Dev 2007;74(4):497–501.

[509] Salvati G, Genovesi G, Marcellini L, et al. Effects of Panax ginseng C.A. Meyer saponins on male fertility. Panminerva Med 1996;38(4):249–54.

[510] Park HJ, Choe S, Park NC. Effects of Korean red ginseng on semen parameters in male infertility patients: a randomized, placebo-controlled, double-blind clinical study. Chin J Integr Med 2016;22(7):490–5.

[511] Robaire B, Henderson NA. Actions of 5-alpha-reductase inhibitors on the epididymis. Mol Cell Endocrinol 2006;250(1–2):190–5.

[512] Gauthaman K, Ganesan AP. The hormonal effects of Tribulus terrestris and its role in the management of male erectile dysfunction – an evaluation using primates, rabbit and rat. Phytomedicine 2008;15(1–2):44–54.

[513] Neychev VK, Mitev VI. The aphrodisiac herb Tribulus terrestris does not influence the androgen production in young male. J Ethnopharmacol 2005;101(1–3):319–23.

[514] Khaleghi S, Bakhtiari M, Asadmobini A, et al. Tribulus terrestris extract improves human sperm parameters in vitro. J Evid Based Complementary Altern Med 2017;22(3):407–12.

[515] Asadmobini A, Bakhtiari M, Khaleghi S, et al. The effect of Tribulus terrestris extract on motility and viability of human sperms after cryopreservation. Cryobiology 2017;75:154–9.

[516] Protich M, Tsvetkov D, Nalbanski B, et al. Clinical trial of a tribestan preparation in infertile men. Akush Ginekol (Sofiia) 1983;22(4):326–9.

[517] Kumanov F, Bozadzhieva E, Platonova M, et al. Clinical testing of Tribestan. Savr Med 1982;4:2115. Available from: http://www.functionalmedicine.org. [Accessed 17 September 2010]. Institute for Functional Medicine. National Standards Monograph.

[518] Adimoelja A. Phytochemicals and the breakthrough of traditional herbs in the management of sexual dysfunctions. Int J Androl 2000;23(S2):82–4.

[519] Kamenov Z, Fileva S, Kalinov K, et al. Evaluation of the efficacy and safety of Tribulus terrestris in male sexual dysfunction – a prospective, randomized, double-blind, placebo-controlled clinical trial. Maturitas 2017;99:20–6.

[520] Santos CA Jr, Reis LO, Destro-Saade R, et al. Tribulus terrestris versus placebo in the treatment of erectile dysfunction: a prospective, randomized, double-blind study. Actas Urol Esp 2014;38(4):244–8.

[521] Roaiah MF, Elkhayat YI, Saleh SF, et al. Prospective analysis on the effect of botanical medicine (Tribulus terrestris) on Serum testosterone level and semen parameters in males with unexplained infertility. J Diet Suppl 2017;14(1):25–31.

[522] Salgado RM, Marques-Silva MH, Gonçalves E, et al. Effect of oral administration of Tribulus terrestris extract on semen quality and body fat index of infertile men. Andrologia 2017;49(5).

[523] Neychev V, Mitev V. Pro-sexual and androgen enhancing effects of Tribulus terrestris L.: fact or fiction. J Ethnopharmacol 2016;179:345–55.

[524] Arletti R, Benelli A, Cavazzuti E, et al. Stimulating property of Turnera diffusa and Pffafia paniculata extracts on the sexual behavior of male rats. Psychopharmacology (Berl) 1999;144:15–19.

[525] Estrada-Reyes R, Ortiz-López P, Gutiérrez-Ortíz J, et al. Turnera diffusa wild (Turneraceae) recovers sexual behavior in sexually exhausted males. J Ethnopharmacol 2009;123(3):423–9.

[526] Zhao J, Dasmahapatra A, Khan S, et al. Anti-aromatase activity of the constituents from damiana (Turnera diffusa). J Ethnopharmacol 2008;120(3):387–93.

[527] Hong CY, Ku J, Wu P. Astragalus membranaceus stimulates human sperm motility in vitro. Am J Chin Med 1992;20(3–4):289–94.

[528] Tripathi YB, Upadhyay AK. Antioxidant property of Mucuna pruriens. Curr Sci 2001;80:1377–8.

[529] Ahmad MK, Mahdi AA, Shukla KK, et al. Effect of Mucuna pruriens on semen profile and biochemical parameters in seminal plasma of infertile male. Fertil Steril 2008;90:627–35.

[530] Shukla KK, Mahdi AA, Ahmad MK, et al. Mucuna pruriens improves male fertility by its action on the hypothalamus–pituitary–gonadal axis. Fertil Steril 2009;92:1934–40.

[531] Gupta A, Mahdi AA, Ahmad MK, et al. A proton NMR study of the effect of Mucuna pruriens on seminal plasma metabolites of infertile males. J Pharm Biomed Anal 2011;55(5):1060–6.

[532] Ahmad MK, Mahdi AA, Shukla KK, et al. Withania somnifera improves semen quality by regulating reproductive hormone levels and oxidative stress in seminal plasma of infertile males. Fertil Steril 2009;94(3):989–96.

[533] Ambiye VR, Langade D, Dongre S, et al. Clinical evaluation of the spermatogenic activity of the root extract of Ashwagandha (Withania somnifera) in oligospermic males: a pilot study. Evid Based Complement Alternat Med 2013;2013:571420.

[534] Gupta A, Mahdi AA, Shukla KK, et al. Efficacy of Withania somnifera on seminal plasma metabolites of infertile males: a proton NMR study at 800 MHz. J Ethnopharmacol 2013;149(1):208–14.

[535] Mahdi AA, Shukla KK, Ahmad MK, et al. Withania somnifera improves semen quality in stress-related male fertility. Evid Based Complement Alternat Med 2011;2011.

[536] Shukla KK, Mahdi AA, Mishra V, et al. Withania somnifera improves semen quality by combating oxidative stress and cell death and improving essential metal concentrations. Reprod Biomed Online 2011;22(5):421–7.

[537] Kolahdooz M, Nasri S, Modarres SZ, et al. Effects of Nigella sativa L. seed oil on abnormal semen quality in infertile men: a randomized, double-blind, placebo-controlled clinical trial. Phytomedicine 2014;21(6):901–5.

[538] Mahdavi R, Heshmati J, Namazi N. Effects of black seeds (Nigella sativa) on male infertility: a systematic review. J Herb Med 2015;5(3):133–9.

[539] Dai JB, Wang ZX, Qiao ZD. The hazardous effects of tobacco smoking on male fertility. Asian J Androl 2015;17(6):954.

[540] Taha EA, Ez-Aldin AM, Sayed SK, et al. Effect of smoking on sperm vitality, DNA integrity, seminal oxidative stress, zinc in fertile men. Urology 2012;80(4):822–5.

[541] Wright C, Milne S, Leeson H. Sperm DNA damage caused by oxidative stress: modifiable clinical, lifestyle and nutritional factors in male infertility. Reprod Biomed Online 2014;28(6):684–703.

[542] Prentki Santos E, López-Costa S, Chenlo P, et al. Impact of spontaneous smoking cessation on sperm quality: case report. Andrologia 2011;43(6):431–5.

[543] Sharma R, Harlev A, Agarwal A, et al. Cigarette smoking and semen quality: a new meta-analysis examining the effect of the 2010 World Health Organization laboratory methods for the examination of human semen. Eur Urol 2016;70(4):635–45.

[544] Fronczak CM, Kim ED, Barqawi AB. The insults of illicit drug use on male fertility. J Androl 2012;33(4):515–28.

[545] Christou MA, Christou PA, Markozannes G, et al. Effects of anabolic androgenic steroids on the reproductive system of athletes

and recreational users: a systematic review and meta-analysis. Sports Med 2017;47(9):1869–83.

[546] Alvarez S. Do some addictions interfere with fertility? Fertil Steril 2015;103(1):22–6.

[547] du Plessis SS, Agarwal A, Syriac A. Marijuana, phytocannabinoids, the endocannabinoid system, and male fertility. J Assist Reprod Genet 2015;32(11):1575–88.

[548] Mruk DD, Cheng CY. Environmental contaminants: is male reproductive health at risk? Spermatogenesis 2011;1(4):283–90.

[549] Lewis RC, Minguez-Alarcón L, Meeker JD, et al. Self-reported mobile phone use and semen parameters among men from a fertility clinic. Reprod Toxicol 2017;67:42–7.

[550] Schauer I, Al-Ali BM. Combined effects of varicocele and cell phones on semen and hormonal parameters. Wien Klin Wochenschr 2018;130(9–10):335–40.

[551] Adams JA, Galloway TS, Mondal D, et al. Effect of mobile telephones on sperm quality: a systematic review and meta-analysis. Environ Int 2014;70:106–12.

[552] Liu K, Li Y, Zhang G, et al. Association between mobile phone use and semen quality: a systemic review and meta-analysis. Andrology 2014;2(4):491–501.

[553] Yildirim ME, Kaynar M, Badem H, et al. What is harmful for male fertility: cell phone or the wireless internet? Kaohsiung J Med Sci 2015;31(9):480–4.

[554] Kamali K, Atarod M, Sarhadi S, et al. Effects of electromagnetic waves emitted from 3G+ wi-fi modems on human semen analysis. Urologia 2017;84(4).

[555] Sun J, Yu G, Zhang Y, et al. Heavy metal level in human semen with different fertility: a meta-analysis. Biol Trace Elem Res 2017;176(1):27–36.

[556] Buck Louis GM, Barr DB, Kannan K, et al. Paternal exposures to environmental chemicals and time-to-pregnancy: overview of results from the LIFE study. Andrology 2016;4(4):639–47.

[557] Broe A, Pottegård A, Hallas J, et al. Association between use of phthalate-containing medication and semen quality among men in couples referred for assisted reproduction. Hum Reprod 2018;33(3):503–11.

[558] Gaskins AJ, Mendiola J, Afeiche M, et al. Physical activity and television watching in relation to semen quality in young men. Br J Sports Med 2015;49(4):265–70.

[559] Vaamonde D, Da Silva-Grigoletto ME, García-Manso JM, et al. Physically active men show better semen parameters and hormone values than sedentary men. Eur J Appl Physiol 2012;112(9):3267–73.

[560] Eisenberg ML, Kim S, Chen Z, et al. The relationship between male BMI and waist circumference on semen quality: data from the LIFE study. Hum Reprod 2014;29(2):193–200.

[561] Lalinde-Acevedo PC, Mayorga-Torres BJ, Agarwal A, et al. Physically active men show better semen parameters than their sedentary counterparts. Int J Fertil Steril 2017;11(3):156.

[562] Maleki BH, Tartibian B. Moderate aerobic exercise training for improving reproductive function in infertile patients: a randomized controlled trial. Cytokine 2017;92:55–67.

[563] Maleki BH, Tartibian B, Chehrazi M. The effects of three different exercise modalities on markers of male reproduction in healthy subjects: a randomized controlled trial. Reproduction 2017;153(2):157–74.

[564] Maleki BH, Tartibian B. High-intensity exercise training for improving reproductive function in infertile patients: a randomized controlled trial. J Obstet Gynaecol Can 2017;39(7):545–58.

[565] Hajizadeh Maleki B, Tartibian B. Combined aerobic and resistance exercise training for improving reproductive function in infertile men: a randomized controlled trial. Appl Physiol Nutr Metab 2017;42(12):1293–306.

[566] Rosety MÁ, Diaz A, Rosety JM, et al. Exercise improved semen quality and reproductive hormone levels in sedentary obese adults. Nutr Hosp 2017;34(3).

[567] Vaamonde D, Garcia-Manso JM, Hackney AC. Impact of physical activity and exercise on male reproductive potential: a new assessment questionnaire. Rev Andal Med Deport 2017;10(2):79–93.

[568] World Health Organization. WHO laboratory manual for the examination of human semen and sperm–cervical mucus interaction. 4th ed. Geneva: WHO; 1999.

APPENDIX 11.1

Fertility chart

Fertility Chart (Celsius)

Age _____

Fertility cycle # _____

Last 12 cycles: _____   longest: _____   shortest: _____   month: _____   year: _____   this cycle length: _____

Route of temperature: oral / vaginal / rectal / underarm

cycle day

date

time temperature normally taken

Temperature rises by 1 place every hour

Ovulation detected by temperature rise of 4 spaces

WAKING TEMPERATURE

Ovulation test

pregnancy test

	1	2	3	4	5	6	7	8	9	10	11	12	13	14	15	16	17	18	19	20	21	22	23	24	25	26	27	28	29	30	31	32	33	34	35	36	37	38	39	40
Circle intercourse on cycle day																																								
ovulation pain																																								
CERVICAL FLUID ASSESSMENT																																								
VISUAL ASSESSMENT																																								
larger amount																																								
medium amount																																								
small amount																																								
dry, spotting or PERIOD																																								
infertile phase and PEAK day																																								
CERVICAL FLUID DESCRIPTION																																								
eggwhite																																								
slippery, will usually stretch																																								
clear/streaked/opaque																																								
lube, wet or humid feeling																																								
creamy																																								
lotiony, milky, smooth																																								
usually white or yellow																																								
wet, moist or cold feeling																																								
sticky																																								
pasty, crumbly, opaque																																								
rubber-cement																																								
dry or sticky feeling																																								
VAGINAL SENSATION																																								
CERVIX POSITION ASSESSMENT																																								
cervix position and opening																																								
diagnostic tests and procedures																																								
herbal medicines and/or medications																																								
exercise																																								
breast self-exam							BSE																																	
miscellaneous																																								
travel																																								
illness																																								
headaches																																								
nausea/vomiting																																								
bowel																																								
skin																																								
breasts																																								
fluid retention																																								
fatigue/energy levels																																								
emotional state																																								
food cravings																																								
sexual desire																																								

APPENDIX 11.2

Timeline of embryonic development

LMP ×/52	LMP ×/7	Post ovulation ×/7	Extra-embryonic	Embryonic	Ultrasound scan	Physical relationship to maternal tissue	Endocrine relationship
2/52	15	1	Pronuclear zygote			FT:AIJ	E2 still dominant
	16	2	2-cell, cleavage				
	17	3	4-cell: compaction	Does not require embryonic transcription			
	18	4	8-cell				
	19	5	Morula			Entry to uterus	P4 dominant
	20	6	Blastocyst; trophoblast	Inner cell mass (eccentric – polarity defined)			
3/52	21	7	Expanded blastocyst Trophectoderm: syncytiotrophoblast + cytotrophoblast	Ectoderm + endoderm = embryonic disk		Hatching, opposition, attachment	hCG
	22	8		Ectoderm forms amnion: amniotic cavity defined		Penetration, completes implantation	
	23	9				Lytic encounter Histiotrophic nutrition from glands	
	24	10				Pre-decidual reaction starts – decidua, endoderm, amnion	
	25	11	Endoderm forms Heuser's membrane Extra-embryonic coelem Extra embryonic mesoderm + trophoblast = chorion	Primary yolk sac			
	26	12	Trophoblast lacunae	Endoderm: prochordal plate, 'cranially', A/P axis defined		Spiral arterial blood flow into lacunar spaces via venous sinuses	
	27	13					

Continued

LMP ×/52	LMP ×/7	Post ovulation ×/7	Extra-embryonic	Embryonic	Ultrasound scan	Physical relationship to maternal tissue	Endocrine relationship
4/52	28	14	Chorion + amnion defined (=syncytiotrophoblast + cytotrophoblast + chorionic mesoderm)	Secondary yolk sac/connecting stalk		Decidual reaction advances	Relaxin, prolactin
	29	15	Cytotrophoblasto columns = primary villi	Gastrulation: primitive streak (caudal), embryonic mesoderm			Missed menses
	30	16				Decidua basalis, capsularis, parietalis (= d. serotina, d. reflexa, d. vera)	
	31	17	Secondary villi	Embryonic disk trilaminar and pear-shaped Hensen's node, blastopore, notochord cloacal membrane caudally			
	32	18	Extra-embryonic blood cells and vessels	Notochordal plate at roof of yolk sac; germ cells in yolk sac endoderm			
	33	19		Neurulation: neural plate and groove			
	34	20		First somite from paraxial mesoderm	Sac 2 mm		
5/52	35	21	Villi with blood vessels	Heart: straight and beating slowly		Placental circulation	
	36	22		Head and tail folding commences	Yolk sac 2 mm		
	37	23		Foregut and hindgut			
	38	24		Pronephros (vest.)			
	39	25		Buccal membrane opens	HR 60 beats/minute		
	40	26		20 somites			
	41	27		Mesonephros			

LMP ×/52	LMP ×/7	Post ovulation ×/7	Extra-embryonic	Embryonic	Ultrasound scan	Physical relationship to maternal tissue	Endocrine relationship
6/52	42	28	Cytotrophoblast shell complete			Syncytiotrophoblast giant cells enter myometrium	
	43	29		28 somites	CR length 5 mm		
	44	30		Neural pores close, completing 5 neurulation			
	45	31		Limb buds obvious			
	46	32		Metanephric duct	HR 120 beats/minute		
	47	33		Germ cells reach genital ridges			
	48	34		Labioscrotal swellings, genital tubercle			
7/52	49	35	Cotyledons developed		CR length 10 mm		
	50	36		Müllerian ducts begin to develop (both sexes)			
	51	37					
	52	38					
	53	39					
	54	40		Cloaca faces caudally			
	55	41		Urorectal septum divides cloaca			
8/52	56	42		Testes differentiate	CR length 16 mm		Fetal testosterone Predominantly α-chains synthesised
	57	43		Metanephric vesicles			
	58	44		Cloacal membrane opens			
	59	45		Sclerotome, dermatome and myotome			
	60	46		Migration done			
	61	47					
	62	48					
9/52	63	49		Ovaries differentiate	CR length 24 mm		
10/52		56		Mesonephric duct disappears in females	CR length 33 mm		

Continued

LMP ×/52	LMP ×/7	Post ovulation ×/7	Extra-embryonic	Embryonic	Ultrasound scan	Physical relationship to maternal tissue	Endocrine relationship
11/52		63		Müllerian ducts have fused; disappearing in males	CR length 44 mm		
12/52		70	Amniotic cavity displaces extraembryonic coelem	Male external genitalia differentiate	CR length >50 mm		Intact LH and FSH synthesised and released
13/52		77		Palatal fusion; organogenesis complete			
14/52		84	D. capsularis villi gone				Hypothalamus: 5α-reductase and aromatase present (until 18/52)
15/52		91		Body wall complete			
16/52		98	Cytotrophoblast disappears				hCG levels falling
17/52							
18/52							GnRH neurones in contact with primitive mantle plexus
19/52							
20/52							
21/52							
22/52							FSH and LH maximal (higher in females and comparable to menopausal adults), until 30/52
Birth							FSH and LH levels secondary rise, then fall to a nadir in early childhood

APPENDIX 11.3

hCG interpretation

hCG testing

Human chorionic gonadotrophin (hCG) is a hormone secreted from the placenta into the maternal circulation with a role in the maintenance of a viable pregnancy. The serum concentration of hCG is used to detect and monitor pregnancy and some malignant conditions.

hCG during pregnancy

During the first weeks of pregnancy, hCG serum concentrations rise rapidly, with a doubling time of about 2 days. This rate of rise then slows, and the peak hCG concentration is reached between 8 and 12 weeks of gestation. The concentration then falls to a plateau, which persists over the second and third trimesters. After delivery, hCG falls, with a half-life of 1–2 days.

High levels may be found in patients with twin or multiple pregnancies or with gestational trophoblastic disease. Low levels may be a marker of non-viable pregnancy (e.g. ectopic pregnancy).

A doubling time of less than 2 days should arouse suspicion of either a possible ectopic pregnancy or a non-viable intrauterine pregnancy. Gynaecological opinion should be sought in this instance. hCG is usually detectable in ectopic pregnancies, but this is not a universal finding.

At hCG concentrations >2500 U/L, a normal intrauterine pregnancy should be visible on a transvaginal ultrasound scan. Note that hCG levels should never be used in isolation for diagnosis of any of the above conditions.

TABLE A11.3 Interpretation of quantitative serum hcg results			
Reference ranges		**Serum hCG (U/L)**	
Weeks since last menstrual period	Approximate hCG range (U/L)		Comment
Women	Premenopausal	<2.0 U/L	
	Postmenopausal	<2.0–10 U/L	
Men		<2.0 U/L	
PREGNANCY TEST			
	Serum hCG (U/L)	Interpretation	
	<2 U/L	Negative (if taken after first missed period)	
	2–25 U/L	Borderline result (suggest repeat in 48 hours)	
	>25 U/L	Consistent with pregnancy (Note: most laboratories will request a repeat assessment if reading is <100 U/L)	
PREGNANCY STAGING			
3–4	0–130		Week prior to first missed period
4–5	75–2600		Week after first missed period
5–6	850–20 800		
6–7	4000–200 000		
7–12	11 500–289 000		
12–16	18 300–37 000		
16–29	1400–3000		Second trimester
29–41	940–60 000		Third trimester

APPENDIX 11.4

General IVF protocol

Step 1: controlled ovarian stimulation

1 Optional: oral contraceptive prescription prior to embarking on stimulating cycle to regulate and control timing.

2 Serum E2, P4 and LH to confirm new cycle.
3 Stimulate the ovaries with injections of FSH.
  (a) A small amount of LH will be included in the preparation for follicle development and proper development of the egg.
  (b) Dose of FSH will be calculated based on the woman's weight to prevent hyperstimulation: dose range 100 U (40 kg) to 450 U (120 kg).
  (c) Objective will be to stimulate a small number of recruits, as only one follicle will be used per cycle (ideally).

(d) Aim for an FSH level of 8–12 U/L 24 hours after injection.

(e) Repeat serum E2 to assess that dose of FSH is appropriate.

(f) Repeat serum E2 and ultrasound scan to determine how many follicles are developing.

4 Prevent the surge of LH with either a GnRH agonist or a GnRH antagonist.

(a) GnRH agonists accentuate the duration of action of GnRH by downregulating the response.

(b) Newer GnRH antagonists block the effect of GnRH.

5 Replace the LH surge at midcycle with a 'trigger' injection of hCG.

(a) Dose is calculated according to the woman's weight: <50 kg, 2500 U; 50–60 kg, 3000 U; 60–90 kg, 5000 U; 90–100 kg, 7000 U; >100 kg, 10 000 U.

(b) Ovulation can be expected in just over 38 hours, and therefore egg retrieval is typically scheduled for 36 hours after hCG injection.

6 Support the receptive state of the endometrium in the luteal phase with hCG or progesterone.

(a) <5 mature follicles: hCG 1500 U at 4 and 8 days.

(b) >5 mature follicles: progesterone pessaries 100 mg b.i.d. until pregnancy test.

7 Monitor ovaries by means of blood tests and ultrasound scans.

(a) In general the goal is to have at least two follicles with a mean diameter of 17–18 mm, ideally accompanied by a few others of diameter 14–16 mm, and a serum E2 concentration that is consistent with the overall size and maturity of the cohort (approximately 200 pg/mL per follicle measuring ≥14 mm).

Step 2: egg retrieval

Egg retrieval is the culmination of ovarian stimulation and monitoring, and is scheduled for approximately 36 hours after the hCG trigger. Eggs are retrieved by the aspiration of the fluid from the immediately preovulatory follicles in which the eggs have detached themselves from the wall of the follicle, are surrounded by a mature cumulus and are at the secondary oocyte stage, and thus are able to be fertilised.

Step 3: sperm retrieval

Unless any sperm abnormalities are detected, standard fresh sperm collection by the man is typically conducted on the same day as egg retrieval so that a fresh sample can be used. Frozen samples are also appropriate.

Step 4: micromanipulation of gametes

Micromanipulation of gametes may be implemented based on the results of other testing.

Sperm

ICSI will be used if oligospermia, azoospermia or other barriers to fertilisation such as sperm antibodies are observed.

Oocytes

Blastocyst culture is maintained to enable growth from a 3-day to a 5-day embryo.

Embryo biopsy for PGD or assisted hatching if warranted.

Step 5: IVF fertilisation

1 50 000–100 000 motile sperm are left with the collected egg.

2 Contact with sperm soon disperses the cumulus.

3 By the next day, approximately 15 hours after introducing the sperm to the eggs, the eggs are checked to see if they have fertilised by examining them for evidence of pronuclei.

4 Day 2: embryos will have divided twice, containing four cells.

5 Day 3: there will be eight cells (PGD may be done if necessary).

6 Day 4: embryo consists of 16 or more cells (morula).

7 Day 5: blastulation – the embryo is now a blastocyst.

Step 5b: ICSI fertilisation

The same process as above, but with the following slight variations:

1 Cumulus is extracted from the outer egg.

2 One selected sperm is injected into the collected egg.

3 Steps (1) to (7) as above.

Step 6: embryo transfer

After successful fertilisation, the day-5 embryo is transferred with guided ultrasound assistance.

Step 7: post-implantation endometrial support

The endometrium is supported in the luteal phase with hCG or progesterone if endometrial thickness is poor, implantation success is doubted or if pregnancy success is questioned based on βhCG and P4 assessments.

APPENDIX 11.5

WHO criteria – semen analysis[568]

Understanding semen analysis (WHO criteria)

TABLE A11.5.1 Macroscopic semen characteristics		
Source	**Volume**	**Characteristics**
Urethral and bulbourethral glands	0.1-0.2 cc	Viscous, clear
Testes, epididymides, vasa deferentia	0.1-0.2 cc	Sperm present
Prostate	0.5-1.0 cc	Acidic, watery
Seminal vesicles	1.0-3.0 cc	Gelatinous, fructose positive
Complete ejaculate	2.0-5.0 cc	Liquefies in 20–25 min

TABLE A11.5.2 Commonly used normal semen parameters (WHO)	
Volume	>2.0 ml
pH	7.2-7.8
Concentration	$>20\times10^6$/ml
Motility	>50%
Morphology	>30% with normal morphology
WBC	$< 1\times10^6$/ml

TABLE A11.5.3 Gradation of sperm motility (WHO)			
Type of motility	**Score**	**Classes of spermatozoa motility**	**Normal value**
No movement	0	Rapid progressive Class **A**	>25%
Movement, none forward Occasional movement of a few sperm Slow, undirected	1 1+ 2	Progressive Class **B** Class **A+B** Non progressive Class **C**	>25% >50% <50%
Slow, directly forward movement	2+	Immotile or static Class **D**	<50%
Fast, but undirected movement Fast, directed forward movement	3– 3	Class **C+D**	<50%
Very fast forward movement Extremely fast forward movement	3+ 4		

TABLE A11.5.4 Nomenclature for semen variables (WHO)	
Normozoospermia	Normal ejaculate as defined in tables 1, 2 and 3.
Oligozoospermia	Sperm concentration fewer than 20×10^6/ml
Asthenozoospermia	Fewer than 50% spermatozoa with forward progression (categories A and B) or fewer than 25% spermatozoa with category A movement
Teratozoospermia	Fewer than 30% spermatozoa with normal morphology
Oligoasthenoteratozoospermia	Signifies disturbance of all three variables (combination of only two prefixes can be used)
Azoospermia	No spermatozoa in the ejaculate
Aspermia	No ejaculate

APPENDIX 11.6

WHO *Guidelines for Semen Analysis* (2010, 5th edition)[59]

| TABLE A11.6 Lower reference limits (5th centiles and their 95% confidence intervals) for semen characteristic ||
Parameter	Lower reference limit
Semen volume (ml)	1.5 (1.4–1.7)
Total sperm number (100 per ejaculate)	39 (33–46)
Sperm concentration (100 per ml)	15 (12–16)
Total motility (PR+NP, %)	40 (38–42)
Progressive motility (PR, %)	32 (31–34)
Vitality (live spermatozoa, %)	58 (55–63)
Sperm morphology (normal forms, %)	4 (3.0–4.0)
Other consensus threshold values	
pH	≥7.2
Peroxidase-positive leucocytes (100 per ml)	<1.0
MAR test (motile spermatozoa with bound particles, %)	<50
Immunobead test (motile spermatozoa with bounds beads, %)	<50
Seminal zinc (μmol/ejaculate)	≥2.4
Seminal fructose (μmol/ejaculate)	≥13
Seminal neutral glucosidase (mU/ejaculate)	≥20

Miscarriage

12

Angela Hywood

OVERVIEW AND DEFINITION

Recurrent miscarriages are post-implantation failures in natural conception; they are also termed as habitual abortions, spontaneous miscarriages or recurrent pregnancy losses. Spontaneous pregnancy loss or miscarriage is the most frequent complication of early pregnancy and represents the major loss for all pregnant women.

A miscarriage refers to the loss of a confirmed pregnancy before 20 weeks of gestation. The physical experience of miscarriage can vary greatly between an early miscarriage and a late miscarriage. An early miscarriage is the loss of a pregnancy before the 12th week of gestation (trimester 1); a late miscarriage occurs between 12 and 20 weeks of gestation (trimester 2).

Recurrent miscarriage is defined as three consecutive pregnancy losses prior to 20 weeks from the last menstrual period, and affects approximately 1–2% of women.[1] In up to 50% of couples affected by recurrent pregnancy loss, no identifiable cause is established.[2]

A miscarriage is legally differentiated from a stillbirth by the week of the loss of pregnancy. A stillbirth refers to the birth of a baby who has died prior to delivery after 20 weeks of gestation. If the length of the pregnancy is unknown, a baby born with no signs of life and weighing less than 400 g is considered a miscarriage.[3]

Pregnancy loss is always heartbreaking to the couple involved and to the treating practitioner. The loss of a pregnancy is both physically and emotionally stressful for couples, especially when faced with the devastation of recurrent pregnancy loss. Feelings of loss, grief, fear, guilt, anger and disappointment are all very common, and the psychology and mental health of those affected can suffer greatly. Tender loving care, counselling and reassurance are to be the very first points of consideration when meeting these couples in our clinical practices.

Most women who have experienced miscarriage will more than likely go on to have a healthy pregnancy in the future. The prognosis is good. The predicted success rate, often confirmed in cohort trials,[4] is 70% despite two or three prior losses.

Pregnancy loss is an area of medicine that has been extensively researched, from aetiology to management of spontaneous miscarriage and recurrent pregnancy loss.

STATISTICS

Spontaneous pregnancy loss is a surprisingly common occurrence, with approximately 12–15% of all clinically recognised pregnancies resulting in miscarriage. Thirty per cent of these pregnancies are lost between implantation and the sixth week.[1,5]

Miscarriage is challenging to study because risk varies markedly by risk factors such as number of weeks of gestation, detection of heartbeat, fetal heart rate, maternal age, paternal age and number of prior miscarriages.[6] Approximately 70% of conceptions fail prior to live birth, with most losses occurring prior to implantation or before the missed menstrual period.[7] In Australia, up to 1 in 4 confirmed pregnancies end in miscarriage before 20 weeks, but many other women miscarry without having confirmation or realising that they are indeed pregnant. Women who smoke cigarettes or drink alcohol moderately are probably at higher risk.[4]

A biochemical pregnancy occurs when an initial pregnancy test is positive, but it does not progress into a clinical pregnancy. Biochemical pregnancy is indeed a conception and is actually a very early miscarriage. This occurs when hormone human chorionic gonadotropin (HCG) is detectable and pregnancy is positive; however, the pregnancy demises prior to implantation or shortly after implantation, resulting in bleeding that occurs around the time of the expected period. Biochemical pregnancies account for 50–75% of all miscarriages.[8]

Recurrent miscarriage (recurrent pregnancy loss), defined as the loss of three or more consecutive pregnancies, affects 1% of couples trying to conceive.[9]

Recurrent miscarriage, defined as the loss of three or more consecutive pregnancies, affects 1% of couples trying to conceive.[9] Based on the incidence of spontaneous pregnancy loss, the incidence of recurrent miscarriage should be approximately 1 in 300 pregnancies. However, epidemiological studies have revealed that 1–2% of women experience recurrent pregnancy loss.[7] Based on the incidence of sporadic pregnancy loss, the incidence of recurrent pregnancy loss should be approximately 1 in 300 pregnancies. However, epidemiological studies have revealed that 1–2% of women experience recurrent pregnancy loss.[7]

The risk of miscarriage after two consecutive losses is 17–25%, and the risk of miscarrying a fourth pregnancy after three consecutive losses is between 25% and 46%. The evidence suggests higher frequency of spontaneous miscarriages among subfertile couples and a higher prevalence of subfertility in women with recurrent spontaneous miscarriages when compared with the general population.[5]

RISK OF MISCARRIAGE BY NUMBER OF WEEKS OF GESTATION OF PREGNANCY

Miscarriage risks are seen to drop as the pregnancy progresses. The risk is highest early in the first trimester. Miscarriages rates decline between 6 and 10 weeks, according to a study of 697 pregnancies with a confirmed fetal heartbeat[10] (see Table 12.1), and by 14 weeks, for most women, the chance of a miscarriage is less than 1%.

In a large prospective study of 4887 women trying to conceive, 4070 became pregnant. Their rate of miscarriage was 4–5% in week 6. By week 7, this risk fell to 2.5%. Rates hovered around 2% per week until week 13, when chances of a miscarriage dipped below 1%.[11] See Fig. 12.1.

A similar study of 668 pregnancies with a confirmed fetal heartbeat between 6 and 10 weeks found a similar decline in miscarriage risk by week. See Table 12.2.

RISK OF MISCARRIAGE BY MATERNAL AGE

Maternal age is positively correlated with miscarriage rates. Advanced maternal age (>35 years of age) is considered to be a risk factor, even after confirmation of a fetal heartbeat. Miscarriage risk to 12 weeks and beyond remains high for women greater than 40 years of age to 12 weeks and beyond, according to a study of 384 women 35 and older.[4] A 40-year-old woman has twice the risk of miscarriage as a 20-year-old woman in euploid as well as certain aneuploid pregnancies.[12] Recurrence risks are slightly higher for older women, for those who smoke cigarettes or drink alcohol and for those exposed to high levels of selected chemical toxins.[4] See Table 12.3.

In those women of an advanced maternal age, a healthy normal ultrasound result from 7 weeks is a promising sign. Women who entered the study in their 4th to 5th week of pregnancy had around a 35% risk of miscarriage. However, women who entered the study later, and who therefore had a normal ultrasound and heartbeat at 7–10 weeks, had a risk under 10%. After 7 weeks, the fetal heart rate was at or above 120 beats per minute for almost all ongoing pregnancies.[12]

TABLE 12.1 Risk of miscarriage by number of weeks of gestation of pregnancy

Week of pregnancy	Miscarriage rates with confirmed fetal heartbeat
6/40	9.4%
7/40	4.6%
8/40	1.5%
9/40	0.5%
10/40	0.7%

TABLE 12.2 Risk of miscarriage by number of weeks of gestation of pregnancy

Week of pregnancy	Miscarriage rates with confirmed fetal heartbeat
6/40	10.3%
7/40	7.9%
8/40	7.4%
9/40	3.1%

Source: Ammon Avalos L, Galindo C, Li DK. A systematic review to calculate background miscarriage rates using life table analysis. *Birth Defects Research Part A: Clinical and Molecular Teratology* 2012;94(6):417–23.

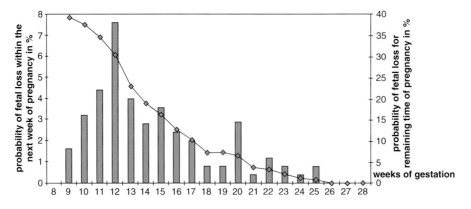

FIGURE 12.1 Probability of pregnancy loss by week of pregnancy

Simpson J, Carson S. Genetic and nongenetic causes of pregnancy loss. *Glob Libr Women's Med* 2013;3(3).

TABLE 12.3 Risk of miscarriage by maternal age

Maternal age	Percentage risk miscarrying by 12/40
35–37	2.8
38–39	7.5
40+	10.8

Source: Cohen-Overbeek TE, den Ouden M, Pijpers L, et al. Spontaneous abortion rate and advanced maternal age: consequences for prenatal diagnosis. *The Lancet* 1990;336(8706):27–9.

TABLE 12.4 Aetiology of pregnancy loss

Aetiology	Statistics
Genetic factors	2–5%
Anatomical factors	10–15%
Autoimmune factors	20%
Infection factors	0.5–5%
Endocrine factors	17–20%
Unexplained, including on APS thrombophilia factors	40–50%

Source: Ford HB, Schust DJ. Recurrent pregnancy loss: etiology, diagnosis, and therapy. *Rev Obstet Gynecol* 2009;2(2):76–83.

FETAL HEART RATE AS MISCARRIAGE RISK DETERMINANT[13]

Fetal heartbeat can indicate a healthy, viable pregnancy. But a fetal heart rate that is too slow can indicate a possible risk of miscarriage or deterioration of fetal health.

AETIOLOGY OF MISCARRIAGES

The causes of miscarriage and recurrent pregnancy loss include chromosomal abnormalities, autoimmunity such as untreated hypothyroidism and diabetes mellitus, uterine anatomical abnormalities, heritable thrombophilia, infections and environmental factors.[1,7] See Table 12.4. From a medical point of view, the management of miscarriages can often be an unsolved problem; up to 50% of cases of recurrent losses will not have a clearly defined aetiology.[5]

Anatomical aetiologies

Anatomical abnormalities account for 10–15% of cases of recurrent pregnancy loss and are generally thought to cause miscarriage by interrupting the vasculature of the endometrium, prompting abnormal and inadequate placentation. Although more readily associated with second-trimester losses or preterm labour, congenital

uterine anomalies also play a part in recurrent miscarriage.[1] See Table 12.5.

A study of 188 women with recurrent pregnancy loss found the prevalence of anatomical anomalies was 41.5% (n = 78).[15] See Table 12.6. The study identified the anatomical factor as the unique cause of recurrent pregnancy loss in 35.6% (n = 67) of cases.[15]

Women with recurrent pregnancy loss have a 3.2–6.9% likelihood of having a major uterine anomaly, and a 1–16.9% chance of having an arcuate uterus. Ultrasound is a quick, readily available and economical way to investigate, with a huge upside benefit of no radiation exposure. In addition, 3D ultrasound has 95% accuracy in identifying uterine anomalies.[5,16]

Some authors consider the combination of hysteroscopy and laparoscopy to be the gold standard in evaluating congenital uterine anomalies; however, these are costly and invasive, with many women underestimating the recovery time involved with laparoscopic surgery.

CERVICAL INCOMPETENCE

Cervical health and structural integrity are important in the development and sustenance of a pregnancy. Cervical insufficiency is a difficult condition to diagnose and can lead to preterm birth, miscarriage or perinatal infant morbidity and mortality. The non-pregnant cervix is normally composed of a dense, collagenous, fibroconnective tissue with small amounts of smooth muscle. In pregnancy, the increased vascularity in the cervix, along with hormonal changes, leads to a softening of the cervix. Throughout pregnancy, the cervix and lower uterine segment change but maintain a 'functionally intact' internal os. If the internal os of the cervix dilates or effaces during pregnancy, this can be a bad sign.

In the beginning of pregnancy, cervical dilation associated with some bleeding is known as an 'inevitable miscarriage'. In later pregnancy, cervical dilation or effacement associated with lower abdominal cramps or pressure is a sign of preterm labour (prior to 37 weeks).

Incompetent cervix is defined as a painless dilation or effacement of the cervix, usually occurring between the mid second trimester (about 20 weeks' gestation) to the early third trimester (about 27–30 weeks). Pregnancy losses at progressively earlier gestational ages often reflect an incompetent cervix. This can give way earlier with each subsequent pregnancy. The causes of cervical incompetence can be congenital or acquired and include:

- Congenital abnormality in the composition of the cervix, with a relative deficiency in the tougher collagenous fibroconnective material or relative increase in concentration of the less tough smooth muscle.
- Congenital hypoplasia (underdevelopment) of the cervix, such as with in utero exposure to diethylstilboestrol (DES).
- Trauma to the cervix, such as with mechanical dilators for dilation and curettage (D+C), cervical cone or extensive biopsy and precipitous labours or cervical lacerations during labour and delivery.

TABLE 12.5 Anatomical abnormality assocated with miscarriage risk		
Anatomical abnormality	**Types**	**Complications**
Congenital uterine anomalies	Uterine septum Müllerian anomalies – unicornuate, didelphic and bicornuate uteri Arcuate uterus	The uterine septum is the congenital uterine anomaly most closely linked to RPL, with as much as a 76% risk of spontaneous pregnancy loss among affected patients. Other Müllerian anomalies, including unicornuate, didelphic and bicornuate uteri, have been associated with smaller increases in the risk for RPL.
Intrauterine adhesions	Asherman's syndrome	Intrauterine adhesions, sometimes associated with Asherman's syndrome, may significantly impact placentation and result in early pregnancy loss.
Uterine fibroids	Intramural fibroids larger than 5 cm Submucosal fibroids of any size	Location of leiomyomas is probably more important than size. Intramural fibroids larger than 5 cm, as well as submucosal fibroids of any size, can cause RPL. Postulated mechanisms leading to pregnancy loss include: 1 thinning of the endometrium over the surface of a submucous leiomyoma, predisposing to implantation in a poorly decidualised site 2 rapid growth caused by the hormonal milieu of pregnancy, compromising the blood supply of the leiomyoma and resulting in necrosis ('red degeneration') that, in turn, leads to uterine contractions and eventually fetal expulsion 3 encroachment of leiomyomas on the space required for the developing fetus, leading to premature delivery Surgical procedures to reduce leiomyomata may occasionally be warranted in women experiencing repetitive second-trimester abortions.
Endometrial polyps		Endometrial polyps are a relatively common finding in infertility patients. They can distort the endometrial cavity, may have a detrimental effect on endometrial receptivity and increase the risk of implantation failure. Although treatment seems to be safe and easy, this may not always be the case if endometrial polyps are diagnosed after starting an in vitro fertilisation cycle.[14]
Cervical insufficiency	Cervical amputation Cervical lacerations Forceful cervical dilation Cervical conisation	An intact cervix is an obvious prerequisite for a successful pregnancy. Aetiology may be genetic, for example perturbations of a connective tissue gene (e.g. collagen, fibrillin).

RPL = recurrent pregnancy loss
Sources: Ford HB, Schust DJ. Recurrent pregnancy loss: etiology, diagnosis, and therapy. Rev Obstet Gynecol 2009;2(2):76–83; Berghella V, Rafael TJ, Szychowski JM, et al. Cerclage for short cervix on ultrasonography in women with singleton gestations and previous preterm birth: a meta-analysis. Obstetrics and Gynecology 2011;117(3):663–71.

TABLE 12.6 Anatomical anomaly and related miscarriage risk	
The type of anatomical anomaly	**Percentage**
Cervical weakness	15.9% ($n = 30$)
Septate uterus	11.7% ($n = 22$)
Uterine synechiae	9.6% ($n = 18$)
Endometrial polyps	1.6% ($n = 3$)
Bicornuate uterus	1.1% ($n = 2$)
Arcuate uterus	0.5% ($n = 1$)
Didelphic uterus	0.5% ($n = 1$)
Submucosal myoma	0.5% ($n = 1$)

The cerclage, also known as a cervical stitch, is a surgical treatment to strengthen the cervix, and is to date, medically, the only treatment option. This surgery involves the placement of a suture of the cervix to hold it closed. In appropriately selected women, the improvement of pregnancy outcome with a cerclage is seemingly impressive. Generally, 80–90% of women with cervical incompetence as their cause of recurrent pregnancy loss will deliver a viable live baby born following cerclage placement.

Cervical cerclage shows more benefits in the maternal and neonatal outcomes than vaginal progesterone therapy for women with an asymptomatic short cervix and prior preterm birth history, while cervical cerclage and vaginal progesterone therapies show similar effectiveness for women with an asymptomatic short cervix but without a history of preterm birth.

From the naturopathic perspective, focusing on supporting collagen and connective tissue integrity can be useful in the 4 months of preconception interval and during pregnancy.[17]

Genetics

Around 10–15% of clinically recognised pregnancies result in miscarriage; of these, 50% result from a chromosomal abnormality.[18] Genetic causes of miscarriage can include chromosomal abnormalities, karyotyping abnormalities and MTHFR polymorphisms leading to methylation defects. Trisomies are the most frequently detected anomalies (61.2%), followed by triploidies (12.4%), monosomy X (10.5%), tetraploidies (9.2%) and structural chromosome anomalies (4.7%).[18]

The incidence of fetal chromosomal abnormalities, which is identified in 29–60% of women with recurrent pregnancy loss, decreases as the number of miscarriages increases, suggesting that other mechanisms may play a role in pregnancy loss.[19]

Laboratory studies with IVF patients have found that a very large percentage of oocytes harbour chromosome abnormalities (the leading cause of miscarriage), and one study found that in natural cycles, about 22% of all conceptions never complete implantation.[7] Considering such evidence, some scientists have speculated that factoring in fertilised eggs that do not implant, along with pregnancies that end in miscarriage, around 70–75% of conceptions end up miscarrying. But whether these failed implantations can be defined as a 'miscarriage' is a matter of opinion.

CHROMOSOMAL ABNORMALITIES

Chromosomal abnormalities relate most strongly to first-trimester pregnancy losses. Fetal losses are more likely to be cytogenetically normal (85%) when occurring after the first trimester.[4] The prevalence of chromosomal abnormalities in women facing a single sporadic miscarriage is 45%. Approximately 50–60% of early spontaneous miscarriages are associated with a chromosomal anomaly of embryo or fetus. The most common abnormality is aneuploidy, with autosomal trisomy accounting for more than 50% of chromosomal abnormality. The 30–50% of first-trimester miscarried fetuses that show no chromosomal abnormalities could still have occurred as a result of other genetic aetiologies.

A strong family history of recurrent miscarriage or genetic anomaly suggests a parental karyotypic abnormality, and a chromosomal analysis of the affected partner is a current medical routine investigation. However, parental karyotyping is not predictive of a subsequent miscarriage.[5]

Chromosomal analysis of the miscarriage can offer an explanation in at least 50% of cases. Parental karyotyping is not predictive of a subsequent miscarriage.[5]

From the naturopathic perspective, implementing genetic counselling, in additional to a thorough maternal and paternal preconception healthcare plan, involving detoxification, methylation support, nutritional and botanical treatment and diet and lifestyle interventions for at least 4 months prior to the next conception remains the best strategy for supporting optimal chromosomal health of oocytes, sperm and, hence, the embryo.

Types of chromosomal abnormalities

MORPHOLOGICALLY ABNORMAL

Establishing an aetiology for preimplantation and preclinical losses is not easy, but the one proven explanation is morphological abnormalities in the early embryo. It is presumed that most are due to chromosomal abnormalities. Abnormal embryos presumably should not implant; however, if implantion is achived, they generally would not survive long, leading to very early pregnancy loss.[4]

Morphologically abnormal embryos in humans most likely result from genetic causes.

MONOSOMES

A monosome (a chromosome having no homologue, especially an unpaired X chromosome) is usually miscarried around the time of implantation (4–5 days after conception).[4]

Monosomy X is the single most common chromosomal abnormality among spontaneous abortions, accounting for 15–20% of miscarriages. Monosomy X embryos usually consist of only an umbilical cord stump.[4] Trisomies usually survive longer but rarely to term.[4]

ANEUPLOIDY

Aneuploidy is the second major category of chromosome abnormalities in which the chromosome number is abnormal. An aneuploidy is defined as the condition of having an abnormal number of chromosomes in a haploid set.[20]

The aneuploidy rate can be as high as 50% in morphologically normal embryos. Aneuploidy is said to be present in 6% of sperm from apparently normal men and in 20% of oocytes of apparently normal women.[4]

Autosomal trisomy abnormalities

Second-trimester losses often involve autosomal chromosomal abnormalities such as trisomies 13, 18 and 21; monosomy X; and sex chromosomal polysomies. Autosomal trisomies comprise the largest (approximately 50%) single class of chromosomal complements in cytogenetically abnormal spontaneous miscarriage, the most common being trisomy 16. The risk of most trisomies increases with maternal age.

Trisomies incompatible with life predictably show slower growth than trisomies compatible with life.[4] This also holds among losses after 20 gestational weeks (stillborn infants), in which the frequency of chromosomal abnormalities is approximately 8–13%.[4]

Sex chromosomal polysomy (X or Y)

The 47 XXY and 47 XYY polysomies each occur in about 1 per 800 live born male births; the 47 XXX polysomy occurs in 1 per 800 female births. X or Y polysomies are only slightly more common in miscarried embryos than in live borns. In pregnancies conceived by intracytoplasmic sperm injection (ICSI), the frequency of 47 XXX and 47 XXY embryos and fetuses seems to be increased.[21]

Age

The age of both parents has a significant role as the risk of an adverse pregnancy outcome is increased if the parents are 35 years or older, and it is 50% higher if the mother is 42 years of age.[22]

INHERITED THROMBOPHILIAS

Inherited maternal hypercoagulable states are strongly associated with increased fetal losses, especially in the second trimester of pregnancy. Evidence is less strong for an association between inherited thrombophilias and recurrent early (<10 weeks' gestation) pregnancy loss. These include:

- factor V Leiden (Q1691G→A)
- prothrombin 2021G→A
- homozygosity for methylene tetrahydrofolate reductase gene (MTHFR) 677C→T in the methylene tetrahydrofolate reductase gene (MTHFR)
- compound heterozygosity for methylene tetrahydrofolate reductase gene (MTHFR) 677C→T and 1298A→C.[4]

FACTOR V LEIDEN AND PROTHROMBIN 2021G→A

Factor V Leiden mutation and the prothrombin 2021G→A mutation association is stronger for fetal deaths, such as stillbirths after 20 weeks' gestation, than it is for recurrent early losses. Most recommend testing for factor V Leiden, activated protein C resistance, fasting homocysteine, antiphospholipid antibodies and the prothrombin gene.[4,23]

The potential association between miscarriage and inherited thrombophilias is based on the theory that impaired placental development and function secondary to venous and or arterial thrombosis could lead to miscarriage. Based on studies that have shown maternal blood to begin flowing within the intervillous spaces of the placenta at approximately 10 weeks of gestation, the link between thrombophilias and pregnancy losses at greater than 10 weeks of gestation is more widely accepted than a link to those that occur prior to 10 weeks of gestation.

Evidence that the transfer of nutrition from the maternal blood to the fetal tissues depends on uterine blood flow, and thus may be affected by thrombotic events occurring there, suggests a role for thrombophilias in pregnancy losses regardless of gestational age.[1]

The heritable thrombophilias most often linked to recurrent pregnancy loss include hyperhomocysteinaemia resulting from MTHFR mutations, activated protein C resistance associated with factor V Leiden mutations, protein C and protein S deficiencies, prothrombin promoter mutations and antithrombin mutations.[24]

The prothrombin gene mutation 2021G→A is a hereditable (autosomal-dominant) thrombophilic mutation that results in an increase of around 30% in levels of prothrombin activity. It occurs more commonly in Caucasians, with approximately 2–5% of the Australian population being heterozygous carriers, and is rare in people of Asian or African descent. It has been detected in 5–10% of patients with venous thromboembolism. It has a variable, relatively weak, effect on thrombophilic risk, with heterozygous carriers having approximately a four-fold increased risk. Women who are heterozygous carriers and who are taking the oral contraceptive pill have a moderately increased seven-fold risk.

Patients who are homozygous for the prothrombin gene mutation, or who have combined heterozygosity with factor V Leiden, have up to a 20-fold or more increased risk. Interestingly, the relatively rare homozygous patients have a very variable risk, with around 40% never having any thrombotic events.[25,26]

MTHFR

MTHFR is an important enzyme in the metabolism of folic acid and is crucial for reproductive function. Variation in the sequence of MTHFR has been implicated in subfertility, but definitive data has been lacking.

In a recent study,[27] a detailed analysis of two common MTHFR polymorphisms (c.677C→T and c.1298A→C) was performed. Several striking discoveries were made:

- Maternal MTHFR c.1298A→C genotype strongly influences the likelihood of a pregnancy occurring, with the 1298C allele being significantly overrepresented among women who have undergone several unsuccessful assisted reproductive treatments.
- Parental MTHFR genotypes were shown to affect the production of aneuploid embryos, indicating that MTHFR is one of the few known human genes with the capacity to modulate rates of chromosome abnormality.[28]
- An unusual deviation was noted for the c.677C→T polymorphism in subfertile patients, especially those who had experienced recurrent failure of embryo implantation or miscarriage, potentially explained by a rare case of heterozygote disadvantage.

Despite new evidence and emergent research, testing for MTHFR is still considered unnecessary within the medical gynaecology and obstetrics profession. Routine testing is not done. Even if a couple is tested and diagnosed with MTHFR polymorphisms, and this is taken into clinical consideration, the intervention prescription of 400 micrograms folic acid is considered medical standard. Patients carrying MTHFR polymorphisms have limited genetic capacity to metabolise folic acid and require intervention to be customised with appropriate doses of activated forms of methylated folate, such as folinic acid or L-5-methyltetrahydrofolate. See Chapter 7: Methylation for more information.

PATERNAL GENETIC CONTRIBUTION

Fetal and maternal factors may be equally important in the establishment and maintenance of the placental/maternal arteriovenous circulation. The inheritance of thrombophilia-related genes may be an important factor in recurrent pregnancy loss cases. The vast majority of the research on recurrent pregnancy loss, especially recurrent pregnancy loss related to thrombophilia, has focused on maternal factors, but little is known about the paternal contribution.

A study has found evidence of an association between the paternal carriage of factor V Leiden and prothrombin gene mutation and the partner's predisposition to recurrent pregnancy loss, thereby supporting the hypothesis that genetic contributions from both parents are essential factors.[2]

Immune aetiologies

ALLOIMMUNE

Because a fetus is not genetically identical to its mother, there are immunological events that are critical to occur to allow the mother to carry the fetus throughout gestation without rejection. The immune system needs to quickly recognise the fetus as a non-threat; hence, immune modulation needs to occur and be sustained through the duration of the pregnancy. Human leukocyte antigen (HLA) compatibility plays an important role in this recognition (HLA-A, B, C, DR, DQ and DP).

If the father's HLA markers too closely resemble the mother's HLA, then permission to implant will not be granted, resulting in a spontaneous miscarriage or implantation failure in the cases of couples failing to conceive, either naturally or via IVF.[29]

When the woman becomes pregnant, her immune system should recognise the paternal HLA as different from her own and protect the leukocytes in her uterus by producing protective, 'blocking antibodies'. These antibodies coat the fetal cells, protecting them from rejection by natural killer (NK) cells. When the couple has similar HLA, there may be an inability to detect the differences that trigger the production of the blocking antibodies; therefore, the developing embryo is rejected. Medical treatment involves immunisation of women with concentrates of their partner's leukocytes to amplify the HLA signal and increase the production of blocking antibodies.[30]

Suggested mechanisms of alloimmune-mediated miscarriage include the presence of cytotoxic antibodies, absence of maternal blocking antibodies, inappropriate sharing of human leukocyte antigens and disturbances in NK cell function and distribution.[31]

HLA-G is a unique HLA that is expressed by placental cells. The HLA-G identifier is vital to the maternal tolerance of the fetus and functions as an immunosuppressant. HLA-G serves as a defence mechanism to protect the placenta (embryo) from the maternal NK cells. When the sperm and the woman hosting the pregnancy share several HLA antigens (e.g. HLA- B, C, DR, DQ or DP), there is a breakdown in normal HLA-G-related cytokine signalling and, hence, blocking. As a result, an imbalance occurs between Th-1 (T-helper 1) and Th-2 (T-helper 2), with Th-1 cytokines predominating. This often causes progressive or sudden implantation (trophoblastic) failure, most commonly manifesting as recurrent miscarriages and sometimes as unexplained IVF failure.

Due to the inappropriate production of cytokines, the immune system fails to switch to the Th-2 (T-helper 2) immune response during pregnancy. The Th-1 (T-helper 1) immune response involves a strong and rapid removal or rejection of infection or foreign tissues (in this case, the embryo or fetus), while the Th-2 immune response is a less aggressive response that occurs at the placenta level to protect and prevent rejection of the fetus. Progesterone has been shown to favour the production of Th-2 cytokines.[30,32,33]

Therefore, abnormalities in these intricate immunological mechanisms could lead to both sporadic and recurrent pregnancy loss. Experimental therapies such as paternal leukocyte immunisation, intravenous immune globulin, third-party donor cell immunisation and trophoblastic membrane infusions are currently being studied to research if there indeed are any clinical benefits.

Proposed medical therapies for alloimmune-related pregnancy loss include leukocyte immunisation and intravenous immune globulin.[31]

AUTOIMMUNE

An association between second-trimester pregnancy loss and certain autoimmune diseases is well accepted; however, for first-trimester pregnancy losses, autoimmune factors are less relevant as most are aetiologically associated with chromosomal abnormality.

The spectrum of antibodies found in women with pregnancy loss includes nonspecific antinuclear antibodies, phospholipids antibodies, histones antibodies and double- or single-stranded DNA antibodies.[1]

Acquired thrombophilia

ANTIPHOSPHOLIPID SYNDROME (APS)

Antiphospholipid syndrome (APS) is the only proven thrombophilia that is associated with adverse pregnancy outcomes.[34] APS is an autoimmune disease with the presence of antiphospholipid autoantibodies (aPLs) formed against the person's own tissues. These autoantibodies interfere with coagulation. The positive test may be triggered by a preceding infection, such as syphilis, Lyme disease, Epstein–Barr virus, cytomegalovirus, HIV or hepatitis C virus.[5]

Of women with recurrent miscarriage, 5–15% have clinically significant antiphospholipid antibody titres, compared with 2–5% of unselected obstetrics patients.[35] Recurrent pregnancy loss often will also test positive for aPLs – the actual reported range varies between 8% and 42%.[5]

APS has been clearly linked with many poor obstetric outcomes, including miscarriage, with the treatment of the APS, along with the correction of endocrine disorders, shown to be effective in preventing miscarriage.[7]

The primary antigenic determinant is β_2-glycoprotein, which has an affinity for phospholipids. APS encompasses:
- lupus anticoagulant (LAC) antibodies
- anticardiolipin antibodies (aCL)
- anti-β_2-glycoprotein.[24]

Values for the latter two should be greater than the 99th percentile of moderate or higher titres. Initially, descriptive studies seemed to show increased aCL antibodies in women with first-trimester pregnancy losses.[1]

International consensus classification criteria for diagnosis of APS is based on the presence of at least one of the laboratory criteria and one of the clinical criteria. Laboratory criteria includes the presence of:
- lupus anticoagulant (LA)
- anticardiolipin (aCL) antibody of IgG and/or IgM isotype in serum or plasma, present in medium or high titre

- anti-β_2 glycoprotein-I antibody of IgG and/or IgM isotype in serum or plasma on two or more occasions, at least 12 weeks apart, measured by a standardised enzyme-linked immunosorbent assay (ELISA) tesing. Clinical criteria include:
- vascular thrombosis
- pregnancy morbidity
- one or more unexplained deaths of a morphologically normal fetus at or beyond the 10th week of gestation
- severe pre-eclampsia or eclampsia
- recognised features of placental insufficiency before 34 weeks' gestation
- three or more unexplained consecutive spontaneous abortions before the 10th week of gestation.

The presence of any one of these clinical features plus an abnormal laboratory test diagnose APS (evidence level I).[5]

NATURAL KILLER CELLS

Peripheral natural killer (pNK) and uterine NK (uNK) cells have been associated with miscarriage. Abnormally functioning immunocompetent cells, including natural killer (NK) cells, in the endometrium are thought to be responsible.

In one study, CD56+ CD16+ uK cells were predominant in the decidua specimens of the studied women with repeated miscarriage. A significant association was found between the presence of CD56+ CD16+ uK cells in the studied decidua specimens and unexplained repeated miscarriage.[36]

Many studies have suggested that women with recurrent miscarriages have signs of generally exaggerated inflammatory immune responses, both before and during pregnancy, and signs of breakage of tolerance to autoantigens and fetal antigens.

High exposure to bisphenol A has been associated with natural killer cell (NK) activity.[37]

INFECTIONS

Infections are known aetiology of late fetal losses and logical causes of early fetal losses. However, the role of infectious agents in recurrent loss is less clear, with a proposed incidence of 0.5–5%. See Box 12.1. Unless untreated, infections as a cause of repeated losses seems less likely.

In healthy women, the normal genital tract flora consists for the most part of *Lactobacillus* spp. bacteria.[38] Potentially infective organisms, such as *Gardnerella vaginalis*, group B streptococci, *Staphylococcus aureus*, *Ureaplasma urealyticum* or *Mycoplasma hominis* occasionally displace lactobacilli as the predominant organisms in the vagina, a condition known as bacterial vaginosis (BV).[39] BV is present in 24–25% of women of reproductive age. Links between BV and miscarriage have been suggested. However, it is medically most accepted that BV is associated with preterm delivery in the second and third trimesters.

Of the many organisms implicated in recurrent pregnancy loss, *U. urealyticum* and *M. hominis* seem the most plausibly related to repetitive spontaneous miscarriage as they can persist in an asymptomatic state.

BOX 12.1 Microorganisms associated with spontaneous abortion and stillbirths

- Cytomegalovirus
- Chlamydia trachomatis
- Variola
- Mycoplasma hominis
- Listeria
- Salmonella typhi
- Vibrio fetus
- Gardnerella vaginalis
- Malaria
- Parvovirus B19
- Varicella

Source: Giakoumelou S, Wheelhouse N, Cuschieri K, et al. The role of infection in miscarriage. *Human Reproduction Update* 2016;22(1): 116–33.

It is recommended that pregnant patients are screened for infections as early as practical in pregnancy care, if indeed they have not been screened during the preconception period.[4] These infections are linked to pelvic inflammatory disease (PID). Hence, asking the patient questions about any history of PID symptoms or diagnosis will be of clinical value.[40]

Endocrine aetiologies

Polycystic ovarian syndrome (PCOS), luteal phase defect, hyperprolactinaemia, diabetes mellitus and thyroid disease (hypothyroidism, Hashimoto's thyroiditis, hyperthyroidism and Graves' disease) are among the endocrine disorders implicated in approximately 17–20% of miscarriage and recurrent pregnancy loss.[1]

POLYCYSTIC OVARY SYNDROME (PCOS)

Polycystic ovary syndrome (PCOS) is the most commonly identified ultrasound abnormality among women with recurrent miscarriages. The prevalence of PCOS is 40% among women with recurrent miscarriage.[5]

Hypersecretion of luteinising hormone (LH)

It has been reported that hypersecretion of basal luteinising hormone with or without PCOS is a risk factor for miscarriage. Women with elevated luteinising hormone, a frequent feature of the PCOS, are at increased risk for miscarriage after either spontaneous or assisted conception.[5]

LUTEAL PHASE DEFECT

Luteal phase defect results from inadequate production of progesterone (i.e. progesterone levels are low) by the corpus luteum and the resultant insufficient endometrial maturation for healthy placentation. Implantation into an inhospitable endometrium is an accepted explanation for pregnancy loss.

Luteal phase defect is diagnosed when there is a persistent lag of longer than 2 days in the histological development of the endometrium compared with the day of the menstrual cycle.[1]

Progesterone acts as an immmunomodulator and shifts proinflammatory Th-1 cytokine responses to anti-inflammatory Th-2 cytokine responses, which are ideal and protective of the pregnancy. Dihydrogesterone is a potential immunomodulator; it produces progesterone-induced blocking factors – protein produced by pregnancy lymphocytes following exposure to progesterone. Progesterone-induced blocking factors inhibit cell-mediated cytotoxicity and natural killer cell activity. Hence, optimal endogenous progesterone levels, necessary for a healthy ovulation and luteal phase, are immunoprotective for pregnancy.[5]

Some studies have noted abnormal elevations in luteinising hormone or in androgens, both clinical features of PCOS, among patients experiencing miscarriages. These abnormalities result in premature ageing of the oocyte and/or disrupted maturation of the endometrial lining.[1,41]

HYPERPROLACTINAEMIA

Hyperprolactinaemia is the presence of abnormally high circulating levels of prolactin. Idopathic hyperprolactinaemia is the term used when no cause of prolactin hypersecretion can be identified, and it is causally related to the development of miscarriage in pregnant women, especially women who have a history of recurrent miscarriage.

A possible mechanism is that high levels of prolactin affect the function of the ovaries, resulting in a luteal phase defect and miscarriage. Dopamine agonists are used to treat by lowering prolactin levels and restoring gonadal function.[42]

INSULIN RESISTANCE AND DIABETES

Insulin resistance plays a significant role in recurrent pregnancy loss and is an independent risk factor for spontaneous miscarriage in spontaneous (naturally conceived) pregnancy. It is not always associated with PCOS and can exist as an independent aetiology. Recent meta-analysis concluded that insulin resistance is associated with the susceptibility to recurrent miscarriages, and it may contribute to the occurrence of recurrent miscarriages. Therefore, insulin resistance might be one of the direct causes that lead to recurrent miscarriage.[1,43]

Patients with insulin resistance should be counselled and taught how to improve their insulin sensitivity through lifestyle changes, in addition to naturopathic and medical intervention, for 4 months prior to conceiving again or before pursuing infertility treatment to reduce their risk of spontaneous miscarriage.

Diabetes is also problematic when it comes to miscarriage risks. Poorly controlled diabetes mellitus results in increased risk for fetal loss. Women whose glycosylated haemoglobin level was greater than four standard deviations above the mean showed higher pregnancy loss rates than women with lower glycosylated haemoglobin levels. Subsequent analysis of this dataset confirmed increased loss at glycaemic extremes.[4] Well-controlled or subclinical diabetes should not be considered a cause of early miscarriage.

OBESITY

Obesity has become a major health problem worldwide and is also associated with adverse pregnancy outcome. Obesity is defined as body mass index (BMI) >30 kg/m². Healthy BMI for fertility is 20–24 kg/m².

Obesity may also lead to a poor pregnancy outcome, such as sudden and unexplained intrauterine death.

The risk of miscarriage in the first trimester increases from 12% to 15% in normal-weight women (under 37 years old) to 31% for BMI >35 kg/m². The rate of recurrent miscarriage increases four-fold in obese women.[44]

Obese women had a significantly higher incidence of early and recurrent early miscarriages compared with the woman of a healthy BMI.[45] Weight management is a vital part of preconception care for women preparing to conceive.

HYPOTHYROIDISM AND THYROID ANTIBODIES

Untreated hypothyroidism is associated with spontaneous miscarriage and recurrent pregnancy loss.[1] Decreased conception rates and increased fetal losses are consequences of overt hypothyroidism or hyperthyroidism. Pregnancy loss was higher in thyroid peroxidase negative women whose TSH was 2.5–4 mIU/L compared to those whose TSH was <2.5 mIU/L (6.1% vs. 3.6%).[4]

A consensus is emerging that TSH values >2.5 mIU/L are outside the normal range. Thyroid hormone requirements in early pregnancy are known to be higher than for women who are not pregnant. The clinical aim is to maintain baseline TSH less than 2.5 mIU/L during pregnancy.

Increased frequency of thyroid antibodies, even in the absence of elevated TSH, has also been observed in several series, and some consider autoimmune thyroid disease to be associated with increased risk of miscarriage.[5]

Environmental aetiologies

Links between sporadic and/or recurrent pregnancy loss and occupational and environmental exposures to organic solvents, medications, ionising radiation and toxins have been suggested, although the studies performed are difficult to draw strong conclusions from because they tend to be retrospective and confounded by alternative or additional environmental exposures.

X-RAY IRRADIATION AND CHEMOTHERAPEUTIC AGENTS

Irradiation and antineoplastic agents in high doses are acknowledged abortifacients. Of course, therapeutic x-rays or chemotherapeutic drugs are administered during pregnancy only to seriously ill women whose pregnancies often must be terminated for maternal indications.[1,4]

RADIATION – IONISING, NON-IONISING AND ELECTROMAGNETIC FIELD

Radiation is ubiquitous, and it is estimated that in 1 month of our present day lives, we are exposed to the equivalent amount our great-grandparents experienced in their lifetime. More and more studies show clear detrimental effects on reproductive health, with significant reduction in viable sperm, oocytes and embryonic development. Radiation exposure is also linked to DNA fragmentation.[46]

A study in Australia found significant morphology abnormalities and a greater than four-fold increase in miscarriage with paternal lower abdominal or back x-ray in the previous 2 years.[47]

Protection from unnecessary x-rays, particularly of the lower body, is essential for both prospective parents. Mobile phone storage on the body has also been shown to reduce sperm count and quality by 8–30%.

ALCOHOL

Alcohol consumption should be avoided during pregnancy for many reasons. Although maternal alcoholism (or frequent consumption of intoxicating amounts of alcohol) is consistently associated with higher rates of spontaneous pregnancy loss, a connection with more moderate ingestion remains tenuous. Studies linking moderate alcohol intake with pregnancy loss have shown an increase in risk when more than three drinks per week are consumed during the first trimester (odds ratio [OR] 2.3) or more than five drinks per week are consumed throughout pregnancy (OR 4.8).[1,4]

SMOKING

It seems logical that cigarette smoking could increase the risk of spontaneous abortion based on the ingestion of nicotine, a strong vasoconstrictor that is known to reduce uterine and placental blood flow.[1,4]

CAFFEINE CONSUMPTION

Caffeine, even in amounts as low as three to five cups of coffee per day, may increase the risk of spontaneous pregnancy loss with a dose-dependent response.[1,4]

High doses of caffeine intake (>200 mg/day) during pregnancy increase the risk of miscarriage, independent of pregnancy-related symptoms.[48] A study of over 1000 women who consumed two standard cups of coffee per day found they had double the risk of miscarriage compared with total caffeine avoidance.[48] An association between pregnancy losses and caffeine ingestion greater than 300 mg daily (1.9-fold increase) was also reported.

One confounding problem is the difficulty in taking into account the effects of nausea, which not only decrease caffeine ingestion but seem to be more common in successful pregnancies. In general, reassurances can be given concerning moderate caffeine exposure and pregnancy loss.

CHEMICAL EXPOSURE

Protecting against exposure to or ingestion of toxins in chemicals is important for pregnant women. Many chemicals have been claimed to be associated with fetal losses, including anaesthetic gases, arsenic, aniline dyes, benzene, solvents, ethylene oxide, formaldehyde, pesticides and heavy metals such as lead, mercury and cadmium.[49]

Heavy metals can enter the human body through ingestion via food and water, inhalation including particulate matter, pharmaceutical medications, dental amalgams and personal care products including make-up. Heavy metals are sequestered in tissue in the body and are difficult to detoxify. Challenge testing utilises a variety of chelating agents, including dimercaptosuccinic acid (DMSA), dimercaptopropane sulfonate (DMPS) and ethylenediaminetetraacetic acid (EDTA). The agents are given by a variety of routes of administration. In integrative medicine, a provoked challenge urine test is considered gold standard when investigating heavy metal toxicity. Mineral hair analysis is unreliable due to hair care products and colouring or dyeing agents often being used by women and men, but it can give a good reflection of stored heavy metal exposure provided the above considerations are acknowledged.

A study of 111 women, with a history of recurrent miscarriage, on the impact of heavy metals on ovarian and pituitary function and induction of immunological changes found that heavy metal contamination, as determined through urinary excretion, was correlated with changes in immunological (NK cells, T-cell subpopulations) and hormonal (progesterone, oestradiol, prolactin, TSH) parameters, which are all important factors in the pathogenesis of repeated miscarriage.[50]

Foresight, the UK preconception care organisation, has included heavy metal diagnosis and elimination as a fundamental cornerstone of its programs for over 30 years. While its studies are now considered to be old and outdated, the results are outstanding for resolution of infertility and prevention of miscarriage and poor infant health.[51]

Male factors

Sperm samples from recurrent pregnancy loss couples show an increase in sperm DNA fragmentation. Therefore, it is of utmost importance to screen the male in couples for sperm DNA fragmentation.

In one study, sperm chromatin structure assay (SCSA®), also known as sperm chromatin integrity test (SCIT), was determined as a prediction for male infertility.[52] A chromosomal abnormality was found in 15.2% men with azoospermia and in 2.3% non-azoospermic men. Male factors abnormality is a significant cause for recurrent pregnancy loss after assisted conception.[53]

THE SPERM CHROMATIN STRUCTURE ASSAY (SCSA®) AND DNA FRAGMENTATION

The SCSA is a pioneering assay for the detection of damaged sperm DNA and altered proteins in sperm nuclei. The SCSA® is considered to be the most precise and repeatable test, providing very unique, dual-parameter data.[54]

Studies have described an association between sperm with DNA damage and a history of recurrent miscarriage.

In a retrospective study between 2008 and 2013, couples with a history of recurrent miscarriage (≥3 first-trimester miscarriages) were investigated comprehensively for known causes (karyotype, uterine, APS, thrombophilia) and also by semen analysis, including DNA fragmentation (SCSA®). In couples experiencing recurrent miscarriage, 30% of men had sperm with high levels of DNA fragmentation (DFI >15%), suggesting that this is a contributing factor to the clinical syndrome of recurrent miscarriage.[55]

Sperm quality critically depends on the amount of damage to the sperm DNA, or DNA fragmentation. It is remarkable that this testing technology exists for men. However, to date, no such testing technology is available to assess the DNA integrity of a woman's oocytes.

Sperm DNA fragmentation has little to nothing to do with the parameters that are measured on the routine semen analysis. Rather, it is a completely independent variable.

Men with otherwise seemingly normal semen analyses as set by the World Health Organization can have a high degree of DNA damage, and men with what was called very poor spermatozoa quality can have very little DNA damage.[56]

More importantly, what has also been demonstrated is that the degree of DNA fragmentation correlates very highly with the inability of the sperm to initiate a birth regardless of the type of conception, be it natural, IVF or ICSI technologies. Spermatozoa with high DNA fragmentation may fertilise an oocyte, but subsequent embryo development stops before implantation, or it may even initiate a pregnancy, but there is a significantly higher likelihood that it will result in miscarriage.

The causes of DNA fragmentation are chemical and toxin exposure, heat exposure, testicular varicoeles, infection, advanced paternal age, smoking, testicular cancer, radiation exposure and any other factors that cause elevation in free radical level in semen.

It is known that the egg has the capacity to repair some DNA damage in the sperm. However, extensive DNA fragmentation most likely cannot be repaired by the egg, and the spontaneous miscarriage rate is approximately two times higher if a man has more than 30% of sperm showing DNA fragmentation. DNA fragmentation is an excellent marker for exposure to potential reproductive toxicants and a diagnostic/prognostic tool for potential male infertility.[57]

Social and dietary toxins such as alcohol, caffeine and trans fatty acids (hydrogenated oils) need to be completely avoided in order to improve sperm health.

Alcohol consumption in men has been shown to be associated with poor sperm parameters. From a naturopathic perspective, all alcohol should be excluded from the diet for a minimum of 4 months prior to conceiving for both partners when they are trying to conceive, particularity for those who have experienced miscarriage.

Excessive consumption of refined processed sugars, trans fats, caffeine and sugar are pro-inflammatory and risk increased oxidative stress. Oxidative stress is a proposed aetiology of fragmentation of sperm DNA.

For more information, please refer to Chapter 11: Fertility – Female and Male.

Recommended investigations

The causes of miscarriage are broad and varied, coming from both maternal and paternal factors. A comprehensive approach to investigation is always absolutely necessary.

Naturopathically, we respect that our reproductive system is not isolated and is affected by our diet, lifestyle, emotions, thoughts and environment. No system can be considered in isolation, especially the immune system.[58]

Thorough investigations are said to have mental and emotional benefit for couples who experience the heartbreak of miscarriage. Patients are frantically looking for answers to the 'why?', as opposed to simply being told their miscarriage was due to simply 'misfortune'. Currently, the patient's doctor or specilaist will only investigate when the patient has experienced 2–3 prior miscarriages. It is warranted to investigate after only one miscarriage. Miscarriage can be preventable if the problems can be identified and treated. A thorough investigation often will identify multifaceted issues, giving clarity to treatment direction. See Table 12.7, Table 12.8 and Table 12.9.

TREATMENT APPROACHES

Tender love, extended emotional and clinical care

A cause for recurrent miscarriage can be identified approximately 50–60% of the time, and as we know, there is immense psychological impact of either spontaneous or recurrent miscarriage.[5]

Psychological support is a foremost treatment priority. Frequent discussions, referral to specialised psychological care and sympathetic counselling can reduce anxiety and help couples persevere on their path to parenthood, despite their grief and feelings of hopelessness.

Couples with unexplained spontaneous or recurrent miscarriage should be offered abundant emotional support and reassurance. Referral to a recurrent miscarriage clinic and expert advice help to identify any aetiologies that may be modifiable, therefore improving the chances of a full-term, healthy pregnancy. Holistic support therapy such as flower essences, emotional freedom technique (EFT) and neuro-emotional technique (NET) may also help the emotional terrain.

Lifestyle modification and stress reduction should be emphasised by pointing out that a healthier lifestyle free from tobacco, alcohol, illicit drugs and undue stress cannot hurt, and may significantly improve, the couple's chances for a successful pregnancy.

Therapeutic objectives

1 Address deficiencies and provide nutrient repletion to restore nutrient pathways.
2 Improve potential to carry pregnancy to full term.

Text continued on p. 358

TABLE 12.7 Miscarriage screen: female blood tests		
Assessment	**Test**	**Reference range**
Immunological		
	Lupus anticoagulant	24–38 s
	Immunoglobulin A (IgA)	0.69–30.9 g/L
	Anti-gliadin antibodies IgA	<34 U/mL
	Anti-gliadin antibodies IgG	<20 U/mL
	Antinuclear antibodies (ANA)	Negative
	Transglutaminase antibodies	<7 U/mL
	Endomysial antibodies	Negative
	Anti-dsDNA	Not detected
	Immunophenotypes: natural killer (NK) cells	Normal
	Thyroid peroxidase antibody (TPO Ab)	<30 IU/mL Ideally undetectable
	Thyroglobulin antibody (TG Ab)	<30 IU/mL Ideally undetectable
	Thyroid stimulating hormone receptor antibody (TR Ab) or TSH receptor antibodies	Ideally undetectable
Thrombotic factors		
	Protein C	70–160%
	Protein S	50–140%
	Anti thrombin III	Functional assay 80–120% Immunological assay 75–140%
	APC resistance	Normal: >2.2 Equivocal: 2–2.2
Mucosal immunity		
	Immunoglobulin A IgA	0.8–4 g/L
	Tissue transglutaminase antibodies (TTG)	Not detected
	Anti-endomysial IgA	Not detected
	Anti-gliadin IgA	Not detected
	Anti-gliadin IgG	Not detected
Infective		
	Mycoplasma hominis (S) PCR	Not detected
	Ureaplasma PCR	Not detected
	Listeria monocytogenes PCR	Not detected
	Chlamydia PCR	Not detected
	Toxoplasmosis PCR	Not detected
	Syphilis	Not detected
	Hep B	Not detected
	Hep C	Not detected
	HIV	Not detected
	Rubella	Immune >40 IU/mL

TABLE 12.7 Miscarriage screen: female blood tests—cont'd

Assessment	Test	Reference range
Endocrine		
	Female hormone tracking FSH, LH, E_2, prolactin, P4	Various
	Fasting insulin	4–10 mU/L
	Fasting glucose	3–5.4 mmol/L
	Glucose tolerance test	<5.5 mmol/L and at 2 hours <7.8 mmol/L
	Haemoglobin A1c, A1C (HbA_{1c})	Traditional units – 4–6% SI (IFCC) units – 20–42 mmol/mol
	Human chorionic gonadotropin (hCG)	Women of reproductive age <5 U/L non pregnant Its peak concentration in blood occurs at about 10 weeks' gestation, with concentrations as high as 250 000 U/L. After that, the concentration falls until about 20 weeks. After 20 weeks, the concentration remains stable. 1st day of missed period (4/40) – mean hCG 100 U/L Gestational sac becomes visible on ultrasound (5/40) – 1000 U/L Peak hCG level 9–10/40–120 000 U/L
	Total testosterone Free testosterone FAI	0.5–3.2 nmol/L 3–37 pmol/L Free androgen index = 100 × total testosterone/SHBG
	Sex hormone binding globulin (SHBG)	Adult female (non-pregnant) 20–110 nmol/L
	Prolactin	Adult female <530 mIU/L
	TSH	Adults 0.4–3.5 mIU/L In pregnancy (mIU/L) 0–6 weeks 0.4–3.2 7–12 weeks 0.1–2.8 13–18 weeks 0.1–2.5 19–term weeks 0.3–2.9
	Free T4	Non pregnant 9–25 pmol/L In pregnancy (pmol/L) 0–6 weeks 11–17 7–12 weeks 11–19 13–18 weeks 10–16 19–term weeks 9–14
	Free T3	Non pregnant 2–6 pmol/L In pregnancy (pmol/L) 0–6 weeks 3.5–5.9 7–12 weeks 3.5–6.3 13–18 weeks 3.6–5.9 19 weeks–full term 3.4–5.6
	Metsyn or IR risk assessment BMI calculation Hip to waist ratio	18.5–25 ≥88 cm in European/North American women; ≥80 cm in Asian, Middle Eastern/Mediterranean, Sub-Saharan African; Central and South American women
Genetics		
	MTHFR polymorphism 1298C-A 667C-T	Does not carry
	Extended karyotping	46 XX Female
	Factor V Leiden (FVq506)	Does not carry Arg506 (normal 'wild type')
	HLA-DQ2 or HLA-DQ8	Does not carry

Continued

Assessment	Test	Reference range
TABLE 12.7 Miscarriage screen: female blood tests—cont'd		
	Prothrombin gene mutation	The prothrombin gene mutation G20210A is a hereditable (autosomal-dominant) thrombophilic mutation that results in an increase of around 30% in levels of prothrombin activity. It occurs more commonly in Caucasians, with approximately 2–5% of the Australian population being heterozygous carriers, and is rare in people of Asian or African descent. It has been detected in 5–10% of patients with venous thromboembolism, especially those under 50 years of age, and in up to 15% of patients investigated for thrombophilia.
Biochemical		
	Plasma zinc	12–20 micromols/L
	Serum copper	12.5–24 micromols/L
	Red cell folate	>650 nmol/L
	Caeruloplasmin	0.24–0.58 g/L
	Vitamin B_{12} (cobalamin)	180–790 pmol/L
	Holotranscobalamin (active B_{12})	>35 pmol/L deficiency unlikely 23–35 pmol/L equivocal <23 pmol/L deficiency likely
	Vitamin D (calciferol)	≥75 nmol/L Optimal target for preventing chronic diseases
	Red cell selenium	Plasma 0.7–1.4 micromols/L
	Iron studies	Serum iron 5–30 micromols/L Transferrin 2–3 g/L Transferrin saturation 10–45% Ferritin 3–160 micrograms/L Transferrin saturation
	Fasting homocysteine	5–13 micromols/L
	Cancer antigen 125	<45 U/mL (pre-menopausal) (usually expressed as 99th percentile)
	Full blood count	Normal ranges
	Biochemistry	Normal ranges
	Liver function tests	Normal ranges
	Blood Group	O A B AB
	Blood group antibodies	O – anti A, anti B A – anti B B – anti A AB – none
	Rh antigen	The blood group antibody screen is performed prior to or during pregnancy. The red cell antibody screen is to detect allo-antibodies; that is, antibodies formed due to exposure to a blood group antigen not present in the patient. Allo-antibodies may be due to previous pregnancy, for example, anti-D, or previous blood transfusion, for example, anti-Jk[a]. This test is not designed to detect ABO antibodies, which are detected in the blood group test; that is, 'reverse blood group'. Red cell antibodies detected in pregnant patients may mean the baby will develop haemolytic anaemia and subsequently even death in utero, or anaemia at birth. Repeated monitoring of the allo-antibody levels, as well as close assessment of fetal wellbeing in a fetal medicine clinic, are appropriate.
Toxicity		
	Chelation challenge Provocation test to investigate heavy metal toxicity	Variable

TABLE 12.8 Miscarriage screen: female Ultrasounds and procedures

Assessment	Test	Reference range
Uterine abnormalities	Hysterosalpingography (hy-co-sy)	Hysteroscopic resection of intrauterine adhesions and intrauterine septa are indicated if these abnormalities are identified. Patients undergoing successful hysteroscopic septum resection seem to enjoy near-normal pregnancy outcomes, with term delivery rates of approximately 75% and live birth rates approximating 85%. Myomectomy should be considered in cases of submucosal fibroids or any type fibroids larger than 5 cm. Resection has been shown to significantly improve live birth rates from 57% to 93%.[6] Myomectomy can be performed via open laparotomy, laparoscopy or hysteroscopy.
	Hysteroscopy	No abnormalities detected
	Laparoscopy	No abnormalities detected
	Trans vaginal pelvic ultrasound	No abnormalities detected
Vaginal/cervical swab		
	Gardnerella vaginalis Group B streptococcus β-haemolytic streptococcus *Staphylococcus aureus* *Staphylococcus milleri* *Candida* spp.	Not detected
Endometrial biopsy	Endometrial T-cell subsets	CD56+ (uterine) NK cells and CD57+ cells present in endometrial stromal cell density (as a percentage)

TABLE 12.9 Miscarriage screen: male

Assessment	Test	Reference range
Semen assessments WHO 5th[56]		Lower limit reference
	Semen volume	1.4–1.7 mL
	Total sperm number (10⁶ per ejaculate)	39 (33–46)
	Sperm concentration (10⁶ per mL)	15 (12–16)
	Total motility (PR + NP, %)	40 (38–42)
	Progressive (PR, %)	32 (31–34)
	Vitality (live spermatozoa, %)	58 (55–63)
	Sperm morphology (normal forms, %)	4 (3–4)
	pH	>7.2
	Peroxidase positive leukocytes (10⁶ per mL)	<1
	MAR test (Motile spermatozoa with bound particles, %)	<50
	Immunobead test (Motile spermatozoa with bound beads, %)	<50
	Seminal zinc	>2.4 micromols/ejaculate
	Seminal fructose	>13 micromols/ejaculate
	Seminar neutral glycosidase (mU/ejaculate)	>20
	Sperm chromatin structure assay (SCSA®) or sperm chromatin integrity test (SCIT) for DNA fragmentation index	A normal sample has less than 15% of the sperm with DNA damage. Men with poor fertility potential have greater than 30% of their sperm damaged. A DFI between 16% and 29% is considered good to fair fertility potential, but becomes poorer as it approaches 27%.

Continued

	TABLE 12.9 Miscarriage screen: male—cont'd	
Assessment	**Test**	**Reference range**
Genetics		
	Extended karyotype	
	MTHFR polymorphism 1298C-A 667C-T	Does not carry
	Prothrombin gene mutation G20210A	Does not carry
Biochemical		
	Plasma zinc	12–20 micromols/L
	Serum copper	12.5–24 micromols/L
	Red cell folate	>650 nmol/L
	Caeruloplasmin	0.24–0.58 g/L
	Vitamin B_{12} (cobalamin)	180–790 pmol/L
	Holotranscobalamin (active B_{12})	>35 pmol/L deficiency unlikely 23–35 pmol/L equivocal <23 pmol/L deficiency likely
	Vitamin D (calciferol)	≥75 nmol/L Optimal target for preventing chronic diseases
	Red cell selenium	Plasma 0.7–1.4 micromols/L
	Fasting homocysteine	5–13 micromols/L
	Full blood count	Normal ranges
	Biochemistry	Normal ranges
	LFT	Normal ranges
	Rh antigen	The blood group antibody screen is performed prior to or during pregnancy. The red cell antibody screen is to detect allo-antibodies; that is, antibodies formed due to exposure to a blood group antigen not present in the patient. Allo-antibodies may be due to previous pregnancy, for example, anti-D, or to previous blood transfusion, for example, anti-Jk^a. This test is not designed to detect ABO antibodies, which are detected in the blood group test; that is, 'reverse blood group'. Red cell antibodies detected in pregnant patients may mean the baby will develop haemolytic anaemia and subsequently even death in utero, or anaemia at birth. Repeated monitoring of the allo-antibody levels, as well as close assessment of fetal wellbeing in a fetal medicine clinic, are appropriate.
Toxicity		
	Chelation challenge Provocation test to investigate heavy metal toxicity	Variable

3 Address aetiological factors after investigation, such as immune management, thrombosis management, infections, hormonal factors, genetic polymorphisms, toxicity and stress.

4 Improve first line defence

5 Decrease autoantibody production

6 Address male aetiological factors involved in spontaneous or recurrent miscarriage such as DNA fragmentation, nutritional deficiency, inherited thrombophilias and genetics.

7 Provide antioxidants to reduce oxidation influence on gametes and embryo/fetus.

8 Support communication between the endocrine and reproductive systems.

9 Encourage optimal eliminatory pathways.

10 Support optimal general health.

11 Ensure emotional psychological support to address grief and coming to terms with pregnancy loss. Provide referrals for specialist psychology care if required.

12 Provide appropriate referrals for physical investigations and medical specialist primary care management.

Complete preconception care for both male and female partners

From the naturopathic viewpoint, the best prevention for miscarriage is thorough investigation to identify any modifiable risks, followed by implementation of a treatment plan for both male and female partners for 4 months prior to conceiving again. This may include the use of co-prescribed pharmaceuticals from a medical specialist should allo-immune, autoimmune or thrombotic factors be involved.

Preconception health care for both parents for a *minimum* of 4 months prior to the next conception is extremely important. It has been shown to significantly improve conception rates and increase the chances of a healthy, full-term pregnancy; a natural, intervention-free birth; uninterrupted bonding with reduced risks of postnatal depression; successful and long-term breastfeeding; and finally, the growth and development of healthy children.

For preconception care recommendations, refer to Chapter 11: Fertility – Female and Male.

Treatment during pregnancy to prevent miscarriage is often clinically challenging, as the safety profile of many botanicals is limited in pregnancy and no time is afforded to work with any modifiable risk factors.

THERAPEUTIC RATIONALE FOR BOTANICAL MEDICINES

Amino acids

GLUTAMINE

Glutamine plays an important role in GIT health and subsequent management of autoimmune disease. It has been shown to decrease intestinal permeability in animal models.[44]

α-lipoic acid (ALA)

α-lipoic acid (ALA) is an antioxidant found in virtually all cells of the body. Oxidative stress has a detrimental effect on pregnancy,[59] and due to its potent antioxidant potential, ALA can be expected to play a protective role. ALA is also beneficial in the management of blood glucose metabolism and gestational diabetes.[44]

N-ACETYLCYSTEINE (NAC)

Taking 600 mg of NAC boosts the chances of pregnancy continuing past 20 weeks by 190%.

Pregnancy could be associated with a state of oxidative stress that could initiate and propagate a cascade of changes that may lead to miscarriage. This process of oxidative stress may be suppressed by the antioxidant effect of NAC. A study aimed to evaluate the effect of NAC therapy in patients diagnosed with unexplained recurrent miscarriage. A group of patients with history of recurrent unexplained miscarriage were treated with NAC 0.6 g + folic acid 500 micrograms/day and compared with an aged-matched group of patients treated with folic acid 500 micrograms/day alone. NAC + folic acid compared with folic acid alone caused a significantly increased rate of continuation of a living pregnancy up to and beyond 20 weeks (OR = 2.9). NAC + folic acid was associated with a significant increase in the take-home baby rate compared with folic acid alone (OR = 1.98). NAC is a well-tolerated amino acid treatment that could be a potentially effective treatment in patients with unexplained recurrent miscarriage.[60]

NAC protects pregnancy from maternal inflammation. Maternal infection or inflammation may induce fetal inflammatory responses and potentially fetal brain injury. NAC, a known anti-inflammatory, may modulate the fetal cytokine response to maternal lipopolysaccharide (an endotoxin injected to create a strong immune response). NAC before lipopolysaccharide injection significantly reduced the fetal IL-6 and IL-1 beta response. Fetal IL-10 was not attenuated by any treatment. NAC attenuated both maternal pro- and anti-inflammatory responses to lipopolysaccharide injection. Maternal NAC suppressed fetal and maternal inflammatory responses. These results suggest that prophylactic NAC may protect the fetus from maternal inflammation and subsequently lower risks of miscarriage.[61]

Glutathione peroxidase is lower in women who miscarry. Red cell and plasma glutathione peroxidase activities of women who had had a miscarriage were significantly lower than in both normal pregnancies and the control group (NAC is a precursor to glutathione peroxidase). The decreased activities of the antioxidant enzymes, red cell and plasma glutathione peroxidase may play an important role in the aetiology of miscarriage.[62]

NAC also helps prevent diabetes-induced birth defects and miscarriage.[63]

CYSTEINE

The cysteine-rich secretory proteins are found in a remarkable range of organisms spanning each of the animal kingdoms and show expression bias to the reproductive tract and immune tissues.

These superfamily proteins are most often secreted and have an extracellular endocrine or paracrine function, and are involved in processes including the regulation of extracellular matrix and branching morphogenesis, potentially as either proteases or protease inhibitors, in ion channel regulation in fertility.

Catabolite activator protein's (CAP) roles in reproduction include spermatogenesis, epididymal maturation and sperm capacitation, and sperm and egg fusion.

Genetic studies associate single nucleotide polymorphisms (SNPs) with reduced fertility.[64]

Cysteine improves glutathione levels, which is important for maturation and embryo development.[65]

METHIONINE

Methionine is critical for optimal methylation, sulphation pathways and overall endocrine regulation. These factors all impact on reproductive outcome.

FISH OIL – OMEGA-3 ESSENTIAL FATTY ACIDS

It was been shown that 5.1 g DHA/EPA lowered miscarriage odds to just 9% in women with APS. Twenty-two patients with persistent APS associated with recurrent miscarriage were treated with fish oil, equivalent to 5.1 g eicosapentaenoic acid (EPA) and docosahexaenoic acid (DHA), at a ratio of 1.5 EPA to DHA. Twenty-two patients had 23 pregnancies (one patient had two pregnancies) over a period of 3 years. There was only one intrauterine fetal death at the 27th week associated with preeclampsia. Twenty-one pregnancies, 19 of which ended after the 37th week, produced a baby. Two pregnancies ended with caesarean births for preeclampsia at 30th and 35th week of gestation and one is ongoing at 32nd week. All babies are well. The weight at birth of babies delivered at term was always >2500 g.[66]

VITAMINS

The use of a general multivitamin can lower miscarriage risk by 57%.[67]

Vitamin A

Vitamin A is an antioxidant required for cell growth and differentiation, which is especially pertinent for the development of the embryo. It is required for gene expression and cell differentiation in organogenesis and embryonic development. It is also required for immunity, regulatory functions and epithelial tissue integrity.[44]

The levels of reduced glutathione, vitamin A, vitamin E and beta carotene were significantly lower in women with habitual miscarriage than in controls. However, the plasma levels of lipid peroxidation, alkaline phosphatase, glucose and blood haemoglobin were significantly higher in habitual miscarriage than in controls. According to the results of this study, it was observed that the levels of lipid peroxidation were increased and plasma levels of vitamin A, vitamin E and beta carotene were decreased in habitual miscarriage.[68]

A full discussion regarding vitamin A safety and pregnancy is given in Chapter 13: Pregnancy and Labour.

Vitamin E

Vitamin E levels are lower in cases of miscarriage with autoimmune, luteal phase defect and unexplained aetiology. Women with recurrent miscarriage were divided into four subgroups according to the aetiology: autoimmune, luteal phase defect, anatomical defect and unexplained. Plasma levels of vitamin C and vitamin E were significantly decreased in autoimmune, unexplained and luteal phase defect subgroups than those in two control groups and the anatomical defect group. Copper levels showed a decline in autoimmune and unexplained subgroups compared to controls, anatomical defect and luteal phase defect aborters. It is suggested that decreased concentrations of plasma, vitamin C and vitamin E in unexplained, autoimmune and luteal phase defect reflect the increased oxidative stress, expressing a progress of the condition. Also, the imbalance between antioxidant defence and free radical activity is more evident in the autoimmune subgroup. As a conclusion, although impaired antioxidant defence may be responsible for recurrent miscarriage, the recurrent miscarriages may also result in oxidative stress and depletion and weakness of antioxidant defence.[69]

Vitamin E is effective in preventing miscarriage not caused by thrombophilia. Considering the potential adverse effects of anticoagulation in miscarriage treatment, researchers investigated whether antioxidants might exert the same immunoprotection. Although the fertility properties of vitamin E have been associated with its antioxidant capacity, its effect on cytokine balance during pregnancy is still unknown. Vitamin E (15 mg/day) was seen to decrease miscarriage rate and to increase IL-6 placental levels, while increasing vascular endothelial growth factor (VEGF) placental levels. Vitamin E was not only able to prevent fetal wastage but also to balance IL-6 and VEGF placental levels, presenting a new potential therapeutic alternative for patients with recurrent miscarriage not associated with thrombophilias.[70]

Vitamin D

Vitamin D is a lipid-soluble vitamin which acts as a potent immunomodulator and can support skeletal health in both the mother and the developing fetus. The active form of vitamin D, 1-25-dihydroxyvitamin D_3, has been shown to regulate the transcription and function of genes associated with placental invasion, normal implantation and angiogenesis. Specifically, its application is best considered in incidences of miscarriage, implantation issues or general infertility.[44]

Vitamin D_3 can be seen as an immunomodulatory agent in treatment of recurrent miscarriage. Different mechanisms have been proposed to account for the immunosuppressive effect of 1-alpha, 25-dihydroxy-vitamin-D_3. A portion of the vitamin D activity involves the downregulation of IL-2, IFN-gamma and TNF-α genes transcription. Because the immunomodulatory effects of vitamin D are very similar to IL-10 effects (downregulates the expression of Th1 cytokines), vitamin D may be valuable as an immunotherapy in the treatment of recurrent miscarriage cases.[71]

Vitamin D reduces inflammation associated with miscarriage. Elevated placental proinflammatory cytokine release is associated with miscarriage, preterm labour and preeclampsia. Specifically, TNF-α-induced cytokines may threaten pregnancy outcome. Since trophoblasts produce calcitriol, a hormone with strong immunosuppressive properties, the effects of this secosteroid on inflammatory cytokines induced in trophoblasts was assessed by challenge with TNF-α. Vitamin D inhibited the expression profile of inflammatory cytokine genes in a dose–response manner. These data show that vitamin D prevents TNF-α induction of inflammatory cytokines through a process likely to be mediated by the vitamin D receptor.[72]

Vitamin C and bioflavonoids

It is important to mimic nature and it is recommended to always prescribe vitamin C with concurrent bioflavonoids. Bioflavonoids have been shown to strengthen capillaries and help prevent miscarriage and breakthrough bleeding.

Low vitamin C levels have been observed in miscarriage with autoimmune, luteal phase or unexplained causes. In one study, plasma levels of vitamin C and vitamin E were significantly decreased in autoimmune recurrent miscarriage, unexplained recurrent miscarriage and luteal phase defect recurrent miscarriage subgroups than those in two control groups and the anatomical defect recurrent miscarriage group. It was suggested that decreased concentrations of plasma vitamin C and vitamin E in unexplained, autoimmune and luteal phase defect recurrent miscarriage reflect the increased oxidative stress, expressing a progress of the condition. Also, the imbalance between antioxidant defence and free radical activity was more evident in the autoimmune recurrent miscarriage subgroup. Although impaired antioxidant defence may be responsible for recurrent miscarriage, the recurrent miscarriage may also result in oxidative stress and depletion and weakness of antioxidant defence.[69]

INOSITOL

Inositol is of benefit for managing insulin resistance and inflammation, which are both linked to increased risks of miscarriage.

Myo-inositol lowers glucose levels, low density lipoproteins (LDLs) and C-reactive protein. The effects of increased serum plasmalogen levels, induced by 2-week administration of myo-inositol treatment, on several clinical and biochemical parameters were examined in 17 hyperlipidaemic subjects, including some with metabolic syndrome. After myo-inositol treatment, significant increases in plasmalogen-related parameters, particularly ChoPlas, and significant decreases in atherogenic cholesterols including small dense LDL were observed. Among the hyperlipidaemic subjects treated with myo-inositol, compared to subjects without metabolic syndrome, subjects with metabolic syndrome had a significant increase in plasmalogens and a tendency towards reduced small dense LDL, high-sensitivity C-reactive protein and blood glucose levels. Correlation analyses between the measured parameters showed that plasmalogens, as well as HDL, function as beneficial factors, and that small dense LDL is a very important risk factor that shows positive correlations with many other risk factors. Inositol also may be of benefit in cases of recurrent miscarriage linked to insulin resistance and PCOS.[73]

MINERALS

Zinc

Zinc is an essential trace element that is known to play an important role in all human living cells, including the transcription of RNA, and the replication of DNA, as well as the synthesis of protein, all of which are crucial for reproduction and fertility and pregnancy outcomes.

In one study, the risk of miscarriage increased when both serum zinc decreased and copper concentrations increased. Methionine-supplemented cows had a higher risk of fetal loss compared with zinc-methionine-supplemented cows (odds ratio = 2.98). Cows that received no supplements had a higher risk for miscarriage than did zinc-methionine-supplemented cows. Results suggest that inflammation and zinc status may play an important role in miscarriage.[74]

Magnesium

Magnesium functions as a cofactor in over 300 enzyme systems within the human body. Magnesium is also critical for blood sugar metabolism, calcium metabolism, mitochondrial health and cardiovascular health of mother and fetus.

Studies observe that low magnesium is associated with miscarriage. Some studies suggest that magnesium deficiency may play a role in miscarriage of diabetic women, in fetal malformations and in the pathogenesis of neonatal hypocalcaemia of the infants of diabetic mothers.

Low calcium, iron, zinc and magnesium are associated with higher rate of miscarriage. Female rats received a control or a 50% mineral-restricted diet for 12 weeks, by which time mineral-restricted rats had lower plasma iron, zinc, magnesium and calcium concentrations. Following mating with control males, a third of the mineral-restricted dams were shifted to the control diet from parturition. Pregnant mineral-restricted dams had a higher miscarriage rate, and body weights of their pups at birth and weaning were lower.[44,75]

Chromium

Chromium improves insulin sensitivity and is of benefit for patients with concurrent insulin resistance and history of recurrent miscarriage.[76]

Maternal undernutrition is linked with an elevated risk of diabetes mellitus in offspring regardless of the postnatal dietary status. This is also found in maternal micronutrition deficiency, especial chromium, which is a key glucose regulator. DNA methylation profiling of offspring livers revealed 935 differentially methylated genes in livers of the maternal chromium restriction diet group. Pathway analysis identified the insulin-signalling pathway was the main process affected by hypermethylated genes.[77]

Iodine

Iodine is critical for healthy thyroid hormone metabolism and adequate intake of iodine is crucial for full-term healthy pregnancy outcomes. It is an essential component of the thyroid hormones T3 and T4 and is required for human growth and development throughout the body and of a fetus.

Maternal subclinical hypothyroidism and thyroid autoimmunity in early gestation are associated with increased risk of miscarriage. One of the factors involved is related to iodine deficiency.[78]

The increased incidence of pregnancy loss in pregnant women with TSH levels between 2.5 and 5 mIU/L provides strong physiological evidence to support redefining the TSH upper limit of normal in the first trimester to 2.5 mIU/L.[79]

Selenium

Selenium is a trace mineral required for healthy function of the thyroid gland. Supplementation may help reduce the risk of miscarriage, such as in thyroid autoimmunity, which may be linked to recurrent miscarriage and infertility.

Selenoproteins play an important role in antioxidant defence systems, such as the action of glutathione peroxidase (GPx), that occur within the cells.

Taking 200 micrograms/day selenium reduced antibodies by 21%. Selenium supplementation (200 micrograms/day) resulted in significant reduction of serum anti-TPO levels during the first 6 months (by 5.6% and 9.9% at 3 and 6 months, respectively). An overall reduction of 21% was seen after 1 year.[80]

Selenium reduces inflammatory cytokines in autoimmune thyroid patients, and is therefore relevant to spontaneous or recurrent miscarriage cases exhibiting positive thyroid antibodies. A study was conducted to compare the effect of selenomethionine on monocyte and lymphocyte cytokine release and systemic inflammation in patients with Hashimoto's thyroiditis. Selenomethionine inhibited lymphocyte release of IL-2, interferon-γ and TNF-α, which was accompanied by a reduction in plasma C-reactive protein levels. Selenomethionine exhibits a systemic antiinflammatory effect in euthyroid females with Hashimoto's thyroiditis. This action, which correlates with a reduction in thyroid peroxidase antibody titres, may be associated with clinical benefits in the prevention and management of Hashimoto's thyroiditis, particularly in subjects receiving both agents.[81]

METHYLATION

For more information regarding methylation support, refer to Chapter 7: Methylation.

PROBIOTICS

Stress affects maternal adaptation to pregnancy and subsequently impedes feto-maternal tolerance. Probiotics have a positive effect on the stress-induced signalling cascade, linking the disequilibrium of the endogenous microflora to immune activation and pregnancy loss. The stress signalling cascade utilises the presence of lipopolysaccharide (LPS), which acts as a danger signal via Toll-like receptor 4.

Modulating the intestinal flora by probiotic bacteria, and in turn, the intestinal barrier function, may be enhanced and mediators of immune tolerance may be restored (i.e. in the context of reproduction and pregnancy outcomes).[82]

Probiotics are also of benefit in HLA and immune tolerance in pregnancy.[83] For more information regarding microbiome support, refer to Chapter 6: Microbiome.

NUTRITIONAL MEDICINE (DIETARY)

Therapeutic objectives

1   Provide nutritional sustenance to encourage health in preconception and for the duration of the pregnancy.

2   Avoid dietary factors that compound miscarriage including caffeine, alcohol and trans fatty acids. Encourage general wholefood dietary principles.

3   Address macro- and micronutrient deficiencies with a focus on folate, B_{12} and vitamin D.

Dietary inclusions

OILY FISH

Adequate intake of omega-3 fatty acids is required to ensure stable cell membrane fluidity and energy production for the developing embryo. Ensure the consumption of small oily fish and avoid larger fish known to contain higher levels of heavy metals such as methylmercury.

WHOLEFOOD DIET

A healthy diet undertaken by both partners in the preconception period and continued for the mother during pregnancy provides a wide variety of nutrients required for the development and maturation of an embryo and fetus. A wholefood diet based on a broad variety of fresh, seasonal foods, organic where possible, will contain a blend of synergistic nutrients required for a healthy full-term pregnancy. See Tables 12.10–12.13.

THERAPEUTIC RATIONALE FOR NUTRITIONAL MEDICINES

Glycyrrhiza glabra (liquorice)

Liquorice is described traditionally as an adrenal agent and adrenocorticotropic (which herbalists now regard as adrenal tonic). It is indicated for primary adrenocortical insufficiency and has anti-inflammatory, immune modulatory and corticosteroid-like activity.

Liquorice is protective against the side effects of adrenal atrophy common to the medium- to long-term corticosteroid drugs, which may be prescribed by reproductive immunologist specialists to manage autoimmune-mediated miscarriage cases, such as those with elevated NK cells.

Liquorice is well indicated for adrenal depletion to aid the recovery of the adrenal cortex. It can be used to support adrenal cortex function in times of high stress and also for fatigue, anxiety, sleeplessness or reduced immune function during periods of prolonged stress and for chronic illness and chronic autoimmune diseases.

Glycyrrhiza glabra root contains triterpenoid saponins, especially glycyrrhizin, which is present in the form of potassium and calcium salts. Glycyrrhetinic acid is the aglycone of glycyrrhizin.

Liquorice used in herbal products usually contains about 1.5% glycyrrhizin (weight/weight of dried root). However, products can be made with high-grade extracts. High-grade liquorice extracts contain about 3% glycyrrhizin. For example, a product with a maximum daily dose of 6 g of standard quality liquorice root would provide about 90 mg/day of glycyrrhizin. A product with a maximum daily dose of 3 g of high-grade liquorice root would also provide about 90 mg/day of glycyrrhizin. When

TABLE 12.10 Sample daily diet

Breakfast	Nourishing green quinoa bowl Steamed quinoa served with lightly sauteed broccoli, edamame, avocado, pumpkin seeds, a poached/boiled egg sprinkled with black sesame seeds (Can be prepped the night before to be more time efficient in the morning)	Broccoli, edamame and avocado are all excellent sources of folate. Higher intake of folate is associated with reduced risk of spontaneous abortion.[85] Greater than 730 micrograms/day of folate, compared to none, was associated with a 20% reduced risk of spontaneous abortion.[85] It is suggested that for every 42 women who go from taking 400 micrograms/day of folate to 730 micrograms/day, one spontaneous abortion could be prevented.[85] The addition of pumpkin seeds and eggs provides high-quality protein and zinc. Zinc is essential for cell division, production of hormones and regulation of the immune system. Maternal zinc deficiency may result in embryo/fetal death, intrauterine growth retardation and teratogenesis.[86]
Lunch	Brown lentil salad with roasted butternut pumpkin, pomegranate, zucchini noodles and microgreens sprinkled with dulse flakes	A wholefood diet rich in fruits, vegetables, whole grains and fish may be protective against pregnancy loss.[87] Emphasis should be on ample green vegetables and a variety of fruits since dietary patterns that are low in green vegetables and fruit and high in saturated fats are associated with an increased risk of miscarriage.[88] Since chromosomal abnormalities are implicated in the case of about 50% of all clinical pregnancy losses[89] and antioxidants assist in protecting chromosomes from damage, antioxidant-rich foods such as pomegranate are advocated. The addition of dulse flakes provides a source of iodine. Moderate-to-severe iodine deficiency during pregnancy increases rates of spontaneous abortion.[90] Iodine is also essential for healthy thyroid function. Miscarriage rates are higher in those with thyroid disease.[91]
Dinner	Black bean spaghetti with lean beef strips, baby spinach, fresh basil and heirloom tomatoes	Black beans are an excellent source of fibre and consumption is associated with an increase in antioxidant status. A number of studies suggest that suboptimal vitamin B_6 status and elevated homocysteine concentrations (a marker of poor folate or vitamin B_{12} status) may increase the risk of spontaneous abortion.[92,93] Spinach is a source of folate. Increasing consumption of folate-containing foods has been shown to reduce homocysteine levels. A diet emphasising foods rich in vitamins B_6 and B_{12} (found in red meat) is also important.
Snack	Dandelion tea Fresh fruit, smoothies, vegetable juices, nuts and seeds	Caffeine intake during early pregnancy is associated with increased miscarriage rates; thus water, herbal teas and juices are preferable. A meta-analysis of 26 studies encompassing approximately 15 000 cases of miscarriage from over 180 000 women found that for every 100 mg/day increase in caffeine intake in early pregnancy, the risk of spontaneous abortion increased by 14% (in a relatively linear fashion).[94] Concentrated source of antioxidants. Antioxidant status has been found to be low in women who have just had a miscarriage.[95]

administered for a short period of time (e.g. a few days to a week), the dosage of glycyrrhizin can be higher than 90 mg/day.

CAUTIONS AND CONTRAINDICATIONS

Liquorice is contraindicated in hypertension (including women who are prone to hypertension in pregnancy), oedema and in those taking thiazide or loop diuretics. In pregnancy, the lowest dosage is recommended for short periods only.[99–101]

Rehmannia glutinosa (Rehmannia)

Rehmannia glutinosa unprocessed root is used in traditional Chinese medicine (TCM) to reduce heat in the blood, nourish yin and promote the production of body fluid. Indications for this type of rehmannia include febrile diseases, general debility, to prolong life and to prevent senility.

In Western herbal medicine, rehmannia is regarded as an adrenal tonic, due mainly to the activity demonstrated in experimental studies.[100]

Rehmannia may be beneficial for the treatment of conditions that involve the immune system, and in the case of autoimmune-mediated recurrent miscarriage, can prove to be a well-indicated herb, including for those who have been prescribed steroids for management of antibodies involved in miscarriage.

Rehmannia treatment has also prevented or reversed morphological changes in the pituitary and adrenal cortex, appearing to antagonise the suppressive effect of glucocorticoids on the hypothalamic–pituitary–adrenal axis.[102]

Oral administration (10–500 mg/kg) of several fractions from the ethanol extract of rehmannia had an immune-modulating effect in an experimental model.[103]

Paeonia lactiflora (paeonia)

In China, Korea and Japan, a decoction of the dried root without bark of *Paeonia lactiflora* has been used in the treatment of inflammatory autoimmune diseases and dysmenorrhoea for more than 1200 years.

A water/ethanol extract of the root is now known as total glucosides of peony (TGP), which contains more than

Text continued on p. 374

TABLE 12.11 Miscarriage management treatment approaches

		Female	
Aetiology	Medical management Rx	Naturopathic treatment Rx Preconception phase	Naturopathic treatment Rx In pregnancy
Immunological		Complementary to medical management	Complementary to medical management
Lupus anticoagulant	Low-dose steroid therapy Heprin Enoxaparin sodium (clexane) Aspirin[96]	*Glycyrrhiza glabra* (liquorice) extract equivalent to dry root 1.75–3.5 g per day or liquorice root 1:1 extract 2.14–5.7 mL per day *Rehmannia glutinosa* (rehmannia) extract equivalent to dry root 350–1400 mg per day or rehmannia root 1:2 extract 4.2–8.5 mL per day *Bupleurum falcatum* (bupleurum) extract equivalent to dry root 700–2800 mg per day or bupleurum root 1:2 extract 3.5–8.5 mL per day *Hemidesmus indicus* (hemidesmus) extract equivalent to dry root 500–2000 mg per day or hemidesmus root 1:2 extract 3.5–8.5 mL per day *Paeonia lactiflora* (paeonia) extract equivalent to dry root 800–3200 mg per day Vitamin D 1000–5000 IU per day dependent on results of 25-OH-D blood tests	*Glycyrrhiza glabra* (liquorice) extract equivalent to dry root 1.75–3.5 g per day or liquorice root 1:1 extract 2.14–5.7 mL per day *A *Rehmannia glutinosa* (rehmannia) extract equivalent to dry root 350–1400 mg per day or rehmannia root 1:2 extract 4.2–8.5 mL per day *B3 *Bupleurum falcatum* (bupleurum) extract equivalent to dry root 700–2800 mg per day or bupleurum root 1:2 extract 3.5–8.5 mL per day *B1 *Hemidesmus indicus* (hemidesmus) extract equivalent to dry root 500–2000 mg per day or hemidesmus root 1:2 extract 3.5–8.5 mL per day *Paeonia lactiflora* (paeonia) extract equivalent to dry root 800–3200 mg per day or paeonia root extract 1:2 4.2–8.5 mL per day Vitamin D 1000–5000 IU per day dependent on results of 25-OH-D blood tests

Anti-gliadin antibodies IgA Anti-gliadin antibodies IgG Transglutaminase antibodies Endomysial antibodies	No treatment unless biopsy confirmed coeliac disease If coeliac, gluten-free diet	Gluten-free diet Gut repair anti-inflammatory protocol Glutamine 2000–4000 mg per day Ulmus rubra stem bark inner powder 500–2000 mg per day Probiotics multi-strain 30 billion colony-forming units Such as: Bifidobacterium longum BB536 Bifidobacterium breve M-16V Bifidobacterium infantis M-63 Bifidobacterium lactis Bi-04 Bifidobacterium lactis HN019 Lactobacillus rhamnosus HN001 Lactobacillus paracasei Lpc-37 Lactobacillus salivarius Ls-33 Lactobacillus casei Lc-11 Curcumin phospholipid complex containing curcumin 90 mg 500–1000 mg per day *A Glycyrrhiza glabra (liquorice) extract equivalent to dry root 1.75–3.5 g per day or liquorice root 1:1 extract 2.14–5.7 mL per day	Gluten-free diet Gut repair anti-inflammatory protocol Glutamine 2000–4000 mg per day Ulmus rubra stem bark inner powder 500–2000 mg per day *A Probiotics multi-strain 30 billion colony-forming units Such as: Bifidobacterium longum BB536 Bifidobacterium breve M-16V Bifidobacterium infantis M-63 Bifidobacterium lactis Bi-04 Bifidobacterium lactis HN019 Lactobacillus rhamnosus HN001 Lactobacillus paracasei Lpc-37 Lactobacillus salivarius Ls-33 Lactobacillus casei Lc-11 Curcumin phospholipid complex containing curcumin 90 mg 500–1000 mg per day *A Glycyrrhiza glabra (liquorice) extract equivalent to dry root 1.75–3.5 g per day or liquorice root 1:1 extract 2.14–5.7 mL per day *A

Continued

TABLE 12.11 Miscarriage management treatment approaches—cont'd

Female

Aetiology	Medical management Rx	Naturopathic treatment Rx Preconception phase	Naturopathic treatment Rx In pregnancy
Immunological		Complementary to medical management	Complementary to medical management
Antinuclear antibodies (ANA)	Oral prednisolone	Glycyrrhiza glabra (liquorice) extract equivalent to dry root 1.75–3.5 g per day or liquorice root 1:1 extract 2.14–5.7 mL per day Rehmannia glutinosa (rehmannia) extract equivalent to dry root 350–1400 mg per day or rehmannia root 1:2 extract 4.2–8.5 mL per day Bupleurum falcatum (bupleurum) extract equivalent to dry root 700–2800 mg per day or bupleurum root 1:2 extract 3.5–8.5 mL per day Hemidesmus indicus (hemidesmus) extract equivalent to dry root 500–2000 mg per day or hemidesmus root 1:2 extract 3.5–8.5 mL per day Paeonia lactiflora (paeonia) extract equivalent to dry root 800–3200 mg per day or paeonia root extract 1:2 4.2–8.5 mL per day Vitamin D 1000–5000 IU per day dependent on results of 25-OH-D blood tests	Glycyrrhiza glabra (liquorice) extract equivalent to dry root 1.75–3.5 g per day or liquorice root 1:1 extract 2.14–5.7 mL per day *A Rehmannia glutinosa (rehmannia) extract equivalent to dry root 350–1400 mg per day or rehmannia root 1:2 extract 4.2–8.5 mL per day *B3 Bupleurum falcatum (bupleurum) extract equivalent to dry root 700–2800 mg per day or bupleurum root 1:2 extract 3.5–8.5 mL per day *B1 Hemidesmus indicus (hemidesmus) extract equivalent to dry root 500–2000 mg per day or hemidesmus root 1:2 extract 3.5–8.5 mL per day Paeonia lactiflora (paeonia) extract equivalent to dry root 800–3200 mg per day or paeonia root extract 1:2 4.2–8.5 mL per day Vitamin D 1000–5000 IU per day dependent on results of 25-OH-D blood tests

		Anti-thrombotic protocol	Anti-thrombotic protocol
Peripheral natural killer (pNK) and uterine NK (uNK)	Oral prednisolone Intravenous immunoglobulins Mechanisms of possible efficacy of high dose of intravenous immunoglobulin therapy for recurrent miscarriage may include enhancement of CD94 expression and subsequent suppression of NK cell cytotoxicity. The Cochrane review analysed various strategies including paternal cell immunisation, third-party donor leukocytes, trophoblast membranes and intravenous immune globulin. One of these interventions proved beneficial over placebo in improving the live birth rate. Meta-analysis showed that IVIG increased the rates of live birth in secondary recurrent miscarriage, but there was insufficient evidence for its use in primary recurrent miscarriage.[5]	*Glycyrrhiza glabra* (liquorice) extract equivalent to dry root 1.75–3.5 g per day or liquorice root 1:1 extract 2.14–5.7 mL per day *Rehmannia glutinosa* (rehmannia) extract equivalent to dry root 350–1400 mg per day or rehmannia root 1:2 extract 4.2–8.5 mL per day *Bupleurum falcatum* (bupleurum) extract equivalent to dry root 700–2800 mg per day or bupleurum root 1:2 extract 3.5–8.5 mL per day *Hemidesmus indicus* (hemidesmus) extract equivalent to dry root 500–2000 mg per day or hemidesmus root 1:2 extract 3.5–8.5 mL per day *Paeonia lactiflora* (paeonia) extract equivalent to dry root 800–3200 mg per day or paeonia root extract 1:2 4.2–8.5 mL per day Curcumin phospholipid complex containing curcumin 90 mg 500–1000 mg per day Vitamin D$_3$ 1000–5000 IU per day, based on blood test results for 25-OH-D	*Glycyrrhiza glabra* (liquorice) extract equivalent to dry root 1.75–3.5 g per day or liquorice root 1:1 extract 2.14–5.7 mL per day *A *Rehmannia glutinosa* (rehmannia) extract equivalent to dry root 350–1400 mg per day or rehmannia root 1:2 extract 4.2–8.5 mL per day *Bupleurum falcatum* (bupleurum) extract equivalent to dry root 700–2800 mg per day or bupleurum root 1:2 extract 3.5–8.5 mL per day *Hemidesmus indicus* (hemidesmus) extract equivalent to dry root 500–2000 mg per day or hemidesmus root 1:2 extract 3.5–8.5 mL per day *B1 *Paeonia lactiflora* (paeonia) extract equivalent to dry root 800–3200 mg per day or paeonia root extract 1:2 4.2–8.5 mL per day Curcumin phospholipid complex containing curcumin 90 mg 500–1000 mg per day *A Vitamin D$_3$ 1000–5000 IU per day, based on blood test results for 25-OH-D

Inherited thrombophilia		Anti-thrombotic protocol	Anti-thrombotic protocol
Antithrombin activity Protein C activity, Protein S levels Factor V Leiden (F5) and/or prothrombin G20210A (F2)	Low-dose steroid therapy Heparin Enoxaparin sodium (clexane) Aspirin[96]	Vitamin E 500 IU per day as mixed tocopherols Garlic *Allium sativum* (garlic) extract equivalent to fresh bulb 3.6–7.2 g per day or garlic bulb 1:1 fresh plant extract 5.7–11.4 mL per day *Ginkgo biloba* (ginkgo) extract equivalent to dry leaf 3–6 g per day standardised to contain ginkolides & bilobalides & ginkgo flavonglycosides or ginkgo leaf 2:1 extract contains 9.6 mg/mL ginkgo flavone glycosides 3–4 mL per day Ubiquinol (active CoQ10) 150 mg per day Alpha lipoic acid 400–800 mg per day NAC 1–2 g per day Fish oil 2–3 g per day	Vitamin E 500 IU per day as mixed tocopherols Garlic *Allium sativum* (garlic) extract equivalent to fresh bulb 3.6–7.2 g per day or garlic bulb 1:1 fresh plant extract 5.7–11.4 mL per day *A *Ginkgo biloba* (ginkgo) extract equivalent to dry leaf 3–6 g per day standardised to contain ginkolides & bilobalides & ginkgo flavonglycosides or ginkgo leaf 2:1 extract contains 9.6 mg/mL ginkgo flavone glycosides 3–4 mL per day *B1 Ubiquinol (active CoQ10) 150 mg per day Alpha lipoic acid 400–800 mg per day NAC 1–2 g per day Fish oil 2–3 g per day

Continued

TABLE 12.11 Miscarriage management treatment approaches—cont'd

Female

Aetiology	Medical management Rx	Naturopathic treatment Rx Preconception phase	Naturopathic treatment Rx In pregnancy
Haematological disorders		Anti-thrombotic protocol	Anti-thrombotic protocol
Antiphospholipid syndrome	Low doses of acetylsalicylic acid + low-molecular-weight heparin (LMWH). This treatment combination of low-dose aspirin and low-molecular-weight heparin reduces the miscarriage rate by 54%, but remains controversial.[97] Glucocorticoids should not be given in APS without connective tissue disorder. Prednisone does not prevent recurrent fetal death in women with APS.	Vitamin E 500 IU per day as mixed tocopherols Garlic *Allium sativum* (garlic) extract equivalent to fresh bulb 3.6–7.2 g per day or garlic bulb 1:1 fresh plant extract 5.7–11.4 mL per day *Zingiber officinale* (ginger) extract equivalent to dry root 150–600 mg per day *Ginkgo biloba* (ginkgo) extract equivalent to dry leaf 3–6 g per day standardised to contain ginkolides & bilobalides & ginkgo flavonglycosides or ginkgo leaf 2:1 extract contains 9.6 mg/mL ginkgo flavone glycosides 3–4 mL per day Ubiquinol (active CoQ10) 150 mg per day Alpha lipoic acid 400–800 mg per day NAC 1–2 g per day Fish oil 2–3 g per day	Vitamin E 500 IU per day as mixed tocopherols Garlic *Allium sativum* (garlic) extract equivalent to fresh bulb 3.6–7.2 g per day or garlic bulb 1:1 fresh plant extract 5.7–11.4 mL per day *A *Zingiber officinale* (ginger) extract equivalent to dry root 150–600 mg per day *A *Ginkgo biloba* (ginkgo) extract equivalent to dry leaf 3–6 g per day standardised to contain ginkolides & bilobalides & ginkgo flavonglycosides or ginkgo leaf 2:1 extract contains 9.6 mg/mL ginkgo flavone glycosides 3–4 mL per day *B1 Ubiquinol (active CoQ10) 150 mg per day Alpha lipoic acid 400–800 mg per day NAC 1–2 g per day Fish oil 2–3 g per day

Genetics

MTHFR mutation	High-dose folic acid (5 mg) and vitamin B$_{12}$ (0.5 mg) once daily has been reported to reduce levels of homocysteine; however, a randomised-controlled trial on the effect of variable doses of both vitamins on pregnancy has yet to be conducted.	Heterozygous on either polymorphism Folinic acid 250–500 mg per day in conjunction to complete B vitamin compound Heterozygous for both polymorphisms Or homozygosity on either polymorphism Riboflavin (as Riboflavin 5'-phosphate sodium) 90–180 mg per day Vitamin B$_6$ (as pyridoxal 5'-phosphate) 45–90 mg per day Folate (as L-5-methyltetrahydrofolate) 500–1000 mg per day Vitamin B$_{12}$ (as methylcobalamin) 3–6 mg per day	Heterozygous on either polymorphism Folinic acid 250–500 mg per day in conjunction to complete B vitamin compound Heterozygous for both polymorphisms Or homozygosity on either polymorphism Riboflavin (as Riboflavin 5'-phosphate sodium) 90–180 mg per day Vitamin B$_6$ (as pyridoxal 5'-phosphate) 45–90 mg per day Folate (as L-5-methyltetrahydrofolate) 500–1000 mg per day Vitamin B$_{12}$ (as methylcobalamin) 3–6 mg per day
Other	In vitro fertilisation (IVF) plus prenatal genetic testing is a suggested strategy in the management of couples with chromosomal abnormalities and recurrent miscarriages	Comprehensive nutritional & botanical preconception care	Comprehensive nutritional prenatal care

Endocrine

IR and or/ diabetes mellitus	Metformin Non-randomised studies have shown that the reduction in insulin levels with metformin in insulin-resistant individuals may reduce miscarriage risk by restoring normal haemostasis and improving the endometrial milieu. Metformin is not recommended as a treatment of recurrent miscarriage[98] Insulin	Chromium 150–600 micrograms per day Gymnema sylvestre (gymnema) extract equivalent to dry leaf – standardised to contain gymnemic acids 3–12 g per day or Gymnema leaf 1 : 1 extract 3.5–10.7 mL per day Zinc 15–30 mg per day ALA 200–300 mg per day Magnesium 100–400 mg per day Manganese 2–4 mg per day Probiotics multi-strain 30 billion colony-forming units Such as: *Bifidobacterium longum* BB536 *Bifidobacterium breve* M-16V *Bifidobacterium infantis* M-63 *Bifidobacterium lactis* Bi-04 *Bifidobacterium lactis* HN019 *Lactobacillus rhamnosus* HN001 *Lactobacillus paracasei* Lpc-37 *Lactobacillus salivarius* Ls-33 *Lactobacillus casei* Lc-11	Chromium 150–600 micrograms per day *Gymnema sylvestre* (gymnema) extract equivalent to dry leaf – standardised to contain gymnemic acids 3–12 g per day or Gymnema leaf 1 : 1 extract 3.5–10.7 mL per day Zinc 15–30 mg per day ALA 200–300 mg per day Magnesium 100–400 mg per day Manganese 2–4 mg per day Probiotics multi-strain 30 billion colony-forming units Such as: *Bifidobacterium longum* BB536 *Bifidobacterium breve* M-16V *Bifidobacterium infantis* M-63 *Bifidobacterium lactis* Bi-04 *Bifidobacterium lactis* HN019 *Lactobacillus rhamnosus* HN001 *Lactobacillus paracasei* Lpc-37 *Lactobacillus salivarius* Ls-33 *Lactobacillus casei* Lc-11

Continued

TABLE 12.11 Miscarriage management treatment approaches—cont'd

Female

Aetiology	Medical management Rx	Naturopathic treatment Rx Preconception phase	Naturopathic treatment Rx In pregnancy
Endocrine			
Luteal phase defect	Progesterone supplementation Human chorionic gonadotropin Administration of progesterone to women with sporadic miscarriages is ineffective. However, in patients with three or more consecutive miscarriages immediately preceding their current pregnancy, empiric progestogen administration may be of some potential benefit. Most commonly used regimen is micronised progesterone tablets 400 mg daily. The route of administration may be either vaginal or oral. The argument for use of progesterone is that there is no evidence of harm and some evidence of benefit, although not coming from huge multicentric trials.[5]	*Vitex agnus-castus* (chaste tree) extract equivalent to dry fruit 500–2000 mg per day or chaste tree fruit 1 : 2 extract 0.85–4.2 mL per day *Paeonia lactiflora* (paeonia) extract equivalent to dry root 800–3200 mg per day or paeonia root extract 1 : 2 4.2–8.5 mL per day Shatavari root 1 : 2 extract 4.2–8.5 mL per day *B2 Pyridoxal 5-phosphate 10–40 mg per day	*Vitex agnus-castus* (chaste tree) extract equivalent to dry fruit 500–2000 mg per day or chaste tree fruit 1 : 2 extract 0.85–4.2 mL per day *B1 *Paeonia lactiflora* (paeonia) extract equivalent to dry root 800–3200 mg per day or paeonia root extract 1 : 2 4.2–8.5 mL per day Shatavari root 1 : 2 extract 4.2–8.5 mL per day *B2 Pyridoxal 5-phosphate 10–40 mg per day
Hyperprolactinaemia	Dopamine agonists Human chorionic gonadotropin Normalisation of prolactin levels with a dopamine agonist improved subsequent pregnancy outcomes in patients with recurrent pregnancy loss Hyperprolactinaemia is treated with dopamine agonist drugs	*Vitex agnus-castus* (chaste tree) extract equivalent to dry fruit 500–2000 mg per day or chaste tree fruit 1 : 2 extract 0.85–4.2 mL per day Pyridoxal 5-phosphate 10–40 mg per day	*Vitex agnus-castus* (chaste tree) extract equivalent to dry fruit 500–2000 mg per day or chaste tree fruit 1 : 2 extract 0.85–4.2 mL per day *B1 Pyridoxal 5-phosphate 10–40 mg per day
Hypothyroidism TSH values more than 2.5 mIU/L are outside the normal range. The aim is to maintain baseline TSH <2.5 mIU/L.[5]	Levothyroxine 50–200 micrograms daily[5]	*Withania somnifera* (withania) extract equivalent to dry root 250–1000 mg per day or withania root 2 : 1 extract contains a minimum of 4 mg/mL of withanolides 1.4–4.2 mL per day Tyrosine 500–2000 mg per day Inositol 300–1200 mg per day Nicotinic acid 5–20 mg per day Nicotinamide 30–120 mg per day Pyridoxal 5-phosphate 10–40 mg per day Zinc 10–40 mg per day Iodine 100–225 micrograms per day Selenium 150–300 micrograms per day	*Withania somnifera* (withania) extract equivalent to dry root 250–1000 mg per day or withania root 2 : 1 extract contains a minimum of 4 mg/mL of withanolides 1.4–4.2 mL per day *B1 Tyrosine 500–2000 mg per day Inositol 300–1200 mg per day Nicotinic acid 5–20 mg per day Nicotinamide 30–120 mg per day Pyridoxal 5-phosphate 10–40 mg per day Zinc 10–40 mg per day Iodine 100–225 micrograms per day Selenium 150–300 micrograms per day

Thyroid peroxidase antibody (TPO Ab) Thyroglobulin antibody (TG Ab)	Levothyroxine 50 micrograms daily for women with raised TPO antibodies, with normal TSH as suggested intervention[5]	Selenium 150–300 micrograms per day Quercetin 500–2000 mg per day Rutin 400–1600 mg per day Bromelain 125–600 mg per day Ascorbic acid 50–1000 mg per day Probiotics multi-strain 30 billion colony-forming units Such as: *Bifidobacterium longum* BB536 *Bifidobacterium breve* M-16V *Bifidobacterium infantis* M-63 *Bifidobacterium lactis* Bi-04 *Bifidobacterium lactis* HN019 *Lactobacillus rhamnosus* HN001 *Lactobacillus paracasei* Lpc-37 *Lactobacillus salivarius* Ls-33 *Lactobacillus casei* Lc-11	Selenium 150–300 micrograms per day Quercetin 500–2000 mg per day Rutin 400–1600 mg per day Bromelain 125–600 mg per day Ascorbic acid 50–1000 mg per day Probiotics multi-strain 30 billion colony-forming units Such as: *Bifidobacterium longum* BB536 *Bifidobacterium breve* M-16V *Bifidobacterium infantis* M-63 *Bifidobacterium lactis* Bi-04 *Bifidobacterium lactis* HN019 *Lactobacillus rhamnosus* HN001 *Lactobacillus paracasei* Lpc-37 *Lactobacillus salivarius* Ls-33 *Lactobacillus casei* Lc-11

Infections

Bacterial vaginosis	Antibiotic therapy – oral clindamycin early in the second trimester significantly reduces the rate of late miscarriage and spontaneous preterm birth.[5]	*Saccharomyces boulardii* 5–20 billion CFU per day Probiotics multi-strain 30 billion colony-forming units Such as: *Bifidobacterium longum* BB536 *Bifidobacterium breve* M-16V *Bifidobacterium infantis* M-63 *Bifidobacterium lactis* Bi-04 *Bifidobacterium lactis* HN019 *Lactobacillus rhamnosus* HN001 *Lactobacillus paracasei* Lpc-37 *Lactobacillus salivarius* Ls-33 *Lactobacillus casei* Lc-11 Garlic *Allium sativum* (garlic) extract equivalent to fresh bulb 3.6–7.2 g per day or garlic bulb 1:1 fresh plant extract 5.7–11.4 mL per day *Echinacea angustifolia* (echinacea) extract equivalent to dry root 600–1200 mg per day or *Echinacea angustifolia* root 1:2 extract Contains a minimum of 1.6 mg/mL alkylamides 2.8–5.7 mL per day	*Saccharomyces boulardii* 5–20 billion CFU per day Probiotics multi-strain 30 billion colony-forming units Such as: *Bifidobacterium longum* BB536 *Bifidobacterium breve* M-16V *Bifidobacterium infantis* M-63 *Bifidobacterium lactis* Bi-04 *Bifidobacterium lactis* HN019 *Lactobacillus rhamnosus* HN001 *Lactobacillus paracasei* Lpc-37 *Lactobacillus salivarius* Ls-33 *Lactobacillus casei* Lc-11 Garlic *Allium sativum* (garlic) extract equivalent to fresh bulb 3.6–7.2 g per day or garlic bulb 1:1 fresh plant extract 5.7–11.4 mL per day *A *Echinacea angustifolia* (Echinacea) extract equivalent to dry root 600–1200 mg per day or *Echinacea angustifolia* root 1:2 extract Contains a minimum of 1.6 mg/mL alkylamides 2.8–5.7 mL per day *A

Continued

TABLE 12.11 Miscarriage management treatment approaches—cont'd

Female

Aetiology	Medical management Rx	Naturopathic treatment Rx Preconception phase	Naturopathic treatment Rx In pregnancy
	Surgery	Pre- and post-surgery protocol	Fibroid growth acceleration prevention for pregnancy
Fibroids or any other defects that will involve surgical correction		*Centella asiatica* (Gotu kola) extract equivalent to dry leaf 2.5–10 g per day or Gotu kola herb 1:1 extract contains 20 mg/mL triterpenes 1.8–5.7 mL per day *Ginkgo biloba* (ginkgo) extract equivalent to dry leaf 3–6 g per day standardised to contain ginkolides & bilobalides & ginkgo flavonglycosides or ginkgo leaf 2:1 extract contains 9.6 mg/mL ginkgo flavone glycosides 3–4 mL per day *Zingiber officinale* (ginger) extract equivalent to dry root 150–600 mg per day or ginger rhizome 1:2 extract 0.71–2.14 mL per day Bromelains 100–400 mg per day Quercetin 250–1000 mg per day Ascorbic acid (vitamin C) 200–1000 mg per day Curcumin phospholipid complex containing curcumin 90–180 mg Equ to 500–1000 mg per day *Brassica oleracea* var. *italica* (broccoli) extract equivalent to fresh sprout 7–14 g per day Cysteine 125–250 mg per day Methionine 125–250 mg per day Iodine 225 micrograms per day Vitamin D₃ 1000–5000 IU per day, dependent on 25-OH-D blood test results Selenium 50–150 micrograms per day Vitamin A 1000–2000 IU per day	*Brassica oleracea* var. *italica* (broccoli) extract equivalent to fresh sprout 7–14 g per day Cysteine 125–250 mg per day Methionine 125–250 mg per day Iodine 225 micrograms per day Vitamin D₃ 1000–5000 IU per day, dependent on 25-OH-D blood test results Selenium 50–150 micrograms per day Vitamin A 1000–2000 IU per day NAC 1 g per day

Cervical weakness/incompetence	Cervical cerclage	In preconception, if history of any cervical incompetence or cervical cone biopsy/trauma	In pregnancy
		Centella asiatica (Gotu kola) extract equivalent to dry leaf 2.5–10 g per day or Gotu kola herb 1:1 extract contains 20 mg/mL triterpenes 1.8–5.7 mL per day Bromelains 100–400 mg per day Quercetin 250–1000 mg per day Ascorbic acid (vitamin C) 200–1000 mg per day Vitamin D₃ 1000–5000 IU per day, dependent on 25-OH-D blood test results Vitamin A 1000–2000 IU per day	*Centella asiatica* (Gotu kola) extract equivalent to dry leaf 2.5–10 g per day or Gotu kola herb 1:1 extract contains 20 mg/mL triterpenes 1.8–5.7 mL per day *B1 Bromelains 100–400 mg per day Quercetin 250–1000 mg per day Ascorbic acid (vitamin C) 200–1000 mg per day Vitamin D₃ 1000–5000 IU per day, dependent on 25-OH-D blood test results Vitamin A 1000–2000 IU per day

*References to Australian TGA guidelines codes for safety in pregnancy, Table 12.12.
Source: Mills S, Bone, K. *The essential guide to herbal safety*. London: Elsevier Health Sciences; 2005.

TABLE 12.12 Australian TGA guidelines codes for safety in pregnancy	
Category A	Drugs that have been taken by a large number of pregnant women and women of childbearing age without any proven increase in the frequency of malformations or other direct or indirect harmful effects on the fetus having been observed.
Category B1	Drugs that have been taken by only a limited number of pregnant women and women of childbearing age, without an increase in the frequency of malformation or other direct or indirect harmful effects on the human fetus having been observed. Studies in animals have not shown evidence of an increased occurrence of fetal damage.
Category B2	Drugs that have been taken by only a limited number of pregnant women and women of childbearing age, without an increase in the frequency of malformation or other direct or indirect harmful effects on the human fetus having been observed. Studies in animals are inadequate or may be lacking, but available data show no evidence of an increased occurrence of fetal damage.
Category B3	Drugs that have been taken by only a limited number of pregnant women and women of childbearing age, without an increase in the frequency of malformation or other direct or indirect harmful effects on the human fetus having been observed. Studies in animals have shown evidence of an increased occurrence of fetal damage, the significance of which is considered uncertain in humans.
Category C	Drugs that, owing to their pharmacological effects, have caused or may be suspected of causing, harmful effects on the human fetus or neonate without causing malformations. These effects may be reversible. Accompanying texts should be consulted for further details.
Category D	Drugs that have caused, are suspected to have caused or may be expected to cause an increased incidence of human fetal malformations or irreversible damage. These drugs may also have adverse pharmacological effects. Accompanying texts should be consulted for further details.
Category X	Drugs that have such a high risk of causing permanent damage to the fetus that they should not be used in pregnancy or when there is a possibility of pregnancy.

Source: Leung HY, Saini B, Ritchie HE. Medications and pregnancy: the role of community pharmacists – a descriptive study. *PloS One* 2018;13(5):e0195101.

15 components. Paeoniflorin is the most abundant ingredient and accounts for the pharmacological effects observed with TGP in both in vitro and in vivo studies. The direct anti-inflammatory effects of TGP were observed in animal models of both acute and subacute inflammation, by inhibiting the production of prostaglandin E_2, leukotriene B4 and nitric oxide, and by suppressing the increase of intracellular calcium ion concentration. TGP was also reported to have protective effects of cells against oxidative stress. In vitro, dual effects of TGP were noted on the proliferation of lymphocytes, differentiation of Th/Ts lymphocytes, and the production of proinflammatory cytokines and antibodies. In vivo, TGP inhibited the delayed-type hypersensitivity in immunoactivated mice, and enhanced the delayed-type hypersensitivity in immunosuppressed mice. In adjuvant arthritis rats, paeoniflorin exerted immunosuppressive effects.[104]

In the context of autoimmune-mediated miscarriage cases, paeonia is useful for immune modulation in autoimmune recurrent miscarriage cases, while also supporting hormonal homeostasis.[104]

Bupleurum falcatum (bupleurum)

Bupleurum falcatum is the main Chinese herb used for liver disharmony. Bupleurum is anti-inflammatory, adaptogenic, hepatoprotective, antitussive and a mild sedative. It is also important for debility. The main constituents are the triterpenoid saponins known as saikosaponins. Injection of saikosaponin a and saikosaponin d in rats demonstrated anti-inflammatory activity, potentiated the activity of cortisone and stimulated ACTH secretion from the pituitary, thereby indicating stimulation of endogenous production of cortisol. Anti-inflammatory activity has also been demonstrated from oral administration of saikosaponins (100 mg/kg). Adrenal gland weight increased in proportion to the dosage of saikosaponins (by injection). Injection of saikosaponins increased protein synthesis in the liver. Saikosaponins have shown an inhibitory effect on prostaglandin E_2 production. (PGE_2 promotes inflammation in the body.) Bupleurum has been found useful in experimental immune damage to kidneys. Bupleurum has a slight sedative effect in some patients, and can occasionally cause nausea and reflux. It may also increase bowel movements and flatulence.

The following uses are based on both pharmacological studies and traditional knowledge:
- chronic inflammatory disorders, especially autoimmune
- acute infections, common cold and with chills and fever, chronic cough. A possible immune-enhancing activity may also be involved in these applications
- irregular menstruation.

Used in the management of miscarriage cases, bupleurum plays an important role in immune modulation and inflammatory management for autoimmune-mediated

TABLE 12.13 Miscarriage management treatment approaches

Male

Aetiology	Medical management Rx	Naturopathic treatment Rx Preconception phase
Sperm DNA fragmentation Duration of treatment 3–4 months PRIOR to attempting conception		Complementary to medical management
	No treatment available	*Vitis vinifera* (grape seed) extract equivalent to dry seed 6–24 g per day *Camellia sinensis* (green tea) extract equivalent to dry leaf 4–16 g per day *Curcuma longa* (turmeric) extract equivalent to dry rhizome 2–8 g per day *Rosmarinus officinalis* (rosemary) extract equivalent to dry leaf 1–4 g per day *Fallopia japonica* (giant knotweed) extract equivalent to dry root 8–30 g per day *Silybum marianum* (St Mary's thistle) extract equivalent to dry seed 4–16 g per day Vitamin D 1000–5000 IU per day dependent on results of 25-OH-D blood tests Vitamin E as mixed tocopherols 500 IU per day Cysteine 20–60 mg per day Glycine 150–500 mg per day Taurine 200–800 mg per day Glutamine 100–500 mg per day Methionine 100–500 mg per day Choline bitartrate 200–800 mg per day Ascorbic acid 20–2000 mg per day Citrus bioflavonoids extract 30–1200 mg per day Selenium 50–200 micrograms per day Zinc 10–50 mg per day Iodine 225 micrograms per day Calcium folinate equiv. folinic acid or methyfolate 50–500 micrograms per day Cyanocobalamin (vit. B_{12}) 500 micrograms 1 mg per day Glutathione 20–100 micrograms per day *Brassica oleracea* var. *italica* (broccoli) 1.5–3 g per day NAC 1–2 g per day Lycopene 6–18 g per day RS-alpha lipoic acid 50–200 mg per day Coenzyme Q10 as ubiquinol 150–300 mg per day

recurrent miscarriage cases, and is very helpful as an adaptogen to assist in adrenal recovery to overcome debility associated recurrent pregnancy loss.[99,100,105]

Hemidesmus indicus (hemidesmus)

Hemidesmus indicus root is regarded in Ayurvedic medicine as a depurative and tonic. Its main action is the depression (immunosuppressive action) of the immune function. In a series of tests, oral administration of ethanol extract of hemidesmus decreased both the cell-mediated and the humoral components of the immune system in mice. In the context of miscarriage cases, this activity would be of benefit in autoimmune-mediated miscarriage cases.[100,105,106]

Curcuma longa (turmeric)

Turmeric is a potent broad spectrum anti-inflammatory and antioxidant agent. The core researched active components are the yellow-coloured pigments, the curcuminoids, found in the turmeric rhizome.

CURCUMIN: KEY MECHANISMS OF ACTION

The main properties of curcumin are antioxidant, anti-inflammatory and anticancer. The underlying mechanisms of its effects, elucidated via thousands of studies, are diverse and involve the regulation of many molecular targets, including:

- transcription factors such as nuclear factor-κB (NFκB), signal transducer and activator of transcription (STAT) proteins, nuclear factor erythroid 2-related factor 2 (Nrf2)
- growth factors such as vascular endothelial cell growth factor
- inflammatory cytokines such as tumour necrosis factor alpha (TNF-α), interleukin 1 (IL-1) and IL-6
- protein kinases such as mitogen-activated protein kinases (MAPKs) and Akt
- other enzymes closely associated with anti-inflammatory and chemo-preventive effects such as cyclooxygenase 2 (COX2), haem oxygenase-1 (HO-1, which is induced via Nrf2 activation) and NAD(P)H: quinone oxidoreductase 1 (NQO1)

In the treatment planning for miscarriage cases, if the patients exhibit autoimmune or inflammatory markers, turmeric is an excellent herb to consider within the treatment plan.

SAFETY

Due to increased bioavailability, caution is advised in patients taking drugs with a narrow therapeutic window and/or antiplatelet or anticoagulant drugs. Monitor anti-inflammatory drugs if used concurrently with turmeric.[100,107]

Allium sativum L. (garlic)

Garlic is an agent that increases perfusion and is used traditionally in the treatment of circulatory disorders. The anti-infective and antibacterial properties of garlic were well known throughout history. Both of these actions are of benefit in miscarriage cases, where microvascular circulation and prevention of infection may need to be taken into therapeutic consideration.

The main compounds in garlic cloves are the organic sulfur compounds. Of these, the most important is allicin. When a garlic clove is crushed, the odourless precursor alliin is broken down by the enzyme alliinase and is converted to the bioactive allicin compound.

Garlic has a wide range of pharmacological activities, including the ability to enhance phase II detoxification by inducing enzymes such as glutathione S-transferase, quinone reductase and epoxide hydrolase. Added antioxidant protection plays a beneficial role to the developing embryo/fetus.

ANTIOXIDANT ENZYMES

In uncontrolled trials, administration of garlic:
- increased the activity of superoxide dismutase and glutathione peroxidase in erythrocytes
- increased the glutathione concentration in circulating erythrocytes, and produced a decreasing trend for the ratio of oxidised glutathione to total glutathione, which is indicative of decreased oxidative stress.

BLOOD FLOW, PERIPHERAL ARTERIAL DISEASE

Several studies have shown that garlic increases blood flow to the periphery and to the internal organs, including the uterus.

ANTIPLATELET AND ANTITHROMBOTIC ACTIVITY

Reducing platelet aggregation may be of benefit in conditions where there is impaired blood flow or perfusion, such as in thrombotic factor miscarriage cases.

In addition to having a beneficial effect on disordered function, garlic may also affect platelet function in the normal or healthy state. The majority of clinical studies indicate an antiplatelet effect for garlic.

Therefore, in the context of miscarriage management, patients who exhibit aetiologies of coagulation factors, oxidative stress and poor phase 2 liver detoxification capacity may benefit from garlic as an addition to their treatment plan.[100,108]

Ginkgo biloba (ginkgo)

Ginkgo has a long history of use in treating blood disorders and shows positive effects on microcirculation. Laboratory studies have shown that ginkgo improves blood circulation by opening up blood vessels and making blood less coagulated. It is also an antioxidant.

Studies show that ginkgo fresh plant extract significantly increased the number of blood cell-perfused nodal points, the venular streaming flow and the local haematocrit in treated participants compared to control participants and compared to values on day 0. The ginkgo preparation also increased microcirculation in the liver, and possessed antioxidative properties that resulted in significant increases in the amount of the radical scavenger glutathione in treated participants.

Ginkgo fresh plant extract increased the microcirculation significantly, and at the same time improved the radical scavenging capacity and was also very well tolerated. This extract is an interesting adjuvant treatment option for patients suffering from impaired microcirculation.

In miscarriages cases, gingko can be used to improve maternal fetal microcirculation in those patients with coagulation factors involved.

In addition, standardised extract of *G. biloba* (EGb) has been demonstrated to possess remarkable antioxidant activity in both cell lines and animals. Phase 2 enzymes play important roles in the antioxidant system by reducing electrophiles and reactive oxygen species (ROS). *G. biloba* was testified to induce the phase 2 genes through the Keap1-Nrf2-ARE signalling pathway, which is (or part of) the antioxidant mechanism of *G. biloba*.[109–111]

Vitex angus-castus (chaste tree berry)

Chaste tree is one of the most archetypal of all female reproductive herbs. It is of benefit in the treatment plan for miscarriage associated with corpus luteum defect or low progesterone resultant from luteal phase defect.

Chaste tree has been beneficial in the treatment of luteal phase defects due to latent hyperprolactinaemia. A placebo-controlled trial found treatment (equivalent to 20 mg/day of dried fruit for 3 months) reduced prolactin release, normalised shortened luteal phases and corrected luteal phase progesterone deficiencies. Two women receiving the herb became pregnant.[100]

In an uncontrolled trial, clinical results in patients with luteal phase defect and infertility were better in those women with hyperprolactinaemia. The number of these women with luteal phase defect and infertility decreased. Chaste tree extract (equivalent to 40 mg/day of dried fruit) was taken for 6 months.[100]

Constituents of the fruit of chaste tree include essential oil, diterpenes of the labdane- and clerodane-type (including rotundifuran), flavonoids (such as casticin) and iridoid glycosides (including aucubin and agnuside).[112]

Some of the effects of chaste tree can be explained by its effect on dopamine. Latent hyperprolactinaemia can cause disturbances of the menstrual cycle, breast tenderness/pain, corpus luteal insufficiency and infertility. Prolactin can be elevated premenstrually and/or by minor stress or during deep sleep at night. Prolactin secretion by the pituitary cells is inhibited by dopamine via the dopamine D2 receptors. Chaste tree extracts, and the diterpenes in particular, have confirmed dopaminergic activity in vitro – inhibition of prolactin secretion from pituitary cells by binding to D2 receptors. The activity by chaste tree is selective; that is, the release of luteinising hormone (LH) and follicle-stimulating hormone (FSH) directly from pituitary cells is not affected.[100]

This dopaminergic mechanism of action supersedes a previous hypothesis: that chaste tree corrected oestrogen excess or relative progesterone deficiency by acting on the pituitary to increase LH and decrease FSH.[100] Instead, chaste tree may correct progesterone deficiency by supporting the normal development of the corpus luteum once the inhibiting effect of elevated prolactin is removed.

Chaste tree caused a dose-dependent increase of melatonin secretion, especially during the night, in healthy volunteers (placebo-controlled trial).[113] Melatonin may contribute to improved oocyte quality in women who cannot fall pregnant because of poor quality oocytes or those who suffer recurrent early pregnancy loss due to poor oocyte quality.[114]

Asparagus racemosus (shatavari)

Shatavari means 'who possesses a hundred husbands or acceptable to many'.[115] It is considered both a general tonic and a female reproductive tonic. In Ayurveda, this herb is known as the 'Queen of herbs'.

It is beneficial in female infertility as it increases libido, reduces inflammation and moistens dry tissues of the reproductive organs, enhances folliculogenesis and ovulation, prepares the womb for conception, prevents miscarriages and acts as a postnatal tonic by increasing lactation and normalising the uterus and changing hormones. This herb is highly effective in problems related to the female reproductive system, leukorrhoea and menorrhagia, and also has important immunomodulatory activities.

A study of ancient classical Ayurvedic literature claimed several therapeutic attributes for the root of *A. racemosus*. It has been specially recommended in cases of threatened abortion and as a galactogogue.[115]

The major active constituents of *A. racemosus* are steroidal saponins (shatavarins I–IV) that are present in the roots. Shatavarin IV has been reported to display significant activity as an inhibitor of core Golgi enzyme transferase in cell free assays and recently to exhibit immuno-modulation activity against specific T-dependent antigens in immunocompromised animals.[9] It is also considered a powerful adaptogen.[116]

EFFECT ON UTERUS

In spite of the cholinergic activity of *A. racemosus*, in one study, extract of the root blocked spontaneous motility of the virgin rat's uterus. The extract also inhibited contraction induced by spasmogens and was found to produce a specific block of pitocin-induced contraction, confirming that shatavari can be used as a uterine sedative. Further, a glycoside, shatavarin 1, isolated from the roots of *A. racemosus*, has been found to be responsible for the competitive block of oxytocin-induced contraction of rat, guinea pig and rabbit uteri, in vitro as well as in vivo.[116]

In Ayurveda, *A. racemosus* has been described as absolutely safe for long-term use, even during pregnancy and lactation.[116]

Withania somnifera (withania)

Withania somnifera, also known as ashwagandha, Indian ginseng and winter cherry, has been an important herb in the Ayurvedic medical systems for over 3000 years. Historically, the plant has been used as an aphrodisiac, liver tonic, anti-inflammatory agent and astringent.

Withania is of benefit for miscarriage cases due to the immunoregulatory, thyrotropic and adaptogenic and relaxant nervine activity.

Chronic stress can result in a number of adverse physiological conditions including cognitive deficit, immunosuppression and sexual dysfunction.[117,118]

Echinacea spp. (echinacea)

Echinacea is of benefit in miscarriage for immune modulation and anxiolytic potential, given its mode of action on the endocannabinoid system.[119] Studies suggests that gestational use of echinacea during organogenesis is not associated with an increased risk for major malformations.[120]

Centella asiatica (Gotu kola)

Gotu kola has several pharmacological actions, based primarily on in vivo experiments. After oral and topical administration in rats, increased cellular hyperplasia and collagen production were noted at the site of injury, measured by increased granulation tissue levels of DNA, protein, total collagen and hexosamine.

More rapid maturation and cross-linking of collagen were seen in animals treated with the herbal extract, as evidenced by elevated stability of acid-soluble collagen and increases in aldehyde content and tensile strength. Compared to control wounds, rats treated with Gotu kola had a higher degree of epithelialisation and a significantly more rapid rate of wound contraction.[121,122]

Integrity of collagen in the cervix is integral to a successful full-term pregnancy. Gotu kola may therefore assist cases of cervical incompetence. In addition to improving wound healing, Gotu kola may also have an effect on connective tissue of varicosities. Gotu kola is also of great benefit for keloid and scar management, which is beneficial pre and post surgery to correct issues such a fibroids or structural abnormalities involved in the aetiology of miscarriage.[123]

Other benefits include Gotu kola's sedative and anxiolytic properties. In Indian literature, Gotu kola is described as possessing CNS benefits such as being a stimulatory-nervine tonic and a rejuvenant, sedative, tranquilliser and intelligence-promoting property. These effects are postulated mainly due to the brahmoside and brahminoside constituents, while the anxiolytic activity is considered to be in part due to binding to cholecystokinin receptors (CCK_B), a group of G-protein-coupled receptors which bind the peptide hormones cholesystokinin (CCK) or gastrin, and are thought to play a potential role in modulation of anxiety.[124]

Zingiber officinale (ginger)

Ginger is reported to decrease age-related oxidative stress markers and improve microvascular circulation. Ginger consumption has also been reported to decrease lipid peroxidation and normalise the activities of superoxide dismutase and catalase, as well as GSH and glutathione peroxidase, glutathione reductase and glutathione-S-transferase. Ginger supplementation before ischaemia/reperfusion resulted in a higher total antioxidant capacity (i.e. normalised glutathione peroxidase and superoxide dismutase activities) and lower total oxidant (lower tissue malondialdehyde, NO and protein carbonyl contents) status levels compared to an untreated group.[125]

Researchers have hypothesised that the anti-inflammatory effects of ginger might be related to its ability to inhibit prostaglandin and leukotriene biosynthesis. Some others have showed that gingerols actively inhibit arachidonate 5-lipoxygenase, an enzyme of leukotriene biosynthesis. [8]-gingerol, but not [6]-gingerol, was shown to inhibit cyclooxygenase-2 (COX-2) expression, which is induced during inflammation to increase formation of prostaglandins. Ginger extract suppresses the activation of TNF-α and expression of COX-2 in human synoviocytes. Proinflammatory cytokines such as TNF-α, interleukin (IL)-1β and IL-12, which are produced primarily by macrophages, play an important role in sepsis, ischaemia/reperfusion injury and transplant rejection.[125]

Sample liquid herbal formulae

MISCARRIAGE MANAGEMENT PRECONCEPTION FORMULA

Autoimmune autoantibody formula

Hemidesmus indicus (hemidesmus) 1:2	40 mL
Echinacea spp. (echinacea) 1:2	20 mL
Curcuma longa (turmeric) 1:2	40 mL
Paeonia lactiflora (paeonia) 1:2	40 mL
Zingiber officinale (ginger) 1:2	10 mL
Bupleurum falcatum (bupleurum) 1:2	25 mL
Rehmannia glutinosa (rehmannia) 1:2	25 mL
TOTAL	200 mL

Dose: 6 mL t.d.s.

MISCARRIAGE MANAGEMENT PREGNANCY FORMULA

Autoimmune autoantibody formula

Hemidesmus indicus (hemidesmus) 1:2	40 mL
Echinacea spp. (echinacea) 1:2	30 mL
Paeonia lactiflora (paeonia) 1:2	40 mL
Zingiber officinale (ginger) 1:2	10 mL
Bupleurum falcatum (bupleurum) 1:2	40 mL
Rehmannia glutinosa (rehmannia) 1:2	40 mL
TOTAL	200 mL

Dose: 4 mL t.d.s.

MISCARRIAGE MANAGEMENT PRECONCEPTION FORMULA

Anti-thrombotic formula

Hemidesmus indicus (hemidesmus) 1:2	60 mL
Curcuma longa (turmeric) 1:2	60 mL
Zingiber officinale (ginger) 1:2	10 mL
Ginkgo biloba (ginkgo) 2:1	70 mL
TOTAL	200 mL

Dose: 4 mL t.d.s.

MISCARRIAGE MANAGEMENT PREGNANCY FORMULA

Anti-thrombotic formula

Hemidesmus indicus (hemidesmus) 1:2	95 mL
Zingiber officinale (ginger) 1:2	10 mL
Ginkgo biloba (ginkgo) 2:1	95 mL
TOTAL	200 mL

Dose: 2 mL t.d.s.

MISCARRIAGE MANAGEMENT LUTEAL PHASE DEFECT PRECONCEPTION FORMULA

Vitex agnus-castus (chaste tree) 1:2	20 mL
Paeonia lactiflora (paeonia) 1:2	60 mL
Asparagus racemosus (shatavari) 1:2	90 mL
Cimicifuga racemosa (black cohosh) 1:2	30 mL
TOTAL	200 mL

Dose: 5 mL t.d.s.

CASE STUDY
Miscarriage

This case represents a specifically structured miscarriage prevention healthcare treatment plan based on specific findings ascertained through assessment at the start of treatment. Both partners presented with specific reproductive health concerns.

OVERVIEW

CASE PRESENTATION

Female HR age 32 and male IL aged 33 presented with an overwhelmingly sad history of two stillborn babies and one subsequent trimester 1 miscarriage.

Pregnancy 1:

Conceive naturally after 4 months of trying in 2013

Gestation reached, 22/40.

Baby boy was delivered stillborn March 2014.

At 20-week ultrasound, the parents where advised that fetal growth was very slow with both baby and placenta very small for date.

After consulting with perinatalogist, they were counselled to expect baby wouldn't survive.

Blood flow to baby from umbilical cord very poor with no rational explanation. HR was prescribed enoxaparin sodium for 7 days by injection, but before she could complete the week, baby passed away.

Pregnancy 2:

Towards the end of 2014, the couple conceived again. Natural conception after 2 months of attempts.

HR was closely obstetrically monitored. Pregnancy was healthy, 20/40 wk ultrasound normal, under care of perinatologist, after 30 weeks saw growth was slowing but was not concerned.

At 31+6/40 weeks, the mother noticed no fetal movement, was alarmed. Returned to hospital for examination. The ultrasound showed neither fetal movement nor heartbeat. Baby had died. HR was induced and a stillborn female baby was delivered 32/40.

No enoxaparin sodium nor any other pharmaceutical intervention was advised or given during the pregnancy. The baby was 1.5 kg, small for date at 8 months. Placenta was small for that gestational age at 32/40.

The collective results of both babies' autopsies reported:

The two losses were probably related in so far as the placentas were both in fifth percentile for their gestational age. In the first, there was irregular villous maturation and in the second, the placenta was appropriately mature.

The difficulty with diagnosing irregular villous maturation is that it can be patchy and subjective. We only know about the accelerated maturation as being a response to utero placental hypoxia. Delayed villous maturation is associated with maternal diabetes, rhesus isoimmunisation, syphilis and Down syndrome. HR did not have maternal gestational diabetes on review of results.

The autopsy reports suggested that poor placentation and some epigenetic phenomenon were not picked up with the array of cytogenics.

Both babies were anatomically and genetically normal in autopsy findings.

Infections were ruled out.

No further investigations were carried out. HR was advised to commence low-dose aspirin and try to conceive again. Little emotional support and counselling were offered to the couple to help them through the grief of two stillborn babies.

Pregnancy 3:

Naturally conceived after 8 months of trying, in 2015.

Pregnancy miscarried at 13/40.

Placentation was normal, genetics normal.

The couple where so deeply grief-stricken by this point in their journey, they took some time away to process their grief and seek more advanced management of their stillborns and miscarriage.

They presented for naturopathic preconception care and advanced investigation and specialist referrals.

FEMALE HR AGED 32

- Nervous: anxiety and depression. Related to losses of the pregnancies.
- Gastrointestinal: normal healthy bowel motions.
- Menstrual: cycle regular (28 days), with a moderate bleed on days 1–3 and a complete ceasing of flow after 7 days (period seems long for her – recent changes have been noted); premenstrual spotting, consisting of dark brown rusty-coloured discharge; premenstrual cravings (chocolate, sugar, fruit for 5 days prior to bleed). No pain or congestion.
- Fertility: capacity to conceive easily. Capacity to carry a pregnancy to full term was the issue at hand.
- Previous contraception: combined oral contraceptive use from age 23 to 30 years; current contraception – nil.
- Diet: the Brahman diet was followed.
  - Meat not allowed.
  - Eggs not allowed.
  - Milk and milk products are permitted – butter, yoghurt, cream.
  - Cheese must not be coagulated with rennet.
  - Stimulants – coffee, tea not allowed.
  - Alcohol – not allowed.
- Lifestyle: corporate tertiary-educated woman, works long hours. Practises yoga and meditation to cope.
- Other: non-smoker; no recreational drugs.
- Height 154 cm; weight: 69 kg; BMI: 29.1 (overweight range).
- Supplement and medication at intake:
  - over-the counter-prenatal (Elevit), 1 per day
  - aspirin 100 mg per day.

TREATMENT PROTOCOL
Initial appointment

The initial appointment consisted of a thorough assessment and detailed intake. Referral for required investigations was organised.

Both partners were requested to complete a dietary and lifestyle diary for a 2-week period.

Treatment

Treatment focus at the initial consultation was on digging deeper into investigations and trying to find some answers to help this couple with their grief and put a treatment plan in place for at least 4–6 months prior to trying to conceive again. We reviewed all past results, stillborn autopsy reports and blood tests.

Discussion regarding lifestyle factors in line with general preconception healthcare were discussed, including diet, toxicity, radiation, environmental impact and chemical xposure.

Referrals to a leading reproductive immunologist were arranged and up-to-date medical treatments were explained, in addition to aetiologies of pregnancy loss explained thoroughly.

SECOND CONSULTATION

Results review and discussion.
Treatment plan and strategy implemented.

INVESTIGATIONS AND RESULTS AT INITIAL CONSULTATION

Pathology, female, HR		
Assessment	**Test**	**Findings**
Immnological		
	Lupus anticoagulant	Negative
	Immunoglobulin A (IgA)	Negative
	Anti-gliadin antibodies IgA	Negative
	Anti-gliadin antibodies IgG	Negative
	Antinuclear antibodies (ANA)	Negative
	Transglutaminase antibodies	Negative
	Endomysial antibodies	Negative
	Anti dsDNA	Not detected
	Immunophenotypes: NK cells	Negative
	Thyroid peroxidase antibody (TPO Ab)	Low positive 26 (ref <60 micromols/L)
	Thyroglobulin antibody (TG Ab)	Low positive 34 (ref <60 micromols/L)
	Thyroid-stimulating hormone receptor antibody (TR Ab) or TSH receptor antibodies	Negative
Thrombotic factors		
	Protein C	Within normal limits
	Protein S	Within normal limits
	Anti-thrombin III	Within normal limits
	APC resistance	Within normal limits
Mucosal immunity		
	Immunoglobulin A IgA	Negative
	Tissue transglutaminase antibodies (TTG)	Not detected
	Anti-endomysial IgA	Not detected
	Anti-gliadin IgA	Not detected
	Anti-gliadin IgG	Not detected
Infections		
	Mycoplasma hominis (S) PCR	Not detected
	Ureaplasma PCR	Not detected
	Listeria monocytogenes PCR	Not detected
	Chlamydia PCR	Not detected

Assessment	Pathology, female, HRs—cont'd	
	Test	**Findings**
	Toxoplasmosis PCR	Not detected
	Syphilis	Not detected
	Hep B	Not detected
	Hep C	Not detected
	HIV	Not detected
	Rubella	Immune
Endocrine		
	Female hormone tracking FSH, LH, E_2, prolactin, P4	All within normal fertile limits
	Fasting insulin	Significantly elevated 22 mU/L
	Fasting glucose	Borderline high 5.2 mmol/L
	Haemoglobin A1c, A1C (HbA$_{1c}$)	Normal
	Total testosterone Free testosterone FAI	All within normal limits
	Sex hormone binding globulin (SHBG)	Normal
	Prolactin	Normal
	TSH	3.23 mIU/L Elevated
	Free T4	Non pregnant 19.2 pmol/L Within range
	Free T3	Non pregnant 5 pmol/L Within range
	Metsyn or IR risk assessment BMI calculation Hip to waist ratio	29.1 Overweight Waist; ≥89 cm
Genetics		
	MTHFR polymorphism	Homozygous 1298C-A
	Extended karyotping	46 XX female Normal
	Factor V Leiden (FVq506)	Does not carry
	HLA-DQ2 or HLA-DQ8	Does not carry
	Prothrombin gene mutation	Does not carry
Biochemical		
	Serum zinc	9 micromols/L Significantly clinically deficient
	Serum copper	21 micromols/L High
	Red cell folate	Normal
	Caeruloplasmin	Normal

Continued

Pathology, female, HR—cont'd		
Assessment	**Test**	**Findings**
	Vitamin B$_{12}$ (cobalamin)	118 pmol/L LOW
	Vitamin D (calciferol)	22 nmol/L Significanly clinically deficient
	Red cell selenium	Normal
	Iron studies	Serum iron 8 micromols/L Transferrin 2–3 g/L Transferrin saturation 22% Ferritin 18 micrograms/L Significant clinical anaemia Transferrin saturation
	Fasting homocysteine	10.23 micromols/L Elevated
	Cancer antigen 125	Negative
	Full blood count	Low Hg Low MCV Low RCD
	Biochemistry	Normal ranges
	Liver function tests	Normal ranges
	Blood group	O
	Blood group antibodies	O – anti A, anti B
	Rh antigen	Negative
Toxicity		
	Chelation challenge Provocation test to investigate heavy metal toxicity	Nothing detected
Vaginal/cervical swab		
	Gardnerella vaginalis Group B streptococcus β-haemolytic streptococcus *Staphylococcus aureus* *Staphylococcus milleri* *Candida* spp.	Not detected
Referrals		
Referral to reproductive immunologist	Alloimmune	
	HLA compatibility issues	Positiive
	NK cell uterine biopsy	Positiive
		Negative

SUMMARY OF FINDINGS

Female HR was found to have a number of factors that increase risks of miscarriage and stillbirths:

- Overweight
- Insulin resistance metabolic syndrome
- Homozygous 1298C-A MTHFR
- Low B$_{12}$
- Low vitamin D
- Low iron – clinically anaemic
- Low zinc with elevated copper
- HLA compatibility issues with partner, indicative of alloimmune diagnosis
- Treatment with intravenous immunoglobulin (IVIg) therapy was commenced under management of reproductive immunologist.

TREATMENT PLAN

Female HR		
Nutrient/botanical	**Dose**	**Rationale**
B complex Including: L-5-methyltetrahydrofolate Vitamin B$_{12}$ (as methylcobalamin) 3–6 mg per day	2 capsules per day L-5-methyltetrahydrofolate 1000 mg per day Methylcobalamin 3 mg per day	Metabolism of carbohydrates, glucose metabolism, hormonal regulation, B vitamin repletion prior to conception To address deficiency Correct metabolically active isomers of folate and B$_{12}$ for homozygosity of 1298A-C gene polymorphism
Magnesium	600 mg per day	Improved insulin signalling and blood sugar regulation, energy production and anxiety support
Chromium	300 micrograms per day	Improved insulin signalling and blood sugar regulation, energy production
Zinc	50 mg per day	To address deficiency hormonal regulation, pregnancy preparation
Iron	75 mg per day	To address deficiency To improve red cell quality and capacity to carry oxygen To improve microvascular circulation
Vitamin D$_3$	10 000 IU/day*	To address deficiency Blood sugar regulation Inflammation management Immune modulation Thyroid hormone management
Tyrosine	1500 mg per day	Adrenal health Blood sugar regulation Thyroid health
Selenium	200 micrograms per day	Thyroid autoantibody management
Alpha lipoic acid	200 mg per day	Improved insulin signalling and blood sugar regulation, energy production Supports mitochondrial function
Vitamin C and bioflavonoids	Quercetin 1000 mg per day Rutin 500 mg per day Bromelain 300 mg per day Ascorbic acid 2000 mg per day	To address adrenal health Assists with uptake of iron Assists with microcirculation
Fish oil Despite dietary preference, fish oil was agreed upon due to preferential concentration sources of EPA and DHA required for healthy pregnancy outcomes	3 g per day	Improvement of microvascular circulation and inflammation management
Gymnema leaf 1:1 extract 3.5–10.7 mL per day	2.5 mL twice a day	Improved insulin signalling and blood sugar regulation
Ginkgo leaf 2:1 extract contains 9.6 mg/mL ginkgo flavone glycosides 3–4 mL per day	4 mL per day	To improve microvascular microcirculation and blood flow
Probiotics multi-strain 30 billion colony-forming units *Bifidobacterium longum* BB536 *Bifidobacterium breve* M-16V *Bifidobacterium infantis* M-63 *Bifidobacterium lactis* Bi-04 *Bifidobacterium lactis* HN019 *Lactobacillus rhamnosus* HN001 *Lactobacillus paracasei* Lpc-37 *Lactobacillus salivarius* Ls-33 *Lactobacillus casei* Lc-11	1 capsule twice per day	Immune regulation Microbiome support
Aspirin	100 mg per day	Recommended to maintain this medication by reproductive immunologist

*10 000 IU prescription requires close management and monitoring. It is only advised in acute bursts followed with repeat screening to assess uptake.

MALE PARTNER: IL AGED 33

- Nervous: depression. Circumstantial. No medication. No counselling to date.
- Gastrointestinal: sluggish bowel, foul flatulence, boating. Related to poor eating habits, dehydration and refined carbohydrate intake.
- Previous medical history: appendicitis age 18; hypertension and hyperlipidaemia since age 26. Strong family history.
- Diet: the Brahman diet was followed.
  - Meat not allowed.
  - Eggs not allowed.
  - Milk and milk products are permitted, butter, yoghurt, cream.
  - Cheese must not be coagulated with rennet.
  - Stimulants – coffee, tea not allowed.
  - Alcohol – not allowed.
- Lifestyle: corporate tertiary-educated man, works long hours in legal firm. Practises yoga and meditation to cope with stress.
- Other: non-smoker; no recreational drugs.
- Height 187 cm; Weight: 102 kg; BMI: 29.2 (overweight range).
- Supplement and medication at intake:
  - supplements – nil
  - long-term use of statin drugs for familial history and personal hyperlipidaemia.

INVESTIGATIONS

Assessment	Test	Reference range
Semen analysis WHO 5th criteria	Semen volume	Normal
	Total sperm number (10^6 per ejaculate)	Normal
	Sperm concentration (10^6 per mL)	Normal
	Total motility (PR + NP, %)	26 (38–42) Low
	Progressive (PR, %)	21 (31–34) Low
	Vitality (live spermatozoa, %)	56 (55–63) Normal
	Sperm morphology (normal forms, %)	3 (3–4) Low
	pH	Normal
	Peroxidase positive leukocytes (10^6 per mL)	Normal
	MAR test (motile spermatozoa with bound particles, %)	Normal
	Immunobead test (motile spermatozoa with bound beads, %)	Normal
	Sperm chromatin structure assay (SCSA®) or sperm chromatin integrity test (SCIT) for DNA fragmentation index	16% Normal
Male hormones		FSH 3 Normal LH 3 Normal Prolactin 133 Normal Testosterone total 10.3 nmol/L Low
Genetics		
	Extended karyotype	Normal
	MTHFR polymorphism	Homozygous 1298C-A
	Prothrombin gene mutation G20210A	Does not carry

Assessment	Test	Reference range
Biochemical		
	Serum zinc	11 micromols/L Low
	Serum copper	16 micromols/L Normal
	Red cell folate	Normal
	Caeruloplasmin	Normal
	Vitamin B$_{12}$ (cobalamin)	188 Borderline low
	Vitamin D (calciferol)	<20 nmol/L Significantly clinically low
	Red cell selenium	Normal
	Fasting homocysteine	18 mol/L High
	Full blood count	Low red cells
	Biochemistry	Normal ranges
	LFT	Normal ranges
	Fasting insulin	18 Elevated
Toxicity		
	Chelation challenge provocation test to investigate heavy metal toxicity	Negative

SUMMARY OF FINDINGS FOR MALE IL

- Poor sperm healthy despite DNA fragmentation being in acceptable limits
  - Reflective of poor diet, stressful lifestyle, being overweight and overt nutritional deficiencies
- Low androgens. Low testosterone – this will be impacting on sperm health.
- Low serum zinc

- Homozygous for 1298C-A MTHFR
- Low B$_{12}$
- Elevated homocysteine
- Significantly clinically deficient vitamin D
- Low red blood cell count, consequential to poor B$_{12}$ status and traditional diet
- Fasting insulin elevated – IR metabolic syndrome
- Overweight, BMI 29.2

TREATMENT PLAN

Male IL		
Nutrient/botanical	**Dose**	**Rationale**
B complex Including: L-5-methyltetrahydrofolate Vitamin B$_{12}$ (as methylcobalamin 3–6 mg per day)	2 capsules per day L-5-methyltetrahydrofolate 1000 mg per day Methylcobalamin 3 mg per day	Metabolism of carbohydrates, glucose metabolism, hormonal regulation, B vitamin repletion prior to conception To address deficiency Correct metabolically active isomers of folate and B$_{12}$ for homozygosity of 1298A-C gene polymorphism
Magnesium	600 mg per day	Improved insulin signalling and blood sugar regulation, energy production and anxiety support
Chromium	300 micrograms per day	Improved insulin signalling and blood sugar regulation, energy production
Zinc	50 mg per day	To address deficiency hormonal regulation, pregnancy preparation

Continued

Male IL—cont'd		
Nutrient/botanical	**Dose**	**Rationale**
Vitamin D₃	10 000 IU/day	To address deficiency Blood sugar regulation Inflammation management Immune modulation Thyroid hormone management
Selenium	200 micrograms per day	Sperm health Antioxidant
Alpha lipoic acid	200 mg per day	Improved insulin signalling and blood sugar regulation, energy production Supports mitochondrial function
Fish oil Despite dietary preference, fish oil was agreed upon due to preferential concentration sources of EPA and DHA required for healthy pregnancy outcomes.	3 g per day	Improvement of microvascular circulation and inflammation management Availability of fat-soluble vitamins (vitamin D) and assists with normalisation of ferritin levels
Vitamin E	1000 IU per day	Sperm health To improve testosterone synthesis Antioxidant Improvement of microvascular circulation and inflammation management
CoQ10 as ubiquinol	300 mg per day	Improvement to fertility parameters Cardiovascular health Microcirculation
Vitamin C and bioflavonoids	Quercetin 1000 mg per day Rutin 500 mg per day Bromelain 300 mg per day Ascorbic acid 2000 mg per day	To address adrenal health Assists with uptake of iron Assists with microcirculation
Gymnema leaf 1:1 extract 3.5–10.7 mL per day	2.5 mL twice a day	Improved insulin signalling and blood sugar regulation
Tribulus terrestris (tribulus) extract equivalent to dry herb (aerial parts) 13.5 g standardised to contain furostanol saponins as protodioscin 110 mg	2 tablets twice per day	Sperm health Hormonal regulation, improvement to fertility parameters
Fallopia japonica (giant knotweed) extract equivalent to dry root 8 g standardised to resveratrol 36 mg *Vitis vinifera* (grape seed) extract equivalent to dry seed 4.8 g standardised to contain procyanidins 38 mg 4.2 g standardised to flavanolignans calculated as silybin 48 mg *Panax ginseng* (Korean ginseng) extract equivalent to dry root 250 mg standardised to ginsenosides calculated as Rg1, Re, Rb1, Rc, Rb2 & Rd 4.2 mg	1 tablet three times a day	Antioxidant to sperm Sperm health Cardiovascular health Microcirculation Hormonal regulation, improvement to fertility parameters

Male IL—cont'd		
Nutrient/botanical	**Dose**	**Rationale**
Probiotics multi-strain 30 billion colony-forming units *Bifidobacterium longum* BB536 *Bifidobacterium breve* M-16V *Bifidobacterium infantis* M-63 *Bifidobacterium lactis* Bi-04 *Bifidobacterium lactis* HN019 *Lactobacillus rhamnosus* HN001 *Lactobacillus paracasei* Lpc-37 *Lactobacillus salivarius* Ls-33 *Lactobacillus casei* Lc-11	1 capsule per day	Immune regulation

NUTRITIONAL MEDICINE (DIETARY) FOR THE COUPLE

- Increase hydration – calculated according to body weight (2.5 L/day minimum).
- Avoid sugar, refined carbohydrates and excess fruit in order to assist treatment of blood sugar issues and metabolic syndrome.
- Increase and optimise protein intake and absorption (educate regarding sugar cravings correlating with blood sugar fluctuations and protein insufficiency).
- Encourage organic, wholefood dietary principles, with optimal protein, vegetables and complex carbohydrates.
- Avoid preservatives, colourings, additives, etc.
- Include fermented foods for gut health.
- Include a herb-rich diet including nigella seeds for blood sugar regulation, turmeric and allium family.
- Introduce coconut oil as anti-inflammatory.
- Despite their dietary choices, they were willing to take fish oil in their treatment plan.

OUTCOME

- The couple completed 6 months of treatment under the collaborative care of myself and an excellent specialist in reproductive immunology.
- They also embarked on a specialist psychology care plan to help process their grief and come to terms with their baby losses.
- During this time, monthly intralipid therapy was undertaken, alongside the integrative treatment plan.
- Regular repeat pathology was facilitated to ensure parameters were returning to normal range and deficiencies were overcome.
- Their health, both physical and emotional, improved tremendously during this time. Both partners effortlessly lost weight with dietary changes implemented and regular commitment to exercise and meditation.
- The couple conceived in their second month of trying to conceive. Mother and baby were under the care of a new high-risk obstetrician specialist, monitored extremely closely and given a great deal of extended tender loving care by this specialist during the course of the pregnancy. Enoxaparin sodium was administered daily by injection for the duration of the pregnancy.
- HR went into spontaneous labour and vaginally delivered a healthy baby girl at 39+4/40.

CONCLUSION

Although spontaneous or recurrent pregnancy loss is devastating, it can be helpful and reassuring for both us as the clinician and our patient to keep in mind the relatively high likelihood that the next pregnancy will be successful.

The likelihood of a full-term pregnancy will increase exponentially after rigorous investigation, allopathic and integrative treatment intervention and, most importantly, thorough preconception diet, lifestyle and nutritional preparation for 4 months prior to conception, involving both the female and the male partner.

Psychological support in all forms and frequent discussion, acknowledgement and sympathetic counselling are crucial to the successful evaluation and treatment of the anxious and emotionally taxed couple. We cannot underestimate the power of counselling to allay stress, which is so counterproductive to fertility and pregnancy.

One study showed that when no aetiological factor is identified and no treatment started, a 60–80% full-term pregnancy rate can be expected. Therefore, couples with unexplained recurrent miscarriage should be offered appropriate emotional support and reassurance.[84]

From a naturopathic management perspective, this may also involve flower essence therapy massage, acupuncture and additional prescription of herbals and nutritionals to treat adrenal and stress factors.

It must be stressed that couples with recurrent miscarriage should be referred to a reproductive endocrinologist/+reproductive immunologist or obstetric gynecologist for primary care management, as specialist-level investigations and concurrent medical treatments may be required in order to help the couple achieve full-term pregnancy and the resultant birth of their long-awaited healthy baby.

REFERENCES

[1] Ford HB, Schust DJ. Recurrent pregnancy loss: etiology, diagnosis, and therapy. Rev Obstet Gynecol 2009;2(2):76–83.

[2] Udry S, Aranda FM, Latino JO, et al. Paternal factor V Leiden and recurrent pregnancy loss: a new concept behind fetal genetics? J Thromb Haemost 2014;12(5):666–9.

[3] Gordon A, Jeffery HE. Classification and description of stillbirths in New South Wales, 2002–2004. Med J Aust 2008;188(11):645–8.

[4] Simpson J, Carson S. Genetic and nongenetic causes of pregnancy loss. Glob Libr Women's Med 2013;3(3).

[5] Jeve YB, Davies W. Evidence-based management of recurrent miscarriages. J Hum Reprod Sci 2014;7(3):159.

[6] Mukherjee S, Edwards DR, Baird DD, et al. Risk of miscarriage among black women and white women in a US Prospective Cohort Study. Am J Epidemiol 2013;177(11):1271–8.

[7] Amodio G, Canti V, Maggio L, et al. Association of genetic variants in the 3' UTR of HLA-G with recurrent pregnancy loss. Hum Immunol 2016;77(10):886–91.

[8] Annan JJK, Gudi A, Bhide P, et al. Biochemical pregnancy during assisted conception: a little bit pregnant. J Clin Med Res 2013;5(4):269.

[9] Schaeffer AJ, Chung J, Heretis K, et al. Comparative genomic hybridization – array analysis enhances the detection of aneuploidies and submicroscopic imbalances in spontaneous miscarriages. Am J Hum Genet 2004;74(6):1168–74.

[10] Tong S, Kaur A, Walker SP, et al. Miscarriage risk for asymptomatic women after a normal first-trimester prenatal visit. Obstet Gynecol 2008;111(3):710–14.

[11] Doubilet PM, Benson CB. Embryonic heart rate in the early first trimester: what rate is normal? J Ultrasound Med 1995;14(6):431–4.

[12] Cohen-Overbeek TE, den Ouden M, Pijpers L, et al. Spontaneous abortion rate and advanced maternal age: consequences for prenatal diagnosis. Lancet 1990;336(8706):27–9.

[13] Ammon Avalos L, Galindo C, Li DK. A systematic review to calculate background miscarriage rates using life table analysis. Birth Defects Res A Clin Mol Teratol 2012;94(6):417–23.

[14] Alansari LM, Wardle P. Endometrial polyps and subfertility. Hum Fertil 2012;15(3):129–33.

[15] Medrano-Uribe FA, Enríquez-Pérez MM, Reyes-Muñoz E. Prevalence of uterine anatomical anomalies in Mexican women with recurrent pregnancy loss (RPL). Gac Med Mex 2015;152(2):163–6.

[16] Ludwin A, Ludwin I, Banas T, et al. Diagnostic accuracy of sonohysterography, hysterosalpingography and diagnostic hysteroscopy in diagnosis of arcuate, septate and bicornuate uterus. J Obstet Gynaecol Res 2011;37(3):178–86.

[17] Wang SW, Ma LL, Huang S, et al. Role of cervical cerclage and vaginal progesterone in the treatment of cervical incompetence with/without preterm birth history. Chin Med J 2016;129(22):2670.

[18] Soler A, Morales C, Mademont-Soler I, et al. Overview of chromosome abnormalities in first trimester miscarriages: a series of 1,011 consecutive chorionic villi sample karyotypes. Cytogenet Genome Res 2017;152(2):81–9.

[19] Ogasawara M, Aoki K, Okada S, et al. Embryonic karyotype of abortuses in relation to the number of previous miscarriages. Fertil Steril 2000;73(2):300–4.

[20] Griffiths AJF, Miller JH, Suzuki DT, et al. An introduction to genetic analysis. 7th ed. New York: W. H. Freeman; 2000.

[21] Bonduelle M, Liebaers I, Deketelaere V, et al. Neonatal data on a cohort of 2889 infants born after ICSI (1991–1999) and of 2995 infants born after IVF (1983–1999). Hum Reprod 2002;17:671.

[22] Maconochie N, Doyle P, Prior S, et al. Risk factors for first trimester miscarriage – results from a UK-population-based case-control study. BJOG 2007;114(2):170–86.

[23] Wu X, Zhao L, Zhu H, et al. Association between the MTHFR C677T polymorphism and recurrent pregnancy loss: a meta-analysis. Genet Test Mol Biomarkers 2012;16(7):806–11.

[24] Strauss JF III, Barbieri RL. Yen & Jaffe's reproductive endocrinology: physiology, pathophysiology, and clinical management. Philadelphia: Saunders; 2013.

[25] Bosler D, et al. Phenotypic heterogeneity in patients with homozygous prothrombin G20210A genotype. J Mol Diagn 2006;8:420–5.

[26] Foy P, Moll S. Thrombophilia: 2009. Curr Treat Options Cardiovasc Med 2009;11(2):114–28.

[27] Enciso M, Sarasa J, Xanthopoulou L, et al. Polymorphisms in the MTHFR gene influence embryo viability and the incidence of aneuploidy. Hum Genet 2016;135(5):555–68.

[28] Tara SS, Ghaemimanesh F, Zarei S, et al. Methylenetetrahydrofolate reductase C677T and A1298C polymorphisms in male partners of recurrent miscarriage couples. J Reprod Infertil 2015;16(4):193.

[29] Kolte AM, Steffensen R, Nielsen HS, et al. Study of the structure and impact of human leukocyte antigen (HLA)-GA, HLA-GB, and HLA-G-DRB1 haplotypes in families with recurrent miscarriage. Hum Immunol 2010;71(5):482–8.

[30] Kwam-Kim J, Kim JW, Gilman Sachi A. Immunology and pregnancy: losses HLA autoantibodies and cellular immunity. Immunology of Pregnancy. New York: Springer Publishers; 2006. p. 303–5.

[31] Porter TF, Scott JR. Alloimmune causes of recurrent pregnancy loss. Semin Reprod Med 2000;18(4):393–400.

[32] Perez-Sepulveda A, Torres MJ, Khoury M, et al. Innate immune system and preeclampsia. Front Immunol 2015;5:244. doi:10.3389/fimmu.2014.00244.

[33] Raghupathy R, Al-Azemi M. Modulation of cytokine production by the dydrogesterone metabolite dihydrodydrogesterone. Am J Reprod Immunol 2015;74(5):419–26.

[34] McNamee K, Dawood F, Farquharson R. Recurrent miscarriage and thrombophilia: an update. Curr Opin Obstet Gynecol 2012;24(4):229–34.

[35] Silver RM, Branch DW, Goldenberg R, et al. Nomenclature for pregnancy outcomes: time for a change. Obstet Gynecol 2011;118(6):1402–8.

[36] Farghali MM, El-kholy AL, Swidan KH, et al. Relationship between uterine natural killer cells and unexplained repeated miscarriage. J Turk Ger Gynecol Assoc 2015;16(4):214.

[37] Sugiura-Ogasawara M, Ozaki Y, Sonta SI, et al. Exposure to bisphenol A is associated with recurrent miscarriage. Hum Reprod 2005;20(8):2325–9.

[38] Ma B, Forney LJ, Ravel J. The vaginal microbiome: rethinking health and diseases. Annu Rev Microbiol 2012;66:371.

[39] Giakoumelou S, Wheelhouse N, Cuschieri K, et al. The role of infection in miscarriage. Hum Reprod Update 2016;22(1):116–33.

[40] Haggerty CL, Totten PA, Tang G, et al. Identification of novel microbes associated with pelvic inflammatory disease and infertility. Sex Transm Infect 2016;92(6):441–6.

[41] Rai R, Backos M, Rushworth F, et al. Polycystic ovaries and recurrent miscarriage – a reappraisal. Hum Reprod 2000;15(3):612–15.

[42] Chen H, Lina H. Dopamine agonists for preventing future miscarriage in women with idiopathic hyperprolactinemia and recurrent miscarriage history. Cochrane Database Syst Rev 2016;(7):CD008883.

[43] Li ZL, Xiang HF, Cheng LH, et al. Association between recurrent miscarriages and insulin resistance: a meta analysis. Zhonghua Fu Chan Ke Za Zhi 2012;47(12):915–19.

[44] Hechtman L. Clinical naturopathic medicine. Chatswood. NSW: Elsevier Health Sciences; 2013.

[45] Lashen H, Fear K, Sturdee DW. Obesity is associated with increased risk of first trimester and recurrent miscarriage: matched case-control study. Hum Reprod 2004;19(7):1644–6.

[46] Durairajanayagam D, Agarwal A, Ong C. Causes, effects and molecular mechanisms of testicular heat stress. Reprod Biomed Online 2015;30(1):14–27.

[47] Ferguson LR, Ford JH. Overlap between mutagens and teratogens. Mutat Res 1997;396:1–8.

[48] Weng X, Odouli R, Li DK. Maternal caffeine consumption during pregnancy and the risk of miscarriage: a prospective cohort study. Am J Obstet Gynecol 2008;198(3):279.e1–8.

[49] Wong EY, Ray RM, Gao DL, et al. Dust and chemical exposures and miscarriage risk among women textile workers in Shanghai, China. Occup Environ Med 2009;66(3):161–8.

[50] Windham B. Mercury and toxic metal effects on kidneys, urinary system & fertility. Available from: https://mercuryexposure.info/wp-content/uploads/2011/03/k2_attachments_The_Effects_of_Mercury_and_Toxic_Metals_on_the_Kidneys_Urinary_System_and_Fertility.pdf.

[51] Ward N, Eaton K. Preconceptional care and pregnancy outcome. J Nutr Environ Med 1995;5(2):205–8.

[52] Ribas-Maynou J, Fernández-Encinas A, García-Peiró A, et al. Human semen cryopreservation: a sperm DNA fragmentation study with alkaline and neutral Comet assay. Andrology 2014;2(1):83–7.

[53] Dul EC, van Echten-Arends J, Groen H, et al. Chromosomal abnormalities in azoospermic and non-azoospermic infertile men: numbers needed to be screened to prevent adverse pregnancy outcomes. Hum Reprod 2012;27(9):2850–6.

[54] Evenson DP. Sperm chromatin structure assay (SCSA®). In: Carrell D, Aston K, editors. Spermatogenesis, vol. 927. Methods in molecular biology (methods and protocols). Totowa, NJ: Humana Press; 2013. p. 147–64.

[55] Leach M, Aitken RJ, Sacks G. Sperm DNA fragmentation abnormalities in men from couples with a history of recurrent miscarriage. Aust N Z J Obstet Gynaecol 2015;55(4):379–83.

[56] Menkveld R. Clinical significance of the low normal sperm morphology value as proposed in the fifth edition of the WHO Laboratory Manual for the Examination and Processing of Human Semen. Asian J Androl 2010;12(1):47–58.

[57] Evenson DP, Wixon R. Environmental toxicants cause sperm DNA fragmentation as detected by the sperm chromatin structure assay (SCSA. Toxicol Appl Pharmacol 2005;207(2):532–7.

[58] Koeman M. Miscarriage antibodies – fertility problems from an immunological perspective. Mod Phytotherapist 1999;5(2):9.

[59] Jauniaux E, Poston L, Burton GJ. Placental-related diseases of pregnancy: involvement of oxidative stress and implications in human evolution. Hum Reprod Update 2006;12(6):747–55.

[60] Amin AF, Shaaban OM, Bediawy MA. N-acetyl cysteine for treatment of recurrent unexplained pregnancy loss. Reprod Biomed Online 2008;17(5):722–6.

[61] Beloosesky R, Weiner Z, Khativ N, et al. Prophylactic maternal n-acetylcysteine before lipopolysaccharide suppresses fetal inflammatory cytokine responses. Am J Obstet Gynecol 2009;200(6):665.e1–5.

[62] Zachara BA, Dobrzyński W, Trafikowska U, et al. Blood selenium and glutathione peroxidases in miscarriage. BJOG 2001;108(3):244–7.

[63] Gäreskog M, Cederberg J, Eriksson UJ, et al. Maternal diabetes in vivo and high glucose concentration in vitro increases apoptosis in rat embryos. Reprod Toxicol 2007;23(1):63–74.

[64] Foster JA, Gerton GL. Autoantigen 1 of the guinea pig sperm acrosome is the homologue of mouse Tpx-1 and human TPX1 and is a member of the cysteine-rich secretory protein (CRISP) family. Mol Reprod Dev 1996;44(2):221–9.

[65] De Matos DG, Furnus CC. The importance of having high glutathione (GSH) level after bovine in vitro maturation on embryo development: effect of β-mercaptoethanol, cysteine and cysteine. Theriogenology 2000;53(3):761–71.

[66] Rossi E, Costa M. Fish oil derivatives as a prophylaxis of recurrent miscarriage associated with antiphospholipid antibodies (APL): a pilot study. Lupus 1993;2(5):319–23.

[67] Hasan R, Olshan AF, Herring AH, et al. Self-reported vitamin supplementation in early pregnancy and risk of miscarriage. Am J Epidemiol 2009;169(11):1312–18.

[68] Şimşek M, Naziro-lu M, Şimşek H, et al. Blood plasma levels of lipoperoxides, glutathione peroxidase, beta carotene, vitamin A and E in women with habitual abortion. Cell Biochem Funct 1998;16(4):227–31.

[69] Vural P, Akgül C, Yildirim A, et al. Antioxidant defence in recurrent abortion. Clin Chim Acta 2000;295(1):169–77.

[70] Junovich G, Dubinsky V, Gentile T, et al. Comparative immunological effect of anticoagulant and antioxidant therapy in the prevention of abortion in mice. Am J Reprod Immunol 2011;65(2):104–9.

[71] Bubanovic I. 1α, 25-dihydroxy-vitamin-D3 as new immunotherapy in treatment of recurrent spontaneous abortion. Med Hypotheses 2004;63(2):250–3.

[72] Díaz L, Noyola-Martinez N, Barrera D, et al. Calcitriol inhibits TNF-α-induced inflammatory cytokines in human trophoblasts. J Reprod Immunol 2009;81(1):17–24.

[73] Maeba R, Hiroshi HARA, Ishikawa H, et al. Myo-inositol treatment increases serum plasmalogens and decreases small dense LDL, particularly in hyperlipidemic subjects with metabolic syndrome. J Nutr Sci Vitaminol 2008;54(3):196–202.

[74] Graham TW, Thurmond MC, Gershwin ME, et al. Serum zinc and copper concentrations in relation to spontaneous abortion in cows: implications for human fetal loss. J Reprod Fertil 1994;102(1):253–62.

[75] Venu L, Harishankar N, Krishna TP, et al. Does maternal dietary mineral restriction per se predispose the offspring to insulin resistance? Eur J Endocrinol 2004;151(2):287–94.

[76] Anderson RA. Chromium and insulin resistance. Nutr Res Rev 2003;16(02):267–75.

[77] Zhang Q, Sun X, Xiao X, et al. Dietary chromium restriction of pregnant mice changes the methylation status of hepatic genes involved with insulin signaling in adult male offspring. PLoS ONE 2017;12(1).

[78] Pearce EN. Maternal subclinical hypothyroidism and thyroid autoimmunity in early gestation are associated with increased risk of miscarriage. Clin Thyroidol 2014;26(9):235–7.

[79] Negro R, Schwartz A, Gismondi R, et al. Increased pregnancy loss rate in thyroid antibody negative women with TSH levels between 2.5 and 5.0 in the first trimester of pregnancy. J Clin Endocrinol Metab 2010;95(9):E44–8.

[80] Mazokopakis EE, Papadakis JA, Papadomanolaki MG, et al. Effects of 12 months treatment with L-selenomethionine on serum anti-TPO levels in patients with Hashimoto's thyroiditis. Thyroid 2007;17(7):609–12.

[81] Krysiak R, Okopien B. The effect of levothyroxine and selenomethionine on lymphocyte and monocyte cytokine release in women with Hashimoto's thyroiditis. J Clin Endocrinol Metab 2011;96(7):2206–15.

[82] Friebe A, Arck P. Causes for spontaneous abortion: what's the bugs 'gut' to do with it? Int J Biochem Cell Biol 2008;40(11):2348–52.

[83] Hunt JS, Petroff MG, McIntire RH, et al. HLA-G and immune tolerance in pregnancy. FASEB J 2005;19(7):681–93.

[84] Stray-Pedersen B, Stray-Pedersen S. Etiologic factors and subsequent reproductive performance in 195 couples with a prior history of habitual abortion. Am J Obstet Gynecol 1984;148(2):140–6.

[85] Gaskins AJ, Rich-Edwards JW, Hauser R, et al. Maternal prepregnancy folate intake and risk of spontaneous abortion and stillbirth. Obstet Gynecol 2014;124(1):23–31.

[86] Uriu-Adams JY, Keen CL. Zinc and reproduction: effects of zinc deficiency on prenatal and early postnatal development. Birth Defects Res B Dev Reprod Toxicol 2010;89(4):313–25.

[87] Twigt JM, Bolhuis ME, Steegers EA, et al. The preconception diet is associated with the chance of ongoing pregnancy in women undergoing IVF/ICSI treatment. Hum Reprod 2012;27(8):2526–31.

[88] Di Cintio E, Parazzini F, Chatenoud L, et al. Dietary factors and risk of spontaneous abortion. Eur J Obstet Gynecol Reprod Biol 2001;95:132–6.

[89] Cramer DW, Wise LA. The epidemiology of recurrent pregnancy loss. Semin Reprod Med 2000;18:331–9.

[90] Zimmermann MB. The role of iodine in human growth and development. Semin Cell Dev Biol 2011;22(6):645–52.

[91] Lepoutre T, Debièye F, Gruson D, et al. Reduction of miscarriages through universal screening and treatment of thyroid autoimmune diseases. Gynecol Obstet Invest 2012;74(4):265–73.

[92] Murphy MM, Fernandez-Ballart JD. Homocysteine in pregnancy. Adv Clin Chem 2011;53:105–37.

[93] Micle O, Muresan M, Antal L, et al. The influence of homocysteine and oxidative stress on pregnancy outcome. J Med Life 2012;5(1):68–73.

[94] Greenwood DC, Thatcher NJ, Ye J, et al. Caffeine intake during pregnancy and adverse birth outcomes: a systematic review and dose-response meta-analysis. Eur J Epidemiol 2014;29:725–34.

[95] Omeljaniuk WJ, Socha K, et al. Antioxidant status in women who have had a miscarriage. Adv Med Sci 2015;60(2):329–34.

[96] Petri M. Systemic lupus erythematosus and pregnancy. Rheum Dis Clin North Am 1994;20(1):87–118.

[97] Empson M, Lassere M, Craig J, et al. Prevention of recurrent miscarriage for women with antiphospholipid antibody or lupus anticoagulant. Cochrane Database Syst Rev 2005;(2):CD002859.

[98] Carrington B, Sacks G, Regan L. Recurrent miscarriage: pathophysiology and outcome. Curr Opin Obstet Gynecol 2005;17(6):591–7.

[99] Mills S, Bone K. The essential guide to herbal safety. London: Elsevier Health Sciences; 2005.

[100] Mills S, Bone K. Principles and practice of phytotherapy: modern herbal medicine. London: Elsevier Health Sciences; 2013.

[101] Ota H, Fukishima M. Stimulation by Kanpo prescriptions of aromatase activity in rat follicle cell cultures. Recent advances in the pharmacology of Kanpo (Japanese herbal) Medicines. Amsterdam: Excerpta Medicine; 1998.

[102] Zha LL. Experimental effect of Rehmannia glutinosa on the pituitary and adrenal cortex in a glucocorticoid inhibition model using rabbits. Zhong Xi Yi Jie He Za Zhi 1988;8(2):95.

[103] Chang HM, But PP, Yao SC. Pharmacology and applications of Chinese materia medica, vol. 1. Singapore: World Scientific; 1986.

[104] He DY, Dai SM. Anti-inflammatory and immunomodulatory effects of Paeonia lactiflora Pall., a traditional Chinese herbal medicine. Front Pharmacol 2011;2:10.

[105] Bone K, Morgan M. Clinical applications of ayurvedic and Chinese herbs: monographs for the Western herbal practitioner. Warwick: Phytotherapy Press; 1996.

[106] Sarris J, Wardle J. Clinical naturopathy: an evidence-based guide to practice. Chatswood. NSW: Elsevier Health Sciences; 2014.

[107] Schaffer M, Schaffer PM, Bar-Sela G. An update on Curcuma as a functional food in the control of cancer and inflammation. Curr Opin Clin Nutr Metab Care 2015;18(6):605–11.

[108] Bayan L, Koulivand PH, Gorji A. Garlic: a review of potential therapeutic effects. Avicenna J Phytomed 2014;4(1):1–14.

[109] Jung F, Mrowietz C, Kiesewetter H, et al. Effect of Ginkgo biloba on fluidity of blood and peripheral microcirculation in volunteers. Arzneimittelforschung 1990;40(5):589–93.

[110] Suter A, Niemer W, Klopp R. A new ginkgo fresh plant extract increases microcirculation and radical scavenging activity in elderly patients. Adv Ther 2011;28(12):1078–88.

[111] Liu XP, Goldring CE, Copple IM, et al. Extract of Ginkgo biloba induces phase 2 genes through Keap1-Nrf2-ARE signaling pathway. Life Sci 2007;80(17):1586–91.

[112] Blumenthal M. Therapeutic guide to herbal medicines. US: American Botanical Council; 1998.

[113] Dericks-Tan JSE, Schwinn P, Hildt C. Dose-dependent stimulation of melatonin secretion after administration of Agnus castus. Exp Clin Endocrinol Diabetes 2003;111(01):44–6.

[114] Takasaki A, Nakamura Y, Tamura H, et al. Melatonin as a new drug for improving oocyte quality. Reprod Med Biol 2003;2(4):139–44.

[115] Sharma K. Asparagus racemosus (Shatavari): a versatile female tonic. Int J Pharm Biol Arch 2011;2(3):855–63.

[116] Alok S, Jain SK, Verma A, et al. Plant profile, phytochemistry and pharmacology of Asparagus racemosus (Shatavari): a review. Asian Pac J Trop Dis 2013;3(3):242–51.

[117] Mishra LC, Singh BB, Dagenais S. Scientific basis for the therapeutic use of Withania somnifera (ashwagandha): a review. Altern Med Rev 2000;5(4):334–46.

[118] Singh G, Sharma PK, Dudhe R, et al. Biological activities of Withania somnifera. Ann Biol Res 2010;1(3):56–63.

[119] Haller J, Freund TF, Pelczer KG, et al. The anxiolytic potential and psychotropic side effects of an echinacea preparation in laboratory animals and healthy volunteers. Phytother Res 2013; 27(1):54–61.

[120] Gallo M, Sarkar M, Au W, et al. Pregnancy outcome following gestational exposure to echinacea: a prospective controlled study. Arch Intern Med 2000;160(20):3141–3.

[121] Suguna L, Sivakumar P, Chandrakasan G. Effects of Centella asiatica extract on dermal wound healing in rats. Indian J Exp Biol 1996;34(12):208–11.

[122] Shetty BS, Udupa SL, Udupa AL, et al. Effect of Centella asiatica L (Umbelliferae) on normal and dexamethasone-suppressed wound healing in Wistar Albino rats. Int J Low Extrem Wounds 2006;5(3):137–43.

[123] MacKay DJ, Miller AL. Nutritional support for wound healing. Altern Med Rev 2003;8(4):359–78.

[124] Gohil K, Patel J, Gajjar A. Pharmacological review on Centella asiatica: a potential herbal cure-all. Indian J Pharm Sci 2010;72(5):546.

[125] Bode AM, Dong Z. The amazing and mighty ginger. Herbal medicine: biomolecular and clinical aspects. Boca Raton: CRC Press; 2011.

13

Pregnancy and labour

Jane Hutchens

INTRODUCTION

Pregnancy is the period from the implantation of a fertilised ovum to birth and takes approximately 40 weeks, roughly divided into three trimesters: trimester 1, weeks 1–13; trimester 2, weeks 14–27; and trimester 3, weeks 28–40. The due date is calculated as 40 weeks from the first day of the last normal menstrual period, or 38 weeks from conception. A baby is considered preterm if it is born before 37 weeks, post-term (or post-dates) if born after 42 weeks, and term if born between 37 and 42 weeks. A pregnancy may be single or multiple (two or more developing fetuses, e.g. twins or triplets). Risks of complications for both mother and baby increase the earlier and the later the child is born. The goal for all women is a healthy pregnancy, which can be defined as one where the mother is physically and psychologically well during pregnancy and the postpartum period and that results in the birth of a healthy baby. Ideally, naturopathic support commences in the preconception period; however, it may start once pregnancy has been confirmed or even later. Thus the level of support and intervention required will vary.

While pregnancy and childbirth are natural events, at times medical intervention is required for the safety of mother and child. Women who are older, have pre-existing medical conditions, have a multiple pregnancy or live in isolated areas may require additional support. Pregnancy is an immeasurably important time for a woman, but the pregnancy and birth of the child also impact on the father, the family and loved ones and care delivery needs to consider these relationships. Furthermore, a woman may be in a heterosexual or a homosexual relationship or be single, the baby may have been conceived naturally or using assisted reproductive technologies, the egg and sperm could be the birth parents' or donated, and the pregnancy may have been planned or unplanned. These relationships and contextual issues are not explored in this chapter, but it is necessary to be mindful of each patient's unique circumstances and to avoid assumptions.

EPIDEMIOLOGY

In 2013 in Australia 304 777 women gave birth to 309 489 babies, a 20% increase from 2003. The crude rate of birth per woman in 2013 was 63.4 per 1000 women aged 15–44 years. The total fertility rate in Australia has remained relatively steady since the late 1970s and it is projected that it will remain at around the 2013 rate of 1.9 births per woman.[1]

Live births and stillbirths

A stillbirth is defined variously in different countries. In Australia it is understood to mean the loss of a pregnancy of at least 20 weeks gestation or weighing at least 400 g at birth.[2] The number of stillbirths has increased since 2002, but the rate is relatively stable (7.1 stillbirths per 1000 births in 2003 and 2013, or 1 in every 135 births) and the increase reflects an increase in total births.[2,3] The rate of stillbirths differs across ages, with the rate in mothers aged 40 or older falling from 12.7 to 10.6 per 1000 births between 1991 and 2009, but the rate for teenage mothers rising from 9.5 to 15.0 per 1000 births for the same period.[2] It is usual for slightly more males than females to be born and this is true for 2013, where males represented 51.4% of births. The mean gestational age in 2013 was 38.7 weeks and 90.9% of babies were born at term (defined in this data set as between 37 and 41 weeks).

Maternal age and parity

Maternal age is a key risk factor for both maternal and infant morbidity and mortality, with both ends of the age spectrum representing the greatest risk. In Australia, the number of older mothers is increasing while the number of younger mothers is decreasing. In 2013 the age of mothers ranged from less than 15 years to 56 years, with a mean age of 30.1 except for Indigenous mothers, who had a mean age of 25.3 years. The proportion of mothers aged 40 years and over has been steadily increasing: 4.4% of women who gave birth in 2013 were aged over 40 compared to 3.2% 10 years earlier. The overall proportion of teenage mothers fell from 4.6% in 2003 to 3.3% in 2013.

Mothers born overseas

Australia is a multicultural community and in 2013 31.6% (94 697) of mothers were born overseas.[3] Indigenous and overseas-born mothers may have specific requirements in order for maternal care to be culturally appropriate and religion-sensitive, and practitioners working within culturally diverse communities will need to apprise themselves of the different practices, beliefs and possible impact of healthcare delivery.[3]

Gestation and birth weight

Gestation and birth weight are key health indicators for mother and infant. In 2013 the average gestational age for babies was 38.7 weeks for live births and 26.9 weeks for stillbirths, with 8.6% of babies preterm (before 37 weeks gestation) and less than 1% post-term (42 weeks or more).[4] This incorporates a 12% increase in preterm births from 1994 to 2004 and the pre-term cohort includes late preterm (34–37 weeks) induction of labour and caesarean section for women identified as low risk.[5] In 2011, 6.3% of live birth babies had a low birth weight (less than 2500 g) and this nearly doubled (11.2%) for women who smoked during pregnancy.[4] In 2010, babies born to Indigenous mothers were twice as likely as those born to non-Indigenous mothers to be of low birth weight (12% compared with 6%).[6]

MODELS OF ANTENATAL CARE

There are various models of antenatal care in different countries, most notably between developing and developed nations, where there is also a stark disparity in perinatal morbidity and mortality rates. Within Australia there is variance in the range of options available for women living in affluent areas of cities compared to lower income areas as well as for city versus regional rural and remote areas.

In Australia an expectant mother receives antenatal care through one or a combination of obstetrician, midwife, shared-care GP and doula, with obstetricians and midwives available in both public and private health systems. In 2013 most mothers gave birth in a hospital labour ward (97%, 296 611), with a small percentage giving birth in a birth centre (2.0%, 6085), at home (0.3%, 958) or in other settings including in transit to the hospital (0.3%, 984).[4]

The majority of Australian women have vaginal deliveries but the proportion of caesarean sections is high and continuing to rise: in the period 1991–2011 caesareans rose from 18% to 32% and vaginal births without intervention fell from 70% to 56%.[6] In comparison, in 2011 the average rate of caesareans was 25.7% for Organisation for Economic Co-operation and Development (OECD) countries, 23.7% for the UK, 32.3% for the US, 14.3% for the Netherlands and 15.7% for Finland.[7]

THE ROLE OF THE NATUROPATH

Obstetricians, midwives and shared-care GPs are the primary maternity service providers and this can be augmented by complementary therapists such as naturopaths, bodyworkers and doulas. Ideally naturopathic care is established in the preconception period, but it may be commenced at any point, including in the postnatal period. The role of the naturopath includes:

- Performing ongoing assessment and monitoring of the patient using clinical observation and assessment, appropriate pathology tests and other tools and questionnaires as indicated
- Evaluating the outcomes of interventions and adjusting treatment accordingly

- Providing education and referral to best meet desired patient outcomes
- Enhancing the patient's nutritional status
- Treating common conditions of pregnancy
- Preparing for labour
- Optimising the patient's overall health and thereby supporting fetal health and development
- Providing advice regarding the safety of herbs and nutritional supplements in pregnancy
- Providing therapeutics as indicated.

There has been a lack of comprehensive information on the use of professional consultations with naturopaths, herbal medicine practitioners, nutritionists and other complementary therapists for pregnancy-related health conditions.[8] A recent review in Australia has begun to provide insight: a survey completed by 1835 women found that 49.4% had consulted a complementary and alternative medicine (CM) practitioner for pregnancy-related health conditions, yet only 7.2% had consulted a naturopath.[9] The use of CM therapies including herbal medicine and nutritional supplements is far in excess of the number of women who consult professionals qualified in these areas. The prevalence for the use of herbal medicine is difficult to quantify as there are geographical and other differences; however, it ranges from 34% in Australia[10] to 58% in the UK,[11] 40% in Norway,[12] 8% in the US[13] and 9% in Canada.[14,15] In addition to the disparity between use of CM and consultation with a CM professional are questions regarding the level of training and supervision of practitioners who are working with pregnant women.[8] Furthermore, there are few clinical guidelines for CM in general, including as relates to pregnancy care, and while there is an increasing and rich body of evidence for the importance of nutrition and nutrients in pregnancy, there is a paucity of research into the safety and efficacy of herbal medicines and other modalities such as meditation.

MODES OF DELIVERY

There are several ways in which a woman may give birth and broadly they can be categorised as normal vaginal delivery (NVD), assisted/instrumented birth and caesarean birth. An NVD may be at home or in the labour ward and can include assorted pain relief as well as CalmBirth and relaxation techniques. Increasingly it is apparent that most women are able to have a NVD after having had a prior caesarean birth and this is known as vaginal birth after caesarean (VBAC). An assisted/instrumented birth may involve an episiotomy or vacuum extraction or be forceps-assisted.

A caesarean birth may be planned or unplanned (emergency) when trial of labour has not progressed, the baby is getting distressed or another problem requires intervention. A caesarean is major surgery and women need additional support following the procedure. Each year some 1.5 million women have a caesarean birth and in countries like Australia that number is increasing.[16] However, there is also an increase in the number of women wishing to try a VBAC, a practice previously not encouraged. A large review spanning 40 years has concluded that while women attempting VBAC have an increased risk of uterine rupture in trial of labour, an increased requirement for blood transfusion and higher overall maternal and perinatal mortality, overall these risks were low and VBAC is a safe option for most women.[16] A Cochrane Review on planned elective caesarean versus vaginal birth after a previous caesarean found that both options have risks and benefits and there is no statistically significant difference between planned caesarean birth and planned vaginal birth.[17]

While most naturopaths are not directly involved in childbirth, it is helpful to know of resources and programs that women and their partners can use. These may be antenatal classes at hospital, meditation and relaxation classes specific to pregnancy and birth, or pregnancy yoga and exercise classes. A recently published study that is the first randomised controlled trial in Australia in this area investigated the effectiveness of a birth preparation course, integrating multiple complementary medicine techniques, for the support of natural birth for first-time mothers.[18] The intervention incorporated six evidence-based complementary medicine techniques: acupressure, visualisation and relaxation, breathing, massage, yoga and facilitated partner support. The treatment group attended a 2-day antenatal education program plus standard care, while the control group received standard care alone. The results include reduced use of epidural in the treatment group (23.9% vs 68.7%), reduced rate of augmentation (e.g. requiring oxytocin), reduced rate of caesarean section, reduced length of second stage labour and perineal trauma, and reduced requirement for resuscitation of the newborn. There were no differences between the two groups for spontaneous onset of labour, use of narcotic analgesia, postpartum haemorrhage, major perineal trauma or admission to high-dependency care for the infant.

EMOTIONAL AND PSYCHOLOGICAL WELLBEING

Pregnancy can be a very positive event but it may also be fraught with negative emotions, trauma, anxiety and depression and it may even act as a memory trigger for prior abuse. Recent research indicates that perinatal anxiety is more prevalent than postnatal depression (and indeed may be the antecedent); thus this needs to be monitored throughout a woman's pregnancy.[19] Establishing and maintaining open communication and trust are essential, as is not making assumptions about the woman's wellbeing. Use of relaxation techniques, meditation and exercise and referral to a specialist counsellor or psychologist may be required, especially if there is a history of trauma, previous stillbirth or grief.

In some relationships, pregnancy appears to be a trigger for domestic violence, which presents serious risks to the woman (including breast and genital injury, miscarriage, antepartum haemorrhage and infection, blunt or penetrating abdominal trauma and death) and to the baby (including fetal fractures, low birth weight, injury, suppressed immune system).[20–22] In the Australian Personal Safety Survey of 2012, 22% of women said that they had experienced physical violence during pregnancy from their current partner and 25% had experienced violence during pregnancy at the hands of their previous partner.[23] In addition, for 25% of women who experienced violence from a previous partner, pregnancy was the first episode of violence. In a further survey of 400 pregnant Australian women, 20% experienced violence during pregnancy.[20] The figures for Australia are not unique and intimate partner violence is a known crisis worldwide.[21] A 2014 Cochrane Review of interventions to reduce intimate partner violence during pregnancy was unable to recommend any strategy, but it is important for practitioners to be aware of the issue and of available resources and referral options for counselling and refuge.[24]

EPIGENETICS AND THE ORIGINS OF DISEASE

In recent years an increasing body of evidence has demonstrated that the preconception, prenatal and postnatal environments influence the health of offspring in adulthood. This concept was first articulated by the late Sir David Barker and hence was known as the Barker Hypothesis; it was later known as Fetal Programming, Fetal Origins of Adult Disease and most recently Developmental Origins of Adult Health and Disease (DOHaD).[25] This last iteration is important because it contains recognition that perinatal environmental influences can enhance, as well as diminish, health in the offspring, and this is indeed the goal of excellent preconception, prenatal and postnatal care.

Influences that may change the fetal phenotype include under- and overnutrition, exposure to environmental toxins and exposure to hormones such as cortisol.[26] Initially it was presumed that these changes were limited to the prenatal period and thus were only influenced by the mother; however, it is apparent that paternal health, nutrition and risks also influence fetal programming.[27] The preconception period and early prenatal period are especially important in establishing the health and functioning of the child, as this is a time of critical development and plasticity. Exposure at this time can modulate the course of development and alter phenotypic outcomes.[27–30] Epigenetic changes may occur from the outset, even before implantation, with the fertilised ovum and blastocyst responding to the environment and nutrient quality within the fallopian tubes.[28] For the first 10 weeks of gestation, while the placenta is still developing, the embryo/fetus is nourished by fluid secreted by the endometrial glands and it is during this time that key organogenesis occurs.

Epigenetic changes alter the expression of a gene without altering the DNA sequence and these changes are heritable.[31] That is, non-genetic factors (such as folate intake) can alter the function of a gene. The changes may be passed on for many future generations via epigenetic imprinting, or they may be erased and not passed on. Changes can occur in the adult, but they are most critical in germ cells in early development in a process called epigenetic reprogramming, where the germline resets genomic potential and erases epigenetic memory, reiterating the unique plasticity of this stage.[32]

One mechanism for epigenetic changes is alteration in methylation, including DNA methylation. Factors that can influence fetal DNA methylation include fetal in-utero exposure to toxins (e.g. cigarette smoke, alcohol), obesity of the mother, nutritional status and stress.[31] Adverse outcomes of epigenetic changes include increased risk of developing chronic diseases in the adult offspring, such as type 2 diabetes, metabolic syndrome, heart disease and neurological conditions.

SAFETY ISSUES IN PREGNANCY

Medication and CM use

The use of over-the-counter (OTC) medicines and nutritional supplements is common in pregnancy and often occurs without professional advice or guidance. The use of CM products including herbal medicine is seen across cultures, although the specific herbs used vary. For instance, studies have found that 20% of perinatal women in China use herbal medicine[33] and 40% of Palestinian women use herbal medicine during pregnancy,[34] as do 69% of Russian women, 58% of British women[11] and 34% of Australian women.[10] Many women chose CM because of the perception that it is 'natural' and therefore 'safe', as well as for reasons of tradition, wanting to be healthy and wanting autonomy and convenience. Unfortunately, many women seek advice on these products from unqualified family and friends, magazines and blogs. This is a concern as all medicines, including nutritional supplements and herbal medicines, have the potential to cause harm to the mother and especially to the developing fetus. A substance may be present in endometrial and fallopian tube fluid or it may cross the placental barrier.

Reviews of supplement use in Australia have found that the most common nutritional supplement is folic acid; however, only 23% of women take it for at least 4 weeks prior to conception and 79% who take it during pregnancy primarily take it only for the first trimester.[35] Other supplements taken include iron (52%), calcium (24%), vitamin B_6 (14%), pregnancy multivitamins (35%) and zinc (7%). The most commonly used herbal preparations are ginger (20%) and raspberry leaf (9%).[36] A Canadian study found that up to 92.8% of women take B vitamins (including folate) in early pregnancy and 89% take them in late pregnancy.[37] However, the combination and doses of nutrients are inadequate, as is dietary intake – for example, 87% of women have inadequate choline intake.

Women who do not follow the recommended guidelines to take folic acid are more likely to be smokers, have a low income and be pregnant with other than their first child.[35] A study in Maryland (US) found that the most common reasons for folic acid non-use are 'not planning pregnancy' (61%) and 'didn't think needed to take' (41%).[38] Use of CM therapies has been associated with increased maternal age, primigravida and having a tertiary/college education, but these are not strong predictors of use.[39] Disclosure of CM use to midwives and medical staff is variable (1–72%) and may be incomplete, such as disclosing having acupuncture or massage but not disclosing use of herbal medicine.[36,39] Non-disclosure of consulting a naturopath and taking CM therapies compromises the quality of communication and information that all healthcare providers caring for the woman are working with. This incomplete information increases the risk of adverse events and drug–herb/supplement interactions, missing the opportunity to forge constructive professional relationships, and contributes to the under-reporting of side effects and adverse outcomes.

Safety

Prescribing for a pregnant woman is far more complex, nuanced and lacking in evidence than prescribing for a non-pregnant woman. Clinical trials cannot be performed on pregnant women due to safety and ethical issues and often information is extrapolated from case studies and in vitro research. Potential teratogenic outcomes include spontaneous abortion, structural malformations, intrauterine growth retardation, fetal death, functional impairment, neuropsychological and behavioural abnormalities, transplacental carcinogenesis and neonatal withdrawal (notably in narcotic use).[40]

Teratogens are agents that can disturb the development of an embryo or a fetus resulting in spontaneous abortion or structural or functional defects. Teratogens can be categorised into four types: physical agents, metabolic conditions, infection, and drugs and chemicals. Sources of exposure to these agents include contaminated air, water, soil, food, beverages, household items and medicines (including pharmaceutical and complementary medicines).[41] Mechanisms of teratogenesis include damage to DNA, membranes, protein and mitochondria; enzyme inhibition; and hormonal interference.[41] The effect of the teratogenic substance will be limited by a number of factors, and combined these result in a relatively low level of teratogenic effect in exposed individuals. These factors include the dose and duration of exposure, the genetic susceptibility of the embryo/fetus, the timing of the exposure (during the critical period of development or not), the route of exposure, the specific mode of action of the teratogen, and the nutritional and disease status of the mother–baby unit.[40,42] There is little evidence of teratogenicity for most nutrient supplementation, the exception being high-dose vitamin A (>10 000 IU) in the first trimester, although adverse effects are also noted for deficiency in vitamin A and other nutrients.[43]

Birth defects affect approximately 3% of babies born in the US and Australia.[44,45] This figure does not include pregnancies that were terminated or ended in miscarriage. In the majority of cases the cause of the defect is unknown.[45] Pharmaceutical use is not considered a major contributor to the incidence of birth defects, as fewer than 1% of cases can be attributed to drug use.[46] Given the lack of reported cases it is likely that CM use in Western countries is a far less important factor than pharmaceuticals.

Critical periods in human development

A critical period is a time during development when the organism is more vulnerable to environmental influences or stimuli. In human development this critical period begins before implantation, when the gametes and zygote are induced by the fallopian tube and endometrial environment. In this period, the most likely consequence of adverse influence is non-survival. If the embryo does survive, the risk of congenital structural malformations to the embryo is greatest 17–70 days post-conception (weeks 4–8), which is the critical stage for all major organ development.[42] Medicines taken later in pregnancy may still have an adverse effect but they are less likely to cause major structural anomalies – although they may induce functional changes that may not be overt until the child is older.[42] The central nervous system, eyes, teeth and external genitalia are the last to fully develop and continue to mature until the baby reaches full term, and thus remain vulnerable.

Box 13.1 outlines some guidelines for prescribing during pregnancy.

Herbal medicines in pregnancy

Classes of herbs to avoid in pregnancy include emmenagogues (avoid in the first trimester and use only under professional supervision at later stages), abortifacients, herbs high in volatile oil and resin, toxic herbs, herbs containing thujone and hormonally acting herbs (see Box 13.2).[47–49] Anthraquinone-containing herbs should be avoided if possible (especially in the first trimester) and need to be used with care.

Pregnancy is not a predictable physiological event and the usual interpretation of the clinical picture, pathology and prescription is complicated. Pharmokinetics and pharmacodynamics are altered and this affects optimal dosing as well as the interpretation of plasma concentration measurements. Briefly, key changes include the following:
- Most substances cross the placenta, especially lipophilic drugs and those with low plasma protein binding
- Active membrane transporters affect drug/substance transfer: reduced albumin concentrations reduce the availability of protein-binding carriers, which may increase the amount of medicine available to exert its effect
- Gastric emptying is delayed, potentially delaying reaching peak drug concentrations after ingestion
- Gastric pH is increased, which may affect the bioavailability of some substances
- Reduced gastrointestinal motility may increase total absorption potential
- Nausea and vomiting may reduce or increase the use of therapeutic agents and affect their absorption
- The increase in total body water and fat stores and the reduction in plasma albumin increase the volume of distribution of many drugs
- Increased cardiac output increases the speed at which distribution of the therapeutic agent or nutrient occurs

BOX 13.1 Guidelines for prescribing during pregnancy

- Assess or reassess the need for treatment in any woman planning a pregnancy or who becomes pregnant; use a safety/risk assessment matrix to quantify risk
- Consider whether dietary and/or lifestyle strategies may be an effective alternative to supplements/herbal medicine
- Determine whether the treatment is likely to be effective
- Review the medical history, obstetric history and personal/family history of malformations
- Balance the risks of medication against the benefit of treatment/non-treatment on the mother and fetus
- Consider the safety of the supplement/herb (stage of pregnancy, route of administration, dose)
- Avoid medicines in the first trimester, if possible (with the exception of the essential nutrients such as folic acid)
- Always assess risks and benefits on an individual patient basis
- Review the evidence and ensure that the most up-to-date information is being used
- Prescribing should be performed by an appropriately qualified naturopath
- Provide patient counselling regarding drug exposure during pregnancy
- Communicate with other health professionals about any intervention.
  If treatment is required:
- Minimise exposure during critical development times
- Use the lowest effective dose
- Use the least toxic substance
- Use for the shortest period of time
- Monitor for efficacy and adverse effects.

Source: Adapted from Stephens S, Wilson G. Prescribing in pregnant women: guide to general principles. Prescriber 2009;20(23–24):1–4. Braun L, Cohen M. Herbs and Natural supplements: an evidence-based guide. 4th edn. Sydney: Elsevier; 2015.

- Hepatic blood flow is increased in the third trimester and there is increased activity of some enzymes (e.g. CYP2A6, CYP2C9, CYP2D6 and CYP3A4 and uridine 5′-diphospho-glucuronosyltransferases) and reduced activity of others (e.g. CYP1A2 and CYP2C19)
- Increased glomerular filtration rate (GFR) enhances excretion of renally excreted substances, including water-soluble vitamins.[50]

These changes are variable throughout pregnancy, so the effects of any given therapeutic agent may alter depending on gestation. Animal studies have limited applicability to humans because of species-specific effects, and clinical trials in pregnancy are only undertaken in special circumstances.

See the interaction table for Chapter 13 in the appendices at the end of this book.

NUTRITIONAL ASSESSMENT

The goal of nutritional assessment is to optimise nutritional status and pregnancy outcomes. Nutritional

BOX 13.2 Herbs contraindicated or to be used with caution in pregnancy

Herbs contraindicated in pregnancy

Achillea millefolium (Yarrow)
Aconitum napellus (Aconite)
Actaea racemosa (Black Cohosh)
Aloe vera (Aloe)
Andrographis paniculata (Andrographis)
Angelica polymorpha (Dong Quai)
Arctostaphylos uva-ursi (Bearberry)
Armoracia rusticana (Horseradish)
Artemisia absinthium (Wormwood)
Artemisia vulgaris (Mugwort)
Berberis vulgaris (Barberry)
Caulophyllum thalictroides (Blue Cohosh)
Commiphora molmol (Myrrh)
Corydalis ambigua (Corydalis)
Fucus vesiculosus (Bladderwrack)
Hydrastis canadensis (Goldenseal)
Hyssopus officinalis (Hyssop)
Juniperus communis (Juniper)
Justicia adhatoda (Adhatoda)
Mahonia aquifolium (Oregon Grape)
Mentha pulegium (Pennyroyal)
Panax notoginseng (Tienchi Ginseng)
Phytolacca decandra (Poke Root)
Piscidia piscipula (Jamaican Dogwood)
Pulsatilla anemone (Pasque Flower)
Ruta graveolens (Rue)
Salvia miltiorrhiza (Danshen)
Salvia officinalis (Sage)
Schisandra chinensis (Schisandra)
Scutellaria baicalensis (first trimester only)
Tabebuia avellanedae (Pau d'arco)
Tanacetum vulgare (Tansy)
Thuja occidentalis (Thuja)
Trifolium pratense (Red Clover)
Uncaria tomentosa (Cat's Claw)
Vitex agnus-castus (Chaste Tree)

Herbs to be used with caution in pregnancy

Aloe vera (Aloes Resin)
Capsella bursa-pastoris (Shepherd's Purse)
Cassia spp (Senna)
Cinnamomum cassia (Cinnamon)
Leonurus cardiaca (Motherwort)
Rehmannia glutinosa (Rehmannia)
Rhamnus purshiana (Cascara)
Rheum palmatum (Rhubarb)
Rubus idaeus (Raspberry), best used in second and third trimesters
Zingiber officinalis (Ginger)

Source: Adapted from Braun L, Cohen M. Herbs and Natural supplements: an evidence-based guide. 4th edn. Sydney: Elsevier; 2015. Bone K, Mills S. Principles and practice of phytotherapy: modern herbal medicine. 2nd edn. Philadelphia: Churchill Livingstone; 2013. Mills S, Bone K. The essential guide to herbal safety. Philadelphia: Elsevier; 2005. Romm A. Botanical medicine for women's health. Philadelphia: Elsevier; 2010.

assessment in pregnancy is similar to a general nutritional assessment, with some adjustment for increased requirements for energy and specific nutrients and the probable omission of body composition and skin-fold testing. In addition, consideration of pregnancy-related symptoms and complications (e.g. nausea and vomiting, gastro-oesophageal reflux disease [GORD] and anaemia) is required when assessing the patient, developing the treatment plan and making suggestions for dietary modifications. The nutritional assessment needs to be revisited at each consultation as the physiological demands, common symptoms and complications, and nutritional requirements change over the course of the pregnancy, thus necessitating changes to the nutritional plan.

The objectives of nutritional assessment in pregnancy are as follows:

- Assess and evaluate diet adequacy (preconception and currently)
- Determine health and nutritional risks for mother and fetus
- Compare to benchmarks and nutritional guidelines where applicable, including gestational weight gain guidelines
- Identify factors that may impact on nutrient intake, absorption and metabolism
- Consider the impact of existing and past chronic diseases on nutritional status and capacity
- Review any nutrition-related issues in previous pregnancies
- Provide appropriate and effective nutritional advice suitable to the stage and health of the pregnancy
- Improve maternal and fetal nutritional and health status and prevent undernutrition and/or disease
- Monitor progress and adjustment treatment as indicated
- Identify leverage points and obstacles for making changes.

Nutritional intake may be affected by aversions to particular flavours or aromas, nausea and vomiting and lack of knowledge of dietary guidelines (e.g. for five or more serves of vegetables). Absorption of nutrients may be enhanced by normal physiological changes of pregnancy (e.g. intestinal calcium absorption doubles) or reduced by chronic illnesses such as inflammatory bowel disease.[51] The metabolism of a nutrient may be impacted, for example, by lack of essential co-factors or genetic single nucleotide polymorphisms (SNPs). Chronic illnesses that may impact on nutritional status include diabetes, hyper- and hypothyroidism, malabsorption disorders and renal disease, as well as chronic systemic inflammation as is seen in conditions such as rheumatoid arthritis.

For multiparous women it is important to review the nature, impact and outcomes of any nutrition-related issues in previous pregnancies. Common issues include gestational diabetes, inadequate or excess weight gain, iron-deficiency anaemia, nausea and vomiting, hyperemesis and pica. The impact may have been minor (e.g. mild nausea for a few weeks) to severe, such as requiring hospitalisation for rehydration, and the outcomes may range from little or no negative consequence to severe, such as neural tube defects in the child. In addition to learning about these nutrition-related issues in previous pregnancies, it is an opportunity to assess how much the patient understands about the condition, what changes they have made to their diet and/or lifestyle and how relevant they see it in the current pregnancy, as well as using the experience as a teaching opportunity (especially if knowledge levels are low).

Aspects of the nutritional assessment

Mindful of the potential for creating anxiety and shame with anthropometric assessments it remains important to monitor weight in pregnancy as it is a key tool in predicting fetal growth, viability and risk of poor outcomes. Relevant biochemical data and medical tests include a full blood count (FBC), urea and creatinine, vitamin D status, iron studies, red blood cell (RBC) folate and methylene tetrahydrofolate reductase (MTHFR) polymorphisms. A core component is the dietary evaluation and nutrition-related history including current food intake, diet in previous pregnancies and postnatally, estimated nutrient requirements, individual preferences, religious and cultural influences on dietary choices, nutrition and food knowledge, and risk of undernutrition and micronutrient deficiencies. Essentially, is the patient consuming enough to meet her basic plus pregnancy-specific requirements and what factors influence her food choices? A number of approaches can be used such as diet recall, keeping a food diary and food frequency assessments.

When reviewing diet it is important to explicitly ask about the use of nutritional supplements and herbal medicines, as the patient may not consider these important and may thus omit including them in the history, especially if they were not prescribed by a practitioner. In addition, it is necessary to identify patterns of usage such as dosage, frequency and duration as well as timing in relation to other supplements or nutrients (e.g. inhibitory co-administration of iron and calcium) and food. Finally, specifically identify whether the patient uses laxatives and/or diuretics, as these can impact on nutritional status as well as posing a risk for the fetus.

WEIGHT IN PREGNANCY

Gestational weight

Weight Gain During Pregnancy: Reexamining the Guidelines published by the Institute of Medicine (IOM; renamed the Health and Medicine Division in 2016) is the widely accepted reference for weight gain in singleton pregnancies (see Table 13.1).[52] For most women a gain of 1–2 kg is expected for the first trimester, then approximately 400 g per week thereafter, with some adjustment based on preconception weight.

The components of weight gain are as follows:
- Increase in breast size = 900 g
- Increase in mother's fluid volume = 1.8 kg
- Placenta = 700 g

TABLE 13.1 Recommended weight gain for singleton pregnancies

Pre-pregnancy BMI	Total weight gain Range (kg)	Rate of weight gain: 2nd and 3rd trimesters Mean (range) (kg/week)
Underweight (<18.5 kg/m²)	12.5–18	0.51 (0.44–0.58)
Normal weight (18.5–24.9 kg/m²)	11.5–16	0.42 (0.35–0.50)
Overweight (25.0–29.9 kg/m²)	7–11.5	0.28 (0.23–0.33)
Obese (≥30.0 kg/m²)	5–9	0.22 (0.17–0.27)

Source: Institute of Medicine (IOM). Weight gain during pregnancy: reexamining the guidelines. Washington: National Academies Press; 2009, pp. 1–2.

TABLE 13.2 Additional energy requirements per trimester

Trimester	Additional energy intake
1st trimester	None
2nd trimester	1.4 kJ (340 cal) per day
3rd trimester	1.9 kJ (450 cal) per day

Source: Australian Government Department of Health and NZ MoH. Nutrient reference values. [Cited 10 November 2016. Available from www.nrv.gov.au/dietary-energy.]

- Increased blood supply = 1.8 kg
- Amniotic fluid = 900 g
- Infant at birth = 3.5 kg
- Increase in uterus and muscles = 900 g
- Mother's fat stores = 3.2 kg.[55]

The additional energy intake required for this weight gain is modest (see Table 13.2). For example, the additional 1.4 kJ can be met by consuming a slice of multigrain toast with peanut butter or a 200 mL tub of full-fat yoghurt and an apple. The focus should be on ensuring nutrient density and swapping low-nutrient kilojoule-dense foods with nutrient-dense foods.[28]

Obese women still need some weight gain, and importantly need a nutrient-dense diet which may be difficult to achieve with a low-calorie diet. A large retrospective study of gestational weight loss (GWL) in 709 575 singleton births found that there was a decreased risk of pregnancy complications, including preeclampsia and non-elective caesarean section, in overweight and obese women compared to healthy weight women, but that this benefit was outweighed by a significant increase (odds ratio [OR] 1.68) in the risk of preterm delivery and small-for-gestational-age (SGA) births, especially for women with a BMI of 30–39.9 kg/m².[53] In women with a BMI over 40 kg/m² there was no increased risk. The study concluded that the risks of GWL outweigh the benefits. This finding is supported by a systematic review, which found that obese women with GWL had higher odds of small-for-gestational-age infants in the <10th percentile, and even though they also had a reduced risk of large-for-gestational-age (LGA) infants, the risk of low birth-weight babies was greater and weight loss could not be recommended.[54]

EXCESSIVE AND INADEQUATE GESTATIONAL WEIGHT GAIN

A prospective study of 664 Australian women tracked their weight gain from 20 to 36 weeks gestation and found that 36% gained weight that met the recommended levels, 26% gained inadequate weight and 38% gained weight in excess of the recommended levels.[57] That is, only about one-third were at the optimal weight. Women who were overweight at conception were more likely to exceed gestational weight gain (GWG) recommendations, with 56% gaining excess weight compared to 30% for those who were a healthy weight at conception, meaning that the problem of excess weight was compounded in pregnancy. The research also found that many women did not know how much weight they should gain and 62% of the study participants reported that the health professionals caring for them during the pregnancy either 'never' or 'rarely' advised them about weight gain.[57]

This lack of knowledge was also demonstrated in a New Zealand study, which asked 644 pregnant women (11–14 weeks gestation) to nominate their body size based on their BMI (underweight: BMI 18.5 kg/m²; normal weight: 18.5–24.9 kg/m²; overweight: 25–29.9 kg/m²; and obese: >30 kg/m²) and what they understood to be the recommended GWG.[58] Two-thirds estimated their BMI correctly but only 31% knew what their recommended GWG was. Overweight and obese women were more likely to suggest excessive GWG, and normal weight and younger women were more likely to suggest GWG below the recommended level. A further Australian study across five hospitals in New South Wales of 326 pregnant women also found poor levels of knowledge about recommended GWG and specific dietary recommendations, as well as a significant proportion of women commencing pregnancy overweight (25.2%) or obese (23.6%).[59]

Ideally weight should be optimised prior to attempting conception, although this is not always possible. Many developed nations are experiencing increasing levels of overweight and obesity which hold significant reproductive risks. The IOM established the first pregnancy weight guidelines in 1990 and updated them in 2009 in the light of the significant increase in rates of overweight and obesity. Furthermore, the issue is not simply weight at the time of conception for GWG; it is about adequate nutritional intake and status, and the intake of macro- and micronutrients, without which the woman and the fetus are at risk of short- and long-term negative health outcomes.

Excessive maternal preconception weight and/or gestational weight gain

Patterns of adult weight prior to conception influence perinatal health risks and behaviours. In the US,

approximately 30% of adults are overweight and this rate remains stable; however, the rate of obesity has nearly tripled, with 35% of adults obese in 2013.[60] Australia has similar figures, with 35.5% of adults overweight and 27.5% obese in 2011–2012.[61] In England in 2014, 39% of adults were overweight and 25.6% were obese, and as with Australia and the US, the rate of overweight is reasonably stable but the rate of obesity is steadily climbing.[62] Rates of obesity are frequently higher in minority groups and lower socioeconomic groups, which also have lower rates of health prevention measures, health literacy and dietary quality. A study in the UK reviewed the health costs of obesity in pregnancy and found that infants born to obese mothers had a mean health services cost 72% higher than for infants of healthy-weight women.[63]

Excessive GWG is associated with postpartum weight retention, regardless of preconception BMI, and with entering the next pregnancy at a higher BMI, compounding the risks for mother and fetus.[60,64] One study found that the lower the preconception BMI, the greater the percentage of weight that was retained (women with a BMI of 22 kg/m² had a 3% increase in body fat and retention of 5.6 kg compared with a 0.58% increase in fat and retention of 2.06 kg for women with a BMI of 30 kg/m²).[64] It is critical to exercise caution when reducing energy intake so as to not reduce nutrient intake in this group, who are already probably undernourished. The risk of excess weight gain is associated not only with preconception weight and diet, but also the effects of low or no exercise.

Risks to the mother of excessive GWG include:
- Nutritional deficiencies and their consequences (e.g. vitamin D, folate)[65,66]
- Increased risk of retaining pregnancy weight and long-term obesity[28,59,60,64]
- Gestational diabetes[28,59,60,67]
- Hypertension and preeclampsia[28,60,67]
- Spontaneous abortion[60]
- Increased risk of labour and delivery problems, instrumentation or operative delivery[60,67]
- Increased likelihood of caesarean delivery[28,60,68,69]
- Perinatal mortality[67]
- Postpartum thromboembolism, perinatal anaemia and infections[60]
- Increased risk of early (<3 months) weaning in women who were overweight or obese before conception.[70]

Risks for the infant include:
- Poorer fetal outcomes[60]
- Preterm birth[68]
- Increased risk of infant and childhood obesity[28,59,67]
- Increased risk of developing chronic diseases later in life[59]
- Fetal macrosomia/large for gestational age[28,67,69,71,72]
- Congenital abnormalities (e.g. shoulder dystocia)[60]
- Adversely effects the early infant intestinal microbiome.[73]

LGA infants have an increased risk of cardiac anomalies, neural tube defects (NTDs), shoulder dystocia, fetal demise, caesarean delivery, neonatal intensive care unit (NICU) admission and long-term obesity.[72]

Underweight preconception and/or inadequate gestational weight gain

The risks of inadequate GWG include:
- Increased risk of early (<3 months) weaning in women who were underweight preconception[70]
- SGA baby[28,60,68,71,72]
- Fetal hypoglycaemia[67]
- Increased perinatal mortality[60]
- Increased weight retention postnatally[60,64]
- Preterm delivery.[60]

SGA infants have an increased risk of low Apgar scores, meconium aspiration, seizures, respiratory complications and long-term problems such as metabolic syndrome, type 2 diabetes, hypertension, stroke and neurological deficits.[28,72] The risk of developing impaired glucose tolerance of type 2 diabetes is four times higher in those who were SGA compared to normal weight.[28]

Multiple pregnancy weight guidelines

Multiple gestation increases the risk of low birth weight, premature delivery and maternal pregnancy complications including gestational diabetes and preeclampsia. For a twin pregnancy, the IOM recommends a GWG of 16.8–24.5 kg for women of normal weight, 14.1–22.7 kg for women who are overweight and 11.3–19.1 kg for obese women.[52] The IOM does not currently make recommendations for triplets or higher-order pregnancies due to lack of data. A systematic review on GWG and twin pregnancies and maternal and child health outcomes found that the existing studies are inadequate and methodologically weak, highlighting the need for more rigorous studies.[74] The analysis did find consistent evidence of a positive association between GWG and fetal size.

A study of 87 sets of triplets sought to review the impact of weight gain[75]: 72% of the women were overweight or obese and their mean weekly gain was 0.54 kg compared with 0.73 kg for women with a normal BMI. Using the mean as a reference point, mothers who gained less than the mean weekly weight gain for their BMI status (normal weight/overweight) had a significantly increased risk of any triplet requiring neonatal intensive care admission (adjusted OR). In addition, they were less likely to deliver at or after 34 weeks gestation and less likely to have an infant of average birth weight. In the absence of guidelines, studies such as this provide some interim reference.

Another study on triplet pregnancies used retrospective data and found no association between preeclampsia or preterm delivery and increasing weight gain in triplet pregnancies; rather, any risk was associated with the woman's baseline BMI. Based on their study the researchers were unable to define a recommended range for GWG.[76] The Cochrane Collaborative also attempted to conduct a literature review to evaluate the effects of specialised diets or nutritional advice for women with multiple pregnancies, but was unable to due to lack of appropriate trials.[77]

The lack of research on multiple pregnancies and guidelines for GWG and nutritional requirements are a significant gap in current knowledge. This is increasingly important when the rate of multiple pregnancies is increasing. For example, in the US the twin birth rate rose by 76% from 1980 to 2009, from 18.9 to 33.3 per 1000 births.[78] Only a third of this increase can be attributed to increasing maternal age (twinning increases by 200% in women over 40 years of age) and other factors include ovarian stimulation and assisted reproductive technology (ART) practices of transferring multiple embryos. Australia has an ageing maternal cohort, but multiple pregnancy rates have remained stable at 1.5–1.7% of total confinements for the past decade.[79] Of note, the Australian guidelines for ART clinics recommends the transfer of single embryos only, not multiples.[80]

Energy and nutrient intake is higher for multiple pregnancies and the needs of each woman should be assessed individually. The increased requirements for nutrients (e.g. iron, folate, vitamin B_{12}, calcium, zinc, docosahexaenoic acid [DHA] and vitamin D) are unlikely to be met by standard prenatal supplements and thus supplementation needs to be tailored to the woman's specific requirements.

NUTRITIONAL MEDICINE – DIETARY

Vegetarians and vegans

A balanced vegetarian diet can provide the nutrients and energy required for a healthy pregnancy.[60,81] Evidence of nutritional deficits is varied and reflects diversity among vegetarians just as similar surveys reflect differences among omnivores. A systematic review found no study that reported an increase in severe adverse outcomes or major malformations except one report of increased hypospadias in infants of vegetarian mothers.[82] Low birth weight was reported in five studies and high birth weight in two studies. Gestation length was comparable between vegan-vegetarians and omnivores. There are nine studies on micronutrients and these suggest that vegan-vegetarian women may be at risk of vitamin B_{12} and iron deficiencies. A careful review of the usual dietary intake will inform decision making regarding the need for additional supplementation, especially for protein, iron, vitamin B_{12} and folate, calcium, zinc and essential fatty acids.

Teenage mothers

Teenage mothers often face additional physical and social challenges in pregnancy. The Australian rate of teen pregnancies was 15 live births per 1000 females in 2008, comparable to the OECD average of 16, but markedly higher than the rate of 4.3 in Switzerland and 4.8 in Japan and Italy.[83]

In the US 17% of teenage girls are obese and probably undernourished, and are thus subject to the risks and concerns of overweight and obesity in pregnancy.[60] Teenagers are more likely to be nutritionally at-risk and have diets higher in saturated fats and carbohydrates and low in essential nutrients.[84] A study of 193 pregnant adolescents in the US found that at birth 21% of neonates were anaemic and 25% had low ferritin (to a greater degree if the mother had low stores).[85]

Teenager mothers are more likely to be single parents, live in areas of greater disadvantage, smoke and have lower levels of education including regarding pregnancy and nutrition.[83,84] Teenagers tend to be present-focused and so may not consider the long-term consequences of their behaviour (including nutrition, smoking and alcohol use) during pregnancy; in addition, they may not believe that risks affect them.[84] Infants born to teenage mothers have an increased risk of preterm birth and low birth weight. Furthermore, the factors that often contribute to teenage pregnancy, if unchanged, mean the young mother is less likely to receive the support she needs during the pregnancy and postnatally.

Interpartum interval

Spacing between pregnancies is essential to allow the mother to restore depleted nutrient levels, especially if she is breastfeeding. Closely spaced pregnancies are associated with an increased risk of preterm birth, intrauterine growth restriction and maternal morbidity and mortality.[60,86,87]

A large retrospective review of 645 529 deliveries in California (US) grouped interpregnancy intervals at <6 months, 6–17 months and 18–50 months.[88] Women who conceived within 6 months of delivery had a significantly higher prevalence of early preterm birth (<34 weeks), low birth weight (<2500 g), neonatal complications, neonatal mortality and severe maternal complications than women with either a 6–17 month or an 18–50 month interval. Interestingly, women who had an interpregnancy interval of 6–17 months had an increased prevalence of preterm births compared with women with an 18–50 month interval but they also had fewer maternal complications, complicated deliveries and stillbirths. This is consistent with another large study which found that the risk of congenital anomalies appears to increase with both short and long interpregnancy intervals, with the lowest rate of issues seen in the those with an interpregnancy interval of 12–17 months.[89]

Food foundations

Dietary inadequacy is common in developed and developing nations, albeit for different reasons. In Australia the average intake of vegetables is approximately 2–2½ serves/day (compared against the recommended intake of 5 serves/day) and only 9–13% of women meet the recommended intake of 2 serves of fruit per day. The Australian Longitudinal Study on Women's Health (n = 606) found that no pregnant woman met the recommendations for all food groups and critically there were micronutrient deficiencies including folate and iron.[90] A study of 58 pregnant women attending an Australian metropolitan antenatal clinic found that only 8% of healthy weight and 36% of overweight mothers knew the recommended daily number of fruit and vegetable serves.[91] For the overweight women, knowledge didn't translate into behaviour as they were less likely than healthy weight women to eat the recommended fruit intake (4% vs 8%), were more likely to drink soft drinks and cordial (55% vs 43%) and were more likely to eat

TABLE 13.3 Food foundations in pregnancy	
Food foundation	**Rationale**
Follow five and two	Consistent intake of vegetables and fruit for nutritional value, water and fibre content
Eat nutrient-dense not kilojoule-dense diet	Energy requirements increase modestly compared to micronutrient requirements
Ensure food variety (as able if nausea and vomiting)	Increases the range of nutrients and reduces the likelihood of omitting any given nutrient; reduces overexposure to one food that may have heavy pesticide residues
Choose wholefoods	Provide vitamin, mineral, macronutrient and phytonutrient richness and complexity; lower GI, higher fibre, less processing, more nutrient dense
Balance macronutrient intake	Ensures adequate protein, fats and low GI carbohydrates
Decrease exposure to toxic substances: eat organic where possible	Avoid caffeine, fast foods, alcohol, mercury and other heavy metals, smoking, plastics (BPA) Wash fruit and vegetables
Notice cravings	Cravings may indicate a nutritional deficiency or metabolic issue: • Craving for ice/dirt (pica), consider iron deficiency • Craving salt, consider electrolytes, monitor BP • Craving sugar/carbs, review protein and fat intake and review blood sugar level • Craving bitter, consider digestive and gall bladder function

takeaway/fast foods more than once a week (37% vs 25%). Only 4% of all women ate the recommended 5 serves of vegetables per day.

These examples highlight the combined issues of low intake of nutrient-dense foods and excess intake of nutrient-poor foods that themselves deplete micronutrients in digesting them (e.g. increased B vitamins are required to metabolise the excess carbohydrates). This dietary inadequacy reinforces the need to improve and optimise diet as the priority and to augment with supplementation, not just to rely on supplements to counter a poor diet. Table 13.3 briefly summarises food foundations in pregnancy.

Dietary foundations

FISH AND MERCURY

Methylmercury accumulates in the aquatic food chain and is considered the most harmful of all forms of mercury. It deposits and is stored in the nervous system of the developing fetus, infants and children, and the primary health effect is impaired neurological development. Children exposed to methylmercury while in utero have demonstrated impairment in cognitive thinking, memory, attention, language and fine motor and visual spatial skills. Methylmercury exposure in utero can result from the mother's consumption of fish and shellfish preconception and during pregnancy. The current Australian and New Zealand recommendation is for pregnant women to eat large fish such as shark (flake), broadbill, marlin and swordfish no more than once a fortnight and not to eat any other fish during that fortnight. Orange roughy (perch) and catfish should be eaten no more than once per week and no other fish should be eaten during that week.[92] The current recommendation in the US is to avoid shark, swordfish, king mackerel and tilefish and sets restrictions for the amount of other fish to be consumed.[93]

CAFFEINE AND COFFEE

Research on the effects of caffeine and coffee has been somewhat inconsistent and this is compounded by the variability in caffeine content of different beverages (depending on coffee source, processing, preparation of the coffee). More recent research has shown increasingly convincing evidence to recommend a reduction or to avoid coffee in pregnancy. Caffeine increases cellular cyclic adenosine monophosphate (cAMP) levels and this can negatively affect cell growth and fetal development.[94] Novel research based on the structural similarities between caffeine and adenine and guanine found that caffeine may be incorporated into DNA during mitosis, thereby causing chromosomal anomalies.[95] Caffeine clearance is slower in pregnant women compared to non-pregnant women and the fetus (which can be exposed via amniotic fluid or placental transfer) has little ability to metabolise and clear the caffeine. Caffeine, especially at higher intakes, has been associated with an increased risk of delayed conception, chromosomal anomalies, spontaneous miscarriage, fetal growth restriction and low birth weight.[96]

A 2015 study found that compared to women who did not drink coffee, women who drank ≥4 servings/day had a 20% increased risk of spontaneous miscarriage.[97] Interestingly, there was no difference in the association between caffeinated and decaffeinated coffee and risk of miscarriage. Women who drank caffeinated tea or caffeinated soda had no increased risk of miscarriage. The risk of miscarriage among women who drank coffee was greatest between 8 and 19 weeks gestation. A meta-analysis involving 26 studies attempted to distinguish between caffeine and coffee (given the variable levels): after adjustment, both caffeine (OR 1.32) and coffee (OR 1.11) consumption was associated with an increased risk of pregnancy loss.[96] The greater the amount of caffeine consumed, the higher the risk of miscarriage, the risk increasing by 19% for every increase in caffeine intake of 150 mg/day and by 8% for every increase in coffee intake of 2 cups per day.

PROTEIN

Protein is essential for fetal, placental and maternal tissue growth. Over the course of a singleton pregnancy an average of 925 g of protein is stored for use in tissue development.[60] Maternal protein synthesis is upregulated to facilitate blood plasma and blood volume expansion, as well as uterine and breast development. The fetal and placental proteins are synthesised by amino acids transferred from the mother. In the first trimester there is little need for additional protein; however, the need for additional protein consistently increases as the pregnancy increases, with one-third of weight gain occurring in the second trimester and two-thirds in the third trimester. The recommended intake of protein in the second and third trimesters is 1–1.2 g/kg per day.[56]

ESSENTIAL FATTY ACIDS

Essential fatty acids (EFAs) cannot be synthesised by the body and are a vital component of neural tissue, phospholipids and the retina. The fetus relies on maternal dietary intake and normal placental function for its EFAs and supplementation is known to increase maternal and fetal DHA status.[98,99] Omega-3 and omega-6 fatty acids and arachidonic acid are required for the normal development and metabolism of phospholipid cell membranes, as well as for maintaining appropriate membrane fluidity and permeability. They are needed in the metabolism of proteins and carbohydrates and in the regulation of gene expression, and they are the precursors of prostacyclins, prostaglandins, thromboxanes and leukotrienes.[100] Omega-3 and omega-6 fatty acids are anti-inflammatory.

Having balance between inflammatory and anti-inflammatory responses is critical for the initiation of labour. The feto-placental unit is supplied with omega-3 and omega-6 fatty acids via the maternal dietary intake and endogenous synthesis; the prostaglandins derived from arachidonic acid within the utero-placental unit is counteracted by the utero-placental omega-3 fatty acids. The balance between these fatty acids and the metabolites of omega-3 and omega-6 fatty acids contributes to the maintenance of a normal gestational length and is critical to cervical ripening and the initiation of labour. If the arachidonic levels are excessive and/or the omega-3 levels are too low, this may induce premature ripening of the cervix and uterine contractions, leading to premature birth.[101] Maternal plasma levels of EFAs increase in the first and second trimesters and then decreases in the third trimester. EFA stores progressively decrease during pregnancy due to increasing fetal demands. This is exacerbated if the mother had poor preconception nutritional status and low dietary intake of fish.[102]

Evidence is mixed regarding length of gestation, birth weight and EFA, but recent analyses demonstrate that omega-3 supplementation during pregnancy increases the mean duration of gestation and is associated with a 40–50% reduction in early preterm birth (<34 weeks gestation).[101] An analysis of 19 studies involving 151 880 women found that dietary fish intake was associated with a lower risk of preterm birth and higher infant birth weight and this effect was greatest in obese women and smokers.[103] In addition to EFAs, fish contains a good source of protein as well as micronutrients such as selenium and zinc. On the other hand, it may also contain contaminants such as heavy metals and together these factors make it difficult to quantify the effect of EFAs alone.

Omega-3 fatty acids have an anti-inflammatory and vasodilatory effect and supplementation is associated with reduced risk of hypertension of pregnancy, premature birth and fetal growth restriction.[104] A study involving women with unexplained recurrent pregnancy loss and restricted uterine blood flow found that low-dose aspirin and omega-3 fatty acid supplementation improved uterine blood flow and may improve pregnancy outcomes.[104] Another cause of infertility and recurrent pregnancy loss is antiphospholipid syndrome and a small study found that supplementation with omega-3 fish oil derivatives was as efficacious as low-dose aspirin in preventing miscarriage.[105] Fetal benefits of adequate omega-3 fatty acids are broad, including normal neurocognitive development and retinal development, improved cognitive performance in childhood, reduced atopy (specifically eczema and asthma) and better hand–eye coordination.[60,106]

Omega-3 fatty acids are known to be beneficial in depression in adults but there have been mixed results in studies on perinatal and postnatal depression. It is probable that decreased omega-3 fatty acids in the postnatal period cause an inflammatory environment that is associated with depression.[107] One study found that

lower omega-3 and relatively higher omega-6 was associated with prenatal but not postnatal anxiety and there was no impact on depression.[108] A Japanese study looked at omega-3 fatty acids in relation to perinatal and postnatal depression and found that women with psychological distress had lower levels of eicosapentaenoic acid (EPA), DHA and total omega-3s than controls.[109] Another recent study measured omega-3 and omega-6 fatty acids and found no association between the types of omega-6 fatty acids (including arachidonic acid) but lower serum concentrations of DHA, EPA and docosapentaenoic acid (DPA) and a higher omega-6/omega-3 ratio at each trimester was associated with a higher risk of depressive symptoms throughout pregnancy.[110]

Dose

RDI: DHA 220 mg, EPA 220 mg[56]
Therapeutic dose: EPA 800 mg, DHA 400 mg
Supplementation of EPA/DHA up to 3 g/day appears to be safe during pregnancy, with no increases in bleeding or haemorrhage either before or after birth.[111]

SAMPLE DAILY DIET

BREAKFAST

| 2 scrambled eggs with toast + ½ avocado | Two large eggs provide approximately 300 mg of choline. Choline supply to pregnant women reduces hippocampal apoptosis, increases neuron size and improves learning and visual-spatial and auditory memory in offspring. Avocado is a rich source of folate (approx. 120 micrograms in one small avocado) and is also required for cell division and closure of the neural tube in the early stages of pregnancy. |

LUNCH

| Tinned salmon with baby spinach, ½ avocado, green beans, potato and grated carrot | Maternal intake of omega-3 fatty acids during pregnancy may reduce the incidence of IgE-mediated allergic disease in their offspring. Tinned salmon not only provides a source of omega-3 fatty acids, but is a source of calcium, requirements of which also increase in pregnancy. Baby spinach and avocado provide further folate and fibre to reduce constipation associated with pregnancy. |

DINNER

| Slow-cooked beef brisket with mushrooms and polenta served with steamed greens drizzled with lemon juice | Beef is a source of iron and zinc, requirements for which increase dramatically in pregnancy. Deficiency of iron causes hypomyelination, permanent deficiency in the number of dopamine receptors and alterations with neurotransmission that may be permanent. Beef can be cooked in the slow cooker, requiring minimal preparation and making it useful for women who are feeling tired. Serve drizzled with lemon juice to further enhance absorption of iron. The meal is low-GI and high in fibre, designed to reduce glucose intolerance in pregnancy. |

SNACKS

Ginger tea	Ginger may reduce nausea and vomiting associated with pregnancy.
Smoothie	A smoothie can be sipped slowly for women suffering from reflux or used to maintain fluid intake for those who vomit frequently.
Nori chips	Nori provides an excellent source of iodine. Pregnant women are at increased risk of iodine deficiency as iodine requirements double during pregnancy. A low iodine maternal diet reduces the level of free T4 and may result in brain damage in the unborn child.

Source: Comerford KB, Ayoob KT, Murray RD, et al. The role of avocados in maternal diets during the periconceptional period, pregnancy, and lactation. Nutrients 2016;8(5):313. doi:10.3390/nu8050313. Best KP, Gold M, Kennedy D, et al. Omega-3 long-chain PUFA intake during pregnancy and allergic disease outcomes in the offspring: A systematic review and meta-analysis of observational studies and randomized controlled trials Am J Clin Nutr 2016; 103(1):128–43. doi:10.3945/ajcn.115.111104.

Micronutrients

Assessment of micronutrient status can be complex due to a range of issues, including variable availability of accurate testing, lack of research on specific nutrient functions and requirements in pregnancy, as well as interpersonal physiological variance. Thus the safest approach uses laboratory data when available, thorough clinical assessment, thorough health and nutritional assessment and ongoing review of each of these to tailor treatment plans to the individual's specific needs. When reviewing laboratory results, the following factors need to be considered:

- Maternal metabolism is altered by hormones that mediate the redirection of nutrients to the placenta, fetus and mammary gland, lowering the amount available and hence measurable in the mother.[112]
- Maternal plasma volume expands by up to 50% commencing at 6 weeks gestation and continuing until it peaks at weeks 30–34.[112,113]
- A 15–20% expansion in red cell mass adds to the increased plasma volume but does not match the degree of increase and the result is haemodilution, reducing the concentration of plasma constituents including nutrients (e.g. iron).[112,113]
- There is a reduction in serum albumin levels, which reduces the amount of protein-binding carrier.[113]
- Increased maternal fat mobilisation increases serum triglycerides, cholesterol and fat-soluble vitamin levels.[112]
- Some nutrient absorption is upregulated in pregnancy (e.g. calcium).[114]
- Renal function is upregulated to manage the clearance of both fetal and maternal metabolic waste. Increased GFR and increased renal plasma flow result in increased excretion of glucose, amino acids and water-soluble nutrients (e.g. folate).[112,113]

NUTRITIONAL MEDICINE – SUPPLEMENTATION

Just as there are some challenges in accurately assessing nutrient status, there are challenges in determining the exact nutrient requirements during pregnancy. Nutrient reference values are calculated using population models and are typically developed by adding an increment to the value for non-pregnant women that is considered to meet the requirements of fetal growth and the associated changes in maternal tissue metabolism. The difficulty is in incorporating aspects of altered maternal metabolism (including changes in the absorption, utilisation and elimination of nutrients) and individual physiology.[112] A simple way to consider the possible risk of deficiency and the possible need for supplementation is to consider these four main pathways to deficiency:

1 Inadequate intake
2 Impaired absorption
3 Increased (and unmet) requirements
4 Excessive loss (including interactions).

Nutrients are best sourced from food; this allows for synergistic actions between compounds and a complexity of food sources, reduces the risk of excess dosing, is cheaper and can simply be part of healthy living. During pregnancy some supplementation is essential (e.g. folate) for all women, and some women may need more extensive support depending on the findings of the nutritional and health assessment. Factors that affect the requirements for micronutrient supplementation include:

- The nutritional value of food: freshness, growing conditions and use of pesticides, long-term storage of foods, food choices, intake of refined foods
- The bioavailability of nutrients: inherent nutrient qualities plus dietary patterns (e.g. low iron absorption is further reduced by a diet high in phytates)
- The nutrient cycle: whether it is stored and/or recycled or has a short period of usability (e.g. thiamine)
- The quantity or dose required to fulfil the additional physiological roles of pregnancy
- Inborn errors of metabolism that may affect micronutrient absorption, use or excretion
- Gastrointestinal (GI) conditions (e.g. inflammatory bowel disease) that may reduce the absorption and increase the use and elimination of nutrients
- Lifestyle (e.g. smoking, alcohol consumption, recreational drug use – past and present)
- Exercise: additional requirements to support more intense or lengthy exercise and reduce oxidative damage
- Pharmaceutical drugs: may affect absorption, bioavailability, use and elimination of nutrients and interactions may reduce or enhance the effect of the pharmaceutical
- Environmental factors such as contaminants in air or water, heavy metals and chemical exposure.

Vitamin B complex

The metabolic pathways for individual B vitamins require other B vitamins and cofactors; thus it is important to provide a B complex, especially if prescribing B vitamins individually. B vitamins are indicated from preconception to the postnatal period and are not only required preconception and in the first trimester.

THIAMINE (B_1)

The active form is thiamine pyrophosphate (TPP), which acts as an essential coenzyme in carbohydrate and branched-chain amino acid metabolism and energy production. Thiamine is required for the synthesis of neurotransmitters, including gamma-aminobutyric acid (GABA) and acetylcholine, and is involved in neurotransmission, the blood–brain barrier and muscle function. In addition, thiamine is required for the synthesis of nucleotide precursors.

Thiamine deficiency in the mother and thus embryo/fetus results in impaired metabolism and adenosine triphosphate (ATP) production in the brain, which in turn causes alterations in neurotransmitters, impaired neural functioning, oxidative stress, inflammation, compromised blood–brain barrier and neurodegeneration.[115] Such cerebral changes in a developing fetus are clearly undesirable and combined with the importance of thiamine in cellular proliferation and differentiation, hormonal function in pregnancy and general energy production a deficiency may be associated with increased risk of congenital abnormalities (e.g. orofacial cleft, impaired neurodevelopment), miscarriage and stillbirth.[116–118]

Women most at risk of thiamine deficiency are those with poor dietary intake, hyperemesis gravidarum, eating disorders, excess alcohol intake or impaired intestinal absorption (e.g. inflammatory bowel disease). In addition, overweight and obese women may be deficient, with one study on women seeking bariatric surgery indicating that between 15.5% and 29% were thiamine deficient.[119] Furthermore, due to thiamine's role in metabolism and energy production, women with diets high in carbohydrate use more thiamine and are therefore at risk of deficiency if requirements exceed intake. TPP is regenerated via the donation of a proton from the reduced form of nicotinamide adenine dinucleotide (NADH). Folate is required for dihydrofolate reductase to regenerate NADH from its oxidative form, enabling NADH to then regenerate thiamine. Therefore a deficiency of B_3 or folic acid leads to a secondary thiamine deficiency, since it cannot be activated and regenerated.

Dose

RDI: 1.4 mg[56]
Therapeutic dose: 5–150 mg[43]

RIBOFLAVIN (B₂)

Riboflavin is essential for metabolism, redox reactions and ATP production and it is an integral component of two coenzymes, flavin mononucleotide (FMN) and flavin adenine nucleotide (FAD), which function as cofactors for methionine synthase reductase (MTRR) and MTHFR, respectively.[120] Riboflavin promotes normal tissue growth, assists in the synthesis of steroids, is required for immune function and supports normal red blood cell life, as well as participating in the conversion of B_6 and folate into their active forms and the conversion of tryptophan to B_3.[43]

Animal studies indicate that riboflavin deficiency can cause impaired embryonic growth and congenital heart defects such as ventral septal defects.[120] A human study of mothers consuming a diet high in saturated fat and low in riboflavin showed an increased risk of congenital heart defects in the offspring.[121] The influence of riboflavin deficiency on the development of preeclampsia is less clear, with some research showing no impact[122] and other studies showing that high-dose supplementation (15 mg/day) led to an approximately 75% reduction in the number of cases of severe preeclampsia.[123]

Dose

RDI: 1.4 mg[56]
Therapeutic dose: 10–200 mg[43]

NIACIN (B₃)

The term 'niacin' refers to nicotinic acid and nicotinamide, which are precursors to the coenzymes nicotinamide adenine dinucleotide (NAD) and nicotinamide adenine dinucleotide phosphate (NADP). NAD is involved in the oxidation of carbohydrates, protein, fats and energy production and NADH contributes to reductive biosynthesis of fatty acids and sterols. NAD is also important in the synthesis and repair of DNA and is involved in neurotransmitter synthesis and transduction and in the conversion of folic acid to tetrahydrofolate (THF). A deficiency can therefore impair DNA stability and function and cause a secondary folate deficiency with potential detrimental effects on the developing fetus.

Mouse studies show that nicotinamide reduces preeclampsia and intrauterine growth retardation.[124] Another mouse study identified that high-dose nicotinamide supplementation (4 g/kg) was associated with DNA hypomethylation and epigenetic changes in the fetus, lower birth weight and increased fetal death rate. Interestingly, this effect was partially or completely prevented by concurrent supplementation with betaine (2 g/kg).[125] A 2016 human study of 497 mothers identified that higher levels of maternal serum nicotinamide and metabolites late in pregnancy were associated with a reduced risk of atopic eczema in babies at 12 months.[126]

Dose

RDI: 18 mg[56]
Therapeutic dose: 25–50 mg

PANTOTHENIC ACID (B₅)

Pantothenic acid exists in most foods as part of two protein complexes – coenzyme A (CoA) (85%) and acyl carrier protein (ACP) – and is essential for numerous biochemical reactions including: lipid, protein and carbohydrate metabolism; fatty acid synthesis and oxidation; and cholesterol and other sterols synthesis. It is also required for the synthesis of substances including haem, acetylcholine and N-acetylglucosamine (essential for connective tissue growth and repair). In addition it is required for vitamin D synthesis and adrenal cortex function.

Animal studies have found that lower levels of pantothenic acid in the amniotic fluid of pregnant mice were associated with increased risk of cleft lip and palate (also seen with lower thiamine and folate levels).[127] A prospective cohort study in Scotland found that deprivation was associated with preterm birth and that low birth weight was more common in women consuming diets low in vitamin C, riboflavin, pantothenic acid and sugars.[128]

Dose

RDI: 5 mg[56]
Therapeutic dose: 5–20 mg[43]

PYRIDOXINE (B₆)

Pyridoxine has a diverse range of actions and is important for a healthy pregnancy and child. It is required for the synthesis of haem, serotonin, dopamine, noradrenaline, GABA, prostaglandins and phospholipids and in the regulation of steroid hormones, vitamins A and D and thyroid hormones.[43] Pyridoxine is needed for the metabolism of amino acids and fats and glycogenolysis and is a necessary cofactor for the enzymes delta-5 and delta-6 desaturase that are crucial in the metabolism of omega-3 and omega-6 fatty acids, which are vital in embryonic and fetal development. Furthermore, pyridoxine catalyses the interconversion of serine and glycine for the production of DNA and RNA and is required for the conversion of tryptophan to niacin and the metabolism of carnitine and folate. Conversion of pyridoxine vitamers to the active forms is reliant on the riboflavin-dependent enzyme pyridoxal phosphate oxidase. Therefore, riboflavin deficiency may lead to a reduction in the conversion of B_6 to its active forms.

In one-carbon metabolism a carbon unit from serine or glycine is transferred to THF to form methylene-THF, and the biologically active form of B_6, pyridoxal phosphate (PLP), acts as a coenzyme for the interconversion of glycine and serine, and the transsulfuration pathway. In homocysteine metabolism pyridoxine acts as a cofactor for cystathionine beta-synthase, which mediates the conversion of homocysteine to cysteine. Alterations to one-carbon metabolism can have significant detrimental effects on cell proliferation, growth and function and thus negatively affect the health of the mother, impair the growth and reprogram the metabolism of the developing fetus, cause long-term morbidity in the offspring and potentially affect miscarriage risk.[129]

A 2012 systematic review evaluated the risks and benefits of interventions with vitamins B_6, B_{12} and C during pregnancy on maternal, neonatal and child health and nutrition outcomes and found that vitamin B_6 supplementation had a significant positive effect on birth weight but did not significantly impact other neonatal outcomes, including preterm birth, low birth weight and perinatal morbidity and mortality.[130] Vitamin B_6 supports progesterone production and is required for normalisation of homocysteine levels and thus reduces the risk of miscarriage. Low levels of vitamin B_6 are associated with nausea and vomiting of pregnancy and hyperemesis gravidarum. Preconception and prenatal low B_6 is associated with miscarriage, low Apgar scores, preeclampsia, gestational carbohydrate intolerance and neurological disease of the offspring; however, there is a need for further research.[131–133]

There is a gradual decline of plasma B_6 levels during pregnancy and activated B_6 (P5P) may be more accurate.[134] Also consider kryptopyrrole status to determine biochemical need. Chronic vitamin B_6 deficiency may precipitate microcytic hypochromic anaemia. Vitamin B_6 is safe in pregnancy and lactation at recommended doses.[43]

Dose

RDI: 1.9 mg[56]
Therapeutic dose: 150 mg[43]

FOLATE (B₉)

Folate is a methyl donor essential for DNA and RNA synthesis, gene expression and stability, cell division and replication, and protein synthesis – all critical for normal fetal and placental development. It also has antioxidant functions and is required for phase II liver detoxification pathways. Deficiency can lead to megaloblastic anaemia, neurological changes and neuropathy and, specifically in

pregnancy, preeclampsia, impaired cognitive development, neural tube closure and neural development of the fetus. In addition, folate may protect against autism spectrum disorder.[135] Folate deficiency interferes with DNA methylation and stability and increases homocysteine levels, which is associated with poor embryo quality and viability and increases placental oxidative damage.[136,137]

MTHFR mutations are known to be associated with adverse pregnancy outcomes including early and late fetal loss, preeclampsia, intrauterine growth retardation, placental abruption and neural tube defects.[138] Research has shown that the MTHFR C677T genotype is associated with increased risk of recurrent pregnancy loss for Asians yet not for Caucasians[138] and preeclampsia in both Asians and Caucasians.[139] A meta-analysis of the MTHFR A1298C polymorphism showed a significant increase in recurrent pregnancy loss.[140] Fetal loss associated with MTHFR mutation may be seen in the absence of high homocysteine. (For further discussion of MTHFR polymorphisms see Chapter 4 in *Clinical Naturopathic Medicine* and Chapters 7 and 8 in this volume.)

In recognition of the importance of folate in reproduction, in 2006 the World Health Organization and the Food and Agricultural Organization of the United Nations published guidelines for the target, minimum and maximum fortification level of folic acid to be used to fortify flour.[141] The implementation of folic acid fortification programs is variable; globally, 86 countries have legislated to mandate fortification of at least one industrially milled cereal grain, although that may be with one or a combination of nutrients including folate, iron and other nutrients.[142] Many European countries (e.g. the UK and Ireland) permit the addition of folic acid and other nutrients to foods on a voluntary basis whereas others prohibit fortification of any kind (e.g. Denmark) or specifically limit fortification with folic acid (e.g. The Netherlands).[143] In the US mandatory fortification of enriched cereal grain products with folic acid was implemented in 1998, adding 140 micrograms of folic acid per 100 g of enriched cereal grain product; it is estimated to provide 100–200 micrograms of folic acid per day to women of childbearing age.[144] New Zealand has allowed voluntary fortification of bread and other foods with folic acid since 1996 and in 2012 the government confirmed that it would continue with voluntary rather than mandated fortification.[145]

Australia introduced mandatory fortification with 200–300 micrograms of folic acid per 100 g of all wheat flour used for making bread (except organic) in September 2009 with the aim of increasing folate intake in women of reproductive years. This was in recognition of the potential for poor intake of folate, the occurrence of unplanned pregnancies and thus a lack of preconception supplementation in the early stage of pregnancy for neural tube closure.[146] It was anticipated that fortification would reduce the rate of NTDs by 4–16%. A review in 2011 reported that approximately 1030 babies were born with NTD between 2007 to 2011 (these statistics exclude Victoria) and the prevalence of NTDs following fortification was 10.9% lower than it was prior to fortification.[146]

Another way to evaluate the efficacy of fortification programs is to measure blood folate concentrations. Homocysteine levels may be considered a functional indicator of folate status in conjunction with blood folate.[144] While it is evident that folic acid reduces the incidence of NTDs, the specific blood level to achieve the greatest reduction is not known. An Irish study found that the greatest reduction in NTDs was produced when blood folate levels were much higher than those set to exclude folate deficiency (approximately serum <7 nmol/L, red cell <360 nmol).[147] This suggests that avoidance of folate deficiency may be inadequate to prevent NTDs and that supplementation is still required.[143] This dose-response between RBC folate concentrations and NTD risk matched an analysis of the Chinese folic acid intervention study (see below). In their analysis, Crider and colleagues stated that the NTD risk was substantially reduced at RBC folate concentrations >1000 nmol/L, nearly three times the level to exclude deficiency.[148] Their results suggest that an RBC folate concentration of approximately 1000–1300 nmol/L may achieve optimal prevention of folate-sensitive NTDs. In 2015 the WHO released guidelines recommending that at the population level, RBC folate concentrations should be >906 nmol/L in women of reproductive age to achieve the greatest reduction of NTDs.[149]

Early research on the use of folic acid supplementation included two landmark studies. The first was a randomised, controlled trial comparing periconceptional multivitamin (including folic acid) supplementation with supplementation with trace minerals alone. The frequency of NTDs was zero in 2471 women receiving 800 micrograms per day of folic acid compared with 6 cases in 2391 women not receiving folic acid.[150] The second study was a large public health initiative in China, including a northern region with known high rates of NTDs, involving 130 142 women who took 400 micrograms of folic acid at any time before or during their pregnancy and 117 689 women who did not take folic acid.[151] The reduction in NTDs varied based on region, existing prevalence of NTDs and consistency of use of folic acid. Women from the northern region who had the highest risk and who took folic acid more than 80% of the time showed an 85% reduction in risk for NTDs. Women in the southern region who already had a lower prevalence had a 41% reduction in risk. Multiple studies have repeated these findings, as outlined in a 2006 Cochrane Review.[152] Serum folate levels have also been found to have a negative association with blood mercury levels, with mercury a known neurotoxicant related to adverse pregnancy outcomes.[153]

Given the widespread recommendation for supplementation with folic acid pre-conception and in early pregnancy at the very least, the response remains inadequate. A 2007 survey by the Center for Disease Control found that among all women of childbearing age only 40% reported taking folic acid daily, even though 81% reported awareness of folic acid and 12% reported knowing that folic acid should be taken before pregnancy.[154] A prospective observational study of 42 362 women in Ireland reported that 43.9% took periconceptional folic acid, 49.4% took postconceptional folic acid and 6.6% took no folic acid.[155] Those most likely to take folic acid were those who planned their pregnancy, were over 30 years old, were non-obese, were Irish-born and were employed professionally; the women with the lowest rates of folic acid supplementation were multiparous and obese, who indeed had higher requirements.

RBC folate levels remain constant throughout the life span of the cell and are more reliable in measuring tissue stores of folate than serum folate, which is affected by recent dietary intake. Low RBC folate levels may be due to poor folate intake as well as vitamin B_{12} deficiency, alcohol, anticonvulsant medications and long-term oral contraception use. Low folate levels should be assessed in conjunction with blood film (and any megaloblastic changes), homocysteine concentrations and MTHFR polymorphisms. RBC folate initially increases slightly then declines during pregnancy, returning to baseline by 6 weeks postpartum.

Dose

RDI: 600 micrograms[56]

Therapeutic dose: 600–5000 micrograms[43]

High intake of folate supplements (not dietary) can mask a B_{12} deficiency by preventing macrocytic changes, though data is lacking on incidence in relation to supplementation for pregnancy. Preconception supplementation is necessary and the critical period for neural tube development is 17–30 days' gestation. Dosage needs to be adjusted based on RBC folate, whether the mother is an older woman, history of pregnancy loss, history of previous pregnancy with NTD, genetic risks, multiple pregnancy and MTHFR SNPs and homocysteine levels. Obese women (BMI > 29 kg/m²) have a higher risk of having a baby with NTDs than women with a lower BMI despite similar periconception supplementation, and this risk is increased in obese smokers.[156] It is unclear why obese women have lower serum levels of folate; it has been suggested that it is related to higher serum glucose rather than a frank deficiency of folic acid.[65]

A 2015 randomised controlled trial investigated whether 5-methylenetetrahydrofolate is more effective than folic acid supplementation in the treatment of recurrent pregnancy loss in MTHFR gene C677T and A1298C polymorphism.[157] Two hundred and twenty women who had suffered three or more idiopathic miscarriages were randomly allocated to receive either 1 mg of folic acid or 1 mg of 5-MTHFR, which they took from at least 8 weeks prior to conception until week 20 of the pregnancy. The results showed no difference in the rate of miscarriage between the two groups and that both had significantly increased serum folate levels, with the 5-MTHFR being highest. Plasma homocysteine decreased significantly in both groups without any significant difference between the two.

CYANOCOBALAMIN (B_{12})

Vitamin B_{12} is required for methyl transfer reactions and is a cofactor in the enzyme methionine synthase in the transmethylation cycle, folate metabolism and lowering of homocysteine. Methylcobalamin is required by methionine synthase, which transfers a methyl group from the inactive methyl folate to homocysteine to produce methionine and activate the folate. The methionine is then converted to S-adenosyl-methionine (SAMe), which is important for protein synthesis and methylation reactions and the availability of choline and betaine. In conjunction with folate it is required for the synthesis of RNA and DNA and the formation of erythrocytes and is essential for the growth, reproduction and division of all cells, particularly those that are rapidly dividing. Vitamin B_{12} is also required for the synthesis of myelin sheath and other fatty acids and the development and function of the nervous system. It contributes to the metabolism of carbohydrates, protein and fat and in the production of ATP.

Because folate and B_{12} are required for cell division and reproduction via DNA and RNA synthesis, a deficiency may increase the risk of fetal injury, malformations and pregnancy loss.[158] Animal studies have shown that low levels of folate and vitamin B_{12} are associated with increased visceral fat, inflammation (including elevated tumour necrosis factor α [TNF-α], leptin and interleukin-6) and dyslipidaemia in the offspring.[159]

While there is an awareness of low vitamin B_{12} intake and serum levels in pregnant women, most research has focused on the outcomes of low levels rather than the effect of supplementation. Low levels of vitamin B_{12} are associated with elevated homocysteine levels, inflammation, preeclampsia and low birth weight.[28,160,161] A 2015 review of research on perinatal vitamin B_{12} found that low levels were associated with adverse maternal and neonatal outcomes, including developmental anomalies (including but not limited to NTDs), spontaneous abortions, preeclampsia and low birth weight.[162] Low maternal intake during pregnancy is associated with low infant vitamin B_{12} status at birth and possibly affects infant cognitive development.[162] Other research has shown that higher maternal intake of one-carbon nutrients (folate, vitamins B_2, B_6 and B_{12} and methionine) is associated with lower rates of childhood acute lymphocytic, lymphoblastic and acute myeloid leukaemia.[163] Recent research has found an association between low maternal B_{12} and gestational diabetes.[164]

Additional dietary and supplemental B_{12} recommendations address both fetal growth requirements and the extra metabolic demands of the mother. B_{12} is the largest and most complex vitamin and it is more reliant on optimal GI function for absorption than other nutrients. The primary natural dietary sources of B_{12} are animal products: B_{12} is synthesised by bacteria and is only found in foods that have been bacterially fermented and in animal tissue. Plant foods are generally poor sources of vitamin B_{12} and are not well recognised by gastric intrinsic factor. While it is understood that women with low or no animal products in their diet (vegetarians and vegans) require careful supplementation to ensure adequate intake, it is important to recognise that insufficient levels of vitamin B_{12} are also noted in women who are not vegetarians.[161] Serum B_{12} levels decrease during pregnancy and they include both active and inactive B_{12}; testing for active B_{12} holotranscobalamin may be more accurate. Other assessments of B_{12} include homocysteine levels and blood film (checking for megaloblastic changes).

Dose

RDI: 2.6 micrograms[56]

Therapeutic dose: 1000–2000 micrograms/day is required to correct deficiency with the aim of prescribing 1:1 with folate prescription. If the woman is on very high folate supplementation (e.g. 5 g/day), an additional 1000 micrograms of vitamin B_{12} is indicated. There is no upper level of intake due to lack of evidence of adverse effects.

Forms

Vitamin B_{12} is available is several forms:

- Cyanocobalamin is a synthetic form and is commonly found in supplements. It has low bioavailability and requires hepatic conversion to be biologically active
- Hydroxycobalamin is commonly used in parenteral preparations and more recently in Australia is available in oral preparations
- Methylcobalamin and adenosylcobalamin are the two coenzymatically active forms.[43,165]

Methylcobalamin is the cofactor of the enzyme methionine synthase, which participates in the metabolic homocysteine pathway, converting homocysteine into methionine (along with vitamin B_6 and folate). The homocysteine pathway is also critical in the regeneration of the methyl donor SAMe and failure to do so limits available SAMe, which affects DNA synthesis and cell replication, especially intense division such as fetal development and erythropoiesis.[165,166]

Adenosylcobalamin is the cofactor of the methylmalonyl-CoA mutase enzyme. Where methylcobalamin is found and active in the cytosol, adenosylcobalamin is active within the mitochondria, in the metabolism of carbohydrates, branched-chain amino acids and fatty acids. The shortage of adenosylcobalamin leads to an accumulation of the intermediate molecule methylmalonic acid. Neuron myelin sheaths are highly dependent on fatty acid metabolism and the low bioavailability of adenosylcobalamin can lead to damage of the myelin sheath and subsequent impairment of nerve transmission.[165,166] In fetal development myelination begins early in the third trimester, with the most rapid period of myelination occurring in the first 2 years of life.

Cyanocobalamin and hydroxycobalamin are provitamin forms that require activation into the cofactor forms of methylcobalamin or adenosylcobalamin before they can be used by the cells.[165]

ANTIOXIDANTS

Oxidation is a physiological process and in health it is balanced by antioxidant activity so that excess free radical damage and inflammation are avoided. Antioxidant status (measured by oxygen radical absorbance capacity [ORAC] and superoxide radical-eliminating ability [SREA]) changes over the course of pregnancy, notably dropping at the critical periods of early pregnancy and peripartum. This may reflect the increased oxidative activity at these times and highlights the importance of antioxidant intake to protect the pregnancy and the mother.[167]

In pregnancy, oxidation and inflammation may have adverse effects on embryogenesis, fetal development and placental health and function. Consequences of excessive oxidative damage may include fetal growth restriction, placental dysfunction, preeclampsia, premature birth and pregnancy loss, as well as increasing the risk of chronic disease in adulthood.[168] ART may increase oxidative activity and a small study of women using ART found that low plasma antioxidant status in early normal gestation was associated with later development of pregnancy complications.[169] Importantly, this study also reviewed diet and found that high consumption of foods of vegetable origin was associated with high plasma levels of phenolic compounds and higher antioxidant status. Antioxidants work synergistically and are best taken as wholefoods and in combination supplements, and many studies on the role, levels and supplementation of antioxidants include more than one antioxidant.

As part of the international Screening for Pregnancy Endpoints (SCOPE) study, pre-morbid antioxidant serum levels of 244 women (15 weeks gestation) who later developed preeclampsia and 472 matched controls who did not were analysed.[170] The results were increased copper and caeruloplasmin in women with preeclampsia, but no significant difference in serum zinc, selenium and manganese, although there was no discussion on the ratio of zinc to copper. A further study examining maternal and cord levels of endogenous antioxidants (malondialdehyde, superoxide dismutase, glutathione peroxidase and glutathione) at 16–20 weeks, 26–30 weeks and delivery found that early antioxidant status was associated with the later development of preeclampsia, suggesting that oxidative damage may alter placental development and lead to fetal programming of adult non-communicable disease in the offspring.[171]

A meta-analysis of observational studies that measured maternal blood levels of non-enzymatic antioxidants (vitamins A, C and E and carotenoids) found that lower serum levels of vitamins A, C and E were significantly associated with overall preeclampsia, but not for mild or severe preeclampsia subtypes, and that evidence for SGA was inconclusive.[172] However, these studies were small and there were methodological imperfections, highlighting the need for more rigorous research. Women who may require additional antioxidant support include those who smoke, are older, are obese, have diabetes (pre-existing or gestational diabetes mellitus [GDM]), have used ART, have chronic illnesses or have a history of pregnancy loss and placental abnormalities including preeclampsia and placental abruption. A study of 9969 women (4993 of whom received vitamins C and E and 4976 who received a placebo) found that vitamin C and E supplementation was associated with more than 40% reduction in placental abruption and greater than 30% reduction in preterm birth among smokers.[173] A study examining placental endoplasmic reticulum (ER) stress in women with well-controlled GDM found low-grade ER stress was in all of the control groups, but this was amplified with a glucose challenge. The addition of vitamins C and E reduced the ER stress.[174]

A Cochrane Review on vitamin C found a 36% relative reduction in placental abruption in women given vitamin C supplements (eight studies over 15 700 women); this was rated as high-quality evidence, albeit some of the studies coadministered vitamin E and this may have influenced the results (i.e. the combined antioxidant effect as opposed to solely vitamin C).[175] For women given vitamin C only, there was a reduction in pre-labour rupture of the membranes (PROM) occurring either preterm or at term, but for women receiving both vitamin E and C there was an increased risk of PROM. Another study on antioxidants and preeclampsia found that in preeclamptic women, leptin was significantly increased and haem oxygenase and CoQ10 were significantly decreased.[176]

As with most nutrient supplements, excessive supplementation (not dietary) of antioxidants may be harmful. For example, an in vitro study found that high levels of vitamins C and E decreased cell viability and secretion of human chorionic gonadotrophin (hCG) by cytotrophoblasts and increased production of TNF-α.[177] There was no discussion of the intake required to reach the cellular amounts in the study, which is an important consideration given the limited absorption of vitamin C at any given time.

VITAMIN A

The term 'vitamin A' refers to any compound with the biological activity of vitamin A including preformed vitamin A retinoids, which are found in foods of animal origin, and provitamin A carotenoids, which are found in plant foods, the most active of which is beta-carotene. Vitamin A is required for gene expression, cell differentiation, organogenesis and embryonic development, and deficiency increases the risk of miscarriage and birth defects. In addition, vitamin A is essential for fetal growth, the growth and repair of mucous membranes and epithelial cells, immune function and RBC production, and retinaldehyde is also essential for vision.[43] Vitamin A is required for neurogenesis in the embryo and control of neural patterning and plasticity.[178] Studies have shown that lower levels of vitamin A in the placenta and fetus are associated with intrauterine growth retardation and premature birth[179]; however, supplementation with 1000 micrograms RE (the RDI) has not been shown to affect gestational age.[180] A Cochrane Review found that prenatal vitamin A supplementation reduces maternal night blindness and anaemia for women who live in areas where vitamin A deficiency is common or who are HIV-positive, as well as resulting in a probable reduction in maternal infection.[181] Vitamin A is also an important antioxidant and may be associated with reduced inflammation and adverse outcomes.

Plasma retinol is not a sensitive indicator of underlying vitamin A status, but concentrations lower than 0.7 micromol/L indicate deficiency. Serum levels gradually decrease in pregnancy due to haemodilution; however, this effect may be reduced due to increased mobilisation of fat stores (as fat-soluble vitamins), which occurs from the end of the first trimester.

Cautions

Large doses (>10 000 IU) may be teratogenic, especially in the first trimester. Avoid excessive supplementation and rich food sources (organ meat, cod liver oil, pâté). Beta-carotene has not been found to be teratogenic.[28,43]

Dose

RDI: 800 micrograms/2600 IU[56]
Therapeutic dose: up to 10 000 IU[43]

VITAMIN C

Vitamin C is the primary water-soluble, non-enzymatic antioxidant in plasma and tissues. It protects proteins, lipids, carbohydrates and nucleic acids (DNA and RNA) and regenerates vitamin E from its oxidised form. In addition, it is essential for the production of collagen, which forms all connective tissue, it increases the bioavailability of iron from foods and is a cofactor for neurotransmitter synthesis. Vitamin C is also an important immune stimulant, modulating lymphocytes and phagocytes, enhancing natural killer cells and protecting neutrophils from auto-oxidative damage.[43] Low levels of vitamin C lead to oxidative damage, which may inhibit the action of luteinising hormone and block steroidogenesis and may be implicated in luteal phase and early miscarriage. However, one randomised controlled trial found no improvement in pregnancy outcomes with supplementation.[182]

Dose

RDI: 60 mg[56]
Therapeutic dose: up to 3000 mg[43] in divided doses

VITAMIN D

Vitamin D is an essential hormone-like fat-soluble vitamin and the active form is 1,25-dihydroxyvitamin D_3 (calcitriol). Within the cell calcitriol binds with a nuclear transcription factor called vitamin D receptor and then joins to another nuclear receptor, retinoic acid X receptor. Together they bind short sequences of DNA and regulate the expression of hundreds of genes involved in skeletal and other biological functions. Core functions in pregnancy include calcium homeostasis, bone mineralisation, cell differentiation, immune function and stimulation and blood pressure regulation.

For the mother, vitamin D is critical for normal hormone synthesis, receptor site uptake and gene regulation, as well as having a positive influence on insulin production and offering protection against gestational diabetes. Vitamin D's positive influence on immune function is relevant to protect against bacterial and viral infections, including bacterial vaginosis and streptococcus B, which are implicated in premature birth.[183] Vitamin D is essential to ensure adequate maternal calcium absorption and homeostasis, as well as skeletal development in the fetus, with approximately 25–30 g of calcium being transferred from the mother to the fetus during pregnancy.[28] Low vitamin D may be an independent risk factor for preeclampsia; supplementation to increase serum 25-hydroxyvitamin D (25(OH)D) at term may reduce the risk of preeclampsia, low birth weight and preterm birth.[184–186] A large clinically validated trial in Ireland (the SCOPE study) has provided evidence for the positive impact of vitamin D on uteroplacental dysfunction as indicated by preeclampsia and SGA.[187] The study followed 1768 low-risk nulliparous women, and the risk of preeclampsia and SGA combined was 13.6% lower in women with a serum vitamin D of >75 nmol/L. Furthermore, there were no adverse effects with serum 25(OH)D levels of >125 nmol/L.

A large 2016 study in the Netherlands measured vitamin D concentrations in 7098 mothers and their babies.[188] Women whose serum 25(OH)D was in the lowest quartile had an increased risk of preterm birth (OR 1.62) and the newborn was twice as likely to be SGA. The authors assessed that 25(OH)D levels of <50 nmol/L increased the population risk of preterm birth by 17.3% and SGA by 22.6%.[188] A prospective cohort study of 1683 pregnant women in Denmark assessed serum 25(OH)D before 22 weeks gestation and the risk of subsequent miscarriage.[189] In the first trimester the research showed a slight reduction in the risk of miscarriage with higher serum vitamin D, but importantly it found that there was a greater than two-fold increase in miscarriage when serum vitamin D was less than 50 nmol/L. There was no significant impact on second trimester pregnancy loss. A study of 792 women with singleton pregnancies reviewed second trimester serum vitamin D and the risk for SGA and found that compared to serum 25(OH)D concentrations of less than 30 nmol/L, women whose levels were 50–74 nmol/L and 75 nmol/L or greater were associated with 43% and 54% reductions in risk of SGA, respectively.[186] Furthermore, Caucasian women with serum vitamin D of >50 nmol/L had a 68% reduction in SGA risk compared to women with levels of <50 nmol/L; there was no association between vitamin D status and risk of SGA in African American women.

For the developing embryo/fetus, maternal vitamin D is critical for implantation and angiogenesis, and is required for skeletal and tooth formation and growth, gene regulation and development of the brain and immune system. Babies with low vitamin D have an increased risk of low birth weight and lowered immune function. Recent preliminary research suggests that autism rates are lower in siblings of children with autism where vitamin D supplementation occurred during pregnancy and early childhood.[190] This research is supported by the findings of a large study of 4229 women and their offspring in the Generation R study.[191] In this study researchers analysed maternal serum zinc and neonatal cord blood mid-gestation and at birth and found that low maternal and fetal vitamin D levels were strongly associated with autism traits in the child at 6 years of age. Low fetal vitamin D may influence fetal programming and affect neuro-programming, immune function and the development of chronic disease, including allergies, autoimmune diseases, cardiovascular diseases, multiple sclerosis,[192] diabetes, bronchiolitis and other respiratory infections, schizophrenia[193] and some cancers.[60,194,195]

Maternal vitamin D deficiency is one of the main risk factors for deficiency in the offspring; in the first 6–8 weeks of life newborns are dependent on the vitamin D transferred across the placenta while in utero. The 25(OH)D levels in the newborn correspond to 60–89% of maternal values and thus will be impacted by maternal deficiency.[195] Maternal supplementation with 2000 IU of vitamin D during pregnancy has been found to increase vitamin D in breastmilk for more than 2 months postpartum[196]: at 2 weeks the women who took vitamin D had nearly one and a half times the vitamin D of those who took nothing or 1000 IU vitamin D and at 2 months the women who took 2000 IU had approximately 35% higher levels of vitamin D. Of note, women who took 1000 IU of vitamin D had similar breast vitamin D activity as those who took no supplementation.

Vitamin D deficiency is common but is more common in obese women and women with dark skin.[66] Deficiency is determined by serum levels of 25(OH)D, although there is ongoing review about these levels with suggestions that higher levels may be indicated in some conditions.[195,197] In addition, there is the question about whether 25(OH)D calcidiol or 1,25-dihydroxyvitamin D_3 (25(OH)D_3) is a more accurate measure, as this is the active form, after final renal hydroxylation, and may be a more accurate reflection of biologically active vitamin D. Research into vitamin D and pregnancy has shown mixed results and some of the issue may be the assay used, not controlling for ethnicity, age and, importantly, weight, the stage of gestation tested and, as relates to GDM, the diagnostic criteria for GDM.[198,199] An example of different results based on whether serum 25(OH)D or 25(OH)D_3 concentrations were used showed that only 25(OH)D_3 levels were significantly associated with GDM risk.[200] A 16 nmol/L increase in 25(OH)D_3 concentration was associated with a 14% decrease in GDM risk, with women in the lowest quartile for 25(OH)D_3 levels having double the risk for GDM.

In Australia vitamin D adequacy is considered to be ≥50 nmol/L at the end of winter (the level may need to be 10–20 nmol/L higher at the end of summer to allow for seasonal decrease), mild deficiency is 30–49 nmol/L, moderate deficiency is 12.5–29 nmol/L and severe deficiency is <12.5 nmol/L.[197] In its 2011 report the IOM recommends that a serum 25(OH)D concentration of 50 nmol/L is adequate for calcium absorption and bone health in adults, including pregnant women, that insufficiency is 25–49 nmol/L and severe deficiency is <25 nmol/L.[201] In contrast, the guidelines from the American Endocrine Society define vitamin D deficiency as a 25(OH)D <50 nmol/L, and vitamin D insufficiency as 50–75 nmol/L.[202] The Endocrine Society reports that if we use the IOM guideline of severe deficiency as 25(OH)D <25 nmol/L, then anywhere between 20% and 100% of people would be classed as deficient. In Australia the AusDiab study found that 4% of the general population had levels <25 nmol/L and 31% had levels <50 nmol/L (22% of men and 39% of women).[203] Other

studies have shown rates of 76% of postnatal women with deficiency[204] and in England, levels of less than 25 nmol/L have been found in 47% of Indian Asian women, 64% of Middle Eastern women, 58% of black women and 13% of Caucasian women.[198,205]

It is difficult to achieve the required levels of vitamin D with diet and sunlight alone and supplementation to achieve optimal levels may be required. Any intestinal absorption, renal or hepatic compromise may impair absorption and hyroxylation to the active form, and obese women are at a higher risk of low vitamin D levels. Vitamin D metabolism is significantly altered in pregnancy. The mother decreases urinary excretion of calcium and increases calcium absorption in early pregnancy, reaching a peak in the last trimester.[195] Maternal plasma levels of calcitriol increase in early pregnancy, also peaking in the third trimester and returning to normal during lactation. The mechanism for the increased synthesis of calcitriol is unique in pregnancy as parathyroid hormone, calcium and phosphorus levels are largely unchanged in pregnancy and a pregnant woman can reach supra-physiological levels of calcitriol (up to 700 nmol/L) without exhibiting hypercalciuria or hypercalcaemia.[206]

Dosage discussion

Two randomised controlled trials evaluating vitamin D deficiency and dose of vitamin D supplementation found that hypertensive disorders of pregnancy, gestational diabetes, infection and preterm labour and birth showed statistically significant differences between the higher risk (lower serum vitamin D) women in the control group (400 IU group) compared with both the 2000 IU and 4000 IU groups.[206,207] Indeed, Hollis and colleagues found that there was no significant difference in achieving a serum 25(OH)D level of ≥80 nmol/L within 1 month between the 2000 IU and 4000 IU groups, but there was a significant difference between 2000 IU and 400 IU (RR 1.52) and 4000 IU and 400 IU (RR 1.60).[206] There were no significant differences between the 400, 2000 and 4000 IU groups for any safety measure and there were no adverse events attributed to vitamin D for any group or individual.[206,207] There was a direct correlation between serum 25(OH)D and vitamin D_3 intake.

A study of ethnically diverse women in South Carolina (US) found that supplementing with the recommended 400 IU of vitamin D made no impact on serum vitamin D and was no different from not taking any supplementation.[207] Hollis and colleagues also found that consuming the recommended 400 IU would have meant that >50% of their total cohort and >80% of African American women in their cohort would be vitamin D deficient and they recommended a serum 25(OH)D concentration of >100 nmol/L for optimal renal and/or placental production of 1,25(OH)$_2$D.[206]

Dose

RDI: 5 micrograms/200 IU[56]
Therapeutic dose: up to 4000 IU daily is considered to be safe.[60,206,207]

VITAMIN E

Vitamin E is an important and potent fat-soluble antioxidant and it protects and stabilises cell membranes against lipid peroxidation, especially polyunsaturated fatty acids (PUFAs) and low-density lipoproteins (LDLs).[43] Vitamin E is regenerated by vitamin C and protects vitamin A. In addition, vitamin E is important for immune competence (humoral and cell-mediated, and increasing natural killer cell [NKC] activity and TNF production). Vitamin E has anti-inflammatory actions, suppressing arachidonic acid production, and by inhibiting protein kinase C activity it prevents vascular smooth-muscle cell proliferation and regulates enzymes acting on vascular function. Vitamin E is also important in gene regulation, in particular in pathways involved with normal vascular function, cell growth and regulation, as well as having a role in cell signalling.[43] These combined effects may account for evidence of reduced placental abruption with vitamin E supplementation.[209] Most research on vitamin E supplementation has been in combination with at least one other nutrient and antioxidant, although deficiency appears associated with miscarriage, preterm birth, preeclampsia and intrauterine growth retardation.[28] In pregnant women in rural Bangladesh, low plasma α-tocopherol was associated with increased risk of miscarriage, and low γ-tocopherol was associated with decreased risk of miscarriage; thus maternal vitamin E status in the first trimester may influence the risk of early pregnancy loss.[210] Vitamin E is not stored to the same degree as other fat-soluble nutrients and toxicity is relatively rare.[43] With fat mobilisation, serum concentration increases from the second trimester onwards.

Dose

RDI: 7 mg/10 IU[56]
Therapeutic dose: 150–1200 IU/day

VITAMIN K

Dietary vitamin K exists primarily as phylloquinone from plants and as a mix of menaquinones found in animal products and provided by colonic bacteria. Vitamin K is a fat-soluble vitamin required for the synthesis of clotting factors II, VII, IX and X, bone mineralisation, the prevention of blood vessel mineralisation and the regulation of various cellular functions including via vitamin K-dependent growth arrest-specific gene 6 protein (Gas6), which regulates cell proliferation. In pregnancy the primary interest is in relation to the cellular growth regulation factor with cell-signalling activities. In women with infertility and/or recurrent pregnancy loss it is important to consider vitamin K levels. Vitamin K deficiency is rare, but newborns are at risk due to low intestinal synthesis, low placental transfer and low breast milk vitamin K.[211]

Dose

RDI: 60 micrograms[56]
Therapeutic dose: 75 micrograms

BIOTIN (B$_7$)

Water-soluble biotin (vitamin B$_7$) is a cofactor for five carboxylases that are critical for fatty acids, glucose and amino acid metabolism, assisting in the regulation of blood sugar levels and hepatic gluconeogenesis and lipid metabolism. Biotin works with vitamin B$_{12}$ and folate for cell division and DNA replication, and it regulates gene expression and chromatin structure.

Deficiency of biotin is thought to be common during pregnancy. While it may be physiological or pathological, deficiency is associated with birth defects and NTDs, and deficiency in mice and other animals is known to be highly teratogenic.[212] Studies have shown that biotin deficiency affects the functions of adaptive immune T- and NK cells, and in vitro research suggests that biotin deficiency enhances the inflammatory response of dendritic cells.[213] Research is scant, with a recent study evaluating biotin intake and levels in pregnant and lactating women being the first human pregnancy study to control for dietary biotin intake.[214] This research confirms earlier findings that marginal biotin deficiency occurs in a substantial proportion of women during normal pregnancy, but also shows that there is reasonable evidence to suggest that a biotin intake of at least two to three times the recommended average daily nutrient intake is probably needed to meet the requirements of pregnancy.[214,215]

Dose

RDI: 30 micrograms[56]
Therapeutic dose: 100–500 micrograms

CHOLINE

Choline is an essential micronutrient and methyl donor and plays a key role in fetal development. With other B vitamins (i.e. folate, B$_{12}$, B$_6$ and B$_2$), choline is required for the metabolism of nucleic acids and amino acids and for the generation of SAMe. The interrelationship of these methyl factors means that deficiency of folate or methionine increases the demand for choline.[216] Choline is also a precursor for betaine, which in addition to its role in methylation is needed for glomerular function and possibly mitochondrial function.[216]

In addition, choline is a precursor for the phospholipid phosphatidylcholine, which is the main constituent of cell membranes and lipoproteins and contributes to the formation of bile and surfactants.[60,217] Choline is required for normal brain function and structure, and is critical for cell division and growth and myelination of neural cells. While organogenesis is largely complete by the eighth week of gestation, brain development and growth are markedly rapid in the third trimester and the need for choline is particularly high at this time (and until around 5 years of age).[217] Adequate choline is required for normal fetal neurological structural development and function and is thought to be essential for hippocampal memory in fetal development and early childhood; levels can have a lifelong impact on memory and cognition.[60,216,217]

Women with low-choline diets have more babies with orofacial clefts and are up to four times as likely to have a baby with a NTD, whereas higher choline diets are associated with improved signalling mechanisms associated with placental angiogenesis and may attenuate some of the pathological processes leading to preeclampsia.[216] Higher choline intake is also associated with altered expression of placental corticotropin-releasing hormone and this may be protective against injury from fetal and maternal stress.[216]

Choline also appears to protect the fetus from injury due to alcohol. In animal studies the offspring of rats treated with choline had fewer deficits associated with alcohol exposure, such as fetal death, reduced birth weight and brain weight, and behavioural and developmental impairment (this was not due to lowering of the alcohol, but through other neuroprotective mechanisms).[216] It is postulated that choline induces synthesis of phospholipids for nerve cell growth and myelination, enhancement of acetylcholine and epigenetic changes.[218]

In the third trimester maternal triglyceride synthesis is increased and it is important that this is metabolised and cleared. Choline is central to this process and inefficient metabolism can induce non-alcoholic fatty liver disease in pregnancy. Phosphatidylcholine and its derivative sphingomyelin yield cell-signalling molecules that have roles in fetal development.[217] Choline is also required for the synthesis of the neurotransmitter acetylcholine, which in the placenta may modulate cellular proliferation and division as well as influencing parturition.[217] Production of phosphatidylcholine includes the incorporation of DHA into the phosphatidylcholine, which may further influence fetal neural development.[216] The fetus and the placenta are reliant on maternal choline and maternal synthesis is upregulated in pregnancy, in part modulated by increased oestrogen. Choline is transported across the placenta and fetal concentrations are about 14 times that of maternal blood. Neonates are born with three times maternal blood levels, highlighting how important this nutrient is to the fetus.[216,217] Maternal choline comes from food sources, de novo synthesis and supplementation.

Animal studies demonstrate that high choline intake improves attention, learning and memory in the offspring, whereas deficiency induces NTDs and impaired cognitive development.[65,216] Dietary inadequacy for choline is common, and combining choline deficiency with the marked increased requirements in pregnancy and lactation mean that many women will benefit from supplementation and that current recommended levels may be too low.[216,217]

Dose

RDI: 440 mg[56]
Therapeutic dose: upper limit 3000 mg/day.

Calcium

Calcium is particularly important in pregnancy in two key areas: ossification of the fetal skeleton and protection of maternal bones; and to reduce the risk of hypertension, preeclampsia and premature birth.[60] Supplementation is not routinely recommended, but this is based on the mother consuming the recommended 1000 mg per day – and this is frequently not the case, especially if she does not consume dairy.

Calcium metabolism is altered in pregnancy: calcium absorption and urinary calcium excretion are approximately doubled during pregnancy compared to non-pregnant metabolism.[219] For optimal calcium absorption and to prevent or minimise bone turnover, vitamin D intake needs to be adequate too, so concurrent supplementation is advisable. The RDI for calcium in pregnancy is 1000 mg but teenagers need 1300 mg as they themselves are still growing. Fetal calcium requirements increase significantly in the second half of the pregnancy when more than 90% of fetal growth occurs. During pregnancy approximately 25–30 g of calcium are transferred to the fetus, with the fetus using around 300 mg/day in the last 2–3 months.[60,220]

Calcium supplementation to prevent hypertension is most effective for women with low calcium intake.[60] Two Cochrane Reviews on calcium and hypertension have been conducted and they provide a combined analysis of 21 randomised controlled trials involving more than 19 000 pregnant women from both developed and developing countries.[221–223] In the studies calcium supplementation ranged from 300 mg to 2000 mg, with the majority of studies commencing supplementation at 20 weeks gestation. Compared to the placebo group, all women who took calcium supplementation reduced their risk of preeclampsia by an average of slightly more than half and this was irrespective of the baseline risk of developing hypertension and calcium intake status. Unsurprisingly, women identified at risk of developing a hypertensive disorder had a much greater reduction in their risk, with an average 78% reduction compared to women with a lower baseline risk of developing hypertension, who had a risk reduction of 41%.[222] In a 2014 update of the Cochrane Review including 12 trials and 15 470 women the average risk of hypertension was reduced with calcium supplementation by 35% compared with the placebo. In addition, there was also a significant reduction in the risk of preeclampsia and the average risk of preterm birth was reduced by 34%.[221]

A 2014 Cochrane Review on calcium for non-hypertension related benefits found no significant difference between the placebo group and the calcium group in reducing the risk of premature birth; however, it did find an increase in birth weight for the supplemented group (mean difference 64.66 g), although the results overall were mixed and the significance of this result was not clear.[223] Other applications for calcium in pregnancy include potential protection against lead and other heavy metal toxicity to the fetus. If the mother has inadequate calcium and/or vitamin D, this increases the risk of maternal bone turnover and liberation of heavy metals stored in the bone.[220]

Cautions

Calcium supplementation has been found to increase the risk of HELLP (haemolysis, elevated liver enzymes, low platelet count) syndrome compared to women who do not use supplements, but both a Cochrane Review and the WHO note that the benefit of supplementing outweighs the risk, especially due to the small numbers of women affected by HELLP.[221,222] Calcium supplementation in pregnancy does not increase the risk of nephrolithiasis.[224]

Dose

RDI: 1000 mg (1300 mg 14–18 years)[56]
Therapeutic dose: 1000–2000 mg/day
Adequate absorption and retention of calcium requires sufficient vitamin D. If the mother is also supplementing with iron, it is necessary to separate the doses.

Chromium

Chromium's main action is in glycaemic control, with a lesser antioxidant function.[43] Stable blood sugar is important for hormone function and is especially relevant in women with a history of polycystic ovary syndrome. In pregnancy there is increased insulin resistance and an apparent increased excretion of chromium. There is little research on chromium levels or supplementation in pregnancy. An early prospective cohort study involving 425 women found no difference in chromium levels in the 396 women who did not develop GDM and the 29 who developed GDM.[225] This study excluded women with known type 2 diabetes or known GDM. A later study of 30 women with known GDM and 60 matched controls found that women with GDM had lower levels of serum chromium than pregnant women without GDM.[226] Supplementation of chromium may be of benefit in reducing GDM, although more trials are required.[43]

Dose

RDI: 30 micrograms[56]
Therapeutic dose: 50–200 micrograms

Iodine

Iodine is an essential trace element, primarily due to its role in the synthesis of thyroid hormone. Thyroxine regulates the cellular metabolism of all tissues, the metabolic rate, thermogenesis and oxidation and affects growth and maturation. In the fetal and early infancy periods, thyroxine is necessary for neuronal migration, myelination of the central nervous system (CNS), and synaptic transmission and plasticity, and thus insufficient intake can have devastating consequences on neural and cognitive development.[28,227] Around 70–80% of iodine is concentrated in the thyroid gland where it is used to produce thyroxine (T4) and triiodothyronine (T3).[228] Maternal production of T4 increases by 50%:

approximately 50 micrograms/day of iodine is transferred to the fetus in the form of thyroxine, necessitating increased maternal iodine intake.[28]

The developing fetal thyroid gland begins to concentrate iodine and produce thyroid hormone (T3 and T4) around the 10th to 12th week of gestation, which coincides with when the fetus begins to synthesise thyroid-stimulating hormone (TSH). It takes until weeks 18–20 of gestation before meaningful fetal thyroid hormone synthesis occurs, so the placental transfer of maternal thyroid hormone is essential until then.[28,227,229] In addition to the marked increase in demand, during pregnancy there is increased plasma volume (causing haemodilution), increased urinary excretion of iodine and increased iodine degradation due to increased activity of utero-placental deiodinases.[43]

Major dietary sources of iodine include bread and milk. Iodine intake has decreased in recent decades due to reduced intake of iodised table salt, bread and cow's milk. Iodine (as iodide) is widespread in the environment but distribution is uneven based on geography and on leaching due to flooding and erosion: mountainous regions, such as the Himalayas, the Andes and the Alps, and flooded river valleys such as the Ganges are among the most severely iodine-deficient areas in the world.[228] There is also a seasonal variance in iodine levels in dairy products, and research in the UK has found the highest levels in winter. This variance means that particular care may need to be taken if preconception and early pregnancy occurs during low iodine periods.[230] Finally, iodine bioavailability is reduced by goitrogens such as soy, and iodine use requires cofactors of selenium and iron, so if a woman is replete with iodine she may still have impaired thyroid function if she is deficient in iron or selenium.

According to the WHO guidelines (see Table 13.4), a median urinary iodine concentration (MUIC) of <100 micrograms/L represents iodine deficiency in children and adults, but a MUIC of <150 micrograms/L indicates iodine deficiency in pregnant women. The corresponding iodine intake to meet these levels is 150 micrograms for non-pregnant adults and 250 micrograms for pregnant

TABLE 13.4 WHO assessment of urinary iodine status and oral intake requirements for pregnant women

Median urinary iodine concentration (MUIC) (micrograms/L)	Status of iodine intake
<150	Insufficient
150–249	Adequate
250–499	More than adequate
≥500	No added health benefit expected

Source: Andersson M, De Benoist B, Delange F, Zupan J. Prevention and control of iodine deficiency in pregnant and lactating women and in children less than 2 years old: conclusions and recommendations of the Technical Consultation WHO Secretariat on behalf of the participants to the Consultation. Public Heal Nutr 2007;10(12A):1606–11.

women.[231,232] While public health measures of food fortification and supplementation have improved people's iodine status worldwide, iodine is still low in women of reproductive years and in infants. It is estimated that as many as 30% of pregnant Americans have low iodine levels (<100 micrograms/L); as in other countries, there is variance depending on location and ethnicity.[28] A study in the UK surveyed iodine levels at weeks 12, 20 and 35 of gestation and found that the MUIC from urine samples collected at all time points was 56.8 micrograms/L, indicating iodine deficiency. In addition, only 3% of women were taking iodine-containing prenatal supplements.[230] A large survey in Norway of 61 904 pregnant women also found inadequate iodine levels, with a mean combined food/supplement intake of 166 micrograms/day, well below the WHO recommendation of 250 micrograms/day.[233]

An early Australian survey of 802 pregnant women in Melbourne found that 48.4% of Caucasians, 38.4% of Vietnamese and 40.8% of Sri Lankan and Indian women had a urinary iodine level of <50 micrograms/L, which is consistent with other surveys and is significantly lower than the WHO guidelines.[234] A more recent survey in northwestern Sydney of 367 women attending their first antenatal visit between 7 and 11 weeks gestation found the median iodine concentration was 81 micrograms/L and that 71.9% had a MUIC of <150 micrograms/L.[235] Of note, there was no change in the serum TSH or T4 levels at the time and this was prior to the fortification of bread. A South Australian study assessing the impact of iodine supplementation and food fortification found that they were inadequate to meet the needs of pregnant women[236]: 196 women had their urinary iodine tested at the beginning of their pregnancy, at 12, 18, 30 and 36 weeks gestation, and at 6 months postpartum. The MUIC was within the mildly deficient range in women not taking supplements (<90 micrograms/L), while women who were taking iodine-containing multivitamins had a MUIC within the WHO recommendations for sufficiency (150–249 micrograms/L). The fortification of bread with iodised salt has increased the MUIC from 68 micrograms/L to 84 micrograms/L; however, this is still in the iodine-deficient range and supplementation is required.

Maternal risks of inadequate iodine include goitre and hypothyroidism, hypertension and increased perinatal mortality, miscarriage and stillbirth. The risks to the embryo/fetus range from irreversible mild to fatal damage, and the risk is greatest in the first 8 weeks of gestation. Fetal consequences include brain damage, impaired neuropsychological development and lower intelligence, hypothyroidism, goitre, congenital abnormalities, cretinism and motor skill and hearing problems.[28,43,230]

Most studies have focused on perinatal and neonatal impacts of low iodine, with fewer analysing long-term impacts, including for mild to moderate deficiency, although one such study was a longitudinal study in Tasmania during a period of mild iodine deficiency in the population, with the children subsequently growing up in an iodine-replete environment. The researchers used local and national assessment tools for the 9-year-olds and found that children whose mothers had a MUIC <150 micrograms/L had reductions of 10.0% in spelling, 7.6% in grammar and 5.7% in English-literacy performance compared with children whose mothers' MUIC was 150 micrograms/L, indicating long-term adverse impacts on fetal neurocognition that are not amended by iodine sufficiency during childhood.[237] A meta-analysis (n = 12 291 children) in China found that maternal iodine deficiency was associated with a drop in IQ of 8–12 points in the child and that supplementation after 6–8 weeks was ineffective in reducing this effect.[28,238]

Excessive iodine is also problematic. Excessive iodine intake (up to 12.5 mg/day) has been associated with rare cases of congenital hyperthyroidism[239] and congenital cardiac defects.[239] With excess iodine exposure the thyroid gland actively inhibits the incorporation of iodine into thyroglobulin for the production of thyroid hormone by an autoregulatory mechanism known as the acute Wolff–Chaikoff effect.[240] In addition, excessive iodine is associated with maternal postpartum thyroiditis and hypothyroidism.[241,242]

Given the importance of iodine and the persistent inadequate levels for many pregnant women, health professionals have a critical role in educating women about their diet and appropriate supplementation during preconception, pregnancy and lactation. A study of 199 midwives and 277 obstetricians in the US found that while they were aware of the importance of iodine, they rarely or never recommended supplementation in pregnancy (66% and 67.1%, respectively) and when iodine supplementation was recommended it was below the recommended dose.[243] This represents a critical opportunity for naturopaths to improve health outcomes for pregnant women and their babies. This need is echoed in findings from a South Australian study, which found that women had poor knowledge regarding the role and sources of dietary iodine in pregnancy and lactation.[244]

Dose

RDI: 220 micrograms[56]
WHO RDI: 250 micrograms, upper limit 500 micrograms[231]
Therapeutic dose: 220–500 micrograms/day
Multiparous women, older women and women with short interpregnancy intervals need higher doses.
Caution: Monitor patients with thyroid antibodies closely; for those with elevated thyroid peroxidase (TPO) antibodies it may not be appropriate to give iodine supplementation.

Iron

Iron deficiency is the largest single-nutrient deficiency worldwide and pregnant women are particularly vulnerable.[65] Contributing factors include food shortages and lack of dietary intake, malabsorption, chronic blood loss and anaemia of chronic illness, and failure to meet the increased demands of pregnancy. The mother's iron stores at the time of conception are strongly predictive of the risk of iron deficiency and anaemia in pregnancy. The background (non-pregnant) incidence of iron deficiency and iron deficiency anaemia varies, with rates ranging from 12% in the US to 43% in developing nations, and for pregnant women it is around 18% in the US and up to 75% for women in developing nations.[28]

Iron has a broad range of essential functions, including as the transport proteins haemoglobin and myoglobin, which are essential for oxygen and carbon dioxide transport, normal immunity, energy production, the synthesis of collagen and elastin and the production of DNA and RNA. Iron also has roles in hormone (e.g. thyroxine) and neurotransmitter production, as well as broad enzyme functions including cytochrome P450 and liver metabolism. Within pregnancy there is an increased iron requirement to meet the growth demands of the fetus and placenta, to accommodate fetal iron deposition in the third trimester, to support increased maternal production of red blood cells and to reduce the impact of blood loss during pregnancy and labour. In a normal singleton pregnancy 450 mg of iron is delivered to the maternal bone marrow, 300 mg is delivered to the fetus and 250 mg is lost during pregnancy and parturition, meaning a total of approximately 1000 mg iron is required. The majority is required in the second and third trimesters for the increase in maternal red cell mass (by 20–30%) and the developing fetus and placenta.[28,245]

Lower haemoglobin levels and iron deficiency are associated with fetal growth restriction and low birth weight, prematurity and maternal and infant mortality.[28,65] Anaemia leads to adverse outcomes due to poor infant stores and fetal brain development and cognitive functioning.[28] Additionally, a study on late preterm infants (≥34 weeks) who had latent in utero iron deficiency found that they had abnormal auditory neural maturation compared with infants with normal in utero iron status.[246] This supports previous studies with similar findings.[247]

A more recent area of research is the association between high maternal serum iron and GDM. An Indian study of 1033 healthy women with singleton pregnancies found there was a relationship between early pregnancy maternal serum iron and gestational diabetes.[248] This was supported by a study of 3976 women from the Nurses' Health Study II cohort, which identified 641 cases of GDM and found that women with the highest intake of iron had a 1.64-fold increased risk of developing GDM compared to the lowest iron intake.[249] A further study implicates elevated iron stores in early pregnancy (as measured by hepcidin and ferritin) as being involved in the development of GDM from the first trimester, which is earlier than when GDM is usually thought to begin to develop, and this highlights the need for accurate individual assessment prior to prescribing supplementation.[250] High haemoglobin due to pathology (e.g. haemochromatosis or failure of normal blood plasma volume expansion in pregnancy) or excess supplementation is associated with increased blood viscosity, maternal hypertension, preeclampsia and diabetes.[65]

A mild drop in haemoglobin may be physiological due to the increase in circulation blood volume and it is possible that the effective dilution of the blood reduces viscosity and thus facilitates placental transfer of blood

and therefore oxygen.[28] It is important to assess iron studies and a full blood count before or early in the pregnancy and to monitor throughout. Evaluation needs to consider the range of parameters, including Hb, ferritin, transferrin saturation and haematocrit, with supplementation adjusted according to need. See the section on iron deficiency anaemia for further discussion.

Dose

RDI: 27 mg; vegetarians and vegans up to 80% higher[56]
Therapeutic dose: 10–100 mg/day[251,252]
Excessively low bioavailable sources can cause nausea and constipation and high doses can limit the absorption of zinc, copper, chromium, molybdenum, manganese and magnesium.

Magnesium

Magnesium is involved in a diversity of fundamental biological roles, including as a cofactor in more than 300 essential enzyme reactions, and it is especially important in energy metabolism and the production of ATP. Other roles include neuromuscular function, vascular tone, DNA synthesis and degradation, glucose utilisation and insulin signalling, and as a calcium antagonist. Within pregnancy serum magnesium is lower in women with mild or severe preeclampsia.[253] Magnesium sulfate is administered intravenously in the management of preeclampsia.[43] In healthy pregnancies magnesium-responsive genes are upregulated; in pregnancies complicated by preeclampsia there is an alteration in magnesium homeostasis.[254] It is suggested that magnesium-sensitive genes affect blood pressure and it is likely that magnesium effects are produced in unison with other nutritional factors such as calcium, vitamins and beta-carotene.[254,255]

Magnesium supplementation of 250 mg/day among women with existing GDM has shown beneficial effects on metabolic status and pregnancy outcomes.[256] This includes positive changes in fasting plasma glucose, serum insulin, serum triglycerides and high-sensitivity C-reactive protein (CRP), as well as a lower incidence of newborn hyperbilirubinaemia and newborn hospitalisation. This is supported by a study that found lower levels of magnesium in women with abnormal glucose tolerance tests and GDM.[257] A further study showed that in pregnancy, women with abdominal obesity and lower plasma magnesium are more likely to have abnormal glucose tolerance test results and that insulin resistance, inflammatory response and oxidative stress are exaggerated in these women.[258] Leg cramps are common in pregnancy and a recent study over 4 weeks involving 80 women found that oral magnesium supplementation significantly reduced their frequency and intensity.[259]

Dose

RDI: 350 mg/day[56]
Therapeutic dose: 300–600 mg/day[43]

Selenium

Selenium is an essential trace element and it is a constituent of more than two dozen selenoproteins that play critical roles in reproduction, thyroid hormone metabolism and reduction of thyroid antibodies, DNA synthesis, immunomodulation; it is also a chemopreventive and powerful antioxidant.[43] Selenium requirements increase in pregnancy and lactation. Selenoenzyme iodothyronine deiodinases are required for the conversion of T4 to the biologically active T3 and selenium deficiency can exacerbate iodine deficiency and hypothyroidism, a significant risk in pregnancy. Selenium is an antioxidant and it regenerates other antioxidants and it is likely that many of its effects in pregnancy, excluding those relating to thyroid function, are due to its antioxidant and anti-inflammatory actions.

Deficiency of selenium is associated with recurrent miscarriage and NTDs. A study of 230 women in the UK with known low selenium found that selenium supplementation significantly reduced the odds ratio for preeclampsia and pregnancy-induced hypertension (OR 0.30).[260] A further study showed that low plasma selenium was associated with SGA infants, possibly mediated through antioxidant effects.[261] A Japanese study found that serum selenium levels (and not copper or zinc) were lower in infants and significantly lower in mothers of premature infants and that maternal serum selenium was positively correlated to birth weight.[262] Low serum selenium has also been associated with an increased risk of GDM.[263,264] Red blood cell levels and plasma levels are poor reflectors of selenium levels unless there is severe deficiency.

Dose

RDI: 65 micrograms/day[56]
Therapeutic dose: minimum 150–400 micrograms/day
Monitor patients on thyroid medication with concurrent supplementation.

Zinc

Zinc is an essential trace mineral that is important for all human cells. Zinc has a key role in the transcription of RNA, the replication of DNA and protein synthesis. Zinc is responsible for the regulation of chromatin structure and function and thus gene expression of embryogenesis. Insufficient zinc during embryogenesis may adversely affect the final phenotype of all organs.[265] Zinc also affects hormone metabolism, including oestrogen and progesterone, prostaglandins and nuclear receptor sites. Zinc is a metalloenzyme involved in up to 200 reactions; it is involved in carbohydrate metabolism and digestion, aids in glycaemic control, is essential for healthy immune function and is an antioxidant.[43,60,266] Zinc is important in cognitive function and mental health and in the fetus it contributes to the regulation of neurogenesis, neuronal migration and differentiation, influencing cognitive development and brain health.[267] Finally, zinc is important in epithelial cell health and healing and is critical for postpartum recovery.

Maternal zinc deficiency can compromise fetal and placental development, as low plasma zinc concentrations reduce placental zinc transport and thus reduce the supply of zinc to the developing fetus.[266] The immune role of zinc means a deficiency may predispose to systemic and intrauterine infections, both of which are major risk factors for preterm birth and pregnancy loss. Zinc deficiency also changes circulating levels of hormones associated with the onset of labour and so may lead to a prolonged labour and associated risks. Low zinc may lead to intrauterine growth retardation, teratogenesis, miscarriage (early or late), postpartum haemorrhage, post-term delivery and SGA babies.[60,268] Low zinc is also known to be associated with increased levels of depression and anxiety, significant issues both prenatally and postnatally.[269–271]

The additional zinc needed for pregnancy is estimated to be about 100 mg, and the additional daily need during the last half of pregnancy when fetal growth is most rapid is about 0.6 mg/day.[268] In the last trimester, maternal transfer of zinc to the fetus is up to 1.5 mg/kg per day.[265] Of the pregnancy-gained 100 mg of zinc, 57% is accrued in the fetus, 6.5% in the placenta, <1% in the amniotic fluid, 24% in the uterus, 5% in mammary tissue and 6.5% in the expanded maternal blood volume.[268,272] Pregnant women need 18–36% more zinc per day compared to non-pregnant women, but most women do not achieve this increase and it is possible that homeostatic adjustment (upregulated intestinal absorption and placental uptake) may accommodate dietary inadequacy.[272]

Studies on zinc supplementation in pregnancy have been inconsistent. Variances may be influenced by location and food sources, study design and lack of consistency across study methods, widely varying doses, inadequate dosages, variable timing and duration of zinc supplementation, background undernutrition, multiple nutrient supplementation, maternal weight and age, GI disease/function, dietary factors affecting zinc bioavailability, the age of the study, a lack of sensitive biomarkers of zinc status and a lack of agreed understanding on adequate baseline levels.[266,268,272] One study of 117 mothers found that women who had premature births and low birth-weight (LBW) infants had lower serum zinc than controls.[273] However, a systematic review in 2012 found that only the reduced risk of preterm birth reached statistical significance (relative risk [RR] 0.86), and that supplementation did not affect any parameter of fetal growth.[268] This 14% relative risk reduction for preterm births was also found by a 2015 Cochrane Review.[274] A meta-analysis found that serum zinc levels were significantly lower in women with preeclampsia compared to healthy controls, an effect possibly mediated by zinc's role as a coenzyme for super-oxide dismutase and other antioxidants.[275] One paper suggested that low maternal zinc affects embryonic development of the GI tract, which in turn increases the risk of neurological disorders such as autism, where it has been found that affected infants have low zinc levels and GI symptoms.[267]

Dose

RDI: 11 mg/day (vegetarians and vegans require an additional 50% due to phytates in plant sources that bind with zinc and reduce absorption)[56,60]
Therapeutic dose: 25–60 mg/day[43]

Undertake careful review of pathology markers to determine correct dose. Women prescribed higher doses of iron may need additional zinc, as iron competes with zinc for absorption (separate doses).[60] Compare serum zinc and copper levels, aiming for a 1:1 ratio. Also review caeruloplasmin and consider kryptopyrrole status to determine the biochemical need and form of zinc required. Plasma zinc levels decline progressively through the pregnancy due in part to the increase in blood volume, and a decrease in albumin which binds zinc.[265]

Coenzyme Q10

Coenzyme Q10 (CoQ10) is an abundant endogenous enzyme cofactor and fat-soluble antioxidant that effects all cells and is essential for the health of all tissues. CoQ10 is a vital electron and proton carrier and is important in oxidative phosphorylation and the synthesis of ATP in the mitochondria. As an antioxidant CoQ10 regenerates the radical form of vitamin E back to its reduced form, where it can continue to function as an antioxidant, stabilises cell membranes and is antihypertensive, anti-atherogenic and neuroprotective.[43,176] CoQ10 also has immunostimulant properties and targets the expression of several genes, in particular those involved with cell signalling, intermediary metabolism, transport and inflammation.[43] CoQ10 is slowly and poorly absorbed due to its hydrophobicity, limited solubility in lipids and large molecular weight and it is better absorbed when consumed with lipids/fats.

Dose

150–300 mg day

R-alpha lipoic acid

Alpha lipoic acid (ALA) is a unique endogenous antioxidant in that it is both lipid- and water-soluble. ALA is reduced to dihydrolipoic acid (DHLA) within cells, but DHLA can leak into the extracellular medium, meaning that protection is afforded to both intracellular and extracellular environments. ALA regenerates other antioxidants (vitamins C and E, glutathione, CoQ10), importantly increasing intracellular glutathione levels. It is neuroprotective and chelates metal ions such as iron, copper, mercury and cadmium, which are highly toxic to the developing embryo and fetus. ALA is also involved in mitochondrial energy metabolism, modulates cell signalling, improves endothelial function and is anti-inflammatory, which is likely to be beneficial to both the fetus and the placenta.[43]

Dose

100–300 mg day

Probiotics

Probiotics modulate immune function at systemic and mucosal levels, increase the secretion of immunoglobulin IgA, are anti-inflammatory, enhance GI barrier integrity and are chemopreventive.[43] In the mother probiotics may improve intestinal transit time and reduce constipation.[43] One study found that probiotic use plus dietary

counselling reduced postpartum central adiposity, an important marker for ongoing health, especially for the health of the mother and child in future pregnancies.[276] Prenatal and postnatal supplementation with probiotics may play a role in immune regulation and the prevention of allergies in the infant. A meta-analysis showed a reduced risk of atopic eczema in children aged 2–7 years but only for lactobacillus strains.[277] The World Allergy Organization suggests the use of probiotics for women at high risk of having an allergic child, for women who breastfeed infants at high risk of developing allergy and for infants at high risk of developing allergy.[278] Vaginal or oral application of lactobacilli improves the therapeutic results of bacterial vaginosis (associated with premature birth) and dysbiosis and is beneficial in infant colonisation.[279]

Other areas where probiotics may be beneficial include regulating unbalanced microflora composition seen in obesity and diabetes, in a protective role in preeclampsia, in GDM, in vaginal infections and in maternal and infant weight gain.[280] Furthermore, recent awareness of microbial colonisation of the previously thought to be sterile placenta and infant intestine will lead to further study areas and possible novel applications for probiotics in pregnancy.

TRIMESTER 1

The following summary is a very brief overview of embryo development. Fertilisation, cleavage, implantation, placentation and embryogenesis are extraordinarily complex and sophisticated and occur within a brief time frame. To enable this, the mother's nutritional status needs to be replete and her immune system needs to downregulate to enable implantation and to prevent immune-mediated miscarriage (at any stage of the pregnancy). Maternal coagulation abnormalities, endocrine dysfunction and other pathologies can cause pregnancy loss (and the presence of these conditions may not be known prior to pregnancy).

Fetal development
WEEKS 1–2

The first step in pregnancy is fertilisation of the oocyte with the spermatozoa, creating the zygote. The three key functions of fertilisation are the transmission of genes from both parents to the offspring via 23 chromosomes from each parent (gamete), restoration of the diploid number of chromosomes that reduced to haploid gametes during meiosis, and initiation of development in the offspring. Fertilisation may occur through intercourse or with ART such as in vitro fertilisation (IVF). In natural conception the oocyte is viable and able to be fertilised 12–24 hours post-ovulation and typically occurs in the fallopian tube.

After approximately 24–36 hours the zygote begins rapidly dividing in a process known as cleavage, dividing into 2 cells, 4 cells, 8 cells and so on to convert the single-celled zygote into a multi-celled embryo. The zygote continues to travel down the fallopian tube and by day 4 it forms a cluster of 12–16 cells and is classified as a morula, which leaves the tube and moves further towards the uterus. By day 5 it has grown to around 100 cells and is classed as a blastocyst; this is the stage when cell differentiation begins. The outer cell mass (trophoblast cells) becomes the placental cells and the inner cell mass (embryoblast cells) becomes the initial embryonic cells and contains the developmental layers for the fetus: the endoderm, the mesoderm and the ectoderm. By day 6 it is classed as an expanded blastocyst and hatches from the zona pellucida of the oocyte and implants in the endometrium.

Implantation

Implantation describes the stages of attachment, invasion and embedding of the blastocyst in the uterine endometrium. For implantation to be successful there must be synchronous morphological and functional changes to both the invading blastocyst and the receiving endometrium. The first stage is apposition (or adplantation), which involves placement of the hatched blastocyst so that it can loosely adhere to the endometrial epithelium. This must occur at the time of maximum endometrial receptivity to the blastocyst (the implantation window), which in a 28-day cycle corresponds to days 20–23, or 6 days after the peak of luteinising hormone. The blastocyst then slows in motility, rolls on the surface of the endometrium so that it aligns with the inner cell mass closest to the epithelium and stops. The next stage is adhesion, when the blastocyst strengthens the attachment by penetrating the endometrium with microvilli from the trophoblast cells, and this is a time of significant communication and coordination between the blastocyst and the endometrium. The final stage is invasion, when the blastocyst differentiates further: the outer trophoblast cells form the syncytiotrophoblast and cytotrophoblast layers and the embryoblast cells form the epiblast and hypoblast layers. The syncytiotrophoblast layer is crucial: it secretes proteolytic enzymes that cause apoptosis of the endometrial epithelial cells, allowing passage of the blastocyst into the endometrial wall, and totally surround the blastocyst. The syncytiotrophoblast cells phagocytise the apoptotic decidual cells and resorb the nutrients they contained, generate spaces that fill with maternal blood lacunae and secrete hCG, which maintains the decidua and corpus luteum (later in development the placenta will secrete hCG). A plug of acellular material (the coagulation plug) seals the small hole where the blastocyst penetrated the endometrial epithelium by day 12.

The most common site for implantation is the posterior uterus, but anterior, superior and lateral implantation can also occur. Abnormal implantation sites are 'ectopic' and occur outside the uterine cavity. The most common ectopic site is the fallopian tube, but implantation can occur on the exterior surface of the uterus, the ovary, the bowel, the mesentery and the peritoneal wall and these sites are not viable.

hCG

The initial functions of hCG are to support the maternal ovarian corpus luteum, which in turn supports the endometrial lining and therefore maintains pregnancy:

- Promotion of corpus luteal progesterone production
- Uterine angiogenesis
- Differentiation of the cytotrophoblast layer and stimulation of metalloproteinases of the cytotrophoblast cell, enabling full endometrial penetration
- Immunosuppression and prevention of phagocytosis of invading trophoblast cells
- Growth of uterus in line with fetal growth
- Calming of uterine muscle contraction, thus reducing the risk of expulsion of the embryo
- Promotion of growth and differentiation of fetal organs
- Umbilical cord growth and development
- Stimulation of the onset of fetal gonadal steroidogenesis.[281,282]

hCG is found in sperm with receptors in the fallopian tubes, suggesting pre-implantation signalling and communication to the uterus. hCG receptors in the adult hippocampus, hypothalamus and brainstem may be implicated in pregnancy nausea and vomiting.

The hCG level increases rapidly in the first 8 weeks of gestation and then decreases steadily until 20 weeks, when it plateaus. Maternal weight and parity affect hCG levels.

WEEK 3

The endometrium is converted into the decidua and forms three distinct anatomical layers: the decidua basalis (implantation site), the decidua capsularis (enclosing the conceptus) and the decidua parietalis (the remainder of the uterus). As the decidua advances at day 14, relaxin and prolactin are secreted. The decidua capsularis and parietalis fuse eventually and the uterine cavity is lost by 12 weeks. The implanted blastocyst (now called an embryo) is like a ball of cells, about 4 mm in diameter. The cells clump together on one side of the ball, continuing to multiply and differentiate before making a linear formation that creates a flat disc with three distinct layers: the endoderm, which becomes the internal organs (lungs, liver, bowel and bladder); the mesoderm, which becomes the skeleton, sex organs, muscles and heart; and the ectoderm, which becomes the skin, hair, eyes, ears, brain and spinal cord.

The placenta

Cells that don't contribute to the developing embryo develop into the placental tissues. The outside of the blastocyst divides into two layers to start forming the life support systems for the blastocyst (embryo). The outer layer (the chorion) grows villi that penetrate the rich endometrium to obtain nourishment from the mother's blood and this is the beginnings of the placenta. The inner layer (the amnion) becomes the amniotic sac, which slowly fills with amniotic fluid that surrounds the embryo, enabling it to move freely, as well as regulating the temperature of the embryonic environment and acting as a shock absorber to protect the growing embryo. The placenta grows throughout pregnancy. Development of the maternal blood supply to the placenta is complete by the end of the first trimester (approximately 12–13 weeks).

WEEK 4

A dense, protective mucus plug forms and fills the endocervical canal, helping to prevent ascending infection, a common cause of preterm labour. The mucus plug is continually renewed throughout pregnancy and it is shed prior to childbirth.[283] In the developing placenta the trophoblast forms a two-layered chorion that secretes βhCG, which in turn signals the corpus luteum to continue to produce progesterone (P4) until the placenta can secrete oestradiol (E2) and P4, stopping the menstrual period.

This is a critical time for the embryo, which is approximately 1.5 mm in size. The thyroid tissue begins to thicken in the floor of the pharynx and it is the beginning of organogenesis when specific tissues and systems differentiate from the trilaminar embryo.

- *Neural tube (ectoderm):* Neurulation is when the neural tube is transformed into the primitive structures that will later develop into the CNS. It begins when the notochord induces the formation of the CNS by signalling the ectoderm germ layer above it to form the thick and flat neural plate. The neural plate folds in upon itself to form the neural tube and the neural tube then differentiates to form the spinal cord and brain, and eventually the CNS. Closure of the neural tube at day 27 is dependent on adequate folic acid
- *Cardiogenesis (mesoderm):* Begins as paired heart tubes that fuse to form a single heart tube in week 3. Growth and folding of the embryo moves the heart ventrally and downwards into the final anatomical position. The heart begins to beat by day 22/23 of gestation and is the first functioning embryonic organ formed
- *Umbilical cord and yolk sac (endoderm):* The endoderm balloons out the front of the embryo at chest level to form a yolk sac, which provides some nourishment and is eventually reabsorbed to form the embryo's bowel, liver, lungs and bladder. The yolk sac is also where the embryo will start producing its own blood supply. A body stalk protrudes from the embryo's waistline, which is the beginning of the umbilical cord.

WEEK 5

The embryo measures 2–4 mm crown-rump length (CRL). The brain and spinal cord begin to develop; the spinal cord grows faster than the body and has a tail-like appearance. Within cardiovascular development septation starts forming the atrial and ventricular septa and three vascular systems are extensively remodelled: systemic, placental and vitelline (ovarian). In the developing respiratory system left and right lung buds push into the pericardioperitoneal canals (primordia of pleural cavity) and within the ears the cochlear part of the otic (auditory) vesicle elongates. The embryo floats in amniotic fluid and attaches to the placenta via early blood vessels that will form the umbilical cord. The umbilical cord develops three vessels containing two arteries and one vein and nutrients; oxygen and waste products pass through the developing umbilical cord.

WEEK 6

The embryo measures about 5 mm CRL. The digestive and renal systems begin to form and the oesophagus, stomach, bowel and kidneys are being defined. The respiratory system continues to develop, with the two small buds that will form the lungs. The heart has four chambers in rudimentary form and beats at a regular rhythm of 90–200 bpm and can be detected on ultrasound. In the nervous system a ridge of tissue forms down the length of the embryo, which will later develop into the brain and spinal cord. The brain develops into five areas and cranial nerves are visible.

Pituitary structural development commenced in week 4 continues and the connecting stalk between the hypophyseal pouch and the oral cavity degenerates. The parathyroid gland begins to form more tissue mass with dorsal cell proliferation and the thymus begins to form more tissue mass with ventral cell proliferation. The adrenal cortex forms from the mesothelium and the medulla neural crest cells form from adjacent sympathetic ganglia. The facial features (eye and ear structures) begin to form. Vertebrae and other bones form and limb buds begin to develop and become visible. Limb bones form by endochondrial ossification and throughout embryo replacement of cartilage with bone occurs.

WEEK 7

The embryo measures about 13 mm (at least >10 mm) CRL. The brain and spinal cord are nearly complete and the limb buds are now arms and legs; fingers and toes are developing and can be identified. Facial features are observable, nasal pits present and the inner ears and tongue are forming. The upper jaw and palate are fusing and the eyes have an optic cup, retina and lens. The embryo has a blood type that is distinct from the mother's. Organogenesis continues: the growing liver prevents the heart and lungs from descending and bile ductile and biliary capillaries develop. The kidneys and lungs continue to develop, and the appendix and the beginnings of the reproductive organs are present. In the pancreas the first endocrine cells appear; these are insulin-expressing cells and they remain the most prevalent endocrine cell type during the first trimester. The umbilical cord is visible on ultrasound and the heartrate is detectable at 110–170 bpm. The gestational age can now be determined by ultrasound.

WEEK 8

The embryo measures 15 mm CRL. The head is rounded and accounts for about 25% of the embryo. Facial features become defined, showing cheeks, mouth, lips, nose and chin. Eyelids develop, although they will remain fused until weeks 24–26. The intestines are growing and the brain and lungs continue to develop. The embryo is surrounded by a sac filled with amniotic fluid. There is more advanced development of the upper limbs and growth in overall length. The limbs rotate and towards the end of week 8 the elbows, knees, shoulders and hips are more pronounced. The fingers and toes further develop with the loss of cells by apoptosis between the digits.

WEEK 9 (THE BEGINNING OF THE FETAL PERIOD)

The fetus measures 2.5 cm CRL and starts to move. Nail beds are forming, and the webbing between the fingers and toes has completely disappeared. In the heart the formation of the four chambers is completed through a process of cardiac folding, remodelling and partitioning. The opening in the interatrial septum, the foramen ovale, remains and serves as an important right-to-left shunt during fetal life. The mitral and aortic valves begin to form, as do pulmonary blood vessels, which direct blood flow to and from the body and lungs via the umbilical cord.

The liver metabolic pathways for bilirubin and bile salts remain underdeveloped at term, with the placenta being the main eliminatory route; however, the liver is now producing blood cells before this is undertaken in the bone marrow. The lungs are growing bronchi tunnels and the pancreas continues to increase hormone secretion that began around week 7 and increases until week 20. The joints continue to develop and refine, the bones are still soft and flexible, and the face is well formed. The ovaries or testes are well developed and internal reproductive organs start to develop.

WEEK 10

The fetus measures 3.5 cm CRL and this is the final week for organ development. Primitive reflexes are present and the facial features including eyes and ears continue to be refined. The heart is almost completely developed and fetal blood is oxygenated through the placenta. The musculoskeletal system continues to develop and the nervous system is more responsive. Between weeks 10 and 14 hCG stimulates testosterone production and within the testis mesenchyme interstitial cells (Leydig cells) secrete testosterone and androstenedione.

WEEK 11

The fetus measures 4.3 cm CRL. The genitalia in both sexes look identical. The senses of hearing and smell, as well as balance, develop. The eyes are nearly fully developed. Nearly all organs are formed and begin to function, GI contractions are present, the limbs are elongated and the head is half the size of the fetus.

WEEK 12

The fetus measures 7.6 cm CRL, the skeleton is hardening and all major organs are formed.

Maternal changes

Breast tenderness and enlargement are early changes noticed by many women and these are due to increased oestrogen and progesterone, which begin to prepare the breasts for lactation. The areola enlarges and darkens and may have small white bumps (Montgomery's tubercles, sweat glands). The veins of the breast may become more visible and the breasts may feel heavy. The increased oestrogen may increase vaginal and cervical secretions. Maternal plasma volume begins to increase at 6–8 weeks, which causes an increase in cardiac output and therefore an increase in the GFR. This causes increased urination,

exacerbated by the growing uterus pressing on the bladder. Nausea and vomiting are common, as is fatigue.

The level of hCG increases rapidly, peaking at weeks 9–10 and declining at week 20. Progesterone levels increase and help keep the cervix closed, relax the myometrium, aid the expansion of the uterus and reduce GI motility, which increases nutrient absorption and encourages maternal fat deposition. Oestrogen also increases, preventing menses and enabling the continued implantation of the embryo/fetus, as well as affecting fluid retention and thyroid function.

The fetal thyroid gland does not become fully effective until the second trimester, so the maternal thyroid production increases to 150%. This increase is enabled by an increase in thyroxine-binding globulin (TBG) secondary to the effect of oestrogens on the liver; the stimulatory effect of hCG on the thyroid-stimulating hormone (TSH) receptor; high concentrations of type 3 iodothyronine deiodinase (D3), which degrades thyroxine and triiodothyronine to inactive compounds; and the supply of iodine available to the thyroid gland.[284] A healthy thyroid is able to accommodate this significant shift in production and metabolism and is able to maintain thyroid hormone levels within a healthy range during pregnancy. However, the increased demand may also reveal an underlying abnormality and subclinical condition (e.g. chronic low-grade Hashimoto's disease) and low iodine status, resulting in elevated TSH and hypothyroidism, which pose a risk to both the mother and the pregnancy.[245,281–287]

Trimester 1 screening and assessments

Table 13.5 outlines components (and a brief rationale) of the general history required for pregnant women.[288]

OBSTETRIC HISTORY

The obstetric history will help assess the risks associated with the current pregnancy and influence the care plan, monitoring schedule and referral to other health professionals, especially an obstetrician. The history may reveal an increased risk of prenatal and postnatal anxiety and depression, especially if there has been trauma and/or loss. Issues to cover in the obstetric history include:

- Gravida and para: gravida is the number of pregnancies and para is the number of children
- Previous pregnancies and the outcomes: miscarriage, stillbirth, termination or live birth
- Mode of delivery of previous births
- Poor outcome of previous pregnancies or pregnancies requiring intensive fetal monitoring
- Multiple pregnancies
- History of early preterm (prior to 34 weeks) or late preterm (34–37 weeks) delivery
- Intra uterine growth restriction (IUGR)
- Gestational diabetes
- Preeclampsia
- Previous uterine surgery including caesarean section, myomectomy, endometrial ablation and cone biopsy of cervix

TABLE 13.5 General history in trimester 1	
Area	**Comment**
Age	Mothers <18 years and >35 years of age associated with fetal and maternal risk factors; additional support and referrals may be required.
Anxiety, depression	Review medications; may require referral to prescriber and consideration of changing or ceasing treatment. Assess for risk of prenatal and postnatal anxiety and depression.
Asthma and eczema	For inflammatory atopic conditions, review medications and inflammatory status and current/previous steroid requirements.
Autoimmune disease	Rheumatoid arthritis and systemic lupus erythematosus may be treated with medications contraindicated in pregnancy; refer to prescriber.
Coagulopathies	Antiphospholipid antibodies, haemophilia, factor V deficiency and others are associated with miscarriage, increased risk of DVT and pulmonary embolism in mother.
Congenital cardiac disease, coronary artery disease	May benefit from genetic assessment, increased homocysteine monitoring and increased methylation nutrients. Refer to cardiologist as may need closer monitoring and/or treatment during pregnancy.
Diabetes	Aim to achieve good blood sugar control before pregnancy; may require closer monitoring during pregnancy; appropriate diet is essential to avoid risks associated with diabetes and GDM.
Drug and alcohol use, smoking	Risk of fetal alcohol syndrome and addiction and other adverse outcomes.
Genetic	Knowledge of personal or family history of hereditary conditions may warrant referral for genetic counselling.
GI function and disease	Inflammatory bowel disease treatment may include drugs contraindicated in pregnancy, thus refer back to prescriber. Aim to optimise GI function and reduce spasm and inflammation in all GI conditions. Assess for antibiotic use and pre- and probiotic use.
Hypertension	Increased risk of preeclampsia. Refer to prescribing doctor if on antihypertensive as some are associated with congenital abnormalities (e.g. ACE inhibitors).
Malignancy	Particularly oestrogen-dependent cancers.
Renal disease	Increases the risk of preeclampsia.
Rubella titre	To assess immune status.
Seizure disorders	Refer to prescriber for review of medications (may consider weaning off if no seizure in >2 years); risk of dysmorphic structural malformation syndromes from some anti-seizure medication; close serum monitoring is required during pregnancy. Higher dose folic acid (>4 mg) may be required to decrease risk of NTDs.
Sexual infections	Assess risk of sexually transmitted infections (STIs) and HIV; refer as indicated.
Social	Support and financial considerations. Intimate partner violence may occur for the first time during pregnancy and represents a significant danger to the mother and fetus.
Thyroid	Hypothyroid and hyperthyroid conditions, and autoimmune conditions hold risk of pregnancy complications and miscarriage.
Toxin exposure	Mercury, lead, cadmium and other toxins are neurotoxic and increase the risk of low birth weight and premature birth. Plastics, including BPAs, are associated with adverse effects on the developing fetus.
Weight	Assess pre-pregnancy health and provide guidance on recommended GWG.

Source: Adapted from Gregory KD, Ramos DE, Jauniaux ERM. Preconception and prenatal care. In: Gabbe S, Niebyl J, Simpson J et al. (eds). Obstetrics: normal and problem pregnancies. 7th edn. Philadelphia: Elsevier; 2017.

- Infertility requiring surgery or fertility medication
- Previous infant with major congenital anomaly and/or inherited disorder, or family history of genetic conditions.

It is also pertinent to establish whether the current pregnancy was planned, natural or with ART, and how the woman feels about being pregnant, her expectations and any concerns. A summary of investigations relevant to trimester 1 is provided in Table 13.6.

DATING SCAN (ULTRASOUND) AT 6–8 WEEKS

The dating scan is performed to establish the gestational age and thus the estimated due date of the pregnancy. In addition it can identify the number of fetuses and gestation sacs, the presence of a heartbeat, the size of the fetus (from which the gestational age is estimated), unusual features of the uterus such as a bicornuate uterus

TABLE 13.6 Trimester 1 investigations	
Trimester 1 investigations	**Integrative medicine consideration**
Full blood count	Serum folate and active B$_{12}$
Iron studies	MTHFR
Blood group and atypical antibody screen	Fasting homocysteine
STIs and HIV	Thyroid panel and antibodies
Rubella titre	Vitamin D$_3$
Hepatitis B surface antigen and hepatitis C antibodies	Plasma zinc, serum copper and caeruloplasmin
Random blood glucose	Spot urinary iodine and creatinine
Diabetes screening as indicated	If history of miscarriage: cardiolipin, phospholipid antibodies, ANA
Pap smear (if not done within 2 years)	Infections (if not screened in preconception): toxoplasmosis, CMV, parvovirus, varicella

or the presence of fibroids, and a non-viable pregnancy (e.g. blighted ovum or ectopic pregnancy).

PRENATAL SCREENING AND DIAGNOSTIC TESTS

Screening tests are used to detect early disease or risk factors for disease in large numbers of apparently healthy individuals, while diagnostic tests seek to establish the presence (or absence) of disease as a basis for treatment decisions in symptomatic or screen-positive individuals (confirmatory test). That is, screening tests rule out a disease, whereas diagnostic tests confirm or rule in the presence of disease. Screening tests have lower accuracy than diagnostic tests and consideration of risk factors, as well as acknowledgement of the need to follow up with further investigations if indicated, is essential. Diagnostic tests tend to be invasive and this is true in prenatal diagnostics as well.

The key objective for conducting prenatal screening and diagnostic testing is to confirm (or exclude) the diagnosis of fetal abnormality. This objective can be then expanded to:

- Obtain an accurate diagnosis as early as possible in the pregnancy
- Provide information on prognosis for the current pregnancy and the likelihood of recurrence in future pregnancies
- Provide counselling to the prospective parents, including expected pregnancy outcomes, possible treatment options, termination and perinatal and delivery recommendations.
  Screening (non-invasive) tests comprise:
- Fetal ultrasound
- Combined first trimester nuchal and serum screening (free βhCG and PAPP-A)
- Circulating fetal DNA (cell-free).
  Diagnostic (invasive) tests comprise:
- Karyotyping and aneuploidy screening (FISH or QF-PCR)
- Chorionic villus sampling (CVS) at 10–14 weeks
- Amniocentesis at 15–18 weeks
- Cordocentesis (umbilical cord sampling).

Prenatal testing for aneuploidies

Aneuploidy is a category of chromosomal mutation where there is an abnormal number of chromosomes in a cell. The most common aneuploidy seen in live infants is trisomy 21 (Down syndrome), where there are three chromosomes on chromosome 21 instead of two. Trisomy 21 accounts for about 50% of aneuploidies detected in the prenatal period and together with trisomy 18 and trisomy 13 they account for 80% of prenatal aneuploidies. Testing technology and sophistication is rapidly evolving and the screening recommendations change as more accurate assessments and combinations of assessments evolve.

CELL-FREE DNA

Cell-free DNA (cfDNA) is of placental origin and is detectable in the plasma of pregnant women from early in the first trimester. Screening can be performed from 10 weeks gestation. cfDNA has the highest sensitivity and specificity of all screening tests for trisomy 21, but it is not covered by Medicare or private health insurance rebates in Australia and the cost is prohibitive to many women.

COMBINED FIRST TRIMESTER SCREENING

Combined first trimester screening (CFTS) is performed at 11+0 to 11+6 weeks of gestation and includes assessment of maternal age, ultrasound measurement of the fetal nuchal translucency and maternal serum marker levels to produce an estimate of the likelihood of trisomy 21. (Trisomy 13 and trisomy 18 can also be incorporated into the calculations.) CFTS has an 85% sensitivity and 95% specificity for trisomy 21 screening.[289]

- *Maternal age:* The likelihood of trisomy 21 in a newborn is 1 : 300 for a 35-year-old woman, increasing to 1 : 100 for a 40-year-old woman[289]
- *Nuchal translucency (NT) screening:* NT uses ultrasound to measure the subcutaneous fluid between the soft tissue of the cervical spine and the skin in a fetus. The risk of associated anomalies increases with wider NT, including structural anomalies such as cardiac defects, diaphragmatic hernia, omphalocele and skeletal anomalies. Further risks associated with a widened NT are numerous genetic syndromes, and discordant NT measurements may predict twin-to-twin transfusion syndrome in monochorionic twins[290]
- *Free-βhCG:* This is elevated in trisomy 21 and normal in NTDs
- *Pregnancy-associated plasma protein-A (PAPP-A).* PAPP-A is the largest of the pregnancy-associated proteins produced by both the embryo and the placenta and its functions include preventing recognition of the fetus by the maternal immune system, matrix mineralisation and angiogenesis. Levels of PAPP-A rise from initial detection at about 32 days after ovulation, increasing rapidly (doubling every 3 days) and finally rising more slowly until term. Elevated levels of PAPP-A indicate an increased risk of trisomy 21 and reduced levels indicate a risk of trisomy 18. A low PAPP-A (<0.4 MoM) is associated with an increased risk of adverse outcomes.[291,292]

Screening no longer recommended by the Royal Australian and New Zealand College of Obstetricians and Gynaecologists includes the double test (maternal age, alpha-fetoprotein and β-hCG), the triple test (maternal age, alpha-fetoprotein, β-hCG and unconjugated oestriol) and NT alone.[289]

MTHFR

Dysfunctions in folate metabolism can result in DNA hypomethylation and abnormal chromosome function. Two common polymorphisms of the MTHFR enzyme (C677T and A1298C) reduce its activity, and while associations have been made with infertility, NTDs and pregnancy loss, there is some inconsistency in the literature.[293] MTHFR polymorphisms are associated with low serum folate and raised homocysteine, known risk factors for NTDs and other adverse pregnancy outcomes. MTHFR testing is not currently routine medical practice but it is included in naturopathic assessment.

FIRST TRIMESTER TESTING: CHORIONIC VILLUS SAMPLING

If CFTS indicates an increased risk of fetal aneuploidy, a prenatal diagnostic test is usually recommended: chorionic villus sampling (CVS) or amniocentesis. CVS can be performed from 11 weeks and allows for early genetic diagnosis. It can be performed using a transabdominal or a transvaginal approach depending on patient preference, the position of the placenta or the presence of genital herpes. The types of genetic tests performed on cells obtained from CVS or amniocentesis include convention (G-banded) karyotyping, rapid aneuploidy tests such as fluorescent in situ hybrid (FISH), quantitative fluorescent polymerase chain reaction (QF PCR), BACs-on-beads (BoBs) and chromosomal microarray analysis.[294] The safety and associated risks of the procedure are both patient and doctor/technician related. A review of CVS performed on 1906 fetuses in Hong Kong (China) reported that the miscarriage rate adjusted for background loss was 0.17%. Pregnancies with reduced PAPP-A carried an increased risk of miscarriage, irrespective of whether they had undergone a CVS.[295]

NAUSEA AND VOMITING

Nausea and vomiting in pregnancy (NVP) is one of the most common symptoms, affecting 50–85% of women during the first half of their pregnancy.[296] Symptoms can start as early as 4 weeks and may persist over the day, not just during the morning; they typically resolve by weeks 18–20.[296–298] For most women NVP is physiological and self-limiting and they are able to manage with dietary and lifestyle modifications. Their symptoms are often mild to moderate and they don't lose weight, become dehydrated or develop electrolyte or nutritional imbalances.

For some women with NVP the symptoms can become pathological and severe, the most extreme form being hyperemesis gravidarum (HG), which occurs in 0.3–1.0% of pregnancies.[296] HG is the most common cause of hospital admissions during the first trimester and can have significant social, emotional and financial implications for the woman and her family. Women with HG report higher levels of anxiety and stress.[296] HG is characterised by:

- Severe nausea and intractable vomiting
- Dehydration
- Electrolyte imbalances including hyponatraemia, hypocalcaemia and hypokalaemia
- Nutritional deficiencies
- Weight loss (>5% of pre-pregnancy weight)
- Otherwise unexplained ketonuria
- Dysgeusia and thirst
- Hypovolaemia: dry mucous membranes, poor skin turgor, orthostatic hypotension or hypotension and increased haematocrit
- Mallory-Weiss syndrome (oesophageal tear from vomiting)
- Metabolic imbalances, ketosis
- Abnormal liver function tests: elevations of the serum aminotransferases.[296–298]

Risk factors

Risk factors for HG are variable and include first pregnancy, multiple gestation, molar pregnancy, prior unsuccessful pregnancy, prior HG, singleton female fetus, gestational trophoblastic disease, hydrops fetalis and fetal karyotypical abnormalities including triploidy and trisomy 21.[297,298]

Aetiology

The pattern of prevalence of NVP and HG indicates a multifactorial pathogenesis and risk factors range from physiological to biochemical, social, geographical and age-related. For example, women in Western countries and Japan experience NVP more commonly than women in Africa, Asia and Alaska (among Native Americans) where it is rare.[298] Theories and possible contributing factors include:

- hCG: serum hCG level peaks when HG is most severe, and the level is higher in patients with HG than in other pregnant patients
- Elevated oestrogen of pregnancy
- Hyperthyroidism[297]
- First pregnancy
- Younger age
- Stress, anxiety, depression
- Fewer than 12 years of education
- Non-smoking status
- Obesity
- Family history of NVP[298]
- Prostaglandin E2: levels are elevated during symptomatic episodes
- *Helicobacter pylori*: some mixed results in the research
- An evolutionary adaptation: protecting the woman and fetus from potentially toxic and harmful foods
- Gastric arrhythmias: delayed emptying and altered peristaltic contractions correlate with the symptoms of NVP
- Altered gastric motility and gastro-oesophageal reflux appear to contribute to the mechanisms of nausea and vomiting in pregnancy
- Liver disease, fatty liver

- Lack of vitamin supplementation in early pregnancy, especially thiamine and pyridoxine
- Gestational thyrotoxicosis (HG not NVP)
- Wernicke's encephalopathy in severe HG.[296,298–301]

Diagnosis

NVP and HG are diagnoses of exclusion, although HG has the additional weight loss and metabolic disturbances that can be objectively measured. Differential diagnoses include GI disorders and liver disease, metabolic and endocrine disorders, neurological disorders, emotional/psychological conditions (including eating disorders), urinary conditions, drug toxicity or intolerance and pregnancy-related conditions such as molar pregnancy.[296,302] See Appendix 13.1 for a summary of assessment tools for NVP. Nausea and vomiting may be triggered by low blood sugar and skipping meals, stress and emotional factors, fatigue, motion and travel, strong smells and tastes, rich fatty or spicy foods, caffeine, alcohol and animal foods.

Consequences

Women with NVP were traditionally thought to have better pregnancy outcomes, with fewer miscarriages and congenital abnormalities in the offspring, although there was little research on this.[297] A 2014 systematic review found a consistent favourable effect of NVP on rates of miscarriage, congenital malformations, prematurity and developmental achievements.[303] A further review as part of the large Norwegian Mother and Child Cohort Study ($n = 51\,675$) found that NVP was associated with significantly reduced odds for unfavourable birth outcomes such as LBW infants and SGA infants. However, women with NVP had significantly increased odds for hypertension and preeclampsia compared to women with no symptoms.[299] More severe NVP is associated with increased anxiety and stress for the mother, social isolation and potentially occupational and financial stress. Hyperemesis, especially if untreated or undertreated, can have serious adverse outcomes.

A recent review found that women with HG were more likely to have a LBW baby (<2500 g) that was SGA and born prematurely.[284] Furthermore, severe HG has been associated with Wernicke's encephalopathy and fetal death.[301]

A Swedish review found that women who had HG in the first trimester had only a slightly increased risk of preeclampsia but women who presented with HG for the first time in the second trimester had more than double the risk of early preeclampsia (<37 weeks), a three-fold risk of placental abruption and a 39% increased risk for SGA birth.[305] Preeclampsia with an early onset has been linked to abnormal endometrial spiral artery modelling and the increased risk of preterm preeclampsia in the second trimester suggests that HG could be associated with abnormal placentation.

Management

Most women experiment with dietary adjustments to manage their NVP and often this is all that is required; however, some women will need additional support regarding dietary and lifestyle measures, as well as supplementation, to manage their NVP. Women with reduced oral intake or with a restricted diet lacking the recommended foods may feel anxious that they are harming their developing fetus; while this is a risk in HG, it is unlikely to be an issue in managed NVP and HG.

Initial interventions are dietary including the avoidance of triggers (which may vary over time). Taking adequate rest and employing techniques and seeking support to manage anxiety and stress are also helpful. Not taking vitamin supplementation in the first trimester is associated with an increased risk of developing NVP and an increased risk of adverse outcomes.[290] It should not be assumed that women are taking supplements, with findings showing that 67% of women with HG in the US and as many as 90% of women with HG in the UK are not being prescribed vitamins (including pyridoxine and thiamine) during the critical period of fetal development when HG commonly presents.[301] In addition, supplements may have triggered the nausea, so a review of the patient's supplementation and providing supplements that don't exacerbate symptoms is essential. Taking supplements with food and later in the day may be helpful.

GINGER

Ginger rhizome is a pungent aromatic herbal medicine (and culinary spice) with a long history of use for nausea, including NVP. The key constituents of ginger are volatile oils (1–3%) including zingiberene, zingiberol, sesquiphellandrene and beta-bisabolene and the pungent principles (1–2.5%), particularly gingerol and shogaol.[47] Ginger increases gastric tone and motility and may increase gastric emptying due to anticholinergic and antiserotonergic actions.[300] Recent studies have also found that the pungent constituents of ginger (shogaol, gingerol and zingerone) non-competitively inhibit serotonin 5-HT responses in a dose-dependent manner, which is the same mechanism of common antiemetic pharmaceuticals such as ondansetron.[306,307]

Trials of ginger are heterogeneous with treatment including teas, powders, tablets/capsules, dried and fresh root, and liquid extracts and using various methodologies.[308] In addition, the trials often do not provide detail on the provenance and analysis of the ginger used, which could significantly alter the outcomes given the variability of constituents and their actions.[47] A systematic review of 12 randomised controlled trials (1278 pregnant women) found that ginger significantly improved the symptoms of nausea when compared to a placebo but did not significantly reduce the number of vomiting episodes during NVP when compared to a placebo.[300] Ginger was not associated with an increased risk of spontaneous abortion compared to a placebo nor did it increase reports of heartburn.

Ginger has a low toxicity profile, and while some constituents have been found to be mutagenic, others have been found to be antimutagenic. High doses (≥4 g per day) should be prescribed with caution in those with thrombophilias or using anticoagulants. Ginger has been used during pregnancy by a large number of women over many years and there have been no proven adverse effects on the fetus.[47] A daily dose of 2 g of dried ginger should not be exceeded in pregnancy.[47] The dose most commonly used in studies is 1000 mg per day. Given the variance in the level of constituents in the different forms of ginger, including fresh ginger, it is difficult to quantify ginger equivalence to 1000 mg. Preparations used in clinical trials include fresh grated rhizome, ginger syrup, ginger tea (½ teaspoon of grated ginger steeped for 5–10 minutes), ginger ale, crystallised ginger and ginger extract. Ginger biscuits can also be helpful. Women may find capsules or tablets easier to tolerate than fresh ginger preparations or extracts.

VITAMIN B₆

Vitamin B_6 has been found to be effective when taken preventively and as an intervention once nausea has started.[290] While studies have been of mixed quality and a large randomised controlled trial has yet to be conducted, based on current research vitamin B_6 appears to be helpful in reducing NVP, especially in early pregnancy and for those with more severe symptoms.[43,296,308] Of note, some studies used doses as low as 5 mg twice daily while studies using higher doses (50 mg plus) resulted in a greater improvement in NVP symptoms.[296] Recommended doses include 10–25 mg every 6 hours[290] and in clinical practice monitored doses of 150 mg have been used.[43]

IN THE KITCHEN

Maintaining hydration is essential and liquid-based meals (smoothies, soups and juices) may help, as can drinking most liquids separately from meals (see Box 13.3). Sipping small amounts of fluids frequently is preferable to having large volumes every few hours, and sucking on ice chips and including ice blocks, frozen yoghurt and ice-creams may help.

In addition to ginger, including the following herbs as infusions or in cooking may be beneficial: Matricaria chamomilla, Mentha x piperita, Mentha spicata, Filipendula ulmaria, Melissa officinalis, Pimpinella anisum, Carum carvi and Syzygium aromaticum. Taraxacum officinalis (radix) tea may assist digestion and reduce NVP. Note: Mentha x piperita may relax the oesophageal sphincter, although this is largely seen with the use of non-enteric-coated supplements, so careful use or avoidance is appropriate if GORD is present.[47]

BOX 13.3 Dietary and lifestyle strategies for managing NVP

- Snacking on dry crackers, fruit
- Eating small amounts frequently (including having a small snack on hand next to the bed for overnight snacking if required)
- Eating slowly
- Avoiding triggers, strong smells and tastes
- Including adequate protein, especially in the evening
- Eating in a well-ventilated space or outdoors
- Drinking fluids in-between meals
- Brushing teeth.

INFECTIONS

Pregnancy requires immune adjustments to prevent the mother from rejecting the fetus (50% of the DNA is paternal). Cell-mediated immune function is reduced and there is a shift towards T-helper 2 dominance and an increased susceptibility to and severity of some infections, such as Listeria and Toxoplasmosis. Additional food-borne infective agents include Campylobacter, Cryptosporidium, E. coli, Hepatitis A, Salmonella, Giardia and Botulinum. Box 13.4 outlines good food hygiene practices to reduce the risk of foodborne disease. Note: sprouts (e.g. alfalfa sprouts, onion sprouts, radish sprouts, mung bean sprouts) have been associated with serious food-borne illness including death from E. coli and should be avoided.

Listeriosis

Listeria monocytogenes is a Gram-positive bacillus that while widespread in nature uncommonly causes illness in healthy people; pregnant women and their fetus, newborns and those who are immunocompromised are at greater risk of infection.[309,310] Listeriosis can cause meningitis, encephalitis, bacteraemia and gastroenteritis. The bacteria cross the intestinal wall at Peyer patches to invade the mesenteric lymph nodes and blood and then can cross the placenta and in rare cases cause miscarriage, premature birth or stillbirth.[309]

BOX 13.4 Good food hygiene practices to reduce the risk of foodborne disease

- Thoroughly wash hands with warm soapy water and dry hands before preparing food
- Keep your refrigerator clean and operate it below 5°C
- Wash knives, cutting boards, food preparation surfaces and kitchen appliances and dry thoroughly after handling raw food
- Thoroughly wash and dry raw fruit and vegetables before eating or juicing
- Scrub the surface of melons such as rockmelon and rinse and dry before cutting
- Thaw ready-to-eat frozen food in the refrigerator – don't thaw at room temperature
- Thoroughly cook all raw meat, chicken and fish
- Don't leave foods to cool on the bench or stove top – put them into the refrigerator as soon as the steam has gone
- If you are keeping food hot, keep it very hot (60°C or hotter)
- Keep cold food cold (5°C or colder)
- Thoroughly reheat food until it is steaming hot
- Keep stored foods covered
- Store raw meat separately from cooked and ready-to-eat foods in the refrigerator. Store it below other foods so that there is no chance that blood or juices will drip onto the other foods.

Source: Adapted from Food Standards Australia and New Zealand. Listeria and food: advice for people at risk. [Cited 18 November 2016. Available from www.foodstandards.gov.au/publications/pages/listeriabrochuretext.aspx.]

Symptoms of listeriosis can be mild and most commonly include flu-like symptoms of fever, headache, tiredness, aches and pains with GI complaints less commonly experienced. Severe infection may progress to septicaemia, meningitis or pneumonia. Diagnosis is most accurate if blood cultures are taken while the woman is febrile. Women who have been exposed to *Listeria monocytogenes*, who have a temperature over 38.1°C, who have signs and symptoms consistent with listeriosis and where other pathology has been excluded should be simultaneously tested and treated for presumptive listeriosis.[310] Placental cultures should be obtained in the event of miscarriage or stillbirth. Treatment is with antibiotics.

Strategies for the prevention of listeriosis include:
- Preparing, storing and handling food hygienically
- Avoiding certain foods that have a higher risk of listeria contamination and being careful about eating food prepared by others
- Eating freshly cooked or freshly prepared foods, and washing fruit and vegetables
- Cooking foods thoroughly
- Reheating foods to 'steaming' hot, and only keeping leftovers for a day and reheating them thoroughly
- Avoiding perishable foods (need to be refrigerated) that have been prepared well in advance and are to be eaten without further cooking
- Only buying ready-to-eat hot food if it is steaming hot
- If eating out, ordering hot meals
- Avoiding foods that are past their 'best before' or 'use by' date
- Avoiding ready-to-eat food from salad bars, sandwich bars, delicatessens and smorgasbords.[309,310]

High-risk foods for pregnant women include the following:
- Cold meats and chicken: unpackaged ready-to-eat from delicatessen counters, sandwich bars and so on and packaged, sliced ready-to-eat hot dogs
- Pâtés, meat spreads and terrines
- Pre-prepared or pre-packaged salads (e.g. from salad bars)
- Chilled seafood: raw (e.g. oysters, sashimi or sushi), smoked ready-to-eat, ready-to-eat peeled prawns (cooked) such as in prawn cocktails, sandwich fillings and prawn salads
- Cheese: soft, semi-soft and surface-ripened cheeses (pre-packaged and delicatessen) such as brie, camembert, ricotta, feta and blue
- Dairy: soft-serve ice-cream and unpasteurised dairy.[309,310]

Toxoplasmosis

Toxoplasma gondii is a protozoan parasite that occurs worldwide and infection is very common. The parasite has three distinct forms: (1) trophozoite, (2) cyst and (3) oocyst. Cats are the only host for the oocyst: the oocyst is formed in the cat's intestine and is subsequently excreted in the faeces. Mammals such as cows, pigs, sheep and kangaroos ingest the oocyst, which is disrupted in the animal's intestine, releasing the invasive trophozoite, which is disseminated throughout the body, ultimately forming cysts in the brain and muscle.[310,311] The cyst is destroyed by heat: human infection occurs when raw or undercooked infected meat is ingested or when food is contaminated by cat faeces via flies, cockroaches or fingers. Infection rates are highest in areas of poor sanitation and crowded living conditions.

Most infections are asymptomatic but clinical disease may develop after a long period of asymptomatic infection. Symptoms, if present, resemble glandular fever. Infection in an immunocompromised person can be severe. Congenital infection occurs in about 40% of neonates born to a mother who had an acute toxoplasmosis during pregnancy.[310] The incubation period is 5–23 days and the diagnosis is made on serological and histological testing. Prenatal diagnosis of congenital toxoplasmosis is via ultrasound and CVS or amniocentesis. Treatment is with antibiotics.

To prevent toxoplasmosis in pregnant women:
- Avoid eating, and minimise handling of, raw meat
- Cook all meat thoroughly and wash hands and utensils after handling raw meat
- Wash all vegetables thoroughly before eating, especially salad vegetables
- Use gloves when emptying cat litter trays. Trays can be disinfected with boiling water. Cysts need more than 24 hours to become infectious after being passed in the faeces, so clean litter trays daily. Cover sandpits when not in use to prevent cats from using them as a litter tray
- Feed cats dry, canned or cooked food and discourage pet cats from hunting
- Wear gloves when gardening. Wash hands thoroughly with soap and warm running water after contact with soil.[311]

FATIGUE

Fatigue is a very common symptom in the first trimester and may co-present with NVP. Fatigue is associated with fluctuating blood sugar levels and hormonal changes, especially increased progesterone. While some women remain fatigued for the duration of their pregnancy, most see a return of energy at 14–16 weeks that lasts until into the third trimester. A recent review of 909 pregnant women found that 77.9% experienced first-trimester fatigue; other studies have found the rate as high as 83.3–96.6%.[312]

Fatigue can impact on the overall experience of pregnancy and contribute to low mood, require time away from work (with associated employment and financial stress) and affect the ability to attend to household activities and raise other children, as well as affecting relationships. While some fatigue is normal, it is necessary to eliminate any pathological causes of fatigue, including thyroid disease, anaemia, cardiovascular disease (subclinical disease may become apparent only with the added demands of pregnancy), respiratory disease, infection, systemic diseases, depression, severe NVP and HG. Other factors that may influence fatigue levels include stress, emotional and psychological distress, overwork, poor quality sleep, lack of physical fitness, environmental factors (including air quality and temperature) and poor nutritional status.

Assess the causes, seek further investigation as indicated (e.g. thyroid panel) and treat as indicated. The most important intervention in managing fatigue is to rest.

- Increase sleep, including naps
- Rest after activities (housework, exercise, shopping)
- Gentle exercise helps build stamina; extreme exercise will deplete it further
- Review and reduce excess activities and commitments as able; seek support
- Support stress management through counselling, meditation, yoga, rest, massage, nutrition and herbal medicine
- Eat regular small meals to ensure adequate energy intake, including ensuring low GI carbohydrates and protein with all meals
- Nutrients for energy production:
  - B complex
  - Magnesium 150–400 mg
  - Iron, if indicated, 15–30 mg
  - Lipoic acid 100–400 mg
  - Coenzyme Q10 50–200 mg
  - Vitamin C 100–1000 mg
- *Eleutherococcus senticosus* (Siberian ginseng) is a mildly stimulating adaptogen, immune-modulator and tonic, and is safe in pregnancy.[47]

BLEEDING AND CRAMPING

Bleeding and cramping can occur at any stage of pregnancy. Bleeding may be caused by implantation bleed, sex, friable cervix, uterine and cervical polyps, and fluctuating hormone levels (especially low progesterone). Possible causes of cramping include gastrointestinal issues (IBS, constipation), stretching of the round ligament, nutritional deficiencies (in particular calcium and magnesium), urinary tract infection and miscarriage.

It is essential that the patient is fully assessed by a midwife or an obstetrician. Once miscarriage or other problems are excluded, simple support measures may be helpful – for example, calcium, magnesium, stretching, yoga and pregnancy massage for cramps and discomfort; avoiding sex, heavy lifting and strenuous activity for a few days after bleeding and cramping stop; and ensuring adequate vitamin B$_6$ for progesterone support. See Chapter 12 for further discussion.

TRIMESTER 2

The second trimester is often the most enjoyable: the fatigue and NVP of the first trimester resolve and the discomfort, GORD, sleep disturbance and fatigue of the additional weight in the third trimester have yet to occur.

Fetal development

WEEKS 13–14

The fetus grows from 7.6 to 9 cm head to toe and the placenta is now fully functional. The soft flexible bones are hardening, facial remodelling begins – including development of the nose and nasal passages – and toenails

appear. By 100 days primary follicles are present in female fetuses. Taste buds begin to develop, a gag reflex is present and the intestines experience peristalsis and fill with meconium.

WEEKS 15–16

The fetus measures 15 cm head to toe, the umbilical cord is completely mature and for the first time the fetus is bigger than the placenta. The fetal weight is about 120 g and while the head is still large, overall it is becoming more proportional. An increase in amniotic fluid increases the size of the uterus and allows the fetus to move around. Pancreatic glucagon is present in fetal plasma, the vocal cords are formed and the initial sucking and Moro reflexes are present. The pituitary adenohypophysis is fully differentiated. Lanugo begins to grow – a soft downy hair that insulates the fetus until it gains enough body fat.

WEEKS 17–18

The fetus measures 19 cm head to toe and weighs around 280 g. Lanugo growth continues and vernix caseosa (creamy white protective substance) covers the skin and lanugo. The mother can feel fetal movement as the fetus moves about exploring in the uterus. The nervous system begins functioning.

WEEKS 19–21

The fetus measures 22 cm head to toe and weighs around 340 g. The bone marrow starts to produce blood cells and the liver produces secretions. Aural bony and neural development are complete, enabling the fetus to hear, and permanent teeth form behind the baby teeth. Fingernails form and fingerprints are visible. Pituitary growth hormone levels peak at 20–24 weeks and then decrease.

WEEKS 22–23

The fetus measures 25 cm head to toe and weighs around 500 g. The nervous system is complete and retinas are fully developed. Hair follicles begin to pigment and eyelashes and eyebrows grow; the eyelids remain fused. The placenta provides 1000 mL of blood an hour and spleen development continues. The lower airways develop but there is no surfactant.

WEEKS 24–25

The fetus measures 28 cm and weighs around 600 g. Sweat glands develop, an initial fine layer of fat is deposited and the vernix is thick. The fetus develops sleep and wake cycles and REM sleep. Alveoli develop and the lungs produce surfactant.

WEEKS 26–27

The fetus measures 33 cm head to toe and weighs around 800 g. The eyelids are no longer fused and the fetus responds to bright light by blinking. The fetus recognises voices and responds to music and touch. It continues to move and has a heart rate of 120–160 bpm.

Maternal changes

The placenta is functional so the corpus luteum now degenerates. Increased production of progesterone relaxes smooth muscle, stimulates maternal respiration, inhibits lactation and acts as a placental immunosuppressant.

Increased steroid production is required to meet the need for an increase in maternal production of oestrogen and cortisol as well as for fetal growth. There are increases in serum levels of aldosterone, deoxycorticosterone, corticosteroid-binding globulin (CBG), adrenocorticotropic hormone (ACTH), cortisol and free cortisol, causing a state of physiological hypercortisolism.[245] By the end of the second trimester plasma concentration of CBG doubles due to hepatic stimulation by oestrogen and this results in increased total plasma cortisol. Elevated free cortisol levels are associated with an increase in hypothalamic corticotropin-releasing hormone (CRH), which stimulates the production of ACTH in the pituitary and from the placenta. In addition, in pregnancy CRH is also produced by the placenta and fetal membranes and is secreted into the maternal circulation. Despite the elevated cortisol level in pregnancy, it appears physiological and Cushing's syndrome is uncommon.[245]

Prolactin production, which began around weeks 5–8, now increases, largely produced by the decidua, to prepare the breasts for lactation. Human chorionic somatomammotropin (hCS) is produced by the placenta and is similar in structure and function (though weaker) to growth hormone. hCS helps moderate maternal insulin sensitivity and use to ensure adequate fetal glucose; it also increases maternal lipolysis, thereby making free fatty acids available for the mother and protecting fetal glucose fuel levels. These actions appear to be one way in which fetal nutrition is secured even during times of maternal undernutrition and illness. hCS has a similar structure to prolactin, although its role in human lactation is unclear.

Nutrient transport to the growing fetus causes significant changes in the mother's carbohydrate metabolism. The increased requirement for insulin causes hypertrophy and hyperplasia of the insulin-producing β-cells of the islets of Langerhans. Some alteration to glucose metabolism occurs in all women, although mostly the changes are mild. Pregnancy results in fasting hypoglycaemia, postprandial hyperglycaemia and hyperinsulinaemia and is considered to be a diabetogenic state.[245,313]

Placental production of oestrogen increases significantly and relies on its aromatising capacity and use of circulating androgens as the precursor substrate, the main one being maternal dehydroepiandrosterone sulphate (DHEAS). The ovaries of non-pregnant women don't secrete oestriol but in pregnancy oestriol accounts for more than 90% of the oestrogen in the maternal urine. Unlike oestradiol and oestrone, oestriol has a very low affinity for sex hormone–binding globulin and is cleared much more rapidly from the circulation. The increased oestrogen levels increase uterine blood flow, facilitating delivery of oxygen and nutrients that stimulate uterine and fetal growth and breast development.[314] The increased oestrogen causes the gums to become spongy so that they may bleed after tooth brushing and nasal congestion may be present. Increased oestrogen also increases vaginal discharge and lowers the pH, increasing the chance of vaginal candidiasis.

The peptide hormone relaxin peaks in concentration by the end of the first trimester but its effects begin to be felt in the second trimester. Relaxin is involved in collagen remodelling, which causes increased flexibility of the pubic symphysis, softening of the cervix and inhibition of uterine contractility. It may also contribute to the increase in backaches at this stage.

As the fetus grows the mother increases weight and her pregnancy becomes more visible. The abdominal swelling may stretch abdominal and pelvic ligaments and cause aching. GI motility slows, enhancing nutrient absorption but predisposing to constipation and discomfort and increasing the chance of haemorrhoids. Gastric hydrochloric acid production is reduced but reflux increases due to changes in sphincter function and the growing fetus compressing the stomach.

The increase in maternal plasma and total blood volume that began around week 6 reaches significant levels in trimester 2 before plateauing around week 30. For a singleton pregnancy the average increase in blood volume is 40–50%; the blood plasma volume increases by around 50% and this represents approximately 1200–1300 mL.[245] The increased blood volume leads to an increase in cardiac output of about 50% by weeks 30–34. In twin pregnancies the blood volume increases by a greater amount and cardiac output increases an additional 20% above singleton pregnancies. By 12 weeks gestation the rise in cardiac output is 34–39% above non-pregnant levels. Cardiac output probably peaks in the second trimester even though blood volume increases until around weeks 30–34.[245]

Second trimester investigations

Investigations and assessments are based on individual requirements and in conjunction with tests arranged by the midwife, GP or obstetrician. Common tests include a full blood count, iron studies, vitamin D_3, urinary iodine, fasting glucose, glucose tolerance test (GTT) and HbA_{1c}. In addition, plasma zinc, copper and other tests may be indicated. Discussion of emotional wellbeing takes place at each consultation; however, it may also be appropriate to use the Edinburgh Postnatal Depression Scale questionnaire (see Appendix 13.2).

DENTAL REVIEW

A dental examination is recommended during trimester 2. Periodontal disease is associated with gum and tooth loss as well as systemic bacteraemia and cardiovascular disease, but it has specific significance in pregnancy. A systematic review found that periodontal disease was modestly but significantly associated with low birth weight and preterm birth.[315] A further meta-analysis found that periodontal disease increased the risk of GDM by 66%.[316] Excellent dental hygiene is to be promoted and immune support provided as required. There is some evidence that CoQ10 topically and internally may be beneficial in periodontal disease.[43]

AMNIOCENTESIS

Amniocentesis is a prenatal diagnostic test usually performed from 15 weeks gestation onwards, by which time the amount of fluid is adequate (approximately 150 mL) to remove 22 mL for analysis. A needle is inserted through the maternal abdomen into the amniotic sac which contains cells from the fetus: these are tested for the same range of chromosomal analysis as CVS. The advantage of amniocentesis compared to CVS is that amniocentesis is slightly safer and associated with a lower miscarriage rate: 0.33–0.5% for amniocentesis compared with 1% for CVS.[294,317] The disadvantage of amniocentesis compared to CVS is that amniocentesis is performed later, limiting the window for termination of the pregnancy if that is elected. Most amniocentesis results are available within 2 weeks, with rapid FISH testing available within 48 hours.

QUADRUPLE TEST

Second trimester screening for aneuploidy is typically the quadruple test, which has 75% sensitivity and 95% specificity.[289] This test considers maternal age in combination with the four tests of alpha-fetoprotein, β-hCG, unconjugated oestriol and inhibin A. Inhibin A is produced by the feto-placental unit throughout pregnancy and higher levels may be associated with trisomy 21.

MID-TRIMESTER MORPHOLOGY SCAN

By mid-trimester (18–20 weeks) the fetus is developed and the uterus has risen from the pelvis, making scanning easier. Findings from the scan can provide diagnostic information that may facilitate the management of problems that arise in later pregnancy and the scan can be performed early enough to conduct further investigations or terminate the pregnancy. The scan enables assessment of placental position, accurate diagnosis of the number of fetuses and cervical measurement. In addition, abnormalities of fetal growth can be detected and a baseline established for further monitoring and comparison. It is estimated that the mid-trimester scan detects more than half of major malformations and anomalies before 24 weeks gestation.[289] Disadvantages include that it doesn't detect all abnormalities, including structural heart disease, small abdominal wall defects, meningomyelocele, early hydrocephalus and oesophageal atresia, and the quality of the scan is dependent on the equipment and operator expertise.

PRENATAL DIAGNOSIS CONSIDERATIONS

Prenatal screening is conducted largely to afford the option to abort an abnormal fetus (in the absence of accessible and effective fetal interventions) but for some people this is unacceptable for religious and ethical reasons. Furthermore, prospective parents may feel pressured to terminate a pregnancy against their will. On the other hand, if the parents continue with the pregnancy, having this information early allows time to prepare for any additional requirements if the infant has special needs.

Screening tests are low risk, but if a diagnostic procedure such as CVS or amniocentesis is required, it involves additional risk to both the mother and the fetus. Screening, diagnostic tests and interventions should be based on informed consent, but this may pose challenges when working with individuals who have mental health problems or who are developmentally delayed. Other issues include does terminating the 'known imperfect' fetus invalidate and devalue to 'living imperfect' in society?

Screening and diagnostic tests do not cover all possible causes of abnormalities and this may not be clear to prospective parents. For genetic conditions, prenatal screening and diagnostic procedures may reveal information that affects one or more third parties (e.g. siblings): this may be undesirable and fraught with ethical issues. Screening needs to be provided in the context of appropriate counselling: unfortunately, currently it is not clear how the availability and quality of counselling is measured, monitored and regulated. Enhanced screening, especially combining biochemistry, clinical history and ultrasound, can significantly reduce the number of women requiring invasive diagnostic procedures, reducing anxiety, risk and cost.

Maternal conditions

HEARTBURN AND GORD

Heartburn is very common in pregnancy, with estimates that up to 80% of women experience heartburn at some stage.[297,298] The prevalence and severity of GORD increases during pregnancy and typically resolves after birth. A recent review found that the prevalence of GORD was 16.9% in the first trimester, 25.3% in the second trimester and 51.2% in the third trimester compared to 6.3% in the control group.[318] Earlier studies found a higher prevalence, although it is unclear whether this difference reflects a reduction in prevalence, improved management or different diagnostic criteria and methodology.[297,298]

Aetiology

GORD is probably a result of the increasing upward pressure on the stomach by the growing fetus and uterus, delayed gastric emptying and progesterone increasing relaxation of the lower oesophageal sphincter. Stress may predispose to GORD or increase sensitivity to symptoms. Symptoms of GORD are as for non-pregnant patients and the woman may present with substernal burning, epigastric discomfort, dyspepsia, mild dysphagia and regurgitation, as well as extra-oesophageal symptoms including chronic cough, hoarseness, sore throat and asthma.[298,318]

Management

Management is as for non-pregnant patients. This includes eating small frequent meals; chewing food well; avoiding fatty and spicy foods; avoiding caffeine, tomatoes, alcohol and chocolate; avoiding cigarette smoke; avoiding drinking large amounts of fluid with meals; and avoiding eating within a few hours of bedtime, elevating the head of the bed 15 cm and sleeping on the left side. Peppermint may increase lower oesophageal sphincter relaxation and should be avoided. Ginger may not cause reflux but should it occur ginger can increase burning sensation. Chewing gum half an hour after eating can aid in salivation and alkalises the oesophagus.

Ulmus rubra (slippery elm) and *Althea officinalis radix* (marshmallow root) have demulcent, anti-inflammatory, antioxidant and soothing nutritive vulnerary properties and can be helpful in GORD and heartburn.[43,47,49] Preparations include powder and capsules. For slippery elm take 1–2 capsules (150 mg each) after each meal and when needed for symptom relief or ½ teaspoon mixed into a slurry with water or yoghurt taken after meals and as required for symptom relief.[43,47]

HYPERTENSION AND PREECLAMPSIA

Hypertension may have been present before pregnancy (chronic hypertension) or it may develop for the first time during pregnancy, typically after 20 weeks gestation.[319,320] Hypertension is diagnosed as blood pressure ≥140 mmHg systolic or ≥90 mmHg diastolic and severe hypertension is blood pressure at least 160 mmHg systolic and/or at least 110 mmHg diastolic.[319] Gestational hypertension is new-onset hypertension in the absence of proteinuria. If preeclampsia does not develop and blood pressure normalises within 12 weeks after birth, the diagnosis of transient hypertension in pregnancy is ascribed.

Preeclampsia is hypertension plus proteinuria and occurs on a spectrum. A woman may have any of the additional pathology noted in Table 13.7. Eclampsia is the occurrence of seizures that cannot be attributed to other causes in a woman with preeclampsia. Preeclampsia occurs in approximately 4% of pregnancies that extend beyond the first trimester.[320] In healthy women preeclampsia is usually mild and not associated with significant fetal risk, and in 75% of cases it develops near term or during labour.[319] Preeclampsia is a heterogeneous syndrome and the pathogenesis may vary among women.[319] For instance, a nulliparous woman may have a different pathogenesis to a multiparous woman with vascular disease or diabetes. Furthermore, early-onset preeclampsia may have a different origin to late or term preeclampsia.[319] Preeclampsia has both maternal and fetal presentations and consequences.

- Maternal features include hypertension, proteinuria, epigastric pain, visual disturbance, nausea and vomiting, facial and pulmonary oedema, ascites, pleural effusion, HELLP syndrome, renal failure, disseminated intravascular coagulation (DIC) and CNS symptoms (e.g. headache, dizziness, tinnitus, drowsiness, altered respiration, tachycardia).
- Fetal features include placental dysfunctional and abruption, fetal growth restriction and inadequate amniotic fluid levels, oligohydramnios and stillbirth due to vascular problems.

Risk factors for preeclampsia

Risk factors for preeclampsia include:
- Nulliparity, with two-thirds of all cases occurring in nulliparous women[320]
- Multiple pregnancy
- Previous preeclampsia
- Mother aged 40 years or older
- ART pregnancy
- Interpregnancy interval >7 years
- Mother born SGA
- Obesity
- GDM
- Poor outcome of previous pregnancy
- Fetal growth restriction, placental abruption, fetal death
- Pre-existing disease – chronic hypertension, renal disease, antiphospholipid antibody syndrome, systemic lupus erythematosus (SLE), diabetes mellitus, thrombophilia
- Factor V Leiden mutation

TABLE 13.7 Comparison of hypertensive disorders of pregnancy			
Clinical feature	**Chronic hypertension**	**Gestational hypertension**	**Preeclampsia**
Onset	<20 weeks	>20 weeks	Typically third trimester
Severity of hypertension	Mild or severe	Mild	Mild or severe
Proteinuria	Absent	Absent	Usually present
Cerebral or visual symptoms	May be present	Absent	Present in 30%
Haemoconcentration	Absent	Absent	May be present
Thrombocytopenia	Absent	Absent	May be present
Hepatic dysfunction	Absent	Absent	May be present
Fetal growth restriction	Absent	Absent	May be present
Pulmonary oedema or cyanosis	Absent	Absent	May be present

Source: Sibai BM. Preeclampsia and hypertensive disorders. In: Gabbe S, Niebyl J, Simpson J et al. (eds). Obstetrics: normal and problem pregnancies. 7th edn. Philadelphia: Elsevier; 2017. Markham KB, Funai EF. Pregnancy-related hypertension. In: Creasy RK, Resnik R, Iams JD et al. (eds). Creasy and Resnik's maternal-fetal medicine: principles and practice. 7th edn. Philadelphia: Elsevier; 2014.

- Race (including Hispanic, African American, Native American)
- Smoking
- Lower socioeconomic status and unmarried.[319,320]

Pathophysiology

The pathophysiology is heterogeneous and not fully understood, although it is widely agreed that abnormal placentation is central to the development of preeclampsia, itself a vascular disorder resulting in placental ischaemia.[168,321] The ischaemic placenta is thought to cause a hypoxia-induced release of placental factors that cause vascular and endothelial dysfunction and an imbalance in angiogenic factors that then cause hypertension.[321] Theories include abnormal trophoblast invasion or poor implantation, imbalance in angiogenesis, coagulopathies, vascular endothelial damage, cardiovascular maladaptation, immunological maladaptation, genetic predisposition, exaggerated inflammatory response and increased oxidative stress.[319,321] Preeclampsia is also associated with hyperhomocysteinaemia, increased inflammation and reversible hypercholesterolaemia.[322]

Oxidative stress may be both a cause and a consequence of preeclampsia.[323] Studies on serum antioxidant status and preeclampsia have been inconsistent, with similar methodological issues as previously discussed.[170,172] A systematic review found a tendency towards lower vitamin E and C levels in cases of preeclampsia and SGA, and lower vitamin A levels in preeclampsia, but concluded that the substantial heterogeneity of results warrants cautious interpretation.[172] A study on micronutrient status and preeclampsia found that copper and caeruloplasmin concentrations were significantly increased in women who subsequently developed preeclampsia compared with controls, but zinc, selenium and manganese were not significantly different.[170] Another study evaluated haem oxygenase, leptin, CoQ10, zinc, copper, total iron-binding capacity (TIBC), ferritin and uric acid in women who developed preeclampsia.[176] The main finding showed that compared to the control group, women with preeclampsia had a significant increase in ferritin, TIBC, copper and leptin, and a significant decrease in haem oxygenase, CoQ10 and zinc. In short, there was an increase in pro-inflammatory and oxidative factors and a reduction in antioxidant factors.

Low magnesium and/or altered magnesium homeostasis has been seen in preeclampsia and magnesium supplementation may lower blood pressure.[43,254] As with other interventions, studies have been inconsistent. A 2014 Cochrane Review did not find enough evidence to support the use of magnesium.[324] Low calcium is also associated with hypertension and preeclampsia. A systematic review found that calcium supplementation during pregnancy reduced the risk of preeclampsia by 52% and severe preeclampsia by 25% and was associated with a significant reduction in the risk of maternal mortality and severe morbidity.[325] Calcium supplementation during pregnancy was also associated with a significant reduction in the risk of preterm birth.

Consequences of preeclampsia

The consequences of preeclampsia are due to the preeclampsia itself as well as the contributing risk factors and underlying conditions (e.g. obesity, SLE). Adverse maternal outcomes include progression to eclampsia and seizures, increased rates of caesarean section, thromboembolism, stroke, haemorrhage, HELLP syndrome, hepatic and renal failure and maternal death. Adverse fetal outcomes include fetal growth restriction, neonatal respiratory difficulties, placental abruption, preterm birth and fetal death.[326] Outcomes are dependent on gestational age at onset and age at birth, multiple gestation, the severity of preeclampsia and the presence of comorbidities such as diabetes, renal disease and thrombophilia. The most severe conditions usually occur in women with early (<32 weeks) development of preeclampsia but the severity of disease is also dependent on maternal age.[319]

Management

A woman with preeclampsia will typically be under the care of a multidisciplinary team including an obstetrician, a cardiologist and a renal doctor.

NATUROPATHIC TREATMENT OBJECTIVES

- Lower the blood pressure
  - Ideally a healthy weight will be achieved preconception, as obesity is a significant risk factor. Aim to meet the recommended gestational weight gain and energy intake guidelines during pregnancy
  - Ensure a high polyunsaturated fat intake (>7.5% of total energy intake)
  - Eat a high-fibre diet
  - Follow a Mediterranean diet[327]
  - Consider the following supplements:
    - > Magnesium: regulates blood pressure via several mechanisms including modulation of vascular tone and reactivity, improving endothelial function and reducing insulin resistance.[43] Low serum magnesium levels increase smooth muscle contraction, which can increase vasospasm leading to increased blood pressure. Women with preeclampsia may have lower magnesium levels, especially those who develop preeclampsia earlier. A trial of 300 mg of oral magnesium citrate given to primigravida women from week 25 onwards found that the women who took magnesium had significantly lower diastolic blood pressure at 37 weeks[328]
    - > Calcium: the newborn skeleton holds approximately 20–30 g of calcium, 80% of which is acquired during the third trimester when the skeleton is rapidly mineralising, and the increased demands of pregnancy may not be met by dietary intake. A 2014 Cochrane Review found that calcium supplementation (≥1 g/day) is associated with a significant reduction in the risk of preeclampsia, particularly for women with low-calcium diets.[329] Furthermore, women

who took calcium supplementation had a reduced risk of maternal morbidity and mortality due to preeclampsia and a reduced rate of preterm birth. WHO recommends supplementing with 1.5–2 g of elemental calcium if a woman has a low calcium intake, especially if there are other risk factors for preeclampsia[222]

> Potassium: may influence blood pressure regulation via modulation of the renin-angiotensin-aldosterone system, natriuresis, increasing vasodilation and reducing vasoconstrictive sensitivity to catecholamines.[330] A study of 150 women with preeclampsia found that the incidence of severe preeclampsia was reduced with a low-sodium and high-potassium intake, and birth weight and gestational age were also higher in this group[331]

> Omega-3 fatty acids: via anti-inflammatory and antioxidant functions, alter eicosanoid synthesis, which reduces arachidonic acid, reducing platelet and leukocyte reactivity and stimulating nitric oxide and vasodilation.[332] Low omega-3 intake has been associated with preeclampsia, although trial results have been mixed

> Vitamin B_2: important in methylation and maintenance of normal homocysteine levels. Low levels are associated with mitochondrial dysfunction and increased oxidative stress

> Vitamin D: deficiency increases the risk of mild and severe forms of preeclampsia.[185] Supplementation may reduce the risk of preeclampsia[184]

> Arginine: studies of arginine supplementation have found a reduction in blood pressure, including for preeclampsia[333]

– Exercise: some research indicates an increased risk if women with preeclampsia exercise, but it is clear that preconception fitness and exercise are protective. One review found that exercise was consistently reported to reduce preeclampsia by up to 35%.[334] Medical clearance and guidelines should be obtained for women who already have preeclampsia.

• *Reduce elevated homocysteine.* Elevated homocysteine in early pregnancy is associated with abnormalities of the placental vasculature, which increases the risk of both pregnancy loss and preeclampsia.[322] A randomised controlled trial found high-dose (5 mg) folic acid reduced homocysteine in pregnant women.[138] Key nutrients are B_2, B_6, folic acid and B_{12}; consider MTHFR polymorphisms

• *Reduce oxidative stress.* CoQ10, zinc, vitamins C and E, ALA supplementation

• *Support stress management.* Nutrients as above will be useful for stress and anxiety (especially zinc, magnesium and omega-3 fatty acids); also consider counselling, meditation and relaxation techniques, yoga (with medical clearance) and herbal medicine.

HERBAL MEDICINE CONSIDERATIONS

• Antihypertensives
  – *Crataegus* spp. (hawthorn): mild hypotensive, mild cardiotonic, cardioprotective, antioxidant, collagen stabilising, antiarrhythmic. In trials, hawthorn did not have adverse effects in embryonic rats.[335] It is not contraindicated in pregnancy[47,49]
  – *Viburnum opulus* (cramp bark)/*Viburnum prunifolium* (black haw): hypotensive, antispasmodic (especially uterine), mild sedative. Long traditional use in pregnancy for hypertension and the prevention of premature labour. It is not contraindicated in pregnancy[49]

• Nervines
  – *Lavandula officinalis* (lavender): anxiolytic, sedative, carminative. It is not contraindicated in pregnancy[43]
  – *Avena sativa* (oats): nervine relaxant, antioxidant, anti-atherogenic, helps stabilise blood sugar levels (BSLs), antihypertensive. It is not contraindicated in pregnancy[43]

• Adaptogen
  – *Withania somnifera* (ashwagandha): tonic, anxiolytic, anti-inflammatory, cardioprotective. Early Ayurvedic writing suggested that *Withania* was an abortifacient, but this has been shown to be incorrect in more recent reviews and studies.[43,47]

TREATMENT SUMMARY

• Magnesium (500–750 mg)
• Calcium (1000 mg)
• Potassium (3–6 g)
• Omega-3 fatty acids (total 2 g/d)
• Antioxidants: zinc (40–80 mg), vitamin E (400 IU), vitamin C (1 g), CoQ10 (100–150 mg), ALA (20–100 mg), beta-carotenes (10–30 mg)
• Vitamin D (1000–4000 IU)
• Arginine (up to 4 g/day based on trials)
• Activated B complex, adequate B_2, B_6, B_9 and B_{12}.

THIRD TRIMESTER

The third trimester is characterised by significant fetal growth and physiological preparation for labour.

Fetal development

WEEK 28

The fetus measures up to 37 cm and weighs around 1100 g. While a neonate may survive if born earlier, it is now considered viable. Respiratory bronchioles proliferate and the immune system develops. The fetus is yawning, sucking and drinking amniotic fluid and is able to distinguish between light and dark.

WEEKS 29–33

The fetus measures 35–45 cm and weighs about 1500–1700 g. It now significantly increases its fat stores. Between 16 and 32 weeks the average amniotic fluid volume increases from 250 mL to 800 mL.[336] The respiratory system continues to develop and bronchioles end in alveolar ducts and sacs. The fetus practises breathing and some rhythmic breathing movements occur. The testes begin to descend. The skeleton is formed but still pliable and muscle bulk and strength increase. Erythropoiesis is more evident in the bone marrow. CNS control continues, the fetus begins to regulate its temperature and myelination is established. There is an increased uptake of iron and calcium in preparation for birth and the fetus may reposition and engage (descend into the pelvis). Hearing sensitivity and ability to distinguish sounds continue.

WEEKS 34–40

By week 36 the average fetus weighs 2800 g and is about 50 cm in length. The growing fetus occupies more of the uterus and there is less room to move; thus, the mother may be less aware of fetal movement. Amniotic fluid decreases to 500 mL at term. The foramen ovale closes leaving a fossa ovalis. TSH, T3 and T4 levels increase then decline to normal levels within the first postnatal week. Toenails reach the tip of the toes. During this period the lanugo starts to fall off as there is increasing body fat to insulate the fetus. The fetus is considered to be 'term' by 37 weeks. Vernix coats the fetus to help prevent excessive heat loss after birth. All organs are developed and functional and the lungs continue to mature until birth. The fetus can suck its thumb and cry.

Maternal changes

The maternal changes reflect the significant increase in fetal size and weight gain. Increased intraabdominal pressure causes reduced lung and gastric capacity, creates pressure on the bladder, increases varicosities and, if pressing on major vessels, may cause a lowering in maternal blood pressure. The woman may experience constipation, GORD, dyspepsia and urinary frequency. Hormonal stimulation may cause hair growth on her face and arms. Fetal temperature increases maternal temperature. The increased plasma volume may cause oedema and can increase the risk of carpal tunnel syndrome if the nerve is compressed by oedematous tissue. Colostrum may begin to leak from the nipples in preparation for breastfeeding, and libido may increase. Leucorrhoea may increase. Backache, abdominal stretching pain and leg cramps are more frequent. Stretch marks may appear or worsen and the skin may be dry with increased pigmentation (chloasma), especially on sun-exposed parts of the face. Fatigue and sleep disturbance are common. Anxiety about childbirth and motherhood may be more pronounced.

Assessments

There is a continued review of symptoms, concerns, weight and nutritional intake. Monitor blood pressure and BSL. Urinalysis is performed to detect glucose and protein (indicative of urinary tract infection [UTI] or preeclampsia). Midwife assessments include fundus measurement, fetal heart rate and movements, and the position, growth and development of the fetus via palpation. Physical assessment may be augmented with ultrasound or Doppler assessment to evaluate placental blood flow and fetal heart rate. A review of mental health issues is warranted at every visit but particularly in the third trimester. Review birth plans, support, postnatal support and contraception, labour and postnatal plans. Routine pathology may include FBC, electrolytes, lung function tests [LFTs], CRP, iron studies, folate and B_{12}, zinc and copper, homocysteine, vitamin D_3, fasting glucose, lipid profile, thyroid function tests and vaginal swab for group B streptococcus (GBS, 35–37 weeks).

Nutrition

The expansion of blood plasma continues until weeks 30–34, resulting in haemodilution of plasma constituents including nutrients (notably iron). In addition, serum albumin levels are lower, reducing the amount of protein-binding carrier available. As the fetus increases its nutrient demand to support growth and to lay down stores for the first 6 months postnatally, there is a reduction in maternal concentration of nutrients. Furthermore, the increased cardiac output increases the GFR and urinary excretion of nutrients including glucose, amino acids and water-soluble micronutrients. Maternal fat mobilisation causes an increase in circulating triglycerides, cholesterol levels and fat-soluble nutrients.

Specific nutrients to monitor regarding intake and status include:
- Vitamin D (critical for calcium metabolism and mineralisation of the fetal skeleton; low levels are associated with preeclampsia)
- Calcium (bone health and to prevent preeclampsia)
- Magnesium (muscle relaxation and to prevent preeclampsia)
- Selenium (to reduce preeclampsia risk)
- Folate (to reduce preeclampsia)
- Iron (the infant is dependent on stores laid down at the end of the third trimester to provide iron for the first 6 months postnatally)
- Protein (to support basic tissue growth and energy requirements and to stabilise BSL)
- Iodine (to prevent irreversible congenital defects and provide stores for the first 6 months postnatally)
- Essential fatty acids (for neurological development and reduction in atopy).

GROUP B STREPTOCOCCUS

GBS infection is caused by the bacterium *Streptococcus agalactiae*, a Gram-positive encapsulated coccus that produces β-haemolysis when grown on blood agar.[310] Between 15% and 25% of pregnant women have GBS in their lower genital tract and rectum.[310,337] GBS is an important cause of early-onset neonatal infection. While the maternal carriage is high, less than one-third of vaginally delivered neonates are colonised with GBS, with one in every 200–400 developing bacteraemia.[337] The neonatal rate of GBS infection in the US is about 0.5 per 1000 live births, with approximately 10 000 cases of early-onset GBS sepsis (EOGBS) annually.[310] EOGBS commonly presents as respiratory symptoms and pneumonia and is associated with a 14–25% mortality rate, with preterm infants at higher risk.[310,337] Late-onset neonatal GBS infection more commonly presents with meningitis, septicaemia and pneumonia and has a lower mortality rate of around 5% for both term and premature infants.[310]

Risk factors for early-onset GBS include preterm labour (especially associated with premature rupture of the membranes), intrapartum maternal fever >38°C, a prolonged period after rupture of the membranes before birth (>18 hours), previous infant with EOGBS, GBS bacteriuria during the current pregnancy, known carriage of maternal GBS in the current pregnancy, clinical diagnosis of chorioamnionitis, twin with EOGBS, maternal youth (<18 years of age) and black or Hispanic ethnicity.[310,337] Diagnosis is made via culture of a vaginal swab (+/– anal swab).

Maternal complications of GBS include increased risk of obstetric infections such as chorioamnionitis, postpartum endometritis, caesarean wound infection and UTI. Fetal risks include respiratory compromise, pneumonia, meningitis, preterm delivery and death. Maternal symptoms comprise fever, abdominal swelling, uterine and bladder tenderness. Fetal symptoms are respiratory distress, fever, lethargy, floppiness, poor feeding, irritability and seizures.

Management

Most countries have prevention as the main goal and undertake routine vaginal swabbing for GBS in late pregnancy (35–37 weeks). If GBS is detected, the first line of treatment is antibiotics (penicillin), ideally at least 4 hours prior to birth. In some circumstances an elective caesarean may be considered.[310,337]

NATUROPATHIC SUPPORT

Naturopathic support will be included in addition to medical management and is focused on supporting the immune function of the mother (see Chapter 11 of *Clinical Naturopathic Medicine* for further discussion of immune function) as well as supporting maternal GI microbiota in the presence of antibiotic treatment. Sample immune support protocol:

- *Echinacea* spp, 1:2: 2–4 mL per day
- Vitamin C: 500–2000 mg per day in divided doses
- Zinc: 10–40 mg per day
- Vitamin E: 200–500 IU per day
- Vitamin A: 1000–2500 IU, with or without beta-carotene (6–15 mg) as a precursor (with appropriate caution with vitamin A dose, especially if it is in a prenatal supplement as well)
- Selenium: 25–50 micrograms per day
- Iron: 15–40 mg per day if iron studies indicate requirement (excess iron is inflammatory and to be avoided)
- Multi-strain probiotics and *Saccharomyces cerevisiae* (*S. boulardii*)
- Fermented foods and prebiotic foods
- Probiotics topically – a small study assessing the vaginal pH and microbes of women who wore panty liners impregnated with the probiotic strain *Lactobacillus plantarum* LB931 found that high

numbers of lactobacilli was associated with a low vaginal pH and lower numbers of group B streptococci.[338]

PRURITIC URTICARIAL PAPULES AND PLAQUES OF PREGNANCY

Also known as polymorphic eruption of pregnancy (PEP), pruritic urticarial papules and plaques of pregnancy (PUPPP) is the most common urticarial dermatosis of pregnancy and affects between 1 in 130 and 1 in 300 women.[339] PUPPP usually commences in the third trimester and resolves within 10–15 days postpartum. Less commonly it may present a few days postpartum. PUPPP is most common in primigravidas and while it may recur in subsequent pregnancies it is less severe.[340,341] The lesions usually first appear within abdominal striae and spare the periumbilical region in most cases.[339] The rash is varied and can involve erythematous papules, plaques, urticarial lesions, vesicular lesions and targetoid lesions reminiscent of erythema multiforme or pemphigoid gestationis.[339] The lesions may join to form larger wheals on the abdomen; it can also spread to the limbs, neck, breasts, back and buttocks but rarely involves the face.[339,341]

Aetiology and pathogenesis

The pathogenesis is not established, but the immunohistological profile of skin lesions is suggestive of a delayed hypersensitivity reaction (antigen unknown). PUPPP is up to 10 times more common in multiple gestations; another theory is that the rapid growth of the abdominal wall triggers an inflammatory reaction, especially as PUPPP is more common in maternal obesity, excess GWG and fetal macrosomia.[339] Multiple pregnancy is not just associated with larger size, but also with increased hormone levels, including oestrogen and progesterone, and progesterone may aggravate inflammation. Fetal DNA has been found in biopsies of PUPPP lesions but the significance of this is unclear.

Differential diagnoses include erythema multiforme, drug eruptions, pemphigoid gestationis, contact dermatitis, urticaria and insect bites. PUPPP is not associated with maternal or fetal morbidity or mortality; however, the itch can be intense and distressing and disturb sleep and it may increase stress.

Management

Topical ointments and salves may be contraindicated as they can increase the sensation of heat in the skin and tinctures may sting. Cooling lotions, compresses, gels, sprays and baths are more appropriate. Topical application needs to be repeated throughout the day.

NATUROPATHIC SUPPORT

Topical anti-inflammatory herbs to consider include the following:

- *Aloe vera*: soothing, cooling gel – safe as a topical agent, contraindicated for internal use in pregnancy
- *Avena sativa* (oats): baths and compresses
- *Hamamelis virginiana* (witch hazel): cooling compresses, taking care as it is astringent

- *Matricaria chamomilla* (chamomile): baths, lotions, compresses and herbal infusions
- *Scutellaria baicalensis* (baikal skullcap): used in traditional Chinese medicine to clear heat and dampness, or inflammation – safe as a topical agent, contraindicated for internal use in pregnancy
- *Hypericum perforatum* (St John's wort): vulnerary and anti-inflammatory
- *Centella asiatica*: vulnerary, collagen and microcirculation support – use in lotion/creams
- *Stellaria media* (chickweed): antipruritic – use in lotion/creams.
- Liquid formula: it may be helpful to include nervines, anti-inflammatories and adaptogens to help ease the itch and support the nervous system and aid sleep. Supplementation:
- Omega-3 fatty acids: 800 mg EPA and 400 mg DHA
- Consider zinc status and zinc:copper ratio – anecdotal evidence shows a correlation
- Zinc picolinate 60 mg
- P5P 50 mg plus B complex
- Evening primrose oil 1 g BD.
  Results should be seen rapidly but this depends on the deficiency state, absorption and the stage of pregnancy.

INTRAHEPATIC CHOLESTASIS OF PREGNANCY

The prevalence of intrahepatic cholestasis of pregnancy (ICP) is around 1 in 140 women.[342,343] ICP is more common in winter although the reason for this is not clear. ICP is more common in multiple pregnancies and in women older than 35 years of age; the recurrence rate is 60–90%.[343]

Aetiology and pathogenesis

ICP has a complex pathogenesis. Genetic influences are apparent, as demonstrated by the high rates in some racial groups (e.g. Indigenous Araucanian people of Chile) and in familial clustering.[344] Mutations that have been identified and may be causative include the *ABCB4* and *ATP8B1* genes that encode phospholipid transporters and the *ABCB11* gene that encodes the principal bile salt transporter and the main bile acid receptor.[342] In addition, there is an association with defects in the *multidrug resistance type 3 (MDR-3)* gene. Endocrine factors may include the markedly elevated oestrogen levels in women with ICP, with oestrogen known to have a cholestatic effect, as well as the effects of elevated progesterone as sulfated progesterone metabolites are also known to be cholestatic. Other factors include the presence of hepatitis C, severe NVP in the first pregnancy, Gilbert's syndrome and a history of Epstein Barr virus.

Presentation

ICP usually presents in the third trimester with symptoms of severe pruritus and signs of deranged serum liver tests. The pruritus typically most severely affects the palms and soles of the feet (spared in PUPPP) and flares at night.[344] ICP is presumed in cases of pruritus in the absence of a rash. Pathology findings include raised transaminases (ALT), typically several-fold, raised bilirubin, raised serum bile acids (common), in severe cases >40 micromol/L,[342]

and jaundice in about 10% of cases.[344] There is also an increased risk of GDM and elevated GTT.[344]

Outcomes

Maternal risk is not significant and while the itch can be severe it usually resolves completely with birth. ICP does increase the risk of postpartum cholelithiasis and if steatorrhoea is present there is an increased risk of vitamin K deficiency and postpartum haemorrhage.[344] The risks to the fetus are much more significant, including an increased risk of poor outcomes such as fetal distress, meconium ileus, asphyxia, premature delivery or stillbirth.

Management

If severe, labour is often induced at 37 weeks.[344] Rest is important for the mother and additional adaptogen and nervine support may be required.

HERBAL MEDICINE

Herbal medicine to support normal hepatic function is relevant. Tablets or capsules are more appropriate than alcohol extracts. Herbs to consider include:
- *Silybum marianum* (St Mary's thistle)
- *Taraxacum officinalis radix* (dandelion)
- *Arctium lappa* (burdock)
- *Cynara scolymus* (globe artichoke)
- Topical agents, adaptogens and nervines as described for PUPPP.
  Supplementation:
- Antioxidants: beta-carotenes, vitamins C and E, zinc, CoQ10, ALA
- Adequate choline in diet and supplementation
- Review methylation and treat accordingly
- Dietary modifications to promote liver health: for example, include bitter vegetables (e.g. radicchio), lemon juice in warm water, avoid excessive fatty foods, eat small amounts frequently, avoid excess simple carbohydrates, and avoid caffeine and alcohol.

GESTATIONAL DIABETES

Gestational diabetes is the most common dysglycaemia of pregnancy and the rate is increasing alongside increasing rates of type 1 and type 2 diabetes, metabolic disturbances and obesity. GDM is defined as glucose intolerance with onset or first recognition during pregnancy. GDM affects approximately 8–10% of pregnancies in Australia[345] and 9.2% in the US[346] but perhaps surprisingly is reported as being as low as 3.5% in England and Wales.[347] Many countries have revised their definitions and thresholds for diagnosis and this impacts on data consistency across time and location. It may also be difficult to distinguish previously undiagnosed type 2 diabetes from GDM until postnatal assessment.

Aetiology and pathogenesis

The pathophysiology of GDM in usually similar to that of type 2 diabetes where there is an inability to maintain an adequate insulin response, in this case because of the significant decreases in insulin sensitivity with advancing gestation.[348] Late pregnancy is considered to be a diabetogenic state due to the progressive increase in postprandial glucose levels and increased insulin response.[313] Early pregnancy, in contrast, is viewed as an anabolic state due to the increases in maternal fat stores and decreases in free fatty acid (FFA) concentration, particularly in normal weight and obese women. This increase in FFA reduces insulin requirements for the mother and at this time there is increased insulin sensitivity, although this changes as the pregnancy progresses. Maternal fasting hepatic glucose production may increase by as much as 30% in late gestation, despite increasing insulin levels, suggesting a hepatic insulin insensitivity, especially in obese women.[313] In addition to altered glucose metabolism in pregnancy and especially GDM there are changes to protein and lipid metabolism. First-trimester maternal protein synthesis is comparable to that of a non-pregnant woman but this increases by 15% during the second trimester, and a further increase of about 25% is seen in the third trimester.[313]

Risk factors

Risk factors for developing GDM include:
- Previous GDM
- Previously elevated blood glucose levels
- Ethnicity: South and Southeast Asian, Aboriginal, Pacific Islander, Māori, Middle Eastern, Indian, non-Caucasian African
- Age ≥40 years
- Family history of diabetes mellitus (first-degree relative with diabetes mellitus or sister with GDM)
- Overweight or obese, especially BMI >35 kg/m²
- High or low birth-weight infant
- Previous macrosomia (baby with birth weight >4500 g or >90th percentile)
- Polycystic ovary syndrome
- Insulin resistance (before and in early pregnancy)
- Medications: corticosteroids, antipsychotics.[313,349]

Assessment

Most women will be asymptomatic (a few may have the classic triad of polydipsia, polyphagia and polyuria) and routine testing with a 75 g oral glucose tolerance test (OGTT) is recommended at 24–28 weeks gestation.[349] Women with one or more risk factors may be screened earlier and more often. The International Association of Diabetes and Pregnancy Study Group Consensus Panel A provides threshold values for the diagnosis of GDM as shown in Table 13.8: a diagnosis is made on any one of the following values.[350]

Complications

Maternal complications of GDM include infertility, hypoglycaemia or hyperglycaemia, later development of type 2 diabetes, spontaneous abortion, preeclampsia and caesarean birth (due to macrosomia). Infant complications include macrosomia, physical and mental abnormalities, hypoglycaemia, respiratory distress, death, shoulder dystocia, bone fracture, nerve palsy and increased risk of developing metabolic and cardiovascular disease in adulthood.

TABLE 13.8 Threshold values for the diagnosis of GDM

Glucose measure	mmol/L
Fasting plasma glucose	≥5.1
1-hour plasma glucose	≥10.0
2-hour plasma glucose	≥8.5

Source: International Association of Diabetes and Pregnancy Study Groups Consensus Panel, Metzger BE, Gabbe SG, et al. International Association of Diabetes and Pregnancy Study Groups recommendations on the diagnosis and classification of hyperglycemia in pregnancy. Diabetes Care 2010;33(3): 676–82.

Management

Prevention is clearly the best approach and this is where preconception planning and care are critical. Normalising glucose control, exercising regularly and achieving a healthy weight are core preconception goals. Pregnancy goals are to stabilise blood glucose levels and prevent complications of poorly controlled GDM.

MEDICAL MANAGEMENT

Medical management includes dietary and lifestyle advice and pharmaceutical agents, typically metformin and glibenclamide oral preparations and subcutaneous insulin. Because of the increased risk of developing type 2 diabetes – especially if risk factors of advanced maternal age, obesity and ethnicity are present – a postnatal OGTT is recommended at 6–12 weeks postpartum and thereafter every 1–2 years. Alternatively, a HbA_{1c} may be performed.[349]

Glycaemic targets in GDM:
- Fasting capillary BSL: ≤5.0 mmol/L
- 1 hour after commencing meal BSL: ≤7.4 mmol/L
- 2 hours after commencing meal BSL: ≤6.7 mmol/L.[349]

NATUROPATHIC MANAGEMENT

Naturopathic management includes excellent preconception care to optimise maternal health and reduce the risk of developing GDM. Dietary support is central to effective management of GDM and is as per type 2 diabetes dietary management:
- Provide dietary and nutritional support to ensure that GWG guidelines are met
- Follow low GI diet/Mediterranean-style diet
- Undertake regular moderate exercise (e.g. 30-minute walk daily)
- Ensure adequate fibre intake (satiation and aids in reducing excessive peaks in BSL)
- Ensure low saturated fats and transfatty acids
- Provide food sources of omega-3 fatty acids such as sardines.

A Mediterranean-style diet has been shown to reduce the risk of GDM.[351] A 2015 systematic review found that a dietary pattern rich in fruit, vegetables, whole grains and fish, and low in red and processed meat (fewer than 3 serves per week), refined grains and high-fat dairy reduced the risk of developing GDM, although it did not quantify dairy serves or forms.[351]

Supplementation:
* Zinc 25–60 mg
* Chromium picolinate 200 micrograms
* Magnesium 400–800 mg
* Selenium 50–100 micrograms
* Natal formula/B complex
* EFAs, 400–600 mg each of EPA and DHA
* ALA 300–400 micrograms
* Protein: 1.2 g/kg
* Vitamin B_{12} – metformin lowers total (not storage) of B_{12} so supplementation is suggested[352]
* Vitamin D_3 1000–4000 IU, dependent of blood tests
* Probiotics.

An increasing number of studies are investigating the role of probiotics in GDM management and a recent study found that supplementing with probiotics (probiotic capsules of four bacterial strains each of >4 × 10^9 CFU *Lactobacillus acidophilus LA-5*, *Bifidobacterium BB-12*, *Streptococcus thermophilus STY-31* and *Lactobacillus delbrueckii bulgaricus LBY-27*) over 6 weeks lowered fasting blood glucose, reduced weight gain in the last 2 weeks of the 6-week study and reduced insulin resistance.[353]

Low B_{12} has been associated with increased adiposity and insulin resistance and a recent study in the UK found that obese women were at risk of B_{12} deficiency; this in turn was associated with a two-times probability of developing GDM.[164]

A recent randomised controlled trial assessed the effects of omega-3 supplementation on inflammatory and oxidative markers in women with GDM. The women received 1000 mg of omega-3 fatty acid supplements (containing 180 mg eicosapentaenoic acid and 120 mg docosahexaenoic acid) or placebo for 6 weeks. This produced a significant decrease in hsCRP and plasma malondialdehyde and resulted in lower rates of infant hyperbilirubinaemia and hospitalisation.[354] A study on selenium supplementation (200 micrograms) for 6 weeks commencing between 24 and 28 weeks gestation resulted in a significant reduction in fasting plasma glucose and serum insulin levels and an increase in insulin sensitivity.[355] In addition, there was a reduction in hsCRP, thus showing an overall improvement in blood glucose management and a reduction in markers of oxidative stress. A study using a supplement of 250 mg of magnesium for 6 weeks similarly found improvements in glucose control, insulin levels, triglycerides and hsCRP and fewer hospitalisations for newborns.[256]

HERBAL MEDICINE

Gymnema sylvestre traditionally has been used to lower BSL, but there is no research on GDM and no safety data to assess. *Cinnamon* spp have been shown to be effective in type 2 diabetes but are contraindicated in pregnancy.[43]

IRON DEFICIENCY ANAEMIA OF PREGNANCY

Iron is essential for normal fetal development and some adverse effects caused by deficiency cannot be reversed by later addition to the diet. Iron deficiency is a common nutritional deficiency and studies on pregnant women consistently show iron deficiency and iron deficiency anaemia in pregnant women. A review of 1224 women as part of the US National Health and Nutrition Examination Survey (NHANES) 1999–2006 found that iron deficiency prevalence in pregnant women increased significantly with each trimester: 6.9% in trimester 1, 14.3% in trimester 2 and 29.5% in trimester 3. Women with two or more children and women with short interpregnancy intervals had the highest prevalence of iron deficiency.[356] Many women enter pregnancy with marginal iron stores (due to menstrual loss, poor intake and absorption, or other reasons) and the additional demands of pregnancy cannot be met.

In a normal singleton pregnancy a total of 1000 mg of iron is required, with approximately 300 mg being delivered to the fetus, which preferentially obtains iron, folate and vitamin B_{12} from the mother. Maternal iron is transferred to the fetus via serum transferrin, which binds to receptors on the apical surface of the placental syncytiotrophoblast. Iron is then released from these receptors and binds to ferritin in placenta cells, where it is transferred to apotransferrin, which enters into the fetal circulation as holotransferrin.[357] If maternal iron levels are low, the placenta increases the number of transferrin receptors to facilitate more uptake of iron in an attempt to protect the fetus from depletion, which further reduces maternal levels.

Iron levels are affected by both iron intake and haemodilution. Starting around week 6 the maternal blood volume progressively increases until about 30 weeks, when it plateaus. For a singleton pregnancy the average increase in blood volume is 40–50%. The blood plasma volume also increases progressively from around week 6 until week 30, when it too plateaus. Blood plasma volume increases by around 50% and this represents approximately 1200–1300 mL.[245] RBC mass begins to increase around week 10 and continues to rise until delivery. RBC mass increases around 18% by term: supplementing can increase this to 30%. The plasma volume increases to a greater degree than the RBC mass and then plateaus at week 30, so the maternal haematocrit falls, most notably around weeks 30–34. After this time, the reduction in haematocrit may lessen as the RBC mass continues to grow and the plasma volume plateaus.[28,245] This may not represent a pathological state, but rather normal maternal physiology. In a normal pregnancy and uncomplicated birth, if the mother has adequate iron stores her haematocrit and haemoglobin levels return to normal by 6 weeks postpartum.[358] The average blood loss in a normal vaginal delivery is 500 mL, which equates to around 250 mg of elemental iron and a ferritin level of 30 micrograms/L. Women who have a caesarean section have double the blood and iron loss.[251]

Aetiology

Around 75% of anaemia in pregnancy is due to iron deficiency (1 mL of erythrocytes contains 1.1 mg iron). Other causes include excessive haemodilution, deficiency in folate and B_{12}, bleeding, haemolytic disorders, bone marrow suppression, chronic blood loss and haematological malignancies. Without supplementation, deficiency may occur in up to 50% of women.

Risk factors

In addition to the known causes above (e.g. blood loss), the following are risk factors for iron deficiency anaemia:

- Previous anaemia
- Known haemoglobinopathy
- Multiparity (3 or more)
- Interpartum spacing <12 months
- Vegetarian or vegan
- Teenager
- Recent history of bleeding or high risk of bleeding
- Aboriginal or Torres Strait Islander
- Jehovah's Witness.[251,252]

Consequences

Maternal consequences of iron deficiency anaemia include exacerbation of underlying cardiorespiratory disease, increased perinatal haemorrhage and mortality, compromised immune function and increased risk of postnatal depression. Infant consequences include low birth weight, premature birth, reduced immune function, psychomotor and cognitive abnormalities and brain developmental and neurocognition problems.

Clinical features

Clinical features of iron deficiency anaemia are as for non-pregnant adults: reduced exercise tolerance and stamina, shortness of breath, pale skin and conjunctiva, fatigue, dizziness, light-headedness and pica. Prenatal assessment may indicate intrauterine growth restriction. Assessment should include careful interpretation of iron studies (as above), serum folate and vitamin B_{12}.

Assessment

For women at risk of low iron, iron studies should be performed in the first trimester at 24–28 weeks and 36 weeks gestation.[359] Anaemia in pregnancy is usually determined to be when the Hb drops to less than 100 g/L or the haematocrit is less than 32%.[359] A serum iron concentration less than 10 mmol/L with a less than 16% transferrin saturation (normal: 20–50%) is suggestive of iron deficiency. Due to delays in depleting serum iron as well as the short-term effects of supplementing, it is necessary to review the whole iron panel and to repeat the test.[245]

Typical findings in iron deficiency anaemia are low iron, transferrin saturation, and ferritin, as well as increased iron-binding capacity and soluble transferrin receptor. It should be noted that up to 15% of pregnant women who do not have iron deficiency anaemia will show an increase in iron-binding capacity and that serum ferritin levels can fluctuate as much as 25% from one day to the next, although a significant decrease is indicative of iron deficiency.[358] Ferritin may also be elevated in the presence of inflammation and/or infection. In addition, blood film will indicate microcytic hypochromic erythrocytes.

Management

Ensuring adequate iron stores before conception is ideal. During the first trimester no additional iron is usually required, but if the mother had low or marginal levels and then has very poor intake of food for a lengthy period due to NVP, the risk of early deficiency increases. Pregnant women require a ferritin level of at least 60 micrograms/L for labour to manage the blood loss associated with childbirth, and the target range for ferritin at term is 60–100 micrograms/L.[251]

The RDI for iron is 27 mg per day and supplementation requires individual assessment and prescription. High-dose iron supplementation without assessment can cause an inadvertent overload of iron, which is associated with increased nausea, excessive coagulation and oxidation as well as hypertension. Most pregnancy nutrient formulas contain a low dose of iron and this may be adequate, but full assessment is required to exclude the risk of deficiency. One review found a 73% reduction in anaemia at term with daily iron supplementation.[360]

SUPPLEMENTATION

The following guidelines (see also Table 13.9) are provided for supplementation.

- Ferritin:
    - ≥100–150 micrograms/L may indicate possible haemochromatosis – no supplementation and possible further investigation (based on clinical history)
    - 60–100 micrograms/L no supplementation necessary
    - 30–60 micrograms/L indicates that increasing reserves will require a supplement of 40 mg/day of ferrous iron
    - <30 micrograms/L may require a supplement of 80–100 mg/day of ferrous iron.[251,252]

If a therapeutic dose of iron supplementation is required, the co-factors to support erythropoiesis should also be supplied, such as protein, vitamin B_2, vitamin B_6, folate, vitamin B_{12}, vitamin A and zinc. Encourage dietary

TABLE 13.9 Interpretation of haemoglobin and ferritin in pregnancy	
Results	**Response**
Hb >110 g/L and ferritin >30 micrograms/L	Monitor; iron-rich diet and education (for all women)
Hb >110 g/L and ferritin ≤30 micrograms/L	65 mg elemental iron daily
Hb >70 g/L and ≤ 110 g/L and ferritin >30 micrograms/L	Reassess
Hb >70 g/L and ≤110 g/L and ferritin ≤30 micrograms/L	Commence 100 mg elemental oral iron daily Consider IV Fe if birth is imminent
Hb <70 g/L, irrespective of ferritin	Urgent haematologist/obstetrician review (and may require Fe infusion or blood transfusion)

Source: King Edward Memorial Hospital. Anaemia in pregnancy: clinical guideline. Perth: Govt Western Australia, Dept Health; 2013.

iron intake and educate on factors that enhance absorption (e.g. acids such as ascorbic acid and vinegar) and factors that reduce absorption (e.g. calcium).

PERINEAL MASSAGE

Prenatal perineal massage is associated with a reduction in the incidence of trauma requiring suturing, a requirement for episiotomy and ongoing perineal pain; however, this effect is greatest in primigravida mothers.[361,362] The mother commences perineal massage at 36 weeks and uses vitamin E oil massaged along the perineum and stretching vaginal opening front to back and side to side.

LABOUR AND CHILDBIRTH

As full term approaches the myometrium starts to develop contractions in response to the release of oxytocin. Prostaglandins are synthesised to increase the myometrial contractility and the mother experiences pain, anxiety and uterine contractions that increase cardiac output, tachycardia and hypertension. These all aid the birth process by giving the mother the force, respiration and blood volume needed during birth. The three stages of labour are:

- First stage: dilation of the cervix
- Second stage: birth
- Third stage: placenta delivery.

Some say that birth is not complete until the baby attaches to the mother's breast.

Labour preparations

RUBUS IDAEUS (RED RASPBERRY LEAF)

Raspberry leaf has long been used as a partus preparator but there is little quality research to support this tradition.[363] In one retrospective study, participants took raspberry leaf from 1 to 32 weeks duration, but they also used different doses and the preparations weren't standardised.[364] The findings were no adverse effects from the raspberry leaf and a slightly shortened labour, as well as a suggestion that the women who ingested raspberry leaf might be less likely to receive an artificial rupture of their membranes or require a caesarean section, forceps or vacuum birth than the women in the control group. As well as the study's methodological issues it was small (108 women: 57 who took raspberry leaf and 51 who did not). A follow-up randomised controlled trial with 192 women who took 1.2 g of raspberry leaf tablets twice a day from 32 weeks until labour sought to examine the effects on maternal blood loss and blood pressure, meconium-stained fluid, Apgar score at 5 minutes of age, birth weight and transfer of baby to special care.[365] No significant differences were seen between the raspberry leaf group and the control, including in length of gestation, medical augmentation of labour and analgesia requirements during labour. The second stage of labour was 9.6 minutes shorter in the raspberry leaf group, but the difference was not statistically significant.

Raspberry leaf is used to facilitate delivery by increasing the efficiency of uterine contractions, shortening the duration of labour, reducing the risk of haemorrhage during labour, reducing the incidence of post-term pregnancy and inducing labour. Dosage is 4–8 g of dried leaf as an infusion three times a day or liquid extract 1 : 1, 4–8 mL up to three times a day or 2.4 g tablet daily from 34 weeks gestation onwards.

OTHER PREPARATIONS

Although the following preparations may be mentioned in the literature as being used in labour preparation, they are contraindicated:

- *Caulophyllum thalictroides*: risk of teratogenic effects, fetal tachycardia[366]
- *Actaea racemosa* (black cohosh)
- *Hydrastis canadensis* (goldenseal)
- *Ricinus communis* (castor oil): possibly effective but unclear safety profile.

NATUROPATHIC SUPPORT

Labour can be exceptionally demanding on the mother so being nutritionally replete, well-fed and well-hydrated will help her through the process. Easy-to-eat protein and carbohydrate snacks (e.g. a fruit smoothie with protein powder or LSA, bliss balls with nut butter and dates) and salty snacks (pretzels or salty crackers) are helpful. A labour-aid drink with salt and glucose is also helpful:

Recipe
¼ cup honey or maple syrup
½ teaspoon sea salt
⅓ cup lemon, grape, apple or pineapple juice
1 crushed calcium tablet (or powder)
1 crushed magnesium tablet (or powder)
Mix ingredients into 1 L of pure water, herbal infusion such as *Rubus idaeus* or diluted coconut water.[367]

Continue supplementation and review doses as required, especially of zinc, iron, magnesium, calcium, essential fatty acids, probiotics and CoQ10. Low zinc is associated with both preterm and postdate pregnancy and prolonged labour.[368] Zinc is sequestered into the placenta in increased amounts in the third trimester and additional supplementation may be beneficial.

The stages of labour and options for support are outlined in Table 13.10.[369]

FOURTH TRIMESTER: THE POSTNATAL PERIOD

Maternal changes

The process by which the uterus and the other reproductive organs return to their pre-pregnant state is called involution and it starts with the delivery of the placenta. The pregnant-term uterus weighs approximately 1000 g and by 5–6 weeks following delivery it recedes to 50–100 g. Within the first fortnight the uterine fundus goes from palpable at or near the level of the maternal umbilicus back into the true pelvis. While the uterus reduces it never returns to quite the pre-pregnant size. Involution commences more rapidly following vaginal birth than caesarean birth.

The decidua (endometrium) rapidly degenerates and by 1 week endometrial glands are already evident. By just after 2 weeks the endometrium is restored except at the site of placental attachment. Immediately after delivery, contractions of the arterial smooth muscles and compression of the vessels by contraction of the myometrium ('physiological ligatures') result in haemostasis. The size of the placental bed decreases by half, and changes in the placental bed are reflected in the quantity and quality of the lochia that is experienced.

TABLE 13.10 Stages of labour and support options		
Body changes	**Sensation and responses**	**Naturopathic support**
Pre-labour		
Baby's head in the pelvis	Backache, period pain or cramping, heavy pelvic pressure	Continue eating and drinking
Lightening: baby's head engages	Waters may break	Herbal medicines, homeopathics, magnesium, general nutritional regimen
Muscles relax under the influence of hormones	Constipation or diarrhoea, +/− vomiting or nausea	Swim, walk, exercise, perineal massage/Epi-No, TENS
Cervix begins to thin and soften, starts to open to 2–3 cm	Mild-to-moderate regular or irregular contractions	Baths, showers, heat packs
Early phase of first stage of labour		
Contractions become closer, more regular and intensify	Show – mucus plug; vaginal discharge may be clear, pink or bright red	Hydrate after every contraction; electrolytes; nourish with food
Cervix opens to 3–4 cm	Membranes may rupture	Homeopathics, magnesium
Contractions last 45–60 seconds	Need to use deeper breaths during contractions	Essential oils, showers, heat packs
Baby's head moves further into pelvis		Visualisation, breathing, massage; watch for regularity of contractions
Active phase/established first stage of labour		
Cervix opening from 4 cm to 7–8 cm	Membranes may rupture	Ice cubes and electrolytes between contractions; empty bladder every 2 hours
Contractions stronger, longer (≥45–60 seconds) and closer together	'Show' with blood may pass	Homeopathics, magnesium (dermal)
Baby's head moving lower	Contractions require full attention	Essential oils, shower, heat packs
	Focus moves inwards	Visualisation, breathing, massage, pelvic rocking, change positions frequently
Transition/end of first stage of labour		
Cervix opens from 7–8 to 10 cm or fully dilated	Leg cramps and shaking; nausea +/− vomiting; need to open bowels; hot and perspiring or cold and shivering	Bath or shower; ice cubes and electrolytes between contractions
Contractions very strong and close together (1–2 minutes apart or back to back)	Heavy bloodstained show	Magnesium gel
Contractions last mostly 60–70 seconds	Pressure in bottom, lower back	Essential oils massaged into feet
	Feels like everything too much, 'not wanting to do this anymore', out of control	Homeopathic gelsemium
Resting phase of second stage of labour		
Cervix fully dilated	No urge to push = rest and wait	Bath or shower, ice cubes and electrolytes between contractions
Baby descends and rotates in the pelvis		Essential oils massaged into feet; magnesium gel
Contractions 5+ minutes apart		Homeopathic gelsemium

	TABLE 13.10 Stages of labour and support options—cont'd	
Body changes	**Sensation and responses**	**Naturopathic support**
Pushing phase of second stage of labour		
Baby moves out of the uterus, through the pelvis and down the vagina	Urge to push	Relax between pushes; use gravity, bath, shower and position
Pushing for 20 minutes to 2 hours	May open bowels	Ice cubes and electrolytes between contractions
Baby's head crowns	Burning and stretching as baby's head crowns	Listen to body cues for timing of pushes to prevent tearing
Birth of the baby		
Third stage of labour		
Uterus contracts, placenta separates and comes down and out of the vagina	Mild contractions/afterpains	Remain in upright position to assist with placental detachment
Delivery of placenta usually within 5–30 minutes	Some bleeding	Give gentle pushes with a contraction or cramping
	Sore bottom, perineum, vagina	Put baby to breast to stimulate placental release from suckling

Source: Adapted from Hechtman L. Pregnancy intensive seminar: the fundamentals for health professionals. Sydney: Integria; 2014.

Lochia rubra is the blood loss straight after birth; it is red and often of significant volume until contractions and haemostasis of the placental attachment site occurs. Once haemostasis is achieved, the flow rapidly decreases and progressively changes to brownish red with a more watery consistency – this is known as lochia serosa. Finally, the discharge diminishes and becomes more yellow – this is known as lochia alba. Lochia lasts for about 6 weeks. Some women may experience an increase in bleeding 7–14 days postnatally: this is due to the eschar of the placental site sloughing off and this time represents the biggest risk for postpartum haemorrhage (PPH).

PPH is a serious condition and can become an emergency. It is characterised by a notable increase in bleeding, clots, fever, cramping, hypotension and signs of blood loss. It may be due to bleeding at the placental site or retained placental tissue and infection. The woman needs to attend the emergency department of the closest hospital and will probably require antibiotics, dilation and evacuation of retained tissue, intravenous fluids and possibly blood or iron transfusion.

The cervix rapidly returns to its pre-pregnancy state, although it never fully returns to a nulliparous state. By 7 days the external os is largely closed. The vagina likewise regresses but never fully returns to a nulliparous state. The increased vascularity and oedema of pregnancy and labour resolve within 3–4 weeks and vaginal rugae reappear in non-lactating women. Women who are breastfeeding will have reduced oestrogen, which may cause vaginal dryness and discomfort during sex, so use of a lubricant is recommended. Sex is discouraged until 6 weeks postnatally to allow healing and reduce the risk of infection and trauma.

The perineum is stretched and traumatised during vaginal birth and may be torn or an episiotomy performed. In birth without significant tears or cuts the swollen and engorged vulva rapidly resolves and returns to normal by about 2 weeks. Most of the muscle tone is regained within 6 weeks, with the remainder of improvement more gradual over the following months. The rate of recovery is dependent on pre-labour muscle tone and the degree of trauma to soft tissue, muscle, nerve and connecting walls.

AFTERPAINS

The uterus will be painful due to the work of labour; it is also still contracting during involution and this may be more painful than expected.

Treatment

- Antispasmodics/uterine tonics: *Mitchella repens* (squaw vine), *Viburnum opulus* (cramp bark), *Viburnum prunifolium* (black haw), *Leonurus cardiaca* (motherwort), *Rubus idaeus* (raspberry leaf) – these herbs do not cause excess uterine laxity that would exacerbate bleeding, but rather improve tone and reduce uncoordinated contractions and pain.[49]
- Haemostatics: *Achillea millefolium* (yarrow), *Mitchella repens* (squaw vine), *Capsella bursa-pastoris* (shepherd's purse)
- Adaptogenic: *Withania somnifera* (ashwagandha)
- Nutritive: *Urtica dioica folia* (nettle leaf), *Rubus idaeus* (raspberry leaf)
- Magnesium and calcium for muscle cramps.

PERINEAL CARE

Sitz baths, sprays, ice blocks and compresses are very effective to soothe and cool swollen and often hot tissue and the following herbs are applicable:

- Astringents: *Achillea millefolium, Hamamelis virginiana*
- Vulnerary: *Calendula officinalis, Centella asiatica*
- Antiseptics: *Commiphora mol mol, Salvia officinalis*
- Analgesics: *Lavandula angustifolia.*

The pelvic floor will be affected regardless of the method of delivery due to the effect of fetal growth and stretching of ligaments, increased intra-abdominal pressure and hormones such as relaxin. A referral to a physiotherapist or continence nurse consultant can provide additional assessment, education and support for women postnatally. The resumption of ovarian function and ovulation is determined by lactation. The average time to resume ovarian activity in a non-breastfeeding woman is around 8 weeks.

EXHAUSTION

Fatigue is inevitable and care should be taken to ensure that the fatigue is not excessive or due to pathology such as infection, hypothyroidism or anaemia. In addition to excellent nutritional support, herbal medicine to support adrenal function, the nervous system and energy can be very valuable. Herbs to consider include: *Withania somnifera, Urtica dioica, Angelica polymorpha, Codonopsis pilosa, Verbena officinalis, Rhodiola rosea, Eleutherococcus senticosus, Avena sativa, Centella asiatica* and *Melissa officinalis.*

CAESAREAN SECTION

A caesarean birth involves major abdominal surgery. In addition to postnatal considerations, the mother will benefit from regular postoperative strategies to support wound healing and reduce the risk of infection. Surgical procedures have associated risks of infection, wound breakdown, formation of abdominal adhesions, haemorrhage, anaesthetic complications and reactions, injury to other organs, uterine atony, placenta praevia and placenta accreta, extended hospital stay and recovery time and increased maternal mortality. An emergency caesarean has higher risks than an elective procedure. A caesarean birth may also be the only way a distressed neonate can be delivered alive and a haemorrhaging mother saved.[370] The incidence of placenta praevia and placenta accreta has increased in frequency corresponding with the increased rate of caesarean births, and for caesarean hysterectomy, placenta accreta may be the most common indication.[370]

A further aspect for the mother may be a sense of failure and of becoming redundant when she is unable to birth vaginally. This feeling may influence the development or severity of postnatal depression.[371] In addition, after a caesarean birth there is often a lengthy delay in skin-to-skin contact between mother and infant.[372] A Cochrane Review reported that skin-to-skin contact is associated with longer duration of breastfeeding, helps the newborn's cardiorespiratory stability, decreases infant crying and may enhance the relationship between mother and infant.[373] A further review found that skin-to-skin contact may increase breastfeeding initiation, reduce formula supplementation in hospital, increase bonding and maternal satisfaction, support the newborn's temperature and reduce newborn stress.[374] It is still possible in many instances to have skin-to-skin contact after a caesarean, but it will take a significant change of practice for it to become routine.[372]

Risks for offspring born via caesarean section are becoming more apparent with increased incidence and research. One particular area of interest is the lack of transfer of vaginal microbiota to the infant during delivery and the subsequent impact on the development of intestinal microbiota.[375] Recent findings include the following:

- Caesarean delivery may contribute to the pathogenesis of disease by deferring the establishment of the infant microbiota, thereby affecting the microbiota's central role in metabolism and immune maturation including switching from T-helper 2–dominated to T-helper 1–dominated cellular immunity. Administration of antibiotics before and during surgery adds another component to the risk that is yet to be fully explored. Infants born vaginally have a greater proportion of *Bifidobacterium* and *Bacteroides* than those born surgically, who have higher levels of *Clostridium* and *Staphylococcus*[376]
- Caesarean birth has been associated with a greater risk of asthma, diabetes and cancer later in life and research has identified epigenetic changes in newborn haematopoietic stem cells following caesareans. It has been proposed that epigenetic changes include altered methylation processing involved with immunoglobulin synthesis, regulation of glycolysis and ketone metabolism and regulation of the response to food[377]
- There is an increased risk of overweight and obesity for offspring born by caesarean delivery. A study of 10 219 children (926 born by caesarean section) found that caesarean delivery was consistently associated with adiposity at 6 weeks of age and this association was even stronger if the children were born from obese mothers. Additionally, by age 11 these children were 1.83 times more likely to be overweight or obese[378]
- There is a moderate but significantly increased risk of developing inflammatory bowel disease.[379] A 2014 meta-analysis confirmed the increased risk of Crohn's disease but not ulcerative colitis.[380] The mechanism may be influenced by disturbances to the microbiota of the child, compromised barrier function and altered immune function[381]
- A retrospective study of 1950 children found an increased risk of Coeliac disease for children born by caesarean delivery[382]
- There is an increased risk of asthma and atopy with caesarean delivery[376]
- Autism spectrum disorder (ASD), a neurological condition, is associated with GI symptoms and early microbiome disruption may be implicated. Elevated

inflammatory markers (reflective of microbiota composition) are also a feature of ASD. Animal studies show that exposure to *Bifidobacterium* or *Lactobacillus* species modulate behaviour.[376]

Post-caesarean recovery

- Nutrients to support tissue healing: vitamin A, zinc, vitamin C, protein
- Anti-inflammatory and antioxidant nutrients: vitamin C, CoQ10, ALA, vitamin A, vitamin C, vitamin E and turmeric
- Herbal medicines to reduce inflammation, infection and support tissue healing: *Curcuma longa, Centella asiatica, Calendula officinalis* and *Echinacea* spp.

Vaginal seeding

Vaginal seeding is the postnatal transfer of vaginal fluid from the mother to the newborn birthed via caesarean section and has been shown to enhance the microbiota profile of the newborn. Long-term outcomes have yet to be observed but theoretically this practice could reduce some of the negative effects of caesarean birth.[383]

PERINATAL DEPRESSION

While most research and focus is on postnatal depression (PND) and anxiety, it is important to recognise that these issues are significant during pregnancy and indeed may predict postnatal mental health issues. Furthermore, depression and anxiety are a concern for up to 10% of fathers.[384] Neither the International Classification of Diseases 10 (ICD-10) nor the Diagnostic and Statistical Manual of Mental Disorders, Fifth Edition (DSM-5) recognises postnatal depression as a discrete diagnosis. According to the DSM-5 the diagnosis is based on meeting the criteria for a major depressive episode and with a perinatal onset (during pregnancy or within 4 weeks of childbirth).[385] The DSM-5 criteria for a major depressive episode are as follows:

a Five or more out of the following 9 symptoms (including at least one of depressed mood and loss of interest or pleasure) in the same 2-week period. Each of these symptoms represents a change from previous functioning and needs to be present nearly every day:
  1 Depressed mood (subjective or observed); can be irritable mood in children and adolescents, most of the day
  2 Loss of interest or pleasure, most of the day
  3 Change in weight or appetite. Weight: 5% change over 1 month
  4 Insomnia or hypersomnia
  5 Psychomotor retardation or agitation (observed)
  6 Loss of energy or fatigue
  7 Worthlessness or guilt
  8 Impaired concentration or indecisiveness or
  9 Recurrent thoughts of death or suicidal ideation or attempt.
b Symptoms cause significant distress or impairment.
c Episode is not attributable to a substance or medical condition.
d Episode is not better explained by a psychotic disorder.
e There has never been a manic or hypomanic episode. Exclusion e) does not apply if a (hypo)manic episode was substance-induced or attributable to a medical condition.

Other sources identify that PND may commence up to 1 year after childbirth.[386] There is lack of agreement about the definition or duration of the postpartum period and it appears that the peak of PND episodes is around 90 days or 13 weeks, outside both the DSM-5 and ICD-10 time frames.[387]

The prevalence of perinatal depression varies, but it has been assessed to be 12.7% during pregnancy and 21.9% postnatally, making PND a major and common complication of pregnancy and childbirth.[387]

Pathogenesis and aetiology

Depression, including perinatal depression, is complex and multifactorial. Genetic factors, acute and/or chronic stress, trauma and loss, and biochemical and hormonal balances may all contribute. A summary of possible pathological pathways follows:

- Dysregulation and volume reduction in critical brain areas such as the anterior cingulate cortex, the amygdala and the hippocampus, possibly due to increased levels of glucocorticoids which they are sensitive to[388]
- HPA axis dysregulation due to elevated cortisol and corticotropin-releasing hormone, and reduced serotonin[388]
- Elevated TSH and lower thyroxine[389,390]; late pregnancy elevated TBG is a strong predictor of PND[391] – TBG concentrations increase markedly during pregnancy and may be an index of sensitivity to elevated oestrogen levels
- A hormone-sensitive phenotype in whom reproductive hormone fluctuations trigger affective dysregulation[392]
- Increased amygdala activation, low serotonin, low melatonin, autoimmunity and increased systemic inflammation[108]
- Low omega-3 fatty acid intake – associated with major depressive episodes and PND.

Risk factors

Psychosocial and genetic factors and medical and reproductive history are related to the risk for PND. The most significant risk is a personal history of depression. A family history of depression and a lack of partner support also increase the risk of postpartum depression.

WHO identifies the following factors that increase the risk of poor maternal mental health, especially in under-resourced settings: poverty and chronic social adversity, crowded living conditions, gender-based violence, lack of autonomy to make sexual and reproductive decisions, unintended pregnancy (especially among adolescent women), lack of empathy from partner and gender stereotypes about the division of household work and infant care, excessive workload and severe occupational fatigue, lack of emotional and practical support or criticism, gender discrimination and devaluing of women, negative reproductive outcomes and poor physical health.[393] Some groups of women at greater risk due to social, economic and political factors include Aboriginal or Torres Strait Islander women, women from culturally and linguistically diverse backgrounds, refugees – including those who have resettled under a refugee program – women living in regional, rural or remote areas, adolescent mothers and homeless women.[384]

Other risk factors include pregnancy ill-health and complications, negative birth experience, unsettled/unwell baby, medical condition (including low thyroid function, chronic autoimmune disease, anaemia), unrealistic expectations about motherhood and perfectionism, pessimism and low resilience, use of ART, postpartum fatigue and sleeplessness, and pregnancy loss.

Assessment

The most commonly used scale to assess for PND is the validated brief Edinburgh Postnatal Depression Scale (EPDS), which a set of 10 questions where symptoms are rated (see Appendix 13.2). This scale can be used prenatally and postnatally and should be repeated during this period. Assess the presence of risk factors and identify and treat other causes for the presenting symptoms (e.g. anaemia). Hypothyroidism is a particular risk and has overlapping symptoms with PND.

Clinical features

In addition to the features listed in the DSM-5, specialist postnatal services identify the following clinical features of PND:
- Change in appetite: under- or overeating
- Sleep problems unrelated to the baby's needs
- Extreme lethargy – a feeling of being physically or emotionally overwhelmed and unable to cope with the demands of chores and looking after the baby
- Memory problems or loss of concentration ('brain fog')
- Loss of confidence and lowered self-esteem; feeling a failure as a parent
- Constant sadness or crying
- Withdrawal from friends and family
- Fear of being alone with the baby
- Intrusive thoughts of self-harm or of harming the baby
- Irritability and/or anger
- Increased alcohol or drug use
- Loss of interest in sex or previously enjoyed activities
- Thoughts of death or suicide
- Agoraphobia
- Fatigue
- The development of obsessive or compulsive behaviours.[384]

Naturopathic approach

A naturopathic approach to managing PND included the following:
- Appropriate assessment
- Supporting the nervous system and maintaining balanced neurotransmitter levels (synthesis, release, receptor binding, intracellular signalling)
- Reducing stress (and thus excessive cortisol and HPA dysregulation)
- Supporting adrenal gland function
- Ensuring adequate sleep and supporting melatonin secretion
- Supporting nutritional intake and correcting deficiencies
- Addressing biochemical imbalances/deficiencies
- Maintaining stable BSL (to ensure optimal neuronal ATP production and stabilise energy levels)
- Ensuring adequate hydration
- Supporting continued breastfeeding, as required
- Supporting and referring, as required, for psychological intervention.

Nutrition

Nutritional status, particularly low levels of EFAs, folate and B_{12}, has been shown to affect depression. Membrane phospholipids mediate the entrance of neurotransmitters into the cell and low levels of omega-3 fatty acids may impede this process.[394] Furthermore, low levels of serotonin, dopamine and noradrenaline may reduce the synthesis of SAMe, a universal methyl donor that contributes to the production of membrane phospholipids and the synthesis of neurotransmitters. Elevated homocysteine is associated with inflammation, as are low omega-3 fatty acids. Omega-3 fatty acids increase neuronal membrane fluidity, decrease inflammation and inflammatory cytokines, and increase the production of brain-derived neurotrophic factor and thus the synthesis, binding and uptake of neurotransmitters. Depression is associated with inflammation, so avoidance of inflammatory foods (red meat, burnt foods, sugar, caffeine, alcohol) and an increase of anti-inflammatory foods (oily fish, fresh fruit and vegetables, nuts and seeds) is recommended.

SUPPLEMENTATION

The following guidelines are provided for supplementation:
- Omega-3 fatty acids – research in pregnancy has been mixed but has shown requirements for higher doses of DHA and EPA[395]: 2–3 g EPA/DHA daily plus a reduction in omega-6 intake
- SAMe may reduce prolactin therefore use with caution – there is evidence of efficacy in non-pregnancy related depression, but a paucity of research for PND. Ensure you consider the patient's methylation status prior to prescribing
- B complex
- Zinc
- Vitamin D.

HERBAL MEDICINE

There is scant research specific to the use of herbal medicine to manage PND. If prescribing herbal medicine while the mother is lactating, ensure there are no contraindications.
- Antidepressants: *Hypericum perforatum*, *Melissa officinalis*, *Passiflora incarnate*, *Lavandula officinalis*, *Crocus sativa*

- Adaptogens/adrenals: *Withania somnifera, Rehmannia glutinosa, Eleutherococcus senticosus, Glycyrrhiza glabra*
- Nervines: *Avena sativa, Verbena officinalis, Matricaria chamomilla, Leonurus cardiaca, Scutellaria lateriflora*
- Anxiolytics: *Lavandula officinalis, Leonurus cardiaca, Scutellaria lateriflora*
- Blood tonics: *Urtica dioica, Angelica polymorpha, Withania somnifera, Rehmannia glutinosa.*

PHARMACEUTICAL TREATMENT

Women may be apprehensive about disclosing anxiety and depression due to stigma, fear and concerns regarding pharmaceutical intervention. It is important to establish trust and rapport and to encourage open communication. Some pharmaceuticals have been linked to adverse infant outcomes (birth defects, low Apgar scores, neonatal pulmonary hypertension) – this includes anticonvulsants (may be used in severe depression), selective serotonin reuptake inhibitors, lithium and benzodiazepines. The risk may be primarily in utero or via breastmilk. The need for pharmaceutical intervention is made on a case-by-case basis and may be essential in severe cases, especially if a woman has suicidal ideation.[386]

POSTPARTUM THYROIDITIS

Postpartum thyroiditis (PPT) is defined as transient thyroid dysfunction in the first year after childbirth in women who were euthyroid before pregnancy.[284] The incidence of PPT is 4–9% and it is more common in women with type 1 diabetes.[396] In most cases it is an autoimmune disorder, a variant of Hashimoto's disease, but it can also occur in the absence of antibodies.[396]

Risk factors

Risk factors include a history of PPT in a prior pregnancy (69% recurrence rate during the subsequent pregnancy) and being thyroid peroxidase antibody positive at the end of the first trimester (up to 50%).[397] Other risk factors include high titres of TPOAb in the first trimester, a family or personal history of thyroid disease, the presence of a goitre, and smoking.[284]

Aetiology

The aetiology in most cases is autoimmune chronic (Hashimoto's) thyroiditis, with a few cases due to hypothalamic or pituitary lesions.[284] It is possible that the shift in immune function postpartum – with enhanced TH1 cell function, loss of tolerance for fetal alloantigens and enhanced immunoglobulin G (IgG) secretion and autoantibody secretion, which may be triggered by the marked drop in protective oestrogen and progesterone – is contributory.[396] The diagnosis is not always clear but is based on abnormal TSH levels (suppressed or elevated) during the first postpartum year, thyroid antibodies (antithyroid peroxidase, antithyroglobulin in particular), an enlarged thyroid gland and the possible presence of a toxic nodule.

Presentation

The clinical course of PPT is variable, but the 'classical' presentation is a transient hyperthyroid phase at 6 weeks to 6 months postpartum (median time of onset, 13 weeks) followed by a hypothyroid phase (median time of onset, 19 weeks) that may persist for up to 1 year after delivery before returning to the euthyroid state.[396] The variance in the course of PTT is seen in a review that showed that only 26% of patients presented in this classic manner and that most patients presented with hyperthyroidism alone (38%) or hypothyroidism alone (36%).[396] Symptoms of hyperthyroidism (anxiety, insomnia, palpitations, fatigue, weight loss and irritability) are often less overt than the subsequent symptoms of hypothyroidism (fatigue, weight gain, constipation, dry skin, depression and poor exercise tolerance).

Assessment considerations

The hyperthyroid phase may present as anxiety and the hypothyroid phase may present very similarly to depression and anaemia, thus using the EPDS and reviewing pathology are important. Assessments include thyroid antibodies (anti-TPO, anti-TG, TSH-receptor antibodies), thyroid function tests, a full blood count, iron studies, urinary iodine, red cell selenium, plasma zinc and copper.

Naturopathic management

The goal is to ameliorate symptoms, reduce autoimmune activity and support normal thyroid function. Specific interventions will be dependent on the symptoms, the pathology and the rest of the clinical history (including whether the woman is breastfeeding).

a Hyperthyroid/thyrotoxic phase
  – To normalise immune function: *Echinacea* spp., *Rehmannia glutinosa, Hemidesmus indicus*
  – To reduce hyperthyroid activity: *Melissa officinalis, Leonurus cardiaca*
  – To support the nervous system: *Withania somnifera, Passiflora incarnata*
  – Nutrients essential for normal thyroid function: selenium, zinc, iron
  – Avoid iodine and include goitrogens.

b Hypothyroid phase
  – To normalise immune function: *Echinacea* spp., *Rehmannia glutinosa, Hemidesmus indicus*
  – To support the nervous system: *Withania somnifera, Passiflora incarnata*
  – Nutrients essential for normal thyroid function: selenium, zinc, iron, iodine, tyrosine
  – Avoid soy, gluten and other goitrogens.

THE PREGNANCY CARE PLAN

The pregnancy care plan (see Table 13.11) provides a guide as to how appointments may be scheduled and should be adapted to practitioner and patient requirements.

TABLE 13.11 The pregnancy care plan		
Investigations and referrals	Intervention	Education
Appointment 1: week 4		
• Initial pregnancy screen – General history, obstetric history, emotional wellbeing – Nutritional assessment – Pathology (iron studies, thyroid etc.) – Urinalysis – Baseline: BP, weight, appearance, tongue, nails, hair, skin, digestion • Pregnancy care options – Referrals and recommendations – Overview of the pregnancy care plan	• Initial prescriptions – Essential nutrients – Additional support for NVP as required – Additional support to reduce risk of miscarriage, as indicated • Dietary – Listeria precautions and food hygiene – Meal planning – Pregnancy dos and don'ts	• Embryo development and critical periods • Embryo goals • Maternal goals • Risks and safety • Miscarriage signs, symptoms and advice • Initial pregnancy counselling and education • Prenatal testing • Infective screening awareness • Lifestyle – Exercise, topical preparations and exposure and cautions – Medications, smoking, alcohol, back care, drugs, emotional, occupational, financial and resources
Appointment 2: week 8		
• Review results • Assessments: BP, weight, fundal height • Update on other consultations (O&G, midwife, GP) and any assessments, scans and prescriptions	• Additional support for NVP, as required • Additional support to reduce risk of miscarriage, as indicated • Symptom support • Treatment adjustments as required based on pathology results	• Embryology education • Tips to deal with NVP and fatigue • Milestones of trimester 1 for mother and baby • General pregnancy counselling • Emotional support
Appointment 3: week 12		
• Assessments: BP, weight • Refer for further investigations, as required • Retest any pathology that was abnormal at initial assessment (e.g. vitamin D, iron) • Check sleep habits • Update on other consultations (O&G, midwife, GP) and any assessments and prescriptions	• Adjustments for trimester 2 – Dietary: calcium, vitamin D, iron, protein, EFAs, magnesium, iodine, choline, vitamin C, B vitamins, zinc – Prescriptions, as required – Lifestyle	• Trimester 2 education – Fetal goals – Maternal goals – Weight management in pregnancy – Advice re dental visit – General pregnancy counselling – Emotional support
Appointment 4: week 18		
• Assessments: BP, weight • Random blood glucose in clinic • Review thyroid symptoms • Emotional assessment, EPDS • Update on other consultations (O&G, midwife, GP) and any assessments and prescriptions	• Treatment review and adjustments, as required • Dietary: calcium, EFAs, iron, zinc, protein • Symptomatic support • Condition-specific support (PRN) • Assessment of need to adjust treatment to prevent weeks 19–24 potential issues (e.g. assess vitamin B status, especially B_{12}, EFAs)	• General review, counselling and education • Prevention for weeks 19–24 potential issues • Prenatal classes and resources
Appointment 5: week 24		
• Assessments: BP, weight • Pathology: FBC, iron studies, glucose/GTT, vitamin D, iodine and others, as indicated • Update on other consultations (O&G, midwife, GP) and any assessments and prescriptions	• Treatment review and adjustments, as required • Symptomatic support • Condition-specific support (e.g. blood glucose management) • Dietary: calcium, EFAs, iron, zinc, protein, magnesium	• General review, counselling and education • Dietary and lifestyle influences on BSL • Healthy weight management

TABLE 13.11 The pregnancy care plan—cont'd

Investigations and referrals	Intervention	Education
Appointment 6: week 28		

• Assessment: BP, weight, urinalysis
• Update on other consultations (O&G, midwife, GP) and any assessments and prescriptions
• Review of digestion and symptoms
	• Treatment adjustments for trimester 3 maternal and fetal growth, including accounting for zinc sequestration and copper retention
	• Prevention of restless legs; electrolyte assessment and education
	• GORD, constipation
	• Dietary: zinc, protein, iron, calcium, EFA, magnesium, vitamin D, folate/B vitamins, iodine
		• Trimester 3 education
		  – Fetal goals
		  – Maternal goals
		  – Birthing education; reading and resources
		  – Dietary guidelines
		  – Immune preparation (maternal and infant immunity, exposure, vaccinations)
		  – Advice to carry Maternity Record Card

Appointment 7: week 32		

• Assessment: BP, weight, urinalysis, emotional assessment, EPDS
• Pathology, review if already taken, consider:
  – FBC, blood type
  – UEC, LFT, ESR, CRP
  – Iron studies
  – Folate and B_{12}
  – Serum zinc/copper
  – Fasting homocysteine
  – 25 OHD_3
  – Fasting glucose
  – Thyroid function
	• Phase 1 birth treatment
	  – Partus preparator
	  – General review, counselling and treatment adjustments
		• Phase 1 birth education
		  – Partus preparator
		  – Creating a birth plan
		  – Cord blood banking
		  – When to clamp the cord
		  – Physiological vs active third stage of labour
		  – Vaginal seeding

Appointment 8: week 36		

• Assessment: BP, weight
• Pathology: review based on week 32 investigations and results
• Vaginal swab for group B streptococcus (with GP, midwife or O&G)
• Review sleep, anxiety, fatigue
	• Phase 2 birth treatment
	  – Labour preparation
	  – Anxiety and labour support
	  – General review, counselling and treatment adjustments
		• Phase 2 birth education:
		  – Labour preparation
		  – Anxiety and labour support
		  – Checklist for hospital for mother and baby
		  – Checklist for home for mother and baby
		  – Postpartum recovery diet

Appointment 9: week 38		

• Assessment: BP, weight
• Review sleep, anxiety, fatigue
	• Phase 3 birth treatment
	  – Breastfeeding preparation
	  – Final pre-labour review
	  – General review, counselling and treatment adjustments
		• Phase 3 birth education:
		  – Breastfeeding preparation
		  – Final pre-labour review
		  – Review and educate regarding PND and anxiety
		  – Trimester 4 resources and support

As required: weeks 38–40/42		
Phone support before and after birth, as required Call day 3–5 • Birth experience, debrief • Analgesia, afterpains • Perineal trauma and care; caesarean section • Blood loss, breastfeeding – lactation consultant, breastfeeding support services		
Appointment 10: 2 weeks postpartum		

• Assessment:
  – Emotional wellbeing
  – Support available and required
  – Baby health
  – Referrals to other clinicians and for investigations, as required
  – EPDS
	• Fourth trimester support and treatment
	  – Postpartum review: mode of birth, lochia, breastfeeding support
	  – Neonatal review: weight gain, feeding, sleeping, nappies (urine and faeces)
		• Fourth trimester education
		  – Breastfeeding
		  – Neonatology
		  – Normalise, counsel and support
		  – Listen to birth story
		  – Connect to local community and support network (mothercraft nurse etc.)
		  – Fatigue and exhaustion

Continued

TABLE 13.11 The pregnancy care plan—cont'd		
Mother	**Infant**	**Education**
Appointment 11: 6 weeks postpartum		

• Postpartum check-up
  – Diastasis rectis assessment[a]
  – Uterine retraction[a]
  – Lochia cessation
  – Breastfeeding
  – Contraception
  – Sleep deprivation
  – Mood and attachment
  – Labour/pregnancy trauma
  – Pathology review, if indicated
    (thyroid, BSL, Fe, FBC)
  – Provide referral for investigations
    before 3/12 postpartum review
	• Neonatal check-up
	  – Sleep
	  – Digestion
	  – Temperament
	  – Reflexes[b]
	  – Measurements: weight, height,
	    length[b]
	  – Feeding
		• Pelvic floor education
		• Tips for newborns, including support options
		  and services
		• Baby formula guide if formula feeding or
		  complementary feeding
		• Emotional support and network
		• Refer for Pap smear, if indicated
		• Nourishing the mother; dietary, lifestyle,
		  social, emotional and spiritual
		• Vaccination education and resources
		• Sexual activity, contraception, lubrication

Appointment 12: 12 weeks postpartum		

• Postpartum check-up
  – Review pathology results and
    nutritional status
  – Pelvic floor
  – Mood and support; EPDS
  – Breastfeeding/formula feeding
	• Infant check up
	  – Sleep
	  – Digestion
	  – Temperament
	  – Reflexes[b]
	  – Measurements: weight, height,
	    length[b]
	  – Feeding
		• Introduction of solids education and
		  preparation
		• Pelvic floor
		• Maternal reproductive health
		• Planning for next pregnancies and fertility
		  generally; pregnancy spacing
		• Vaccination discussion

Note: [a]These assessments are performed by the midwife, child and family health nurse, GP or obstetrician. [b]These assessments are performed by the child and family health nurse or GP.
Source: Adapted from Hechtman L. Pregnancy intensive seminar: the fundamentals for health professionals. Sydney: Integria; 2014.

CASE STUDY 1: ECZEMA AND GDM

OVERVIEW

RP was 38 years old and 22 weeks pregnant with her second child; she presented for assistance managing her blood glucose and to reduce the likelihood of her second child having atopic conditions that she, her husband and her first child had.

RP had previously sought assistance in managing her eczema, which was now well controlled (only occasional mild flares during periods of significant stress). Her diet was a healthy balance of nutrients and was rich in fruit and vegetables, and she exercised regularly. She was taking a pregnancy formula and an omega-3 EFA supplement, which she commenced about 10 weeks before conception. Her first pregnancy was uncomplicated and she delivered a healthy daughter at term via NVD.

Her past history included eczema, which affected her face, torso and arms and was severe enough to impact on her ability to work and fulfil her ADLs. Her preconception BMI was 26.9 kg/m² and she did not retain any of the 13 kg GWG from her first pregnancy. Her husband PB had hay fever and no other medical conditions.

INVESTIGATIONS

All of RP's pathology testing had been within the normal range, although her recent GTT (performed at 20 weeks) was borderline, as follows:

	20 weeks results	**GDM threshold**
Fasting glucose	4.9 mmol/L	≥5.0 mmol/L
1-hour glucose	9.6 mmol/L	≥10.0 mmol/L
2-hour glucose	8.4 mmol/L	≥8.5 mmol/L

These results were within the normal range but very close to exceeding the threshold so her obstetrician referred her to an endocrinologist and the pregnancy diabetes clinic, and a repeat GTT was scheduled for 28 weeks. In addition to wanting to avoid developing GDM and the associated risks, RP was anxious to avoid requiring insulin injections as she had a fear of needles.

MANAGEMENT

RP attended the diabetes clinic and kept a diet diary and monitored her blood glucose at home. She continued to attend group exercise (modified for pregnancy) twice a week and aimed to walk 30–50 minutes on the remaining days. Her diet was already nutritious and varied so the main adjustment was to ensure she was getting adequate protein (approximately 1.2 g/kg) and that her carbohydrates were low GI.

SAMPLE DAILY DIET

Breakfast	Scrambled eggs, mushrooms, tomato and gluten-free toast Smoothie made with dairy or almond milk and frozen berries, LSA, baby spinach, whey protein powder, dessertspoon of nut butter and ice Homemade baked beans and poached egg Mixed grain porridge with home-made stewed pears
Lunch	Large mixed salad with chicken and dressed with olive oil and lemon juice Leftover roast vegetables, hummus, cannellini beans, pepitas and pesto Lamb, red lentil and vegetable stew
Dinner	Mixed steamed vegetables with fish, chicken or beef Stir-fry with bok choy, capsicum, mushrooms, garlic, onion, corn, zucchini, chicken and brown basmati rice Barbeque with mixed salads
Snacks	Rye crackers with nut butter Occasional chocolate Fruit with natural yoghurt Mixed nuts and seeds Small smoothie Nut butter on toast
Drinks	Water Herbal tea

Supplementation

RP wanted to minimise the number of tablets/capsules she had to take but was keen to support her pregnancy as best she could. In addition, while she had previously taken both liquid and tablet forms of herbal medicine with good effect, she wanted to be extra cautious in this pregnancy and did not want herbal medicine now. The naturopath recommended the following supplements for RP:

- Prenatal formula
- Zinc: 30 mg
- Magnesium: 600 mg
- Selenium: 50 micrograms
- EFAs: DHA 400 mg, EPA 600 mg
- Vitamin D_3: 2000 IU
- Probiotics containing *Lactobacillus rhamnosus LGG* 2 billion CFU plus other strains including *Acidophilus* and *Bifidobacterium*, totalling more than 25 billion CFU.

The zinc, selenium, vitamin D and probiotics could be added to food, reducing the number of tablets/capsules RP

needed to take. The prenatal formula contains adequate folate and B_{12}. Specifically, magnesium supports glucose metabolism and was to reduce the occasional leg cramps RP experienced. Selenium is an important antioxidant and has been shown to reduce plasma glucose, insulin and CRP and is also helpful in atopy. EFAs support glucose metabolism, reduce inflammation and atopy and are routine inclusions in pregnancy supplementation. Vitamin D is important in immune system development and function in the fetus, including reducing atopy. Probiotics may reduce GDM as well as reducing atopy and allergies in the offspring.

FOLLOW-UP

RP attended for review every 4–6 weeks during her pregnancy and gained a total of 12.6 kg. Her GTT at 28 weeks was a follows:

	28 weeks	20 weeks	GDM threshold
Fasting glucose	4.1 mmol/L	4.9 mmol/L	≥5.0 mmol/L
1-hour glucose	8.2 mmol/L	9.6 mmol/L	≥10.0 mmol/L
2-hour glucose	6.3 mmol/L	8.4 mmol/L	≥8.5 mmol/L

Due to the reduction in GTT and normal random glucose test results (with the exception of one result after eating birthday cake) the obstetrician did not repeat the GTT and relied on fasting and random glucose for the remainder of the pregnancy, all of which were normal.

RP gave birth via NVD at 38 weeks to a healthy daughter and had normal blood glucose when checked in the 20 months since birth. She lost most of her GWG and continued to eat a balanced diet. At 20 months her daughter showed no evidence of the eczema that was pronounced with her older sister.

CASE STUDY 2: WEIGHT MANAGEMENT AND NVP

OVERVIEW

LB first presented for preconception care. She and her husband CS were healthy, in their late 20s and neither had any diagnosed medical conditions. LB had always been slim (as are her mother and sisters) until she spent 12 months doing volunteer aid work in developing nations, during which time her weight dropped significantly and her BMI was 17.1 kg/m². All of her pathology results were normal and bio-impedance assessment showed a body fat of 18% and lean muscle mass at the lower end of normal. LB increased her intake of nutrient and kilojoule-dense foods and added strength training to the jogging and yoga she was already doing. As a result her weight and muscle mass increased moderately prior to conception.

LB attended at 9 weeks into her pregnancy and had nausea and vomiting all day. While that was unpleasant, she was more concerned about her baby not receiving adequate nutrition and about losing weight. LB was vomiting 2–4 times a day with the main triggers being the smell of coffee and raw animal products (fish, poultry, meat). She took prenatal nutrient supplements and these did not appear to worsen her nausea.

MANAGEMENT

LB had good preparation for pregnancy, including a nutrient-dense diet, and this probably provided some protection against the fetus suffering nutrient deficiency; knowing this reassured her.

Dietary strategies

- All food preparation that involved animal products (except eggs, which LB could cook without problems) was undertaken by her husband and LB ensured that she was as far away from cooking smells as possible – for instance, she often went for a walk or had a shower while her husband cooked
- LB had small snacks every 1–2 hours, including having crackers and cheese on her bedside table which she could eat when she regularly woke feeling nauseated at about 3 am. She also had a small snack before getting up in the morning
- LB ate kilojoule- and nutrient-dense foods like avocado, nut butter, eggs and protein balls (including dates, mixed nut butters, pepitas, coconut and sometimes ginger)
- LB also drank ginger tea and chamomile tea.

Supplementation

In addition to the prenatal formula and omega-3 EFAs, LB took:
- vitamin B$_6$ 50 mg three times a day
- *Zingiber officinalis* tablets 400 g of dried root two to three times a day, as required.

FOLLOW-UP

LB's NVP reduced significantly to a mild nausea in the morning before breakfast and resolved completely by 14 weeks gestation. LB gained a total of 1.4 kg in the first trimester (1–2 kg is normal weight gain for this trimester). The remainder of her pregnancy was uncomplicated and she gained a total of 14.6 kg and delivered a healthy baby at term. She maintained a healthy weight postnatally and breastfed for 18 months.

CASE STUDY 3: POSTNATAL ANXIETY AND DEPRESSION

OVERVIEW

ME was 32 years old and presented with postnatal anxiety and depression 3 months after the birth of her son. ME had a history of anxiety in her early 20s and at that time consulted a psychologist for several months who provided effective support and strategies. ME had not experienced any significant anxiety or depression until 2 months postnatally, at

which time her partner DF took ME to her GP for review, as she was concerned about ME. The GP diagnosed PND and anxiety, recommended antidepressants and provided a referral to a psychologist. ME discussed with the GP and her partner that she wanted to try counselling support before commencing on medication as she had had a positive response previously. The GP, ME and DF agreed to trial this and ME was to return for review in 2 weeks or sooner, if required. ME denied suicidal ideation.

ME's pregnancy was her third, with two previous terminations. Her son was conceived via IVF using donor sperm from a friend and conception was achieved on the second attempt. Her diet was mixed during her pregnancy with low intake of vegetables and only intermittent intake of a prenatal supplement. She had a caesarean birth as labour was not progressing after 28 hours and the baby was showing signs of distress. Her immediate postnatal and postoperative recovery was uncomplicated. ME struggled with breastfeeding and her baby was exclusively bottle-fed. ME was an auditor and had 12 months maternity leave; DF was a computer technician and had 4 weeks off after the birth before going back to work full-time.

ME's previous history included a motor vehicle accident and fractured femur at the age of 21 and occasionally mild seasonal hay fever. ME experienced headaches when over-tired and/or dehydrated. She reported that she was told all of her blood tests and scans during pregnancy were normal.

ASSESSMENT

ME was sleeping poorly, on average 3–4 hours of broken sleep per night and occasional short naps during the day, and had very poor energy levels. Her son slept for 6–8 hours overnight and was very settled, but ME felt she should check on him very frequently. DF provided support when she was home and although they had several friends who might be able to help ME was reluctant to accept that she needed assistance and support. She felt inadequate and anxious that she would fail to raise her son safely and competently. She thought other mothers were 'naturals at motherhood' and that she was some kind of fraud. She felt 'stuck' and couldn't find the motivation to do the washing or to shower and get dressed into day clothes. She also felt a bit numb and did not want to leave the house or see people, and DF felt that ME was shutting down and shutting her out.

ME had little interest in food and only ate 'because she had to', which was a significant change from before her pregnancy when dining out and cooking were enjoyable pastimes. Her diet was lacking in essential fatty acids, complex carbohydrates, fruit and vegetables, and protein; she ate processed cereal and milk for breakfast, toast with margarine and jam or chocolate spread for lunch and pasta or steak and vegetables for dinner. She snacked on biscuits and sweets and drank 4–6 cups of espresso coffee per day. She drank no water and rarely ate fruit or nuts and seeds. Most nights ME and DF shared at least a bottle of red wine to help them unwind and get to sleep.

ME's hair was lank and her skin mildly pale and a bit sallow. Her nails were soft and her gums bled when she brushed her teeth. Her BP was 126/72 and her pulse was 62 and regular. ME gained 21 kg during her pregnancy and so far had lost 5 kg. She was a healthy body weight before her pregnancy. She reported her urine as being a bit concentrated and that her bowels opened every 2–3 days with the stool hard and pebble-like.

Pathology

FBC, EUC, LFT, MTHFR: nil abnormalities detected
TSH: 2.89 mIU/L
Urinary iodine: 83 micrograms/L
Serum copper:zinc ratio: 1.67
Serum vitamin D: 38 nmol/L
Serum iron: 27 micromol/L
Ferritin: 28 pmol/L
hsCRP: 11 mg/L

TREATMENT GOALS

- Improved nutritional status
- Reduced/eliminated symptoms of depression and anxiety
- Improved sleep
- Improved energy
- Normal thyroid, adrenal and nervous system function
- Reduced/eliminated inflammation
- Regular bowel motions and normal stool.

TREATMENT STRATEGIES

ME was referred to a psychologist who specialised in perinatal mental health and who had also given ME contacts for PND support groups and online resources. ME had not seen a dentist since before she was pregnant and planned to do so.

ME and DF were encouraged to spend time outdoors – for example, walking around the river path, having lunch in the park and going for walks. ME was encouraged to go for a 30-minute walk every day. ME wanted to get back into yoga so investigated online options and DF offered to stay home with their baby so ME could attend classes. Both ME and DF were encouraged to keep connected with their family and friends and to accept offers of help if appropriate.

DIETARY SUGGESTIONS

It was important not to increase ME's sense of not coping by recommending a complex and difficult meal plan and to not unnecessarily draw on her limited energy. Where possible DF cooked the evening meal and some meals were batch-prepared and frozen for the times when both were too tired to cook or had run out of fresh food. A home-delivery service was used to obtain fresh fruit and vegetables, eggs, nuts and seeds. This enabled one or both of them to shop once a fortnight for other supplies such as meat, and DF picked up milk on the way home from work. They tried a home-delivery meal service for a short period but didn't like the choices and restrictions. ME was advised to drink water consistently during the day and she did this by ensuring that she drank a glass of water whenever she fed her son. The diet focused on low-GI foods (and removing sweets to help stabilise blood glucose and energy levels), having nutrient-dense wholefoods and adequate protein and essential fatty acids.

It was recommended that ME have no alcohol, but if she wanted to drink it was to be reduced to 2 nights per week and a maximum of 2 standards drinks at one sitting (i.e. about 200 mL).

SAMPLE DAILY DIET

Breakfast	Fresh fruit, natural yoghurt, mixed chopped nuts and seeds Eggs on toast Smoothie with banana, LSA, chia seeds and egg or protein powder Natural muesli with natural yoghurt and fruit Avocado on wholegrain toast
Lunch	Homemade vegetable and chicken/lamb soup with lentils or chickpeas Salad bowl: mixed green leaves, tomato, cucumber, onion, avocado, capsicum, sweet potato, boiled egg and tuna dressed with walnut or olive oil and lemon juice or vinegar and sprinkled with pepitas or tamari-baked seeds Leftovers
Dinner	Slow-cooked meals: e.g. lamb shanks and vegetables, tagines, curries Vegetable curry with dhal and brown basmati rice Fish with steamed vegetables Roast chicken and vegetables
Snacks	Mixed nuts and seeds with a few cranberries Fresh fruit Nut butter on rye or veg sticks Boiled egg Natural yoghurt with granola or prunes on top
Drinks	>1.5 L of water per day Coffee reduced to 2 cups per day, none after 3 pm

Nutritional supplementation

Nutritional deficiencies were addressed through diet and supplementation. Iodine, zinc, selenium and iron were provided to support normal thyroid function, to reduce the risk of auto-antibody production and to support energy production. Selenium, zinc, vitamin C and EFAs were provided for their antioxidant and anti-inflammatory effects and iron was provided to correct the iron deficiency. Iron and zinc doses were not at the higher end of the therapeutic range as they may have been lower due to the inflammation that was present. It was unclear whether the ferritin level was elevated due to inflammation and thus would normally be lower. Zinc was also indicated in the management of anxiety and depression and to correct the imbalance in the copper:zinc ratio (aiming for a ratio of 1 : 1). Vitamin D supplementation was supplied to correct the deficiency and for its role in inflammation, immune function and mental health and cognitive function. No specific supplement was given for constipation as it was hoped that this would be resolved through diet and exercise. Vitamin C was included for adrenal function and gum health and a methylated B

CASE STUDY CONTINUED

complex was added for neurological function, energy production and liver support.

- Iron: 30 mg/day (with vitamin C and bioflavonoids)
- Vitamin D: 4000 IU/day
- Zinc: 30 mg/day
- Omega-3: EFA, 3 mg, including 1020 mg EPA and 720 mg DHA
- Selenium: 200 micrograms/day
- Iodine: 150 micrograms/day
- Vitamin C: 1000 mg/twice daily
- Methylated B complex/day.

Herbal medicine

Herbal medicine was used to modulate the GABA pathway and reduce anxiety (*Piper methysticum*, *Passiflora incarnata*), to modulate monamines (*Hypericum perforatum*, *Rhodiola rosea*), as a traditional anxiolytic for women (*Leonurus cardiaca*), as an adrenal tonic and anti-inflammatory (*Glycyrrhiza glabra*) and as an adaptogen/tonic (*Withania somnifera*, *Rhodiola rosea*). *Withania* also supports the conversion of T4 to T3. *Gentiana lutea* was added as a bitter digestive and hepatic and to stimulate appetite. A separate sleeping aid was not provided initially as ME wanted to first try the relaxation techniques provided by the psychologist. If one was required, the recommendation was for a simple preparation of *Piper methysticum* extract as it aids sleep and is anxiolytic.

- Herbal formula
  - *Rhodiola rosea* 2 : 1 60 mL
  - *Withania somnifera* 2 : 1 50 mL
  - *Leonurus cardiaca* 1 : 2 30 mL
  - *Passiflora incarnata* 1 : 2 40 mL
  - *Gentiana lutea* 1 : 2 20 mL dose 5 mL tds
  - *Hypericum perforatum* tablets, 1.8 g 1 tablet extract tds
- Tisanes: ME was advised to drink 2 or more cups of herbal tisanes a day, including a blend of *Passiflora incarnata*, *Verbena officinalis* and *Glycyrrhiza glabra* (which also sated the desire for a sweet taste).

FOLLOW-UP

ME returned 2 weeks later having been 75% compliant with her supplements and herbal medicine and having significantly improved her diet. She had only been for a walk twice, as she was not confident enough to go without DF. Her anxiety was reduced but still impacting her life, as was her depression. She was less constipated and was sleeping 4–5 hours per night. The plan was to continue the current regimen and encourage her to walk with friends and to continue the relaxation techniques provided by the psychologist. The regimen was reduced as her symptoms and health improved and her pathology results normalised over the following months, with omega-3 fatty acid and a B complex as the only long-term supplements required.

REFERENCES

[1] Australian Government. 2015 intergenerational report: Australia in 2055. Commonwealth of Australia; 2015. Available from www.treasury.gov.au/PublicationsAndMedia/Publications/2015/2015 -Intergenerational-Report.

[2] Australian Institute of Health and Welfare (AIHW), Hilder L, Li Z, et al. Stillbirths in Australia, 1999–2009. Perinatal Statistics Series no. 29. Cat. no. PER 63. Canberra: AIHW National Perinatal Epidemiology and Statistics Unit; 2014. Available from www.aihw. gov.au/WorkArea/DownloadAsset.aspx?id=60129548877.

[3] Australian Institute of Health and Welfare (AIHW). Perinatal data portal. Available from www.aihw.gov.au/perinatal-data. [Cited 24 September 2016].

[4] Australian Institute of Health and Welfare (AIHW). Australia's mothers and babies, 2013: in brief. Perinatal Statistics Series no. 31. Cat no. PER 72. Canberra: AIHW; 2015.

[5] Australian Health Ministers' Conference. National Maternity Services Plan 2010. Canberra; 2010.

[6] Australian Institute of Health and Welfare (AIHW). Australia's health 2014. Australia's Health Series no.14. Cat. no. AUS 178. Canberra: AIHW; 2014.

[7] OECD. Health at a glance 2011: OECD indicators. Paris: OECD Publishing; 2011.

[8] Steel A, Adams J. The role of naturopathy in pregnancy, labour and post-natal care: broadening the evidence base. Complement Ther Clin Pract 2011;17(4):189–92.

[9] Steel A, Adams J, Sibbritt D, et al. Utilisation of complementary and alternative medicine (CAM) practitioners within maternity care provision: results from a nationally representative cohort study of 1835 pregnant women. BMC Pregnancy Childbirth 2012;12(1):146.

[10] Frawley J, Adams J, Sibbritt D, et al. Prevalence and determinants of complementary and alternative medicine use during pregnancy: results from a nationally representative sample of Australian pregnant women. Aust NZ J Obstet Gynaecol 2013;53(4):347–52.

[11] Holst L, Wright D, Haavil S, et al. Safety and efficacy of herbal remedies in obstetrics: review and clinical implications. Midwifery 2011;27(1):80–6.

[12] Nordeng H, Bayne K, Havnen GC, et al. Use of herbal drugs during pregnancy among 600 Norwegian women in relation to concurrent use of conventional drugs and pregnancy outcome. Complement Ther Clin Pr 2011;17(3):147–51.

[13] Birdee GS, Kemper KJ, Rothman R, et al. Use of complementary and alternative medicine during pregnancy and the postpartum period: an analysis of the National Health Interview Survey. J Womens Health (Larchmt) 2014;23(10):824–9.

[14] Moussally K, Oriachi D, Berard A. Herbal products used during pregnancy: prevalence and predictors. Pharmacoepidemiol Drug Saf 2009;18(6):454–61.

[15] Kennedy DA, Lupattelli A, Koren G, et al. Safety classification of herbal medicines used in pregnancy in a multinational study. BMC Complement Altern Med 2016;16:2012.

[16] Guise JM, Eden K, Emeis C, et al. Vaginal birth after cesarean: new insights. Evid Rep Technol Assess 2010;191:1–397.

[17] Dodd JM, Crowther CA, Huertas E, et al. Planned elective repeat caesarean section versus planned vaginal birth for women with a previous caesarean birth. Cochrane Database Syst Rev 2013;(12):CD004224.

[18] Levett KM, Smith CA, Bensoussan A, et al. Complementary therapies for labour and birth study: a randomised controlled trial of antenatal integrative medicine for pain management in labour. BMJ Open 2016;6(7):e010691.

[19] Fairbrother N, Janssen P, Antony M, et al. Perinatal anxiety disorder prevalence and incidence. J Affect Disord 2016;200:148–55.

[20] Walsh D. The hidden experience of violence during pregnancy: a study of 400 pregnant Australian women. Aust J Prim Heal 2008;14(1):97–105.

[21] Bailey BA. Partner violence during pregnancy: prevalence, effects, screening, and management. Int J Womens Health 2010;2:183–97.

[22] Hoang TN, Van TN, Gammeltoft TW, et al. Association between intimate partner violence during pregnancy and adverse pregnancy outcomes in Vietnam: a prospective cohort study. PLoS ONE 2016.

[23] Australian Bureau of Statistics. Personal Safety Survey, Australia, 2012. Canberra: Australian Bureau of Statistics; 2013.

[24] Jahanfar S, Howard LM, Medley N. Interventions for preventing or reducing domestic violence against pregnant women. Cochrane Database Syst Rev 2014;(11):CD009414.

[25] Rosenfeld CS. Homage to the 'H' in developmental origins of health and disease. J Dev Orig Heal Dis 2017;8(1):8–29.

[26] Guardino CM, Schetter CD, Saxbe DE, et al. Diurnal salivary cortisol patterns prior to pregnancy predict infant birth weight. Heal Psychol 2016;35(6):625–33.

[27] Hocher B. More than genes: the advanced fetal programming hypothesis. J Reprod Immunol 2014;104–105:8–11.

[28] Lowensohn R, Stadler D, Naze C. Current concepts of maternal nutrtition. Obstet Gynecol Surv 2016;71(7):413–26.

[29] Marques AH, O'Connor TG, Roth C, et al. The influence of maternal prenatal and early childhood nutrition and maternal prenatal stress on offspring immune system development and neurodevelopmental disorders. Front Neurosci 2013;7(120).

[30] Vickers MH. Early life nutrition, epigenetics and programming of later life disease. Nutrients 2014;6(6):2165–78.

[31] Geraghty AA, Lindsay KL, Alberdi G, et al. Nutrition during pregnancy impacts offspring's epigenetic status: evidence from human and animal studies. Nutr Metab Insights 2015;8(Suppl. 1):41–7.

[32] von Meyenn F, Reik W. Forget the parents: epigenetic reprogramming in human germ cells. Cell 2015;161(6):1248–51.

[33] Zeng Y, Zhou Y, Chen P, et al. Use of complementary and alternative medicine across the childbirth spectrum in China. Complement Ther Med 2014;22(6):1047–52.

[34] Al-Ramahi R, Jaradat N, Adawi D. Use of herbal medicines during pregnancy in a group of Palestinian women. J Ethnopharmaco 2013;150(1):79–84.

[35] Forster DA, Wills G, Denning A, et al. The use of folic acid and other vitamins before and during pregnancy in a group of women in Melbourne, Australia. Birth 2009;25(2):134–46.

[36] Maats FH, Crowther CA. Patterns of vitamin, mineral and herbal supplement use prior to and during pregnancy. Aust NZ J Obs Gynaecol 2002;42(2):494–6.

[37] Masih SP, Plumptre L, Ly A, et al. Pregnant Canadian women achieve recommended intakes of one-carbon nutrients through prenatal supplementation but the supplement composition, including choline, requires reconsideration. J Nutr 2015;145(8):1824–34.

[38] Bixenstine PJ, Cheng TL, Cheng D, et al. Folic acid supplementation before pregnancy: reasons for non-use and association with preconception counseling HHS public access. Matern Child Heal J 2015;19(9):1974–84.

[39] Strouss L, Mackley A, Guillen U, et al. Complementary and alternative medicine use in women during pregnancy: do their healthcare providers know? BMC Complement Altern Med 2014;14(85):1–9.

[40] Stephens S, Wilson G. Prescribing in pregnant women: guide to general principles. Prescriber 2009;20(23–24):1–4.

[41] Kovacic P, Somanathen R. Mechanism of teratogenesis: electron transfer, reactive oxygen species, and antioxidants. Birth Defects Res C Embryo Today 2006;78(4):308–25.

[42] Freyer AM. Drug-prescribing challenges during pregnancy. Obstet Gynaecol Reprod Med 2008;18(7):180–6.

[43] Braun L, Cohen M. Herbs and Natural supplements: an evidence-based guide. 4th ed. Sydney: Elsevier; 2015.

[44] Centres for Disease Control and Prevention (CDC). Birth defects. Available from www.cdc.gov/ncbddd/birthdefects/index.html. [cited 20 November 2016].

[45] Abeywardana S, Sullivan EA. Congenital anomalies in Australia 2002–2003. Birth Anomalies Series no. 3. Cat. no. PER 41. Sydney; 2002.

[46] Webster WS, Freeman JAD. Is this drug safe in pregnancy? Reprod Toxicol 2001;15(6):619–29.

[47] Bone K, Mills S. Principles and practice of phytotherapy: modern herbal medicine. 2nd ed. Philadelphia: Churchill Livingstone; 2013.

[48] Mills S, Bone K. The essential guide to herbal safety. Philadelphia: Elsevier; 2005.

[49] Romm A. Botanical medicine for women's health. Philadelphia: Elsevier; 2010.

[50] Thomas SHL, Yates LM. Prescribing without evidence: pregnancy. Br J Clin Pharmacol 2012;74(4):691–7.

[51] Kovacs CS, Ralston SH. Presentation and management of osteoporosis presenting in association with pregnancy or lactation. Osteoporos Int 2015;26(9):2223–41.

[52] Institute of Medicine (IOM). Weight gain during pregnancy: reexamining the guidelines. Washington: National Academies Press; 2009. p. 1–2.

[53] Beyerlein A, Schiessl B, vonKries R. Associations of gestational weight loss with birth-related outcome: a retrospective cohort study. BJOG 2011;118(1):55–61.

[54] Kapadia MZ, Park CK, Beyene J, et al. Weight loss instead of weight gain within the guidelines in obese women during pregnancy: a systematic review and meta-analyses of maternal and infant outcomes. PLoS ONE 2015;10(7):e0132650.

[55] Institute of Medicine (IOM). Weight gain during pregnancy: reexamining the guidelines. Washington: National Academies Press; 2009.

[56] Australian Government Department of Health and NZ MoH. Nutrient reference values. Available from www.nrv.gov.au/dietary-energy. [Cited 10 November 2016].

[57] De Jersey SJ, Nicholson JM, Callaway LK, et al. A prospective study of pregnancy weight gain in Australian women. Aust NZ J Obstet Gynaecol 2012;52(6):545–51.

[58] Jeffs E, Haszard J, Sharp B, et al. Pregnant women lack accurate knowledge of their BMI and recommended gestation weight gain. NZ Med J 2016;129(1439):37–45.

[59] Bookari K, Yeatman H, Williamson M. Australian pregnant women's awareness of gestational weight gain and dietary guidelines: opportunity for action. J Pregnancy 2016.

[60] Horvitz West E, Hark L, Catalano P. Nutrition during pregnancy. In: Gabbe S, Niebyl J, Simpson J, et al, editors. Obstetrics: normal and problem pregnancies. 7th ed. Philadelphia: Elsevier; 2017.

[61] Australian Bureau of Statistics. Overweight and obesity. 4338.0 Profiles of Health, Australia, 2011–13. Canberra: ABS; 2013.

[62] Craig R, Fuller E, Mindell J. Health Survey for England 2014: health, social care and lifestyles. London; 2014.

[63] Morgan KL, Rahman MA, Hill RA, et al. Obesity in pregnancy: infant health service utilisation and costs on the NHS Centre for the Development and Evaluation of Complex Interventions for Public Health Improvement. BMJ Open 2015;5:e008357.

[64] Widen EM, Whyatt RM, Hoepner LA, et al. Excessive gestational weight gain is associated with long-term body fat and weight retention at 7 y postpartum in African American and Dominican mothers with underweight, normal, and overweight prepregnancy BMI. Am J Clin Nutr 2015;102(6):1460–7.

[65] Stotland NE, Bodnar LM, Abrams B. Maternal nutrition. In: Creasy RK, Resnik R, Iams JD, et al, editors. Creasy & Resnik's maternal-fetal medicine: principles and practice. 7th ed. Philadelphia: Elsevier; 2014.

[66] McAree T, Jacobs B, Manickavasagar T, et al. Vitamin D deficiency in pregnancy: still a public health issue. Matern Child Nutr 2013;9(1):23–30.

[67] Shub A, Huning EY, Campbell KJ, et al. Pregnant women's knowledge of weight, weight gain, complications of obesity and weight management strategies in pregnancy. BMC Res Notes 2013;6(278).

[68] Drehmer M, Duncan BB, Kac G, et al. Association of second and third trimester weight gain in pregnancy with maternal and fetal outcomes. PLoS ONE 2013.

[69] Godoy AC, do Nascimento SL, Garanhani Surita F. A systematic review and meta-analysis of gestational weight gain recommendations and related outcomes in Brazil. Clin (San Paulo) 2015;70(11):758–64.

[70] Castillo H, Santos I, Matijasevich A. Maternal pre-pregnancy BMI, gestational weight gain and breastfeeding. Eur J Clin Nutr 2016;70:431–6.

[71] Park S, Sappenfield WM, Bish C, et al. Assessment of the Institute of Medicine recommendations for weight gain during pregnancy: Florida, 2004–2007. Matern Child Health J 2011.

[72] Simas TAM, Waring ME, Liao X, et al. Prepregnancy weight, gestational weight gain, and risk of growth affected neonates. J Womens Health (Larchmt) 2011;21(4):410–17.

[73] Lemas DJ, Young BE, Baker PR, et al. Alterations in human milk leptin and insulin are associated with early changes in the infant intestinal microbiome. Am J Clin Nutr 2016;103(5):1291–300.

[74] Bodnar LM, Pugh SJ, Abrams B, et al. Gestational weight gain in twin pregnancies and maternal and child health: a systematic review. J Perinatol 2014;34(4):252–63.

[75] Bacak S, Zozzaro-Smith P, Glantz J, et al. Impact of weight gain in triplet pregnancies on perinatal outcomes. Am J Obstet Gynecol 2015;212(1):S275–6.

[76] Johnston RC, Erfani H, Shamshirsaz A, et al. Optimal weight gain in triplet pregnancies. J Matern Fetal Neonatal Med 2017;31(6):1–22.

[77] Bricker L, Reed K, Wood L, et al. Nutritional advice for improving outcomes in multiple pregnancies. Cochrane Database Syst Rev 2015;(11):CD008867.

[78] Martin JA, Hamilton BE, Osterman MJK. Three decades of twin births in the United States, 1980–2009. Atlanta: Centers for Disease Control and Prevention; 2012. p. 1–8.

[79] Australian Bureau of Statistics. Births. 3301.0 Births, Australia. 2015. Available from www.abs.gov.au/AUSSTATS. [Cited 18 November 2016].

[80] Fertility Society of Australia. Code of Practice for Assisted Reproductive Technology Units. South Melbourne: Fertility Society of Australia; 2014.

[81] Craig WJ, Mangels AR, American Dietetic Association. Position of the American Dietetic Association: vegetarian diets. J Am Diet Assoc 2009;109:1266–82.

[82] Piccoli GB, Clari R, Vigotti FN, et al. Vegan-vegetarian diets in pregnancy: danger or panacea? A systematic narrative review. BJOG 2015;122(5):623–33.

[83] Australian Institute of Health and Welfare (AIHW). Risk factors: teenage pregnancy. Canberra: AIHW; 2016.

[84] Montgomery KS. Improving nutrition in pregnant adolescents: recommendations for clinical practitioners. J Perinat Educ 2003;12(2):22–30.

[85] Lee S, Guillet R, Cooper EM, et al. Prevalence of anemia and associations between neonatal iron status, hepcidin, and maternal iron status among neonates born to pregnant adolescents. Pediatr Res 2016;79(1–1):42–8.

[86] Ball SJ, Pereira G, Jacoby P, et al. Re-evaluation of link between interpregnancy interval and adverse birth outcomes: retrospective cohort study matching two intervals per mother. Br Med J 2014;69(12):717–19.

[87] Gemmill A, Lindberg L. Short interpregnancy intervals in the United States. Obs Gynecol 2013;122(1):64–71.

[88] Cofer FG, Fridman M, Lawton E, et al. Interpregnancy interval and childbirth outcomes in California, 2007–2009. Matern Child Heal J 2016;20(Suppl. 1):43–51.

[89] Chen I, Jhangri GS, Chandra S. Relationship between interpregnancy interval and congenital anomalies. Am J Obs Gynecol 2014;210(6):564.e1–8.

[90] Hure A, Young A, Smith R, et al. Diet and pregnancy status in Australian women. Public Health Nutr 2008;12(6):853–61.

[91] de Jersey SJ, Nicholson JM, Callaway LK, et al. An observational study of nutrition and physical activity behaviours, knowledge, and advice in pregnancy. BMC Pregnancy Childbirth 2013;13:115.

[92] Food Standards Australia and New Zealand. Mercury in fish. Available from www.foodstandards.gov.au/consumer/chemicals/mercury/Pages/default.aspx. [Cited 30 November 2016].

[93] US Food & Drug Administration. What you need to know about mercury in fish and shellfish. Available from www.fda.gov/food/resourcesforyou/consumers/ucm110591.htm. [Cited 30 November 2016].

[94] Grosso LM, Bracken MB. Caffeine metabolism, genetics, and perinatal outcomes: a review of exposure assessment considerations during pregnancy. Ann Epidemiol 2005;15(6):460–6.

[95] Ebrahimi A, Habibi-Khorassani M, Akher FB, et al. Caffeine as base analogue of adenine or guanine: a theoretical study. J Mol Graph Model 2013;42:81–91.

[96] Li J, Zhao H, Song J-M, et al. A meta-analysis of risk of pregnancy loss and caffeine and coffee consumption during pregnancy. Int J Gynecol Obstet 2015;130:116–22.

[97] Gaskins AJ, Rich-Edwards JW, Williams PL, et al. Pre-pregnancy caffeine and caffeinated beverage intake and risk of spontaneous abortion. Eur J Nutr 2018;57(1):105–7.

[98] Victoria Escolano-Margarit M, Campoy C, Carmen Ramírez-Tortosa M, et al. Effects of fish oil supplementation on the fatty acid profile in erythrocyte membrane and plasma phospholipids of pregnant women and their offspring: a randomised controlled trial. Br J Nutr 2016;109:1647–56.

[99] Meher A, Randhir K, Mehendale S, et al. Maternal fatty acids and their association with birth outcome: a prospective study. PLoS ONE 2016;11(1):e0147359.

[100] Bobiński R, Mikulska M. The ins and outs of maternal-fetal fatty acid metabolism. Acta Biochim Pol 2015;62(3):499–507.

[101] Makrides M, Best K. The role of DHA in the first 1000 days: docosahexaenoic acid and preterm birth. Nutr Metab 2016;69:30–4.

[102] Pinto TJP, Farias DR, Rebelo F, et al. Lower inter-partum interval and unhealthy life-style factors are inversely associated with n-3 essential fatty acids changes during pregnancy: a prospective cohort with Brazilian women. PLoS ONE 2015;10(3):e0121151.

[103] Leventakou V, Roumeliotaki T, Martinez D, et al. Fish intake during pregnancy, fetal growth, and gestational length in 19 European birth cohort studies. Am J Clin Nutr 2014;99(3):506–16.

[104] Lazzarin N, Vaquero E, Exacoustos C, et al. Low-dose aspirin and omega-3 fatty acids improve uterine artery blood flow velocity in women with recurrent miscarriage due to impaired uterine perfusion. Fertil Steril 2009;92(1):296.

[105] Carta G, Iovenitti P, Falciglia K. Recurrent miscarriage associated with antiphospholipid antibodies: prophylactic treatment with low-dose aspirin and fish oil derivates. Clin Exp Obs Gynecol 2005;32(1):49–51.

[106] Swanson D, Block R, Mousa SA. Omega-3 fatty acids EPA and DHA: health benefits throughout life. Adv Nutr 2012;3:1–7.

[107] Anderson G, Maes M. Postpartum depression: psychoneuroimmunological underpinnings and treatment. Neuropsychiatr Dis Treat 2013;9:277–87.

[108] Chong MF, Ong YL, Calder PC, et al. Long-chain polyunsaturated fatty acid status during pregnancy and maternal mental health in pregnancy and the postpartum period: results from the GUSTO study. J Clin Psychiatry 2015;76(7):e848–56.

[109] Hamazaki K, Harauma A, Otaka Y, et al. Serum n-3 polyunsaturated fatty acids and psychological distress in early pregnancy: Adjunct Study of Japan Environment and Children's Study. Transl Psychiatry 2016;6:e737.

[110] Pinto TJ, Vilela AA, Farias DR, et al. Serum n-3 polyunsaturated fatty acids are inversely associated with longitudinal changes in depressive symptoms during pregnancy. Epidemiol Psychiatr Sci 2016.

[111] Makrides M, Duly L, Olsen SF. Marine oil, and other prostaglandin precursor, supplementation for pregnancy uncomplicated by pre-eclampsia or intrauterine growth restriction. Cochrane Database Syst Rev 2006;(3):CD003402.

[112] Lapido OA. Nutrition in pregnancy: mineral and vitamin supplements. Am J Clin Nutr 2010;72(1):280s–90s.

[113] Gabbe S, Niebyl J, Simpson J, et al, editors. Obstetrics: normal and problem pregnancies. 7th ed. Philadelphia: Elsevier; 2017.

[114] Grieger JA, Clifton VL. A review of the impact of dietary intakes in human pregnancy on infant birthweight. Nutrients 2015;7:153–78.

[115] Abdou E, Hazell AS. Thiamine deficiency: an update of pathophysiologic mechanisms and future therapeutic considerations. Neurochem Res 2014;40(2):353–61.

[116] Bâ A. Comparative effects of alcohol and thiamine deficiency on the developing central nervous system. Behav Brain Res 2011;225(1):235–42.

[117] Bâ A. Alcohol and B1 vitamin deficiency-related stillbirths. J Matern Fetal Neonatal Med 2009;22(5):452–7.

[118] Krapels IPC, Van Rooij IALM, Ocké MC, et al. Maternal dietary B vitamin intake, other than folate, and the association with orofacial cleft in the offspring. Eur J Nutr 2004;43(1):7–14.

[119] Kerns JC, Arundel C, Chawla LS. Thiamin deficiency in people with obesity. Adv Nutr 2015;6:147–53.

[120] Chan J, Deng L, Mikael LG, et al. Low dietary choline and low dietary riboflavin during pregnancy influence reproductive outcomes and heart development in mice. Am J Clin Nutr 2010;91(4):1035–43.

[121] Smedts HPM, Rakhshandehroo M, Verkleij-Hagoort AC, et al. Maternal intake of fat, riboflavin and nicotinamide and the risk of having offspring with congenital heart defects. Eur J Nutr 2008;47(7):357–65.

[122] Neugebauer J, Zanre Y, Wacker J. Riboflavin supplementation and preeclampsia. Int J Gynaecol Obs 2006;93(2):136–7.

[123] Molina L, Rivas V, Sanchez R, et al. PROPER: a pilot study of the role of riboflavin supplementation for the prevention of preeclampsia. Int J Biol Biomed Eng 2012;6(1):43–50.

[124] Li F, Fushima T, Oyanagi G, et al. Nicotinamide benefits both mothers and pups in two contrasting mouse models of preeclampsia. Proc Natl Acad Sci 2016;113(47):13450–5.

[125] Tian Y-J, Luo N, Chen N-N, et al. Maternal nicotinamide supplementation causes global DNA hypomethylation, uracil hypo-incorporation and gene expression changes in fetal rats. Br J Nutr 2014;111(9):1594–601.

[126] El-Heis S, Crozier S, Robinson S, et al. Higher maternal serum concentrations of nicotinamide and related metabolites in late pregnancy are associated with a lower risk of offspring atopic eczema at age 12 months. Europe PMC Funders Group. Clin Exp Allergy 2016;46(10):1337–43.

[127] Scheller K, Röckl T, Scheller C, et al. Lower concentrations of B-vitamin subgroups in the serum and amniotic fluid correlate to cleft lip and palate appearance in the offspring of A/WySn mice. J Oral Maxillofac Surg 2013;71(9).

[128] Haggarty P, Campbell DM, Duthie S, et al. Diet and deprivation in pregnancy. Br J Nutr 2009;102(10):1487–97.

[129] Kalhan S. One carbon metabolism in pregnancy: impact on maternal, fetal and neonatal health. Mol Cell Endocrinol 2016;435:48–60.

[130] Dror DK, Allen LH. Interventions with vitamins B6, B12 and C in pregnancy. Paediatr Perinat Epidemiol 2012;26(Suppl. 1):55–74.

[131] Ronnenberg AG, Venners SA, Xu X, et al. Preconception B-vitamin and homocysteine status, conception, and early pregnancy loss. Am J Epidemiol 2007;166(3):304–12.

[132] Hovdenak N, Haram K. Influence of mineral and vitamin supplements on pregnancy outcome. Eur J Obstet Gynecol Reprod Biol 2012;164:127–32.

[133] Agarwal N, Dora S, Kriplani A, et al. Response of therapy with vitamin B_6, B_{12} and folic acid on homocysteine level and pregnancy outcome in hyperhomocysteinemia with unexplained recurrent aborts. Int J Gynecol Obstet 2012;119(3):S759.

[134] Cikot RJ, Steegers-Theunissen RP, Thomas CM, et al. Longitudinal vitamin and homocysteine levels in normal pregnancy. Br J Nutr 2001;85(1):49–58.

[135] Suren P, Roth C, Bresnahan M, et al. Association between maternal use of folic acid supplements and risk of autism spectrum disorders in children. J Am Med Assoc 2013;309(6):570–7.

[136] Laanpere M, Altmae S, Stavreus-Evers A, et al. Folate-mediated one-carbon metabolism and its effect on female fertility and pregnancy viability. Nutr Rev 2010;68(2):99–113.

[137] Sayyah-Melli M, Ghorbanihaghjo A, Alizadeh M, et al. The effect of high dose folic acid throughout pregnancy on homocysteine (Hcy) concentration and pre-eclampsia: a randomized clinical trial. PLoS ONE 2016;11(5):1–11.

[138] Wu X, Zhao L, Zhu H, et al. Association between the MTHFR C677T polymorphism and recurrent pregnancy loss: a meta-analysis. Genet Test Mol Biomarkers 2012;16(7):806–11.

[139] Wu X, Yang K, Tang X, et al. Folate metabolism gene polymorphisms MTHFR C677T and A1298C and risk for preeclampsia: a meta-analysis. J Assist Reprod Genet 2015;32(5):797–805.

[140] Nair RR, Khanna A, Singh R, et al. Association of maternal and fetal MTHFR A1298C polymorphism with the risk of pregnancy loss: a study of an Indian population and a meta-analysis. Fertil Steril 2013;99(5):1311–18.

[141] Allen L, De Benoist B, Dary O, et al, editors. Guidelines on food fortification with micronutrients. Geneva: WHO; 2006.

[142] Food Fortification Initiative. Global progress. Available from www.ffinetwork.org/global_progress/index.php. [Cited 11 November 2016].

[143] Bailey LB, Stover PJ, Mcnulty H, et al. Biomarkers of Nutrition for development: folate review. J Nutr 2015;145(7):1–45.

[144] Crider KS, Bailey LB, Berry RJ. Folic acid food fortification: its history, effect, concerns, and future directions. Nutrients 2011;3(3):370–84.

[145] New Zealand Ministry of Health. Folate/folic acid. Available from www.health.govt.nz/our-work/preventative-health-wellness/nutrition/folate-folic-acid#current_polic. [Cited 6 June 2017].

[146] National Perinatal Unit. Neural tube defects in Australia, 2007–2011. Canberra: Commonwealth of Australia; 2011.

[147] Daly LE, Kirke PN, Molloy A, et al. Folate levels and neural tube defects: implications for prevention. JAMA 1995;274(21):1698–702.

[148] Crider KS, Devine O, Hao L, et al. Population red blood cell folate concentrations for prevention of neural tube defects: bayesian model. BMJ 2014;349:g4554.

[149] World Health Organization. Guideline optimal serum and red blood cell folate concentrations in women of reproductive age for prevention of NTD. World Heal Organ 2015;1542:33–6.

[150] Czeizal AE, Duda I. Prevention of the first occurence of neural-tube defects by periconceptional vitamin supplementation. N Engl J Med 1992;327(10):685–91.

[151] Berry RJ, Li Z, Erickson JD, et al. Prevention of neural-tube defects with folic acid in China. English J 1999;341(20):1485.

[152] De-Regil LM, Fernández-Gaxiola AC, Dowswell T, et al. Effects and safety of periconceptional folate supplementation for preventing birth defects. Cochrane Database Syst Rev 2014;2(10):1–135.

[153] Kim H, Kim K-N, Hwang J-Y, et al. Relation between serum folate status and blood mercury concentrations in pregnant women. Nutrition 2013;29(3):514–18.

[154] Centres for Disease Control and Prevention. Folic acid: data and statistics. Available from www.cdc.gov/NCBDDD/folicacid/data.html. [Cited 11 November 2016].

[155] McKeating A, Farren M, Cawley S, et al. Maternal folic acid supplementation trends 2009–2013. Acta Obs Gynecol Scand 2015;94(7):727–33.

[156] Pre-Conception Health Special Interest Group. Micronutrient (folic acid, iodine and vitamin D) supplements pre-conception and during pregnancy. Melbourne: Fertility Society Australia; 2016, p. 1–4.

[157] Hekmatdoost A, Vahid F, Yari Z, et al. Methyltetrahydrofolate vs folic acid supplementation in idiopathic recurrent miscarriage with respect to methylenetetrahydrofolate reductase C677T and A1298C polymorphisms: a randomized controlled trial. PLoS ONE 2015;10(12):1–12.

[158] Gernand AD, Schulze KJ, Stewart CP, et al. Micronutrient deficiencies in pregnancy worldwide: health effects and prevention HHS Public Access. Nat Rev Endocrinol 2016;12(5):274–89.

[159] Kumar KA, Lalitha A, Pavithra D, et al. Maternal dietary folate and/or vitamin B_{12} restrictions alter body composition (adiposity) and lipid metabolism in Wistar rat offspring. J Nutr Biochem 2013;24(1):25–31.

[160] Jamshed Siddiqui M, Sze Min C, Kumar Verma R, et al. Role of complementary and alternative medicine in geriatric care: a mini review. Pharmacogn Rev 2014;8(16):81–7.

[161] Sukumar N, Rafnsson SB, Kandala NB, et al. Prevalence of vitamin B_{12} insufficiency during pregnancy and its effect on offspring birth weight: a systematic review and meta-analysis. Am J Clin Nutr 2016;103(5):1232–51.

[162] Finkelstein JL, Layden AJ, Stover PJ. Vitamin B_{12} and perinatal health. Adv Nutr 2015;6(5):552–63.

[163] Singer AW, Selvin S, Block G, et al. Maternal prenatal intake of one-carbon metabolism nutrients and risk of childhood leukemia. Cancer Causes Control 2016;27(7):929–40.

[164] Sukumar N, Wilson S, Venkataraman H, et al. Low vitamin B_{12} in pregnancy is associated with maternal obesity and gestational diabetes. Endocr Abstr 2015;39:206.

[165] Rizzo G, Laganà AS, Maria A, et al. Vitamin B_{12} among vegetarians: status, assessment and supplementation. Nutrients 2016;8(767):1–23.

[166] Thakkar K, Billa G. Treatment of vitamin B_{12} deficiency-methylcobalamine? Cyancobalamine? Hydroxocobalamin? Clearing the confusion. Eur J Clin Nutr 2015;69(1):1–2.

[167] Furukawa S, Nakajima A, Sameshima H. The longitudinal change of extracellular antioxidant status during pregnancy using an electron spin resonance method. J Matern Fetal Neonatal Med 2016;18:2994–9.

[168] Mistry HD, Williams PJ. The importance of antioxidant micronutrients in pregnancy. Oxid Med Cell Longev 2011:841749.

[169] Ramiro-Cortijo D, Herrera T, Rodríguez-Rodríguez P, et al. Maternal plasma antioxidant status in the first trimester of pregnancy and development of obstetric complications. Placenta 2016;47:37–45.

[170] Mistry HD, Gill CA, Kurlak LO, et al. Association between maternal micronutrient status, oxidative stress, and common genetic variants

in antioxidant enzymes at 15 weeks gestation in nulliparous women who subsequently develop preeclampsia. Free Radic Biol Med 2015;78:147–55.

[171] D'Souza V, Rani A, Patil V, et al. Increased oxidative stress from early pregnancy in women who develop preeclampsia. Clin Exp Hypertens 2016;38(2):225–32.

[172] Cohen JM, Beddaoui M, Kramer MS, et al. Maternal antioxidant levels in pregnancy and risk of preeclampsia and small for gestational age birth: a systematic review and meta-analysis. PLoS ONE 2015;10(8):e0135192.

[173] Gandley R, Abramovic A. PP170. Prenatal vitamin C and E supplementation is associated with a reduction in placental abruption and preterm birth in smokers. Pregnancy Hypertens 2012;2(3):331–2.

[174] Yung H-W, Alnaes-Katjavivi P, Jones CJP, et al. Placental endoplasmic reticulum stress in gestational diabetes: the potential for therapeutic intervention with chemical chaperones and antioxidants. Diabetologia 2016;59:2240–50.

[175] Rumbold A, Ota E, Nagata C, et al. Vitamin C supplementation in pregnancy. Cochrane Database Syst Rev 2015;(9):CD004072.

[176] Abo-Elmatty DM, Badawy EA, Hussein JS, et al. Role of heme oxygenase, leptin, coenzyme Q10 and trace elements in pre-eclamptic women. Indian J Clin Biochem 2012;27(4):379–84.

[177] Guan Z, Li HF, Guo LL, et al. Effects of vitamin C, vitamin E, and molecular hydrogen on the placental function in trophoblast cells. Arch Gynecol Obstet 2015;292(2):337–42.

[178] Shearer KD, Stoney PN, Morgan PJ, et al. A vitamin for the brain. Trends Neurosci 2012;35(12):733–41.

[179] Agarwal K, Dabke AT, Phuljhele NL, et al. Factors affecting serum vitamin A levels in matched maternal-cord pairs. Indian J Pediatr 2008;75(5):443–6.

[180] Christian P, Klemm R, Shamim AA, et al. Effects of vitamin A and beta-carotene supplementation on birth size and length of gestation in rural Bangladesh: a cluster-randomized trial. Am J Clin Nutr 2013;97(1):188–94.

[181] McCauley ME, van den Broek N, Dou L, et al. Vitamin A supplementation during pregnancy for maternal and newborn outcomes. Cochrane Database Syst Rev 2015;(10):CD008666.

[182] Shah D, Nagarajan N. Luteal insufficiency in first trimester. Indian J Endocrinol Metab 2013;17(1):44–9.

[183] Weinert LS, Silveiro SP. Maternal-fetal impact of vitamin D deficiency: a critical review. Matern Child Health J 2014;19(1):94–101.

[184] De-Regil LM, Palacios C, Lombardo LK, et al. Vitamin D supplementation for women during pregnancy. Cochrane Database Syst Rev 2016;(1):CD008873.

[185] Baca K, Simhan HN, Platt RW, et al. Low maternal 25-hydroxyvitamin D concentration increases the risk of severe and mild preeclampsia. Ann Epidemiol 2016;26(12):853–7.

[186] Gernand AD, Simhan HN, Caritis S, et al. Maternal vitamin D status and small-for-gestational-age offspring in women at high risk for preeclampsia. Obstet Gynecol 2014;123(1):40–8.

[187] Kiely ME, Zhang JY, Kinsella M, et al. Vitamin D status is associated with uteroplacental dysfunction indicated by pre-eclampsia and small-for-gestational-age birth in a large prospective pregnancy cohort in Ireland with low vitamin D status. Am J Clin Nutr 2016;104(2):354–61.

[188] Miliku K, Vinkhuyzen A, Blanken LM, et al. Maternal vitamin D concentrations during pregnancy, fetal growth patterns, and risks of adverse birth outcomes. Am J Clin Nutr 2016;103(6):1514–22.

[189] Andersen LB, Jorgensen JS, Jensen TK, et al. Vitamin D insufficiency is associated with increased risk of first trimester miscarriage in the Odense Child Cohort. Am J Clin Nutr 2015;102(3):633–8.

[190] Stubbs G, Henley K, Green J. Autism: will vitamin D supplementation during pregnancy and early childhood reduce the recurrence rate of autism in newborn siblings? Med Hypotheses 2016;88:74–8.

[191] Vinkhuyzen AAE, Eyles DW, Burne TH, et al. Gestational vitamin D deficiency and autism-related traits: the Generation R Study. Molec Psychiatr 2018;doi:10.1038/mp.2016.213. advance online publication 29 November 2016.

[192] Munger KL, Aivo J, Hongell K, et al. Vitamin D Status during pregnancy and risk of multiple sclerosis in offspring of women in the Finnish maternity cohort. JAMA Neurol 2016;73(5):515–19.

[193] McGrath JJ, Burne TH, Féron F, et al. Developmental vitamin D deficiency and risk of schizophrenia: a 10-year update. Schizophr Bull 2010;36(6):1073–8.

[194] Belderbos ME, Houben ML, Wilbrink B, et al. Cord blood vitamin D deficiency is associated with respiratory syncytial virus bronchiolitis. Pediatrics 2011;127:e1513–20.

[195] Urrutia-Pereira M, Solé D. Vitamin D deficiency in pregnancy and its impact of the fetus, the newborn and in childhood. Rev Paul Pediatr 2015;33(1):104–13.

[196] Wall CR, Stewart AW, Camargo CA, et al. Vitamin D activity of breast milk in women randomly assigned to vitamin D3 supplementation during pregnancy. Am J Clin Nutr 2015;103(2):382–8.

[197] Nowson CA, McGrath JJ, Ebeling PR, et al. Vitamin D and health in adults in Australia and New Zealand. Med J Aust 2012;196(11):686–7.

[198] Royal College of Obstetricians & Gynecologists. Vitamin D in pregnancy. Scientific Impact Paper no. 43. London; 2014.

[199] Burris HH, Camargo CA. Vitamin D and gestational diabetes mellitus. Curr Diab Rep 2014;14(1):451.

[200] Arnold DL, Enquobahrie DA, Qiu C, et al. Early pregnancy maternal vitamin D concentrations and risk of gestational diabetes mellitus. Paediatr Perinat Epidemiol 2015;29(3):200–10.

[201] Institute of Medicine (IOM), Ross AC, Taylor CL, et al, editors. Dietary reference intakes for calcium and vitamin D. Washington, DC: The National Academies Press; 2011.

[202] Holick MF, Binkley NC, Bischoff-Ferrari HA, et al. Evaluation, treatment, and prevention of vitamin D deficiency: an Endocrine Society clinical practice guideline. J Clin Endocrinol Metab 2011;96(7):1911–30.

[203] Daly RM, Gagno C, Lu ZX, et al. Prevalence of vitamin D deficiency and its determinants in Australian adults aged 25 years and older: a national, population-based study. Clin Endocrinol (Oxf) 2012;77(1):26–35.

[204] Mohammad KI, Kassab M, Shaban I, et al. Postpartum evaluation of vitamin D among a sample of Jordanian women. J Obs Gynaecol 2016;18.

[205] Yu CK, Sykes L, Sethi M, et al. Vitamin D deficiency and supplementation during pregnancy. Clin Endocrinol 2009;70:685–90.

[206] Hollis BW, Johnson D, Hulsey TC, et al. Vitamin D supplementation during pregnancy: double blind, randomized clinical trial of safety and effectiveness. Women's Heal 2012;8(3):323–40.

[207] Hamilton SA, McNeil R, Hollis BW, et al. Profound vitamin D deficiency in a diverse group of women during pregnancy living in a sun-rich environment at latitude 32N. Int J Endocrinol 2010.

[208] Thomas CE, Guillet R, Queenan RA, et al. Vitamin D status is inversely associated with anemia and serum erythropoietin during pregnancy. Am J Clin Nutr 2015;102(5):1088–95.

[209] Rumbold A, Ota E, Hori H, et al. Vitamin E supplementation in pregnancy. Cochrane Database Syst Rev 2015;(9):CD004069.

[210] Shamim AA, Schulze K, Merrill RD, et al. First-trimester plasma tocopherols are associated with risk of miscarriage in rural Bangladesh. Am J Clin Nutr 2015;101(2):294–301.

[211] Lippi G, Franchini M. Vitamin K in neonates: facts and myths. Blood Transfus 2011;9(1):4–9.

[212] Mock D. Marginal biotin deficiency is common in normal human pregnancy and is highly teratogenic in mice. J Nutr 2009;139(1):154–7.

[213] Agrawal S, Agrawal A, Said HM. Biotin deficiency enhances the inflammatory response of human dendritic cells. Am J Physiol Cell Physiol 2016;311(3):C386–91.

[214] Perry CA, West AA, Gayle A, et al. Pregnancy and lactation alter biomarkers of biotin metabolism in women consuming a controlled diet. J Nutr 2014;144:1977–84.

[215] Mock D. Adequate intake of biotin in pregnancy: why bother? J Nutr 2014;144(12):1885–6.

[216] Zeisel SH. Nutrition in pregnancy: the argument for including a source of choline. Int J Wom Health 2013;5(1):193–9.

[217] Caudill M. Pre- and postnatal health: evidence of increased choline needs. J Am Diet Assoc 2010;10(8):1198–206.

[218] Wozniak JR, Fuglestad AJ, Eckerle JK, et al. Choline supplementation in children with fetal alcohol spectrum disorders: a randomized, double-blind, placebo-controlled trial. Am J Clin Nutr 2015;102(5):1113–25.

[219] Grieger JA, Clifton VL. A review of the impact of dietary intake in human pregnancy on infant birthweight. Nutrients 2015;7:153–78.

[220] Ettinger AS, Lamadrid-Figueroa H, Téllez-Rojo MM, et al. Effect of calcium supplementation on blood lead levels in pregnancy: a randomized placebo-controlled trial. Environ Health Perspect 2009;117(11):26.

[221] Hofmeyr GJ, Lawrie TA, Atallah AN, et al. Calcium supplementation during pregnancy for preventing hypertensive disorders and related problems. Cochrane Database Syst Rev 2014;(6):CD001059.

[222] World Health Organization (WHO). Guideline: calcium supplementation in pregnant women. Geneva: WHO; 2013. Available from: www.who.int/about.

[223] Buppasiri P, Lumbiganon P, Thinkamrop J, et al. Calcium supplementation (other than for preventing or treating hypertension) for improving pregnancy and infant outcomes. Cochrane Database Syst Rev 2011;(10):CD007079.

[224] Berry C, Atta MG. Hypertensive disorders in pregnancy. World J Nephrol 2016;5(5):418–28.

[225] Woods SE, Ghodsi V, Engel A, et al. Serum chromium and gestational diabetes. J Am Board Fam Med 2008;21(2):153–7.

[226] Sundararaman PG, Sridhar GR, Sujatha V, et al. Serum chromium levels in gestational diabetes mellitus. Indian J Endocrinol Metab 2012;16:S70–3.

[227] Skeaff SA. Iodine deficiency in pregnancy: the effect on neurodevelopment in the child. Nutrients 2011;3(2):265–73.

[228] Zimmermann MB. The role of iodine in human growth and development. Semin Cell Dev Biol 2011;22:645–52.

[229] Gallego G, Goodall S, Eastman CJ. Iodine defiency in Australia: is iodine supplementation for pregnant and lactating women warranted? Med J Aust 2010;192(8):461–3.

[230] Bath SC, Furmidge-Owen VL, Redman CWG, et al. Gestational changes in iodine status in a cohort study of pregnant women from the United Kingdom. Am J Clin Nutr 2015;1180–7.

[231] Andersson M, De Benoist B, Delange F, et al. Prevention and control of iodine deficiency in pregnant and lactating women and in children less than 2 years old: conclusions and recommendations of the Technical Consultation WHO Secretariat on behalf of the participants to the Consultation. Public Heal Nutr 2007;10(12A):1606–11.

[232] Eastman CJ. Screening for thyroid disease and iodine deficiency. Pathology 2012;44(2):153–9.

[233] Brantsæter AL, Abel MH, Haugen M, et al. Risk of suboptimal iodine intake in pregnant Norwegian women. Nutrients 2013;5(2):424–40.

[234] Hamrosi MA, Wallace EM, Riley MD. Iodine status in pregnant women living in Melbourne differs by ethnic group. Asia Pac J Clin Nutr 2005;14(1):27–31.

[235] Blumenthal N, Byth K, Eastman CJ. Iodine intake and thyroid function in pregnant women in a private clinical practice in northwestern Sydney before mandatory fortification of bread with iodised salt. J Thyroid Res 2012.

[236] Clifton VL, Hodyl NA, Fogarty PA, et al. The impact of iodine supplementation and bread fortification on urinary iodine concentrations in a mildly iodine-deficient population of pregnant women in South Australia. Nutr J 2013;12:1.

[237] Hynes KL, Otahal P, Hay I, et al. Mild iodine deficiency during pregnancy is associated with reduced educational outcomes in the offspring: 9-year follow-up of the gestational iodine cohort. J Clin Endocrinol Metab 2013;98(5):1954–62.

[238] Qian M, Wang D, Watkins WE, et al. The effects of iodine on intelligence in children: a meta-analysis of studies conducted in China. Asia Pacific J Clin Nutr 2005;14(1):32–43.

[239] Connelly KJ, Boston BA, Pearce EN, et al. Congenital hypothyroidism caused by excess prenatal maternal iodine ingestion. J Pediatr 2012;161(4):760–2.

[240] Thaker VV, Leung AM, Braverman LE, et al. Iodine-induced hypothyroidism in full-term infants with congenital heart disease: more common than currently appreciated? J Clin Endocrinol Metab 2014;99(10):3521–6.

[241] Sun X, Shan Z, Teng W. Effects of increased iodine intake on thyroid disorders. Endocrinol Metab 2014;29(3):240–7.

[242] Guan H, Li C, Fan C, et al. High iodine intake is a risk factor of post-partum thyroiditis: result of a survey from Shenyang, China. J Endocrinol Invest 2005;28(10):876–81.

[243] De Leo S, Pearce EN, Braverman LE. Iodine supplementation in women during preconception, pregnancy and lactation: current clinical practice by US obstetricians and midwives. Thyroid 2017;27(3):434–9.

[244] Charlton K, Yeatman H, Lucas C, et al. Poor knowledge and practices related to iodine nutrition during pregnancy and lactation in Australian women: pre- and post-iodine fortification. Nutrients 2012;4:1317–27.

[245] Antony KM, Racusin DA, Aagaard K, et al. Maternal physiology. In: Gabbe S, Niebyl J, Simpson J, et al, editors. Obstetrics: normal and problem pregnancies. 7th ed. Philadelphia: Elsevier; 2017.

[246] Choudhury V, Amin SB, Agarwal A, et al. Latent iron deficiency at birth influences auditory neural maturation in late preterm and term infants. Am J Clin Nutr 2015;102(5):1030–4.

[247] Amin SB, Orlando M, Eddins A, et al. In utero iron status and auditory neural maturation in premature infants as evaluated by auditory brainstem response. J Pediatr 2010;156(3):377–81.

[248] Behboudi-Gandevani S, Safary K, Moghaddam-Banaem L, et al. The relationship between maternal serum iron and zinc levels and their nutritional intakes in early pregnancy with gestational diabetes. Biol Trace Elem Res 2013;154(1):7–13.

[249] Bao W, Chavarro JE, Tobias DK, et al. Long-term risk of type 2 diabetes in relation to habitual iron intake in women with a history of gestational diabetes: a prospective cohort study. Am J Clin Nutr 2016;103(2):375–81.

[250] Rawal S, Hinkle SN, Bao W, et al. A longitudinal study of iron status during pregnancy and the risk of gestational diabetes: findings from a prospective, multiracial cohort. Diabetologica 2016;1–9.

[251] Kidson-Gerber G, Zheng S. Iron deficiency in pregnancy: what you need to know. MedicineToday 2016;17(4):41–6.

[252] Pavord S, Myers B, Robinson S, et al. UK guidelines on the management of iron deficiency in pregnancy. Br J Haematol 2012;156(5):588–600.

[253] Jafrin W, Mia AR, Chakraborty PK, et al. An evaluation of serum magnesium status in pre-eclampsia compared to the normal pregnancy. Mymensingh Med J 2014;23(4):649–53.

[254] Rylander R. Magnesium in pregnancy blood pressure and pre-eclampsia: a review. Pregnancy Hypertens 2014;4:146–9.

[255] Nestler A, Rylander R, Kolisek M, et al. Blood pressure in pregnancy and magnesium sensitive genes. Pregnancy Hypertens 2014;4:41–5.

[256] Asemi Z, Karamali M, Jamilian M, et al. Magnesium supplementation affects metabolic status and pregnancy outcomes in gestational diabetes: a randomized, double-blind, placebo-controlled trial. Am J Clin Nutr 2015;102:222–9.

[257] Goker TU, Tasdemir N, Kilic S, et al. Alterations of ionized and total magnesium levels in pregnant women with gestational diabetes mellitus. Gynecol Obs Invest 2015;79(1):19–24.

[258] Mostafavi E, Nargesi AA, Asbagh FA, et al. Abdominal obesity and gestational diabetes: the interactive role of magnesium. Magnes Res 2015;28(4):116–25.

[259] Supakatisant C, Phupong V. Oral magnesium for relief in pregnancy-induced leg cramps: a randomised controlled trial. Matern Child Nutr 2015;11(2):139–45.

[260] Rayman MP, Bath SC, Westaway J, et al. Selenium status in UK pregnant women and its relationship with hypertensive conditions of pregnancy. Br J Nutr 2015;113:249–58.

[261] Mistry HD, Kurlak LO, Young SD, et al. Maternal selenium, copper and zinc concentrations in pregnancy associated with small-for-gestational-age infants. Matern Child Nutr 2014;10(3):327–34.

[262] Tsuzuki S, Morimoto N, Hosokawa S, et al. Associations of maternal and neonatal serum trace element concentrations with neonatal birth weight. PLoS ONE 2013;8(9):e75627.

[263] Kong FJ, Ma LL, Chen SP, et al. Serum selenium level and gestational diabetes mellitus: a systematic review and meta-analysis. Nutr J 2016;15(94):1–10.

[264] Askari G, Iraj B, Salehi-Abargouei A, et al. The association between serum selenium and gestational diabetes mellitus: a systematic review and meta-analysis. J Trace Elem Med Biol 2015;29:195–201.

[265] Terrin G, Canani RB, Di Chiara M, et al. Zinc in early life: a key element in the fetus and preterm neonate. Nutrients 2015;7:10427–46.

[266] Darnton-Hill I. Zinc supplementation during pregnancy: biological, behavioural and contextual rationale. Available from www.who.int/elena/bbc/zinc_pregnancy/en. [Cited 18 November 2016].

[267] Vela G, Stark P, Socha M, et al. Zinc in gut–brain interaction in autism and neurological disorders. Neural Plast 2015:972791.

[268] Chaffee BW, King JC. Effect of zinc supplementation on pregnancy and infant outcomes: a systematic review. Paediatr Perinat Epidemiol 2012;26(Suppl. 1):118–37.

[269] Vashum KP, McEvoy M, Milton AH, et al. Dietary zinc is associated with a lower incidence of depression: findings from two Australian cohorts. J Affect Disord 2014;166:249–57.

[270] Roomruangwong C, Kanchanatawan B, Sirivichayakul S, et al. Lower serum zinc and higher CRP strongly predict prenatal depression and physio-somatic symptoms, which all together predict postnatal depressive symptoms. Mol Neurobiol 2016; 1–10.

[271] Swardfager W, Herrmann N, Mazereeuw G, et al. Zinc in depression: a meta-analysis. Biol Psychiatry 2013;74(15):872–8.

[272] Donangelo CM, King JC. Maternal zinc intake and homeostatic adjustments during pregnancy and lactation. Nutrients 2012;4:782–98.

[273] Khadem N, Mohammadzadeh A, Farhat A, et al. Relationship between low birth weight neonate and maternal serum zinc concentration. Iran Red Crescent Med J 2012;14(4):240–4.

[274] Ota E, Mori R, Middleton P, et al. Zinc supplementation for improving pregnancy and infant outcome. Cochrane Database Syst Rev 2015;(2):CD000230.

[275] Ma Y, Shen X, Zhang D. The relationship between serum zinc level and preeclampsia: a meta-analysis. Nutrients 2015;7(9):7806–20.

[276] Ilmonen J, Isolauri E, Poussa T, et al. Impact of dietary counselling and probiotic intervention on maternal anthropometric measurements during and after pregnancy: a randomized placebo-controlled trial. Clin Nutr 2011;30(2):156–64.

[277] Doege K, Grajecki D, Zyriax BC, et al. Impact of maternal supplementation with probiotics during pregnancy on atopic eczema in childhood: a meta-analysis. Br J Nutr 2016;10:1–6.

[278] Fiocchi A, Pawankar R, Cuello-Garcia C, et al. World Allergy Organization-McMaster University Guidelines for Allergic Disease Prevention (GLAD-P): probiotics. WAO J 2015;8(4):1–13.

[279] Mendling W. Vaginal microbiota. Adv Exp Med Biol 2016;902:83–93.

[280] Nuriel-Ohayon M, Neuman H, Koren O. Microbial changes during pregnancy, birth, and infancy. Front Microbiol 2016;7(1031):1–13.

[281] Cole LA. hCG, the wonder of today's science. Reprod Biol Endocrinol 2012;10(24):1–18.

[282] Cole LA. Biological functions of hCG and hCG-related molecules. Reprod Biol Endocrinol 2010;8(102):127–35.

[283] Critchfield AS, Yao G, Jaishankar A, et al. Cervical mucus properties stratify risk for preterm birth. PLoS ONE 2013;8(8):e69528.

[284] Mestman JH. Thyroid and parathyroid diseases in pregnancy. In: Gabbe S, Niebyl J, Simpson J, et al, editors. Obstetrics: normal and problem pregnancies. 7th ed. Philadelphia: Elsevier; 2017.

[285] Burton GJ, Sibley CP, Jauniaux ERM, et al. Placental anatomy and physiology placental physiology 12. In: Gabbe S, Niebyl J, Simpson J, et al, editors. Obstetrics: normal and problem pregnancies. 7th ed. Philadelphia: Elsevier; 2017.

[286] Kim JH, Shin MS, Yi G, et al. Serum biomarkers for predicting pregnancy outcome in women undergoing IVF: human chorionic gonadotropin, progesterone, and inhibin A level at 11 days post-ET. Clin Exp Reprod Med 2012;39(1):28–32.

[287] Pan FC, Brissova M. Pancreas development in humans. Curr Opin Endocrinol Diabetes Ob 2014;21(2):77–82.

[288] Gregory KD, Ramos DE, Jauniaux ERM. Preconception and prenatal care. In: Gabbe S, Niebyl J, Simpson J, et al, editors. Obstetrics: normal and problem pregnancies. 7th ed. Philadelphia: Elsevier; 2017.

[289] The Royal Australian and New Zealand College of Obstetricians and Gynaecologists. Prenatal screening and diagnosis of chromosomal and genetic conditions in the fetus in pregnancy. East Melbourne; 2016.

[290] Bromley B, Shipp TD. First-trimester imaging. In: Creasy RK, Resnik R, Iams JD, et al, editors. Creasy and Resnik's maternal-fetal medicine: principles and practice. 7th ed. Philadelphia: Elsevier; 2014.

[291] Park SY, Jang IA, Lee MA, et al. Screening for chromosomal abnormalities using combined test in the first trimester of pregnancy. Obs Gynecol Sci 2016;59(5):357–66.

[292] Gagnon A, Wilson RD, Audibert F, et al. Obstetrical complications associated with abnormal maternal serum markers analytes. J Obs Gynaecol Can 2008;30(10):918–49.

[293] Enciso M, Sarasa J, Xanthopoulou L, et al. Polymorphisms in the MTHFR gene influence embryo viability and the incidence of aneuploidy. Hum Genet 2016;135(5):555–68.

[294] Wapner RJ. Prenatal diagnosis of congenital disorders. In: Creasy RK, Resnik R, Iams JD, et al, editors. Creasy and Resnik's maternal-fetal medicine: principles and practice. 7th ed. Philadelphia: Elsevier; 2014.

[295] Wah YM, Leung TY, Cheng YK, et al. Procedure-related fetal loss following chorionic villus sampling after first-trimester aneuploidy screening. Fetal Diagn Ther 2016;41(3):184–90.

[296] O'Donnell A, McParlin C, Robson SC, et al. Treatments for hyperemesis gravidarum and nausea and vomiting in pregnancy: a systematic review and economic assessment. Heal Technol Assess 2016;20(74):1–268.

[297] Cappell MS. Gastrointestinal disorders during pregnancy. In: Gabbe S, Niebyl J, Simpson J, et al, editors. Obstetrics: normal and problem pregnancies. 7th ed. Philadelphia: Elsevier; 2017.

[298] Kelly TF, Savides TJ. Gastrointestinal disease in pregnancy. In: Creasy RK, Resnik R, Iams JD, et al, editors. Creasy and Resnik's maternal-fetal medicine: principles and practice. 7th ed. Philadelphia: Elsevier; 2014.

[299] Chortatos A, Haugen M, Iversen O, et al. Pregnancy complications and birth outcomes among women experiencing nausea only or nausea and vomiting during pregnancy in the Norwegian Mother and Child Cohort Study. BMC Pregnancy Childbirth 2015;15:138.

[300] Viljoen E, Visser J, Koen N, et al. A systematic review and meta-analysis of the effect and safety of ginger in the treatment of pregnancy-associated nausea and vomiting. Nutr J 2014;13(1):20.

[301] Goodwin TM, Poursharif B, Korst LM, et al. Secular trends in the treatment of hyperemesis gravidarum. Am J Perinatol 2008;25(3):141–7.

[302] Quinlan JD, Hill DA. Nausea and vomiting of pregnancy. Am Fam Physician 2003;68(1):121–8.

[303] Koren G, Madjunkova S, Maltepe C. The protective effects of nausea and vomiting of pregnancy against adverse fetal outcome: a systematic review. Reprod Toxicol 2014;47:77–80.

[304] Veenendaal M, van Abeelen A, Painter R, et al. Consequences of hyperemesis gravidarum for offspring: a systematic review and meta-analysis. BJOG 2011;118:1302–13.

[305] Bolin M, Åkerud H, Cnattingius S, et al. Hyperemesis gravidarum and risks of placental dysfunction disorders: a population-based cohort study. BJOG 2013;120(5):541–7.

[306] Walstab J, Krüger D, Stark T, et al. Ginger and its pungent constituents non-competitively inhibit activation of human recombinant and native 5-HT3 receptors of enteric neurons. Neurogastroenterol Motil 2013;25(5):439–47.

[307] Jin Z, Lee G, Kim S, et al. Ginger and its pungent constituents non-competitively inhibit serotonin currents on visceral afferent neurons. Korean J Physiol Pharmacol 2014;18:149–53.

[308] Matthews A, Haas DM, O'Mathúna DP, et al. Interventions for nausea and vomiting in early pregnancy. Cochrane Database Syst Rev 2015;(9):CD007575.

[309] Food Standards Australia and New Zealand. Listeria and food: advice for people at risk. Available from www.foodstandards.gov.au/publications/pages/listeriabrochuretext.aspx. [Cited 18 November 2016].

[310] Duff P, Birsner M. Maternal and perinatal infection in pregnancy: bacterial. In: Gabbe SG, Niebyl JR, Simpson JL, et al, editors. Obstetrics: normal and problem pregnancies. 7th ed. Philadelphia: Elsevier; 2017.

[311] SA Health. Toxoplasma infection: including symptoms, treatment and prevention. Available from www.sahealth.sa.gov.au/wps/wcm/

connect/public+content/sa+health+internet/health+topics. [Cited 18 November 2016].

[312] Nazik E, Eryilmaz G. Incidence of pregnancy-related discomforts and management approaches to relieve them among pregnant women. J Clin Nurs 2014;23(11–12):1736–50.

[313] Landon MB, Catalano PM, Gabbe SG. Diabetes mellitus complicating pregnancy. In: Gabbe SG, Niebyl JR, Simpson JL, et al, editors. Obstetrics: normal and problem pregnancies. 7th ed. Philadelphia: Elsevier; 2017.

[314] Liu JH. Endocrinology of pregnancy. In: Creasy RK, Resnik R, Iams JD, et al, editors. Creasy & Resnik's maternal-fetal medicine: principles and practice. 7th ed. Philadelphia: Elsevier; 2014.

[315] Ide M, Papapanou PN. Epidemiology of association between maternal periodontal disease and adverse pregnancy outcomes: systematic review. J Clin Periodontol 2013;(Suppl. 14):S181–94.

[316] Abariga SA, Whitcomb BW. Periodontitis and gestational diabetes mellitus: a systematic review and meta-analysis of observational studies. BMC Pregnancy Childbirth 2016;16(344).

[317] Moeindarbari S, Tara F, Lotfalizadeh M. The effect of diagnostic amniocentesis and its complications on early spontaneous abortion. Electron Physician 2016;8(8):2787–92.

[318] Malfertheiner M, Malfertheiner P, Costa SD, et al. Extraesophageal symptoms of gastroesophageal reflux disease during pregnancy. J Gastroentero 2015;53(9):1080–3.

[319] Sibai BM. Preeclampsia and hypertensive disorders. In: Gabbe S, Niebyl J, Simpson J, et al, editors. Obstetrics: normal and problem pregnancies. 7th ed. Philadelphia: Elsevier; 2017.

[320] Markham KB, Funai EF. Pregnancy-related hypertension. In: Creasy RK, Resnik R, Iams JD, et al, editors. Creasy and Resnik's maternal-fetal medicine: principles and practice. 7th ed. Philadelphia: Elsevier; 2014.

[321] Hariharan N, Shoemaker A, Wagner S. Pathophysiology of hypertension in preeclampsia. Microvasc Res 2017;13(2):33–7.

[322] Zeng Y, Li M, Chen Y, et al. Homocysteine, endothelin-1 and nitric oxide in patients with hypertensive disorders complicating pregnancy. Int J Clin Exp Pathol 2015;8(11):15275–9.

[323] Bilodeau JF. Maternal and placental antioxidant response to preeclampsia: impact on vasoactive eicosanoids. Placenta 2014;28:S32–8.

[324] Makrides M, Crosby DD, Bain E, et al. Magnesium supplementation in pregnancy. Cochrane Database Syst Rev 2014;(4):CD000937.

[325] Imdad A, Bhutta ZA. Effects of calcium supplementation during pregnancy on maternal, fetal and birth outcomes. Paediatr Perinat Epidemiol 2012;(Suppl. 1):138–52.

[326] Mustafa R, Ahmed S, Gupta A, et al. A comprehensive review of hypertension in pregnancy. J Pregnancy 2012.

[327] Schoenaker D, Soedamah-Muthu S, Callaway L, et al. Prepregnancy dietary patterns and risk of developing hypertensive disorders of pregnancy: results from the Australian Longitudinal Study on Women's Health. Am J Clin Nutr 2015;102(1):94–101.

[328] Bullarbo M, Ödman N, Nestler A, et al. Magnesium supplementation to prevent high blood pressure in pregnancy: a randomised placebo control trial. Arch Gynecol Obs 2013;288(6):1269–74.

[329] Hofmeyr GJ, Lawrie TA, Atallah AN, et al. Calcium supplementation during pregnancy for preventing hypertensive disorders and related problems. Cochrane Database Syst Rev 2010;(8):CD001059.

[330] Haddy FJ, Vanhoutte PM, Feletou M. Role of potassium in regulating blood flow and blood pressure. Am J Physiol Regul Integr Comp Physiol 2006;290(3):R546–52.

[331] Yilmax MI, Solak Y, Covic A, et al. Renal anemia of inflammation: the name is self-explanatory. Blood Purif 2011;32(3):220–5.

[332] Jensen CL. Effects of omega 3 fatty acids during pregnancy and lactation. Am J Clin Nutr 2006;83(6):S1452–7.

[333] Dorniak-Wall T, Grivell RM, Dekker GA, et al. The role of L-arginine in the prevention and treatment of pre-eclampsia: a systematic review of randomised trials. J Hum Hypertens 2014;28(4):230–5.

[334] Dignon A, Reddington A. The physical effect of exercise in pregnancy on pre-eclampsia, gestational diabetes, birthweight and type of delivery: a structured review. Available from www.rcm.org.uk/learning-and-career/learning-and-research/ebm-articles/the-physical-effect-of-exercise-in-pregnancy.

[335] Yao M, Ritchie HE, Brown-Woodman PD. A reproductive screening test of hawthorn. J Ethnopharmacol 2008;118(1):127–32.

[336] Ross MG, Gore Ervin M. Fetal development and physiology. In: Gabbe S, Niebyl J, Simpson J, et al, editors. Obstetrics: normal and problem pregnancies. 7th ed. Philadelphia: Elsevier; 2017.

[337] The Royal Australian and New Zealand College of Obstetricians and Gynaecologists. Maternal Group B Streptococcus in pregnancy: screening and management. East Melbourne; 2016.

[338] Rönnqvist PD, Forsgren-Brusk UB, Grahn-Håkansson E. Lactobacilli in the female genital tract in relation to other genital microbes and vaginal pH. Acta Obs Gynecol Scand 2006;85(6):726–38.

[339] Wang AR, Kroumpouzos G. Skin disease and pregnancy. In: Gabbe S, Niebyl J, Simpson J, et al, editors. Obstetrics: normal and problem pregnancies. 7th ed. Philadelphia: Elsevier; 2017.

[340] Jurecka W. Pregnancy dermatoses. In: Lebwohl MG, Heymann WR, Berth-Jones J, et al, editors. Treatment of skin disease: comprehensive therapeutic strategies. 4th ed. Philadelphia: Elsevier; 2014.

[341] Rapini RP. The skin and pregnancy. In: Creasy RK, Resnik R, Iams JD, et al, editors. Creasy and Resnik's maternal-fetal medicine: principles and practice. 7th ed. Philadelphia: Elsevier; 2014.

[342] Dixon PH, Williamson C. The pathophysiology of intrahepatic cholestasis of pregnancy. Clin Res Hepatol Gastroenterol 2016;40(2):141–53.

[343] Williamson C, Mackillop L, Heneghan M. Diseases of the liver, biliary system, and pancreas. In: Creasy RK, Resnik R, Iams JD, et al, editors. Creasy and Resnik's maternal-fetal medicine: principles and practice. 7th ed. Philadelphia: Elsevier; 2014.

[344] Cappell MS. Hepatic disorder during pregnancy. In: Gabbe S, Niebyl J, Simpson J, et al, editors. Obstetrics: normal and problem pregnancies. 7th ed. Philadelphia: Elsevier; 2017.

[345] Moses RG, Morris G, Petocz P, et al. Impact of the potential new diagnostic criteria on the prevalence of gestational diabetes mellitus in Australia. Med J Aust 2011;194:338–40.

[346] DeSisto CL, Kim SY, Sharma AJ. Prevalence estimates of gestational diabetes mellitus in the United States, Pregnancy Risk Assessment Monitoring System (PRAMS), 2007–2010. Prev Chronic Dis 2014;11.

[347] McGovern A, Butler L, Jones S, et al. Diabetes screening after gestational diabetes in England: a quantitative retrospective cohort study. Br J Gen Pr 2014;64(618):e17–23.

[348] Moore T, Haugel-De Mouzon S, Catalanon P. Diabetes in pregnancy. In: Creasy RK, Resnik R, Iams JD, et al, editors. Creasy & Resnik's maternal-fetal medicine: principles and practice. 7th ed. Philadelphia: Elsevier; 2014.

[349] Nankervis A, Conn J. Gestational diabetes mellitus: negotiating the confusion. Aust Fam Phys 2013;42(8):528–31.

[350] International Association of Diabetes and Pregnancy Study Groups Consensus Panel, Metzger BE, Gabbe SG, et al. International Association of Diabetes and Pregnancy Study Groups recommendations on the diagnosis and classification of hyperglycemia in pregnancy. Diabetes Care 2010;33(3):676–82.

[351] Schoenaker DA, Mishra GD, Callaway LK, et al. The role of energy, nutrients, foods, and dietary patterns in the development of gestational diabetes mellitus: a systematic review of observational studies. Diabetes Care 2016;39:16–23.

[352] Gatford KL, Houda CM, Lu ZX, et al. Vitamin B_{12} and homocysteine status during pregnancy in the metformin in gestational diabetes trial: responses to maternal metformin compared with insulin treatment. Diabetes Obes Metab 2013;15(7):660–7.

[353] Dolatkhah N, Hajifaraji M, Abbasalizadeh F, et al. Is there a value for probiotic supplements in gestational diabetes mellitus? A randomized clinical trial. J Heal Popul Nutr 2015;33:25.

[354] Jamilian M, Samimi M, Kolahdooz F, et al. Omega-3 fatty acid supplementation affects pregnancy outcomes in gestational diabetes: a randomized, double-blind, placebo-controlled trial. J Matern Fetal Neonatal Med 2016;29(4):669–75.

[355] Asemi Z, Jamilian M, Mesdaghinia E, et al. Effects of selenium supplementation on glucose homeostasis, inflammation, and oxidative stress in gestational diabetes: randomized, double-blind, placebo-controlled trial. Nutrition 2015;31:1235–42.

[356] Mei Z, Cogswell ME, Looker AC, et al. Assessment of iron status in US pregnant women from the National Health and Nutrition Examination Survey (NHANES). Am J Clin Nutr 2011;93:1312–20.

[357] Kilpatrick SJ. Anemia and pregnancy. In: Creasy RK, Resnik R, Iams JD, et al, editors. Creasy & Resnik's maternal-fetal medicine: principles and practice. 7th ed. Philadelphia: Elsevier; 2014.

[358] Samuels P. Hematologic complications of pregnancy. In: Gabbe S, Niebyl J, Simpson J, et al, editors. Obstetrics: normal and problem pregnancies. 7th ed. Philadelphia: Elsevier; 2017.

[359] King Edward Memorial Hospital. Anaemia in pregnancy: clinical guideline. Perth: Govt Western Australia, Dept Health; 2013.

[360] Yakoob MY, Bhutta ZA. Effect of routine iron supplementation with or without folic acid on anemia during pregnancy. BMC Public Health 2011;11(Suppl. 3):S21.

[361] Demirel G, Golbasi Z. Effect of perineal massage on the rate of episiotomy and perineal tearing. Int J Gynaecol Obs 2015;131(2):183–6.

[362] Beckman MM, Stock OM. Antenatal perineal massage for reducing perineal trauma. Cochrane Database Syst Rev 2013;(4):CD005123.

[363] Holst L, Haavik S, Nordeng H. Raspberry leaf: should it be recommended to pregnant women? Complement Ther Clin Pract 2009;15(4):204–8.

[364] Parsons M, Simpson M, Ponton T. Raspberry leaf and its effect on labour: safety and efficacy. Aust Coll Midwives Inc J 1999;12(3):20–5.

[365] Simpson M, Parson M, Greenwood J, et al. Raspberry leaf in pregnancy: its safety and efficacy in labor. J Midwif Wom Heal 2001;46(2):51–9.

[366] Hall HG, McKenna LG, Griffiths DL. Complementary and alternative medicine for induction of labour. Women Birth 2012;25(3):142–8.

[367] Price C, Robinson S. Birth: conceiving, nurturing and giving birth to your baby. Sydney: MacMillan; 2004.

[368] Wang H, Hu YF, Hao JH, et al. Maternal serum zinc concentration during pregnancy is inversely associated with risk of preterm birth in a Chinese population. J Nutr 2016;146(3):509–12.

[369] Hechtman L. Pregnancy intensive seminar: the fundamentals for health professionals. Sydney: Integria; 2014.

[370] Berghella V, Mackeen D, Jauniaux ER. Cesarean delivery. In: Gabbe SG, Niebyl JR, Simpson JL, et al, editors. Obstetrics: normal and problem pregnancies. 7th ed. Philadelphia: Elsevier; 2017.

[371] Bayes S, Fenwick J, Hauck Y. Becoming redundant: Australian women's experiences of pregnancy after being unexpectedly scheduled for a medically necessary term elective cesarean section. Int J Childbirth 2012;2(2):73–84.

[372] Stevens J, Schmied V, Burns E, et al. A juxtaposition of birth and surgery: providing skin-to-skin contact in the operating theatre and recovery. Midwifery 2016;37:41–8.

[373] Moore ER, Anderson GC, Bergman N, et al. Early skin-to-skin contact for mothers and their healthy newborn infants. Cochrane Database Syst Rev 2012;(5):CD003519.

[374] Stevens J, Schmied V, Burns E, et al. Immediate or early skin-to-skin contact after a caesarean section: a review of the literature. Matern Child Nutr 2014;10(4):456–73.

[375] Neu J, Rushing J. Cesarean versus vaginal delivery: long-term infant outcomes and the hygiene hypothesis. Clin Perinatol 2011;38(2):321–31.

[376] Arrieta MC, Stiemsma LT, Amenyogbe N, et al. The intestinal microbiome in early life: health and disease. Front Immunol 2014;5:427.

[377] Almgren M, Schlinzig T, Gomez-Cabrero D, et al. Cesarean delivery and hematopoietic stem cell epigenetics in the newborn infant: implications for future health? Am J Obs Gynecol 2014;211(5):502.e1–8.

[378] Blustein J, Attina T, Liu M, et al. Association of caesarean delivery with child adiposity from age 6 weeks to 15 years. Int J Obes 2013;37:900–6.

[379] Bager P, Simonsen J, Nielsen NM, et al. Cesarean section and offspring's risk of inflammatory bowel disease: a national cohort study. Inflamm Bowel Dis 2012;18(5):857–62.

[380] Li Y, Tian Y, Zhu W, et al. Cesarean delivery and risk of inflammatory bowel disease: a systematic review and meta-analysis. Scand J Gastroenterol 2014;49(7):834–44.

[381] Vindigni SM, Zisman TL, Suskind DL, et al. Therapeutic advances in gastroenterology. Ther Adv Gastroenterol 2016;9(4):606–25.

[382] Decker E, Hornef M, Stockinger S. Cesarean delivery is associated with celiac disease but not inflammatory bowel disease in children. Gut Microbes 2011;2:91–8.

[383] Dominguez-Bello MG, De Jesus-Laboy KM, Shen N, et al. Partial restoration of the microbiota of cesarean-born infants via vaginal microbial transfer. Nat Med 2016;22(3):250–3.

[384] Perinatal Anxiety & Depression Australia (PANDA). Perinatal anxiety & depression Australia. Available from www.panda.org.au/practical-information/information-for-men. [Cited 24 November 2016].

[385] American Psychiatric Association. Diagnostic and statistical manual of mental disorders: DSM-V. Washington, DC: American Psychiatric Publishing; 2013.

[386] Austin MP, Highet N, Guidelines Expert Advisory Committee. Clinical practice guidelines for depression and related disorders — anxiety, bipolar disorder and puerperal psychosis — in the perinatal period: a guideline for primary care health professionals. Melbourne: beyondblue; 2011.

[387] Wisner KL, Sit DKY, Bogen DL, et al. Mental health and behavioral disorders in pregnancy. In: Gabbe S, Niebyl J, Simpson J, et al, editors. Obstetrics: normal and problem pregnancies. 7th ed. Philadelphia: Elsevier; 2017.

[388] Yonkers KA. Management of depression and psychoses in pregnancy and in the puerperium. In: Creasy RK, Resnik R, Iams JD, et al, editors. Creasy & Resnik's maternal-fetal medicine: principles and practice. 7th ed. Philadelphia: Elsevier; 2014.

[389] Pedersen CA, Johnson JL, Silva S, et al. Antenatal thyroid correlates of postpartum depression. Psychoneuroendocrinol 2007;32(3):235–45.

[390] Bunevicius R, Kusminskas L, Mickuviene N, et al. Depressive disorder and thyroid axis functioning during pregnancy. World J Biol Psychiatr 2009;10(4):324–9.

[391] Pedersen C, Leserman J, Garcia N, et al. Late pregnancy thyroid-binding globulin predicts perinatal depression. Psychoneuroendocrinol 2016;65:84–93.

[392] Edler Schiller C, Meltzer-Brody S, Rubinow DR. The role of reproductive hormones in postpartum depression. CNS Spectr 2015;20(1):48–59.

[393] World Health Organization (WHO). Maternal mental health and child health and development in resource-constrained settings. Report of a UNFPA/WHO International Expert Meeting: The Interface Between Reproductive Health and Mental Health. Geneva: WHO; 2009.

[394] Rechenberg K, Humphries D. Nutritional interventions in depression and perinatal depression. Yale J Biol Med 2013;86(2):127–37.

[395] Rees AM, Austin MP, Parker GB. Omega-3 fatty acids as a treatment for perinatal depression: randomized double-blind placebo-controlled trial. Aust NZ J Psychiatry 2008;42(3):199–205.

[396] Nader S. Thyroid disease and pregnancy. In: Creasy RK, Resnik R, Iams JD, et al, editors. Creasy & Resnik's maternal-fetal medicine: principles and practice. 7th ed. Philadelphia: Elsevier; 2014.

[397] Lazarus JH. The continuing saga of postpartum thyroiditis. J Clin Endocrinol Metab 2011;96:614.

APPENDIX 13.1

Tools to assess NVP

Tool	Description
PUQE: Pregnancy-Unique Quantification of Emesis and Nausea	Three questions regarding nausea, vomiting and retching during previous 12 or 24 hours For each component: 0 = no symptoms, 5 = worst possible symptoms Maximum score = 15 Score ≥13 indicates severe symptoms
RINVR: Rhodes Index of Nausea, Vomiting and Retching	Eight questions about duration, amount, frequency and distress caused by symptoms of nausea, vomiting and retching For each component: 0 = no symptoms, 5 = worst possible symptoms Maximum score = 40 Score ≥33 indicates severe symptoms
McGill Nausea Questionnaire	Measures nausea only using a nausea rating index that has nine sets of words that describe sensory, affective, evaluative and miscellaneous afferent feelings related to nausea that women rank An overall nausea index: 0–5, where 0 = no symptoms, 5 = excruciating symptoms Plus a VAS: 0 cm = no nausea, 10 cm = extreme nausea
NVPI: Nausea and Vomiting of Pregnancy Instrument	Three questions relating to nausea, retching and vomiting over the past 7 days For each component: 0 = no symptoms, 5 = worst possible symptoms Maximum score = 15 Score ≥8 indicates severe symptoms
VAS: Visual Analogue Scale	Patients rate their symptoms on a scale of 0–10, where 0 = no symptoms and 10 = extreme symptoms

Source: Adapted from O'Donnell A, McParlin C, Robson SC, Beyer F, Moloney E, Bryant A et al. Treatments for hyperemesis gravidarum and nausea and vomiting in pregnancy: a systematic review and economic assessment. Heal Technol Assess 2016;20(74).

APPENDIX 13.2

Edinburgh Postnatal Depression Scale (EPDS)

Question	Score

1. I have been able to laugh and see the funny side of things
  ☐ As much as I always could
  ☐ Not quite so much now
  ☐ Definitely not so much now
  ☐ Not at all
	0
	1
	2
	3

2. I have looked forward with enjoyment to things
  ☐ As much as I ever did
  ☐ Rather less than I used to
  ☐ Definitely less than I used to
  ☐ Hardly at all
	0
	1
	2
	3

3. I have blamed myself unnecessarily when things went wrong
  ☐ Yes, most of the time
  ☐ Yes, some of the time
  ☐ Not very often
  ☐ No, never
	3
	2
	1
	0

4. I have been anxious or worried for no good reason
  ☐ No, not at all
  ☐ Hardly ever
  ☐ Yes, sometimes
  ☐ Yes, very often
	0
	1
	2
	3

5. I have felt scared or panicky for no very good reason
  ☐ Yes, quite a lot
  ☐ Yes, sometimes
  ☐ No, not much
  ☐ No, not at all
	3
	2
	1
	0

Question	Score
6. Things have been getting on top of me	
□ Yes, most of the time I haven't been able to cope at all	3
□ Yes, sometimes I haven't been coping as well as usual	2
□ No, most of the time I have coped quite well	1
□ No, I have been coping as well as ever	0
7. I have been so unhappy that I have had difficulty sleeping	
□ Yes, most of the time	3
□ Yes, sometimes	2
□ Not very often	1
□ No, not at all	0
8. I have felt sad or miserable	
□ Yes, most of the time	3
□ Yes, quite often	2
□ Not very often	1
□ No, not at all	0
9. I have been so unhappy that I have been crying	
□ Yes, most of the time	3
□ Yes, quite often	2
□ Only occasionally	1
□ No, never	0
10. The thought of harming myself has occurred to me	
□ Yes, quite often	3
□ Sometimes	2
□ Hardly ever	1
□ Never	0

Source: Murray D, Cox J. Screening for depression during pregnancy with the Edinburgh Depression Scale (EDDS). J Reprod Infant Psych 1990;8(2):99–107.

Scoring

0–9: Scores in this range may indicate the presence of some symptoms of distress that may be short-lived and are less likely to interfere with day-to-day ability to function at home or at work. However, if these symptoms have persisted more than a week or two, further enquiry is warranted.

10–12: Scores within this range indicate the presence of symptoms of distress that may be discomforting. Repeat the EDS in 2 weeks time and continue monitoring progress regularly. If the scores increase to above 12, assess further and consider referral as needed.

13 +: Scores above 12 require further assessment and appropriate management as the likelihood of depression is high. Referral to a psychiatrist/psychologist may be necessary.

Item 10: Any woman who scores 1, 2 or 3 on item 10 requires further evaluation before leaving the office to ensure her own safety and that of her baby.

14

Breastfeeding

Dawn Whitten

INTRODUCTION

Breastfeeding is the biological norm. It facilitates an extra-uterine link between mother and child.[1] As such, breastfeeding continues many of the functions of the placenta, including protection of the infant from illness, nutritional nourishment and promoting and regulating development. Furthermore, it supports neural–hormonal homeostatic regulation, promotes bonding and is a source of comfort and even pain relief for the infant.[2–4] Breastfeeding also has health and neuroprotective functions for mothers, many of which have been under-realised until recently. Suboptimal breastfeeding in the US is estimated to be the cause of 3340 maternal deaths (due to myocardial infarction, breast cancer and diabetes) and 721 paediatric deaths annually.[5] When practitioners work to protect the breastfeeding dyad, they support the short- and long-term health of the mother and child.

Each mother–baby breastfeeding relationship (or dyad) is unique, and many mothers experience challenges during breastfeeding despite breastfeeding being normal and natural. There are a range of social–cultural and physiological factors that can contribute to breastfeeding challenges which will be explored in this chapter alongside practical and naturopathic strategies that can be utilised to help resolve them.

There are three key health professional areas of competency that are fundamental to supporting mothers with breastfeeding challenges:

1   good knowledge of human lactation physiology, including an appreciation for what is normal in breastfeeding
2   good referral practices that ensure mothers are connected with appropriate services and support to help them to resolve challenges quickly.
3   Sensitive and responsive communication skills enabling the communication of accurate information while remaining sensitive to the mother's needs. A core aspect of this is being sensitive to where a mother 'is at' in her breastfeeding and motherhood journey, and endeavouring to meet her there.

THE WORLD HEALTH ORGANIZATION RECOMMENDATIONS FOR BREASTFEEDING

The World Health Organization (WHO) recommends 6 months exclusive breastfeeding, followed by continued breastfeeding for the first 2 years or beyond.[6] These recommendations are made for all countries,[7] as breastfeeding is a significant determinant of health in both affluent and economically disadvantaged countries. Exclusive breastfeeding means oral ingestion of only breast milk, with the exception of required medications. No water, juices, breast milk substitutes or solid foods are given.[6]

The WHO estimates that globally only 38% of infants are exclusively breastfed for 6 months.[8] Data from Australia, Canada and the US show that these countries fare worse than the global average, with less than 25% of infants exclusively breastfed to the age of 6 months.[9–11] Furthermore, the 2010 National Health Survey found that only 1% of UK infants were exclusively breastfed to 6 months.[12] Interestingly, breastfeeding initiation rates are quite promising in Australia, with rates ranging up to 90%.[10] However, by 4 months only half of infants are receiving any breast milk. In the US and the UK, a similar pattern is evident, with an national initiation rate of 81%, followed by a substantial drop in both exclusive and any breastfeeding, according to recent surveys in both countries.[11,12] Furthermore, only 33% and 5% of Australian 9-month-olds and 24-month-olds, respectively, receive any breast milk.[10]

Based on the data available, it would appear that most children in these countries are not being breastfed according to WHO recommendations, and that there is a steady decline in breastfeeding and breastfeeding exclusivity following promising initiation rates. This prompts the question: why is this the case in these comparatively well-resourced countries?

HISTORICAL CONTEXT

While challenges with breastfeeding efficacy have existed throughout the ages, there are some unique aspects to the challenges and barriers for mothers today. During the past century we have seen a rise in the use of breast milk substitutes, owing to the successful marketing of these substitutes through direct promotion to the public and through strong relationships with hospitals and health professionals.[13,14]

In the early 1970s, breastfeeding hit an all-time low, with only 25% of babies being breastfed beyond 1 week of age in the US[15] and 36% being breastfed on discharge from hospital in Australia.[13] This means that many new mothers today have not been breastfed themselves or have been breastfed partially for only a short period. Furthermore, it means that the important support people in a new mother's life such as her own mother, in-laws, aunties and significant health professionals may often not have been breastfed, and are likely to have received inaccurate and unhelpful advice on breastfeeding. Unfortunately, mothers today still receive advice, such as feed scheduling resembling formula-feeding practices (author's observation from clinical practice), which is detrimental to breastfeeding success. Another consequence of the low breastfeeding rates of the 1970s and 1980s is that many mothers today have not had the opportunity to learn about normal breastfeeding behaviour through passive exposure.

Since the 1970s, there has been a steady effort directed at restoring and developing breastfeeding-friendly culture and practices in hospitals, the community and the work place.[14]

The WHO International Code of Marketing of Breast milk Substitutes was developed in 1981 and all United Nations member states were encouraged to include the code in their legislation. The aim of this code is to protect and promote breastfeeding and to limit the use of breast milk substitutes to only situations where they are medically necessary, by preventing aggressive advertising of breast milk substitutes.[16] Two key elements of the code include: 1) prohibiting the marketing of formula, artificial teats or bottles to parents or the general public; and 2) not allowing the practice of giving free formula samples to parents, pregnant women, health professionals or health services and hospitals. Interestingly, a recent Hong Kong (China) study found that when hospitals switched to paying market price and no longer accepted free formula, in-hospital exclusive breastfeeding rates increased from 17.9% to 41.4%.[17]

Currently, only 70% of countries have taken on at least some elements of the WHO code, including the UK, Iran, Brazil and Papua New Guinea.[18] In the US, industry adherence to the WHO code is voluntary as the WHO code is in conflict with the US's free trade legislation. Canada has only implemented a small portion of the elements. In Australia, a self-regulating industry agreement is in place, the Marketing in Australia of Infant Formulas (MAIF) Agreement, that encompasses only some aspects of the code and relies on voluntary adherence by industry signatories.[16]

The Baby-Friendly Hospital Initiative (BFHI) was launched in 1991 by the WHO and UNICEF as a key strategy to protect and promote breastfeeding.[19] The BFHI requires hospitals to put in place 'Ten Steps' (see Box 14.1), key components being: avoiding the use of artificial teats, avoiding formula supplementation in hospitals unless it is medically indicated, keeping mothers and babies together and supporting access to ongoing breastfeeding support. BFHI-certified hospitals are required to adhere to the WHO code, including paying market price for infant formula.

While there have been many positive outcomes owing to these efforts, there still remain challenges in these areas. Australia and the US have not signed the WHO code.[18] Some hospital practices still negatively impact on breastfeeding, and there are issues with compliance among BFHI-certified hospitals.[21] Ultimately, it is the combination of the hospital policies and the staff attitude and culture around breastfeeding that will determine the care experienced by mothers and babies. It is unfortunate that many hospitals claim to be too resource poor to maintain the 10 steps for infants in neonatal intensive care and special care units (NICUs), commonly neglecting to facilitate mothers being able to stay with their infants despite a growing body of evidence demonstrating the value of NICUs being designed to facilitate parents' '24-hour' presence with regards to infant stress, maternal

---

BOX 14.1 BFHI ten steps by WHO and UNICEF[19]

1. Have a written breastfeeding policy that is routinely communicated to all healthcare staff.
2. Train all healthcare staff in the skills necessary to implement this policy.
3. Inform all pregnant women about the benefits and management of breastfeeding.
4. Revised in 2009 to: Place babies in skin-to-skin contact with their mothers immediately following birth for at least an hour. Encourage mothers to recognise when their babies are ready to be breastfed and offer help if needed.[20] It is preferable that babies be left even longer than an hour, if feasible, as they may take longer than 60 minutes to breastfeed. (Previously Step 4 stated: Help mothers initiate breastfeeding within a half-hour of birth.)
5. Show mothers how to breastfeed and how to maintain lactation, even if they should be separated from their infants.
6. Give newborn infants no food or drink other than breast milk, unless medically indicated.
7. Practise rooming-in: allow mothers and infants to remain together 24 hours a day.
8. Encourage breastfeeding on demand.
9. Give no artificial teats or pacifiers to breastfeeding infants.
10. Foster the establishment of breastfeeding support groups and refer mothers to them on discharge from the hospital or clinic.

confidence, reduced pharmacological interventions, reduced sepsis and better breastfeeding rates.[22,23]

Pressures to return to work, community attitudes towards breastfeeding in public and difficulties accessing breastfeeding help all continue to challenge the return of a breastfeeding-friendly culture.

BREASTFEEDING: BARRIERS AND ENABLERS

Factors that impact on breastfeeding outcomes for mothers and babies

If practitioners can develop an understanding of the barriers and enabling factors (outlined in Tables 14.1 and 14.2) that may impact on the breastfeeding dyad and breastfeeding success, then this can help them to have insight into some of the less visible obstacles mothers face. This can also assist the clinician to keep a big picture view, where each mother is seen as part of a cultural web of influence, and we avoid seeing the mother at fault when breastfeeding does not work out. Importantly, an awareness of the social–cultural and maternal-centred barriers that impede breastfeeding confidence can prompt tailored preventive interventions.

TAILORED INTERVENTIONS TO ADDRESS BREASTFEEDING BARRIERS

- Unpacking the family stories around breastfeeding when there are negative beliefs within the family. Explanations about breastfeeding physiology can help bring insight to why previous family members had trouble, and how poor breastfeeding advice such as feed scheduling may have jeopardised breastfeeding.
- Building rapport and working to educate fathers and partners so they are more likely to be supportive of breastfeeding.
- Exploring creative options to reduce return-to-work pressure and/or to find solutions around continued breastfeeding while working.
- Connecting women with breastfeeding-friendly communities both locally and through social media.
- Being on the lookout for signs of perinatal depression and pre-emptively providing support to work through body image issues.

HEALTHCARE PRACTICES THAT ACT AS BREASTFEEDING BARRIERS AND ENABLERS

Numerous healthcare practices can have an impact on breastfeeding (see Table 14.2). Hence, promoting parental access to appropriate perinatal support and education is an important aspect of protecting breastfeeding. When birth becomes more complicated, it is invaluable for parents and birth support people to have an understanding of how to protect breastfeeding under these circumstances.

Key actions the naturopath can undertake during the prenatal period to protect breastfeeding include:

- Encourage parental access to prenatal breastfeeding education.
- Connect mothers with good breastfeeding support within their local area, including peer support services (through organisations such as the Australian Breastfeeding Association and La Leche League) and International Board Certified Lactation Consultants.
- Encourage mothers to get help early when challenges arise, such as pain or discomfort with breastfeeding, from the above organisations and health professionals.
- Encourage parents to explore their birth preparation and birth support options.
- Encourage parents to write a breastfeeding plan that includes requests to hospital and birth support people for immediate uninterrupted skin-to-skin contact and the avoidance, where possible, of separation, artificial feeds, use of teats and dummies and the minimisation of strong odours. Draft breastfeeding plans are available from the Australian Breastfeeding Association website.
- Reinforce the value of skin-to-skin contact both immediately following birth and during the early weeks of life. Skin-to-skin contact:
  – promotes maternal infant attachment
  – promotes infant cardiovascular and thermal regulation[75]
  – reduces pain for the infant[80]
  – supports maternal milk supply and effective attachment
  – reduces artificial milk supplementation[57,75]

For the mother and infant who have experienced early separation time, skin-to-skin contact is especially important.

Social–cultural barriers and enablers, maternal factors and healthcare practices create the context in which a mother's breastfeeding journey begins. All of these factors will have an impact on her breastfeeding intent and breastfeeding self-efficacy. Breastfeeding self-efficacy can be described as the mother's belief and confidence that she will resolve breastfeeding challenges, and her drive to experiment and find solutions to breastfeeding problems that may arise. The breastfeeding obstacles that are most frequently cited as the reason for early discontinuation of breastfeeding are outlined in Table 14.3. These include perceived low milk supply, breast or nipple pain and having a fussy or unsettled baby.[25,81,82]

WORKING WITH NEW MOTHERS – THE ROLE OF THE NATUROPATH

Maternal intention to breastfeed and self-efficacy are influenced by the many factors discussed above. Becoming a mother is a profound life-altering experience, and sensitivity to this is imperative in the provision of health support. Three early transitional postnatal phases were described by Rubin in the 1960s, and provide a model for understanding some aspects of early mothering behaviour and needs[91] (see Box 14.2). More contemporary understanding of the motherhood transition suggests that

TABLE 14.1 Social–cultural and maternal factors that present barriers to breastfeeding[9,24–30]

Social–cultural barriers

Mother was not breastfed
Grandmother's attitude may be a particularly potent determinant. A 2016 systematic review found that a grandmother's negative views of breastfeeding was associated with a 70% decrease in the likelihood of breastfeeding.[26] The family stories and a mother's exposure to breastfeeding prior to being pregnant are likely to influence her sense of breastfeeding self-efficacy.

Friends and family did not breastfeed
This is a widely reported trend.[25,27,31] A 2016 study provides some interesting insight, finding that feeding advice from those regarded as important support people influenced breastfeeding outcomes. Further advice that promoted breastfeeding, formula feeding or mixed feeding matched the feeding experiences of the provider.[27]

Partner/father not supportive
Paternal support and greater paternal breastfeeding education increases breastfeeding initiation rates.[32,33]

Lower education level
Lack of tertiary education in particular.[34]

Lower socioeconomic status

Maternal age
Generally younger maternal age is associated with poorer breastfeeding outcomes; however, findings are inconsistent, and in some populations, older first-time mothers have poorer breastfeeding outcomes than younger mothers.

Race and ethnicity
There are racial differences in breastfeeding rates that frequently echo socioeconomic patterns. In the US, African Americans, North American Indians and Hispanics have breastfeeding rates substantially lower than the national average.[35,36] Conversely, mothers with Black or Asiatic ethnicity have better breastfeeding rates in the UK.[12] In Australia, Aboriginal and Torres Strait Islander people have poorer breastfeeding rates than the national average, particularly in rural and regional areas.[37]

Early return-to-work pressure
Lack of paid maternity leave is associated with lower breastfeeding initiation and lower rates of exclusive breastfeeding, indicating that return-to-work pressure may impact on early breastfeeding decisions.[9,34,38,39] Flexible arrangements for return to work (including reduced hours and work from home options) that are compatible with breastfeeding may have further protective effects of longer-term breastfeeding outcomes.[40]
Attitudes towards breastfeeding in the workplace also appear to impact on breastfeeding.[40]

Mode of conception
The use of assisted reproductive technology (ART) is associated with exposure to a number of risk factors that predict poorer breastfeeding outcomes, including higher risk or preterm birth, caesarean birth, thyroid disease, polycystic ovary syndrome (PCOS) and higher risk of perceived lactational insufficiency.[41–43] One study found ART users had twice the rate of caesarean births and that caesarean births in this population predicted poor breastfeeding outcomes.[42]

Maternal factors

Obesity
Obesity is a risk factor for premature cessation of breastfeeding. This is thought to be multifactorial. A recent Australian study found that obese woman anticipated social discomfort both breastfeeding in public and with close friends and family.[44] Obesity can also be associated with delayed lactogenesis II, low supply and less intention to breastfeed.[45] The latter may be associated with anticipated social discomfort. Newby et al.suggest that interventions during pregnancy that address body image issues in relation to breastfeeding may support and facilitate breastfeeding success for obese mothers and their infants.[44]

Perinatal depression
An association between postnatal depression symptoms (PDS) and breastfeeding problems is well established.[46,47] Some studies have found that breastfeeding difficulties and premature cessation of breastfeeding may also be causal and/or a multiplier for PDS,[46,48,49] suggesting there is a two-way street between PDS and breastfeeding cessation. Sense of overwhelm may contribute to risk of breastfeeding cessation.[50] Bascom et al., in a US study of 1271 women with PDS, found that the presence of postnatal depression symptoms was associated with 'too many household chores' as a primary reason for breastfeeding cessation prior to 6 months.[50]

these phases are not distinct, but that mothers display aspects of them at different timepoints.[92] A more recent view has been put forward that pregnancy and early motherhood is a state of continual transformation.[93]

Maternal support, stress and mental health state are factors that modify adaptation and attainment of maternal self-efficacy.[94] Unfortunately current social constructs mean that many new mothers are isolated, with limited or deficient access to both practical and emotional support.[95] First-time mothers can benefit from peer support from other new mothers to help normalise some of the challenging feelings they experience.[93,96] Traumatic birth experiences can add an under layer of post-trauma stress. In the US, up to 45% of mothers describe their birth as traumatic, 18% display symptoms of post-traumatic stress and 3.5–7.5% have symptoms consistent with

TABLE 14.2 Healthcare practices that act as breastfeeding barriers and enablers

Barriers	Enablers
Birth interventions Caesarean birth (planned and emergency) Labour induction with synthetic oxytocin[51] Pethidine[52,53] Epidural,[52,54,55] especially when infant not fully rooming in[55] Traumatic birth experiences[56] Note: a long labour or stressful birth experience may also impact on breastfeeding independent of birth interventions **Separation of mother and baby**[57–60] **Delayed first breastfeed**[61] **Supplemental feeds given in hospital**[61–64] Note: judicious use of supplemental feeds does not appear to impair breastfeeding rates according to preliminary studies.[65,66] However reasons for in-hospital supplementation are frequently in conflict with evidence[24,67] (i.e. not judicious). **Use of artificial teats, bottles and dummies/pacifiers**[61,68] **Limited breastfeeding support after hospital discharge**[25] **Conflicting advice from healthcare practitioners**[69,70] **Poor advice and lack of encouragement from health professionals due to health professional knowledge deficit**[70,71] **Being born on a Saturday**[72]; hence, limited access to in-hospital breastfeeding support	**Prenatal breastfeeding education**[73] **Birth support –** continuity of midwifery care and doula support[74] Note: these factors also have a protective effect on breastfeeding when interventions such as instrument and caesarean birth have occurred – maternal support and empowerment in these scenarios protects breastfeeding. **Skin-to-skin contact –** mother and baby skin-to-skin contact immediate and uninterrupted after birth[24,57–59] Skin-to-skin contact immediately after caesarean birth increases breastfeeding successes[75] **Delay weighing** and other routine procedures for at least an hour after birth and until after the baby has had first breastfeed **Mother and baby rooming in**[19,76] **Consistent advice given by health professionals with good breastfeeding knowledge**[69,70,76] Health professionals supportive of breastfeeding[71,73] **Continued breastfeeding support after discharge**[19] Connection to breastfeeding peer-support groups[73,77,78] Medicare-reimbursed lactation support after discharge[79]

TABLE 14.3 Common reasons mothers give for premature cessation of breastfeeding

Perceived insufficient milk supply[24,25,81,83–85] (see page 491)

Baby is fussy/unsettled – see *Clinical Natural Medicine* Chapter 23 section 'The unsettled and unsoothable infant'. Note: babies who are unsettled are at greater risk of supplementation as this prompts parents to perceive the mother has insufficient milk.[86–88]

Nipple or breast pain[82] (see page 503 and 507)

Baby 'had trouble sucking or latching'[83,84]

Anticipating returning to work[85,89]

Maternal fatigue perceived to be related to breastfeeding[85]

Mother taking medication – ceases breastfeeding because of own concern or on advice of health professional[90] (see page 514)

BOX 14.2 Rubin's puerperal change model

Taking-in phase (1–2 days following birth) – mothers are often vulnerable. She accepts help from others, accepts being cared for, reacts passively to advice and often has a need to talk through her birth experience to help her process it. She is in the immediate stage of physical recovery from the birth.

Taking-hold phase – mother's focus turns to mothering. She is focused on the present, often self-critical and impatient with self to learn. She displays a high level of focus on her infant and may be anxious about her infant's care.

Letting-go phase – mother experiences identity adjustment: *loss of old self* (which may be associated with some unexpected grief) *and beginning of new self as mother*. She accepts the permanence of the infant as a person in her life.

---

post-traumatic stress disorder.[95] By contrast, studies of Swedish mothers found that 9% described their birth as traumatic and 1.3% had symptoms consistent with post-traumatic stress disorder.[95] Practitioners' alertness to the possibility of birth trauma, and where appropriate, referral to appropriate support services, may facilitate mothers' recovery from these experiences. Kendall-Tackett suggests that the most important message practitioners can give mothers is that these 'difficult beginnings don't have to be a blueprint for the rest of their mothering career and don't have to dictate what subsequent births are like'.[95]

New mothers are experiencing changes in many spheres: physical, practical, hormonal, sense of self and emotional change. As they transition this period, they often report a sense of overwhelm which is exacerbated by the common experience of receiving conflicting advice from health professionals.[69,70]

To ensure that naturopathic support doesn't contribute to this sense of overload, practitioners can:

- Devote time to listening to the mother's concerns.
- Ask the mother about the advice she has been given by other health professionals.
- Reinforce the aspects of this advice that seems helpful and try to avoid giving conflicting advice.
- Encourage the mother to experiment and see what works for her and her baby.
- Keep treatment suggestions simple and doable.

- Provide simple written information.
- Ensure that the mother's immediate concerns are addressed even if they do not seem the highest priority to the practitioner.

The naturopath is well placed to capture opportunities to protect and promote breastfeeding. These sometimes brief interactions may have a profound impact on a mother and baby's breastfeeding journey and on a mother's subsequent breastfeeding journeys. One of the most important roles the naturopath can play is identifying when referral for breastfeeding support is appropriate.

The value of good referral practice

The importance of referring women who are having breastfeeding difficulties to experienced certified lactation consultants and breastfeeding support services cannot be emphasised enough. When challenges are addressed and resolved quickly, breastfeeding is more likely to continue. In some cases, a team approach including the involvement of a paediatrician, paediatric speech pathologist, lactation consultant and naturopath/herbalist may be indicated. The team approach works well when practitioners are aware of their area of expertise and their limitations. One of the factors hindering effective health professional support of breastfeeding women is the contradictory advice they receive, especially from practitioners with inadequate training in lactation physiology.[69]

Another important role the naturopath can play is to reassure mothers about normal breastfeeding and infant behaviour and to help the mother to access accurate information.

When it comes to providing accurate information about the risks of breastfeeding cessation and the introduction of breast milk substitutes, health professionals often feel a tension between supporting parents to make an informed choice (informed consent), on the one hand, and wanting to avoid exacerbating the mother's feeling of guilt or judgment.[97] This is delicate territory, not least because parents do have a right to accurate information. Sometimes the impact of this can be softened by celebrating the breastfeeding outcomes that the mother and baby have had, rather than focusing entirely on the negative implications of a feeding choice. Sometimes it is helpful to remind mothers that it does not need to be an all-or-nothing decision. Any breastfeeding has value. Mothers might find shorter breastfeeding goals more within their coping capacity. When a mother of a newborn is experiencing significant challenges, she may find thinking about a goal of exclusively breastfeeding for the next 6 months is impossible and discouraging. She may, however, find setting a goal to exclusively breastfeed for the next 4 days or a week is manageable. From this place, a new goal can be set based on how breastfeeding is going.

Practitioners need to be aware of their own story. Studies indicate that health professionals' own breastfeeding experiences influence the care and advice they provide mothers.[98,99]

When the practitioner has a sense of the historical and cultural breastfeeding context, including the many enabling and inhibiting factors at play, it may assist them to hold a broad view of each presentation related to breastfeeding and to 'meet the mother where she is at'; that is, apply a rather dynamic approach to breastfeeding promotion by sensing and communicating in a responsive way to the mother.

FUNCTIONS OF BREASTFEEDING

Breastfeeding is an integral part of the reproductive process, and the functions it has for the mother and child continue to be uncovered. The role human milk plays in providing nourishment for the infant is well appreciated, as is to a lesser extent its role in immune protection (discussed in detail below). Less appreciated are the many other functions of breastfeeding, which have far-ranging lifelong effects on the health of mothers and children (see Table 14.4). The functions of breastfeeding in most cases are 'dose dependent'. In other words, there is a direct correlation between breastfeeding duration (as well as duration of exclusive breastfeeding) and the functional health effects for the mother and child.

Immune protection as a primary function

Contemporary perspectives informed by evolutionary science suggest that the primary function of mammalian milk is actually protection from infection, and that over time, additional secondary functions, including nutrition, have evolved. The mammary gland is thought to have evolved from an ancestral apocrine-like gland associated with hair follicles.[103] The earliest form of lactation may have been by the synapsids in the form of antimicrobial substances secreted from skin to protect soft egg shells from microbial growth. The modified hair follicles seen in monotremes, such as the platypus, further support this concept.[133] Many of the nutritional components in breast milk have anti-microbial actions and have their molecular origin based on immune defence compounds, further suggesting an initial function of protection.[103,133]

This proposition, that the function of protection came first, frames the value of breastfeeding differently from when it is seen primarily as nutrition. It could be argued that part of the infant's immune system resides in its mother, and the breast is the connection between the mother and the offspring. Hence the concept of the maternal–infant hybrid immune system.

THE MATERNAL–INFANT HYBRID IMMUNE SYSTEM

Turfkruyer et al. proposed that the infant immune system is only complete in the presence of breast milk.[134] See Figure 14.1. Breast milk contains non-specific defence in the form of: immune cells, probiotic bacteria, prebiotic components, bacterial and viral blocking agents (human milk oligosaccharides, glycolipids and glycoproteins)[100,101] and antimicrobial agents (lactoferrin, lysozymes, fatty acids,

TABLE 14.4 Functions of breastfeeding for mother and child

Functions for child	Examples
Protection from infection	**Mother–baby hybrid immune system** – **Non-specific immune defences** > Bacterial and viral blocking agents[100,101] > Antimicrobial agents[102] > Non-specific immune cells[103] – **Specific antibody defence** > Specific antibodies > Immune cell pathogen-primed responses[103]
Establishment and nourishment of gut microbiota	**Hypothesis that bacteria are selectively sampled and transferred from mother's colon to breast milk**[104] **Breast milk contains numerous probiotic bacteria**[105–108] **Prebiotic human oligosaccharides with a unique pattern from each mother**[101] **Other factors in breast milk shape the microbiota, including:** lactoferrin,[100,102] lysozymes,[102] lactose,[109,110] haptocorrin (vitamin B_{12}-binding protein), bile salt-stimulated lipase, κ-casein and human milk mucins,[102,111] glycolipids, glycoproteins and glycopeptides[101]
Developmental programming	**Epigenetic modulators program development for a number of systems:** • **Gastrointestinal –** mucosa maturation, reduced permeability, maturation of the enteric nervous system, promoting immune tolerance • **Immunological** • **Neurological** • **Vascular –** breast milk contains angiopoietins Breast milk components involved include: stem cells, immune cells, growth factors, cytokines, hormones, gangliosides and neurotrophic factors[112–114]
Nutrition and hydration	Nutrients are supplied in a highly bioavailable form.[1,115] Furthermore, the compositions of preterm milk, colostrum and transitional milk are different from mature milk, reflecting the higher needs for protein and some nutrients[116] Fat and carbohydrate composition of the breast milk changes during a feed, during the day and over the course of lactation[117] Composition is dynamic and responsive to feeding frequency,[117] providing a means of adapting to the hydration and nutritional needs of the infant Breast milk contains amylase[118] and bile salt-stimulated lipase,[119,120] which assist with the digestion of starches and lipids
Hormonal regulation	Metabolic regulation and imprinting[121] Circadian rhythm – hormonal input[122]
Comfort, stress reduction and pain relief	Breastfeeding before and during immunisations reduces pain according to a systematic review of 10 studies[3] One study found that breastfeeding was associated with better cortisol recovery following stress exposure[2] Cholecystokinin hormone is released in response to suckling to a lipid-rich breastfeed, and promotes digestion as well as satiety, relaxation and pain relief[123,124]
Neurocognitive development[125–127]	Exposure to oxytocin and breastfeeding behaviour, such as maternal eye contact and tactile sensory input, are thought to contribute to neurocognitive development and learnt capacity to recognise and respond to social cues[125–128]
Orthodontic and facial structural development	Breastfeeding appears to be associated with healthy orofacial development. But this may be mediated by longer breastfeeding duration, reducing non-nutritive sucking of fingers and dummies[129]
Functions for mother	Examples
Support recovery from pregnancy and birth	Reduced postnatal blood loss, supports uterine return to normal size, lactational amenorrhoea facilitating child spacing and building of iron stores, prevents anaemia[130]
Neuro-protective	Maternal hormones – support adaptation to motherhood[48]
Metabolic regulation	Lactation suggested to provide 'a reset' to the adverse metabolic profile women are exposed to during pregnancy[131] Oxytocin may mediate cardiovascular regulatory effects[132]
Reproductory hormone exposure regulation	Low oestrogen profile balances the high oestrogen and oncogenic exposure period of pregnancy and potentially provides normalised oestrogen exposure from a life span perspective.

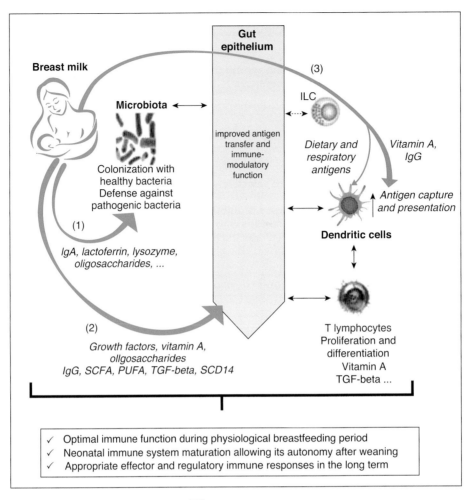

FIGURE 14.1 Breast milk – neonatal immune system[134]

actoperoxidase).[102] Human milk also contains specific immune protection through antibodies and leukocytes, providing protection from pathogens to which the mother and infant are exposed.[103] Interestingly, a rise in breast milk leukocytes has been observed when mothers are asymptomatic but the infant has an infection, including respiratory infection, gastrointestinal infection or roseola infantum,[103] suggesting that the maternal immune system is responsive to the infant's state of health. Highlighting the immune system role of the breast, a 4-month-old infant consumes on average 75 mg of secretory immunoglobulin A (SIgA) per kg of body weight per 24 hours. This is almost twice the amount a non-lactating adult produces per kg of body weight.[133]

Summary of other known functions for the infant

Human milk provides tailored nutrition and hydration to the infant, which adapts depending on the age of the infant[116] and time of day.[116] The composition of milk at the beginning and the end of a feed is different, with more fat being present as the breast is comparatively 'emptier'.[116] Nutrients are delivered in highly bioavailable forms. Breast milk provides the complete nutritional needs, including hydration, until around 6 months of age, at which point

complementary foods are needed to meet the iron and zinc needs of the infant.[135–137] Breast milk continues to be the most nutritionally complete food in an infant's diet for the remainder of the first and during the second year of life.[136] When co-ingested, breast milk may assist with the digestibility of solid foods via the presence of amylase[118] and bile salt-stimulated lipase[119,120] in breast milk. Furthermore, it promotes tolerance to dietary proteins via the presence of SIgA and other factors in milk.[138] Maternal nutrient status impacts on some aspects of breast milk composition, while many components, macronutrients in particular and some minerals, are regulated independent of maternal status (see Tables 14.7–14.9).

Breast milk contains species-specific growth and neurotrophic factors and stem cells that promote and regulate the development of the gastrointestinal mucosa, the enteric nervous system, the infant's immune system, the neurological system and the vascular system.[112–114] Hormonal factors present in milk support the regulation of circadian and metabolic systems.[121,122,139,140] Breastfeeding promotes neurocognitive and social development,[125–128,141] provides comfort and pain relief[3] and is a rich source of sensory nourishment for the infant. Furthermore, it may support the healthy development of the orofacial muscles and oral cavity.[142] And not least, breastfeeding helps to establish and nourishes a healthy infant gut microbiota (see below).

Functions for mothers and the mother–baby dyad

For the mother–baby dyad, breastfeeding promotes bonding and synchronised care. Breastfeeding has neuroprotective and maternal adaptation and resilience-promoting effects on the mother,[143,144] largely thought to be mediated by oxytocin exposure.[145] Hence, breastfeeding provides a protective buffer for the maternal brain during a major life transition, and as such, is associated with reduced risk and reduced severity of mood and depressive disturbances for the mother.[143,145,146] Breastfeeding also protects against maternal infant neglect.[147]

Through promoting lactational amenorrhoea, breastfeeding provides an opportunity for mothers to re-establish iron stores from pregnancy.[130] Oxytocin release during breastfeeding initiation assists with uterine contraction and reducing postnatal blood loss.[130]

What is probably least appreciated about breastfeeding is its role in the metabolic and hormonal health of the mother. The breastfeeding state provides a period of lower oestrogen exposure that may balance the higher oestrogen states of pregnancy and ovulational cycling. Breastfeeding also primes women for the maintenance of healthy insulin sensitivity in later years.[131] Breastfeeding is theorised to provide a reproductive hormone and metabolic 'reset phase' that balances the unfavourable metabolic,[131] and potentially the oncogenic, profile women are exposed to during pregnancy. Further breastfeeding exposes the breast to breast milk factors such as HAMLET (a human milk complex of alpha-lactalbumin and oleic acid), which appear to induce tumour cell death.[148] Hence, for the duration of breastfeeding, the breast may be bathed in an anti-cancer milieu.

RISKS ASSOCIATED WITH SUBOPTIMAL BREASTFEEDING FOR INFANTS

The risks to infants who are suboptimally breastfed are numerous (see Table 14.5). For this reason, promotion and protection of breastfeeding is arguably one of the most important health interventions. Accordingly, a recent systematic review found that breastfeeding was the nutrition-related factor that made the biggest difference to long-term health outcomes.[149] A 2016 systematic review predicted that globally, 13.8% (823 000) of annual deaths in children under the age of two would

TABLE 14.5 Risks associated with insufficient breastfeeding for mothers and children (based mostly on data from economically advantaged countries such as Australia, the US, Germany and the UK) Updated from[158]

Child		Mother
Child mortality (all causes) [150–153]	**Maternal child abuse and neglect** [147]	**Postnatal anaemia** [195,196]
SIDS [150,159,160]	**Child, adolescent and adult mental health problems** [141,177]	**Increased anxiety and depression** (in mothers with pre-existing postnatal depression and anxiety) [146]
Hospitalisation [150,154,155,161–163]	**Attention deficit hyperactivity disorder and autism** [178,179]	Longer duration breastfeeding gives greater protection against:
Lower respiratory tract infection [153,161]	**Developmental delay** [180,181]	**Ovarian cancer** [197–201]
Wheeze [164]	**Poorer motor development adolescence** [182]	**Endometrial cancer** [202,203]
Gastroenteritis [161]	**Reduced IQ or related measure** [126,127,150,183]	**Breast cancer** [150,204–206]
Otitis media [150,165,166]	**Depression in adulthood** [184]	**Breast cancer mortality** [207,208]
Urinary tract infection [167]	**Obesity** [150,173,185,186]	**Thyroid cancer** [209]
Inflammatory bowel disease[168] **Coeliac disease** [169–171]	**Cardiovascular disease** [173,187]	**Vascular calcification** [210]
Childhood leukaemia [172,173]	**Diabetes types 1 and 2** [188–190]	**Myocardial infarction** [204]
Necrotising enterocolitis [174–176]	**Snoring** [191]	**Type 2 diabetes** [211–214]
	Dental malocclusion [142,192]	**Metabolic syndrome** [215–217]
	Primary enuresis [193]	**Hypertension** [132]
	Delayed spontaneous enuresis [194]	**Osteoporotic fracture** [178,204,218,219]
		Rheumatoid arthritis [220,221]

not occur if breastfeeding neared the WHO recommendations.[150] The myth that insufficient breastfeeding is only life-threatening in developing countries has been dispelled by data collected over the past decade, showing that premature cessation and insufficient exclusive breastfeeding are associated with increased risk of child mortality, severe infection and hospitalisation in countries such as Australia, the UK and the US.[5,151–157]

RISKS ASSOCIATED WITH SUBOPTIMAL BREASTFEEDING FOR MOTHERS

The risk to mothers who do not breastfeed, or who prematurely cease breastfeeding, are arguably under-appreciated (see Table 14.5). Suboptimal breastfeeding in the US is estimated to be the cause of 3340 maternal deaths (due to myocardial infarction, breast cancer and diabetes).[5] Hence, Batrick et al. argue that breastfeeding is just as much a women's health issue as it is a child health issue.[5] Suboptimal breastfeeding increases the risk of the other reproductive cancers, both ovarian[197] and uterine.[202] Furthermore, suboptimal breastfeeding is a risk factor for anxiety and postnatal depression, with this association being bi-directional.[46,48,49]

Establish and nourish the infant microbiome

Breast milk nourishes and fosters the development of a healthy gastrointestinal microbiome. The microbiome of the exclusively breastfed infant is dominated by several *Bifidobacterium* spp. and has been coined the milk-oriented microbiome (MOM) because of the composition characteristics.[222] The MOM assists in protecting the infant from infection through competitive inhibition of pathogenic bacteria[222] and promotes a healthy intestinal barrier function. It is thought to be integral in preventing necrotising enterocolitis. The MOM interacts with the host in myriad ways, supporting healthy immune development, oral tolerance[223] and metabolic regulation, and may play a role in neurocognitive development.[100,224–226]

Breast milk as a source of bacteria

Accumulating evidence indicates that breast milk is an important source of bacteria, some of which appear to colonise the infant's intestine, including species from the *Bifidobacterium, Lactobacillus, Staphylococcus, Faecalibacterium, Bacteroides* and *Roseburia* genera. Identical strains from these genera have been isolated from the milk of mothers and their infant's faeces.[105–108] Jost et al. found matched strains across 10 different genera in maternal faeces, breast milk and infant faeces.[106] Colonisation persistence of the infant at 6 months of age has been observed for *Bifidobacterium* maternal/infant matched strains.[105] One study indicated that breast milk is a reservoir for *Bifidobacterium* strains, but suggested that there was a possibility that some of these strains are initially shared from the newborn to the breast milk microbiota, as they were detected in some infants' faeces

prior to breast milk.[107] This same study detected *Bifidobacterium* strains in some newborns' meconium stools on the first day of life, suggesting their initial inoculation occurred either in utero or following vaginal delivery. However, *Bifidobacterium* strains have been identified in colostrum samples prior to any breastfeeding by other researchers.[224,227]

The entero–mammary pathway

It has been postulated that an entero–mammary pathway exists whereby bacteria are selectively sampled from the mother's colon and transported via mononuclear immune cells to the breast.[104] The presence of multiple matched strains in maternal faeces, breast milk and infant faeces[105,106] supports this hypothesis, as does animal evidence from both mouse and cow models.[228] Other studies have found that maternal ingestion of some specific bacterial strains (*L. reuteri* strain Protectus, *L. rhamnosus* GG, *L. fermentum* CECT5716) was associated with detection of these same strains in infant stool[229] and/or breast milk.[230,231] Transfer into breast milk appears to be strain specific as other probiotic strains administered to lactating women have not been detected in infant faeces after maternal administration.[229]

Given the probable presence of the entero–mammary pathway,[104] the maternal intestinal microbiome may determine some aspects of the breast milk microbiota and the species and strain composition available to the infant. This suggests a mechanism by which the maternal intestinal microbiome influences the health of the infant. In support of this are the findings of Grönlund et al., showing that maternal intestinal bifidobacteria status correlated with bifidobacteria colonisation of the infant at age 1 year and 6 months.[232]

Breast milk prebiotics

There are multiple prebiotics present in human milk. Human milk oligosaccharides (HMOs) are a group of diversely structured sugar molecules that are probably the most well-known prebiotics in human milk. *Bifidobacterium* strains, in particular, appear to utilise HMOs.[233,234] Each mother has a genetically determined unique set of HMOs in her milk which in turn uniquely cultivate bacteria in the infant's gut.[101] HMOs are the third most abundant component in breast milk, present at a concentration of 5–15 g per litre. To date, 200 different HMOs have been identified, and it has been suggested that the characterisation of further HMOs is limited by the constraints of analytical technology.[101] Of interest, the presence of some types of HMOs (produced by women positive for the Lewis gene which regulates one type of sugar linkage present in some HMOs) may protect infants from neonatal group B streptococcus infection.[235]

Other important prebiotic components include glycolipids, glycoproteins and glycopeptides.[101] Furthermore, lactose is a conditional prebiotic, and undigested lactose in the infant's colon may support the growth of bifidobacteria and lactobacilli[109,110] and be associated with suppressed growth of *Bacteroides* and *Clostridia* spp.[109]

Other factors that favourably influence the infant's microbiome

Breast milk includes other bioactive components that also support the development of a healthy microbiome. Lactoferrin holds iron in a form that prevents bacteria from utilising it.[100] Free iron has the potential to cause dysbiosis and mucosal inflammation and increase the risk of bacterial infection.[236,237] Lactoferrin also has bactericidal effects – it binds to Gram-negative bacteria and disrupts their cellular membranes. Lysozymes (another bioactive breast milk protein) work in concert with lactoferrin, entering the bacterial cells lactoferrin has disrupted and

effectively killing the bacteria. One study found that lactoferrin was active against *Streptococcus mutans*, *Streptococcus pneumoniae*, *Escherichia coli*, *Vibrio cholerae*, *Pseudomonas aeroginosa* and *Candida albicans*.[102] HMOs prevent mucosa attachment of potential pathogens as well as being prebiotics.[100] Several other components in breast milk are active against unfavourable bacteria including: haptocorrin (vitamin-B_{12}-binding protein), bile salt-stimulated lipase, κ-casein and human milk mucins.[102,111] Many of the bioactive compounds in human milk work together synergistically. Furthermore, these components are able to resist digestion and are found in infant faeces.[102]

See Table 14.6.

TABLE 14.6 Bioactive components of human milk (mature)		
Components	**Sub-components**	**Functions**
Cells (10 000–13 million cells/mL)[103]	Stem cells	**Developmental programming:** Secrete growth factors including vascular endothelial growth factor, hepatocyte growth factor[238] Transferred and integrated into different tissues of the breast-fed offspring[239]
	Leukocytes 200–260 000 leukocytes/mL Bacteria	**Immunomodulatory effects –** defence, immune system programming[103,240] **Seeding for the infant** including transfer from maternal gastrointestinal system **Mammary protection**
Growth factors	Many	**Developmental and metabolic programming** Examples include: neurotrophic factors – brain-derived neurotrophic factor (BDNF), glial cell line-derived neurotrophic factor (GDNF), glial fibrillary acidic protein (GFAP), fibroblast growth factor 21 (FGF21), lysophosphatidic acid (LPA) and autotaxin (ATX)[112]
Hormones	Many	**Developmental and metabolic programming** Examples include: melatonin, growth hormone, leptin, insulin, adiponectin, ghrelin, resistin, obestatin, peptide YY, glucagon-like peptide 1, calcitonin, somato-statin[121,139,140,241]
Cytokines and chemokines	Many	**Immunomodulation and inflammation regulation**
Carbohydrates	Lactose 7 g/100 mL Human milk oligosaccharides 0.5 to 1.5 g/100 mL	**Conditional prebiotic**[109,110] **Prebiotic** The combination and specific structures are genetically determined. HMOs also function as surface-protecting decoys preventing bacterial and viral infections in the gut, respiratory tract and urinary tract[242,243]
Lipids	Galactolipids Gangliosides	Prebiotic and viral bacterial receptor binding[243] Support neonatal brain development and myelination[244]
Proteins Note: the human milk proteome includes 976 identified proteins and many of these have immune-related properties[240]	Alpha-lactalbumin Human lactoferrin SlgA IgG Lysozyme and actoperoxidase microRNAs	Part of HAMLET promotes tumour cell apoptosis[245,246] Highly bio-available form of iron, bacteriostatic[247,248] May support cognitive development[249] Immune protection, promotion of tolerance, reduced allergen exposure[134,250] Antimicrobial protection[102] These enter the systemic circulation and exert tissue-specific immunoprotective and developmental functions[251]

Note: This is a list of examples, not an exhaustive list.

Allergy prevention

Breastfeeding is thought to promote tolerance via a number of mechanisms including: nourishing the infant's microbiome, supporting healthy barrier function,[223] and antibody and cytokine tolerance promotion.[250,252] A 2015 systematic review that included 89 studies concluded that longer duration of breastfeeding was associated with less asthma at 5–18 years.[253] In addition, the studies found some evidence (while not as strong) for protection against eczema and allergic rhinitis.[253] A greater effect was seen in low- and middle-income countries. It was suggested that protection from infection was an important mechanism for reducing asthma development. Breastfeeding during solid introduction, in particular while introducing potential allergens, has the potential to promote tolerance.[254–257]

NUTRITIONAL CONSIDERATIONS FOR THE BREASTFEEDING MOTHER

As with pregnancy, the special care of certain nutrients is important for the health of both the mother and the child. From a practical perspective, the time to discuss breastfeeding nutrition is during the third trimester. Some clearly written recommendations can go a long way, providing information that can be referred back to and reduces 'consultation overload' during the busy early weeks postnatally. Breastfeeding mothers need healthy food fast. The ideal situation is to have support with meals for the early weeks. Short of this, mothers will benefit by preparing and freezing some healthy meal bases ahead of time, and by having some simple wholesome meal and snack ideas (see the Sample meal plan below).

Sample meal plan

Meal	Menu	Meal is a rich source of:
Breakfast	Breakfast bowl • 2 tablespoons ground organic flaxseeds • 1 tablespoon chia seeds • 2 teaspoons lecithin • ¼ to ½ cup organic berries (thawed frozen or fresh) • ½ cup yoghurt containing prebiotics (i.e. *L. rhamnosus* GG) • Handful of organic almonds and 2 Brazil nuts • Additional chopped fruit as desired	Calcium, polyphenols and other antioxidants, prebiotics, choline, vitamin E, protein, probiotics, alpha-linolenic acid, potassium
Morning snack	Avocado on sourdough bread or wholegrain gluten-free alternative	Vitamin E, carotenoids, folate, potassium
Lunch	Lunch Buddha bowl • ½ to 1 cup of the cooked mix mung bean rice mix (see below) • 2 cups of leafy greens (e.g. dark green and red lettuce leaves) • 1 tablespoon pumpkin seeds • A drizzle of tahini • A drizzle of apple cider vinegar • A handful of cherry tomatoes • Top with a poached or fried egg (DHA-rich source) Mung bean and rice preparation Precook brown rice and mung beans and store in fridge. To prepare, mix ½ cup of red or brown rice with ½ cup of mung beans. Add 3 cups of water, bring to the boil and simmer on low heat for about 30 minutes. Stir occasionally. Once cooled, store in the fridge and use as a base.	Protein, resistant starch, polyphenols, folate, calcium, magnesium, vitamin C, B group vitamins, choline, DHA, carotenoids, potassium Greens considered lactogenic[31]
Afternoon snack	Sardines on whole crackers and piece of fruit	EPA, DHA, calcium, protein
Alternative snack	Raw carrot and hummus	Vitamin C, fibre, polyphenols etc.
Dinner	Slow-cooked root vegetable stew Add to a slow cooker: sweet potato, potato, red quinoa, purple carrots, beetroot, a protein source (tofu, legume or clean meat option), herbs and spices – in particular, consider carminative spices such as coriander, cumin, turmeric. Fifteen minutes prior to serving up, add sliced fennel and other leafy greens. Serve and add drizzle of olive oil and cracked pepper to taste	Protein, resistant starch, polyphenols, carotenoids, potassium, folate, B vitamins Note: root vegetables and fennel vegetable traditionally considered lactogenic[31]
After-dinner snack	Fruit	Vitamin C, fibre, polyphenols etc.

Note: ideally new parents have help with meals during the first 4 weeks postnatally. Some will have eager friends who organise meal rosters and friends and families who make elaborate celebratory meals that are left at the door without expectation of visiting. The meals above are designed for minimal preparation and maximum effect. Some young infants may be sensitive to allium family foods and raw cruciferous vegetables.

With regard to breastfeeding nutrition, nutrients are divided into two categories: group 1 and group 2 (see Tables 14.7–14.9). The breast milk concentration of group 1 nutrients are dependent on maternal status, while the group 2 nutrients are regulated independently of maternal status. There are some nutrients for which poor maternal status is common and others that may

be tightly regulated with some consequences to the mother's nutrient stores. These are considered *priority nutrients* (listed in Table 14.7 and detailed in Tables 14.8–14.9), and with a few exceptions they tend be similar to the nutrients that need special care during pregnancy.

Text continued on p 482

TABLE 14.7 Group 1 and group 2 nutrients for lactating mothers

Group 1 nutrients (dependent on maternal status)	Maternal inadequate intake common	Group 2 nutrients (regulated independent of maternal status)	Maternal inadequate intake common
Vitamin A Vitamin C Vitamin D Vitamin E Thiamine Riboflavin Vitamin B$_6$ Vitamin B$_{12}$ Choline Iodine Selenium DHA	Vitamin D Vitamin B$_{12}$ Choline Iodine Selenium DHA	Folate Calcium Zinc Iron Magnesium Copper	Folate Zinc Calcium

More detail relating to each nutrient is included in Tables 14.8 and 14.9. It is prudent to supplement mothers with all of the nutrients listed in the lower row unless dietary sources are adequate. Some mothers may have insufficient intake of other nutrients listed above.

TABLE 14.8 Group 1 nutrients for lactating women – maternal intake or status correlates with breast milk content

Nutrient information (group 1 nutrients)	Maternal intake/ dosage recommendations
Vitamin A Fetal hepatic liver stores accumulate throughout pregnancy, and particularly during the third trimester with increased placental transfer.[258] The vitamin A content of breast milk is greater during the early months of lactation,[259] probably to facilitate the development of neonatal liver stores. A dynamic relationship between maternal hepatic stores and breast milk vitamin A appears to exist. Maternal vitamin A stores begin replenishing from 6 months postnatally, yet hepatic stores do not correlate with breast milk, suggesting that vitamin A in breast milk is at least partially regulated independently of maternal status.[259] Nevertheless, Vitamin A is considered a group 1 nutrient because maternal deficiency (which is common in developing countries) results in lower breast milk vitamin A.[258] The preterm infant has a greatest risk of vitamin A deficiency owing to shorter gestation and subsequent inadequate hepatic stores.[258] In addition, some findings suggest that preterm breast milk may have lower vitamin A content than term milk.[258] Of note, hind milk has a higher vitamin A content because the vitamin is present in the lipid fraction of the milk.[260] Hence, milk sample collection technique may be a confounding factor with these and other findings. Maternal vitamin A supplementation can influence breast milk vitamin A, but only at higher-end doses. Most of the research in this area has been done in resource-poor countries where a single mega-dose is the most feasible option. While this is probably not the most ideal dosage regimen, a systematic review of 11 studies found that a single mega-dose of 200 000 IU increases breast milk vitamin A concentrations,[261] and breast milk vitamin A concentrations seem to be maintained for at least the first 4 weeks.[262] Interestingly, a 2016 Cochrane systematic review found that there were no benefits to maternal or child morbidity or mortality with this practice.[263] Furthermore, rises in breast milk vitamin A may be in part related to correction of maternal vitamin A deficiency. A maternal daily dose of 5000 IU over the first month of lactation would appear a reasonable strategy to maintain good breast milk vitamin A if maternal vitamin A insufficiency is suspected. It is prudent to keep the portion supplied by retinol to 3000 IU to be in keeping with a dosage range that would be acceptable (in terms of perceived risk) in the event of an unexpected pregnancy. Of interest, the WHO recommends 10 000 IU of retinol vitamin A daily to pregnant women suspected of deficiency.[264] The RDIs for lactating women set by the US Institute of Medicine (IOM) and National Health and Medical Reserch Council (NHMRC) are 1110 IU[265] and 840–900 IU[266] per day, respectively.	Individualise Ensure dietary sources When dietary sources are inadequate, supplement with 5000 IU daily comprising a maximum of 3000 IU direct vitamin A (retinol)

Continued

TABLE 14.8 Group 1 nutrients for lactating women – maternal intake or status correlates with breast milk content—cont'd	
Nutrient information (group 1 nutrients)	**Maternal intake/ dosage recommendations**
Vitamin C Maternal vitamin C intake consistently correlates with breast milk vitamin C, according to several observation studies.[267–269] One study found that vitamin C from dietary sources had a greater effect on breast milk vitamin C than that from supplements, and correlated with lower risk of atopy.[269] However, this may equally have been related to higher maternal fruit and vegetable consumption. Another study found that supplementing 500 mg of vitamin C along with 100 IU of vitamin E per day improved the antioxidant capacity of breast milk.[270] Breast milk vitamin C would appear to be easily maintained with a diet rich in fresh fruit and vegetables, or with supplementation in the order of 500 mg of vitamin C daily for mothers on restrictive diets.	Supplement with 500 mg/day of vitamin C when maternal fresh fruit and vegetable intake is restricted
Vitamin D Breast milk vitamin D content reflects maternal vitamin D intake.[271] Some researchers propose that because most transfer of vitamin D is in the parent form cholecalciferol (vitamin D_3), daily dosing of vitamin D_3 or, alternatively, tri-weekly maternal adequate UVB exposure may be necessary to ensure good breast milk transfer of vitamin D.[271,272] However, not all clinical study findings support the need for daily exposure to the parent compound.[273] For clinical purposes, it seems appropriate to both maintain daily vitamin D (through supplementation or tri-weekly adequate sun exposure when this is acceptable and feasible) and obtain optimal maternal status. An RDI of 400 IU for infants has been derived in part for protection against rickets, for which the dose is 400 IU.[274] In some countries, it is recommended to give all exclusively breastfed infants 400 IU daily from birth. Maternal vitamin D supplementation is arguably preferable to infant vitamin D supplementation. Infant vitamin D supplementation may undermine the mother's confidence in her breast milk adequacy, it exposes the immature gastrointestinal tract of the infant to excipients and furthermore treating the mother also provides maternal protection from vitamin D deficiency. Findings from clinical studies based in the US indicate that daily maternal supplementation of 6400 IU of vitamin D_3 raises breast milk vitamin D concentrations sufficiently to meet the infant's RDI.[272,275] In addition, infant serum vitamin D levels were no different when groups receiving maternal dose of 6400 IU were compared to infants supplemented directly with 400 IU.[272] A study utilising 2000 IU daily improved breast milk vitamin D content, but did not raise the mean concentration to a level that would supply the infant RDI.[276] Hollis and colleagues found that a maternal dose of 4000 IU came closer than 2000 IU to supplying the infant RDI, providing the infant with a daily intake of 135 IU and 70 IU, respectively.[277] Thiele et al. compared a maternal vitamin D dose of 3800 IU to 400 IU, both given throughout pregnancy and lactation, and found 4–6-week-old exclusively breastfed infants in the active and control group had an average status of 62 nmol/L and 42.5 nmol/L, respectively.[278] Interestingly, vitamin D levels of all infants were lower at 4–6 weeks than they were at birth.[278] Variations relating to geographical location, season, lifestyle, sun exposure and skin pigmentation should be taken into consideration when extrapolating these findings to the individual. An additional consideration is that breast milk vitamin D content may be underestimated because, like vitamin A, breast milk vitamin D is present in the lipid fraction of the mother's milk. Extrapolating from the study by Wagner et al.,[275] a maternal 25-hydroxyvitamin D status of >110 nmol/L appears to be associated with adequate breast milk vitamin D concentrations. It appears prudent to maintain maternal status between 110 and 130 nmol/L to ensure vitamin D sufficiency in the infant and avoid the potential for adverse effects. The IOM proposes there is a potential for adverse effects at a status greater than >150 nmol/L, and that levels over 500 nmol/L are toxic.[279] **Note on optimal vitamin D status** The optimal vitamin D range is still debated, with different sufficiency values proposed by different organisations. The respective sufficiency values proposed for the IOM, Endocrine Society and Vitamin D Council are >50 nmol/L,[280] >75 nmol/L[281] and >100 nmol/L[282] respectively. Based on physiological parameters including adequate breast milk transfer and appropriate suppression of parathyroid hormone, disease prevention and approximated values likely to represent evolutionary equivalency, Baggerly et al. propose an optimal status of 120 nmol/L (but not greater).[283]	Individualise to achieve status >100 nmol/L and < 130 nmol/L Appropriate maintenance dose may range from 2000 IU to 6000 IU and needs to be triturated based on status and the factors discussed

TABLE 14.8 Group 1 nutrients for lactating women – maternal intake or status correlates with breast milk content—cont'd

Nutrient information (group 1 nutrients)	Maternal intake/ dosage recommendations
Vitamin E During pregnancy, placental transfer of vitamin E is limited. Consequently, the neonate has minimal stores at birth and depends entirely on breast milk as a source.[284] Vitamin E concentrations are highest in colostrum and reduce as breast milk transitions to mature milk. Infants consume larger volumes of mature milk; hence, daily infant vitamin E intake may be similar. While maternal stores may impact on breast milk vitamin E status, maternal serum levels and habitual daily dietary intake do not correlate with breast milk levels.[284,285] However, a single 400 IU vitamin E dose was associated with increased colostrum and transitional milk vitamin E concentration 24 hours later.[284,286] It is not clear whether this indicates that higher-dose vitamin E may influence breast milk concentration overall or that this effect is specific to the colostrum and transitional breast milk phase. These studies also found that natural vitamin E was more effective at raising colostrum levels than synthetic vitamin E.[284,286] One study found that a 100 IU/day dose of vitamin E (form not available) combined with 500 mg/day of vitamin C improved the antioxidant capacity of breast milk indirectly.[270] Based on the current data, it would seem that including dietary sources that supply natural tocopherols and maintain maternal vitamin E status is adequate for most women. For women with poor nutrient intake, supplementation with a natural form of vitamin E is prudent. The IOM and the NHMRC set the RDI and AI at 28.4 IU[265] and 16.4 IU[266] respectively. Ensuring intake is adequate to also contribute to maternal stores may be more appropriate, such as 100 IU in the form of natural alpha tocopherol and mixed tocopherols obtained through diet or supplementation, if necessary.	Ensure good dietary sources When dietary intake is insufficient, consider supplementation with 100 IU/day in a natural form containing mixed tocopherols
Thiamine Thiamine is actively transported into breast milk. Supplementation increases breast milk concentration in deficient women but not in replete women.[287] The IOM RDA for thiamine during lactation is 1.4 mg/day.[288] Given there are a range of dietary factors that can reduce thiamine bioavailability,[289] it may be prudent to aim for a daily intake higher than the RDI during pregnancy and lactation.	5 mg daily
Riboflavin Breast milk levels strongly correlate with dietary intake. Breast milk riboflavin is present in the coenzyme form flavin adenine dinucleotide (54%), as well as free riboflavin (39%).[288] Supplementation of riboflavin increases free riboflavin but not flavin adenine dinucleotide.[287] The IOM and the NHMRC have both set the RDI for lactation at 1.6 mg/day.[265,266] However, a dose of 1.8 mg daily did not result in sufficient breast milk levels in a population of riboflavin-deficient mothers.[287] Based on this finding, a dosage of 10 mg/day may be more appropriate when maternal riboflavin insufficiency is suspected. Note: riboflavin supplementation can result in yellow colouring of infant's urine, which could be confused with signs of dehydration or insufficient breast milk intake.	When dietary intake is insufficient, consider supplementation of 10 mg daily
Vitamin B$_6$ Following pyridoxine hydrochloride supplementation, there is a rapid increase in breast milk pyridoxal, pyridoxamine and pyridoxal phosphate, occurring over a 3- to 8-hour period.[288] Pyridoxal 5 phosphate (the biologically active form) is also present in breast milk in comparatively low levels.[290] The vitamin B$_6$ RDI set by the NHMRC for lactation is 2 mg per day.[266] To promote good breast milk transfer, a daily intake of 10–15 mg is recommended.[288] A mix of pyridoxine hydrochloride and pyridoxal 5 phosphate may be the most appropriate B$_6$ supplement option, to ensure both bioavailability and maternal access to the active form in the case of inborn errors in metabolism.[291]	15 mg daily

Continued

TABLE 14.8 Group 1 nutrients for lactating women – maternal intake or status correlates with breast milk content—cont'd

Nutrient information (group 1 nutrients)	Maternal intake/ dosage recommendations
Vitamin B$_{12}$ Infantile Vitamin B$_{12}$ deficiency infers risk of anaemia and severe impaired neurological development at a critical time point.[292] Maternal deficiency is associated with low breast milk B$_{12}$ concentrations. Furthermore, low maternal status during pregnancy results in poor infant vitamin B$_{12}$ stores at birth. Classic maternal risk factors are vegan, vegetarian or low-animal-food diet, malabsorption issues and pernicious anaemia. However, a 2016 systematic review found that vitamin B$_{12}$ insufficiency is also common in non-vegetarian populations.[293] Additionally, a recent UK study found that 12% of pregnant women had low serum B$_{12}$ levels.[294] Maternal supplementation with 250 micrograms daily throughout pregnancy and breastfeeding is associated with improved breast milk vitamin B$_{12}$ levels.[295] In light of how common vitamin B$_{12}$ insufficiency is, prudent supplementation of vitamin B$_{12}$ during pregnancy and breastfeeding is recommended. An oral dose of 1000 micrograms appears to be sufficient in individuals with pernicious anaemia,[296] indicating that a dose of this order overcomes malabsorption barriers. Ensuring the adequacy of vitamin B$_{12}$ dose is a priority in this population. Serum B$_{12}$ assay has limited value in predicting B$_{12}$ status.[297] Due to the complexities of cobalamin physiology, a full panel of markers is necessary for accurate status assessment and would suggest sufficiency when serum B$_{12}$ is >300 pmol/L, total serum holo-transcobalamin is 40–125 pmol/L, plasma homocysteine is <13 micromols/L and methylmalonic acid is <250 nmol/L.[297] See Chapter 7 for further information on the assessment of B$_{12}$ status. Until adequate maternal status is certain, supplementation is recommended with a dose sufficient to overcome potential absorption issues. As stated previously, a daily dose of 1000 micrograms overcomes absorption issues in most people. A formula containing methylcobalamin 500 micrograms and adenosylcobalamin 500 micrograms is recommended, as these two active forms are not known be cross-converted,[298] and both may be necessary for neurological development and myelin formation.[298,299]	500–1000 micrograms daily until adequate maternal status confirmed and monitored Ideally, this is made up with a combination of methylcobalamin and adenosylcobalamin
Choline Choline is present in breast milk mostly as phosphocholine and glycerophosphocholine, with smaller amounts of free choline, phosphatidylcholine and sphingomyelin.[288] The IOM adequate intake (AI) for choline in lactation is set at 550 mg/day. Folate-mediated enzyme pathway polymorphisims may reduce maternal endogenous choline synthesis and altered partitioning of dietary choline through the enzymatic pathways. For these women, a greater need for exogenous choline either via the diet or through supplementation is needed to prevent choline insufficiency and further to promote appropriate biotransformation of choline and protect betaine synthesis.[300] Maternal choline supplementation of 960 mg and of 750 mg per day as phosphatidylcholine have been shown to increase breast milk choline, betaine and other choline metabolites in breast milk.[301,302] Ganz et al. found that 960 mg/day choline appeared to support normal choline dynamics in women with folate-mediated enzyme pathway polymorphisims.[300] Fischer et al.'s finding suggests that intake above 750 mg/day choline may not alter breast milk further.[302] Studies in the US and Canada suggest that the majority of pregnant and breastfeeding women do not meet the AI for choline.[303,304] Dietary intake correlates with breast milk concentration.[302] The inclusion of eggs in the diet has a positive effect on maternal choline status.[303]	750 mg from dietary or supplementary sources
Iodine Iodine deficiency may cause stunting and impairs neurological development in infants. Insufficient maternal iodine intake and status are both relatively common and are associated with lower breast milk iodine content.[305] The mammary gland has some capacity to concentrate breast milk iodine content via active transport mechanisms.[305] Hence, it is advisable to avoid excessive maternal iodine. The IOM and the NHMRC have set iodine RDIs for lactating women at 290 and 270 micrograms, respectively.[305,306] Data suggests this predicts appropriate breast milk iodine levels of >100 micrograms per L.[305] When supplementing lactating mothers with iodine, consider their dietary intake of iodine, which will depend on regional iodine soil levels and dietary patterns, in particular the consumption of iodine-fortified foods such as salt and bread.[307–309] The IOM and the NHMRC recommend supplementing lactating women with 150 micrograms of iodine per day, expecting that the remaining iodine will come from dietary intake.[305,310] Cautions: women with a history of Graves' disease may experience a Graves' episode with iodine even with relatively low doses, in the order of 50 micrograms daily. Close monitoring of thyroid hormones and collaboration with medical practitioners is necessary. Excess maternal iodine intake may cause thyroid disruption and disease in mothers[311] and infants.[312] In infants, this may impair growth and development. When iodine needs are not met by the diet, gradual introduction of iodine supplementation may reduce the risk of thyroid disruption occurring. Note: long-term iodine deficiency may cause higher susceptibility to thyroid disruption in response to iodine supplementation.[313] Starting with a dose of 100 micrograms for 2–3 weeks and gradually increasing to the desired dosage level over a 6-week period is ideal. When lactating women have been taking iodine throughout pregnancy, this graduation is not necessary. Sea vegetables may be an unpredictable and unreliable source of iodine because iodine content can vary from inadequate to excessive.[314]	Individualise daily supplemental dose to cover dietary gap Typically 150–250 micrograms Gradual increase of dose to meet target over 4- to 6-week period Caution: history of Graves' disease or other thyroid disease

TABLE 14.8 Group 1 nutrients for lactating women – maternal intake or status correlates with breast milk content—cont'd	
Nutrient information (group 1 nutrients)	Maternal intake/ dosage recommendations
Selenium Breast milk selenium levels appear to correlate with maternal selenium status.[315] Furthermore, low population breast milk selenium correlates with regional selenium soil-deficiency patterns.[315–317] Selenium is present in breast milk in organic forms. Glutathione peroxidase represents 4–32% of total selenium according to one source, and the other forms are present in decreasing order > selenocystamine > selenocystine > selenomethionine.[317] Selenium concentration in colostrum is twice as high as in mature milk.[318] It has been suggested that the mammary complexing of selenium with amino acids places some rate-limiting control of the passage of selenium into breast milk.[317] Older studies suggest that breast milk glutathione capacity is reached with a daily intake of 100 micrograms per day.[317] Organic forms appear to be better utilised.[317] The current RDI set by most countries is 75 micrograms daily.[318] Preliminary data suggests that selenium methionine at a dose of 200 micrograms reduces the risk of postnatal thyroiditis.[319,320] Hence, it would appear prudent to ensure women obtain 100–200 micrograms daily from combined sources. Supplementation should be tailored to regional soil status and based on maternal dietary intake. For women living in selenium deficient regions, supplementing 100 micrograms/day selenomethionine would seem justified.	Supplement when dietary intake suspected to be inadequate 100 micrograms daily as selenomethionine or other organic form
Docosahexaenoic acid (DHA) It is well established that breast milk DHA correlates with maternal intake.[321–323] Furthermore, it has been proposed that DHA (and potentially arachidonic acid [AA]) is conditionally essential for the young infant who may not be able to manufacture sufficient levels for optimal neurological development.[324] Recently, Jackson et al. suggested that a breast milk DHA target should be set of at least 0.3%, and potentially up to 1% of the total breast milk fatty acids.[325] The latter is said to reflect the breast milk DHA levels of populations with lifelong intake of fish. Sanders et al. proposed that vegans are particularly at risk of low DHA, finding the mean DHA of vegan Hindu women was 0.49%, compared to omnivores 1.36% and vegetarians 1.25%.[326] How generalisable this data is to other vegan populations is uncertain. While maternal DHA 400 mg supplementation substantially increases the DHA concentration of breast milk,[322] the potential for this intervention to have favourable effects on neurodevelopment is yet to be clarified. A 2015 Cochrane review of eight studies (including a total of 1567 breastfeeding women) investigating various long-chain polyunsaturated fatty acids (LCPUFA)-based supplements containing DHA concluded that maternal LCPUFAs supplementation had no effect on neurodevelopment, visual acuity or growth.[327] It did, however, find weak evidence for improvement of child's attention at age 5 years.[327] It has been proposed that some of the differences in outcomes may be related to the dietary patterns of the participants, and there may be a threshold DHA supplementary dose that is no longer beneficial.[321] Delgado-Noguera et al. did not analyse the systematic review findings for this possibility. Cohort studies looking at breast milk fatty acid profiles and maternal dietary patterns suggest that higher breast milk DHA supports neurological or motor development.[127,321,328,329] Regular thrice weekly intake of dietary oily fish appears to be fairly consistently correlated with higher breast milk DHA,[267] and it has been suggested that this may have more favourable neurocognitive implications.[321] However, high fish intake, especially of higher-order fish, increases mothers' mercury exposure (see Environmental Pollutants and Contaminants below). Dietary DHA may be more safely boosted through maternal intake of DHA-rich eggs and smaller fish such as sardines, where they are tolerated. A DHA supplement may be considered depending on dietary preferences and access to these foods. Supplementing vegans with 400 mg is probably warranted.	Dietary manipulation and or supplementation of 400 mg/day.

RDI = recommended daily intake; AI = adequate intake

TABLE 14.9 Group 2 nutrients for lactating women – breast milk concentration is maintained independently of maternal status and intake

Nutrient information (group 2 nutrients)	Maternal intake/dosage recommendations
Folate L-5-methyltetrahydrofolate (L-5-MTHF) is the predominant form found in breast milk.[288] However, folic acid is the main form found in most prenatal multivitamins and in many fortified foods. One North American study on a population exposed to folic acid fortification found that unmetabolised folic acid made up on average 8% of the folate content of breast milk.[330] Another study found that folic acid supplementation was associated with increased breast milk folic acid with no significant effect on breast milk L-5-MTHF or total folate levels.[331] Note: ensure that the mother's methylation is properly assessed prior to prescribing the methylated form, and consider the activated form if indicated. The current view is that maternal intake of folic acid or L-5-MTHF has minimal impact on breast milk total folate levels.[330] However, maternal folate stores may decrease if dietary intake is inadequate,[288] which may be to the detriment of future pregnancies. Hence, maintaining maternal folate status is vitally important. Houghton et al. found that a dose of 416 micrograms of L-5-MTHF was at least equally effective at maintaining maternal red blood cell folate levels as 400 micrograms of folic acid.[332]	Promote dietary folate intake to obtain 400 micrograms per day supplement with L-5-MTHF/day when a gap is suspected
Iron Unlike pregnancy, breastfeeding is typically a time of lower maternal iron requirements.[333] The healthy term infant is born with iron stores, and breast milk represents only a small source of iron. Breast milk iron is regulated independently of maternal iron status to protect the infant from deficiency and iron excess.[334,335] Iron is present in breast milk bound to lactoferrin.[335] Interestingly, breast milk iron concentration may increase during the weaning period.[334] While maternal iron supplementation has no effect on breast milk iron concentrations,[333] poor maternal iron status does have bearing on maternal health and wellbeing, and health of future pregnancies.[336] During the week following birth, maternal iron stores increase due to iron salvaging from haemoglobin following the reduction in blood volume and the return to pre-pregnancy red blood cell numbers.[336] Hence, the majority of women will have adequate iron. However, as many as 14–24% of women have iron deficient anaemia at 1 week postnatally, which is associated with having iron deficiency during pregnancy and higher blood losses at parturition and during the postnatal period.[336,337] Postnatal anaemia following haemorrhage will typically be managed prior to discharge with high-dose iron therapy (oral or IV) combined with erythropoietin, and, in severe cases, with blood transfusion.[338] The ideal iron status for women is still to be clarified. High normal maternal ferritin is associated with increased risk of both type 2 diabetes[339] and gestational diabetes.[340,341] Note: the associations between ferritin and inflammation were largely controlled by the studies included in these systematic reviews. Balancing the risks of high/normal versus inadequate stores, especially in light of the potential for future pregnancies, a target serum ferritin level between 40 micrograms/L and 75 micrograms/L would appear appropriate. Ferritin is an acute phase reactant which can be raised in inflammatory states independent of iron status.[336] Therefore, serum ferritin needs to be considered in the context of the iron panel. This panel congruently suggests iron deficiency when serum ferritin and serum transferrin saturation are low and serum soluble transferrin receptor is raised. During the first week postnatally serum iron rises, serum transferrin receptor levels decrease, and consequently transferrin saturation increases; hence, the latter is a poor indicator of iron status at this time point. Ferritin, however, typically stays consistent from 1 to 8 weeks postnatally, suggesting this marker is reasonably reliable during the early postnatal period so long as inflammatory processes are not at play.[336] Serum ferritin should be viewed with a full blood count, allowing red blood cell indices and haemoglobin concentration to be evaluated. From 2 weeks postnatally, the iron panel can be evaluated similarly to that of a non-lactating woman. Note: in the unusual scenario that postnatal iron deficiency occurs in the patient with haemochromatosis, iron supplementation is usually avoided or very carefully tailored in consultation with the patient's medical practitioner. Where iron supplementation is indicated, iron bisglyconate appears to be the preferred form. As such, several studies indicate that iron bisglycinate may be more bioavailable than iron sulphate, facilitating similar improvements to iron status with lower-dose therapy and with less side effects.[342–344] One study found that iron bisglycinate was as effective as iron sulphate at half the dose.[344] The dose and dosing interval need to be considered with regard to the woman's ferritin status. In the context of the breastfeeding amenorrhoeic iron-deficient mother with a ferritin value between 8 and 15 micrograms/L, 2-week treatment with daily alternating dose of 25 and 50 mg iron bisglycinate, followed by 2–4 weeks of treatment of 25 mg, is typically sufficient to restore iron status. Follow-up iron studies 4 weeks following treatment initiation are important to avoid oversupplementation and ensure appropriate response to treatment. Alternative causes of iron deficiency such as malabsorption and/or occult loss should be investigated when iron deficiency persists. Once iron stores are restored and during the period of lactational amenorrhoea, breastfeeding mothers have lower iron requirements than menstruating women. As such, the 2016 Italian Consensus Document recommends a daily intake of 11 mg during the lactational amenorrhoea period and 18 mg after the resumption of menstruation.[337] These amounts are usually easily obtained from dietary sources alone.	Individualise based on maternal iron status as indicated by blood iron panel Target serum ferritin level of 40–75 micrograms/L In most cases, iron supplementation is not required

TABLE 14.9 Group 2 nutrients for lactating women – breast milk concentration is maintained independently of maternal status and intake—cont'd	
Nutrient information (group 2 nutrients)	**Maternal intake/ dosage recommendations**
Copper Breast milk copper is maintained independent of maternal intake and status.[334,345] Similarly to zinc, copper breast milk levels are highest in early lactation.[345] The NHMRC has set the AI for copper during lactation at 1.5 mg/day.[266] Most women will have adequate copper status, although intake varies depending on factors such as soil content, agricultural practices, household plumbing, water source and zinc intake.[346] Some populations may be at risk of excess copper. Preliminary observational studies have found that mean serum copper levels are higher in women with a history of postnatal depression compared to control groups.[347] This may be in part related to inflammatory processes. Further zinc supplementation and improvement of the zinc/ copper ratio was associated with improvement of anxiety levels in one small study (not during lactation).[348] Currently there is no consensus on the appropriate way to assess copper status. Serum and plasma copper levels are considered appropriate for assessing population status, but do not appear to consistently respond to copper depletion and repletion diets,[346] and are reported to only indicate extremes of copper status.[349] Copper is, on the one hand, an essential nutrient, and on the other, a potential driver of inflammation and toxicity, and appropriate intake is still being debated.[346] Avoiding copper excess via maintaining healthy zinc intake (see below) is prudent. Note that zinc supplementation greater than 50 mg elemental long term may lead to maternal copper deficiency and associated adverse outcomes.	Individualised supplementation is rarely required. Copper excess could be harmful
Zinc Breast milk zinc levels are considerably higher than maternal serum zinc levels, indicating that zinc is actively transported and concentrated in the breast milk. Breast milk transfer gradually declines over the first 6–9 months. Zinc breast milk transfer starts at 2–3 mg per day during the first month, decreasing to 1 mg per day by 3 months, and 0.5 mg per day by 6 months.[350] Maternal requirements are thought to increase by 4 mg daily. Some of this may be achieved through increased maternal zinc absorption and recycling of zinc from involuting uterine tissue.[350] Breast milk zinc transfer appears to be largely regulated independent of maternal status. However, data in this area is mixed, suggesting that zinc deficiency and low intake may influence breast milk transfer partially.[335,350,351] There are an array of zinc transporters and mechanisms at play to maintain breast milk zinc homeostasis. As with iron, infants are born with some zinc stores. Clinicians should also be aware that there is a very rare genetic trait that results in impaired zinc transfer to breast milk.[335] Emerging insights indicate that zinc may play a critical role in mammary gland development, maintaining tissue integrity and functional aspects including cell signalling and protein synthesis.[352] The mammary gland accumulates and concentrates zinc, and it is suggested that this is for both supplying the infant and maintaining the functional integrity of the mammary gland.[352] Hence, maintaining good zinc status during adolescence, pregnancy and lactation may benefit mammary development and function. Regarding evaluating maternal zinc status: dietary assessment has been suggested as the most reliable method to assess this.[353] Clinical signs of zinc deficiency correlate reasonably well with low zinc status (such as frequent infections, poor wound healing and fatigue), although many are non-specific. The utility of plasma zinc levels for reflecting zinc status is still debated.[353,354] This is principally because plasma zinc represents only 1% of total zinc, and a number of factors other than status can modify this marker including infection, inflammation, collection technique, diurnal effects and haemodilution of pregnancy.[353,354] In zinc-replete women, maternal plasma zinc concentrations tend to return to pre-pregnancy levels within the first few weeks postnatally.[350] Despite such limitations, plasma zinc can be a useful tool that may reveal more severe zinc deficiency, but it may not reflect more mild deficiency[353] and should be used in conjunction with clinical presentation and dietary history. Of import, low plasma zinc have been associated with postnatal depression in one observational study.[355] Furthermore, low serum zinc may be a marker of major depression[356] and anxiety in conjunction with raised serum copper levels.[348] Although these findings are of a preliminary nature, nonetheless they do suggest that protecting zinc status and promoting optimal zinc–copper balance may assist with maternal mental wellbeing. The IOM and the NHMRC have set the RDIs for zinc in lactation at 13 mg and 12 mg, respectively.[265,266] Given the daily zinc output associated with breastfeeding and that inadequate intake is common, maternal maintenance of zinc status via supplementation seems prudent, especially during the first 6 months postnatally. A dose of 20–30 mg should ensure adequacy, without causing copper deficiency.[349,353] The forms zinc glycinate,[357] zinc gluconate, zinc citrate[357] and zinc sulphate[358] have evidence of good bioavailability, while zinc oxide has more limited bioavailability.[357]	Consider supplementation of 20 mg/day elemental zinc in a well-absorbed form for at least the first 6 months postnatally

Continued

TABLE 14.9 Group 2 nutrients for lactating women – breast milk concentration is maintained independently of maternal status and intake—cont'd	
Nutrient information (group 2 nutrients)	Maternal intake/ dosage recommendations
Calcium Breast milk calcium is maintained independently of maternal intake.[359] Maternal calcium conservation strategies such as increased intestinal absorption and decreased urinary loss may assist with meeting calcium requirements.[359] However, during the first 6 months of lactation, calcium mobilisation from bone appears to occur regardless of maternal intake, although not all findings are congruent.[359] Bone mineral loss is recovered during the latter stages of breastfeeding and following weaning.[359] Maternal skeletal calcium mineralisation is returned at least to the pre-lactation state at the time of weaning, with some findings indicating greater mineralisation compared to baseline.[359] While there have been mixed findings with regards to breastfeeding and osteoporosis risk, a recent meta-analysis of 12 studies found that longer duration of breastfeeding is associated with reduced maternal osteoporotic fracture risk.[218] The skeletal mobilisation that occurs during the third trimester and lactation can result in higher plasma lead, particularly in women with higher maternal lead burden.[360] Fetal transfer via the placenta is a concern. Lead transfer to breast milk is limited, but still worthy of prevention. Supplementation with 1200 mg of calcium (as calcium carbonate) daily was associated with a 5–16% decrease in breast milk lead levels in a population with high maternal skeletal lead burden.[361,362] Depending on maternal dietary calcium intake, and maternal lead exposure history, supplementing with 600 mg once or twice daily may be beneficial to ensure a daily intake of 1200 mg from all sources.	1200 mg/daily from a combination of dietary and supplementary sources
Magnesium Maternal magnesium intake does not appear to influence breast milk magnesium.[363] As with calcium, skeletal mobilisation liberates magnesium from bone.[363] High calcium intake does not appear to impact breast milk magnesium.[363] Maintaining good dietary intake and supplementing when there is a risk of inadequate magnesium intake would seem prudent. Interestingly, the NHMRC RDI is 320 mg daily,[266] which is the same as for a non-lactating women. Independent of lactation, some women may have higher magnesium requirements due to higher activity or stress levels. When negative magnesium balance is suspected, supplement with 150 mg of elemental magnesium once to twice daily. Choose a well-absorbed form, such as magnesium citrate, over magnesium oxide, which appears to be poorly absorbed.[364]	350–400 mg/day obtained from a combination of dietary sources and supplementation where needed. Supplement in 150 mg increments.

RDI = recommended daily intake

Framing nutritional advice positively is important so that women don't feel concerned about their breast milk nutrient adequacy. It can be helpful to explain that this is a time of high needs, and hence there are a few nutrients that need to be taken care of during this period.

Impact of maternal diet on macronutrients

Overall, the evidence indicates that total fat, carbohydrate and protein intake in breast milk is maintained independently of maternal intake.[267] Furthermore, the lactose content of breast milk is not altered by changes in maternal dietary protein, fat or carbohydrate intake.[267]

While maternal dietary patterns don't appear to impact on the overall macronutrient composition of breast milk, some aspects of the lipid profile may be modified by diet.[267] The lactocyte manufactures medium chain fatty acids (MCFAs), which represent 4–27% of the total fatty acids in breast milk. Higher levels of MCFAs occur when women are consuming a low-fat, carbohydrate-rich diet and they have low plasma triglycerides.[267] Maternal diet appears to influence breast milk long-chain polyunsaturated fatty acid (LCPUFA) composition, although there are inconsistent findings among the many studies, and an array of different dietary patterns have been assessed.[267] The maternal dietary omega-3:omega-6 fat intake consistently modifies the ratios of these fats in breast milk,[321] and breast milk DHA correlates with maternal intake (see Table 14.8 for more detail on DHA). Moreover, maternal dietary eicosapentaenoic acid (EPA) and DHA intake during the third trimester also correlate with breast milk content,[365] suggesting that some of the breast milk fatty acids reflect those that are in the maternal fat stores.[321,365]

General maternal dietary themes and outcomes in offspring

A Mediterranean-style diet rich in fruit, vegetables, fish and vitamin D sources appears to be the one consistent theme in terms of health-promoting dietary patterns during lactation (and pregnancy).[366] In particular, this dietary pattern is associated with reduced allergies.[366] Higher maternal dietary fish consumption also appears to correlate with improved neurological development.[127,328]

FISH OIL SUPPLEMENTATION: YES OR NO?

The question as to whether maternal fish oil supplementation has a favourable effect on infant health is debated. With regard to prevention of allergies, it is difficult to separate the findings associated with fish oil given prenatally to that given postnatally.[367] Some aspects of allergy susceptibility may be modified with fish oil supplementation. However, evidence is of a very preliminary nature[367] and dietary manipulation may be more influential than supplementation. Supplementation with a DHA-rich fish oil, or a vegan alternative, certainly seems warranted if dietary manipulation is not feasible, and even many non-vegan individuals may not obtain the DHA RDI without supplementation.[368]

ANTIOXIDANTS

A Mediterranean-style diet may also in part mediate favourable health effects through rich exposure to a diverse range of antioxidants. In particular, dietary patterns impact on carotenoids in breast milk[369,370] (including lutein, beta-carotene,[371] alpha-carotene, beta-cryptoxanthin,[369] zeaxanthin[372] and lycopene[370]). Of note, there appears to be mammary regulation of carotenoids that prevents the displacement of carotenoids such as lutein and zeaxanthin by beta-carotene.[372] Aromatic compounds from herbs and spices, being of small molecular weight and lipophilic, are also likely to find their way into breast milk. Polyphenols are present in breast milk at low levels, depending on maternal intake.[373]

Breastfeeding is associated with a greater range of taste acceptance in children,[374] which is theorised to be related to the exposure to subtle flavour changes from maternal diet through breast milk.[375,376]

The breast milk microbiome

The breast milk microbiome is thought to play a critical role in the health of the infant and breast health throughout lactation.[224,377] Key proposed functions of the breast milk microbiome include:

- seeding the infant with bacteria
- improving infant intestinal barrier function
- modulating infant immune function
- supporting the development of oral tolerance
- enhancing nutritional quality of breast milk
- protecting the breast from infection.

The diversity of the breast milk microbiota is yet to be fully established. Breast milk samples have been reported to include 100–600 species,[378,379] with the potential of multiple strains of these species being present. A 2016 systematic review including 12 studies from various geographical locations that utilised culture-independent methods indicated that 47 genera were detected across these studies.[380] The reviewers concluded that inter-individual variation in genera representations was high. Several genera, however, were represented in the findings of the majority of these studies. These included *Streptococcus*, *Lactobacillus*, *Staphylococcus* and *Bifidobacterium*.[380] Reports on the breast milk bacteria cell count range from 10^3 to 10^6/mL,[379] the latter probably being more accurate due to improved analysis technique.[379] Based on this range, an infant would ingest approximately 8.0×10^8 bacteria per day (from 800 mL of breast milk) and would be exposed to a diverse range of bacteria.

Urbaniak et al. found that among 39 Caucasian Canadian mothers, 47 genera were represented, with half of these being present in all samples.[381] However, these studies are based on small samples in industrialised countries and may be different from the microbial composition of the breast milk of women consuming traditional diets and living in rural or wild landscapes without antibiotic exposure. A further consideration is the variety of detection methods utilised by studies.

Factors such as maternal antibiotic exposure, stress, mode of delivery of infant, gestational age, diet, maternal obesity, geographical location and stage of lactation all appear to impact on the breast milk microbiota[377,382,383] (see Table 14.10).

TABLE 14.10 Maternal factors impacting on the breast milk microbiota[377,382–384]

Antibiotic exposure
Antibiotics during pregnancy or lactation may be associated with risk of bifidobacteria or lactobacilli absence in breast milk[385]

Intestinal microbiome

Specific probiotic strain supplementation
Through an indirect mechanism:
VSL#3 supplementation during trimester 3 and while breastfeeding increased breast milk bifidobacteria and lactobacilli of women birthing vaginally but not by caesarean[386]
Through direct transfer to breast milk:
Table 14.11 lists probiotic strains that have some evidence of transfer to breast milk

Mode of delivery and gestational age
Caesarean and preterm birth have been associated with reduced breast milk bifidobacteria,[382] although not all study findings are congruent.[381]

Lactation stage
The microbiota increases in diversity during the last trimester of pregnancy; this is maintained until weaning, at which point the diversity rapidly declines.[387]

Geographical location

Dietary factors

Maternal obesity

TABLE 14.11 Probiotic strains with evidence of transfer to human milk		
Strain	**Evidence**	**Potential therapeutic indication**
Lactobacillus reuteri Protectis Strain synonym names: American-type culture collection (ATCC) 55730	RDBPCT study *n* = 232 mothers. Administered to mothers from 36 weeks of gestation until delivery. Culturing technique used to identify the bacteria in colostrum within 3 days of delivery. Identified in 12% of probiotic group. Note: the detection method used is likely to underestimate the presence of this bacteria as would delayed assay.[230]	May reduce infant gastrointestinal dysmotility (see Chapter 23 in *Clinical Naturopathic Medicine*).
Lactobacillus rhamnosus GG (LGG)	RDBPCT – probiotic milk containing LGG and 2 other strains was administered to mothers from 36 weeks of gestation and for 3 months postnatally while breastfeeding. Only LGG colonised the infants at 10 days and 3 months of age.[229]	May increase neonatal intestinal bifidobacteria (Note: research looked at perinatal maternal administration, so this effect may be mediated through breast milk and/or vaginal exposure).[388] Allergy prevention.[389] Maternal or infant antibiotic exposure (to reduce the adverse effects on the microbiome of infant and mother).
Lactobacillus fermentum CECT5716	RCT with three arms (two probiotic arms and one antibiotic arm) *n* = 352. After 3 weeks of treatment, the administered probiotics were detected in the breast milk of the corresponding probiotic group. Assay method used: species-specific PCR and 16S rRNA sequencing.[231]	Consider for the prevention of mastitis recurrence or when breast milk dysbiosis is suspected. May have immunoprotective benefits for the infant including reduced URTI and GIT infections.[390,391]
Lactobacillus salivarius CECT5713	RCT with three arms (two probiotic arms and one antibiotic arm, as described above) *n* = 352. After 3 weeks treatment, the administered probiotics were detected in the breast milk of the corresponding probiotic group. Assay method used: species-specific PCR and 16S rRNA sequencing[231] RCT *n* = 20. After 4 weeks supplementation, both probiotics were identified in 60% of the treated women at day 30 of the study. Assay method used: species-specific PCR and 16S rRNA sequencing.[392]	Consider for the prevention of mastitis recurrence or when breast milk dysbiosis is suspected.
Lactobacillus gasseri CECT5714	As above in[392]	Consider for the prevention of mastitis recurrence or when breast milk dysbiosis is suspected.

RDBPCT: random double blind placebo controlled trial; RCT: random controlled trial

The entero–mammary pathway hypothesis suggests that maternal intestinal microbiome will impact on the breast milk microbiome during late pregnancy and throughout lactation, and have flow-on effects to infant health and breast health, including susceptibility to mastitis.[239] The maternal breast milk microbiota may be favourably modified by positively affecting the gastrointestinal microbiota (see Chapter 6 for strategies) and using specific therapeutic probiotic strains (see Table 14.11). Optimising the maternal microbiome, including the gastrointestinal, skin, oral, breast milk and vaginal regions, is an important consideration preconceptionally, during pregnancy and lactation.

The breast milk microbiota includes commensal bacteria and may contain some potentially pathogenic bacteria. In a healthy scenario, potential pathogens are suppressed by the numerous antimicrobial components in breast milk and through commensal bacteria's competitive inhibition.[393] Interestingly, there may be some cooperation between commensal bacteria in their defence tactics against potential mastitis pathogens.[394] When dysbiotic, the breast milk microbiota may be a factor contributing to recurrent mastitis (see Table 14.23).[224,394]

ANATOMY AND PHYSIOLOGY OF LACTATION

The mammary gland is a highly adaptive organ which has the ability to change its structure dramatically to meet physiological requirements.[395] The basic component of the mature mammary gland is the alveoli (see Fig. 14.2). This is a grape-like sack lined with columnar cells called lactocytes which secrete milk into the lumen. Surrounding the alveolar are myoepithelial cells and capillaries. The alveoli are grouped in bunches called lobules; each lobule is drained via a duct (lactiferous duct), which makes its way to the nipple. Some of the lactiferous ducts join on their way to the nipple. The myoepithelial cells, which also line the ducts, contract

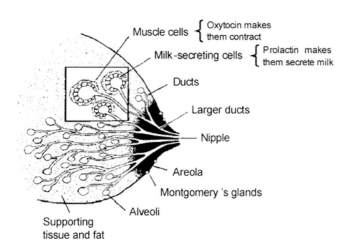

FIGURE 14.2 Anatomy of the breast[130]

under *the influence of oxytocin*, promoting milk ejection from the alveoli and duct.

Mammogenesis

The basic stages of mammogenisis are depicted in Fig. 14.3. The neonate has the beginnings of mammary development with a simple ductal system. Some newborns secrete a small amount of 'witches milk' in response to maternal hormones in the days following birth, indicating the capacity for some functional response under these hormonal influences. Throughout childhood, mammary development is restricted to general growth.[396]

At the onset of puberty oestrogen, epidermal growth factor and insulin-like growth factor are thought to drive glandular development and increased fat deposition in the mammary stroma.[397] The ducts elongate and branch, and the terminal buds develop into terminal ductal lobular units (TDLUs). As puberty progresses, the number of buds in the TDLUs increase. With each ovulatory menstrual cycle, greater differentiation occurs under the influence of

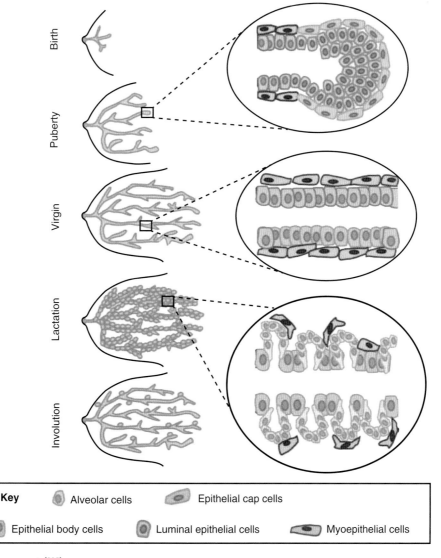

FIGURE 14.3 Mammogenesis[395]

progesterone and prolactin.[396] This development peaks at the end of the luteal phase, then regresses partially and continues again with the next menstrual cycle. With each cycle, further development occurs.[395] Lack of ovulatory cycles may impact on breast development for some women, but for most such women, this is overcome by the continued glandular development that occurs during pregnancy.

During the first trimester, proliferation of epithelial cells (which later become milk-producing cells called lactocytes) and ductal growth are stimulated by an interplay of placental hormones (oestrogen, progesterone and placental lactogen) and other hormones (growth hormone, insulin, insulin-like growth factor, prolactin and thyroid hormones). By the 16th week, mammary development is sufficient to the point that loss of the pregnancy will usually result in the initiation of lactation.[396]

During the second half of the pregnancy, the hormones prolactin and progesterone are thought to have the strongest influence on lobulo-alveolar growth. The nipples and areolae also grow and darken. Also the Montgomery follicles present in the areola become more active, secreting lubricating, protective substances and pheromones that will assist the infant to locate the areola.

Secretory differentiation (lactogenesis I) describes mammary epithelial cell differentiation into lactocytes with the capacity to synthesise unique milk constituents.[398] Secretory differentiation and the formation of colostrum typically occurs between 16 and 20 weeks of gestation. However, colostrum doesn't usually leak and isn't easily expressed until later in the pregnancy.[396]

The volume ingested by the neonate during the first few days is comparatively small. One older study found a mean total intake of 37 g on the first day, with a range of 7–122 g.[399] The Academy of Breastfeeding Medicine (ABM) estimates an average of 2–10 mL, 5–15 mL and 15–30 mL colostrum intake *per feed* during the first, second and third 24 hours, respectively.[400]

This initial period is thought to be an important stage in establishing surface protection. Colostrum contains high concentrations of protective proteins such as lactoferrin and SIgA, as well as oligosaccharides, which protect the surfaces of the respiratory and gastrointestinal tracts[398] and promote the growth of bifidobacteria.[222] Components within colostrum also promote the passage of meconium. Compared to mature milk, colostrum has low lactose and higher sodium concentrations.[396]

During this phase, the tight junctions between lactocytes are not properly formed, allowing for paracellular transfer of ions (such as sodium) and small molecules between the blood and milk compartments.[401,402]

Secretory activation (lactogenesis II) describes the onset of copious milk production. This phase is initiated 30–40 hours following birth, in response to the delivery of the placenta and the subsequent drop in progesterone. Until this point, the presence of progesterone is thought to inhibit secretory activation through inhibiting prolactin stimulus to the lactocyte.[396,398] The drop in progesterone also promotes the closure of the epithelial tight junctions in the breasts, which completes around 72 hours

postnatally, facilitating a change in milk production and composition.[401,402]

At around 36 hours postnatally, copious milk secretion is initiated. This increases 10-fold over the next 36 hours.[396]

FACTORS THAT MAY IMPEDE SECRETORY ACTIVATION

A retained portion of placenta may delay or prevent secretory activation by continuing to release progesterone. Risk of delayed secretory activation is also associated with obesity, gestational diabetes, a stressful labour, high-intervention labour and the antenatal use of corticosteroids.[403–406]

It is worth noting that the maternal experience of feeling the 'milk coming in' is thought to be an 'over-shoot' in production that results in a temporary state of engorgement until milk synthesis adjusts based on milk removal representing the infant's need. The time point that women experience the 'milk coming in' varies, with some women experiencing successful lactation without sensing this. However, not sensing the milk coming in can be an indication of delayed secretory activation.[398]

Prolactin in established lactation

During established lactation, prolactin is often described as permissive. Its presence is necessary for milk production, but the way it interacts with prolactin receptors is modulated by other factors. Suckling stimulates the release of prolactin from the anterior pituitary (see Fig. 14.4). Prolactin release is greatest 30 minutes after the initiation of a feed,[130] and levels are higher in response to night-time feeding. This is one explanation why night-time feeding can be important for maintaining milk supply and for maintaining lactational amenorrhoea.[130] Prolactin reaches the breast and stimulates the prolactin receptors on lactocytes, which stimulates the synthesis of milk.

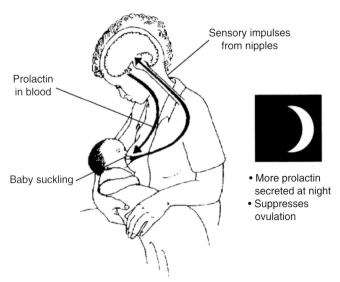

Sensory impulses from nipples

Prolactin in blood

Baby suckling

- More prolactin secreted at night
- Suppresses ovulation

Secreted after feed to produce next feed

FIGURE 14.4 Prolactin in established lactation[130]

BOX 14.3 *Vitex agnus-castus*: further discussion of anti-galactagogue potential

While there are some mixed findings with regards to the effect of *Vitex agnus-castus* (VAC) on prolactin, the evidence overall suggests that VAC may suppress prolactin. Suppression of prolactin and progesterone promotion are likely to have a negative effect on breast milk production in early lactation and are unlikely to assist with low supply in established lactation. Hence, it would appear prudent to avoid this herb in women with low supply, and particularly during early lactation. Additionally, it is plausible that VAC use during pregnancy (especially the second half) may negatively impact on the functional breast development that occurs in part in response to high circulating prolactin.

Studies on *Vitex agnus-castus* relating to prolactin and lactation

Two older studies are sometimes cited in support of low-dose VAC having a galactagogue effect.[408] The methodology of these studies has been criticised.[409,410] One of the studies appeared to be an unblinded case series, the findings being unclear.[410] The other study[411] was an inadequately blinded study (n = 817) that appeared to correlate VAC (by Agnolyt, Madaus equivalent to approximately 180 mg of dried fruit) with greater milk production at 20 days postnatally. The milk volumes reported in the study were, however, very small (430 mL versus 275 mL), suggesting that some of the infants were receiving supplemental formula, which would be a major confounding factor that would drive down breast milk supply. It would also appear that women in the VAC group may have had lower milk production on days 1 to 3, and a return of menses during the early postnatal period.

Some authors propose that the effect of VAC on prolactin may be dose related. This is based on the findings of a study conducted on healthy men that found a lower dose (120 mg) of a concentrated extract BP1095E1 (16:1 extract; solvent not identified) was associated with prolactin-promoting effects, and a higher dose of this same extract (480 mg) was associated with prolactin-suppressing effects.[412]

This study does provide an interesting proposition for a U-shaped effect. However, two other studies and two case reports detail findings consistent with prolactin suppression in women associated with relatively low-dose VAC extracts.

Forty women with hyperprolactinaemia received either 3 months of treatment with Agnucaston (3.2 mg–4.8 mg extract equivalent to 40 mg dried VAC) or bromocriptine (a dopamine agonist). Prolactin levels dropped by 44% in the Agnucaston group and 51% in the bromocriptine group, with no significant difference between these treatments.[413]

Another study (n = 52) investigated the effects of a VAC extract (Strontan, 3 mg of a 10–16:1 ethanolic extract, equivalent to 20 mg dried VAC) on women with latent hyperprolactinaemia and found that 3 months of treatment was associated with decreased prolactin release in response to thyroid-releasing hormone.[414]

Two case reports[410,415,416] reported prolactin reduction by 27% after 3 months of treatment with liquid extract of VAC in women with hyperprolactinaemia. The daily dose described in one of these cases was 15 drops of a 1:10 tincture.

When might *Vitex agnus-castus* be appropriate?

The potential hormonal actions of VAC (promoting progesterone and suppressing prolactin levels)[414] prompt careful consideration of its possible impact on lactation. According to current concepts in lactation physiology, once lactation is established, prolactin's role is permissive rather than regulatory, and progesterone no longer suppresses lactation,[417] or at least not to the same extent as it does in early lactation. Consequently, the hormonal effects of VAC may be less likely to cause low supply in established lactation, and the cautious prescription of this herb may be appropriate in occasional instances. Furthermore, in the years preceding conception, VAC may play a role in preventing lactational insufficiency in women with luteal phase defects, as it is understood that healthy luteal phase progesterone levels are important for breast development.[418,419]

Certainly there is sufficient data to indicate that VAC has the potential to negatively impact on lactation during the early months of lactation and prompt an earlier return of menses. The latter may deprive women of some of the health benefits associated with the lower levels of circulating oestrogen during lactation. In addition, the use of VAC in the second half of pregnancy may negatively impact on the functional breast development that occurs in part in response to high circulating prolactin.

There is a theory that more frequent breastfeeding during the early weeks of breastfeeding results in a greater number (or sensitivity) of prolactin receptors, and helps to promote good milk supply in the future. It has also been proposed that multiparous mothers have a higher number of receptors present and therefore a greater response to prolactin.[407] Prolactin receptor sensitivity may also be altered by hormonal factors[407] and/or local effects at the breast. There may be some interplay with genetics also.

Caution is warranted with the use of any herbs that might antagonise prolactin, including *Vitex agnus-castus*. See Box 14.3 for a further discussion on *V. agnus-castus*.

Oxytocin and the milk ejection reflex

The milk ejection reflex (MER) is a neuroendocrine reflex (see Fig. 14.5). The reflex is initiated both in response to neural stimulation and as a conditioned response. Tactile stimulus of the areola and nipple triggers a neural impulse that initiates the release of oxytocin from the posterior pituitary. Oxytocin travels via the circulatory system to the breast and stimulates contraction of the myoepithelial cells which surround the alveoli, causing milk ejection.[420] The MER lasts from 45 seconds to 3.5 minutes.[420] This reflex is also triggered by visual, audio and tactile cues and thoughts. The MER may be initiated as the mother

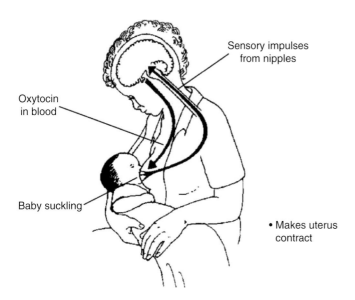

Works before or during a feed to make the milk flow

FIGURE 14.5 The milk ejection reflex[130]

TABLE 14.12 Infant feeding cues	
Early cues	Change in breathing pattern Opening and closing mouth Stirring Turning head Seeking/rooting
Mid cues	Stretching Increased physical movement Hand to mouth
Late cues	Crying Agitated movements Turning red

(adapted from[425])

prepares to breastfeed and then further with the tactile stimulation of breastfeeding. Hearing her infant cry, touching and smelling her infant and having loving thoughts towards her infant are all cues that may trigger oxytocin release and support the MER.[130] On the other hand, high anxiety, pain and embarrassment,[130] as well as alcohol intake,[421] can dull the MER. Disruption to the nerve pathways that carry this impulse causes an impaired or absence of an oxytocin and prolactin response to tactile stimulus. This may be caused by surgery, depending on the incision line.[396] When the other breast is not affected, the MER can be stimulated by breastfeeding initially on that side.[396] Of note, some nerve repair can occur following surgery and the number of years since surgery may be a factor determining the extent of repair.

Oxytocin is a neuroprotective hormone. Greater exposure is linked to positive parenting behaviour, including affectionate touch, duration of breastfeeding and early life care.[145,422,423] Higher plasma levels of oxytocin have also been associated with resilience, including fewer depressive symptoms and maintenance of positive parenting behaviour following psychological stress.[145] Oxytocin receptor genotypes may modify maternal responses to oxytocin.[422]

Galactopoiesis: maintenance of good milk supply

Maintaining good milk supply is dependent upon adequate removal of milk from the breast and adequate stimulation of the breast. This means frequent breastfeeds of adequate duration (and/or frequent expressing) with effective milk transfer. The breasts are under autocrine control, so the rate of milk synthesis is directly affected by the rate of milk removal. The baby's attachment, more gently described as their 'fit and hold' by Douglas,[424] needs to be

effective to ensure adequate milk transfer. When milk remains in the breast, milk synthesis inhibitory factors accumulate and decrease milk synthesis. Removal of milk from the breast removes these inhibitors, thereby causing accelerated milk synthesis.[425]

Storage capacity

Storage capacity varies enormously between women. In a small study, Daly et al. found that breast milk storage capacity varied from 192 to 787 mL.[426] However, daily breast milk production of women with different storage capacities was similar. Women with smaller storage capacities fed their infants more frequently and milk synthesis was more rapid. This illustrates the individuality of the mother–baby dyad. Women with smaller storage capacity must feed more frequently to deliver the quantity of milk required to meet their baby's needs. The mother–baby dyad is dependent on responsiveness to feeding cues (see Table 14.12). It is important to remember that crying is a late hunger cue which often hinders effective feeding due to the effects of exhaustion and elevated stress hormones.[425]

BREASTFEEDING INITIATION

The WHO guidelines state:

> *Babies should be placed in skin-to-skin contact with their mothers immediately following birth for at least an hour and mothers should be encouraged to recognise when their babies are ready to breastfeed, offering help if needed.*[20]

A strong evidence base indicates that early uninterrupted skin-to-skin contact between mothers and babies following birth improves breastfeeding outcomes,[58,59] as well as promoting cardiorespiratory, temperature and blood glucose regulation for the newborn.[58,427] One study found that skin-to-skin contact reduced maternal pain during episiotomy repair.[58] Conversely, interruption of mother–baby skin-to-skin contact is associated with increased risk of infants not breastfeeding during the first 2 hours following birth.[428]

To avoid disrupting this contact, routine procedures and medical checks should be delayed at least until after the baby has had their first breastfeed. Where possible, any medical interventions should be done with the baby kept in physical contact with their mother.

Following birth, neonates have an alert period, enabling them to be ready to breastfeed for the first time. Placed prone on their mother's bare chest, most newborns will respond with a similar sequence of behaviour that leads them to self-attach and breastfeed. This phenomenon has been called the 'breast crawl'.[429] Most infants will orientate and attach within an hour after birth. It has been proposed that allowing the infant to go through this behaviour sequence promotes early self-regulation and orientation at the breast.[430] Guided by their reflexes and with gravity's assistance, the neonate typically attaches deeply. It is thought that this has an imprinting effect which supports effective breastfeeding attachment in subsequent breastfeeds. A small number of studies show that the breast crawl is associated with better short-term breastfeeding outcomes and lower risk of breastfeeding attachment issues.[430]

During the first 6 weeks, the newborn infant retains this set of innate breast-seeking behaviours that are elicited when placed prone on their mother's chest.[429] This baby-led attachment often supports a more effective and wider latch.[429] These neonatal feeding behaviours are further enhanced when mothers and babies are in skin-to-skin contact. Svensson et al. found that regular skin-to-skin time with breastfeeding support was more effective than only breastfeeding support to resolve severe latching issues in mother–baby pairs 1–16 weeks postnatally.[431] There has been recent interest in encouraging mothers to experiment with breastfeeding in a reclining position, for the reasons discussed above. This is often described as 'laid back nursing' or 'biological nurturing', as coined by Colson. Colson encourages the phrasing 'baby led, mother guided' to acknowledge that the mother is part of this exchange, supporting the infant's innate search for the breast.[432] Douglas et al. have described the gestalt breastfeeding method that also works with the mother in a supported reclining position, with the baby prone on the mother, as a way of assisting mother–baby pairs who have experienced difficulty with positioning and breast attachment. Colson suggests that mothers maintaining a semi-reclined posture, rather than a fully supine posture, supports the infant's torso angle in a way that promotes airway stability.[432] Additionally, the line of sight between mother and baby is maintained so that the mother can monitor the infant's breathing.

The natural odours of the breast assist the infant in finding the breast and promote breast-seeking behaviour.[433] This seeking is easier for babies when mothers refrain from washing their breasts during the first 24 hours after birth. Also, strong scents and perfumes are best kept away from babies as these can be disruptive.

Practitioners can encourage parents to write a breastfeeding plan that is aligned with the BFHI ten steps (see page 466). Along with requests around uninterrupted skin-to-skin contact, parents may also include strategies to reduce disruption of olfactory cues.

BREASTFEEDING SUPPORT

The breastfeeding dyad shifts and changes over time. Practitioners working with breastfeeding mothers and babies need to have a clear sense of what infant behaviours may be normal and what maternal and infant manifestations may be flags that require support or a more urgent intervention. Table 14.13 outlines a guide of key age-related patterns of infant and maternal behaviour and has flags to look for. A number of common breastfeeding concerns are discussed in the following section.

Problems with positioning and attachment are common for new mothers. When left unresolved, these lead to problems such as nipple injury, mastitis, unsettled behaviour in infants and poor supply, all of which can have serious consequences for breastfeeding longevity. For these reasons, women should be strongly encouraged to seek help from a lactation consultant or breastfeeding counsellor if they have any pain or discomfort while breastfeeding.

COMMON BREASTFEEDING CHALLENGES

Perceived and true lactation insufficiency

Careful assessment and consideration of history is required to distinguish true lactation insufficiency from perceived insufficiency. Many women will assume there are problems with their milk supply when their baby is unsettled and/or cries, when their baby wants to feed more often, when their baby wakes more frequently in the night, when their breasts feel smaller or softer and/or when minimal milk can be expressed.[436] While some of these may be present when milk supply is low, none of these signs is a clear indicator of low milk supply. These signs may be present when babies are unwell, in pain and/or in a period of accelerated growth. Changes in breast fullness are often associated with the normal change from oversupply to supply matching the need of the baby that frequently occurs when the baby is 2–4 months old. The MER is often reduced in response to a pump, so pumped milk volume does not reliably represent milk available to a breastfeeding baby. See Figure 14.6.

Unfortunately, inappropriate management of perceived lactation insufficiency often leads to true lactation insufficiency. For example, concern about milk supply will often lead to the use of supplementary artificial feeds.[437] Giving supplementary feeds satiates the baby, so the baby takes less milk from the breast, and consequently breast milk production declines.[417] When the supplement is given in a bottle, exposure to the artificial teat often leads to nipple confusion, resulting in breast refusal, which further compounds the problem.

When responding to a mother's concern about milk supply, it is important to understand why she feels her milk supply is low and find out key information to assess her individual case. First, it needs to be determined if her baby is receiving sufficient milk through careful assessment of the baby's stool and urination history, as

TABLE 14.13 Breastfeeding behaviour and key infant feeding features during the first 24 months of life[434]

Age range	Key infant features	Breastfeeding behaviour	Refer for breastfeeding help
0 to 2 weeks	Infant's stomach capacity 5–7 mL on day one 22–27 mL on day three 45–60 mL at 1 week	Frequent feeding is needed: because of small stomach capacity; to promote good milk supply and the laying down of prolactin receptors Infants typically feed most of the time they are awake	Nipple or breast pain Low stool or urine output Jaundice Breastfeeding concerns
2 weeks to 12 weeks	Stomach capacity increases Infant becoming more alert Infants can be unsettled Many have periods of crying Infant has sensory needs met by walks outside; outings; social contact; being held	Feeding frequency varies between mother/baby pairs based on breast storage capacity and infant hunger and satiety Most infants cluster feed in the evening (feed very frequently) Night feeding is important for maintaining supply	Frequent falling asleep early stages of feed Nipple or breast pain Frequent falling asleep during early stage of feed Unsettled baby Low stool or urine output Breastfeeding concerns
3 to 6 months	Wide variance of infant sleep needs 9–18 hours/24 hours Crying and unsettled periods begin to decrease for most infants	Infants may have longer intervals between feeds Feeding frequency varies based on breast storage capacity and infant hunger and satiety Most infants cluster feed in the evening (feed very frequently). Night feeding is important for maintaining supply	Nipple or breast pain Frequent falling asleep during early stage of feed Unsettled baby Low urine output Breastfeeding concerns
6 to 9 months	At around 6 months infants are ready for solids	Breast milk intake remains stable and may even increase a little. Infants add to the breast milk intake with solids/complementary foods. Breastfeeding prior to offering solids avoids displacing breast milk from the diet	Nipple or breast pain Low urine output Breastfeeding concerns
9 to 12 months	Infant's intake of solids varies	Breastfeeding frequency and intake varies	Nipple or breast pain Low urine output Breastfeeding concerns
12 to 18 months	Solids start to become the main nutrition for most infants. Breast milk continues to contribute valuable nutrition[136] and provides back-up nutrition in times of illness or emergency[435] Infant's intake of solids varies	Breastfeeding frequency and intake varies. Immune factors continue to be available to the infant through breastfeeding even when infant feeds infrequently[136] Breastfeeding frequency increases when infants are unwell or during developmental transitions	Nipple or breast pain Low urine output Breastfeeding concerns
18 to 24 months and beyond	As above	As above	As above

well as growth and development (see Table 14.14). How often and for how long is her baby feeding? Is her baby having night feeds (which are important for maintaining supply)? Has she seen a qualified and experienced lactation consultant? Have the baby's latch and other baby-related health issues that may impact on milk transfer been assessed? Table 14.15 gives a summary of the possible causes of lactation insufficiency. In the case of true low milk supply, all efforts to avoid exposing the baby to artificial teats should be made. In most cases, any necessary supplementation can be administered via a lactation aid which allows babies to receive this additional milk at the breast, keeping them accustomed to receiving milk at the breast and ensuring some breast stimulation (discussed further below). Cup feeding is another method used that avoids the use of artificial teats.[6] When supplementary feeds have been deemed necessary, it is important that strategies are in place to resolve breastfeeding challenges, improve maternal milk supply and phase out supplementation whenever possible. All health professionals should be aware of the WHO order of preferences for supplementary feeds (see Table 14.19).

How to increase supply

It is vital that the two most common reasons for insufficient milk intake and low supply are addressed. These are:

1 **Inadequate feeding frequency** and **feeding duration**, which commonly occur: with scheduled feeding; when feeds are terminated before the baby lets go (reduces access to kilojoule-dense hind milk); when breast milk substitutes are given; or when babies are drowsy due to prematurity, illness, exposure to birth medications or due to exhausting hunger crying.

AVERAGE MILK INTAKE 1–6 MONTHS
ABOUT 900 mL PER DAY

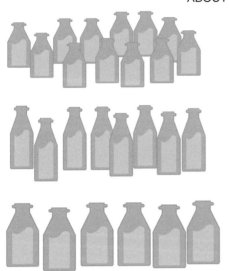

- Baby often takes from both breasts
- Needs many feeds per day to gain weight well
- Must wake often at night to feed
- You may never double pump > 120 mL

You may have a SMALL STORAGE CAPACITY
~75 mL × 12 feeds = 900 mL

- Baby may take from one or both breasts
- Needs 7–8 feeds per day to gain weight well
- Needs some night feedings
- You may double pump ~120 mL with missed feed, ~60 mL ~60 min. after feed

You may have a MEDIUM STORAGE CAPACITY
~110 mL × 8 feeds = 900 mL

- Baby often takes from one breast, is done quickly
- Needs fewer feeds per day to gain weight well
- May sleep for longer stretches at night
- You often double pump > 120 mL

You may have a LARGE STORAGE CAPACITY
~ 150 mL × 6 feeds = 900 mL

IF FED ON CUE, BABIES CAN THRIVE WITH ANY STORAGE CAPACITY:

But because the amount of milk they get per feed varies by so much, to get the milk they need per 24 hours, their feeding patterns must vary

FIGURE 14.6 Storage capacity from Mohrbacher 2014 – a useful infogram for mothers

TABLE 14.14 Signs of insufficient milk intake by baby (from Whitten)[158,438]

Fewer than 3 stools/day in babies 4 days old or more
- after 4–6 weeks, not reliable – stool frequency varies

Fewer than 6 wet nappies per day in babies 6 days old or more (fewer than 5 very wet disposables)
- strong odour and/or yellow staining

Persistent/increasingly painful nipples
- pain while breastfeeding

Pinched or misshapen nipple immediately after feeding (not so easy to assess – refer to LC)

No audible or visible swallowing from the baby (sometimes difficult to assess – refer to LC)

Slow weight gain or weight loss
- Equal to or greater than 7% weight loss over the first week post birth indicates a need for careful assessment of the breastfeeding dyad and could indicate insufficient breast milk intake.[400] Noel-Weiss and colleagues suggested that baseline birth weights are better assessed 24 hours post birth to allow for initial fluid loss.[439] They found that higher urinary output was associated with greater weight loss over this 24-hour period, indicating that weight loss in the first 24 hours is not an accurate indication of intake. Furthermore, increased maternal IV fluid and maternal fluid status may be a factor influencing 24-hour weight loss.[440,441] Weight loss after 24 hours correlates more closely with poor intake.
- Not regaining birth weight by 2 weeks.
- Weight crossing percentiles downwards in first 3 months (it can be normal to cross percentiles downwards after 3 months of age); flat growth curve at any age. Note: breastfed babies should be assessed according to WHO growth charts which have been constructed using data from babies fed according to WHO recommendations. Multiple measurements spaced adequately in time are needed to obtain useful data.[417]
- Caution: weighing errors are very common and occur with poor weighing technique, use of different scales, scale faults and varied timing of weighing (e.g. in relation to bowel movement or large void).[442] With overly frequent weighing, there is a risk that variations do not reflect true weight change.
- Weight loss may be due to illness (if this is the case, prescription of breast milk substitutes will expose the baby to further illness risk).

Referral to an International Board Certified Lactation Consultant and other relevant health professionals is recommended if any of these signs are observed; LC = lactation consultant

2 **Poor latch and associated ineffective milk transfer** is a commonly overlooked hindrance to supply. Hence, assessment of latch by an experienced lactation consultant or breastfeeding counsellor is essential for all women with suspected low milk supply.[425,436]

Maximising skin-to-skin contact is also important.[425] This can be encouraged by suggesting bath breastfeeds and cosy topless time with baby. When low supply is suspected, offering both breasts at each feed will ensure that breast milk synthesis inhibitors are drained from both breasts.

TABLE 14.15 Causes of lactation insufficiency	
Poor lactation management (most common)	Early postnatal care: • separation of mother and baby • lack of skin-to-skin contact • delayed first feed; reduced frequency of feeds • supplementary feeds given Ongoing care: • scheduled feeds (not frequent or long enough) • not feeding according to baby's cues • supplementary feeds given • lack of appropriate support to identify and resolve challenges

Infant-related challenges (common)	• Poor latch:
	  – poor early lactation management
	  – cleft palate
	  – prematurity (and late preterm birth)
	  – Down syndrome
	  – classic tongue tie (ankyloglossia) – caution about over-diagnosis
	• Heart defect

Hormonal or drug effects (moderately common)	• Effect of birth interventions • Thyroid disease • Insulin resistance (PCOS, gestational diabetes, diabetes mellitus) • ↑ Progesterone (retained placenta; contraceptives; pregnancy) • ↑ Glucocorticoids (stressful labour; administered in premature labour; administered to treat asthma during pregnancy) • Obesity (may lower initial prolactin response; may also impact latch) • Pituitary disease (uterine haemorrhage → pituitary shock) • Other drugs (progestins, oestrogens, alcohol, nicotine, pseudoephedrine, dopamine agonists)
Structural (unusual)	• Insufficient glandular tissue (previously estimated to occur in 0.01% of women)*may be on the rise due to an increase in hormone-related factors. *Many women who receive poor breastfeeding management are erroneously told they have insufficient glandular tissue.* • Nipple abnormality
Structural due to surgery or trauma	• Severed 4th intercostal nerve (interferes with MER) • Breast reduction (may affect supply, but with appropriate support many such women are able to fully or partly breastfeed)

[425,436]*Many texts incorrectly quote a figure of 5% referencing a 1938 BMJ article, or a secondary reference originating from this source.[425] However, in this article, the 5% figure includes cleft palate and other infant-related challenges that hinder lactation success.[443] With the rise in the use of ART, there is the potential for an associated rise in the incidence of true insufficient glandular tissue, as some health conditions that pose as fertility obstacles are associated with insufficient glandular tissue. However, several studies have found that ART users are also at higher risk of preterm birth, prenatal corticosteroid exposure and caesarean birth,[41,42,444] which may then expose them to higher risk of post-birth separation and artificial supplementation. Additionally, this group tends to be more susceptible to perceived lactational insufficiency.[41] One study found that many of the determinants of poor breastfeeding outcomes in a population of ART users were modifiable and could be overcome by ensuring consistent breastfeeding advice.[444]
(updated from Whitten[158])[407,425,436]

HERBAL GALACTAGOGUES

Herbal galactagogues may be used to help support milk supply. It is essential to continue to address all factors that may be impacting milk supply and specifically ensure there is frequent effective removal of milk from the breast and that the breasts are receiving adequate stimulation. Without these measures, herbal galactagogues are likely to have limited impact.

Information on how herbal galactagogues work is of a preliminary nature and there are multiple theories. Tables 14.16 and 14.17 list some commonly prescribed herbal galactagogues, mostly from the Western Herbal Materia Medica. For more information on the clinical trial data for herbal galactagogues, a systematic review is available.[445] Table 14.18 provides some information on some potential anti-galactagogues.

Possible mechanisms for herbal galactagogue action include[448,453,489,490]:

- Enhancing prolactin levels through dopamine receptor antagonism in the same way that the pharmaceutical galactagogues domperidone and metoclopramide appear to work.[475]
- Modulation of other hormone receptors, affecting sensitivity to insulin, progesterone and oestrogens.[407,491]
- Directly increasing the amount of functional breast tissue.
- Positively influencing infant feeding behaviour through altering the taste or exerting carminative actions via constituents transferred to the breast milk.
- Diaphoretic action based on the idea of the mammary alveoli being a modified sweat gland.
- Improving mammary blood flow.

- Exerting anxiolytic and thymoleptic actions which may support the improvement of breastfeeding confidence and allow effective milk ejection reflex and prolactin response by reducing inhibitory stress hormones.

Nervine actions may be particularly important for breastfeeding mothers, as anxiety and depression frequently occur in this population, and ironically worry about milk supply may in itself inhibit MER and over time lead to poor milk supply. Education on breast physiology and the use of relaxation techniques particularly while feeding may be useful for some women.

Individualising herbal galactagogue prescription allows herbal treatment to be tailored to suit the woman's situation and improve efficacy. The herbalist may include galactagogues with nervine properties when stress is suspected to be a significant factor or herbs that improve insulin sensitivity when impaired glucose tolerance is suspected.

Common problems with galactagogue clinical trial methodology

While there are a growing number of small clinical trials assessing the efficacy of herbal galactagogues, the results of these studies need to be assessed cautiously. Many studies have methodological limitations.[445,461,492]

TABLE 14.16 Information on some core herbal galactagogues from the Western Herbal Materia Medica

Core galactagogues	Actions*/daily dosage suggestion/ cautions	Traditional information	Contemporary information	Clinical trial data
Pimpinella anisum Aniseed *Foeniculum vulgare* Fennel**	**Actions that may support galactagogue effect:** Carminative Selective oestrogen Receptor modulator? **Daily dosage suggestions:** 5–30 g crushed seed as infusion (higher end of dosage when used as a simple) **Cautions:** Internal use of the essential oils of either of these herbs may not be safe during lactation due to the presence of the potential toxin oestragole. Infusions of *F. vulgare* seed within the recommended dosage range are unlikely to deliver excessive amounts of oestragole.[446] Additionally, there is some evidence that other constituents present in *F. vulgare* infusions may inactivate oestragole.[447] *P. anisum* may occasionally be substituted with the potentially toxic *Illicium anisatum* (Japanese star anise).	***F. vulgare* references:** There are many references to the use of *F. vulgare* in traditional texts[448–451] Decocted in barley water to 'draw down the milk'[449] 'From a very early period of medical history, fennel seed has been credited with the power of increasing the secretion of milk, (galactagogue) … leading physicians of many countries ascribe to it excellent power in this direction. The infusion of the seed may be used without limitation.'[450] 'The leaves or seed boiled in barley water and drank are good for nurses, to increase their milk and make it more wholesome for the child.'[452] ***P. anisum* references:** Aniseed biscuits are a traditional gift for new mothers in the Netherlands to ensure 'bountiful milk'.[453] 'breeds milk'[454]	*P. anisum* and *F. vulgare* contain trans-anethole which has structural similarity to dopamine and is theorised to act as a dopamine receptor antagonist.[448] One study found *F. vulgare* leaf had considerably greater concentrations of trans-anethole and lower concentrations of oestragole than the fruit.[455] One report describes four cases of premature thelarche and raised oestradiol levels in children who had received *F. vulgare* tea (one 5-month-old and three children under the age of 6). The dose and characteristics of the tea were not supplied. Thelarche resolved and oestradiol levels returned to normal range 3–6 months after ceasing the tea.[456] Further investigation into the potential effect of *F. vulgare* on serum oestrogen is warranted. One small study found lactating cows treated with a combination of *F. vulgare* and *Nigella sativa* seed (information on dose and preparation not available) had greater mean milk yield compared to controls after 1 week (15.4%) and 24 days (16.9%) of treatment (P <0.003).[457]	Two human studies investigating herbal complexes containing fennel were found. One older unblinded Bulgarian study (n = 5) observed an increase in milk volume after 10 days of treatment with a herbal formula containing fennel compared to baseline. Many details of the study are unavailable.[458,459] Turkyılmaz and colleagues compared outcomes for women drinking Humana® tea (reported to contain fennel extract (600 mg per day) and fennel essential oil (20 mg per day), as well as five other herbal ingredients including hibiscus 7.8 g/day, rooibos 600 mg/day, vervain 600 mg/day, raspberry leaf 600 mg/day, fenugreek 300 mg/day, goat's rue 300 mg/day, and also vitamin C) to 'apple tea' and no treatment (n = 66). Humana® tea group had: • higher mean volume of expressed breast milk at 3 days postnatally: 73.2 mL compared to 38.8 mL (apple tea) and 31.1 mL (no tx), P <0.05 • lower mean infant weight loss in the first week: 5.7% compared to 6.6% (apple tea) and 8.3% (no tx), P <0.05 • faster regain of their birth weight: 6.7 days compared to 7.3 days (apple tea) and 9.9 days (no tx), P <0.05.[460]

Continued

TABLE 14.16 Information on some core herbal galactagogues from the Western Herbal Materia Medica—cont'd				
Core galactagogues	Actions*/daily dosage suggestion/ cautions	Traditional information	Contemporary information	Clinical trial data
Trigonella foenum-graecum Fenugreek	**Actions that may support galactagogue effect:** Demulcent Diaphoretic Nutritive Hypoglycaemic (depending on dose and delivery) **Daily dosage suggestions:** 3.5–10 g crushed seed **Safety:** Generally well tolerated according to the Academy of Breastfeeding Medicine. Diarrhoea and maple syrup odour of sweat and urine are the most common reported adverse effects.[461] **Caution: possible peanut and other Fabaceae allergen cross sensitivity**[461,462] Huggins[463] (who allegedly has experience with greater than 1200 lactating women using fenugreek) reports: • observing two or three cases of diarrhoea resolved with reduced dose or discontinuation of herb • two asthmatic mothers reported aggravated asthma symptoms • no reported side effects in infants.	Allegedly used in Ancient Egypt as a galactagogue.[464] There are ethnobotanical references to its use as a galactagogue in Sudan, Africa, Iraq, Egypt and Argentina.[465]	Huggins (lactation consultant, claiming to have observed the response of 1200 women over a 6-year period), reports that 'nearly all' women who took fenugreek report an increase in milk production within 24–72 hours of taking the herb. The dosage prescribed in her clinic is 1200–1800 mg of encapsulated ground seed 3 times/day (t.d.s.). She recommends discontinuation of herbal treatment when milk production is at sufficient level and maintaining supply through adequate breast stimulation and emptying of the breast.[463] Of note is that the dosage recommended by Huggins is greater than the dose that appears to have been used in some of the small clinical studies. A survey of lactation consultants in the US found that 49% of the 124 respondents reported using fenugreek to 'promote lactation'.[466] One small study on the effect of fenugreek on lactating goats suggested that fenugreek treatment increased growth hormone – growth hormone being one of the hormones involved in lactation.[467]	Three small clinical trials have delivered mixed results and had methodological limitations. In an open label study ($n = 10$), the 24-hour mean breast milk volumes of women after 1 no-treatment week were compared to volumes after 1 week of fenugreek supplementation (1830 mg encapsulated ground seed Natures Way t.d.s.). Mean 24-hour breast milk volumes were significantly greater after 1 week of fenugreek treatment (mean daily volume 464 mL) compared to 1 week of no treatment (207 mL) $P = 0.004$.[468] Another study found no significant differences in pump volume or prolactin levels between women given placebo or fenugreek (three capsules of unreported quantity/extract per day) for 21 days postnatally.[469] In a third study, two cycles of 30-day fenugreek treatment (600 mg of ground seed 3 t.d.s.) was compared to two other active treatment arms Molocco+B$_{12}$ (vitamin B$_{12}$ and placenta extract) or a traditional Bataknese medicinal soup containing *Coleus amboinicus*). At no point was the 24-hour infant breast milk intake of the fenugreek group different to that of the Molocco+B$_{12}$. The 24 hour breast milk intake of the infants in the traditional Bataknese soup group was significantly greater than both the other active treatments.[470] Additionally, one study (see above under Fennel for a description of the study on Humana® tea) reported to deliver a daily fenugreek dose of 300 mg per day in combination with several other herbs.[460]

TABLE 14.16 Information on some core herbal galactagogues from the Western Herbal Materia Medica—cont'd

Core galactagogues	Actions*/daily dosage suggestion/ cautions	Traditional information	Contemporary information	Clinical trial data
Silybum marianum St Mary's thistle	**Actions that may support galactagogue effect:** May improve insulin sensitivity[471] Hepatoprotective **Daily dosage suggestions:** >420 mg silymarin (dose based on study) **15 g of ground seed ingested** Extrapolation from absorption studies on phospholipid silymarin preparations[472,473] suggests a potential for co-prescription of lecithin to improve bioavailability of silymarin from the ground seeds. **Cautions:** Asteraceae allergy	Mary's milk said to have splashed on the leaves. Traditionally seen as a food for breastfeeding mothers, the whole plant being boiled after the spikes were removed.[474] Ingestion of the whole herb would have facilitated the absorption of actives with poor water solubility.	The galactagogue effect may occur via dopamine receptor antagonism according to one study.[475] This is based on findings of a rat study. 14-day treatment with micronised silymarin extract BIO-C® was associated with a dose-dependent increase in serum prolactin levels. The dopamine D2 receptor agonist bromocriptine given at an oral dose of 1 mg/kg significantly reduced the high serum prolactin levels in the BIO-C®-treated group. The researchers propose that dopamine D2 receptor antagonism may be at least a partial mechanism for the effect of BIO-C® on female rat prolactin levels. Another study (randomised controlled) was conducted on 30 dairy cows treated with 10 g of silymarin extract reported to contain 49.1% silybin.[476] From 10 days prior to expected calving date until 15 days postnatally, 15 of 30 cows were given silymarin extract. Treated cows reached their average lactation peak 1 week prior to control cows and maintained a higher milk yield throughout lactation. Milk yield of treated cows was greater than controls on days 21 and 30 by 14.6% and 15%, respectively (P <0.05).	Three human studies are summarised below. Peila et al. conducted a placebo-controlled study using BIO-C® 420 mg on preterm mothers of infants 10+ days old and found no difference in milk production measurements between the two arms.[477] Di Pierro et al. conducted a controlled study (randomised or investigator blinding was not reported) investigating the effect of 63 days of treatment with micronised silymarin extract BIO-C® 420 mg per day on women (n = 50) diagnosed with low milk supply, defined as producing less than 700 mL breast milk per day.[478] Milk production was assessed over a 24-hour period by weighing infants before and after feeding, and measuring milk pumped after each feed to quantify milk retained in the breast. 24-hour breast milk production was assessed on days 0, 30 and 63. After 30 days, the treatment group had a mean observed increase in breast milk volume of 64.4%, and the placebo group of 22.5% (P <0.01). After 63 days, the treatment and placebo groups had a mean increase from baseline of 85.9% and 32.1%, respectively (P <0.01). Zecca et al. utilised an extract containing both silymarin-phosphatidylserine and *Galega officinalis* (otherwise poorly described extract) and compared to placebo reported an increase in expressed breast milk of exclusively pumping mothers (n = 50) of preterm infants.[479] Of note, expressing practices and frequency were not recorded.

Continued

	TABLE 14.16 Information on some core herbal galactagogues from the Western Herbal Materia Medica—cont'd			
Core galactagogues	Actions*/daily dosage suggestion/ cautions	Traditional information	Contemporary information	Clinical trial data
Galega officinalis Goat's rue	**Actions that may support galactagogue effect:** Diaphoretic May improve insulin sensitivity **Daily dosage suggestions:** Recommendations vary: 5–30 g/day or equivalent of the dried leaves and flowers. Dried leaves and flowers. Note: this herb is subject to quality issues which can have marked effect on efficacy (author's clinical observation). Ensure high-quality starting material with at least good organoleptic indicators of quality and a low proportion of stem. **Cautions:** Humphrey[453] cautions against use of the fresh plant.	Several references to its traditional use as a galactagogue used on goats and cows in France[448,480,481] Suggested root for *Galega* from Greek: *Gala* = milk, *agein* = to drive.[448] 'stimulate the lactiferous vessels to an increased secretion during the period of lactation',[451] although this is followed by a reference to its lack of use at the time.		As above – Zecca et al.[479] Additionally, one study (see above under Fennel for a description of the study on Humana® tea) reported to deliver a daily goat's rue dose of 300 mg per day in combination with several other herbs.[460]
Cnicus benedictus Blessed Thistle	**Actions that may support galactagogue effect:** Thymoleptic Anxiolytic Digestive bitter tonic Diaphoretic Emmenagogue (could suggest oxytocic effect) **Daily dosage suggestions:** 6 g tea (or tincture) may be more effective than solid doses **Cautions:** Avoid in pregnancy; strong emmenagogue	Referred to as a galactagogue by Sayre[481] in his US pharmacognosy text, who also states that the cold infusion is a bitter tonic and the hot infusion a diaphoretic and emetic in larger doses. Perhaps if the galactagogue effect is linked to the diaphoretic action a warm infusion may be more effective. Cook states, 'It slowly promotes nearly all the secretions'[450] (Not sure if breast milk is included in his list of secretions) According to Weed,[482] it is 'Famed for its ability to increase milk supply' and it 'removes suicidal feelings and lifts depression'.		No studies identified

TABLE 14.16 Information on some core herbal galactagogues from the Western Herbal Materia Medica—cont'd

Core galactagogues	Actions*/daily dosage suggestion/cautions	Traditional information	Contemporary information	Clinical trial data
Verbena officinalis Vervain	**Actions that may support galactagogue effect:** Thymoleptic Nutritive **Daily dosage suggestions:** 5–10 g **Cautions:** None known	'a remedy for sore breasts'[452]		No studies identified apart from one where vervain was used in combination with a number of other herbs (see above under Fennel for a description of the study on Humana® tea), reported to deliver a daily vervain dose of 600 mg per day in combination with several other herbs[460]

*Actions that may relate to or support its use as a galactagogue; **Also consider other carminatives of the Apiaceae family such as *Anethum graveolens*, dill, and *Coriandrum sativum*, Coriander; tx treatment
(updated from Whitten[158])

TABLE 14.17 Supportive galactagogues

Supportive galactagogues	Specific information
Urtica dioica Nettle	Nutritive
Althaea officinalis Marshmallow root	Nutritive, moistening
Medicago sativa Alfalfa	Nutritive
Lavandula angustifolia Lavender	Nervine, thymoleptic, carminative May be useful when MER is diminished
Chamomilla recutita Chamomile	Nervine, carminative May be useful when MER is diminished
Nepeta cataria Catnip	Nervine, thymoleptic May be useful when MER is diminished
Asparagus racemosus Shatavari	Nervine, female reproductory tonic
Hibiscus sabdariffa Rosella	Diuretic, mild hypotensive
Humulus lupulus Hops	Strong nervine traditionally used when MER impaired. Use low dose only (up to 1 g per day in divided doses). Avoid over-sedating mother and baby.
Zingiber officinalis Ginger	May support milk production in the immediate postnatal period.[483] Traditional use from Thailand.

MER = milk ejection reflex
(updated from Whitten[158,409,448,453])

A NOTE ON RELACTATION

Many women and health workers are not aware that relactation is possible. Relactation is the recommencement of lactation months or even years after breastfeeding has ceased.[493–495] Relactation is encouraged via regular stimulation of the breast, and is usually easier when less time has lapsed. However, case studies attest to the potential for successful relactation and return to exclusive breastfeeding after longer intervals.[496–498] The support of family and health workers can contribute substantially. Mothers who continue to need to supplement can benefit from using a supply line to support breast stimulation and normalise feeding at the breast for the infant. **Adoptive lactation** (also called induced lactation) is also possible, where a woman who may, or may not, have lactated previously can stimulate the production of milk.[461,498,499] This also requires regular stimulation and may be assisted by hormonal medications and galactagogues.[496]

The use of breast milk substitutes

The ABM and the WHO provide clear guidelines on the appropriate use of breast milk substitutes.[130,400] The first priority is to understand why the mother seeks a breast milk substitute and explore the reason with her. One of the most common reasons for mothers to introduce a breast milk substitute is because of perceived low milk supply (see above). A number of other reasons are common, including concerns related to returning to work and the belief that supplementation will improve their infant's sleep (see below). Very occasionally the mother requires a medication that is contraindicated in breastfeeding (see below). For most medication classes, there are options that are compatible with breastfeeding.

In many cases, when the reasons for supplementing are explored, education, reassurance and referral for lactation support can result in the continuation of breastfeeding and

TABLE 14.18 Potential anti-galactagogues	
Herb	**Potential mechanism**
Salvia officinalis Sage	Long tradition of use as anti-galactagogue
Ephedra **spp.**	Contains pseudoephedrine Anecdotal reports and one small clinical study indicate that the drug pseudoephedrine may suppress lactation, possibly in part through prolactin suppression[484]
Mucuna pruriens **Velvet Bean**	Contains L-Dopa[485]; therefore, may diminish prolactin release
Vicia faba **Broad bean, fava bean**	Contains L-Dopa[485]; therefore, may diminish prolactin release **Caution:** A principle in *V. faba* can trigger haemolytic anaemia and hyperbilirubinaemia in babies with Glucose 6-phosphate dehydrogenase (G6PD) deficiency[425,486]
Mentha **spp.** **Mint**	Low to moderate dose of *Mentha* spp. as tea or extract is unlikely to cause anti-galactagogue effect. High dose peppermint and/or use of the essential oil topically may have an anti-galactagogue effect Some women have reported reduction in milk supply after consuming peppermint essential oil or lollies containing menthol and/or using toothpastes with these ingredients[487]
Petroselinum crispum **Parsley**	Traditionally seen as a herb/food that lowers milk supply. Women report reduction in breast milk supply after consuming large amounts such as would be obtained from eating tabouleh.[453] Small intake is unlikely to impact on lactation. Culpepper discusses its use topically for engorgement.[452]
Vitex agnus-castus **Chaste tree**	Theoretical anti-galactagogue via dopaminergic action and potential to suppress prolactin (see Box 14.1) There is, however, divided opinion among herbalists regarding its effect on lactation. There appears to be some traditional evidence for use as a galactagogue.[409,449] **Caution:** may cause early return of menses, which may deprive mothers of some of the health benefits associated with lactational amenorrhoea as well as delayed fertility. Use during the second half of pregnancy could theoretically have a negative effect on pregnancy-related breast development.[453,488]

Note: this is not an exhaustive list; some reactions may be idiosyncratic, observe for individual reactions to herbal preparations. (updated from Whitten[158])

TABLE 14.19 Feeding preference in order of safety for the infant[6,501]		
Preference	**Feeding option**	**Considerations**
1st	Mother's own milk direct from her breast	The biological norm
2nd	Mother's own expressed breast milk	Depending on the timing of the expressed milk and period of storage, this milk may not confer the same immune protection as mother's milk direct from the breast Appropriate handling and storage methods are important[400]
3rd	Donor milk from a known and safe source	Obtain from a milk bank (these will be screened and pasteurised) or from a known donor who is confirmed free of transmissible infections such as HIV. Appropriate handling, transportation and storage procedures are important[400]
4th	Commercially made breast milk substitute (formula)	Ensure the composition complies with the international standards. Appropriate preparation techniques are important to reduce the risk of pathogenic bacteria exposure[400]
5th	Unimproved non-human mammalian milk and homemade formula	These options pose the greatest risk to the infant and are strongly discouraged (see below).

the avoidance of breast milk substitutes. Practitioners being alert and ready to meet women at these crossroads can have a profound and long-lasting effect on the health of mother and child. Of course, ensuring any breastfeeding concern is appropriately assessed by a lactation consultant or breastfeeding counsellor and that the infant is

adequately nourished is essential (see Table 14.14) and a duty of care. Informing parents of the order of feeding preference in terms of the safest to least safe options for their infant (see Table 14.19) is arguably also a duty of care. This needs to be done in a sensitive manner with an awareness of the mother's situation. It is also important for practitioners to be aware that it is in conflict with the WHO code to promote breast milk substitutes to mothers, including providing samples.[500]

When a supplementary feed is necessary (expressed breast milk or formula), this can be delivered via a number of methods. Minimising exposure to artificial teats reduces the risk of infants developing a preference for these and learning sucking techniques that impact on effective milk transfer at the breast. Mothers who are partially breastfeeding and needing to supplement because of supply issues can benefit from using a lactation aid or supply line, which allows babies to receive this additional milk at the breast. This keeps the infant accustomed to receiving milk at the breast and ensures breast stimulation.[400] Some mothers who are exclusively supplementing may choose to use a supply line for the physical closeness it provides and for the more normative orthodontic implications. Cup feeding is another method that avoids the use of artificial teats.[6] Two 2016 Cochrane reviews found that using cup feeding for any necessary supplementation of late preterm infants had a protective effect on breastfeeding initiation and duration compared to bottle feeding.[502]

The supplementing device most culturally expected is of course the bottle. Noted concerns are the distinct difference in infant tongue and jaw movement, milk flow rate and potential long-term developmental concerns.[400] The use of bottles is associated with greater risk of dental caries[503] and is a dose-dependent risk factor for obesity, with higher frequency of use causing greater risk.[504] Recently, it has been suggested that a 'responsive bottle feeding' or 'baby-led' method is preferable for infants who are bottle fed,[505,506] the idea being that feeding is responsive to the infant's interest, therefore promoting infant recognition of satiety and theoretically reducing some of the obesogenic effects of formula feeding.[505] The latter is yet to be tested. Other suggestions are to ensure parents alternate sides and hold their infant close so they continue to experience the physical closeness and social engagement of feeding.

Any supplementation is likely to lead to lowered breast milk supply. The infant becomes satiated from the supplement and takes less milk from the breast in the following period. The breast down-regulates production in response to reduced milk removal. This initiates a perpetuating cycle that often leads to premature cessation of breastfeeding[400]; hence the value of the involvement of a lactation consultant or breastfeeding counsellor to help the mother with strategies to protect her supply.

The WHO considers donor milk as the third-safest option for feeding, after direct breastfeeding and the feeding of the mother's expressed breast milk.[6,501] When mothers ask 'which formula is the best', explaining how donor milk (from a known and safe source) is a safer option than formula can help to put formula in perspective. This may also help the mother to more highly value her own milk, and knowing that women are giving her their breast milk may encourage her to continue breastfeeding. Interestingly, a 2016 systematic review found that receipt of donor milk was associated with longer duration of breastfeeding but not exclusivity

compared to formula milk supplementing.[507] However, at least one study has shown a beneficial effect on exclusivity.[508]

Any discussion of donor milk as an option needs to be accompanied with an explanation of how to ensure its safety. The most reliable source of donor milk is from a milk bank or from a friend or relative of the mother who is known, trusted and in good health and who has had recent tests for HIV and other infectious diseases. Walker suggests four pillars of safe milk sharing: informed consent, donor self-exclusion, health and lifestyle communication, and blood testing.[509] Both donor milk and the mother's own milk need to be expressed, handled, stored and transported in an appropriate way. Some straightforward guidelines are available from the ABM.[510]

When an infant is partially or fully supplemented with formula, the question arises as to how to reduce the health impact of this. Numerous health claims and nutrition content claims are made by commercial formula companies,[511,512] and frequently these claims are promoted in ways that are in conflict with the WHO code.[512] Companies may vie for certain markets through health concepts related to 'special' ingredients or characteristics such as prebiotics, DHA, low lactose content and being certified organic. Formula is frequently promoted as being close to human milk in composition,[512] which is of course a fallacy. It has been suggested that from a marketing perspective, human milk is the leading 'brand', and formula companies strive to be seen as second or similar to this leading 'brand'. More recently, advertising has developed the rather cunning strategy of appealing to mothers who feel shamed or socially excluded because they are not breastfeeding.[513]

Infant formula marketing provides no real information on which formula will be least harmful to an infant. Some issues relating to formula selection are worth discussing, however. Lactose-free formulas are not recommended unless the infant has a congenital lactase deficiency (which is an extremely rare life-threatening condition apparent during the first week postnatally). Lactose is the predominant sugar present in breast milk and has prebiotic[109,110] and immune-modulating effects.[514] When a formula-fed infant is suspected to have a cow's milk allergy, a partially or extensively hydrolysed whey or casein[515] formula should be selected. Of note, a recent Cochrane systematic review concluded that hydrolysed formulas do not reduce the risk of allergies,[516] suggesting that precautionary use of hydrolysed formulas in formula-fed infants at risk of allergies may not provide any benefit.

DANGERS OF HOMEMADE FORMULA

Motivated by a healthy cynicism for the formula industry, practitioners may be inclined to guide parents to make homemade breast milk substitutes (homemade formula) and/or recommend the use of unmodified non-human mammalian milks. These options are strongly discouraged by the authors of this text book because of the potential for devastating effects to the infant and the medico–legal risks to the practitioner. The younger the infant is, the more vulnerable they are to adverse effects, with infants under the age of 4 months being particularly at risk. All infants are at risk, however.

Human infants have limited capacity to excrete solutes[517]: they display digestive[119,518] and xenobiotic metabolic immaturity.[519] Accordingly, breast milk has a lower solute load than other mammalian milks.[517,520] The solute load of artificial breast milk substitutes needs to be specifically defined to avoid electrolyte disturbances and renal strain. Hence, appropriate levels of specific electrolytes and proteins as well as overall solute concentration need to be maintained.[517,520,521]

Commercial infant formula will never be able to resemble the adaptive living tissue that is breast milk. However, for the most part, commercial infant formula maintains the basic essential nutrients within tight limits to minimise toxicity and deficiency and provide for the basic nutritional needs of the infant. The composition of infant formula is regulated by national bodies in most developed countries including the US and Australia.[522] These regulatory bodies draw on global recommendations for formula composition created by the Codex Alimentarius Commission, which seeks advice from experts in infant physiology; namely, the European Society for Paediatric Gastroenterology, Hepatology and Nutrition (EPSGAN).[521] With these nutrient composition guidelines in place, infant formula is the fourth choice in order of safety, and is assuredly ahead of homemade options.

Homemade formula is at high risk of providing both toxic excesses and inadequate levels of essential nutrients. The consequences of either during the critical window in infant development can be devastating in both the short and the long term. Homemade formula recipes available on the internet recommend the inclusion of ingredients such as chicken livers, bone broth and carrot juice. Analysis of one homemade formula showed levels equal to or in excess of 500% the RDI for infants of vitamin A, iron and sodium, and 200% the recommended protein intake.[523] A further consideration is the potential for lead exposure from bone broth.[524] Raw milks, or raw animal ingredients, may also expose infants to pathogens that they are particularly vulnerable to due to the infant's higher gastric pH,[518] increased intestinal permeability[525] and lowered natural immune resistance compared to breastfed infants.[526]

Several case studies show severe consequences associated with feeding infants homemade formula or whole milks such as goat's milk and cow's milk. One case study associated homemade formula based on goat's milk with macrocytic anaemia secondary to severe folate deficiency.[527] Another report describes methaemoglobinaemia secondary to nitrate exposure from a silverbeet decoction that was added to commercial formula.[528] Another case study linked fresh goat's milk feeding to the development of severe hypernatraemia, azotaemia and intracranial infarctions.[529] Yet another report describes a 1-week-old infant who developed metabolic acidosis after being fed goat's milk exclusively from 2 days of age.[530] A further example found severe anaemia and hypoproteinaemia with associated oedema in

a 19-month-old who had been consuming approximately 800 mL whole cow's milk from the age of 9 months.[531]

Commercially formulated goat's milk formula is a safer option for parents wanting to avoid a cow's-milk-based formula.[520] However, the effort used looking into breast milk substitutes could be better directed towards obtaining a safe source of donor milk and ensuring that access to breastfeeding support has been provided. Attempts at homemade formula and the use of whole non-human milk place infants at unnecessary risk.

INTERVENTIONS THAT MAY BE HELPFUL FOR FORMULA-FED INFANTS

When an infant is receiving commercial formula, there may be some scope for the addition of agents that have the potential to modify some of the specific health concerns for these infants; namely, heightened risk of infection and of derangement of the gut microbiota. In keeping with the principle of *first do no harm*, there are two broad considerations for the practitioner:

1 *Avoiding actions that may further disrupt breastfeeding.* When a mother is partially breastfeeding, the addition of substances viewed as therapeutic to the formula may inadvertently promote the formula over breastfeeding. The mother may become concerned with her infant receiving the 'medicines' in the formula and preference this over breastfeeding. Conversely, treating through the mother is likely to strengthen the mother's breastfeeding intentions.

2 *Avoiding the addition of any substance that has the potential to cause harm to the infant.* For most developed countries, a set of composition standards on vitamin and mineral content is adhered to by formula manufacturers. The further addition of vitamins or minerals to infant formula may result in excessive exposure to the infant. Infants have immature digestion, gut immune defence, renal function and xenobiotic metabolism. They are therefore vulnerable to adverse effects from bacterial contaminants, potential allergens and any substances that puts a renal or toxic load on their system.

Addition of the following agents may be worth considering for the exclusively formula-fed infant.

1 Prebiotics. A variety of prebiotic compounds have been trialled in formula-fed infants. While these agents may have favourable effects on the altered and potentially dysbiotic microbiota of the formula-fed infant, they are structurally different to and certainly do not display the diverse nature of HMOs. Hence they are unlikely to mimic some of the structure-specific effects of HMOs.[532] However, it is worth considering their addition to formula given the potential for benefit. Initially, it would seem prudent to introduce only one prebiotic at the clinically trialled dose. As this is tolerated, the clinician may suggest adding a second prebiotic. Note that some formulas may contain one of these agents at a therapeutic or sub-therapeutic concentration, which needs to be considered in dosing:

– Galacto-oligosaccharides at a dose of 4 g/L may have a bifidogenic and lactogenic effect and be associated with lower clostridium in formula-fed infants, bringing their microbiota closer to that of breastfed infants.[533]

– Galacto-oligosaccharides/fructo-oligosaccharide in a 9 : 1 ratio given in feed at a dose of 6–8 g/L may help to reduce allergies in formula-fed infants.[534] It also appears to promote both bifidobacteria and lactobacilli growth and have a stool-softening effect.[535]

– Orafti Synergy1 (50 oligofructose:50 FOS) at a dose of 4 to 8 g per litre promotes bifidobacteria and lactobacilli growth and has a stool softening effect in formula-fed infants[535,536]

2 Probiotics. The judicious selection of strains with evidence of safety and efficacy is an ethical responsibility considering the vulnerability of this population. The following are some examples of probiotic strains that have evidence for their efficacy and safety in formula-fed infants:

– *Lactobacillus fermentum* CECT 5716 has clinical evidence of efficacy in preventing common respiratory and gastrointestinal infections in both 1- to 5- and 6- to 12-month-old formula-fed infants.[537]

– *Lactobacillus rhamnosus* GG (LGG) may have several therapeutic benefits in formula-fed infants. LGG may promote cow's milk tolerance in cow's milk allergic infants and promote butyrate production in the bowel when combined with an extensively hydrolysed casein formula compared to soy-based formula.[515,538] Furthermore, it may help to resolve blood in the stool and bowel inflammation in allergic colitis.[539]

– *Combination LGG* and *Bifidobacterium lactis* Bb-12-treated (versus placebo-treated) formula-fed infants had roughly half as many episodes of acute otitis media, acute upper respiratory infections and courses of antibiotics prescriptions according to one study.[540]

3 Long-chain polyunsaturated fatty acids (LCPUFAS). Practitioners should be cautious about adding LCPUFAs to formula because altering their ratios may have detrimental effects:

– Docosahexaenoic acid (DHA) – has gained attention as a fatty acid important for neurological development. However, when it is added to formula in excess of arachidonic acid (AA), it may be detrimental to infant neurodevelopment.[541] Breast milk DHA correlates with maternal intake, yet remains below breast milk AA levels. In contrast, breast milk AA levels remain stable[541] and the AA:DHA ratio is >1 even when mothers are supplemented with 400 mg of DHA.[322] It has been proposed that these nutrients may be conditionally essential for the young infant who may not be able to manufacture sufficient levels for optimal development. Not all infant formula contains DHA (and AA)[522]; hence, naturopaths may be inclined to recommend the addition of DHA to formula. The ratio of DHA to AA may be particularly important for the young infant's brain development.[541,542]

Infant formula with DHA in excess of AA fed to baboons resulted in impaired transfer of AA to parts of the brain.[541] One study found that DHA in excess of AA was associated with poorer language skills at age 14 months but not 39 months compared to formula with DHA and AA combined or controlled unenriched formula.[543,544] Another study found that the highest dose of DHA with unmatched AA was associated with poorer performance on a number of cognitive tests compared to controls and groups receiving lower DHA than AA.[545] A 2013 meta-analysis concluded that DHA added to formula at a rate greater than 0.3% of the fat content of the formula and equal to or less than the AA would be sufficient to promote optimal visual acuity.[546] Until further research clarifies the importance of the DHA to AA ratio, it seems prudent to dose in line with current guidelines. Current composition requirements globally indicate that DHA and AA are to be added to infant formula, stipulating that the AA levels should be higher than the DHA levels.[542]

– Further recommendations about PUFAs ratios in infant formula. The World Association of Perinatal Medicine, Early Nutrition Academy and Child Health Foundation recommends that eicosapentaenoic acid (EPA) does not exceed DHA[547] and that AA is at least equal to DHA. Both linoleic acid and α-linolenic acid (ALA) should be present in infant formula as they cannot be manufactured.[547] The WHO recommends DHA in infant formula be maintained at 0.2–0.5% of fats, and further states that given that breast milk DHA can approach 1.5% of the total fat content, this is the upper-limit for infants.[547]

Nipple pain

Nipple pain is a red flag for a feeding attachment issue and warrants fast referral to a lactation consultant or breastfeeding counsellor. Trauma due to breastfeeding attachment issues can predispose women to secondary causes of nipple pain, including: bacterial or fungal infections, dermatitis and vasospasm.[548] Hence, an attachment issue needs to be considered as a potential predisposing factor. Furthermore, poor attachment at the breast results in poor milk transfer, increased risk of mastitis and risk of low supply.

Some of the common and less common causes of nipple pain are outlined in Table 14.20. Frequently, the aetiology can be difficult to distinguish and two or more conditions may coexist such as: physical injury, atopic dermatitis, psoriasis, blocked duct and/or superficial infection. Resolving attachment issues and trialling some initial measures such as small doses of sunshine and topical expressed breast milk is a good starting point in these cases. In most cases direct breastfeeding at the breast with attention to positioning to support comfort should be encouraged. The exceptions are herpes simplex lesion, and potentially herpes zoster lesions, where the infant needs to avoid contact with the lesion and the milk from that breast until the lesion has healed.[82] The infant can continue to breastfeed from the other breast and the mother should express milk from the affected breast to protect her milk supply and prevent mastitis.

Careful consideration needs to be given to the use of any topical treatments as the baby will be exposed to these even if they are mostly wiped off. Components may have harmful effects on the immature gastrointestinal system of the infant, promote allergy and may cause breast aversion due to their taste.

Pain with breastfeeding increases the risk of breastfeeding discontinuation and the use of supplementary feeds.[82] Mothers may space feeds due to fear of pain; this can lead to engorgement and mastitis and can reduce milk supply. Breastfeeding pain may contribute to postnatal depression, and this interaction may further predicate breastfeeding cessation.[557]

TABLE 14.20 Differential diagnosis of nipple pain[549]			
Diagnosis	**Considerations**	**Presentation**	**Treatment/action**
Trauma	Caused by attachment/positioning issue or breastpump misuse This needs to be ruled out as it is frequently the primary cause	Pain or pinching sensation during a feed Note: sometimes pain for the first 10 seconds of breastfeeding that then subsides can be normal, especially during the first 2 weeks	Refer to lactation specialist or breastfeeding counsellor for assessment of breastfeeding positioning
Vasospasm	Nipple trauma is frequently an underlying cause of vasospasm	Following a breastfeed the nipple blanches and the mother often describes extreme pain associated with this. Vasospasm is often triggered by exposure to cold	Refer to lactation specialist or breastfeeding counsellor for assessment of breastfeeding positioning Treatment: encourage breastfeeding in a warm environment and utilising a heat pack immediately following feeding Internal treatments often recommended by lactation consultants include up to 600 mg/day of elemental magnesium in divided doses and fish oil Herbal treatments include a combination of peripheral vasodilatory herbs such as *Zanthoxylum americanum*, *Viburnum opulus*, *Zingiber officinale* and the antioxidant *Pinus pinaster* Sometimes the pharmaceutical nifedipine is necessary
Bleb/milk blister	A duct that is blocked near the nipple	Typically very painful. A white spot or blister is evident on the nipple. Mastitis is a common sequela. Blebs often recur	Refer to lactation specialist or breastfeeding counsellor Prevention strategies as for mastitis
Infections: bacterial superficial	Secondary to skin trauma	Persistent cracks, yellow crusting, weeping, redness Keep an eye out for cellulitis.	Refer to lactation specialist or breastfeeding counsellor and breastfeeding-knowledgeable GP if infection signs persist. Treatment: small doses of direct (2–5 minutes) sunshine Consider: thyme tea or lemon myrtle tea compress after feeds (made with 2 tablespoons dried herb per cup boiling water) Topical direct expressed breast milk Direct sunshine in small doses (2 to 5 minutes) Spending some time each day with the breasts uncovered Caution: breast pads can be a source of re-infection and can create a moist environment
Infections: *Candida*	This condition is over-diagnosed May occur following maternal antibiotics. Considered plausible when mother has vaginal candidiasis or there are clear indicators of oral thrush in infant (*Clinical Naturopathic Medicine* Chapter 15)	Pink shiny nipple area (can also be due to poor attachment) Burning pain; shooting breast pain	Refer to lactation specialist or breastfeeding counsellor for assessment of breastfeeding positioning Treatment: maternal oral *Lactobacillus rhamnosus* LGG (selected because there is evidence of breast milk transfer and anti-*Candida* activity) Direct sunshine in small doses (2–5 minutes) Topical expressed breast milk Consider: thyme tea compress after feeds as described above. Spending some time each day with the breasts uncovered Caution: breast pads can be a source of re-infection and can create a moist environment

TABLE 14.20 Differential diagnosis of nipple pain[549]—cont'd			
Diagnosis	**Considerations**	**Presentation**	**Treatment/action**
Infection: viral herpes simplex (HSV)	Exposure to herpes simplex virus can have severe consequences to the infant	Extremely painful small cluster of vesicles and/or small ulcer(s)	Refer to lactation specialist or breastfeeding counsellor for assessment and for advice on maintaining supply Refer to doctor with good breastfeeding knowledge for swab and diagnostic confirmation Prevent contact between lesion and infant (i.e. until the lesion has healed avoid breastfeeding or feeding an infant the expressed breast milk from the affected breast). Continue to express (and discard) milk from the affected side until the lesion heals to protect the milk supply and avoid mastitis Pharmaceutical anti-viral medication may be warranted to reduce the time period of breastfeeding disruption Naturopathic treatment Facilitate action plan to ensure mother is able to get adequate support to assist her in recovering Botanical approach: immune support and adaptogen (*Echinacea* spp., *Withania somnifera*, *Piper longum*), galactagogue, anti-viral (topical) Ensure maternal nutrient sufficiency including the priority nutrients vitamin D and zinc. Employ first-principle naturopathic treatments for herpes virus, factoring in breastfeeding suitability Topical treatment: options are less restrictive as the infant will not be in contact with the lesion. Treatment needs to be individualised based on lesion sensitivity and stage of healing: *Lavendula officinalis* essential oil is typically well tolerated neat and will dry the lesion, and is often effective in the early stages The following essential oils have anti-herpes action.[550] They can be added to a therapeutic ointment or carrier oil and generally can be tolerated at the stated concentrations: *Syzygium aromaticum* 10–20 drops per 100 mL, *Origanum vulgare* hirtum 10 drops (only) per 100 mL or *Thymus officinalis* 10 drops only per 100 mL; *Melissa officinalis* 5% Other topical considerations based on their vulnerary or anti-viral actions include: green tea,[551–553] zinc sulphate (4% solution)[554] and *Croton lechleri* sap[555]
Infection: viral herpes zoster	Maternal herpes zoster (shingles) affecting dermatome 4 may result in lesions on the breast. Direct exposure to herpes zoster lesions theoretically could cause primary varicella (chickenpox) in the infant. Severity may be attenuated via maternal antibodies	Pain and vesicular rash following a dermatome. The rash typically starts close to the spinal column This needs to be differentiated from HSV as the consequences of HSV exposure to the infant are severe	Refer to doctor with good breastfeeding knowledge for management and for swab and diagnostic confirmation Refer to lactation specialist for specific lactation support. Decisions about breastfeeding on the affected side should be made on a case-by-case basis Topical treatments compatible with breastfeeding include *T. vulgaris* leaf and green tea leaf compress Internal treatments for the mother as above. For persistent neuralgia, consider agents that are neuroprotective, including lipoic acid[556] and curcumin in a bioavailability enhanced form,[556] and herbal treatments compatible with breastfeeding. Herbal aims include immune modulation, adaptagen support and neuroprotective. First-principle nutrition should be applied as above
Dermatitis: contact	May be triggered by traces of food present in infant's mouth or in response to topical treatments such as lanolin, antibiotics, antifungals and/or breastfeeding equipment, breast pads, laundry detergents Infection and trauma may predispose		Focus on identifying trigger Caution: topical treatments may exacerbate Trial: direct sunshine in small doses (2–5 minutes)
Psoriasis	Mother may have a history of psoriasis in other areas Flare typically occurs >6 weeks postnatally Trauma may predispose	Erythematous plaques Border clearly demarcated Scale (fine silvery)	UVB treatment is highly effective Topical vitamin D (avoid infant ingesting this) Trial purified lanolin as emollient Consider internal treatments appropriate with breastfeeding including nervous system support

Continued

	TABLE 14.20 Differential diagnosis of nipple pain[549]—cont'd		
Diagnosis	**Considerations**	**Presentation**	**Treatment/action**
Dermatitis: atopic	Consider when an atopic tendency is present		Small doses of direct sunlight Trial purified lanolin as emollient Consider internal treatments appropriate with breastfeeding including nervous system support
Mammary Paget's disease (Paget's disease of the nipple)	Carcinoma affecting interductal tissue Mimics dermatitis Occasionally occurs in younger women (more common women >60 years old)	Suspect with unilateral slowly progressing nipple eczema that persists >3 weeks, especially if associated with palpable mass	Refer for medical assessment by a physician with good breastfeeding knowledge

Tongue tie

An undiagnosed classic tongue tie which involves a membranous connection tethering the neonate's tongue, preventing movement, may impact on breastfeeding attachment, resulting in nipple trauma. For most infants, this will be identified in the days following birth, and severing this translucent membranous tissue is a quick and a relatively minor resolution. A recent shift in practice has resulted in a marked increase in infants who have been labelled with related tongue restriction diagnoses that are quite controversial. Some of these are said to lack a convincing evidence base, including posterior tongue tie and top lip tie.[558] A growing number of clinicians argue that these are actually part of the diversity of normal physiology and are perfectly compatible with breastfeeding, and attest to the successful resolution of nipple pain through improving positioning to support breastfeeding attachment.[558] Unnecessary laser surgery has significant risk to the infant including trauma and oral aversion, and to the mother–baby breastfeeding dyad. Professionally this can be a delicate and difficult situation for clinicians who need to find professionals in their area who are rigorous and not biased towards these often default diagnoses. When mothers have been recommended these treatments, supporting them to seek a second opinion may help to prevent unnecessary surgery and harm.

Breast milk stasis, blocked ducts and mastitis

Milk stasis, blocked ducts and mastitis are conditions that exist along a continuum that develop when there is inefficient removal of milk from the breast.[559] Mastitis is an inflammatory condition of the breast that may or may not be associated with infection.[559] The onset of fever indicates that there has been a breakdown in the integrity of the blood–breast barrier and that *either* milk *or* bacteria components are acting as pyrogens. Hence, fever and other systemic symptoms do not necessarily or reliably indicate the presence of infection.[560] Typically, however, non-infective mastitis left unresolved leads to infective mastitis because of disruption of the blood–breast barrier,

TABLE 14.21 Signs and symptoms of mastitis
Local signs and symptoms • tender, painful area on breast • redness • increased Na & Cl in breast milk (salty breast milk) • blood and pus may be in breast milk

Systemic signs and symptoms
• elevated temperature/fever
• flu-like symptoms:
  – body aches
  – headache
  – nausea and vomiting
  – fatigue
• *flu in a breastfeeding mother is mastitis until proven otherwise*

and if left to progress, infective mastitis can lead to breast abscess.

Mastitis is a common reason for premature cessation for breastfeeding,[82] especially when it is recurrent. Hence, it is imperative that mothers receive effective treatment and education on prevention. Mothers who overcome mastitis typically become skilled at noticing early warning signs and implementing strategies to prevent recurrence. However, the adage *flu in a breastfeeding mother is mastitis until proven otherwise* is important clinically, as mothers are busy and may not connect their symptoms of breast tenderness with systemic symptoms, especially if they have not experienced mastitis previously. (See Table 14.21 for the signs and symptoms of mastitis.) Furthermore, the flu-like symptoms and 'bone tiredness' may manifest before breast tenderness in some cases.

The WHO estimates that around a third of breastfeeding women experience at least one bout of mastitis.[561] Mastitis prevalence is high during the first 6 weeks postnatally.[559] One recent Australian study found that 20% of women experienced mastitis in the first 8 weeks postnatally,[562] with 6% of women experiencing more than one episode during this period.[562] Aside from the early weeks, mastitis often occurs as infants are getting older because breastfeeding frequency may be altered by factors such as: maternal return to work, greater lengths of maternal infant separation, sleep changes and infant distractibility at the breast.

TABLE 14.22 Types of mastitis

Main categories	Sub-categories
Milk stasis (non-infective)	Engorgement 1st week postnatally (see below) (i.e. oedema, milk stasis + inflammation) Milk stasis after 1st week (e.g. blocked milk duct)
Infective	Generalised or localised? Breast abscess
Other	Ductal carcinoma Inflammatory breast cancer Trauma

TABLE 14.23 Predisposing factors for mastitis

Factors that cause milk stasis[559]
- **Reduction in breastfeeding frequency**
  - breast refusal, rapid weaning, sleeping through, spacing feeds, separation
- **Ineffective removal of milk from the breast**
  - latch/positioning issue (assess in all cases)
- **Pressure on breast**
  - ill-fitting bra, tight clothing, heavy breast, sleeping prone, trauma from breast pump
  - recent history of mastitis episode and remaining focal point prone to obstruction
- **Oversupply of milk (caution as mastitis can cause undersupply)**
- **Elevated stress hormones**
  - impaired oxytocin release → diminishes milk ejection reflex
    > short-term can cause milk stasis[563]
    > long-term reduced milk supply

Factors impacting on immune resilience
- **Mental–emotional stress**
  - may impact on mammary immunity[563]
  - mastitis could be a flag[563,564]
- **Poor micronutrient status**
  - consider at-risk nutrients in this population that are important for immunity and breast health (vitamin D, zinc, selenium, iodine)
- **Inadequate support**
  - inadequate rest[559]
- **Maternal illness**
- **Immune system dysfunction**
  - such as SIgA deficiency[565]

Breast milk dysbiosis
- Maternal antibiotic exposure[566]
- Topical antifungal treatments?[566]

Nipple injury (may allow bacteria entry?)[559]

When clinically assessing a woman presenting with mastitis, it is important to have a sense of the broad causal categories and the possible differentials (see Table 14.22). Less common, but serious, causes such as breast abscess and carcinoma need to be considered. Typically, mastitis responds to treatment within 24 hours with full recovery within 3 days. Carcinoma needs to be ruled out when mastitis is protractive and unresponsive to treatment or is recurrent. It is also valuable to make the distinction between mastitis occurring in the first week postnatally (during the secretory activation stage of lactation, discussed below) and mastitis occurring in established lactation as there are some differences with the aetiology and management.

Predisposing factors collectively tend to be things that cause milk stasis, reduce immune resistance or promote dysbiosis of the breast (see Table 14.23). Attending to these factors is essential for preventing recurrence.

THE MAMMARY DEFENCE SYSTEM

The breasts have several defence strategies. These include:
- local immune defence in the form of bactericidal and receptor-blocking agents such as lactoferrin, lysozymes, HMOs and antibodies[100][101]
- macrophages and neutrophils that phagocytose pathogens[103]
- breast milk commensal bacteria that compete with potential pathogens. Numerous breast milk bacteria are active against *S. aureus*[394,567]
- flushing effect of frequent removal of breast milk.

MANAGEMENT OF MASTITIS

The critical central treatment strategy for mastitis is frequent and effective drainage of the breast (see Table 14.24). Failing to attend to this is likely to result in further worsening of the condition despite the use of other therapies. Other important strategies include ensuring adequate rest and support, as well as employing topical heat and gentle massage techniques to help clear blockages (see Table 14.24). Some women find alternating heat and cold applications effective. Heat prior to breastfeeding can support the MER and help the breast to clear more easily.

After ensuring all the above strategies are in place, in particular frequent effective milk removal, naturopathic treatments can be added. Herbal medicine can be a wonderful adjunct to the above. A herbal formula tailored to the individual may include agents with the following actions: immune modulation, restorative, adaptogenic, nervine, lymphatic, circulatory stimulant, anti-inflammatory, antioxidant and antibacterial (see Table 14.25 and Box 14.4). The value of topical applications such as a herbal cream should not be underestimated. A therapeutic cream can be massaged into the affected area, and a heat pack can be used to help the therapeutic agents penetrate (see Box 14.5). Care needs to be taken to avoid the nipple area and to prevent the infant from ingesting the cream or residue.

It should be noted that the primary aim of management is to overcome the acute episode. Therefore, therapies focused on this should be prioritised. Stage two is working to prevent recurrence (see below).

A NOTE ON PROBIOTICS IN ACUTE MASTITIS

It has been proposed that probiotics could be an alternative to antibiotics for the treatment of infective mastitis based on the results of a comparator study.[231] However, the antibiotics employed in this study varied and many would be deemed unsuitable for the treatment of

TABLE 14.24 Core management strategies for mastitis

Ensure frequent effective milk removal
- Suggest a goal of draining the affected breast every 2 hours during the day and ensuring the breast is drained several times overnight as well
- Breastfeed affected side first:
  - if it is painful to feed on this side, start on the non-affected side and switch to the affected side
- Express to further drain breast as required (hand express)
- Gentle self-breast massage during breastfeed
- Gentle vibration over lump
- Assess latch/positioning (refer to an IBCLC lactation consultant)
  - nipple discomfort an indication of problems with latch
  - poor latch means ineffective milk removal (this needs to be ruled out)

Note: it is safe to feed the well full-term infant from a mastitis-affected breast[559]
- *The infant is often best at draining the breast*
- ***Exception*** – *mothers who are HIV positive are more likely to transmit the virus to their infant during a mastitis episode (from the affected breast)*

Key supportive measures recommended by the Academy of Breastfeeding Medicine
- **Heat**
  - Heat packs, showers
  - Heat pack prior to feeds
  - Some women find:
    - > cold packs after feeds help with pain
    - > alternating hot and cold applications assists with recovery generally
- **Rest**
  - Bed rest (support needed with baby and home)

TABLE 14.25 Herbal medicines as adjunctive treatment for mastitis

Immune support
- *Echinacea* spp., *Piper longum*, *Andrographis paniculata* (some suggest caution)

Lymphatics – to support effective lymphatic drainage of the breast
- *Echinacea* spp., low-dose *Phytolacca decandra*, *Calendula officinalis*, *Galium aparine*

Circulatory stimulants – work in tandem with the lymphatics
- *Zingiber officinale*, *Origanum vulgare* ssp. *hirtum*, *Piper longum*, *Curcuma longa*, *Zanthoxylum clava-herculis*

Nervine-building herbs
- Rationale for including nerviness:
  - stress response can play a role in mastitis pathophysiology
  - nervines may assist with MER
  - nervines may be especially useful for preventing recurrence
- *Verbena officinalis*, *Withania somnifera*, *Lavandula angustifolia*, *Chamomilla recutita*, *Leonorus cardiaca*

Antimicrobial herbs
- *Origanum vulgare* ssp. *hirtum*, *Allium sativum* – fresh where maternal ingestion is tolerated by the infant

Contraindications
- **Generally avoid use of herbs that reduce milk supply**
  - *Salvia officinalis*
- **Caution with use of strong galactagogues**
  - *Trigonella foenum-graecum*
  - *Foeniculum vulgare*
  - *Pimpinella anisum*
  - *Galega officinalis*

BOX 14.4 Example herbal formulas

Herbal formula for mastitis example 1

When stress and exhaustion appear to be part of the history.

Echinacea	40 mL
Oregano	15 mL
Lavender	10 mL
Ginger	5 mL
Shatavari	25 mL

Dose: 5–7.5 mL four t.d.s. until symptoms are at least 75% better (typically within 24–48 hours), then taper down. *When convenient take after breastfeeding*

Herbal formula for mastitis example 2

History suggests prolonged milk stasis due to recent history of infrequent breastfeeding.

Echinacea	35 mL
Calendula	15 mL
Turmeric	35 mL
Ginger	7.5 mL
Long pepper	7.5 mL

Similar dosage recommendations to above

BOX 14.5 Example herbal cream ingredients

Herbal cream for mastitis example

Ginger (1 : 2) tincture 10%
Poke root (1 : 10) tincture 10%
Lavender essential oil 3%
    In an olive oil and beeswax base

Recommendations

Apply with massage to affected area four times daily after a breastfeeding
For prevention of recurrence, massage once daily

Caution

Prevent infant ingestion by:
- avoiding areola
- allowing time to soak in before little hands get to it
- applying heat to increase penetration

mastitis. So it has been argued that the study did not adequately test the hypothesis.[568] Interestingly, the efficacy of antibiotics for the treatment of mastitis has not been established, according to a 2013 Cochrane review.[569] Arroyo found that 3 weeks of treatment with probiotics appeared to be superior to antibiotic treatment.[569] While acceptable in chronic breast pain, this treatment timeframe is completely unacceptable in acute mastitis. Probiotics should be viewed as a useful adjunct, but their efficacy in acute mastitis is yet to be established as they may not be

BOX 14.6 Proposed practice guidelines for referral of women with mastitis

Refer to a doctor with good breastfeeding knowledge to discuss antibiotics when:

Severe:

- especially if present for more than 12–24 hours
- redness spreading, persistent high fever

Poor response to treatment:

- no improvement within 24–48 hours of comprehensive treatment
- getting worse within 12–24 hours despite comprehensive treatment

Note: when antibiotics are prescribed, it is critical that an appropriate antibiotic is selected as the common mastitis pathogens are penicillin resistant.

Follow-up within 12–24 hours is essential during the acute stage of mastitis.

sufficiently rapid in their action. They are, however, highly valuable in the prevention of mastitis recurrence (see below), and depending on the mother's budget, they can be commenced during the acute phase of mastitis.

FOLLOW-UP AND LIMITS OF THERAPY

Appropriate follow-up is a duty of care in this scenario. The clinician needs to make contact at least every 12–24 hours during the acute phase of the condition to assess response to treatment and the need for referral for antibiotics. While in most cases antibiotics can be avoided, it is important to have a clear clinical framework to avoid putting women at risk of damage to the breast, breast abscess or, in the worst-case scenario, septicaemia.

The ABM recommends antibiotic treatment if the woman is not improving within 24 hours or if she is acutely unwell.[559] Given the potential negative sequelae associated with antibiotic treatment, it could be argued that there is scope for allowing a little more time prior to considering antibiotics. Particularly so if the core aspects of treatment are combined with a herbal medicine approach. A proposed practice guideline for naturopaths is set out in Box 14.6.

INFECTIVE VERSUS NON-INFECTIVE MASTITIS

Distinguishing between infective and non-infective mastitis is difficult. The relevance of fever in mastitis is commonly misunderstood. As discussed previously, fever in mastitis means that pyrogens have entered the blood stream, and in the case of mastitis, this may be milk proteins or bacteria products. Culturing of breast milk is not valid for diagnosing infective mastitis because of skin flora contamination and the normal bacteria present in breast milk. Kvist et al. found that women with mastitis symptoms were more likely to have positive cultures for common mastitis pathogens *Staphylococcus aureus* (45% vs 31% $P = 0.001$) and group-B streptococci (GBS) (21% vs 10% $P < 0.001$) than healthy women.[570] It is notable that a large

proportion of women without mastitis symptoms had positive cultures for these potential pathogens. Additionally, the authors found there was no correlation with *S. aureus* counts and severity of mastitis symptoms, or risk of abscess, and many women with high counts of *S. aureus* recovered with good lactation advice and supportive treatments alone. Kvist et al. recommended daily assessment of symptoms to decide on the need for antibiotics.[570]

COMPLICATIONS OF MASTITIS

Poorly managed mastitis can result in numerous complications (outlined below). Hence, prompt effective management is of primary importance.

Premature cessation of breastfeeding

Mastitis can be an extremely painful and debilitating experience for mothers, which may drive them to considering abrupt discontinuation of breastfeeding. Effective frequent breastfeeding is the most important treatment for mastitis. Abrupt weaning may cause a progression of the condition and may increase the risk of abscess formation. Support from both health professionals and family to enable mothers to continue breastfeeding is a necessity.[559] A mother's experience of mastitis may impact on her future breastfeeding decisions.

Breast abscess

Breast abscess typically occurs when milk stasis is not adequately addressed. It occurs in approximately 3% of women with mastitis. An abscess should be suspected when there is a well-defined area of the breast that remains hard, tender and red. Diagnostic ultrasound reveals a collection of fluid. Note that breast abscess can present atypically. Sometimes there will be no apparent preceding signs and symptoms of milk stasis. Occasionally, it may present bilaterally. The typical treatment is antibiotic therapy and ultrasound-guided fine-needle aspiration.[571] A catheter drain and surgery may be indicated for very large abscesses. Breastfeeding is encouraged. When there is a drain, the baby's mouth needs to be kept clear of it. A culture and antibiotic sensitivity of the exudate should be obtained to guide antibiotic selection.[559]

Breast tissue damage and lowered milk supply

Damage to the breast tissue can result in loss of functional glandular tissue and reduced capacity to synthesise breast milk. Additionally, disruption of the integrity of the breast tissue predisposes the mother to recurrent infections.

Septicaemia

The extreme worst-case scenario of untreated mastitis is the progression to infective mastitis and further progression to septicaemia.

PREVENTING MASTITIS RECURRENCE

After an episode of mastitis, many women appear to be susceptible to recurrence. This is particularly apparent for

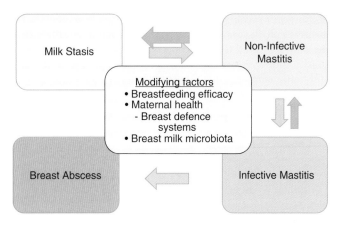

FIGURE 14.7 Progression of mammary inflammation and modifying factors

women who progress to develop infective mastitis. It is notable that some women can be exposed to milk stasis, and this easily resolves without sequelae, while other women will find even a relatively mild episode of milk stasis very quickly progresses to severe mastitis, and potentially infective mastitis. It would appear that multiple factors contribute to resilience in the mammary system (see Fig. 14.7). Hence, prevention of recurrence is about both helping mothers to avoid/minimise episodes of milk stasis as well as boost the general mammary resistance.

The following strategies promote mammary resilience and prevent recurrence.

Maintain a high level of vigilance to ensure the breast is well drained

- Refer to a lactation consultant:
  - to identify and resolve issues with positioning and attachment that may be impacting on breast milk transfer and predisposing the woman to mastitis
  - for guidance regarding expressing technique, including: ensuring the mother knows how to hand express; utilising expressing when the breast is engorged to assist with infant attachment; utilising expressing when the infant does not relieve breast fullness; assessment of the fit of any equipment to prevent pump-induced breast trauma.
- Ensure breastfeeds are not restricted so that the breast is well drained at each feed.

Prompt recognition of milk stasis

- Encourage mothers to check for redness, lumps and/or tender areas and immediately begin actions to help resolve stasis (see Table 14.24).
- Consider having a herbal formula on hand and commence taking this if there are any signs of milk stasis.
- If symptoms have not resolved within 24 hours, suggest she contacts her healthcare provider.

Maintain herbal treatments for precautionary period

When there is a history of mastitis recurrence it is prudent to continue a maintenance herbal treatment. If this is in a tincture form, consider keeping the dose to 5 mL twice a day to lower the alcohol exposure level.

Promote a healthy breast milk microbiota

Probiotic supplementation is particularly indicated when there is a history of infective mastitis and when maternal antibiotic exposure has occurred. A healthy breast milk microbiota may reduce susceptibility to infective mastitis.[394] To ensure mothers are receiving evidence-based care, it is important to utilise strains with proven therapeutic efficacy:

- *L. fermentum* CECT5716 *and L. salivarius* CECT5713 have both been shown to reduce mastitis recurrence compared to placebo.[231] *L. fermentum* CECT5716 also appears to reduce breast milk *Staphylococcus* load and reduce breast pain.[572]
- *L. salivarius* PS2 also has clinical evidence for efficacy in preventing mastitis recurrence.[573]
- Promoting a favourable maternal intestinal microbiome may positively influence the breast milk microbiota. See Chapter 6: The Microbiome for further information.

Ensure optimal maternal nutrient status

Naturopathic first principles suggest addressing any nutritional inadequacies. Several nutrients may be particularly important for protection against recurrent infective mastitis:

- Vitamin D. Evidence from bovine models suggests higher susceptibility to infective mastitis with vitamin D deficiency.[574] Vitamin D may support local mammary immune defence against mammary pathogens.[575]
- Iodine. Iodine insufficiency is common in breastfeeding mothers who live in soil-deficient regions.[576] Iodine is actively transferred into breast milk,[307] and preliminary data suggest that iodine may have some efficacy in non-lactational fibrocystic breast disease[577] and mastalgia.[578] These phenomena suggest that normative maternal iodine status may be important for breast health, and hence it is theoretically plausible that normal iodine status modulates mastitis susceptibility. Note: excess iodine intake may cause harm to mother and child (see Table 14.8).
- Selenium. Evidence from animal models[579,580] suggests higher susceptibility to clinical mastitis with selenium deficiency and increased inflammatory lesions after *S. aureus* exposure.[581] Selenium may support local mammary antioxidant defence systems and reduce injury to breast tissue in the event of infective mastitis.
- Other nutrients. Optimal zinc, essential fatty acid and antioxidant status may also help prevent recurrent infective mastitis given the impact of these factors on immunity and inflammation.

Explore ways for mothers to rest more and draw on support networks

Fatigue is a well-known factor contributing to mastitis susceptibility.[559] Hence, working with mothers to explore ways they can get more rest is valuable. New mothers typically need to have a nap or a lie down during the day to compensate for the night-time parenting. Drawing on more family support with household tasks can help prevent the mother's desire to see these jobs done from competing for her need for rest.

Promote emotional and mental wellbeing

Psychological stress is associated with increased risk of inflammatory breast disease during lactation.[564] High levels of stress may lead to milk stasis through dulling of the oxytocin response.[564] Further stress may impact on mammary immune defence.[563,564] Hence, promoting maternal wellbeing through access to meaningful social contact, physical exercise and the use of herbal mood support may all help to prevent mastitis recurrence. Additionally, the need for further psychological support or therapy needs to be considered. Recurrent mastitis may be a flag for underlying postnatal dysphoria.[564]

Lecithin

Anecdotal evidence suggests that lecithin may assist with reducing blocked ducts[582] and hence assist in preventing milk stasis. Increased maternal intake of choline results in an increase in breast milk choline up to a threshold (see Table 14.8). Improving breast milk choline, and in particular, phosphatidylcholine, may impact on the way fat globules adhere to the mammary membrane and prevent mastitis.[582] Or alternatively, choline may have anti-inflammatory actions that assist in preventing blocked ducts.[582] A dose of 5 g of lecithin once per day is typically prescribed by lactation consultants. This would provide 450 mg of choline daily, which is well below the upper tolerable limit of choline in lactation set by the NHMRC and the New Zealand Ministry of Health (7500 mg per day).[582]

ENGORGEMENT MASTITIS OCCURRING DURING THE FIRST WEEK POSTNATALLY

During the secretory activation stage of lactation, there is a sudden increase in milk synthesis. This can be associated with some swelling, inflammation and lymphatic and vascular congestion, which causes interstitial oedema. Some degree of this is normal, and typically begins and then peaks at 2 and 5 days postnatally, respectively.[583] This is the scenario most suited to the traditional use of cold cabbage leaves. The cold cabbage leaves may assist in reducing the inflammation in the interstitial tissue.

Excessive engorgement may occur when other factors contribute to either milk stasis or oedema of the breast. Ineffective milk removal (due to poor latch, separation, restricted feeds or supplementation)[583] causes milk stasis, creating backflow pressure in the breasts. Intrapartum IV fluid[584] and the antidiuretic actions of Syntocinon[585] may both contribute to breast oedema. When there is a build-up of fluid in the interstitial tissue, this can cause compression to the milk ducts, further exacerbating milk stasis. A cycle of inflammation, interstitial oedema and milk stasis ensues that ultimately can lead to damage to breast tissue. This can cause milk supply issues due to damaged ductal areas. Infective mastitis may occur as a result of prolonged milk stasis and inflammatory disruption of the blood–milk barrier in the breast, facilitating bacteria entry to the parenchymal tissue.

A woman's breasts will feel hard and sore but she may have trouble expressing milk because of the pressure on the ductal system. In addition, breast pain and anxiety may dull the milk ejection reflex. The oedema in the breast and around the areola in particular make it difficult for the infant to latch deeply, which both impairs milk transfer and causes nipple damage.

Prevention and treatment strategies for early postnatal engorgement include:

- Frequent feeding with good attachment, including responding to early hunger cues and gently rousing sleepy newborns to feed to avoid extended gaps between breastfeeds. Ideally the newborn avoids gaps of longer than 2–3 hours; newborns are nocturnal and may naturally have one longer sleep period during the day.
- When the baby is not effectively transferring milk, hand or careful pump expressing is necessary.
- Reverse pressure softening helps to shift the fluid away from the areola so the infant can latch effectively.[583,585]
- Gentle lymphatic drainage massage gently shifts fluid towards the axilla.
- Cold compresses or cold cabbage leaves applied after feeding can help reduce the interstitial inflammation.[583]
- Some women find warm compresses prior to feeding helpful to promote the MER, potentially by aiding oxytocin uptake.[583]

Dysmorphic milk ejection reflex (DMER)

For most mothers, the MER is accompanied by feelings of connection and calmness. A very small number of women experience the opposite. DMER describes an abrupt emotional 'drop' that appears at the time of the MER and lasts for no more than a few minutes.[586] This can be experienced as 'whimsical' to deep self-loathing or despair. It has been postulated that this phenomenon is mediated through a drop in dopamine. One case report associated *Rhodiola rosea* with some relief from DMER.[586]

Breast refusal (nursing strike)

Breast refusal describes the scenario where the infant refuses to nurse. This may be for some feeds or it may be complete refusal to breastfeed for a short or prolonged

TABLE 14.26 Causes of breast refusal	

Oral discomfort
• Teething
• Oral infections (herpes[589]; scarlet fever; hand, foot and mouth; oral thrush)
• Oral aversion after oral surgery, suctioning, oral examination
• Allergy
Positional instability
• The infant feels physically uncomfortable and/or unstable in the breastfeeding position that is adopted
Other discomfort
• Peristalsis and defecation urge may be stimulated when breastfeeding and cause digestive discomfort
• Due to injury – if positioning causes pressure to the injured part
• Torticollis (stiff neck) may cause one-sided breast refusal
• Nasal congestion – infants are obligate nose breathers while feeding
Distractibility
• Frequently developmental and confused with self-weaning
Nipple confusion
• Infant has become accustomed to a bottle teat that requires a different sucking action and may have a faster flow
Frustration
• Due to slower let-down response:
  – Maternal anxiety
  – Maternal alcohol ingestion
  – Natural evolution of lactation
• Infant's sympathetic nervous system is dialled up and they can't relax to feed
• Reduced breast milk supply due to reduction in number of feeds
	Taste change
	• Maternal mastitis may cause the milk to taste salty due to increased sodium ions in milk[590]
	• During menstruation, breast milk flavour may change and/or supply may dip a little
	• Maternal dietary change
	• Deodorant change or use of perfume
	• Maternal medications
	Forceful MER
	• The infant may find the flow rate difficult to keep up with
	  – Allowing the milk to spray into a towel until the flow rate has settled to a pace that the infant can manage can assist
	Biting
	• A mother's reaction to a bite may be frightening for the infant and the infant may associate this reaction with breastfeeding rather than biting[591]
	  – Infants appear to have an urge to clench their gums together when teething

period, including days or weeks. The underlying cause should always be sought (see Table 14.26). Unfortunately, many parents and caregivers confuse breast refusal with self-weaning. Given the WHO recommendations and the American Academy of Pediatrics[587] and the NHMRC guidelines and the growing body of evidence indicating the continued functions of breastfeeding into the second year of life and beyond (immune protection, nutrition, developmental programming, mental health and shaping of the microbiota as discussed above), infants' refusal or disinterest in the breast prior to 12 months, and arguably prior to 18–24 months, should be described and treated as breast refusal rather than self-weaning. A 2008 US study found that 27% of women reported their reason for not meeting their breastfeeding goal of at least 8 months was because their infant self-weaned.[588] Another study found that 47% of mothers indicated self-weaning as the reason for ceasing breastfeeding at or prior to 9 months of age.[83] These findings potentially reflect poor understanding and management of this phenomenon. Prompt referral of the mother to a breastfeeding counsellor or lactation consultant is important to identify the possible cause and to find strategies to gently encourage the infant to return to the breast. During this period, it is important for mothers to protect their breast milk supply through expressing. Obtaining a hospital grade pump may be worthwhile, depending on how prolonged the breast refusal episode is.

Weaning

Based on archaeological evidence and interspecies comparisons utilising dentition and anthropometric indices, it has been suggested that the natural weaning age is between 2.5 and 7 years of age.[136] Several more recent archaeological findings have indicated weaning was completed after 4 years.[592–594]

The age of weaning is a decision for each mother and child to navigate based on emotional, social and physical needs. Breastfeeding continues to have functional benefits regardless of the child's age. Having insight into the potential age range of natural weaning may be reassuring for mothers who feel pressured to wean before they are ready. Many mothers conceal breastfeeding beyond 12 months.[595] Unfortunately, this can lead to social isolation.[596] Brockway describes a social coercion to wean by 12 months, whereby societal norms result in a withdrawal of support or even the expressing of negative views about breastfeeding beyond 12 months.[595,597] Unfortunately women also perceive negative attitudes among health professionals.[596,597]

In the ideal scenario, weaning happens gradually over a period of months, allowing the child to adapt and the breasts to gradually involute. A gradual transition is also important for avoiding mastitis or breast tissue disruption.[396] Weaning may be child led, or mother led, depending on what the mother chooses. Occasionally, women need to wean abruptly for medical reasons.

Child-led weaning means that the mother supports the child to determine the course of weaning. (Note: when there is a loss of interest in breastfeeding in a child under 18 months, this is more accurately described as breast refusal – see above). The child becomes increasingly engaged in the world, which typically results in a gradual reduction in breastfeeding interest, until he or she stops all together. Parents choosing this path may sometimes be pressured by family to wean. They will benefit from positive attitudes from healthcare providers.

Strategies for gentle mother-led weaning include the 'don't offer, don't refuse' approach. Parents may be able to distract the child with other activities, keep them full and hydrated, and their interest in breastfeeding may gradually reduce. Typically, infants can feel anxious and want to feed more frequently when they are refused the breast. Hence, the advantage of the 'don't offer, don't refuse' approach, which provides a strategy for the mother to reduce child anxiety and distress.

Parents may be keen to night wean their infants. Prior to the age of 9 months, this can be detrimental to maternal milk supply. Typically, after the age of 12 months infants are more able to understand concepts such as the 'breasts going to sleep' and are increasing their intake of solid foods.

Abrupt weaning for medical reasons presents a challenge to both the mother and the child. This can be a source of profound grief for mothers. Seeking a second opinion from a physician with good breastfeeding knowledge is warranted. When abrupt cessation is necessary, women should be referred to a lactation consultant or breastfeeding counsellor for assistance with the weaning process. Strategies to minimise the risk of mastitis should be implemented. The use of herbal anti-galactagogues such as *Salvia officinalis*, along with anxiolytics, may be of benefit.

WEANING AND MATERNAL EMOTIONAL RESPONSES

Women may experience a range of emotions following weaning. Some women may experience both positive feelings and feelings of sadness. Weaning is associated with hormonal shifts in mothers and these, along with some of the psychological responses to breastfeeding cessation, may affect maternal mental health. Women with pre-existing anxiety or depression may be at risk of exacerbation following breastfeeding cessation, according to cohort study findings.[146,598] Furthermore, several published case studies suggest that abrupt weaning may be a trigger for major depression[599] or mania[600] in susceptible women. This has been theorised to be linked to the fall in prolactin[599] and the abrupt rise in dopamine levels.[600]

Breastfeeding and family planning

CHILD SPACING RECOMMENDATIONS

One of the positive health effects attributed to breastfeeding is its association with a prolonged birth to pregnancy interval. The WHO recommends a birth to pregnancy interval of 2 years.[601] Data, mostly from low- and middle-income countries, associates an interval of less than 18 months with increased risk of miscarriage, fetal growth restriction, preterm birth and fetal death.[601,602] One older study found that mothers in Scotland with a shorter birth interval had higher risk of uterine haemorrhage, anaemia, hypertension and maternal mortality.[603] The findings of a more recent Australian study questioned the evidence for a causal link between short birth intervals and preterm birth.[601]

LACTATIONAL AMENORRHOEA METHOD

The average postnatal amenorrhoea period is longer in women who exclusively breastfeed and who feed during the night. According to a 2015 systematic review, 50–80% of exclusively breastfeeding women had amenorrhoea at 6 months,[604] while another systematic review of studies on non-lactating mothers found that the mean first ovulation day occurred between 1.5 months and 3 months postnatally,[605] and there was a small number of women who ovulated before 6 weeks postnatally.[605] The lactational amenorrhoea method (LAM) of contraception is said to be 98% effective.[606] This method requires *all* of the following circumstances[606]:

- The infant is younger than 6 months.
- The infant is exclusively breastfed.
- The infant has unrestricted access to breastfeeding.
- The infant breastfeeds at night.
- The mother has amenorrhoea.

A 2015 Cochrane systematic review found that the LAM method ranged in efficacy from 92.5% to 99%.[604] The authors noted that exclusive breastfeeding (with amenorrhoea) was as effective as following the full LAM criteria.[604] They suggested that defining amenorrhoea as no menstrual bleeding after 10 days postnatally would improve contraceptive efficacy.[604]

BREASTFEEDING THROUGH A PREGNANCY AND TANDEM FEEDING

Many mothers breastfeed through pregnancy. The intensity of breastfeeding varies between mother–infant dyads. In some cases, the breastfeeding will contribute a fairly minimal nutritional load to the child, and in other cases, breastfeeding continues to make a reasonable nutritional contribution. In both cases, but in particular the latter, some additional attention to maternal nutritional support is appropriate. Given that many pregnancies are unplanned, strategies to maintain maternal status of priority pregnancy nutrients should be a matter of course.

Two studies found there was no increase in the risk of preterm or spontaneous birth associated with breastfeeding throughout pregnancy.[607,608] This is a commonly expressed concern of both mothers and health professionals.[607]

Mothers may choose to continue breastfeeding through pregnancy and continue on to tandem breastfeed because they feel that their child is not ready to wean, and/or they feel that breastfeeding will assist the child through the transition of adjusting to siblinghood and facilitate bonding between siblings. On the other hand, some parents may decide to gently wean their breastfeeding child midway through the pregnancy because they prefer not to tandem feed. Some children self-wean during pregnancy because of taste and supply changes. Nipple tenderness during pregnancy is experienced by some mothers.

Mothers planning to tandem feed will benefit from a session with a lactation consultant or breastfeeding counsellor. An obvious consideration is the newborn's priority access to breast milk. An individualised approach is necessary, taking into consideration the unique and changing features of the breastfeeding dyad including maternal milk supply and storage capacity, as well as differences in feeding patterns and developmental capacity of the older child. Some mothers find allocating a breast to each child works well, while other mothers feed their newborn first, and mothers who have an abundant milk supply find they can feed their older child freely. These mothers often find the older child's ability to drain the breasts provides helpful prevention and treatment for milk stasis and mastitis.

MEDICATIONS/DRUGS AND BREASTFEEDING

Contrary to popular belief, for most medications, the amount of drug transfer to breast milk is relatively small, unlike placental transfer.[609] Also, for most medications, breast milk transfer is considered clinically insignificant, especially when balanced against the risks associated with premature breastfeeding cessation.[610] Current evidence indicates that only a small number of medications are contraindicated in breastfeeding.[609,610]

Unfortunately, many women discontinue breastfeeding because of the perceived risk of pharmaceutical medications to their infant, or because they have been advised to do so by a health professional.[611] The risks of breastfeeding cessation and interruption (see Table 14.5) in these scenarios are often underappreciated. Some mothers feed their infants formula and 'pump and dump' their breast milk for the duration of drug treatment, as advised by some health professionals, which presents a major obstacle to breastfeeding continuation. A 2015 systematic review showed that at least 34% of women take a pharmaceutical medication while they are breastfeeding,[611] indicating this dilemma is a common one for mothers and health professionals.

Several questions need to be considered in the clinical context of breastfeeding and the use of medication, and some of these also apply to the clinical reasoning around the use of herbal and other natural medicines. These include:

1   What is the nature of the maternal health issue?
    –   How important is the treatment to the mother's short- and long-term health?
    –   What are the risks associated with no treatment?
    –   Is the treatment offered evidence-based and with a good probability of efficacy?

TABLE 14.27 Databases with high-quality information on pharmaceutical drugs and breastfeeding	
LactMed	Peer-reviewed database with information on numerous medications and breastfeeding: http://toxnet.nlm.nih.gov
Medications and Mothers' Milk Online	Regularly updated database compiled by clinical pharmacologist Dr Thomas Hale and colleague Dr Hilary Rowe: http://www.medsmilk.com/

2   How likely is the drug to have an effect on the infant?
    –   Underpinning this are the factors of breast milk transfer (see Table 14.27), drug bioavailability, infant-related factors (see below) and drug pharmacological effects.
3   How does the risk of drug exposure compare to the health risks associated with premature cessation of breastfeeding?
4   Is there an alternative acceptable treatment (including a different drug) that is more compatible with breastfeeding?

Familiarity with reliable resources that provide accurate information to mothers on medications and breastfeeding can assist them to make an informed decision (see Table 14.27). Many drug monographs are not up-to-date. There is a tendency for them to blanketly advise against breastfeeding women using the medication for medico-legal reasons, and potentially because of a lack of appreciation of the risks associated with premature cessation of breastfeeding.

Most drugs transfer between the plasma and breast milk as a result of passive diffusion from an area of high concentration to one of low concentration. Active transport of drugs into breast milk is rare. Iodine (including radioactive iodine) is a rare exception. Some medications have specific data on them with regards to breast milk transfer. However, pharmacokinetic principles can aid in the prediction of drug transfer based on the chemical characteristics of the drug (see Table 14.28). In most clinical circumstances, there will be several drugs to choose from, and some will be better suited to breastfeeding based on their minimal transfer to breast milk, low oral bioavailability and tolerability data.

Infant factors

Rowe et al. described three infant risk categories (low, moderate or high risk):

1   The lowest risk category includes healthy infants aged 6–18 months. At this age, infants have a greater capacity to metabolise most xenobiotics more safely. Furthermore, the volume of breast milk they receive per kg of bodyweight is less than that of a younger baby,[609] and hence the per kg drug exposure will be less.
2   Infants at moderate risk are healthy term infants between the age of 2 weeks and 20 weeks.

3   The high-risk category includes infants aged less than 2 weeks, premature infants and infants with health conditions that make them more vulnerable to the medication effects or cause them to have less capacity to clear medications (e.g. renal dysfunction).[609] Consistent with these guidelines, a 2016 review of reported adverse reactions to maternal medications found that the majority of severe reactions occurred in infants less than 1 month old.[612]

TABLE 14.28 Factors influencing transfer of medications and drugs into breast milk[609,610]

Characteristic	Explanation
Molecular weight	The higher the molecular weight, the less transfer to breast milk
Maternal plasma level	The higher the plasma level, the higher the transfer to breast milk
CNS active agents	Substances that pass into the brain compartment are also more readily transferred in human milk
Protein binding	A high level of protein binding means less transfer to breast milk
PK_a	Some drugs with a PK_a >7.2 become ionised and trapped in the breast milk
Drug half-life	Higher maternal plasma levels may be maintained for a longer duration
Lipophilic	Lipophilic drugs are transferred more readily into breast milk than lipophobic drugs
Poor oral bioavailability	Usually poorly transferred into breast milk. Further bioavailability to the infant is likely to be low

PK_a is the pH at which a drug is equally ionic and non-ionic.

RELATIVE INFANT DOSE (RID)[612,613]

Calculating relative infant dose (RID), compared to the maternal dose, can be a useful tool to aid risk assessment. An RID of greater than 10% is generally considered an indication of concern.[609] The RID is calculated by dividing the dose transferred to the infant via breast milk (mg/kg daily) by the mother's weight-adjusted dose (mg/kg daily). To do this calculation, it is necessary to know the concentration of drug in the breast milk and the volume of milk taken by the infant. Information on drug concentration is not always available, but data on a growing number of drugs is accumulating. Similarly the daily breast milk volume intake of an infant is often unknown; an estimate of 150 mL/kg/day is often used for exclusively breastfed infants.

Maternal antibiotics and breastfeeding

The capacity for antibiotics to transfer to breast milk varies considerably. Table 14.29 looks at a number of commonly prescribed antibiotics and breast milk transfer.

Obviously, it is preferable to avoid any potential antibiotic exposure. Hence, antibiotics should always be prescribed judiciously to lactating mothers. In most cases, when an antibiotic is necessary, a drug with minimal breast milk transfer can be selected. Accordingly, the transfer of such antibiotics into the breast milk is very small, often representing less than 1% of the relevant infant dose. Theoretically, even this low level of exposure could have the potential to impact on the microbiome of the infant. However, the numerous prebiotic components within breast milk are likely to buffer these effects. Maternal anxiety about the potential for the antibiotic to cause harm to the infant may result in premature breastfeeding cessation, or temporary exposure to formula,

TABLE 14.29 Breast milk transfer and estimated RID of some commonly prescribed antibiotics[614]

Antibiotic	Indication	Data on transfer to breast milk	Estimated relative infant dose (RID)*
Amoxicillin	Respiratory tract infections Many other infections	After a maternal dose of 1 g, peak breast milk levels occurred at 4 and 5 hours (range 0.39–1.3 mg/L was detected in breast milk)	Standard maternal dose of 500 mg t.d.s. would result in infant exposure of approximately 0.1 mg/kg/day, reflecting an estimated RID of 0.25–0.5%
Cephalexin	Urinary tract infection Infective mastitis	Maternal dose of 500 mg q.i.d. estimated to deliver 112 micrograms/kg daily to the infant	RID of 0.001–0.005%
Dicloxacillin	Mastitis	After a single oral dose of 250 mg of dicloxacillin, milk levels ranged from 0.2 to 0.3 mg/L between 2 and 4 hours after the dose. The drug was undetectable in milk at 1 and 6 hours after the dose	RID of 0.2%
Erythromycin	Skin infections Respiratory tract infections Chlamydia	With a maternal dose of 500 mg, breast milk level at 2, 4 and 6 hours was 1, 1.2 and 1.1 mg/L, respectively	RID in the order of 0.6% Note: maternal erythromycin use in the first 2 weeks postnatally is associated with an increased risk of pyloric stenosis in the infant.[615]

*RID calculation based on typical maternal prescribed dose for a 60 kg mother.

both of which have a far greater risk of causing harm to both the infant and the mother (see Table 14.5).

Alcohol and breastfeeding

The implications of alcohol in breastfeeding are quite different from alcohol in pregnancy.[618] Alcohol enters (and exits) breast milk via passive diffusion, entering the breast milk 30–60 minutes following ingestion. The amount of alcohol the infant is exposed to is roughly 5–6% of the maternal weight-adjusted dose.[618] Combined findings from multiple studies indicate that it takes approximately 2–2.5 hours for the alcohol from one standard drink[10] to be completely cleared from breast milk, and an additional 2–2.5 hours for each subsequent drink to be cleared.[618] Haastrup et al. estimated the possible exposure an infant could obtain from a mother who drank four standard drinks (assuming the infant drank a reasonable volume from the breast when the alcohol was at its peak plasma level) as 0.005%; that is, one-tenth the blood alcohol level acceptable to drive in most European countries.[618] Therefore, based on biological plausibility, occasional moderate alcohol intake of one to two standard drinks is proposed to have minimal physiological effect on the infant,[618] and arguably far less risk than formula supplementation.

Due to ethical constraints, investigation into the effect of maternal chronic alcohol use on infants is limited. Surprisingly, two small studies found that infants had less active sleep in the 3.5-hour period after being exposed to the very low levels of alcohol expected from maternal consumption of 1.5 standard drinks.[619,620] The effect of daily maternal drinking ≥2 standard drinks is largely unknown and findings are mixed,[618][621] but some evidence suggests the possibility of delayed psychomotor development.[622][623] Newborns metabolise alcohol at approximately half the rate of adults,[618] suggesting some possibility of accumulation.

Alcohol does have the potential to have negative effects on lactation physiology. Acute alcohol exposure equivalent to 1.8 to 2.5 standard drinks substantially blunts the oxytocin release and the MER, and reduces the volume of milk available to an infant at a feed, possibly by 10% or more.[618] Hence, regular moderate alcohol consumption could impact on breast emptying and have a small effect on milk supply.

The obvious concern with maternal alcohol ingestion is the impact this may have on bed sharing safety (see below) and risk of abuse or neglect.

Recreational drugs and breastfeeding

For an excellent overview of the issues relating to drug use and breastfeeding, refer to the ABM Clinical Protocol #21 on this topic.[621]

Herbal medicines and breastfeeding

Prescribing herbal medicine to breastfeeding mothers requires both consideration of the dosage form and the breastfeeding compatibility of the herbal ingredients.

DOSAGE FORMS (TINCTURES, HERBAL TEAS AND SOLID DOSAGE FORMS)

A number of factors may affect the dosage form selected by herbalists including safety, affordability, quality issues, ability to individualise the prescription and convenience for the patient. Herbal tinctures allow for individualised prescriptions and are relatively convenient for the patient. However, the consequences of exposing mothers and babies to alcohol need to be considered. The alcohol delivered in a 5 mL dose of tincture will vary according to the prescription. A 5 mL dose of a 50% alcohol tincture will contain approximately 2 g of alcohol (assuming a specific gravity of 0.8) and deliver approximately 20% of a standard drink. By comparison, a 10 mL dose of a 65% alcohol tincture would deliver approximately 56% of a standard drink. Some mothers may be consuming alcoholic beverages, and tinctures represent an additional source of alcohol, and some mothers may take more than the recommended dose of prescribed tinctures.

Alcohol exposure to the infant can be reduced by using a lower dose, and a low dosing frequency, and by suggesting mothers take their tincture just after feeding. However, any instructions on the timing of the dose in relation to breastfeeding need to be given cautiously as delaying breastfeeding could have a negative effect on breast milk supply and the infant's wellbeing. Additionally, a therapeutic dose of the herbs needs to be obtained.

Herbal teas and decoctions have economic advantages, allow for individualisation and are alcohol free, but may not appeal to some patients due to their taste and preparation requirements. Some of these factors can be overcome through suggesting practical solutions such as making a large batch of tea to be drunk over the course of 1 or 2 days and careful formulation for palatability.

While they are convenient and alcohol free, solid dosage forms do not allow for individualised prescriptions, and it may be difficult to evaluate the quality of the extracts they contain.

SAFETY CONSIDERATIONS FOR HERBS AND BREASTFEEDING

The considerations for prescribing herbal medicines during breastfeeding are distinctly different from prescribing during pregnancy. Unfortunately, reference material usually provides collective recommendations for pregnancy and breastfeeding. Additionally, the age of the infant and stage of lactation should be borne in mind with any prescribing decision (see 'Infant factors' in the 'Medications/drugs and breastfeeding' section above). Some of the principles associated with pharmaceutical medications can be applied to the prescription of herbal medicines in breastfeeding. These include:

- assessing the need for treatment and the consequences of no treatment
- the age and health status of the infant and lactation stage
- the potential for herbal agents to transfer through the milk. For example, herbal constituents that act on the central nervous system (CNS) may be more likely to

TABLE 14.30 Safety considerations relevant to prescribing herbal medicines during lactation[616]

Safety consideration	Examples
Anti-galactagogue potential	*Salvia officinalis*, *Ephedra* spp., *Mucuna pruriens* (velvet bean), *Vicia faba* (broad bean, fava bean), *Vitex agnus-castus*, *Mentha* x *piperita* (essential oil), *Lycopus* spp.[453,485] See Table 14.18 for more details
Toxic	*Phytolacca* spp. (a dose below 0.2 mL/day of 1:10 dried plant tincture may be acceptable) Herbs containing aristolochic acid and pyrrolizidine alkaloids *Mentha pulegium* (pennyroyal) *Caulophyllum thalictroides* *Artemisia absinthium* *Tanacetum vulgare* Warning: maternal consumption of broad or faba beans (*V. faba*) can trigger haemolytic anaemia and hyperbilirubinaemia in babies with glucose 6-phosphate dehydrogenase (G6PD) deficiency[425,486]
Strong herbal sedative or CNS-acting herbs	*Piper methysticum* *Humulus lupulus* (caution with higher dosage)[616]
Potential to affect drug pharmacokinetics	*Schisandra chinensis* *Piper longum* *Piper nigrum* *Hypericum perforatum* Berberine-containing herbs[617]

Note: this is not an exhaustive list.

pass through the blood–breast barrier. Similarly, small-molecular-weight constituents and lipophilic constituents are theoretically more likely to enter the breast milk.

Other considerations relating to the safety of herbal prescriptions include avoiding herbs that have: anti-galactagogue potential, toxicity risk, stronger sedative or CNS-acting potential, and/or the potential to affect drug pharmacokinetics and therefore plasma levels of any medications the mother is taking (see Table 14.30). Specifically relating to toxicity risk, Humphrey warns against herbs containing aristolochic acid and pyrrolizidine alkaloids.[409] Mills et al. warn against higher dosages of herbs containing potentially toxic volatile constituents, such as *Artemisia absinthium* and *Tanacetum vulgare*, as well as the use of any essential oils internally.[616]

A perhaps easily overlooked consideration is the importance of mitigating the risk of exposure to herbal adulterants that may have toxic potential. Appropriate botanical verification methods are not always applied within the herbal product industry,[624] and recommended verification methods are sometimes not adequate for detecting adulteration.[625] Therefore, practitioners need to cautiously select any product they utilise and ensure any herbal medicines prescribed have been botanically verified. Humphrey suggests particular caution with herbs with known toxic substitutes such as *Scutellaria lateriflora*,[409] which has been substituted with hepatotoxic species *Teucrium canadense* and *Teucrium chamaedrys*.[626]

Environmental pollutants and contaminants

Breast milk is an easily obtainable fluid for research purposes, and hence is often utilised as a way of measuring population exposure to chemical contaminants.[627,628] Knowledge of human exposure gained via breast milk analysis rightfully encourages policy change that helps to reduce the exposure of future generations.[628]

Media coverage of findings can undermine breastfeeding[628] when breast milk is viewed as 'contaminated'.[629] While contaminants in breast milk do represent a potential concern, these risks need to be considered with an appreciation of the risks associated with breastfeeding cessation.[627] Consequently, messages about chemical exposure need to be carefully communicated both in the media and within clinical practice. Furthermore, there is high probability of contaminant exposure from breast milk substitutes.[629]

The WHO monitors exposure levels and campaigns for nations to reduce human exposure to harmful pollutants. For example, the WHO conducted a global survey and risk assessment of digoxin-like compounds in human milk.[627] It noted regional differences in breast milk levels of these compounds, finding that many of these chemicals were above potentially toxic thresholds, particularly in poorer countries. The WHO issued a plea to nations to reduce exposure levels. It also concluded that the benefits of breastfeeding far outweigh the potential risks associated with polychlorinated dibenzo-p-dioxins (PCDDs), polychlorinated dibenzofurans (PCDFs) and polychlorinated biphenyls (PCBs) in human milk.[627]

The principles that govern the transfer of drugs to breast milk apply similarly to the transfer of contaminants, in that the character of the chemical determines the degree of transfer. Accordingly, the transfer of many contaminants in breast milk is regulated or limited, yet still unwanted. Observational studies have difficulty separating the implications of exposure of the offspring during pregnancy from that of lactation. The deleterious effects of exposure during pregnancy tend to be more significant, both because placental transfer is greater than breast milk transfer and because of the developmental vulnerability of the fetus.[627] In regions with contaminated water, breastfeeding protects infants from some contaminants as the concentration of most contaminants in breast milk is far lower than formula prepared with contaminated water.[630–632] There are examples of contaminants that are sequestered into breast milk, however.[633] The WHO and the Centers for Disease Control and Prevention (CDC) both give guidelines for heavy-metal-exposed mothers and breastfeeding, providing specific information about threshold levels and appropriate actions. It is extremely rare that maternal contaminants status warrants breastfeeding interruption. In these scenarios, it is important that a full risk balance assessment is done, as the risks of breastfeeding cessation need to be weighed in appropriately.

Some considerations for the reduction of exposure of specific heavy metals include:

- Arsenic. A protective physiological mechanism brings about a rise in maternal arsenic methylation during pregnancy and lactation. Methylated arsenic has very limited capacity to transfer to breast milk.[360] Hence, breastfed infants have lower arsenic status than formula-fed infants when arsenic is present in tap water.[632] Practitioners may further reduce the risk of arsenic exposure via supporting maternal methylation pathways. Additionally, maintaining optimal selenium status may provide some protection against arsenic toxicity.[634]
- Lead. Lead mobilisation from maternal bone may be reduced by calcium supplementation.[360] Greater amounts of dietary and environmental lead are absorbed by mothers who are iron deficient. Pregnant and breastfeeding women should minimise exposure to lead by avoiding: kajal eyeliner, lead-containing ceramic crockery, PVC, lead in plumbing, occupational exposure to agriculture products and exposure to the sanding or renovating activity of older buildings.[360,635]
- Cadmium. Maternal maintenance of healthy iron status reduces maternal cadmium absorption from the environment. Maternal maintenance of optimal vitamin D status may reduce infant exposure to cadmium.[360]
- Mercury. Maternal avoidance of predatory fish will minimise exposure to methylmercury. High breast milk mercury levels have been found in the women of the Seychelles islands in accordance with their fish-eating habits. Additionally, maintaining optimal selenium status may provide some protection against mercury toxicity.[634]

BREASTFEEDING AND HIV

The current United Nations HIV recommendation regarding feeding of infants of HIV-positive mothers is: 'where replacement feeding is acceptable, feasible, affordable, sustainable, and safe, avoidance of all breastfeeding is recommended, otherwise exclusive breastfeeding is recommended for the first few months of life'.[636] Hence, in high-income countries, HIV-positive

mothers are advised not to breastfeed their infants.[636] Levison et al. and Johnson et al. have recommended encouraging an open dialogue with HIV-positive mothers on feeding decisions and educating them on milk replacement options (see above section) and risk-reduction strategies if they are choosing to breastfeed.[636,637]

In low-income countries, the WHO recommendations for HIV-infected mothers and their infants are: exclusive breastfeeding for 6 months and continued breastfeeding until 12 months, combined with triple maternal anti-retroviral therapy.[638] Infants of HIV-positive mothers who are formula fed have higher mortality risk in resource-poor countries than those who are exclusively breastfed, even without ART.[639] HIV transmission attributed to exclusive breastfeeding was 4% for infants between the ages of 6 weeks and 6 months, with mixed feeding doubling the risk of transmission, according to one controlled study.[639,640] Breast milk has a number of anti-viral components which may help to reduce breast milk transmission of HIV.[641] Once the infant commences solids, or is given a breast milk substitute, the risk of infection rises steeply. This is thought to be caused by multiple factors including: 1) increased HIV viral load in breast milk occurring with weaning and other disruptions to continuous breastfeeding[639]; 2) HIV viral-blocking components in breast milk may be diluted with the introduction of other foods; and 3) a loss of barrier function occurs due to micro-injuries caused by exposure to foods other than breast milk.[639] The use of maternal ART substantially reduces the risk of infant transmission from pregnancy, birth and breastfeeding to less than 5%.[642]

MATERNAL INFANT SLEEP AND BREASTFEEDING

The popular view is that breastfeeding is associated with reduced parental sleep. Consequently, mothers may be advised by friends, family or even caregivers to introduce night-time formula and commence solids to improve parental sleep.[643] Maternal beliefs and expectations around sleep can both contribute to parental anxiety and predict parents' likelihood of introducing formula and/or early solid introduction.[643] Surprisingly, several studies have found that on average, exclusively breastfeeding mothers get the same number of hours of sleep[644] or slightly more[644,645] than mothers who are supplementing with some formula or exclusively formula feeding. Sleep fragmentation is also the same.[24,645]

Interestingly, poor maternal sleep and poor daytime functioning may lead mothers to perceive their infants to have a sleep problem.[646] Hence, employing strategies to help mothers get more rest and helping parents to have realistic expectations of infants' sleep may reduce parental anxiety and improve maternal wellbeing.

The sleep architecture of a breastfeeding mother is different from that of mothers not breastfeeding. Breastfeeding is associated with a marked increase in slow-wave sleep (SWS).[644] This is suspected to be modulated by prolactin. It has been suggested that supplementing the infant may blunt the mother's prolactin levels overnight, and result in a reduction in SWS and overall sleep quality.[644]

Many parents are concerned about their infant's sleep, and may be told not to let their infant fall asleep at the breast and/or to limit the number of night feeds. Infants have a wide variation in sleep needs,[647,648] and night-time feeding patterns may vary and fluctuate based on factors such as maternal breast milk storage capacity and the need to stimulate milk supply, growth and development stages of the infant and the infant's state of health. Infants typically increase their night-time feeding when they are unwell, teething or going through a growth or developmental shift.

Parents may be reassured to hear that night waking is normal, and that it may even help protect infants from sudden infant death syndrome (SIDS) while their neurorespiratory mechanisms are immature.

Infant sleep location and safety

The evidence clearly indicates that parental room sharing protects infants from SIDS.[649–652] However, the evaluation of bed-sharing safety is complex due to different variables that are not always clearly delineated by researchers.[653]

From an evolutionary perspective, an infant's close proximity to a caregiver (usually their mother) has been important for survival.[653]

Breastfeeding infants and mothers interact while they sleep and wake through the night. The co-rousing that occurs has been proposed to assist the immature nervous system of the infant to maintain cardiorespiratory function.[654,655] The sleeping behaviour of non-breastfeeding mothers and infant pairs is distinctly different.[655]

Some modern factors such as parental smoking, alcohol consumption, drug use, obesity and sofa sleeping alter the risk profile of bed sharing.[653] However, bed sharing of breastfeeding mothers and term infants when these factors are not present does not increase the risk compared to separate surface sleeping, according to an analysis of pooled SIDS studies,[653] and it may decrease the risk of SIDS in infants over the age of 3 months.[653] This could be because of the effect of bed sharing on exclusive breastfeeding. Mothers who co-sleep with their infants are more likely to exclusively breastfeed[656] and to continue breastfeeding for longer.[657] The bidirectional relationship between breastfeeding and bed sharing needs to be considered when parents are counselled about their infant's sleeping arrangements. Furthermore, because breastfeeding at night can be tiring, mothers who are getting up to feed in a chair or on a sofa are at risk of falling asleep with their infant. Hence, by actively trying to avoid bed sharing, these mothers may put their infants at greater risk.

Many parents may intentionally or unintentionally end up bed sharing[658] because it makes night-time parenting easier.[659] Hence, it is recommended that clinicians actively inform parents about how they can more safely bed share, whether or not parents intend to do it (see Box 14.7 Safe Sleep Seven).

BOX 14.7 Summary of *The Safe Sleep Seven* for safer bed sharing, from La Leche League International[660]

If the mother is:
1. breastfeeding
   and all present in the bed are:
2. non-smokers
3. sober (no alcohol or drugs)
   and her baby is:
4. healthy
5. on his/her back
6. lightly dressed and unswaddled
7. and they share a safe sleep surface:
   – firm and simple flatbed surface
   – avoid: sofas, recliners, pets in the bed, extra pillows, very soft beds, cords or tangling items, heavy comforters, spaces between headboards and walls where baby could get caught
   – ensure: bed is not too high from the ground
   When all of these are applied, the baby's risk of SIDS is no greater than in a crib or cot.

CONCLUSION

While herbal and nutritional support can play an important part in supporting women with breastfeeding concerns, it may be the knowledge, attitude, support and referral skills of the practitioner that make the biggest difference to their patients' breastfeeding outcomes. Naturopaths, like other health professionals, can play a pivotal role in determining women's likelihood of initiating and continuing to breastfeed. Health professionals' knowledge of lactation physiology and the risks associated with premature breastfeeding cessation, and their ability to refer women to specialised practitioners and breastfeeding peer support groups are key determinants in the successful promotion of breastfeeding.

REFERENCES

[1] Rautava S, Walker WA. Academy of Breastfeeding Medicine Founder's Lecture 2008: breastfeeding – an extrauterine link between mother and child. Breastfeed Med 2009;4(1):3–10.

[2] Beijers R, Riksen-Walraven JM, de Weerth C. Cortisol regulation in 12-month-old human infants: associations with the infants' early history of breastfeeding and co-sleeping. Stress 2013;16(3): 267–77.

[3] Harrison D, Reszel J, Bueno M, et al. Breastfeeding for procedural pain in infants beyond the neonatal period. Cochrane Database Syst Rev 2016;(10):CD011248.

[4] Johnson K. Maternal–infant bonding: a review of literature. Int J Childbirth Educ 2013;28(3).

[5] Bartick MC, Schwarz EB, Green BD, et al. Suboptimal breastfeeding in the United States: maternal and pediatric health outcomes and costs. Matern Child Nutr 2017;13(1).

[6] World Health Organization. Infant and young child feeding: model chapter for textbooks for medical students and allied health professionals. WHO; 2009.

[7] World Health Organization. Exclusive breastfeeding for six months best for babies everywhere; 2011. Available from https://

www.who.int/mediacentre/news/statements/2011/
breastfeeding_20110115/en/.

[8] World Health Organization. Global Health Observatory: early
     initiation and exclusive breastfeeding; 2013. Available from
     www.who.int/gho/child_health/prevention/breastfeeding_text/en/
     index.html.

[9] Al-Sahab B, Lanes A, Feldman M, et al. Prevalence and predictors
     of 6-month exclusive breastfeeding among Canadian women: a
     national survey. BMC Pediatr 2010;10:20.

[10] Australian Bureau of Statistics. Australian Health Survey: Health
     Service Usage and Health Related Actions, 2011–2012: Australian
     Bureau of Statistics; 2013 [updated April 2013; cited 2013].
     Available from http://www.abs.gov.au/ausstats/abs@.nsf/
     Latestproducts/6664B939E49FD9C1CA257B39000F2E4
     B?opendocument.

[11] Centers for Disease Control and Prevention. Breastfeeding report
     card progressing towards national breastfeeding goals United
     States 2016. CDC 2016.

[12] McAndrew F, Thompson J, Fellows L, et al. Infant feeding survey
     2010. Leeds: Health and Social Care Information Centre; 2012.

[13] Smith J. The contribution of infant food marketing to the
     obesogenic environment in Australia. Breastfeed Rev
     2007;15(1):23–35.

[14] Stevens EE, Patrick TE, Pickler R. A history of infant feeding. J
     Perinat Educ 2009;18(2):32–9.

[15] Fomon SJ. Infant feeding in the 20th century: formula and Beikost.
     J Nutr 2001;131(2):409S–20S.

[16] Smith J, Blake M. Infant food marketing strategies undermine
     effective regulation of breast-milk substitutes: trends in print
     advertising in Australia, 1950–2010. Aust N Z J Public Health
     2013;37(4):337–44.

[17] Tarrant M, Lok KYW, Fong DYT, et al. Effect on baby-friendly
     hospital steps when hospitals implement a policy to pay for infant
     formula. J Hum Lact 2016;32(2):238–49.

[18] World Health Organization. Country implementation of the
     International Code of Marketing of Breast-Milk Substitutes: status
     report 2011; 2013. Available from https://apps.who.int/iris/
     bitstream/handle/10665/85621/9789241505987_eng.pdf;jsessionid=
     7B51D76DB9050B1BDEF3602E69DE950A?sequence=1.

[19] Pérez-Escamilla R, Martinez JL, Segura-Pérez S. Impact of the
     Baby-Friendly Hospital Initiative on breastfeeding and child health
     outcomes: a systematic review. Matern Child Nutr 2016;12(3):
     402–17.

[20] World Health Organization, UNICEF. Baby-Friendly Hospital
     Initiative: revised, updated and expanded for integrated care
     2009.

[21] Hawkins SS, Stern AD, Baum CF, et al. Compliance with the
     Baby-Friendly Hospital Initiative and impact on breastfeeding
     rates. Arch Dis Child Fetal Neonatal Ed 2014;99(2):F138–43.

[22] Flacking R, Thomson G, Ekenberg L, et al. Influence of NICU
     co-care facilities and skin-to-skin contact on maternal stress
     in mothers of preterm infants. Sex Reprod Healthc 2013;4(3):
     107–12.

[23] Lester BM, Hawes K, Abar B, et al. Single-family room care and
     neurobehavioral and medical outcomes in preterm infants.
     Pediatrics 2014;134(4):754–60.

[24] Pierro J, Abulaimoun B, Roth P, et al. Factors associated with
     supplemental formula feeding of breastfeeding infants during
     postpartum hospital stay. Breastfeed Med 2016;11(4):196–202.

[25] Oniwon O, Tender JAF, He J, et al. Reasons for infant feeding
     decisions in low-income families in Washington, DC. J Hum Lact
     2016;32(4):704–10.

[26] Negin J, Coffman J, Vizintin P, et al. The influence of grandmothers
     on breastfeeding rates: a systematic review. BMC Pregnancy
     Childbirth 2016;16:91.

[27] Schafer EJ, Williams NA, Digney S, et al. Social contexts of infant
     feeding and infant feeding decisions. J Hum Lact 2016;32(1):132–
     40. doi:10.1177/0890334415592850.

[28] Dubois L, Girard M. Social inequalities in infant feeding during the
     first year of life. The Longitudinal Study of Child Development in
     Québec (LSCDQ 1998–2002). Public Health Nutr 2003;6(8):773–83.

[29] Atchan M, Foureur M, Davis D. The decision not to initiate
     breastfeeding – women's reasons, attitudes and influencing factor –
     a review of the literature. Breastfeed Rev 2011;19(2):9–17.

[30] Magarey A, Kavian F, Scott JA, et al. Feeding mode of Australian
     infants in the first 12 months of life. J Hum Lact
     2016;32(4):NP95–104.

[31] Jacobson H. Mother food for breastfeeding mothers. New York: St
     Martin's Press; 2004.

[32] Maycock B, Binns CW, Dhaliwal S, et al. Education and support for
     fathers improves breastfeeding rates: a randomized controlled trial.
     J Hum Lact 2013;29(4):484–90.

[33] Mitchell-Box KM, Braun KL. Impact of male-partner-focused
     interventions on breastfeeding initiation, exclusivity, and
     continuation. J Hum Lact 2013;29(4):473–9.

[34] Dagher RK, McGovern PM, Schold JD, et al. Determinants of
     breastfeeding initiation and cessation among employed mothers:
     a prospective cohort study. BMC Pregnancy Childbirth 2016;16:
     194.

[35] Jones KM, Power ML, Queenan JT, et al. Racial and ethnic
     disparities in breastfeeding. Breastfeed Med 2015;10(4):186–96.

[36] Bartick MC, Jegier BJ, Green BD, et al. Disparities in breastfeeding:
     impact on maternal and child health outcomes and costs. J Pediatr
     2017;181:49–55.

[37] Helps C, Barclay L. Aboriginal women in rural Australia; a small
     study of infant feeding behaviour. Women Birth
     2015;28(2):129–36.

[38] Mirkovic KR, Perrine CG, Scanlon KS, et al. Maternity leave
     duration and full-time/part-time work status are associated with US
     mothers' ability to meet breastfeeding intentions. J Hum Lact
     2014;30(4):416–19.

[39] Mirkovic KR, Perrine CG, Scanlon KS. Paid maternity leave and
     breastfeeding outcomes. Birth 2016;43(3):233–9.

[40] Majee W, Jefferson UT, Goodman LR, et al. Four years later: rural
     mothers' and employers' perspectives on breastfeeding barriers
     following the passage of the Affordable Care Act. J Health Care
     Poor Underserved 2016;27(3):1110–25.

[41] Wiffen J, Fetherston C. Relationships between assisted reproductive
     technologies and initiation of lactation: preliminary observations.
     Breastfeed Rev 2016;24(1):21–7.

[42] Fisher J, Hammarberg K, Wynter K, et al. Assisted conception,
     maternal age and breastfeeding: an Australian cohort study. Acta
     Paediatr 2013;102(10):970–6.

[43] Michels KA, Mumford SL, Sundaram R, et al. Differences in infant
     feeding practices by mode of conception in a United States cohort.
     Fertil Steril 2016;105(4):1014–22.e1.

[44] Newby RM, Davies PSW. Antenatal breastfeeding intention,
     confidence and comfort in obese and non-obese primiparous
     Australian women: associations with breastfeeding duration. Eur J
     Clin Nutr 2016;70(8):935–40.

[45] Turcksin R, Bel S, Galjaard S, et al. Maternal obesity and
     breastfeeding intention, initiation, intensity and duration: a
     systematic review. Matern Child Nutr 2014;10(2):166–83.

[46] Dias CC, Figueiredo B. Breastfeeding and depression: a systematic
     review of the literature. J Affect Disord 2015;171:142–54.

[47] Woolhouse H, James J, Gartland D, et al. Maternal depressive
     symptoms at three months postpartum and breastfeeding rates at
     six months postpartum: implications for primary care in a
     prospective cohort study of primiparous women in Australia.
     Women Birth 2016;29(4):381–7.

[48] Figueiredo B, Canário C, Field T. Breastfeeding is negatively
     affected by prenatal depression and reduces postpartum
     depression. Psychol Med 2014;44(05):927–36.

[49] Ystrom E. Breastfeeding cessation and symptoms of anxiety and
     depression: a longitudinal cohort study. BMC Pregnancy Childbirth
     2012;12:36.

[50] Bascom EM, Napolitano MA. Breastfeeding duration and primary
     reasons for breastfeeding cessation among women with
     postpartum depressive symptoms. J Hum Lact 2016;32(2):282–91.

[51] Garcia-Fortea P, Gonzalez-Mesa E, Blasco M, et al. Oxytocin
     administered during labor and breast-feeding: a retrospective
     cohort study. J Matern Fetal Neonatal Med 2014;27(15):
     1598–603.

[52] Adams J, Frawley J, Steel A, et al. Use of pharmacological and
     non-pharmacological labour pain management techniques and
     their relationship to maternal and infant birth outcomes:
     examination of a nationally representative sample of 1835
     pregnant women. Midwifery 2015;31(4):458–63.

[53] Fleet J, Belan I, Jones MJ, et al. A comparison of fentanyl with pethidine for pain relief during childbirth: a randomised controlled trial. BJOG 2015;122(7):983–92.

[54] Herrera-Gómez A, García-Martinez O, Ramos-Torrecillas J, et al. Retrospective study of the association between epidural analgesia during labour and complications for the newborn. Midwifery 2015;31(6):613–16.

[55] Zuppa AA, Alighieri G, Riccardi R, et al. Epidural analgesia, neonatal care and breastfeeding. Ital J Pediatr 2014;40:82.

[56] Machado MCM, Assis KF, Oliveira FdCC, et al. Determinants of the exclusive breastfeeding abandonment: psychosocial factors. Rev Saude Publica 2014;48(6):985–94.

[57] Moore ER, Anderson GC, Bergman N, et al. Early skin-to-skin contact for mothers and their healthy newborn infants. Cochrane Database Syst Rev 2012;(5):CD003519.

[58] Sharma A. Efficacy of early skin-to-skin contact on the rate of exclusive breastfeeding in term neonates: a randomized controlled trial. Afr Health Sci 2016;16(3):790–7.

[59] Moore ER, Bergman N, Anderson GC, et al. Early skin-to-skin contact for mothers and their healthy newborn infants. Cochrane Database Syst Rev 2016;(11):CD003519.

[60] Crenshaw JT. Healthy birth practice #6: keep mother and baby together – it's best for mother, baby, and breastfeeding. J Perinat Educ 2014;23(4):211–17.

[61] DiGirolamo AM, Grummer-Strawn LM, Fein SB. Effect of maternity-care practices on breastfeeding. Pediatrics 2008;122(Suppl. 2):S43–9.

[62] Nguyen TT, Withers M, Hajeebhoy N, et al. Infant formula feeding at birth is common and inversely associated with subsequent breastfeeding behavior in Vietnam. J Nutr 2016;146(10):2102–8.

[63] Parry JE, Ip DKM, Chau PYK, et al. Predictors and consequences of in-hospital formula supplementation for healthy breastfeeding newborns. J Hum Lact 2013;29(4):527–36.

[64] Zakarija-Grković I, Šegvić O, Bozinović T, et al. Hospital practices and breastfeeding rates before and after the UNICEF/WHO 20-hour course for maternity staff. J Hum Lact 2012;28(3):389–99.

[65] Flaherman VJ, Aby J, Burgos AE, et al. Effect of early limited formula on duration and exclusivity of breastfeeding in at-risk infants: an RCT. Pediatrics 2013;131(6):1059–65.

[66] Straňák Z, Feyereislova S, Černá M, et al. Limited amount of formula may facilitate breastfeeding: randomized, controlled trial to compare standard clinical practice versus limited supplemental feeding. PLoS ONE 2016;11(2):e0150053.

[67] Boban M, Zakarija-Grković I. In-hospital formula supplementation of healthy newborns: practices, reasons, and their medical justification. Breastfeed Med 2016;11(9):448–54.

[68] Buccini GdS, Pérez-Escamilla R, Paulino LM, et al. Pacifier use and interruption of exclusive breastfeeding: systematic review and meta-analysis. Matern Child Nutr 2016;13(3).

[69] Hauck YL, Graham-Smith C, McInerney J, et al. Western Australian women's perceptions of conflicting advice around breast feeding. Midwifery 2010;27(5):e156–62.

[70] Laanterä S, Pölkki T, Pietilä A-M. A descriptive qualitative review of the barriers relating to breast-feeding counselling. Int J Nurs Pract 2011;17(1):72–84.

[71] Ekström AC, Thorstensson S. Nurses and midwives professional support increases with improved attitudes – design and effects of a longitudinal randomized controlled process-oriented intervention. BMC Pregnancy Childbirth 2015;15:275.

[72] Fitzsimons E, Vera-Hernández M. Breast feeding and the weekend effect: an observational study. BMJ Open 2016;6(7):e010016.

[73] Balogun OO, O'Sullivan EJ, McFadden A, et al. Interventions for promoting the initiation of breastfeeding. Cochrane Database Syst Rev 2016;(11):CD001688.

[74] Nommsen-Rivers LA, Mastergeorge AM, Hansen RL, et al. Doula care, early breastfeeding outcomes, and breastfeeding status at 6 weeks postpartum among low-income primiparae. J Obstet Gynecol Neonatal Nurs 2009;38(2):157–73.

[75] Stevens J, Schmied V, Burns E, et al. Immediate or early skin-to-skin contact after a Caesarean section: a review of the literature. Matern Child Nutr 2014;10(4):456–73.

[76] Burgio MA, Laganà AS, Sicilia A, et al. Breastfeeding education: where are we going? A Systematic Review Article. Iran J Public Health 2016;45(8):970–7.

[77] Bergman M, Nygren-Brunell O, Vilakati D, et al. Prolonged exclusive breastfeeding through peer support: a cohort study from a community outreach project in Swaziland. J Community Health 2016;41(5):932–8.

[78] Kaunonen M, Hannula L, Tarkka M-T. A systematic review of peer support interventions for breastfeeding. J Clin Nurs 2012; 21(13–14):1943–54.

[79] Wouk K, Chetwynd E, Vitaglione T, et al. Improving access to medical lactation support and counseling: building the case for medicaid reimbursement. Matern Child Health J 2016;1–9.

[80] Johnston C, Campbell-Yeo M, Fernandes A, et al. Skin-to-skin care for procedural pain in neonates. Cochrane Database Syst Rev 2014;(1):CD008435.

[81] Newby RM, Davies PSW. Why do women stop breast-feeding? Results from a contemporary prospective study in a cohort of Australian women. Eur J Clin Nutr 2016;70(12):1428–32.

[82] Buck ML, Amir LH, Cullinane M, et al. Nipple pain, damage, and vasospasm in the first 8 weeks postpartum. Breastfeed Med 2014;9(2):56–62.

[83] Li R, Fein SB, Chen J, et al. Why mothers stop breastfeeding: mothers' self-reported reasons for stopping during the first year. Pediatrics 2008;122(Suppl. 2):S69–76.

[84] Declercq ER, Sakala C, Corry MP, et al. Major survey findings of listening to mothers III: new mothers speak out: report of national surveys of women's childbearing experiences conducted October–December 2012 and January–April 2013. J Perinat Educ 2014;23(1):17–24.

[85] Brown CR, Dodds L, Legge A, et al. Factors influencing the reasons why mothers stop breastfeeding. Can J Public Health 2014;105(3):e179–85.

[86] Segura-Millán S, Dewey KG, Perez-Escamilla R. Factors associated with perceived insufficient milk in a low-income urban population in Mexico. J Nutr 1994;124(2):202–12.

[87] Scott J, Colin W. Breastfeeding: reasons for starting, reasons for stopping and problems along the way. Breastfeed Rev 2002;10(2):13.

[88] Gatti L. Maternal perceptions of insufficient milk supply in breastfeeding. J Nurs Scholarsh 2008;40(4):355–63.

[89] Attanasio L, Kozhimannil KB, McGovern P, et al. The impact of prenatal employment on breastfeeding intentions and breastfeeding status at one week postpartum. J Hum Lact 2013; 29(4):doi:10.1177/0890334413504149.

[90] Varalda A, Coscia A, Di Nicola P, et al. Medication and breastfeeding. J Biol Regul Homeost Agents 2012;26(3 Suppl.):1–4.

[91] Sleutel MR. Intrapartum nursing: integrating Rubin's framework with social support theory. J Obstet Gynecol Neonatal Nurs 2003;32(1):76–82.

[92] Martell LK. Heading toward the new normal: a contemporay postpartum experience. J Obstet Gynecol Neonatal Nurs 2001;30(5):496–506.

[93] Darvill R, Skirton H, Farrand P. Psychological factors that impact on women's experiences of first-time motherhood: a qualitative study of the transition. Midwifery 2010;26(3):357–66.

[94] Leahy-Warren P, McCarthy G. Maternal parental self-efficacy in the postpartum period. Midwifery 2011;27(6):802–10.

[95] Kendall-Tackett K. Childbirth-related posttraumatic stress disorder: symptoms and impact on breastfeeding. Clin Lact 2014;5(2):51–5.

[96] Neves PR, Salim N, Soares GCF, et al. Experiences of women in a pregnant group: a descriptive study. Online Braz J Nurs 2013;12(4):862–71.

[97] Berry NJ, Gribble KD. Breast is no longer best: promoting normal infant feeding. Matern Child Nutr 2008;4(1):74–9.

[98] Brodribb W, Fallon A, Jackson C, et al. The relationship between personal breastfeeding experience and the breastfeeding attitudes, knowledge, confidence and effectiveness of Australian GP registrars. Matern Child Nutr 2008;4(4):264–74.

[99] Sattari M, Levine D, Neal D, et al. Personal breastfeeding behavior of physician mothers is associated with their clinical breastfeeding advocacy. Breastfeed Med 2013;8(1):31–7.

[100] Collado MC, Cernada M, Baüerl C, et al. Microbial ecology and host-microbiota interactions during early life stages. Gut Microbes 2012;3(4):352–65.

[101] Pacheco AR, Barile D, Underwood MA, et al. The impact of the milk glycobiome on the neonate gut microbiota. Annu Rev Anim Biosci 2015;3:419–45.

[102] Lonnerdal B. Bioactive proteins in breast milk. J Paediatr Child Health 2013;49(Suppl. 1):1–7.

[103] Hassiotou F, Geddes DT. Immune cell–mediated protection of the mammary gland and the infant during breastfeeding. Adv Nutr 2015;6(3):267–75.

[104] Rodríguez JM. The origin of human milk bacteria: is there a bacterial entero-mammary pathway during late pregnancy and lactation? Adv Nutr 2014;5(6):779–84.

[105] Milani C, Mancabelli L, Lugli GA, et al. Exploring vertical transmission of bifidobacteria from mother to child. Appl Environ Microbiol 2015;81(20):7078–87.

[106] Jost T, Lacroix C, Braegger CP, et al. Vertical mother-neonate transfer of maternal gut bacteria via breastfeeding. Environ Microbiol 2014;16(9):2891–904.

[107] Makino H, Martin R, Ishikawa E, et al. Multilocus sequence typing of bifidobacterial strains from infant's faeces and human milk: are bifidobacteria being sustainably shared during breastfeeding? Benef Microbes 2015;6(4):563–72.

[108] Martín V, Maldonado-Barragán A, Moles L, et al. Sharing of bacterial strains between breast milk and infant feces. J Hum Lact 2012;28(1):36–44.

[109] Francavilla R, Calasso M, Calace L, et al. Effect of lactose on gut microbiota and metabolome of infants with cow's milk allergy. Pediatr Allergy Immunol 2012;23(5):420–7.

[110] Szilagyi A, Shrier I, Heilpern D, et al. Differential impact of lactose/lactase phenotype on colonic microflora. Can J Gastroenterol 2010;24(6):373–9.

[111] Liu B, Newburg DS. Human milk glycoproteins protect infants against human pathogens. Breastfeed Med 2013;8(4):354–62.

[112] Li R, Xia W, Zhang Z, et al. S100B protein, brain-derived neurotrophic factor, and glial cell line-derived neurotrophic factor in human milk. PLoS ONE 2011;6(6):e21663.

[113] Velasco I, Santos C, Limón J, et al. Bioactive components in human milk along the first month of life: effects of iodine supplementation during pregnancy. Ann Nutr Metab 2016;68(2):130–6.

[114] Palmano K, Rowan A, Guillermo R, et al. The role of gangliosides in neurodevelopment. Nutrients 2015;7(5):3891–913.

[115] Lönnerdal B. Nutritional and physiologic significance of human milk proteins. Am J Clin Nutr 2003;77(6):1537S–43S.

[116] Gidrewicz DA, Fenton TR. A systematic review and meta-analysis of the nutrient content of preterm and term breast milk. BMC Pediatr 2014;14:216.

[117] Hassiotou F, Hepworth AR, Williams TM, et al. Breastmilk cell and fat contents respond similarly to removal of breastmilk by the infant. PLoS ONE 2013;8(11):e78232.

[118] Dewit O, Dibba B, Prentice A. Breast-milk amylase activity in English and Gambian mothers: effects of prolonged lactation, maternal parity, and individual variations. Pediatr Res 1990;28(5):502–6.

[119] Lindquist S, Hernell O. Lipid digestion and absorption in early life: an update. Curr Opin Clin Nutr Metab Care 2010;13(3):314–20.

[120] Hamosh M, Henderson TR, Ellis LA, et al. Digestive enzymes in human milk: stability at suboptimal storage temperatures. J Pediatr Gastroenterol Nutr 1997;24(1):38–43.

[121] Çatli G, Olgaç Dündar N, Dündar BN. Adipokines in breast milk: an update. J Clin Res Pediatr Endocrinol 2014;6(4):192–201.

[122] Illnerová H, Buresová M, Presl J. Melatonin rhythm in human milk. J Clin Endocrinol Metab 1993;77(3):838–41.

[123] Uvnäs-Moberg K, Marchini G, Winberg J. Plasma cholecystokinin concentrations after breast feeding in healthy 4 day old infants. Arch Dis Child 1993;68(1 Spec No):46–8.

[124] Gribble KD. Mental health, attachment and breastfeeding: implications for adopted children and their mothers. Int Breastfeed J 2006;1:5.

[125] Straub N, Grunert P, Northstone K, et al. Economic impact of breast-feeding-associated improvements of childhood cognitive development, based on data from the ALSPAC. Br J Nutr 2016;2016:1–6.

[126] Jedrychowski W, Perera F, Jankowski J, et al. Effect of exclusive breastfeeding on the development of children's cognitive function in the Krakow Prospective Birth Cohort Study. Eur J Pediatr 2012;171(1):151–8.

[127] Belfort MB, Rifas-Shiman SL, Kleinman KP, et al. Infant feeding and childhood cognition at ages 3 and 7 years: effects of breastfeeding duration and exclusivity. JAMA Pediatr 2013;167(9):836–44.

[128] Krol KM, Monakhov M, Lai PS, et al. Genetic variation in CD38 and breastfeeding experience interact to impact infants' attention to social eye cues. Proc Natl Acad Sci USA 2015;112(39):E5434–42.

[129] Agarwal SS, Sharma M, Nehra K, et al. Validation of association between breastfeeding duration, facial profile, occlusion, and spacing: a cross-sectional study. Int J Clin Pediatr Dent 2016;9(2):162–6.

[130] World Health Organization. Infant and young child feeding: A model chapter for medical students and allied health professionals 2009. Available from http://www.who.int/nutrition/publications/infantfeeding/9789241597494/en/.

[131] Perrine CG, Nelson JM, Corbelli J, et al. Lactation and maternal cardio-metabolic health. Annu Rev Nutr 2016;36(1):627–45.

[132] Stuebe AM, Schwarz EB, Grewen K, et al. Duration of lactation and incidence of maternal hypertension: a longitudinal cohort study. Am J Epidemiol 2011;174(10):1147–58.

[133] McClellan HL, Miller SJ, Hartmann PE. Evolution of lactation: nutrition v. protection with special reference to five mammalian species. Nutr Res Rev 2008;21(2):97–116.

[134] Turfkruyer M, Verhasselt V. Breast milk and its impact on maturation of the neonatal immune system. Curr Opin Infect Dis 2015;28(3):199–206.

[135] National Health and Medical Research Council. Infant feeding guidelines: information for health workers 2012. Canberra: Australia National Health and Medical Research Council; 2013.

[136] Mortensen K, Tawia S. Sustained breastfeeding. Breastfeed Rev 2013;21(1):22.

[137] Tawai S. Iron and exclusive breastfeeding. Breastfeed Rev 2012;20(1):35–47.

[138] Mosconi E, Rekima A, Seitz-Polski B, et al. Breast milk immune complexes are potent inducers of oral tolerance in neonates and prevent asthma development. Mucosal Immunol 2010;3(5):461–74.

[139] Savino F, Liguori SA. Update on breast milk hormones: leptin, ghrelin and adiponectin. Clin Nutr 2008;27(1):42–7.

[140] Katzer D, Pauli L, Mueller A, et al. Melatonin concentrations and antioxidative capacity of human breast milk according to gestational age and the time of day. J Hum Lact 2016;32(4):NP105–10.

[141] Schwarze CE, Hellhammer DH, Stroehle V, et al. Lack of breastfeeding: a potential risk factor in the multifactorial genesis of borderline personality disorder and impaired maternal bonding. J Personal Disord 2014;29(5):610–26.

[142] Sanchez-Molins M, Grau Carbo J, Lischeid Gaig C, et al. Comparative study of the craniofacial growth depending on the type of lactation received. Eur J Paediatr Dent 2010;11(2):87–92.

[143] Montgomery SM, Ehlin A, Sacker A. Breast feeding and resilience against psychosocial stress. Arch Dis Child 2006;91(12):990–4.

[144] Kendall-Tackett K. The new paradigm for depression in new mothers: current findings on maternal depression, breastfeeding and resiliency across the lifespan. Breastfeed Rev 2015;23(1):7–10.

[145] Zelkowitz P, Gold I, Feeley N, et al. Psychosocial stress moderates the relationships between oxytocin, perinatal depression, and maternal behavior. Horm Behav 2014;66(2):351–60.

[146] Ystrom E. Breastfeeding cessation and symptoms of anxiety and depression: a longitudinal cohort study. BMC Pregnancy Childbirth 2012;12(1):36–41.

[147] Strathearn L, Mamun AA, Najman JM, et al. Does breastfeeding protect against substantiated child abuse and neglect? A 15-year cohort study. Pediatrics 2009;123(2):483–93.

[148] Franca-Botelho ADC, Ferreira MC, Franca JL, et al. Breastfeeding and its relationship with reduction of breast cancer: a review. Asian Pac J Cancer Prev 2012;13(11):5327–32.

[149] Zalewski BM, Patro B, Veldhorst M, et al. Nutrition of infants and young children (one to three years) and its effect on later health: a systematic review of current recommendations (EarlyNutrition project). Crit Rev Food Sci Nutr 2017;57(3):489–500.

[150] Victora CG, Bahl R, Barros AJD, et al. Breastfeeding in the 21st century: epidemiology, mechanisms, and lifelong effect. Lancet 2016;387(10017):475–90.

[151] Bartick M, Reinhold A. The burden of suboptimal breastfeeding in the United States: a pediatric cost analysis. Pediatrics 2010;125(5):e1048–56.

[152] Chen A, Rogan WJ. Breastfeeding and the risk of postneonatal death in the United States. Pediatrics 2004;113(5):e435–9.

[153] Ma P, Brewer-Asling M, Magnus J. A case study on the economic impact of optimal breastfeeding. Matern Child Health J 2013;17(1):9–13.

[154] Ladomenou F, Moschandreas J, Kafatos A, et al. Protective effect of exclusive breastfeeding against infections during infancy: a prospective study. Arch Dis Child 2010;95(12):1004–8.

[155] Smith JP, Thompson JF, Ellwood DA. Hospital system costs of artificial infant feeding: estimates for the Australian Capital Territory. Aust N Z J Public Health 2002;26(6):543–51.

[156] Duijts L, Ramadhani MK, Moll HA. Breastfeeding protects against infectious diseases during infancy in industrialized countries. A systematic review. Matern Child Nutr 2009;5(3):199–210.

[157] Quigley MA, Kelly YJ, Sacker A. Breastfeeding and hospitalization for diarrheal and respiratory infection in the United Kingdom Millennium Cohort Study. Pediatrics 2007;119(4):e837–42.

[158] Whitten D. A precious opportunity: supporting women with concerns about their breastmilk supply. Aust J Herb Med 2013;25(3):112.

[159] Vennemann MM, Bajanowski T, Brinkmann B, et al. Does breastfeeding reduce the risk of sudden infant death syndrome? Pediatrics 2009;123(3):e406–10.

[160] Byard RW. Breastfeeding and sudden infant death syndrome. J Paediatr Child Health 2013;49(4):E348–354E.

[161] Quigley MA, Kelly YJ, Sacker A. Breastfeeding and hospitalization for diarrheal and respiratory infection in the United Kingdom Millennium Cohort Study. Pediatrics 2007;119(4):e837–42.

[162] Ajetunmobi OM, Whyte B, Chalmers J, et al. Breastfeeding is associated with reduced childhood hospitalization: evidence from a Scottish birth cohort (1997–2009). J Pediatr 2015;166(3):620–5.e4.

[163] Kaur A, Singh K, Pannu MS, et al. The effect of exclusive breastfeeding on hospital stay and morbidity due to various diseases in infants under 6 months of age: a prospective observational study. Int J Pediatr 2016;2016:7647054.

[164] Verduci E, Banderali G, Peroni D, et al. Duration of exclusive breastfeeding and wheezing in the first year of life: a longitudinal study. Allergol Immunopathol (Madr) 2017;45(4):316–24.

[165] Sabirov A, Casey JR, Murphy TF, et al. Breast-feeding is associated with a reduced frequency of acute otitis media and high serum antibody levels against NTHi and outer membrane protein vaccine antigen candidate P6. Pediatr Res 2009;66(5):565–70.

[166] Kørvel-Hanquist A, Koch A, Niclasen J, et al. Risk factors of early otitis media in the Danish national birth cohort. PLoS ONE 2016;11(11):e0166465.

[167] McNiel ME, Labbok MH, Abrahams SW. What are the risks associated with formula feeding? A re-analysis and review. Breastfeed Rev 2010;18(2):25–32.

[168] Gearry RB, Richardson AK, Frampton CM, et al. Population-based cases control study of inflammatory bowel disease risk factors. J Gastroenterol Hepatol 2010;25(2):325–33.

[169] Kemppainen KM, Lynch KF, Liu E, et al. Factors that increase risk of celiac disease autoimmunity following a gastrointestinal infection in early life. Clin Gastroenterol Hepatol 2017;15(5):694–702.

[170] Radlovic NP, Mladenovic MM, Lekovic ZM, et al. Influence of early feeding practices on celiac disease in infants. Croat Med J 2010;51(5):417–22.

[171] Akobeng AK, Ramanan AV, Buchan I, et al. Effect of breast feeding on risk of coeliac disease: a systematic review and meta-analysis of observational studies. Arch Dis Child 2006;91(1):39–43.

[172] Bener A, Hoffmann GF, Afify Z, et al. Does prolonged breastfeeding reduce the risk for childhood leukemia and lymphomas? Minerva Pediatr 2008;60(2):155–61.

[173] Smith JP, Harvey PJ. Chronic disease and infant nutrition: is it significant to public health? Public Health Nutr 2010;14(2):279–89.

[174] Quigley MA, Henderson G, Anthony MY, et al. Formula milk versus donor breast milk for feeding preterm or low birth weight infants. Cochrane Database Syst Rev 2007;(4):CD002971.

[175] Henderson G, Craig S, Brocklehurst P, et al. Enteral feeding regimens and necrotising enterocolitis in preterm infants: a multicentre case-control study. Arch Dis Child Fetal Neonatal Ed 2009;94(2):F120–3.

[176] Lambert DK, Christensen RD, Henry E, et al. Necrotizing enterocolitis in term neonates: data from a multihospital health-care system. J Perinatol 2007;27(7):437–43.

[177] Oddy WH, Kendall GE, Li J, et al. The long-term effects of breastfeeding on child and adolescent mental health: a pregnancy cohort study followed for 14 years. J Pediatr 2010;156(4):568–74.

[178] Chapman DJ. Longer cumulative breastfeeding duration associated with improved bone strength. J Hum Lact 2012;28(1):18–19.

[179] Boucher O, Julvez J, Guxens M, et al. Association between breastfeeding duration and cognitive development, autistic traits and ADHD symptoms: a multicenter study in Spain. Pediatr Res 2017;81(3):434–42.

[180] Quigley MA, Hockley C, Carson C, et al. Breastfeeding is associated with improved child cognitive development: a population-based cohort study. J Pediatr 2012;160(1):25–32.

[181] Sacker A, Quigley MA, Kelly YJ. Breastfeeding and developmental delay: findings from the millennium cohort study. Pediatrics 2006;118(3):e682–9.

[182] Grace T, Oddy W, Bulsara M, et al. Breastfeeding and motor development: a longitudinal cohort study. Hum Mov Sci 2017;51:9–16.

[183] Kafouri S, Kramer M, Leonard G, et al. Breastfeeding and brain structure in adolescence. Int J Epidemiol 2013;42(1):150–9.

[184] Peus V, Redelin E, Scharnholz B, et al. Breast-feeding in infancy and major depression in adulthood: a retrospective analysis. Psychother Psychosom 2012;81(3):189–90.

[185] Shi Y, De Groh M, Morrison H. Perinatal and early childhood factors for overweight and obesity in young canadian children. Can J Public Health 2013;104(1):e69–74.

[186] Wallby T, Lagerberg D, Magnusson M. Relationship between breastfeeding and early childhood obesity: results of a prospective longitudinal study from birth to 4 years. Breastfeed Med 2017;12:48–53.

[187] Ravelli AC, van der Meulen JH, Osmond C, et al. Infant feeding and adult glucose tolerance, lipid profile, blood pressure, and obesity. Arch Dis Child 2000;82(3):248–52.

[188] Owen CG, Martin RM, Whincup PH, et al. Does breastfeeding influence risk of type 2 diabetes in later life? A quantitative analysis of published evidence. Am J Clin Nutr 2006;84(5):1043–54.

[189] Taylor JS, Kacmar JE, Nothnagle M, et al. A systematic review of the literature associating breastfeeding with type 2 diabetes and gestational diabetes. J Am Coll Nutr 2005;24(5):320–6.

[190] Patelarou E, Girvalaki C, Brokalaki H, et al. Current evidence on the associations of breastfeeding, infant formula, and cow's milk introduction with type 1 diabetes mellitus: a systematic review. Nutr Rev 2012;70(9):509–19.

[191] Brew BK, Marks GB, Almqvist C, et al. Breastfeeding and snoring: a birth cohort study. PLoS ONE 2014;9(1):e84956.

[192] Kobayashi HM, Scavone H Jr, Ferreira RI, et al. Relationship between breastfeeding duration and prevalence of posterior crossbite in the deciduous dentition. Am J Orthod Dentofacial Orthop 2010;137(1):54–8.

[193] de Oliveira DM, Dahan P, Ferreira DF, et al. Association between exclusive maternal breastfeeding during the first 4 months of life and primary enuresis. J Pediatr Urol 2016;12(2):95.e1–e6.

[194] Sancak EB, Oguz U, Aykac A, et al. The effect of breastfeeding on spontan resolution of monosymptomatic enuresis. Int Braz J Urol 2016;42(3):550–7.

[195] Bodnar LM, Siega-Riz AM, Miller WC, et al. Who should be screened for postpartum anemia? An evaluation of current recommendations. Am J Epidemiol 2002;156(10):903–12.

[196] Rioux FM, Savoie N, Allard J. Is there a link between postpartum anemia and discontinuation of breastfeeding? Can J Diet Pract Res 2006;67(2):72–6.

[197] Sung HK, Ma SH, Choi J-Y, et al. The effect of breastfeeding duration and parity on the risk of epithelial ovarian cancer: a systematic review and meta-analysis. J Prev Med Public Health 2016;49(6):349–66.

[198] Titus-Ernstoff L, Rees JR, Terry KL, et al. Breast-feeding the last born child and risk of ovarian cancer. Cancer Causes Control 2010;21(2):201–7.

[199] Jordan SJ, Siskind V, Green A, et al. Breastfeeding and risk of epithelial ovarian cancer. Cancer Causes Control 2010;21(1):109–16.

[200] Danforth KN, Tworoger SS, Hecht JL, et al. Breastfeeding and risk of ovarian cancer in two prospective cohorts. Cancer Causes Control 2007;18(5):517–23.

[201] Li D-P, Du C, Zhang Z-M, et al. Breastfeeding and ovarian cancer risk: a systematic review and meta-analysis of 40 epidemiological studies. Asian Pac J Cancer Prev 2014;15(12):4829–37.

[202] Zhan B, Liu X, Li F, et al. Breastfeeding and the incidence of endometrial cancer: a meta-analysis. Oncotarget 2015;6(35):38398–409.

[203] Wang L, Li J, Shi Z. Association between breastfeeding and endometrial cancer risk: evidence from a systematic review and meta-analysis. Nutrients 2015;7(7):5697–711.

[204] Stuebe A. The risks of not breastfeeding for mothers and infants. Rev Obstet Gynecol 2009;2(4):222–31.

[205] Shinde SS, Forman MR, Kuerer HM, et al. Higher parity and shorter breastfeeding duration: association with triple-negative phenotype of breast cancer. Cancer 2010;116(21):4933–43.

[206] Lambertini M, Santoro L, Del Mastro L, et al. Reproductive behaviors and risk of developing breast cancer according to tumor subtype: a systematic review and meta-analysis of epidemiological studies. Cancer Treat Rev 2016;49:65–76.

[207] Connor AE, Visvanathan K, Baumgartner KB, et al. Pre-diagnostic breastfeeding, adiposity, and mortality among parous Hispanic and non-Hispanic white women with invasive breast cancer: the Breast Cancer Health Disparities Study. Breast Cancer Res Treat 2016;161(2):321–31.

[208] Lööf-Johanson M, Brudin L, Sundquist M, et al. Breastfeeding associated with reduced mortality in women with breast cancer. Breastfeed Med 2016;11(6):321–7.

[209] Yi X, Zhu J, Zhu X, et al. Breastfeeding and thyroid cancer risk in women: a dose-response meta-analysis of epidemiological studies. Clin Nutr 2016;35(5):1039–46.

[210] Schwarz EB, McClure CK, Tepper PG, et al. Lactation and maternal measures of subclinical cardiovascular disease. Obstet Gynecol 2010;115(1):41–8.

[211] Stuebe AM, Rich-Edwards JW, Willett WC, et al. Duration of lactation and incidence of type 2 diabetes. JAMA 2005;294(20):2601–10.

[212] Schwarz EB, Brown JS, Creasman JM, et al. Lactation and maternal risk of type 2 diabetes: a population-based study. Am J Med 2010;123(9):863.e1–6.

[213] Gunderson EP, Hurston SR, Ning X, et al. Lactation and progression to type 2 diabetes mellitus after gestational diabetes: a prospective cohort study. Ann Intern Med 2015;163(12):889–98.

[214] Aune D, Norat T, Romundstad P, et al. Breastfeeding and the maternal risk of type 2 diabetes: a systematic review and dose–response meta-analysis of cohort studies. Nutr Metab Cardiovasc Dis 2014;24(2):107–15.

[215] Schwarz EB, Ray RM, Stuebe AM, et al. Duration of lactation and risk factors for maternal cardiovascular disease. Obstet Gynecol 2009;113(5):974–82.

[216] Gunderson EP, Jacobs DR Jr, Chiang V, et al. Duration of lactation and incidence of the metabolic syndrome in women of reproductive age according to gestational diabetes mellitus status: a 20-Year prospective study in CARDIA (coronary artery risk development in young adults). Diabetes 2010;59(2):495–504.

[217] Gunderson EP, Lewis CE, Wei GS, et al. Lactation and changes in maternal metabolic risk factors. Obstet Gynecol 2007;109(3):729–38.

[218] Duan X, Wang J, Jiang X. A meta-analysis of breastfeeding and osteoporotic fracture risk in the females. Osteoporos Int 2017;28(2):495–503.

[219] Schnatz PF, Barker KG, Marakovits KA, et al. Effects of age at first pregnancy and breast-feeding on the development of postmenopausal osteoporosis. Menopause 2010;17(6):1161–6.

[220] Karlson EW, Mandl LA, Hankinson SE, et al. Do breast-feeding and other reproductive factors influence future risk of rheumatoid arthritis? Results from the Nurses' Health Study. Arthritis Rheum 2004;50(11):3458–67.

[221] Pikwer M, Bergstrom U, Nilsson JA, et al. Breast feeding, but not use of oral contraceptives, is associated with a reduced risk of rheumatoid arthritis. Ann Rheum Dis 2009;68(4):526–30.

[222] Goldsmith F, O'Sullivan A, Smilowitz JT, et al. Lactation and intestinal microbiota: how early diet shapes the infant gut. J Mammary Gland Biol Neoplasia 2015;20(3):149–58.

[223] Mikami K, Kimura M, Takahashi H. Influence of maternal bifidobacteria on the development of gut bifidobacteria in infants. Pharmaceuticals (Basel) 2012;5(6):629–42.

[224] LaTuga MS, Stuebe A, Seed PC. A review of the source and function of microbiota in breast milk. Semin Reprod Med 2014;32(1):68–73.

[225] Sherman MP, Zaghouani H, Niklas V. Gut microbiota, the immune system, and diet influence the neonatal gut-brain axis. Pediatr Res 2015;77(1–2):127–35.

[226] Diaz Heijtz R. Fetal, neonatal, and infant microbiome: perturbations and subsequent effects on brain development and behavior. Semin Fetal Neonatal Med 2016;21(6):410–17.

[227] Cabrera-Rubio R, Collado MC, Laitinen K, et al. The human milk microbiome changes over lactation and is shaped by maternal weight and mode of delivery. Am J Clin Nutr 2012;96(3):544–51.

[228] Young W, Hine BC, Wallace OAM, et al. Transfer of intestinal bacterial components to mammary secretions in the cow. PeerJ 2015;3:e888.

[229] Dotterud CK, Avershina E, Sekelja M, et al. Does maternal perinatal probiotic supplementation alter the intestinal microbiota of mother and child? J Pediatr Gastroenterol Nutr 2015;61(2):200–7.

[230] Abrahamsson TR, Sinkiewicz G, Jakobsson T, et al. Probiotic lactobacilli in breast milk and infant stool in relation to oral intake during the first year of life. J Pediatr Gastroenterol Nutr 2009;49(3):349–54.

[231] Arroyo R, Martín V, Maldonado A, et al. Treatment of infectious mastitis during lactation: antibiotics versus oral administration of Lactobacilli isolated from breast milk. Clin Infect Dis 2010;50(12):1551–8.

[232] Grönlund M-M, Grześkowiak L, Isolauri E, et al. Influence of mother's intestinal microbiota on gut colonization in the infant. Gut Microbes 2011;2(4):227–33.

[233] Davis JCC, Totten SM, Huang JO, et al. Identification of oligosaccharides in feces of breast-fed infants and their correlation with the gut microbial community. Mol Cell Proteomics 2016;15(9):2987–3002.

[234] Asakuma S, Hatakeyama E, Urashima T, et al. Physiology of consumption of human milk oligosaccharides by infant gut-associated bifidobacteria. J Biol Chem 2011;286(40):34583–92.

[235] Andreas NJ, Al-Khalidi A, Jaiteh M, et al. Role of human milk oligosaccharides in Group B Streptococcus colonisation. Clin Transl Immunology 2016;5(8):e99.

[236] Jaeggi T, Kortman GAM, Moretti D, et al. Iron fortification adversely affects the gut microbiome, increases pathogen abundance and induces intestinal inflammation in Kenyan infants. Gut 2015;64(5):731–42.

[237] Kortman GAM, Dutilh BE, Maathuis AJH, et al. Microbial metabolism shifts towards an adverse profile with supplementary iron in the TIM-2 in vitro model of the human colon. Front Microbiol 2015;6:1481.

[238] Kaingade PM, Somasundaram I, Nikam AB, et al. Assessment of growth factors secreted by human breastmilk mesenchymal stem cells. Breastfeed Med 2015;11(1):26–31.

[239] Bode L, McGuire M, Rodriguez JM, et al. It's alive: microbes and cells in human milk and their potential benefits to mother and infant. Adv Nutr 2014;5(5):571–3.

[240] Hassiotou F, Geddes DT, Hartmann PE. Cells in human milk. J Hum Lact 2013;29(2):171–82.

[241] Andreas NJ, Hyde MJ, Gale C, et al. Effect of maternal body mass index on hormones in breast milk: a systematic review. PLoS ONE 2014;9(12):e115043.

[242] Zivkovic AM, German JB, Lebrilla CB, et al. Human milk glycobiome and its impact on the infant gastrointestinal microbiota. Proc Natl Acad Sci USA 2011;108(Suppl. 1):4653–8.

[243] Bode L. The functional biology of human milk oligosaccharides. Early Hum Dev 2015;91(11):619–22.

[244] McJarrow P, Schnell N, Jumpsen J, et al. Influence of dietary gangliosides on neonatal brain development. Nutr Rev 2009;67(8):451–63.

[245] Hallgren O, Aits S, Brest P, et al. Apoptosis and tumor cell death in response to HAMLET (human α-lactalbumin made lethal to tumor cells). In: Bösze Z, editor. Bioactive components of milk. New York, NY: Springer New York; 2008. p. 217–40.

[246] do Carmo França-Botelho A, Ferreira MC, França JL, et al. Breastfeeding and its relationship with reduction of breast cancer: a review. Asian Pac J Cancer Prev 2012;13(11):5327–32.

[247] Queiroz VAdO, Assis AMO, R. Júnior HdC. Efeito protetor da lactoferrina humana no trato gastrintestinal. Rev Paul Pediatr 2013;31:90–5.

[248] Rai D, Adelman AS, Zhuang W, et al. Longitudinal changes in lactoferrin concentrations in human milk: a global systematic review. Crit Rev Food Sci Nutr 2014;54(12):1539–47.

[249] Wang B. Molecular determinants of milk lactoferrin as a bioactive compound in early neurodevelopment and cognition. J Pediatr 2016;173(Suppl.):S29–36.

[250] Munblit D, Verhasselt V. Allergy prevention by breastfeeding: possible mechanisms and evidence from human cohorts. Curr Opin Allergy Clin Immunol 2016;16(5):427–33.

[251] Alsaweed M, Hartmann PE, Geddes DT, et al. MicroRNAs in breastmilk and the lactating breast: potential immunoprotectors and developmental regulators for the infant and the mother. Int J Environ Res Public Health 2015;12(11):13981–4020.

[252] Tawia S. Development of oral tolerance to allergens via breastmilk. Breastfeed Rev 2015;23(3):35–9.

[253] Lodge CJ, Tan DJ, Lau MXZ, et al. Breastfeeding and asthma and allergies: a systematic review and meta-analysis. Acta Paediatr 2015;104:38–53.

[254] Vajpayee S, Sharma SD, Gupta R, et al. Early infant feeding practices may influence the onset of symptomatic celiac disease. Pediatr Gastroenterol Hepatol Nutr 2016;19(4):229–35.

[255] Minniti F, Comberiati P, Munblit D, et al. Breast-milk characteristics protecting against allergy. Endocr Metab Immune Disord Drug Targets 2014;14(1):9–15.

[256] Henriksson C, Boström A-M, Wiklund IE. What effect does breastfeeding have on coeliac disease? A systematic review update. Evid Based Med 2013;18(3):98–103.

[257] Sansotta N, Piacentini GL, Mazzei F, et al. Timing of introduction of solid food and risk of allergic disease development: understanding the evidence. Allergol Immunopathol (Madr) 2013;41(5):337–45.

[258] Souza G, Dolinsky M, Matos A, et al. Vitamin A concentration in human milk and its relationship with liver reserve formation and compliance with the recommended daily intake of vitamin A in pre-term and term infants in exclusive breastfeeding. Arch Gynecol Obstet 2015;291(2):319–25.

[259] Fujita M, Shell-Duncan B, Ndemwa P, et al. Vitamin A dynamics in breastmilk and liver stores: a life history perspective. Am J Hum Biol 2011;23(5):664–73.

[260] Tanumihardjo SA, Russell RM, Stephensen CB, et al. Biomarkers of nutrition for development (BOND) – vitamin A review. J Nutr 2016;146(9):1816S–48S.

[261] Caminha MdFC, Batista Filho M, Fernandes TFdS, et al. Suplementação com vitamina A no puerpério: revisão sistemática. Rev Saude Publica 2009;43:699–706.

[262] Bezerra DS, de Araújo KF, Azevêdo GMM, et al. A randomized trial evaluating the effect of 2 regimens of maternal vitamin A supplementation on breast milk retinol levels. J Hum Lact 2010;26(2):148–56.

[263] Oliveira JM, Allert R, East CE. Vitamin A supplementation for postpartum women. Cochrane Database Syst Rev 2016;(3):CD005944.

[264] McGuire S. WHO guideline: vitamin A supplementation in pregnant women. Geneva: WHO, 2011; WHO guideline: vitamin A supplementation in postpartum women. Geneva: WHO, 2011. Adv Nutr 2012;3(2):215–16.

[265] Ares Segura S, Arena Ansótegui J, Marta Díaz-Gómez N. The importance of maternal nutrition during breastfeeding: do breastfeeding mothers need nutritional supplements? An Pediatr (Barc) 2016;84(6):347.e1–e7.

[266] National Health and Medical Research Council, Ministry of Health. Nutrient reference values for Australia and New Zealand. Canberra: NHMRC, MOH; 2005.

[267] Bravi F, Wiens F, Decarli A, et al. Impact of maternal nutrition on breast-milk composition: a systematic review. Am J Clin Nutr 2016;104(3):646–62.

[268] Tawfeek HI, Muhyaddin OM, al-Sanwi HI, et al. Effect of maternal dietary vitamin C intake on the level of vitamin C in breastmilk among nursing mothers in Baghdad, Iraq. Food Nutr Bull 2002;23(3):244–7.

[269] Hoppu U, Rinne M, Salo-Vaananen P, et al. Vitamin C in breast milk may reduce the risk of atopy in the infant. Eur J Clin Nutr 2004;59(1):123–8.

[270] Zarban A, Toroghi MM, Asli M, et al. Effect of vitamin C and E supplementation on total antioxidant content of human breastmilk and infant urine. Breastfeed Med 2015;10(4):214–17.

[271] Thiele DK, Senti JL, Anderson CM. Maternal vitamin D supplementation to meet the needs of the breastfed infant: a systematic review. J Hum Lact 2013;29(2):163–70.

[272] Hollis BW, Wagner CL, Howard CR, et al. Maternal versus infant vitamin D supplementation during lactation: a randomized controlled trial. Pediatrics 2015;136(4):625–34.

[273] Oberhelman SS, Meekins ME, Fischer PR, et al. Maternal vitamin D supplementation to improve the vitamin D status of breastfed infants: a randomized control trial. Mayo Clin Proc 2013;88(12):1378–87.

[274] Munns CF, Shaw N, Kiely M, et al. Global Consensus recommendations on prevention and management of nutritional rickets. J Clin Endocrinol Metab 2016;101(2):394–415.

[275] Wagner CL, Hulsey TC, Fanning D, et al. High-dose vitamin D3 supplementation in a cohort of breastfeeding mothers and their infants: a 6-month follow-up pilot study. Breastfeed Med 2006;1(2):59–70.

[276] Wall CR, Stewart AW, Camargo CA, et al. Vitamin D activity of breast milk in women randomly assigned to vitamin D3 supplementation during pregnancy. Am J Clin Nutr 2016;103(2):382–8.

[277] Hollis BW, Wagner CL. Vitamin D requirements during lactation: high-dose maternal supplementation as therapy to prevent hypovitaminosis D for both the mother and the nursing infant. Am J Clin Nutr 2004;80(6):1752S–8S.

[278] Thiele DK, Ralph J, El-Masri M, et al. Vitamin D3 supplementation during pregnancy and lactation improves vitamin d status of the mother–infant dyad. J Obstet Gynecol Neonatal Nurs 2017;46(1):135–47.

[279] Vitamin D Fact Sheet for Health Professionals [Internet]. U.S. Department of Health & Human Services 2016. Available from https://ods.od.nih.gov/factsheets/VitaminD-HealthProfessional/.

[280] Ross AC, Manson JE, Abrams SA, et al. The 2011 report on dietary reference intakes for calcium and vitamin D from the Institute of Medicine: what clinicians need to know. J Clin Endocrinol Metab 2011;96(1):53–8.

[281] Holick MF, Binkley NC, Bischoff-Ferrari HA, et al. Evaluation, treatment, and prevention of vitamin D Deficiency: an Endocrine Society clinical practice guideline. J Clin Endocrinol Metab 2011;96(7):1911–30.

[282] Bouillon R, Van Schoor NM, Gielen E, et al. Optimal vitamin D status: a critical analysis on the basis of evidence-based medicine. J Clin Endocrinol Metab 2013;98(8):E1283–304.

[283] Baggerly CA, Cuomo RE, French CB, et al. Sunlight and vitamin D: necessary for public health. J Am Coll Nutr 2015;34(4):359–65.

[284] Lima MSR, Dimenstein R, Ribeiro KDS. Vitamin E concentration in human milk and associated factors: a literature review. J Pediatr (Rio J) 2014;90(5):440–8.

[285] Martysiak-Żurowska D, Szlagatys-Sidorkiewicz A, Zagierski M. Concentrations of alpha- and gamma-tocopherols in human breast milk during the first months of lactation and in infant formulas. Matern Child Nutr 2013;9(4):473–82.

[286] Clemente HA. Avaliação da suplementação com vitamina E, na forma natural ou sintética, em mulheres no pós-parto imediato e sua concentração no colostro 2013.

[287] Hampel D, Shahab-Ferdows S, Adair LS, et al. Thiamin and riboflavin in human milk: effects of lipid-based nutrient supplementation and stage of lactation on vitamer secretion and contributions to total vitamin content. PLoS ONE 2016;11(2):e0149479.

[288] Allen LH. B Vitamins in breast milk: relative importance of maternal status and intake, and effects on infant status and function. Adv Nutr 2012;3(3):362–9.

[289] Frank LL. Thiamin in clinical practice. JPEN J Parenter Enteral Nutr 2015;39(5):503–20.

[290] Israel-Ballard KA, Abrams BF, Coutsoudis A, et al. Vitamin content of breast milk from HIV-1-infected mothers before and after flash-heat treatment. J Acquir Immune Defic Syndr 2008;48(4):444–9.

[291] Stover PJ, Field MS. Vitamin B-6. Adv Nutr 2015;6(1):132–3.

[292] Quentin C, Huybrechts S, Rozen L, et al. Vitamin B12 deficiency in a 9-month-old boy. Eur J Pediatr 2012;171(1):193–5.

[293] Sukumar N, Rafnsson SB, Kandala N-B, et al. Prevalence of vitamin B-12 insufficiency during pregnancy and its effect on offspring birth weight: a systematic review and meta-analysis. Am J Clin Nutr 2016;103(5):1232–51.

[294] Sukumar N, Adaikalakoteswari A, Venkataraman H, et al. Vitamin B(12) status in women of childbearing age in the UK and its relationship with national nutrient intake guidelines: results from two National Diet and Nutrition Surveys. BMJ Open 2016;6(8):e011247.

[295] Siddiqua TJ, Ahmad SM, Ahsan KB, et al. Vitamin B12 supplementation during pregnancy and postpartum improves B12 status of both mothers and infants but vaccine response in mothers only: a randomized clinical trial in Bangladesh. Eur J Nutr 2016;55(1):281–93.

[296] Chan CQH, Low LL, Lee KH. Oral vitamin B12 replacement for the treatment of pernicious anemia. Front Med (Lausanne) 2016;3:38.

[297] Hannibal L, Lysne V, Bjørke-Monsen A-L, et al. Biomarkers and algorithms for the diagnosis of vitamin B(12) deficiency. Front Mol Biosci 2016;3:27.

[298] Thakkar K, Billa G. Treatment of vitamin B12 deficiency. Methylcobalamine? Cyancobalamine? Hydroxocobalamin? – Clearing the confusion. Eur J Clin Nutr 2015;69(1):1–2.

[299] Thakkar K, Billa G. Response to: 'Methylcobalamine is effective in peripheral neuropathies'. Eur J Clin Nutr 2015;69(4):534–5.

[300] Ganz AB, Shields K, Fomin VG, et al. Genetic impairments in folate enzymes increase dependence on dietary choline for phosphatidylcholine production at the expense of betaine synthesis. FASEB J 2016;30(10):3321–33.

[301] Davenport C, Yan J, Taesuwan S, et al. Choline intakes exceeding recommendations during human lactation improve breast milk choline content by increasing PEMT pathway metabolites. J Nutr Biochem 2015;26(9):903–11.

[302] Fischer LM, da Costa KA, Galanko J, et al. Choline intake and genetic polymorphisms influence choline metabolite concentrations in human breast milk and plasma. Am J Clin Nutr 2010;92(2):336–46.

[303] Lewis ED, Subhan FB, Bell RC, et al. Estimation of choline intake from 24 h dietary intake recalls and contribution of egg and milk consumption to intake among pregnant and lactating women in Alberta. Br J Nutr 2014;112(1):112–21.

[304] Boeke CE, Gillman MW, Hughes MD, et al. Choline intake during pregnancy and child cognition at age 7 years. Am J Epidemiol 2013;177(12):1338–47.

[305] Fisher W, Wang J, George NI, et al. Dietary iodine sufficiency and moderate insufficiency in the lactating mother and nursing infant: a computational perspective. PLoS ONE 2016;11(3):e0149300.

[306] Mackerras DE, Eastman CJ. Estimating the iodine supplementation level to recommend for pregnant and breastfeeding women in Australia. Med J Aust 2012;197(4):238–42.

[307] Azizi F, Smyth P. Breastfeeding and maternal and infant iodine nutrition. Clin Endocrinol (Oxf) 2009;70(5):803–9.

[308] Huynh D, Condo D, Gibson R, et al. Comparison of breast-milk iodine concentration of lactating women in Australia pre and post mandatory iodine fortification. Public Health Nutr 2017;20(1):12–17.

[309] Osei J, Andersson M, van der Reijden O, et al. Breast-milk iodine concentrations, iodine status and thyroid function of breastfed infants aged 2–4 months and their mothers residing in a South African township. J Clin Res Pediatr Endocrinol 2016;8(4):381–91.

[310] Forehan S. Thyroid disease in the perinatal period. Aust Fam Physician 2012;41:578–81.

[311] Aakre I, Bjøro T, Norheim I, et al. Excessive iodine intake and thyroid dysfunction among lactating Saharawi women. J Trace Elem Med Biol 2015;31:279–84.

[312] Aakre I, Strand TA, Bjøro T, et al. Thyroid function among breastfed children with chronically excessive iodine intakes. Nutrients 2016;8(7):398.

[313] Bürgi H. Iodine excess. Best Pract Res Clin Endocrinol Metab 2010;24(1):107–15.

[314] Teas J, Pino S, Critchley A, et al. Variability of iodine content in common commercially available edible seaweeds. Thyroid 2004;14(10):836–41.

[315] Björklund KL, Vahter M, Palm B, et al. Metals and trace element concentrations in breast milk of first time healthy mothers: a biological monitoring study. Environ Health 2012;11:92.

[316] Zachara BA, Pilecki A. Selenium concentration in the milk of breast-feeding mothers and its geographic distribution. Environ Health Perspect 2000;108(11):1043–6.

[317] Dorea JG. Selenium and breast-feeding. Br J Nutr 2002;88(5):443–61.

[318] Kipp AP, Strohm D, Brigelius-Flohé R, et al. Revised reference values for selenium intake. J Trace Elem Med Biol 2015;32:195–9.

[319] Negro R, Greco G, Mangieri T, et al. The influence of selenium supplementation on postpartum thyroid status in pregnant women with thyroid peroxidase autoantibodies. J Clin Endocrinol Metab 2007;92(4):1263–8.

[320] Reid SM, Middleton P, Cossich MC, et al. Interventions for clinical and subclinical hypothyroidism in pregnancy. Cochrane Database Syst Rev 2010;(7):CD007752.

[321] Innis SM. Impact of maternal diet on human milk composition and neurological development of infants. Am J Clin Nutr 2014;99(3):734S–41S.

[322] Sherry CL, Oliver JS, Marriage BJ. Docosahexaenoic acid supplementation in lactating women increases breast milk and plasma docosahexaenoic acid concentrations and alters infant omega 6:3 fatty acid ratio. Prostaglandins Leukot Essent Fatty Acids 2015;95:63–9.

[323] Lauritzen L, Carlson SE. Maternal fatty acid status during pregnancy and lactation and relation to newborn and infant status. Matern Child Nutr 2011;7:41–58.

[324] Carlson SE. Docosahexaenoic acid and arachidonic acid in infant development. Semin Neonatol 2001;6(5):437–49.

[325] Jackson KH, Harris WS. Should there be a target level of docosahexaenoic acid in breast milk? Curr Opin Clin Nutr Metab Care 2016;19(2):92–6.

[326] Sanders TA, Reddy S. The influence of a vegetarian diet on the fatty acid composition of human milk and the essential fatty acid status of the infant. J Pediatr 1992;120(4 Pt 2):S71–7.

[327] Delgado-Noguera MF, Calvache JA, Bonfill Cosp X, et al. Supplementation with long chain polyunsaturated fatty acids (LCPUFA) to breastfeeding mothers for improving child growth and development. Cochrane Database Syst Rev 2010;(12): CD007901.

[328] Luxwolda MF, Kuipers RS, Boersma ER, et al. DHA status is positively related to motor development in breastfed African and Dutch infants. Nutr Neurosci 2014;17(3):97–103.

[329] Lassek WD, Gaulin SJC. Linoleic and docosahexaenoic acids in human milk have opposite relationships with cognitive test performance in a sample of 28 countries. Prostaglandins Leukot Essent Fatty Acids 2014;91(5):195–201.

[330] Houghton LA, Yang J, O'Connor DL. Unmetabolized folic acid and total folate concentrations in breast milk are unaffected by low-dose folate supplements. Am J Clin Nutr 2009;89(1): 216–20.

[331] West AA, Yan J, Perry CA, et al. Folate-status response to a controlled folate intake in nonpregnant, pregnant, and lactating women. Am J Clin Nutr 2012;96(4):789–800.

[332] Houghton LA, Sherwood KL, Pawlosky R, et al. [6S]-5-Methyltetrahydrofolate is at least as effective as folic acid in preventing a decline in blood folate concentrations during lactation. Am J Clin Nutr 2006;83(4):842–50.

[333] Miller EM. The reproductive ecology of iron in women. Am J Phys Anthropol 2016;159:172–95.

[334] Domellöf M, Lönnerdal B, Dewey KG, et al. Iron, zinc, and copper concentrations in breast milk are independent of maternal mineral status. Am J Clin Nutr 2004;79(1):111–15.

[335] Lönnerdal B. Trace element transport in the mammary gland. Annu Rev Nutr 2007;27(1):165–77.

[336] Milman N. Postpartum anemia I: definition, prevalence, causes, and consequences. Ann Hematol 2011;90(11):1247.

[337] Marangoni F, Cetin I, Verduci E, et al. Maternal diet and nutrient requirements in pregnancy and breastfeeding. An Italian Consensus Document. Nutrients 2016;8(10):629.

[338] Milman N. Postpartum anemia II: prevention and treatment. Ann Hematol 2012;91(2):143–54.

[339] Kunutsor SK, Apekey TA, Walley J, et al. Ferritin levels and risk of type 2 diabetes mellitus: an updated systematic review and

meta-analysis of prospective evidence. Diabetes Metab Res Rev 2013;29(4):308–18.

[340] Fu S, Li F, Zhou J, et al. The relationship between body iron status, iron intake and gestational diabetes: a systematic review and meta-analysis. Medicine (Baltimore) 2016;95(2):e2383.

[341] Bowers KA, Olsen SF, Bao W, et al. Plasma concentrations of ferritin in early pregnancy are associated with risk of gestational diabetes mellitus in women in the Danish national birth cohort. J Nutr 2016;146(9):1756–61.

[342] Ferrari P, Nicolini A, Manca ML, et al. Treatment of mild non-chemotherapy-induced iron deficiency anemia in cancer patients: comparison between oral ferrous bisglycinate chelate and ferrous sulfate. Biomed Pharmacother 2012;66(6):414–18.

[343] Pineda O, Ashmead HD. Effectiveness of treatment of iron-deficiency anemia in infants and young children with ferrous bis-glycinate chelate. Nutrition 2001;17(5):381–4.

[344] Milman N, Jønsson L, Dyre P, et al. Ferrous bisglycinate 25 mg iron is as effective as ferrous sulfate 50 mg iron in the prophylaxis of iron deficiency and anemia during pregnancy in a randomized trial. J Perinat Med 2014;42(2):197–206.

[345] Choi YK, Kim J-M, Lee J-E, et al. Association of maternal diet with zinc, copper, and iron concentrations in transitional human milk produced by Korean mothers. Clin Nutr Res 2016;5(1): 15–25.

[346] Bost M, Houdart S, Oberli M, et al. Dietary copper and human health: current evidence and unresolved issues. J Trace Elem Med Biol 2016;35:107–15.

[347] Crayton JW, Walsh WJ. Elevated serum copper levels in women with a history of post-partum depression. J Trace Elem Med Biol 2007;21(1):17–21.

[348] Russo AJ. Decreased zinc and increased copper in individuals with anxiety. Nutr Metab Insights 2011;4:1–5.

[349] Gaetke LM, Chow-Johnson HS, Chow CK. Copper: toxicological relevance and mechanisms. Arch Toxicol 2014;88(11):1929–38.

[350] Donangelo CM, King JC. Maternal zinc intakes and homeostatic adjustments during pregnancy and lactation. Nutrients 2012;4(7):782–98.

[351] Dumrongwongsiri O, Suthutvoravut U, Chatvutinun S, et al. Maternal zinc status is associated with breast milk zinc concentration and zinc status in breastfed infants aged 4–6 months. Asia Pac J Clin Nutr 2015;24(2):273–80.

[352] McCormick NH, Hennigar SR, Kiselyov K, et al. The biology of zinc transport in mammary epithelial cells: implications for mammary gland development, lactation, and involution. J Mammary Gland Biol Neoplasia 2014;19(1):59–71.

[353] King JC, Brown KH, Gibson RS, et al. Biomarkers of nutrition for development (BOND) – zinc review. J Nutr 2016;146(4): 858S–85S.

[354] Wieringa FT, Dijkhuizen MA, Fiorentino M, et al. Determination of zinc status in humans: which indicator should we use? Nutrients 2015;7(5):3252–63.

[355] Wojcik J, Dudek D, Schlegel-Zawadzka M, et al. Antepartum/postpartum depressive symptoms and serum zinc and magnesium levels. Pharmacol Rep 2006;58(4):571–6.

[356] Styczeń K, Sowa-Kućma M, Siwek M, et al. The serum zinc concentration as a potential biological marker in patients with major depressive disorder. Metab Brain Dis 2017;32(1):97–103.

[357] DiSilvestro RA, Koch E, Rakes L. Moderately high dose zinc gluconate or zinc glycinate: effects on plasma zinc and erythrocyte superoxide dismutase activities in young adult women. Biol Trace Elem Res 2015;168(1):11–14.

[358] Zekavat OR, Karimi MY, Amanat A, et al. A randomised controlled trial of oral zinc sulphate for primary dysmenorrhoea in adolescent females. Aust N Z J Obstet Gynaecol 2015;55(4):369–73.

[359] Olausson H, Goldberg GR, Ann Laskey M, et al. Calcium economy in human pregnancy and lactation. Nutr Res Rev 2012;25(1): 40–67.

[360] Rebelo FM, Caldas ED. Arsenic, lead, mercury and cadmium: toxicity, levels in breast milk and the risks for breastfed infants. Environ Res 2016;151:671–88.

[361] Ettinger AS, Téllez-Rojo MM, Amarasiriwardena C, et al. Influence of maternal bone lead burden and calcium intake on levels of lead in breast milk over the course of lactation. Am J Epidemiol 2006;163(1):48–56.

[362] Hernandez-Avila MM. Dietary calcium supplements to lower blood lead levels in lactating women: a randomized placebo-controlled trial. Epidemiology 2003;14(2):206–12.

[363] Dórea JG. Magnesium in human milk. J Am Coll Nutr 2000;19(2):210–19.

[364] Walker AF, Marakis G, Christie S, et al. Mg citrate found more bioavailable than other Mg preparations in a randomised, double-blind study. Magnes Res 2003;16(3):183–91.

[365] Nishimura RY, Barbieiri P, de Castro GSF, et al. Dietary polyunsaturated fatty acid intake during late pregnancy affects fatty acid composition of mature breast milk. Nutrition 2014;30(6):685–9.

[366] Netting MJ, Middleton PF, Makrides M. Does maternal diet during pregnancy and lactation affect outcomes in offspring? A systematic review of food-based approaches. Nutrition 2014;30(11–12):1225–41.

[367] Gunaratne AW, Makrides M, Collins CT. Maternal prenatal and/or postnatal n-3 long chain polyunsaturated fatty acids (LCPUFA) supplementation for preventing allergies in early childhood. Cochrane Database Syst Rev 2015;(7):CD010085.

[368] Jia X, Pakseresht M, Wattar N, et al. Women who take n-3 long-chain polyunsaturated fatty acid supplements during pregnancy and lactation meet the recommended intake. Appl Physiol Nutr Metab 2015;40(5):474–81.

[369] Canfield LM, Clandinin MT, Davies DP, et al. Multinational study of major breast milk carotenoids of healthy mothers. Eur J Nutr 2003;42(3):133–41.

[370] Lipkie TE, Morrow AL, Jouni ZE, et al. Longitudinal survey of carotenoids in human milk from urban cohorts in China, Mexico, and the USA. PLoS ONE 2015;10(6):e0127729.

[371] Haftel L, Berkovich Z, Reifen R. Elevated milk β-carotene and lycopene after carrot and tomato paste supplementation. Nutrition 2015;31(3):443–5.

[372] Lietz G, Mulokozi G, Henry JCK, et al. Xanthophyll and hydrocarbon carotenoid patterns differ in plasma and breast milk of women supplemented with red palm oil during pregnancy and lactation. J Nutr 2006;136(7):1821–7.

[373] Khymenets O, Rabassa M, Rodriguez-Palmero M, et al. Dietary epicatechin is available to breastfed infants through human breast milk in the form of host and microbial metabolites. J Agric Food Chem 2016;64(26):5354–60.

[374] Shim JE, Kim J, Mathai RA. Associations of infant feeding practices and picky eating behaviors of preschool children. J Am Diet Assoc 2011;111(9):1363–8.

[375] Hausner H, Nicklaus S, Issanchou S, et al. Breastfeeding facilitates acceptance of a novel dietary flavour compound. Clin Nutr 2010;29(1):141–8.

[376] Cooke L, Fildes A. The impact of flavour exposure in utero and during milk feeding on food acceptance at weaning and beyond. Appetite 2011;57(3):808–11.

[377] Gomez-Gallego C, Garcia-Mantrana I, Salminen S, et al. The human milk microbiome and factors influencing its composition and activity. Semin Fetal Neonatal Med 2016;21(6):400–5.

[378] Hunt KM, Foster JA, Forney LJ, et al. Characterization of the diversity and temporal stability of bacterial communities in human milk. PLoS ONE 2011;6(6):e21313.

[379] Boix-Amorós A, Collado MC, Mira A. Relationship between milk microbiota, bacterial load, macronutrients, and human cells during lactation. Front Microbiol 2016;7:492.

[380] Fitzstevens JL, Smith KC, Hagadorn JI, et al. Systematic review of the human milk microbiota. Nutr Clin Pract 2016;32(3): 354–64.

[381] Urbaniak C, Angelini M, Gloor GB, et al. Human milk microbiota profiles in relation to birthing method, gestation and infant gender. Microbiome 2016;4:1.

[382] Khodayar-Pardo P, Mira-Pascual L, Collado MC, et al. Impact of lactation stage, gestational age and mode of delivery on breast milk microbiota. J Perinatol 2014;34(8):599–605.

[383] Cabrera-Rubio R, Mira-Pascual L, Mira A, et al. Impact of mode of delivery on the milk microbiota composition of healthy women. J Dev Orig Health Dis 2016;7(1):54–60.

[384] Garcia-Mantrana I, Collado MC. Obesity and overweight: impact on maternal and milk microbiome and their role for infant health and nutrition. Mol Nutr Food Res 2016;60(8):1865–75.

[385] Soto A, Martín V, Jiménez E, et al. Lactobacilli and bifidobacteria in human breast milk: influence of antibiotherapy and other host and clinical factors. J Pediatr Gastroenterol Nutr 2014;59(1):78–88.

[386] Mastromarino P, Capobianco D, Miccheli A, et al. Administration of a multistrain probiotic product (VSL#3) to women in the perinatal period differentially affects breast milk beneficial microbiota in relation to mode of delivery. Pharmacol Res 2015;95–96:63–70.

[387] Fernández L, Langa S, Martín V, et al. The human milk microbiota: origin and potential roles in health and disease. Pharmacol Res 2013;69(1):1–10.

[388] Gueimonde M, Sakata S, Kalliomaki M, et al. Effect of maternal consumption of lactobacillus GG on transfer and establishment of fecal bifidobacterial microbiota in neonates. J Pediatr Gastroenterol Nutr 2006;42(2):166–70.

[389] Rautava S, Kainonen E, Salminen S, et al. Maternal probiotic supplementation during pregnancy and breast-feeding reduces the risk of eczema in the infant. J Allergy Clin Immunol 2012;130(6):1355–60.

[390] Gil-Campos M, López MÁ, Rodriguez-Benítez MV, et al. Lactobacillus fermentum CECT 5716 is safe and well tolerated in infants of 1–6 months of age: a randomized controlled trial. Pharmacol Res 2012;65(2):231–8.

[391] Maldonado J, Canabate F, Sempere L, et al. Human milk probiotic Lactobacillus fermentum CECT5716 reduces the incidence of gastrointestinal and upper respiratory tract infections in infants. J Pediatr Gastroenterol Nutr 2012;54(1):55–61.

[392] Jiménez E, Fernández L, Maldonado A, et al. Oral Administration of lactobacillus strains isolated from breast milk as an alternative for the treatment of infectious mastitis during lactation. Appl Environ Microbiol 2008;74(15):4650–5.

[393] Reid G, Brigidi P, Burton JP, et al. Microbes central to human reproduction. Am J Reprod Immunol 2015;73(1):1–11.

[394] Ma Z, Guan Q, Ye C, et al. Network analysis suggests a potentially 'evil' alliance of opportunistic pathogens inhibited by a cooperative network in human milk bacterial communities. Sci Rep 2015;5:8275.

[395] Inman JL, Robertson C, Mott JD, et al. Mammary gland development: cell fate specification, stem cells and the microenvironment. Development 2015;142(6):1028–42.

[396] Brodribb W. Breastfeeding management in Australia. 4th ed. East Malvern: Australian Breastfeeding Association; 2012.

[397] Anderson SM, Rudolph MC, McManaman JL, et al. Key stages in mammary gland development. Secretory activation in the mammary gland: it's not just about milk protein synthesis! Breast Cancer Res 2007;9(1):204.

[398] Pang WW, Hartmann PE. Initiation of human lactation: secretory differentiation and secretory activation. J Mammary Gland Biol Neoplasia 2007;12(4):211–21.

[399] Saint L, Smith M, Hartmann PE. The yield and nutrient content of colostrum and milk of women from giving birth to 1 month post-partum. Br J Nutr 1984;52(1):87–95.

[400] ABM Clinical Protocol #3: hospital guidelines for the use of supplementary feedings in the healthy term breastfed neonate, revised 2009. Breastfeed Med 2009;4(3):175–82.

[401] Owens MB, Hill ADK, Hopkins AM. Ductal barriers in mammary epithelium. Tissue Barriers 2013;1(4):e25933.

[402] Stelwagen K, Singh K. The role of tight junctions in mammary gland function. J Mammary Gland Biol Neoplasia 2014;19(1):131–8.

[403] Dewey KG, Nommsen-Rivers LA, Heinig MJ, et al. Risk factors for suboptimal infant breastfeeding behavior, delayed onset of lactation, and excess neonatal weight loss. Pediatrics 2003;112(3):607–19.

[404] Nommsen-Rivers LA, Chantry CJ, Peerson JM, et al. Delayed onset of lactogenesis among first-time mothers is related to maternal obesity and factors associated with ineffective breastfeeding. Am J Clin Nutr 2010;92(3):574–84.

[405] Nommsen-Rivers LA, Dolan LM, Huang B. Timing of stage ii lactogenesis is predicted by antenatal metabolic health in a cohort of primiparas. Breastfeed Med 2011;7(1):43–9.

[406] Henderson JJ, Hartmann PE, Newnham JP, et al. Effect of preterm birth and antenatal corticosteroid treatment on lactogenesis ii in women. Pediatrics 2008;121(1):e92–100.

[407] Marasco LA. Unsolved mysteries of the human mammary gland: defining and redefining the critical questions from the lactation consultant's perspective. J Mammary Gland Biol Neoplasia 2014;19(3):271–88.

[408] Weiss R. Herbal medicine. Beaconsfield: Beasonsfield Publishers; 1956.

[409] Humphrey SR. Breastfeeding and botanical medicine. In: Romm A, editor. Botanical medicine for women's health. London: Churchill Livingstone; 2010. p. 433–55.

[410] Anonymous. Chasteberry. LactMed 2013.

[411] Mohr H. Clinical studies in increase of lactation. Dtsch Med Wochenschr 1954;79(41):1513–16.

[412] Merz PG, Gorkow C, Schrodter A, et al. The effects of a special Agnus castus extract (BP1095E1) on prolactin secretion in healthy male subjects. Exp Clin Endocrinol Diabetes 1996;104(6):447–53.

[413] Kilicdag EB, Tarim E, Bagis T, et al. Fructus agni casti and bromocriptine for treatment of hyperprolactinemia and mastalgia. Int J Gynaecol Obstet 2004;85(3):292–3.

[414] Milewicz A, Gejdel E, Sworen H, et al. [Vitex agnus castus extract in the treatment of luteal phase defects due to latent hyperprolactinemia. Results of a randomized placebo-controlled double-blind study]. Arzneimittelforschung 1993;43(7):752–6.

[415] Tamagno G, Burlacu MC, Daly AF, et al. Vitex agnus castus might enrich the pharmacological armamentarium for medical treatment of prolactinoma. Eur J Obstet Gynecol Reprod Biol 2007;135(1):139–40.

[416] Gallagher J, Lynch FW, Barragry J. A prolactinoma masked by a herbal remedy. Eur J Obstet Gynecol Reprod Biol 2008;137(2):257–8.

[417] Riordan JWK, editor. Breastfeeding and human lactation. 4th ed. Canada: Jones and Bartlett Publishers; 2010.

[418] Robinson GW, Hennighausen L, Johnson PF. Side-branching in the mammary gland: the progesterone–Wnt connection. Genes Dev 2000;14(8):889–94.

[419] Arbour MW, Kessler JL. Mammary hypoplasia: not every breast can produce sufficient milk. J Midwifery Womens Health 2013;58(4):457–61.

[420] Gardner H, Kent JC, Lai CT, et al. Milk ejection patterns: an intra-individual comparison of breastfeeding and pumping. BMC Pregnancy Childbirth 2015;15(1):156.

[421] Imani B. Alcohol and lactation. Asia Pac J Med Toxicol 2014;3(Suppl. 1):14.

[422] Tombeau Cost K, Unternaehrer E, Plamondon A, et al. Thinking and doing: the effects of dopamine and oxytocin genes and executive function on mothering behaviours. Genes Brain Behav 2017;16(2):285–95.

[423] Bell AF, Erickson EN, Carter CS. Beyond labor: the role of natural and synthetic oxytocin in the transition to motherhood. J Midwifery Womens Health 2014;59(1):35–42.

[424] Douglas P. Tongues tied about tongue-tie. Available from https://pameladouglas.com.au/sites/default/files/pdf/Tongues%20tied%20about%20tongue-tie_0.pdf.

[425] Riordan JWK, editor. Breastfeeding and human lactation. 4th ed. Sudbury, MA: Jones and Bartlett Publishers; 2010.

[426] Daly SE, Owens RA, Hartmann PE. The short-term synthesis and infant-regulated removal of milk in lactating women. Exp Physiol 1993;78(2):209–20.

[427] Ferreira M, Vaz T, Aparício G, et al. OC20 – skin-to-skin contact in the first hour of life. Nurs Child Young People 2016;28(4):69–70.

[428] Robiquet P, Zamiara P-E, Rakza T, et al. Observation of skin-to-skin contact and analysis of factors linked to failure to breastfeed within 2 hours after birth. Breastfeed Med 2016;11(3):126–32.

[429] Schafer R, Genna CW. Physiologic breastfeeding: a contemporary approach to breastfeeding initiation. J Midwifery Womens Health 2015;60(5):546–53.

[430] Widström AM, Lilja G, Aaltomaa-Michalias P, et al. Newborn behaviour to locate the breast when skin-to-skin: a possible method for enabling early self-regulation. Acta Paediatr 2011;100(1):79–85.

[431] Svensson KE, Velandia MI, Matthiesen A-ST, et al. Effects of mother-infant skin-to-skin contact on severe latch-on problems in older infants: a randomized trial. Int Breastfeed J 2013;8(1):1.

[432] Colson S. Does the mother's posture have a protective role to play during skin-to-skin contact? Research observations and theories. Clin Lact 2014;5(2):41–50.

[433] Doucet S, Soussignan R, Sagot P, et al. The 'smellscape' of mother's breast: effects of odor masking and selective unmasking on

neonatal arousal, oral, and visual responses. Dev Psychobiol 2007;49(2):129–38.

[434] Cleugh F, Langseth A. Fifteen-minute consultation on the healthy child: breast feeding. Arch Dis Child Educ Pract Ed 2016;102(1):8–13.

[435] Carothers C, Gribble K. Infant and young child feeding in emergencies. J Hum Lact 2014;30(3):272–5.

[436] Amir LH. Breastfeeding – managing 'supply' difficulties. Aust Fam Physician 2006;35(9):686–9.

[437] Gatti L. Maternal perceptions of insufficient milk supply in breastfeeding. J Nurs Scholarsh 2008;40(4):355–63.

[438] Hurst NM. Recognizing and treating delayed or failed lactogenesis II. J Midwifery Womens Health 2007;52(6):588–94.

[439] Noel-Weiss J, Woodend AK, Peterson WE, et al. An observational study of associations among maternal fluids during parturition, neonatal output, and breastfed newborn weight loss. Int Breastfeed J 2011;6:9.

[440] Okumus N, Atalay Y, Onal EE, et al. The effects of delivery route and anesthesia type on early postnatal weight loss in newborns: the role of vasoactive hormones. J Pediatr Endocrinol Metab 2011;24(1–2):45–50.

[441] Chantry CJ, Nommsen-Rivers LA, Peerson JM, et al. Excess weight loss in first-born breastfed newborns relates to maternal intrapartum fluid balance. Pediatrics 2011;127(1):e171–9.

[442] Sachs M, Dykes F, Carter B. Weight monitoring of breastfed babies in the UK – centile charts, scales and weighing frequency. Matern Child Nutr 2005;1(2):63–76.

[443] Spence JC. Decline of breast-feeding. BMJ 1938;2(4057):729–33.

[444] Hammarberg K, Fisher JRW, Wynter KH, et al. Breastfeeding after assisted conception: a prospective cohort study. Acta Paediatr 2011;100(4):529–33.

[445] Mortel M, Mehta SD. Systematic review of the efficacy of herbal galactagogues. J Hum Lact 2013;29(2):154–62.

[446] Raffo A, Nicoli S, Leclercq C. Quantification of estragole in fennel herbal teas: implications on the assessment of dietary exposure to estragole. Food Chem Toxicol 2011;49(2):370–5.

[447] Gori L, Gallo E, Mascherini V, et al. Can estragole in fennel seed decoctions really be considered a danger for human health? A Fennel Safety Updat. Evid Based Complement Alternat Med 2012;1–10.

[448] Bruckner C. A survey on herbal galactagogues used in Europe. Medicaments eT Aliments; L'Approche Ethnopharmacologique; 1993. Available from http://horizon.documentation.ird.fr/exl-doc/pleins_textes/pleins_textes_6/colloques2/010005528.pdf.

[449] Dioscorides. De Materia Medica 64CE. Available from www.cancerlynx.com/dioscorides.html.

[450] Cook W. The physiomedical dispensary; 1869.

[451] Lloyd F. King's American dispensatory; 1808.

[452] Culpeper N. Culpeper's complete herbal: a book of natural remedies for ancient ills. Great Britain: The Wordsworth Collection Reference Library; 1653. 1995.

[453] Humphrey S. The nursing mother's herbal. Minneapolis: Fairview Press; 2003.

[454] Salmon W. Botanologia; 1710.

[455] Miguel MG, Cruz C, Faleiro L, et al. Foeniculum vulgare essential oils: chemical composition, antioxidant and antimicrobial activities. Nat Prod Commun 2010;5(2):319–28.

[456] Türkyılmaz Z, Karabulut R, Sönmez K, et al. A striking and frequent cause of premature thelarche in children: foeniculum vulgare. J Pediatr Surg 2008;43(11):2109–11.

[457] Torabi Gudarzi M, Faramarz QGL, Abu Al-Fazl Y, et al. Investigation on to the effect of fennel (Foeniculum vulgare) and nigella (Nigella sativa) on production in milking cow. Qom Agricultural and Natural Resources Research Center, Qom (Iran) 2008;25.

[458] Nikolov P, Avramov NR. Investigations on the effect of Foeniculum vulgare, Carum carvi, Anisum vulgare, Crataegus oxyacanthus, and Galga officinalis on lactation. Izv Meditsinskite Inst Bulg Akad Naukite Sofia Otd Biol Meditsinski Nauki 1951;1:169–82.

[459] Fennel Lactmed [Internet] 2013 [cited 2013]. Available from http://toxnet.nlm.nih.gov/cgi-bin/sis/search/f?./temp/~8T1mrA:1.

[460] Turkyilmaz C, Onal E, Hirfanoglu IM, et al. The effect of galactagogue herbal tea on breast milk production and short-term catch-up of birth weight in the first week of life. J Altern Complement Med 2011;17(2):139–42.

[461] ABM Clinical Protocol #9: use of galactagogues in initiating or augmenting the rate of maternal milk secretion (first revision January 2011). Breastfeed Med 2011;6(1):41–9.

[462] Fæste CK, Namork E, Lindvik H. Allergenicity and antigenicity of fenugreek (Trigonella foenum-graecum) proteins in foods. J Allergy Clin Immunol 2009;123(1):187–94.

[463] Huggins KE. Fenugreek: one remedy for low milk production. Breastfeeding online. Available from http://www.breastfeedingonline.com/fenuhugg.shtml.

[464] Toppo FA, Akhand R, Pathak A. Pharmacological actions and potential uses of Trigonella foenum-graecum: a review. Asian J Pharm Clin Res 2009;2(4):30.

[465] Bingel F. Higher plants as potential sources of galactagogues. Econ Med Plant Res 1991;6:1–54.

[466] Schaffir J, Czapla C. Survey of lactation instructors on folk traditions in breastfeeding. Breastfeed Med 2012;7:230–3.

[467] Alamer MBG. Feeding effects of fenugreek seeds (Trigonella foenum-graecum L.) on lactation performance, some plasma constituents and growth hormone levels in goats. Pak J Biol Sci 2005;8(11):1553–6.

[468] Swafford B. Effect of fenugreek on breast milk volume. ABM News Views 2000;6(3):21.

[469] Reeder C, Legrand A, O'Conner-Von SK. The effect of fenugreek on milk production and prolactin levels in mothers of premature infants. J Hum Lact 2011;27(1):75.

[470] Damanik R, Wahlqvist M, Wattanapenpaiboon N. Lactagogue effects of Torbangun, a Bataknese traditional cuisine. Asia Pac J Clin Nutr 2006;15:267–74.

[471] Suksomboon N, Poolsup N, Boonkaew S, et al. Meta-analysis of the effect of herbal supplement on glycemic control in type 2 diabetes. J Ethnopharmacol 2011;137(3):1328–33.

[472] Abrol S, Trehan A, Katare OP. Comparative study of different silymarin formulations: formulation, characterisation and in vitro/in vivo evaluation. Curr Drug Deliv 2005;2(1):45–51.

[473] Song Y, Zhuang J, Guo J, et al. Preparation and properties of a silybin-phospholipid complex. Pharmazie 2008;63(1):35–42.

[474] Grieve M. A modern herbal. New York: Dover Publications; 1931.

[475] Capasso R, Aviello G, Capasso F, et al. Silymarin BIO-C, an extract from Silybum marianum fruits, induces hyperprolactinemia in intact female rats. Phytomedicine 2009;16(9):839–44.

[476] Tedesco D, Tava A, Galletti S, et al. Effects of silymarin, a natural hepatoprotector, in periparturient dairy cows. J Dairy Sci 2004;87(7):2239–47.

[477] Peila C, Coscia A, Tonetto P, et al. Evaluation of the galactagogue effect of silymarin on mothers of preterm newborns (<32 weeks). Pediatr Med Chir 2015;37(3).

[478] Di Pierro F, Callegari A, Carotenuto D, et al. Clinical efficacy, safety and tolerability of BIO-C (micronized Silymarin) as a galactagogue. Acta Biomed 2008;79(3):205–10.

[479] Zecca E, Zuppa AA, D'Antuono A, et al. Efficacy of a galactagogue containing silymarin-phosphatidylserine and galega in mothers of preterm infants: a randomized controlled trial. Eur J Clin Nutr 2016;70(10):1151–4.

[480] Remington W. Dispensatory of the United States of America; 1918.

[481] Sayre LE. A manual of organic materia medica; 1917.

[482] Weed S. Wise woman herbal for the childbearing year. New York: Ash Tree Publishing; 1986.

[483] Paritakul P, Ruangrongmorakot K, Laosooksathit W, et al. The effect of ginger on breast milk volume in the early postpartum period: a randomized, double-blind controlled trial. Breastfeed Med 2016;11(7):361–5.

[484] Aljazaf K, Hale TW, Ilett KF, et al. Pseudoephedrine: effects on milk production in women and estimation of infant exposure via breastmilk. Br J Clin Pharmacol 2003;56(1):18–24.

[485] Brauckmann BM, Latte KP. L-Dopa deriving from the beans of Vicia faba and Mucuna pruriens as a remedy for the treatment of Parkinson's disease. Schweiz Z Ganzheits Medizin 2010;22(5):292.

[486] Ahmed SN. Do favic patients resume fava beans ingestion later in their life, a study for this, and a new hypothesis for favism etiology. Hematol Oncol Stem Cell Ther 2013;6(1):9–13.

[487] Marasco W. The breastfeeding mothers guide to making more milk. Sydney: McGraw Hill; 2009.

[488] Dugoua J-J, Seely D, Perri D, et al. Safety and efficacy of chaste tree (Vitex agnus-castus) during pregnancy and lactation. Can J Clin Pharmacol 2008;15(1):e74–9.

[489] Abascal K, Yarnell E. Botanical galactagogues. Altern Complement Ther 2008;14(6):288–94.

[490] Westfall E. Galactagogue herbs: a qualitative study and review. Can J Midwifery Res Pract 2003;2(2):22.

[491] Luecha P, Umehara K, Miyase T, et al. Antiestrogenic constituents of the Thai medicinal plants Capparis flavicans and Vitex glabrata. J Nat Prod 2009;72(11):1954–9.

[492] Anderson PO, Valdes V. A critical review of pharmaceutical galactagogues. Breastfeed Med 2007;2(4):229–42.

[493] Marquis GS, Diaz J, Bartolini R, et al. Recognizing the reversible nature of child-feeding decisions: breastfeeding, weaning, and relactation patterns in a shanty town community of Lima, Peru. Soc Sci Med 1998;47(5):645–56.

[494] Patwari AK, Satyanarayana L. Relactation: an effective intervention to promote exclusive breastfeeding. J Trop Pediatr 1997;43(4):213–16.

[495] Lommen A, Brown B, Hollist D. Experiential perceptions of relactation. J Hum Lact 2015;31(3):498–503.

[496] Muresan M. Successful relactation – a case history. Breastfeed Med 2011;6(4):233–9.

[497] Kayhan-Tetik B, Baydar-Artantas A, Bozcuk-Guzeldemirci G, et al. A case report of successful relactation. Turk J Pediatr 2013;55(6):641–4.

[498] Szucs KA, Axline SE, Rosenman MB. Induced lactation and exclusive breast milk feeding of adopted premature twins. J Hum Lact 2010;26(3):309–13.

[499] Gribble KD. The influence of context on the success of adoptive breastfeeding: developing countries and the west. Breastfeed Rev 2004;12(1):5–13.

[500] Grawey AE, Marinelli KA, Holmes AV, et al. ABM Clinical Protocol #14: breastfeeding-friendly physician's office: optimizing care for infants and children, revised 2013. Breastfeed Med 2013;8(2):237–42.

[501] Bertino E, Giuliani F, Baricco M, et al. Benefits of donor milk in the feeding of preterm infants. Early Hum Dev 2013;89(Suppl. 2):S3–6.

[502] Flint A, New K, Davies MW. Cup feeding versus other forms of supplemental enteral feeding for newborn infants unable to fully breastfeed. Cochrane Database Syst Rev 2016;(8):CD005092.

[503] Avila WM, Pordeus IA, Paiva SM, et al. Breast and bottle feeding as risk factors for dental caries: a systematic review and meta-analysis. PLoS ONE 2015;10(11):e0142922.

[504] Ventura AK. Developmental trajectories of bottle-feeding during infancy and their association with weight gain. J Dev Behav Pediatr 2016;38(2):109–19.

[505] Shloim N, Vereijken CMJL, Blundell P, et al. Looking for cues – infant communication of hunger and satiation during milk feeding. Appetite 2017;108:74–82.

[506] Ventura AK, Mennella JA. An experimental approach to study individual differences in infants' intake and satiation behaviors during bottle-feeding. Child Obes 2017;13(1):44–52.

[507] Williams T, Nair H, Simpson J, et al. Use of donor human milk and maternal breastfeeding rates: a systematic review. J Hum Lact 2016;32(2):212–20.

[508] Arslanoglu S, Moro Guido E, Bellù R, et al. Presence of human milk bank is associated with elevated rate of exclusive breastfeeding in VLBW infants. J Perinat Med 2012;41(2):1–3.

[509] Walker S, Armstrong M. The four pillars of safe breast milk sharing. Midwifery Today Int Midwife 2012;101:34–7.

[510] ABM Clinical Protocol #8: human milk storage information for home use for full-term infants (original protocol March 2004; revision #1 March 2010). Breastfeed Med 2010;5(3):127–30.

[511] Belamarich PF, Bochner RE, Racine AD. A critical review of the marketing claims of infant formula products in the United States. Clin Pediatr (Phila) 2016;55(5):437–42.

[512] Berry NJ, Gribble KD. Health and nutrition content claims on websites advertising infant formula available in Australia: a content analysis. Matern Child Nutr 2016;13(4):e12383.

[513] Rosen-Carole C. Breastfeeding medicine physicians blogging about breastfeeding [Internet] 2015. Available from https://bfmed .wordpress.com/2015/06/16/two-lies-and-a-truth-formula-feeding -campaign-is-off-base/.

[514] Cederlund A, Kai-Larsen Y, Printz G, et al. Lactose in human breast milk an inducer of innate immunity with implications for a role in intestinal homeostasis. PLoS ONE 2013;8(1):e53876.

[515] Berni Canani R, Nocerino R, Terrin G, et al. Formula selection for management of children with cow's milk allergy influences the rate of acquisition of tolerance: a prospective multicenter study. J Pediatr 2013;163(3):771–7.e1.

[516] Boyle RJ, Ierodiakonou D, Khan T, et al. Hydrolysed formula and risk of allergic or autoimmune disease: systematic review and meta-analysis. BMJ 2016;352:i974.

[517] Michaelsen KF, Greer FR. Protein needs early in life and long-term health. Am J Clin Nutr 2014;99(3):718S–22S.

[518] Kaye J. Review of paediatric gastrointestinal physiology data relevant to oral drug delivery. Int J Clin Pharm 2011;33(1):20–4.

[519] Yokoi T. Essentials for starting a pediatric clinical study (1): pharmacokinetics in children. J Toxicol Sci 2009;34(Special): SP307–12.

[520] Baur LA, Allen JR. Goat milk for infants: yes or no? J Paediatr Child Health 2005;41(11):543.

[521] Koletzko B, Baker S, Cleghorn G, et al. Global standard for the composition of infant formula: recommendations of an ESPGHAN coordinated international expert group. J Pediatr Gastroenterol Nutr 2005;41(5):584–99.

[522] Kent G. Regulating fatty acids in infant formula: critical assessment of U.S. policies and practices. Int Breastfeed J 2014;9(1):2.

[523] Brodribb WE. Substitutes for breastmilk –weighing the risks. Breastfeed Med 2015;10(5):28.

[524] Monro JA, Leon R, Puri BK. The risk of lead contamination in bone broth diets. Med Hypotheses 2013;80(4):389–90.

[525] Le Huërou-Luron I, Blat S, Boudry G. Breast- v. formula-feeding: impacts on the digestive tract and immediate and long-term health effects. Nutr Res Rev 2010;23(1):23–36.

[526] Kramer MS, Kakuma R. Optimal duration of exclusive breastfeeding. Cochrane Database Syst Rev 2012;(8):CD003517.

[527] Ziegler DS, Russell SJ, Rozenberg G, et al. Goats' milk quackery. J Paediatr Child Health 2005;41(11):569–71.

[528] Moro PA, Benedetti M, Biban P, et al. A case of severe methemoglobinemia in a baby fed homemade decoction of silverbeet. Int J Case Rep Med 2013;2013.

[529] Basnet S, Schneider M, Gazit A, et al. Fresh goat's milk for infants: myths and realities – a review. Pediatrics 2010;125(4):e973–7.

[530] Hendriksz CJ, Walter JH. Feeding infants with undiluted goat's milk can mimic tyrosinaemia type 1. Acta Paediatr 2004;93(4):552–3.

[531] Hamrick HJ. Whole cow's milk, iron deficiency anemia, and hypoproteinemia: an old problem revisited. Arch Pediat Adolesc Med 1994;148(12):1351–2.

[532] Musilova S, Rada V, Vlkova E, et al. Beneficial effects of human milk oligosaccharides on gut microbiota. Benef Microbes 2014;5(3):273–83.

[533] Giovannini M, Verduci E, Gregori D, et al. Prebiotic effect of an infant formula supplemented with galacto-oligosaccharides: randomized multicenter trial. J Am Coll Nutr 2014;33(5):385–93.

[534] Osborn DA, Sinn JKH. Prebiotics in infants for prevention of allergy. Cochrane Database Syst Rev 2013;(3):CD006474.

[535] Veereman-Wauters G, Staelens S, Van de Broek H, et al. Physiological and bifidogenic effects of prebiotic supplements in infant formulae. J Pediatr Gastroenterol Nutr 2011;52(6):763–71.

[536] Closa-Monasterolo R, Gispert-Llaurado M, Luque V, et al. Safety and efficacy of inulin and oligofructose supplementation in infant formula: results from a randomized clinical trial. Clin Nutr 2013;32(6):918–27.

[537] López-Huertas E. Safety and efficacy of human breast milk Lactobacillus fermentum CECT 5716. A mini-review of studies with infant formulae. Benef Microbes 2015;6(2):219–24.

[538] Berni Canani R, Sangwan N, Stefka AT, et al. Lactobacillus rhamnosus GG-supplemented formula expands butyrate-producing bacterial strains in food allergic infants. ISME J 2016;10(3):742–50.

[539] Baldassarre ME, Laforgia N, Fanelli M, et al. Lactobacillus GG improves recovery in infants with blood in the stools and presumptive allergic colitis compared with extensively hydrolyzed formula alone. J Pediatr 2010;156(3):397–401.

[540] Rautava S, Salminen S, Isolauri E. Specific probiotics in reducing the risk of acute infections in infancy – a randomised, double-blind, placebo-controlled study. Br J Nutr 2008;101(11):1722–6.

[541] Hadley KB, Ryan AS, Forsyth S, et al. The essentiality of arachidonic acid in infant development. Nutrients 2016;8(4):216.

[542] Koletzko B, Carlson SE, van Goudoever JB. Should infant formula provide both omega-3 DHA and omega-6 arachidonic acid? Ann Nutr Metab 2015;66(2–3):137–8.

[543] Scott DT, Janowsky JS, Carroll RE, et al. Formula supplementation with long-chain polyunsaturated fatty acids: are there developmental benefits? Pediatrics 1998;102(5):e59.

[544] Auestad N, Scott DT, Janowsky JS, et al. Visual, cognitive, and language assessments at 39 months: a follow-up study of children fed formulas containing long-chain polyunsaturated fatty acids to 1 year of age. Pediatrics 2003;112(3):e177–83.

[545] Colombo J, Carlson SE, Cheatham CL, et al. Long-term effects of LCPUFA supplementation on childhood cognitive outcomes. Am J Clin Nutr 2013;98(2):403–12.

[546] Qawasmi A, Landeros-Weisenberger A, Bloch MH. Meta-analysis of LCPUFA supplementation of infant formula and visual acuity. Pediatrics 2013;131(1):e262–72.

[547] Tai EKK, Wang XB, Chen Z-Y. An update on adding docosahexaenoic acid (DHA) and arachidonic acid (AA) to baby formula. Food Funct 2013;4(12):1767–75.

[548] Kent J, Ashton E, Hardwick C, et al. Nipple pain in breastfeeding mothers: incidence, causes and treatments. Int J Environ Res Public Health 2015;12(10):12247.

[549] Berens P, Eglash A, Malloy M. ABM Clinical Protocol #26: persistent pain with breastfeeding. Breastfeed Med 2016;11(2):46–53.

[550] Lai W-L, Chuang H-S, Lee M-H. Inhibition of herpes simplex virus type 1 by thymol-related monoterpenoids. Planta Med 2012;78(15):1636–8.

[551] Yiannakopoulou E. Recent patents on antibacterial, antifungal and antiviral properties of tea. Recent Pat Antiinfect Drug Discov 2012;7(1):60–5.

[552] Cantatore A, Randall SD, Traum D, et al. Effect of black tea extract on herpes simplex virus-1 infection of cultured cells. BMC Complement Altern Med 2013;13:139.

[553] de Oliveira A, Adams SD, Lee LH, et al. Inhibition of Herpes Simplex Virus type 1 with the modified green tea polyphenol palmitoyl-epigallocatechin gallate. Food Chem Toxicol 2013;52:207–15.

[554] Mahajan BB, Dhawan M, Singh R. Herpes genitalis – topical zinc sulfate: an alternative therapeutic and modality. Indian J Sex Transm Dis 2013;34(1):32–4.

[555] Jones K. Review of sangre de drago (Croton lechleri) – a South American tree sap in the treatment of diarrhea, inflammation, insect bites, viral infections, and wounds: traditional uses to clinical research. J Altern Complement Med 2003;9(6):877–96.

[556] Çakici N, Fakkel TM, van Neck JW, et al. Systematic review of treatments for diabetic peripheral neuropathy. Diabet Med 2016;33(11):1466–76.

[557] Brown A, Rance J, Bennett P. Understanding the relationship between breastfeeding and postnatal depression: the role of pain and physical difficulties. J Adv Nurs 2016;72(2):273–82.

[558] Douglas PS. Rethinking 'posterior' tongue-tie. Breastfeed Med 2013;8(6):503–6.

[559] Amir LH. ABM Clinical Protocol #4: mastitis, revised March 2014. Breastfeed Med 2014;9(5):239–43.

[560] Fetherston C. Mastitis in lactating women: physiology or pathology? [corrected] [Published erratum appears in Breastfeed Rev 2001 Jul;9(2):21.]. Breastfeed Rev 2001;9(1):5–12.

[561] World Health Organization. Mastitis. Causes and management. Geneva, Switzerland: World Health Organization; 2000.

[562] Cullinane M, Amir LH, Donath SM, et al. Determinants of mastitis in women in the CASTLE study: a cohort study. BMC Fam Pract 2015;16:181.

[563] Wöckel A, Abou-Dakn M, Beggel A, et al. Inflammatory breast diseases during lactation: health effects on the newborn – a literature review. Mediators Inflamm 2008;2008(1):1–7.

[564] Wöckel A, Beggel A, Rücke M, et al. Predictors of inflammatory breast diseases during lactation – results of a cohort study. Am J Reprod Immunol 2010;63(1):28–37.

[565] Fetherston CM, Lai CT, Hartmann PE. Recurrent blocked duct(s) in a mother with immunoglobulin A deficiency. Breastfeed Med 2008;3(4):261–5.

[566] Mediano P, Fernández L, Rodríguez JM, et al. Case-control study of risk factors for infectious mastitis in Spanish breastfeeding women. BMC Pregnancy Childbirth 2014;14:195.

[567] Heikkila MP, Saris PE. Inhibition of Staphylococcus aureus by the commensal bacteria of human milk. J Appl Microbiol 2003;95(3):471–8.

[568] Amir LH, Griffin L, Cullinane M, et al. Probiotics and mastitis: evidence-based marketing? Int Breastfeed J 2016;11:19.

[569] Jahanfar S, Ng CJ, Teng CL. Antibiotics for mastitis in breastfeeding women. Cochrane Database Syst Rev 2013;(2):CD005458.

[570] Kvist LJ, Larsson BW, Hall-Lord ML, et al. The role of bacteria in lactational mastitis and some considerations of the use of antibiotic treatment. Int Breastfeed J 2008;3:1–7.

[571] Fahrni M, Schwarz EI, Stadlmann S, et al. Breast Abscesses: diagnosis, treatment and outcome. Breast Care (Basel) 2012;7(1):32–8.

[572] Maldonado-Lobón JA, Díaz-López MA, Carputo R, et al. Lactobacillus fermentum CECT 5716 reduces staphylococcus load in the breastmilk of lactating mothers suffering breast pain: a randomized controlled trial. Breastfeed Med 2015;10(9):425–32.

[573] Fernandez L, Cardenas N, Arroyo R, et al. Prevention of infectious mastitis by oral administration of Lactobacillus salivarius PS2 during late pregnancy. Clin Infect Dis 2016;62(5):568–73.

[574] Nelson CD, Reinhardt TA, Lippolis JD, et al. Vitamin D signaling in the bovine immune system: a model for understanding human vitamin D requirements. Nutrients 2012;4(3):181–96.

[575] Alva-Murillo N, Téllez-Pérez AD, Medina-Estrada I, et al. Modulation of the inflammatory response of bovine mammary epithelial cells by cholecalciferol (vitamin D) during Staphylococcus aureus internalization. Microb Pathog 2014;77:24–30.

[576] Nazeri P, Mirmiran P, Shiva N, et al. Iodine nutrition status in lactating mothers residing in countries with mandatory and voluntary iodine fortification programs: an updated systematic review. Thyroid 2015;25(6):611–20.

[577] Ghent WR, Eskin BA, Low DA, et al. Iodine replacement in fibrocystic disease of the breast. Can J Surg 1993;36(5):453–60.

[578] Kessler JH. The effect of supraphysiologic levels of iodine on patients with cyclic mastalgia. Breast J 2004;10(4):328–36.

[579] Zigo F, Farkasova Z, Elecko J, et al. Effect of parenteral administration of selenium and vitamin E on health status of mammary gland and on selected antioxidant indexes in blood of dairy cows. Pol J Vet Sci 2014;17(2):217–23.

[580] Kommisrud E, Østerås O, Vatn T. Blood selenium associated with health and fertility in Norwegian dairy herds. Acta Vet Scand 2005;46(4):229–40.

[581] Gao X, Zhang Z, Li Y, et al. Selenium deficiency facilitates inflammation following S. aureus infection by regulating TLR2-related pathways in the mouse mammary gland. Biol Trace Elem Res 2016;172(2):449–57.

[582] McGuire E. Case study: white spot and lecithin. Breastfeed Rev 2015;23(1):23–5.

[583] Mangesi L, Zakarija-Grkovic I. Treatments for breast engorgement during lactation. Cochrane Database Syst Rev 2016;(6):CD006946.

[584] Kujawa-Myles S, Noel-Weiss J, Dunn S, et al. Maternal intravenous fluids and postpartum breast changes: a pilot observational study. Int Breastfeed J 2015;10:18.

[585] Cotterman KJ. Reverse pressure softening: a simple tool to prepare areola for easier latching during engorgement. J Hum Lact 2004;20(2):227–37.

[586] Heise AM, Wiessinger D. Dysphoric milk ejection reflex: a case report. Int Breastfeed J 2011;6:6.

[587] Cunniff A, Spatz D. Mothers' weaning practices when infants breastfeed for more than one year. MCN Am J Matern Child Nurs 2016;42(2):88–94.

[588] Odom EC, Li R, Scanlon KS, et al. Reasons for earlier than desired cessation of breastfeeding. Pediatrics 2013;131(3):e726–32.

[589] Mathers LJ, Mathers RA, Brotherton DR. Herpes zoster in the T4 dermatome: a possible cause of breastfeeding strike. J Hum Lact 2007;23(1):70–1.

[590] Yoshida M, Shinohara H, Sugiyama T, et al. Taste of milk from inflamed breasts of breastfeeding mothers with mastitis evaluated using a taste sensor. Breastfeed Med 2014;9(2):92–7.

[591] Winchell K. Nursing strike: misunderstood feelings. J Hum Lact 1992;8(4):217.

[592] Ventresca Miller A, Hanks BK, Judd M, et al. Weaning practices among pastoralists: new evidence of infant feeding patterns from Bronze Age Eurasia. Am J Phys Anthropol 2016;162(3):409–22.

[593] Tsutaya T, Shimomi A, Nagaoka T, et al. Infant feeding practice in medieval Japan: stable carbon and nitrogen isotope analysis of human skeletons from Yuigahama-minami. Am J Phys Anthropol 2015;156(2):241–51.

[594] Bourbou C, Fuller BT, Garvie-Lok SJ, et al. Nursing mothers and feeding bottles: reconstructing breastfeeding and weaning patterns in Greek Byzantine populations (6th–15th centuries AD) using carbon and nitrogen stable isotope ratios. J Archaeol Sci 2013;40(11):3903–13.

[595] Brockway M, Venturato L. Breastfeeding beyond infancy: a concept analysis. J Adv Nurs 2016;72(9):2003–15.

[596] Tomori C, Palmquist AEL, Dowling S. Contested moral landscapes: negotiating breastfeeding stigma in breastmilk sharing, nighttime breastfeeding, and long-term breastfeeding in the U.S. and the U.K. Soc Sci Med 2016;168:178–85.

[597] Dowling S, Brown A. An exploration of the experiences of mothers who breastfeed long-term: what are the issues and why does it matter? Breastfeed Med 2012;8(1):45–52.

[598] Figueiredo B, Canário C, Field T. Breastfeeding is negatively affected by prenatal depression and reduces postpartum depression. Psychol Med 2014;44(5):927–36.

[599] Sharma V, Corpse CS. Case study revisiting the association between breastfeeding and postpartum depression. J Hum Lact 2008;24(1):77–9.

[600] Schmidt KA, Palmer BA, Frye MA. Mixed mania associated with cessation of breastfeeding. Int J Bipolar Disord 2016;4(1):18.

[601] Ball SJ, Pereira G, Jacoby P, et al. Re-evaluation of link between interpregnancy interval and adverse birth outcomes: retrospective cohort study matching two intervals per mother. BMJ 2014;349:g4333.

[602] Cleland J, Conde-Agudelo A, Peterson H, et al. Contraception and health. Lancet 2012;380(9837):149–56.

[603] Smith GCS, Pell JP, Dobbie R. Interpregnancy interval and risk of preterm birth and neonatal death: retrospective cohort study. BMJ 2003;327(7410):313.

[604] Van der Wijden C, Manion C. Lactational amenorrhoea method for family planning. Cochrane Database Syst Rev 2015;(10):CD001329.

[605] Jackson E, Glasier A. Return of ovulation and menses in postpartum nonlactating women: a systematic review. Obstet Gynecol 2011;117(3):657–62.

[606] Fabic MS, Choi Y. Assessing the quality of data regarding use of the lactational amenorrhea method. Stud Fam Plann 2013;44(2):205–21.

[607] Ishii H. Does breastfeeding induce spontaneous abortion? J Obstet Gynaecol Res 2009;35(5):864–8.

[608] Shaaban OM, Abbas AM, Abdel Hafiz HA, et al. Effect of pregnancy-lactation overlap on the current pregnancy outcome in women with substandard nutrition: a prospective cohort study. Facts Views Vis Obgyn 2015;7(4):213–21.

[609] Rowe H, Baker T, Hale TW. Maternal medication, drug use, and breastfeeding. Child Adolesc Psychiatr Clin N Am 2015;24(1):1–20.

[610] Sachs HC, Frattarelli DAC, Galinkin JL, et al. The transfer of drugs and therapeutics into human breast milk: an update on selected topics. Pediatrics 2013;132(3):e796–809.

[611] Saha MR, Ryan K, Amir LH. Postpartum women's use of medicines and breastfeeding practices: a systematic review. Int Breastfeed J 2015;10:28.

[612] Anderson PO, Manoguerra AS, Valdés V. A review of adverse reactions in infants from medications in breastmilk. Clin Pediatr (Phila) 2016;55(3):236–44.

[613] Brown A, Angus D, Chen S, et al. Costs and outcomes of chiropractic treatment for low back pain (structured abstract). Health Technol Assess Database 2005;2:88. http://www.cadth.ca/en/products/health-technology-assessment/publication/525.

[614] de Sá Del Fiol F, Barberato-Filho S, de Cássia Bergamaschi C, et al. Antibiotics and breastfeeding. Chemotherapy 2015;61(3):134–43.

[615] Lund M, Pasternak B, Davidsen RB, et al. Use of macrolides in mother and child and risk of infantile hypertrophic pyloric stenosis: nationwide cohort study. BMJ 2014;348:g1908.

[616] Mills S, Bone K. The essential guide to herbal safety. Chatswood. NSW: Elsevier Health Sciences; 2005.

[617] Gurley BJ, Fifer EK, Gardner Z. Pharmacokinetic herb–drug interactions (part 2): drug interactions involving popular botanical dietary supplements and their clinical relevance. Planta Med 2012;78(13):1490–514.

[618] Haastrup MB, Pottegård A, Damkier P. Alcohol and breastfeeding. Basic Clin Pharmacol Toxicol 2014;114(2):168–73.

[619] Mennella JA, Garcia-Gomez PL. Sleep disturbances after acute exposure to alcohol in mothers' milk. Alcohol 2001;25(3):153–8.

[620] Mennella JA, Gerrish CJ. Effects of exposure to alcohol in mother's milk on infant sleep. Pediatrics 1998;101(5):e2.

[621] Reece-Stremtan S, Marinelli KA. ABM Clinical Protocol #21: guidelines for breastfeeding and substance use or substance use disorder, revised 2015. Breastfeed Med 2015;10(3):135–41.

[622] May PA, Hasken JM, Blankenship J, et al. Breastfeeding and maternal alcohol use: prevalence and effects on child outcomes and fetal alcohol spectrum disorders. Reprod Toxicol 2016;63:13–21.

[623] Giglia RC. Alcohol and lactation: an updated systematic review. Nutr Diet 2010;67(4):237–43.

[624] Booker A, Jalil B, Frommenwiler D, et al. The authenticity and quality of Rhodiola rosea products. Phytomedicine 2016;23(7):754–62.

[625] Mudge EM, Betz JM, Brown PN. The importance of method selection in determining product integrity for nutrition research. Adv Nutr 2016;7(2):390–8.

[626] Metzman HL. Monograph of scutellaria lateriflora. J Am Herb Guild 2007;7(1):4–18.

[627] van den Berg M, Kypke K, Kotz A, et al. WHO/UNEP global surveys of PCDDs, PCDFs, PCBs and DDTs in human milk and benefit–risk evaluation of breastfeeding. Arch Toxicol 2017;91(1):83–96.

[628] Arendt M. Communicating human biomonitoring results to ensure policy coherence with public health recommendations: analysing breastmilk whilst protecting, promoting and supporting breastfeeding. Environ Health 2008;7(Suppl. 1):S6.

[629] Dórea JG. Alkylphenols and other pollutants contaminate human milk as well as cow's milk: formula feeding cannot abate exposure in nursing infants. Environ Int 2009;35(2):451.

[630] Mandour RA, Ghanem A-A, El-Azab SM. Correlation between lead levels in drinking water and mothers' breast milk: dakahlia, Egypt. Environ Geochem Health 2013;35(2):251–6.

[631] Castro F, Harari F, Llanos M, et al. Maternal–child transfer of essential and toxic elements through breast milk in a mine-waste polluted area. Am J Perinatol 2014;31(11):993–1002.

[632] Carignan CC, Karagas MR, Punshon T, et al. Contribution of breast milk and formula to arsenic exposure during the first year of life in a US prospective cohort. J Expo Sci Environ Epidemiol 2016;26(5):452–7.

[633] Mannetje A, Coakley J, Mueller JF, et al. Partitioning of persistent organic pollutants (POPs) between human serum and breast milk: a literature review. Chemosphere 2012;89(8):911–18.

[634] Gaxiola-Robles R, Labrada-Martagon V, Celis de la Rosa Ade J, et al. Interaction between mercury (Hg), arsenic (As) and selenium (Se) affects the activity of glutathione S-transferase in breast milk; possible relationship with fish and shellfish intake. Nutr Hosp 2014;30(2):436–46.

[635] Shawahna R, Zyoud A, Dwikat J, et al. Breast milk lead levels in 3 major regions of the West Bank of Palestine. J Hum Lact 2016;32(3):455–61.

[636] Levison J, Weber S, Cohan D. Breastfeeding and HIV-infected women in the United States: harm reduction counseling strategies. Clin Infect Dis 2014;59(2):304–9.

[637] Johnson G, Levison J, Malek J. Should providers discuss breastfeeding with women living with HIV in high-income countries? An ethical analysis. Clin Infect Dis 2016;63(10):1368–72.

[638] World Health Organization. Guideline: updates on HIV and infant feeding: the duration of breastfeeding, and support from health services to improve feeding practices among mothers living with HIV. Geneva: World Health Organization; 2016.

[639] Coovadia HM, Rollins NC, Bland RM, et al. Mother-to-child transmission of HIV-1 infection during exclusive breastfeeding in the first 6 months of life: an intervention cohort study. Lancet 2007;369(9567):1107–16.

[640] Palma P. Human breast milk: is it the best milk to prevent HIV transmission? J Virus Erad 2016;2(2):112–13.

[641] Wahl A, Baker C, Spagnuolo RA, et al. Breast milk of HIV-positive mothers has potent and species-specific in vivo hiv-inhibitory activity. J Virol 2015;89(21):10868–78.

[642] Altan AMD, Taafo F, Fopa F, et al. An assessment of option B implementation for the prevention of mother to child transmission in Dschang, Cameroon: results from the DREAM (Drug Resource Enhancement against AIDS and Malnutrition) cohort. Pan Afr Med J 2016;23:72.

[643] Rudzik AEF, Ball HL. Exploring maternal perceptions of infant sleep and feeding method among mothers in the United Kingdom: a qualitative focus group study. Matern Child Health J 2016;20(1):33–40.

[644] Blyton DM, Sullivan CE, Edwards N. Lactation is associated with an increase in slow-wave sleep in women. J Sleep Res 2002;11(4):297–303.

[645] Doan T, Gay CL, Kennedy HP, et al. Nighttime breastfeeding behavior is associated with more nocturnal sleep among first-time mothers at one month postpartum. J Clin Sleep Med 2014;10(3):313–19.

[646] Loutzenhiser L, Ahlquist A, Hoffman J. Infant and maternal factors associated with maternal perceptions of infant sleep problems. J Reprod Infant Psychol 2011;29:doi:10.1080/02646838.2011.653961.

[647] Rudzik AE. Normal infant sleep and parental expectations. Int J Birth Parent Educ 2015;2(2):7–10.

[648] Galland BC, Taylor BJ, Elder DE, et al. Normal sleep patterns in infants and children: a systematic review of observational studies. Sleep Med Rev 2012;16(3):213–22.

[649] Keene Woods N. 'Same room, safe place': the need for professional safe sleep unity grows at the expense of families. J Prim Care Community Health 2017;8(2):94–6.

[650] Carlin RF, Moon RY. Risk factors, protective factors, and current recommendations to reduce sudden infant death syndrome: a review. JAMA Pediatr 2017;171(2):175–80.

[651] Whittingham K, Douglas P. Optimizing parent–infant sleep from birth to 6 months: a new paradigm. Infant Ment Health J 2014;35(6):614–23.

[652] Moon RY, Darnall RA, Feldman-Winter L, et al. SIDS and other sleep-related infant deaths: updated 2016 recommendations for a safe infant sleeping environment. Pediatrics 2016;138(5).

[653] Fleming P, Pease A, Blair P. Bed-sharing and unexpected infant deaths: what is the relationship? Paediatr Respir Rev 2015;16(1):62–7.

[654] McKenna JJ, Mosko S, Dungy C, et al. Sleep and arousal patterns of co-sleeping human mother/infant pairs: a preliminary physiological study with implications for the study of sudden infant death syndrome (SIDS). Am J Phys Anthropol 1990;83(3):331–47.

[655] McKenna JJ, Gettler LT. There is no such thing as infant sleep, there is no such thing as breastfeeding, there is only breastsleeping. Acta Paediatr 2016;105(1):17–21.

[656] Smith LA, Geller NL, Kellams AL, et al. Infant sleep location and breastfeeding practices in the United States, 2011–2014. Acad Pediatr 2016;16(6):540–9.

[657] Ball HL, Howel D, Bryant A, et al. Bed-sharing by breastfeeding mothers: who bed-shares and what is the relationship with breastfeeding duration? Acta Paediatr 2016;105(6):628–34.

[658] Ateah CA, Hamelin KJ. Maternal bedsharing practices, experiences, and awareness of risks. J Obstet Gynecol Neonatal Nurs 2008;37(3):274–81.

[659] Kendall-Tackett K, Cong Z, Hale TW. Mother–infant sleep locations and nighttime feeding behavior: US data from the Survey of Mothers' Sleep and Fatigue. Clin Lact 2010;1(1):27–31.

[660] La Leche League International. The Safe Sleep Seven for safer bed sharing 2018. Available from https://www.llli.org/the-safe-sleep-seven/.

15

Infancy

Tabitha McIntosh, Dawn Whitten, Helen Padarin

INTRODUCTION

Infants are inextricably connected to their mothers or main caregivers, and the significance of the first year of life out of the womb is exceptional, and formative of future health outcomes. A mother's instinct when it comes to her own child's needs provides the healthcare provider with valuable information, and it is important to validate a mother or father's concerns about their infant, if concerns arise. Infants respond very well to subtle naturopathic treatment, in particular when treatment is delivered via the breastfeeding mother. A collaborative approach when caring for an infant is necessary as naturopaths do not have the specific clinical training necessary for acute infant care. Immediate referral to a GP or emergency department is paramount for any acute presentation of the infant, and for that reason we discuss in this chapter potential red flags to be aware of.

Infants are also inextricably connected to their immediate environment, and can be sensitive to the surrounding energy/emotions/pace of life. For further reading on neonates' and infants' exquisite vulnerability to environmental chemicals in their local environment, refer to Chapter 2: Environmental Medicine.

Early life experiences such as mode of delivery, breastfeeding and nutrition are cornerstones of lifelong health, and have long-lasting impacts throughout life. Promoting and protecting breastfeeding is a priority intervention for the health of the infant and the mother[1,2] (see Chapter 14: Breastfeeding). The infant who is suboptimally breastfed is at greater risk of infection, chronic disease and poorer neurocognitive function.[2-4]

Educating new parents on healthy eating practices and lifestyle choices, and the appropriate introduction of solid foods will impact on health outcomes of these future adults. In the case of suboptimal health or illness, breastfeeding support, a naturopathic approach and specific dietary guidance can have profound effects on the infant's recovery. Treatments must always be tailored to be suitable for infants, keeping in mind that infants are not just little adults. Infants have different nutritional needs to cope with the rapid adaptation, growth and development that occurs particularly in the first year of life, as well as immature digestive and metabolic capacity, and throughout this chapter we will discuss appropriate foods to introduce and nourish growing infants.

GOOD REFERRAL PRACTICE

Infants lack the cardiorespiratory and metabolic reserves of adults and older children, and hence they can quickly decompensate and become critically unwell. Prompt referral practice is essential in the provision of care to infants. Failure to appropriately refer can be devastating. The traffic light tool created by The National Institute for Health and Care Excellence (NICE) (see Table 15.1) for the assessment of febrile infants provides a good base for clinical decisions about referral for both febrile and non-febrile infants. Any infant displaying signs consistent with the middle and far right (orange and red) column should be referred to a medical practitioner or emergency department, respectively. Febrile infants under the age of 3 months need to be referred for medical assessment that day because the risk of a serious cause is high. Urinary tract infections should be ruled out in any infant who is febrile. Parental perception that something is wrong is an important red flag and correlates with higher likelihood of serious illness.[6,7]

Children with any features from the middle column should be referred to a medical practitioner and those from the far right should be referred to an accident and emergency department. Any infant with a fever should be assessed for a urinary tract infection, even in the absence of features from the middle and right-hand column.

Neonates (infants less than 1 month old) are at the highest risk of mortality. Clinical presentations can relate to congenital or acquired causes. Preterm birth (<37 weeks) and low-birth-weight (<2500 g) infants are even more vulnerable, with greater risk of mortality and long-term morbidity.[8]

Practitioners also need to be on the lookout for evidence of inadequate intake (see Box 15.1) and/or feeding issues (see also Chapter 14) that require prompt referral to a lactation consultant or paediatrician. A detailed history of stool and urinary output is of value, particularly because poor weight gain does not necessarily indicate poor intake or poor breast milk supply. When assessing weight gain and growth the World Heath Organization's (WHO) charts are the appropriate

TABLE 15.1 Traffic light table for assessing risk of serious illness in feverish children aged <5 years old

	Green – low risk	Amber – intermediate risk	Red – high risk
Colour (of skin, lips or tongue)	Normal colour	Pallor reported by parent or carer	Pale, mottled, ashen or blue
Activity	Responds normally to social cues Content or smiles Stays awake or awakens quickly Strong normal cry or not crying	Not responding normally to social cues No smile Wakes only with prolonged stimulation Decreased activity	No response to social cues Appears ill to a healthcare professional Does not wake, or if roused, does not stay awake Weak, high-pitched or continuous cry
Respiratory		Nasal flaring Tachypnoea: respiratory rate (RR) >50 breaths/min at ages 6–12 months RR >40 breaths/min at ages >12 months Oxygen saturation ≥95% in air Crackles in the chest	Grunting Tachypnoea: RR >60 breaths/min Moderate or severe chest indrawing
Circulation and hydration	Normal skin and eyes Moist mucous membranes	Tachycardia: >160 beats/min at age <12 months >150 beats/min at age 12–24 months >140 beats/min at age 2–5 years Capillary refill time ≥3 seconds Dry mucous membranes Poor feeding in infants Reduced urine output	Reduced skin turgor
Other	None of the amber or red symptoms or signs	Temperature ≥39°C at ages 3–6 months Fever for ≥5 days Rigors (see definitions box) Swelling of limb or joint Non-weight-bearing limb or not using an extremity	Temperature ≥38°C at age >3 months Non-blanching rash Bulging fontanel Neck stiffness Status epilepticus Focal neurological signs Focal seizures

Source: Fields E, Chard J, Murphy MS, et al. Assessment and initial management of feverish illness in children younger than 5 years: summary of updated NICE guidance. BMJ 2013;346:f2866.[5]

BOX 15.1 Assessing infant intake

Stool and urinary output: 'what goes in must come out'.

In breastfed infants greater than 5 days old, good intake is indicated by:

- Stool output:
  - 2–3+ substantial (at least 3 cm^2) runny or loose yellow stools/24 hours[9]

  or
  - stools with most feeds[10]

  Note: after 4–6 weeks, this is no longer a good indicator, with some thriving exclusively breastfed infants going only once every 10 days.

- Urinary output:*
  - 5+ disposable (or 6–8 very wet cloth) nappies/24 hrs
  - pale and odourless[10]

  Note: maternal ingestion of riboflavin (B$_2$) can cause yellow pigmentation of breastfed infants' urine

  Growth and appropriate weight gain:
- WHO growth charts needs to be used – these are based on breastfed babies' growth patterns (see Figs 15.1–15.4)
- Poor weight gain could be due to illness or weighing error (see Box 15.2)

*Urinary output is a particularly reliable sign of intake.

---

standard as they are based on breastfeeding populations (see Figs 15.1–15.4; these are available from http://www.who.int/childgrowth/standards/height_for_age/en/). In addition to infants with poor weight gain, infants with growth in length disproportionate to weight (e.g. 90th percentile for length and 20th for weight or 50th for length and 3rd for weight) should be referred for assessment.[10]

Poor weighing technique (see Box 15.2) is a frequent cause of erroneously diagnosed poor weight gain, which unfortunately may result in inappropriate use of breast milk substitutes. Further, poor weight gain may be secondary to other causes such as allergy, infection and congenital heart defect. These may impact infants' feeding efficacy, energy utilisation, or result in malabsorption.

Text continued on p. 538

Weight-for-age GIRLS

Birth to 2 years (percentiles)

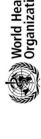
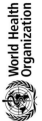

World Health Organization

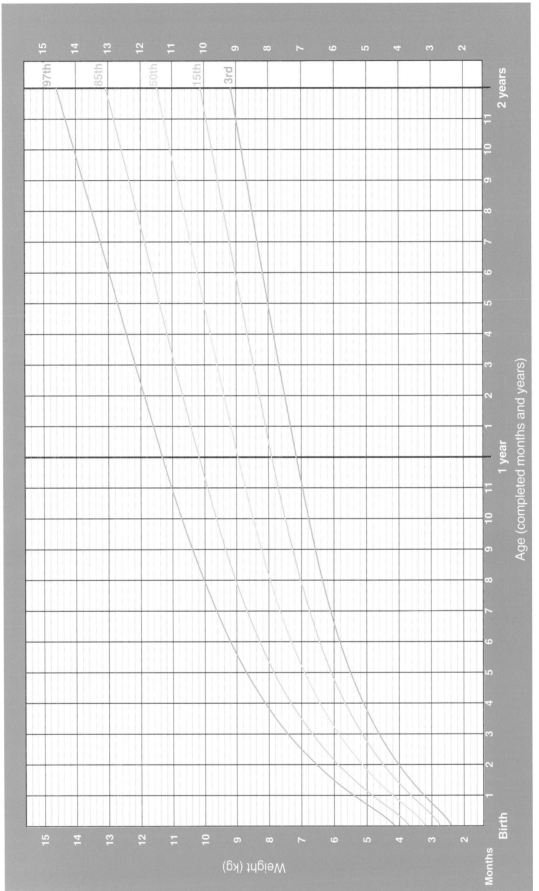

WHO Child Growth Standards

FIGURE 15.1 Weight-for-age girls

http://www.who.int/childgrowth/standards/cht_wfa_girls_p_0_2.pdf?ua=1

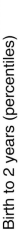

Weight-for-age BOYS

Birth to 2 years (percentiles)

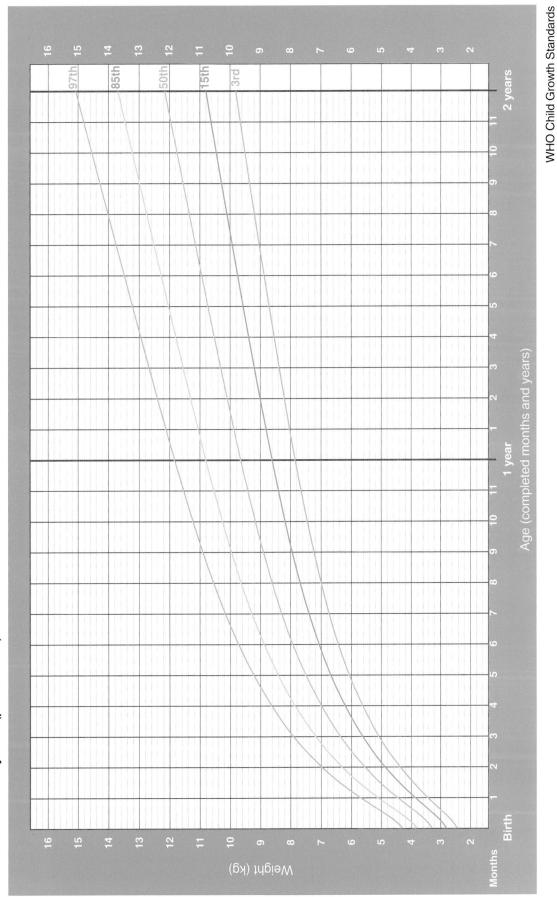

FIGURE 15.2 Weight-for-age boys

http://www.who.int/childgrowth/standards/cht_wfa_boys_p_0_2.pdf?ua=1

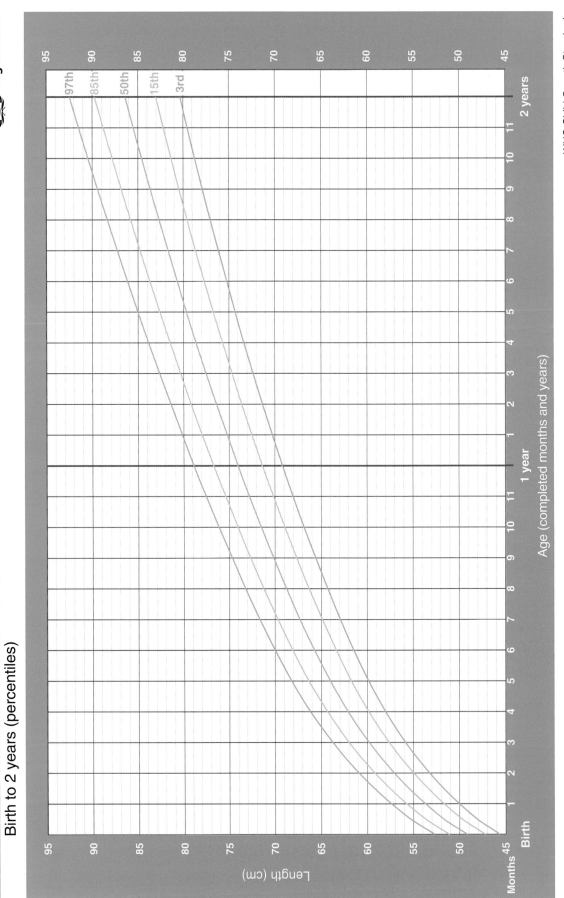

Length-for-age GIRLS
Birth to 2 years (percentiles)

FIGURE 15.3 Length-for-age girls

http://www.who.int/childgrowth/standards/cht_lfa_girls_p_0_2.pdf?ua=1

Length-for-age BOYS

Birth to 2 years (percentiles)

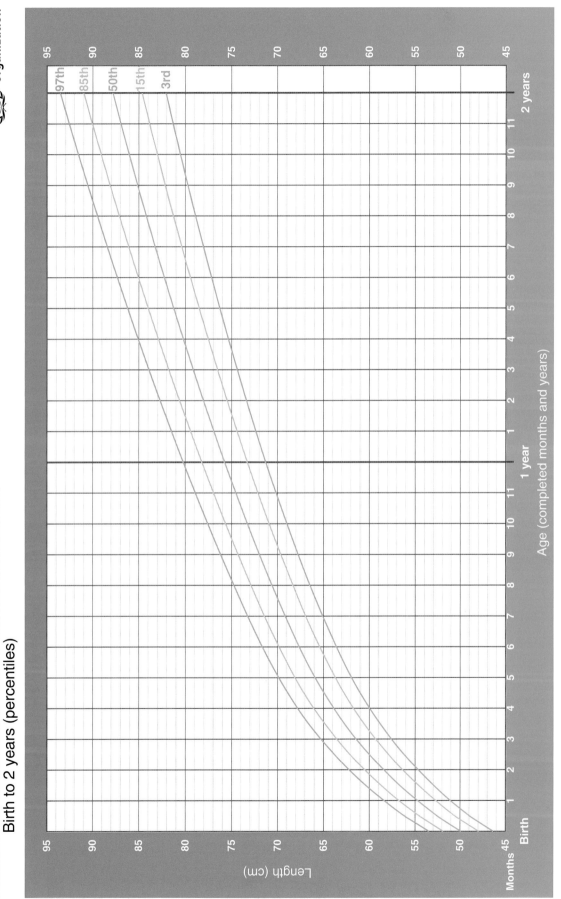

FIGURE 15.4 Length-for-age boys
http://www.who.int/childgrowth/standards/cht_lfa_boys_p_0_2.pdf?ua=1

Developmental milestones give an approximate guide to normal infant development (see Table 15.2 and discussion below). Any infant who is not meeting these developmental milestones should be sensitively referred for assessment to a paediatrician. Table 15.3 summarises referral guidelines relating to different clinical presentations.

BOX 15.2 Common causes of weighing errors

Weighing errors

- Causes of error include[11,12]:
  - Use of different scales
  - Poor weighing technique
  - Scale faults (common)
  - Varying timing of weighing in relation to feeding, bowel movement or void
    - > A large void and stool combination may weigh 100 g
  - Weighing more often than fortnightly carries the risk that variations do not reflect true weight change
- Scale measurements need to be considered in the context of the infant's total health picture
- Other indicators of intake need to be considered (urinary and stool output) and visual assessment

---

THE FOURTH TRIMESTER: THE NEWBORN 0–3 MONTHS

The first 3 months postnatally are often referred to colloquially as the 'fourth trimester'. This time presents a unique opportunity for the infant to bond with parents/family/siblings, and for the establishment of a sense of parental confidence with understanding and responding to baby's cues, cries and rhythms (if any). This time immediately postnatally is also pivotal to nurturing the development and composition of the residing microbes at different body sites such as the gastrointestinal system and the skin. For this reason, minimal intervention in terms of bathing and washing with commercially available baby products (baby shampoos, fragranced wipes, baby soaps and bubble baths), which may disrupt the skin or genitourinary microbiome, is recommended.

The human infant is born developmentally immature compared to many other mammals. The fourth trimester describes an 'extra-uterine trimester' where there is rapid neurodevelopment and social learning. Breastfeeding provides an extra-uterine link between the mother and

---

TABLE 15.2 Developmental milestones 0–5			
Communication and language milestones	**Average age**	**Developmental milestones (tasks)**	**Average age**
Social smile	6 weeks	Sits without support	5–8 months
Cooing	3 months	Crawls	6–9 months
Turns to voice	4 months	Puts everything into mouth	4–8 months
Babbles	6–9 months	Pulls to standing position	6–10 months
'Mamma'/'Dadda' (no meaning)	8–9 months	First tooth	6–9 months
'Mamma'/'Dadda' (with meaning)	10–18 months	Walks holding on	7–13 months
Understands several words	1 year	Drinks from cup	10–15 months
Speaks single words	12–15 months	Waves goodbye	8–12 months
Points to body parts	14–22 months	Climbs stairs	14–20 months
Able to name one body part	18 months	Turns pages	2 years
Combines two words	14–24 months	Scribbles	1–2 years
Speaks six or more words	12–20 months	Uses a spoon	14–24 months
Able to name five body parts	2 years	Puts on clothing	21–26 months
Has 50-word vocabulary	2 years	Buttons up	30–42 months
Uses pronouns (me, you, I)	2 years	Jumps on spot	20–30 months
Developmental milestones (tasks)	**Average age**	Rides a tricycle	21–36 months
Follows eyes past the midline	6 weeks	Bowel control	18 months–4 years
Smiles	6 weeks	Bladder control (day)	18 months–4 years
Bears weight on legs with support	3–7 months	Clear hand preference	2–5 years
Sits with support	4–6 months		

Source: Oberklaid F, Drever K. Is my child normal? Milestones and red flags for referral. *Australian Family Physician* 2011;40:666–70.[13]

TABLE 15.3 Referral guideline summary for different clinical presentations

Presentation	Refer to
ANY signs of being acutely unwell: • Fever in <12-week-old • Traffic light signs (see Table 15.1) • Bulging or sunken fontanel • Drowsy; low tone or 'floppy baby' • High-pitched, prolonged screaming • Projectile vomiting • Breathing difficulty • Altered skin tones (pale/ashen/mottled) • Parent concerned something is wrong	Hospital emergency department (or immediate appointment with paediatrician or child-focused doctor) • URGENT – within hours
Signs of inadequate milk intake: • Low number of stools or voids • Mother reports nipple pain • Poor weight gain/slowed growth Evidence of feeding difficulties – always needs to be ruled out	Lactation consultant (International Board Certified Lactation Consultant) • FAST – within a day or two
Delay to meet milestones Poor weight gain/slowed growth	GP or paediatrician (with breastfeeding knowledge) • Prompt – timing based on severity

child, maintaining immune protection and developmental programming (see Chapter 14). The newborn human infant is often soothed by experiences that are womb-like, and maintains better cardiorespiratory stability[14] and lower stress hormone profiles[15] when in physical contact with their parent.

Baby wearing provides infants with many of the womb comforts and further supports good breast milk supply, sensory nourishment of the infant and parental freedom and mobility. The rhythmic motion the infant experiences through parental walking has a direct calming effect on the infant and is thought to support neurodevelopment.[16,17] Providing information on safe baby wearing may help parents feel more confident to initiate this.

Parents can be reassured by having a concept of the range of normal when it comes to infant sleeping, feeding and crying behaviour. The stomach volume of the newborn is approximately 20 mL,[18] and this volume grows over the early weeks. The average intake per feed on days one and three is 2–10 mL and 30–60 mL, respectively.[19] Because of small stomach capacity and the digestibility of breast milk, newborns feed frequently to meet their needs, and often feed most of their waking hours during the early weeks.[18] It has been proposed that the newborn stomach volume, digestibility and transit time of breast milk, cholecystokinin release and sleep cycle length indicate that it is normal for newborns to feed at least hourly.[18] Many infants cluster feed, particularly in the evening, feeding frequently for a period of time usually prior to having a longer sleep. Cluster feeding may enable the infant to access more lipid-rich hind milk, stimulate greater

cholecystokinin release in the infant and stimulate maternal milk supply. The infant feeds more effectively when early feeding cues are responded to (see Chapter 14). Frequent feeding is also important for establishing maternal milk supply, and more frequent feeding during the early weeks correlates with better milk supply in established lactation.[20]

Sleep needs of infants vary widely[21,22] and change based on development, sensory nourishment, illness and in relation to the breastfeeding dyad. Night-time parenting can be a source of anxiety for parents, and many parents may perceive their infants to have sleeping problems based on cultural beliefs (for further discussion see Chapter 14). Infant crying and fussing is discussed later in this chapter.

ARRIVAL

According to the Australian Institute of Health and Welfare,[23] the average gestational age for all Australian babies is 38.7 weeks, with the vast majority (91%) born at term (37–41 weeks).

On average, less than 10% of babies are born pre term, with most of these births occurring at gestational ages of between 32 and 36 completed weeks. Pre-term birth (before 37 completed weeks of gestation) is associated with a higher risk of adverse neonatal outcomes.[23]

Multiple pregnancies represent approximately 1.5% of all pregnancies, almost all (98%) of which are twins. A small proportion (2%) are other multiples (i.e. triplets, quadruplets or higher). The proportion of multiple pregnancies increases with maternal age and use of assisted reproductive technology (ART). For example, the proportion of multiple pregnancies in 2013 among mothers who received ART was seven times higher than for mothers who did not receive ART treatment (8.4% compared to 1.2%).[23]

A baby's birth weight is a key indicator of future infant health and a determinant of a baby's chances of survival and health later in life. In 2013, the mean birth weight of live born babies was 3355 g, with the vast majority of babies born in the normal-birth-weight range (92%); less than 7% of babies tend to be low birth weight; and a smaller proportion again (less than 2%) tend to be high birth weight.[23]

GROWTH AND DEVELOPMENT

After arrival, the first 3 months of life are primarily characterised by intensely rapid growth and adaptation. From the moment of birth, the neonate is thrust into a variable environment – hot and cold, dark and light, hunger and satiety – in contrast to the heavily regulated environment in the uterus. This places great stress on the infant, an important aspect of development, as all the organ systems learn to adapt to an ever-changing environment.

The Academy of Breastfeeding Medicine (ABM) states that in the days following birth, 'The normal maximal weight loss is 5.5–6.6% of birth weight in optimally exclusively breastfed infants.'[19] This may occur as a function of fluid loss. According to the ABM, equal to or greater than 7% weight loss over the first week post birth indicates a need for careful assessment of the breastfeeding dyad and could indicate insufficient breast milk intake.[19] Refer to Chapter 14 for more on this.

Noel-Weiss et al. suggested that baseline birth weights are better assessed 24 hours post birth to allow for initial fluid loss.[24] They found that higher urinary output was associated with greater weight loss over this 24-hour period, indicating that weight loss in the first 24 hours is not an accurate indication of intake. Further, increased maternal IV fluid may be a factor influencing 24-hour weight loss.[25] Weight loss after 24 hours correlates more closely with poor intake.

Two weeks into life an infant's weight gain should be at least 500 g per 4 weeks, averaging 15–30 g per day, although gains will vary week to week over each month. Brodribb indicates that average gain of less than 105 g per week, or any unexplained weight loss, in infants aged 2–12 weeks should prompt quick referral to a lactation specialist (to assess for feeding issues including latch and supply) and GP or paediatrician to assess for underlying health issues[10] (see above referral guidelines). Similarly, infants dropping down growth chart percentile lines and/or with disproportionately low weight for height should be assessed.

Weight gain can be variable, erratic and very individual, and to compound this, there is much room for error with the weighing process (see Box 15.2). Weighing infants more often than fortnightly increases the risk of weight variations not reflecting true weight change and can cause undue worry for the parents. Furthermore, other indicators of intake and health need to be considered alongside weight gain as discussed above and in Box 15.1. It is appropriate to use the WHO growth charts when assessing weight and growth in infants as these have been developed using breastfeeding populations (see Figs 15.1–15.4). Breastfed infants have different growth patterns from formula-fed infants. Interestingly, some breastfed infants will gain weight more rapidly during the first few months of life, with weight gains as high as 800 g per week, and then slow their gain at around 3–4 months of age.[10] WHO data indicate that birth weight of breastfed infants doubles at 4 months and triples at 13 and 15 months in boys and girls, respectively.[26] The WHO growth charts are considered the normative standard, and hence are an appropriate standard for assessing the growth of both breastfed and formula-fed infants.[27] Formula feeding should aim to promote a similar growth pattern to breastfeeding. The accelerated weight gain observed in some formula-fed infants is considered a deviation from normative growth, and may contribute to the development of obesity.[28]

In the first month of life, jerky primitive reflexes dominate movement, with little or no purposeful movement. Limbs are flexed and fists will clench around anything put into the hand. By the end of the first month, movements will begin to become smoother and a little coordinated.

Around 3 months of age, an infant will begin to raise their head and chest and then support their upper body with their arms when lying on their stomach. Movements become much more coordinated. Physical growth continues rapidly – rolling and briefly sitting at 6 months, pivoting with support of arms while on stomach at 7 months, crawling on stomach and pulling self to standing between 7 and 9 months. Vision is close to fully developed at 8 months. Development of fine motor skills begins from 9 months with acquiring the skill of the pincer grip. At 10 months, most infants competently crawl on hands and knees and are able to walk with the aid of furniture or with hands being held.

By 12 months of age, an infant can usually stand upright without support and may begin to walk unassisted. They begin to use words meaningfully and attempt simple conversation (babble!).

SHAPING THE EARLY INTESTINAL MICROBIOTA

There is a growing recognition that the development and composition of the human microbiome in infants may have important consequences for human health, immune capacity and tolerance, and disease susceptibilities later in life.[29] Infants' skin, gastrointestinal systems and genitourinary systems are colonised with microbial communities that undergo dynamic change during development, with the most dramatic changes in composition believed to occur throughout infancy and early childhood.

The healthy microbiota of the infant gastrointestinal tract (GIT) acts as a physical barrier between the host and the external environment as well as a contact point for pathogenic organisms in the digestive tract, competitively inhibiting the colonisation of pathogenic microorganisms.[30] Other functions of the microbiota include modulation of the immune system, potentially protection against atopic development, and up-regulating non-specific immunity and immunoglobulin A (IgA) production. Health and diversity of the infant microbiota is also critical to improving nutritional status via the production of enzymes, vitamins (especially B vitamins and biotin), enhancing absorption of minerals and polyunsaturated fatty acids, the pre-digestion of foods and regulation of gut-associated lymphoid tissue (GALT) among other major endocrine, neurological and immunological functions.[31,32]

Both genetic and environmental factors shape the infant's unique gut microbiota. The dogma that the fetus resides in a sterile environment is being challenged by recent findings and with the advancement of microbial gene sequencing assessment techniques. For decades, it was believed that the uterine environment was sterile – that the amniotic sac, and the fluid that surrounded the embryo/fetus, was a uniquely pristine environment devoid of any bacteria in order to protect the growing embryo/fetus, which still does not have a fully developed immune system. The conventional wisdom was that the baby's first exposure to bacteria began during the birth process, from the mother's birth canal, and continued through the infant's skin-to-skin contact with the mother and from its

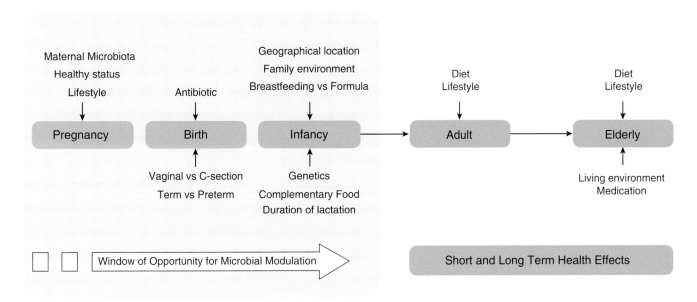

FIGURE 15.5 Factors influencing the infant gut microbiota development and the adult and elderly microbiota.

Rodríguez JM, Murphy K, Stanton C, et al. The composition of the gut microbiota throughout life, with an emphasis on early life. Microbial ecology in health and disease 2015;26.[33]

new environment. But in recent years, this understanding has been challenged – scientists have been able to detect small amounts of bacteria in the amniotic fluid and in the placenta, and even in the fetus' intestines. Meconium, which was previously presumed sterile, has been found to harbour a complex microbial community, supporting the idea that the baby's microbiome actually begins establishing itself before birth.[33] See Fig. 15.5.[33]

The first 3 years of life represents the most critical period for dietary interventions aimed at microbiota modulation to improve child growth and development and positively affect health.

The infant microbiome is particularly impressionable and highly variable. A baby's gut microbiota, for example, can be influenced by mode of birth delivery, hospitalisation, nature of feeding, antibiotic and other pharmaceutical exposures, environmental chemical exposures, introduction of solids and quality of diet. All of these factors plus more can have an impact on an infant's immune expression and health outcomes.[29]

Children born by caesarean have been shown to have significantly different counts of faecal bacterial species, most notably a reduction in bifidobacteria, and slowness for these bacteria to eventually colonise. This is most likely to be a result of bypassing direct exposure to maternal microbes through the birthing process, as well as the potential use of prophylactic antibiotics.[34] Infants born via caesarean are predominantly colonised with microbes associated with the skin and the hospital environment.

Some 60–90% of the faecal microbiota in breastfed infants consist of bifidobacteria.[35] Several studies confirm that bifidobacteria are the predominant bacteria in the infant gut.[36,37] This is largely a result of the presence of *Bifidobacterium* spp. in the breast milk itself, as well as the presence of human milk oligosaccharides in the breast

milk – an abundant carbohydrate in human milk which functions similarly to a prebiotic, stimulating the growth of *Bifidobacterium* spp. – thereby selectively altering microbial composition in the establishment of infantile intestinal microbiota.[29,38,39]

Exclusive breastfeeding during the first months after birth is associated with lower asthma rates during childhood. The effect, caused by immunomodulatory qualities of breast milk, avoidance of allergens or a combination of these and other factors, strengthens the advantage of breastfeeding, especially if a family history of atopy is present.[40] The proliferation of beneficial microbes supported by breastfeeding may provide protection from disorders such as allergies,[39] neonatal diarrhoea,[41] necrotising enterocolitis,[42] obesity[43] and type 2 diabetes.[44] For a more in-depth discussion on breast milk composition and beneficial immune- and growth-stimulating factors, see Chapter 14.

Following birth, the gut microbial composition undergoes remarkable alterations: increasing in diversity and stability, maturing over the first years of life to resemble the microbiota of adult individuals by approximately the age of 3 years old.[45] As such, the first 3 years of life represent the most critical period for dietary interventions to improve child growth and development. Alteration of the intestinal microbiota during this period has the potential to profoundly affect host health and development.[46]

Factors that disrupt/harm the infant gut microbiota include the use of antibiotics during the birth process or by direct exposure orally to the infant. Antibiotic therapy leads to rapid shifts in composition of the intestinal microbiota and a decline in microbial diversity. After cessation of antibiotic therapy, some communities may never return to their original diversity. The remainder of

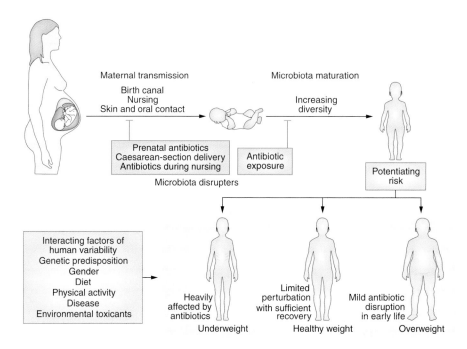

FIGURE 15.6 A model of microbiota transmission, maturation and perturbation in the first years of life and possible effects on weight.[49]

Cox LM, Blaser MJ. Antibiotics in early life and obesity. Nature Reviews Endocrinology 2015;11:182–90.[49]

the microbiome may take months or even years to recover.[47,48]

The response of the gut microbiome to antibiotics, and its potential link to the development of disease, is especially complex to study in the changing infant gut. However, based on the evidence that the microbiota can participate in metabolic signalling and nutrient extraction, changes in early life due to antibiotic exposure may result in metabolic derangements, including excessive weight gain or stunted development, if chronic (see Fig. 15.6).

Preterm birth also has potential to perturb the optimal development of the infant microbiota. In preterm infants, the microbiota is characterised by reduced diversity, higher levels of potentially pathogenic bacteria and lower numbers of *Bifidobacterium* and *Bacteroides* spp. compared with full-term infants.[50] Preterm birth is often confounded with both caesarean delivery and antibiotic usage, since these three factors are often associated (see Table 15.4).

INFANT GASTROINTESTINAL DEVELOPMENT

The infant has distinctly different gastrointestinal anatomy and physiology from that of an older child or adult. To safely and effectively derive nutrition from solid foods, significant developmental changes occur. From an anatomical perspective, the infant has a shorter neck and there is limited space in the oropharynx due to buccal fat pads and the tongue filling the mouth.[63] This enables an effective latch while breastfeeding. The epiglottis and soft palate approximate protecting the infant's airway while they nurse.[63] Furthermore, there is typically a lack of

TABLE 15.4 Factors that disrupt the infant microbiome

Antibiotic exposure
Prenatal; intrapartum and direct to infant[51,52]
Maternal exposure prior to pregnancy

Proton pump inhibitors[53]
Direct to infant. Also alter the microbiota of lung and gastric secretions[54]
Maternal exposure likely to alter horizontal transfer of bacteria species

Caesarean birth[51]

Preterm birth[55]
This is multifactorial relating to: higher medications exposure; risk of supplementation; risk of not receiving breast milk[55]; higher caesarean birth population, lack of or limited skin-to-skin contact and environmental exposure to unfavourable microbes[56]

Lack of skin-to-skin contact at birth
Limited research on this at this stage but it is plausible that immediate contact with hospital surfaces rather than a parent's skin could result in differed colonisation affecting the skin gut and other areas

Lack of breastfeeding[57,58]
Formula feeding and the absence or proportional reduction in breast milk all negatively impact on the infant gut microbiota. Note: human milk prebiotics play a major role in shaping the infant's intestinal microbiome (see Chapter 14).

Iron supplementation
Supplementation[59,60] and use of iron-fortified foods[61]

Dietary factors
Maternal high-fat, low-fibre and low-prebiotic diet[62]
Infant early food exposure

teeth. Feeding reflexes and the oral musculature are adapted to breastfeeding. The tongue protrusion reflex expels non-liquids from the mouth.[64] The gastrointestinal motility tends to be more irregular and the intestinal transit time is longer.[65]

The human infant gut is immune naïve and depends on the immune input from human milk including antibodies, immune factors, prebiotics, immune cells and cytokines for protection from infection. The infant also has greater intestinal mucosal permeability and immature intestinal barrier function. The neonate gut is especially permeable.[66] Breast milk components assist with the development of the barrier both[67] directly and via the promotion of a healthy microbiome.[57,68] The infant who is not breastfed has greater intestinal permeability, especially in the first month of life.[69] Exposure to substances other than breast milk, including food, cow's milks and formula, prior to developmental readiness appear to cause inflammation,[70] and in some cases, micro-bleeding,[71] and dilute the functions of breast milk.[70,72,73] (See also Chapter 14: Breastfeeding – Table 14.4 Functions of breastfeeding for mother and child.)

Protein digestion

The neonate has a fasting gastric pH of 6–7, contrasting markedly with the adult pH range of 1–3.5.[65] The infant's gastric pH gradually decreases each month and matches that of an adult by age 20–30 months.[65] Furthermore, the infant secretes fewer gastric and pancreatic proteolytic enzymes and the enzymes have lower activity than that of adults.[74] This is thought to be a strategy to protect the developing intestinal mucosal cells.

The combination of reduced proteolytic action (through higher stomach pH, lower enzyme levels and activity) and increased gastrointestinal permeability results in infants absorbing greater amounts of intact proteins.

Carbohydrate digestion

Infant lactase activity surpasses that of adults. However, the neonate has a pancreatic amylase level 0.2–5% of an adult. At around 4–6 months of age, pancreatic amylase matches adult levels.[74] Breast milk also contains amylase[75] and therefore may assist with the digestion of co-ingested starches.

Lipid digestion

Infants secrete minimal pancreatic triglyceride lipase and have lower bile production. Human milk contains bile salt-stimulated lipase,[76,77] which assists with the digestion of lipids in breast milk lipid digestion and may assist with the co-ingested fats.

Xenobiotic metabolism and renal function

Human infants have limited capacity to excrete solutes.[78] Accordingly, breast milk has a lower solute load than other mammalian milks.[78,79] The solute load of artificial breast milk substitutes needs to be specifically defined to avoid

electrolyte disturbances and renal strain. Infants also display xenobiotic metabolic immaturity, making them more vulnerable to accumulation and toxicity.[80]

NUTRITIONAL REQUIREMENTS 0–12 MONTHS

Due to the exceptional rate of growth and development in the first year of life, the meeting of nutritional needs during this time plays a formative role in the long-term health potential of the infant. Numerous epidemiological studies, animal models and clinical trials have highlighted the importance of early nutrition on adult health.[32,81,82]

Breast milk is a unique and beneficial, robust and reliable source of nutrition to the infant. Exclusive breastfeeding for the first 6 months comprehensively caters for the developmental needs of an infant.[70,83] At around 6 months of age, infants have a need for iron- and zinc-rich complementary foods. Some at-risk infants may exhaust their iron stores prior to 6 months (as discussed below).

The breast milk concentrations of most nutrients are regulated independently to maternal status, including protein, carbohydrates, calcium, magnesium, zinc, folate and iron,[84–89] while concentrations of some nutrients are affected by maternal status, including vitamin D, choline, vitamin B_{12} and iodine.[90–95] Hence, nutritional strategies that optimise maternal nutrition are an important aspect of caring for the infant (see Chapter 14).

When parents are considering supplementing infant feeds with formula, it is valuable to seek to understand and explore the reason. In many cases, when the motivations for supplementing are explored, education, reassurance and referral for lactation support can result in the continuation of breastfeeding and the avoidance of breast milk substitutes. If a substitute is to be used, the feasibility of the mother's own expressed milk or that of a safe donor human milk source should be considered. After these options, commercial formula is the next choice in order of safest to least safe (considered the fourth choice coming after: 1) direct breastfeeding; 2) mother's own expressed breast milk; and 3) donor milk from a safe source, as per the WHO guidelines).[96] Commercial formulas are fortified to contain recommended dietary intakes (RDIs) of infant vitamins, minerals and trace minerals, and the composition is regulated by national bodies in most developed countries including the US and Australia.[97] Some strategies that may improve the health outcomes of formula-fed infants are outlined in Chapter 14.

The authors of this chapter **strongly discourage** the use of home-made breast milk substitutes (home-made formula) and/or the use of unmodified non-human mammalian milks because of the potential for devastating effects to the infant and the medico-legal risks to the practitioner. The younger the infant is, the more vulnerable they are to adverse effects, with infants under the age of 4 months being particularly at risk. All infants are at risk, however. For further discussion of these risks please see Chapter 14.

The infant who is receiving donor milk, or formula, is best fed in a way that physically resembles breastfeeding; that is, held close and with a gentle, responsive, passive feeding style. This close cuddle time is important for neurosocial development, facilitates bonding and promotes oxytocin release in the parent and the infant. It is recommended that the parents alternate the holding position rather than feeding on the same side. A supply-line supplementer is a system that enables supplementary feeds to be provided at the breast, supporting orofacial development and closeness and stimulating maternal milk supply.

INTRODUCTION OF SOLIDS

Once an infant has reached an appropriate level of gastrointestinal and immune maturity, solid foods may be introduced. This is usually between the beginning of the 6th month and the beginning of the 7th month of life (or around 6 months[98]). In the weeks prior to being ready, the infant may watch with anticipation, and even mimic the chewing actions of their parents. The introduction of solids can be a venture faced by new parents with a mixture of enthusiasm and anxiety because of conflicting advice from various health professionals and well-meaning friends and family. Food labelling messages often conflict with the WHO and government recommendations, causing further confusion.[99] As the science continues to update, guidelines have certainly shifted as to the most optimal timing of solids and most appropriate first foods. The push and pull between the European Society for Paediatric Gastroenterology, Hepatology and Nutrition (ESPGHAN) and the WHO has been evident regarding timing of introduction of solids. The former was criticised for having strong ties with the baby food industry and for not being systematic in its appraisal of the evidence following its 2008 recommendations to commence solids at 4 months.[100] Since then, ESPGHAN has updated its policy to be closer to the WHO guidelines. The WHO guidelines state:

> Infants should be exclusively breastfed for the first six months of life to achieve optimal growth, development and health. Thereafter, to meet their evolving nutritional requirements, infants should receive nutritionally adequate and safe complementary foods, while continuing to breastfeed for up to two years or beyond.[101]

The ESPGHAN recommends:

> Exclusive or full breast-feeding should be promoted for at least 4 months (17 weeks, beginning of the fifth month of life) and exclusive or predominant breast-feeding for around 6 months (26 weeks, beginning of the seventh month) is a desirable goal. Complementary foods (i.e. solid foods and liquids other than breast milk or infant formula) should not be started before four months but should not be delayed beyond six months. Breast-feeding should continue as complementary foods are introduced.[102]

The 2017 *Australian Consensus on Infant Feeding Guidelines to Prevent Food Allergy: Outcomes from the Australian Infant Feeding Summit* represent a welcome clarification of feeding advice. These are the recommendations that came out of two round-table discussions attended by allergy specialists and infant feeding stakeholders in Australia and included representatives from the WHO, the National Health and Medical Research Council (NHMRC), the ABM and the Australasian Society of Clinical Immunology and Allergy (ASCIA).[103] The guidelines state:

> 1 When your infant is ready, at around 6 months, but not before 4 months, start to introduce a variety of solid foods, starting with iron-rich foods, while continuing breast-feeding.
> 2 All infants should be given allergenic solid foods including peanut butter, cooked egg, dairy, and wheat products in the first year of life. This includes infants at high risk of allergy.
> 3 Hydrolyzed (partially or extensively) infant formula is not recommended for the prevention of allergic disease.[103]

The influence of the baby food industry, often labelling foods 'from 4+ months' or 'suitable for 4–6 months', further muddies the waters, as parents can feel that they might be lagging behind if they are not feeding solids from 4 months of age. Often, first-time mothers find that waiting until 6 months was challenging, despite knowledge of the WHO recommendations and an initial desire to comply with its guidelines. Research highlights a parental belief that complementary foods will assist the infant's weight gain, sleeping patterns and enjoyment at meal times. Barriers preventing parents complying with the recommendations include subjective and group norms, peer influences, infant cues indicating early readiness and food labelling inconsistencies.[99,104]

In fact, early introduction of solids before an infant is developmentally ready has potential to displace nutrient-dense breast milk, and a recent Cochrane review states that 'for infants at four to six months, we found no evidence of benefit from additional foods ... and ... we found no evidence to disagree with the current International recommendations that healthy infants exclusively breastfeed for the first six months'.[75,83] It becomes the unique opportunity of the healthcare provider/naturopath to reassure, remind and encourage each parent on an individual basis of the most current WHO recommendations.

Despite the most current recommendation from just about every major health body, including the American Academy of Pediatrics (AAP), the ESPGHAN, the WHO and the NHMRC, to delay solids introduction until 6 months of age, parents may continue to receive different advice from healthcare providers. Some clinicians may still be practising based on the former and now outdated 2008 ASCIA recommendations of 4–6 months being the best 'window of tolerability'. Concerns with this previous recommendation/approach include displacing nutrient-dense and developmentally appropriate breast milk and dilution of functional effects of breastfeeding, including immune protection. Clinicians must tread carefully in these scenarios and remain sensitive to individual needs of each mother–infant dyad.

Another challenge with the introduction of solids is the changeable and often conflicting advice from government and specialist groups surrounding early introduction of potentially allergenic foods (eggs, seafoods, nuts, dairy, wheat/barley/rye and other gluten-containing grains) versus abstinence/delayed introduction to enhance digestive maturity. This is discussed below.

Considering the delicate and newly developing infant's gastrointestinal system, judicious introduction of solids is strongly recommended so as not to displace nutrient-dense breast milk, and so as not to overload the infant's gastrointestinal system with solids. While there are many digestive and immune functions to breast milk, including particular antibodies, enzymes, live bacteria, prebiotic factors and bioavailable nutrients, these functions do not extend to solid foods. An appropriate level of gastrointestinal and immune maturity must be present in the infant prior to introduction of solids to ensure optimal tolerance.

Infants differ in the age when they are developmentally ready for solid foods. While infants may watch with eager anticipation as people around them eat for some weeks prior to being ready for solids, signs that an infant may be developmentally ready to start solids include:

- being able to sit relatively unaided
- loss of the tongue-thrust reflex that pushes food back out, ability to move food from the front to the back of the mouth
- ability to hold mouth around a spoon
- the child's own initiation – reaching out, grabbing food and eating it.

Interpretation of these signs is obviously varied and advice is best given after individualised assessment of all presenting infants.

Iron requirements

At birth, the neonate has a relatively high concentration of haemoglobin (around 170 g/L) having adapted to the lower oxygen environment of the womb.[71] Over the first 4 weeks of life, haemoglobin levels reduce to around 120 g/L, and iron is salvaged from this process. Consequently, the 4-week-old infant has dramatically increased their ferritin levels from birth, with typical values around 350 micrograms/L.[71] By the age of 6 months, ferritin levels have declined to around 30 micrograms/L. Breast milk iron is highly bioavailable, yet only present at low levels. Hence, the infant relies largely on iron stores to maintain healthy iron status until the point that iron is derived from complementary foods.

Certain factors predispose infants to have inadequate iron stores and/or increased risk of iron deficiency. These include low birth weight,[105] preterm birth, immediate cord clamping[106,107] and above median weight gain since birth,[105] as well as factors such as low socioeconomic status and/or immigrant status,[106] high cow's milk intake and low intake of iron-rich complementary foods.[71] Interestingly, findings are conflicting with regards to the relationship between maternal perinatal iron deficiency

and iron status in infancy.[108,109] In susceptible infants, exclusive breastfeeding for 6 months compared to 4 months has been associated with iron deficiency anaemia (IDA).[110] A 2015 meta-analysis found that introduction of solids at 4 months improved iron status but had no effect on growth, both in developed and developing countries, and no effect on haemoglobin status of infants in developed countries.[111] Additionally, a 2016 study found that when gender, birth weight and inflammation were controlled for, exclusive breastfeeding to 6 months decreased IDA in a resource-poor setting.[112] The impact of earlier complementary foods on haematological health is not clear. However, any potential benefits to iron status afforded by earlier introduction of solids needs to be balanced with the increased infection disease risk associated with this action.[70] Hence, most health advisory bodies (including the WHO,[113] the AAP,[114] the NHMRC,[98] Nordic Nutrition Recommendations[115] and the Cochrane reviews of this area[70,83]) continue to recommend exclusive breastfeeding for 6 months.

Nevertheless, iron deficiency is the most common micronutrient deficiency worldwide, and young children, even in affluent societies, are a special risk group because their rapid growth leads to high iron requirements.[106] Therefore, careful consideration of the infant's iron status is important. The healthy full-term infant with a birth weight greater than 3000 g, delayed cord clamping (≥3 minutes)[116] and exclusively breastfed for 6 months will typically have sufficient iron stores for at least 6, and up to 8, months.[117,118] The commencement of iron-rich solid foods at 6 months maintains iron stores and prevents iron deficiency. At-risk infants should be closely monitored (see Box 15.3) and iron assessment may be warranted. Iron status assessment should also be considered in infants with reduction in milestone achievement, reduction in growth and who have frequent infections.

Routine iron supplementation is not recommended as a method of preventing iron deficiency. Cautious iron supplementation in collaboration with a medical

---

BOX 15.3 Factors that increase the risk of iron deficiency in infancy

Immediate cord clamping at birth[107]
Preterm and late preterm birth[119]
Birth weight <3000 g[105]
Above median weight gain since birth[105]
Male gender[105] (when combined with other above factors)
Whole cow's milk intake[71]:

- can cause gut micro-bleeding as well as competitive inhibition and iron displacement

Consuming high volumes of complementary foods with low iron content:

- some food components may impair absorption of breast milk iron and cause gastrointestinal irritation[71]

Gastrointestinal bleeding
Coeliac disease[71]

practitioner may be appropriate in confirmed iron deficiency. Iron bisglyconate may be a more bioavailable and better tolerated form of iron,[120] and based on data from adults, it may be effective at lower doses than other iron forms.[121]

The frequency of iron deficiency in infancy has prompted iron fortification of food products and use of iron supplements in many populations.[110] It is widely advised that from the age of 6 months, all infants and toddlers should receive iron-rich (complementary) foods, including meat products and/or iron-fortified foods.

IRON FORTIFICATION

The appropriateness of iron-fortified foods is subject to debate. Preliminary evidence suggests that iron-fortified foods may cause oxidative stress, inflammation, dysbiosis and increased risk of gastrointestinal infections in infants.[61,122] Findings in this area are mixed, however, with one study finding that non-fortified cereal, iron-fortified cereal and meat all increased reactive oxygen species similarly.[123] The post hoc analysis of this study also found that the iron-fortified cereal group had higher faecal calprotectin levels, suggesting greater intestinal inflammation. Where acceptable, meat may be preferable to iron-fortified foods. Haem iron (from animal products) and lactoferrin-bound iron (from breast milk) both have greater bioavailability than non-haem forms (found in formula, iron-fortified cereals and plants foods). Furthermore, meat is iron dense, enabling sufficient iron load with a small intake of solid foods.[71] Vegetarian families may be able to increase the bioavailability of iron from legumes via traditional germination and fermentation techniques[124,125] (uttapam, tempeh). However, for some infants, these strategies may not be sufficient to meet their requirements. Iron-rich foods include egg yolk, slow cooked grass-fed meats (lamb, beef, pork), poultry (in particular the thigh), sardines, legumes, greens, sprouted mungbeans, buckwheat and millet.[106,126]

Unmodified cow's milk should not be fed as the main milk drink to infants before the age of 12 months, and intake should be limited to <500 mL/day in toddlers to minimise the risk of iron deficiency due to its low iron content and high calcium content, which can competitively inhibit iron absorption. It is important to ensure that this dietary advice reaches high-risk groups such as socioeconomically disadvantaged families and immigrant families.[106] Iron deficiency in infants and children is associated with functional impairments affecting cognitive development, immune mechanisms and developmental milestones.[127] This is discussed in detail in Chapter 16: Paediatrics and Adolescence.

Other developmental needs

When foods are introduced into the diet, it is important the food choices are nutrient-dense in order to provide adequate macro- and micronutrients for the rapidly growing infant. Besides iron, fat and cholesterol are of particular importance to a developing infant; 50–60% of kilojoules in breast milk from a healthy mother are derived from fat,[128] almost half of which comprises saturated fatty acids. The breast milk fatty acid composition is influenced by maternal diet (see Chapter 14). Saturated fatty acids are critical for the production of myelin in the brain and spinal cord.[129] The cholesterol intake from breast milk is almost six times the amount most adults consume in a day[128] and is required for the development of the brain and vision. Several studies have shown that infants and children on low-fat and low-cholesterol diets fail to grow and develop properly, with significant deficits in neurological function, including depressed IQ, and visual deficits.[130,131] Nutrient-dense, high-fat foods (partially cooked egg yolk, meats, ghee, unprocessed fats and oil such as cod liver oil, coconut oil, olive oil) should be encouraged.

The long-chain polyunsaturated fatty acids (LCPUFAs), docosahexaenoic acid (DHA) and eicosapentaenoic acid (EPA) are of particular importance for infants.[132,133] These two fatty acids play critical roles in visual development and are essential building blocks for the sophisticated and delicate process of continued neurodevelopment and brain function. They have a structural role in membranes, skin and mucous membranes. These polyunsaturated fatty acids are precursors of biologically active 'messengers' in the body, such as prostaglandins, and are involved with hormone and neurotransmitter production and function. In particular, DHA omega-3 forms a structural component of growing brains and retinas throughout infancy, which is vital to normal development and both qualitatively and quantitatively important.[134]

For example, the DHA status of the newborn and breast-fed infant varies widely and depends on the maternal intake of DHA. The standard Australian diet is particularly low in omega-3 fatty acids, including plant-based alpha-linolenic acid (ALA) and DHA, which is found mainly in oily fish. Epidemiological studies have linked low maternal DHA to increased risk of poor child neural development.[135] Several studies have demonstrated positive associations between blood DHA levels and improvements on tests of cognitive and visual function in healthy children, and intervention studies have shown that improving maternal DHA nutrition decreases the risk of poor infant and child visual and neural development.[136]

There is also evidence that mothers who use EPA and DHA supplementation during pregnancy and breastfeeding may protect their children against allergies. This may be due to the fact that fish-oil supplementation has been associated with decreased levels of the body cells associated with inflammation and immune response.[137]

Increasing DHA intake in pregnant women, breastfeeding mothers, infants and children should be a primary goal for optimising health, behaviour, neurocognition, IQ and vision. Formula, however, needs to have the appropriate balance of DHA to arachidonic acid (see Chapter 14).

When we consider that the introduction of solids to an infant is a 'sampling of the environment', both *moderation* and *diversity* are key. The numerous and overwhelming benefits of continued breastfeeding (with no outer limit on duration) extend to maximising tolerance to new food antigens introduced and providing protection against the development of allergic disease.[138–141]

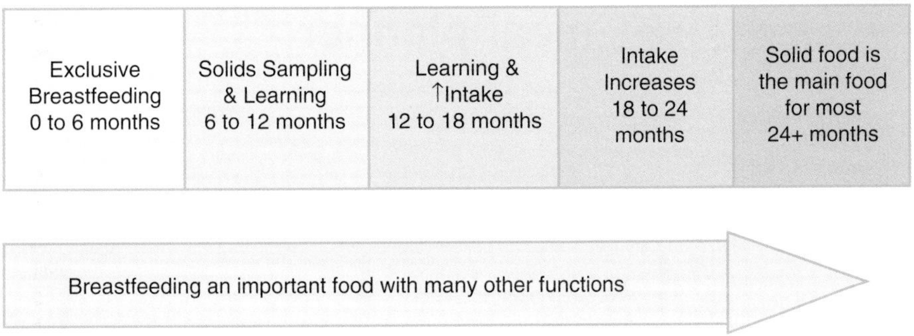

FIGURE 15.7 Solids introduction timeline

Practical aspects to commencing solids

The saying 'before 1 year old, food is mostly just for fun' is worth imparting to parents. The commencement of solids ideally occurs gradually (see Fig. 15.7). The aim is to allow infants to explore and enjoy food as they develop this new skill and to partake in the social aspect of sharing meals with the family. Parents sometimes need to find strategies to help them relax about the messy exploration that happens and focus more on enjoying watching their infant discover new things. The baby-led weaning (BLW) approach often lends itself to the infant's relaxed participation in family meals (see further discussion below).

Breastfeeding prior to offering solid food throughout the day is encouraged for a number of reasons:

- It is much easier for the infant to learn when they are not ravenously hungry.
- It ensures breast milk is not displaced from the diet.
- The presence of breast milk may improve the immune tolerability and digestibility of the food.

Healthy appetite regulation is also important to foster. Hence, parents should be encouraged to respond to their infant's cues and avoid the temptation of trying to encourage them to eat more than they are interested in, or finish off the serving of food. This is one of the advantages of the BLW method, which allows infants to be in full control of their intake through self-feeding of hand-held foods. Many parents feed their infants with a mixed style, including both infant self-feeding of hand-held foods and responsive assisted spoon feeding. Infants have preferences for feeding styles too, with some infants needing to have full control of any food entering their mouths and other infants wanting help to get the food in.

First foods should be easily digestible and nutrient dense and provide nourishment for the infant's microbiome. Nut butters; avocado; meats and egg yolk from pasture-raised animals; small wild fish; and non-genetically modified, cold-pressed, plant-based oils such as olive oil (as a part of a balanced diet) provide good quality fat, cholesterol and fat soluble vitamins, which are necessary for neurological, visual, immune and digestive development (see Fig. 15.8). Egg yolks, cooked organic red meats ensure adequate intake of protein iron and zinc in addition to breast milk or formula.[142]

While diversity and moderation are key, individual assessment and guidance are important (as per naturopathic philosophy), and it is advisable that each infant's food sampling is in alignment with 'family foods' and the family's own cultural practices. Infants need to be observed while eating at all times.

For recommended foods to introduce to young infants between 6 and 12 months of age, see Table 15.5.

Introduction of solids may be one of the most critical factors involved in creating compositional change and diversity in the paediatric microbiome.[144] The introduction of solid foods is followed by a large shift in phyla abundances within the infant's microbiome, in addition to increased bacterial loads and short-chain fatty acids levels. While there is a clear increase in complexity of the intestinal microbiota with the introduction of solids, it has been shown that the quality of the initial inoculation at birth is a predetermining factor for future microbial colonisation in the gut.[144] Gut microbiota diversity increases following introduction of solid food, with enhanced colonisation of butyrate producers.[144,145]

FOOD ALLERGY AND INTOLERANCE IN INFANTS

Food allergy is an important public health problem, affecting infants, children and adults, and may be increasing in prevalence.[146,147] Symptoms of adverse food reactions range right across all body systems, from the skin (rash, eczema, cradle cap), to digestive (visceral hypersensitivity, dysmotility, oesophagitis, food-protein-induced enterocolitis syndrome [FPIES], allergic proctocolitis), to immune compromise (frequent ear infections), to respiratory and cardiometabolic (anaphylaxis). Common food allergens include egg, milk, peanut, tree nuts, wheat, crustacean shellfish and soy. Despite the risk of severe allergic reactions and even death, there is no current treatment for food allergy – it is predominantly managed by allergen avoidance or treatment of symptoms. The diagnosis and management of food allergy also may vary from one clinical practice setting to another.

BABY 6–12m meal **planner**

week starting:

	sample foods offered after breastmilk	sample foods offered after breastmilk	sample foods offered after breastmilk	sample foods offered after breastmilk
MONDAY	Rolled quinoa porridge made with breastmilk	Avocado hummus and sweet potato mash	Slow cooked Moroccan beef stew	Sourdough Spelt rusks
TUESDAY	Apple and prune puree with a millet porridge	Organic chicken and preservative-free dried apricot mash	Sweet potato and coconut flesh/milk puree	Banana
WEDNESDAY	Poached pear and banana with millet porridge	White bean, cauliflower and leek soup or mash with sprinkle of chia seeds	Snapper, brown rice with broccoli and zucchini mash	A few table-spoons of natural tub-set yoghurt with prune puree
THURSDAY	Egg yolk mash	Brown rice, slow cooked chicken thigh and vegetables	Aduki bean and pumpkin casserole	Poached pear and millet porridge with blueberry mash
FRIDAY	Brown rice porridge with coconut milk and blueberries	Broccoli, pumpkin and puree with extra virgin olive oil	Purple carrot and spinach mash with 1/4 tsp organic unsalted butter for taste	Oat biscuits with roast beetroot mash dip
SATURDAY	Natural tub-set yoghurt with banana mash	Green pea, mint mash with and cottage cheese	Lentil and organic beef bolognese with sweet potato mash	Baked sweet potato fingers
SUNDAY	Oat porridge with preservative-free dried apricots	Wild salmon, avocado and spinach mash	Lamb shoulder slow cooked with roast sweet potato mash	Sourdough rye toast fingers with avocado mash

FIGURE 15.8 Sample meal planner of introduction of solids 6–12 months

Types of adverse food reactions can be classified as shown in Fig. 15.9.

Non-allergic food reaction, such as food intolerance, has much higher prevalence than food allergy, and prevalence also seems to be increasing. In response to concern around the increasing prevalence, the National Institute of Allergy and Infectious Diseases, working with 34 professional organisations, federal agencies and patient advocacy groups, led the development of clinical guidelines for the diagnosis and management of food allergy. These guidelines are intended for use by a wide variety of healthcare professionals and include a consensus definition for food allergy, discuss comorbid conditions often associated with food allergy and focus on both IgE-mediated and non-IgE-mediated reactions to food. Having a family history of atopy and the presence of atopic dermatitis in an infant are risk factors for the development of both sensitisation to food and confirmed food allergy. Exerting caution is advised when introducing specific foods that are known allergens, particularly when an infant is at high risk of developing allergy (i.e. infants with at least one first-degree relative [parent or sibling] with allergic disease). Some research shows that approximately one-third of children with refractory, moderate–severe atopic dermatitis have IgE-mediated clinical reactivity to food proteins.[149] The prevalence of food allergy in this population is significantly higher than in the general population, and an evaluation for food allergy should be considered in these infants. Patients with atopic dermatitis who developed severe dermatitis within the first 3 months of age most often had sIgE to milk, egg and peanut, suggesting that this group is at risk for manifesting IgE-mediated food allergy.[150]

It has been demonstrated that the majority of infant patients allergic to peanut have atopic dermatitis.[151] Egg allergy is very common in peanut-allergic patients, and sesame seeds should perhaps be considered one of the major food allergens.

TABLE 15.5 Sample staged introduction of solids		
0–6 months	**6 to 8+ months**	**8 to 12+ months**
Breast milk, donor milk or infant formula	Iron-rich foods at least daily Examples • Pureed meat • Organic liver (1–2 teaspoon once a week only to avoid risk of hypervitaminosis A, ensure well cooked to minimise risk of food borne illness, preference duck or chicken over larger animals) • Well-cooked egg yolk • Mung beans have low phytate level (pre-sprouting and cooking well improves iron bioavailability)[124] • Tempeh Small amounts of the following foods may also be given: Pureed vegetables (carrots, fresh beetroot, sweet potato, zucchini, pumpkin, squash, parsnips) mixed with breast milk, or extra virgin olive oil Pureed stewed fruit (apricot, peaches, pears, apples, berries) Mashed raw fruits (banana, mangoes, papaya, avocado, blueberries) Parents following BLW approach carefully select foods that present low choking hazard (see below)	Avocado chunks Banana pieces Soaked and well-cooked legumes Soaked and well-cooked grains, including quinoa porridge, millet porridge, brown rice porridge, buckwheat, wheat, rye, barley and oat porridge Boiled or steamed nuts – then pureed (to reduce allergenicity) Nut butters such as salt-free peanut butter, almond butter, cashew butter, tahini (boiling raw peanuts reduces allergenicity, while roasting increases it[143]) Herbs for seasoning Cooked whole egg Citrus fruit (depending on child's dexterity, peel skin from segment) Small amounts of full-fat dairy from pasture-fed animals, starting with true yoghurt, aged cheese and kefir

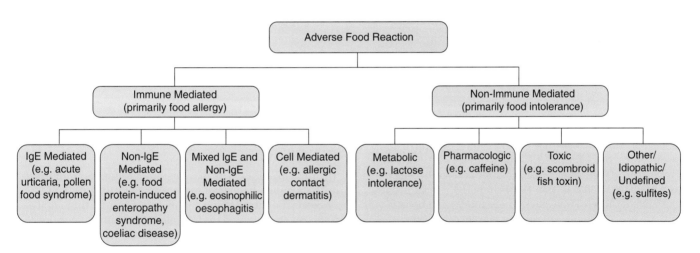

FIGURE 15.9 Types of adverse food reactions

From Boyce JA, Assa'ad A, Burks AW et al. Guidelines for the diagnosis and management of food allergy in the United States: report of the NIAID-sponsored expert panel. *The Journal of Allergy and Clinical Immunology* 2010;126(6 Suppl.):S1–58[146]; copied from ASCIA.[148]

Previous strategies to prevent food allergy through allergen avoidance during pregnancy, breastfeeding and infancy have more recently been called into question.[101] Current evidence does not support a major role for maternal dietary restrictions during pregnancy or lactation. At present, there are insufficient data to document a protective effect of any dietary intervention beyond 6 months of age for the development of atopic disease.[152] Scientific evidence has mounted to show no clinical benefit in delayed introduction of solids beyond 6 months of age.[153] Some research suggests that sensitisation to allergens occurs through environmental exposure via pregnancy and mother's breast milk, and consumption of that food allergen induces oral tolerance.[133] Alternative hypotheses such as the hygiene hypotheses, the impact of the state of one's microbiome, lack of immune-modulating

vitamin D, disrupted skin barrier function and impacts of food processing all may play a role in increasing incidence of food allergy and intolerance.[154]

Despite guidelines recommending avoidance of peanuts during infancy in the UK, Australia and until recently, North America, peanut allergy continues to increase in these countries. Peanut is introduced earlier and is eaten more frequently and in larger quantities in Israel than in the UK, yet research has demonstrated that Jewish children in the UK have a prevalence of peanut allergy that is 10-fold higher than that of Jewish children in Israel. This difference is not accounted for by differences in atopy, social class, genetic background or peanut allergenicity. Israeli infants consume peanut in high quantities in the first year of life (typically boiled rather than roasted[155]), whereas UK infants avoid peanuts. These findings raise the question of whether early introduction of peanut during infancy, rather than avoidance, will prevent the development of peanut allergy.[156] A decline in the age of first peanut reaction may be attributable to earlier exposure.[151]

Breastfeeding may offer protection against the development of coeliac disease. Coeliac disease is a multifactorial condition, originating from the interplay of genetic and environmental factors. Breastfeeding during the introduction of dietary gluten and increasing duration of breastfeeding have been associated with reduced risk of developing coeliac disease.[157] It is not clear whether breastfeeding provides a permanent protection against coeliac disease or just delays the onset. Long-term prospective cohort studies are required to investigate further the relationship between breastfeeding and coeliac disease.[158]

Regular fish consumption before age 1 also appears to be associated with a reduced risk of allergic disease and sensitisation to food and inhalant allergens during the first 4 years of life.[159]

Most children with food allergy eventually will tolerate milk, egg, soy and wheat; far fewer will eventually tolerate tree nuts and peanut. The time course of food allergy resolution in children varies by food and may occur as late as the teenage years.[146] Despite the above, there are many gaps in the current scientific knowledge that need to be addressed through future research.[146]

Another consideration when introducing solids to infants is avoiding damaging, nutrient-poor foods such as white starches, refined cereals and grains, juice, added sugar and sugar substitutes (such as honey, high-fructose corn syrup), food additives (colours, preservatives, flavour enhancers), processed or packaged foods, condiments (such as added salt, salted butter, commercial bone broths with salt added, sauces, jams, etc.). These foods are nutrient void and are unsuitable for infants, as they may adversely impact on the oral and digestive microbiota and will place considerable strain on the baby's immature kidneys and digestive capacity.

As discussed in detail in Chapters 2 and 13, infants and babies are uniquely vulnerable to the vast array of environmental contaminants that are ubiquitous with modern life. As such, throughout infancy, choosing to prioritise organic animal and fresh produce when possible is advisable to reduce exposure to pesticide residues, which may be developmentally harmful,[160] in addition to keeping food packaging chemicals low and avoiding reheating foods in plastic in microwaves.

Choking hazards also need to be avoided: small hard foods, such as items that cannot be mashed on the roof of the mouth with the tongue (e.g. popcorn, whole nuts, grapes, peas, raisins, raw apple, carrot); leaves (such as spinach, rocket, basil); raw and under-ripe fruit; fruit and vegetable skins that may stick to the roof of baby's mouth; and cooked food cut too large, such as sausages cut into round 'coins' or crackers that may potentially occlude airways. Some of these foods are well tolerated when steamed or mashed to ideal texture.

See Box 15.4 for a list of foods to avoid for infants.

> ## BOX 15.4 Foods that should be avoided when introducing solids to babies (adapted from[161])
>
> - Small hard foods – such as popcorn, whole nuts, peas, celery, raisins, raw apple, carrot
> - Leaves, such as spinach, rocket, basil (unless cooked and pureed)
> - Whole grapes
> - Hard, under-ripe fruit
> - Fruit and vegetable skins that may stick to roof of baby's mouth
> - Cooked foods cut too large, like sausages cut into round 'coins'
> - Crackers and wafers that may potentially occlude airways
>   (all above are choking risks)
> - White starches, refined cereals and grains
> - Juice, cordial, soft drinks
> - Added sugar and sugar substitutes such as honey, high-fructose corn syrup
> - Food additives – colours, preservatives, flavour enhancers
> - Processed or packaged foods
> - Condiments – added salt, salted butter, sauces, jams
> - Bone broths due to potential lead risks and added salt

BABY-LED WEANING (BLW) (OR BABY-LED INTRODUCTION OF SOLIDS)

The principle of BLW is that the infant self-feeds from the beginning with hand-held foods. Parental spoon feeding is avoided. The infant shares family foods at meal times and is responsively breastfed (or formula fed) to ensure nutritional needs are met while learning to eat solids. BLW is based on the premise that if the infant is not ready they will not eat, and the infant will direct their intake based on their readiness and appetite. The parent decides which foods to offer and the infant decides what and how much to eat.

Prior to offering foods, the infant needs to be capable of sitting on their own with minimal support. They should be around 6 months and showing a keen interest in food. Being able to sit upright rather than slumping or reclining gives the infant the control they need to minimise the risk of choking. As outlined above, it is recommended that the infant is breastfed prior to offering food so that they are not ravenous.[162] The aim is to avoid frustration or excessive solid intake that displaces breast milk. As with all early feeding, the infant needs to be closely supervised at all times throughout the meal, and parents need to be equipped to understand when their infant may need help and when their infant is managing.[162]

BLW aims to cultivate lifelong healthy attitudes to food including appetite self-regulation, preventing neophobia and encouraging healthy socialising at meal times.[163] It also ensures the transition to solid foods is paced by the infant and tends to support longer duration of breastfeeding.[163,164] To date, one study investigating BLW found this method was associated with greater satiety responsiveness at 18–24 months and decreased risk of young children being overweight.[165] Another study found that the BLW method meant that infants were more likely both to participate in family meals and to be exclusively breastfed to 6 months.[164] The BLW approach often frees up parents to eat while their infant explores the new wonders of food at the dinner table, which can be very entertaining.

Another virtue of the BLW method is the oral and neurodevelopment that occurs via exposure to textures and learning to manipulate foods in the mouth. Infants who have delayed exposure to lumpy foods beyond 9 months may be more likely to develop texture aversion.[166]

The two main questions that arise in relation to BLW are the nutritional adequacy and perceived greater infant choking risk as discussed below.

Nutritional adequacy

There is a concern that the BLW method may put some infants at nutritional risk and potentially increase the risk of growth faltering.[161] Some infants may be offered a higher proportion of unhealthy foods, depending on the dietary habits of the family, including hot chips, fast foods and sweet biscuits. More health-conscious families may offer infants only fruits and vegetables, and infants may miss out on more energy-, iron- and zinc-dense foods that they require.[161,164] When parents are engaged and educated, they are well placed to offer their infants hand-held foods that are nutritionally appropriate, including energy- and iron-dense options. The BLISS guidelines below provide a helpful framework to ensure BLW infants have access to optimal nutrition. Infants with developmental issues impacting on coordination are probably not suited to exclusive BLW method, as they may lack the dexterity to derive adequate nutrition from finger foods and may be at greater risk of choking.

Choking

Parents and health professionals worry that choking risk may be higher with the BLW method. The gag reflex is triggered further forward on the tongue at 6 months than it is at 1 year (i.e. it moves back).[167] BLW theory suggests that this heightened and proximal gag reflex protects the airway while infants are learning to manipulate food in their mouth. All parents, whether undertaking the BLW method or conventional feeding methods, should obtain first-aid training so that they are equipped to recognise and appropriately respond to choking events, and so they can distinguish between gagging and choking.

Proponents suggest that choking is no more likely with BLW than it is in spoon-fed infants providing the infant is: 1) around 6 months at initiation; 2) in an upright seating position; 3) in full control of what is put into their mouth; and 4) fully supervised.[163]

The limited research to date suggests that BLW is not associated with more choking than conventional feeding methods. One recent study investigating a modified BLW method called the BLISS method found that choking incidence was not different between BLISS and conventional solid introduction methods.[168] One difficulty is distinguishing between gagging and choking. As such, a survey of 20 mothers using BLW found that 30% reported at least one choking event.[167] In all cases, the infant dealt with it by expelling the food from their mouth. Parents stated that they were less anxious about choking as time went on and they felt they could more confidently distinguish between gagging and choking.

The BLISS approach is a variation on BLW that aims to reduce the risk of low-iron- and low-energy-dense food intake and decrease the risk of choking.

The essential characteristics of BLISS are[161]:

1 Offer foods that the infant can pick up and feed themselves (i.e. follow a BLW approach)
2 Offer one high-iron food at each meal.
3 Offer one high-energy food at each meal.
4 Offer food prepared in a way that is suitable for the infant's developmental age to reduce the risk of choking, and avoid offering foods listed as high-choking-risk foods.
   – Advised to test foods before they are offered to the infant to make sure they are soft enough to mash with the tongue on the roof of the mouth.
   – Provided with a list of specific foods to avoid (e.g. raw apple).
   – Advised to also avoid: foods that form a crumb in the mouth, hard foods, small foods and circular (coin)-shaped foods.
   – Educated on safety around eating including how to differentiate between gagging and choking, and what to do if choking occurs.

An example of the BLISS guide for parents is available from Daniels L, Heath A-LM, Williams SM et al. Baby-Led Introduction to SolidS (BLISS) study: a randomised controlled trial of a baby-led approach to complementary feeding. *BMC Pediatrics* 2015;15:179. https://www.ncbi.nlm.nih.gov/pmc/articles/PMC4643507/figure/Fig2/.

The foods listed in Box 15.5 are usually well managed by most infants. General recommendations to parents for introducing solids are listed in Box 15.6.

BOX 15.5 Foods that typically hold together well and are suitable for infant self-feeding, depending on infant dexterity

Foods that hold together well (many have longitudinal fibres):
- Steamed parsnips
- Longitudinal sliced cucumber
- Rind of organic rockmelon or honeydew
- Celery
- Steamed quince
- Steamed broccoli and cauliflower florets
- Larger strawberries (ensure they are ripe)
- Raspberries – mush up nicely in mouths
- Beetroot – can be a little challenging
- Banana and avocado as dexterity improves

BOX 15.6 General recommendations to parents for introducing solids

- Introduction of solid foods according to what the family usually eats, regardless of whether the food is considered to be a common food allergen. There is some evidence that the introduction of common allergenic foods (including cooked egg, peanuts, nuts, wheat, fish) should not be delayed. However, further evidence is required to clarify optimal timing for each food.
- You may choose to introduce one new food at a time so that if a reaction occurs, the problem food can be more easily identified. If a food is tolerated, continue to give this as a part of a varied diet. Moderation and diversity are key.
- If possible, continue to breastfeed while you introduce foods to your infant. There is some evidence that this may reduce the risk of allergies developing, and there are many other health benefits of continued breastfeeding.
- Cow's milk or soy milk (or their products, such as cheese and yoghurt) can be used in cooking or with other foods if dairy products/soy are tolerated.
- There is good evidence that for infants with severe eczema and/or egg allergy, regular peanut intake before 12 months of age can reduce the risk of developing peanut allergy. If your child already has an egg allergy or other food allergies or severe eczema, you should discuss how to do this with your doctor.
- There is moderate evidence that introducing cooked egg (raw egg is not recommended) into an infant's diet before 8 months of age, where there is a family history of allergy, can reduce the risk of developing egg allergy.
- When introducing foods that other family members are allergic to, it is important to follow risk minimisation strategies to prevent cross-contamination of allergens for those who are allergic to the foods.
- It is important to understand that the facial skin in babies is very sensitive and that many foods (including citrus, tomatoes, berries, other fruit and Vegemite) can irritate the skin and cause redness on contact – this is not food allergy. Smearing food on the skin will not help to identify possible food allergies.
- Some infants will develop food allergies. If there is any allergic reaction to any food, that food should be stopped and you should seek advice from a doctor with experience in food allergy. If an adverse food reaction occurs:
  - The suspected food should be avoided until the infant is reviewed by their medical practitioner.
  - Continue to introduce other new foods.
  - Referral to a clinical immunology/allergy specialist may be necessary.

NATUROPATHIC MANAGEMENT OF COMMON INFANTILE PRESENTATIONS

Treating through the mother

The gastrointestinal developmental vulnerability and lowered xenobiotic metabolic capability of the infant makes them particularly at risk of ill effects from the oral ingestion of medicines, supplements and herbal medicines. Ill effects may be caused by the medicine or by the excipients present. Bacterial contaminants are also greater risk to young infants as they lack the defences afforded by low stomach pH, and their gastrointestinal immune defence is immature.

The authors strongly recommend exercising caution in administering nutritional supplements or herbal medicines directly to the infant below 12 months of age and **avoiding direct supplementation in infants under the age of 6 months who are exclusively breastfed**. A superior and safer strategy is to treat the infant primarily via the mother. The younger the infant, the greater the risk of adverse events with direct supplementation due to immature and poorly established regulatory mechanisms in the infant.

Some examples of effective therapeutic treatment of the infant via the mother are outlined in Tables 15.6 and

TABLE 15.6 Probiotic treatments through breast milk

Intervention	Relevant therapeutic evidence
Lactobacillus rhamnosus GG (LGG)	Studies in infants and children suggest LGG clinical efficacy: Reducing antibiotic-associated side effects[169–171] (from maternal or infant exposure) Food allergy – accelerates tolerance to cow's milk[172–174] Improving gut barrier function[175] Decreased infection – GIT[176] and upper respiratory tract[177,178] Evidence of breast milk transfer[179] Animal evidence suggests LGG may reduce visceral hypersensitivity[180]
Lactobacillus reuteri Protectis	*L. reuteri* MM53 – decreased the potentially inflammatory cytokine TGF-beta2 in breast milk.[181] Note: the role of TGF-beta2 and TGF-beta1 is still being established[182] May have some beneficial effects on gastrointestinal health Evidence of breast milk transfer[183]
Lactobacillus fermentum CECT5716	Studies in infants: Decreased respiratory and gastrointestinal infection in infants[184] Decreased infective mastitis recurrence[185] Evidence of breast milk transfer[185] Animal evidence suggests this strain has gastrointestinal anti-inflammatory and immunomodulatory effects[186]

TABLE 15.7 Nutritional and herbal interventions via breast milk

Nutritional interventions	Breast milk change associated with the intervention
Fructooligosaccharides	Increase regulatory cytokines in breast milk when maternally administered at a dose of 4 g twice daily[187]
EPA/DHA (dietary and supplementary)	Increasing EPA and DHA content increases omega-3 to omega-6 ratio and reduces the risk of asthma in the infant[188]
Maternal vitamin D status of 120 nmol/L	Daily vitamin D supplementation (or thrice weekly maternal UVB exposure) that is sufficient to maintain maternal levels at 100–120 nmol/L ensures breast milk vitamin D meets the RDI for the infant[90,189,190] (see Table 14.7 for more information) Optimal vitamin D supports maternal mental health[191–193] Not all findings corroborate[171] One study found maternal vitamin D supplementation decreased infection rates in infants[194] Additional studies directly testing the effect of improved maternal vitamin D status on infantile lower respiratory tract infection and growth in resource-poor settings are currently underway[195,196] Studies relating to infants' vitamin D status suggest maternal supplementation may: • reduce respiratory infection[197] • reduce aeroallergen sensitisation and asthma[198] • prevent food allergy[199]
General maternal nutrition optimisation	See Tables 14.7 and 14.8 in Chapter 14.

Herbal interventions	Indications and rationale
Maternal mood support	Supporting maternal mood may translate into mothers more happily engaging in parenting. Maternal wellbeing promotes maternal infant synchrony and responsiveness to infant cues.[200] Depression has been associated with higher breast milk levels of the potentially inflammatory TGF-β2[201] Suitable herbs include: *Chamomilla recutita* (German chamomile), *Nepeta cataria* (catnip), *Lavandula angustifolia* (English lavender), *Asparagus racemosus* (shatavari), *Verbena officinalis* (vervain), *Withania somnifera* (withania), *Leonorus cardiaca* (motherwort), *Melissa officinalis* (lemon balm) Consider high-quality teas where possible as a means to minimising alcohol exposure via breast milk to the infant
Carminatives	Small volatile components may be transmitted via the breast milk and could exert carminatives effects to the infant, thereby assisting with the passage of trapped wind and easing digestive discomfort Suitable herbs include: *Chamomilla recutita* (German chamomile), *Nepeta cataria* (catnip), *Lavandula angustifolia* (English lavender), *Melissa officinalis* (lemon balm), *Pimpinella anisum* (aniseed), *Foeniculum vulgare* (fennel), *Carum carvi* (caraway seed), *Zingiber officinalis* (ginger rhizome), *Anethum graveolens* (dill seeds)
Curcuma longa (or curcumin phytosome)	May have gut healing and anti-inflammatory effects via mother Consider maternal supplementation when there is evidence of gastrointestinal inflammation such as mucus present in stool

15.7. When treating through the mother, some therapeutic effects may occur via passage of the agent, such as vitamin D and some specific probiotic strains, through breast milk. Other effects may occur secondary to the influence of the therapy on the mother's wellbeing, such as nervines that may help mothers to engage more happily with parenting. This may also exert a positive effect through the breast milk as improved mental wellbeing may promote both higher levels of relaxing hormones and immunoregulatory cytokine patterns.

When treating via the mother is not possible

The exclusively formula-fed infant under the age of 6 months is also highly vulnerable to ill effects from herbs, nutritional supplements and probiotics (see Chapter 14).

Probiotics in <6-month-old formula-fed infants

Carefully selected specific probiotics strains and characterised prebiotics may be suitable to administer to the exclusively formula-fed infant with the goal of modifying some of the specific health concerns for these infants – namely, heightened risk of infection and derangement of the gut (see Chapter 14).

Most of the studies assessing the safety and efficacy of probiotics in infants <6 months old have been conducted on formula-fed infants. This population is different from breastfed infants in numerous ways, including having greater risk of infectious disease,[73,202,203] and consequently, probiotics may be more likely to have a beneficial effect in formula-fed infants. Hence, these effects cannot necessarily be generalised to breastfed infants as the risk to benefit ratio is different for this population.

Supplementation with probiotics will expose infants to excipients (such as fillers, growth medium) and, potentially, flavouring and sweetening agents. In some countries including Australia, not all of these ingredients have to be listed.[204] Microbial contamination is a serious concern, and studies have confirmed this is an issue.[205,206] Unfortunately, independent post-marketing surveillance is limited, which may increase the risk of manufacturer complacency. Microbial contamination poses a serious threat to the young infant. Contamination may also occur once the product is opened, and this may pose a particularly high risk in the hospital environment. The use of a capsule may reduce the risk of home or hospital bacterial contamination. The capsule can be opened and mixed into pre-warmed formula.

If a practitioner chooses to prescribe a probiotic in an infant under the age of 6 months, judicious choice of a strain with evidence of efficacy is essential. Strains with evidence of safety and efficacy (mostly relating to reduced infection) in formula-fed infants include *Lactobacillus rhamnosus* GG (LGG),[207,208] *Lactobacillus fermentum* CECT 5716[184,209] and *Bifidobacterium lactis* Bb-12 in combination with LGG[210] or *L. reuteri* Protectis.[211] Selection of an appropriate strain does not ensure safety, however, for the reasons discussed above.

Two cases of neonatal *Saccharomyces cerevisiae* fungaemia have been related to the use of directly administered *S. cerevisiae* probiotic preparations.[212] It may be prudent to avoid direct supplementation of *Saccharomyces* spp. in the infant under 6 months.

When an infant is partially breastfed, it is preferable to treat via the mother to avoid inadvertently promoting the formula as medicinal, and thereby risking parents preferencing this over breastfeeds, to ensure the infant accesses the prescribed medicines. Treating through the mother is likely to strengthen the mother's breastfeeding intentions.

Infants older than 6 months

For the infant older than 6 months, cautious direct administration of some natural medicines, as outlined in each condition's section, may be appropriate. Evaluation of the individual infant is important, and consideration must be given to the adjusted age of premature infants. Fried's rule provides a guide to dosage of herbal preparations based on age in months[213] and can be cautiously applied (see Fig. 15.10). Consideration of the infant's exposure to alcohol when applying this guide is also important. Treating through the mother is the central preferred treatment mode during the first year of life or more, and aspects of this approach continue to be of value beyond 12 months. Topical applications may be an alternative method of treatment in some cases. Given the comparatively smaller volume to surface area ratio of infants, immature

$$\frac{\text{Age in months} \times \text{adult dose}}{150} = \text{child's dose}$$

FIGURE 15.10 Fried's rule dosage calculations for children under 1–2 years of age[213]

skin barrier and metabolic capability, it is important to be very cautious with the use of essential oils as there is toxicity potential. This text provides some condition-specific suggestions for their use highly diluted in well-tolerated carrier oils.

Fever

A normal temperature in an infant is between 36.5°C and 37.2°C. Fever is the result of a complex immunological response to infection. Fever is an important component of the immune system's defence mechanism against pathogens, where prostaglandins mediate a rise in temperature, creating a hostile environment for viruses and bacteria, inhibiting certain enzymes and the ability of viruses and bacteria to replicate. Fever management therefore needs to focus on keeping the child comfortable throughout the fever and carefully assessing the need for medical referral.

While axillary measurement of fever with a digital thermometer is the most frequently advised method of assessing temperature,[214] it is generally recommended to 'treat the child, not the fever'. An infant's whole presentation needs to be considered – their colour, vital signs, respiratory function, behaviour, signs of dehydration, normal feeding, urinary output and so on. This has been formalised in an approach named the traffic light tool (refer to Table 15.1).

An infant under the age of 3 months with a temperature ≥38°C is at high risk of serious illness and needs immediate referral. Infants between the ages of 3 and 12 months with a fever ≥39°C are at high risk of serious illness and also should be referred immediately. Immediate intervention is also necessary if any of the red flags is present, and an infant should be referred immediately to the GP or emergency if fever persists for longer than 24 hours. When fever persists, the cause must be identified.

Viral infections are very common; the majority of these are upper respiratory infections such as tonsillitis and otitis media. A mild fever may also present after routine childhood immunisations. Fever should not be blamed on teething.[215]

Other relevant questioning and considerations include the duration and degree of fever, past medical history, any known contact with family members who are unwell, recent travel and so on. An infant with an unexplained fever of 38°C or higher lasting for more than 24 hours should have a urine sample tested to rule out urinary tract infection as system cause of fever, particularly when there is no other obvious cause of fever.[216]

Often there is a parental desire or pressure from other family members to 'do something'. The use of physical interventions such as cool bathing, exposure to cold air, rubbing the body with alcohol or using ice is not recommended.[214] The use of such methods can cause an increase in core body temperature owing to superficial vasoconstriction.[214,217] Limited, lukewarm sponging, however, is not associated with adverse effects. However, even this action may cause distress to the infant. If any antipyretics are used, the ideal is in the form of herbal tea, such as the traditional YEP blend of yarrow, elderflower and peppermint, in an infant older than 6 months of age. This, in addition to *frequent* breastfeeding, is also a good way to keep fluids up to prevent dehydration during fever. Additionally, sips of warm water may be appropriate for the older infant.

Fever can cause significant worry and concern for parents, particularly in the case of febrile convulsions. Although paracetamol and ibuprofen can reduce fever, they have not been shown to prevent febrile convulsions.[214] Febrile convulsions, although extremely frightening for parents, generally have no adverse effect on the child.[217]

Every year there are numerous cases of over- and under-dosing with antipyretic pharmaceuticals.[218] Overdoses of antipyretic drugs have been associated with increased frequency of fever and can have severe adverse effects. If paracetamol or ibuprofen are administered, it is important that ibuprofen not be given to a child under the age of 6 months, and that either drug is dosed by weight, rather than age of the child. The NSW government's guidelines for dosage are: paracetamol 15 mg/kg given up to 4 hourly, with a maximum of 4 doses per 24 hours; ibuprofen 5–10 mg/kg/dose given every 6–8 hours (preferably with food).[219]

Paracetamol use in infancy has been linked with increased risk of asthma. The association is more significant in genetically susceptible infants and may be mediated by antioxidant glutathione depletion and eosinophilic inflammation.[220]

Hopefully most parents can be dissuaded from using paracetamol through education of the negative effects and unlikely benefit, despite the common belief that it is a necessary part of fever management.

SUMMARY OF FEVER MANAGEMENT

1   An infant younger than 3 months with fever should be immediately referred to a medical practitioner or emergency facility.

2   Assess the need for medical referral according to the traffic light tool (see Table 15.1) for all infants. Any infant displaying signs consistent with the middle and far right (orange and red) column should be referred to a medical practitioner or emergency department, respectively.

3   Monitor hydration status carefully and **refer if there are signs of dehydration**. Aim to prevent dehydration by encouraging fluid intake via very frequent breastfeeding, and in the older infant, some additional sipping of water or antipyretic YEP herbal tea (see below).

4   Disinterest in feeding for an infant is a red flag, and immediate referral to a medical practitioner or emergency department is indicated if the infant is too drowsy to feed.

5   Monitor and allow the fever to run its natural completion so that it is resolved as quickly as possible.

6   Refer the infant immediately to a medical practitioner or emergency department if fever persists for longer than 24 hours. When fever persists, the cause must be identified.

7   Never use aspirin. Never use ibuprofen for infants under 6 months old. Never mix ibuprofen and paracetamol. Antipyuretics such as paracetamol are only recommended when the infant is distressed. The level of severity indicates the need for medical referral and work-up.[221]

Fever-support tea blend (only in infants beyond 6 months of age)

*   10 g yarrow – febrifuge
*   10 g elderflower – febrifuge
*   10 g peppermint – febrifuge
*   10 g echinacea – immune support
*   10 g chamomile – calms a distressed or upset infant

Blend together and store in glass jar. Use 1 teaspoon per cup of boiling water. Infuse for 10 minutes before administering, ensuring that tea has cooled adequately first. Suitable for infants above 6 months of age; begin on 30 mL 3 times a day. All the herbs in this tea blend are very safe to consume in large amounts.

Well-appearing children with an apparent source of fever may be treated via the mother with specific therapy according to the source. Treating via the mother to maximise immune capacity with a low-sugar diet, plenty of rest, zinc adequacy and use of probiotics is indicated.

Reducing infection rates in the exclusively formula-fed infants

The exclusively, and partially, formula-fed infant is in effect immunosuppressed,[67] and consequently, experiences a greater number of infections with greater severity.[73,202,203] Some strains of probiotics have been investigated for their efficacy in reducing severity and duration of fever in exclusively formula-fed infants. Healthy term infants, aged 4–10 months, in childcare were fed a formula supplemented with *L. reuteri* Protectis or *B. lactis* BB12 as a part of a large double-blinded, randomised, controlled clinical trial in Israel. The infants fed formula with probiotics *L. reuteri* Protectis *or B. lactis* BB12 (dose 1 billion CFU daily) had a significant decrease of number of days with fever, clinic visits, childcare absences and antibiotic prescriptions.[211] Other strains that have evidence of efficacy with regards to decreasing infection rates and severity in formula-fed infants include LGG[176–178] and *L. fermentum* CECT5716.[184]

The unsettled and unsoothable infant
BACKGROUND

One in 5 infants are perceived by their parents to cry excessively.[222–224] A meta-analysis of 24 studies looking at parental crying diaries suggested the average crying at weeks 6 and 10–12 is around 110 minutes and 70 minutes, respectively.[225,226] Five per cent of infants presenting with excessive crying have an organic disease cause identified, and urinary tract infection is the most frequent cause in this group[227] (see Table 15.8). While this low proportion is reassuring, there is unfortunately an association between excessive crying in the early months and behavioural

TABLE 15.8 Serious underlying causes of crying in infants in the first few months of life

Abdominal	Appendicitis, malrotation/midgut volvulus, intussusception, incarcerated/strangulated hernia, peritonitis, choledocholithiasis, pancreatitis, intestinal obstruction
Cardiac	Myocarditis, congestive heart failure, supraventricular tachycardia
Chest	Hypoxia, hypercarbia, pneumonia, bronchiolitis, acute airway obstruction (croup, foreign body, asthma)
General	Bacteraemia, sepsis, hypovolaemia, hyperbilirubinaemia
Genitourinary	Testicular/ovarian torsion, genital tourniquet, UTI, nephrolithiasis
Head, eyes, ENT	Foreign body
Haematological	Sickle-cell disease, malignancy, neutropenia, thrombocytopenia, anaemia
Skin/ musculoskeletal	Septic arthritis, osteomyelitis, digital tourniquet, fracture, dislocation, subluxation, non-accidental trauma, cellulitis
Neurological	Bacterial meningitis, encephalitis, intracranial haemorrhage, hydrocephalus, cerebral oedema, epilepsy, degenerative condition
Toxic metabolic	Prenatal drug use, toxic ingestion, electrolyte abnormality, inborn error of metabolism, hyperthyroidism

Source: Reproduced with permission from Freedman SB, et al. The crying infant: Diagnostic testing and frequency of serious underlying disease. *Pediatrics* 2009;123:841–8. Copyright 2013 APP.

issues and ADHD diagnosis in childhood.[228,229] These findings indicate, on the one hand, that crying during the first 3 months is a common phenomenon and that most infants transition out of this, and on the other hand, that excessive crying in infancy is not benign and should be addressed. Communicating the potential associations with behavioural and developmental challenges to parents may not be helpful, however, as this may raise parental anxiety, which is a known risk factor for excessive crying.[230]

Frequently, parents go on a journey which involves seeing multiple practitioners in a quest to soothe the infant's crying, exposing parents to many sources of conflicting advice. Infants who cry excessively are often tagged with a range of diagnostic labels (see below) and are at greater risk of medical or pharmaceutical interventions.[231,232] They are also more likely to be prematurely weaned and given breast milk substitutes.[233–235] Postnatal depression correlates strongly with excessive infant crying.[236] Sadly, excessive crying is associated with a higher risk of infant head trauma via parental shaking.[237,238]

Parenting practices may influence infant crying frequency and duration. The influence of maternal carrying while walking on infant crying and neurophysiology has recently been investigated.[17,239] Walking compared to sitting with the infant soothes infant crying. Infants also stop voluntary movements and have a rapid decrease in heart rate, which is associated with parasympathetic changes. This suggests the relaxation effect is both a physiological and a behavioural response.[17] This phenomenon is observed in humans as well as other mammals. A study by James-Roberts et al. found that proximal parenting (which involves carrying [or wearing] the infant, spending most of the time in close contact, responding promptly to the infant's cues, and co-sleeping) was associated with 50% less crying per 24 hours compared to more typical Western parenting practices (holding the baby less, separate sleeping arrangements and delayed responses to the infant). However, babies in both groups had bouts of unsoothable crying.[240]

Responsiveness to crying may modify crying as a risk factor for later negative mental health outcomes. One study found that rapid parental response to crying was associated with reduced risk of depression later in life.[241] While parental responsiveness may support child mental emotional resilience, prolonged crying may be a trigger for uncontrolled parental abuse behaviour (such as shaking an infant), so parents need strategies to keep their infant safe in the event that they sense they are not coping with prolonged crying or unsettled behaviour.

NEURO-ENDOCRINE MODEL UNSOOTHABLE CRYING

One explanatory model for persistent unsoothable crying is a positive neurohormonal feedback loop that is triggered by physical discomfort or perceived threat. This model suggests that an initial stimulus causes sympathetic nervous system (SNS) arousal and adrenaline release, which triggers a crying response.[242] The crying response causes further SNS arousal and the release of cortisol and adrenaline. Crying continues even after the initial stimulus for crying has been removed. A sensitised stress response may develop in some infants resulting in the infant more easily entering this unsoothable crying state. Douglas et al. propose that unrecognised feeding problems may be a major initiating and maintaining factor, causing a sensitised stress response.[242] Unsoothable crying spells resolve at around 4 months for most infants, in line with neuroendocrine maturation.[242]

COMMON DIAGNOSTIC LABELS APPLIED TO UNSETTLED INFANTS

Colic

Colic describes the extreme end of unsettled crying behaviour. Previously, it has been defined as the rule of threes: crying for 3 hours or more, 3 or more days of the week, for 3 weeks or more in an infant that is less than 3 months of age in the absence of organic disease.[232,243] The Rome IV criteria has reclassified colic as being consistent with 'the prolonged, hard to soothe and unexplained nature of (the) crying behaviour'.[243] Colic by definition does not describe a particular cause for the crying. However, frequently the term 'colic' is used loosely as a term to describe what is perceived to be wind pain in the infant. It is important to consider this possibility in context of the broader discussion of infant physiology and infant–parental and environmental interactions presented here.

GORD

Based on current evidence, gastro-oesophageal reflex disease (GORD) is an *unlikely* cause of infant crying.[244,245] Despite this, infants who cry excessively are frequently tagged with the diagnostic label of 'reflux', and some go on to be prescribed proton pump inhibitors, which is at odds with current evidence and general practice recommendations.[246–249] An Australian-population-based study involving 4674 infants found that 23% of parents reported their infant had reflux, and more than half of the infants who were taken to a medical practitioner were prescribed acid-suppressing medication.[231] This amounted to 8% of the total population. Similarly, other studies have shown a dramatic increase in the prescriptions of acid-suppressing medications in infants.[248,250,251]

REFLUX AND NORMAL PHYSIOLOGY

All infants have physiological reflux (or GOR), which is the passage of stomach contents into the oesophagus,[249] and most babies exhibit regurgitation (the passive movement of stomach contents into the pharynx or mouth).[245] Infants have a greater number of daily physiological reflux events due to having a comparatively shorter oesophagus than adults, having an immature lower oesophageal sphincter[252] and being on a liquid diet. Regurgitation occurs in 60–85% of 2-month-old infants[253] and peaks at age 4 months, with 40% of infants regurgitating with most feeds.[254] By the age of 12 months, only 5% of infants regurgitate.[253]

Note: vomiting, which is the *forceful* movement of stomach contents through the mouth, needs to be distinguished from regurgitation. Vomiting, particularly when it is projectile, occurring more than twice requires investigation and may indicate the presence of pyloric stenosis. Vomiting can also be a sign of acute illness or allergy.

GORD occurs when GOR causes troublesome symptoms or damage. The ESPGHAN has clearly stated that there is no symptom or symptom complex that is diagnostic of GORD or that predicts response to therapy.[246] Despite this, many symptoms are often inappropriately attributed to GORD (see Box 15.7). The main reason that true GORD is very uncommon in infants is that most refluxate in infants is non-acidic.[258] Infants produce proportionally less stomach acid than adults.[258] The presence of breast milk or formula in the stomach has a buffering effect for 2 hours after feeds; this is the period when most reflux events occur (73%). Outside this period, refluxate is still non-acidic one-third of the time.[259] Further, reflux events occur less frequently during sleep.[260] Note: GOR may coincide with a crying spell because crying causes oesophageal spasm and may alter stomach motility.[255]

Based on current physiological understandings, the frequent nature of infant feeding means that refluxate is buffered most of the time, particularly when infant feeding is cue-based. Hence, exposure to acid GOR is

infrequent at most, and the potential for repeated acid GOR producing GORD is remote.

A 2015 systematic review found that acid-suppressing medications are no better than placebo for treating symptoms ascribed to GORD in infants.[247] It was noted that in both the treatment and no treatment groups, there was an improvement in symptoms over time.[247] This, along with placebo effects, means that empirical observations can be misleading when it comes to gauging the effectiveness of these treatments. There is a growing appreciation of the potential of acid-suppressing medications to cause harm, including increased risk of allergy, coeliac disease, dysbiosis, lower and upper respiratory tract infections, gastrointestinal infections and acid rebound.[53] Further flora alterations in lung and gastric secretions have been identified in paediatric populations with a history of acid-suppressing medication exposure.[54] The ESPGHAN and the NASPGHAN clinical practice guidelines state that there is no evidence for the empirical use of acid-suppressing medications in infants,[246] which is further supported by Gieruszczak-Białek et al.'s more recent systematic review findings.[247]

Cow's milk protein allergy can cause dysmotility, which may result in enhanced GOR and, potentially, GORD.[261] Further allergy may manifest as oesophageal irritation, including eosinophilic oesophagitis in a small number of infants.[262] However, most infants have physiological GOR that is unrelated to their crying. Infants with oesophageal atresia or cystic fibrosis and neurologically handicapped children are more likely to suffer from true GORD.[245]

LACTOSE INTOLERANCE

Congenital lactose intolerance is an extremely rare life-threatening condition that becomes apparent on the second or third day of life. It is associated with severe

---

BOX 15.7 Non-specific signs often erroneously used to support diagnosis of GORD (i.e. not evidence based)[255,256]

1. Back arching and crying or fussing during feeds:
   Frequently related to postural instability (positioning and attachment issue)[232]
   Response to slow or fast milk ejection reflex
   Defecation urge[257] or uncomfortable peristalsis stimulated by suckling
2. Irritability
3. Cries unless held
   Normal infant behaviour
4. Coughing, choking and gagging when feeding
   Frequently due to fast milk ejection
   Babies who display breathing difficulties when feeding should be assessed by a paediatrician
   May indicate tracheomalacia or heart defect
5. Poor weight gain
   Non-specific sign
   Intake needs to be assessed (see Box 15.1)
   Weighing errors are common (see Box 15.2)

TABLE 15.9 Types of lactose intolerance

Developmental	Neonates born before 34 weeks of gestation have decreased enzyme due to gut immaturity: Early feeding with human milk promotes gut maturation and increased lactase enzyme[264]
Congenital	A rare condition that becomes apparent on the 2nd or 3rd day of life: Only a few cases described in the literature[263] Severe watery diarrhoea, dehydration, malnutrition and electrolyte disturbances[263] Life-threatening, requiring immediate withdrawal of lactose from the diet[263]
Primary	Does not occur in infants: Lactase non-persistence occurs after weaning for 75% of the population worldwide Typically this does not occur before age 6 or 7 years[265,266]
Secondary	A temporary condition resulting from villi damage: Caused by allergy; infection; inflammatory bowel disease; coeliac disease; antibiotic use[266,267]; and may or may not be temporary after bowel surgery. Depending on the underlying cause, infant may exhibit signs of failure to thrive
Lactose overload	Relatively common and easily resolved with breastfeeding support: Feeding issue results in lower lipid intake, causing faster transit time and increased large bowel exposure to lactose. Infants are typically thriving, but can be unsettled with explosive stools and large volumes of intestinal gas[255]

watery diarrhoea, dehydration, electrolyte disturbances and malnutrition.[263] Only a few cases have been described, mostly from Finland.[263] This is not a presentation that the naturopath is ever likely to see in the community.

Secondary lactose intolerance occurs as a result of villi damage through allergy, infection and bowel surgery. An infant with secondary lactose intolerance may present with frothy, greenish, watery stools and meteorism. Depending on the cause and the duration of exposure, they may have associated signs of dehydration, including lowered urinary output and poor weight gain. Mucus may be present in the stool. Referral for appropriate medical work-up to identify the underlying cause and for monitoring of hydration status is important. Lactose intolerance associated with viral gastroenteritis typically resolves within a week.

Lactose in breast milk will not harm the gut, and breast milk is important for gut mucosal repair and protection from infection. Breastfeeding should be encouraged and protected. Even for formula-fed infants, lactose-free formulas are not recommended for extended periods as it is physiologically normal for infants to have a high lactose intake.

See Table 15.9 for types of lactose intolerance.

LACTOSE OVERLOAD

Feeding issues can give rise to lower lipid intake, faster transit time and increased large bowel lactose exposure, resulting in lactose fermentation and gas production.[255] This is a potential cause of infant discomfort. Decreased stool pH results can give rise to skin irritation in the nappy area.[267] This phenomenon is called *lactose overload*. It can be corrected with breastfeeding assistance that ensures effective drainage of the breast and that the infant accesses the breast milk lipids, which are more available as the breast empties.[255,267] Simplistic regimented strategies such as block feeding may cause further breastfeeding problems, including low supply. Cue-based feeding, allowing comfort nursing and cluster feeding, gives infants the opportunity to access the lipid-rich hind milk.[255] A lactation consultant or breastfeeding counsellor can give individualised guidance. The main goals are to ensure effective positioning and attachment at the breast, support breast milk removal and give the infant greater access to lipid-rich hind milk.

LACTOSE MALABSORPTION TESTING IN BREASTFED INFANTS

The high concentration of lactose in breast milk means that some lactose resists digestion and absorption in the small intestine. Hence, the majority of healthy breastfed infants test positive to reducing sugars in the stool,[268–270] making this test unreliable for assessing lactose malabsorption.[270]

OTHER POTENTIAL CAUSAL FACTORS
Postnatal maternal mood disorders

Maternal anxiety and mood dysphoria and infant crying appear to have a bidirectional association. Caring for an infant with high levels of crying and fussing increases the risk of postnatal depression.[271] Unsurprisingly, postnatal depression also appears to increase the risk of higher levels of crying in infant offspring.[236]

Frequent bouts of unsoothable crying are particularly difficult for parents to bear. Several studies have found an association with parents' reports of unsoothable or prolonged crying and postnatal depression.[271,272] An aspect of this is the parents' feeling of helplessness when their infant cries. Increased rates of postnatal depression continue for months after the crying has resolved.[271]

Maternal depression as assessed in the first weeks postnatally is associated with increased risk of excessive infant crying later.[236] This is particularly the case when there is altered parental attachment that impacts on parental responsiveness to infant cues, which may lead to infant dysregulation.[236] Three main factors may underpin altered parental attachment: 1) maternal depression reduces maternal attentiveness and response behaviour to infant crying[273,274]; 2) parents report fears of spoiling their infant by responding to their cries or holding them too much, which may consciously override their instinct to respond[230]; and 3) a generational knock-on effect may occur via learnt behaviour from the mother's experiences as an infant.[200,275] Aside from altered attachment, parental mood may have a direct influence on an infant's sense of ease.

Parental anxiety may be heightened by fearing high levels of crying indicate something is wrong with their infant, and the pursuit of an answer and receipt of a high level of conflicting advice may further contribute to anxiety.

Early life stress

Stressful experiences such as birthing difficulties, separation, medical interventions and high parental anxiety may heighten the newborn infant's stress response and make them more prone to bouts of unsoothable crying.[242] Dysregulation of maternal–infant synchrony is also a proposed source of infant stress.[242]

Sensory hunger

Infants have a need for positive sensory stimulation, and this can be important not only for their neurocognitive development, but also plays a role in growth, weight gain and psychomotor development.[276] It is postulated that positive sensory stimulation may assist with down regulating the SNS (dialling down infant stress levels).[277] Types of stimulation thought to support neurocognitive development include those experienced: while breastfeeding (or feeding in physically close contact); when in skin-to-skin contact; during responsive social interactions; while rhythmic walking[16]; and through being outdoors in natural environments.[277,278] It has been proposed that lack of sensory stimulation (or boredom) may be one of many potential triggers for crying in the young infant.[277]

Visceral hypersensitivity

The infant may be more vulnerable to visceral hypersensitivity occurring secondary to dysbiosis, immaturity, food allergy or infection. Interestingly, Eutamène et al. found that the luminal contents of 'colicky' infants induced visceral hypersensitivity in mice, while that of 'non-colicky' infants did not.[279] They also found that visceral hypersensitivity correlated with the presence of *Bacteroides vulgatus* counts,[279] supporting a dysbiosis hypothesis.

Dysbiosis

Dysbiosis has the potential to induce a chronic low-grade inflammatory response, resulting in the release of inflammatory cytokines and causing sensitisation of local nervous tissue (visceral hypersensitivity).[280] The relative abundance of gas-producing bacteria types may also cause gastrointestinal discomfort.[281] A 2017 systematic review of studies utilised DNA sequencing techniques to compare intestinal microbiota characteristics between infants defined as 'colicky' (displaying high levels of infant crying) and 'non-colicky controls'. Between-study similarities included high levels of crying associated with greater numbers of *Klebsiella* and *Escherichia* genus species, and lower levels of *Actinobacteria* and *Firmicutes* phyla including lactobacilli and bifidobacteria.[280] They also found lower diversity was a risk factor for greater crying. Dysbiosis does seem a plausible explanation for gastrointestinal discomfort for infants.

Gastrointestinal food allergy

As discussed above, food allergy can contribute to visceral hypersensitivity and dysmotility.[282] More severe presentations may result in malnutrition and acute hypovolaemic shock. These more severe presentations are typically restricted to the formula-fed infant.[283] Table 15.10 describes the clinical features of gastrointestinal allergy in infants. Infants with any of these clinical presentations require medical assessment by a paediatrician. It is worth noting that the non-IgE allergy disorders will *not* be detected via skin prick or RAST testing. Allergic proctocolitis, while thought to be a relatively common presentation, is often not considered within a differential diagnosis. This condition is typically diagnosed based on exclusion of other causes for blood streaks in the stool (see Table 15.11) in the thriving breastfed infant.[284]

Migraine

It has been proposed that migraine is a possible cause for inconsolable infant crying.[286] This theory arose based on case control studies finding that children and adolescents with a history of high levels of infant crying are 6.6–7 times more likely to experience migraines.[287] Further, maternal migraine is a risk factor for high levels of infant crying.[288]

CLINICAL APPROACH TO THE UNSETTLED AND UNSOOTHABLE INFANT

The clinical presentation of an infant with a history of excessive crying and/or 'unsettledness' needs to be considered in two domains: 1) considering the possible cause for distress including ruling out serious disease; and 2) considering the stress experienced by the parent in both caring for an unsettled infant and worrying that something may be seriously wrong with their infant. The interaction between infant crying and parental mental health needs to be considered, and the potential for a bidirectional relationship appreciated and factored into the care provided. Further, an appreciation of the multifactorial nature of cry-fuss problems provides a useful context for understanding this presentation, including consideration of the cultural, biological, psychosocial and environmental influences.

The first priority, as with any infant-related presentation, is to identify and/or rule out serious causes of infant distress. See the traffic light tool for signs of acute illness, and further consider other indications for concern and referral, such as signs of inadequate intake (see Table 15.1), and/or being slow to reach development milestones (see Table 15.3), or blood and/or mucus in stool (see Table 15.11). A frequently unidentified cause of infant distress is a feeding problem[255] (see Box 15.8). Hence, referral to a lactation consultant or breastfeeding counsellor is important to identify and rule out this as the cause or contributing factor.

Feeding issues: lipids and cholecystokinin

When feeding difficulties are present, this may result in infants accessing less fat, or 'cream', at the breast. This is

		TABLE 15.10 Gastrointestinal allergic disorders in infancy[283]		
Disorder	**Mechanism**	**Site affected, clinical features**	**Immune mechanisms**	**Common allergens**
Eosinophilic gastroenteropathies	Mixed IgE/non-IgE	GIT Vomiting and diarrhoea hours to days after exposure	Eosinophilic infiltration of GIT	Multiple foods
Food-protein-induced enteropathy	Non-IgE	GIT vomiting and diarrhoea – moderate failure to thrive Symptoms delayed 40–72 hours (Typically infants 2–24 months; majority resolves by 2–3 years)		Cow's milk, soy, grains Does not occur in breastfed infant
Food-protein-induced proctocolitis	Non-IgE	Blood-streaked stools in infants Mucus occurring 6–72 hours after exposure (infant normal weight gains) (Typically infant <6 months; resolves by 12 months)	Eosinophilic infiltration in the colon This is possibly a milder version of FPIES – occurring in the breastfed infant	Allergen exposure trace amounts via breast milk Cow's milk, egg, soy are commonly reported; a wide variety of food allergens may be involved
Food-protein-induced enterocolitis syndrome (FPIES)	Non-IgE	GIT Profuse repeated vomiting 2–6 hours after ingesting allergen, often with bloody diarrhoea (fluid shift, dehydration, failure to thrive). Chronic presentation occurs in some infants/toddlers – very rarely in exclusively breastfed infants Prognosis depends on allergy: 25% soy and 40% cow's milk; resolve by 2 years, respectively	Mechanism unclear – T cell mediated? ↑TNFα ↓TNFβ	Cow's milk (40% of cases), soy milk, egg, and corn proteins. Wide range of foods can be implicated in the infant eating solid foods, including grains (rice, oat), meats, fish, egg and vegetables Very rarely in exclusively breastfed infants

TABLE 15.11 Differential diagnosis of rectal infantile food protein-induced enterocolitis syndrome (FPIES)	
Severe	Necrotising enterocolitis Sepsis Hirschsprung's disease Intussusception Volvulus
Mild/moderate	Anal fissure Perianal dermatitis/excoriations Gastrointestinal infection (*Salmonella*, *Shigella*, *Campylobacter*, *Yersinia* spp., parasites) Coagulation disorders Vitamin K deficiency FPIAP

FPIAP = food-protein-induced allergic proctocolitis
Source: Nowak-Węgrzyn A, editor Food protein-induced enterocolitis syndrome and allergic proctocolitis. *Allergy and Asthma Proceedings* 2015;36(3):172–84.[285]

BOX 15.8 Evidence of feeding difficulties[277]

Nipple pain or damage

The most common cause of nipple pain is an attachment/latch issue. Ineffective attachment leads to insufficient milk transfer, which may risk maternal supply and/or result in inadequate intake (see Chapter 14). As part of taking the history, it is important to ask about nipple pain, including asking if breastfeeding is comfortable.

Frequent crying and fussing at breast

This includes back arching at the breast. Fussing and back arching at the breast may represent the infant's response to a range of issues, including positional instability, infant oral–motor issue,[98,278] forceful let down, slow let down or low supply, infant wants the other breast, feeding stimulates the urge to defecate or urinate.[100]

Any indication of insufficient intake (see Box 15.1)

because there is a higher proportion of lipid content as the breast empties which may not be accessed with poor attachment, for example. Hence, in this scenario, there may be lower cholecystokinin release. Cholecystokinin is a hormone that promotes satiety and relaxation after a feed.[289] One small study showed that infants with higher levels of crying had lower pre- and 1-hour postprandial cholecystokinin levels than controls.[290]

Lower fat concentration also means breast milk travels through the digestive tract more quickly, reducing the time available for lactose digestion. Hence, a greater lactose load reaches the large bowel, resulting in greater gas production (lactose overload as discussed previously).

OVERVIEW OF CAUSES OF INFANT CRYING

Once immediate safety concerns have been ruled out and feeding issues have been addressed, it is valuable to consider the infant with an appreciation of normal physiology and infant behaviour, and to have an understanding of the many reasons infants cry and how crying is typically a signal indicating an unmet need or a perception of threat. Box 15.9 lists the potential immediate triggers for an infant crying episode. Following this, it can be helpful to consider a broader view of why an infant may be more prone to excessive crying (see Table 15.12). It is worth considering the different domains and the potential interaction between these. One proposed model is the possums approach, which has produced some promising initial findings.[278]

Possums approach

The possums approach has been developed by a multidisciplinary clinic in Australia. This involves

addressing five domains of infant and maternal wellbeing: mother's health, baby's health, feeding, sleeping and sensation. The model involves utilising cued care and encourages mothers to continue with activities that they enjoy, including social activity and exercising with their infant. The aim is promoting sensory nourishment for the infant through exposure to varied healthy, nourishing environments that are also enjoyable for mothers.[289] An overarching goal is synchronised maternal–infant attachment and responsiveness in a context that makes the mother's life easier, not harder.[242] This model aims to upregulate oxytocic, dopaminergic and parasympathetic nervous systems and downregulate SNS and neuroendocrine anxiety-inducing activity in infants and mothers.[242] Preliminary research on this model has suggested that it has favourable effects on infants' day and night crying time and on mothers' mental wellbeing.[278]

Naturopathic treatments that may be of benefit are discussed in Table 15.13. It must be highlighted that good referral practice is a crucial part of naturopathic management. Considering the wellbeing of the infant in the context of the mother/parent–baby dyad and greater family is another important goal. Accordingly, naturopathic strategies may be focused on maternal and parental emotional wellbeing as well as infant gastrointestinal health and immune regulation. Treating through the mother is recommended when working with the exclusively breastfed infant.

COMMON INFANTILE PRESENTATIONS

Oral thrush

Candida spp. are both commensal organisms and potential pathogens. Oral *Candida* colonisation appears to occur in 10–20% of infants aged 0–1 year.[306] Importantly, infants who are colonised with *Candida* do not necessarily develop

---

> **BOX 15.9 Immediate causes of infant crying**
>
> Startled/ frightened
>   Call for help
> - To be close to parent to be safe
> - To nurse
>   Hunger
> - Early hunger cues may have been missed
>   Feeding difficulty
>   Boredom
> - Sensory needs not being met
>   Processing stimuli
> - Overwhelm
> - Changing experience of the world
>   Tired – needing help to transition into sleep
>   Need to urinate or defecate
>   Pain or discomfort
>   Reaction to parental stress?
>   Can signal serious injury or illness

TABLE 15.12 Causes of excessive crying and distress in infants (serious illness excluded)		
Neurobiological	**Feeding issue**[255]	**GIT distress**
Signalling to parent	Attachment issues	Visceral hypersensitivity[291]
• To be carried	Positional instability	Secondary to
• Safety/neuro-calming	Scheduling	• Immature gut
• Need for suckling	Cues missed	• Stress
Sensory deprivation/boredom	• Greater stress with feeds	• Intolerance or allergy[282]
• Need for change of scene	• Hunger	• Inflammation
• Need for more sensory input – observe activity; skin to skin; outside	Lack of 'dessert feeds'	• Dysbiosis[279]
Sensory overload/overwhelm	• Reduced lipids, reduced cholecystokinin[255]	When needs to defecate?
• Stress release response	• Lactose overload	Dysmotility – reflux
		Secondary to
Pregnancy stress/birth trauma/separation trauma		• Food allergy[282]
• Stress		• Dysbiosis
• Musculoskeletal impact		Oesophagitis
Parental anxiety/depression[292]		Secondary to
• Baby/parent feedback		• Food allergy[262]
		• Acid reflux (very rare)
		Secondary lactose intolerance

oral thrush (also termed acute pseudomembranous candidosis) or other manifestations of infection. While transmission to the infant occurs via intranatal vaginal exposure,[307,308] extra-maternal sources appear to account for some colonisation.[309] Dummies and bottle teats can act as reservoirs for *Candida* and *Staphylococcus* spp., for example.[310,311] Interestingly, lactoferrin concentration in breast milk has an inverse relationship with *Candida* colonisation in the infant.[306] Maternal prenatal and intranatal antibiotics and neonatal antibiotic exposure increase the risk of neonatal *Candida* infection.[312] The preterm and low-birth-weight infant is at greater risk of buccal inflammation and systemic *Candida* infection.[313] Malnutrition increases the risk of *Candida* carriage and infection,[314] as does HIV infection.[314] Corticosteroids and other immune-suppressing medications also increase the risk of *Candida* infection.[315] In the healthy newborn, oral thrush is self-limiting; however, because it can lead to feeding problems, it should be treated. Thrush developing in the older infant may be an indication of immunosuppression, coexisting health issue and/or nutritional deficiency.

TABLE 15.13 Naturopathic treatments for excessive crying in infancy	
Essentials	
• Rule out serious health issue (see Table 15.1)	– Refer for medical work-up
• Address feeding issues	– Refer to lactation consultant
Initial treatments (phase I)	
Probiotics via the breastfeeding mother	*Lactobacillus rhamnosus* GG (LGG) Has the potential to reduce allergy risk,[293] promote tolerance to food allergens[172–174] and may reduce visceral sensitivity[180] and intestinal inflammations.[294] Furthermore, there is evidence that it passes through the breast milk.[179] *Lactobacillus reuteri* Protectis (*L. reuteri* MM53 and *L. reuteri* DSM 17938) There is evidence of breast milk transfer[183] (see Table 14.11). Maternal administration is associated with decreased inflammatory cytokine TGF-beta2 in breast milk.[295] One study in infants indicated that it may have utility for reducing regurgitation events.[296] A 2015 meta-analysis including six RCTs found that crying time had decreased by after 2 weeks and more than halved after 3 weeks of treatment, but by the fourth week crying time was not different to controls.[297] This may be related to the gastrointestinal maturation and neurological development that drives improvement with time. Treatment via the mother is the preferred option in the infant under 6 months. When the infant is exclusively formula-fed probiotics, can be added to formula.
Prebiotics	Breast milk is a rich source of a large array of prebiotic foods that selectively nourish the infant microbiome (see Chapter 14); hence, prebiotic supplementation is not indicated. The formula-fed infant may benefit from galactooligosaccharides at 0.4 g/100 mL of formula.[298] Maternal supplementation with fructooligosacharides 4 g BD may increase the regulatory cytokine IL-27 in breast milk according to one human study.[187]
Support maternal healthy microbiome	Maternal healthy microbiota likely to influence infant microbiota via the entero–mammary transfer of bacteria.[299] Optimise the maternal intestinal and mammary microbiome through dietary interventions that ensure a diverse intake, or dietary prebiotics and selective supplementation with prebiotics and probiotics, and where indicated select probiotics with evidence of transfer to the breast milk, including LGG, *L. reuteri* Protectis and *L. fermentum* CECT5716 (see Table 14.11).
Lifestyle suggestions	• Supporting sensory nourishment and 'dialling' down of the infant and maternal nervous system – Responsive cue-based feeding – Baby wearing and carrying[16] – Walks – Outdoor pleasant sensory experiences Enjoyable social contact for parents with baby in tow[289]
Herbal treatment through the mother	Carminatives Selecting those with a thymoleptic or anxiolytic action such as *Chamomilla recutita* and *Lavendula officinalis* may support dual benefit Nervines A nourishing herbal approach to the mother which has a mood lifting and gentle adaptogenic effect, and is also likely to have a positive influence on the infant by improving the wellbeing of the mother. Consider herbs such as *C. recutita*, *Lavendula officinalis*, *Asparagus racemosa*, *Withania somnifera*, *Verbena officinalis* and *Leonorus cardiaca*. Anti-inflammatory Turmeric has a range of actions that may be of benefit including supporting mood and neuroprotective, anti-inflammatory and carminative actions.

TABLE 15.13 Naturopathic treatments for excessive crying in infancy—cont'd

Initial treatments (phase I)

Support infant defecation and passage of wind	Many infants appear to be more settled after defecation and passage of gas. Elimination communication One strategy to support defecation and the passage of flatus is the traditional practice of elimination communication or a modified form of this.[257] In essence, this involves holding the infant in a supported squat position over a collecting vessel without any restriction to the abdomen, as may occur with clothing and nappies. Typically, the infant's back is supported against the parent's abdomen. Parents may find their infant displays behaviour such as wriggling and fussing while feeding that they then come to link with their infant's need to defecate, pass wind or urinate.[257] Abdominal massage with carminative oils *Pimpinella anisum* (aniseed) and *Foeniculum vulgare* (fennel) contain primarily the volatile oil anethole. *Anethum graveolens* (dill) is high in carvone and *Carum carvi* (caraway) is rich in d-carvone.[300] *Pimpinella anisum* has been shown to have relaxant and antispasmodic effects on smooth muscle of rats by inhibiting acetylcholine-induced contraction.[301] Due to these oils being the main active constituent, these herbs can be used topically by diluting the essential oils into a base oil to be massaged gently into the abdomen in a clockwise direction, or the mother can drink them as a tea. Specific herbal medicines include: *P. anisum* (aniseed), *F. vulgare* (fennel), *C. carvi* (caraway seed), *Zingiber officinalis* (ginger rhizome), *Matracaria recutita* (chamomile flowers), *A. graveolens* (dill seeds) Essential oils If using essential oil, use 3 drops maximum for a 0–2-month-old and up to 5 drops for a 2–12-month-old per 30 mL base oil. Dilute 1 drop each of 3–5 essential oils of the herbs listed above into 30 mL base oil, such as olive oil. Mix well and use as a massage oil for the abdomen (clockwise motions), legs and feet (massaging towards the heart).
A conversation about relactation	The reintroduction of breast milk promotes gastrointestinal healing and the return of the many functions for maternal and infant health, including intestinal mucosal development and maturation, protection from gastrointestinal infections and dysbiosis. Relactation may be a welcome possibility for some mothers, many of whom are unlikely to know that this is a genuine possibility.

Phase II (earlier when specifically indicated based on history)

Osteopathy and cranial sacral therapy	Musculoskeletal restrictions associated with birth and rapid growth, along with heightened pain perception, have been theorised to be a potential cause of infant distress,[302] and occasionally, feeding difficulties. Referral to an osteopath or cranial sacral practitioner with paediatric training accreditation is another avenue to consider. This therapy may help resolve restrictions, particularly when the birth has been traumatic. A systematic review of clinical studies in this area suggests that these treatments may be beneficial, although there were some limitations with the quality of the included studies.[303]

Infant maternal elimination diets	Food allergy is suspected when:
	  – there is a strong family history of atopy
	  – signs of gastrointestinal inflammation such as mucus or blood in the stool (other causes ruled out)
	  – when infantile eczema or asthma is present[282]
	  – when the infant has very dry skin.
	The dietary triggers that have been more commonly reported in association with excessive crying in infancy include: cow's milk protein (which commonly cross-reacts with goat's and sheep's milk protein), eggs, peanuts, tree nuts, wheat, soy and fish. One unblinded study found that maternal dietary elimination of these foods was associated with reduced crying after 1 week compared to control group.[304] A reduction in symptoms should be apparent after 2 weeks of exclusion.[282] In the formula-fed infant, a 2 week trial of a partially or extensively hydrolysed whey or casein formula is worthwhile.[208]
	While evidence of food allergy suggests that an elimination diet may assist with symptom reduction, in the absence of clear evidence of moderate to severe allergic response, the benefits of allergen avoidance need to be weighed against the potential risks associated with this approach. Elimination diets can place an already stretched family under greater stress. They may also deprive infants of the potential to develop tolerance by limiting exposure during a critical window, and predispose them to developing a more severe food allergy.[305] One overarching goal is to promote oral tolerance.

CLINICAL PRESENTATION

Oral *Candida* infection (thrush) appears as white plaques on the tongue, inside the cheek and inside the lips. When the plaque is removed or rubbed off, a red area is revealed that may bleed. The general area is often red and inflamed. Oral thrush can be overdiagnosed through misinterpreting normal milk residue in the infant's mouth or the presence of benign features such as Ebstein's pearls[316] and/or breastfeeding keratosis.[317] Nipple pain is more likely to be related to a breastfeeding attachment issue than *Candida* infection, although trauma associated with the former may predispose the area to fungal or bacterial infection.[318]

Note: medical assessment is recommended for any lesion that has blisters, when the infant is unwell and/or when the lesion fails to resolve. Concerning diagnoses include malignancy and herpes infection.[319]

TREATMENT OF ORAL THRUSH

Prior to treatment, rule out other causes of mouth lesions (see above). When *Candida* infection is present, both the baby's mouth and the mother's breast need to be simultaneously treated (see Chapter 14). Carefully select treatments that will have lowest risk to the infant's health considering the infant's age. Maternal administration of a probiotic strain with proof of efficacy in preventing or treating *Candida* infection and colonisation, such as *L. rhamnosus* GG and *L. reuteri* Protectis, is recommended.[170,320] These strains are also suitable because there is evidence they are transferred to maternal milk.[179,183] Higher-end maternal dosages are recommended to facilitate breast milk transfer. Oral candidiasis is a condition where topical application of these probiotics is potentially justified if there is not improvement after several days. The newer probiotic oil preparations are probably the most suitable for direct application to the infant. Where this is not available, the mother can place a quarter teaspoon of probiotic powder in a clean dish and then gradually into the infant's mouth using a clean finger. Two to three drops of a cooled thyme tea can be applied to the infant's mouth 2–3 times daily at a separate time to the probiotics. The infusion can be prepared by steeping in a covered vessel 2 teaspoons of dried thyme leaves to half a cup of boiling water for 30 minutes, and allowing this to cool before using it for the day.

The infant's condition should be resolved or at least markedly better within a week of treatment. If the infant's symptoms are worsening, prompt referral to a medical practitioner is recommended. Referral is also recommended when the symptoms have not markedly improved within a week.

Nappy rash

Nappy rash (or diaper dermatitis) is a common issue for infants. Immature skin barrier function increases the infant's vulnerability to irritants. The skin of the infant nappy area is often exposed to prolonged moisture contact, friction, pH alterations, faecal bacteria, bacterial enzymes, nappy materials and/or washing residues. Furthermore, many infants may be exposed to irritants in baby wipes, creams and talcum powder. Of note, preliminary epidemiology evidence has linked perianal talcum powder use with increased ovarian cancer risk.[321]

Coughlin et al. suggested that it is useful to consider three broad categories of nappy rash: 1) skin conditions that are caused by the presence of a nappy; 2) rashes exacerbated by the presence of a nappy; and 3) rashes or eruptions that are present irrespective of the presence of a nappy[322] (see Table 15.14). Of note, irritation caused by a nappy can cause skin barrier breakdown predisposing to infection, most commonly with *Candida* spp. but also with *Streptococcus* spp. and *Staphylococcus* spp. When nappy rash persists for longer than 3 days, a secondary infection should be considered.[322] A rash that follows the nappy elastic line is suggestive of allergic contact dermatitis.

TREATMENT

Once serious causes of the rash have been ruled out, often simple treatment steps are fairly universally effective:

TABLE 15.14 Quick guide to eruptions in the nappy area			
Subgroup	**Eruption**	**Morphology**	**Distribution in the nappy area**
Skin conditions caused by the presence of the nappy	Irritant diaper dermatitis	Redness, papules, scaling, superficial erosions; less commonly elevated papules or nodules	Skin under the nappy
	Allergic diaper dermatitis	Redness, oedema, vesicles, superficial erosions	Skin in contact with the nappy
	Miliaria	Erythematous papules, occasionally small pustules	Occluded skin in the nappy area
Rashes exacerbated by the nappy (but not directly caused by it)	*Candida albicans* diaper dermatitis	Bright-red patches with satellite macules or pustules, collarettes of scale	Intertriginous folds
	Streptococcal nappy dermatitis	Bright red patches, some maceration, no satellitosis	Perianal or inguinal creases
	Staphylococcal diaper dermatitis	Small red papules, pustules, fragile blisters, folliculitis, less commonly furuncles or abscesses	Skin under the nappy
	Seborrhoeic dermatitis	Red patches, some scale	Intertriginous folds, gluteal cleft
	Psoriasis (nappy psoriasis)	Red patches, some scale	Buttocks, legs, abdomen, neck, face
	Psoriasiform id reaction	Red patches and papules, some scale	
Eruptions present irrespective of the presence of the nappy	Infantile haemangiomas	Erythematous papules, plaques and nodules	Skin under the nappy
	Langerhans cell histiocytosis	Scale, crusting, barely palpable haemorrhagic papules resembling petechiae, atrophy, deep ulcerations	Inguinal creases
	Zinc deficiency (including acrodermatitis enteropathica)	Red patches and plaque with accentuated scale (golden brown to mahogany colour) at the margin	Periorificial
	Kawasaki disease	Erythema, desquamation	Perianal
	Coxsackie virus infection (especially the A6 strain)	Vesicles, bullae, punched-out erosions, purpura, petechiae, Gianotti–Crosti-like papules	Buttocks, groin

Source: Coughlin CC, Eichenfield LF, Frieden IJ. Diaper dermatitis: clinical characteristics and differential diagnosis. *Pediatric Dermatology* 2014;31:19–24.[322]

- Nappy-free time as much as possible/feasible.
- Change nappies frequently to avoid prolonged contact with urine or faeces.
- Avoid baby wipes – instead use soft flannelette cloths (from washed old sheets rather than from new fabric which has chemical residue) and filtered water for washing.
- Use a natural barrier cream with simple ingredients such as beeswax and olive oil, shea butter or purified lanolin (avoid coconut oil and almond oil because of allergy risk, which is heightened on damaged skin).
- Topical breast milk can assist with reducing inflammation (and is as effective as corticosteroids according to one study[323]) and has antimicrobial and antifungal actions.
- If *Candida* or bacterial overgrowth is suspected, the following treatments can be trialled:
  - Application of a cream made in a pure olive oil and beeswax base (can be made with 1 part beeswax to 4 parts olive oil) with 3% lavender essential oil, 10% zinc oxide and 20% *Calendula-officinalis*-infused oil (in pure olive oil). Note: *Calendula officinalis* tincture has a high ethanol percentage which may be an irritant.
  - An infusion of *Origanum vulgare hirtum* (Greek oregano) leaf or *Thymus vulgaris* leaf (3 tablespoons of leaf steeped in a litre of boiling water in a covered vessel for half an hour). Add this to a bath containing at least 1 additional litre of water, allowing the infant's bottom to sit in the water. Following the bath, apply the above cream or a more simple barrier cream.

Cradle cap

Otherwise called infantile seborrhoeic dermatitis, cradle cap is suspected to have several causative factors. Dysfunction of the sebaceous glands appears to play a role as well as potentially lingering effects of placental hormones.[324] Additionally, the yeasts of the genus *Malassezia* are associated with cradle cap, particularly *M. furfur*.[325] Cradle cap has a higher incidence in families with a history of allergy or asthma.[326] Furthermore, severe cradle cap may precede atopic eczema. Older studies have linked impaired functioning of delta-6-desaturase with the development of cradle cap.[327] Tollesson et al. found that topical treatment with gamma-linoleic-acid (GLA)-rich borage seed oil was effective for cradle cap.[327] When cradle cap becomes severe and widespread, the infant should be investigated for immune suppression and other causes, including Leiner's disease.

SIGNS AND SYMPTOMS

Inflammatory eruptions of the scalp (and sometimes upper face) with redness and greasy-looking, yellowish scales and flakes.[326]

THERAPEUTIC TREATMENT

Scraping off the scales can cause bleeding and infection risk. A topical scalp treatment made to the following recipe can be used:

Oreganum officinalis leaf 2 tsp
Chamomilla recutita 2 tsp
Infused in ¾ cup of boiling water
Add 1 tablespoon of raw honey when water still warm
Add 2 tablespoons of apple cider vinegar
Spray or apply carefully to the scalp area once to twice daily
Make a fresh batch of the solution up every second day
Alternative treatment 2% lavender oil in olive oil used to soften the scales and for antifungal effect – massage scalp once a week.

Treat through the mother to improve essential fatty acid profile and optimal vitamin D status (see Chapter 14) and employ strategies to prevent the development of atopic disease, including maternal LGG supplementation.

Allergy in infancy

Infantile allergy typically manifests as eczema (see Chapter 16 in *Clinical Naturopathic Medicine* [CNM]) or gastrointestinal allergy (see Table 15.10). Asthma (refer to Chapter 14 in CNM) is less common in infancy. The first sign of allergy potential is often very dry skin in the newborn, and promoting optimal barrier function is a key strategy for allergy prevention. This and other important strategies are outlined in Chapter 16. Key strategies at birth may further promote healthy barrier function. These include immediate skin-to-skin contact, preservation of the infant's vernix and delay of the first bath, all of which may assist with promoting healthy skin flora colonisation and protect against acquiring potentially harmful species from hospital surfaces. Infants should be bathed in filtered water, and soaps should be avoided. Furthermore, avoidance of baby products that include anything but gentle plant-based ingredients is also advised.[328] Unnecessary ingredients, such as antiseptics (such as triclosan, found in some wipes and hand sanitisers), foaming agents (such as sodium lauryl sulphate, found in some commercial infant shampoos and bubble baths), fragrance and preservatives, should be diligently avoided as they can disturb the skin barrier and balance.[329–331]

Teething

The mean age for the first tooth to erupt is 8 months,[332] with a wide range including, rarely, infants being born with teeth. The current view is that localised symptoms of teething vary, but severe systemic upsets are unrelated to teething.[333] Importantly, studies investigating the cause of fever in children who are teething have found that other serious causes for the fever were present, most commonly urinary tract infections or gastrointestinal infections.[332] Hence, it is recommended that the traffic light referral guidelines (see Table 15.1) are followed despite the coexistence of apparent teething. Many parents believe that diarrhoea and fever can be caused by teething, which runs the risk of trivialising these signs to the point that parents do not seek assistance when they otherwise would.[333]

TREATMENT

Natural approaches can support infants with the local discomfort and with the associated emotional hardship. Topical treatments need to be age-appropriate. For the infant under 6 months, it is preferable to avoid these. Treatments that may assist include:

- *Breastfeeding.* Systematic review evidence indicates that breastfeeding is an effective form of pain relief for infants.[334] This may be due to pain relieving hormones, the soothing effect of suckling and the associated comfort. Ensuring deep attachment can reduce any biting or bearing down while teething. Other techniques may also be provided by a breastfeeding counsellor or lactation consultant.
- *Cuddle therapy* (responsive and tactile comforting of the infant) and use of distractions such as book reading, singing and playing.[335]
- *Gentle gum massage* by the mother using a clean finger.[335]
- *Teething toys* that are made of untreated non-toxic materials such as wood.
- *Safe foods* such a celery sticks and mango seeds that do not present a choking hazard in the infant who is eating solids.
- *Herbal medicines.* For the infant over 6 months, a topical gel containing 10% *Syzygium aromaticum* 1:2 tincture and 90% glycerol can be rubbed over the gums. Nervine herbs such as chamomile and lemon balm are excellent choices for distress associated with teething in the older infant. Blend the two dried herbs together and use 1 teaspoon to make a 100 mL infusion, and offer the older infant sips throughout the day. A therapeutic chewing cloth can be prepared by moistening the cloth in *Syzygium aromaticum* decoction (1 tablespoon of buds simmered in 1 cup of water for 10 minutes) and cooling it in the freezer.

CAUTIONS ABOUT PHARMACEUTICAL TEETHING GELS

Some over-the-counter teething gels contain salicylate compounds, which are contraindicated in children and infants because of the risk of developing Reye's syndrome.[336] Infants are particularly at risk of accumulation due to their comparatively slower metabolism of these compounds. Accordingly, several cases of salicylate toxicity from teething gels have been reported in the literature.[337] Following these reports, Bonjela has replaced the salicylate compounds with lidocaines in the UK and Australia. The safety of lidocaine exposure in infants is also dubious, with toxicity causing seizures in children.[338] In 1 year, the FDA reported 22 cases of serious adverse reactions, including death, in infants and young children aged 5 months to 3.5 years who were given oral viscous lidocaine 2% solution to treat mouth pain, including teething, or had accidental ingestion.[339] Popular brands are using a lower concentration; however, risks appear to outweigh the benefit of this treatment. Benzocaine is also not recommended because of case reports linking it to methaemoglobinaemia, a rare life-threatening condition.[340]

Infantile constipation

Considerable variation in 'normal' bowel habit in infants is accepted, and stool frequency is also age dependent.[341] Until 4–6 weeks of age, breastfeeding infants should pass a stool the size of their palm at least twice daily (see Table 15.1).

Bowel habits of the breastfed infant can shift at 4–6 weeks of age, following which the vast majority of infants will pass a bowel motion between 3 times a day and every second day.[342] Despite these common outcomes, a healthy infant beyond 6 weeks of age may go up to 10 days without passing a movement – highlighting the extent of the variation of 'normal'.[343]

A difference in stool frequency is widely observed between breastfed and bottle-fed babies,[344] but time to first stool after passage of meconium remains the same in both groups.[344] Stool colour is commonly yellow at 4 weeks and changes to brown by 6 months.[345] The introduction of solids at around 6 months of age will have an impact on the infant's microbiome, stool frequency and stool odour.

The wide variation in normal defecation patterns in infants discussed above makes it difficult to define constipation. Constipation can be divided into two categories: organic and functional. Organic causes of constipation include Hirschsprung's disease, anorectal malformation, hypothyroidism and spina bifida,[346] and are significantly less common.[347] Functional constipation is usually caused by one or a combination of the following: dehydration, dysbiotic bowel flora, food sensitivity, inadequate fibre intake (in an infant older than 6 months of age), anal fissures (cause and effect) and some medications.[348]

Functional constipation in a child has been defined by the Rome III criteria[349] as having two or more of the following features occurring at least once a week for the duration of at least 2 months before diagnosis: two or fewer stools per week, either hard or painful stools, a passage of very large stool, stool retention and a history of large faecal mass in rectum.[346] Screaming on defecation and severe stool withholding manoeuvres are also features of infantile constipation.[350]

Constipation and subsequent faecal retention behaviour often begins soon after an infant has experienced a painful evacuation. The diagnosis of constipation requires careful history taking and interpretation. A simple cause may be insufficient fluid intake, or insufficient fibre intake in a baby older than 6 months on solid foods.[348] When infants transition rapidly from exclusive breastfeeding to a high intake of solids, they are also at risk of constipation.

Cow's milk allergy is shown to be a significant aetiological factor for constipation in infants and young children. Serum levels of IgE to cow's milk proteins are helpful, although not definitive, for diagnosis.[351] Formula-fed infants with a strong family history of cow's milk protein intolerance, or raised eosinophil count, and elevated specific IgE to cow's milk, may benefit from a trial of cow's-milk-protein-free diet and, in infants, a hydrolysed formula.[351] A trial of cow's-milk-protein-free diet is also merited for non-IgE-mediated cow's milk protein intolerance in those with a suggestive history; for example, if constipation started on switching from breast- to formula-feeding.[352] Sensitively exploring the option of continued breastfeeding or relactation is also worthwhile.

It has been shown there are significant differences in bowel flora populations in constipated compared to non-constipated individuals and that this dysbiosis can also be an effect of rather than a cause of constipation.[353] Treatment time for constipation can range from a few days in simple cases to 12 months in more severe cases.[346]

SIGNS AND SYMPTOMS

- Large, hard stools
- Small, dry, pellet-like stools
- Painful defecation
- Infrequent bowel motions
- Skinny stools (indicates compacted faeces around the lumen, with only a narrow passage for overflow faeces to move through)
- Withholding behaviours (infants may withhold bowel motion to avoid pain of passing stool)
- Encopresis
- Overspill syndrome where watery stool will pass by compacted faeces in the rectum, giving the appearance of diarrhoea
- Straining, often indicated by whole body tensing and reddening of the face
- Haemorrhoids

TREATMENT OF INFANTILE CONSTIPATION

Ensuring adequate fluid intake, and in an infant older than 6 months of age established on solids, ensuring daily consumption of gentle fibres from plant foods, can be effective.[354]

Specific foods such as ground flaxseeds, ground chia seeds, prunes and kiwi fruit may be useful in increasing defecation frequency in infants over 6 months of age established on solids.[354,355]

Testing for cow's milk allergy and coeliac disease can be useful if suspected, and if other avenues have been exhausted.

Gut microbiota are clearly associated with GI motility,[356] and some probiotic bacteria have been shown to stimulate intestinal motility and peristalsis and decrease transit time, which is helpful to treat slow-transit constipation.[357,358] Probiotic supplementation is a predominantly simple and safe treatment option for infantile constipation. Probiotic powders may be given straight to the mouth of the older infant, applied to the breast nipple or added to expressed breast milk or formula after it has been warmed. Specific probiotic strains that have been shown to have a beneficial effect on bowel motion frequency and oro–faecal transit time include:

- *Bifidobacterium lactis* Bb-12 and DN-173 010[359,360]
- *Bifidobacterium lactis* HN019[361]
- *Lactobacillus casei* Shirota[362,363]
- *Lactobacillus casei rhamnosus* Lcr35[364]
- *Lactobacillus reuteri* MM53.[365]

For an infant older than 6 months already established on solids, the highly absorbent slippery elm may act as bulking and softening agent, at around 1–1.25 g per dose, between 1 and 3 times daily. Beyond about 9 months of age, ground chia seeds or ground flax meal may also be trialled in small amounts (e.g. 1 teaspoon per day). This increased bulk stimulates peristalsis, initiating a soft but formed bowel motion. These bulking agents also contain valuable prebiotics – substrates for healthy bacteria to feed off. Psyllium husks are slightly more abrasive and may not be suitable to infants under 12 months of age. It is important that the infant's breast milk and fluid intake is encouraged for the bulking agent to work effectively.

Slippery elm powder – up to 1.25 g per dose – is recommended mixed into sufficient water per day for infants up to 1 year old. It can be mixed into a paste with a little breast milk, formula or water and then mixed into mashed banana or pureed food. Often, a combination of slippery elm and probiotic quickly resolves almost all cases of minor constipation and greatly helps to establish regular bowel motions in chronic and severe constipation.

When dietary measures do not provide adequate relief, the osmotic laxative lactulose is usually effective and has ancillary prebiotic benefit – dose of 2–5 mL per day in infants between 6 and 12 months. Typically, the dose needs to be gradually increased to continue to be effective as the intestinal microbiota shift to utilise greater amounts of this prebiotic sugar. This is generally well tolerated by infants, but a few may experience bloating and increased flatulence. An excessive dose may cause diarrhoea.[366]

Other osmotic laxative agents may be prescribed by a GP or paediatric gastroenterologist, short term, to help loosen impacted faeces for evacuation. Possible adverse events when using common conventional osmotic and stimulant laxatives for the management of paediatric constipation include flatulence, abdominal pain, nausea and diarrhoea.[367]

HERBAL MEDICINE FOR MOTHERS WITH CONSTIPATION

Anthroquinone-containing laxative herbs are to be avoided in breastfeeding mothers and infants due to their habit-forming consequences and compromise to bowel tone. Prolonged use of laxatives – drug or herbal – can result in laxative dependence. Digestive bitters, cholagogues and hepatostimulant herbs for the breastfeeding mother may improve digestion and increase bile production, often resulting in softer stools.

Suitable herbal medicine for the breastfeeding mother if she is constipated include:

- *Taraxacum officinale radix* (dandelion root)
- *Glycyrrhiza glabra* (liquorice)
- *Mentha* x *piperita* (peppermint)
- *Matricaria recutita* (chamomile)
- *Foeniculum vulgare* (fennel)
- *Melissa officinalis* (lemon balm)
- *Gentiana lutea* (gentian)

EXAMPLE PROTOCOL

Supplementation

- Probiotic of suitable strains (mentioned above) at a dose of 5–10 billion CFU per day via breastfeeding mother, or directly to infant older than 6 months.
- From 6 months of age, gentle introduction of organic soaked prunes, peeled mashed kiwi fruit and slippery elm powder 1.25 g, up to 3 times a day added to meals (in small amounts).
- From 9 months of age, ground chia seeds or flax seeds, 1 teaspoon daily, mixed into a little water/breast milk/formula/mushy food.

> ### Constipation and safety
>
> Constipation can present as a medical emergency. Refer to Table 15.1 for assessing risk of serious illness and immediately refer to a GP or paediatric emergency in instances of any 'amber' or 'red' light presentations such as concomitant fever, respiratory changes or tachycardia.

Infantile diarrhoea

Diarrhoea is defined as the frequent passage of loose, watery stools. Acute diarrhoea is defined as that which lasts less than 2 weeks, while chronic diarrhoea is defined as that which lasts longer than 2 weeks. Diarrhoea in breastfed infants can be hard to diagnose as it is normal for these infants to have frequent loose stools. In this situation, diagnosis would be made by a change of these habits to even more frequent and watery stools.

THERAPEUTIC CONSIDERATIONS

Causes of diarrhoea range from the less common congenital, autoimmune illnesses and illness that affects pancreatic function (such as cystic fibrosis) to more common factors such as infections (viral, bacterial or parasitic), medication related (e.g. antibiotic-associated diarrhoea, AAD) or initial stages of chronic diarrhoea such as inflammatory bowel disease (Crohn's disease or ulcerative colitis), coeliac disease, food allergy or food intolerance. Copious green frothy stools and 'meteorism' in an otherwise thriving breastfed infant, particularly with persistent nappy rash, suggest that the breastfeeding dyad should be assessed as lactose overload may be present (see Table 15.9).

The most common cause of childhood diarrhoea is viral gastroenteritis (rotavirus infection).[368–370] Enteropathogenic *E. coli* can also cause chronic diarrhoea. Diarrhoea also occurs more frequently when there are urinary tract or respiratory tract infections.[369] Prophylactic use of probiotics during respiratory infections has been shown to reduce the incidence of secondary diarrhoea.[369]

The primary concern of acute infantile diarrhoea is the possibility of resultant dehydration. It is important for any infant with diarrhoea to have constant breast milk or fluid intake. In infants with acute diarrhoea, maintaining adequate blood volume and correcting fluid and electrolyte imbalances take priority over the identification of the causative agent. Dehydration of 3% (of estimated body weight loss of fluid) is undetectable, whereas dehydration of 10% or more is often fatal.[369] If dehydration starts to become apparent medical assistance should be sought (see Table 15.1).

In addition to the resultant dysbiosis caused with diarrhoea, diarrhoea may cause microtrauma to the mucosa of the digestive tract, creating inflammation and a reduction in digestive enzymes. This can result in malabsorption of macro- and micronutrients. This is of particular concern when chronic diarrhoea is present, as it can lead to failure to thrive and/or long-lasting secondary health concerns owing to multiple nutrient deficiencies during critical stages of growth and development.

It is well established that the risk of infant morbidity is negatively associated with the duration of breastfeeding, and breastfeeding is medically recommended for its protective effects against acute infections and diarrhoea. The risk of having diarrhoea is significantly reduced even when infants are partially breastfed for 6 months.[371]

Cohort studies of mother–infant pairs show that a significant amount of hospital admissions of infants with diarrhoea could be prevented with exclusive breastfeeding. Breastfeeding, particularly when exclusive and prolonged, protects against severe morbidity. A population-level increase in exclusive, prolonged breastfeeding would considerably reduce the disease burden of infantile diarrhoea and other infectious diseases.[372]

ANTIBIOTIC-ASSOCIATED DIARRHOEA (AAD) IN INFANCY

Ingestion of antibiotics has a disruptive effect on the intestinal microbiome. Antibiotics are prescribed frequently to infants and children, and antibiotic-associated diarrhoea (AAD) is common in this population. Breastfeeding supports microbiome resilience in the face of antibiotic exposure[52,373] through an array of prebiotics, including the human milk oligosaccharides and maternally derived probiotics.[373–375] Mothers typically feel reassured to know that their milk is providing their infant with some protection against the disruptive effects of antibiotics. Specific probiotic strains may assist in preventing AAD when given via the mother, and potentially co-administered to the infant over 6 months. Most likely, separating doses of antibiotics and probiotics by 2 hours is wise to maximise outcomes.

Probiotic strains with the most promising evidence for the prevention of AAD include LGG and *Saccharomyces boulardii* CNCM I-745 at 5–40 billion CFU/day). Adverse events are very rare.[376–380] Separating the dose of the probiotic by 2 hours seems appropriate.

A 2015 systematic review investigating the efficacy of probiotics in the prevention of paediatric AAD concluded that there is moderate quality of evidence to support efficacy without increase in adverse events.[377,381] Although adverse events in otherwise healthy children are very rare, serious adverse events have been observed in severely debilitated or immunocompromised children with underlying risk factors including central venous catheter use and disorders associated with bacterial/fungal translocation. Until further research has been conducted, probiotic use should be avoided in paediatric populations at risk for adverse events.[377] Among the various probiotics evaluated, LGG and *S. boulardii* (strain not stated) each had three and four studies respectively suggesting their efficacy in paediatric populations.[377]

TREATMENT OF INFANTILE DIARRHOEA

Regular intake of fluids is essential to maintain adequate hydration. Breast milk is ideal for infants as a rehydration solution. Coconut water is not a suitable rehydration fluid in the case of diarrhoea because it is not electrolyte matched. It is prudent to avoid artificial colours and flavours in a commercial electrolyte solution to minimise food chemical reactions in compromised infants (see Table 15.11).

With acute diarrhoea in infants who are not breastfed, changing to a lactose-free diet may result in earlier resolution of acute diarrhoea and reduce treatment failure.[382]

Nutritional medicine (supplementation)

There has been extensive research into the effect of probiotics on prevention and treatment of infantile diarrhoea. Dysbiosis is almost guaranteed in the case of any type of diarrhoea, and due to inflammatory effects of diarrhoea leading to disruptions in function of mucosal immunity, immune support is always warranted. Breast milk provides surface protection via immune cells, antibodies, human milk oligosaccharides and antiviral and selectively antimicrobial compounds such as lactoferrin, lysozymes, prebiotics and maternal transferred probiotics.[373–375,383] Additional probiotic treatment via the mother or direct to the infant older than 6 months may provide further protection. Careful prescription of specific bacterial strains may help to prevent and treat diarrhoea in the infant who is not breastfed. Specific probiotics strains with demonstrated efficacy address diarrhoeal diseases by a number of functions, including providing physical support to the gastrointestinal mucosal barrier (preventing pathogenic microbes from making contact), competitively inhibiting adhesion of pathogenic microbes to intestinal wall and stimulating non-specific host resistance to pathogenic microbes.[384] Numerous studies show that probiotics can be used successfully prophylactically, while others have identified specific strains for use in different types of diarrhoeal illnesses. Acute viral diarrhoea has been successfully treated with *L. acidophilus* LB, *L. reuteri* Protectis, LGG and *S. boulardii* CNCM I-745.[385–390] Antibiotic- and bacterial-induced diarrhoea can be successfully treated with LGG and *S. boulardii* CNCM I-745.[169,391] Persistent diarrhoea that follows acute gastroenteritis is best treated with *S. boulardii* CNCM I-745.[392]

Glutamine is a non-essential amino acid and a primary fuel source for enterocytes. Glutamine becomes conditionally essential during times of illness or injury and is required for rapidly dividing immune cells.[393] Hence, providing glutamine supplementation is thought to be an avenue of protection.[393] However, studies investigating the efficacy of glutamine in infantile diarrhoeal disease have produced inconclusive findings.[394,395] A once-daily dose of 500 mg of glutamine, along with a gentle soluble fibre such as slippery elm, in an infant over 6 months of age with mild diarrhoea may be gentle and supportive in helping to repair the inflamed mucosa of the infant intestinal mucosa.

Zinc depletion has been noted in children with dehydrating diarrhoea.[396] Zinc reduces the incidence and duration of diarrhoea in children due to its impact on digestive and immune function.[397] The mechanisms by which zinc reduces occurrence and duration of diarrhoea are not totally understood, but are believed to be due to its roles in improving water and electrolyte absorption in the intestines, rapid regeneration of gut mucosa, production of pancreatic and brush border enzymes and involvement in immune response.[397]

In areas where the prevalence of zinc deficiency or the prevalence of moderate malnutrition is high, zinc may be of benefit in children aged 6 months or more. The WHO guidelines on the clinical management of diarrhoea include routine use of zinc supplementation, at a dosage of 10–20 mg per day for infants older than 6 months, for 10–14 days duration following acute gastroenteritis.[398,399] Doses this high are significantly over the NHMRC RDI for zinc of 3 mg for an infant older than 6 months, which is reflective of breast milk zinc concentrations from a nutritionally replete mother,[400] so caution is advised. Zinc supplementation increases the risk of vomiting,[401] potentially via irritation of the stomach, which is probably more likely with higher doses. In children with persistent diarrhoea, zinc supplementation probably shortens the average duration of diarrhoea by around 16 hours.[402] A dose of 5 mg of elemental zinc (as gluconate or sulphate form) per day for 10–14 days in an infant older than 6 months, mixed into breast milk, food or electrolyte rehydration solution, may be helpful in reducing the frequency of diarrhoeal episodes and duration, and aiding recovery.[403] Zinc is mainly excreted in the faeces. In infants with persistent diarrhoea (greater than 2 weeks' duration) there is depletion of zinc with the progression of the disease, and oral zinc administration may improve zinc status.[404] The current evidence does not support the use of zinc supplementation in children below 6 months of age.[401]

Herbal medicine

For infants older than 6 months, vulnerary, anti-inflammatory and demulcent herbs are useful for soothing and healing gastrointestinal inflammation associated with diarrhoea. Slippery elm powder absorbs excess water in the bowel and the mucilage content is soothing to the GIT, helping to reduce inflammation. Other suitable herbs include calendula, mullein, chamomile, lemon balm and marshmallow. These can be used as a tea of herb extract in infants over 6 months of age.

Diarrhoea and safety

Diarrhoea can present as a medical emergency. If diarrhoea persists for more than 6 hours in infants under 6 months or 12 hours in an infants over 6 months, seek medical advice. Refer to Table 15.1 for assessing risk of serious illness and immediately refer to a general practitioner or paediatric emergency in instances of any 'amber' or 'red' light presentations such as concomitant fever, respiratory changes or tachycardia.

REFERENCES

[1] Zalewski BM, Patro B, Veldhorst M, et al. Nutrition of infants and young children (one to three years) and its effect on later health: a systematic review of current recommendations (Early Nutrition project). Crit Rev Food Sci Nutr 2017;57(3):489–500.

[2] Bartick MC, Schwarz EB, Green BD, et al. Suboptimal breastfeeding in the United States: maternal and pediatric health outcomes and costs. Matern Child Nutr 2017;13(1):e12366.

[3] Victora CG, Bahl R, Barros AJD, et al. Breastfeeding in the 21st century: epidemiology, mechanisms, and lifelong effect. Lancet 2016;387(10017):475–90.

[4] Stuebe A. The risks of not breastfeeding for mothers and infants. Rev Obstet Gynecol 2009;2(4):222–31.

[5] Fields E, Chard J, Murphy MS, et al. Assessment and initial management of feverish illness in children younger than 5 years: summary of updated NICE guidance. BMJ 2013;346:f2866.

[6] Van den Bruel A, Haj-Hassan T, Thompson M, et al. Diagnostic value of clinical features at presentation to identify serious infection in children in developed countries: a systematic review. Lancet 2010;375(9717):834–45.

[7] Thompson M, Van den Bruel A, Verbakel J, et al. Systematic review and validation of prediction rules for identifying children with serious infections in emergency departments and urgent-access primary care. Health Technol Assess 2012;16(15):1–100.

[8] Sidebotham P, Fraser J, Covington T, et al. Understanding why children die in high-income countries. Lancet 2014;384(9946):915–27.

[9] Cleugh F, Langseth A. Fifteen-minute consultation on the healthy child: breast feeding. Arch Dis Child Educ Pract Ed 2017;102:8–13.

[10] Brodribb W. Breastfeeding management in Australia. 4th ed. East Malvern: Australian Breastfeeding Association; 2012.

[11] Sachs M, Dykes F, Carter B. Weight monitoring of breastfed babies in the UK – centile charts, scales and weighing frequency. Matern Child Nutr 2005;1(2):63–76.

[12] Newman J. Is my baby getting enough milk? 2009. Available from: http://www.breastfeedinginc.ca/content.php?pagename=doc-IMB.

[13] Oberklaid F, Drever K. Is my child normal? Milestones and red flags for referral. Aust Fam Physician 2011;40(9):666–70.

[14] Stevens J, Schmied V, Burns E, et al. Immediate or early skin-to-skin contact after a Caesarean section: a review of the literature. Matern Child Nutr 2014;10(4):456–73.

[15] Gitau R, Modi N, Gianakoulopoulos X, et al. Acute effects of maternal skin-to-skin contact and massage on saliva cortisol in preterm babies. J Reprod Infant Psychol 2002;20(2):83–8.

[16] Esposito G, Setoh P, Yoshida S, et al. The calming effect of maternal carrying in different mammalian species. Front Psychol 2015;6:445.

[17] Esposito G, Yoshida S, Ohnishi R, et al. Infant calming responses during maternal carrying in humans and mice. Curr Biol 2013;23(9):739–45.

[18] Bergman NJ. Neonatal stomach volume and physiology suggest feeding at 1-h intervals. Acta Paediatr 2013;102(8):773–7.

[19] ABM Clinical Protocol #3: hospital guidelines for the use of supplementary feedings in the healthy term breastfed neonate, revised 2009. Breastfeed Med 2009;4(3):175–82.

[20] Marasco LA. Unsolved mysteries of the human mammary gland: defining and redefining the critical questions from the lactation consultant's perspective. J Mammary Gland Biol Neoplasia 2014;19(3):271–88.

[21] Rudzik AE. Normal infant sleep and parental expectations. Int J Birth Parent Educ 2015;2(2):7–10.

[22] Galland BC, Taylor BJ, Elder DE, et al. Normal sleep patterns in infants and children: a systematic review of observational studies. Sleep Med Rev 2012;16(3):213–22.

[23] Australian Institute of Health and Welfare. Australia's mothers and babies 2013 – in brief. Canberra: AIHW; 2015.

[24] Noel-Weiss J, Woodend AK, Peterson WE, et al. An observational study of associations among maternal fluids during parturition, neonatal output, and breastfed newborn weight loss. Int Breastfeed J 2011;6:9.

[25] Okumus N, Atalay Y, Onal EE, et al. The effects of delivery route and anesthesia type on early postnatal weight loss in newborns: the role of vasoactive hormones. J Pediatr Endocrinol Metab 2011;24(1–2):45–50.

[26] Onis M. WHO Child Growth Standards based on length/height, weight and age. Acta Paediatr 2006;95(S450):76–85.

[27] De Onis M. World Health Organization Reference Curves. The EOCG's ebook on child and adolescent obesity; 2015. Available from: https://ebook.ecog-obesity.eu/content/.

[28] Koletzko B, von Kries R, Monasterolo RC, et al. Can infant feeding choices modulate later obesity risk? Am J Clin Nutr 2009;89(5):1502S–8S.

[29] Johnson CL, Versalovic J. The human microbiome and its potential importance to pediatrics. Pediatrics 2012;129(5):950–60.

[30] Salminen SJ, Gueimonde M, Isolauri E. Probiotics that modify disease risk. J Nutr 2005;135(5):1294–8.

[31] Kolida S, Saulnier DM, Gibson GR. Gastrointestinal microflora: probiotics. Adv Appl Microbiol 2006;59:187–219.

[32] Neu J, Hauser N, Douglas-Escobar M, editors. Postnatal nutrition and adult health programming. Semin Fetal Neonatal Med 2007;12:78–86.

[33] Rodríguez JM, Murphy K, Stanton C, et al. The composition of the gut microbiota throughout life, with an emphasis on early life. Microb Ecol Health Dis 2015;26.

[34] Chen J, Cai W, Feng Y. Development of intestinal bifidobacteria and lactobacilli in breast-fed neonates. Clin Nutr 2007;26(5):559–66.

[35] Favier CF, Vaughan EE, De Vos WM, et al. Molecular monitoring of succession of bacterial communities in human neonates. Appl Environ Microbiol 2002;68(1):219–26.

[36] Bjorksten B, Sepp E, Julge K, et al. Allergy development and the intestinal microflora during the first year of life. J Allergy Clin Immunol 2001;108(4):516–20.

[37] Ouwehand A, Isolauri E, Salminen S. The role of the intestinal microflora for the development of the immune system in early childhood. Eur J Nutr 2002;41(Suppl. 1):I32–7.

[38] Isolauri E, Salminen S. Probiotics, gut inflammation and barrier function. Gastroenterol Clin North Am 2005;34(3):437–50, viii.

[39] Gronlund MM, Gueimonde M, Laitinen K, et al. Maternal breast-milk and intestinal bifidobacteria guide: the compositional development of the Bifidobacterium microbiota in infants at risk of allergic disease. Clin Exp Allergy 2007;37(12):1764–72.

[40] Gdalevich M, Mimouni D, Mimouni M. Breast-feeding and the risk of bronchial asthma in childhood: a systematic review with meta-analysis of prospective studies. J Pediatr 2001;139(2):261–6.

[41] Ruiz-Palacios GM, Calva JJ, Pickering LK, et al. Protection of breast-fed infants against Campylobacter diarrhea by antibodies in human milk. J Pediatr 1990;116(5):707–13.

[42] McGuire W, Anthony M. Donor human milk versus formula for preventing necrotising enterocolitis in preterm infants: systematic review. Arch Dis Child Fetal Neonatal Ed 2003;88(1):F11–14.

[43] Owen CG, Martin RM, Whincup PH, et al. Effect of infant feeding on the risk of obesity across the life course: a quantitative review of published evidence. Pediatrics 2005;115(5):1367–77.

[44] Owen CG, Martin RM, Whincup PH, et al. Does breastfeeding influence risk of type 2 diabetes in later life? A quantitative analysis of published evidence. Am J Clin Nutr 2006;84(5):1043–54.

[45] Yatsunenko T, Rey FE, Manary MJ, et al. Human gut microbiome viewed across age and geography. Nature 2012;486(7402):222–7.

[46] Borre YE, Moloney RD, Clarke G, et al. The impact of microbiota on brain and behavior: mechanisms & therapeutic potential. Adv Exp Med Biol 2014;817:373–403.

[47] Jernberg C, Löfmark S, Edlund C, et al. Long-term impacts of antibiotic exposure on the human intestinal microbiota. Microbiology 2010;156(1):3216.

[48] Vangay P, Ward T, Gerber JS, et al. Antibiotics, pediatric dysbiosis, and disease. Cell Host Microbe 2015;17(5):553–64.

[49] Cox LM, Blaser MJ. Antibiotics in early life and obesity. Nat Rev Endocrinol 2015;11(3):182–90.

[50] Barrett E, Kerr C, Murphy K, et al. The individual-specific and diverse nature of the preterm infant microbiota. Arch Dis Child Fetal Neonatal Ed 2013;98(4):F334–40.

[51] Mueller NT, Bakacs E, Combellick J, et al. The infant microbiome development: mom matters. Trends Mol Med 2015;21(2):109–17.

[52] Azad MB, Konya T, Persaud RR, et al. Impact of maternal intrapartum antibiotics, method of birth and breastfeeding on gut microbiota during the first year of life: a prospective cohort study. BJOG 2016;123(6):983–93.

[53] Stark CM, Nylund CM. Side effects and complications of proton pump inhibitors: a pediatric perspective. J Pediatr 2016;168: 16–22.

[54] Rosen R, Amirault J, Liu H, et al. Changes in gastric and lung microflora with acid suppression: acid suppression and bacterial growth. JAMA Pediatr 2014;168(10):932–7.

[55] Cong X, Xu W, Janton S, et al. Gut microbiome developmental patterns in early life of preterm infants: impacts of feeding and gender. PLoS ONE 2016;11(4):e0152751.

[56] Groer MW, Gregory KE, Louis-Jacques A, et al. The very low birth weight infant microbiome and childhood health. Birth Defects Res C Embryo Today 2015;105(4):252–64.

[57] Goldsmith F, O'Sullivan A, Smilowitz JT, et al. Lactation and intestinal microbiota: how early diet shapes the infant gut. J Mammary Gland Biol Neoplasia 2015;20(3):149–58.

[58] Davis EC, Wang M, Donovan SM. The role of early life nutrition in the establishment of gastrointestinal microbial composition and function. Gut Microbes 2017;4(8):143–71.

[59] Kortman GAM, Dutilh BE, Maathuis AJH, et al. Microbial metabolism shifts towards an adverse profile with supplementary iron in the TIM-2 in vitro model of the human colon. Front Microbiol 2015;6:1481.

[60] Kortman GAM, Raffatellu M, Swinkels DW, et al. Nutritional iron turned inside out: intestinal stress from a gut microbial perspective. FEMS Microbiol Rev 2014;38(6):1202–34.

[61] Jaeggi T, Kortman GAM, Moretti D, et al. Iron fortification adversely affects the gut microbiome, increases pathogen abundance and induces intestinal inflammation in Kenyan infants. Gut 2015;64(5):731–42.

[62] Chu DM, Meyer KM, Prince AL, et al. Impact of maternal nutrition in pregnancy and lactation on offspring gut microbial composition and function. Gut Microbes 2016;7(6):459–70.

[63] Matsuo K, Palmer JB. Anatomy and physiology of feeding and swallowing: normal and abnormal. Phys Med Rehabil Clin N Am 2008;19(4):691–707, vii.

[64] Delaney AL, Arvedson JC. Development of swallowing and feeding: prenatal through first year of life. Dev Disabil Res Rev 2008;14(2):105–17.

[65] Kaye J. Review of paediatric gastrointestinal physiology data relevant to oral drug delivery. Int J Clin Pharm 2011;33(1):20–4.

[66] Le Huërou-Luron I, Blat S, Boudry G. Breast- v. formula-feeding: impacts on the digestive tract and immediate and long-term health effects. Nutr Res Rev 2010;23(01):23–36.

[67] Turfkruyer M, Verhasselt V. Breast milk and its impact on maturation of the neonatal immune system. Curr Opin Infect Dis 2015;28(3):199–206.

[68] Mikami K, Kimura M, Takahashi H. Influence of maternal bifidobacteria on the development of gut bifidobacteria in infants. Pharmaceuticals (Basel) 2012;5(6):629–42.

[69] Catassi C, Bonucci A, Coppa GV, et al. Intestinal permeability changes during the first month: effect of natural versus artificial feeding. J Pediatr Gastroenterol Nutr 1995;21(4):383–6.

[70] Kramer MS, Kakuma R. Optimal duration of exclusive breastfeeding. Cochrane Database Syst Rev 2012;(8):CD003517.

[71] Tawai S. Iron and exclusive breastfeeding. Breastfeed Rev 2012;20(1):35–47.

[72] Coovadia HM, Rollins NC, Bland RM, et al. Mother-to-child transmission of HIV-1 infection during exclusive breastfeeding in the first 6 months of life: an intervention cohort study. Lancet 2007;369(9567):1107–16.

[73] Quigley MA, Carson C, Sacker A, et al. Exclusive breastfeeding duration and infant infection. Eur J Clin Nutr 2016;70(12):1420–7.

[74] Blackburn S. Maternal, fetal, & neonatal physiology: a clinical perspective. St Louis: Saunders Elsevier; 2007.

[75] Dewit O, Dibba B, Prentice A. Breast-milk amylase activity in English and Gambian mothers: effects of prolonged lactation, maternal parity, and individual variations. Pediatr Res 1990;28(5):502–6.

[76] Lindquist S, Hernell O. Lipid digestion and absorption in early life: an update. Curr Opin Clin Nutr Metab Care 2010;13(3):314–20.

[77] Hamosh M, Henderson TR, Ellis LA, et al. Digestive enzymes in human milk: stability at suboptimal storage temperatures. J Pediatr Gastroenterol Nutr 1997;24(1):38–43.

[78] Michaelsen KF, Greer FR. Protein needs early in life and long-term health. Am J Clin Nutr 2014;99(3):718S–22S.

[79] Baur LA, Allen JR. Goat milk for infants: yes or no? J Paediatr Child Health 2005;41(11):543.

[80] Yokoi T. Essentials for starting a pediatric clinical study (1): pharmacokinetics in children. J Toxicol Sci 2009;34(Special): SP307–12.

[81] Demmelmair H, von Rosen J, Koletzko B. Long-term consequences of early nutrition. Early Hum Dev 2006;82(8):567–74.

[82] Koletzko B. Early nutrition and its later consequences: new opportunities. Adv Exp Med Biol 2005;569:1–12.

[83] Smith HA, Becker GE. Early additional food and fluids for healthy breastfed full-term infants. Cochrane Database Syst Rev 2016;(8):CD006462.

[84] Dórea JG. Magnesium in human milk. J Am Coll Nutr 2000;19(2):210–19.

[85] Olausson H, Goldberg GR, Ann Laskey M, et al. Calcium economy in human pregnancy and lactation. Nutr Res Rev 2012;25(1):40–67.

[86] Bravi F, Wiens F, Decarli A, et al. Impact of maternal nutrition on breast-milk composition: a systematic review. Am J Clin Nutr 2016;104(3):646–62.

[87] Houghton LA, Yang J, O'Connor DL. Unmetabolized folic acid and total folate concentrations in breast milk are unaffected by low-dose folate supplements. Am J Clin Nutr 2009;89(1):216–20.

[88] Domellöf M, Lönnerdal B, Dewey KG, et al. Iron, zinc, and copper concentrations in breast milk are independent of maternal mineral status. Am J Clin Nutr 2004;79(1):111–15.

[89] Lönnerdal B. Trace element transport in the mammary gland. Annu Rev Nutr 2007;27(1):165–77.

[90] Thiele DK, Senti JL, Anderson CM. Maternal vitamin D supplementation to meet the needs of the breastfed infant: a systematic review. J Hum Lact 2013;29(2):163–70.

[91] Fisher W, Wang J, George NI, et al. Dietary iodine sufficiency and moderate insufficiency in the lactating mother and nursing infant: a computational perspective. PLoS ONE 2016;11(3):e0149300.

[92] Davenport C, Yan J, Taesuwan S, et al. Choline intakes exceeding recommendations during human lactation improve breast milk choline content by increasing PEMT pathway metabolites. J Nutr Biochem 2015;26(9):903–11.

[93] Fischer LM, da Costa KA, Galanko J, et al. Choline intake and genetic polymorphisms influence choline metabolite concentrations in human breast milk and plasma. Am J Clin Nutr 2010;92(2):336–46.

[94] Siddiqua TJ, Ahmad SM, Ahsan KB, et al. Vitamin B12 supplementation during pregnancy and postpartum improves B12 status of both mothers and infants but vaccine response in mothers only: a randomized clinical trial in Bangladesh. Eur J Nutr 2016;55(1):281–93.

[95] Quentin C, Huybrechts S, Rozen L, et al. Vitamin B12 deficiency in a 9-month-old boy. Eur J Pediatr 2012;171(1):193–5.

[96] World Health Organization. Infant and young child feeding: a model chapter for medical students and allied health professionals; 2009. Available from: http://www.who.int/nutrition/publications/infantfeeding/9789241597494/en/.

[97] Kent G. Regulating fatty acids in infant formula: critical assessment of U.S. policies and practices. Int Breastfeed J 2014;9(1):2.

[98] National Health and Medical Research Council. Infant feeding guidelines: information for health workers 2012. Canberra: Australia National Health and Medical Research Council; 2013.

[99] Walsh A, Kearney L, Dennis N. Factors influencing first-time mothers' introduction of complementary foods: a qualitative exploration. BMC Public Health 2015;15:939.

[100] Cattaneo A, Williams C, Pallás-Alonso CR, et al. ESPGHAN's 2008 recommendation for early introduction of complementary foods: how good is the evidence? Matern Child Nutr 2011;7(4):335–43.

[101] World Health Organization. Infant and young child feeding: model chapter for textbooks for medical students and allied health professionals. Switzerland: WHO; 2009.

[102] Fewtrell M, Bronsky J, Campoy C, et al. Complementary feeding: a position paper by the European Society for Paediatric Gastroenterology, Hepatology, and Nutrition (ESPGHAN) Committee on nutrition. J Pediatr Gastroenterol Nutr 2017;64(1):119–32.

[103] Netting MJ, Campbell DE, Koplin JJ, et al. An Australian consensus on infant feeding guidelines to prevent food allergy: outcomes from the Australian infant feeding summit. The journal of allergy and clinical immunology. In Pract 2017;5(6):1617–24.

[104] Walsh A, Kearney L, Dennis N. Factors influencing first-time mothers' introduction of complementary foods: a qualitative exploration. BMC Public Health 2015;15:939.

[105] Yang Z, Lönnerdal B, Adu-Afarwuah S, et al. Prevalence and predictors of iron deficiency in fully breastfed infants at 6 mo of age: comparison of data from 6 studies. Am J Clin Nutr 2009;89(5):1433–40.

[106] Domellof M, Braegger C, Campoy C, et al. Iron requirements of infants and toddlers. J Pediatr Gastroenterol Nutr 2014;58(1):119–29.

[107] McDonald SJ, Middleton P, Dowswell T, et al. Effect of timing of umbilical cord clamping of term infants on maternal and neonatal outcomes. Cochrane Database Syst Rev 2013;(7):CD004074.

[108] Terefe B, Birhanu A, Nigussie P, et al. Effect of maternal iron deficiency anemia on the iron store of newborns in Ethiopia. Anemia 2015;2015:808204.

[109] Paiva Ade A, Rondó PHC, Pagliusi RA, et al. Relationship between the iron status of pregnant women and their newborns. Rev Saude Publica 2007;41:321–7.

[110] Gondolf UH, Tetens I, Michaelsen KF, et al. Iron supplementation is positively associated with increased serum ferritin levels in 9-month-old Danish infants. Br J Nutr 2013;109(1):103–10.

[111] Qasem W, Fenton T, Friel J. Age of introduction of first complementary feeding for infants: a systematic review. BMC Pediatr 2015;15:107.

[112] Uyoga MA, Karanja S, Paganini D, et al. Duration of exclusive breastfeeding is a positive predictor of iron status in 6- to 10-month-old infants in rural Kenya. Matern Child Nutr 2017;13(4):e12386.

[113] World Health Organization. Exclusive breastfeeding for six months best for babies everywhere. Switzerland: WHO; 2011.

[114] Eidelman AI, Schanler RJ, Johnston M, et al. Breastfeeding and the use of human milk. Pediatrics 2012;129(3):e827–41.

[115] Hornell A, Lagstrom H, Lande B, et al. Breastfeeding, introduction of other foods and effects on health: a systematic literature review for the 5th Nordic Nutrition Recommendations. Food Nutr Res 2013;57.

[116] Kc A, Rana N, Målqvist M, et al. Effects of delayed umbilical cord clamping vs early clamping on anemia in infants at 8 and 12 months: a randomized clinical trial. JAMA Pediatr 2017;171(3):264–70.

[117] Dewey KG. The challenge of meeting nutrient needs of infants and young children during the period of complementary feeding: an evolutionary perspective. J Nutr 2013;143(12):2050–4.

[118] Dewey KG, Chaparro CM. Session 4: mineral metabolism and body composition Iron status of breast-fed infants: symposium on 'Nutrition in early life: new horizons in a new century'. Proc Nutr Soc 2007;66(3):412–22.

[119] Akkermans MD, Uijterschout L, Abbink M, et al. Predictive factors of iron depletion in late preterm infants at the postnatal age of 6 weeks. Eur J Clin Nutr 2016;70(8):941–6.

[120] Pineda O, Ashmead HD. Effectiveness of treatment of iron-deficiency anemia in infants and young children with ferrous bis-glycinate chelate. Nutrition 2001;17(5):381–4.

[121] Milman N, Jønsson L, Dyre P, et al. Ferrous bisglycinate 25 mg iron is as effective as ferrous sulfate 50 mg iron in the prophylaxis of iron deficiency and anemia during pregnancy in a randomized trial. J Perinat Med 2014;42(2):197–206.

[122] Ma J, Sun Q, Liu J, et al. The effect of iron fortification on iron (Fe) status and inflammation: a randomized controlled trial. PLoS ONE 2016;11(12):e0167458.

[123] Qasem W, Azad MB, Hossain Z, et al. Assessment of complementary feeding of Canadian infants: effects on microbiome & oxidative stress, a randomized controlled trial. BMC Pediatr 2017;17(1):54.

[124] Bains K, Uppal V, Kaur H. Optimization of germination time and heat treatments for enhanced availability of minerals from leguminous sprouts. J Food Sci Technol 2014;51(5):1016–20.

[125] Gibson RS, Perlas L, Hotz C. Improving the bioavailability of nutrients in plant foods at the household level. Proc Nutr Soc 2006;65(2):160–8.

[126] Iron needs of babies and children. Paediatr Child Health 2007;12(4):333–4.

[127] Abbaspour N, Hurrell R, Kelishadi R. Review on iron and its importance for human health. J Res Med Sci 2014;19(2):164–74.

[128] Jensen RG. Lipids in human milk. Lipids 1999;34(12):1243–71.

[129] Enig MG. Know your fats: the complete primer for understanding the nutrition of fats, oils and cholesterol. Silver Spring, MD: Bethesda Press; 2000.

[130] Hardy SC, Kleinman RE. Fat and cholesterol in the diet of infants and young children: implications for growth, development, and long-term health. J Pediatr 1994;125(5):S69–77.

[131] Shahidi F, Senanayake SPJN. Fatty acids A2. In: Heggenhougen HK, editor. International encyclopedia of public health. Oxford: Academic Press; 2008. p. 594–603.

[132] Lien VW, Clandinin MT. Dietary assessment of arachidonic acid and docosahexaenoic acid intake in 4–7 year-old children. J Am Coll Nutr 2009;28(1):7–15.

[133] Ryan AS, Astwood JD, Gautier S, et al. Effects of long-chain polyunsaturated fatty acid supplementation on neurodevelopment in childhood: a review of human studies. Prostaglandins Leukot Essent Fatty Acids 2010;82(4–6):305–14.

[134] Bourre JM. Roles of unsaturated fatty acids (especially omega-3 fatty acids) in the brain at various ages and during ageing. J Nutr Health Aging 2004;8(3):163–74.

[135] Heaton AE, Meldrum SJ, Foster JK, et al. Does docosahexaenoic acid supplementation in term infants enhance neurocognitive functioning in infancy? Front Hum Neurosci 2013;7:774.

[136] Innis SM. Dietary omega 3 fatty acids and the developing brain. Brain Res 2008;1237:35–43.

[137] Swanson D, Block R, Mousa SA. Omega-3 fatty acids EPA and DHA: health benefits throughout life. Adv Nutr 2012;3(1):1–7.

[138] Vajpayee S, Sharma SD, Gupta R, et al. Early infant feeding practices may influence the onset of symptomatic celiac disease. Pediatr Gastroenterol Hepatol Nutr 2016;19(4):229–35.

[139] Minniti F, Comberiati P, Munblit D, et al. Breast-milk characteristics protecting against allergy. Endocr Metab Immune Disord Drug Targets 2014;14(1):9–15.

[140] Henriksson C, Boström A-M, Wiklund IE. What effect does breastfeeding have on coeliac disease? A systematic review update. Evid Based Med 2013;18(3):98–103.

[141] Sansotta N, Piacentini GL, Mazzei F, et al. Timing of introduction of solid food and risk of allergic disease development: understanding the evidence. Allergol Immunopathol (Madr) 2013;41(5):337–45.

[142] Krebs NF. Dietary zinc and iron sources, physical growth and cognitive development of breastfed infants. J Nutr 2000;130(2):358S–60S.

[143] Beyer K, Morrowa E, Li X-M, et al. Effects of cooking methods on peanut allergenicity. J Allergy Clin Immunol 2001;107(6):1077–81.

[144] Koenig JE, Spor A, Scalfone N, et al. Succession of microbial consortia in the developing infant gut microbiome. Proc Natl Acad Sci USA 2011;108(Suppl. 1):4578–85.

[145] Fallani M, Young D, Scott J, et al. Intestinal microbiota of 6-week-old infants across Europe: geographic influence beyond delivery mode, breast-feeding, and antibiotics. J Pediatr Gastroenterol Nutr 2010;51(1):77–84.

[146] Boyce JA, Assa'ad A, Burks AW, et al. Guidelines for the diagnosis and management of food allergy in the United States: report of the

NIAID-sponsored expert panel. J Allergy Clin Immunol 2010; 126(6 Suppl.):S1–58.

[147] Branum AM, Lukacs SL. Food allergy among children in the United States. Pediatrics 2009;124(6):1549–55.

[148] Australasian Society of Clinical Imunology and Allergy. Food allergy clinical update; 2016.

[149] Eigenmann PA, Sicherer SH, Borkowski TA, et al. Prevalence of IgE-mediated food allergy among children with atopic dermatitis. Pediatrics 1998;101(3):E8.

[150] Hill DJ, Hosking CS, de Benedictis FM, et al. Confirmation of the association between high levels of immunoglobulin E food sensitization and eczema in infancy: an international study. Clin Exp Allergy 2008;38(1):161–8.

[151] Green TD, LaBelle VS, Steele PH, et al. Clinical characteristics of peanut-allergic children: recent changes. Pediatrics 2007;120(6):1304–10.

[152] Greer FR, Sicherer SH, Burks AW. Effects of early nutritional interventions on the development of atopic disease in infants and children: the role of maternal dietary restriction, breastfeeding, timing of introduction of complementary foods, and hydrolyzed formulas. Pediatrics 2008;121(1):183–91.

[153] Zutavern A, Brockow I, Schaaf B, et al. Timing of solid food introduction in relation to atopic dermatitis and atopic sensitization: results from a prospective birth cohort study. Pediatrics 2006;117(2):401–11.

[154] Lack G. Epidemiologic risks for food allergy. J Allergy Clin Immunol 2008;121(6):1331–6.

[155] Levy Y, Broides A, Segal N, et al. Peanut and tree nut allergy in children: role of peanut snacks in Israel? Allergy 2003;58(11):1206–7.

[156] Du Toit G, Katz Y, Sasieni P, et al. Early consumption of peanuts in infancy is associated with a low prevalence of peanut allergy. J Allergy Clin Immunol 2008;122(5):984–91.

[157] Silano M, Agostoni C, Guandalini S. Effect of the timing of gluten introduction on the development of celiac disease. World J Gastroenterol 2010;16(16):1939–42.

[158] Akobeng AK, Ramanan AV, Buchan I, et al. Effect of breast feeding on risk of coeliac disease: a systematic review and meta-analysis of observational studies. Arch Dis Child 2006;91(1):39–43.

[159] Kull I, Bergstrom A, Lilja G, et al. Fish consumption during the first year of life and development of allergic diseases during childhood. Allergy 2006;61(8):1009–15.

[160] Smith-Spangler C, Brandeau ML, Hunter GE, et al. Are organic foods safer or healthier than conventional alternatives?: a systematic review. Ann Intern Med 2012;157(5):348–66.

[161] Cameron SL, Taylor RW, Heath A-LM. Development and pilot testing of Baby-Led Introduction to SolidS – a version of baby-led weaning modified to address concerns about iron deficiency, growth faltering and choking. BMC Pediatr 2015;15:99.

[162] Daniels L, Heath A-LM, Williams SM, et al. Baby-Led Introduction to SolidS (BLISS) study: a randomised controlled trial of a baby-led approach to complementary feeding. BMC Pediatr 2015;15:179.

[163] Rapley G. Baby-led weaning: transitioning to solid foods at the baby's own pace. Community Pract 2011;84(6):20–3.

[164] Morison BJ, Taylor RW, Haszard JJ, et al. How different are baby-led weaning and conventional complementary feeding? A cross-sectional study of infants aged 6–8 months. BMJ Open 2016;6(5):e010665.

[165] Brown A, Lee MD. Early influences on child satiety-responsiveness: the role of weaning style. Pediatr Obes 2015;10(1):57–66.

[166] Coulthard H, Harris G, Emmett P. Delayed introduction of lumpy foods to children during the complementary feeding period affects child's food acceptance and feeding at 7 years of age. Matern Child Nutr 2009;5(1):75–85.

[167] Cameron SL, Heath A-LM, Taylor RW. Healthcare professionals' and mothers' knowledge of, attitudes to and experiences with, Baby-Led Weaning: a content analysis study. BMJ Open 2012;2(6).

[168] Fangupo LJ, Heath A-LM, Williams SM, et al. A baby-led approach to eating solids and risk of choking. Pediatrics 2016;138(4).

[169] Szajewska H, Kołodziej M. Systematic review with meta-analysis: Lactobacillus rhamnosus GG in the prevention of antibiotic-associated diarrhoea in children and adults. Aliment Pharmacol Ther 2015;42(10):1149–57.

[170] Hu H-J, Zhang G-Q, Zhang Q, et al. Probiotics prevent Candida colonization and invasive fungal sepsis in preterm neonates: a systematic review and meta-analysis of randomized controlled trials. Pediatr Neonatol 2017;58:103–10.

[171] Gould JF, Anderson AJ, Yelland LN, et al. Association of cord blood vitamin D at delivery with postpartum depression in Australian women. Aust N Z J Obstet Gynaecol 2015;55(5):446–52.

[172] Cosenza L, Nocerino R, Scala CD, et al. Bugs for atopy: the Lactobacillus rhamnosus GG strategy for food allergy prevention and treatment in children. Benef Microbes 2015;6(2):225–32.

[173] Berni Canani R, Sangwan N, Stefka AT, et al. Lactobacillus rhamnosus GG-supplemented formula expands butyrate-producing bacterial strains in food allergic infants. ISME J 2015;10(3): 742–50.

[174] Berni Canani R, Di Costanzo M, Pezzella V, et al. The potential therapeutic efficacy of Lactobacillus GG in children with food allergies. Pharmaceuticals (Basel) 2012;5(6):655–64.

[175] Nermes M, Kantele JM, Atosuo TJ, et al. Interaction of orally administered Lactobacillus rhamnosus GG with skin and gut microbiota and humoral immunity in infants with atopic dermatitis. Clin Exp Allergy 2011;41(3):370–7.

[176] Szajewska H, Wanke M, Patro B. Meta-analysis: the effects of Lactobacillus rhamnosus GG supplementation for the prevention of healthcare-associated diarrhoea in children. Aliment Pharmacol Ther 2011;34(9):1079–87.

[177] Liu S, Hu P, Du X, et al. Lactobacillus rhamnosus GG supplementation for preventing respiratory infections in children: a meta-analysis of randomized, placebo-controlled trials. Indian Pediatr 2013;50(4):377–81.

[178] Luoto R, Ruuskanen O, Waris M, et al. Prebiotic and probiotic supplementation prevents rhinovirus infections in preterm infants: a randomized, placebo-controlled trial. J Allergy Clin Immunol 2013;133(2):405–13.

[179] Dotterud CK, Avershina E, Sekelja M, et al. Does maternal perinatal probiotic supplementation alter the intestinal microbiota of mother and child? J Pediatr Gastroenterol Nutr 2015;61(2): 200–7.

[180] Kannampalli P, Pochiraju S, Chichlowski M, et al. Probiotic Lactobacillus rhamnosus GG (LGG) and prebiotic prevent neonatal inflammation-induced visceral hypersensitivity in adult rats. Neurogastroenterol Motil 2014;26(12):1694–704.

[181] Bottcher MF, Abrahamsson TR, Fredriksson M, et al. Low breast milk TGF-beta2 is induced by Lactobacillus reuteri supplementation and associates with reduced risk of sensitization during infancy. Pediatr Allergy Immunol 2008;19(6):497–504.

[182] Oddy WH, Rosales F. A systematic review of the importance of milk TGF-β on immunological outcomes in the infant and young child. Pediatr Allergy Immunol 2010;21(1 Pt I):47–59.

[183] Abrahamsson TR, Sinkiewicz G, Jakobsson T, et al. Probiotic lactobacilli in breast milk and infant stool in relation to oral intake during the first year of life. J Pediatr Gastroenterol Nutr 2009;49(3):349–54.

[184] Maldonado J, Canabate F, Sempere L, et al. Human milk probiotic Lactobacillus fermentum CECT5716 reduces the incidence of gastrointestinal and upper respiratory tract infections in infants. J Pediatr Gastroenterol Nutr 2012;54(1):55–61.

[185] Arroyo R, Martin V, Maldonado A, et al. Treatment of infectious mastitis during lactation: antibiotics versus oral administration of Lactobacilli isolated from breast milk. Clin Infect Dis 2010;50(12):1551–8.

[186] Rodriguez-Nogales A, Algieri F, Vezza T, et al. The viability of Lactobacillus fermentum CECT5716 is not essential to exert intestinal anti-inflammatory properties. Food Funct 2015;6(4):1176–84.

[187] Kubota T, Shimojo N, Nonaka K, et al. Prebiotic consumption in pregnant and lactating women increases IL-27 expression in human milk. Br J Nutr 2014;111(4):625–32.

[188] Yang H, Xun P, He K. Fish and fish oil intake in relation to risk of asthma: a systematic review and meta-analysis. PLoS ONE 2013;8(11):e80048.

[189] Wagner CL, Hulsey TC, Fanning D, et al. High-dose vitamin d3 supplementation in a cohort of breastfeeding mothers and their infants: a 6-month follow-up pilot study. Breastfeed Med 2006;1(2):59–70.

[190] Hollis BW, Wagner CL, Howard CR, et al. Maternal versus infant vitamin d supplementation during lactation: a randomized controlled trial. Pediatrics 2015;136(4):625–34.

[191] Vaziri F, Nasiri S, Tavana Z, et al. A randomized controlled trial of vitamin D supplementation on perinatal depression: in Iranian pregnant mothers. BMC Pregnancy Childbirth 2016;16:239.

[192] Accortt EE, Schetter CD, Peters RM, et al. Lower prenatal vitamin D status and postpartum depressive symptomatology in African American women: preliminary evidence for moderation by inflammatory cytokines. Arch Womens Ment Health 2016;19(2):373–83.

[193] Fu CW, Liu JT, Tu WJ, et al. Association between serum 25-hydroxyvitamin D levels measured 24 hours after delivery and postpartum depression. BJOG 2015;122(12):1688–94.

[194] Chandy DD, Kare J, Singh SN, et al. Effect of vitamin D supplementation, directly or via breast milk for term infants, on serum 25 hydroxyvitamin D and related biochemistry, and propensity to infection: a randomised placebo-controlled trial. Br J Nutr 2016;116(1):52–8.

[195] Roth DE, Gernand AD, Morris SK, et al. Maternal vitamin D supplementation during pregnancy and lactation to promote infant growth in Dhaka, Bangladesh (MDIG trial): study protocol for a randomized controlled trial. Trials 2015;16:300.

[196] Morris SK, Pell LG, Rahman MZ, et al. Maternal vitamin D supplementation during pregnancy and lactation to prevent acute respiratory infections in infancy in Dhaka, Bangladesh (MDARI trial): protocol for a prospective cohort study nested within a randomized controlled trial. BMC Pregnancy Childbirth 2016;16:309.

[197] Grant CC, Kaur S, Waymouth E, et al. Reduced primary care respiratory infection visits following pregnancy and infancy vitamin D supplementation: a randomised controlled trial. Acta Paediatr 2015;104(4):396–404.

[198] Grant CC, Crane J, Mitchell EA, et al. Vitamin D supplementation during pregnancy and infancy reduces aeroallergen sensitization: a randomized controlled trial. Allergy 2016;71(9):1325–34.

[199] Allen KJ, Koplin JJ, Ponsonby A-L, et al. Vitamin D insufficiency is associated with challenge-proven food allergy in infants. J Allergy Clin Immunol 2013;131(4):1109–16.

[200] Swain JE, Kim P, Spicer J, et al. Approaching the biology of human parental attachment: brain imaging, oxytocin and coordinated assessments of mothers and fathers. Brain Res 2014;1580:78–101.

[201] Kondo N, Suda Y, Nakao A, et al. Maternal psychosocial factors determining the concentrations of transforming growth factor-beta in breast milk. Pediatr Allergy Immunol 2011;22(8):853–61.

[202] Duijts L, Jaddoe VWV, Hofman A, et al. Prolonged and exclusive breastfeeding reduces the risk of infectious diseases in infancy. Pediatrics 2010;126(1):e18–25.

[203] Quigley MA, Kelly YJ, Sacker A. Breastfeeding and hospitalization for diarrheal and respiratory infection in the United Kingdom Millennium Cohort Study. Pediatrics 2007;119(4):e837–42.

[204] Therapeutic Goods Association. Guidelines for the labelling of medicines. Canberra: Australian Government; 2014.

[205] Drago L, Rodighiero V, Celeste T, et al. Microbiological evaluation of commercial probiotic products available in the USA in 2009. J Chemother 2010;22(6):373–7.

[206] Patro JN, Ramachandran P, Barnaba T, et al. Culture-independent metagenomic surveillance of commercially available probiotics with high-throughput next-generation sequencing. mSphere 2016;1(2):e00057-16.

[207] Berni Canani R, Sangwan N, Stefka AT, et al. Lactobacillus rhamnosus GG-supplemented formula expands butyrate-producing bacterial strains in food allergic infants. ISME J 2016;10(3):742–50.

[208] Berni Canani R, Nocerino R, Terrin G, et al. Formula selection for management of children with cow's milk allergy influences the rate of acquisition of tolerance: a prospective multicenter study. J Pediatr 2013;163(3):771–7.e1.

[209] López-Huertas E. Safety and efficacy of human breast milk Lactobacillus fermentum CECT 5716. A mini-review of studies with infant formulae. Benef Microbes 2015;6(2):219–24.

[210] Rautava S, Salminen S, Isolauri E. Specific probiotics in reducing the risk of acute infections in infancy – a randomised, double-blind, placebo-controlled study. Br J Nutr 2008;101(11):1722–6.

[211] Weizman Z, Asli G, Alsheikh A. Effect of a probiotic infant formula on infections in child care centers: comparison of two probiotic agents. Pediatrics 2005;115(1):5–9.

[212] Roy U, Jessani LG, Rudramurthy SM, et al. Seven cases of Saccharomyces fungaemia related to use of probiotics. Mycoses 2017;60(6):375–80.

[213] Harris P, Nagy S, Vardaxis NJ, editors. Mosby's dictionary of medicine, nursing & health professions. Chatswood. NSW: Mosby Elsevier; 2010.

[214] Chiappini E, Principi N, Longhi R, et al. Management of fever in children: summary of the Italian Pediatric Society guidelines. Clin Ther 2009;31(8):1826–43.

[215] Blythe A, Buchan J, editors. Essential primary care. London: Wiley; 2016.

[216] Elhassanien AF, Hesham A-AA, Alrefaee F. Fever without source in infants and young children: dilemma in diagnosis and management. Risk Manag Healthc Policy 2013;6:7–12.

[217] NSW Kids and Families. Children and infants with fever – acute management. North Sydney: NSW Department of Health; 2010.

[218] Kelly M, Sahm LJ, Shiely F, et al. Parental knowledge, attitudes and beliefs regarding fever in children: an interview study. BMC Public Health 2016;16(1):540.

[219] NSW Department of Health. Infants and children: acute management of fever – clinical practice guideline. North Sydney: NSW Department of Health; 2010.

[220] Kang SH, Jung YH, Kim HY, et al. Effect of paracetamol use on the modification of the development of asthma by reactive oxygen species genes. Ann Allergy Asthma Immunol 2013;110(5):364–9.e1.

[221] Green R, Jeena P, Kotze S, et al. Management of acute fever in children: guideline for community healthcare providers and pharmacists. S Afr Med J 2013;103:948–54.

[222] Wake M, Morton-Allen E, Poulakis Z, et al. Prevalence, stability, and outcomes of cry-fuss and sleep problems in the first 2 years of life: prospective community-based study. Pediatrics 2006;117(3):836–42.

[223] van der Wal MF, van den Boom DC, Pauw-Plomp H, et al. Mothers' reports of infant crying and soothing in a multicultural population. Arch Dis Child 1998;79(4):312–17.

[224] Vandenplas Y, Abkari A, Bellaiche M, et al. Prevalence and health outcomes of functional gastrointestinal symptoms in infants from birth to 12 months of age. J Pediatr Gastroenterol Nutr 2015;61(5):531–7.

[225] Wolke D, Samara M, Alvarez Wolke M. Meta-analysis of fuss/cry durations and colic prevalence across countries. In: Proceedings of the 11th international infant cry research workshop. 18–10 June 2011; Zeist, The Netherlands; 2011.

[226] Douglas P, Hill P. Managing infants who cry excessively in the first few months of life. BMJ 2011;343.

[227] Freedman SB, Al-Harthy N, Thull-Freedman J. The crying infant: diagnostic testing and frequency of serious underlying disease. Pediatrics 2009;123(3):841–8.

[228] Santos IS, Matijasevich A, Capilheira MF, et al. Excessive crying at 3 months of age and behavioural problems at 4 years age: a prospective cohort study. J Epidemiol Community Health 2015;69(7):654–9.

[229] Hemmi MH, Wolke D, Schneider S. Associations between problems with crying, sleeping and/or feeding in infancy and long-term behavioural outcomes in childhood: a meta-analysis. Arch Dis Child 2011;96(7):622–9.

[230] Canivet CA, Östergren P-O, Rosén A-S, et al. Infantile colic and the role of trait anxiety during pregnancy in relation to psychosocial and socioeconomic factors. Scand J Soc Med 2005;33(1):26–34.

[231] Hua S, Peters RL, Allen KJ, et al. Medical intervention in parent-reported infant gastro-oesophageal reflux: a population-based study. J Paediatr Child Health 2015;51(5):515–23.

[232] Halpern R, Coelho R. Excessive crying in infants. J Pediatr (Rio J) 2016;92(3, Suppl. 1):S40–5.

[233] Segura-Millán S, Dewey KG, Perez-Escamilla R. Factors associated with perceived insufficient milk in a low-income urban population in Mexico. J Nutr 1994;124(2):202–12.

[234] Scott J, Colin W. Breastfeeding: reasons for starting, reasons for stopping and problems along the way. Breastfeed Rev 2002;10(2):13.

[235] Gatti L. Maternal perceptions of insufficient milk supply in breastfeeding. J Nurs Scholarsh 2008;40(4):355–63.

[236] Akman I, Kuşçu K, Özdemir N, et al. Mothers' postpartum psychological adjustment and infantile colic. Arch Dis Child 2006;91(5):417–19.

[237] Fujiwara T, Yamaoka Y, Morisaki N. Self-reported prevalence and risk factors for shaking and smothering among mothers of 4-month-old infants in Japan. J Epidemiol 2016;26(1):4–13.

[238] Barr RG. Crying as a trigger for abusive head trauma: a key to prevention. Pediatr Radiol 2014;44(4):559–64.

[239] Esposito G, Setoh P, Yoshida S, et al. The calming effect of maternal carrying in different mammalian species. Front Psychol 2015;6:445.

[240] St James-Roberts I, Alvarez M, Csipke E, et al. Infant crying and sleeping in London, Copenhagen and when parents adopt a 'proximal' form of care. Pediatrics 2006;117(6):e1146–55.

[241] Williams CJ, Kessler D, Fernyhough C, et al. The association between maternal-reported responses to infant crying at 4 weeks and 6 months and offspring depression at 18: a longitudinal study. Arch Womens Ment Health 2016;19:401–8.

[242] Douglas PS, Hill PS. A neurobiological model for cry-fuss problems in the first three to four months of life. Med Hypotheses 2013;81(5):816–22.

[243] Koppen IJN, Nurko S, Saps M, et al. The pediatric Rome IV criteria: what's new? Expert Rev Gastroenterol Hepatol 2017;11(3):193–201.

[244] Hegar B, Satari DHI, Sjarif DR, et al. Regurgitation and gastroesophageal reflux disease in six to nine months old Indonesian infants. Pediatr Gastroenterol Hepatol Nutr 2013;16(4):240–7.

[245] Vandenplas Y, Hauser B. An updated review on gastro-esophageal reflux in pediatrics. Expert Rev Gastroenterol Hepatol 2015;9(12):1511–21.

[246] Vandenplas Y, Rudolph CD, Di Lorenzo C, et al. Pediatric gastroesophageal reflux clinical practice guidelines: joint recommendations of the North American Society for Pediatric Gastroenterology, Hepatology, and Nutrition (NASPGHAN) and the European Society for Pediatric Gastroenterology, Hepatology, and Nutrition (ESPGHAN). J Pediatr Gastroenterol Nutr 2009;49(4):498–547.

[247] Gieruszczak-Białek D, Konarska Z, Skórka A, et al. No effect of proton pump inhibitors on crying and irritability in infants: systematic review of randomized controlled trials. J Pediatr 2015;166(3):767–70.

[248] Safe M, Chan WH, Leach ST, et al. Widespread use of gastric acid inhibitors in infants: are they needed? Are they safe? World J Gastrointest Pharmacol Ther 2016;7(4):531–9.

[249] Ferreira CT, Carvalho Ed, Sdepanian VL, et al. Gastroesophageal reflux disease: exaggerations, evidence and clinical practice. J Pediatr (Rio J) 2014;90(2):105–18.

[250] Barron JJ, Tan H, Spalding J, et al. Proton pump inhibitor utilization patterns in infants. J Pediatr Gastroenterol Nutr 2007;45(4):421–7.

[251] Illueca M, Alemayehu B, Shoetan N, et al. Proton pump inhibitor prescribing patterns in newborns and infants. J Pediatr Pharmacol Ther 2014;19(4):283–7.

[252] Marseglia L, Manti S, D'Angelo G, et al. Gastroesophageal reflux and congenital gastrointestinal malformations. World J Gastroenterol 2015;21(28):8508–15.

[253] Czinn SJ, Blanchard S. Gastroesophageal reflux disease in neonates and infants. Paediatr Drugs 2013;15(1):19–27.

[254] Martin AJ, Pratt N, Kennedy JD, et al. Natural history and familial relationships of infant spilling to 9 years of age. Pediatrics 2002;109(6):1061–7.

[255] Douglas PS. Diagnosing gastro-oesophageal reflux disease or lactose intolerance in babies who cry a lot in the first few months overlooks feeding problems. J Paediatr Child Health 2013;49(4):E252–6.

[256] Lightdale JR, Gremse DA. Gastroesophageal reflux: management guidance for the pediatrician. Pediatrics 2013;131(5):e1684–95.

[257] Jordan GJ. Elimination communication as colic therapy. Med Hypotheses 2014;83(3):282–5.

[258] Rosen R. Gastroesophageal reflux in infants: more than just a phenomenon. JAMA Pediatr 2014;168(1):83–9.

[259] Skopnik H, Silny J, Heiber O, et al. Gastroesophageal reflux in infants: evaluation of a new intraluminal impedance technique. J Pediatr Gastroenterol Nutr 1996;23(5):591–8.

[260] Djeddi D-D, Kongolo G, Stéphan-Blanchard E, et al. Involvement of autonomic nervous activity changes in gastroesophageal reflux in neonates during sleep and wakefulness. PLoS ONE 2013;8(12):e83464.

[261] Morais MBd. Signs and symptoms associated with digestive tract development. J Pediatr (Rio J) 2016;92(3, Suppl. 1):S46–56.

[262] Erwin EA, Kruszewski PG, Russo JM, et al. IgE antibodies and response to cow's milk elimination diet in pediatric eosinophilic esophagitis. J Allergy Clin Immunol 2016;138(2):625–8.

[263] Berni Canani R, Pezzella V, Amoroso A, et al. Diagnosing and treating intolerance to carbohydrates in children. Nutrients 2016;8(3):157.

[264] Shulman RJ, Schanler RJ, Lau C, et al. Early feeding, antenatal glucocorticoids, and human milk decrease intestinal permeability in preterm infnats. Pediatr Res 1998;44:519–23.

[265] Di Rienzo T, D'Angelo G, D'Aversa F, et al. Lactose intolerance: from diagnosis to correct management. Eur Rev Med Pharmacol Sci 2013;17(Suppl. 2):18–25.

[266] Vandenplas Y. Lactose intolerance. Asia Pac J Clin Nutr 2015;24(Suppl. 1):S9–13.

[267] Lira C, Tuel S, Goldberg LR. Diagnosing lactose intolerance: how PAs can facilitate breastfeeding. J Am Acad Physician Assist 2013;26(4):21–3.

[268] Counahan R, Walker-Smith J. Stool and urinary sugars in normal neonates. Arch Dis Child 1976;51(7):517–20.

[269] Nitzan M, Rosenfeld Z. Stool sugars and pH in breast-fed neonates. Arch Dis Child 1977;52(4):336–7.

[270] Anderson J. Lactose intolerance and the breastfed baby; 2012. Available from: https://www.breastfeeding.asn.au/bfinfo/lactose.html.

[271] Vik T, Grote V, Escribano J, et al. Infantile colic, prolonged crying and maternal postnatal depression. Acta Paediatr 2009;98(8):1344–8.

[272] Radesky JS, Zuckerman B, Silverstein M, et al. Inconsolable infant crying and maternal postpartum depressive symptoms. Pediatrics 2013;131(6):e1857–64.

[273] Laurent HK, Ablow JC. A cry in the dark: depressed mothers show reduced neural activation to their own infant's cry. Soc Cogn Affect Neurosci 2012;7(2):125–34.

[274] Esposito G, Manian N, Truzzi A, et al. Response to infant cry in clinically depressed and non-depressed mothers. PLoS ONE 2017;12(1):e0169066.

[275] Madden V, Domoney J, Aumayer K, et al. Intergenerational transmission of parenting: findings from a UK longitudinal study. Eur J Public Health 2015;25(6):1030–5.

[276] Avan BI, Raza SA, Kirkwood BR. A community-based study of early childhood sensory stimulation in home environment associated with growth and psychomotor development in Pakistan. Int J Public Health 2014;59(5):779–88.

[277] Douglas P, Shirley B. How to treat: the crying baby. Aust Doct 2013;31–8.

[278] Douglas PS, Miller Y, Bucetti A, et al. Preliminary evaluation of a primary care intervention for cry-fuss behaviours in the first 3-4 months of life ('The Possums Approach'): effects on cry-fuss behaviours and maternal mood. Aust J Prim Health 2015;21(1):38–45.

[279] Eutamène H, Garcia-Rodenas CL, Yvon S, et al. Luminal contents from the gut of colicky infants induce visceral hypersensitivity in mice. Neurogastroenterol Motil 2017;29(4):e12994.

[280] Dubois NE, Gregory KE. Characterizing the intestinal microbiome in infantile colic. Biol Res Nurs 2016;18(3):307–15.

[281] Savino F, Cordisco L, Tarasco V, et al. Antagonistic effect of Lactobacillus strains against gas-producing coliforms isolated from colicky infants. BMC Microbiol 2011;11:157.

[282] Nocerino R, Pezzella V, Cosenza L, et al. The controversial role of food allergy in infantile colic: evidence and clinical management. Nutrients 2015;7(3):2015–25.

[283] Nowak-Węgrzyn A. Food protein-induced enterocolitis syndrome and allergic proctocolitis. Allergy Asthma Proc 2015;36(3):172–84.

[284] ABM Clinical Protocol #24: allergic proctocolitis in the exclusively breastfed infant. Breastfeed Med 2011;6(6):435–40.

[285] Nowak-Węgrzyn A, editor. Food protein-induced enterocolitis syndrome and allergic proctocolitis. Allergy Asthma Proc 2015;36(3):172–84.

[286] Gelfand AA. Infant colic. Semin Pediatr Neurol 2016;23(1):79–82.

[287] Romanello S, Spiri D, Marcuzzi E, et al. Association between childhood migraine and history of infantile colic. JAMA 2013;309(15):1607–12.

[288] Gelfand AA, Thomas KC, Goadsby PJ. Before the headache: infant colic as an early life expression of migraine. Neurology 2012;79(13):1392–6.

[289] Whittingham K, Douglas P. Optimizing parent–infant sleep from birth to 6 months: a new paradigm. Infant Ment Health J 2014;35(6):614–23.

[290] Huhtala V, Lehtonen L, Uvnäs-Moberg K, et al. Low plasma cholecystokinin levels in colicky infants. J Pediatr Gastroenterol Nutr 2003;37(1):42–6.

[291] Inamo Y, Hasegawa M, Saito K, et al. Serum vitamin D concentrations and associated severity of acute lower respiratory tract infections in Japanese hospitalized children. Pediatr Int 2011;53(2):199–201.

[292] Petzoldt J, Wittchen H-U, Wittich J, et al. Maternal anxiety disorders predict excessive infant crying: a prospective longitudinal study. Arch Dis Child 2014;99(9):800–6.

[293] Rautava S, Kainonen E, Salminen S, et al. Maternal probiotic supplementation during pregnancy and breast-feeding reduces the risk of eczema in the infant. J Allergy Clin Immunol 2012;130(6):1355–60.

[294] Baldassarre ME, Laforgia N, Fanelli M, et al. Lactobacillus GG improves recovery in infants with blood in the stools and presumptive allergic colitis compared with extensively hydrolyzed formula alone. J Pediatr 2010;156(3):397–401.

[295] Fatheree NY, Liu Y, Ferris M, et al. Hypoallergenic formula with Lactobacillus rhamnosus GG for babies with colic: a pilot study of recruitment, retention, and fecal biomarkers. World J Gastrointest Pathophysiol 2016;7(1):160–70.

[296] Garofoli F, Civardi E, Indrio F, et al. The early administration of Lactobacillus reuteri DSM 17938 controls regurgitation episodes in full-term breastfed infants. Int J Food Sci Nutr 2014;65(5):646–8.

[297] Xu M, Wang J, Wang N, et al. The efficacy and safety of the probiotic bacterium lactobacillus reuteri dsm 17938 for infantile colic: a meta-analysis of randomized controlled trials. PLoS ONE 2015;10(10):e0141445.

[298] Giovannini M, Verduci E, Gregori D, et al. Prebiotic effect of an infant formula supplemented with galacto-oligosaccharides: randomized multicenter trial. J Am Coll Nutr 2014;33(5):385–93.

[299] Jost T, Lacroix C, Braegger CP, et al. Vertical mother-neonate transfer of maternal gut bacteria via breastfeeding. Environ Microbiol 2014;16(9):2891–904.

[300] Shelef L. Herbs of the umbelliferae. In: Caballero B, Finglas P, Toldra F, editors. Encyclopedia of food sciences and nutrition. Amsterdam: Academic Press; 2003. p. 3090–8.

[301] Tirapelli CR, de Andrade CR, Cassano AO, et al. Antispasmodic and relaxant effects of the hidroalcoholic extract of Pimpinella anisum (Apiaceae) on rat anococcygeus smooth muscle. J Ethnopharmacol 2007;110(1):23–9.

[302] Yao DAN, Deng X, Wang M. Management of musculoskeletal dysfunction in infants. Exp Ther Med 2016;11(6):2079–82.

[303] Dobson D, Lucassen PLBJ, Miller JJ, et al. Manipulative therapies for infantile colic. Cochrane Database Syst Rev 2012;(12):CD004796.

[304] Hill DJ, Roy N, Heine RG, et al. Effect of a low-allergen maternal diet on colic among breastfed infants: a randomized, controlled trial. Pediatrics 2005;116(5):e709–15.

[305] Al Dhaheri W, Diksic D, Ben-Shoshan M. IgE-mediated cow milk allergy and infantile colic: diagnostic and management challenges. BMJ Case Rep 2013;2013:bcr2012007182.

[306] Stecksén-Blicks C, Granström E, Silfverdal SA, et al. Prevalence of oral Candida in the first year of life. Mycoses 2015;58(9):550–6.

[307] Zisova LG, Chokoeva AA, Amaliev GI, et al. Vulvovaginal candidiasis in pregnant women and its importance for Candida colonization of newborns. Folia Med (Plovdiv) 2016;58(2):108–14.

[308] Filippidi A, Galanakis E, Maraki S, et al. The effect of maternal flora on Candida colonisation in the neonate. Mycoses 2014;57(1):43–8.

[309] Payne MS, Cullinane M, Garland SM, et al. Detection of Candida spp. in the vagina of a cohort of nulliparous pregnant women by culture and molecular methods: is there an association between maternal vaginal and infant oral colonisation? Aust N Z J Obstet Gynaecol 2016;56(2):179–84.

[310] Comina E, Marion K, Renaud FNR, et al. Pacifiers: a microbial reservoir. Nurs Health Sci 2006;8(4):216–23.

[311] da Silveira LC, Charone S, Maia LC, et al. Biofilm formation by Candida species on silicone surfaces and latex pacifier nipples: an in vitro study. J Clin Pediatr Dent 2009;33(3):235–40.

[312] Benjamin DK, Stoll BJ, Gantz MG, et al. Neonatal Candidiasis: epidemiology, risk factors, and clinical judgment. Pediatrics 2010;126(4):e865–73.

[313] Khan EA, Choudhry S, Fatima M, et al. Clinical spectrum, management and outcome of neonatal candidiasis. J Pak Med Assoc 2015;65(11):1206–9.

[314] Matee MI, Simon E, Christensen MF, et al. Association between carriage of oral yeasts and malnutrition among Tanzanian infants aged 6–24 months. Oral Dis 1995;1(1):37–42.

[315] Hacimustafaoglu M, Celebi S. Candida infections in non-neutropenic children after the neonatal period. Expert Rev Anti Infect Ther 2011;9(10):923–40.

[316] Heller MM, Fullerton-Stone H, Murase JE. Caring for new mothers: diagnosis, management and treatment of nipple dermatitis in breastfeeding mothers. Int J Dermatol 2012;51(10):1149–61.

[317] Kiat-amnuay S, Bouquot J. Breastfeeding keratosis: this frictional keratosis of newborns may mimic thrush. Pediatrics 2013;132(3):e775–8.

[318] Berens P, Eglash A, Malloy M, et al. ABM Clinical Protocol #26: persistent pain with breastfeeding. Breastfeed Med 2016;11(2):46–53.

[319] Patil S, Rao RS, Majumdar B, et al. Oral lesions in neonates. Int J Clin Pediatr Dent 2016;9(2):131–8.

[320] Romeo MG, Romeo DM, Trovato L, et al. Role of probiotics in the prevention of the enteric colonization by Candida in preterm newborns: incidence of late-onset sepsis and neurological outcome. J Perinatol 2011;31(1):63–9.

[321] Huncharek M, Muscat J. Perineal talc use and ovarian cancer risk: a case study of scientific standards in environmental epidemiology. Eur J Cancer Prev 2011;20(6):501–7.

[322] Coughlin CC, Eichenfield LF, Frieden IJ. Diaper dermatitis: clinical characteristics and differential diagnosis. Pediatr Dermatol 2014;31(s1):19–24.

[323] Farahani LA, Ghobadzadeh M, Yousefi P. Comparison of the effect of human milk and topical hydrocortisone 1% on diaper dermatitis. Pediatr Dermatol 2013;30(6):725–9.

[324] Hengge UR. Topical, non-medicated LOYON® in facilitating the removal of scaling in infants and children with cradle cap: a proof-of-concept pilot study. Dermatol Ther (Heidelb) 2014;4(2):221–32.

[325] Ljubojević S, Skerlev M, Lipozencić J, et al. The role of Malassezia furfur in dermatology. Clin Dermatol 2002;20(2):179–82.

[326] Mimouni K, Mukamel M, Zeharia A, et al. Prognosis of infantile seborrheic dermatitis. J Pediatr 1995;127(5):744–6.

[327] Tollesson A, Frithz A. Borage oil, an effective new treatment for infantile seborrhoeic dermatitis. Br J Dermatol 1993;129(1):95.

[328] Kuller JM. Infant skin care products: what are the issues? Adv Neonatal Care 2016;16(Suppl. 5S):S3–12.

[329] Jakasa I, De Jongh CM, Verberk MM, et al. Percutaneous penetration of sodium lauryl sulphate is increased in uninvolved skin of patients with atopic dermatitis compared with control subjects. Br J Dermatol 2006;155(1):104–9.

[330] Atherton D, Mills K. What can be done to keep babies' skin healthy? RCM Midwives 2004;7(7):288–90.

[331] Afsar FS. Skin care for preterm and term neonates. Clin Exp Dermatol 2009;34(8):855–8.

[332] Does a teething child need serious illness excluding? Arch Dis Child 2007;92(3):266–8.

[333] Owais AI, Zawaideh F, Bataineh O. Challenging parents' myths regarding their children's teething. Int J Dent Hyg 2010;8(1):28–34.

[334] Harrison D, Reszel J, Bueno M, et al. Breastfeeding for procedural pain in infants beyond the neonatal period. Cochrane Database Syst Rev 2016;(10):CD011248.

[335] Memarpour M, Soltanimehr E, Eskandarian T. Signs and symptoms associated with primary tooth eruption: a clinical trial of nonpharmacological remedies. BMC Oral Health 2015;15:88.

[336] Beutler AI, Chesnut GT, Mattingly JC, et al. FPIN's Clinical Inquiries. Aspirin use in children for fever or viral syndromes. Am Fam Physician 2009;80(12):1472.

[337] Williams GD, Kirk EP, Wilson CJ, et al. Salicylate intoxication from teething gel in infancy. Med J Aust 2011;194(3):146–8.

[338] Aminiahidashti H, Laali A, Nosrati N, et al. Recurrent seizures after lidocaine ingestion. J Adv Pharm Technol Res 2015;6(1):35–7.

[339] FDA: don't use lidocaine to treat teething pain. J Mich Dent Assoc 2014;96(9):8.

[340] Balicer RD, Kitai E. Methemoglobinemia caused by topical teething preparation: a case report. ScientificWorldJournal 2004;4:517–20.

[341] Weaver L, Steiner H. The bowel habit of young children. Arch Dis Child 1984;59(7):649–52.

[342] Afzal NA, Tighe MP, Thomson MA. Constipation in children. Ital J Pediatr 2011;37(1):28.

[343] Arias A, Bennison J, Justus K, et al. Educating parents about normal stool pattern changes in infants. J Pediatr Health Care 2001;15(5):269–74.

[344] Metaj M, Laroia N, Lawrence RA, et al. Comparison of breast- and formula-fed normal newborns in time to first stool and urine. J Perinatol 2003;23(8):624–8.

[345] Steer CD, Emond AM, Golding J, et al. The variation in stool patterns from 1 to 42 months: a population-based observational study. Arch Dis Child 2009;94(3):231–3.

[346] Tobias N, Mason D, Lutkenhoff M, et al. Management principles of organic causes of childhood constipation. J Pediatr Health Care 2008;22(1):12–23.

[347] Youssef NN, Di Lorenzo C. Childhood constipation: evaluation and treatment. J Clin Gastroenterol 2001;33(3):199–205.

[348] Afzal NA, Tighe MP, Thomson MA. Constipation in children. Ital J Pediatr 2011;37:28.

[349] Buonavolonta R, Boccia G, Turco R, et al. Pediatric functional gastrointestinal disorders: a questionnaire on pediatric gastrointestinal symptoms based on Rome III criteria. Minerva Pediatr 2009;61(1):67–91.

[350] Loening-Baucke V. Constipation in early childhood: patient characteristics, treatment, and longterm follow up. Gut 1993;34(10):1400–4.

[351] El-Hodhod MA, Younis NT, Zaitoun YA, et al. Cow's milk allergy related pediatric constipation: appropriate time of milk tolerance. Pediatr Allergy Immunol 2010;21(2 Pt 2):e407–12.

[352] du Toit G, Meyer R, Shah N, et al. Identifying and managing cow's milk protein allergy. Arch Dis Child Educ Pract Ed 2010;95(5):134–44.

[353] Khalif I, Quigley E, Konovitch E, et al. Alterations in the colonic flora and intestinal permeability and evidence of immune activation in chronic constipation. Dig Liver Dis 2005;37(11):838–49.

[354] Bae SH. Diets for constipation. Pediatr Gastroenterol Hepatol Nutr 2014;17(4):203–8.

[355] Chang CC, Lin YT, Lu YT, et al. Kiwifruit improves bowel function in patients with irritable bowel syndrome with constipation. Asia Pac J Clin Nutr 2010;19(4):451–7.

[356] Barbara G, Stanghellini V, Brandi G, et al. Interactions between commensal bacteria and gut sensorimotor function in health and disease. Am J Gastroenterol 2005;100(11):2560–8.

[357] Quigley EM. Probiotics in the management of functional bowel disorders: promise fulfilled? Gastroenterol Clin North Am 2012;41(4):805–19.

[358] Miller LE, Ouwehand AC. Probiotic supplementation decreases intestinal transit time: meta-analysis of randomized controlled trials. World J Gastroenterol 2013;19(29):4718–25.

[359] Matsumoto M, Ohishi H, Benno Y. Impact of LKM512 yogurt on improvement of intestinal environment of the elderly. FEMS Immunol Med Microbiol 2001;31(3):181–6.

[360] Meance S, Cayuela C, Turchet P, et al. A fermented milk with a Bifidobacterium probiotic strain DN-173 010 shortened oro-fecal gut transit time in elderly. Microb Ecol Health Dis 2001;13(4):217–22.

[361] Waller PA, Gopal PK, Leyer GJ, et al. Dose-response effect of Bifidobacterium lactis HN019 on whole gut transit time and functional gastrointestinal symptoms in adults. Scand J Gastroenterol 2011;46(9):1057–64.

[362] Koebnick C, Wagner I, Leitzmann P, et al. Probiotic beverage containing Lactobacillus casei Shirota improves gastrointestinal symptoms in patients with chronic constipation. Can J Gastroenterol 2003;17(11):655–9.

[363] Umesaki Y. Effect of L. casei strain Shirota on large intestinal function, bowel movements, and fecal properties. Lactobacillus casei strain Shirota – intestinal flora and human health. Tokyo: Yakult Honsha Co, Ltd; 1999. p. 119–28.

[364] Chmielewska A, Szajewska H. Systematic review of randomised controlled trials: probiotics for functional constipation. World J Gastroenterol 2010;16(1):69–75.

[365] Coccorullo P, Strisciuglio C, Martinelli M, et al. Lactobacillus reuteri (DSM 17938) in infants with functional chronic constipation: a double-blind, randomized, placebo-controlled study. J Pediatr 2010;157(4):598–602.

[366] Vandenplas Y, Alturaiki MA, Al-Qabandi W, et al. Middle East consensus statement on the diagnosis and management of functional gastrointestinal disorders in <12 months old infants. Pediatr Gastroenterol Hepatol Nutr 2016;19(3):153–61.

[367] Gordon M, MacDonald JK, Parker CE, et al. Osmotic and stimulant laxatives for the management of childhood constipation. Cochrane Database Syst Rev 2016;(8):CD009118.

[368] Loo M. Integrative medicine for children. 1st ed. Saint Louis: W.B. Saunders; 2009.

[369] Walker-Smith JA, Murch SH. Diarrhoea in childhood. Medicine (Baltimore) 2003;31(1):41–4.

[370] Chen CC, Walker WA. Probiotics and prebiotics: role in clinical disease states. Adv Pediatr 2005;52:77–113.

[371] Raheem RA, Binns CW, Chih HJ. Protective effects of breastfeeding against acute respiratory tract infections and diarrhoea: findings of a cohort study. J Paediatr Child Health 2017;53(3):271–6.

[372] Quigley MA, Kelly YJ, Sacker A. Breastfeeding and hospitalization for diarrheal and respiratory infection in the United Kingdom Millennium Cohort Study. Pediatrics 2007;119(4):e837–42.

[373] Savino F, Roana J, Mandras N, et al. Faecal microbiota in breast-fed infants after antibiotic therapy. Acta Paediatr 2011;100(1):75–8.

[374] Musilova S, Rada V, Vlkova E, et al. Beneficial effects of human milk oligosaccharides on gut microbiota. Benef Microbes 2014;5(3):273–83.

[375] Bode L. The functional biology of human milk oligosaccharides. Early Hum Dev 2015;91(11):619–22.

[376] Johnston BC, Supina AL, Ospina M, et al. Probiotics for the prevention of pediatric antibiotic-associated diarrhea. Cochrane Database Syst Rev 2007;(2):CD004827.

[377] Goldenberg JZ, Lytvyn L, Steurich J, et al. Probiotics for the prevention of pediatric antibiotic-associated diarrhea. Cochrane Database Syst Rev 2015;(12):CD004827.

[378] Hawrelak JA, Whitten DL, Myers SP. Is Lactobacillus rhamnosus GG effective in preventing the onset of antibiotic-associated diarrhoea: a systematic review. Digestion 2005;72(1):51–6.

[379] Szajewska H, Kołodziej M. Systematic review with meta-analysis: Saccharomyces boulardii in the prevention of antibiotic-associated diarrhoea. Aliment Pharmacol Ther 2015;42(7):793–801.

[380] Szajewska H, Canani RB, Guarino A, et al. Probiotics for the prevention of antibiotic-associated diarrhea in children. J Pediatr Gastroenterol Nutr 2016;62(3):495–506.

[381] Johnston BC, Goldenberg JZ, Parkin PC. Probiotics and the prevention of antibiotic-associated diarrhea in infants and children. JAMA 2016;316(14):1484–5.

[382] MacGillivray S, Fahey T, McGuire W. Lactose avoidance for young children with acute diarrhea. Cochrane Database Syst Rev 2013;(10):CD005433.

[383] Lonnerdal B. Bioactive proteins in breast milk. J Paediatr Child Health 2013;4(Suppl. 1):1–7.

[384] Isolauri E. The role of probiotics in paediatrics. Curr Paediatr 2004;14(2):104–9.

[385] Dinleyici EC, Kara A, Dalgic N, et al. Saccharomyces boulardii CNCM I-745 reduces the duration of diarrhoea, length of emergency care and hospital stay in children with acute diarrhoea. Benef Microbes 2015;6(4):415–21.

[386] Dinleyici EC, Eren M, Ozen M, et al. Effectiveness and safety of Saccharomyces boulardii for acute infectious diarrhea. Expert Opin Biol Ther 2012;12(4):395–410.

[387] Ahmadi E, Alizadeh-Navaei R, Rezai MS. Efficacy of probiotic use in acute rotavirus diarrhea in children: a systematic review and meta-analysis. Caspian J Intern Med 2015;6(4):187–95.

[388] Szajewska H, Urbańska M, Chmielewska A, et al. Meta-analysis: Lactobacillus reuteri strain DSM 17938 (and the original strain ATCC 55730) for treating acute gastroenteritis in children. Benef Microbes 2014;5(3):285–93.

[389] Szajewska H, Ruszczyński M, Kolaček S. Meta-analysis shows limited evidence for using Lactobacillus acidophilus LB to treat acute gastroenteritis in children. Acta Paediatr 2014;103(3): 249–55.

[390] Salazar-Lindo E, Miranda-Langschwager P, Campos-Sanchez M, et al. Lactobacillus casei strain GG in the treatment of infants with acute watery diarrhea: a randomized, double-blind, placebo controlled clinical trial [ISRCTN67363048]. BMC Pediatr 2004; 4:18.

[391] Pozzoni P, Riva A, Bellatorre AG, et al. Saccharomyces boulardii for the prevention of antibiotic-associated diarrhea in adult hospitalized patients: a single-center, randomized, double-blind, placebo-controlled trial. Am J Gastroenterol 2012;107(6):922–31.

[392] Gaon D, Garcia H, Winter L, et al. Effect of Lactobacillus strains and Saccharomyces boulardii on persistent diarrhea in children. Medicina 2003;63(4):293–8.

[393] Fitton N, Thomas JS. Gastrointestinal dysfunction. Surgery 2009;27(11):492–5.

[394] Mok E, Hankard R. Glutamine supplementation in sick children: is it beneficial? J Nutr Metab 2011;2011:617597.

[395] Kamuchaki JM, Kiguli S, Wobudeya E, et al. No benefit of glutamine supplementation on persistent diarrhea in Ugandan children. Pediatr Infect Dis J 2013;32(5):573–6.

[396] Roy SK, Tomkins AM. The impact of experimental zinc deficiency on growth, morbidity and ultrastructural development of intestinal tissue. Bangladesh J Nutr 1989;2(2):1–7.

[397] Hoque KM, Binder HJ. Zinc in the treatment of acute diarrhea: current status and assessment. Gastroenterology 2006;130(7):2201–5.

[398] World Health Organization. Clinical management of acute diarrhoea; 2004. Available from: https://www.who.int/maternal_child_adolescent/documents/who_fch_cah_04_7/en/.

[399] World Health Organization. Implementing the new recommendations on the clinical management of diarrhoea; 2006. Available from: https://www.who.int/maternal_child_adolescent/documents/9241594217/en/.

[400] National Health and Medical Research Council. Zinc; 2014. Available from: https://www.nrv.gov.au/nutrients/zinc.

[401] Lazzerini M, Ronfani L. Oral zinc for treating diarrhoea in children. Cochrane Database Syst Rev 2013;(1):CD005436.

[402] Lazzerini M, Wanzira H. Oral zinc for treating diarrhoea in children. Cochrane Database Syst Rev 2016;(12):CD005436.

[403] Bajait C, Thawani V. Role of zinc in pediatric diarrhea. Indian J Pharmacol 2011;43(3):232–5.

[404] Lukacik M, Thomas RL, Aranda JV. A meta-analysis of the effects of oral zinc in the treatment of acute and persistent diarrhea. Pediatrics 2008;121(2):326–36.

16

Paediatrics and adolescence

Tabitha McIntosh and Helen Padarin

INTRODUCTION

Children have unique nutritional requirements to provide for the exponential growth, adaptation and development that occurs particularly in the first 3 years of life, and beyond into adolescence. Ensuring that they receive all of the necessary building blocks to optimally nourish their bodies, and safeguarding their environment to ensure that it supports their development, can have long-lasting and foundational impacts on the health outcomes of these future adults.

When we look at why early life nutrition is so important, the most obvious feature is the rapid rate of physical growth, development and functional maturation that is intrinsic to childhood and adolescence. Nutritional adequacy is necessary to maintain bodily functions and for continued physical growth and adequate neural development. The development that occurs through childhood to adolescence is significant indeed: blood volume expansion is considerable, skeletal growth is profound and neurodevelopment is unmatched later in life. The benefits of supporting children in establishing healthy eating habits from an early age cannot be underestimated in allowing a child to reach their health potential. Educating parents on healthy eating practices and lifestyle habits that support the various developmental stages, and empowering them to provide highly nutritious school lunches, snacks and meals, is a critical component of preventive health and naturopathic care.

Extending beyond only covering developmental requirements, single nutrients, combinations of nutrients and herbal medicines can be successfully applied as therapeutic tools to support child and adolescent recovery from infection and healing. In the case of acute illness, nutritional supplementation, herbal medicine and specific dietary guidelines can have dramatic positive effects on a child's recovery.

Furthermore, there are many nutritional and environmental health challenges inherent to modern living that have potential to compromise a growing child's health and development. Highly processed convenience foods, heavy marketing of energy-dense packaged drinks and foods, and poor quality diet contribute to the current epidemic of micronutrient deficiencies and obesity in children and adolescents. Significant environmental

chemical exposures provide additional challenges to health and development. These exposures may occur directly via the food chain (persistent organic pollutants, or POPs, organophosphate pesticides, methylmercury), food packaging (phthalates, bisphenol A), drinking water (heavy metals, chlorine byproducts, pesticides), from use of personal care products (fragrance, phthalates, endocrine disrupting chemicals – EDCs), from the child's immediate environments (flame retardants, triclosan, heavy metals) or from the built environment. Due to their biological differences (smaller size, faster metabolic rates, decreased expression of detoxifying enzymes), their proportionately greater exposures based on body weight and the exquisitely delicate windows of development, children in particular are disproportionately vulnerable to the ill effects of environmental exposures.[1]

The body of research is gaining momentum as to how many environmental chemicals (in isolation and in combination) may adversely impact on the gut, brain and the immune axis in developing children. Some of these environmental challenges were not implicated even 50 years ago, so in terms of paediatric environmental medicine, it is a new and expanding discipline awakening us to the profound impact of chemicals and environmental hazards on a child's health.

Using 'food as medicine' in an effort to achieve nutritional adequacy, healthy elimination and a thriving microbiota are valuable goals to optimise resilience and minimise adverse health impacts that these environmental toxin and chemical exposures may bring. There is no doubt that children respond very well to all aspects of naturopathic care. Treatments must always be tailored to be suitable for children, keeping in mind that children are not just little adults.

DOSAGE CALCULATIONS

Child dosage

Calculating the dosage for children can be easily achieved by applying some simple formulas (see Table 16.1). Please note that these methods are only approximates as metabolic changes can interfere. Dosages may need to be adjusted depending on the duration and severity of the child's condition as well as the child's concomitant

TABLE 16.1 Formulas to calculate children's doses

The following are general guidelines for dosing children. Dosages may need to be adjusted depending on the duration and severity of the child's condition, as well as the child's concomitant presentations, weight, diet and lifestyle. Practitioners must use their best clinical judgment when calculating appropriate doses for children, and err on the side of caution.

Clark's rule (based on weight, appropriate for children aged 2–17 years):

$$\text{In kilograms} \quad \frac{\text{weight in kilograms} \times \text{adult's dose}}{\text{divided by 67}} = \text{the child's dose}$$

Young's rule (based on age):

$$\frac{\text{age in years} \times \text{adult's dose}}{\text{divided by child's age} + 12} = \text{the child's dose}$$

Fried's rule (based on age in months, appropriate for infants 12–24 months):

$$\frac{\text{age in months} \times \text{adult's dose}}{\text{divided by 150}} = \text{infant's dose}$$

NB: Calculations stipulate and are based on the assumption of 20 drops per mL.

presentations, weight, diet and lifestyle. Practitioners use their best clinical judgment when calculating appropriate doses for children.

CALCULATING DOSES OF SPECIFIC TREATMENTS

Nutrients

For nutritional dosage requirements for age, see Table 16.1. Dosages for certain nutrients, like proteins and amino acids, are better calculated as mg/kg of body weight.

Herbal medicines

Infants and children have faster resting metabolic rates than adults due to the speed of their growth and development. Therefore, resting metabolic rate as well as body weight needs to be taken into account when prescribing herbal dosages for children (see Table 16.1).

GROWTH AND DEVELOPMENTAL NUTRITION – 12–36 MONTHS – THE TODDLER

Due to the exceptional rate of growth and development in the first few years of life, the meeting of nutritional needs during this time plays a critical role in the long-term health of the individual. Numerous epidemiological studies, animal models and clinical trials have highlighted the importance of early nutrition on health that extends through the lifetime of the individual, and very likely even into subsequent generations.[2–4]

Nutritional status and diet quality in early life certainly have long-term programming effects on health in

adulthood. High energy intake from carbohydrate-based foods, particularly high-glycaemic-index carbohydrates in early life, is associated with hyperinsulinaemia,[3] predisposing the individual to diabetes and obesity later in life. Children with wheezing in the first 3 years of life are more likely to develop asthma later in life. A diet high in omega-3 fatty acids in early infancy is also associated with reduced rates of atopic dermatitis, upper respiratory tract infections (URTIs) and allergic rhinitis.[4]

On the other hand, a poor quality 'Western' diet centred on 'white' foods (grains, sugar, cows milk) and protein calorie restriction is associated with many nutritional deficiencies, particularly for minerals such as iron and trace minerals such as iodine[5] and zinc,[6] which are essential for neurological, gastrointestinal and immunological development. Protein deficiency is implicated in the development of multiple health issues later in life.[7] Protein is required for the structure of all cells; hence, during stages of intense growth, development, illness and repair, protein requirements are always increased. A poor quality 'Western' diet is also deficient in essential fatty acids, which are of central importance for the normal development and functioning of the growing brain, eyes and central nervous system throughout childhood.

Feeding behaviours change dramatically during toddlerhood. It is a time of transition from a direct maternal selection of foods to more self-selection and attempt for increased autonomy. An improvement of motor skills means toddlers learn to use spoons, cups and bottles from about 1 year of age. Often, a fierce independence begins to emerge at this time, and most toddlers enjoy and demand the challenge of feeding themselves. Food preparation should be carried out with this in mind, with the serving of foods that are mushy, soft and in small pieces. Toddlers should always be observed while eating, as risk of choking is high at this age.

Picky or fussy eating is a relatively common problem among children, affecting up to 50% of all 2-year-olds[8,9]; however, prevalence rates vary significantly based on age and various definitions.[10] There is no single widely accepted definition of picky eating, making it difficult to formulate specific reliable assessment tools; hence, we rely on parents and carer feedback to inform us of their concerns. Primary caregivers' (usually mothers') concerns regarding restrictive diets, nutrient deficiencies, the development of eating disorders and adverse health outcomes are legitimate, despite the fact that the body of literature suggests that picky eating is usually a temporary behaviour and is a part of normal development in preschool children.[8]

Children classified as picky eaters generally have a strong preference for a limited variety of low-nutrient-dense foods such as sugary or salty snacks, and refined grains, while avoiding fruits and vegetables, fibre-rich foods and a variety of protein sources. Additionally, picky eaters tend to have special preferences for food texture, colour and combinations. Food preferences and suspicion of new foods in infancy may have had evolutionary benefits[11] in reducing the risk of consuming toxins, but in the modern world, these behaviours can provide a barrier to the acceptance of some food items. Picky eating and food neophobia (reluctance to eat or avoidance of new foods) can prevent dietary and nutrient variety, leading to concern about nutritional compromise. A chronic avoidance of nutrient-rich foods can potentially lead to poor growth rates,[9] micronutrient deficiencies, gastrointestinal issues (e.g. constipation), reduced immunity, sleep disturbances and compromised cognitive and behavioural development.[12]

Picky eaters also place notable stress upon caregivers and family relationships.

Factors contributing to the development of picky eating in children are numerous. Early feeding practices seem to influence the incidence of pickiness in childhood substantially. Early cessation of exclusive breastfeeding and subsequent weaning has been related to pickiness in children, while other research shows that breastfeeding beyond 6 months of age may reduce the odds of picky eating in children.[9] Breastfed infants are less likely to be fussy eaters than formula-fed babies, as they have been exposed to a variety of flavours while being breastfed.[13] Breast milk has the innate ability to take on the flavour of a mother's diet, giving infants who are breastfed greater exposure to various flavours, encouraging willingness to try new foods. Consequently, it is equally important for mothers who are breastfeeding to consume a diet with varied flavours and types of foods in order to avoid preferences for a limited number of food groups.[11] Several studies have identified associations between the mother's liked and disliked food items and those of the child, as well as the frequency of consumption of those items.[14]

Children may exhibit normal exploratory behaviours with new foods such as touching, smelling, playing and putting foods in their mouth and then spitting them out before they are willing to taste and swallow various foods.[15] Repeated taste exposure, or 'familiarisation', and modelling of behaviours in non-coercive fashion have been shown to increase food acceptance.[16] Conversely, pressuring children to eat can cause them to dislike those foods. Studies into food neophobia found that children need to be exposed to a new food or texture multiple times before accepting it; however, many parents incorrectly assume that rejection of a new food indicates dislike. Researchers in a study of 3022 infants found that many caregivers were not aware that their infants and toddlers needed as many as 8–15 exposures to a particular food before they gained acceptance of that food.[10,17] Repeated exposure to familiarise children with new foods is key, and as a new food is introduced, it does not need to be the focus of the meal; rather, only a couple of bites is enough to enhance acceptance of that food. In practice, the 'rule of ten' appears to be effective more often than not. Increased acceptance and consumption of poorly liked food, such as nutrient-rich fruits and vegetables, by children can be achieved by offering children very small tastes of new and previously disliked fruits and vegetables.[18]

Food is also more readily accepted in young children when others around them are eating the same type of food. Such modelling positively highlights the enjoyment of such foods. Praising children for trying new food and giving them small, token (non-food) rewards, such as stickers or time together reading a book, also increases acceptance.[19]

NUTRITIONAL REQUIREMENTS – 12–36 MONTHS – THE TODDLER

Despite growth rates peaking in the first year of life, a relatively high rate of growth and development continues through early childhood. Thus nutritional requirements remain high, and in some cases are higher than adult requirements (e.g. a 3- or 4-year-old toddler has a higher recommended daily intake for iron than a fully grown 30- to 40-year-old man).[20] The toddler and preschool years are generally considered to be the most difficult phase of life to study based on the complexities of controlling for variables such as emotional state, motivation, comprehension of instructions and inability to assess for outcomes of toddler performance such as IQ, which is notably challenging to assess until primary school.[21] Hence, precise information on toddler nutritional requirements and their connection to health outcomes is scarce, and more research is needed.

We do know that this is a time of rapid and dramatic changes in the brain (i.e. brain plasticity), and it is a time for procurement of foundational cognitive, social and interpersonal skills. Vocabulary increases significantly, motor coordination improves and focus and concentration begin to develop. The relationship between nutrition and brain development is complex and there are various mechanisms by which nutrition may influence brain development and behaviour.[21]

Infants and toddlers continue to lay down extensive amounts of neural tissue, and visual development also continues through and beyond age 6 years,[22] reflected in a higher requirement for certain nutrients such as choline, folic acid, zinc, iron and long-chain polyunsaturated fatty acids (PUFAs) AA and DHA.[23] Fat requirements are estimated to be around 50% of energy intake, with a larger requirement for saturated fat than is required later in life.[24] Low-fat products are not suitable for children under two years of age for this reason. For a sample toddler meal planner, refer to Appendix 16.1.

Essential fatty acids

Clean, unprocessed dietary fats with essential fatty acids provide the substrates for docosahexaenoic acid (DHA; which is an omega-3 fatty acid), arachidonic acid (AA; an omega-6 fatty acid) and their metabolites. Of the human brain's dry weight, 60% is comprised of lipids, of which 20% are DHA and AA.[25]

In addition to being basic structural components of neuronal membranes, these fatty acids also modulate membrane fluidity and influence neurotransmitter, receptor and enzyme activities in the brain. Since rapid brain growth occurs during the first years of life (and by the age of 2 the brain reaches 80% of its adult weight),[26] adequate supply of these essential fatty acids is indispensable to visual and cognitive development throughout childhood. This period of life may be particularly sensitive to essential fatty acid deficiencies and imbalances in the diet, affecting the maturation of the central nervous system, which may manifest in children as developmental delay, learning disorder or behavioural disturbance.[7] Several studies have focused on essential fatty acid metabolism in children with behavioural disturbance and ADHD, highlighting that children with lower compositions of total omega-3 fatty acids may have significantly more behavioural problems, temper tantrums and learning, health and sleep problems than those with high proportions of omega-3 fatty acids.[27] Levels of the omega-3 fatty acids docosahexaenoic acid (DHA) and eicosapentaenoic acid (EPA) are often low in the Western diet.[28] Several controlled trials have shown that diets supplemented with EPA and DHA have resulted in reduced incidences of childhood psychiatric disorders.[29]

The richest sources of EPA and DHA include breast milk from a replete mother; fish such as mackerel, wild salmon, herring, sardine, skipjack tuna, rainbow trout, flathead and snapper; grass-fed animal products such as beef and pasture-raised egg yolk; flaxseed oil, walnuts, chia seeds and TGA (Therapeutic Goods Administration)-approved supplements.

Unprocessed dietary fats are a valuable source of fat soluble vitamins and are required for absorption of minerals.[30] Kilojoules from fat are also 'protein sparing', allowing protein to be used for growth and development rather than for energy. In addition to enhancing flavour of a food or meal, unprocessed fats also slow down stomach emptying, allowing for satiety (a sense of fullness/satisfaction) and balanced glycaemic control, thereby preventing hypoglycaemia and hyperinsulinaemia.

Protein requirement remains relatively high, as it is the main structural component of all cells, which are rapidly growing and multiplying in early childhood. It is essential to ensure adequate intake of complete or combined incomplete proteins to ensure an adequate supply of all essential amino acids. Toddler protein requirements are estimated to be between 0.88 g/kg[31] and 1.2 g/kg.[32]

Carbohydrates that are nutrient dense and that have a low glycaemic index and low glycaemic load are recommended for all ages, but are particularly indicated during the highly active years of toddlerhood. Foods with high glycaemic indices can also set up dysfunctional metabolism throughout life. Nutrient-dense and fibre-rich carbohydrate sources ensure that the nutrients required for the digestion of the food are present, and that transit time is adequate to obtain maximum nutrition.

An aspect of healthy diet that most toddlers don't fare well with is achieving recommended daily serves of fruits and vegetables. The 2012–13 Australian Health Survey: Consumption of Food Groups from the Australian Dietary Guidelines[33] assessed the reported food and nutrient intake of children and young people and their physical activity levels, along with their weight, height and waist circumference. The survey was based on a sample of 4487 children and teens, aged between 2 and 16 years, who were randomly selected from across Australia. The study found that children aged 2–18 years averaged 1.8 serves of vegetables per day, and less than 1% usually consumed their recommended number of vegetable serves. The study

also found that the majority of younger children's energy came from milk and cereal foods.

One serve of fruit is 150 grams, which is equal to one medium-sized apple, orange, banana or pear; two smaller pieces of fruit (e.g. apricots, kiwi fruit or plums); 1 cup of chopped fruit; or 1½ tablespoons of dried fruit.

One serve of vegetables is 75 grams, which is equal to ½ cup cooked vegetables, ½ medium potato, 1 cup of salad vegetables or ½ cup cooked legumes (dried or canned beans, chickpeas or lentils) (see Table 16.2).

Achieving daily adequacy for vegetables and fruits during childhood and beyond is critical for healthy growth, development, energy and vitality. Also, the phytochemicals present in our colourful plant foods may reduce risk of many chronic diseases such as heart disease, childhood obesity, hypertension and some forms of cancer.[35] The phytochemicals achieved from eating a variety of colourful, in-season fruits and vegetables may offer protection to DNA[36] and may also selectively nourish healthy strains of bacteria in the developing gastrointestinal tract (GIT) microbiota.[37]

The fibre provided by consuming recommended serves of vegetables and fruits daily is fundamental to ensure healthy bowel transit time and to provide a food source for the evolving microflora of the intestinal tract. As a result of feeding on the fibre and phytochemicals such as polyphenols in plant foods, the microflora produce short-chain fatty acids, some of which are absorbed and much of which are used as the primary fuel source for enterocytes.

The Australian National Health and Medical Research Council (NHMRC) recommends an adequate daily intake of 14 g fibre for toddlers, and an adequate intake of approximately 1 L per day (4 cups) of fluids such as water and milk.[38]

The most commonly studied micronutrients in toddler nutrition are iron, iodine and zinc. All three are essential for development, and deficiencies in any one of them will have implications throughout life.

TABLE 16.2 Recommended daily serves of fruit and vegetables by age[33,34]				
Age	Fruit (girls)	Fruit (boys)	Vegetables (girls)	Vegetables (boys)
1–2	½	½	2–3	2–3
2–3	1	1	2 ½	2 ½
4–8	1 ½	1 ½	4 ½	4 ½
9–11	2	2	5	5
12–18	2	2	5	5 ½

Note: One serve of vegetables is 75 grams (equal to ½ cup cooked vegetables, ½ medium potato, 1 cup of salad vegetables) or ½ cup cooked dried or canned legumes (beans, chickpeas or lentils).
One serve of fruit is 150 grams (equal to 1 medium-sized apple, banana, orange or pear; 2 pieces of smaller fruit (e.g. apricots, kiwi fruit or plums); 1 cup of chopped fruit; ½ cup (125 mL) 100% fruit juice; or 1½ tablespoons dried fruit such as dried aricots or sultanas).
Source: Ministry of Health, NSW Department of Education, Office of Sport, The Heart Foundation. Eat more fruit and vegies 2016.

Iron

In toddlers and children, the relationship between the mineral iron and cognitive development is well researched. The blood–brain barrier, which functions to protect the brain from noxious chemicals, is still functionally developing tight junctions in infants, potentially to allow for maximal uptake of iron into the brain for optimal neurodevelopment.[39] When growing brains are not achieving adequate iron from a mineral-rich diet, we see impaired cognitive development, delayed psychomotor development, decreased resistance to infection, immune deficiencies and slower recovery from infection, poor cognitive function, fatigue, behavioural disturbance, sleep disturbance, and more.[5]

Iron is essential for development, and the effects of iron deficiencies in early childhood may not be reversible, possibly resulting in neurodevelopmental and motor delays.[40,41]

Yet, the prevalence of iron deficiency anaemia is significant – on average, about 20% of the Australian toddler and child population.[42,43] Between 3 and 48% of Australian preschool children have been shown to be deficient in iron, and a further 10–20% have lower than recommended intakes.[44]

Iron deficiency is most problematic in children with a highly processed, poor-quality diet, with low vitamin C food intakes and high levels of milk consumption. Furthermore, iron deficiency reduces a child's innate resilience against environmental chemical exposures, particularly heavy metals such as lead, putting children at greater risk of lead poisoning. Lead is particularly destructive to iron metabolism.[45] Lead is taken up by the same iron absorption machinery and, secondarily, blocks iron through competitive absorption. It interferes with metabolic steps such as haem synthesis, and has been labelled one of the 12 developmental neurotoxins that threaten brain development and IQ. In their paper on developmental toxicity, Dr Phillipe Grandjean and Dr Philip Landrigan discuss the fact that neurodevelopmental disabilities, including autism, attention-deficit hyperactivity disorder, dyslexia and other cognitive impairments, affect millions of children worldwide, with diagnoses increasing in frequency: *'Our very great concern is that children world-wide are being exposed to unrecognised toxic chemicals that are silently eroding intelligence, disputing behaviours, truncating future achievements and damaging societies.'*[46]

In Australia, iron deficiency anaemia is most likely to occur:
- with fussy eating, or with limited or restricted diets
- when young children are raised on a vegetarian- or vegan-style diet, where dietary iron is minimal and not readily absorbed due to high phytate content of a high grain/legume/soy-based diet
- when young children are given large quantities of cow's milk (>600 mL/day), where the calcium content can displace/competitively inhibit opportunistic iron absorption from the diet[47]
- following a pre-term birth, because a substantial amount of iron stores are transferred to newborns from the mother in late pregnancy. Premature babies miss out on this
- with parasitic infection, recurrent gastroenteritis, inflammatory bowel disease, gut inflammation and poorly managed or undiagnosed coeliac disease, where iron assimilation and absorption is compromised or where there are increased losses via the bowel
- with the use of proton pumps inhibitors in infancy for reflux. Drugs like Losec and Zantac – due to their effect on suppressing gastric acid production – impact on iron solubility and mineral status
- with developmental lead exposure from the environment.[48]

Iron-deficient toddlers present with a pale face, purple hue under the eyes, poor concentration, reduced exercise tolerance, increased risk of infection and longer recovery time. Often there are behavioural manifestations such as irritability and sleep disturbance. The nails may be brittle or weak, and pallor of the conjunctiva and the palmar creases can also be assessed for as signs of iron-deficiency anaemia.[47]

Chronic iron-deficiency anaemia can present as poor appetite, slowed growth and development and unusual craving for non-food items, such as ice, dirt, paint or starch. This craving is called pica.[49]

For iron-deficiency anaemia, the cut-off values as set by the World Health Organization are:
- haemoglobin <100 grams per litre for children under 5 years of age
- haemoglobin <115 grams per litre for children between 5 and 11 years of age.[50]

If iron deficiency is suspected, in addition to a full blood count, performing an iron study including serum ferritin (a protein that helps store iron) helps ascertain how much stored iron the body has. In an anaemic child, levels of ferritin below 10–12 micrograms/L is diagnostic of iron store deficiency, and levels between 12 and 30 micrograms/L are highly suggestive.[47] However, ferritin is also an acute-phase protein and is elevated in inflammation, infection, liver disease and malignancy. This can result in misleadingly elevated ferritin levels in iron-deficient patients with coexisting systemic illness. Hence a serum ESR and CRP should be concurrently run to exclude systemic inflammation which could give false positive ferritin results.

If iron deficiency is confirmed, iron supplementation is recommended at a rate of 3–6 mg/kg per day for 4 weeks, followed by re-testing of iron studies.[23]

Dietary opportunities for iron include beef, mussels, lamb, liver, egg yolk, chicken thigh, pork and some fish flesh, while vegetarians can get iron from green leafy vegetables, tempeh, cashews, seeds and some dried fruits such as sulfur-free dried apricots.[51]

Iodine

It is well understood that iodine is critically important in pregnancy for neuropsychological development in the baby during fetal and early postnatal life.[52] This importance continues into the toddler and early childhood years, yet there is much evidence to confirm the alarming existence of inadequate iodine intake extensively throughout the Australian paediatric community.[53] The decline in iodine intake in Australia and some other countries has particularly been detected since the cessation of iodine-based sterilising agents in our commercial dairies, which for decades was a major source of dietary iodine. Chlorine-based sanitisers have replaced iodine-based sanitisers.

The most significant and profound consequences of iodine deficiency are on the developing brain.

Research suggests that iodine deficiency results in a global loss of 10–15 IQ points at a population level, and constitutes the world's greatest single cause of preventable brain damage and mental retardation.[52]

Adequate iodine intake is also thought to be particularly protective against excessive exposures to fluoride, chlorine and bromine. Yet iodine deficiency and suboptimal iodine status has become a huge problem in past decades.[54] Are we an iodine-deficient population or an over-fluorinated and over-chlorinated population? Whichever scenario, it involves children with reduced IQs.[55]

Dietary opportunities for iodine include mackerel, cod, salmon, skipjack tuna, seaweed, dried kelp, dulse, miso soup, small ocean fish, shellfish and iodised salt.

Zinc

Zinc is a co-factor in more than 200 enzymes that regulate diverse metabolic activity. At-risk populations for zinc deficiency include those with a low intake of animal foods, high dietary phytic acid content and increased faecal losses during diarrhoea. Other groups at risk include growing toddlers, children and teens; people with diabetes because of increased zinc losses with glycosuria; people with high intake of processed foods; and especially those of Pacific and Aboriginal and Torres Strait Islander ethnicities.[23]

Infants and toddlers with zinc deficiency may have impaired taste, reduced appetite and food intake, and a textural focus on food. Leukonychia is commonly seen in Australian children and is associated with zinc insufficiency.[56]

Immunodeficiency, frequent respiratory infections, chronic sinus infections, slow skin healing, brittle nails and skin conditions should also prompt a thorough zinc assessment. Zinc supplementation can be useful in reducing the frequency and severity of colds.[57]

Signs of more chronic zinc deficiency in children include abnormal sexual development, growth retardation, weight loss, nausea, vomiting, and also behavioural and mood symptoms like depression and anxiety.[5,58]

Zinc is excreted via faeces, urine and sweat. Zinc losses are increased when there is diarrhoea, so supplementation may need to be considered, particularly as diarrhoea is chronic in nature. The World Gastroenterology Association recommends 20 mg of elemental zinc in all children recovering from acute infectious diarrhoea,[59] alongside oral rehydration therapy. Support from both animal and

human studies shows a relationship between low zinc and particular mental health issues.[60] Promoting a mineral-rich diet can reduce the burden of mental health disorders in the paediatric population.[61]

Dietary opportunities for zinc include beef, oysters, mussels, lamb, kangaroo, eggs, chicken, salmon, wheatgerm, pumpkin seeds, sunflower seeds, pine nuts, cashews and legumes. Because zinc absorption is so profoundly affected by the phytic acid content of some of these seeds, nuts, legumes and grains, it is advised to sprout/soak/ferment plant-based zinc foods to improve zinc bioavailability.[62]

Monitoring growth

Regular growth monitoring during childhood enables the detection of trends in growth, in particular looking to see if a child has fallen off their normal trajectory of growth, and allows for detection of childhood obesity. The NHMRC suggests that Australians use height and weight for age charts (gender specific) from the US Centers of Disease Control and Prevention (CDC) as a clinical tool[63] (see Fig. 16.1).

Childhood obesity

Exclusive intake of nutrient-poor, energy-dense foods has potential to lead to childhood obesity and its comorbid conditions. Obesity is defined as an excessive deposition of adipose tissue, and is usually diagnosed if a child's body fat is greater than 120% of that expected for their age.[64]

The epidemic of childhood obesity is progressing at an alarming rate: childhood obesity rates have doubled between 1995 and 2007, and if the current trajectory continues, we can anticipate over 30% of Australian children being overweight or obese by 2025.[33]

The inflammatory cycle of chronic childhood obesity impacts on every body system.[65]

Comorbid conditions include increased metabolic disease, increased cardiovascular disease (hypertension, hyperlipidaemia, atherosclerosis) and a significant increase in paediatric non-alcoholic fatty liver disease.[66]

Other identified consequences of childhood obesity include a heightened stress response, increased bone and joint disease, more mood disorders, increased allergic and atopic disease, higher incidence of inflammatory bowel disease and autoimmune conditions.[65,67] Increased incidence and this vicious obesogenic cycle strengthen the case for a much stronger emphasis on prevention and resolution of obesity in childhood.

Breaking the cycle of excessive television/screen time is critical in managing childhood obesity, with over 2 hours of screen time a day a useful indicator of children at risk of poor-quality diet and low physical activity.[68–70]

Management focus for childhood obesity is to ensure nutritional adequacy of trace minerals, minerals and vitamins; to restrict high-energy beverages such as soft drinks, juices, cordials and flavoured milks; and to limit energy-dense snack foods. Limiting screen time and ensuring adequate opportunity for exercise/outdoor activity is also crucial to healthy childhood weight.[71] Education around inclusion of an abundance of in-season vegetables (and some fruit) with lean proteins, adequate essential fatty acids, plenty of water and physical activity is key.[72] Whole-family participation is also a helpful and effective strategy.

Finally, the child's environment should always be considered in the management of childhood obesity. The term 'environmental obesogens' has been coined,[73] and EDCs such as phthalates and bisphenol A have been linked in several studies to the childhood obesity epidemic.[74,75]

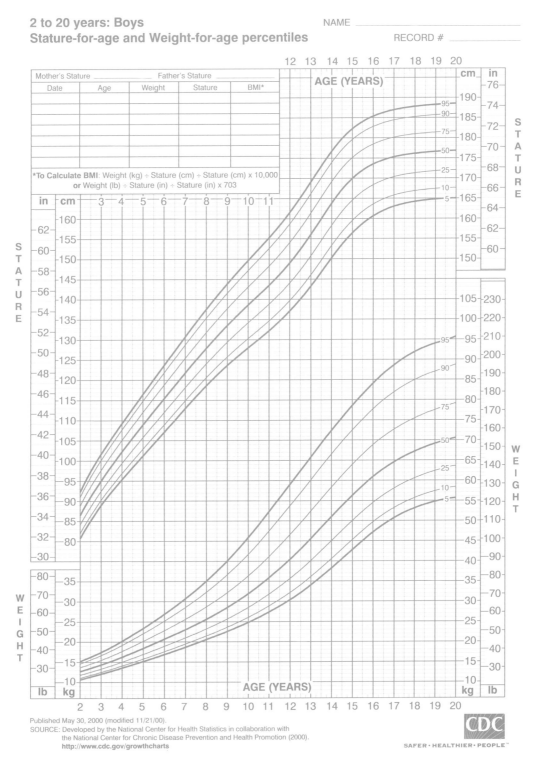

FIGURE 16.1 CDC growth charts for boys and girls: stature-for age-and weight-for-age percentile charts

http://www.cdc.gov/growthcharts/clinical_charts.htm

Continued

2 to 20 years: Girls
Stature-for-age and Weight-for-age percentiles

NAME _____

RECORD # _____

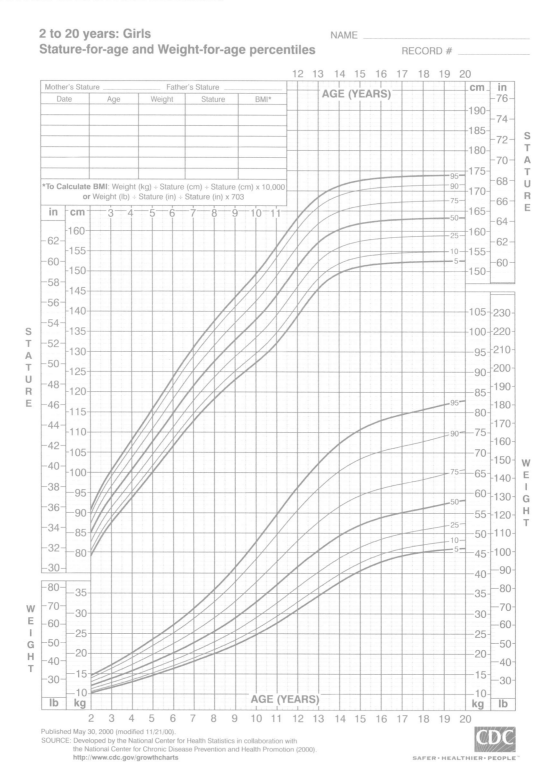

*To Calculate BMI: Weight (kg) ÷ Stature (cm) ÷ Stature (cm) x 10,000
or Weight (lb) ÷ Stature (in) ÷ Stature (in) x 703

Published May 30, 2000 (modified 11/21/00).
SOURCE: Developed by the National Center for Health Statistics in collaboration with
the National Center for Chronic Disease Prevention and Health Promotion (2000).
http://www.cdc.gov/growthcharts

SAFER · HEALTHIER · PEOPLE™

FIGURE 16.1, cont'd

Development of the microbiota of the gastrointestinal tract (GIT) in toddlers

The healthy microbiota of the human GIT acts as a physical barrier between the host and the external environment, as well as a contact point for pathogenic organisms in the digestive tract, preventing the settlement of unwanted microorganisms.[76] Other functions of the microbiota include the production of enzymes, vitamins – especially B vitamins and biotin – minerals and omega-3 and omega-6 PUFAs, the pre-digestion of foods and major endocrine, neurological and immunological functions.[77] Intestinal microbiota play a critical role in cholesterol metabolism and the regulation of gut-associated lymphoid tissue (GALT)[77] and affect production of Th1 and Th2 cytokines.

Both genetic and environmental factors shape the developing paediatric gut microbiota. Recent advances in genome sequencing techniques and metagenomic analysis methods have enabled revolutionary detection of new microbial species, significantly broadening our understanding of the resident paediatric GIT microbiota.[78] These DNA-sequencing/molecular techniques supersede the limited culturing techniques that were used for decades and led to a narrow understanding of the microbiome.

For example, for decades, it was understood that that the uterine environment of a developing infant was sterile – that the amniotic sac, and the fluid that surrounded the baby, was a uniquely pristine environment devoid of any bacteria in order to protect the growing baby, whose immune system was immature. The conventional wisdom was that the baby's first exposure to bacteria began during birth, from the mother's birth canal, and continued through the infant's skin-to-skin contact with the mother and from its new environment. But in recent years, scientists have been able to detect small amounts of bacteria in the amniotic fluid and in the placenta, and even in the fetus' intestines, supporting the idea that the baby's microbiome actually gets established far earlier than thought, in the womb.[79]

The intestinal microbiome undergoes dynamic change during development of infancy and childhood, and is particularly impressionable in the first 3 years of life.[78]

Factors that influence the development of the GIT microbiota include prenatal exposure, gestational age, mode of delivery, feeding type, introduction of solids, dietary prebiotic intake, probiotic use, antibiotic use and host genetics. All of these factors plus more can impact on a child's immune expression and health outcomes.[80]

A toddler's diet profoundly affects the composition of the microbiota, and changes in composition may have important consequences for physiology, immune development and susceptibility to disease.[78,81,82] Increasing whole plant food consumption appears to nourish and up-regulate commensal bacteria, in some case selectively increasing growth of the beneficial bacteria.[83] A diet high in particular fibres and polyphenols can support short-chain fatty acid production in the intestinal lumen and support gut integrity.[84] Besides enhancing gastrointestinal health and immune resilience, this may contribute to the health effects of these foods on other chronic human diseases into adult life, such as cancers and cardiovascular disease.[85]

Antibiotics and the paediatric microbiome

As a function of modern living, the paediatric and adolescent microbiome is overly exposed to antibiotics via their widespread medical prescription, as well as due to their prolific use in farm animals and crops. Microbiome composition can be rapidly altered by exposure to antibiotics, with potential immediate effects on health – impacting on the functioning of our immune system and our ability to resist infection.[86]

Early alterations in the microbiota due to antibiotic use can have significant lifelong implications.[87] Early antibiotic use has been associated with increased risk of asthma,[88] obesity,[89] inflammatory bowel disease[90] and allergic rhinitis.[91]

A naturopathic objective when working with the paediatric community is to optimise immune capacity, and therefore minimise use of pharmaceutical antibiotics. A reduction of microbial diversity is often observed within days of antibiotic ingestion, and complete recovery is not always achieved.[92]

Diversity within the microbiota is a marker of good health, and the reduced diversity of the intestinal microbiome due to widespread antibiotic use may also be placing children at increased risk of atopic conditions, colitis and *Clostridium difficile* infections.[78]

Use of appropriate strains of supplemental probiotics, defined as 'live microorganisms which when administered in adequate amounts confer a health benefit to the host'[78] are believed to assist the transient and resident microbiota in recovering and preventing pathogen adherence.[93]

Despite our understanding that the paediatric microbiome becomes less adaptable after the age of 3, recent metagenomic studies suggest that the gut microbiota of school-aged and adolescent children differ significantly from adults, suggesting that the human microbiome may still be evolving during childhood and adolescence.[94]

GROWTH AND DEVELOPMENTAL NUTRITION – MIDDLE CHILDHOOD – 36 MONTHS– 10 YEARS

Growth during middle childhood occurs in about 3–6 spurts per year. Average yearly weight gain is roughly 3.1 kg, while height increases by roughly 6.3 cm. The primary teeth begin to come out at around 6–7 years of age. Ethmoid sinuses reach adult size. Lymphoid tissue grows beyond adult size at around 6–8 years of age and then reduces to adult size. Middle childhood is a period of rapid bone growth. Children aged between 5 and 11 years are most likely to fracture a bone. Respiratory rate declines and diastolic blood pressure increases to adult levels at around 6 years. Gastric emptying time is still faster than that of an adult, and may affect digestion and absorption of food and nutrients.

Brain development is still significant during this time of life. Myelination of white matter continues (well into young adulthood) and rapid growth of grey matter continues up to 5 years of age, at which point it begins to selectively thin in areas of the most basic sensory perception and movement – an indication of synaptic pruning, which is a sign of maturation process.[95] Results from the National Institutes of Health MRI study of healthy brain development indicate that by 6 years of age, 95% of the brain volume has been achieved.[26]

Neuromotor skills rapidly develop during this time and plateau by 13–15 years of age.[96]

Early childhood marks the end of the egocentric phase of life. At around 6 years of age, children are able to compare themselves with others. At 7–8 years, children can differentiate their own feelings from those of others. Understanding the concept of competition, particularly in regard to sport, begins at around 9 years of age. Between 6 and 11 years, children develop their understanding of moral judgment.[97,98]

Middle childhood is an important time for the development of language and social skills and coincides with a thickening of the grey matter in the cortex of the temporal and frontal lobes.[95] Deficits in these areas, as a result of genetics, nutrition or environment, tend to have lifelong consequences in social settings and ability to earn an income. At around 7–8 years, grammatical skills are learnt and applied. Ability to store memory is matured by 5 years of age, but working memory does not begin until about 6 years of age. Writing becomes fluent for most children at around 6 years of age[99] and is an important part of language development.

NUTRITIONAL REQUIREMENTS – MIDDLE CHILDHOOD – 36 MONTHS–10 YEARS

Nutritional requirements begin to stabilise during middle childhood as speed of growth slows down. Owing to the continued high rate of development of the nervous system and cognitive faculties, and eventual initiation of sexual development, intake of adequate nutrients is still paramount and can affect health in adulthood.

Following on from childhood, the nutrient deficiencies of childhood associated with impaired cognitive function include iron and iodine, zinc and essential fatty acids DHA and EPA.

Impairments as a result of iron deficiency, essential for neurological development, may not be reversible.[24] Signs of iron deficiency can mimic those of lead poisoning, so if present, both should be tested for.[23]

Zinc deficiency may also cause impaired taste and result in self-limited eating. If picky eating continues into middle childhood, particularly past the age of 6 or 7, when picky eating usually abates, zinc deficiency should be

considered. Symptoms of zinc deficiency are very similar to those of anorexia: appetite loss, weight loss, focus on texture, nausea and vomiting, and delayed sexual development.[100] As such, zinc deficiency should also be a primary consideration in the aetiology of eating disorders such as anorexia, which can often start at between 7 and 12 years of age.

Requirements for fat may be reduced to 30–40% of kilojoules; however, data available on fat requirements are conflicting. Children on a low-fat diet are more likely to be deficient in a number of nutrients,[7] including vitamin A. Mild or subclinical vitamin A deficiency is associated with impaired immune function.[24] Owing to the high rate of recurrent infections in childhood, the intake of fats that contain vitamin A becomes an important consideration. Parasitic infections, particularly common in middle childhood, can cause both vitamin A and iron deficiencies[101] and, if suspected, should be treated immediately to prevent long-term consequences of chronic deficiency.

The NHMRC recommends an adequate intake of 18 g of fibre for children between 4 and 8 years of age and 20–24 g of fibre daily for children between 9 and 13 years of age.[38] An adequate intake of approximately 1.2 L per day (5 cups) of fluids such as water and milk for children 4–8 years of age, and 1.4–1.6 L (5–6 cups) for children 9–13 years of age is the guide provided by the NHMRC.[38] However, in addition to that, about a third of a child's water requirement can come from eating the suggested amount of vegetables and fruits.

Essential fatty acids

The importance of dietary omega-3 PUFAs to health is well known. Quality dietary polyunsaturated fats are essential as building blocks for the sophisticated and delicate process of continued neurodevelopment and brain function; they have a structural role in membranes, skin and mucous membranes. These PUFAs are precursors of biologically active 'messengers' in the body such as prostaglandins, and are involved with hormone and neurotransmitter production and function. In particular, docosahexaenoic acid (DHA) omega-3 forms a structural component of growing brains and retinas throughout childhood, which is vital to normal development, and both qualitatively and quantitatively important.[102]

The standard Australian diet is particularly low in omega-3 fatty acids, including plant-based alpha-linolenic acid (ALA), and DHA, which is found mainly in fish. Several studies have demonstrated positive associations between blood DHA levels and improvements on tests of cognitive and visual function in healthy children. Intervention studies have shown that improving maternal DHA nutrition decreases the risk of poor infant and child visual and neural development.[103] Controlled trials have also shown that supplementation with DHA and EPA may help in the management of childhood psychiatric disorders and improve visual and motor function.[29] Increasing DHA intake in our children should be a primary goal for optimising health, behaviour, neurocognition, IQ and vision.

Consumers are faced with a dilemma when it comes to the fact that harmful POPs and methylmercury are also present in some fatty fish, our richest source of DHA. Some medical evidence says that the beneficial effects of omega-3 fatty acids and selenium in fatty fish outweigh and somewhat counteract toxicities of methylmercury and persistent organic pollutants.[104] As part of its 2006 report *Seafood Choices: Balancing Benefits and Risks*, the Institute of Medicine (now called the National Academy of Medicine) reviewed the scientific evidence, and the expert panel concluded that although selenium may diminish some of the toxic effects of some forms of mercury and other heavy metals, the mechanisms for these interactions are poorly understood. In addition, there was little or no evidence showing that selenium affected the toxicity of other seafood contaminants such as polychlorinated biphenyls (PCBs) or dioxins. Therefore, choosing seafood that is highest in omega-3 DHA and lowest in contaminants such as methylmercury and POPs is still the best course of action.[105]

Accompanying/compounding the aforementioned nutrient building blocks required for healthy toddler and childhood development, both vitamin D and the mineral calcium are required in generous amounts for adequate bone mineralisation at such a rapid time of growth, which extends well into adolescence. Bone mass increases about sevenfold from birth to puberty, and a further threefold during adolescence.[106]

Maximising peak bone mineralisation at this crucial time can definitely reduce the risk of adult osteoporosis. Calcium deficiency is quite hard to diagnose due to the large skeletal bank of calcium; however, a thorough diet analysis can shed light on an individual's calcium intake/adequacy.

Calcium

Calcium is required for the normal development and maintenance of the skeleton as well as for the proper functioning of neuromuscular and heart function. The majority of the body's calcium is stored in the teeth and bones where it provides structure and strength. Low intakes of calcium have been associated with low bone density and osteoporosis – which is quite common in Western cultures – often resulting in bone fracture.[107]

Calcium intake throughout life, particularly growth phases, is a major factor affecting the incidence of osteoporosis in adulthood. However, other factors – notably adequate vitamin D status, exercise and diet quality – also play a role.

The NHMRC advises a recommended daily intake of 700 mg of calcium for children 4–8 years of age, 1000 mg of calcium daily for children 9–11 years of age and 1300 mg of calcium daily for children 14–18 years of age.[108]

During the adolescent growth spurt, the required calcium retention is 2–3 times higher than that required for the development of peak bone mass which occurs at the same time as maximum height. It has been demonstrated that adequate calcium intake during growth may influence peak bone mass/density, and may be instrumental in preventing subsequent adulthood/postmenopausal osteoporosis. Calcium intake during adolescence appears to affect skeletal calcium retention directly, and a calcium intake of up to 1600 mg/day may be required to ensure a level of skeletal retention of calcium sufficient for maximal peak bone mass.[109] This is significantly higher than the current RDI for calcium already established for children, adolescents and young adults.

In addition to nutrition, heredity (both parents) and endocrine factors (sexual development) appear to have profound effects on peak bone mass formation, as does weight-bearing exercise for the deposition of calcium into the bone matrix.[110] Most of the skeletal mass will be accumulated by late adolescence, indicating early timing of peak bone mass.[109]

Calcium is found predominantly in milk and dairy-based foods, with smaller amounts in the bones of fish (such as wild salmon, sardines and anchovies), legumes and certain nuts, seeds and fortified soy milk/almond milk beverages. Consumption of vegetarian diets may influence calcium needs because of their relatively high oxalate and phytate content; however, on balance, lacto-ovo-vegetarians appear to have similar calcium intakes to omnivores.[111]

The efficiency of calcium absorption varies across foods as calcium may be poorly absorbed from foods rich in oxalic acid (e.g. spinach, rhubarb and beans) or phytic acid (seeds, nuts, grains, certain raw beans and soy isolates).

Adolescents sometimes become vegetarian for ethical rather than health reasons, raising concern for their mineral intake and development overall.[112]

Vegans have a lower calcium intake than vegetarians and omnivores. However, research has shown that both lactovegetarians and vegans can attain calcium balance, and that a well-selected vegan diet maintains calcium status, at least for a short-term period of 20–30 days.[113]

Despite the lower intake of calcium in vegetarian and vegan diets, the low acid load of these diets can explain the absence of osteoporosis or low bone mineral density (BMD) in some vegans. Low acid load is correlated with lower bone resorption and higher BMD. Low acid load is linked to high intake of potassium-rich nutrients, such as fruits and vegetables, as found in vegetarian diets. This might be an important factor for the protection of vegetarians from osteoporosis.[114] In contrast, the diet of Western-style omnivores has a higher acid load which is associated with lower BMD and higher fracture risk.[114]

Still, it is a major disservice to a growing child to exclude dairy from the diet for longer than 20–30 days without providing structured guidance for achieving calcium requirements from vegan and vegetarian sources.

Vitamin D

Vitamin D is essential for bone growth – deficiency in children has been linked to adverse effects such as growth failure and rickets. Although vitamin D is available in some foods and drinks, recent estimates suggest the prevalence of vitamin D deficiency among infants, children and adolescents is between 12 and 24%.[115,116]

Children with dark skin are at an increased risk and require more skin exposure to sunshine, without the use of sunblock. Epidemiological research, in both children and adolescents, has shown that vitamin D supplementation has beneficial effects on bone mineral augmentation when adequate dietary calcium intake is in place; for example, by decreasing the concentration of bone resorption markers.[117]

Vitamin D adequacy also benefits immune modulation, preventing the development of some autoimmune conditions and susceptibility of microbial infection.[118]

A positive association between lower respiratory tract infection and vitamin D deficiency has been investigated in children,[119] and multiple studies have shown that low serum 25-hydroxyvitamin D levels are associated with a higher risk of upper and lower respiratory infections in children, that low vitamin D status may affect the severity of acute lower respiratory infection[120] and that a shortage of vitamin D may contribute to severity of asthma symptoms.[121–123]

While most healthy children in Australia and New Zealand receive enough sunlight exposure to maintain adequate vitamin D levels, a significant number living in the more temperate zones develop mild vitamin D deficiency during winter.[124]

If children can be encouraged to participate in regular outdoor activities, blanket vitamin D supplementation for children and adolescents may not be warranted.

Children who are dark-skinned, veiled, exposed to reduced sunlight or who have an underlying medical condition should receive 400 IU vitamin D daily to prevent vitamin D deficiency.[125]

Siblings of a child diagnosed with vitamin D deficiency should be screened.[126]

The major source of vitamin D (more than 80%) in Australia and New Zealand is skin exposure to sunlight (UVB radiation).[127]

Balance needs to be struck between sufficient sun exposure to maintain adequate vitamin D_3 production and minimise the risk of skin cancer.

No evidence suggests that daily supplementation of 400 IU of vitamin D is toxic,[128] and it is a simple and cost effective intervention, particularly during the winter months, to optimise childhood development and reduce disease burden.

For a sample lunchbox meal planner, refer to Appendix 16.1.

GROWTH AND DEVELOPMENTAL NUTRITION – ADOLESCENCE – 10 YEARS AND OLDER

During the pre-teen, teenage and young adult years, there are not only rapid and significant changes to physical appearance, but also dramatic changes in physiological, psychological and social functioning. Adolescence is a significant and sensitive developmental period, with research indicating that structural reorganisation, brain and cognitive maturation and – in particular – major developments in the pre-frontal cortex take place during puberty.[5] Adequate adolescent nutrition is critical to the function and optimal outcomes of these hormonally driven, nutrient-hungry physiological changes and the ongoing neurological development that occurs at this time.[129]

At adolescence, there is a marked gain in both weight and height that is referred to as the adolescent growth spurt. On average, the spurt in height begins at 10–11 years in girls, and at 12–13 years in boys, and generally lasts for 2 years.[64] Sexual maturation begins for girls at an average age of 10.9, beginning with breast budding. For boys, sexual maturation begins at an average age of 10.5 years with growth of the penis. These developmental changes follow a fairly predictable pattern of occurrence; however, every child is unique, and individual variations in the timing and pace of development undoubtedly exist.

The adolescent period of development is divided into three phases – early, middle and late adolescence. Each stage is marked by a characteristic set of biological, cognitive and psychosocial milestones (see Table 16.3).

Growth acceleration begins in adolescence, with 15–20% of adult height accrued during puberty.[129]

A number of factors influence physical development at puberty. Besides nutritional and environmental influences such as physical activity and environmental exposures, a child's growth and ultimate height will be influenced by heredity.

Females attain a peak height velocity of 8–9 cm per year at sexual maturity rating 2–3, about 1 year after breast budding, and approximately 6 months before menarche. Menstruation usually starts about 18 months to 2 years after the onset of puberty. On average, the first menses occur just before girls turn 13.[130] Earlier age of menarche has been commonly associated with increased body mass index (BMI) in childhood and adolescence, and a recent body of research has found associations between earlier age of menarche and environmental factors such as exposure to EDCs.[131–133]

Males typically begin their growth acceleration at a later sexual maturity rating stage 3–4, achieve a peak height velocity of 9–10 cm per year later in the course of puberty, and continue their linear growth for approximately 2–3 years after females have stopped growing.[129]

Despite the averages mentioned, children have a tendency to grow in spurts. These individual variations in timing – along with hereditary factors – are largely responsible for the wide variations in size among children the same age.

One-half to two-thirds of total body calcium is laid down during puberty. Bone growth precedes increases in bone mineralisation and bone density, which may increase the adolescent's risk of fracture during times of rapid growth. Since skeletal growth precedes muscle growth, sprains and strains may be more common during this time as well. A child's need for kilojoules rises during times of rapid growth, gradually increasing as they move through middle childhood into puberty.

TABLE 16.3 Milestones in early, middle and late adolescent development[129]			
Variable	**Early adolescence**	**Middle adolescence**	**Late adolescence**
Approximate age range	10–13 years	14–17 years	18–21 years
Sexual maturity rating*	1–2	3–5	5
Physical	• Females: secondary sex characteristics (breast, pubic, axillary hair), start of growth spurt • Males: testicular enlargement, start of genital growth	• Females: peak growth velocity, menarche (if not already attained) • Males: growth spurt, secondary sex characteristics, nocturnal emissions, facial and body hair, voice changes • Change in body composition • Acne	• Physical maturation slows • Increased lean muscle mass in males
Cognitive and moral	• Concrete operations • Egocentricity • Unable to perceive long-term outcome of current decisions • Follow rules to avoid punishment	• Emergence of abstract thought (formal operations) • May perceive future implications, but may not apply in decision making • Strong emotions may drive decision making • Sense of invulnerability • Growing ability to see others' perspectives	• Future-oriented with sense of perspective • Idealism • Able to think things through independently • Improved impulse control • Improved assessment of risk vs reward • Able to distinguish law from morality
Self-concept/ identity formation	• Preoccupied with changing body • Self-consciousness about appearance and attractiveness	• Concern with attractiveness • Increasing introspection	• More stable body image • Attractiveness may still be of concern • Consolidation of identity
Family	• Increased need for privacy • Exploration of dependence/ independence boundaries	• Conflicts over control and independence • Struggle for greater autonomy • Increased separation from the parents	• Emotional and physical separation from family • Increased autonomy • Re-establishment of 'adult' relationship with parents
Peers	• Same-sex peer affiliations	• Intense peer group involvement • Preoccupation with peer culture • Conformity	• Peer group and values recede in importance
Sexual	• Increased interest in sexual anatomy • Anxieties and questions about pubertal changes • Limited capacity for intimacy	• Testing ability to attract partner • Initiation of relationships and sexual activity • Questions of sexual orientation	• Consolidation of sexual identity • Focus on intimacy and formation of stable relationships • Planning for future and commitment

Source: Kleigman R, Stanton B, St Geme J, et al, editors. Nelson Textbook of Pediatrics. 19th ed. Philapdelphia, PA: Elsevier Saunders; 2011.

NUTRITIONAL REQUIREMENTS – ADOLESCENCE – 10 YEARS AND OLDER

Adolescent nutrition is crucial for proper growth and development and is a prerequisite for achieving full developmental potential. Suboptimal nutrition may contribute to delayed and stunted growth[134] as well as impaired development.

Adolescent nutritional health care is challenging compared to that of children and adults, due to adolescents' rapidly evolving physical, intellectual and emotional development. Increasing importance of the peer group (and separation from parents as a part of normal psychosocial development) may have an impact on food and lifestyle choices. Group cohesion and a sense of belonging become important in adolescence. Food eaten will now depend less on family food patterns and more on a variety of other factors, including self-image, media, social expectations, financial cost, access to food outlets and peers. Conformity with peers in manners of behaviour and attitudes towards food and lifestyle may present as adolescents work on establishing their own identity. Similarly, peer pressure may exist. Parents and providers may each work with adolescents to foster good decision making.

Early and middle adolescence are commonly the ages at which poor or distorted body image and eating disorders may develop. Early adolescents undergo rapid physical changes and may experience uncertainty about whether all of these anatomical and physiological changes are progressing normally. Reassurance from adults, including their healthcare providers, may be comforting. As puberty comes to an end and these changes slow, the middle adolescent's preoccupation may shift to whether the adolescent is attractive to others. A strong emphasis on physical appearance during this time is normal. Collaborative clinical care is always required if an eating disorder is suspected.

Protein requirements are moderate to ensure growth in skeletal muscle and availability of adequate building blocks for hormones, neurotransmitters and body structures. The NHMRC recommends 40 g a day of protein for boys aged 9–13 (calculated at 0.94 g per kg of body weight) and 65 g a day for adolescent boys aged 14–18 (calculated at 0.99 g per kg of body weight). For girls, the recommendations are 35 g a day of protein between the ages of 9 and 13 (calculated at 0.87 g per kg of body weight) and 45 g a day for between the ages of 14 and 18 (calculated at 0.77 g per kg of body weight).[135]

The NHMRC recommends an adequate intake of 20–22 g of fibre for girls aged 9–18 and 24–28 g of fibre daily for boys aged 9–18.[136]

Calcium and vitamin D adequacy, as previously discussed, are critical considerations during adolescence to account for the enormous bone accrual at this time.

Iron is also a crucial consideration to account for the haemodilution and considerable blood volume expansion that occurs with the growth in height. Iron is a particularly important consideration for adolescent girls after menarche due to menstrual losses. In addition to a quality diet generous in iron and other minerals, a recent systematic review and meta-analysis, titled *Interventions to Improve Adolescent Health and Nutrition*, found that micronutrient supplementation among adolescents (predominantly females) can significantly decrease anaemia prevalence.[137]

The physiological requirements for zinc peak around the pubertal growth spurt, which generally occurs in girls between 10 and 15 years and in boys between 12 and 15 years.[138,139]

Even marginal zinc deficiency during the pubertal growth spurt has been associated with slower skeletal growth, slower maturation, stunting and reduced bone mineralisation.[140]

As children progress into adolescence, continuing after the growth spurt has ceased, they may require additional zinc to replenish tissue zinc pools depleted during puberty.[140]

As nearly a third of total skeletal mineral is accumulated in the 3–4 year period immediately after the onset of puberty, suboptimal zinc intake may have long-term consequences on bone health.[141–143]

Both zinc and iron deficiency are prevalent[144] among children and adolescents (including in industrialised countries), with associations with immune system dysfunction and restricted physical development.[145]

Children and adolescents are particularly vulnerable to suboptimal zinc and iron status during periods of rapid growth that create increased zinc and iron needs that may not be met.[146,147]

Inadequacies in dietary intakes can be attributed to poor food selection patterns and low energy intakes. Additional exacerbating factors may include high menstrual losses, strenuous exercise, pregnancy, low socioeconomic status and ethnicity. Moreover, if adolescents enter pregnancy with a compromised iron and zinc status, and continue to receive intakes of iron and zinc that do not meet their increased needs, their poor iron and zinc status could adversely affect the pregnancy outcome.[148] Diet quality and mineral adequacy at this time is crucial to accommodate for development.

It should be noted that adolescents sometimes become vegetarian or vegan for ethical rather than health reasons. This may result in health problems if knowledge of nutrition is limited. In support of vegan and vegetarian diets, there is often a higher intake than omnivores of vegetables, legumes and dietary supplements, and lower intakes of cakes, biscuits, candy and chocolate.[112] However, vegetarians and vegans have dietary intakes lower than the average requirements for riboflavin, vitamin B_{12}, vitamin D, calcium, zinc, iron and selenium.[112]

The dietary habits of vegetarians and vegans vary considerably, and thorough education around best management of a vegan diet for growing children and adolescents is critical to ensure intake of recommended requirements for essential nutrients.

Performing a thorough diet review to assess for zinc and other mineral food intake, in combination with a serum/plasma zinc concentration, can help to understand a child or adolescent's status. It is well established that plasma zinc concentration can fall in response to factors unrelated to zinc status or dietary zinc intake, such as infection, inflammation, exercise, stress or trauma.[138]

Beneficial therapeutic responses to zinc have been observed in many paediatric and adolescent conditions, including mood,[149] skin conditions, autoimmune conditions and inflammatory disorders. Besides being a cofactor in the function of many enzyme systems in the body, and being of structural importance, zinc is an intracellular signalling molecule in that it plays an important role in cell-mediated immune functions and oxidative stress.[150]

As iron and zinc are known to compete for absorption, it is possible that high-dose iron supplements may impair child zinc status.[62,138] Separation by at least 2 hours of iron supplementation from zinc supplementation is advised.

SPECIFIC CONDITIONS

Constipation

Bowel movement frequency ranges between children; however, 85% of 1- to 4-year-olds eating a predominantly low-fibre diet open their bowels once or twice a day, and 96% of all children fall within the range of 3 times a day to every second day.[151] The colon transit time of normal healthy children and adolescents is on average 36 hours, and does not appear to be age- or gender-related (above the age of 3 years).[104,152]

The definition of constipation varies from author to author, but can most simply be defined by one or a combination of frequency, size, consistency and ease of elimination.[153] Constipation can be divided into two categories: organic and functional. Organic causes of constipation are the least common and include Hirschsprung's disease, anorectal malformation, hypothyroidism and spina bifida.[153] Functional constipation is usually caused by one or a combination of the following: dehydration, dysbiotic bowel flora, food sensitivity, inadequate fibre intake, anal fissures (cause and effect) and some medications. Reduced physical activity, and fluid losses induced from fever or recent diarrhoea, also promote constipation.[100,154]

Constipation is common in children, peaking between ages 2 and 4.[155] It is the second most referred condition in paediatric gastroenterology practices, accounting for up to 25% of all visits.[156] The diagnosis of constipation requires careful history taking and interpretation. Diagnostic tests are not often needed and are reserved for those who are severely affected. The daily bowel habits of children are extremely susceptible to any changes in routine environment. Constipation and subsequent 'holding', or faecal retention, behaviour often begins soon after a child has experienced a painful evacuation.[99]

It has been shown there are significant differences in bowel flora populations in constipated compared with non-constipated individuals and that this dysbiosis can also be an effect rather than a cause of constipation.[157] Treatment time for constipation can range from a few days, in simple cases, up to 12 months in more severe cases.[158]

Signs and symptoms of constipation include[159]:
- large hard stools
- small, dry, pellet-like stools
- infrequent bowel motions
- skinny stools (indicates compacted faeces around the lumen, with only a narrow passageway for overflow faeces to move through)
- withholding behaviours (infants and toddlers may withhold bowel motion to avoid pain of passing stool)
- encopresis
- over-spill syndrome where watery stool will pass by compacted faeces in the rectum, giving the appearance of diarrhoea
- abdominal pain
- early satiety
- painful defecation
- straining – often indicated by whole body tensing and reddening of the face
- haemorrhoids.

Abdominal pain is one of the most common presenting symptoms for chronic constipation in the toddler years.

Possible dietary contributing factors include:
- low intake of fruits and vegetables and lack of fibre in the diet[159]
- insufficient fluid intake[100]
- cow's milk allergy[160]
- non-coeliac gluten sensitivity or gluten intake in an undiagnosed coeliac.[161]

Possible psychological contributing factors include[155]:
- sexual abuse
- depression
- anorexia nervosa
- anxiety.

CONSTIPATION: TREATMENT

Childhood constipation can be very difficult to treat. It often requires prolonged support by doctors and parents, explanation, medical treatment and, most importantly, the child's cooperation.[104]

Herbal medicine

Digestive bitters, cholagogues and hepatostimulant herbs improve digestion and increase bile production, often resulting in softer stools. Hepatic support is also warranted due to the toxic burden on the liver caused by reabsorption of toxins from the bowel as a result of constipation. Lymphatic herbs also support the process of detoxification and therefore support liver function.

Anthroquinone-containing laxative herbs are to be avoided in infants and children, and used sparingly in adolescence. They can be used short-term for stubborn or severe constipation to help loosen impacted faeces for evacuation. Prolonged use of laxatives – drug or herbal – can result in reduced bowel tone and laxative dependence. If anthroquinone herbs are deemed necessary, it is important to also use carminatives such as peppermint, lemon balm, chamomile or fennel to ease and avoid possible pain of intestinal spasm caused by the laxatives.

Suitable herbal medicine for use in constipation includes:
- *Taraxacum officinale radix* (dandelion root)
- *Rumex crispus* (yellow dock)
- *Glycyrrhiza glabra* (liquorice)
- *Mentha x piperita* (peppermint)
- *Matricaria recutita* (chamomile)
- *Foeniculum vulgare* (fennel)
- *Iris versicolor* (blue flag)
- *Melissa officinalis* (lemon balm)
- *Gentiana lutea* (gentian)

Nutritional medicine (supplementation)

The first avenue of treatment for constipation of all ages is probiotic therapy, and this is one of the most easily administered therapies for children and adolescents, with good compliance. Their excellent safety profile also makes probiotics an attractive option in the treatment of functional constipation.[162] Probiotic powders can be given straight to the mouth of a child as powder or capsule, put into room temperature food, smoothies, yoghurt or water.

Probiotics that have been shown to have a beneficial effect on bowel motion frequency and oro-faecal transit time:
- *Lactobacillus reuteri*[162]
- *Bifidobacterium longum* 46 and 2C[163]
- *Bifidobacterium lactis* HN01, Bb-12, LKM512 and DN-173 010[164,165]
- *Lactobacillus casei* Shirota[166,167]

- *Escherichia coli* Nissle 1917 ('Mutaflor')[168]
- *Bifidobacterium animalis*[165]
- *Lactobacillus rhamnosus*[169]
- *Propionibacterium freudenreichii*[169]
- *Lactobacillus plantarum* SN13T[170]

The highly absorbent slippery elm, chia seeds, psyllium husks and flax meal draw water into the bowel, acting as bulking and softening agents. The increased bulk stimulates peristalsis, initiating a soft but formed bowel motion. The best bulking agents for children are slippery elm powder, chia seed and flax seed meal, followed by psyllium husks. Psyllium husks are slightly more abrasive than flax and slippery elm, and so may not be suitable for all children. All three bulking agents also contain valuable prebiotics – substrates for healthy bacteria to feed off. Encouragement of the infant's fluid intake is important for the bulking agent to work effectively.

Slippery elm is very effective in treating constipation in infants and children from a young age. The increased bulk stimulates peristalsis, while its mucilaginous properties create soft slippery stools, together initiating a soft but formed bowel motion. The author finds that a combination of slippery elm and probiotic, in addition to dietary intervention with adequate plant-based fibre, quickly resolves almost all cases of minor constipation and greatly helps to establish regular bowel motions in chronic and severe constipation.

Freshly ground flax seeds can be added to yoghurt, mashed or stewed fruit or mixed into water to drink. Flax seed meal is mucilaginous and a bulking agent, resulting in slippery, soft, well-formed stools, and has the added benefit of providing essential omega-3 fatty acids. Chia seeds are an effective alternative.

Essential fatty acid supplements – for example, a liquid fish oil or cod liver oil – can be useful interventions, providing 'lubrication' to the bowel, increasing intestinal motility, speeding bowel transit time and increasing defecation.[171]

Absorbable magnesium powders, such as magnesium citrate, alginate, oxalate or amino acid chelate can be used to help relax and promote healthy peristalsis of the smooth muscle of the intestinal tract.

Lactulose can be used as an osmotic laxative, with the dose of 10 mL daily for children aged 1–6 and mL per day for children aged 7–15. Lactulose should be used under clinical supervision, beginning slowly in case of flatulence as a side effect.[172]

As an extreme measure, unabsorbable magnesium sulfate (Epsom salts) provides a useful avenue for initial removal of compacted faeces in very constipated children.[173] Use of Epsom salts to cause loose or diarrhoea-like stools can then be followed up with use of slippery elm bark and probiotics. Fluid intake must be increased.

Nutritional medicine (dietary)

Ensuring adequate fluid intake is key. Ensuring adequate soluble and insoluble fibre in the diet is also essential for regular bowel habits. Dietary requirements can be calculated using the age +5 g rule. Good sources of dietary fibre include guar gum (used in cooking), chia seeds, sweet potato, broccoli and apple (when choking is no longer a hazard). Foods high in prebiotics include globe artichokes, garlic, onion, leeks, asparagus, chives, legumes, peas, fruit and okra. Short-chain fatty acids help feed and fuel the cells of the colon and prevent dysbiosis and inflammation in the gut.[174]

Cow's milk allergy has been shown to be a significant aetiological factor for paediatric and childhood constipation, and if this is suspected withdrawal from cow's milk and dairy products for a 1-month period can be trialled, followed by a cow's milk challenge over 2 weeks to observe changes in bowel transit time. Serum levels of IgE to cow's milk proteins are helpful, although not definitive for diagnosis.[175]

Furthermore, some research suggests that daily kiwi fruit consumption for 4 weeks shortens colon transit time, increases defecation frequency and improves bowel function in individuals suffering from constipation.[176]

Probiotic-rich foods have been shown to positively affect bowel habits. Consuming beneficial bacteria in live food is very effective as the bacteria are active in their food source, and so are accompanied by the building blocks they need to colonise in the gut. Probiotic-rich foods include homemade fermented vegetables, such as sauerkraut; kefir made with dairy, coconut water or filtered sweetened water; probiotic yoghurt; and kombucha.

Fluid intake, in the form of water, water kefir, kombucha, coconut water and herbal tea should also be monitored.

Lifestyle recommendations

Studies show that sedentary and overweight children are more likely to experience constipation. Adequate exercise/activity and healthy eating are important for both weight management and prevention of constipation. In the event of constipation, abdominal massage in a clockwise direction may help promote peristalsis and emptying of the rectal vault. The effect of massage can be amplified with the use of essential oils such as chamomile and lemon balm diluted into 30 mL of carrier oil. See dosages considerations in Appendix 16.2 for how many drops to use.

Sitting on a modern toilet often adds to the difficulty of passing a bowel motion. With the help of an adult, some children may be able to squat with feet on the toilet seat, or platforms can be bought to go around toilet seats for this purpose. Alternatively, encouraging the child to sit in a squat position, with weight on the heels of the feet, applies intra-abdominal pressure and is often effective at initiating urge, promoting bowel movements. The use of a toilet stool can also optimise anatomical position for complete evacuation.

EXAMPLE PROTOCOL

Supplementation

- Probiotic of suitable strains (mentioned above) at a dose of 25 billion CFU daily
- *Ulmus rubra* (slippery elm) powder 1–3 g, 3 times a day – mixed into a little water/juice/yoghurt/food

- *Linum usitatissimum* (flax meal) or chia seeds 10–15 g, once daily – mixed into water/juice/yoghurt/food or made into a chia pudding
- A kiwi fruit daily
- Optional lactulose at 10 mL a day (watch for flatulence).

HERBAL FORMULA

Taraxacum officinale radix (dandelion root)	1:2	40 mL
Iris versicolor (blue flag)	1:2	20 mL
Matricaria recutita (chamomile)	1:2	20 mL
Glycyrrhiza glabra (liquorice)	1:2	20 mL
Total:		100 mL

Dose: Based on an adult dose of 5 mL 2 or 3 times a day, calculate child's dose.

Diarrhoea

As previously mentioned, bowel movement frequency ranges between children, and 96% of all children fall within the range of 3 times a day to every second day.[151] The colon transit time of normal healthy children and adolescents is on average 36 hours, and does not appear to be age or gender related (above the age of 3 years).[104,151]

Diarrhoea is defined as the frequent passage of loose, watery stools. Acute diarrhoea is defined as that which lasts less than 2 weeks, while that which lasts longer than 2 weeks defines chronic diarrhoea.

Causes of diarrhoea range from the less common congenital autoimmune illnesses and illnesses that affect pancreatic function (such as cystic fibrosis) to more common factors such as antibiotic use, food intolerances (such as to lactose in dairy[177]), infections, chronic inflammatory bowel diseases (such as Crohn's disease, coeliac disease or ulcerative colitis) and parasitic infection.[123] Diarrhoea may occur more frequently when there is urinary tract or respiratory tract infection.[178]

Prophylactic use of probiotics during respiratory infections has been shown to reduce the incidence of secondary diarrhoea. The most common cause of childhood diarrhoea is viral gastroenteritis (rotavirus infection).[179,180] Enteropathogenic *Escherichia coli* (*E. coli*) can also cause chronic diarrhoea. Other common pathogens include bacteria *Campylobacter jejuni*, *Salmonella* spp., *Shigella* spp. and *Klebsiella pneumoniae*; and protozoan parasites *Giardia lamblia* and *Cryptosporidium parvum*; and possible pathogenic parasites *Blastocyst* spp. and *Dientamoeba fragilis*.[181–183]

The primary concern of diarrhoea is the possibility of resultant dehydration. Dehydration of 3% (of estimated body weight loss of fluid) is undetectable, whereas dehydration of 10% or more is often fatal.[178]

It is important for any child with diarrhoea to have constant fluid intake, with electrolytes. If dehydration starts to become apparent, medical assistance should be sought. The first sign of dehydration is loss of skin turgor (at 3–5% dehydration), followed by depressed fontanel and slightly sunken eyes (5% dehydration). Severe dehydration is marked by the same symptoms being more pronounced

and the development of a weak rapid pulse and cold blue extremities.[178]

A careful history of the characteristics of the diarrhoea is important in assessing the severity of the illness and in formulating a differential diagnosis. Stool frequency, volume and appearance; the presence of blood or mucus; presence of fever; rash; abdominal pain; and the relationship to feeding or dietary intake should be documented.[184]

Laboratory examination should begin with microbiological studies for bacteria and parasites in the stool. Both stool culture and DNA-sequencing multiplex polymerase chain reaction (multiplex PCR) methodology are of value. *Clostridium difficile* toxin assay can also be performed, especially in the setting of recent antibiotic use.[184]

A common feature of diarrhoea is the microtrauma to the mucosa of the digestive tract, creating inflammation and a reduction in digestive enzymes. This can result in malabsorption of macro- and micronutrients. This is of particular concern when chronic diarrhoea is present as it can lead to failure to thrive and/or long-lasting secondary health concerns owing to multiple nutrient deficiencies during critical stages of growth and development. Temporary lactose intolerance may ensue after acute and chronic diarrhoea, but is reversible after rehabilitation of the GIT mucosa. Post-infection irritable bowel syndrome and post-infectious food intolerance are also potential outcomes after bouts of infectious diarrhoea.[185]

TREATMENT

Objectives of treatment are to ensure optimal hydration, promote gastrointestinal healing and decrease gastrointestinal inflammation. Regular intake of fluids is essential to maintain hydration. Add electrolytes in the form of a touch of natural sea salt and a squeeze of some citrus fruit (citric acid aids absorption of water and electrolytes). For acute diarrhoea, coconut water may be considered as a home oral rehydration solution in well-nourished children in the early stages of mild diarrhoeal diseases[117,186]; however, due to its variable sodium, potassium and glucose content (depending on the stage of development of the coconut), it is not a reliable rehydration option in children who are more than mildly dehydrated.[187] Fruit juice and flat soft drink should be avoided as they can worsen the symptoms of diarrhoea and contribute to dehydration. In cases of moderate to severe dehydration in children, immediate referral to the hospital for IV fluids and oral electrolyte replacement is advised.

Herbal medicine

Slippery elm powder is a herbal demulcent, and absorbs excess water in the bowel. The mucilage content is soothing to the GIT, helping to reduce inflammation.

Astringent herbs can be used to improve integrity of gut mucosa. A tea can be made of dried herb preparations of cranesbill, raspberry leaves, blackberry leaves and pomegranate husk.

Immune-boosting and antimicrobial herbs have an important role to play, particularly in infectious diarrhoea.

Pomegranate husk (*Shi Liu Pi*) has a long history of use as an anti-diarrhoeal. It is antioxidant rich and shows selective antimicrobial effects on pathogens with no impact on beneficial bacteria in in vitro studies.[188]

Vulnerary, anti-inflammatory and demulcent herbs are useful for soothing and healing gastrointestinal inflammation associated with diarrhoea. Suitable herbs include *Calendula officinalis* (calendula), *Verbascum thapsus* (mullein), *Matricaria chamomilla* (chamomile), *Melissa officinalis* (lemon balm) and *Althaea officinalis* (marshmallow). These can be used as a tea of herb extract.

Berberine-containing herbs such as *Hydrastis canadensis* (goldenseal) and *Berberis vulgaris* (barberry) will help address a number of possible infectious pathogens involved in diarrhoea. *Hydrastis canadensis* (goldenseal) may also assist the integrity of the gut mucosa; however, as it is classed as a threatened (near endangered) medicinal plant, choosing a cultivated golden seal or considering an alternative herbal option is recommended. These are challenging prescriptions for children and masking taste or relying on alternatives may be required.

Essential oils

Massage with spasmolytic essential oils can help reduce abdominal pain caused by cramping of intestinal smooth muscle. Suitable oils include *Pimpinella anisum* (aniseed), *Matricaria chamomilla* (Roman chamomile), *Zingiber officinale* (ginger) and *Lavandula angustifolia* (lavender). For infectious diarrhoea, oils of tea tree, lemon, red thyme and oregano can be added to the massage oil formula. If the child is not too sensitive, the oils can be massaged into the abdomen, but if that is not appropriate, the oils can be massaged into feet, legs, hands and arms. Therapeutic effect is still achieved owing to rapid absorption of active constituents through the dermal layers directly into the blood stream. See Appendix 16.2 for more information about application of essential oils.

Nutritional medicine (supplementation)

L-glutamine is a non-essential amino acid and a primary fuel source for enterocytes. L-glutamine becomes conditionally essential during times of illness or injury, and providing glutamine supplementation is an avenue of protection.[178] L-glutamine is also required for rapidly dividing immune cells[178] and is associated with fewer infections.[189] For these reasons, L-glutamine becomes a warranted therapeutic tool in the recovery from gastrointestinal inflammation as a result of diarrhoea to promote gastrointestinal healing. The ideal dose is approximately 0.3–0.5 g per kg of ideal body weight per day. For example, for a 20 kg child, the dose would be 6–10 g per day in recovery phase.[190]

Diarrhoeal disease is one area where there has been intense, extensive study on the effect of probiotics on prevention and treatment. Probiotics address diarrhoeal diseases by a number of functions, including providing physical support to the gastrointestinal mucosal barrier (preventing pathogenic microbes from making contact), stimulating non-specific host resistance to pathogenic microbes.[191] Numerous studies show that probiotics can

be used successfully prophylactically, while others have identified specific strains for use in different types of diarrhoeal illnesses. Acute viral diarrhoea has been successfully treated with *L. acidophilus* LB, *L. reuteri*, *L.* GG, *L. rhamnosus*, *L. casei* GG, *B. lactis* HN019, *B. breve* YIT4064 and *S. thermophiles*.[192,193] Antibiotic and bacterial induced diarrhoea can be successfully treated with *Lactobacillus rhamnosus* GG,[194,195] and *Saccharomyces boulardii*.[179,196]

Lactobacillus rhamnosus (at 5–40 billion colony-forming units/day) or *Saccharomyces boulardii* (at 250 mg b.i.d.) may be appropriate in significantly reducing the risk of persistent diarrhoea on days 3, 6 and 7, and the likelihood of an adverse event is very rare.[195,196]

S. boulardii may be effective in treating giardiasis when combined with metronidazole therapy[196] and has also been shown to have potential beneficial effects in *Blastocystis hominis* infection – reducing symptoms and the presence of parasites – in children.[197]

Zinc depletion has been noted in children with dehydrating diarrhoea.[198] Zinc reduces the incidence and duration of diarrhoea in children due to its impact on digestive and immune function.[199] The mechanisms by which zinc reduces occurrence and duration of diarrhoea is not completely understood, but is believed to be due to its roles in improving water and electrolyte absorption in the intestines, rapid regeneration of gut mucosa, production of pancreatic and brush border enzymes and involvement in immune response.[199] Best results for recovery from acute diarrhoea have been observed with combined use of zinc and electrolyte replacement fluid.

The World Gastroenterology Organisation recommends 20 mg of elemental zinc daily for 14 days in all children with acute infectious diarrhoea.[200]

Lactase deficiency or lactose intolerance as a cause of paediatric diarrhoea must be excluded. If lactose is excluded from the diet long term, lactose-free daily products and other dietary sources of calcium or calcium supplements need to be provided. Digestive enzymes may help to increase breakdown of ingested foods and thereby improve absorption of nutrients, reducing risk of malabsorption as a result of diarrhoea. Improperly digested saccharides (such as lactose) can also contribute to symptoms of diarrhoea, so enhancing digestion may help reduce irritation to gut mucosa caused by maldigested food particles.

Nutritional medicine (dietary)

Persistent diarrhoea is often a result of post-enteritis food sensitivity development. Diarrhoea caused by food sensitivity is also common in children with a family history of Th2-dominant illnesses such as atopy and inflammatory bowel diseases (although these can also have significant Th1 overactivity as well). In light of this, the most commonly reactive foods can be eliminated on a 2-week trial basis to assess which individual foods are contributing to occurrence of diarrhoea. The most common foods are pasteurised and unfermented dairy, wheat, eggs, soy and corn.[179] Often, removal of only dairy can resolve diarrhoea caused by food sensitivity. Lactofermented dairy has been shown to reduce occurrence of diarrhoea.[201]

The diet in general should consist of easily digestible foods, in order to optimise absorption of essential nutrients. Well-cooked (not overcooked) non-starchy vegetables and slow-cooked soups and crock-pot meals are excellent options, particularly if organic chicken bones are used in the cooking of the soup or slow-cooked meal. This will provide easily assimilable minerals and nutrients such as collagen, which is anti-inflammatory and required for healing the gut mucosa.

Foods that support colonic health with prebiotic and prebiotic-like properties should be included in recovery from acute diarrhoea to increase production of short-chain fatty acids which have a trophic effect on both the small and the large bowel. Prebiotic and prebiotic-like foods include blueberries, cooked apple, orange and purple carrots, blackcurrants, brown rice, purple rice, quinoa, flax seeds, hazelnuts, banana, beetroot, fennel, leek, garlic, artichoke, spinach, olives, green peas, green tea and cacao.[202–204]

Prebiotic supplements such as lactulose, galacto-oligosaccharides (GOS), inulin and partially hydrolysed guar gum are also of benefit in selectively stimulating the growth of the beneficial bacteria in the colon.[202]

Sample protocol:
- Electrolyte replacement fluid (sip throughout day)
- Zinc – requirements are best when adult dose is calculated on child's weight (Clark's rule); however, as a general guide the following can be applied:
  - 20 mg (elemental) for 14 days after diarrhoea has resolved for children under 25 kg
  - 30–40 mg for older children and adolescents who are greater than 25 kg
  - Preferably administered before bed/throughout the evening. May be added to electrolyte replacement fluid
- Probiotic with suitable strains for diarrhoea type:
  - *S. boulardii*: 250 mg twice daily for acute diarrhoea, once daily for chronic/persistent.
  - *Lactobacillus rhamnosus* GG: 25 billion CFU twice daily for acute diarrhoea, once daily for chronic/persistent
- Massage oil – applied 1–3 times daily (see Appendix 16.2)
  - 30 mL base of coconut oil
  - Lavender 1 drop
  - Tea tree 1 drop
  - Roman chamomile 1 drop
- Herbal tea – equal proportions of:
  - *Calendula officinalis, Verbascum thapsus, Ulmus fulva, Ulmus rubra* and/or *Rubeus idaeus*
  - When well combined add 1 teaspoon to a cup of boiling water and steep for 15 minutes, or until cool enough. Sweeten with stevia if necessary. Tincture of barberry and goldenseal may be added.

Recurrent and chronic infections

Repeated episodes of infection throughout childhood are required for the development of a competent and robust immune system, and are a standard developmental process. A child's immune system needs to be able to effectively respond to a broad range of microbes, and naturopathic medicine has a generous amount of support it can offer (in both nutritional and herbal medicine) to optimise host immune defences, hasten recovery and build immune resilience in children and adolescents alike.

In addition to experiencing fever, the most common recurrent childhood infections include otitis media; infections of the tonsils and adenoids; respiratory tract, gastrointestinal system or urinary tract infections; and dermatological infections such as warts, molluscum contagiosum and *Staphylococcus aureus*. Recurrent and chronic infections are an indication of compromised or suboptimal immune function.

In terms of a normal spectrum of infections, it is suggested that between 4 and 6 URTIs per year for the first 5 years of life is normal and expected. This number may increase for children in a day care setting or with school-age siblings. For older children, 2–4 URTIs per year is considered normal. Rather than the number of infections, the nature and pattern of infections are important to consider – for example, the severity, how quickly a child resolves the infection, unusual infectious organisms and any complications from infection give more insight into the child's resilience than the total number. Identification of risk factors for recurrent infection helps the management of further risk.[205,206]

In children with recurrent infections, consider these possible pathological causes of immunodeficiency:
- malnutrition, under-nutrition
- malabsorption (coeliac disease, inflammatory bowel disease, parasitic infection)
- malignancies
- primary immunodeficiency.

Clinical history that may indicate primary or secondary immunodeficiency and that further assessment is needed include: 6 new infections within 12 months; 2 months of antibiotics with little effect; need for intravenous antibiotics and/or hospitalisation to clear infections; failure to gain weight or grow normally; skin or oral candidiasis; and family history of immunodeficiency or lymphopenia in infancy.[207]

Many factors have been shown to influence infection risk in children:
- nutrition
- breastfeeding
- passive smoking
- presence of atopy
- chronic inflammation facilitating pathogen adherence to respiratory epithelium
- seasonal patterns of infection
- gastro-oesophageal reflux disease (GORD) and medication for GORD impacting on nutritional status
- obesity: associated with increased risk of acute respiratory tract infections in children
- reduced physical activity: preadolescent children who have low physical exercise are more at risk of recurrent acute respiratory tract infection than children who have moderate and high levels of exercise
- day care attendance
- school-aged siblings
- anatomical defects of upper and lower airways.[208–211]

The impact of a child's or adolescent's diet and nutritional status is well demonstrated. Nutrient deficiencies that impair immune function include protein, zinc, copper, iron, selenium, magnesium, vitamin A, vitamin C, vitamin E, vitamin D, vitamin B_2, vitamin B_6, folic acid, vitamin B_{12}, biotin and omega-3 and omega-6 PUFAs.

Diet modification is an important approach to modulating infection risk. Quality of the diet, its mineral density and the load of sugar (via sweets, soft drinks, juice, breakfast cereals, etc.) all must be considered. Studies have shown that increasing vegetable intake to daily, encouraging lean beef 3 times per week and including full-fat butter for a period of 3 months in children aged 1–6 years old with recurrent respiratory tract infections reported far fewer days with respiratory infection, sub-febrile temperatures and febrile temperatures after the 3-month dietary intervention.[212]

NUTRITIONAL MEDICINE (SUPPLEMENTATION) FOR RECURRENT AND CHRONIC INFECTIONS

Zinc

Zinc is one of the most widely used minerals in the body, used in every cell and involved in more than 200 enzyme pathways. Deficiency of zinc leads to reduced Th1 cytokines and thymic hormone activity,[213–215] atrophy of the thymus, reduction in lymphocyte number and lymphocytopenia, dysfunctions of cell-mediated immunity, lowered production of T cell-dependent antibodies, splenic plaque forming cells, decrease in CD4+ helper cells, decreased activity of natural killer (NK) cells, decreased T-cell cytotoxicity, reduced IL-2 production by lymphocytes and adverse effects of B-cell function.[216] Zinc deficiency also leads to defective wound healing and poor tissue integrity, resulting in lesions in mucous membranes.[216] Zinc supplementation is therefore highly indicated in most immune deficiencies or challenges as such conditions increase the requirements for zinc. A diet low in protein is the most common cause of zinc deficiency.[216] A Cochrane review found that prophylactic zinc supplementation (zinc sulfate 10–15 mg/day) given to children for at least 5 months reduced the incidence of common cold (IRR 0.64), school day absences (–0.66 days) and risk of antibiotic prescriptions (OR 0.27).[217–219] A small double-blinded study showed that zinc picolinate is better absorbed than zinc citrate or gluconate.[220] Picolinic acid increases the absorption of zinc.[221,222]

Vitamin A

An estimated 124 million children around the world are deficient in vitamin A. Vitamin A is essential for growth, mucosal and systemic immune function and maintenance of epithelial tissue. Young children and breastfeeding women are most at risk of vitamin A deficiency, primarily owing to increased requirements.[223] Vitamin A deficiency is linked to compromised immune function (Th1 and Th2 immunity) and increased morbidity and mortality from infections.[224] Subclinical vitamin A deficiency is more common than overt deficiency. Effects include atrophy of lymphoid tissue, loss of CD4+ lymphocytes, reduced B lymphocytes and NK cells in the spleen, decreased goblet cells in mucosa, changes in mucosal T-lymphocytes, epithelial ciliary loss, low secretory IgA and altered cytokine production of the respiratory epithelium and conjunctiva.[225] Viral damage to mucosal membranes is particularly severe in vitamin-A-deficient subjects.[226,227] Vitamin A therapy has shown to be therapeutic even in individuals without vitamin A deficiency,[228,229] especially low-birthweight infants and children with recurrent respiratory infections.[225] Deficiency in vitamin A impairs repair of ruptures in tympanic membrane and can therefore lead to chronic otitis media.[230] Vitamin A helps to counter oxidative damage of the mucous membranes of the inner ear as a result of otitis media.[230] Food sources of vitamin A include cod liver oil and unpasteurised dairy.

Vitamin D

Vitamin D is an immunomodulatory molecule related to innate immunity and it has a regulatory role in adaptive immunity that may contribute to the increased occurrence of acute lower respiratory infection in children.[231] Regarding immunity, vitamin D is involved in macrophage maturation, stimulating macrophage phagocytosis and induction of β-defensin.[232]

Reduced levels of vitamin D are associated with pro-inflammatory cytokines and impaired immune function, including T cell abnormalities.[233,234]

Vitamin D deficiency is common in all age groups. Risk of deficiency is related to the latitude at which someone resides, skin tone, indoor lifestyles and 'sun-safe' policies. Other factors include BMI, malabsorption syndromes and medications. See Table 16.4 for common causes of vitamin D deficiency in children and adolescents.

Measurement of serum 25-hydroxyvitamin D level by blood is a reliable and simple assessment. The Endocrine Society definitions for vitamin D deficiency are[236]:
- Vitamin D deficiency: 25(OH)D <20 ng/mL (<50 nmol/L)
- Vitamin D insufficiency: 25(OH)D 20–30 ng/mL (<50–75 nmol/L).

Low vitamin D is associated with increased risk of upper respiratory tract infection, severity of lower respiratory tract infection, chronic obstructive pulmonary disease and tuberculosis.[231,237]

Supplementing 1200 IU vitamin D to Japanese school children throughout the winter months reduced the incidence of seasonal influenza A.[238]

As vitamin D is a cost-effective intervention, with an excellent tolerability and safety profile, if testing is not possible, the Endocrine Society tolerable upper limit recommendations are[236]:
- 0–6 months: 1000 IU/day
- 6 months–1 year: 1500 IU/day
- 1–3 years: 2500 IU/day
- 4–8 years: 3000 IU/day
- >8 years: 4000 IU/day.

The Endocrine Society recommendations to correct deficiency are[236]:

TABLE 16.4 Causes of vitamin D deficiency in infants and adolescents[235]

Reduced intake or synthesis of vitamin D$_3$

Being born to a vitamin-D-deficient mother; most commonly veiled or dark-skinned women, or women of Asian background who actively avoid exposure to sunlight

Prolonged breastfeeding

Dark skin colour

Reduced sun exposure due to:
• veiled or modest clothing
• chronic illness or hospitalisation
• intellectual disability
• excessive use of sunscreen

Low intake of foods containing vitamin D

Abnormal gut function or malabsorption due to:
• small-bowel disorders (e.g. coeliac disease)
• pancreatic insufficiency (e.g. cystic fibrosis)
• biliary obstruction (e.g. biliary atresia)

Reduced synthesis or increased degradation of 25-OHD or 1,25-(OH)$_2$D due to:
• chronic liver or renal disease
• drugs: rifampicin, isoniazid and anticonvulsants

25-OHD = 25-hydroxyvitamin D or calcidiol.
1,25-(OH)$_2$D = 1,25-dihydroxyvitamin D or calcitriol.

Source: https://www.mja.com.au/journal/2006/185/5/prevention-and-treatment-infant-and-childhood-vitamin-d-deficiency-australia-and#18

• 0–1 years: 2000 IU/day for 6 weeks to achieve >30 ng/mL (75 nmol/L) followed by maintenance therapy of 400–1000 IU/day
• 1–18 years: 2000 IU/day for at least 6 weeks to achieve >30 ng/mL (75 nmol/L).

Cod liver oil provides naturally occurring vitamin D along with vitamin A and anti-inflammatory omega-3 essential fatty acids.

Selenium

Selenium is involved in leucocyte and NK cell function. Deficiencies are associated with increased viral virulence and progression in children with viral infections.[224]

Vitamin C

Vitamin C plays an important role in the recovery from infections including otitis media owing to its antioxidant and immune stimulating effects. Vitamin C boosts glutathione and immunoglobulin levels,[239] influences cytokine production, plays a role in leucocyte production and function (especially of neutrophils, lymphocytes and phagocytes) and decreases free radical production, thereby reducing the severity of the effect of pathogen endotoxins.[224] Vitamin C also has antiallergic and anti-inflammatory effects.[240]

B vitamins

Deficiencies of vitamins B$_1$ (thiamine), B$_3$ (niacin) and B$_6$ (pyridoxine) are associated with increased occurrence of infections.[241,242] B$_6$ is involved in humoral and cellular immunity, and deficiency of this vitamin impairs these functions. B vitamins play crucial roles in the synthesis of ATP, DNA and RNA and the production of both red and white blood cells.[241] As metabolic rate is increased during infection and fever, B vitamin complex supplementation is therefore warranted.

Probiotics

Probiotics, as mentioned earlier, play a key role in mucosal and systemic immunity. Modifying intestinal flora through specific probiotic supplements and prebiotics has demonstrated infection protection for diverse infection sites, not only restricted to the GIT.

Studies have shown that probiotics containing *Lactobacillus* GG, *Streptococcus thermophilus*, *Lactobacillus acidophilus* and *Bifidobacterium* spp. were effective in reducing levels of bacteria in the upper respiratory tract that are associated with otitis media.[243]

Children in day care who were supplemented with *Lactobacillus rhamnosus* GG had reduced: absenteeism (16%), respiratory infections with complications and respiratory tract infections (17%) and antibiotic treatment for respiratory infection (19%).[244]

Lactobacillus acidophilus NCFM and *Bifidobacterium lactis* Bi-07 combination given to 3- to 5-year-old children for 6 months reduced incidence of fever (63%), cough (54%), runny nose (44%), antibiotic use (80%) and number of days with symptoms (30%).[244]

Prebiotics in the diet can also be used to augment non-specific infection prevention and immunity. Just one of the beneficial effects of prebiotics is stimulation of immune system, which can be direct or indirect through increasing population of beneficial microbes in the gut. An important mechanism of action of probiotics and prebiotics, by which they can affect the immune system, is by increasing the expression of anti-inflammatory cytokines, while reducing the expressions of pro-inflammatory cytokines.[245]

Fever

As is now well understood, fever is an important mechanism of the immune system's defence against pathogens. The increased temperature during fever inhibits certain enzymes and the ability of viruses and bacteria to replicate. Fever management therefore needs to focus on keeping the child comfortable throughout the fever.

The most frequently advised method of measurement of fever is axillary measurement using a digital thermometer.[246] Oral and rectal temperature taking may be more accurate, but are best performed in a GP or hospital setting. The use of physical interventions such as cool bathing or sponge baths, exposure to cold air, rubbing the body with alcohol or using ice is not recommended.[246] The use of such methods can cause an increase in core body temperature owing to superficial vasoconstriction.[246,247] Lukewarm sponging, however, is not associated with adverse effects. If any antipyretics are used, the ideal is in the form of herbal tea, such as the traditional YEP blend of yarrow, elderflower and peppermint. This is also a good way to keep fluids up to prevent dehydration during fever. Between 2 and 5% of children experience seizure with fever; 33% of those will have recurrence.[248]

Although paracetamol and ibuprofen can reduce fever, they have not been shown to prevent febrile convulsions.[246] Febrile convulsions, although frightening for parents, in the majority of cases have no lasting adverse effect on the child.[247]

A randomised controlled study of children with chicken pox showed that paracetamol did not relieve the symptoms of fever and may in fact have prolonged the illness.[249] Overdoses of antipyretic drugs have been associated with increased frequency of fever, and can have severe adverse effects. If paracetamol or ibuprofen are administered, it is important that ibuprofen not be given to a child under the age of 6 months and that either drug is dosed by weight, rather than age, of the child. The NSW government's guidelines for dosage are: paracetamol 15 mg/kg given up to 4 hourly, with a maximum of 4 doses per 24 hours; ibuprofen 5–10 mg/kg/dose given every 6–8 hours (preferably with food).[247]

SUMMARY OF FEVER MANAGEMENT

1 Try to identify the cause of fever/location of infection (suspect a UTI if unknown)
2 Monitor and allow the fever to run its natural completion so that it is resolved as quickly as possible.
3 Intervene only if the temperature is over 38.3°C in an infant and 39°C in a child.
4 Assess the child for changes in alertness, breathing difficulties (and use of accessory muscles to breathe), colour (pale/mottled) and decreased fluid intake or urine output. Identify children at risk and seek help from a GP or emergency department if concerned.[247]
5 Never use aspirin. Never use ibuprofen for infants under 6 months old. Never mix ibuprofen and paracetamol. Only use paracetamol if the temperature stays too high for more than 2 hours in an infant or 6 hours in a child, in spite of natural interventions.
6 Monitor and prevent dehydration – give sips of water or preferably YEP (equal blend of yarrow, elderflower and peppermint tea). Commercial rehydration formulas may also be used.
7 Strengthen the immune system in the long term with zinc; vitamin C; cod liver oil; herbs such as echinacea, cat's claw, liquorice and calendula; and nutrient-dense, low-sugar, additive-free foods.
8 Make child comfortable by adding clothing and bedding as desired, and removing clothing as desired once fever resolves.

HERBAL MEDICINE

Fever-support tea blend:
- 10 g *Achillea millefolium* (yarrow) – febrifuge
- 10 g *Sambucus nigra* (elderflower) – febrifuge
- 10 g *Mentha x piperita* (peppermint) – febrifuge
- 10 g *Echinacea purpurea* (echinacea) – immune support

- 10 g *Matricaria chamomilla* (chamomile) – calms a distressed or upset infant

Blend together and store in glass jar. Use 1 teaspoon per cup of boiling water. Infuse for 10 minutes before administering, ensuring that tea has cooled adequately first. Suitable for all ages. Infants and small children can start on 30 mL 3 times a day. All the herbs in this tea blend are very safe to consume in large amounts.

Otitis media

Otitis media (OM) is an infection of the upper respiratory tract, involving middle ear symptoms. OM covers a group of diagnoses including acute otitis media (AOM), recurrent acute otitis media, acute otitis media with effusion (AOME) and chronic suppurative otitis media (CSOM – discharge through ruptured tympanic membrane).[250] OM is a very common condition and a leading cause of healthcare visits, antibiotic prescription[251] and surgery for children in developed countries.[250] It is also associated with absence from school, impaired hearing and learning difficulties.[252,253]

Studies carried out in developed countries show that by their third birthday, 80% of children will have experienced at least one episode of AOM.[254,255]

For most children, OM will self-resolve within 14 days. However, it is important to address the underlying causes, especially if OM becomes recurrent. A number of causes or contributing factors are linked with OM. Bacterial or viral infections can result in OM, although swabs taken are often negative. Pathogens that are known to be possible causes of OM include: *Haemophilus influenzae*, *Aspergillus* spp., *Streptococcus pneumoniae*, β haemolytic *Streptococcus* group G, β haemolytic *Streptococcus* group A, *Moraxella catarrhalis*, *Klebsiella pneumoniae*, *Staphylococcus aureus*, methicillin-resistant *S. aureus*, *Pseudomonas aeruginosa*, *Candida* spp., *Enterococcus faecalis* and *Absidia corymbifera*.[256–259] Other factors linked to OM include certain high allergy and mucus-forming foods (the largest being dairy, wheat, peanuts, soy, corn, oranges and tomatoes),[179,250] atopy, environmental triggers and structural imbalances leading to impaired drainage of the eustachian tubes. Environmental triggers include exposure to cigarette smoke, exposure to air pollution and environmental allergens, all of which can increase upper respiratory tract congestion, providing a breeding ground for bacteria and viruses.[179] Most critically, day care attendance doubles the risk for RAOM.[205]

Congestion can result in negative middle ear pressure and therefore intermittent obstruction of the eustachian tube. Structurally, infants are more prone to OM as they have short and horizontally placed eustachian tubes, which impair drainage. With growth and development, the eustachian tube lengthens and becomes more upright, and is therefore better suited to protect the middle ear from nasopharyngeal secretions. GORD is also associated with increased occurrence of OM. Chronic inflammation of nasopharynx caused by reflux and reflux of gastric contents into the middle ear (due to immature structure of the eustachian tube) are implicated in the pathogenesis of OM.[252]

Even though recent literature states that AOM resolves naturally within 14 days without intervention, conventional treatment of AOM almost always involves antibiotics.[260] Chronic and recurrent OM are often also treated with steroids and surgery (myringotomy with or without the insertion of tympanostomy tubes). Sometimes adenoids are also removed, but several studies show that this is an ineffective approach.[250] OM is one of the most common reasons for antibiotic prescriptions for children, even though there is solid evidence demonstrating limited benefit of antibiotic treatment.[261] Antibiotics may help reduce symptoms of pain and crying by about 1 day, but do not shorten the duration of the illness.[262,263] A number of studies[264] have highlighted the potentially disastrous consequences to the individual, as well as the community, of antibiotic resistance after treatment of URTIs with antibiotics. There is both little and inconclusive evidence that any conventional treatments are effective in treating OM.[265,266] The role of free radicals in the pathogenesis of OM has been reported in a number of studies.[267] Children with OM have been shown to have lower levels of antioxidants such as vitamins A, C and E than do healthy children.[268]

Infection, air pollution, cigarette smoke and death of bacteria as a result of antibiotic use all cause free radical damage in the eustachian tube, leading to increased membrane permeability, oedema, elevated mucus production and reduction of cilia in the middle ear.[230,269,270] Owing to the damaging inflammatory effects of oxidative stress on mucosal integrity and immune function, antioxidants can play an important role in the treatment and prevention of OM.[230]

REDUCING THE RISKS OF OM

Breastfeeding for at least 4 months has been shown to provide the greatest protective mechanisms against OM.[271–274] Some of this protection would arise from the presence of immune factors such as antibodies, lysozyme and lactoferrin – compounds responsible for maintaining microbial balance of the eustachian tube[275] – and on development of mucosal immunity. Infants are born with Th2-dominant mucosal immunity, and breast milk components such as lactoferrin, lysozyme and sIgA help to regulate the shift to a balanced Th2/Th1 function.[276–278] Other important preventive factors include keeping the infant or child away from cigarette smoke and air pollution and addressing immunological defects. Compromised systemic and local immune function has been shown to be common in children with recurring OM, exhibited in part by lower levels of serum antibodies and nasopharyngeal IL-1B, IL-6 and TNF-α.[279] In children with atopy, balance of Th2 immune response is likely to prove beneficial in prevention of OM. Keeping children away from cigarette smoke and excessive air pollution is important for OM prevention. For children with excessive mucus production, avoidance of mucus-forming foods (pasteurised dairy, oranges, soy, corn, peanuts, tomatoes and grain products) can provide successful prevention and treatment.

TREATMENT
Herbal medicine

Stimulation of systemic and mucosal immune function is the primary aim. Herbs such as *Echinacea* spp. and *Uncaria tomentosa* (cat's claw) provide immune stimulation. A small number of atopic children may have an allergy or sensitivity to *Echinacea* spp., generally only if there is known allergy to the *Asteraceae* (daisy) family. If this is suspected, cat's claw is an excellent alternative. Echinacea is immunostimulatory, a topical antiseptic, systemically antiviral (including against *H. influenzae*),[280] antibacterial, lymphatic and vulnerary.

Calendula officinalis (calendula) provides lymphatic support, an important factor considering systemic immune function as well as local immunity via the MALT (mucosa associated lymphoid tissue) in the inner ear. Calendula's astringent and vulnerary properties help to heal the inflamed inner ear and Eustachian tube. Used topically, *Calendula officinalis* (calendula) is also antiseptic and antiviral.

Glycyrrhiza glabra (liquorice) is an immune stimulant, antiviral, demulcent and anti-inflammatory, and often renders a herb mix more palatable for children, an important factor for compliance. The anti-tussive properties of liquorice make it particularly useful if there is a concomitant cough.

Hydrastis canadensis (goldenseal) provies excellent mucous membrane support, can help dry up excess effusions and mucus secretion and is antimicrobial. Elderflower is also an excellent herb for children to dry up excess mucus.

Aqueous extracts of *Verbascum thapsus* (mullein) have been shown to have greater antibacterial effects against *Staphylococcus aureus* and *Klebsiella pneumoniae* than do alcohol extracts.[257] Therefore the use of *Verbascum thapsus* as an infusion or decoction is beneficial to address some of the microbes known to cause OM and respiratory infections. *Verbascum thapsus* also has demulcent and vulnerary actions and is therefore soothing and healing for inflamed mucous membranes. Its expectorant properties make it useful when there is concomitant cough. Infused *Verbascum thapsus* oil has been part of studies showing successful analgesic effects of herbal ear drops.[281]

Small amounts of *Zingiber officinale* (ginger) tincture may be used to increase circulation and create a warming effect to help loosen mucus. It is also anti-inflammatory. *Zingiber officinale* tea sweetened with stevia or xylitol provides a tasty, immune-boosting anti-inflammatory drink for children. Alternatively, a poultice can be made out of warming herbs such as *Zingiber officinale*, *Allium sativum* (garlic), *Thymus vulgaris* (thyme) and onion and placed over the ear and neck to reduce pain. When there is lymphadenopathy present, additional lymphatic herbs such as *Galium aparine* (cleavers) can be used. *Chamomilla recutita* (chamomile) is another particularly useful herb for the treatment of children's infections as it is antimicrobial, anti-inflammatory and soothing to the nervous system.

Pain relief and local treatment can be applied using herbal ear drops, made with either tinctures and/or infused oil of *Calendula officinalis* (calendula), *Hypericum perforatum* (St John's wort), *Allium sativum* (garlic) and *Verbascum thapsus* (mullein). Essential oils can also be added to the ear drop formula. Useful essential oils include *Chamomilla recutita* (German chamomile), *Eucalyptus globulus* (eucalyptus) and *Thymus vulgaris* (thyme). Herbal ear drops were found to be just as effective or more effective at treating pain and duration of OM as pharmaceutical anaesthetic ear drops and more effective than use of antibiotics.[281,282] *Allium sativum* (garlic) has many therapeutic properties: of greatest importance in the treatment of OM and recurrent infections are its antimicrobial (antiviral against influenza B, parainfluenza type 3 and HSV), immunostimulant and circulatory stimulant properties. Allicin and thiosulfinates appear to be the compounds responsible for antiviral activity. *Allium sativum* (garlic) also promotes sweating and so is useful when fever is present.

Physical therapies

Osteopathy and chiropractics can address structural issues implicated with recurrent OM. Craniosacral manipulations are able to support drainage of the eustachian tube, reducing the opportunity for infection.[283] Lymphatic massage around the cervical lymph nodes may also help drainage and will stimulate immune function via promotion of lymphatic drainage. This is a technique that can easily be taught to parents so they can carry on this treatment at home. The addition of suitable essential oils may also increase the effects of lymphatic drainage. Physical manipulations have also shown positive effects on NK cell production, immunoglobulins, CD4 counts, neutrophils and monocytes, thereby stimulating immune function.

Checking for hearing loss after recurrent OM is paramount. CSOM is an important cause of preventable hearing loss, particularly in the developing world,[284] and is a reason of serious concern, particularly in children, because it may have long-term effects on early communication, language development, auditory processing, psychosocial and cognitive development and educational progress and achievement.[285]

Nutritional medicine

Probiotics strains *Lactobacillus rhamnosus* GG and *Bifidobacterium lactis* Bb-12 may reduce the risk of early acute otitis media, antibiotic use and recurrent respiratory infections in infancy and early childhood.[286,287]

Vitamin D supplementation reduces the risk of acute otitis media in otitis-prone children. The administration of vitamin D in a dosage of 1000 IU/day may restore serum values and is associated with a significant reduction in the risk of uncomplicated AOM.[288]

Vitamin A may also be considered as an additional intervention for the medical treatment of AOM, as it plays a role in the prevention of oxidative tissue damage.[289]

Foods known to be common contributing factors of OM should be considered for elimination – dairy (particularly pasteurised dairy), wheat, soy, oranges, corn, tomatoes and egg whites (particularly the former three).

Warming foods such as soups and broths, with good quality protein, are the foods of choice. Protein is required for zinc absorption and metabolism. Meats and liver provide the richest sources of B vitamins and absorbable protein. Liver, being high in vitamin A, is an excellent therapeutic food for immune function. Lightly cooked dark green leafy and cruciferous vegetables are alkalising, inhibiting the growth of many pathogenic microbes.

Naturally lactofermented foods such as homemade sauerkraut or commercial fermented drinks such as Grainfields BE liquid or fermented Lemon and Ginger drink are excellent sources of active beneficial bacteria, enzymes and nutrients required for immune function and infection recovery.

Coconut oil contains lauric acid, a powerful antiviral, antibacterial and antifungal fatty acid. Use in cooking or to make tasty treats.

Xylitol shows very effective actions as an antimicrobial, in particular against *Streptococcus pneumoniae* and *Haemophilus influenzae*,[290] two microbes commonly causing OM. The only adverse effect reported from intake of xylitol is abdominal discomfort or diarrhoea at high doses (45 g/day) due to osmotic effect. Xylitol chewing gum (2 pieces 5 times daily after meals and snacks, providing 8.4 g xylitol) or xylitol syrup (providing 10 g xylitol) were shown to decrease the occurrence and duration of AOM and reduced the prescription rate for antibiotics without gastrointestinal upset. Oral xylitol solution[290,291] showed effective results and was well tolerated in 120 children aged 6–36 months of age at doses of 5 g 3 times a day, and 7.5 g once daily.

EXAMPLE PROTOCOL FOR OM

Herbal medicine

EAR DROPS

Ear drops made with infused oils of calendula, St John's wort, mullein and garlic (equal parts). Add 1 drop each of tea tree oil, lavender and myrrh per 30 mL. Place 1–2 drops in each ear 2–4 times daily. Ears may be gently plugged with some cotton wool to keep oil in. For more information on application of essential oils, see Appendix 16.2.

Herbal formula

Echinacea spp.	1:2	50 mL
Glycyrrhiza glabra	1:1	30 mL
Sambucus nigra	1:2	30 mL
Calendula officinalis	1:2	30 mL
Galium aparine	1:2	50 mL
Zingiber officinale	1:2	10 mL
Total:		200 mL

Adult dose of 5 mL 3–4 times daily. Calculate paediatric dosage.

HERBAL TEA

Verbascum thapsus (mullein), *Zingiber officinale* (ginger) and *Glycyrrhiza glabra* (liquorice) tea – equal parts of each herb. 1 teaspoon steeped in hot water or gently boiled for 10 minutes. Cool. Sweeten with stevia or xylitol if need be. Wait for tea to cool sufficiently and give to infant/child to drink throughout day. (Alternatively, make into a jelly using agar. Colour pink with a few drops of beetroot juice if desired.)

Nutritional medicine (supplementation)

Please use Clark's rule to determine dose with adult doses listed below:

- High vitamin cod liver oil – 1 teaspoon daily. Other cod liver oils – 2 teaspoons daily
- Vitamin D 1000 IU (maximum duration 12 weeks)
- Vitamin A 10 000 IU (maximum duration 6 weeks)
- Zinc: 20 mg elemental zinc per day, in bioavailable forms such as citrate, picolinate, gluconate, diglycinate
- High-quality vitamin C powder, providing 2–6 g of vitamin C per day (or to bowel tolerance)
- Probiotic containing 25 billion CFU *Lactobacillus* GG, *Streptococcus thermophilus*, *Lactobacillus acidophilus* and *Bifidobacterium* spp.

Tonsillitis

Tonsillitis is an acute inflammation of the tonsils, two small masses of lymphoid tissue on either side of the throat. Acute tonsillitis, or 'sore throat', refers to a viral or bacterial tonsillitis with enlargement and reddening of the tonsils, odynophagia (pain when swallowing), possibly also with hoarseness of the voice, tonsillar exudate, cervical lymphadenopathy and fever >38.3°C.[292]

Bacterial and viral infections can cause tonsillitis and, more commonly, viral causes include adenoviruses, *Haemophilus influenzae* viruses, parainfluenza viruses and Epstein–Barr virus (EBV).[292]

Another common cause of acute tonsillitis is infection caused by *Streptococcus pyogenes* (group A streptococci bacteria, often referred to as 'strep throat'). Generally, bacterial causes of tonsillitis cause more rapid symptoms and can result in very high fever, quickly.[292]

A possible complication following streptococci throat infection is a secondary autoimmune illness, such as rheumatic fever, or paediatric autoimmune neurological disease associated with streptococci (PANDAS), where the immune system compromises the brain and causes rapid onset of tics, obsessive-compulsive behaviours and anxiety.[293,294]

To determine the cause of tonsillitis, a general practitioner may perform a throat swab culture or rapid immune test for streptococci antigens to detect if the infection is bacterial, in which case it may respond to a short course of appropriate antibiotics.[292] If the swab for bacteria is negative, it may be assumed that the tonsillitis is caused by a viral infection, which will not respond to antibiotics. Instead, the body will work to clear the infection with supportive therapies such as adequate rest, topical gargles and nutritional support. Nutritional treatment for acute tonsillitis mirrors nutritional treatment discussed above for otitis media.

Tonsillitis can make it hard to swallow solid foods, so herbal teas, soups, broths and homemade natural ice blocks (with coconut water and pureed fruit) are all relevant interventions.

Typical herbal gargles for acute tonsillitis contain solutions with *Salvia officinalis* (sage leaf), *Thymus vulgaris* (thyme) or *Matricaria recutita* (chamomile flower) due to their anti-inflammatory, immune modulatory and lymphatic properties and their ability to maintain the mucous membrane.[295] Many phytotherapeutics may have immunostimulatory effects.[295]

Echinacea spp. (purple cone flower) may enhance cell-mediated immunity by stimulation of macrophages, NK cells and granulocytes, as well as humoral immunity through monokines, interferons and the complement system.[296,297]

Calendula officinalis (calendula) provides lymphatic support, an important factor considering systemic immune function as well as local immunity via the MALT (mucosa-associated lymphoid tissue) in the throat. Calendula's astringent and vulnerary properties help to heal the inflamed throat and, used topically, pharmacological studies reveal that *Calendula officinalis* exhibits antibacterial, antiviral and anti-inflammatory properties.[298]

Phytolacca americana (pokeweed or phytolacca) provides lymphatic support, an important factor considering systemic immune function as well as local immunity via the MALT in the throat. Used topically as a gargle for older children, *Phytolacca americana* is also antiseptic and antiviral.[299]

Glycyrrhiza glabra (liquorice) is an immune stimulant, antiviral, demulcent and anti-inflammatory and often renders a herb mix more palatable for children, an important factor for compliance.

Gargle with salt water may be indicated as a mild antimicrobial – it is important not to swallow the salt water. More traditionally, especially in paediatric populations, a simple *Leptospermum scoparium* (manuka honey), onion and garlic syrup may have been prepared by chopping a clove of garlic, dicing an onion and leaving them macerating in a small bowl of manuka honey to extract the antimicrobial components of the combination ingredients.[300,301] Compliance with this in young patients is reasonable, and it can be stored in the fridge and a spoon added to a warm mug of water to sip on to soothe the sore throat. This preparation may also have some analgesic effects post operatively after a tonsillectomy[302] and may reduce the need for pharmaceutical analgesics in the paediatric population with tonsillitis post tonsillectomy.[303]

EXAMPLE PROTOCOL FOR ACUTE TONSILLITIS

Herbal medicine

HERBAL FORMULA

Echinacea spp.	1:2	50 mL
Glycyrrhiza glabra	1:1	20 mL
Calendula officinalis	1:2	25 mL
Phytolacca americana	1:5	5 mL
Total:		100 mL

Adult dose of 5 mL 3–4 times daily. Calculate paediatric dosage. Possible to gargle and spit, and then take a second dose and swallow.

Recurrent tonsillitis, or recurrent throat infections, refers to recurrences of acute tonsillitis.[304] These are, in contrast to a single attack of acute tonsillitis, usually caused by many different pathogens, and may flare up again a few weeks after cessation of an antimicrobial therapy.[305]

Tonsillectomy (surgical removal of the tonsils) is still one of the most frequent procedures during childhood.[292] Historically, the tonsils have been regarded as a reservoir of pathogenic bacteria[306]; therefore, tonsillectomy was performed to remove an apparent infection focus in recurrent sore throat patients.[306] More contemporary recognition that the lymphoid tissue of the tonsils plays an important role in mucosal immunity and host defence against invading antigens of the upper respiratory tract leaves this common practice in question.[307] Despite this, depending on the frequency and severity of tonsillitis episodes, some medical specialists may see indication for tonsillectomy. Removal of the lymphatic tissue that is normally a protective component of the greater immune system should be considered a last resort treatment option, reserved only for reoccurring bacterial tonsillitis that does not respond to other treatment. Tonsillectomies are associated with the possibility of complications (such as postoperative bleeding, oedema, nausea, vomiting, poor oral intake and pain),[308] and some studies have shown that surgery for tonsillectomy does not provide a decrease in the number of postoperative visits for URTIs – in fact, visits for URTIs decreased over time whether or not a tonsillectomy was performed.[308] There are no nationally accepted guidelines for when to perform a tonsillectomy.[292]

For nutritional treatment of chronic tonsillitis, please refer to 'Nutritional medicine (dietary and supplementation)' for recurrent and chronic infections, above.

Warts

Warts are viral skin lesions/tumours caused by the human papillomavirus (HPV). There are more than 70 known subtypes of HPV. Many people choose not to treat warts as sometimes treatments can be more unpleasant than the wart itself, which is often asymptomatic. Cutaneous warts are known to be recurrent and often resistant to therapy.

Warts are usually self-limiting, but spontaneous resolution may take months to years.[309]

Being of viral origin, warts are a sign of compromised or suboptimal immune function, and so should be treated with appropriate antiviral and immune-stimulating herbs and nutrients.

TREATMENT

Herbal medicine

Herbs with documented systemic antiviral activity include *Echinacea* spp. (echinacea), *Hypericum perforatum* (St John's wort), *Lomatium utriculatum* (lomatium), *Phyllanthus emblica* (phyllanthus), *Pau d'arco* (pau d'arco), *Thuja occidentalis* (thuja) and *Uncaria tomentosa* (cat's claw). Herbs with topical antiviral actions include *Glycyrrhiza glabra* (liquorice), *Calendula officinalis* (calendula), *Hypericum perforatum* (St John's wort), *Humulus lupulus* (hops) and *Melissa officinalis* (lemon balm).

HERBAL FORMULA

Echinacea spp.	1:2	60 mL
Glycyrrhiza glabra	1:1	30 mL
Uncaria tomentosa	1:2	70 mL
Hypericum perforatum	Std Ext	20 mL
Thuja occidentalis	1:5	20 mL
Phytolacca decandra	1:5	10 mL
Total:		200 mL

Based on adult dose of 5 mL 3 times a day, work out the appropriate child dose based on weight or age.

TOPICAL TREATMENT

A blend of the following herbs in equal parts can be mixed into a base cream for topical application, 2–3 times daily: calendula, liquorice, hops, St John's wort and lemon balm. Tea tree essential oil or tea tree solution and coconut oil can also be added.

Nutritional medicine

Zinc deficiency has been shown to cause decreased immunity to cutaneous infections.[310] It also has specific antiviral activity: first, by cross-linking the double helix of viral DNA so that it is unable to undergo the scission necessary for viral replication; and secondly, by inactivating the viral surface glycoproteins, thus interfering with penetration into a susceptible host cell.[311]

Nutrient-dense, unprocessed wholefoods should be the focus – vegetables, meats, soups, broths and 1–2 pieces of fruit per day. Elimination of added sugars is of utmost importance owing to the immunosuppressive effects of sugars. Coconut oil contains lauric acid, a potent antiviral. Coconut oil is excellent for cooking due to the stable saturated fatty acids. Use in the diet and apply topically as a moisturiser. Fresh raw garlic is an excellent antiviral if tolerated, but it is important to note that it is too strong for infants. For children, mix ½–1 clove chopped raw garlic in some raw honey to eat from the spoon once or twice a day.

NUTRITIONAL MEDICINE (SUPPLEMENTATION)

Please use Clark's rule to determine dose with adult doses listed below:

- High vitamin cod liver oil – 1 teaspoon daily. Other cod liver oils – 2 teaspoon daily
- Zinc: 20 mg elemental zinc per day, in bioavailable forms such as citrate, picolinate, gluconate, diglycinate
- High-quality children's multi B vitamin powder – ½ teaspoon twice daily
- High-quality vitamin C powder, providing 1–3 g of vitamin C per day (or to bowel tolerance)
- Probiotic containing *Lactobacillus* GG, *Streptococcus thermophilus*, *Lactobacillus acidophilus* and *Bifidobacterium* spp.

NUTRITIONAL MEDICINE (TOPICAL)

Zinc can be a useful oral or topical treatment modality in common warts. Many studies have demonstrated efficacy of topical zinc in treating warts without significant adverse effects. Apply topical 10–20% zinc sulfate solution, 3 times daily for 4 weeks as an efficacious, painless and safe therapeutic option for wart treatment.[312–314]

Molluscum contagiosum

Molluscum contagiosum is a skin disease caused by molluscum contagiosum virus, a poxvirus. The infection causes firm, small, skin-coloured, papular lesions, often with an umbilicated centre. Lesions may have a region of redness, and can be found anywhere on the body. Lesions may remain for many weeks to months before resolving without treatment; however, in immunocompromised individuals, infection with molluscum contagiosum can cause giant lesions and a large number of lesions that require treatment. Diagnosis is usually made upon visual inspection of the lesions.[315] Extensive and persistent skin infection with the virus can indicate underlying immunodeficiency.

Molluscum contagiosum virus is spread by contact with lesion skin or exudate. Recommendations to prevent the spread of molluscum contagiosum virus on an individual's body or to others may include keeping the lesions covered and not sharing baths, bath towels, clothing, linens, gym equipment or items that may contain lesion exudate.[315,316]

Molluscum contagiosum is considered a benign, self-limiting condition. Individual lesions typically clear within 2 months, and most cases resolve without treatment by 18 months. Sudden disappearance of lesions is possible, and is generally the consequence of a vigorous immune response in healthy people.[317]

Children with eczema often have more extensive lesions, and the research demonstrates a positive association between atopic dermatitis and molluscum contagiosum.[315]

There are several approaches to treating moluscum contagiosum lesions, including physical destruction (cryotherapy, curettage, laser therapy) or use of a topical immunotherapy ointment.

TREATMENT

Herbal medicine

Herbal medicine treatment mirrors above as for warts.

Nutritional medicine (dietary and supplemental)

Nutritional medicine treatment mirrors above as for warts.

Topical treatment

Essential oil of Australian *Backhousia citriodora* (lemon myrtle) has been shown to be effective in the treatment of molluscum contagiosum in children. A specific anti-molluscum blend of essential oil of Australian lemon myrtle oil 10%, in a base of olive oil, applied as a once-daily topical application for 21 days, showed a greater than 90% reduction in the number of lesions.[318]

Furthermore, a twice daily topical application of essential oil of *Melaleuca alternifolia* (tea tree oil) plus iodine (35 micromols) showed benefit after 30 days, with a greater than 90% reduction in the number of lesions. No child discontinued treatment due to adverse events.[319]

Atopy

Atopy refers to the genetic tendency to develop allergic diseases such as atopic dermatitis (eczema), asthma and allergic rhinitis. Atopy is typically associated with heightened immune responses to common allergens, especially inhaled allergens and food allergens.[320]

Children with eczema may go on to develop asthma (15–40%); allergic rhinitis (27–45%) or both (up to 65%). The term 'the allergic march' (also called 'the atopic march') describes this sequential development of allergic disorders and atopic comorbidities.[321] The allergic march is characterised by a typical sequence of immunoglobulin E (IgE) antibody responses and clinical symptoms which may appear early in life and persist over years or decades, and often remit spontaneously with age.[322] Risk is greater with food allergen sensitisation, younger onset and severe eczema.[323–325]

The development of atopic disease in childhood depends on a complex interaction between genetic factors, environmental exposures to allergens, tobacco smoke, air pollution, infections and more.

RISK FACTORS FOR ATOPY

Risk factors for atopy include[326,327]:

Hereditary predisposition:
- A first-degree relative with eczema, allergic rhinitis or asthma

Perinatal factors:
- Perinatal maternal stress[328]
- C-section birth[329]
- Acute maternal atopic symptoms and maternal respiratory infections[330]
- Exposures to breast milk substitutes, such as cow's milk formula, and early introduction of cow's milk[331]

Nutritional factors:
- Early introduction of solids <3 months
- Low plant food
- Low antioxidant status
- High food additive intake, processed foods
- Low omega-3:omega-6 ratio
- Vitamin D deficiency
- Obesity and sedentary lifestyle

Environmental factors:
- Air pollution – car exhaust, cigarette smoke, air pollution in the home[332]
- House dust mite[333]
- Chemical exposure – cutaneous and oral[332]
- Common household chemicals such as cleaning products, phthalates, volatile organic compounds and formaldehyde, and home renovations/construction[334,335]
- Urban living – low microbial diversity environment
- Antibiotics (prenatal, 0–2 years)[88]
- Paracetamol (prenatal, 0–2years)
- Anthelminthic therapy
- Proton pump inhibitors
- Prenatal excessive folic acid supplementation in third and fourth trimester[336]

Protective factors against developing atopy include:
Antenatal factors[326,337]:
- Vaginal birth
- Maternal farm exposure
- Breastfeeding, exclusive breastfeeding for at least 4 months[333,338]

Nutritional (maternal and child) factors[327]:
- Mediterranean diet – high plant food, high fish, low meat intakes
- Vitamin D sufficiency
- Good antioxidant status
- Favourable gut ecology
- Early exposure to potential allergens via breastmilk

Environmental factors[339]:
- Rural living
- Exposure to farm animals
- Owning a furry pet (not consistent in asthma)
- Exposure to a greater variety of microorganisms – older siblings
- Regular physical exercise

Early appropriate management of atopic dermatitis and food intolerance for genetically high-risk groups is important for the prevention of allergic march.[325] For example, manipulation of the maternal diet during pregnancy and a childhood promoting a diet rich in antioxidants and omega-3 fatty acids could be protective for allergic diseases in childhood.[327] Thus, with early intervention it may be possible to interfere with the natural course of allergic disease and prevent allergic disease progressing in childhood.[333]

Atopic dermatitis

Atopic dermatitis (AD) is a chronic inflammatory skin disorder that typically occurs during childhood, especially in the first year of life. In most atopic individuals, AD is the first clinical manifestation of the 'atopic march', with the highest incidence during the first months of life, and the highest period prevalence during the first 3 years of life. AD has the potential to lead to the development of asthma or allergic rhinitis.[321]

AD has variable severity and is characterised by eczematous skin lesions associated with itching. AD can exert a profound impact on the quality of life of patients and their families. Children with eczema may have their sleep disturbed due to the significant itch they suffer. AD has a 10–30% prevalence among young children, and prevalence in adolescence has been estimated to be around 5–15%.[324]

A vicious multifactorial cycle can ensue with skin barrier deficiency and AD, with both environmental factors and persistent skin inflammation further aggravating skin barrier function, driving the immune imbalance and severity of eczema. Understanding how to optimise skin barrier maintenance is one aspect of management.[340]

The literature has pointed towards lower zinc levels in atopic children, with mean serum zinc levels of the AD patients significantly lower than those of the controls. It is unsure whether the decreased plasma zinc concentration in children with eczema is a consequence of the skin barrier change in AD or is a contributing factor.[341] Regardless, a good dietary intake of high biological value protein and zinc is of value to correct the disturbances, especially those which could lead to exaggeration of the allergic conditions.[342]

Increasing long-chain omega-3 PUFAs during pregnancy, lactation, infancy and childhood appears to have a strong protective effect on atopic outcomes in infants and children.[343] Fish intake and fish oil supplementation during pregnancy and lactation or during infancy or childhood results in a higher omega-3 PUFA status in infants and children. Fish oil supplementation may reduce sensitisation to common food allergens and reduce inflammatory cascade by mediating eicosanoid production. The omega-3 PUFA EPA may be involved in this mechanism, as erythrocyte EPA level has a negative association with eczema.[344]

The majority of children usually outgrow eczema by the time they turn 6 years old. Despite this, the increased global prevalence of AD cannot be attributed to genetics alone, suggesting that lifestyle factors and evolving environmental exposures may trigger and/or flare disease in predisposed children. Some interventions that have been shown to interfere with the natural course of allergic disease and prevent allergic disease progressing into later childhood include natural birth. The upturning trend of >30% C-section rates in some regions and hospitals does not appear to always be based on medical indications. A C-section birth may increase the risk of eczema up to 43%.[329,345]

Exclusive breastfeeding for 5–6 months, then continued breastfeeding alongside solid foods for at least a year, may be of benefit in reducing AD. Studies from Scandinavian countries have shown that the longer a child is breastfed, the lower the risk of allergies throughout childhood, and even at 17 years of age the child has a 50% lowered risk.[346]

The use of probotics also offers some protection. *Lactobacillus rhamnosus* GG given to pregnant mothers reduces the risk of eczema in the baby by up to 50%.[347] The protective effect of probiotic strain *Lactobacillus rhamnosus* HN001 against eczema in the first 2 years of life has also been shown to persist to age 4 years.[348]

Furthermore, it appears that the immune system response is modulated by intermittent early exposure, such that introducing small amounts of allergens into the breastfeeding mother's diet and into solids introduction can be of benefit in early sensitisation. Signs of eczema, hives or mucus in the bowel motions are cause to stop.[349]

The immunomodulating effects of vitamin D may have beneficial effects on childhood atopic presentation.[333,350] In addition to playing outdoors and gaining adequate vitamin D via safe sunshine exposure, children who grow up with exposure to a dog or with access to farm animals during the first years of life have reduced risk of asthma at age 6.[351] Compared with a city upbringing, those with early-life farm exposure have less atopic sensitisation due to a higher environmental or microbial biodiversity in early life having beneficial effects on reducing atopy. In urban settings, diversity such as childhood exposure to cats, dogs, day care, bedroom sharing and older siblings also shows some benefit, but to a lesser magnitude than a childhood farm environment.[333,352,353]

The estimated lifetime prevalence of AD has increased 2–3 fold during the past 30 years, especially in urban areas in industrialised countries, emphasising the importance of lifestyle and environment in the pathogenesis of atopic diseases.[354] There is a complex interplay between individual genetic predisposition to atopy/AD and different environmental factors, including the use of personal care products and exposure to pollution, food and other exogenous factors. Avoidance of environmental chemicals that may irritate the immune system and the skin, such as washing powder ingredients, fabric softeners, soaps, shampoos, creams that contain fragrance, phthalates, sodium lauryl sulfates, paraffin and preservatives such as propylene glycol, is also recommended. Apart from disrupting the skin barrier and driving itchiness, these chemicals may disrupt normal hormonal and immunological control of atopic processes.[339] We cannot overlook the influence on AD of various environmental chemicals that we face in everyday life – air pollutants, contact allergens and skin irritants, ingredients in cosmetics and personal care products, and food additives may significantly impact on the prevalence and severity of AD.[354] Hypersensitivity to food additives such as monosodium glutamate, food colours such as carmine and preservatives such as sodium benzoate and sulfites could be particularly aggravating to some AD children.[355,356]

A whole-foods diet with plenty of fresh vegetables, no processed or packaged foods, no additives, that is low in sugar and rich in zinc and essential fats is crucial to the management of AD.

The treatment of eczema in young children with herbal medicines can be a considerable challenge, primarily because of the taste of the medicines and poor compliance that might ensue. For discussion of herbal management of eczema, please refer to Chapter 16 'Dermatology' of *Clinical Naturopathic Medicine*.

TOPICAL TREATMENT

Objectives when managing AD topically in children are to avoid skin irritants and to optimise skin barrier function.

Topical herbal treatments may be useful, particularly when herbal medicines can be mixed into a natural cream base (such as vitamin E cream) or into an emollient base, such as a shea butter. Organic shea butter provides excellent clinical results in children as an emollient, providing a lipid barrier to keep in moisture. Twice daily application can help to seal in moisture, and shea butter can also be used as a base for application of topical herbal medicines. Topical herbal medicines such as calendula, chamomile, St John's wort and liquorice may be mixed into natural cream bases for their healing and vulnerary actions, as well as to help stop the itch cycle. Aloe vera and a few drops of lavender essential oil may also be of use.

Example topical emollient for eczema:
- Base 100 mL *Butyrospermum parkii* (shea butter) (liquid at room temperature on a warm day)
- 3 mL *Glycyrrhiza glabra* (liquorice) 1:1
- 4 mL *Matricaria recutita* (chamomile) 1:2
- 3 mL *Calendula officinalis* (calendula) 1:2
- 2 drops of *Lavandula angustifolia* (lavender) essential oil

Avoidance of skin barrier disruptors, such as chemical irritants (detergents, soap products with sodium lauryl sulfate, baby wipes with fragrance and alcohol, other personal care products with fragrance and preservatives such as parabens) is wise to protect skin. Avoidance or minimising bathing with conventional soaps and bubble baths is also recommended. Choosing hypoallergenic, fragrance-free, petrochemical-free detergents for washing clothes can also make a difference to eczematic skin.

Limiting over-use of standard medical topical treatments such as corticosteroids and petroleum-based emollients is recommended, as skin atrophy may ensue with repeated application, and rebound inflammation can occur post corticosteroid application. Systemic absorption of corticosteroids is another adverse outcome to consider.[357]

CASE STUDY 16.1

OVERVIEW

A 7-year-old girl, CB, presented with eczema (AD), which had begun 4 years ago, on her arms, legs and torso. It was worse each summer, perhaps due to weekly swimming lessons in a chlorinated pool.

The AD was also worse after attending birthday parties and school events where cupcakes and coloured popcorn were given. CB had been prescribed a topical steroid to good effect, but her mother was concerned she was over-using the steroid cream and that it wasn't treating the 'cause'.

Her mother had tried removing dairy from CB's diet, without much success. Diet included excessive consumption of sweet biscuits, cupcakes and pasta.

CB's weight gain was poor, and lab results (provided through GP) showed low ferritin (21 microgram/L; REF 15–200 microgram/L) and low p-Zinc (8 micromol/L; REF 9–19 micromol/L).

Over the previous 6 months, CB had been prescribed multiple courses of antibiotics for URTIs, and she had had disturbed sleep from both coughing at night and also itching/scratching of her AD, particularly on her legs. CB had no pets at home.

CLINICAL EXAMINATION

Nails – leukonychia on three fingernails. Cuticles of nails looked dry and peeling.

Skin – dry, itchy skin, AD worse on legs. Skin showed no sign of secondary infection.

Face and eyes – pale face, dark purple hue under both eyes.

Body – very lean, minimal body fat, slightly distended abdomen.

Provided though GP, lab results showed low ferritin (21 microgram/L; REF 15–200) and low p-Zinc (8 micromol/L; REF 9–19 micromol/L).

INITIAL CONSULTATION TREATMENT PROTOCOL

The following prescription was made:

- Education on avoiding artificial food additives, with a 'no E-numbers' policy. Recipes for simple, nutritious, dairy-free snacks given.
- Meal planner given including iron-rich meals, decreasing grains and increasing colourful vegetables and seasonal fruit.
- Rx 3 mL of liquid fish oil, unflavoured, providing 1000 mg EPA and 400 mg DHA daily with breakfast.
- Rx *Lactobacillus rhamnosus* GG 20 billion CFU daily with breakfast.
- Rx 15 mg of elemental zinc (as glycinate) daily with dinner.
- Rx topical *Butyrospermum parkii* (shea butter) infused with *Calendula officinalis* (calendula) 1 : 2 organic + 2 drops of *Lavandula angustifolia* (lavender) essential oil to be used before the swimming pool, as well as after baths each night.
- Further testing for serum IgE allergy serology, specific IgE ordered for house dust mite (HDM), cat, dog and perennial rye grass.
- Further testing for 25 (OH) vitamin D.

AT FIRST FOLLOW-UP CONSULTATION

After 2 weeks, the skin barrier had improved substantially and CB's face and legs were less red and less itchy.

Sleep quality was better and she hadn't experienced any infections.

PATHOLOGY RESULTS

- 25 (OH) vit D results 43 nmol/L (REF 51–200 nmol/L)
- IgE to HDM returns a positive elevated result of 15.4 kIU/L. Perennial rye grass, cat and dog results of <0.35 kIU/L (REF <0.35 negative)
  The following prescriptions were made:
- Continue Rx as above, adding in more dairy-free, iron-rich recipes to slowly build iron stores

- Vacuum playing area and sleeping area every second day with HEPA filter vacuum to remove dust and particulates. Consider replacing carpets with hard floors.
- Wash sheets and pillowcases weekly in water hotter than 55 degrees C.
- Cover mattress, pillow and quilt with HDM-resistant cases. Cases must be washed every 2 months. Remove sheepskin and woollen underlays.
- Education to leave shoes at the door and to let fresh air inside daily by opening bedroom window each afternoon after school.
- Add in 1000 IU D$_3$ via drops daily, with food, probiotic and liquid omega-3 as per above.
- Also education around safe sun exposure, short snippets of sunshine without SPF to legs and arms, approx. 5 minutes, between 11 am and 4 pm most days.
- Educate family on high-calcium foods (dairy free) such as unhulled tahini, sesame seeds, green leafy veg, parsley and bones in wild salmon and sardines to ensure calcium adequacy for CB's skeletal growth.

AT SECOND FOLLOW-UP CONSULTATION

After a further 4 weeks, CB's skin continued to improve, with only occasional patches of mild eczema, in response to particular food ingredients at birthday parties. With CB and her family's education around E-numbers being a driver for itchy eczema, CB became intrinsically motivated to avoid these colours and preservatives for her own comfort. She now teaches her friends about these.

CB's energy increased, and she was sick less often, so enjoyed playing outdoors, and slowly increased her diet repertoire to include a serve of fermented dairy (natural tub-set yoghurt) several times per week, with no aggravation of her skin. CB endured the following autumn and winter with nothing more than a head cold, and no requirement for antibiotic use.

Asthma

Asthma is the most prevalent chronic respiratory disease in both children and adults, and resembles a complex syndrome rather than a single disease. Risk factors for asthma specifically include genetics, family history of asthma and atopy, infections early in life, allergic diseases and lung function deficits.[358] Asthmatic wheeze may already be observed during early infancy. A majority of 'early wheezers' turn out to be transiently symptomatic, whereas in a minority, the symptoms of wheeze and asthma may persist throughout school age and adolescence. A large proportion of children with asthma lose their symptoms during school age and adolescence.

Besides the risk factors and protective factors described above, food intolerance may play a role in asthma and atopy. Foods can induce a variety of IgE-mediated, skin, gastrointestinal and respiratory reactions. The most common foods responsible for allergic reactions in children are egg, milk, peanut, soy, fish, shellfish and tree nuts. Asthma alone as a manifestation of a food allergy is rare; rather, a food allergy may aggravate underlying respiratory symptoms that already exist, and may induce airway hyper-responsiveness beyond the initial reaction.[359]

Food additives such as sulfite preservatives can cause respiratory reactions. This reaction occurs primarily in patients with underlying asthma, particularly in patients with more severe asthma. Food reactions tend to be more severe or life threatening when they involve the respiratory tract. The presence of a food allergy is a risk factor for the future development of asthma, particularly for children with sensitisation to egg protein. The diagnosis of a food allergy can be useful, and positive testing should be followed by a food-challenge procedure for a definitive diagnosis. Negative testing generally rules out a food allergy.

Antibiotic exposure during infancy may also lead to development of asthma. In a meta-analysis including data from a total of 27 167 children and 3392 asthma cases, it was found that exposure to at least one course of antibiotics in the first year of life appears to be a risk factor for the development of childhood asthma.[88] This may be due to the fact that a healthy human microbiome (i.e. the communities of microbes and their interaction with the host) plays a role in the maintenance of immune homeostasis, and inappropriate microbial community composition and function in both the airway and the GIT are related to atopy and asthma.[360]

Evidence to date suggests that the airway and/or gut microbiome may represent fertile targets for prevention or management of allergic asthma and other diseases in which adaptive immune dysfunction is a prominent feature.[361] Commensal microflora is crucial to maintain inflammatory homeostasis and to induce immune regulation; therefore, the microbiome may play an important role in the development of allergic conditions.[362]

The health of the indoor/domestic/school environment is also critical in asthma/allergy development and exacerbation. Inhalant allergens are also implicated in childhood and adolescent asthma symptoms. Smoking at home and environmental tobacco smoke exposure are closely associated with an increased prevalence of symptoms of asthma and rhinitis in primary-school-aged children.[363] Cats, dust mites and cockroaches have also been found to be causally related to lung inflammation and asthma, aggravating symptoms in children and adolescents.[364]

Over the past few decades, the prevalence of asthma, allergic disease and atopy has increased significantly and in parallel with the increased use of products and materials emitting volatile organic compounds in the indoor environment. Domestic exposure to volatile organic compounds – found in some paints, varnishes, paint stripper, glues/adhesives, upholstery, foam, air fresheners, nail polishes, formaldehydes, dry cleaning chemicals and photocopier chemicals – has been studied in relation to asthma and allergy in children and adults.[335]

Exposure to environmental stressors such as early swimming in chlorinated pools[365] can also contribute to airway epithelium dysfunction, as chlorine is a respiratory toxicant. Chlorinated pool exposure exerts an adjuvant effect on atopy that seems to contribute significantly to the burden of asthma and respiratory allergies among adolescents.[366]

Swimming is often recommended as a sport because of its several benefits to health. It is also recommended in asthmatic children as a sport with a lower potential for prompting exercise-induced asthma. However, there is growing interest in the potentially harmful effects of repeated respiratory tract exposure to chlorinated products, and the problem of possible swimming-related health hazards is gaining importance at international level. It is already known that acute exposure to chlorine gas, as in swimming pool accidents, causes lung damage, and also that elite swimmers may have increased airway inflammation and bronchial hyper-reactivity, probably as a result of repeated exposure to chlorine derivatives. Recently, some studies have been conducted to investigate whether repeated exposure to chlorine byproducts in recreational swimmers might also lead to lung damage.[367,368]

In addition, some studies have been published on the even more debated issue of the possible harmful effects of baby swimming on respiratory health, discussing data from the literature on the effects of chlorine derivatives in different categories of people routinely attending swimming pools. The need for longitudinal studies is emphasised to definitively clarify any role of chlorinated swimming pool attendance in the development of asthma in recreational swimmers.[369]

Rhinitis

Seasonal allergic rhinoconjunctivitis is generally not observed during the first 2 years of life. However, children may develop specific IgE antibodies years before they become manifest[6,7] as a part of the 'allergic march'. In most cases of childhood rhinitis, it is observed together with comorbidity of the lower airways (seasonal asthma), AD and pollen-associated food allergy.

Reflecting the risk factors for above atopic conditions, a family history of atopy, frequent respiratory tract infection, sinusitis, antibiotic use in the first year of life, a cat at home in the first year of life, dampness at home and perianal redness are well understood risk factors for increased risk for allergic rhinitis. Frequent consumption of fruits and vegetables were inversely, and frequent consumption of lollies were positively, associated with allergic rhinitis symptoms.[91]

As discussed above, indoor environment is relevant to allergic rhinitis symptomatology and severity, and environmental tobacco smoke exposure is closely associated with an increased prevalence of symptoms of asthma and rhinitis in primary-school-aged children.[363]

SAMPLE DAILY DIET FOR AN ATOPIC CHILD

BREAKFAST

- Quinoa and oat porridge cooked in coconut milk, natural vanilla essence, topped with ground pepitas and flax seed meal

OR

- Soaked buckwheat pancakes with maple syrup and stewed apple

OR

- Eggs any way and fermented vegetables

OR

- Almond/oat milk smoothie with frozen banana, chia seeds, liquid fish oil and probiotic powder

LUNCH

- Dinner leftovers

OR

- Red salmon patties with lentils and sweet potato, dusted in coconut flour, served with green beans

OR

- Mini chicken satays and vegetables/salad

OR

- Chicken breast salad with greens, avocado, pine nuts

DINNER

- Stuffed capsicum (stuffed with savoury mince) and cooked green vegetables or salad drizzled with olive or flax oil and balsamic vinegar

OR

- Lamb cutlets and roast sweet potato and green vegetables

OR

- Beef bolognaise or black bean vegetarian bolognaise served as tacos, with buckwheat pasta spirals, or as cottage pie with sweet potato mash

SNACKS

- Vegetable sticks and additive-free hummus
- Soaked crunchy sea-salted nuts
- Cashews and fresh fruit, or an apple cut into wedges with cashew butter
- Apple and cinnamon muffin (made with coconut or almond flour)
- Tasty liver meatballs (do not tell them and they will never know there is liver in there!)

BEVERAGES

- Variety of herbal teas, cooled
- Pure water
- Coconut water
- Water kefir

Teenage acne

Particularly in Westernised societies, acne vulgaris is the most common disorder among the adolescent age group, affecting 90–95% of the mid-teen population.[314] This visible skin condition is characterised by a combination of red pimples, white heads and blackheads on the skin, in particular on the face, and can also present on the neck, décolletage, back and arms. It is due to inflamed or infected sebaceous glands. Acne usually occurs during adolescence, commonly starting between ages 10 and 13, but it can persist throughout life and leave permanent scarring on the face. For a more in depth discussion on acne vulgaris, please refer to Chapter 16 'Dermatology' of *Clinical Naturopathic Medicine*.

The reasons for acne development in adolescence are complex. Gender, genetics, nationality, shifts in hormone production and metabolism, diet and lifestyle are all involved in the aetiology. Some of the main drivers include androgen-mediated stimulation of sebaceous gland activity, follicular hyperkeratinisation, colonisation of the bacterium *Propionibacterium acnes* and inflammation.[370]

The astonishing difference in the incidence of adolescent acne between non-Western and Western societies cannot be attributed to genetic differences alone, but rather most likely results from differing environmental factors.[370] The relationship between diet and acne has historically been controversial. In the past decade, however, several studies and increasing evidence have led dermatologists to acknowledge the credibility of the connection between diet quality and acne.[371]

Evidence suggests that components of Western diets, particularly high intakes of carbohydrate and dairy products, may be associated with acne incidence and severity.[372,373]

Compelling evidence shows that a high-glycaemic-index/glycaemic-load diet is positively associated with acne vulgaris.[374,375] Regularly consuming foods with excess energy value has been shown to exacerbate and significantly contribute to the progression of acne in adolescents, with an excess of the normal daily requirements for carbohydrates also significantly affecting the severity of acne.[376]

In addition to the impact of high glycaemic load and glycaemic index on acne, longitudinal studies have also shown positive associations between high intakes of dairy products and acne in adolescence. As such, the 'load' of dairy in a teenager's diet may be a contributing factor[377] to acne aetiology, with some studies implicating consumption of low-fat/skim milk, but not full-fat milk, as positively associated with acne.[378] By way of understanding this mechanism, there is increasing evidence in support of the interplay of growth hormone (GH), insulin and insulin-like growth factor-1 (IGF-1) signalling during puberty, which have a causal role in pathogenesis of acne by influencing adrenal and gonadal androgen metabolism. Typical high intake of hyperglycaemic carbohydrates and insulinotropic dairy in the Western diet may over-stimulate insulin and IGF-1 signalling, activating sebaceous gland activity and sebum production, and aggravating acne symptoms.[379] Conversely, some literature shows that decreased insulin/

IGF-1 signalling (IIS) via dietary adjustments to include more lean protein and high load of plant/vegetable food can exhibit reduced prevalence rates of acne.[380] The influence of nutritional patterns and diet quality on acne aetiology and severity in young adults reveals that there are many areas for clinicians to be aware of in prevention and management of acne in teens.

Lack of zinc in the diet may also affect the severity of the pathological process in severe forms of acne, and can have an impact on the extent of scarring. There seems to be a correlation between the severity and type of acne lesions with serum zinc levels in patients with acne vulgaris, with the mean serum zinc levels consistently measuring lower in acne groups.[381,382] A systematic review of the literature suggests that zinc is of clinical therapeutic value in management of adolescent acne. The evidence suggests zinc has antibacterial and anti-inflammatory effects and that it may decrease sebum production.[383] Success rates for treatment with zinc vary greatly depending on the disease, mode of administration and precise zinc preparation used.[384]

In addition to serum zinc levels, evaluation of serum vitamins A, E and D levels varies according to the severity of acne vulgaris in teens.[385] Lack of vitamin A (retinol) and its provitamin (carotene) may significantly affect the severity of acne, and it has been found in young adolescent men with severe acne that vitamin D deficiency significantly potentiates the inflammatory process.[376] Supportive dietary measures include an abundance of foods rich in vitamin A and E and zinc in the acne prophylaxis and treatment.[385] Supportive treatment with these nutrients supplementally in severe acne may lead to improvements over time. Serum vitamin D levels should also be checked to ensure adequacy. Supplementation is a consideration as direct sunlight exposure on acne-affected areas may worsen scarring.

There are a number of research studies examining the role and relationship between dietary fat and/or omega-3 fatty acids, dietary fibre and antioxidants, yet the evidence is less robust, and more research is needed.[371,375]

Systemic supplementation with probiotics is increasingly being explored as a potential treatment strategy for acne, with acknowledgment of the significant gut–skin axis. Since dysregulation of insulin signalling has been implicated in the pathogenesis of adolescent acne, supplementation with the probiotic strains such as *Lactobacillus rhamnosus* SP1 has been proposed to normalise skin expression of genes involved in insulin signalling and improve the appearance of acne.[386] The ability of oral probiotics and the gut microbiota to influence systemic inflammation, oxidative stress, glycaemic control, tissue lipid content and even mood may have important implications in acne.[387] This intricate relationship between gut microbiota and the skin is also influenced by diet quality.[388]

Typical allopathic treatment of acne is based on local medicines, oral antibiotics, oral retinoids and oral hormonal therapies,[389] but increasingly dietary interventions and medicinal plants are also used. Due to the common allopathic prescription of systemic antibiotics in adolescent acne vulgaris, it is important to note that intolerable side effects may invariably occur (such as digestive upset and vaginal candidiasis). Long-term systemic antibiotic therapy for acne – for example, for over a period of 3–6 months – is without consideration of the downstream effects on the health and diversity of the microbiota. In patients where antibiotic therapy is recommended, probiotics may reduce the side effects imparted by chronic antibiotic use, while working as a therapeutic adjunct for acne vulgaris by providing a synergistic anti-inflammatory effect.[390]

Besides the dietary and nutritional discussion above, for the treatment of acne with herbal and plant medicines, the following properties are valued: antibacterial, anti-inflammatory, antioxidant and anti-androgenic.[391]

For topical use, the inner gel of aloe vera leaves may be a soothing, anti-inflammatory, vulnerary topical agent for mild acne. In addition, aloe vera gel is gently antimicrobial and nutritive, containing vitamins E and C, carotenoids, flavonoids and tannins.[392,393]

Furthermore, aloe vera gel may be used as a carrier substance to carry the smallest amount of eucalyptus or tea tree essential oil, for use directly onto infected spots. A strong antimicrobial effect against *P. acnes* strains is attributed to flavonoids isolated from *Eucalyptus maculata* extract,[394] which would be too strong to apply directly to skin, but could be applied in a small amount (just 1–2 drops of essential oil) mixed in a base of aloe gel.

In the treatment of mild acne, plants with anti-androgen properties can be used to good effect. Evidence about efficacy is beginning to emerge for plant-derived anti-androgens such as in spearmint tea, which may be indicated in the management of both polycystic ovarian syndrome (PCOS) and acne.[395] For example, a randomised clinical trial[396] showed that drinking spearmint tea twice daily for 30 days (as opposed to chamomile tea, which was used as a control) significantly reduced plasma levels of gonadotropins and androgens in patients with hirsutism associated with PCOS.

Green tea is another consideration for mild acne as it contains epigallocatechins and inhibits 5-alpha reductase, thereby reducing the conversion of normal testosterone into the more potent DHT.[395]

TEENAGE ACNE AND SELF-ESTEEM

As acne affects the appearance of the skin, it is likely to bring stress to the adolescent's life regarding sensitivity about their appearance. Apart from managing the clinical manifestations of acne, clinicians should be aware of the psychiatric comorbidities when treating adolescents with acne vulgaris. Especially, low self-esteem, social anxiety and life quality impairment should warn clinicians to predict high social anxiety levels in adolescent acne patients.[397,398]

Acne severity may have a considerable adverse impact on quality of life and self-esteem. Clinicians need to emphasise the psychosocial consequences of severe acne and offer strategies and remedies in the management of this.[399] Acne vulgaris has been found to have a more direct effect on self-esteem, self-confidence and identity, especially in girls. Coping strategies that may be offered to patients and families include reassurance, empowerment and cognitive adaptation.[400]

TREATMENT

Herbal medicine

For the treatment of acne, the following properties are valued: immune-enhancing, anti-inflammatory, vulnerary, lymphatic, depurative, antioxidant and anti-androgenic.

HERBAL FORMULA

Echinacea spp.	1:2	60 mL
Glycyrrhiza glabra	1:1	30 mL
Calendula officinalis	1:2	60 mL
Arctium lappa	1:2	40 mL
Phytolacca decandra	1:5	10 mL
Total		200 mL

Based on adult dose of 5 mL 3 times a day, work out the appropriate adolescent dose based on weight.

Nutritional medicine (dietary)

- Adequate hydration, with plenty of water, herbal teas (such as green tea and spearmint tea), additive-free coconut water, occasional fermented teas such as kombucha.
- Avoidance of fruit juice, soft drink and large volumes of cow's milk.
- Regular meals including lean protein and high load of plant/vegetable foods may be helpful in decreasing insulin signalling, reducing prevalence and severity of acne.[380]
- Avoidance of high-glycaemic-load or high-glycaemic-index foods such as white breads, fruit juice and confectionery.
- Foods rich in zinc to include: lean grass-fed beef, oysters, wheatgerm, pepitas, pine nuts, sunflower seeds, raw or dry roasted cashews.
- Foods rich in betacarotene and vitamin A to include: organic chicken liver, pasture-raised eggs, colourful vegetables (sweet potato, capsicum, kale, carrots, spinach, green leafies, rocket, parsley)
- Foods rich in omega-3 fatty acids to include: oily fish such as salmon, ocean trout and sardines; flathead; snapper; shellfish such as oysters and mussels; plant omega-3 sources such as linseeds, chia seeds, walnuts and seaweeds; and micro-algaes such as spirulina and chlorella.

Nutritional medicine (supplementation)

Please use Clark's rule to determine dose with adult doses listed below:

- High vitamin cod liver oil – 1–2 teaspoons daily, for both the omega-3 and vitamins A and D.
- Zinc: 20–30 mg elemental per day, in bioavailable forms such as citrate, picolinate, gluconate, diglycinate.[314]
- High-quality vitamin C powder, providing 1–3 g of vitamin C per day (or to bowel tolerance).
- Multi-strain, high-dose probiotic containing *Lactobacillus* GG.

SAMPLE DAILY DIET FOR A CHILD OR TEEN WITH ACNE

BREAKFAST

- Savoury frittata with 2 eggs, sweet potato, baby spinach and pine nuts

OR

- Soaked buckwheat pancakes with cashew butter and banana or berries

OR

- Eggs any way with fermented vegetables, cherry tomatoes, rocket

OR

- Natural, fermented brown rice protein powder smoothie with baby spinach, frozen banana, probiotic powder, chia seeds and almond milk

LUNCH

- Dinner leftovers

OR

- Brown rice fried rice, made with coconut oil, including colourful stir-fried vegetables and line-caught skipjack tuna

OR

- Mini chicken satays and vegetables/salad

OR

- Chicken salad with 2–3 cups of colourful salad vegetables

DINNER

- Dhal with brown or basmati rice topped with pine nuts; or chicken, coconut milk and vegetable curry with rice

OR

- Lamb cutlets and vegetables

OR

- Wholemeal buckwheat spiral pasta with pesto, wild salmon, broccolini and cherry tomatoes

OR

- Shepherd's pie with lean beef bolognaise, topped with sweet potato or cauliflower mash

SNACKS

- Vegetable sticks and additive-free hummus
- Soaked, dry roasted, crunchy sea-salted nuts
- Apple and cinnamon muffin (made with almond flour)
- Almond meal cacao coconut bliss balls with a spearmint tea

BEVERAGES

- Water
- Additive-free coconut water
- Spearmint tea
- Green tea
- Kombucha
- Water kefir

CASE STUDY 16.2

OVERVIEW

JR, a 17-year-old male, presented with mild–moderate acne on his face and back, which had been present for the past 3 years. It seemed to worsen after school sport, and JR was a very active basketball player, playing 3–4 games per week, often without showering afterwards.

JR had been prescribed by his GP a topical antibacterial gel, to use each night before bed, and had been told to use the pH-neutral face wash Cetaphil after basketball games and before bed each night.

He was in discussion with the same GP about potential of an oral antibiotic and/or Roaccutane to control his acne, but his mother had brought him in for naturopathic consultation to get a second opinion before beginning medications. JR occasionally picked at his acne and some scarring had begun – JR commented that the lesions were taking several days to heal. JR's acne was bothering him and his mother noted his appearance was adversely impacting on his self-esteem, and he was engaging less with peers for social events.

JR did however enjoy a can of soft drink (Fanta) after each basketball game, and loved salty crisps while studying. He also ate 4–5 apples each day and enjoyed 1 L of cow's milk each day with breakfast. On consultation, it was revealed that JR's water was low, and his vegetable intake was limited to just one serving per day. JR complained of excessive wind and occasional looseness + urgency with his bowels, with BM 2 per day.

CLINICAL EXAMINATION

Nails – leukonychia on eight fingernails
Skin – dry, coarse, peeling in patches, with multiple open and closed comedones, acne worse on his cheeks and chin, as well as upper back. There was some evidence of scarring on his back.
Face and eyes – multiple open and closed comedones. Inflammation was present with some pustules. No evidence of any cysts.
Body – tall, lean, strong, healthy weight, BMI of 24.
JR was a non-smoker and non-drinker (with exams coming up had been socialising very little).

INITIAL CONSULTATION TREATMENT PROTOCOL

The following prescription was made, with the objective of reducing number of comedones/lesions by half, over a period of 4–6 weeks.

A secondary goal of speeding healing time of pimples and reducing scarring was also established.

- Education on significantly increasing zinc foods (lean beef, shellfish, wheatgerm, eggs, pepitas and pine nuts) with appropriate snack ideas and recipes given.
- Education around the role of insulin spikes in aetiology of acne/excess sebum production. Fanta and soft drinks replaced with coconut water. Apples halved to maximum 2 per day, and replaced with vegetable snacks instead.
- Breakfast smoothie recipe given, using almond milk, baby spinach, chia seeds, frozen banana and cacao, to replace

1 L of milk at breakfast. Other dairy products (cheese, natural yoghurt) still encouraged.
- Rx 50 mg of elemental zinc (as glycinate and citrate dihydrate blend) daily with dinner.
- Rx two capsules of sustainably sourced fish oil, providing 1000 mg EPA and 400 mg DHA daily with breakfast.
- Rx multi-strain probiotic, including *Lactobacillus rhamnosus* SP1 40 billion CFU daily with breakfast.
- Rx herbal tonic (see below) dose 7.5 mL b.i.d. before meals.

Echinacea spp.	1:2	60 mL
Glycyrrhiza glabra	1:1	30 mL
Calendula officinalis	1:2	60 mL
Arctium lappa	1:2	40 mL
Phytolacca decandra	1:5	10 mL
Total		200 mL

AT FOLLOW-UP CONSULTATION

After 4 weeks, the skin barrier had improved substantially and JR was motivated by the changes to further improve his diet.

He agreed to six oysters per week with his father, and his basketball performance had also improved.

Cravings for sweet drinks and salty chips had reduced significantly, and JR triumphantly announced that his healing time had sped up significantly to just 3 days for a single pimple. A protein chart was given, as JR was interested in further improving his diet, and gaining more muscle mass.

JR also reported that his bowels were feeling more comfortable and stools more formed, without the urgency. He chose to continue limiting his apple and cow's milk intake.

With the trajectory of improvements in such a short time, JR was feeling less like he wanted to trial oral medication from the GP. JR did however ask about an alternative to the herbal tonic, and also to the topical antibiotic gel he was using.

FOLLOW-UP CONSULTATION TREATMENT PROTOCOL

Protein chart, as above, with goal of attaining 60–80 g of protein daily.

Continued low apple and minimal cow's milk intake.

Same nutritional prescriptions as above, with change of liquid herbal tonic to a commercially available tablet formula.

Topical pure aloe gel prescribed, with pure tea tree essential oil, to be applied: 1 teaspoon of aloe gel, with 3 drops of tea tree essential oil, directly onto spots as needed.

ENVIRONMENTAL CHEMICALS AND PAEDIATRIC AND ADOLESCENT HEALTH

Paediatric environmental medicine covers a tremendously broad amount of topics, and for a more in depth discussion on environmental medicine and health, please refer to Chapter 2.

Many lessons from the past have shown the power of the environment to shape health and disease,[1] and we cannot ignore the fact that the environment is a determinant in health for all of us, in particular children. Looking at things from a historical perspective, over the past 100 years we have seen major changes in the health landscape: major reductions in infectious diseases (due to antibiotics, some immunisations, better hygiene and access to clean water); major increases in life expectancy; and significant increases in chronic paediatric diseases such as atopic conditions, reproductive developmental disorders, childhood leukaemia and brain cancer, neurodevelopmental dysfunction disorders such as autism spectrum disorders, insulin resistance and diabetes, childhood obesity and cardiovascular disease.[401,402]

Not coincidentally, more than 85 000 new chemicals have been developed and released into the global environment over the same period of time. Commercial chemical production has risen exponentially on a global scale, and this dramatic rise has resulted in industrial chemicals being ubiquitous with modern life. Approximately 3000 of these new chemicals are high-production chemicals to which we have daily exposures, and others are produced inadvertently as the byproducts of industrial processes. There is a growing body of evidence suggesting that chemicals present in air, water, soil, our food, the built environment, on our homes, our personal care products and even our clothes are toxicants that contribute to the increasing burden of chronic paediatric illness described above.[403]

Looking at the global landscape, the World Health Organization quotes that 36% of all deaths among children aged 0–14 years of age are attributable to modifiable environmental risk factors.[404]

Profoundly, it is well understood that babies are not born with a clear slate, but rather enter this world with a pre-existing body burden of environmental contaminants, as a result of maternal transfer during gestation. A landmark investigation conducted by the Environmental Working Group in 2005 identified an average of 200 industrial chemicals and pollutants in umbilical cord blood from babies born in US hospitals. A total of 287 chemicals were found in the group – including pesticides, consumer product ingredients and wastes from burning coal, petrol and garbage – exposing that we are, disturbingly, birthing a generation of pre-polluted babies.[405]

We simply cannot ignore the profound impact of chemical and environmental hazards on a child's health, nor the impact of our inevitable chemical body burden on reproduction, human development and the health of the subsequent generations.[403,406] It is further suggested that exposures during critical windows of development and early life exposures are significant contributors to chronic diseases later in life, as well as across generations.[407,408] The intergenerational health implications of this are huge, and it is vital that we develop a better understanding of the mechanisms and interactions between nutrition, genetic predisposition, environmental exposures, timing of exposures and the subsequent immune dysregulation and

oxidative stress caused by chemicals and their metabolites, which are biologically plausibly adding to the increasing burden of chronic disease in our children.[409–411]

While the human body has many protected mechanisms in its own innate intelligence, environmental chemicals are widespread and ubiquitous with modern life. Developing children – both in utero and as infants, toddlers and beyond – have an exquisite vulnerability to many chemicals for myriad reasons.[412] The very nature of children's growth and development creates windows of vulnerability to both nutritional deficiencies and toxicant exposures.[413] There are huge discrepancies in how children handle chemicals compared with adults, driven by several factors:

- Proportionally, children have higher consumption of food and drink per kilogram of body weight – children eat more and drink more per unit body weight than adults.[414]
- Children's behaviours magnify their exposures (mouthing things, being closer to the ground and carpet/dust with flame retardants).[415]
- While ingestion of toxic chemicals is a significant route of exposure for children, dermal and inhalation exposures are also higher than adults. A child's skin is more permeable than an adults, plus infants and children have higher metabolic rates, leading to increased inhalation of toxic air pollutants.[416]
- They are more biologically vulnerable, with decreased expression of detoxification enzymes leading to decreased ability to effectively deal with chemical exposures. For example, the biological half-life of some common organophosphate pesticides such as malathion and parathion is about 6 hours in an adult (it takes approximately 6 hours to get rid of half of an exposure); the half-life for the same pesticides is over 36 hours in a newborn.[417]
- Rapid growth, development and differentiation of vital organ systems in utero, infancy and beyond are delicate developmental processes that can be easily disrupted. Exposure to chemicals during these periods of rapid development could lead to permanent and irreversible damage to organ systems. Some of these chemicals are developmental toxicants (e.g. EDCs that interfere with reproductive development), some are immune toxicants and others interfere with neurological growth. For example, we know that the developing brain is more susceptible to neurotoxicants: if exposures occur at dangerous windows of vulnerability (i.e. during brain cell migration), serious irreversible effects can take place.[418]

While definitive data is lacking on the exact underlying mechanisms by which environmental chemicals impact on paediatric health outcomes, children's exposures to chemicals in the environment are understood to contribute to the causation and exacerbation of certain chronic, disabling diseases including asthma (we know that common household chemicals increase risk of allergy risks in preschool-age children[334]), cancer,[419] testicular dysgenesis syndrome (such as hypospadias[420,421] and cryptorchidism),[422] obesity,[423,424] neurodevelopmental disorders and functional brain impairments.[425]

Over the past five decades in particular, the prevalence of neurodevelopmental disorders such as autism spectrum disorders (ASDs), attention-deficit hyperactivity disorder (ADHD), dyslexia and other cognitive impairments has grown substantially among children. For instance, in 2014, the CDC identified 1 in 68 children (1 in 42 boys and 1 in 189 girls) as having ASD,[426] a deterioration from 1 in 150 children in the year 2000.[427]

Some authors predict that if the incidence of autism continues to increase at the same trajectory, then half of children born in 2032 will be diagnosed with autism – a frightening projection.[428] For a more in depth discussion on ADHD and autism spectrum disorders and their management, please refer to Chapter 18.

Mounting evidence supporting a significant contribution of environmental factors to autism risk is compelling.[429] A number of studies have demonstrated significant increases in ASD risk with estimated exposure to air pollution during the prenatal period, particularly for heavy metals and particulate matter.[430] Industrial chemicals widely disseminated in the environment are important contributors to what researchers have called 'the global silent pandemic of neuro-developmental disorders and toxicity'.[46] For example, systematic reviews published in both 2005[431] and 2014 identified 11 industrial chemicals that injure the growing brain, leading to the current pandemic of developmental neurotoxicity: lead, methylmercury, polychlorinated biphenyls, arsenic, toluene, manganese, fluoride, chlorpyrifos, dichlorodiphenyltrichloroethane, tetrachloroethylene and the polybrominated diphenyl ethers. The authors postulate that even more developmental neurotoxicants remain undiscovered.[46] It is clear that more rigorous exposure assessment and more research is urgently needed to better understand the interactions between genes, nutrition and environmental factors in the development of neurodevelopmental disorders, and that the health impact of these chemical exposures is most evident in paediatric medicine.[432]

Among the environmental toxicants to which children are at risk of exposure are modern, fast-acting pesticides.[433] Conventional food production commonly uses organophosphate pesticides, which are neurotoxins that act on the nervous system of humans by blocking an important enzyme (cholinesterases). Organophosphate pesticide exposure in children and teens is mainly through the diet.[434]

The increasingly wide use of organophosphate pesticides in the world has led to rapidly growing concerns over their health and wellbeing impacts.[435] There is a growing body of in-vitro, in-vivo and human research that suggests that pesticides, such as the widely used organophosphates, have endocrine-disrupting activity and neurotoxic effects at low levels of exposure and during critical windows of development in utero and in infancy and childhood.[46,436,437]

Organic foods are grown without synthetic pesticides (insecticides, herbicides, fungicides), fertilisers or routine use of antibiotics and growth hormones, and many people choose to eat organic food as a precautionary approach to reduce pesticide exposure. Adopting an organic diet appears to be an effective solution for reducing dietary pesticide exposure.[438]

Other environmental exposure risks are EDCs – chemicals that have the capacity to interfere with hormonal signalling systems. EDCs may alter hormonal messaging and feedback systems in the brain, pituitary, reproductive organs, thyroid and other components of the endocrine system, affecting development. EDCs include organochlorine pesticides,[439,440] bisphenol A,[441] phthalates[424] and PCBs. The impacts of EDCs have been described in wildlife populations, and to a more limited extent in humans. It is hypothesised that in utero and early childhood exposures to EDCs may be responsible, at least in part, for decreases in semen quality,[442,443] increasing incidence of congenital malformations of the reproductive organs (such as hypospadias[420,421] and cryptorchidism),[422] increasing incidence of testicular cancer,[419] development of childhood obesity[423,424] and acceleration of onset of puberty in females.[444,445]

The prediction of health risks of these chemicals based on traditional toxicological testing – of no observable adverse effects levels – does not account for real-life exposures to multiple chemicals, where unpredictable, additive and synergistic effects may occur.

It is well known that socioeconomic factors, nutritional factors and health status influence the vulnerability of infants and children to environmental toxicants, and standard toxicological risk assessment also does not account for this variable handling of toxicants. Individual factors such as gender, ethnicity, genetics, GIT microbiota health, diet and nutritional status, medications and comorbidities all influence the risk of adverse health outcomes to chemical exposures.[446]

Evidence exists that nutritional status can modify and reduce absorption of many toxins. Malnourished children may be more vulnerable to adverse health effects of chemical exposures.[447] Suboptimal body stores of iron, calcium, zinc and selenium make individuals more susceptible to toxicity from exposures to heavy metals such as methylmercury, aluminium and pesticides.[448] Anaemic individuals have reduced defences against methylmercury exposures,[449] and those who are not achieving their daily iron and calcium requirement have greater potential than people who are calcium replete to uptake lead from water, paints and car exhaust into their bones. Rebalancing the body's dynamic mineral balance will aid the body in mobilising and excreting heavy metals and will moderate future absorption.[2] The protection of children against environmental toxins is a major challenge to modern society.

Ensuring sufficiency of nutrients critical to development – omega-3 fats, iodine, iron, zinc, calcium and vitamin D – creates an ideal environment for optimal development and functioning. Providing children with a whole-foods diet, rich in minerals and a rainbow of colourful, seasonal vegetables, ensures a good supply of plant phytochemical compounds. Some plant-based foods are rich in 'bio-active' phytochemicals that work synergistically to functionally protect healthy cells and to disable the free radicals produced from toxin break-down processes. Plant foods may provide desirable health benefits beyond basic nutrition to reduce the risk of the development of chronic diseases.[450]

Strategies for building resilience during infancy, childhood and beyond include:

- ensuring all of the nutritional building blocks are available to support optimal development (immune, neurodevelopment and endocrine function)
- supplying an abundance of minerals, trace minerals and plant-based antioxidants that protect against and support the body's handling of inevitable exposures
- maintaining adequate hydration and ensuring bowel clearance daily
- implementing daily lifestyle strategies that support detoxification pathways
- limiting medications that destroy good gut bacteria and addressing GIT dysbiosis and GIT permeability if relevant
- consuming foods daily that nourish the gut and microbiome for optimal digestive function and nutrient assimilation
- choosing to filter tap water to minimise exposures to heavy metals, disinfection chemical byproducts and other particulates and contaminants
- choosing to eat an organic diet to reduce pesticide load from daily food consumption.

Young people and the environment are inseparable. With a double burden of nutrient deficiencies and environmental exposures, a substantial portion of the world's children may never realise their right to optimal health and development. As an urgent attempt to reduce the burden of environmental chemical exposure on paediatric disease, research into environmental risk factors for childhood diseases has grown substantially over the past 15 years. Despite the increasing attention to this topic, our current understanding is still just the tip of the iceberg. Until we better understand the complex, dynamic nature of environmental chemical exposure on paediatric health, avoidance strategies and adoption of a precautionary approach to keep exposures low is paramount,[406] alongside recognition of the unique vulnerability of the developing brain and body.

Frustratingly, environmental chemical assessment is generally overlooked in clinical practice, and development of clinical tools to better assess environmental exposures in paediatric patients (relevant questions, toxicity questionnaires, specific testing) is critical to better handling of this enormous dilemma.[402]

There is also need for a concerted action by patients, parents, educators and society as a whole to better understand the impact of environmental chemicals on human health, and an onus on corporations, policy makers, regulatory authorities and government to better test and control chemicals, minimising the extent to which chemical toxic exposure impacts on current and future generations.[451]

REFERENCES

[1] Landrigan PJ, Etzel RA, editors. Textbook of children's environmental health. Oxford University Press; 2013.

[2] Demmelmair H, von Rosen J, Koletzko B. Long-term consequences of early nutrition. Early Hum Dev 2006;82(8):567–74.

[3] Neu J, Hauser N, Douglas-Escobar M. Postnatal nutrition and adult health programming. Semin Fetal Neonatal Med 2007;12(1):78–86.

[4] Koletzko B. Early nutrition and its later consequences: new opportunities. Adv Exp Med Biol 2005;569:1–12.

[5] Nyaradi A, Li J, Hickling S, et al. The role of nutrition in children's neurocognitive development, from pregnancy through childhood. Front Hum Neurosci 2013;7:97.

[6] Black MM. Zinc deficiency and child development. Am J Clin Nutr 1998;68(2):464S–9S.

[7] Hardy SC, Kleinman RE. Fat and cholesterol in the diet of infants and young children: implications for growth, development, and long-term health. J Pediatr 1994;125(5):S69–77.

[8] Cardona Cano S, Tiemeier H, Van Hoeken D, et al. Trajectories of picky eating during childhood: a general population study. Int J Eat Disord 2015;48(6):570–9.

[9] Taylor CM, Wernimont SM, Northstone K, et al. Picky/fussy eating in children: review of definitions, assessment, prevalence and dietary intakes. Appetite 2015;95:349–59.

[10] Carruth BR, Ziegler PJ, Gordon A, et al. Prevalence of picky eaters among infants and toddlers and their caregivers' decisions about offering a new food. J Am Diet Assoc 2004;104(1 Suppl. 1): s57–64.

[11] Lam J. Picky eating in children. Front Pediatr 2015;3:41.

[12] Green RJ, Samy G, Miqdady MS, et al. How to improve eating behaviour during early childhood. Pediatr Gastroenterol Hepatol Nutr 2015;18(1):1–9.

[13] Mennella JA, Jagnow CP, Beauchamp GK. Prenatal and postnatal flavor learning by human infants. Pediatr 2001;107(6):E88.

[14] Beauchamp GK, Mennella JA. Early flavor learning and its impact on later feeding behavior. J Pediatr Gastroenterol Nutr 2009;48(Suppl. 1):S25–30.

[15] Johnson SL, Bellows L, Beckstrom L, et al. Evaluation of a social marketing campaign targeting preschool children. Am J Health Behav 2007;31(1):44–55.

[16] Hendy HM, Raudenbush B. Effectiveness of teacher modeling to encourage food acceptance in preschool children. Appetite 2000;34(1):61–76.

[17] Dovey TM, Staples PA, Gibson EL, et al. Food neophobia and 'picky/fussy' eating in children: a review. Appetite 2008;50(2–3):181–93.

[18] Horne PJ, Greenhalgh J, Erjavec M, et al. Increasing pre-school children's consumption of fruit and vegetables. A modelling and rewards intervention. Appetite 2011;56(2):375–85.

[19] Addessi E, Galloway AT, Visalberghi E, et al. Specific social influences on the acceptance of novel foods in 2–5-year-old children. Appetite 2005;45(3):264–71.

[20] Australian Government. Iron; 2014. Available from https:// www.nrv.gov.au/nutrients/iron.

[21] Rosales FJ, Reznick JS, Zeisel SH. Understanding the role of nutrition in the brain and behavioral development of toddlers and preschool children: identifying and addressing methodological barriers. Nutr Neurosci 2009;12(5):190–202.

[22] Benjamin W. Borish's clinical refraction. 2nd ed. St Louis Missouri: Butterworth–Heinemann; 2006. p. 1395–460.

[23] Baker R, Baker SS. Toddler and infant nutrition. In: Wyllie R, Hyams W, Kay M, editors. Pediatric gastrointestinal and liver disease. Cleveland, OH: Elsevier Saunders; 2011.

[24] Lawson M. Caballero B, Allen L, Prentice A, editors. Encyclopedia of human nutrition. Amsterdam: Academic Press; 2005.

[25] de Souza AS, Fernandes FS, do Carmo M. Effects of maternal malnutrition and postnatal nutritional rehabilitation on brain fatty acids, learning, and memory. Nutr Rev 2011;69(3):132–44.

[26] Lenroot RK, Giedd JN. Brain development in children and adolescents: insights from anatomical magnetic resonance imaging. Neurosci Biobehav Rev 2006;30(6):718–29.

[27] Burgess JR, Stevens L, Zhang W, et al. Long-chain polyunsaturated fatty acids in children with attention-deficit hyperactivity disorder. Am J Clin Nutr 2000;71(1 Suppl.):327s–30s.

[28] Schuchardt JP, Huss M, Stauss-Grabo M, et al. Significance of long-chain polyunsaturated fatty acids (PUFAs) for the development and behaviour of children. Eur J Pediatr 2010;169(2):149–64.

[29] Ryan AS, Astwood JD, Gautier S, et al. Effects of long-chain polyunsaturated fatty acid supplementation on neurodevelopment

in childhood: a review of human studies. Prostaglandins Leukot Essent Fatty Acids 2010;82(4–6):305–14.

[30] Fallon S, Enig MG. Nourishing traditions: the cookbook that challenges politically correct nutrition and diet dictocrats. Brandywine, Maryland: New Trends Publishing; 2000.

[31] Food and Nutrition Board. Dietary Reference intakes for energy, carbohydrate, fiber, fat, fatty acids, cholesterol, protein, and amino acids (macronutrients). Washington, DC: National Academies Press; 2002.

[32] Bauer J. Guidelines for the use of parenteral and enteral nutrition in adult and pediatric patients. J Parenter Enteral Nutr 2002;26:1–138.

[33] Australian Government. Australian health survey: consumption of food groups from the Australian Dietary Guidelines. Canberra: Australian Bureau of Statistics; 2013. p. 2012–13.

[34] Ministry of Health, NSW Department of Education, Office of Sport, The Heart Foundation. Eat more fruit and vegies; 2016. Available from http://www.healthykids.nsw.gov.au/kids-teens/eat-more-fruit-and-vegies.aspx.

[35] Tomás-Barberán FA, Selma MV, Espín JC. Interactions of gut microbiota with dietary polyphenols and consequences to human health. Curr Opin Clin Nutr Metab Care 2016;19(6):471–6.

[36] Smeriglio A, Barreca D, Bellocco E, et al. Chemistry, pharmacology and health benefits of anthocyanins. Phytother Res 2016;30(8):1265–86.

[37] Morais CA, de Rosso VV, Estadella D, et al. Anthocyanins as inflammatory modulators and the role of the gut microbiota. J Nutr Biochem 2016;33:1–7.

[38] National Health and Medical Research Council. Nutrients & Dietary Energy Calculator; 2014. Available from https://www.nrv.gov.au/nutrients-energy-calculation/nutrients-energy-calc-result-1475522171.

[39] Saunders NR, Liddelow SA, Dziegielewska KM. Barrier mechanisms in the developing brain. Front Pharmacol 2012;3:46.

[40] Lozoff B, Jimenez E, Wolf AW. Long-term developmental outcome of infants with iron deficiency. New Eng J Med 1991;325(10):687–94.

[41] Walter T. Effect of iron-deficiency anemia on cognitive skills and neuromaturation in infancy and childhood. Food Nutr Bull 2003;24(4 Suppl.):S104–10.

[42] Heath DL, Panaretto KS. Nutrition status of primary school children in Townsville. Aust J Rural Health 2005;13(5):282–9.

[43] Karr M, Alperstein G, Causer J, et al. Iron status and anaemia in preschool children in Sydney. Aust N Z J Public Health 1996;20(6):618–22.

[44] Pasricha SR, Flecknoe-Brown SC, Allen KJ, et al. Diagnosis and management of iron deficiency anaemia: a clinical update. Med J Aust 2010;193(9):525–32.

[45] National Heart Blood and Lung Institute. What are the signs and symptoms of iron-deficiency anemia? 2014. Available from https://www.nhlbi.nih.gov/health/health-topics/topics/ida/signs.

[46] Grandjean P, Landrigan PJ. Neurobehavioural effects of developmental toxicity. Lancet Neurol 2014;13(3):330–8.

[47] Grant CC, Wall CR, Brewster D, et al. Policy statement on iron deficiency in pre-school-aged children. J Paediatr Child Health 2007;43(7–8):513–21.

[48] Wasserman G, Graziano JH, Factor-Litvak P, et al. Independent effects of lead exposure and iron deficiency anemia on developmental outcome at age 2 years. J Pediatr 1992;121(5):695–703.

[49] Institute NHBaL. What are the signs and symptoms of iron-deficiency anemia? 2014. Available from https://www.nhlbi.nih.gov/health/health-topics/topics/ida/signs.

[50] World Health Organization. Haemoglobin concentrations for the diagnosis of anaemia and assessment of severity; 2011. Available from https://www.who.int/vmnis/indicators/haemoglobin/en/.

[51] Food Standards Australia and New Zealand. NUTTAB 2010; 2010. Available from http://www.foodstandards.gov.au/science/monitoringnutrients/nutrientables/pages/default.aspx.

[52] Delange F. The role of iodine in brain development. Proc Nutr Soc 2000;59(1):75–9.

[53] Li M, Eastman CJ, Waite KV, et al. Are Australian children iodine deficient? Results of the Australian National Iodine Nutrition Study. Med J Aust 2006;184(4):165–9.

[54] Li M, Ma G, Boyages SC, et al. Re-emergence of iodine deficiency in Australia. Asia Pac J Clin Nutr 2001;10(3):200–3.

[55] Choi AL, Sun G, Zhang Y, et al. Developmental fluoride neurotoxicity: a systematic review and meta-analysis. Environ Health Perspect 2012;120(10):1362–8.

[56] Seshadri D, De D. Nails in nutritional deficiencies. Indian J Dermatol Venereol Leprol 2012;78(3):237–41.

[57] Kurugol Z, Bayram N, Atik T. Effect of zinc sulfate on common cold in children: randomized, double blind study. Pediatr Int 2007;49(6):842–7.

[58] Bhatnagar S, Taneja S. Zinc and cognitive development. Br J Nutr 2001;85(Suppl. 2):S139–45.

[59] Khan WU, Sellen DW. Zinc supplementation in the management of diarrhea; 2011. Available from http://www.who.int/elena/titles/bbc/zinc_diarrhoea/en/.

[60] DiGirolamo AM, Ramirez-Zea M. Role of zinc in maternal and child mental health. Am J Clin Nutr 2009;89(3):940s–5s.

[61] DiGirolamo AM, Ramirez-Zea M, Wang M, et al. Randomized trial of the effect of zinc supplementation on the mental health of school-age children in Guatemala. Am J Clin Nutr 2010;92(5):1241–50.

[62] Lonnerdal B. Dietary factors influencing zinc absorption. J Nutr 2000;130(5S Suppl.):1378s–83s.

[63] Centers for Disease Control and Prevention, National Center for Health Statistics. Clinical growth charts; 2009. Available from http://www.cdc.gov/growthcharts/clinical_charts.htm.

[64] Wahlqvist ML, editor. Food and nutrition. 3rd ed. Crows Nest, NSW: Allen & Unwin; 2011.

[65] Reilly JJ, Methven E, McDowell ZC, et al. Health consequences of obesity. Arch Dis Child 2003;88(9):748–52.

[66] Baker JL, Olsen LW, Sorensen TI. Childhood body mass index and the risk of coronary heart disease in adulthood. Ugeskr Laeger 2008;170(33):2434–7.

[67] Reilly JJ, Kelly J. Long-term impact of overweight and obesity in childhood and adolescence on morbidity and premature mortality in adulthood: systematic review. Int J Obes 2005;35(7):891–8.

[68] Cleland VJ, Schmidt MD, Dwyer T, et al. Television viewing and abdominal obesity in young adults: is the association mediated by food and beverage consumption during viewing time or reduced leisure-time physical activity? Am J Clin Nutr 2008;87(5):1148–55.

[69] Salmon J, Campbell KJ, Crawford DA. Television viewing habits associated with obesity risk factors: a survey of Melbourne schoolchildren. Med J Aust 2006;184(2):64–7.

[70] Spinks A, Macpherson A, Bain C, et al. Determinants of sufficient daily activity in Australian primary school children. J Paediatr Child Health 2006;42(11):674–9.

[71] Leech RM, McNaughton SA, Timperio A. The clustering of diet, physical activity and sedentary behavior in children and adolescents: a review. In J Nutr Phys Act 2014;11:4.

[72] Bailes JR, Strow MT, Werthammer J, et al. Effect of low-carbohydrate, unlimited calorie diet on the treatment of childhood obesity: a prospective controlled study. Metab Syndr Relat Disord 2003;1(3):221–5.

[73] Trasande L, Attina TM, Blustein J. Association between urinary bisphenol A concentration and obesity prevalence in children and adolescents. JAMA 2012;308(11):1113–21.

[74] Calafat AM, Xiaoyun Y, Lee-Yang W, et al. Exposure of the US population to bisphenol A and 4-tertiary-octylphenol: 2003–2004. Environ Health Perspect 2008;116(1):39–44.

[75] Eng DS, Lee JM, Gebremariam A, et al. Bisphenol A and chronic disease risk factors in US children. Pediatrics 2013;132(3):e637–45.

[76] Isolauri E, Salminen S. Probiotics, gut inflammation and barrier function. Gastroenterol Clin North Am 2005;34(3):437–50, viii.

[77] Kolida S, Saulnier D, Gibson G. Gastrointestinal microflora: probiotics. Adv Appl Microbiol 2006;59:187–219.

[78] Johnson CL, Versalovic J. The human microbiome and its potential importance to pediatrics. Pediatrics 2012;129(5):950–60.

[79] Ardissone AN, de la Cruz DM, Davis-Richardson AG, et al. Meconium microbiome analysis identifies bacteria correlated with premature birth. PLoS ONE 2014;9(3):e90784.

[80] Li M, Wang M, Donovan SM. Early development of the gut microbiome and immune-mediated childhood disorders. Semin Reprod Med 2014;32(1):74–86.

[81] Baumler AJ, Sperandio V. Interactions between the microbiota and pathogenic bacteria in the gut. Nature 2016;535(7610):85–93.

[82] Kau AL, Ahern PP, Griffin NW, et al. Human nutrition, the gut microbiome and the immune system. Nature 2011;474(7351):327–36.

[83] Tan J, McKenzie C, Potamitis M, et al. The role of short-chain fatty acids in health and disease. Adv Immunol 2014;121:91–119.

[84] Myers SP. The causes of intestinal dysbiosis: a review. Altern Med Rev 2004;9(2):180–97.

[85] Tuohy KM, Conterno L, Gasperotti M, et al. Up-regulating the human intestinal microbiome using whole plant foods, polyphenols, and/or fiber. J Agric Food Chem 2012;60(36):8776–82.

[86] Langdon A, Crook N, Dantas G. The effects of antibiotics on the microbiome throughout development and alternative approaches for therapeutic modulation. Genome Med 2016;8(1):1.

[87] Francino M. Antibiotics and the human gut microbiome: dysbioses and accumulation of resistances. Front Microbiol 2016;6:1543.

[88] Marra F, Lynd L, Coombes M, et al. Does antibiotic exposure during infancy lead to development of asthma?: a systematic review and metaanalysis. Chest 2006;129(3):610–18.

[89] Trasande L, Blustein J, Liu M, et al. Infant antibiotic exposures and early-life body mass. Int J Obes 2013;37(1):16–23.

[90] Shaw SY, Blanchard JF, Bernstein CN. Association between the use of antibiotics in the first year of life and pediatric inflammatory bowel disease. Am J Gastroenterol 2010;105(12):2687–92.

[91] Tamay Z, Akcay A, Ones U, et al. Prevalence and risk factors for allergic rhinitis in primary school children. Int J Pediatr Otorhinolaryngol 2007;71(3):463–71.

[92] Dethlefsen L, Relman DA. Incomplete recovery and individualized responses of the human distal gut microbiota to repeated antibiotic perturbation. Proc Natl Acad Sci USA 2011;108(Suppl. 1):4554–61.

[93] Servin AL, Coconnier MH. Adhesion of probiotic strains to the intestinal mucosa and interaction with pathogens. Best Prac Res Clin Gastroenterol 2003;17(5):741–54.

[94] Agans R, Rigsbee L, Kenche H, et al. Distal gut microbiota of adolescent children is different from that of adults. FEMS Microbiol Ecol 2011;77(2):404–12.

[95] Toga AW, Thompson PM, Sowell ER. Mapping brain maturation. Trends Neurosci 2006;29(3):148–59.

[96] Largo RH, Fischer JE, Rousson V. Neuromotor development from kindergarten age to adolescence: developmental course and variability. Swiss Med Wkly 2003;133(13–14):193–9.

[97] Hetherington EM, Parke RD, Locke VO. Child psychology: a contemporary viewpoint. New York, NY: McGraw-Hill; 1999.

[98] Rappley KJ. Developmental-behavioral pediatrics. In: Levine MD, Carey WB, Crocker AC, editors. Developmental behavioral practices. 4th ed. Philadelphia, PA: WB Saunders Company; 2009.

[99] Adi-Japha E, Freeman NH. Development of differentiation between writing and drawing systems. Dev Psychol 2001;37(1):101–14.

[100] Bakan R. The role of zinc in anorexia nervosa: etiology and treatment. Med Hypotheses 1979;5(7):731–6.

[101] Wisniewski SL. Child nutrition, health problems, and school achievement in Sri Lanka. World Dev 2010;38(3):315–32.

[102] Bourre JM. Roles of unsaturated fatty acids (especially omega-3 fatty acids) in the brain at various ages and during ageing. J Nutr Health Aging 2004;8(3):163–74.

[103] Innis SM. Dietary omega 3 fatty acids and the developing brain. Brain Res 2008;1237:35–43.

[104] Harris M. The fish paradox: are maternal omega-3 (n-3) DHA and selenium (Se) intake protective against negative effects of methylmercury exposure on infant cognitive development? Vitam Miner 2014;3:e126.

[105] Nesheim MC, Yaktine AL, editors. Seafood choices. Washington DC: National Academies Press; 2006.

[106] Peacock M. Calcium absorption efficiency and calcium requirements in children and adolescents. Am J Clin Nutr 1991;54(1 Suppl.):261s–5s.

[107] Hegsted DM. Fractures, calcium, and the modern diet. Am J Clin Nutr 2001;74(5):571–3.

[108] Australian Government. Nutrient reference values for Australia and New Zealand. Canberra, ACT: Department of Health and Aging; 2005.

[109] Matkovic V. Calcium and peak bone mass. J Intern Med 1992;231(2):151–60.

[110] Hind K, Burrows M. Weight-bearing exercise and bone mineral accrual in children and adolescents: a review of controlled trials. Bone 2007;40(1):14–27.

[111] Reed JA, Anderson JJ, Tylavsky FA, et al. Comparative changes in radial-bone density of elderly female lacto-ovovegetarians and omnivores. Am J Clin Nutr 1994;59(5 Suppl.):1197s–202s.

[112] Larsson CL, Johansson GK. Dietary intake and nutritional status of young vegans and omnivores in Sweden. Am J Clin Nutr 2002;76(1):100–6.

[113] Kohlenberg-Mueller K, Raschka L. Calcium balance in young adults on a vegan and lactovegetarian diet. J Bone Miner Metab 2003;21(1):28–33.

[114] Burckhardt P. The role of low acid load in vegetarian diet on bone health: a narrative review. Swiss Med Wkly 2016;146:w14277.

[115] Gordon CM, Feldman HA, Sinclair L, et al. Prevalence of vitamin D deficiency among healthy infants and toddlers. Arch Pediatr Adolesc Med 2008;162(6):505–12.

[116] Gordon CM, DePeter KC, Feldman HA, et al. Prevalence of vitamin D deficiency among healthy adolescents. Arch Pediatr Adolesc Med 2004;158(6):531–7.

[117] Viljakainen HT, Natri AM, Karkkainen M, et al. A positive dose-response effect of vitamin D supplementation on site-specific bone mineral augmentation in adolescent girls: a double-blinded randomized placebo-controlled 1-year intervention. J Bone Miner Res 2006;21(6):836–44.

[118] Liu PT, Stenger S, Li H, et al. Toll-like receptor triggering of a vitamin D-mediated human antimicrobial response. Science 2006;311(5768):1770–3.

[119] Sismanlar T, Aslan AT, Gulbahar O, et al. The effect of vitamin D on lower respiratory tract infections in children. Turk Pediatri Arsivi 2016;51(2):94–9.

[120] McNally JD, Leis K, Matheson LA, et al. Vitamin D deficiency in young children with severe acute lower respiratory infection. Pediatr Pulmonol 2009;44(10):981–8.

[121] Bozzetto S, Carraro S, Giordano G, et al. Asthma, allergy and respiratory infections: the vitamin D hypothesis. Allergy 2012;67(1):10–17.

[122] Esposito S, Baggi E, Bianchini S, et al. Role of vitamin D in children with respiratory tract infection. Int J Immunopathol Pharmacol 2013;26(1):1–13.

[123] Roth DE, Shah R, Black RE, et al. Vitamin D status and acute lower respiratory infection in early childhood in Sylhet, Bangladesh. Acta Paediatr 2010;99(3):389–93.

[124] Munns CF, Simm PJ, Rodda CP, et al. Incidence of vitamin D deficiency rickets among Australian children: an Australian Paediatric Surveillance Unit study. Med J Aust 2012;196(7):466–8.

[125] Gartner LM, Greer FR. Prevention of rickets and vitamin D deficiency: new guidelines for vitamin D intake. Pediatrics 2003;111(4 Pt 1):908–10.

[126] Robinson PD, Hogler W, Craig ME, et al. The re-emerging burden of rickets: a decade of experience from Sydney. Arch Dis Child 2006;91(7):564–8.

[127] Nowson CA, Margerison C. Vitamin D intake and vitamin D status of Australians. Med J Aust 2002;177(3):149–52.

[128] Casey CF, Slawson DC, Neal LR. Vitamin D supplementation in infants, children, and adolescents. Am Fam Physician 2010;81(6):745–8.

[129] Kleigman R, Stanton B, St Geme J, et al, editors. Nelson textbook of pediatrics. 19th ed. Philadelphia, PA: Elsevier Saunders; 2011.

[130] Remsberg KE, Demerath EW, Schubert CM, et al. Early menarche and the development of cardiovascular disease risk factors in adolescent girls: the Fels Longitudinal Study. JCEM 2005;90(5):2718–24.

[131] Adair LS, Gordon-Larsen P. Maturational timing and overweight prevalence in US adolescent girls. Am J Public Health 2001;91(4):642.

[132] Buttke DE, Sircar K, Martin C. Exposures to endocrine-disrupting chemicals and age of menarche in adolescent girls in NHANES (2003–2008). Environ Health Perspect 2012;120(11):1613.

[133] Euling SY, Selevan SG, Pescovitz OH, et al. Role of environmental factors in the timing of puberty. Pediatrics 2008;121(Suppl. 3):S167–71.

[134] Story M. Textbook of adolescent medicine. In: McAnarney ER, Kreipe RE, Orr DE, et al, editors. Textbook of adolescent medicine. Philadelphia, PA: WB Saunders; 1992. p. 21–34.

[135] Australian Government, National Health and Medical Research Council. Protein; 2014. Available from https://www.nrv.gov.au/nutrients/protein.

[136] Australian Government. Dietary fibre 2014. Available from https://www.nrv.gov.au/nutrients/dietary-fibre.

[137] Salam RA, Hooda M, Das JK, et al. Interventions to improve adolescent nutrition: a systematic review and meta-analysis. J Adolesc Health 2016;59(4s):S29–39.

[138] Moran VH, Stammers AL, Medina MW, et al. The relationship between zinc intake and serum/plasma zinc concentration in children: a systematic review and dose-response meta-analysis. Nutrients 2012;4(8):841–58.

[139] Aksglaede L, Olsen LW, Sorensen TI, et al. Forty years trends in timing of pubertal growth spurt in 157,000 Danish school children. PLoS ONE 2008;3(7):e2728.

[140] King JC. Does poor zinc nutriture retard skeletal growth and mineralization in adolescents? Am J Clin Nutr 1996;64(3):375–6.

[141] Slemenda CW, Reister TK, Hui SL, et al. Influences on skeletal mineralization in children and adolescents: evidence for varying effects of sexual maturation and physical activity. J Pediatr 1994;125(2):201–7.

[142] Bouglé DL, Sabatier JP, Guaydier-Souquières G, et al. Zinc status and bone mineralisation in adolescent girls. J Trace Elem Med Biol 2004;18(1):17–21.

[143] Clark PJ, Eastell R, Barker ME. Zinc supplementation and bone growth in pubertal girls. Lancet 1999;354(9177):485.

[144] Gibson RS, Hess SY, Hotz C, et al. Indicators of zinc status at the population level: a review of the evidence. Br J Nutr 2008; 99(Suppl. 3):S14–23.

[145] Shankar AH, Prasad AS. Zinc and immune function: the biological basis of altered resistance to infection. Am J Clin Nutr 1998; 68(2 Suppl.):447s–63s.

[146] Mayo-Wilson E, Junior JA, Imdad A, et al. Zinc supplementation for preventing mortality, morbidity, and growth failure in children aged 6 months to 12 years of age. Cochrane Database Syst Rev 2014;(5):CD009384.

[147] Moran VH, Stammers A-L, Medina MW, et al. The relationship between zinc intake and serum/plasma zinc concentration in children: a systematic review and dose-response meta-analysis. Nutrients 2012;4(8):841–58.

[148] Gibson RS, Heath AL, Ferguson EL. Risk of suboptimal iron and zinc nutriture among adolescent girls in Australia and New Zealand: causes, consequences, and solutions. Asia Pacific J Clin Nutr 2002;11(Suppl. 3):S543–52.

[149] Lopresti AL. A review of nutrient treatments for paediatric depression. J Affect Disord 2015;181:24–32.

[150] Prasad AS. Impact of the discovery of human zinc deficiency on health. J Am Coll Nutr 2009;28(3):257–65.

[151] Weaver LT, Steiner H. The bowel habit of young children. Arch Dis Child 1984;59(7):649–52.

[152] Velde SV, Notebaert A, Meersschaut V, et al. Colon transit time in healthy children and adolescents. Int J Colorectal Dis 2013;28(12):1721–4.

[153] Tobias N. Management principles of organic causes of childhood constipation. J Pediatr Health Care 2008;22(6):398.

[154] Arnaud MJ. Mild dehydration: a risk factor of constipation? Eur J Clin Nutr 2003;57(Suppl. 2):S88–95.

[155] Rajindrajith S, Devanarayana NM. Constipation in children: novel insight into epidemiology, pathophysiology and management. J Neurogastroenterol Motil 2011;17(1):35–47.

[156] Youssef NN, Di Lorenzo C. Childhood constipation: evaluation and treatment. J Clin Gastroenterol 2001;33(3):199–205.

[157] Khalif IL, Quigley EM, Konovitch EA, et al. Alterations in the colonic flora and intestinal permeability and evidence of immune activation in chronic constipation. Dig Liver Dis 2005;37(11):838–49.

[158] Homsy Y. Dysfunctional voiding disorders and nocturnal enuresis. In: Bellman B, King LR, Kramer SA, editors. Clinical pediatric urology. London: CRC Press; 2002.

[159] Afzal NA, Tighe MP, Thomson MA. Constipation in children. Ital J Pediatr 2011;37(1):1–10.

[160] El-Hodhod MA-A, Hamdy AM, El-Deeb MT, et al. Cow's milk allergy is a major contributor in recurrent perianal dermatitis of infants. ISRN Pediatr 2012;2012:408769.

[161] Elli L, Roncoroni L, Bardella MT. Non-celiac gluten sensitivity: time for sifting the grain. World J Gastroenterol 2015;21(27):8221.

[162] Coccorullo P, Strisciuglio C, Martinelli M, et al. Lactobacillus reuteri (DSM 17938) in infants with functional chronic constipation: a double-blind, randomized, placebo-controlled study. J Pediatr 2010;157(4):598–602.

[163] Pitkala KH, Strandberg TE, Finne Soveri UH, et al. Fermented cereal with specific bifidobacteria normalizes bowel movements in elderly nursing home residents. A randomized, controlled trial. J Nutr Health Aging 2007;11(4):305–11.

[164] Matsumoto M, Ohishi H, Benno Y. Impact of LKM512 yogurt on improvement of intestinal environment of the elderly. FEMS Immunol Med Microbiol 2001;31(3):181–6.

[165] Meance S, Cayuela C, Turchet P, et al. A fermented milk with a Bifidobacterium probiotic strain DN-173 010 shortened oro-fecal gut transit time in elderly. Microb Ecol Health Dis 2001;13(4):217–22.

[166] Koebnick C, Wagner I, Leitzmann P, et al. Probiotic beverage containing Lactobacillus casei Shirota improves gastrointestinal symptoms in patients with chronic constipation. Can J Gastroenterol 2003;17(11):655–9.

[167] Umesaki Y. Effect of L. casei strain Shirota on large intestinal function, bowel movements, and fecal properties. In: Yokokura T, editor. Lactobacillus casei strain Shirota—intestinal flora and human health. Tokyo: Yakult Honsha; 1999. p. 119–28.

[168] Mollenbrink M, Bruckschen E. Treatment of chronic constipation with physiologic Escherichia coli bacteria. Results of a clinical study of the effectiveness and tolerance of microbiological therapy with the E. coli Nissle 1917 strain (Mutaflor). Med Klin (Munich) 1994;89(11):587–93.

[169] Ouwehand AC, Lagstrom H, Suomalainen T, et al. Effect of probiotics on constipation, fecal azoreductase activity and fecal mucin content in the elderly. Ann Nutr Metab 2002;46(3–4):159–62.

[170] Higashikawa F, Noda M, Awaya T, et al. Improvement of constipation and liver function by plant-derived lactic acid bacteria: a double-blind, randomized trial. Nutrition 2010;26(4):367–74.

[171] Jonkers IJ, Ledeboer M, Steens J, et al. Effects of very long chain versus long chain triglycerides on gastrointestinal motility and hormone release in humans. Dig Dis Sci 2000;45(9):1719–26.

[172] Treepongkaruna S, Simakachorn N, Pienvichit P, et al. A randomised, double-blind study of polyethylene glycol 4000 and lactulose in the treatment of constipation in children. BMC Pediatr 2014;14(1):1.

[173] Bothe G, Coh A, Auinger A. Efficacy and safety of a natural mineral water rich in magnesium and sulphate for bowel function: a double-blind, randomized, placebo-controlled study. Eur J Nutr 2015;56(2):491–9.

[174] Fewtrell D, editor. Lecture and notes from MINDD International Forum on Children. 2009.

[175] El-Hodhod MA, Younis NT, Zaitoun YA, et al. Cow's milk allergy related pediatric constipation: appropriate time of milk tolerance. Pediatr Allergy Immunol 2010;21(2 Pt 2):e407–12.

[176] Chang CC, Lin YT, Lu YT, et al. Kiwifruit improves bowel function in patients with irritable bowel syndrome with constipation. Asia Pac J Clin Nutr 2010;19(4):451–7.

[177] Glatstein M, Reif S, Scolnik D, et al. Lactose breath test in children: relationship between symptoms during the test and test results. Am J Ther 2016;25(2):1.

[178] Fitton N, Thomas JS. Gastrointestinal dysfunction. Surgery 2009;27(11):492–5.

[179] Loo M. Integrative medicine for children. 1st ed. Saint Louis: W.B. Saunders; 2009.

[180] Chen CC, Walker WA. Probiotics and prebiotics: role in clinical disease states. Adv Pediatr 2005;52:77–113.

[181] Caeiro JP, Mathewson JJ, Smith MA, et al. Etiology of outpatient pediatric nondysenteric diarrhea: a multicenter study in the United States. Pediatr Infect Dis J 1999;18(2):94–7.

[182] Friesema IH, de Boer RF, Duizer E, et al. Etiology of acute gastroenteritis in children requiring hospitalization in the Netherlands. Eur J Clin Microbiol Infect Dis 2012;31(4):405–15.

[183] Dennehy PH. Acute diarrheal disease in children: epidemiology, prevention, and treatment. Infect Dis Clin North Am 2005;19(3):585–602.

[184] Zella GC, Israel EJ. Chronic diarrhea in children. Pediatr Rev 2012;33(5):207–17, quiz 217–18.

[185] Ericsson CD, Hatz C, DuPont AW. Postinfectious irritable bowel syndrome. Clin Infect Dis 2008;46(4):594–9.

[186] Adams W, Bratt DE. Young coconut water for home rehydration in children with mild gastroenteritis. Trop Geogr Med 1992;44(1–2):149–53.

[187] Vigliar R, Sdepanian VL, Fagundes-Neto U. Biochemical profile of coconut water from coconut palms planted in an inland region. J Pediatr (Rio J) 2006;82(4):308–12.

[188] Ismail T, Sestili P, Akhtar S. Pomegranate peel and fruit extracts: a review of potential anti-inflammatory and anti-infective effects. J Ethnopharmacol 2012;143(2):397–405.

[189] De-Souza DA, Greene LJ. Intestinal permeability and systemic infections in critically ill patients: effect of glutamine. Crit Care Med 2005;33(5):1125–35.

[190] Mittra D, Bukutu C, Vohra S. Complementary, holistic, and integrative medicine: a review of therapies for diarrhea. Pediatr Rev 2008;29(10):349–53.

[191] Isolauri E. The role of probiotics in paediatrics. Curr Pediatr 2004;14(2):104–9.

[192] Isolauri E. Probiotics for infectious diarrhoea. Gut 2003;52(3):436–7.

[193] Szajewska H, Kotowska M, Mrukowicz JZ, et al. Efficacy of Lactobacillus GG in prevention of nosocomial diarrhea in infants. J Pediatr 2001;138(3):361–5.

[194] Donato KA, Gareau MG, Wang YJ, et al. Lactobacillus rhamnosus GG attenuates interferon-{gamma} and tumour necrosis factor-alpha-induced barrier dysfunction and pro-inflammatory signalling. Microbiology 2010;156(Pt 11):3288–97.

[195] Hayes SR, Vargas AJ. Probiotics for the prevention of pediatric antibiotic-associated diarrhea. Explore (NY) 2016;62(3):495–506.

[196] Szajewska H, Skorka A, Dylag M. Meta-analysis: Saccharomyces boulardii for treating acute diarrhoea in children. Aliment Pharmacol Ther 2007;25(3):257–64.

[197] Dinleyici EC, Eren M, Dogan N, et al. Clinical efficacy of Saccharomyces boulardii or metronidazole in symptomatic children with Blastocystis hominis infection. Parasitol Res 2011;108(3):541–5.

[198] Roy SK, Tomkins AM. The impact of experimental zinc deficiency on growth, morbidity and ultrastructural development of intestinal tissue. Bangladesh J Nutr 1989;2:1–7.

[199] Hoque KM, Binder HJ. Zinc in the treatment of acute diarrhea: current status and assessment. Gastroenterology 2006;130(7):2201–5.

[200] World Gastroenterology Organisation. Acute diarrhea in adults and children: a global perspective; 2012. Available from http://www.worldgastroenterology.org/guidelines/global-guidelines/acute-diarrhea/acute-diarrhea-english.

[201] Perdigon G, Nader de Macias ME, Alvarez S, et al. Prevention of gastrointestinal infection using immunobiological methods with milk fermented with Lactobacillus casei and Lactobacillus acidophilus. J Dairy Res 1990;57(2):255–64.

[202] Hawrelak JA. Prebiotics, synbiotics, and colonic foods. In: Pizzorno J, Murray M, editors. Textbook of natural medicine. St Louis: Elsevier; 2013. p. 966–78.

[203] Biesiekierski JR, Rosella O, Rose R, et al. Quantification of fructans, galacto-oligosaccharides and other short-chain carbohydrates in processed grains and cereals. J Hum Nutr Diet 2011;24(2):154–76.

[204] Perez-Jimenez J, Neveu V, Vos F, et al. Identification of the 100 richest dietary sources of polyphenols: an application of the Phenol-Explorer database. Eur J Clin Nutr 2010;64(Suppl. 3):S112–20.

[205] Hughes S, Clark J. Investigation of recurrent infection. Paediatr Child Health 2008;18(11):483–90.

[206] Ballow M. Approach to the patient with recurrent infections. Clin Rev Allergy Immunol 2008;34(2):129–40.

[207] Alkhater SA. Approach to the child with recurrent infections. J Family Community Med 2009;16(3):77–82.

[208] Genoni G, Prodam F, Marolda A, et al. Obesity and infection: two sides of one coin. Eur J Pediatr 2014;173(1):25–32.

[209] Jedrychowski W, Maugeri U, Flak E, et al. Cohort study on low physical activity level and recurrent acute respiratory infections in schoolchildren. Cent Eur J Public Health 2001;9(3):126–9.

[210] Aghamohammadi A, Abolhassani H, Mohammadinejad P, et al. The approach to children with recurrent infections. Iran J Allergy Asthma Immunol 2012;11(2):89–109.

[211] Savastio S, Cadario F, Genoni G, et al. Vitamin D deficiency and glycemic status in children and adolescents with type 1 diabetes mellitus. PLoS ONE 2016;11(9):e0162554.

[212] Steenbruggen TG, Hoekstra SJ, van der Gaag EJ. Could a change in diet revitalize children who suffer from unresolved fatigue? Nutrients 2015;7(3):1965–77.

[213] Fraker PJ, King LE, Laakko T, et al. The dynamic link between the integrity of the immune system and zinc status. J Nutr 2000; 130(5S Suppl.):1399s–406s.

[214] Fraker PJ. Roles for cell death in zinc deficiency. J Nutr 2005;135(3):359–62.

[215] Mocchegiani E, Ciavattini A, Santarelli L, et al. Role of zinc and alpha2 macroglobulin on thymic endocrine activity and on peripheral immune efficiency (natural killer activity and interleukin 2) in cervical carcinoma. Br J Cancer 1999;79(2):244–50.

[216] Beisel W. Zinc and the immune system. In: Ratcliffe M, editor. Encyclopedia of Immunobiology. Oxford, UK: Academic Press; 2004. p. 2515–16.

[217] Singh M, Das RR. Zinc for the common cold. Cochrane Database Syst Rev 2013;(6):CD001364.

[218] Lassi ZS, Haider BA, Bhutta ZA. Zinc supplementation for the prevention of pneumonia in children aged 2 months to 59 months. Cochrane Database Syst Rev 2010;(12):CD005978.

[219] Larson CP, Nasrin D, Saha A, et al. The added benefit of zinc supplementation after zinc treatment of acute childhood diarrhoea: a randomized, double-blind field trial. Trop Med Int Health 2010;15(6):754–61.

[220] Barrie SA, Wright JV, Pizzorno JE, et al. Comparative absorption of zinc picolinate, zinc citrate and zinc gluconate in humans. Agents Actions 1987;21(1–2):223–8.

[221] Salgueiro MJ, Zubillaga M, Lysionek A, et al. Zinc as an essential micronutrient: a review. Nutr Res 2000;20(5):737–55.

[222] Solomons NW. Zinc. In: Caballero B, Trugo LC, Finglas PM, editors. Encyclopedia of food sciences and nutrition. Amsterdam: Elsevier; 2003. p. 6272–7.

[223] Wedner SH, Ross DA. Vitamin A deficiency and its prevention. In: Heggenhougen H, Quah S, editors. International encyclopedia of public health. Boston: Academic Press; 2008. p. 526–32.

[224] Cunningham-Rundles S, McNeeley DF, Moon A. Mechanisms of nutrient modulation of the immune response. J Allergy Clin Immunol 2005;115(6):1119–28, quiz 1129.

[225] Hanekom WA, Hussey GD. Vitamin A and immunity against infections. Clin Immunol Newsletter 1996;16(7):101–6.

[226] Ahmed F, Jones DB, Jackson AA. The interaction of vitamin A deficiency and rotavirus infection in the mouse. Br J Nutr 1990;63(2):363–73.

[227] Stephensen CB, Blount SR, Schoeb TR, et al. Vitamin A deficiency impairs some aspects of the host response to influenza A virus infection in BALB/c mice. J Nutr 1993;123(5):823–33.

[228] Bates CJ. Vitamin A. Lancet 1995;345(8941):31–5.

[229] Semba RD. Vitamin A, immunity, and infection. Clin Infect Dis 1994;19(3):489–99.

[230] Yilmaz T, Kocan EG, Besler HT, et al. The role of oxidants and antioxidants in otitis media with effusion in children. Otolaryngol Head Neck Surg 2004;131(6):797–803.

[231] Inamo Y, Hasegawa M, Saito K, et al. Serum vitamin D concentrations and associated severity of acute lower respiratory tract infections in Japanese hospitalized children. Pediatr Int 2011;53(2):199–201.

[232] Hewison M. An update on vitamin D and human immunity. Clin Endocrinol (Oxf) 2012;76(3):315–25.

[233] Cantorna MT, Zhu Y, Froicu M, et al. Vitamin D status, 1, 25-dihydroxyvitamin D3, and the immune system. Am J Clin Nutr 2004;80(6):1717S–20S.

[234] Willis K, Broughton K, Larson-Meyer D. Vitamin D status and immune system biomarkers in athletes. J Am Diet Assoc 2009;109(9):A15.

[235] Munns C, Zacharin MR, Rodda CP, et al. Prevention and treatment of infant and childhood vitamin D deficiency in Australia and New Zealand: a consensus statement. Med J Aust 2006;185(5):268–72.

[236] Holick MF, Binkley NC, Bischoff-Ferrari HA, et al. Evaluation, treatment, and prevention of vitamin D deficiency: an Endocrine Society clinical practice guideline. J Clin Endocrinol Metab 2011;96(7):1911–30.

[237] Prietl B, Treiber G, Pieber TR, et al. Vitamin D and immune function. Nutrients 2013;5(7):2502–21.

[238] Urashima M, Segawa T, Okazaki M, et al. Randomized trial of vitamin D supplementation to prevent seasonal influenza A in schoolchildren. Am J Clin Nutr 2010;91(5):1255–60.

[239] Werbach MR. Nutritional strategies for treating chronic fatigue syndrome. Altern Med Rev 2000;5(2):93–108.

[240] Jamison J. Clinical guide to nutrition & dietary supplements in disease management. Aust J Herb Med 2003;15(4):153–63.

[241] Field CJ. Infection fever and nutrition. In: Caballero B, Trugo LC, Finglas PM, editors. Encyclopedia of food sciences and nutrition. Amsterdam: Academic Press; 2003. p. 3307–15.

[242] Herrmann W, Obeid R. Functions and deficiencies of B-vitamins (and their prevention). In: Heggenhougen H, Quah S, editors. International encyclopedia of public health. US: Elsevier; 2008. p. 677–82.

[243] Glück U, Gebbers J-O. Ingested probiotics reduce nasal colonization with pathogenic bacteria (Staphylococcus aureus, Streptococcus pneumoniae, and β-hemolytic streptococci). Am J Clin Nutr 2003;77(2):517–20.

[244] Hatakka K, Savilahti E, Ponka A, et al. Effect of long term consumption of probiotic milk on infections in children attending day care centres: double blind, randomised trial. BMJ 2001;322(7298):1327.

[245] Shokryazdan P, Faseleh Jahromi M, Navidshad B, et al. Effects of prebiotics on immune system and cytokine expression. Med Microbiol Immunol 2016;206:1–9.

[246] Chiappini E, Principi N, Longhi R, et al. Management of fever in children: summary of the Italian Pediatric Society guidelines. Clin Ther 2009;31(8):1826–43.

[247] NSW Health. Children and infants with fever – acute management; 2010. Available from https://www1.health.nsw.gov.au/pds/ ActivePDSDocuments/PD2010_063.pdf.

[248] Knoebel EE. Fever: to treat or not to treat. Point. Clin Pediatr (Phila) 2002;41(1):9–11.

[249] Doran TF, De Angelis C, Baumgardner RA, et al. Acetaminophen: more harm than good for chickenpox? J Pediatr 1989;114(6):1045–8.

[250] Morris PS, Leach AJ. Acute and chronic otitis media. Pediatr Clin North Am 2009;56(6):1383–99.

[251] Klein JO. The burden of otitis media. Vaccine 2000;19(Suppl. 1):S2–8.

[252] Kotsis GP, Nikolopoulos TP, Yiotakis IE, et al. Recurrent acute otitis media and gastroesophageal reflux disease in children. Is there an association? Int J Pediatr Otorhinolaryngol 2009;73(10):1373–80.

[253] Usonis V, Jackowska T, Petraitiene S, et al. Incidence of acute otitis media in children below 6 years of age seen in medical practices in five East European countries. BMC Pediatr 2016;16(1):108.

[254] Teele DW, Klein JO, Rosner B. Epidemiology of otitis media during the first seven years of life in children in greater Boston: a prospective, cohort study. J Infect Dis 1989;160(1):83–94.

[255] Vergison A, Dagan R, Arguedas A, et al. Otitis media and its consequences: beyond the earache. Lancet Infect Dis 2010;10(3):195–203.

[256] McIntyre M. Herbal treatment of children. Sydney: Elsevier; 2005. p. 1–320.

[257] Turker AU, Camper N. Biological activity of common mullein, a medicinal plant. J Ethnopharmacol 2002;82(2):117–25.

[258] Ninkovic G, Dullo V, Saunders N. Microbiology of otitis externa in the secondary care in United Kingdom and antimicrobial sensitivity. Auris Nasus Larynx 2008;35(4):480–4.

[259] Oğuz F, Ünüvar E, Süoğlu Y, et al. Etiology of acute otitis media in childhood and evaluation of two different protocols of antibiotic therapy: 10 days cefaclor vs. 3 days azithromycin. Int J Pediatr Otorhinolaryngol 2003;67(1):43–51.

[260] Johnson NC, Holger JS. Pediatric acute otitis media: the case for delayed antibiotic treatment. J Emerg Med 2007;32(3):279–84.

[261] Taylor PS, Faeth I, Marks MK, et al. Cost of treating otitis media in Australia. Expert Rev Pharmacoecon Outcomes Res 2009;9(2):133–41.

[262] Bollag U, Bollag-Albrecht E. Recommendations derived from practice audit for the treatment of acute otitis media. Lancet 1991;338(8759):96–9.

[263] Burke P, Bain J, Robinson D, et al. Acute red ear in children: controlled trial of non-antibiotic treatment in general practice. BMJ 1991;303(6802):558–62.

[264] Chung A, Perera R, Brueggemann AB, et al. Effect of antibiotic prescribing on antibiotic resistance in individual children in primary care: prospective cohort study. BMJ 2007;335(7617):429.

[265] Del Mar C. Childhood otitis media i. general practitioner view. Aust Prescr 1994;17(4).

[266] Morris PS. Upper respiratory tract infections (including otitis media). Pediatr Clin North Am 2009;56(1):101–17.

[267] Aladag I, Guven M, Eyibilen A, et al. Efficacy of vitamin A in experimentally induced acute otitis media. Int J Pediatr Otorhinolaryngol 2007;71(4):623–8.

[268] Cemek M, Dede S, Bayiroğlu F, et al. Oxidant and antioxidant levels in children with acute otitis media and tonsillitis: a comparative study. Int J Pediatr Otorhinolaryngol 2005;69(6):823–7.

[269] Parks RR, Huang CC, Haddad J. Evidence of oxygen radical injury in experimental otitis media. Laryngoscope 1994;104(11):1389–92.

[270] Takoudes TG, Haddad J. Free radical production by antibiotic-killed bacteria in the guinea pig middle ear. Laryngoscope 2001;111(2):283–9.

[271] Blewett HJH, Cicalo MC, Holland CD, et al. The immunological components of human milk. Adv Food Nutr Res 2008;54:45–80.

[272] Duncan B, Ey J, Holberg CJ, et al. Exclusive breast-feeding for at least 4 months protects against otitis media. Pediatrics 1993;91(5):867–72.

[273] Chung M, Raman G, Chew P, et al. Breastfeeding and maternal and infant health outcomes in developed countries. Evid Technol Asses (Full Rep) 2007;153:1–186.

[274] Golding J, Emmett PM, Rogers IS. Does breast feeding protect against non-gastric infections? Early Hum Dev 1997;49:S105–20.

[275] Park K, Lim DJ. Development of secretory elements in murine tubotympanum: lysozyme and lactoferrin immunohistochemistry. Ann Otol Rhinol Laryngol 1993;102(5):385–95.

[276] Cummin AG, Thompson FM. Postnatal changes in mucosal immune response: a physiological perspective of breast feeding and weaning. Immunol Cell Biol 1997;75(5).

[277] Donovan SM. Role of human milk components in gastrointestinal development: current knowledge and future needs. J Pediatr 2006;149(5):S49–61.

[278] Lönnerdal B. Nutritional and physiologic significance of human milk proteins. Am J Clin Nutr 2003;77(6):1537S–43S.

[279] Rynnel-Dagöö B, Ågren K. The nasopharynx and the middle ear. Inflammatory reactions in middle ear disease. Vaccine 2000;19:S26–31.

[280] Sharma S, Anderson M, Schoop S, et al. Bactericidal and anti-inflammatory properties of a standardized Echinacea extract (Echinaforce®): dual actions against respiratory bacteria. Phytomedicine 2010;17(8):563–8.

[281] Sarrell EM, Cohen HA, Kahan E. Naturopathic treatment for ear pain in children. Pediatrics 2003;111(5):e574–9.

[282] Sarrell EM, Mandelberg A, Cohen HA. Efficacy of naturopathic extracts in the management of ear pain associated with acute otitis media. Arch Pediatr Adolesc Med 2001;155(7):796–9.

[283] Erickson K, Shalts E, Kligler B. Case study in integrative medicine: Jared C, a child with recurrent otitis media and upper respiratory illness. Explore (NY) 2006;2(3):235–7.

[284] Berman S. Otitis media in developing countries. Pediatrics 1995;96(1 Pt 1):126–31.

[285] World Health Organization. Chronic suppurative otitis media: burden of illness and management options. Switzerland: WHO; 2004.

[286] Esposito S, Rigante D, Principi N. Do children's upper respiratory tract infections benefit from probiotics? BMC Infect Dis 2014;14(1):1.

[287] Rautava S, Salminen S, Isolauri E. Specific probiotics in reducing the risk of acute infections in infancy – a randomised,

double-blind, placebo-controlled study. Br J Nutr 2009; 101(11):1722–6.

[288] Marchisio P, Consonni D, Baggi E, et al. Vitamin D supplementation reduces the risk of acute otitis media in otitis-prone children. Pediatr Infect Dis J 2013;32(10):1055–60.

[289] Aladag I, Guven M, Eyibilen A, et al. Efficacy of vitamin A in experimentally induced acute otitis media. Int J Pediatr Otorhinolaryngol 2007;71(4):623–8.

[290] Uhari M, Tapiainen T, Kontiokari T. Xylitol in preventing acute otitis media. Vaccine 2000;19:S144–7.

[291] Vernacchio L, Vezina RM, Mitchell AA. Tolerability of oral xylitol solution in young children: implications for otitis media prophylaxis. Int J Pediatr Otorhinolaryngol 2007;71(1): 89–94.

[292] Stelter K. Tonsillitis and sore throat in children. GMS Curr Top Otorhinolaryngol Head Neck Surg 2014;13.

[293] Graziella O, Cardona F, Cox C, et al. Pediatric autoimmune neuropsychiatric disorders associated with streptococcal infections (PANDAS). In: Ferretti J, Stevens D, Fischetti V, editors. Streptococcus pyogenes: basic biology to clinical manifestations. Oklahoma City: University of Oklahoma Health Sciences Center; 2016.

[294] Macerollo A, Martino D. Pediatric autoimmune neuropsychiatric disorders associated with streptococcal infections (PANDAS): an evolving concept. Tremor Other Hyperkinet Mov (N Y) 2013; 25:3.

[295] Ciuman RR. Phytotherapeutic and naturopathic adjuvant therapies in otorhinolaryngology. Eur Arch Otorhinolaryngol 2012;269(2):389–97.

[296] Melchart D, Linde K, Fischer P, et al. Echinacea for preventing and treating the common cold. Cochrane Database Syst Rev 2000;(2):CD000530.

[297] Schoop R, Klein P, Suter A, et al. Echinacea in the prevention of induced rhinovirus colds: a meta-analysis. Clin Ther 2006;28(2):174–83.

[298] Arora D, Rani A, Sharma A. A review on phytochemistry and ethnopharmacological aspects of genus Calendula. Pharmacogn Rev 2013;7(14):179.

[299] Rau E. Treatment of acute tonsillitis with a fixed-combination herbal preparation. Adv Ther 2000;17(4):197–203.

[300] Cowan MM. Plant products as antimicrobial agents. Clin Microbiol Rev 1999;12(4):564–82.

[301] Carter DA, Blair SE, Cokcetin NN, et al. Therapeutic manuka honey: no longer so alternative. Front Microbiol 2016;7.

[302] Ozlugedik S, Genc S, Unal A, et al. Can postoperative pains following tonsillectomy be relieved by honey? A prospective, randomized, placebo controlled preliminary study. Int J Pediatr Otorhinolaryngol 2006;70(11):1929–34.

[303] Boroumand P, Zamani MM, Saeedi M, et al. Post tonsillectomy pain: can honey reduce the analgesic requirements? Anesth Pain Med 2013;3(1):198–202.

[304] Georgalas CC, Tolley NS, Narula A. Recurrent throat infections (tonsillitis). BMJ Clin Evid 2007;June.

[305] Jensen JH, Larsen SB. Treatment of recurrent acute tonsillitis with clindamycin. An alternative to tonsillectomy? Clin Otolaryngol Allied Sci 1991;16(5):498–500.

[306] Hultcrantz E, Ericsson E. Factors influencing the indication for tonsillectomy: a historical overview and current concepts. ORL J Otorhinolaryngol Relat Spec 2013;75(3):184–91.

[307] van Kempen MJ, Rijkers GT, Van Cauwenberge PB. The immune response in adenoids and tonsils. Int Arch Allergy Immunol 2000;122(1):8–19.

[308] Choi HG, Park B, Sim S, et al. Tonsillectomy does not reduce upper respiratory infections: a national cohort study. PLoS ONE 2016;11(12):e0169264.

[309] Sinha S, Relhan V, Garg VK. Immunomodulators in warts: unexplored or ineffective? Indian J Dermatol 2015;60(2):118.

[310] Ibs KH, Rink L. Zinc-altered immune function. J Nutr 2003;133(5 Suppl. 1):1452s–6s.

[311] Fraker PJ, King LE. Reprogramming of the immune system during zinc deficiency. Annu Rev Nutr 2004;24:277–98.

[312] Sharquie KE, Khorsheed AA, Al-Nuaimy AA. Topical zinc sulphate solution for treatment of viral warts. Saudi Med J 2007;28(9):1418–21.

[313] Khattar JA, Musharrafieh UM, Tamim H, et al. Topical zinc oxide vs. salicylic acid-lactic acid combination in the treatment of warts. Int J Dermatol 2007;46(4):427–30.

[314] Gupta M, Mahajan VK, Mehta KS, et al. Zinc therapy in dermatology: a review. Dermatol Res Pract 2014;2014.

[315] McCollum AM, Holman RC, Hughes CM, et al. Molluscum contagiosum in a pediatric American Indian population: incidence and risk factors. PLoS ONE 2014;9(7):e103419.

[316] Sladden MJ, Johnston GA. Common skin infections in children. BMJ 2004;329(7457):95–9.

[317] Chen X, Anstey AV, Bugert JJ. Molluscum contagiosum virus infection. Lancet Infect Dis 2013;13(10):877–88.

[318] Burke BE, Baillie JE, Olson RD. Essential oil of Australian lemon myrtle (Backhousia citriodora) in the treatment of molluscum contagiosum in children. Biomed Pharmacother 2004;58(4):245–7.

[319] Markum E, Baillie J. Combination of essential oil of Melaleuca alternifolia and iodine in the treatment of molluscum contagiosum in children. J Drugs Dermatol 2012;11(3):349–54.

[320] American Academy of Allergy, Asthma & Immunology. Atopy; 2016. Available from https://www.aaaai.org/conditions-and -treatments/conditions-dictionary/atopy.

[321] Schneider L, Hanifin J, Boguniewicz M, et al. Study of the atopic march: development of atopic comorbidities. Pediatr Dermatol 2016;33(4):388–98.

[322] Wahn U. The atopic march; 2015. Available from http:// www.worldallergy.org/professional/allergic_diseases_center/ allergic_march/.

[323] Ricci G, Patrizi A, Giannetti A, et al. Does improvement management of atopic dermatitis influence the appearance of respiratory allergic diseases? A follow-up study. Clin Mol Allergy 2010;8(1):1.

[324] Ricci G, Bellini F, Dondi A, et al. Atopic dermatitis in adolescence. Dermatol Reports 2012;4(1).

[325] Kijima A, Murota H, Takahashi A, et al. Prevalence and impact of past history of food allergy in atopic dermatitis. Allergol Int 2013;62(1):105–12.

[326] Sicherer SH, Sampson HA. Food allergy: epidemiology, pathogenesis, diagnosis, and treatment. J Allergy Clin Immunol 2014;133(2):291–307, quiz 308.

[327] Saadeh D, Salameh P, Baldi I, et al. Diet and allergic diseases among population aged 0 to 18 years: myth or reality? Nutrients 2013;5(9):3399–423.

[328] Mosconi E, Rekima A, Seitz-Polski B, et al. Breast milk immune complexes are potent inducers of oral tolerance in neonates and prevent asthma development. Mucosal Immunol 2010;3(5):461–74.

[329] Bager P, Wohlfahrt J, Westergaard T. Caesarean delivery and risk of atopy and allergic disease: meta-analyses. Clin Exp Allergy 2008;38(4):634–42.

[330] Illi S, Weber J, Zutavern A, et al. Perinatal influences on the development of asthma and atopy in childhood. Ann Allergy Asthma Immunol 2014;112(2):132–9.e1.

[331] Strassburger SZ, Vitolo MR, Bortolini GA, et al. Nutritional errors in the first months of life and their association with asthma and atopy in preschool children. J Pediatr (Rio J) 2010;86(5):391–9.

[332] McFadden JP, Basketter DA, Dearman RJ, et al. The hapten-atopy hypothesis III: the potential role of airborne chemicals. Br J Dermatol 2014;170(1):45–51.

[333] Halken S. Prevention of allergic disease in childhood: clinical and epidemiological aspects of primary and secondary allergy prevention. Pediatr Allergy Immunol 2004;15(Suppl. 16):4–5, 9–32.

[334] Choi H, Schmidbauer N, Sundell J, et al. Common household chemicals and the allergy risks in pre-school age children. PLoS ONE 2010;5(10):e13423.

[335] Tagiyeva N, Sheikh A. Domestic exposure to volatile organic compounds in relation to asthma and allergy in children and adults. Expert Rev Clin Immunol 2014;10(12):1611–39.

[336] Brown SB, Reeves KW, Bertone-Johnson ER. Maternal folate exposure in pregnancy and childhood asthma and allergy: a systematic review. Nutr Rev 2014;72(1):55–64.

[337] von Hertzen L, Haahtela T. Con: house dust mites in atopic diseases. Am J Respir Crit Care Med 2009;180(2):113–19.

[338] Minniti F, Comberiati P, Munblit D, et al. Breast-milk characteristics protecting against allergy. Endocr Metab Immune Disord Drug Targets 2014;14(1):9–15.

[339] Kantor R, Silverberg JI. Environmental risk factors and their role in the management of atopic dermatitis. Expert Rev Clin Immunol 2016;1-12.

[340] Egawa G, Kabashima K. Multifactorial skin barrier deficiency and atopic dermatitis: essential topics to prevent the atopic march. J Allergy Clin Immunol 2016;138(2):350–8.e1.

[341] David T, Wells F, Sharpe T, et al. Low serum zinc in children with atopic eczema. Br J Dermatol 1984;111(5):597–601.

[342] El-Kholy M, Gas AM, El-Shimi S, et al. Zinc and copper status in children with bronchial asthma and atopic dermatitis. J Egypt Public Health Assoc 1989;65(5–6):657–68.

[343] Kremmyda LS, Vlachava M, Noakes PS, et al. Atopy risk in infants and children in relation to early exposure to fish, oily fish, or long-chain omega-3 fatty acids: a systematic review. Clin Rev Allergy Immunol 2011;41(1):36–66.

[344] Kunitsugu I, Okuda M, Murakami N, et al. Self-reported seafood intake and atopy in Japanese school-aged children. Pediatr Int 2012;54(2):233–7.

[345] Renz-Polster H, David MR, Buist AS, et al. Caesarean section delivery and the risk of allergic disorders in childhood. Clin Exp Allergy 2005;35(11):1466–72.

[346] Saarinen UM, Kajosaari M. Breastfeeding as prophylaxis against atopic disease: prospective follow-up study until 17 years old. Lancet 1995;346(8982):1065–9.

[347] Pelucchi C, Chatenoud L, Turati F, et al. Probiotics supplementation during pregnancy or infancy for the prevention of atopic dermatitis: a meta-analysis. Epidemiology 2012;23(3):402–14.

[348] Wickens K, Black P, Stanley TV, et al. A protective effect of Lactobacillus rhamnosus HN001 against eczema in the first 2 years of life persists to age 4 years. Clin Exp Allergy 2012;42(7):1071–9.

[349] Perkin MR, Logan K, Tseng A, et al. Randomized trial of introduction of allergenic foods in breast-fed infants. N Engl J Med 2016;374(18):1733–43.

[350] Bunyavanich S, Rifas-Shiman SL, Platts-Mills TA, et al. Prenatal, perinatal, and childhood vitamin D exposure and their association with childhood allergic rhinitis and allergic sensitization. J Allergy Clin Immunol 2016;137(4):1063–70.e2.

[351] Fall T, Lundholm C, Ortqvist AK, et al. Early exposure to dogs and farm animals and the risk of childhood asthma. JAMA Pediatr 2015;169(11):e153219.

[352] Campbell B, Raherison C, Lodge CJ, et al. The effects of growing up on a farm on adult lung function and allergic phenotypes: an international population-based study. Thorax 2016.

[353] Graham-Rowe D. Lifestyle: when allergies go west. Nature 2011;479(7374):S2–4.

[354] Kim K. Influences of environmental chemicals on atopic dermatitis. Toxicol Res 2015;31(2):89–96.

[355] Kang MG, Song WJ, Park HK, et al. Basophil activation test with food additives in chronic urticaria patients. Clin Nutr Res 2014;3(1):9–16.

[356] Catli G, Bostanci I, Ozmen S, et al. Is patch testing with food additives useful in children with atopic eczema? Pediatr Dermatol 2015;32(5):684–9.

[357] Gutfreund K, Bienias W, Szewczyk A, et al. Topical calcineurin inhibitors in dermatology. Part I: properties, method and effectiveness of drug use. Postepy Dermatol Alergol 2013;30(3):165–9.

[358] Fuchs O, Bahmer T, Rabe KF, et al. Asthma transition from childhood into adulthood. Lancet Respir Med 2016;5(3):224–34.

[359] Beausoleil JL, Fiedler J, Spergel JM. Food Intolerance and childhood asthma: what is the link? Paediatr Drugs 2007;9(3):157–63.

[360] Panzer AR, Lynch SV. Influence and effect of the human microbiome in allergy and asthma. Curr Opin Rheumatol 2015;27(4):373–80.

[361] Fujimura KE, Lynch SV. Microbiota in allergy and asthma and the emerging relationship with the gut microbiome. Cell Host Microbe 2015;17(5):592–602.

[362] Legatzki A, Rosler B, von Mutius E. Microbiome diversity and asthma and allergy risk. Curr Allergy Asthma Rep 2014;14(10):466.

[363] Monteil MA, Joseph G, Chang Kit C, et al. Smoking at home is strongly associated with symptoms of asthma and rhinitis in children of primary school age in Trinidad and Tobago. Rev Panam Salud Publica 2004;16(3):193–8.

[364] Wisniewski JA, Agrawal R, Minnicozzi S, et al. Sensitization to food and inhalant allergens in relation to age and wheeze among children with atopic dermatitis. Clin Exp Allergy 2013;43(10):1160–70.

[365] Bernard A, Nickmilder M, Dumont X. Chlorinated pool attendance, airway epithelium defects and the risks of allergic diseases in adolescents: interrelationships revealed by circulating biomarkers. Environ Res 2015;140:119–26.

[366] Bernard A, Nickmilder M, Voisin C, et al. Impact of chlorinated swimming pool attendance on the respiratory health of adolescents. Pediatrics 2009;124(4):1110–18.

[367] Chowdhury S, Alhooshani K, Karanfil T. Disinfection byproducts in swimming pool: occurrences, implications and future needs. Water Res 2014;53:68–109.

[368] Llana-Belloch S, Priego Quesada JI, Perez-Soriano P, et al. Disinfection by-products effect on swimmers oxidative stress and respiratory damage. Eur J Sport Sci 2016;16(5):609–17.

[369] Uyan ZS, Carraro S, Piacentini G, et al. Swimming pool, respiratory health, and childhood asthma: should we change our beliefs? Pediatr Pulmonol 2009;44(1):31–7.

[370] Toyoda M, Morohashi M. Pathogenesis of acne. Med Electron Microsc 2001;34(1):29–40.

[371] Kucharska A, Szmurlo A, Sinska B. Significance of diet in treated and untreated acne vulgaris. Postepy Dermatol Alergol 2016;33(2):81–6.

[372] Spencer EH, Ferdowsian HR, Barnard ND. Diet and acne: a review of the evidence. Int J Dermatol 2009;48(4):339–47.

[373] Mahmood SN, Bowe WP. Diet and acne update: carbohydrates emerge as the main culprit. J Drugs Dermatol 2014;13(4):428–35.

[374] Cerman AA, Aktas E, Altunay IK, et al. Dietary glycemic factors, insulin resistance, and adiponectin levels in acne vulgaris. J Am Acad Dermatol 2016;75(1):155–62.

[375] Burris J, Rietkerk W, Woolf K. Acne: the role of medical nutrition therapy. J Acad Nutr Diet 2013;113(3):416–30.

[376] Siniavskii Iu A, Tsoi NO. Influence of nutritional patterns on the severity of acne in young adults. Vopr Pitan 2014;83(1):41–7.

[377] Ulvestad M, Bjertness E, Dalgard F, et al. Acne and dairy products in adolescence: results from a Norwegian longitudinal study. J Eur Acad Dermatol Venereol 2016.

[378] LaRosa CL, Quach KA, Koons K, et al. Consumption of dairy in teenagers with and without acne. J Am Acad Dermatol 2016;75(2):318–22.

[379] Kumari R, Thappa DM. Role of insulin resistance and diet in acne. Indian J Dermatol Venereol Leprol 2013;79(3):291–9.

[380] Melnik BC, John SM, Schmitz G. Over-stimulation of insulin/IGF-1 signaling by western diet may promote diseases of civilization: lessons learnt from Laron syndrome. Nutr Metab (Lond) 2011;8:41.

[381] Rostami Mogaddam M, Safavi Ardabili N, Maleki N, et al. Correlation between the severity and type of acne lesions with serum zinc levels in patients with acne vulgaris. Biomed Res Int 2014;2014:474108.

[382] Gupta M, Mahajan VK, Mehta KS, et al. Zinc therapy in dermatology: a review. Dermatol Res Pract 2014;2014:709152.

[383] Brandt S. The clinical effects of zinc as a topical or oral agent on the clinical response and pathophysiologic mechanisms of acne: a systematic review of the literature. J Drugs Dermatol 2013;12(5):542–5.

[384] Bae YS, Hill ND, Bibi Y, et al. Innovative uses for zinc in dermatology. Dermatol Clin 2010;28(3):587–97.

[385] Ozuguz P, Dogruk Kacar S, Ekiz O, et al. Evaluation of serum vitamins A and E and zinc levels according to the severity of acne vulgaris. Cutan Ocul Toxicol 2014;33(2):99–102.

[386] Fabbrocini G, Bertona M, Picazo O, et al. Supplementation with Lactobacillus rhamnosus SP1 normalises skin expression of genes implicated in insulin signalling and improves adult acne. Benef Microbes 2016;1–6.

[387] Bowe WP, Logan AC. Acne vulgaris, probiotics and the gut-brain-skin axis – back to the future? Gut Pathog 2011;3(1):1.

[388] Bowe W, Patel NB, Logan AC. Acne vulgaris, probiotics and the gut-brain-skin axis: from anecdote to translational medicine. Benef Microbes 2014;5(2):185–99.

[389] Rathi SK. Acne vulgaris treatment: the current scenario. Indian J Dermatol 2011;56(1):7.

[390] Jung GW, Tse JE, Guiha I, et al. Prospective, randomized, open-label trial comparing the safety, efficacy, and tolerability of an acne treatment regimen with and without a probiotic supplement and minocycline in subjects with mild to moderate acne. J Cutan Med Surg 2013;17(2):114–22.

[391] Dzialo M, Mierziak J, Korzun U, et al. The potential of plant phenolics in prevention and therapy of skin disorders. Int J Mol Sci 2016;17(2):160.

[392] Radha MH, Laxmipriya NP. Evaluation of biological properties and clinical effectiveness of Aloe vera: a systematic review. J Tradit Complement Med 2015;5(1):21–6.

[393] Hajheydari Z, Saeedi M, Morteza-Semnani K, et al. Effect of Aloe vera topical gel combined with tretinoin in treatment of mild and moderate acne vulgaris: a randomized, double-blind, prospective trial. J Dermatolog Treat 2014;25(2):123–9.

[394] Takahashi T, Kokubo R, Sakaino M. Antimicrobial activities of eucalyptus leaf extracts and flavonoids from Eucalyptus maculata. Lett Appl Microbiol 2004;39(1):60–4.

[395] Grant P, Ramasamy S. An update on plant derived anti-androgens. Int J Endocrinol Metab 2012;10(2):497.

[396] Grant P. Spearmint herbal tea has significant anti-androgen effects in polycystic ovarian syndrome. A randomized controlled trial. Phytother Res 2010;24(2):186–8.

[397] Unal D, Emiroglu N, Cengiz FP. Evaluation of social anxiety, self-esteem, life quality in adolescents with acne vulgaris. Int J Adolesc Med Health 2016.

[398] Dunn LK, O'Neill JL, Feldman SR. Acne in adolescents: quality of life, self-esteem, mood, and psychological disorders. Dermatol Online J 2011;17(1):1.

[399] Hosthota A, Bondade S, Basavaraja V. Impact of acne vulgaris on quality of life and self-esteem. Cutis 2016;98(2):121–4.

[400] Nguyen CM, Koo J, Cordoro KM. Psychodermatologic effects of atopic dermatitis and acne: a review on self-esteem and identity. Pediatr Dermatol 2016;33(2):129–35.

[401] Suk WA, Murray K, Avakian MD. Environmental hazards to children's health in the modern world. Mutat Res 2003;544(2–3):235–42.

[402] Genuis SJ. Evolution in pediatric health care. Pediatr Int 2010;52(4):640–3.

[403] Bijlsma N, Cohen M. Environmental chemical assessment in clinical practice: unveiling the elephant in the room. Int J Environ Res Public Health 2016;13(2):181.

[404] Prüss-Üstün A, Corvalán C. Preventing disease through healthy environments. Towards an estimate of the environmental burden of disease. Geneva: World Health Organization.; 2006.

[405] Environmental Working Group. Body burden: the pollution in newborns; 2005. Available from https://www.ewg.org/research/body-burden-pollution-newborns.

[406] Lantz S, McIntosh T. One bite at a time: reduce toxic exposure and eat the world you want: Self-published; 2016.

[407] Diamanti-Kandarakis E, Bourguignon JP, Giudice LC, et al. Endocrine-disrupting chemicals: an Endocrine Society scientific statement. Endocr Rev 2009;30(4):293–342.

[408] Bergman Å, Heindel J, Jobling S, et al. State-of-the-science of endocrine disrupting chemicals, 2012. Toxicol Lett 2012;211:S3.

[409] Woodruff TJ, Zota AR, Schwartz JM. Environmental chemicals in pregnant women in the United States: NHANES 2003-2004. Environ Health Perspect 2011;119(6):878.

[410] Houlihan J, Kropp T, Wiles R, et al. Body burden: the pollution in newborns. Environmental Working Group; 2005;14.

[411] Landrigan PJ, Schechter CB, Lipton JM, et al. Environmental pollutants and disease in American children: estimates of morbidity, mortality, and costs for lead poisoning, asthma, cancer, and developmental disabilities. Environ Health Perspect 2002;110(7):721.

[412] Falck AJ, Mooney S, Kapoor SS, et al. Developmental exposure to environmental toxicants. Pediatr Clin North Am 2015;62(5):1173–97.

[413] Rice D, Barone S Jr. Critical periods of vulnerability for the developing nervous system: evidence from humans and animal models. Environ Health Perspect 2000;108(Suppl. 3):511.

[414] Landrigan PJ, Claudio L, Markowitz SB, et al. Pesticides and inner-city children: exposures, risks, and prevention. Environ Health Perspect 1999;107(Suppl. 3):431–7.

[415] Moya J, Bearer CF, Etzel RA. Children's behavior and physiology and how it affects exposure to environmental contaminants. Pediatrics 2004;113(4 Suppl.):996–1006.

[416] Landrigan PJ, Kimmel CA, Correa A, et al. Children's health and the environment: public health issues and challenges for risk assessment. Environ Health Perspect 2004;112(2):257.

[417] Eskenazi B, Kogut K, Huen K, et al. Organophosphate pesticide exposure, PON1, and neurodevelopment in school-age children from the CHAMACOS study. Environ Res 2014;134:149–57.

[418] Weiss B. Vulnerability of children and the developing brain to neurotoxic hazards. Environ Health Perspect 2000;108(Suppl. 3):375.

[419] Meeks JJ, Sheinfeld J, Eggener SE. Environmental toxicology of testicular cancer. Urol Oncol 2012;30(2):212–15.

[420] Kalfa N, Paris F, Philibert P, et al. Is hypospadias associated with prenatal exposure to endocrine disruptors? A French collaborative controlled study of a cohort of 300 consecutive children without genetic defect. Eur Urol 2015;68(6):1023–30.

[421] Michalakis M, Tzatzarakis MN, Kovatsi L, et al. Hypospadias in offspring is associated with chronic exposure of parents to organophosphate and organochlorine pesticides. Toxicol Lett 2014;230(2):139–45.

[422] Virtanen HE, Adamsson A. Cryptorchidism and endocrine disrupting chemicals. Mol Cell Endocrinol 2012;355(2):208–20.

[423] Iughetti L, Lucaccioni L, Predieri B. Childhood obesity and environmental pollutants: a dual relationship. Acta Biomed 2015;86(1):5–16.

[424] Tang-Peronard JL, Andersen HR, Jensen TK, et al. Endocrine-disrupting chemicals and obesity development in humans: a review. Obes Rev 2011;12(8):622–36.

[425] Landrigan PJ, Garg A. Chronic effects of toxic environmental exposures on children's health. J Toxicol Clin Toxicol 2002;40(4):449–56.

[426] Christensen DL. Prevalence and characteristics of autism spectrum disorder among children aged 8 years—autism and developmental disabilities monitoring network, 11 sites, United States, 2012. MMWR Surveill Summ 2016;65.

[427] Centers for Disease Control and Prevention. Autism spectrum disorder (ASD); 2016. Available from http://www.cdc.gov/ncbddd/autism/data.html.

[428] Weintraub K. The prevalence puzzle: autism counts. Nature 2011;479(7371):22–4.

[429] Berghuis SA, Bos AF, Sauer PJ, et al. Developmental neurotoxicity of persistent organic pollutants: an update on childhood outcome. Arch Toxicol 2015;89(5):687–709.

[430] Lyall K, Schmidt RJ, Hertz-Picciotto I. Maternal lifestyle and environmental risk factors for autism spectrum disorders. Int J Epidemiol 2014;43(2):443–64.

[431] Grandjean P, Landrigan PJ. Developmental neurotoxicity of industrial chemicals. Lancet 2006;368(9553):2167–78.

[432] Chaste P, Leboyer M. Autism risk factors: genes, environment, and gene-environment interactions. Dialogues Clin Neurosci 2012;14(3):281–92.

[433] Forman J, Silverstein J, Bhatia JJS, et al. Organic foods: health and environmental advantages and disadvantages. Pediatrics 2012;130(5):e1406–15.

[434] Lockie S, Lyons K, Lawrence G, et al. Choosing organics: a path analysis of factors underlying the selection of organic food among Australian consumers. Appetite 2004;43(2):135–46.

[435] Mostafalou S, Abdollahi M. Pesticides and human chronic diseases: evidences, mechanisms, and perspectives. Toxicol Appl Pharmacol 2013;268(2):157–77.

[436] Munoz-Quezada MT, Lucero BA, Barr DB, et al. Neurodevelopmental effects in children associated with exposure to organophosphate pesticides: a systematic review. Neurotoxicology 2013;39:158–68.

[437] Gonzalez-Alzaga B, Lacasana M, Aguilar-Garduno C, et al. A systematic review of neurodevelopmental effects of prenatal and postnatal organophosphate pesticide exposure. Toxicol Lett 2014;230(2):104–21.

[438] Oates L, Cohen M, Braun L, et al. Reduction in urinary organophosphate pesticide metabolites in adults after a week-long organic diet. Environ Res 2014;132:105–11.

[439] Konkel L. Obesogen Holdover: prenatal exposure predicts cardiometabolic risk factors in childhood. Environ Health Perspect 2015;123(10):A265.

[440] Mendez MA, Garcia-Esteban R, Guxens M, et al. Prenatal organochlorine compound exposure, rapid weight gain, and overweight in infancy. Environ Health Perspect 2011;119(2):272–8.

[441] Bhandari R, Xiao J, Shankar A. Urinary bisphenol A and obesity in U.S. children. Am J Epidemiol 2013;177(11):1263–70.

[442] Fathi Najafi T, Latifnejad Roudsari R, Namvar F, et al. Air pollution and quality of sperm: a meta-analysis. Iran Red Crescent Med J 2015;17(4):e26930.

[443] Bergamo P, Volpe MG, Lorenzetti S, et al. Human semen as an early, sensitive biomarker of highly polluted living environment in healthy men: a pilot biomonitoring study on trace elements in blood and semen and their relationship with sperm quality and RedOx status. Reprod Toxicol 2016;66:1–9.

[444] Landrigan P, Garg A, Droller DB. Assessing the effects of endocrine disruptors in the National Children's Study. Environ Health Perspect 2003;111(13):1678.

[445] National Institute of Environmental Health Sciences. Endocrine disruptors; 2016. Available from http://www.niehs.nih.gov/health/topics/agents/endocrine/.

[446] Krewski D, Acosta D Jr, Andersen M, et al. Toxicity testing in the 21st century: a vision and a strategy. J Toxicol Environ Health B Crit Rev 2010;13(2–4):51–138.

[447] Kordas K, Lönnerdal B, Stoltzfus RJ. Interactions between nutrition and environmental exposures: effects on health outcomes in women and children. J Nutr 2007;137(12):2794–7.

[448] Ralston NV, Raymond LJ. Dietary selenium's protective effects against methylmercury toxicity. Toxicology 2010;278(1):112–23.

[449] Grandjean P, Herz KT. Methylmercury and brain development: imprecision and underestimation of developmental neurotoxicity in humans. Mt Sinai J Med 2011;78(1):107–18.

[450] Liu RH. Potential synergy of phytochemicals in cancer prevention: mechanism of action. J Nutr 2004;134(12 Suppl.):3479s–85s.

[451] Bijlsma N, Cohen MM. Environmental chemical assessment in clinical practice: unveiling the elephant in the room. Int J Environ Res Public Health 2016;13(2):181.

APPENDIX 16.1

Dietary planning

TODDLER — meal **planner**

week starting: _____

	breakfast	lunch	dinner	snack
MONDAY	Brown rice or Quinoa flakes Porridge w bananas, apricots	Organic marinated chicken drumstick with 'satay' dipping sauce and celery sticks	Quinoa or brown rice and vegetable stirfry with lamb, green beans and coconut oil.	Chia pudding made with cashew or almond milk
TUESDAY	Pumpkin breakfast muffins with cashew butter.	Homemade spelt Pizza with parmesan cheese, salmon and grilled vegetables	Organic chicken and corn soup with gluten free pasta and dulse flakes.	Spelt toast fingers with avocado or a cashew nut butter
WEDNESDAY	Hardboiled egg with gluten-free bread soldiers	Sustainable tuna, grated carrot and avocado on corn fritters/cakes.	Beef and vegetable bolognese, with zucchini 'pasta' or spelt spirals	Organic goats yoghurt with blueberries or banana
THURSDAY	Banana and blueberry nut milk smoothie	Sweet Zucchini spelt loaf fingers with avocado and white bean puree.	Carrot, pumpkin and coconut soup; with cooked quinoa or gluten-free toast.	A hardboiled egg
FRIDAY	Yoghurt, poached pears, chia seed mix.	Salmon and red lentil patties with a small avocado and grated carrotsalad	Lamb, Oat and Vegetable Stew	Apricot, fig and coconut oil, tahini Iron Bliss balls.
SATURDAY	Zucchini and cheese omelette	Homemade baked beans with scrambled egg.	Spelt flour dusted fish fingers (salmon, flathead, mullet, john dory etc), with cauliflower mash, peas and broccoli.	Mango and coconut homemade ice block
SUNDAY	Banana pancakes with stewed apples	Beef rissoles with cooked / roasted veggies such as sweet potato, carrots, broccoli, peas, asparagus, beans	Kangaroo sausages with blanched broccolini and mashed sweet potato (with minced garlic)	Slightly cooked vegetable sticks with avocado mash or hummus

School lunchbox **meal planner**   week starting:

	Morning Tea	lunch	Afternoon Tea	
MONDAY	1 mandarin + 20g cheese	Homemade-Zucchini Slice and almond/cashew butter	200g yoghurt, 1 tsp chia seeds, strawberries	
TUESDAY	Spelt pumpkin muffin change to GF muffin	A home-made beef rissole, tomato 'sauce' and lettuce to wrap.	Half an avocado with lemon juice and tamari or sea salt. or try GF banana bread	
WEDNESDAY	Yoghurt (100g) with handful blueberries.	Salmon and lentil patties, iceberg lettuce and baby carrots	Banana and almond milk smoothie	
THURSDAY	Apricot, fig, sunflower seed and tahini 'bliss balls'	Wholemeal wrap with turkey, avo, grated carrots, cheese and baby spinach	Rice/corn thins with tahini and honey	
FRIDAY	1 pear + 20g cheese	Mini muffin-sized fritatta with smoked salmon, sweet potato, fetta	Homemade popcorn with coconut oil	
SATURDAY	Apple wedges dipped in ABC nutspread	Brown rice tuna sushi rolls with cucumber, carrot and avocado	'Trail' mix apricots, goji berries, cashews and pumpkin seeds.	
SUNDAY	1/2 mango + popcorn	Baked Falafel with hummus and tabouli	Vege sticks green tahini dip (see recipe)	

APPENDIX 16.2

Essential oils

Essential oils are extremely potent plant extracts and should not be used internally for infants or children. Essential oils are very effective diluted and used topically or added to a diffuser or humidifier.

An approximate guide for essential oil quantities for children is:

- Diffusers: 1–6 drops of oil.
- Humidifiers: 1–9 drops.
- Bath: 1–3 drops added after bath is filled.
- Diluted into 30 mL base oil such as olive, almond or coconut oil for massage:
  - 2 months–12 months old: 3–5 drops
  - 1–5 years: 5–10 drops
  - 5–7 years: 5–12 drops
  - 7–12 years: 5–15 drops
  - Puberty: 10–20 drops.

Tissue or handkerchief: 1 drop – place by pillow, tuck into clothing.

17

Geriatrics

Jane Hutchens

INTRODUCTION

In clinical medicine, the term 'geriatrics' is most commonly used to refer to care of patients 65 years of age or older. The World Health Organization (WHO) classifies people older than age 60 as being 'elderly', because life expectancy is still shorter in many parts of the developing world.[1] With continuing advances in medical care and extended longevity in most developed countries, many would argue that clinical geriatrics now encompasses an even older population, often focused on those aged 70 years and older. However, in many circumstances, chronological age may be a much less important factor than physiological or biological age.[2]

EPIDEMIOLOGY

In 2016 in Australia there were approximately 3.7 million people aged 65 years or older (about 15% of the population) and the number and proportion of older people is expected to grow.[3] Of those older adults, more than 1.8 million live with a disability, including 654 600 with a profound or severe disability.[4] Highlighting the gap between Indigenous and non-Indigenous health and life expectancy, older Indigenous Australians are considered to be those aged over 50 years.[3] The majority of older Australians live in their own home, with 76% owning their home without a mortgage, though this percentage is trending down.[3] In the 2011 Census 37% of people aged 65 and older engaged in either paid or voluntary work or provided unpaid care for a child or older person.[5]

AGEING

The ageing process is referred to as senescence – 'the deteriorative changes with time during postmaturational life that underlie increasing vulnerability to challenges, thereby decreasing the ability of the organism to survive'.[6] That is, ageing is characterised by two simultaneous processes: an increasing decline in physiological reserves and cognitive function, and an increasing vulnerability to illness. The term 'homeostenosis' is used to describe the inevitable ageing-related loss of physiological (homeostatic) reserve capacity that characterises the development of the geriatric syndromes.[7]

Older adults are a large and heterogeneous population. Ageing is experienced at different rates and in different presentations and since it incorporates the preceding child and adult years, it is the accumulation of life's experiences, illnesses and exposures, not an isolated epoch. Ageing is typically viewed negatively – as lost youth, vitality and reduced time before death – but it is important to remember that ageing in and of itself can be positive, neutral (of no consequence to health per se) or negative. For example:

- *Positive:* increased experience and wisdom, reduced anxiety of youth and more confidence
- *Neutral:* hair greying, skin changes
- *Negative:* changes such as the accumulation of oxidative damage that leads to the development of pathology such as atherosclerosis or amyloid plaques in the brain and subsequent outcomes from those changes such as heart attack or Alzheimer's disease.[8]

Ageing is an inevitable result of increasing longevity, and while earlier research focused on the biology of ageing, in recent decades the focus has shifted to 'ageing well'. In a landmark 1980 paper on human life span,[9] Fries hypothesised that it would be possible to compress the number of years of infirmity or chronic ill-health into a shorter time frame, thus enabling older people to live well, enjoy a quality of life and 'to live more successful, productive lives that benefit themselves and society'[10] for a longer period of time. In this sense, he instigated a paradigm shift that is still in place today, where the goal is to delay the onset of any chronic illness, to maintain function and independence and to resist a complacency or impotent sense of inevitability about excessive frailty or illness.

Healthy ageing is defined by WHO as the process of developing and maintaining the functional ability that enables wellbeing in older age.[11] In order to achieve healthy ageing we need to prevent ill-health and frailty; once an older person has diminished reserves, the ability to recover to baseline is significantly reduced. Knowledge of epigenetics makes it apparent that preconception and prenatal influences have a significant role in the development of chronic illness in adults; however, while preventive care could commence then ('primordial prevention'), the focus is on adopting healthy behaviours in early and mid-adult life to improve old age quality of life.[12]

Goals of geriatric medicine are:
- Increase life expectancy
- Maintain or improve quality of life

- Maintain and restore physiological function and reserves
- Prevent or delay the development of geriatric syndromes (e.g. sarcopenia and frailty).

Theories of ageing

Theories about the mechanisms of ageing (and thus factors that may accelerate or delay that process) are diverse and may be generally grouped into one of two categories:
- Error or damage theories
- Program theories.[13,14]

In reality, no one theory is adequate; rather, the multitude of theories reflect the complexity of ageing and explore different aspects of ageing. Damage theories include the effects of chronic inflammation, oxidative damage (especially DNA and mitochondrial), loss of telomere function and genetic instability. Program theories include neuroendocrine and genetic determinants of longevity and programmed cell death, and the Hayflick theory, which states that each cell line has a pre-set limit to the number of cell divisions.[13,14] Indeed, these theories are largely biological and they intersect with sociological and psychological theories of ageing. If the mechanisms that instigate and speed ageing are defined, then the goal is to slow or halt those processes in the emerging field of anti-ageing medicine.

Physiology of ageing

Age-related physiological and functional changes are characterised by a progressive and heterogeneous pattern of decline in all body systems. Changes may be beneficial, neutral or, increasingly with advancing age, pathological. A sound understanding of the physiological changes of ageing enables the practitioner to evaluate the patient's health in context and to be able to provide appropriate care for older adults. There is great diversity in the patterns and rate of ageing among individuals and across age ranges and this is further complicated by the coexistence of single or multiple morbidities. It can be difficult to distinguish what is a physiological change and what is a pathological process, yet this is essential in order to understand the clinical issues and to devise a safe, effective and rational treatment plan.[7,15] Further, understanding age-related physiological changes includes appreciation of the changes to physiological reserves, reduced capacity to maintain homeostasis and the difference in treatment responses that may be expected between a young adult and an elderly adult.

The nervous system

With advancing age there are progressive loss of neurons, changes in dendritic function, alterations in glial cell reactivity and reduced cerebral blood flow and production of neurotransmitters (e.g. noradrenaline [norepinephrine] and dopamine).[7,16] Brain atrophy leads to loss of 5–7% of brain weight; grey matter is more affected by atrophy than white matter and the residual space is filled by increased cerebrospinal fluid.[16,17] The reduction in neural density does not directly correlate with mental functioning, as in younger adults there appears to be neuronal mass in excess of requirements.[16]

In the autonomic nervous system, parasympathetic outflow reduces and sympathetic increases, exacerbating cardiovascular changes. As seen in the cardiovascular and respiratory systems there is a reduced responsiveness to beta-adrenergic stimulation. The changes to sympathetic and parasympathetic nervous function negatively affect thermoregulation, reduce baroreceptor sensitivity and predispose to dehydration. This increases susceptibility to the effects of temperature changes and postural hypotension and syncope.[16] Reflexes progressively diminish, especially the gag reflex, which increases the risk of aspiration of food and drink.[17] Postural sway is increased and there is a slowing of correction for postural swaying.[18] Gait changes are an important factor associated with the incidence of falls in the elderly. Gait consists of two components, equilibrium (maintaining an upright posture) and locomotion (initiating movement and step function), and both of these may be negatively affected by ageing.[18]

There is a reduction of blood flow to the brain by 10–15%, moderated through altered baroreceptor function and age-related physiological changes to the renal and cardiovascular systems.[17] Atherosclerotic changes increase the risk of multiple cerebral infarcts associated with multi-infarct dementia, transient ischaemic attacks (TIAs) and stroke.

Older adults may have increased sensitivity to central nervous system agents such as opiates and anaesthetic and may have reduced metabolic clearance of these substances. Moreover, increasing age is associated with postoperative cognitive dysfunction irrespective of what anaesthetic agent is used.[16] Postoperative cognitive dysfunction is characterised by a continued deterioration of cognitive function following surgery. The key consistent risk factor is advanced age, with postoperative cognitive decline at least twice as common in those aged 60 years or older than in younger adults.[16] It appears that elderly patients diagnosed with cognitive impairment are more vulnerable to postoperative cognitive decline than elderly patients who are not.[19] Cognitive function is associated with a range of abilities that allow us to make sense of our experiences. This includes the ability to comprehend new information, to think abstractly and to execute functions such as decision-making skills, goal-setting, planning and judgment as well as visuospatial skills, numerical ability and verbal fluency. Age-related physiological changes to the brain may result in changes to any of these dimensions but there is significant inter-individual variability – an older person may continue to perform as well as a younger person.[20]

Cognitive changes occur on a spectrum (rather than a continuum) from minimal to mild age-related cognitive decline, cognitive dysfunction and the most severe presentation, dementia.[7,21] Cognitive decline is multifactorial and significant change is not inevitable; rather, it is associated with a neurodegenerative disorder thus reflecting a pathological process.[7] For example, mild deposition of amyloid plaques in the hippocampal and medial temporal structures may be seen as normal age-related changes (and may have little consequence); however, more extensive deposits are pathological and characteristic of Alzheimer's disease.

Cognitive changes do occur more commonly in older people than in younger people, but more recent research proposes that this is a secondary effect of older adults having greater biological ageing through the accumulation of neurological injuries due to inflammation, oxidative stress and vascular and metabolic changes.[21–23] That is, chronological age may not be as important as biological age (a concept that reflects the physiological functioning of essential body systems, physiological reserve, senescence, vigour and viability) and cognitive decline may be seen to be the end product of decades of exposure to, and interrelationships between, environmental, genetic and disease influences.[21]

Practice points

- Changes of ageing may predispose to cardiovascular and renal effects, including reduced baroreceptor function and postural hypotension
- Ageing brings progressive cerebrovascular changes and increases in cerebral infarcts, dementia and stroke
- Altered cognitive function and behavioural changes may be due to a range of disparate causes and all changes should be investigated (and not assumed to be dementia)
- Major decline in cognitive function is not inevitable, though some slowing and memory impairment is common with increasing age.

The cardiovascular system

Cardiovascular disease is the leading single cause of hospitalisation and death in older adults and results in significant reductions in quality of life and autonomy.[24] The changes to the cardiovascular system are complex, comprehensive and evident at the cellular, metabolic, tissue, organ and system levels. Individuals experience different rates of ageing as well as different patterns of ageing for the cardiovascular system and this is further complicated by other disease states and the effects of medications and treatments. The resultant heterogeneous clinical picture for the cardiovascular system can make it a challenge to determine what is normal ageing, what is a normal ageing process that is excessive for the person's chronological age and what is a disease process or a consequence of a disease.

The mitochondrial theory of ageing focuses on the impact of the generation of reactive oxygen species (ROS) as a by-product of the electron transfer chain (ETC) activity.[25] This results in oxidative stress damage to the ETC components and mitochondrial DNA (mtDNA), thus further increasing the production of ROS. mtDNA may be more susceptible to oxidative damage due to the lack of protective histones that are present in other cells. Increased mitochondrial damage reduces the energy available to the myocardium and thus impairs cardiac function as well as increasing oxidative damage and tissue.

Increased mitochondrial damage ultimately alters the structure and reduces the function of myocytes.[25]

With ageing there is a progressive loss of ventricular myocytes and an increase in the volume of the remaining myocytes.[14] Lipofuscin, an intralysosomal lipid-containing pigment residue from the peroxidative destruction of mitochondrial membranes and other oxidative processes, and amyloid, aggregates of structurally and functionally compromised proteins, accumulate in the myocytes.[26] The amount of lipofuscin and amyloid is inverse to longevity and they are considered markers of ageing.

The connective tissue is altered with an increase in fibrinogen and collagen as well as a shift to a greater percentage of non-enzymatic cross-linking increases, such as advanced glycation end products, compared with enzymatic cross-linkages in the collagen.[7,14,27] With age, calcium deposition into the collagen increases and further stiffens myocardial tissue and impedes normal cardiac valve function. The ratio of myocytes to collagen mass is stable due to the increased size of the myocytes and these changes represent hypertrophy rather than hyperplasia of the myocardium.[14] These changes result in reduced elasticity (compliance) and strength, increased rigidity, altered cell signalling and conduction errors, potentially leading to heart failure, arrhythmias and other pathology.

The hypertrophic and functional changes to the myocytes reduce the efficacy of ventricular filling (the left ventricular early diastolic filling rate progressively decreases to 50% of the peak by 80 years of age[14]), lengthen contraction time and reduce the ventricular ejection fraction, leading to a progressive increase in both atrial and ventricular hypertrophy and hypertension.[14–16,28] Decreases in the left ventricular ejection fraction are initially seen primarily in a maximum ejection fraction during upright exercise but over time ageing leads to an overall reduction in ejection fraction.[14] The reduced stroke volume causes a reduced cardiac output and cardiac reserves progressively diminish with age.[14,15]

The resting heart rate does not change significantly, but the maximal achievable heart rate decreases (an 85-year-old can achieve about 70% of the heart rate of a 20-year-old) and thus so does the capacity to respond to exercise or stress.[14] This reduced heart rate variability and responsiveness is a marker of increased risk of cardiac events and all-cause mortality.

The vasculature undergoes significant change as well with calcification and fibrous infiltration of vessel walls, increased elastolytic and collagenolytic activity and deposition of stiff non-enzymatic cross-linked collagen.[15] Arteries become hyperplastic and thickened, reducing compliance and increasing stiffness. The intimal thickness of the carotid artery increases 2–3-fold between 20 and 90 years of age and the progressively rigid large arteries can increase in stiffness by 40–50%.[14,28] Intimal thickening is associated with endothelial dysfunction and the development of atherosclerosis.[7]

Peripheral resistance increases cardiac afterload, which further contributes to left ventricular hypertrophy.[14,15] In younger adults blood pressure is primarily influenced by peripheral vascular resistance but with increasing age the key determinant is central artery stiffness. Systolic blood pressure continues to rise up to the ninth decade but diastolic blood pressure peaks in the sixth decade then declines, hence the common clinical presentation of isolated systolic hypertension.[14,15] The widened pulse pressure (between systolic and diastolic pressure), especially the reduction in diastolic pressure, compromises myocardial perfusion and further reduces overall cardiac function. The extent of the widening (or elevation) of the pulse pressure is a strong predictor of cardiovascular disease.[6,14,28]

The venous system holds 70% of circulating blood volume, thus while ageing changes are not as significant as arterial changes they can still be important.[15] Veins also stiffen, lose compliance and may have weakened peripheral valves and varicosities and thus can influence intravascular pressure.[29] The aortic and mitral valves calcify and valvular heart disease increases with age.[16]

The number of pacemaker cells in the sinoatrial node decreases and there is an increase in surrounding fatty and fibrous tissues.[14,28] A significant loss of pacemaker cells (>50%) increases the risk of atrial arrhythmias, evidenced in the 10-fold increased risk of atrial fibrillation in those aged over 60 years compared with the general population.[14,28]

Impaired baroreceptor sensitivity results from chronic hypertension and reduced arteriole compliance, blunted transductions of stretch signals, altered central neural processing and dysfunction of sympathetic modulation.[14,16,28] The reduced sensitivity and delayed response of baroreceptors lead to labile blood pressure, postural and postprandial hypotension and loss of sinus arrhythmia.[28]

The decreased function of beta-adrenergic receptors reduces the ability of agonists (e.g. adrenaline [epinephrine] and noradrenaline [norepinephrine]) to exert a positive inotropic effect and thereby increase cardiac output as well as impairing chronotropic function and thus altering heart rate and rhythm.[6,14,27] Impaired alpha-adrenergic receptor function further reduces myocardial contractility.[14] This reduction in inotropic and chronotropic responsiveness is amplified by intense exercise and physiological stress and results in a compromised ability to respond to those stressors.[6,27]

Renin is secreted by the glomerular cells in response to changes in renal perfusion and is the initiating step in the renin-angiotensin-aldosterone system (RAAS). The RAAS is a hormone and enzyme cascade that regulates arterial blood pressure, tissue perfusion and extracellular volume, primarily via vasoconstriction and relaxation and mediation of sodium and water retention. Renin secretion is also provoked by sympathetic nervous system stimulation and thus physiological, psychological and emotional stress.[30,31] The RAAS also has pro-inflammatory and pro-fibrotic effects at the cellular and molecular levels and in particular angiotensin II promotes inflammation, cell growth, vascular remodelling and generation of ROS at the cellular and mitochondrial levels. Further, angiotensin II influences energy metabolism and the progression of cell senescence.[30,31] Prolonged and excessive activation of the RAAS is thus associated with increased tissue and mitochondrial oxidative stress, systemic inflammation and cardiovascular disease, including hypertension and atherosclerosis as well as increasing end-organ damage.[30,31]

TABLE 17.1 Summary of physiological changes to the cardiovascular system and clinical presentation	
Physiological changes	**Clinical presentation**
Reduced arterial compliance (increased vascular resistance)	Systolic hypertension, aneurysm, peripheral vascular disease, coronary artery disease, stroke
↓ left ventricular compliance and hypertrophy	Heart failure, coronary artery disease, stroke, atrial fibrillation
↓ resting and maximal cardiac output	↓ haemodynamic reserve ↓ stamina ↓ end-organ perfusion
Reduced inotropic and chronotropic response to beta-adrenergic agonists	↓ maximal heart rate ↓ responsiveness to increased demand (illness, infection, emotional stress, injuries and extreme physical exertion) ↓ response to beta-receptor medication
Endothelial dysfunction	Hypertension, inflammation, atherosclerosis, stroke
Altered myocardial energy metabolism	Impaired mitochondrial capacity to increase ATP, fatigue, reduced exercise tolerance
↓ pacemaker cells in SA node, atrial fibrosis and fatty changes	↑ arrhythmias, especially atrial fibrillation
Degeneration of conducting tissue	Heart block, arrhythmias
Aortic and mitral valve changes	Stenosis, filling defects, murmurs
↓ heart rate response to postural stress	Syncope when change of posture
Impaired autoregulation/ blunted baroreceptor response to postural change	↓ vasoconstriction in response to hypotension Postural hypotension

With progressive age the RAAS activity shifts and increasingly the response to upright posture is reduced or absent and the aldosterone response to sodium restriction is blunted.[15] See Table 17.1 for a summary of physiological changes to the cardiovascular system and the corresponding clinical presentation.

The respiratory system

The effects of ageing on the respiratory system are the result of multiple mechanisms and changes and the cumulative impact of environmental insults. The degree of ageing is highly variable between people and is often under-recognised unless the individual has other disease states or experiences increased respiratory demand through illness or physical exertion. Changes can be categorised as structural, functional or immune, though it

Practice points

- Older adults are at risk of both hypertension and hypotension, in particular postural hypotension; perform supine and erect BP measurements
- Older patients are unlikely to tolerate tachycardia or AF as well as younger patients
- Ageing changes and compromise are more evident during exercise or under stress (e.g. during illness)
- Age-related changes may contribute to earlier decompensation during illness
- A sedentary lifestyle may both worsen ageing changes and obscure the impact as the heart is not placed under extreme conditions
- Lifestyle factors, including exercise and diet, may delay and partially reverse the changes of cardiovascular ageing.

is important to recognise the influence of these categories on each other. Ageing is associated with reduced intervertebral space (more so with osteoporosis) and hyperkyphosis, changed chest shape to more barrel-shape, ossification of costo-cartilage, osteoarthritic pain and spondylitis, which all contribute to reduced movement and compliance and reduced lung volume.[32–34]

A decrease in fast-twitch fatigue-resistant type IIa fibres in the muscles of respiration (diaphragm, intercostal and accessory muscles) combined with a reduction in myosin (a protein that converts chemical energy in the form of ATP to mechanical energy, and is essential for muscle contraction and strength) results in reduced muscle strength and endurance from 50 years of age and an increased reliance on the diaphragm.[32,33] The diaphragm becomes more reactive to stimulation by the phrenic nerve but the amplitude of that reaction (force of diaphragm contraction) is reduced.[32] The fast-twitch muscle fibres also act to maintain airway tension and their reduction increases the premature collapse of small airways.[34]

The alveoli and alveolar ducts dilate, parenchymal tissue is lost and the gaseous exchange surface area reduces by up to 20%.[32,33] There is increased infiltration of airways with altered collagen fibres, which causes a reduced elasticity and dilation (called senile emphysema), and the reduced surface tension leads to an increased propensity of the small airways to collapse with expiration.[33]

Amyloid and increased collagen deposits are noted in the respiratory vasculature and it becomes less elastic and thickens, causing increased resistance to blood flow in the lungs and increased pulmonary artery pressure (pulmonary hypertension). This may occur in conjunction with an increase in, or be increased by, cardiovascular changes.[32,33] There is decreased density of capillaries and reduced capillary volume, which reduces gaseous exchange.

The forced expiratory volume in one second (FEV_1) is reduced, as is the forced vital capacity (FVC) although to a lesser degree. The residual volume (RV) and functional residual capacity (FRC) increase due to loss of recoil and lung collapse, thus older people have higher lung volumes.

The RV as a proportion of total lung capacity is approximately 20% at 20 years of age and 40% at 70 years.[16] This increases the workload of the respiratory muscles and is responsible for respiratory energy expenditure that is up to 120% that of a young adult.[16]

Structural changes that impede elastic recoil and expansion, loss of alveolar surface area and early lung collapse in expiration, combined with reduced capillaries, all contribute to reduce gaseous exchange.[32,33] The early lung collapse leads to ventilation-perfusion (V/Q) mismatch, which lowers resting arterial oxygen tensions. Physiological functional capacity abruptly decreases after age 60–70 years, due to reduced maximal oxygen consumption (VO_2 max) and exercise velocity at the lactate threshold.[28]

In a healthy adult the reduced tidal volume is offset by increasing the respiratory rate. In older adults there may be dysfunction of the chemosensory receptors, thus blunted responses to hypoxia and hypercapnia. As seen in the cardiovascular system, there is reduced beta-adrenoceptor responsiveness, which reduces bronchodilation and responsiveness to beta-agonist medication.[33] Neurological conditions more common with advanced age can impact on central neural control of breathing as well as impairing the cough reflex and swallowing, leading to increased risk of aspiration. Silent reflux is also a risk for aspiration. A combination of the chemosensory function and response, reduced chest wall compliance and reduced awareness of bronchoconstriction contribute to respiratory compromise and also a possible masking of deterioration and thus delay in seeking appropriate intervention and care.

Sleep-associated apnoea and periodic breathing occur more frequently in the elderly, possibly due to impaired neural control.[32] Sleep-disordered breathing increases with age and is compounded by pathology such as cardiovascular disease, obesity and medication. The relationship between conditions such as sleep apnoea and hypertension, cardiovascular and cerebrovascular disease, heart failure and Alzheimer's disease is thought to be bidirectional; that is, both causative and an effect. Diagnosing respiratory issues related to sleep-disordered breathing is often compromised by the common and general nature of symptoms of fatigue and snoring which can readily be ascribed to a range of other pathology, overweight and obesity and medication side effects.

The inevitable exposure to environmental insults results in oxidative stress and a subsequent increase in ROS, a reduction in the volume and efficacy of protease inhibitors (such as alpha-1 antitrypsin), increased epithelial permeability and augmented nuclear factor-kappa beta (NF-κβ), which in turn stimulates the release of inflammatory cytokines and neutrophils. This leads to increased mucus production in the lower airways, plasma leakage and bronchoconstriction, which increases lung consolidation, infection and compromised gaseous exchange.

Intracellular and extracellular superoxide dismutase (SOD) and glutathione levels decrease, leaving the lungs increasingly at risk of oxidative and inflammatory damage. Both innate and acquired immunity are reduced with the key changes noted in Table 17.2. The lung milieu is progressively inflammatory and this affects the cell phenotype and function and, combined with the age-related dampened immune function (immunosenescence), reduces the ability to raise an effective immune response when challenged.[33,34]

The net results of age-related changes to the respiratory system are:

- Reduced respiratory capacity, especially with increased demand
- Reduced responsiveness to hypoxia and hypercapnia
- Increased work of breathing
- Increased risk of respiratory infection and reduced capacity to mount an effective immune response (thus greater mortality)
- Impaired control and regulation of breathing
- Increased risk of aspiration.

Practice points

- The lack of overt respiratory signs and symptoms (especially at rest) does not preclude significant reduction in respiratory capacity
- Symptoms of respiratory compromise and/or disease may be attributed to other causes (e.g. anaemia or cardiovascular problems)
- Responsiveness to medications may be blunted (especially to beta-agonists).

TABLE 17.2 Summary of age-related changes to immune function of the respiratory system

Innate immunity changes	Acquired immunity changes
↓ glandular epithelial cells, thus impaired mucosal barrier (especially large airways)	↑ pro-inflammatory cytokines (IL-6, TNF, IL-1β, PGE$_2$)
↓ cilia and mucociliary clearance	↑ anti-inflammatory mediators (TNF receptors, IL-1 receptor agonists and acute-phase proteins e.g. CRP)
Impaired chemotaxis and phagocytosis	Atrophy of the thymus, altered memory T-cell function, shift from Th1 to Th2 profile
↓ SOD generation	↓ T-cell production, numbers and receptors
↓ chemotactic activity and bactericidal effect of neutrophils	↓ response to antigens, ↓ antibody generation and responsiveness
↑ number of NK cells but decreased NK-cell cytotoxicity	↓ B-cell production
↓ macrophage function, generation of ROS and pro-inflammatory cytokines with infection	

The renal system

Renal function decline with age can vary significantly and may only become evident with illness or side effects from impaired clearance of medications. The ageing kidneys are subject to cumulative cellular and tissue injuries as seen with other systems and organs via increased oxygen radicals and fibrogenic mediators, mitochondrial damage and dysfunction, reduced nitric oxide and antioxidant levels and loss of telomeres.[35] Cross-linkages between proteins, lipids and nucleic acids (advanced glycation end products, AGEs) accumulate with age and cause vascular and tissue damage, thus hyperglycaemia and poorly controlled diabetes accelerate the rate of AGE accumulation and tissue damage.[36]

The renal mass decreases by up to 25% by the ninth decade, but other factors such as the glomerular filtration rate (GFR), gender and body surface area appear to be more strongly correlated with renal mass than age.[15,35] The glomeruli increase in size but reduce in density, change shape and show sclerotic changes with a thickened glomerular basement membrane, which reduces the available surface area for filtration, thus contributing to age-related reduction in GFR.[15,35] There is an increase in glomerular permeability demonstrated by microalbuminuria and proteinuria, the mechanism for which is not agreed upon, though the research focus is increasingly on disturbances of endothelial or podocyte function rather than disturbances of basement membrane function.[15,37]

Renal blood flow reduces by 10% per decade after 30 years of age and there is a reduction in the capacity to vasodilate the afferent renal artery in order to increase renal plasma flow, which results in a reduced GFR. There is a progressive imbalance between the vasoconstrictive and vasodilatory response with age. Renal blood vessels become hyalinised and eventually hyalinising arteriosclerosis develops, leading to further ischaemic injury and loss of nephrons.[14]

The renal tubules shorten and fibrose, resulting in blunted reabsorption and secretion of solutes, leading to electrolyte imbalance. Alterations to the function and interactions between aldosterone, antidiuretic hormone (ADH) and atrial natriuretic peptide (ANP) also contribute to reduced renal function with age.[14] There is a reduced responsiveness to fluid shifts and a diminished responsiveness to a low-sodium diet. This in turn leads to a reduced angiotensin II and aldosterone response and sodium loss, causing hyponatraemia. A diminished responsiveness to ADH leads to reduced urine concentrating ability and increases nocturia.[14]

The reduced renal reserve, mass, functional parenchymal tissue, blood flow and GFR reduce the kidneys' ability to autoregulate in response to changed environment, ischaemia and fluid alterations and increase the vulnerability of the kidneys to acute injury and predispose them to the development of chronic kidney disease (CKD).[15,36]

Renal atrophy, cellular and metabolic changes can lead to a reduction of up to 50% of functional nephrons by 80 years of age and this is reflected in the GFR.[16] The GFR is seen as a key assessment of renal function and this begins to decline by approximately 1–1.5%, or 0.87 mL/minute/year after 30 years of age.[6,14,15,38] There is, however, significant variation in the reduction of GFR in healthy adults, with the Baltimore Longitudinal Study of Aging reporting that roughly one-third of study participants had the predicted linear reduction in GFR, one-third had a more rapid decline and one-third had no reduction, leading many to question whether a reduction in GFR is inevitable.[6,39] Factors other than age that affect GFR may themselves be influenced by age and include nutritional intake (especially refined carbohydrates and protein), weight, diabetes, hypertension, muscle mass, gender, medication use and ethnicity (e.g. elderly African American and Japanese adults appear to have a higher rate of decline in renal function than white Americans).[6,15,38]

While creatinine clearance may be reduced, serum creatinine is typically stable as there is reduced skeletal muscle mass, which means less creatinine is being produced.[14] Regardless of the challenges in assessing renal function accurately, it is estimated that some 26% of adults over 70 years of age have some degree of chronic renal impairment.[34]

Renal changes are likely to be responsible for mild changes to the acid–base balance.[6] A meta-analysis recently countered the belief that acid–base is stable with ageing and found that there is a progressive increase in blood hydrogen ion concentration and a progressive decrease in blood bicarbonate ion and carbon dioxide concentrations. This may be exacerbated by disease states and could both influence and be influenced by medications.[6]

ADDITIONAL KIDNEY FUNCTION: ERYTHROPOIETIN AND VITAMIN D

Erythropoietin (EPO) is primarily synthesised by interstitial cells in the capillary bed surrounding the tubules of the renal cortex, with further amounts being synthesised in the liver. The renal cortex is the location for the greatest proportion of renal shrinkage and the most significant reduction in renal blood flow. Changes to EPO are discussed under 'The haematological system'.

Vitamin D synthesis is a multi-step process starting with the biologically inactive form of ergocalciferol (vitamin D_2) from the diet and cholecalciferol (vitamin D_3) from the skin and some foods, which is hydroxylated in the liver to 25-dihydroxyvitamin D_3 (calcidiol). The final step is hydroxylation of calcidiol in the kidneys to the biologically active form 1,25-dihydroxyvitamin D (1,25[OH]$_2$D), or calcitriol. Age-related changes to the kidneys result in a 50% reduction in the production of calcitriol, though this is moderated to some degree by a compensatory increase in parathyroid function.[40] Vitamin D status is the result of a complex combination of renal, integumentary, gastrointestinal, hepatic, parathyroid and dietary factors and inadequate levels may reduce immune function, bone density, muscle function, cardiovascular reserves, cognition and mood.

LOWER URINARY TRACT

Changes to the bladder structure are associated with functional compromise. Within the bladder wall the ratio of smooth muscle to collagen decreases, reducing contractile strength. The ageing bladder may develop dense bands of sarcolemma and loss of sarcolemma caveolae, which normally contain a range of receptors, second messengers and other molecules that help regulate muscle function. Sensory and motor changes caused by alterations in the epithelium and oxidative stress damage may also occur. These changes are linked to increased involuntary detrusor contractions, changes in contraction strength and velocity and a decrease in elasticity and compliance, affecting bladder storage and emptying function. There are changes to bladder innervation, exacerbated by overactivity or obstruction (e.g. seen with benign prostatic hypertrophy).[41]

There is a reduction in muscle volume and tone in the pelvic floor; however, ageing may not be the prime causative factor – other causes may include obesity and overweight, parity and vaginal delivery, overall lack of muscle tone, medications and prolonged straining (e.g. occupational requirement to lift heavy weights). In women, the loss of oestrogen amplifies these effects and may lead to atrophic urethritis. The bladder and pelvic floor changes predispose older men and women to incontinence and reduced quality of life.[41]

> ### Practice points
> - Significant functional loss and CKD may be present without overt signs and symptoms until there is additional renal insult such as alteration in fluid status, illness, surgery or trauma, or change to medications.
> - Multiple factors influence GFR and these may be more significant than age.
> - Renal impairment can significantly reduce drug elimination, and reduced body water mass may alter drug pharmacokinetics.
> - Reduced thirst and ADH responsiveness predispose to dehydration and electrolyte imbalance.
> - Old age, chronic illness and specifically CKD may cause chronic anaemia, and vitamin D synthesis may be impaired.

The gastrointestinal and hepatobiliary systems

Changes to the gastrointestinal tract (GIT) and to the hepatobiliary system typically accrue gradually and there may be a long period of subclinical change before overt symptomatology or deranged pathology is evident. That said, an Italian study of 3238 people over the age of 60 years attending an outpatient clinic (for any cause) found that 43% experienced some upper gastrointestinal symptoms.[42] Symptoms were more prevalent in females, those with other medical conditions (especially respiratory and psychiatric conditions), smokers, those who were obese and those taking multiple medications. For the healthy older person, the impact of GIT ageing may be modest and may not have significant impact; conversely, a compromised gut and liver can have broad and significant implications for quality of life, morbidity and mortality.

Oral changes, altered dentition, gingival recession and reduced jaw strength may reduce chewing efficacy, affecting swallowing and choice of foods. A loss of taste is common and multifactorial, including smell dysfunction, upper respiratory and sinus infection, head injury, pharmaceutical side effects, the loss of taste buds, reduced saliva and idiopathic causes. The reduced oral function and sense of taste represent a risk factor for developing nutritional deficiencies.

Neuromuscular changes and reduced ability to coordinate complex reflexes in the oesophagus and oropharynx reduce the efficacy and success of swallowing. Reduced muscle strength reduces contraction velocity and desynchronised contraction and relaxation can lead to conditions such as achalasia, spasm and reflux. Motility abnormalities are particularly seen in the cricopharyngeus muscle of the upper oesophageal sphincter and are associated with aspiration, dysphagia and pharyngeal diverticula.[14] Achalasia is characterised by a loss of ganglia in the oesophagus, incomplete relaxation and increased tone of the lower oesophageal sphincter (LOS) and lack of peristalsis of the oesophagus.[2]

Gastro-oesophageal reflux disease (GORD) is a common condition and age-related changes contribute to its development. Risk factors for GORD include reduced LOS relaxation as well as increased transient LOS relaxation, decreased LOS resting pressure, reduced oesophageal peristaltic activity and poor oesophageal acid clearance, a modest delay in gastric emptying, impaired saliva flow and increased oxidative stress, which are all more common with increasing age.[2] The severity of GORD, marked by increased epithelial damage, pre-cancerous changes and silent aspiration, increases with age yet the overt symptoms of reflux and heartburn decrease.[2]

Postprandial hypotension increases with age and poses a cardiovascular, cerebrovascular and falls risk.[2] With exposure to nutrients and stomach distension, blood is shunted to the gut to support digestion. In healthy and younger people, other vessels vasoconstrict in order to maintain blood pressure, but this function is compromised with age.[2,43]

The myenteric plexus arises from the medulla oblongata; it is carried via the vagal nerve to the gut, and provides motor innervation to the gut, having both parasympathetic and sympathetic input, as well as controlling GIT motility. In older people there are fewer neurons in the myenteric plexus and a reduced bowel response to stimulation.[2,7,17] Oxidative stress and mitochondrial dysfunction have been proposed as mechanisms leading to this neuronal loss.[2]

Within the colon mucosal changes are present but have less impact; the main change is an altered bowel wall with thickening of the muscular layers of the colon caused by progressively increasing deposition of collagen and build-up of elastin between myocytes (and not through hypertrophy or hyperplasia of myocytes).[7] Colonic contractions and propulsion are affected and this contributes to constipation, dry stool and faecal impaction, which in turn increase the development of diverticular disease and haemorrhoids and are associated with colorectal cancer.[7] Fibro-fatty changes and thickening of

the internal anal sphincter may predispose to faecal incontinence.[7]

Within the small intestine the villi progressively lose height from 60 years of age, reducing the available absorptive surface area, and normal mucosal parenchyma and smooth muscle cells are replaced by fibrous connective tissue affecting secretion and absorption capacity.[14]

There is a reduced production and changed composition of saliva, with a decrease in the amylase ptyalin and an increase in mucin (lubricating and immune functions) which makes the saliva thicker and more viscous.[14]

The gastric mucosa and glands become atrophic and the epithelial cells regenerate more slowly, causing a reduction in the secretion of mucus, bicarbonate, intrinsic factor and pepsin. Nerve and blood supply to the stomach is compromised and endogenous prostaglandin function altered.[2,44] Endogenous prostaglandins are thought to modulate acid secretion and their release is up-regulated in response to injury, likely as a protective mechanism, thus a gastric environment with reduced baseline prostaglandins may be more vulnerable to damage. Conversely, a critical factor in the extent of inflammatory damage to the gastric mucosa seen with *Helicobacter pylori* infection is the excessive endogenous production of prostaglandin E_2 (PGE_2) and nitric oxide (NO) triggered by the overexpression of cyclooxygenase-2 (COX-2) and inducible nitric oxide synthase (iNOS).[45]

Pernicious anaemia is seen in 0.1% of the general population, increasing to 1.9% in people over the age of 60 years, and accounts for 20–50% of the causes of vitamin B_{12} deficiency in adults.[46] The age-related gastric atrophy (specifically the reduction in intrinsic factor secretion) and altered milieu is a risk factor for developing pernicious anaemia. This effect is amplified by the further destruction of the gastric mucosa by a process of cell-mediated autoimmunity.[46]

Impaired blood flow and oxygen supply, impaired nerve supply, altered hormonal and prostaglandin environment and reduced mucosal defence increase the stomach's susceptibility to damage by ingested substances (including alcohol, aspirin, non-steroidal anti-inflammatory drugs), impair healing, may reduce the efficacy of anti-ulcer pharmaceuticals, increase the risk of ulceration and perforation and may reduce the digestion and absorption of nutrients, especially vitamin B_{12}.[27,45] Reduced digestive capacity may increase sensations of dyspepsia, which can reduce appetite.

The gut has an extensive network of neurons and several neurotransmitters and neuropeptides seen in the brain are also expressed by enteric neurons, as are transmitter and neuropeptide receptors. Enteric neurons synthesise and release not only acetylcholine, substance P, nitric oxide, adenosine triphosphate, vasoactive intestinal polypeptide and 5-hydroxytryptamine but also opioid peptides as their transmitters.[47] Endorphins are endogenous opioid neuropeptides and their release activates opioid receptors on the enteric nerve that control motility and secretion leading to a slowing of gastric emptying, an increase in sphincter tone and inhibition of motor function which, when combined with inhibition of ion and fluid secretion, result in constipation.[47] This effect is seen with both endogenous and exogenous opioids, and elderly people have greater binding of plasma endorphins to intestinal receptors, making them particularly susceptible to these effects.[7]

Over a century ago, Russian embryologist Ilya Ilyich Mechnikov (Élie Metchnikoff) theorised that health could be enhanced and senility could be delayed by manipulating the intestinal microbiota. He had observed Eastern Europeans living simple lives in sometimes harsh conditions, with a largely plant-based diet and regular physical activity and who were typically very long-lived.[48] In particular, he recognised the importance of microbiota for healthy ageing (though his understanding of the mechanisms of actions may be challenged today) and he developed a regimen to suppress 'putrefactive colonic bacteria' that included the use of dietary probiotics in the form of yoghurt or kefir milk drinks cultured using *Bulgarian bacillus* (*Lactobacillus bulgaricus*).[48]

While more than 1000 different species colonise the human gut, they represent a small number of phyla with the most abundant being Firmicutes (includes *Lactobacillus*, *Enterococcus* and *Clostridium* genera), Bacteroidetes (includes *Bacteroides* genus) and Actinobacteria (includes *Bifidobacterium*), with a lesser representation of Proteobacteria (includes *Enterobacter*, *Escherichia* and *Klebsiella* genera), Fusobacteria, Cyanobacteria and Verrucomicrobia.[49,50] Once established, the composition of the intestinal microbiota is relatively stable, but it can be altered (short or long term) by extrinsic factors.[50] There is high inter-individual variability in microbiota composition in adults and this is exaggerated in the elderly.[50] These differences are influenced by age, diet, medications, disease, hormones, co-habitants, stress, genes and geography[49,51] but in healthy adults there is still a core gut microbiota of the four phyla Firmicutes, Actinobacteria, Bacteroidetes and Proteobacteria.[49] Morphological and physiological changes to the gut affect the composition of the intestinal microbiota as do other age-related factors such as dietary changes, reduced mobility, increased bowel transit time, medications, hospitalisation and communal living with other elderly people, infections, antibiotic use and altered immune response.[50,52]

The functions of the gut microbiota are diverse and include polysaccharide digestion, regulation of gut motility, regulation of the gastrointestinal barrier, energy metabolism and mitochondrial function, immune system development, defence against infections, synthesis of vitamins, fat storage, angiogenesis regulation, behaviour development and psychological health.[46,51,53] Of particular interest for ageing is that the gut microbiota may modulate elements of frailty, including changes in innate immunity, sarcopenia and cognitive function.[54]

Key dietary findings include that animal-based diets (higher in fat and protein) increase the proportion of bile-tolerant microorganisms such as *Bacteroides* and decrease the levels of Firmicutes that metabolise dietary plant polysaccharides.[55,56] Microbiota composition appears stable for most people until the eighth decade.[52,53] With the significant number of factors that influence an

individual's microbiota it is challenging to generalise about age-related changes, but there is a general increase in pro-inflammatory bacteria with age while health-promoting *Bifidobacterium* remain relatively stable. The characteristics and composition of an individual's microbiota correlate with the degree of frailty, presence of co-morbidities, nutritional status and level of inflammatory markers.[51]

Studies into the microbiota of elderly people have been inconsistent.[57] A Finnish study found reduced abundance of Firmicutes, Bacteroidetes and Actinobacteria in the elderly compared with younger adults, as did an Irish study.[58,59] Studies by Claesson[59] and Biagi et al.[60] assessed the microbiota composition of elderly Italians and Irish, respectively, and were published at the same time but had notably different results. Interestingly, location and co-habitation appeared more important than age up until very old age and the Italians and Irish had distinctly different bacteria.[52] In the absence of disease, marked microbiota compositional stability was noted until around 80 years of age, which is much older than for other age-related changes; in the Italian study significant changes were only noted in centenarians.[52] The Bacteroidetes component remained unchanged in the Italian population but it increased substantially in the Irish elderly and displaced Firmicutes to become the dominant phylum. Further, the Irish had an abundance of *Faecalibacterium* spp while the Italians had a reduction in this group. For the challenges and inconsistencies between studies, it is generally considered that there is an increase in pro-inflammatory opportunistic bacteria, a decrease in carbohydrate digestion and fermentation and an increase in proteolytic capacity.[51] Another finding by Biagi et al.[52] involved the influence of living environment: 'younger elderly' (average 70 years of age) who lived with their very elderly parents had an increase in the proportion of opportunistic pro-inflammatory bacteria of their parents compared with matched individuals who did not live with their very elderly parents.

LIVER AND GALL BLADDER

Parenchymal atrophy reduces the volume of the liver with age and portal blood flow decreases. Hepatocytes accumulate ageing pigments (such as lipofuscin) and oxidative DNA damage leads to an increase in mutations, particularly within mitochondria. Ageing is associated with reduced metabolic activity of the hepatic parenchyma though in the absence of disease liver function tests (LFTs) may remain within normal parameters.

The reduced metabolic activity of the liver may mean a reduced ability to metabolise, conjugate and detoxify some substances and this makes older adults more susceptible to dose-related side effects that a younger adult would not experience. With age the liver is more prone to stress and inflammatory damage and along with obesity and hyperglycaemia these increase the rate of hepatic ageing. Further, the regenerative and healing capacity of the liver diminishes with age, thereby the elderly are vulnerable to increased hepatic injury and reduced capacity to respond and heal.[16,61]

The capacity to synthesise compounds reduces and may be seen in reduced plasma volume, reduced plasma protein binding and reduced plasma protein.[16] The production and flow of bile decrease with age, increasing the risk of cholelithiasis and cholecystitis as well as negatively impacting on digestion. There is also an increase in the plasma concentration of most pro-coagulant factors, increasing cardiovascular and cerebrovascular risk.

> ### Practice points
> - Older adults are at a higher risk of achalasia and dysphagia, which in turn increases their risk of silent reflux and aspiration
> - There is a high prevalence of digestive symptoms and disorders in older people, including constipation, dyspepsia, GORD, irritable bowel syndrome and coeliac disease
> - Many conditions can be ameliorated through dietary intervention and supported by herbal medicine
> - The reduced hepatic function is particularly important for metabolism of pharmaceutical drugs as well as supplements and herbal medicine; see 'Pharmacotherapy' for further elaboration
> - Dietary intake and nutritional status are paramount in maintaining health into older age, and optimising digestive function is integral to this approach.

The haematological system

With age, and moderated by genetic and environmental factors, there is an increase in bone marrow fat and a reduction in haematologically functional bone marrow tissue.[17,62] The total white cell count is stable but ratios alter, with an increase in the output of myeloid cells and a decrease of B- and T-cell progenitors.[17,62] While the number of neutrophils and monocytes may remain steady, the effectiveness of those cells is blunted, especially when faced with acute infections or trauma, leaving the older person vulnerable to infection.[15,16,63]

Anaemia is common with age but is multifactorial and may be related to indirect causes such as low intake of iron or gastrointestinal bleeding, or more direct renal or bone marrow causes. Regardless, anaemia poses a significant risk when combined with reduced cardiorespiratory capacity.[16] Impaired reticulocytosis leaves the bone marrow unable to respond quickly and effectively to acute blood loss.[15] This may be due to reduced bone marrow tissue and/or increased haematopoietic stem cell resistance to EPO. With age there is an imbalance between EPO need, production and function and this may be exacerbated by inflammatory cytokines that contribute to EPO sensitivity.[64]

Serum EPO increases with age, presumably as a compensatory mechanism for reduced cardiorespiratory effectiveness, subclinical blood loss (e.g. gastric erosion), increased red blood cell turnover or increased EPO resistance of haematopoietic stem cells. With increasing age the renal production of EPO, especially in those with renal impairment (e.g. diabetes), fails to sustain the compensatory increase and ultimately leads to 'anaemia of

old age'.[64] In addition, there is 'anaemia of chronic disease' which is associated with chronic illness and inflammation and mediated by the protein hepcidin, which is synthesised in the liver. Hepcidin regulates the metabolism and transport of iron, and elevated inflammatory cytokines, in particular interleukin-6 (IL-6), cause an increase in hepcidin synthesis leading to increased iron-trapping within macrophages and liver cells and decreased gut iron absorption, thus reducing available circulating iron and causing anaemia.[64,65] Hepcidin production is increased via three main triggers: inflammation, iron overload and, unhelpfully, hypoxia/anaemia. Hepcidin levels are increased in CKD and, when combined with altered EPO production and stem cell EPO-resistance, there is a compounding of effects and inevitable and recalcitrant anaemia.[63,65]

> ### Practice points
> - There is an increased risk of anaemia and subsequent reduced aerobic capacity and exercise tolerance
> - The leucocytic immune response to infection is reduced.

The immune system

Immunosenescence, the age-related changes to the immune system, is qualitative and quantitative and may involve a gradual decline and senescence and/or dysregulation and remodelling of immune cells.[14,66] Changes affect both innate and acquired immunity and are associated with increased vulnerability to infection and a compromised response to immune challenges. Changes to innate immunity include alterations to physical barriers such as reduced mucosal IgA expression and vitamin D synthesis, reduced cell turnover and recovery, and reduced integrity of epidermal and mucosal surfaces.[15] Phagocytosis and chemotaxis of macrophages and neutrophils are compromised, especially macrophage antigen processing and presentation. NK cells increase in number, though exhibit a reduction in cytokine expression and thus cytotoxicity, especially with exposure to stress.[14,15,66] Complement pathway cytolysis, opsonisation and initiation of inflammation in response to infection are dampened.[14]

Bone marrow changes result in reduced production of B- and T-cells and altered proportions of CD4+ and CD8+ naïve T-cells, all of which are increasingly intrinsically damaged, with defects seen in old CD4+ and naïve T-cells that appear to impair their responsiveness to antigenic stimulation. In addition, thymus involution, which starts at birth, is 90% complete by 60 years of age.[15,62,66,67] B-cells have a blunted ability to produce antibodies against new antigenic material.[67]

Cytokine activity is aberrant; there is increased nonspecific activation of cytokines, marked by elevated serum inflammatory mediators, but a reduced efficacy of cytokines such as tumour necrosis factor-α (TNF-α), interleukin-1 (IL-1) and nitric oxide. Recent research proposes that immunosenescence is less age-dependent and more a consequence of a history of exposure to pathogens, in particular cytomegalovirus.[62,67]

Immune function is affected by the presence of chronic illness and inflammation as well as subclinical nutrient deficiencies and combined these make older people more susceptible to infectious diseases as well as chronic diseases where the immune system is involved, such as autoimmune diseases and cancer.[16]

Practice points

- Older people have blunted immune and inflammatory responses, increasing their susceptibility to infections
- There is dysregulation of immune cells and increased prevalence of autoimmune diseases and cancer
- Chronic over-expression and altered function of inflammatory cytokines may influence other disease pathogenesis.

The endocrine system

In a healthy elderly person there is a modest reduction in endocrine function, but many lifestyle factors and other comorbidities may reduce endocrine function to a clinically significant level. While the endocrine glands atrophy to varying degrees and most have a reduction in hormone production, they can still maintain normal function in the absence of triggers or stressors. As seen in other systems there is diminished reserve in endocrine glands so when stressed there is a reduced capacity to respond appropriately and an increased risk of the older adult suffering organ injury. For example, an elderly person maintaining a healthy diet and active lifestyle may maintain a blood glucose level within the normal range, but they would be expected to have a reduced capacity to respond to a glucose load or challenge and thus have a more pronounced and prolonged elevation in blood glucose compared with a younger adult.[7]

Compounding reduced hormone secretion there is reduced end-organ/tissue responsiveness as seen in the increased prevalence of insulin resistance. Changes in cell signalling often relate to post-receptor changes, but may also involve receptor sensitivity and numbers.[15] There is an age-associated reduction in insulin secretion not associated with lifestyle, and progressive glucose intolerance occurs irrespective of lifestyle factors. Importantly, not all endocrine function reduction is absolute, inevitable or severe.[32] Increased insulin resistance, carbohydrate intolerance and testosterone levels (in men) are determined more by diet, obesity and a sedentary lifestyle than by age.[14,15,29,68,69]

A reduction in growth hormone (GH) secretion and decreased serum levels of insulin-like growth factor-1 (IGF-1) are seen in the absence of pituitary pathology. Accompanying the decreased GH is a reduction in GH half-life.[14] Reduced GH is associated with reduced tissue turnover, loss of lean body and bone mass, increased fat mass and reduced healing capacity. GH reduction is a response to falling oestradiol and testosterone levels.[7,14]

The thyroid gland shows increased fibrosis and atrophy, reduced iodine uptake and lower levels of thyroxine and free thyroxine. There is reduced conversion of thyroxine (T_4) to the more biologically active triiodothyronine (T_3) and an increase in the ratio of reverse T_3.[14,29] This may be balanced by reduced clearance of thyroxine with age and for healthy elderly people net thyroid function may not diminish until the ninth decade.[14,70] A moderate increase is seen in thyroid-stimulating hormone (TSH). Both hypothyroidism and hyperthyroidism are seen in older populations, with the most significant increase seen with autoimmune disturbance. Subclinical hyperthyroidism is associated with an increased risk of total mortality, ischaemic heart disease mortality and the incidence of atrial fibrillation, but the clinical presentation may be atypical (see 'Atypical presentation').[71]

Parathyroid hormone is important in maintaining calcium homeostasis and it does this through three main mechanisms involving the bones, kidneys and gut. Parathyroid hormone stimulates the kidneys to increase renal calcium resorption and phosphate excretion; it also stimulates osteoclastic activity on the surfaces of bone trabeculae and converts 25-hydroxyvitamin D to its most active metabolite, 1,25-dihydroxyvitamin D_3 (1,25-$(OH)_2$ D_3, calcitriol), by activation of the enzyme 1-hydroxylase in the proximal tubules. Calcitriol promotes gut absorption of calcium by promoting the formation of calcium-binding protein within the intestinal epithelial cells. These mechanisms increase calcium ion concentration in the blood. Parathyroid hormone levels are increased with ageing and this is implicated in the development of osteopenia and osteoporosis. Parathyroid hormone is normally countered by calcitonin that is produced by the thyroid gland and acts to reduce serum calcium; however, calcitonin levels fall with age.[14]

Menopause and andropause are discussed in Chapters 18 and 19 in *Clinical Naturopathic Medicine*, but briefly, the decline in oestrogen for women leads to a marked increase in cardiovascular risk following menopause. In addition, there is an increased loss of bone density and vasomotor, connective tissue and mood changes.[14] The reduced oestrogen is accompanied by an increase in luteinising hormone (LH) and follicle-stimulating hormone (FSH). For males, cross-sectional and longitudinal studies have reported a decline in serum testosterone concentration, an increase in sex hormone-binding globulin (SHBG) concentration and a decrease in dehydroepiandrosterone (DHEA) and free testosterone with age. Compared with the dramatic reduction in oestrogen for women, the rate of hormone decline for men is typically 1% per annum or less.[70] The rise in SHBG exaggerates the already reduced levels of testosterone. While the decrease in testosterone is linked with reduced Leydig cell function, the decline is not experienced universally across men. Whereas menopause is absolute, testosterone levels in men are influenced by general health and fall with increased adiposity, depression, smoking, inactivity and metabolic syndrome – or they may remain at the levels of a younger man if the elderly man is healthy.[68–70] A 5-year study in Australia measured total testosterone, LH, FSH and SHBG levels of 1588 men with a mean age of 54 years (43–65 years) at recruitment. Testosterone declined in men with ongoing depression, those who were unmarried, had developed a chronic disease, or were obese or smoked, and increased over time in men who were married. Ceasing smoking, becoming obese and depression were inversely related to SHBG change.[68] These results were repeated in a US study of 1653 men,[69] which found that in healthy men there was no decrease in testosterone with increasing age but there was a negative correlation between testosterone and body mass index (BMI) and a positive correlation between testosterone and fitness. Reduced physical fitness can lead to a decreased level of testosterone, and a reduced testosterone level can increase sarcopenia, completing a cycle of decline. This was also seen in a longitudinal study of 2736 men across eight European centres, which found that weight loss was associated with a rise in free testosterone, testosterone and SHBG and a weight gain saw a reduction in the same parameters.[72]

Pregnenolone is the precursor for progestogens, mineralocorticoids, glucocorticoids, DHEA, androgens and oestrogens, as well as the neuroactive steroids that influence synaptic functioning, are neuroprotective and are thought to enhance myelinisation, and levels decline with age.[70] DHEA and its sulfate (DHEA-S) decline with age due to reduced production in the adrenal cortex, and there is a positive correlation between the extent of the decline and the degree of frailty.[14,29] DHEA may be up to five times higher at 30 years of age than at 85 years of age.[29] What is less clear is whether there is benefit in DHEA-S replacement.[29,71]

Ageing is associated with a shift in the diurnal pattern to earlier in the day, with late-day and evening increases in cortisol levels. The earlier increase in maximum cortisol (phase advance) may mean a move from 9.30 am for a younger adult to 6.30 am for an older adult. There is also lower circadian secretion and less orderly cortisol secretion patterns. The pattern, duration and quality of sleep declines, and this sleep disturbance may be exacerbated by other factors such as nocturia, pain and depression. The research is inconsistent and it is not clear whether these alterations reflect or cause ageing-associated reduction in functional ability, cognition and depression.[71] A meta-analysis reviewed hypothalamic-pituitary-adrenal (HPA) axis function and physical performance and ageing and found that a more dynamic HPA axis (greater decline in diurnal levels) was associated with better performance on most measures, irrespective of weight, age or BMI, and was also associated with a better physical performance in later life.[73] The greater diurnal drop (i.e. healthy reduction in cortisol over the day) was associated with better physical performance including faster walking speed and a quicker chair-rise time but there was no association with balance or grip strength. A lack of diurnal decline has been shown to be associated with increased psychosocial stress and a higher BMI.[74]

The Longitudinal Aging Study Amsterdam[75] is a cohort study in a general population of older persons (65 years or older): serum and salivary cortisol was measured in 1181 men and women over a 6/7-year period to evaluate associations with the prevalence of cortisol and chronic disease. The results showed that high salivary cortisol levels were associated with increased mortality risk in older participants. Interestingly, higher morning salivary cortisol levels were associated with increased mortality rate in men, whereas higher night-time salivary cortisol levels were associated with increased mortality rate in women. Both men and women had an increased risk of diabetes and men had an increased risk of hypertension.

Melatonin is secreted by the pineal gland and levels reduce with age.[70] Low nocturnal levels are associated with sleep disturbances in the elderly. Increases in cortisol are typically matched with decreases in melatonin, increasing the impact on sleep disturbance. Melatonin also has effects on the immune system, stimulating immune cell production, especially NK cells and CD4 T-helper lymphocytes, thus impacting on immunosenescence. Melatonin is also an antioxidant and a reduction in melatonin levels potentially increases the rate of ageing via increased oxidative stress. Further, melatonin effects DNA and histone production indicating a potential role in epigenetic modulation. Melatonin increases GH and IGF-1 secretion, meaning a reduced level will also impact on their functions.[70]

Gastrointestinal hormone function and changes are discussed in the section on 'Anorexia'; see Table 17.3 for a summary of other hormonal changes of ageing.

> ### Practice points
> - Subclinical decline in endocrine function may only be evident with stress, infection, illness or injury, but may be detected with thorough assessment
> - Treating subclinical decline may improve morbidity and mortality as well as quality of life
> - While evidence for the decline in hormones such as DHEA and pregnenolone is clear, it is less clear whether replacement therapy is helpful in reducing frailty and improving ageing
> - Decline in endocrine function is strongly influenced by diet, physical activity and adiposity and these should be addressed.

The musculoskeletal system

There is increasing loss of muscle mass, strength and flexibility with age. Sarcopenia is the age-related loss of skeletal muscle mass and strength and is discussed in more detail in the section 'Geriatric syndromes'. Loss of bone mineral density predisposes to osteopenia and osteoporosis, pathological fractures and chronic pain and while this is discussed in Chapter 15 in *Clinical Naturopathic Medicine* it warrants inclusion here due to the significant impact that bony changes can have on quality of life and morbidity.

In addition to basic structural support, organ protection and movement functions, bones have roles in hearing (ossicles), bone marrow blood cell production and storing fatty acids. Metabolically the bones also play a role in the storage and regulation of calcium and phosphorus, and contribute to acid–base balance and storing heavy metals which may play a

TABLE 17.3 Summary of age-related changes to hormone levels

Decreased	Increased	Unchanged/minimal change
Growth hormone	Adrenocorticotrophic hormone (ACTH)	Adrenaline (epinephrine)
Insulin-like growth factor-1	Cortisol	Prolactin
Insulin	Luteinising hormone (male and female)	
Pregnenolone	Follicle-stimulating hormone	
Dehydroepiandrosterone/sulfate	Parathyroid hormone	
Aldosterone	Noradrenaline (norepinephrine)	
Oestrogen (women)	Anti-diuretic hormone (day)	
Testosterone	Thyroid-stimulating hormone	
Triiodothyronine (T3)	Reverse T3	
Antidiuretic hormone (night)		
Vitamin D		
Thyroxine		
Renin		

protective role from the toxic effects of these substances. Age-related changes to bone therefore are more than loss of bone mineral density, though that is critical.

Men lose bone at approximately 1% per year after 50 years of age, compared with women who, after menopause, lose bone at a rate of up to 2%. In addition to age, dietary factors, low levels of weight-bearing exercise and medications may contribute to bone loss, and these are increasingly prevalent with advancing age.[15] Reduced bone density leads to thinning of the vertebrae and there is a concurrent reduction in disc thickness leading to a reduction in height. Over time, the weakened vertebrae are increasingly susceptible to compression and wedge fractures, resulting in pain, postural changes and possible spinal nerve impingement. Nerve impingement may also be secondary to arthritic osteophyte formation. Vertebral fractures may go undiagnosed and are difficult to quantify, whereas hip, pelvis and wrist fractures are more readily identified and counted.

The self-reported prevalence of osteoporosis in Australian adults older than 50 years was 9.4% in 2011–2012,[76] but a more in-depth analysis put this figure much higher. In 2013 it was estimated that 4.74 million Australians over the age of 50 had osteoporosis or poor bone health and that there was one fracture every 3.6 minutes.[77] This is an increase from one fracture every 8.1 minutes in 2001 and less than the one fracture every 2.9 minutes which is predicted by 2022.[76,77] Increasing age increases the likelihood of fractures and worsens outcomes, with increasing morbidity and pain, functional decline, necessity of additional care or transition to an age care facility, and mortality.

Practice points

- Assess bone health, nutrient status and exercise regularly
- Seek further information on under-reported age-related pain as it may indicate low-trauma or pathological fractures
- Include lifestyle and physical activity in treatment plans (in conjunction with the doctor and body movement expert, e.g. exercise physiologist).

The dermatological system

Skin changes are the result of progressive physiological and degenerative changes and are overlayed by environmental effects. Physiological changes include fewer sweat and oil glands, which makes skin more prone to dryness-related conditions such as roughness and itching and impair barrier function. Reduced turnover of the epidermal cells, decreased keratinocyte and fibroblast numbers and reduced vascular networks result in skin atrophy with reduced healing capacity. The dermis may become thicker and capillaries are more readily damaged and telangiectasia may result.[15]

Reduced production of elastin (suppleness) and collagen (dense fibres for strength) leads to wrinkles and skin sagging. At the same time the undulating dermal ridges flatten. The subcutaneous fat pads are reduced and senile lentigines (age or liver spots) are often seen on the upper limbs and face; these are due to a mild localised epidermal hyperplasia, increased melanin production and a clustering of increased numbers of melanocytes.[7,17] A common skin change is actinic (also called senile or solar) keratosis, scaly lesions on sun-damaged skin, considered to be pre-cancerous or an early form of squamous cell carcinoma.[17] The number of mast cells and Langerhans cells is decreased, reducing the immune protection they afford.[7] Finally, there is reduction in vitamin D synthesis which has implications for bone, immune and neurological health.[15]

Physiological changes are exacerbated by ultraviolet light damage, vascular insufficiency (e.g. stasis dermatitis), smoking and environmental exposure such as chemicals used in the workplace. Conditions such as vascular insufficiency and heart failure as well as pharmaceuticals such as steroids exacerbate age-related skin changes (e.g. stasis dermatitis) and there is an increased risk of skin tears and pressure sores with a simultaneous reduction in the capacity to heal. The reduced immune function of ageing leaves the older person vulnerable to skin infections and malignancies.[15]

Practice points

- Maintain skin integrity and practice safe sun exposure.

Metabolism and thermoregulatory changes

The basal metabolic rate (BMR) begins to decline in the third decade, with some estimates suggesting that reduced energy expenditure and physical activity could lead to a 20% reduction in BMR.[28] Factors that affect changes to the BMR include reduced skeletal muscle mass, reduced organ mass and increased fat mass. Age-related anorexia occurs due to impaired taste and smell, faster antral filling and early satiation and leads to reduced dietary energy intake. The weight loss associated with age-related anorexia and other causes further reduces BMR. Additional elements that contribute to the BMR are metabolic factors such as endocrine function (in particular, thyroid), reduced gluconeogenesis, fat oxidation and Na^+/K^+ adenosine triphosphate activity, and altered mitochondrial permeability and function.[28] A higher BMR with advancing age may predict higher multi-morbidity and thus may be indicative of deteriorating health.[78]

A number of age-related physiological changes negatively impact on thermoregulation, though it is unclear whether there is a change to baseline core temperature.[28,79] Changes to sympathetic and parasympathetic nervous function negatively affect thermoregulation.[16] There is reduced skin responsiveness to changes in environmental temperature and reduced vasomotor responses lead to less effective integumentary-based thermoregulation.[6] The shivering reflex is diminished and hepatic thermogenesis is reduced, leading to reduced heat production. An impaired fever response to infection contributes to immunosenescence. Research on 230 patients showed a blunted elevation in temperature with diagnosed bacteraemia.[79] Interestingly, the body temperature of older men continues to rise after they cease exercising, whereas in young men it returns to normal.[6] The net effect is that an older person is less able to compensate for changes to ambient temperature and thus is more vulnerable to injuries from excess heat or cold.

> **Practice points**
> - Dietary adjustment is required based on age, body composition and energy expenditure
> - Altered thermoregulation may distort temperature readings and clinical presentation.

Senses

TASTE AND SMELL

Taste and smell are interrelated and are important to the pleasure of eating as well as for practical issues such as checking for hazards in the environment (e.g. spoiled food, or smoke). There is a reduction in the number of taste buds, and hence taste, particularly after 80 years of age. There may also be a reduced sense of smell, and conditions such as blockage or disease of the olfactory receptors in the upper sinus may be the cause.

Medications, in particular polypharmacy, can also reduce or alter smell and sense of taste.[28]

EYES AND VISION

Changes to fat, muscle and tissue elasticity may lead to the eyes appearing sunken, or to ectropion or entropion. A reduction in the production of tears can predispose to corneal ulceration and keratitis.[17] Vision changes can occur through a number of age-related changes and may be exacerbated by disease, nutritional status, medications and environmental factors. A loss of elasticity and accommodation in the lens results in presbyopia (long-sightedness) and late-onset myopia may be experienced. Sclerosis of the lens leads to cataract formation and age-related macular degeneration may lead to loss of all or part of the central field of vision. Changes in the vitreous humour, iris, lens and macula visual acuity reduce the field of vision and lead to the development of visual floaters.[17] Older people are more sensitive to low light as well as thickening and yellowing of the lens, which causes light diffraction, increased sensitivity to glare, decreased depth perception and more difficulty distinguishing pastel colours, especially blues and greens.

EARS AND HEARING

With ageing there is a decrease in sensitivity to high-frequency tones (presbycusis) and decreased discrimination of similar pitches due to changes in the bones and cochlear hair cells of the inner ear. Otosclerosis and accumulated wax can cause conductive deafness. Otosclerosis and changes to hairs in the semicircular canal can lead to vertigo.[17]

> **Practice points**
> - Sensory changes can significantly reduce quality of life and independence
> - Ensure communication is clear and confirm understanding.

ASSESSMENT

Assessment of older adults includes general adult assessment items, geriatric screening and nutritional assessment and screening. It may involve assessing an acute minor to mild condition such as an upper respiratory tract infection in a 'healthy' 65-year-old at one end of the scale to a full multidimensional, multidisciplinary geriatric assessment in a frail 85-year-old at the other end of the scale. A health assessment of an older adult is not simply the same as an assessment of a younger adult for several reasons, including:
- There is a difference between a healthy older person and a sick older person, albeit that difference is not fully defined and agreed upon[80]
- Older adults may have atypical presentation of diseases (see below)
- Quantifiable pathology tests where an objective numerical value and reference range is provided is

based on the results for a 'normal healthy adult'; that is, not an older adult[80]

- The older the person, the more years of health, ill-health, accidents, motherhood, socioeconomic vicissitudes, psychological stress and environmental exposure as well as an increasing likelihood of epigenetic changes and multi-morbidities (past and present), all of which make attempting simple comparative analysis of a health assessment to someone 30 years younger an ambitious but flawed endeavour.[80,81]

Laboratory reference ranges are based on healthy younger adults and whereas adjustments to reference ranges have been developed for paediatrics there has not been significant development in this area for older adults.[80,82] The question remains regarding how to interpret results in the context of diminished physiological reserves, compensatory mechanisms and single and multiple morbidities.[80] A recent review of reference intervals in the frail elderly found that alanine aminotransferase, phosphate, albumin and sodium were lower and that creatinine and urea were higher in the frail elderly and it was concluded that using conventional reference ranges was misleading and potentially dangerous.[83]

Furthermore, older adults often have highly changeable and fluctuating symptoms, meaning that the timing of the assessment is essential lest the diagnosis be missed; moreover, the broad nature of geriatric syndromes means it is easy to miss or to attribute symptomatology to other causes.[7] That is not to say that there is no place for pathology testing; rather, it should be noted that assessments are most valuable when they are part of a continuum for the individual, marking progress and decline against themselves.[80] Finally, an individual's family, close friends or long-term carers are likely to notice differences earlier than a health professional who has episodic exposure to the person and to some extent uses blunt diagnostic tools[83]; this is particularly so for cognitive changes and early dementia.[84]

A Comprehensive Geriatric Assessment (CGA)[81] is typically performed by aged care specialists from complementary disciplines – for example, geriatrician, occupational therapist, physiotherapist, registered nurse, dietitian and nutritionist, speech therapist, mental health professional and specialist aged care assessor – who determine care needs in the home or residential care placement. While it is not typically the domain of the naturopath to conduct these assessments, it is advisable to be cognisant of the types of assessments and some of the tools used. Of particular note, when determining and assessing the parameters of frailty and reduced quality of life in ageing, the opposite is also defined; that is, the counterpoint to frailty is 'ageing well' and this is an area of preventive healthcare to which naturopaths are particularly well positioned to make an important contribution.

A CGA reviews the current or presenting complaint, identifies risk factors, monitors ongoing management of pre-existing issues (including a medication review and potential de-prescribing), and may assess anaesthetic and surgical risk as well as evaluate care and support needs in the home or the requirement for residential placement.[81] Compared with an assessment for a younger adult which is likely to focus on acute care needs with a lesser component of preventive care, the geriatric assessment has an increased focus on quality of life and functional status and explicitly explores goals of care needs.[81] Within a medical context, discussion about end-of-life preferences and advanced care planning is also essential.[85–87] A full review of geriatric and frailty assessment instruments and scales is beyond the scope of this chapter, but they are available in reviews such as by Rubenstein and Rubenstein[81] and de Vries et al.[88]

'Quality of life' includes the domains of socioeconomic status, environmental factors, health and disease status, and functional status.[81] There are many views on what constitutes quality of life and thus what to include in any measurement tool. Analysis and interpretation can be focused on health, financial, social, spiritual and other domains; however, it is possible to group the domains into two broad dimensions as outlined in a review by the University of Buffalo:

1 Personal or internal (including functional status and health) versus socioenvironmental or external conditions (such as prosthetics)
2 Subjective (e.g. qualitative measures of life satisfaction) versus objective (including income, physical environment and housing) factors.[89]

General quality of life measures (e.g. the WHOQOL tool)[90] as well as health status quality of life measures (e.g. the Medical Outcomes Study Short Form Health Survey, SF-36) are available[91] but increasingly disease-specific measures are being developed as they are considered to have greater specificity and thus relevance. Recent work by Ware et al. has standardised measures across diseases to bring some uniformity.[92]

Assessment components can be summarised as follows:
- Physical examination including inspection of the oral cavity, skin, joints, gait
- Neurological assessment
- Cognitive assessment (e.g. Mini-Mental State Examination, MMSE)[93]
- Vital signs (ideally lying and standing blood pressure measurements to assess postural response)
- Functional assessment
- Mobility and falls risk
- Depression and mood
- Individual disease state and multi-morbidity picture (e.g. using tools such as the Charlson Comorbidity Index)[94]
- Medication review
- Diet and nutrition
- Weight, including changes
- Continence
- Sexual function
- Vision and hearing
- Dentition
- Living situation (e.g. home, residential care)
- Financial concerns
- Support needs
- Spirituality
- Advance care preferences
- Goals of care.

Cognitive assessment

Cognitive assessment can help distinguish between delirium, early cognitive decline and dementia. A common tool is the MMSE, which is a brief 5–10-minute test that evaluates domains affected by dementia, including orientation, registration, attention and calculation, recall, language and ability to follow simple instructions. Scores range from 0 to 30; a score less than 24 is interpreted as evidence of a dementing illness.[93] The Rowland Universal Dementia Assessment Scale (RUDAS) is another brief cognitive screening tool that is administered by a health professional and was designed to minimise the effects of cultural learning and language diversity on the assessment of baseline cognitive performance.[95]

Functional assessment

Functional assessment includes basic activities of daily living (ADLs) and independent activities of daily living (IADLs; see Table 17.4); both can be predictive of current and future health status.[96]

Potential challenges of geriatric assessment

Conducting an assessment of an older adult may present unique challenges for the practitioner and require extended consultation time as well as the input and support of family or close support people, depending on the health and functioning of the individual. Some of the potential challenges include:
- Multiplicity and complexity of complaints and diseases (and varied responses to pharmacotherapy)[17]
- Atypical presentation of disease
- The nonspecific manifestation of disease and the nonspecific nature of geriatric syndromes, e.g. the

presenting complaint may be something like not wanting to eat, or a report by a family member that the patient won't get out of bed[97]
- Delayed presentation and underreporting of illness – the patient may not want to be a burden, may not recognise the problem or may have no access to support or transport; they may also think that having aches, pains, weakness, digestive disturbance or other symptoms is a normal part of getting old and that there is nothing that can be done[17]
- Delayed or reduced quantifiable pathology (e.g. attenuated and delayed rise in white blood cells in bacteraemia)
- Delayed development of overt symptoms (e.g. slow and blunted elevation in temperature)
- Inaccurate self-diagnosis
- The older adult may be a 'poor historian', unable to provide what is considered to be a sequential, cause-and-effect history of the condition or situation
- Cognitive changes including altered memory and dementia
- Language and communication barriers
- Mental health conditions
- The ageist attitude of the practitioner, believing that morbidities are inevitable and investigation and treatment are not warranted.[98]

Strategies to facilitate effective history taking with older adults are provided in Box 17.1.

Atypical presentation of disease

The clinical presentation of disease in older adults may differ from that in younger adults and from that which is typically described in pathophysiology texts (see Table 17.5 for examples). The reasons for this include the reduced physiological reserve and attenuation of homeostatic and immunological responses to injury and disease, as discussed

---

TABLE 17.4 ADLs and IADLs

Activities of daily living (ADLs), basic self-care tasks	Independent ADLs (IADLs), ability to maintain an independent household
• Personal hygiene • Toileting • Maintaining continence • Dressing and grooming • Feeding • Transferring (e.g. chair to standing, and vice versa) • Mobility, walking (independently or with walking aids, but not requiring another person).	• Shopping for groceries and necessities • Driving or using public transport • Using the telephone and/or email • Performing housework and laundry • Preparing meals • Managing own medications • Managing own finances.

Source: Griebling TL. Aging and geriatric urology. In: Wein AJ, Kavoussi LR, Partin AW, et al (eds). Campbell-Walsh urology. 11th edn. Philadelphia: Elsevier; 2012, pp. 2083–102. Morley JE. Function assessment scales. In: Sinclair AJ, Morley JE, Vellas B (eds). Pathy's principles and practice of geriatric medicine. 5th edn. Oxford: Wiley-Blackwell; 2012, pp. i–x.

BOX 17.1 History-taking of older adults

- Slow down the pace; allow time for the person to reflect
- Ensure that the person can hear
- Speak clearly and avoid jargon
- Ask direct questions
- Establish the speed of onset of the illness
- Use the person's previous status as a core measure of change (not norms based on younger adults)
- If the presentation is vague, carry out a systematic enquiry
- Confirm and expand on the history with additional information sources (e.g. family, carer, doctor, nurse)
- If considering further investigations (blood tests, scans), first determine whether the results of those investigations will alter management and, if not, whether they are necessary
- Look beyond the 'classic presentation'
- Reflect on geriatric syndromes
- Confirm understanding – yours and theirs
- Clarify and confirm the person's goals for their health and their requirements from their healthcare provider.

TABLE 17.5 Atypical presentations of disease		
Condition	**Younger person**	**Older adult**
Myocardial infarction	Substernal chest pain, may radiate to left jaw and arm.	Shortness of breath, falls, fatigue, confusion or palpitations. May have vague chest pain, heart failure.
Heart failure	Fatigue, shortness of breath on exertion/at rest, orthopnoea, paroxysmal nocturnal dyspnoea, acute pulmonary oedema, dependent oedema.	Insidious changes e.g. anorexia, changed functional status. Signs of reduced cardiac output (weakness, falls, fatigue, confusion, syncope, insomnia, non-productive cough). Cardiac cachexia, dependent oedema.
Pulmonary oedema	Acute dyspnoea, paroxysmal nocturnal dyspnoea or coughing, generalised oedema.	Confusion, anorexia.
Pneumonia	Shortness of breath, fever, chills, pleuritic chest pain, productive cough (if bacterial).	Confusion may be the only symptom. May also be tachycardic, anorexic, with low-grade fever, cough, vague chest pain.
Diabetes mellitus	Polyuria, polyphagia and polydipsia, weight loss.	Severe dehydration, hyperosmolarity and even coma may develop rapidly in the absence of overt symptoms. If present, polyuria may be attributed to prostatic or urinary diseases. Confusion, delirium, behavioural changes (hypo- or hyperglycaemia).
Lack of insulin, hyperglycaemia	Ketoacidosis, ketone breath, shallow rapid respirations.	Not ketotic, no ketone breath, hyperosmolar, non-ketotic coma.
Hyperthyroidism	Tachycardia, sweats or anxiety states, diarrhoea, hyperactive reflexes, heat intolerance, hyperphagia.	Depressed and apathetic, unanimated, coarse tremor (especially associated with weight loss), new-onset atrial fibrillation.
Hypothyroidism	Fatigue, constipation, slowed memory, sensitivity to cold, lethargy.	Confusion, agitation.
Acute infection	Fever, hot, flushed, perspiring	None or blunted fever response.
Acute appendicitis	Peritoneal signs – abdominal pain localised to right lower quadrant, guarding, Blumberg's sign (rebound tenderness) and nausea, vomiting, fever, leucocytosis.	Confusion, delirium. 'Silent' acute abdomen (no reports of pain). May have generalised abdominal rigidity, decreased bowel sounds, nausea and vomiting.
Urinary tract infection	Dysuria, fever.	Confusion, dizziness, anorexia. Asymptomatic.
GORD	Postprandial heartburn, especially reclining.	Regurgitation, dysphagia, chronic cough, hoarse voice, no pain.
Peptic ulcer disease	Epigastric abdominal pain, may be better (duodenal) or worse (gastric) with eating and drinking.	Bleeding, nausea, vomiting, anorexia, abdominal pain not relieved by eating or drinking (duodenal ulcers).
Cholecystitis	Right upper quadrant pain, Murphy's sign (pain on deep inspiration), radiating pain through to back or shoulder, fever, nausea, vomiting.	Generalised abdominal pain, anorexia, nausea and vomiting. May have low-grade fever.
Depression	Sadness, depressed mood, hypersomnia and insomnia, loss of interest and pleasure, fatigue, sense of hopelessness and worthlessness, clouded cognition, weight gain or loss, suicidal ideation.	May present with dysphoria, diminished concentration, social withdrawal, confusion. Atypical presentation includes somatic complaints (e.g. anorexia, vague GIT symptoms, constipation and sleep disturbances), hyperactivity.
Pain	Verbalises pain, restricted movement, guarding, distress.	Altered sensation of pain and under-reporting, especially with cognitive decline (note this does not mean they have no pain).

Note: this is not a comprehensive list of signs and symptoms for the above conditions but shows examples of specific differences.
Source: Adapted from [17,94,97–101].

earlier. This lack of clarity is compounded by the presence of comorbid conditions and polypharmacy. So-called classic symptoms may be present, absent, diminished or replaced with nonspecific complaints such as fatigue, weight loss or functional decline.[99] For example, an older adult may have a history of falls that could have been triggered by hyponatraemia, post-prandial hypotension, polypharmacy or an undiagnosed urinary tract infection. Another example is myocardial infarction: a younger adult (especially male) would typically have chest pain, whereas 70% of non-diabetic adults aged 70 years and over do not complain of chest pain – instead they may present with shortness of breath, falls, confusion or palpitations.[17]

A study conducted by Grosmaitre et al.[97] regarding atypical presentation of ST-elevation myocardial infarction (STEMI) in emergency departments highlights the dangers of atypical presentations. For the 225 patients aged 75 years or older who had a STEMI, their presenting symptoms were chest pain 41.2%, falls and/or felt faint 15.7%, dyspnoea 9.8%, impaired general condition 6.7% and delirium 5%. Delirium can be attributed to a myriad of causes, as can falls and general decline in function. Compared with older adults whose presenting complaint was chest pain, those who had a STEMI but had other presenting symptoms took longer to present to emergency, had more severe clinical symptoms, waited longer to be triaged and treated, may have not had full treatment and had double the mortality at 1 month. A review of 633 presentations of older adults to emergency departments in Thailand found that 28.6% of presentations were atypical.[100] The top two atypical presentations were failure to develop a fever in conditions known to cause fever (e.g. appendicitis, pneumonia, sepsis) and lack of pain in conditions known to cause pain (e.g. appendicitis, myocardial infarction, renal calculi).[100] The ultimate risks of atypical presentations are missed diagnoses and poor outcomes, including increased risk of death.[99]

Nutritional assessment

Decline in nutritional status is a key feature of functional decline and frailty in older adults and it may be a recent development or the cumulative effects of a lifetime of poor nutrition.[1,102] The overall goal of nutritional assessment is to determine whether intake meets current and ongoing requirements to maintain body weight and composition, physiological function, reduce morbidity and optimise health.[103,104] Assessing nutritional status allows the naturopath (or other health professional) to determine the current status and develop strategies to maintain and improve the nutritional and overall health of their older patients.

COMPONENTS OF THE NUTRITIONAL ASSESSMENT

Nutritional assessment for older adults includes the techniques used for all population groups (see Box 17.2). In addition, specific screening for malnutrition may be used for older and frail adults and for those who have a recent change in health and functional status. To enable contextual interpretation the nutrition assessment should

---

> **BOX 17.2 Aspects of the nutritional assessment**
>
> - Determine the baseline.
> - Determine health and nutritional risks.
> - Compare with benchmarks and nutritional guidelines where applicable.
> - Establish the nature and aetiology of nutrition-based issues.
> - Identify leverage points and obstacles for making changes.
> - Establish priorities.
> - Provide an appropriate and effective treatment plan.
> - Improve nutritional and health status and prevent recurrence of undernutrition and/or disease.
> - Monitor progress.
> - Modify the plan as indicated.

---

not be conducted in isolation.[103,104] Conducting a specific and structured nutrition assessment facilitates consistency and objectivity and allows the practitioner and patient to have a clear record of changes in nutritional status. It is imperative that this information is clearly recorded in the patient's file for accuracy of health records, monitoring and evaluating progress, modifying the nutritional prescription, helping motivate patients and facilitating communication with other healthcare providers.

The dimensions of nutritional assessment can be grouped into the ABCD format and enable a structured and objective approach:

*A*nthropometric parameters
*B*iochemical data and medical test results
*C*linical history
*D*ietary evaluation and nutrition-related history.

Anthropometric measures encompass body weight, height, skinfold measurement, waist and hip circumference and bio-impedance. Weight loss and loss of lean muscle mass are the core measures in predicting the risk of malnutrition. Anthropometric measurements may not be accurate for people who have poorly controlled heart failure and oedema, ascites and other conditions that predispose to significant fluctuations in weight, body water and measurements.[103]

Biochemical data and medical test results include full blood count, urea and creatinine, vitamin D status and other relevant tests. As above, there are limitations in interpreting laboratory results for older adults, and interpreting nutrient levels at the tissue or cellular level is difficult. Serum markers such as serum albumin, transferrin and cholesterol levels are used as nonspecific indicators of nutritional status but interpretation in older adults needs to consider the normal reduction in synthesis of albumin with ageing and that levels of these markers can be affected by hydration status, inflammatory cytokines, physiological stress, recent dietary intake and trauma.[101,103]

Clinical history is included within the general history and assessment, but from a nutrition perspective it is important to ensure a full exploration of factors that may affect eating, swallowing, absorption and use of nutrients – for example, appetite, dentition, gag reflex and swallowing, GORD, bowel disorders, medications, diarrhoea, constipation, liver dysfunction.

Dietary evaluation and nutrition-related history includes current food intake, estimated nutrient requirements, individual preferences and religious and cultural influences on dietary choices. Essentially, is the person consuming enough to meet basic and disease-specific requirements, and what factors influence their food choices? A number of approaches can be used such as diet recall, keeping a diary and food frequency assessments; a combination may be required to best elicit the degree of information required.

Other considerations that may arise from the general assessment are issues of financial status, living arrangements, level of function and independence (especially as relates to shopping and food preparation) and support that is in place or available. Further, it is important to determine who makes the decisions about food and how the practitioner can best support change.

EXERCISE

Some practitioners include a specific review of physical activity with the nutrition assessment (thus making it ABCDE); alternatively it is included in the general health assessment. According to the Australian Bureau of Statistics, in 2014–15 nearly 25% of adults aged 65 years and over exercised for at least 30 minutes on 5 or more days in the week before the survey, while almost 50% undertook no exercise.[105]

Regular exercise helps reduce age-related physiological changes across body systems and is associated with improved morbidity and mortality in the middle and older years.[6,28,106] Exercise is known to improve respiratory peak flow capacity and VO_2 max, improve arterial compliance and endothelial function (including arterial dilation), increase free radical scavenging capacity and fibrinolytic capacity, and help regenerate the endothelium and reduce intima-wall thickness.[28,106] Further, regular exercise improves blood glucose control, reduces the severity and prevalence of musculoskeletal disorders such as osteoporosis and sarcopenia, reduces frailty and improves mental health status.[106]

HYDRATION

Maintaining adequate hydration presents a unique challenge for older people who may be negotiating the conflicting need for hydration with conditions such as arthritis and limited mobility, incontinence and heart failure. Total body water declines with age and regulatory mechanisms such as renal function decline. There is a diminished sense of thirst and hypodipsia is common; for example, it is estimated to be present in up to 30% of residents in nursing homes.[103]

The risks of dehydration include reduced perception of thirst or awareness of intake (e.g. impaired cognitive status), acute illness which may further reduce intake or be associated with GIT loss and diarrhoea, medication dependency (especially diuretics) including requiring assistance to get fluids and to drink, chronic illness, cognitive decline, dementia and delirium.[103] Outcomes of inadequate fluid intake and dehydration can be significant and include increased risk of falls, confusion, postprandial

---

> ### BOX 17.3 Markers of dehydration
>
> - Urine colour (very dark amber)
> - Blood urea nitrogen-to-creatinine ratio (>25:1 mg/dL)
> - Serum osmolarity (>300 mmol/kg)
> - Serum sodium level (>150 mEq/L)
> - Urine specific gravity (>1.029)
> - Low urine output (<800 mL/day)
> - Only as a secondary measure, elevated serum albumen and protein.
>
> Source: Adapted from Johnson LE, Sullivan DH. Malnutrition in Older Adults. In: Fillit HM, Rockman K, Young J (eds). Brocklehurst's textbook of geriatric medicine and gerontology. 8th edn. Philadelphia: Elsevier; 2017, pp. 914–22.

and orthostatic hypotension, renal impairment, altered pharmacokinetics and pharmacodynamics.[103]

Age-related integumentary changes make relying on skin turgor unreliable for assessment of hydration status in older adults. Box 17.3 provides markers for assessing hydration status.

NUTRITIONAL SCREENING FOR MALNUTRITION

Nutritional screening for malnutrition is acknowledged as being valuable in determining the risk of malnutrition, though it is less clear whether it improves outcomes.[103,107] The critical issue is developing an effective plan in response to the findings. The most commonly used screening tools are the Malnutrition Screening Tool (MST)[108], the Mini-Nutritional Assessment (MNA) and the Mini-Nutritional Assessment Short Form (MNA-SF).[109] A recent review of 11 well-studied and widely used tools rated the MST highest in terms of reliability and validity within an acute hospital setting.[103,110] A modified Simplified Nutrition Assessment Questionnaire has been developed for community-dwelling adults aged 65 years and older (SNAQ65+)[111] which looks at weight loss (or if clothes are looser or tighter), arm circumference, appetite and functionality walking up 15 stairs. For further information Hamirudin et al.[107] and Skipper et al.[110] provide useful reviews of validated malnutrition screening tools. A comparison of the main nutritional assessment tools is provided in Table 17.6.

GERIATRIC SYNDROMES

The term 'geriatric syndromes' (previously known as the giants of geriatrics) has been developed to identify and define conditions that are primarily seen in older adults but that do not readily fit within a systems approach to pathophysiology.[112,113] Geriatric syndromes are a heterogeneous group of conditions and while as yet poorly defined, they are associated with reduced quality of life and increased morbidity and mortality.[112,113] There is no universally agreed list of geriatric syndromes but the most commonly cited are frailty, sarcopenia, falls, depression, delirium, functional decline, anorexia of ageing and malnutrition, polypharmacy, dizziness, syncope, urinary incontinence and pressure ulcers.[112]

TABLE 17.6 Comparison of the MNA, MST and SNAQ65+ screening tools			
Screening tool	**Criteria assessed**	**Outcome categories**	**Comments**
MNA	• Weight loss (1–3 kg or >3 kg over the past 3 months) • Appetite • Mobility • Psychological stress of acute illness • Dementia/psychological problems • BMI (or calf circumference if BMI unavailable).	• Malnourished • At risk of malnutrition • Normal nutritional status.	Validated for early detection of undernutrition and frailty in community-dwelling people aged ≥65 years of age.
MST	• Weight loss (1–5 kg, 6–10 kg, 11–15 kg or >15 kg) over the past 6 months • Appetite.	• High risk • Medium risk • Low risk.	Developed and validated for acute hospital, oncology and residential care patients.
SNAQ65+	• Weight loss (>4 kg unintentional loss in the past months) • Mid-upper arm circumference • Appetite and functionality.	• Malnourished • At risk of malnutrition • Normal nutritional status.	Designed for community-living older adults.

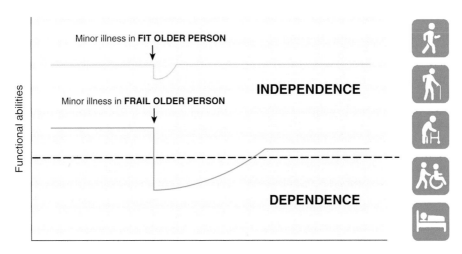

FIGURE 17.1 Reduced reserve and recovery in frail older adults

Common features of geriatric syndromes include their prevalence among adults 65 years and older, especially the frail elderly. There are numerous and compounding contributing factors involving multiple organ systems and shared risk factors including increasing age, cognitive and functional impairment and impaired mobility.[112] In clinical presentation the primary complaint may not represent the specific pathophysiological processes that initiated the decline in health status. For example, a urinary tract infection may not be mentioned as the health complaint, but it may be the underlying event that triggers the presenting complaint of delirium. In this way the two conditions, urinary infection and neurological alteration, illustrate some of the atypical presentations of disease already discussed. This apparent separation between origin and expression of pathology in distinct and distant organs is described by Inouye[112] as 'a disconnect between the site of the underlying physiologic insult and the resulting clinical symptom'. Assessment and diagnosis are not linear, nor do they follow an obvious cause-and-effect model, and the syndromes characteristically involve several body systems and thus professional disciplines.

Frailty

Frailty results from a multi-system reduction in reserve capacity which increases the individual's vulnerability for developing greater dependency, as well as increasing mortality when exposed to a stressor.[114] Avoidance of frailty is a major challenge, yet it represents the best possible outcome as the ability to recover from frailty is limited (see Fig. 17.1). Analyses of studies on the prevalence of frailty average 9% for frailty and 44.2% for pre-frailty.[115] A consensus statement on frailty from European and US societies is noted in Box 17.4.[114]

Frailty results from cumulative decline across multiple physiological systems and is associated with adverse outcomes. It is the end point of physiological decline compounded with environmental insults, multi-morbidity, malnutrition and age. While there is overlap, frailty is not synonymous with disability, which is an inability to perform ADLs; for example, in a study of people diagnosed with frailty, 27% had neither disability nor comorbidity.[39]

BOX 17.4 A consensus statement on frailty

Definition

The consensus definition of physical frailty is 'a medical syndrome with multiple causes and contributors that is characterized by diminished strength, endurance, and reduced physiologic function that increases an individual's vulnerability for developing increased dependency and/or death.'

Screening

- Simple rapid screening tests have been developed and validated, such as the simple FRAIL scale
- All persons older than 70 years and all individuals with significant weight loss (≥5%) due to chronic disease should be screened for frailty.

Intervention

Physical frailty can potentially be prevented or treated with specific modalities, such as:
- Exercise
- Protein-calorie supplementation
- Vitamin D
- Reduced polypharmacy.

Source: Adapted from Morley JE, Vellas B, Abellan van Kan, G et al. Frailty consensus: a call to action. J Am Med Dir Assoc 2013;14(6): 392–7.

ASSESSMENT CRITERIA

Assessment of frailty is based on meeting three of the following five screening criteria:

1. Weight loss: low baseline weight, unintentional weight loss of more than 5% or 4 kg over 12 months
2. Exhaustion: self-report of excess effort required, unusually tired and weak, low rated energy (0–10)
3. Low physical activity
4. Slowness: timed walking 4 m
5. Weakness: grip strength.[7,39,41,116]

Frailty is also characterised by increased levels of inflammatory markers (IL-6, C-reactive protein) and D-dimer and an elevated white cell count.[41] The degree of frailty can be quantified using the Clinical Frailty Scale, shown in Table 17.7.

Malnutrition is one of the key determinants of frailty; it is modifiable to varying degrees and is both a cause and a result of frailty.[102] In particular, known modifiable risks for frailty include protein energy malnutrition and deficiency of vitamin D and selenium.[102,117] A review of the results of 4731 US adults aged 60 years or older from the Third National Health and Nutrition Examination Survey (NHANES) analysed frailty, energy, biomarkers of nutritional status and food insufficiency.[117] Perhaps surprisingly, the prevalence of frailty was highest among people who were obese (20.8%), followed by overweight (18.4%) and normal weight (16.1%) and was lowest among people who were underweight (13.8%); this is indicative of obesogenic sarcopenia. Regardless of BMI, daily energy intake was lowest in people who were frail, followed by

TABLE 17.7 Clinical Frailty Scale

Grade	Plain language descriptor	Common characteristics
1	Very fit	Robust, active, energetic, motivated and fit. Usually exercises regularly and is in the fittest group for their age; commonly describes their health as 'excellent'.
2	Well	Without active or symptomatic disease, but less fit than people in category 1.
3	Well, with treated comorbid disease	Disease symptoms are well controlled compared with those in category 4.
4	Apparently vulnerable	Although not frankly dependent, commonly complains of being 'slowed up' or has disease symptoms or self-rates health as 'fair', at best. If cognitively impaired, they do not meet dementia criteria.
5	Mildly frail	Shows limited dependence on others for IADLs.
6	Moderately frail	Needs help with instrumental and some personal ADLs. Walking commonly is restricted.
7	Severely frail	Completely dependent on others for personal ADLs
8	Terminally ill	Terminally ill.

Source: Adapted from [116].

those who were pre-frail and was highest in people who were not frail, with frail people consuming 9% fewer calories (151 calories) than the not-frail group. In addition, serum albumin, carotenoids and selenium levels were lower in frail adults than in not-frail adults.

Sarcopenia

Sarcopenia is a change in body composition associated with ageing. Specifically, it is a syndrome characterised by progressive and generalised loss of skeletal muscle mass and strength.[15,102,118–120] Sarcopenia in the elderly is an independent predictor of poor gait, falls, fractures and other disability.[121] It is associated with adverse outcomes, reduced QOL, increased complications from hospitalisation and morbidity.[118,119] The prevalence of sarcopenia is reported variably from approximately 30% in people over 60 years of age to around 50% in those aged 75 years or more.[102]

With sarcopenia there is reduced muscle mass, infiltration of muscle with fat and connective tissue, a decrease in muscle fibres (a greater loss of type II fibres than type I fibres), disorganisation of myofilaments, proliferation on endoplasmic reticulum, a decrease in the number of motor units and accumulation of the 'ageing pigment' lipofuscin.[119] At a basic level the loss of muscle mass is partially due to reduced physical activity and in part due to the diminished size, and to a lesser degree the diminished number, of motor neurons.[39] It is estimated that there is a 30% decline in muscle mass from the third to the eighth decade, predominantly type II fibres, resulting in a significant reduction of VO_2 max and force contraction.[15] Age-related changes to collagen fibres within joints contribute to reduced elasticity and movement. Maximum muscle strength decreases by about 20–40% by the seventh to eighth decade due to the large loss of skeletal muscle fibres and concomitant reduction in the number of motor neurons.[7]

As with all geriatric syndromes, the development of sarcopenia is multifactorial. The reduced size and number of motor neurons and loss of skeletal muscle mass is exacerbated by physical inactivity. Other factors that influence sarcopenia development are:

- Neurological decline
- Reduced anabolic hormone levels (testosterone, oestrogens, growth hormone, insulin-like growth factor-1)
- Reduced vitamin D and parathyroid hormone
- Inflammatory pathway activation and increased pro-inflammatory cytokines (especially TNF-α, IL-6)
- Oxidative stress
- Changes in the mitochondrial function of muscle cells
- Chronic illness (reduces physical activity, promotes inflammation)
- Fatty infiltration of muscle
- Protein/energy malnutrition
- Reduced intake of vitamin D.[7,119,122,123]

SARCOPENIC OBESITY

Sarcopenic obesity is the co-occurrence of sarcopenic age-related loss of skeletal muscle and excess body fat. Sarcopenic obesity increases with age, as the metabolic rate continues to fall, lean muscle mass diminishes and there is limited physical activity, all of which both cause and are a result of sarcopenic obesity.[102] Increased weight and reduced strength make these older adults at particular risk of adverse outcomes and functional decline.[102] It has been suggested that sarcopenic obesity can predict disability more than sarcopenia or obesity as independent conditions.[123]

The risk factors for sarcopenic obesity are an overlap of those for obesity and sarcopenia: malnutrition with excess energy intake, insulin resistance, inactivity, low-grade inflammation, and hormonal and peptide influences.[102] The increasing prevalence of overweight and obesity in young and middle-aged adults signals a potential increase in the prevalence of sarcopenic obesity in older adults in the coming decades.

Intervention is complex and the focus needs to be on preventing the development of sarcopenia and sarcopenic obesity. Physical activity, in particular resistance training, is the most effective strategy to maintain and gain lean muscle mass. This can be supported by improving nutritional intake and status, with a particular focus on adequate protein and vitamin D and reducing inflammation.[123]

Falls

Falls are an archetypal geriatric syndrome because they are due to multiple interacting conditions that create and worsen reduced tolerance to any type of external stress that is characteristic of ageing.[124] It is estimated that more than one-third of community-living older adults fall each year and more than half of those have recurrent falls.[125] Falls are associated with significant morbidity and mortality, with 20–30% of falls causing moderate to severe injuries including cuts and head injuries, and approximately 3–5% of falls resulting in fractures.[17,125] Further, falls account for two-thirds of injury-related deaths in those aged 85 years and older and are the leading cause of death from injury in adults aged 65 years and older.[17,125] In Australia in 2011–12, 96 385 people aged 65 and over were hospitalised for a fall-related injury, which is three and a half times as many as for 45–64 year olds. The rate of hospitalisation increases dramatically with age: for women aged 65–69, the age-specific rate of hospitalised falls was 1100 cases per 100 000 population, compared with 9451 cases per 100 000 for women aged 85–89. For men, the equivalent rates were 737 and 6383 per 100 000 men.[125] A fractured hip (neck of femur) has major consequences with increased short- and long-term morbidity: the death rate is up to 24% in the first 3 months post-surgery.[126] In addition, there is loss of mobility and independence and an increased requirement to move to residential care facilities. Risk factors for falls are outlined in Table 17.8.

Interventions for falls are based on a risk management approach. The risks are identified and either eliminated (e.g. occupational therapy review, installation of handrails and removal of rugs) or reduced (e.g. exercise physiology and physiotherapy to improve strength and balance, nutritional enhancement, medications review).

Pain

Pain is not restricted to older adults, but the prevalence is high and it is an important contributor to reduced QOL, reduced mobility and subsequent loss of muscle mass, sarcopenia and increased frailty. In addition, pain is associated with increased need for analgesia and associated risks of polypharmacy. Pain may be under-reported as it is perceived as a normal part of ageing.[7]

Depression

Depression is not exclusive to older adults and is discussed in full in Chapter 21. It is included here as it is a significant and common cause of morbidity and mortality in the elderly and it may be under-diagnosed or misdiagnosed (e.g. as dementia).[7] Depression is a key contributory factor for undernutrition which underpins geriatric syndromes and functional decline.[128] The prevalence of depression is estimated to be 10–19% among those aged 75 or over.[129,130] Residents in aged-care facilities are thought to have a prevalence of depression up to 35%; in addition, anxiety may also be present in 10% of older adults.[129] Assessment tools such as the Geriatric Depression Scale[131] may aid in diagnosis. The risk factors

TABLE 17.8 Falls risk factors

Extrinsic	Intrinsic: physical	Intrinsic: psychological and cognitive
• Living alone (also greater risk of not being able to get help) • Trip and slip hazards, e.g. rugs, uneven flooring, wet floors • Poor lighting • Cluttered walkways • Footwear and clothing • Inappropriate walking aids (or inappropriate use of those devices) • Lack of handrails • Poor stair design.	• Poor mobility • Impaired balance and gait • Visual impairment • Reduced muscle strength • Poor reaction times • A history of falls • Postural hypotension • Incontinence • Polypharmacy, CNS-active medications • Comorbidities, especially cardiovascular and circulatory, COPD, arthritis and neurological disorders • Sedentary behaviour • Nutritional deficiencies, especially vitamin D.	• Fear of falling (a major risk) • Cognitive impairment, even subtle deficits • Confusion • Delirium • Depression.

Source: [124,125,127].

TABLE 17.9 Signs and symptoms of depression in older people

Thoughts	Feelings	Physical symptoms
• Indecisiveness • Apathy • Loss of self-esteem • Persistent suicidal thoughts • Negative comments like 'I'm a failure', 'It's my fault' or 'Life isn't worth living' • Excessive concerns about financial situation • Perceived change of status within the family.	• Moodiness or irritability, which may present as anger or aggressiveness • Sadness, hopelessness or emptiness • Feeling overwhelmed • Feeling worthless or guilty.	• Cognitive problems, including memory problems • Insomnia, hypersomnia • Persistent fatigue • Slowed movements • Somatic symptoms: headaches, backache, pain • Digestive disturbances including changes in bowel habits • Agitation, hand wringing, pacing • Anorexia • Significant weight change.

Source: Beyondblue. Signs and symptoms of anxiety and depression in older people. Beyondblue. [Cited 16 September 2016. Available from www.beyondblue.org.au/who-does-it-affect/older-people/signs-and-symptoms-of-depression-in-older-people.]

for depression in old age are inclusive for a large proportion of older people, as follows:
• Being female (though suicide is higher in men)
• Loss or adverse life events
• Medical disorders such as stroke, cardiovascular disease (conversely, depression is also a recognised risk factor for cardiovascular disease)
• Prior depression or mental illness
• Neurodegenerative disease – three to four times more common with dementia
• Isolation.[9,129,130]

Depression in older people may be under-diagnosed and treatment responses may not be significant or sustained. A review of the course of depression in 285 older people found that almost half (48.4%) of those who were clinically depressed at the commencement of the study also suffered from a depressive disorder 2 years later. Those with more severe symptoms of depression, comorbidities and a younger age of onset were at a higher risk of persistent or recurrent depression.[132] Further, findings showed that late-life depression often has a chronic nature even when treated according to age-specific guidelines.[132] See Table 17.9 for signs and symptoms of depression in older people.

Suicide rates are alarmingly high in older males.[130,133,134] In Australia in 2013, the highest age-specific suicide death rate for males was observed in the 85 years and over age group (38.3 per 100 000 males).[133] The lowest age-specific death rate (outside 0–14-year-olds) for female deaths was in the 80–84 year age group (4.0 deaths per 100 000). Risk factors for suicide include psychological, social and physical factors such as severe depression, loneliness, social isolation and lack of social support; chronic ill-health and pain; and loss of autonomy and reduced QOL.

Delirium

Delirium is an acute neuropsychiatric disorder of attention and cognition.[135] It is characterised by a reduced clarity of awareness of the environment and a decreased ability to focus, maintain or shift attention.[16] While delirium is associated with worsening dementia severity, declining functional status and higher mortality in those with dementia, delirium and dementia are two discrete entities.[135] Table 17.10 compares the features of delirium and dementia.

A common presentation of delirium is postoperatively or with bacteraemia. Estimates of prevalence in hospital settings vary from 10% to 30% of all hospitalised elderly people[16] and up to 50% of older adults in surgical units.[7] The lack of definitive prevalence statistics is due to probable under-reporting and under-diagnosis, including the condition being incorrectly attributed to dementia or drug reactions.[7] That said, polypharmacy and altered pharmacokinetics and pharmacodynamics are key risk

Feature	Delirium	Dementia
TABLE 17.10 Features of delirium compared with dementia		
Onset	Acute (most cases)	Insidious
Course	Fluctuating levels of consciousness over the day, lucid at times	Generally stable (exacerbated by delirium)
Duration	Hours to weeks Reversible	Months to years Irreversible
Alertness	Abnormally low or high, agitated and distracted	Usually normal
Perception	Perceptual disturbance, e.g. visual hallucinations; impaired visuospatial orientation	Usually normal, no hallucinations
Attention	Disorganised, difficulty with concentration, orientation and attention	Normal unless advanced disease
Memory	Immediate and recent memory impaired	Recent and remote memory impaired
Thoughts	Disorganised	Impoverished
Speech	Incoherent, slow or rapid	Word-finding difficulty
Psychomotor activity	Increased, shifting or reduced	Often normal
Physical illness or medication causative	Frequently, e.g. febrile illness, drug toxicity or organ failure	Usually absent

Source: Adapted from Browne W, Nair K. Geriatric medicine. In: Talley NJ, Frankhum B, Currow D (eds). Essentials of internal medicine. 3rd edn. Philadelphia: Churchill Livingstone; 2015, pp. 777–90. Hevesi ZG, Hammel LL. Geriatric disorders. In: Hines LH, Marschall KE (eds). Stoelting's anesthesia and co-existing disease. 6th edn. Philadelphia: Saunders; 2012, pp. 642–54. Heflin MT, Cohen HJ. The Aging Patient. In: Benjamin IJ, Griggs RC, Wing EJ, et al (eds). Andreoli and Carpenter's Cecil essentials of medicine. Philadelphia: Elsevier; 2016. Davis DH, Muniz Terrara G, Keage H, et al. Delirium is a strong risk factor for dementia in the oldest-old: a population-based cohort study. Brain 2012;135(Pt 9):2809–16.

factors for delirium – an estimated 39% of delirium cases are due to medications.[99]

Elder abuse

The WHO defines elder mistreatment as 'a single or repeated act or lack of appropriate action occurring within any relationship where there is an expectation of trust, which causes harm or distress to an older person'.[136] In addition, the US National Research Council definition includes 'failure by a caregiver to satisfy the elder's basic needs or to protect the elder from harm'.[137] See Table 17.11 for categories of elder abuse. The incidence and prevalence of elder abuse is unclear as it is unrecognised, under-reported, insidious and hidden.[7] In 2015 the WHO reported that estimated prevalence rates in high- or middle-income countries ranged from 2% to 14%.[11] In contrast, the Australian Longitudinal Study on Women's Health suggests that neglect could be as high as 20% among women in the older age group.[138] The perpetrator may be a family member and the older person may feel too vulnerable, disempowered and ashamed to disclose abuse.[7] Unlike mandatory reporting for vulnerable children, there are no protective and screening measures in place for vulnerable older people.

A systematic review of risk factors for elder abuse categorised risks according to four domains:
- Factors associated with the older person, such as cognitive impairment, behavioural problems, psychiatric or psychological problems, functional dependency, ill-health, frailty, low income, trauma or past abuse, and ethnicity
- Factors associated with the perpetrator, such as caregiver burden or stress, psychiatric illness or psychological problems
- Factors associated with relationships, including family disharmony, poor or conflictual relationships
- Environmental factors such as low social support and living with others including in residential care.[137,139]

An older person may show evidence of physical trauma or behavioural and cognitive change if subject to abuse; they will become withdrawn, anxious and depressed.

PHARMACOKINETICS, POLYPHARMACY AND POSOLOGY

This section reviews issues relating to pharmaceuticals and older people, including clinical evidence, pharmacokinetics, pharmacodynamics, polypharmacy, adverse reactions and risk management. In the absence of a body of evidence for complementary medicines and older patients, it may be appropriate to extrapolate the learnings from pharmaceuticals to natural therapies.

Epidemiology of medication use and potential issues

An ageing population has an increased prevalence of multiple medical conditions and thus medication use, as pharmacological management may be seen as the most appropriate therapeutic intervention with advancing age.

TABLE 17.11 Categories of elder abuse				
Psychological abuse	**Physical abuse**	**Sexual abuse**	**Financial abuse**	**Neglect**
Inflicting mental stress via actions and threats that cause fear, violence, isolation, deprivation and feelings of shame and powerlessness. Includes: • Verbal abuse • Intimidation • Humiliation • Threats to put the older person into residential care • Social abuse (e.g. isolating from others).	Non-accidental acts that result in physical pain or injury, or physical coercion. Examples include any form of assault such as: • Hitting • Slapping • Shoving • Pushing • Burning • Using physical restraint such as tying a person to a chair or bed • Locking a person in a room.	Unwanted sexual acts, including sexual contact, rape, language or exploitative behaviour where the person's consent was not obtained or where consent was obtained through coercion. Sexual abuse can also include sexually exploitative or shaming acts such as: • Leaving a person in a state of undress • Forced viewing of sexually explicit materials or images • Sexually suggestive comments • Exhibitionism • Inappropriate touching • Uninvited sexual approaches.	The illegal use, improper use or mismanagement of a person's money, property or financial resources. For example: • Taking a loan with a promise of repayment but not paying the money back • Stealing money or using an older person's banking and credit card without consent • Forcefully encouraging changes to a will or other legal document • Sale of any property or assets without authority or consent • Forced transfers of property.	*Active neglect* is the deliberate withholding of basic care or necessities, including: • Leaving an older person in an unsafe place or state • Stopping access to medical treatment • Abandonment • Not providing adequate clothing or sufficient food and liquids • Untreated illnesses • Over- or under-medicating. *Passive neglect* is the failure to provide proper care, due to carer stress, lack of knowledge or ability. It may occur unintentionally and may simply require getting additional support to assist the carer and older person.

Source: Tinker A, Biggs S, Manthorpe J. The mistreatment and neglect of frail older people. In: Fillit HM, Rockwood K, Young J (eds). Brocklehurst's textbook of geriatric medicine and gerontology. 8th edn. Philadelphia: Elsevier; 2017. Seniors Rights Victoria. Your rights: elder abuse. [Cited 20 September 2016. Available from https://seniorsrights.org.au.][140]

People aged 65 years and older are prescribed medications more frequently than any other age group and increasingly will be taking more than one medication. In Australia half of all people aged between 65 and 74 years and two-thirds of those aged 75 years and over report taking five or more medicines daily.[141]

Data from the US National Health and Nutrition Examination Survey (NHANES)[142] for 37 959 adults (20 years and older) showed an 8% increase in overall use of prescription drugs from 1999–2000 to 59% for 2011–2012. In the same period the prevalence of polypharmacy (defined as ≥5 medications) in older adults rose from an estimated 8.2% to 15%. In the US, people aged 65 years and older comprise only 13% of the population, yet account for more than 33% of total outpatient spending on prescription medications. It is anticipated that by 2020 people 65 years and older will account for 50% of all medication use.

In the past decade, the average number of items prescribed for each person per year in England increased by 53.8% from 11.9% in 2001 to 18.3% in 2011.[143] A large Scottish study has confirmed the considerable and increasing prevalence of polypharmacy: 12% of patients were dispensed five or more drugs in 1995, rising to 22% in 2010; and 1.9% of patients were dispensed 10 or more drugs in 1995, rising to 5.8% in 2010.[144] The study also reviewed prescriptions for all 310 000 adult residents in

the Tayside region in 1995 and 2010 and found that the proportion of adults dispensed five or more medications doubled to 20.8%, and the proportion dispensed 10 or more tripled to 5.8%. Increasing age was strongly associated with more medications (especially in the 10 or more group), as was living in socioeconomic disadvantage and living in care facilities. Reflecting the complexity and risks of polypharmacy, those with a greater number of drugs experienced the greater number of drug interactions. While the overall proportion of adverse drug interactions more than doubled to 13% of adults in 2012, this was most likely in those taking a greater number of drugs (10.4% for those on two to four drugs, compared with 80.8% for those taking 15 or more).[144]

In addition to the increasing prevalence of disease states in the aged, medication use is also increasing due to preventive or risk-reduction interventions, especially for cardiovascular and cerebrovascular disease where interventions are aimed at reducing stroke, heart attack and multi-infarct dementias.[143] While an increased level of medication use may be indicated in the management of multiple pathology states, it does not come without risks and it requires methodical and careful monitoring and clinical practice. This statement can also be applied to the use of herbal medicines and nutritional supplements. The potential issues of polypharmacy or of 'polyCM' are exponentially increased if both exist in the same

partially because of the inherent physiological changes in the older person and critically because of the significant knowledge gap of what the impact of the multiplicity of diverse therapeutic agents in the elderly might be.

Clinical trials in the elderly

There is an ever-increasing array of medications available, including for 'anti-ageing' purposes, with 435 new drugs in phase I to phase III trials in the US as of 2015.[145] While most governments have identified the risks of medication use in the elderly and implemented a range of strategies to reduce adverse events, a key area that remains unanswered is the lack of clinical trials involving elderly people. In 2011 the European Medicines Agency published the *EMA Geriatric Medicines Strategy*, a document with a vision statement that included the intention of '... ensuring that medicines used by geriatric patients are of high quality, and appropriately researched and evaluated, throughout the lifecycle of the product, for use in this population'.[146] The Agency produced a plan including audit, education and validation of practice tools, but as yet there is no plan for addressing the issue of appropriate research and evaluation of medication use in the elderly.

There are almost no clinical drug trials on 'old elderly' people (aged 85 years and over) and these are the people most likely to use medications and to use multiple medications. When an older cohort is included in pharmaceutical clinical drug trials it is typically 'young elderly' and usually excludes those with multiple comorbidities and who are taking multiple medications to best control for confounders in the analysis.[147] Further, there may be issues with ethics, frailty and vulnerability, cognitive decline and valid informed consent when including the old elderly in trials. One well-known exception to the exclusion of elderly adults is the Hypertension in the Very Elderly Trial, where participants were over 80 years of age; however, they were 'well elderly' and it was a single-issue trial on hypertension.[148] The main trial was terminated for ethical reasons in 2007 by the Independent Trial Steering Committee, as the independent Data Monitoring Committee noted a significant reduction in all-cause mortality in participants on active treatment at the second interim analysis, and while this can be seen as a good outcome, it does limit the scope of the trial.[149] Interestingly, a later Cochrane Review of treating hypertension in healthy people over 60 years of age found benefit only in those 60–80 years of age, not those who were older.[150]

Clinical trials may fail to accurately identify adverse drug events and drug interactions in older patients and, while necessary, frequently the outcome measures are very restricted and so fail to consider the impact of the medication on QOL measures and personal and social aspects such as care needs.[143] As such, there is often an inadequate analysis of the burden of treatment and the cost–benefits of medication use in the elderly.

Another limitation of most pharmaceutical and health research is that it is focused on single issues and single interventions, thus omitting the multi-morbidity and polypharmacy-prone elderly. Furthermore, this single-disease framework is characteristic of most health services, medical and health education and clinical guidelines developed to inform practice, which therefore fail to incorporate the complexities of progressive ageing.

The paucity of drug trials involving the elderly, and the very limited nature of those trials, raises the question of the generalisability of the study results. For example, can a trial on a new antihypertensive conducted on a cohort of men 50–70 years of age and without multiple comorbidities be extrapolated in a meaningful way for an 80-year-old woman with diabetes, Hashimoto's disease and depression? Further, there is limited research comparing various options for the management of a single clinical condition, thus impacting on a prescriber's ability to make an informed clinical decision – how to choose one over the other.[147]

The lack of research including the elderly in clinical drug trials is echoed by limited post-release surveillance and reporting. That is, how has the medication been tolerated, what is the efficacy, what have the adverse reactions been in a complex and heterogeneous elderly population? Knowledge of adverse events relies upon clinicians writing case reports for publication or presentation and reporting to the relevant regulatory agencies, which is a very passive and inadequate approach. There is a presumed under-reporting of adverse medication events and this is compounded by a lack of information about the denominator population with which to compare outcomes and health status and thus make informed analysis regarding the perceived adverse event.[145,147]

Pharmacokinetics

Pharmacokinetics is the study of tissue sensitivity, drug absorption, distribution, metabolism and excretion. Physiological changes with ageing may impact on each of these processes, are variable and difficult to predict and have varying clinical significance (see Table 17.12).[150,151] Further, alterations in pharmacokinetics may be seen in the aged, but not because of age, but instead due to disease states (e.g. coeliac disease).

The reduction in serum albumin with age (amplified in illness) is due to reduced liver synthesis and to cytokine excess and this can markedly reduce drug binding and thus increase the amount of free circulating drugs. Reduced renal excretion of drugs is a key area of risk for the elderly and even in healthy elderly people there is a reduced renal mass and blood flow and reduced muscle mass (which complicates evaluation of renal function if relying on creatinine clearance). CKD can be insidious as it is possible to lose up to 90% of kidney function before becoming overtly symptomatic, highlighting the importance of assessing renal function regardless of symptoms. Perhaps due to the stealth nature of CKD in the earlier stages, it has a high prevalence in many countries, including Australia where in 2011–2012 the overall prevalence was 10%.[153] This rate increases dramatically with age, with the rate in people 75 years and older at 42%. Polypharmacy affects both CKD and acute renal failure (ARF). In a study of 20 790 patients in Taiwan Province of China the extent and duration of polypharmacy was positively associated with ARF: polypharmacy over 31–90 days had an odds ratio of 1.33 for developing ARF and polypharmacy over 181 days had an odds ratio of 1.65 for

TABLE 17.12 Age-related physiology and stages of pharmacokinetics

Pharmacokinetic function	Age-related changes	Clinical effect
Tissue sensitivity	Alterations in: • Cell receptor numbers and affinity • Nuclear responses • Second messenger function • P-glycoprotein function.	• More or less sensitivity to a given medication.
Absorption	Decrease in: • Intestinal blood flow • Absorptive surface Gastrointestinal motility Increase in: • Gastric pH.	• Least affected by changes associated with ageing, even with stated physiological changes as most oral drugs absorbed by passive diffusion • Most relevant for drugs that require acid environment, e.g. calcium carbonate (thus use Ca citrate) • Some enteric-coated drugs may dissolve more quickly with increased gastric pH.
Distribution	Decrease in: • Total body water • Serum albumin and alpha-1-acid glycoprotein* • Lean body mass Increase in: • Body fat.	• Higher concentration of drugs • Longer elimination half-life of lipid-soluble drugs • More widely distributed fat-soluble and less widely distributed water-soluble drugs.
Metabolism	Decrease in: • Liver volume • Hepatic blood flow • Enzyme activity (cytochrome P450 family).	• Decreased biotransformation and first-pass metabolism • Decreased phase 1 reaction activity and prolonged half-life for some drugs.
Excretion	Decrease in: • Renal perfusion • Glomerular filtration • Tubular secretion.	• Decreased renal elimination of drugs.

*Alpha-1-acid glycoprotein (AGP, also known as AAG or orosomucoid) is an important plasma protein involved in the binding and transport of many drugs, especially basic compounds.[152]

Source: Adapted from Musini VM, Tejani AM, Bassett K, et al. Pharmacotherapy for hypertension in the elderly. Cochrane Database Syst Rev 2009;4. Cepeda OA, Morley JE. Polypharmacy. In: Sinclair AJ, Morley JE, Vellas B (eds). Principles and practice of geriatric medicine. 5th edn. Chichester: John Wiley; 2012, pp. 145–51.

an odds ratio of 1.33 for developing ARF and polypharmacy over 181 days had an odds ratio of 1.65 for developing ARF. The mortality rate for people hospitalised with ARF is approximately 45%.[154]

Cytochrome P450 (CYP450) enzymes are a group of enzymes responsible for the production of cholesterol, steroids, prostacyclins and thromboxane A_2 as well as being responsible for the detoxification of foreign chemicals and the metabolism of drugs. There are more than 50 CYP450 enzymes, but CYP1A2, CYP2C9, CYP2C19, CYP2D6, CYP3A4 and CYP3A5 metabolise 80–90% of drugs. These enzymes are predominantly expressed in the liver, but they also occur in the small intestine (reducing drug bioavailability), lungs, placenta and kidneys.[155,156] Inducers increase CYP450 enzyme activity by increasing enzyme synthesis, inhibitors reduce synthesis and other substances act as substrates. Pharmaceuticals and herbal medicines are known to induce and/or inhibit CYP450 enzymes and this can affect the response to the drug or herbs as well as impact on the body's ability to metabolise other drugs. The extent to which this occurs, and the translation between measureable CYP450 change and clinical significance, is variable. In addition, genetic polymorphisms may affect CYP450 function and ageing reduces CYP450 expression and function.[155,156]

P-glycoprotein (P-gp) is an efflux membrane transporter responsible for limiting cellular uptake and the distribution of xenobiotics and toxic substances. It is widely distributed throughout the body in organs or tissues with an excretory and/or barrier function such as on the surface of hepatocytes, the epithelial cells of the renal tubules, intestine, placenta and testes, and it is highly expressed at the vessel walls of the brain capillaries.[155,157,158] At the blood–brain barrier P-gp extrudes a range of unrelated compounds from the brain and is thus thought to be central to protecting the brain from accumulation of potentially toxic substances, including drugs.[157,158] A gender difference exists for P-gp expression between men and women; for example, hepatic P-gp expression is 2.4-fold lower in females and some of this effect may be due to the influence of oestrogen and progesterone (previously or at the time of study).[158] This, in addition to lean mass, fat mass and water distribution, may determine gender differences in drug efficacy and adverse drug reactions.

Ageing is associated with a decreased P-gp function and may be a key mechanism behind increased sensitivity and drug toxicity and increased CNS side effects of drugs

TABLE 17.13 Summary of key physiological impacts of ageing on medication use		
System	**Age-related physiological changes**	**Implication for medication use**
Renal	• Reduced renal mass and blood flow • Reduced glomerular filtration.	• Reduced excretion • Greater vulnerability to renal insult.
GIT	• Reduced intestinal blood flow • Reduced gastric motility • Decreased mucosal absorptive surface.	• In general, slightly reduced absorption of most drugs • Active transport of some nutrients, glucose, calcium, vitamin B_{12} and leucine is impaired.
Hepatic	• Reduced albumin and protein ingestion and synthesis • Reduced metabolic clearance by the liver.	• Decreased biotransformation and first-pass metabolism • Reduced drug binding and increased free bioactive drug.
Cardiovascular	• Reduced cardiac reserve (including reduced compliance and contractility, hypertension, ventricular hypertrophy) • Decreased function of beta-adrenergic receptors.	• More vulnerable to drugs but less sensitive to drugs acting on beta-adrenergic pathways.
Respiratory	• Reduced elasticity, functional volume and vital capacity • Increased work of breathing.	• Reduced beta-adrenoceptor responsiveness, thus reduced responsiveness to beta-agonist medication
Endocrine	• Decreased insulin sensitivity and secretion and decreased glucose tolerance.	• Impact on renal function and drug excretion.
Neurological	• Reduced brain mass and neurons • Altered calcium homeostasis and receptor function and sensitivity (e.g. GABA receptors) • Reduced functional activity of P-gp efflux pump in the blood–brain barrier.	• Impaired cognition with cholinergics • Exaggerated response to CNS active drugs; increased sedation, increased sensitivity to opioids and general anaesthesia.
Metabolic	• Decreased lean mass and total body water • Increased body fat • Decreased albumin • Decreased gastric and intestinal secretions • Decreased mucosal surface.	• Reduced absorption • Altered distribution of drugs • Reduced creatinine and impact on renal assessment.

Source: Welker KL, Mycyk MB. Pharmacology in the geriatric patient. Emerg Med Clin North Am 2016;34:4469–81. Jansen PAF, Brouwers JRBJ. Clinical pharmacology in old persons. Scientifica (Cairo) 2012;1–32.[160]

that cross the blood–brain barrier as seen in older adults. In addition, the older person may be taking drugs that inhibit or downregulate P-gp function, which further impairs the protective function of P-gp. Reduced P-gp function may increase vulnerability to both exogenous and endogenous neurotoxins (such as amyloid-beta, the protein that accumulates in the brain in Alzheimer's disease); thus it is implicated in the pathogenesis of neurodegenerative diseases of ageing. It is noted that reduced P-gp function is seen to a greater degree in women, which corresponds with the higher prevalence of diseases such as Alzheimer's in women.[157] Table 17.13 outlines the key physiological impacts of ageing on medication use.

Pharmacodynamics

Pharmacodynamics refers to the effect of drugs on the body. It involves receptor sensitivity and binding, post-receptor effects and chemical interactions. That is, whereas pharmacokinetics is the study of how the body affects the drug, pharmacodynamics looks at how the drug affects the body. Both pharmacokinetics and pharmacodynamics influence dosing, drug effects and potential adverse drug effects, though as previously discussed, research on pharmacodynamics in geriatrics is minimal and what research there has been is

difficult to make generalisable.[151,161] There is variability in sensitivity to the effects of drugs as well as inter-individual variability. For example, older people are typically more sensitive to opioids and sedatives but less sensitive to drugs acting on beta-adrenergic pathways.[151]

Pharmacogenetics/ pharmacogenomics

Pharmacogenetics is the study of inherited genetic differences in drug metabolic pathways. Clinical pharmacogenetics describes whether individual variances in the expression of a protein or an enzyme affect the metabolism of a drug. These genetic variances may lead to changes in the levels of active or inactive metabolites, and may inform altered dosing or the use of a different drug.[162] The US Food and Drug Administration (FDA) states that drug labelling with information on genomic biomarkers may describe:
• Drug exposure and clinical response variability
• Risk of adverse events
• Genotype-specific dosing
• Mechanisms of drug action
• Polymorphic drug target and disposition genes.[163]

The FDA provides a list of currently FDA-approved drugs with pharmacogenomics information in their labelling. For example for codeine, the pharmacogenomics biomarker is CYP2D and the specific group affected is CYP2D6 ultrarapid metabolisers, and the boxed warning on the label notes warning and precautions in this group.[163]

Epigenetics

The inter-individual variance in drug response exceeds what can be attributed to pharmacokinetics, pharmacodynamics and pharmacogenetics, especially with the exaggerated variance in the elderly. The term 'epigenetics' describes genetic information that is 'epi' ('beyond' or 'above') the information coded solely by our genetic code. Epigenetics refers to cellular and physiological phenotypic trait variations that result from environmental factors that switch genes on and off and affect cell gene expression.[164] These epigenetic mechanisms are present in all genes and it is believed that the main mechanisms of epigenetics changes are methylation (DNA and protein, especially histones) and microRNA (miRNA) interference in gene expression.[165,166] Such epigenetic mechanisms regulate genomic activity beyond simple transcriptional factor inducer or repressor functions of genes to generate mRNA.[165]

Epigenetic regulation of gene activity is important in maintaining normal phenotypic activity of cells, as disruptions are implicated in ageing as well as having a role in the development of neurodegenerative diseases such as Alzheimer's and cancer.[165,166] In healthy people the tendency is towards global genome hypomethylation but with specific areas of hypermethylation.[166] With age, the shift is towards general hypermethylation of promoter regions and genes regulated by DNA expression tend to reduce their expression; this includes drug metabolising enzymes, drug transporters and drug receptors and other genes involved in drug metabolism and distribution.[166] Environmental factors that may have accelerated ageing may thus effect epigenetic changes, which then affect drug metabolism, therapeutic efficacy and adverse reactions, and these in turn may further accelerate ageing. The area of pharmacogenetics and epigenetics, and similarly nutrigenomics, is subject to increasing investigation and in future may facilitate personalised prescriptions that afford greater therapeutic efficacy and reduced adverse reactions.

Polypharmacy

Polypharmacy is a recognised risk factor for poor clinical outcomes and adverse drug reactions, especially for elderly persons; however, despite agreement that it is a significant risk there is not a consistent and agreed definition of polypharmacy. Definitions range from the use of two medications to the use of nine or more medications.[147] Given that the medications may indeed be essential, the number or quantity of medications alone is not adequate in defining polypharmacy and more recent definitions of polypharmacy also address issues of the quality of

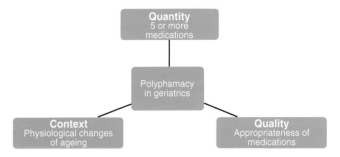

FIGURE 17.2 Aspects of polypharmacy in geriatrics

medications and of prescribing practices (see Fig. 17.2).[167] Further, regardless of the number of medications, some drugs are inherently higher risk (e.g. anticoagulants), have a very narrow therapeutic window (e.g. insulin) or may not be appropriate in the elderly due to known side effects.[38,167] An Australian study by Gnjidic et al.[168] aimed to 'determine an optimal discriminating number of concomitant medications associated with geriatric syndromes, functional outcomes, and mortality in community-dwelling older men'. The review of 51 705 men aged 70 years and older concluded that five or more medications should be used as the numerical definition of polypharmacy when assessing the risk of medication-related adverse outcomes in older people.

While no consensus definition of polypharmacy exists, the most commonly used definition is the use of more than five drugs and/or more medications than required.[167] That said, in the case of chronic and complex care, five medications may be too low, so any definition must have a caveat of individuation applied.[143,145] A British review of polypharmacy and medication safety qualified the term polypharmacy, using the following definitions:

> Appropriate polypharmacy *is defined as prescribing for an individual for complex conditions or for multiple conditions in circumstances where medicines use has been optimised and where the medicines are prescribed according to best evidence.*
> Problematic polypharmacy *is defined as the prescribing of multiple medications inappropriately, or where the intended benefit of the medication is not realised.*[143]

COMPLEMENTARY MEDICINES (CM) AND POLYPHARMACY

Polypharmacy usually refers to prescribed medications, presumably due to the fact that if a medication is restricted to prescription-only it holds greater potential risks. Polypharmacy research and interventions therefore often do not include over-the-counter pharmaceuticals the patient uses, let alone herbal medicines and nutritional supplements.[167] It is currently impossible to quantify the impact of concurrent complementary medicine (CM) use and polypharmacy. It is possible that the additive effects may be significantly deleterious, and it is also possible that the inclusion of CM reduces the dose requirements of pharmaceuticals, thereby reducing the risks associated with polypharmacy and adverse drug reactions while improving outcomes. The innumerable combinations of drugs and herbs and/or supplements are further complicated by the marked inter-individual variability in the physiological effects of ageing on pharmacokinetics and pharmacodynamics in the aged population. This substantial lack of knowledge and clinical evidence about the intersection of polypharmacy and CM use necessitates prudent prescribing by the naturopath.

Reviews from multiple countries identify CM use in the elderly but research is often limited to targeting specific cohorts or single diseases or conditions (e.g. use in menopause or community-dwelling versus residential care). Prevalence is varied and reported to be as high as 53–62.7%.[169,170] A review of 25 papers on CM use in the elderly found that use transcends culture or geography but that the specific therapies chosen are often informed by the individual's cultural or ethnic heritage.[171] For example, a study of 1475 Lebanese elders found that nearly 30% used CM and for this group that meant herbal medicine in 75% of cases.[172] On the other hand a German study found herbal medicines represented only 33% of CM use and dietary supplements represented 35% of CM use.[173]

The specific conditions that CM is used for varies among the aged, as seen in an American review comparing CM use in baby boomers (born 1946–1964) and the so-called silent generation (born 1925–1945).[174] The 'young elderly' baby boomers were more likely to use CM within the past year, 43.1% compared with 35.4% for the 'older elderly', and the baby boomers were more likely to use CM for heart disease, cancer and diabetes. In both groups CM use was associated with chronic pain. Older people chose to use CM for a wide range of reasons including wanting the 'best of both worlds' (using both CM and orthodox pharmaceuticals), desire for autonomy in healthcare decisions and wanting to be active in managing their own health, engagement with traditional knowledge and practices, dislike of the effects of pharmaceuticals, disillusionment with conventional medicine, negative experiences with conventional practitioners, the desire to postpone or minimise age-related deterioration and mortality, and the perception that 'natural products' are safe.[170,175]

The Australian Longitudinal Study of Ageing (ALSA) is an ongoing multidisciplinary prospective study of the older population that commenced in 1992 in South Australia. Data from this study have been analysed on patterns of CM and OTC medication use for 2087 adults aged 65 years and over living in the community or residential aged care facilities.[176] The results show an increase in CM use from 12.8% in 2000–2001 to 17% in 2003–2004. The most commonly used CM in 2003–2004 were vitamins and minerals (14%), herbal medicine (5.5%) – in particular garlic, celery and ginkgo biloba (5.5%) – nutritional supplements (7.6%), especially cod liver oil, fish oil and glucosamine and combination products (5.1%).

A 2011 review by Yen et al.[177] surveyed 2540 Australians aged 50 years and older about consultations with CM practitioners and revealed a disparity between CM use and CM professional consultation. Only 8.8% of respondents reported seeing a CM practitioner in the past 3 months, most commonly for musculoskeletal conditions

(osteoporosis, arthritis), pain or depression/anxiety. The lack of professional advice increases the risk of adverse effects, drug–CM interactions and negative clinical outcomes for the older patient. In addition to not seeking professional advice for CM use from a CM professional, many also did not seek information from other health professionals and only a minority disclosed CM use to their doctor.[171,172] A German study of 400 people aged 70 years and over found that 61.3% used some CM (dietary supplements 35.5%, herbal medicines 33.3% and external preparations 26.8%) and while many said they did not assess or did not know how to assess for drug–CM interactions, 3% identified a drug–CM interaction.[173]

The lack of professional consultations may reflect lack of knowledge, financial limitations, restricted mobility and independence, a lack of perceived need or low health literacy. Health literacy refers to possessing skills and knowledge about health and healthcare, including the ability to identify, understand and communicate health information, seek appropriate care and make informed decisions about healthcare.[169] Systematic reviews of relevant literature conclude that low levels of health literacy are associated with poorer health and treatment outcomes including poor medication compliance, increased admissions to emergency departments, reduced ability to interpret labels and health messages, poorer health status and increased mortality among the elderly.[169] A review of health literacy and CM use in New South Wales found that the three domains that older people performed worst in were appraisal of health information, the ability to find good information and navigating the healthcare system.[169] Conflicting and unreliable information was a notable issue, in particular the media and internet sources. The issue of quality of information extends to professional sources and creates challenges for health professionals and community members alike.[155]

RISK FACTORS FOR RECEIVING POLYPHARMACY

Increasing age is a key risk for polypharmacy, though there is evidence that being on a few medications when younger also increases the risk.[159] Additional factors include:

- Frequent healthcare/doctor visits
- Poor communication
- Having multiple healthcare providers
- Fragmented medical/healthcare
- Poor prescribing practices
- Poor or absent monitoring and reviewing practices.[147]

Other factors are yet to be fully elucidated but include location, practitioner beliefs and the education, race and socioeconomic status of the older person.[144,147,178] For example, a study that compared medication prescriptions in six European cities collected prospective data from 900 consecutive older patients admitted to six university teaching hospitals in Geneva (Switzerland), Madrid (Spain), Ostend (Belgium), Perugia (Italy), Prague (Czech Republic) and Cork (Ireland) and found very high levels of polypharmacy (more than 10 medications), ranging from 4% of patients in regional Perugia to 21% in the city of

Geneva. This finding reflects differences in potentially inappropriately prescribed medicines unrelated to age variations.[178]

RISKS OF POLYPHARMACY

Polypharmacy is associated with increased admissions to hospital, functional and cognitive impairment, geriatric syndromes (delirium, falls or frailty) and mortality. Additional negative consequences are poorer health outcomes (adverse drug reactions, adverse drug withdrawal events, therapeutic failure), declining nutritional status, excessive cost and reduced QOL.[141,145,179] The number of possible drug–drug interactions (and potentially herb–herb and herb–drug interactions) rises sharply with concurrent use of five or more drugs, meaning that the addition of only one more drug can have significant impacts. An Australian prospective 16-week cohort study evaluated drug interactions in 275 patients aged 65 years and older with polypharmacy (>5 drugs) admitted to a community hospital.[178] The prevalence of potential CYP-mediated drug–drug interactions was 80%: the probability of at least one CYP-mediated drug–drug interaction was 50% for people taking 5–9 drugs, 81% for 10–14 drugs, 92% for 15–19 drugs and 100% for 20 or more drugs. Each additional drug introduced to a five-drug regimen conferred a 12% increased risk of a potential CYP-mediated drug–drug interaction.[180]

Polypharmacy is strongly associated with delirium, especially if the elderly person presents to the emergency department with new delirium, with medication found to be the leading cause of delirium in up to 39% of cases.[181] Catic et al.[181] have identified risk factors for developing delirium as follows:

- Nine or more chronic medications
- 12 or more doses of medications per day
- Six or more concurrent chronic dosages
- History of previous drug reactions
- Low body weight
- Age greater than 85 years
- Estimated creatinine clearance <50 mL/min.[182]

Falls are another risk when using multiple medications.[183,184] Different classes of medications clearly have different risks, with central nervous system agents being higher risk than something like paracetamol, for example. One study of 6666 adults aged 50 years and older found that polypharmacy with antidepressants increased the risk of having a fall (RR 1.6) or an injurious fall (RR 1.51), whereas antidepressant use without polypharmacy was not associated with an increased risk of falls – and nor were anti-hypertensives, diuretics and anti-psychotics.[183] Another study compared alcohol use, polypharmacy and falls in 2444 older Americans and found that drinking alcohol was inversely associated with taking any medication but had no statistically significant association with increased falls. Medication use on the other hand was strongly associated with the incidence of falls.[184] A Taiwanese study showed a dose/number of medications-dependent gradient in falls-related fractures in elderly people.[185] A Japanese study also investigated polypharmacy and falls-related fractures but found that polypharmacy alone was not the key issue, rather it was the class of drugs used, including those

prohibited when driving.[186] Falls are associated with significant morbidity and mortality and are an important risk factor to minimise.

Under-prescribing

Under-prescribing is the omission of drug therapy that is indicated for the treatment or prevention of a disease or condition. Paradoxically it appears that both polypharmacy and under-prescribing occur, especially in the elderly, with older people often either being under-treated or having too few medications prescribed to adequately manage their health conditions and symptoms.[143,161,178] Those with greater comorbidity and reduced independence in ADLs are at high risk for under-treatment.[145]

Reasons for under-prescribing may include concerns about over-prescribing and avoidance of polypharmacy, complexity and higher costs of treatment, previous adverse reactions, patient preference, lack of knowledge of evidence-based guidelines where they exist (especially for preventive interventions) and the non-existent evidence base regarding multi-morbidities and polypharmacy efficacy. Further, there may be an ageist attitude leading to a belief that there is no therapeutic benefit in older people or a greater focus on palliation of symptoms rather treating the disease.[143] Indeed, if these factors are influencing prescribing decisions, it is possible that those at highest risk of complications have the lowest likelihood of receiving the recommended medications. Clinical guidelines for the management of complex conditions such as coronary heart disease with type 2 diabetes often recommend the concurrent prescription of multiple medications to improve outcomes (especially in older people) and, if applied correctly, this would be an example of appropriate polypharmacy.[143] Under-prescribing in these circumstances does not follow recommended practice and is likely to worsen clinical outcomes.

The aforementioned study on 900 older patients admitted to six university teaching hospitals in Europe sought to elucidate the prevalence and patterns of inappropriate prescribing, focusing on polypharmacy, but unexpectedly found that almost 60% of participants were not receiving evidence-based medications that are known to have therapeutic or preventive efficacy, including treatments for osteoporosis and preventive cardiovascular interventions.[178] Meid et al.[187] used data from 2714 participants in the German population-based study ESTHER and conducted a longitudinal analysis to examine the association of medication under-use with cardiovascular outcomes and factors associated with medication under-use. The findings were that medication under-use (including under-prescribing and non-adherence) was as high as 69%. This is an interesting study as it begins to define the non-treated outcomes that are often missing from clinical trials in the elderly. See Box 17.5 for suggestions of issues to explore regarding the pattern of medication use. Conditions most commonly under-treated include lack of gastro-protection when using NSAIDs, lack of angiotensin converting enzyme inhibitors in diabetics with proteinuria and no calcium or vitamin D in osteoporosis.[147] The other key area missed by under-prescribing was for the secondary prevention of cardiovascular events (e.g. antihypertensive

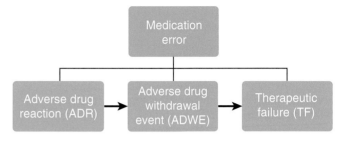

FIGURE 17.3 Categories of adverse outcomes from medication errors

Greene-Naples J, Handler SM, Maher RL, et al. Geriatric pharmacotherapy and polypharmacy. In: Fillit HM, Rockwood K, Young J (eds). Brocklehurst's textbook of geriatric medicine and gerontology. 8th edn. Philadelphia; 2017.

and antiplatelet agents).[187] Other authors have found a similar pattern for classes of drugs most likely to be omitted, including:

- Cardiovascular agents, especially anti-angina medication
- Blood modifiers (e.g. anticoagulants)
- Vitamins and minerals, especially vitamin D and calcium in osteoporosis
- Central nervous system medications (e.g. antidepressants).[145]

Medication errors and adverse events

A medication error can be defined as 'any preventable event that may cause or lead to inappropriate medication use or patient harm while the medication is in the control of the healthcare professional, patient, or consumer'.[188] Medication errors may occur at any or multiple points in the process of medication delivery, including manufacturing, labelling, prescribing, dispensing, communicating, administering and monitoring. Importantly, research to reduce medication risk has identified these points where errors may occur and a range of strategies have been implemented to reduce risk, including labelling regulations, regulations for manufacturing practices and checklists for prescribing and dispensing. However, the area that remains poorly addressed is the level of monitoring of medication use and response.[145] The core responsibility for monitoring lies with the clinician and this applies to naturopaths as well as to medical practitioners.

The adverse outcomes from medication errors can be grouped into the following three categories and it should be noted that while the initial reaction may fall into one category, it is possible that ultimately it may involve two or more categories (see Fig. 17.3). That is, an adverse drug reaction may lead to cessation of the drug and therefore therapeutic failure.

1 *Adverse drug reaction (ADR):* the most common adverse consequence, this is an injury resulting from medical intervention related to a drug; a noxious and unintended response to a drug

2 *Adverse drug withdrawal event (ADWE):* signs and symptoms relating to the withdrawal or cessation of a drug

3 *Therapeutic failure (TF):* the goals of treatment are not met due to inadequate or inappropriate drug therapy.[145]

Adverse drug reactions, adverse withdrawal reaction events and therapeutic failure can also occur with naturopathic therapies and prescriptions for herbal medicines and nutritional supplements. While there is little research in this field, naturopaths should adopt strategies developed for reducing errors in pharmaceutical medication use.

ADVERSE DRUG REACTIONS

Adverse drug reactions are classified based on cause and impact.

- Type A reactions are the most common, are based on the drug's pharmacological properties and are usually dose-dependent (e.g. bleeding with warfarin use).
- Type B reactions are idiosyncratic and as such harder to control for, are not dose-dependent or related to the drug's pharmacological properties but are less common (e.g. anaphylaxis).
- Type C reactions are chronic effects related to long-term drug use, such as analgesic nephropathy.
- Type D reactions are delayed drug effects, such as the development of leukaemia following chemotherapy for another cancer.[155]

Numerous studies have identified the rate of hospitalisation for geriatrics due to ADRs including a recent systematic review of hospitalisations of elderly people from 2000 to 2013, which found that ADRs were implicated in 5–30.4% of admissions.[189] The wide range in the estimates of hospital admissions due to ADRs reflects the challenges in accurately diagnosing the presenting condition and its probable cause. Parameswaran et al.[190] reviewed current evidence on ADR-related hospital admissions in older patients living in the community and found the ADR-related hospital admissions ranged from 6% to 12% in older patients. The main risk factors or predictors of an ADR-related admission were advanced age, polypharmacy, comorbidity and potentially inappropriate medications.

Gurwitz and colleagues have conducted numerous studies on medication use and adverse events and while it is an older study their review on the causes of ADRs in nursing homes in the US remains pertinent.[191] The results showed that over a one-year period 2916 nursing home residents had 546 ADRs; overall nearly 44% of the ADRs were fatal, life-threatening or serious and 51% were preventable. This reflects other research that identifies the greater the loss of independence and thus the greater the degree of frailty, the more vulnerable the individual is to a significant negative outcome.[144,145] Further highlighting the issue of a 'set and forget' approach to prescribing, Gurwitz et al.[192] conducted a later study of ADRs in two large nursing homes and found that 80% of ADRs occurred at the monitoring stage and that 42% of these were preventable.

ADVERSE DRUG WITHDRAWAL EVENTS

The scope of adverse drug withdrawal events is harder to define and quantify as it has not been formally examined and there is no comparative cohort.[145] An adverse drug withdrawal event may involve a physiological withdrawal syndrome (e.g. benzodiazepam withdrawal) or exacerbation of the underlying pathology that the medication was prescribed to treat (e.g. hypertension).[144] The most common classes of medications associated with adverse drug withdrawal events are cardiovascular and central nervous system agents. The duration of medication use and the number of other medications used (and thus presumably the number of comorbidities) increase the risk of an adverse drug withdrawal event.

THERAPEUTIC FAILURE

Therapeutic failure is complex and under-represented in the research. The most common conditions where therapeutic failure is reported are heart failure and chronic obstructive pulmonary disease.[144] Reasons for therapeutic failure may be related to the medication or to the individual, and this includes altered pharmacokinetics in older adults due to the physiological changes of ageing. Briefly, reasons include:

- Inadequate dose
- Inadequate duration of treatment
- Interactions with other medications (and potentially herbs and supplements)
- Drug resistance or non-response
- Inadequate monitoring and adjustment of dose or medication
- Non-compliance (possibly the most significant issue).[145]

Non-compliance includes failure to get the prescription filled, missed doses and irregular medication use. Non-compliance may be intentional (in an attempt to reduce perceived side effects, dislike taking medication etc.) or non-intentional (the individual was ill, forgot to take their medication or missed getting their prescription repeated or filled in a timely manner).[147]

Clinical tools for appropriate prescribing

Acknowledging the need to prescribe according to clinical requirement and disease burden, evidence (as it exists) and

patient preference, focus is increasingly on appropriateness of medication prescription and use, of which the number of medications (polypharmacy) is one aspect. To that end numerous tools have been developed to help the medical practitioner to prescribe safely and with the best clinical outcomes.[143,145,193] Kauffman et al.[193] provide a useful summary of 46 tools to assess inappropriate prescribing with some more applicable to hospital settings and others to community settings.

Some of the most commonly used tools in the literature are the Beers Criteria,[194] STOPP/START[161,195] and the modified Medication Appropriateness Index.[143,196,197] An Australian tool has also been developed, Prescribing Indicators in Elderly Australians (PIEA), but this is not as widely used, though Curtain et al.[198] suggest it may be a useful adjunct to STOPP/START.

The American Geriatric Society's Beers Criteria was most recently updated in 2015.[194] The criteria identify 53 medications or medication classes which are divided into three categories: potentially inappropriate medications (PIMs) and classes to avoid in older adults; potentially inappropriate medications and classes to avoid in older adults with certain diseases and syndromes that the drugs listed can exacerbate; and medications to be used with caution in older adults. A Western Australian study applied the Beers Criteria for 187 616 people (65 years or older) over a 5-year period and found that 74.7% took one or more potentially inappropriate medications, with the most common being Temazepam (a benzodiazepine).[197]

The Screening Tool of Older Persons (STOPP) identifies medications to avoid or use with caution in the elderly and provides criteria and an explanation for potentially inappropriate prescribing in older people.[159,193] Table 17.14 uses examples of classes of drugs identified by the STOPP tool and the Beers Criteria as being of risk for older people and suggests possible alternatives. The Screening Tool to Alert doctors to Right Treatments (START) includes 22 evidence-based prescribing indicators for common conditions in the elderly.[161,195] A Turkish study used STOPP/START in analysing the medications of 374 patients aged 65 and older and found that 41.2% had at least one potentially inappropriate medication and 73.3% had at least one potential prescription omission.[196] The medications most commonly omitted were, as seen elsewhere, calcium and vitamin D in osteoporosis, and statins and antiplatelet therapy in diabetes associated with other risk factors. Potential inappropriate medication prescription in this study was associated with being female, the number of medications prescribed, reduced independence in meeting ADLs and osteoporosis. Potential prescription omissions were associated with age, depression, diabetes, chronic obstructive pulmonary disease, the number of medications and incontinence.

Strategies to reduce medication-related problems in elderly patients

The first step is to ensure that the treatment, be it pharmaceutical, herbal medicine or supplement, is the

TABLE 17.14 Potentially inappropriate medications in geriatrics from the Beers Criteria and STOPP tools

Drug	Class/group	Risk	Advice	Possible alternatives
Citalopram, fluoxetine, paroxetine	SSRIs	Risk of hyponatraemia in the elderly.	Avoid	Omega-3 fatty acids, *Crocus sativus*, *Rhodiola rosea*, *Hypericum perforatum*, counselling, social support.
Ibuprofen, diclofenac, Indocid	NSAIDs	Risk of GI bleeding and peptic u lcer disease, risk of nephrotoxicity, may exacerbate hypertension.	Avoid	*Curcuma longa*, *Boswellia serrata*, anti-inflammatory diet, omega-3 fatty acids.
Promethazine, diphenhydramine	Anticholinergic (anti-histamine)	Anticholinergic effects such as urinary retention, confusion with sedation, dry mouth, constipation and falls. Increased risk of toxicity with age as clearance decreases.	Avoid	*Scutellaria baicalensis*, *Zingiber officinalis*, quercetin.
Alprazolam, diazepam, clonazepam	Benzodiazepines	Increased risk of falls, fractures, cognitive impairment and delirium. (May be indicated if seizure disorder, end-of-life or other.) Do not use for insomnia, agitation or delirium.	Avoid	*Scutellaria lateriflora*, *Leonurus cardiaca*, *Valeriana officinalis*, *Humulus lupulus*, magnesium, adenosine, SAMe (benzodiazepine withdrawal can be an acute medical situation and should only be done under supervision).
Amitriptyline	Tricyclic antidepressants (also used for pain)	Risk of sedation, orthostatic hypotension and anticholinergic effects (urinary retention, confusion, falls etc.).	Avoid	*Scutellaria lateriflora*, *Leonurus cardiaca*, *Crocus sativus*, *Magnolia* spp, *Piscidia erythrina*, *Anemone pulsatilla*, *Corydalis ambigua*, magnesium, anti-inflammatory diet, omega-3 fatty acids, counselling, mindfulness stress reduction programs.
Scopolamine	Antispasmodics	Anticholinergic effects such as urinary retention, confusion or sedation, dry mouth, constipation, falls etc.	Avoid	*Mentha x piperita*, *Chamomilla recutita*, *Dioscorea villosa*, *Viburnum prunifolium/opulus*.

Caveat: if the complementary therapy has similar pharmacodynamics to the pharmaceutical equivalent, the same risks and cautions apply.
Note: this is a brief list of suggested alternatives and is not intended to be comprehensive.
Source: Braun L, Cohen M. Herbs and natural supplements: an evidence-based guide. 4th edn. Sydney: Elsevier; 2015. Compton RD. Polypharmacy concerns in the geriatric population. Osteopath Fam Physician 2013;5:147–52. Bone K, Mills S. Principles and practice of phytotherapy: modern herbal medicine. 2nd edn. Philadelphia: Churchill Livingstone; 2013.

correct one for the patient at that time. The second step is to ensure that the patient is educated on medication usage and risks and to build compliance. When prescribing for older patients the risk of under-treatment/prescribing needs to be balanced against that of over-treatment/problematic polypharmacy and unrealistic expectations.[146] While interventions, tools (e.g. STOPP/START) and education to improve safety are important, a Cochrane Review[200] concluded that it was unclear whether interventions to improve appropriate polypharmacy resulted in clinically significant improvement, even though they appeared to reduce inappropriate prescribing. Further, clinical guidelines are often based on single diseases or scenarios and not multi-morbidity scenarios, thus making their applicability compromised in multi-morbidity and polypharmacy.[143]

Clinical presentation of ADRs in older patients

A combination of physiological changes of ageing, altered pharmacokinetics and pharmacodynamics and polypharmacy means that ADRs may present with ill-defined and nonspecific clinical pictures (see Box 17.6). Practitioners may not recognise that symptoms could be iatrogenic and may inadvertently prescribe new medication to counter the adverse effects of other drugs (known as incremental prescribing or the 'prescribing cascade') and clearly this should be avoided through studious clinical judgment.[143] If the naturopath suspects an ADR to a pharmaceutical medication they should contact or refer the patient back to the prescribing doctor or emergency department, as indicated.

Posology

Posology is the study and determination of the most appropriate dosages of medication and provides a multi-dimensional plan for dosing (see Box 17.7). Calculating dosage for the elderly can be complex and a patient and prudent approach is essential. Dosing based on age alone or even age plus weight is inadequate due to reduced organ reserve (especially hepatic and renal) and specific system

BOX 17.6 Clinical presentation of ADRs in older adults

In addition to common ADRs such as rashes or bleeding when taking anticoagulants, an older patient may present with the following:

- Dizziness
- Falls
- Confusion
- Delirium
- Constipation
- Dry mouth
- Blurred vision
- Hypotension.

Source: Duerden M, Avery T, Payne R. Polypharmacy and medicines optimisation: making it safe and sound. London: The King's Fund; 2013. [Available from www.kingsfund.org.uk.] Pretorius RW, Gataric G, Swedlund SK, et al. Reducing the risk of adverse drug events in older adults. Am Fam Physician 2013;87(5):331–6.[201] Yu YM, Shin WG, Lee J-Y, et al. Patterns of adverse drug reactions in different age groups: analysis of spontaneous reports by community pharmacists. PLoS ONE 2015;10(7): e0132916. http://doi.org/10.1371/journal.pone.0132916.[202]

BOX 17.7 Dimensions of posology

- Dose (e.g. mL, mg, mg/kg, number of specific tablet formulations)
- Frequency of dose (e.g. daily, every 4 hours)
- Duration of use (e.g. for 8 doses, 7 days)
- Maximum number of doses per day/in total
- Route of administration (e.g. oral, topical)
- Advice on discontinuation
- Advice if dose missed
- Dose adjustment (e.g. for acute symptoms)
- Reducing and responding to ADRs
- Intake in relation to food, drink and other medications/herbs/supplements
- Interactions requirements for dose adjustment.

alterations (e.g. increased sensitivity to sedatives).[159] As noted earlier, the addition of each therapy increases the risk of CYP450 interactions and renal insult as well as having unclear clinical value. Not all aspects of the following dimensions will be covered in each consultation, but they do need to be considered for each new prescription.

The following factors make posology a complex area when working with elderly patients:

- Lack of clinical trials on older populations (especially the old-elderly and frail) – the dose may not be appropriate even accounting for the specific requirements or conditions of an individual
- Physiological changes of ageing
- Age-related alterations to pharmacokinetics, pharmacodynamics and epigenetics
- Multi-morbidities, especially involving the liver and kidneys (including diabetes and hypertension)
- Polypharmacy
- Previous ADRs.

In addition, the following factors should be considered when prescribing and determining dosage:

- The patient's age (young-old or old-old)
- Gender (reduced P-gp and CYP450 function, reduced lean mass and surface area for females)
- Height and weight (body surface area)
- Liver and renal function
- Concurrent use of other medications/herbs/supplements and polypharmacy.

Strategies listed in Box 17.9 later in the chapter will help inform the need for dose adjustments with older patients.

A NOTE ON FRAILTY AND PHARMACOTHERAPY

- The lack of research and testing of drugs on the elderly is more pronounced in the frail elderly, with a minimum of pre-marketing research in this group
- Definitions of frailty are inconsistent, thus making interpreting and generalising information from the research fraught with challenges
- Frailty has a clear association with inflammation; inflammation may reduce drug metabolism and transporter pathways, thus exaggerating other age-related impacts on pharmacotherapy
- The elderly are likely to accumulate epigenetic changes that further impact on drug metabolism in a nuanced manner with increased inter-individual variance.[203]

Specific examples of altered function in the frail include downregulated CYP34A in the frail when the old and very old can maintain this pathway; and reduced sulfation of metoclopramide (anti-emetic) and glucuronidation of paracetamol.[203] Phase I pathways may also be affected with reduced esterase activity (except for aspirin) corresponding with increased inflammatory markers (C-reactive protein, IL-6 and TNF-α), though there are conflicting results from the research.[204,205] The reduced effect in metabolic pathways is not universally applied though, again making generalising problematic; for instance, diclofenac is metabolised normally in the frail.[203] When considering dose-adjustment for age, objectivity is paramount, as the elderly are commonly under-prescribed, and this perceived ageism in prescribing is greater in the frail.[205]

ASSESSMENTS TO INFORM POSOLOGY DECISIONS

Clinical treatment and prescribing decisions will be informed by the outcomes of history taking and assessments. The following should be considered in reviewing assessments:

- Drug assay parameters are based on healthy adults, not the elderly, and especially not the old-elderly, and thus may not be generalisable to the elderly[151]
- Liver function tests may not reflect impaired function, especially drug detoxification efficiency
- Assessment of creatinine clearance and eGFR are compromised by age greater than 70 years, ethnicity (e.g. Asian), low muscle mass (e.g. elderly, amputee, malnourished patients), low intake of dietary protein (e.g. vegan) and obesity[206]
- Renal assessment using serum creatinine and renal creatinine clearance is imperfect, and more so in the

elderly and those with a body surface area of less than 1.73 m², albeit it remains the main tool at present.[207,208]

Common formulas to estimate GFR include the Cockcroft-Gault equation, the Chronic Kidney Disease Epidemiology Collaboration (CKD-EPI) equation, the Cystatin C-estimated GFR, the Modification Diet in Renal Disease (MDRD) equation and the Grubb equation. The issue arises in variance between the assessments, with some over-estimating and some under-estimating renal creatinine clearance, thus there will be poor concordance between the results using different equations on the same person.[209] Further, a study of 243 elderly people highlighted the lack of correlation between serum creatinine and reduced renal function, whereby 41% with reduced renal function (cystatin C-estimated GFR <60 mL/min) had a normal serum creatinine.[210]

In addition to the inconsistencies between these equations in general, it is notable that they have largely been developed and validated for younger patients. For instance, the CKD-EPI equation was based on 12 000 people with a mean age of 47 years, while only 13% were aged 65 years or older.[205,208] More recently two equations have been developed out of the Berlin Initiative Study to specifically estimate the GFR of persons aged 70 years or older – BIS1: creatinine-based and BIS2: creatinine and cystatin-C based.[211] These two equations have shown improved precision and accuracy in GFR measurement in the elderly compared with the other equations.[205,211]

In Australia most renal creatinine clearance assessment is performed automatically by pathology services and prescribing software for medical practitioners includes calculators for in-clinic assessment. The tool used is usually the CKD-EPI unless otherwise requested and notation is provided on anticipated levels of reduced clearance based on age.[210] The Royal College of Pathologists of Australasia (RCPA) notes that the eGFR is accurate to +/–30%, a not insignificant range; further, the RCPA and the Best Practice Advocacy Centre New Zealand note that it is not validated for all ethnicities (e.g. Māori, Pacific Islander).[212,213]

The Australian Therapeutic Goods Administration (TGA) and Kidney Health Australia recommend using the Cockcroft-Gault (CG) formula to calculate creatinine clearance in order to estimate renal function in patients being prescribed drugs that are preferentially renally excreted or where the eGFR is below 60 mL/min.[182,207] The TGA notes that the eGFR assumes a body surface area of 1.73 m² and there is the potential to overestimate GFR at low body surface area, which may be more prevalent in malnourished frail aged, especially females.[207] In people with a body surface area of less than 1.73 m² relying on the eGFR for posology considerations could result in an excessive dose being prescribed.[207,214]

Cockcroft-Gault equation

$$\text{Creatinine clearance mL/min} = \frac{140 - \text{age} \times \text{weight (kg)} \times F}{0.815 \times \text{serum creatinine (mmol/L)}}$$

(F = 1 for males and 0.85 for females)[215]

Most agencies do not provide prescriptive formulae for dose adjustment with age and/or renal impairment, rather they provide factors to consider. NPS MedicineWise in

Australia promotes the 'start low, go slow' approach to dosing and provides the broad and flexible recommendation 'Start with half the usual adult dose, adjust based on tolerability and response.'[216] The Best Practice Advocacy Centre New Zealand provides a more prescriptive guide to drug dose adjustment in renal impairment based on the Cockcroft-Gault equation for creatinine clearance (CrCl); for example:

Metformin: CrCl <30 mL/min, avoid; 30–60 mL/min, maximum 1000 mg/day; 60–90 mL/min, maximum 2000 mg/day

Simvastatin: CrCl <30 mL/min, doses above 10 mg daily should be avoided.[213]

Options and implications for clinical naturopathic medicine

As noted above, the issues for pharmacotherapy and the elderly also apply for naturopathic treatments and the above information, including strategies to reduce risk, should be applied in the naturopathic context. Elderly people may be particularly vulnerable to poor-quality information and exploitation through social isolation, cognitive changes, poor health literacy and a desire to avoid the trials of ageing, and it is imperative that practitioners practise in an ethically sound and defensible manner. Practice that will support the health of geriatric patients is based upon informed consent, open communication and respect.[155,169] In Australia naturopaths are compelled to comply with the Code of Conduct for Unregistered Practitioners (Public Health Regulation 2012 – Schedule 3, Code of Conduct, Clause 99)[217], and the key areas that apply to the safe and ethical management of medications, herbal medicines and supplements are outlined in Box 17.8. Two areas of significant potential risk in older patients are variable compliance in following prescribed pharmaceutical (and naturopathic) regimens, and reduced disclosure of use of complementary therapies to the prescribing doctor. A key role the naturopath can play is to facilitate communication between care providers, in particular if an ADR is suspected.

The principles for prescribing herbal medicines and nutritional supplements to older adults are described in Box 17.9.

DIET AND NUTRITIONAL ISSUES

Older people are the single largest demographic group at a disproportionately high risk of inadequate dietary intake and thus undernutrition or malnutrition.[107,218,219] They are particularly vulnerable to nutritional deficiencies due to a complex interplay of physiological, social and psychological factors, chronic illness and reduced physical activity, and this is further exacerbated by polypharmacy and hospitalisations.

The nutritional status and requirements for older people reflect the diversity of their health status as well as the fact that people may be categorised as 'old' (over 65 years) for

BOX 17.8 Safe and ethical management of medications, herbal medicines and supplements

Health practitioners to provide services in safe and ethical manner

1. A health practitioner must encourage his or her clients to inform their treating medical practitioner (if any) of the treatments they are receiving.
2. A health practitioner must have a sound understanding of any adverse interactions between the therapies and treatments he or she provides or prescribes and any other medications or treatments, whether prescribed or not, that the health practitioner is aware the client is taking or receiving.

Appropriate conduct in relation to treatment advice

1. A health practitioner must not attempt to dissuade clients from seeking or continuing with treatment by a registered medical practitioner.
2. A health practitioner should communicate and cooperate with colleagues and other healthcare practitioners and agencies in the best interests of their clients.

Source: Adapted from NSW Government. Code of conduct for unregistered health professionals, 2012. [Available from www.austlii. edu.au/au/legis/nsw/consol_reg/phr2012217/sch3.html.]

BOX 17.9 Principles of prescribing herbal medicines and supplements for older adults

1. Establish whether the herb/supplement is necessary. What is the indication and is there a non-herb/supplement intervention that could be used instead? What are the pros and cons of using the herb/supplement?
2. Understand the pharmacology of the herb/supplement in relation to the patient's age.
3. Assess the patient, in particular renal (eGFR) and hepatic function.
4. Know the adverse effect profile of the herb/supplement in relation to the patient's other medication(s) and disease(s).
5. Start low, go slow. Choose an initial dose and adjust it carefully (doses will often need to be lower in older people).
6. Simplify the regimen whenever possible.
7. Select the least costly option.
8. Establish clear, realistic therapeutic end points.
9. Monitor for adverse drug/herb/supplement reactions at every consultation.
10. Introduce only one herb/supplement at a time whenever possible.
11. Slowly taper medications to prevent or minimise adverse drug withdrawal events.
12. Review the need for treatment at each consultation.
13. Review compliance and barriers to correct usage.
14. Make it clear: provide written and verbal instructions and ensure these are understood.
15. Provide information on possible adverse reactions and how to respond.
16. Use aids as indicated (e.g. dispensing tools).
17. Communicate with other healthcare providers (e.g. doctor, carer).
18. Space the timing of herbs/supplements to reduce interactions.

Source: Adapted from Greene-Naples J, Handler SM, Maher RL, et al. Geriatric pharmacotherapy and polypharmacy. In: Fillit HM, Rockwood K, Young J (eds). Brocklehurst's textbook of geriatric medicine and gerontology. 8th edn. Philadelphia; 2017.

several decades and requirements may change due to a wide range of factors over such a long time period. When considering nutritional adequacy/inadequacy, there are distinct differences between older people living in their own home (community living) and those living in aged care residences (hostels, nursing homes).

In the 2013–2014 financial year 7.8% of Australians aged 65 years an older (or 270 559 people) were in residential care at some point; this may have been permanent care or respite care for a short period.[220] Women represented 69% of those in permanent care at 30 June 2014 and were also older (85.8 years compared with 81.6 years for men). For the same period, 2.4%, or 83 841 older people, received home care at some point, which may include assistance with personal hygiene, housework, shopping, food preparation or medical assistance such as dressing wounds or having blood taken. Another feature of the older population that may influence their nutritional status and dietary habits is their country of origin. In Australia in 2014, 37% of older people were born overseas, 14% from English-speaking countries (the UK, Ireland, New Zealand, Canada, the US and South Africa) and 23% from non–English speaking countries.[3]

Food and nutrient intake of older adults

Many older Australians report eating a variety of foods, albeit at levels below current recommendations. The Australian Bureau of Statistics conducted the 2014–2015

National Health Survey in all states and territories and across urban, rural and remote areas (other than very remote areas) and included around 19 000 people in nearly 15 000 private dwellings, noting the estimated serves of fruit and vegetables for Australian adults as shown in Table 17.15. It is interesting to note the decline in fruit and vegetable consumption in the oldest age bracket for women, whereas men's fruit intake increases.

Alcohol consumption is relevant both as the hypothesised dose-dependent benefit for cardiovascular disease risk reduction and due to the negative impacts on nutritional intake and nutrient status and increased morbidity and mortality if excessive.[221–223] From the 2014–2015 National Health Survey, the proportion of older Australians who exceeded the recommended maximum of two standard drinks (10 g alcohol) per day was 11.2% of

TABLE 17.15 Estimated serves of fruit and vegetables for Australian adults

Recommended serve	All adults >18 years	Adults 65–74 years		Adults 75 years and over	
		Males	Females	Males	Females
Fruit (2 or more serves)	49.8%	52.6%	68.5%	58.8%	62.3%
Vegetables (5 or more serves)	7.0%	6.9%	14.8%	11.0%	9.4%
Fruit and vegetable serves	5.1%	5.6%	10.8%	8.4%	7.5%

Source: Australian Bureau of Statistics. 4364.0.55.001. National health survey: first results, 2014–15; 2015. [Cited 10 September 2016. Available from www.abs.gov.au/ausstats/abs@.nsf/Lookup/by Subject/4364.0.55.001~2014-15~Main Features~Key findings~1.]

women and 26.8% of men aged 65–74 years, falling to 7.9% of women and 15.3% of men aged 75 years and over.[105] The other key risk with alcohol is bingeing or exceeding single occasion drinking recommendations of no more than four drinks in a sitting, and perhaps surprisingly there remained significant risks of this in the older population, especially men aged 65–74 years. As with average alcohol intake, men drank more than women and the rates declined in the oldest cohort, 75 years and older: 9.4% of women and 35.8% of men aged 65–74 years drank four or more drinks in a single occasion and this fell to 3.6% of women and 12.1% of men aged 75 years and over.[105]

Weight

Being either underweight or overweight/obese has negative health consequences for older people. Overweight and obesity may lead to secondary health issues, such as increased load-bearing on arthritic joints, which can result in reduced physical activity that then leads to a raft of other issues including altered insulin sensitivity, dysglycaemia, inflammation and increased risk of cardiovascular disease and cancer. Further, obesity can impair functional status and independence and is associated with poor mental health status. On the other hand, underweight older people have a greater reduction in nutritional and functional reserves and a greater risk of morbidity and mortality than those who are overweight.[128] The apparent protective benefit of the extra weight is conferred in older age and not beforehand. While it is considered beneficial to have additional weight with increasing age, it is not beneficial to have excess weight in younger years and midlife, as this is associated with increasing morbidity and mortality. Obesity and the physiological processes of ageing share metabolic characteristics, and obesity in the mid-years can accelerate ageing and lead to poor outcomes. Progressive dysfunction of adipose tissue is an important feature of the ageing process and in obesity, and contributes to metabolic changes, organ damage and a systemic pro-inflammatory state (referred to as 'inflammageing').[224]

It is predicted that in Australia (and likely elsewhere) the prevalence of midlife obesity will continue to increase, while the prevalence of overweight is likely to remain relatively stable over time and the number of middle-aged people with a normal BMI will decline.[225] The number of persons aged 65 and older who will have a history of

TABLE 17.16 Proportion of obese middle- and older-aged adults who were obese at 50 years of age

Year	65-year-olds who were obese at 50 years of age	85-year-olds who were obese at 50 years of age
2010	22%	8% of males 9% of females
2050 prediction	43% of males 37% of females	36% of males 33% of females

Source: Nepal B, Brown L. Projection of older Australians with a history of midlife obesity and overweight 2010–2050. Obesity 2013.

midlife obesity is projected to increase from less than 500 000 individuals in 2010 to more than 2.8 million in 2050, representing a five-fold increase (see Table 17.16).[225] This increase in the number and proportion of people entering old age overweight and obese means they are also entering old age with pre-existing pathology, and with advancing age they will have a reduced reserve and capacity to recover from or manage their diseases, hence leading to a rise in morbidity and mortality in older age.

The recommended BMI for younger and middle-aged adults is 18.5–24.9 kg/m²[226] but for adults aged over 65 years the recommendation is 22–27 kg/m²[128] or even 25–30 kg/m².[121] While the best life expectancy has been shown to be had with a BMI of 25–27 kg/m², the best BMI for avoiding disability is 24 kg/m².[121] The reasons for improved outcomes with a higher BMI include improved energy reserves for periods of stress, illness and trauma; reduced osteoporosis; and reduced falls risk and subsequent injury.[102] A higher BMI may also act as a surrogate indicator of the absence or reduced impact of the contributing factors to malnutrition, such as depression, polypharmacy and anorexia of ageing. An example of the apparent protective effects is seen in a comparison between outcomes for people with COPD who were either obese or malnourished ($n = 313\ 233$ COPD hospital admissions): the study found that obese patients had a lower in-hospital mortality risk and early re-admittance risk, and the malnourished patients had a much higher risk of death when in hospital (OR = 1.73).[227]

Older people lose weight with ageing and after 50–60 years of age there is an increasingly disproportionate loss of lean body mass compared with fat loss.[103] After 50 years of age an average 3 kg of lean body mass (predominantly skeletal muscle) is lost per decade.[103,121] Further, more people over 75 years of age have a BMI of less than 18.5 kg/m² more than those aged 45–64 years.[121] The difference is not due to overweight and obese people dying younger, thus only leaving the underweight people to grow old, rather it is due to anorexia of ageing and a complex range of physiological, psychological, social and medical factors.

A 16-year study of 1008 Mediterraneans aged 65 and over investigated the relationship between BMI and long-term mortality; the baseline BMI was 26.8 kg/m² and of the 672 deaths recorded the lowest mortality was at a BMI of 30.5 kg/m², which is defined as obese.[228] Men had lower mortality risk with increasing BMI and interestingly cardiovascular disease was associated with higher mortality in the low-BMI category. A BMI less than 21–22 kg/m² is associated with a significant increase in adverse events, but when the BMI falls to less than 18.5 kg/m² the consequences can be severe.[121] A further study of 882 people aged 70–95 years showed a mortality hazard 20% lower for the obese group compared with the normal-underweight group.[229] Further, the mortality hazard was 65% higher for the low-BMI group than for the BMI-stable group. Finally, a meta-analysis investigating the association between BMI and all-cause mortality in 197 940 adults aged 65 years and older found that compared with a BMI of 23.0–23.9 kg/m² there was a 12% greater risk of mortality with a BMI of 21.0–21.9 kg/m² and a 19% greater risk with a BMI of 20.0–20.9 kg/m² and that obesity only began to impact on mortality once it was greater than 33.0 kg/m².[230]

The BMI is recognised as an imperfect tool, but it still has application, especially for public health uses. Further, it is a globally recognised measure and it can be modified to specific sub-populations. For example, while the *ESPEN Consensus Statement* on diagnostic criteria for malnutrition acknowledged that the relevance of the BMI for clinical and care settings may be questioned, that a fixed cut-off of a BMI less than 18.5 kg/m² may not be helpful at an individual level in particular for older adults, and that *changes in weight* may be more relevant than BMI by itself, the statement still kept it as one of two options in diagnosing malnutrition.[231]

WEIGHT LOSS

Weight loss is generally undesirable in older people, especially rapid weight loss, which is associated with increased risks for people of all weights, including the overweight and obese.[128] If weight reduction is necessary due to functional impairment, it should be undertaken cautiously, with support and in conjunction with resistance exercise to maintain lean muscle mass.[128] Appropriately managed weight loss produces improvements in mobility, reduces morbidity and mortality from chronic disease, reduces joint loading and disability and improves QOL.[102]

When older people do lose weight, it is most often unintentional and it includes loss of lean muscle mass. If they then regain the weight, there is a disproportionate gain of fat over muscle; that is, even if the weight returns to the baseline level there is a change in body composition and a net loss of lean muscle mass.[232] If this is repeated, a cycle of weight loss and regain could accelerate sarcopenia.[232,233] Changes in body composition following weight loss and regain are in addition to any age-related loss of lean muscle mass.[233] For example, in a study on postmenopausal women, for every 1 kg of fat mass lost during weight loss, 0.26 kg of lean tissue was lost; however for every 1 kg of fat mass regained in the following 12 months, only 0.12 kg of lean tissue was regained and this disproportionate fat regain was greater the greater the weight loss.[234]

Weight loss cautions

Unintended weight loss, especially significant and/or rapid weight loss, may indicate serious pathology (e.g. cancer, hepatic or renal failure, heart failure) and should be investigated promptly and thoroughly.

The association between a change in weight or BMI and mortality is widely reported. The Systolic Hypertension in the Elderly Program (SHEP) found increased mortality with weight gain and with weight loss, but weight loss was more significant and this effect was even present in those who were obese (BMI >31 kg/m²) at baseline.[235] Participants who had a BMI of <23.6 kg/m² at baseline and who lost more than 1.6 kg per year had a mortality rate of 22.6%, which was extraordinarily nearly 20 times greater than those whose baseline BMI was 23.6–28.0 kg/m² and remained stable.

The Cardiovascular Health Study of 4714 community-living people over 65 years of age found that after 3 years 17% of participants had lost 5% or more of their initial weight and 13% had gained 5% or more. The weight-loss group had more than a two-fold increase in mortality whereas the weight-gain group had no increase in mortality. The increase in mortality was regardless of starting weight.[236]

An Australian study investigated the association between mortality and changes in waist and hip circumference and weight from 1990–1994 to 2003–2007 in a prospective cohort study of 21 298 people aged 40–69 years at baseline.[237] There were 1465 deaths (including 109 cancer, 242 cardiovascular disease) during an average 7.7 years of follow-up. Loss of waist circumference (hazard ratio [HR]: 1.26), weight (HR 1.80) or hip circumference (HR 1.35) was associated with an increased risk of all-cause mortality, particularly for older adults. Weight loss was associated with cardiovascular disease mortality (HR 2.40) but change in body size was not associated with obesity-related cancer mortality.

Further, the Look Ahead study recruited 5145 men and women (aged 45–76 at commencement) who were overweight or obese and who had type 2 diabetes and randomised participants to an intensive lifestyle intervention or to the regular diabetes education only.[238] Over the 8-year follow-up it was demonstrated that although the intervention group who exercised and reduced kilojoules lost significant fat and lean mass loss during the first year of intervention (average 9.4 kg for males and 7.0 kg for females, 70% of which was fat mass), 7 years later 100% of the fat mass was regained and lean mass continued to decline. Of note though, the intervention group tended to have better glycaemic control and used less hypoglycaemic medication, and it is possible that longer term benefits are yet to be realised.

Two studies that used imaging tools to study specific compositional changes had similar results.[233,239] A study using total body (dual-energy x-ray absorptiometry [DeXA]) and thigh (computed tomography [CT]) composition data for 24 adults (aged 65–79 years) 18 months after completion of a 5-month randomised trial comparing resistance training alone with combined resistance training plus kilojoule restriction found that the short-term body composition benefits of the combined intervention may be lost within 18 months of completion of the intervention.[233] This study included evaluation of the thigh muscles and showed a decreased muscle volume and increase in fat around the thigh muscles as well as in intramuscular fat, which is a significant body composition predictor of loss of gait speed and muscle strength and the onset of disability from reduced mobility in older adults. The second study involving 1803 men and women aged 70–79 years tracked compositional changes using DeXA and CT over a 5-year period.[239] In that time, both men and women lost weight, including lean mass and thigh mass and even though they lost body fat overall, they gained intermuscular thigh fat. Of the 995 deaths during the study period, losing thigh muscle mass was associated with an increase in mortality and this effect was strongest for those with a BMI of less than 25 kg/m². Unlike younger adults, changes in visceral fat area were not associated with changes in mortality. These findings support the proposal that maintaining lean muscle mass is more important than losing weight or fat mass for prolonging life and health.

Kilojoule restriction and weight loss therefore are seen as positive in overweight and obese younger and middle-aged adults but not in older adults unless sustained resistance exercise maintains or increases lean muscle mass. In addition to the above risks of weight loss, there is also an increased risk of nutritional deficiencies, for example macronutrients, vitamins, minerals and phytonutrients.[121]

Malnutrition

Malnutrition exists in both community-living and residential care-living people and is often a missed diagnosis and so remains a silent threat.[121,240,241] It is estimated that between 10% and 44% of community-living Australians are at risk of malnutrition.[128] Further, overall malnutrition in older people is estimated to be present in 15% of those who live in the community, 23–62% of those hospitalised and up to 85% of those in residential care.[121] Malnutrition refers to *any* nutritional inadequacy, though it is most commonly understood to mean undernutrition as it is rare to have an excessive intake of a single micronutrient even in the case of overweight and obesity.[128,237] That is, an obese person is most likely to be undernourished (masked malnutrition). The term 'malnutrition' therefore is nonspecific and encompasses

any condition resulting from inadequate, excessive or imbalanced consumption, absorption or use of nutrients and it exists as a dynamic spectrum of disordered nutrition.[103]

Medical and health literature use the terms 'undernutrition' and 'malnutrition' interchangeably and there is no universally accepted definition or diagnostic criteria.[103,128] A 2009 attempt to develop consensus among experts for the definition and criteria for malnutrition failed to achieve full agreement.[242] The majority of experts identified deficiency of energy, deficiency of protein and decrease in fat-free mass as the most relevant elements in the definition of malnutrition. Nevertheless, they disagreed on the relative importance of these three elements as well as the necessity for including age, functional loss, changes to body composition and anthropometric measurements, nutrient deficits, cachexia, anorexia and medical conditions.[242] A Dutch study drawing on expertise of geriatricians agreed upon the following working definition:

> Malnutrition is to be regarded as a geriatric syndrome, resulting from multiple diseases and risk factors.
> Malnutrition in geriatric patients has the following characteristics: involuntary weight loss and/or an acute or chronic discrepancy between nutritional needs and nutritional intake, and loss of function.[243]

This paper also described malnutrition prevalence among hospitalised Dutch geriatrics as ranging from 32% to 61%, noting this to be higher than for other European countries, which ranged from 23% to 39%, and multi-morbidity was nominated as the main cause of the malnutrition.[243]

In 2015 the European Society for Clinical Nutrition and Metabolism (ESPEN) developed a consensus statement for the diagnosis of malnutrition. It uses the following definition from Sobotka/ESPEN that malnutrition due to starvation, disease or ageing is:

> a state resulting from lack of uptake or intake of nutrition leading to altered body composition (decreased free fat mass) and body cell mass leading to diminished physical and mental function and impaired clinical outcome from disease.[244]

This definition is less prescriptive in cause and includes body composition, functional decline and impaired clinical outcomes. The ESPEN criteria include the cut-off for underweight as BMI <18.5 kg/m² as per WHO recommendations, but also include a second option for the diagnosis of malnutrition and inherent in this is the acknowledgment that nutritional status is not simply defined by weight (see Box 17.10).[226,231] For instance, this definition notes the issues associated with rapid and/or significant weight loss, and that a person may conceivably be in a catabolic state, losing more than 10% of their body weight in less than 6 months but still have a 'healthy' BMI.[231] Importantly, the ESPEN criteria also include the desirability for older people to have a higher BMI than younger adults.

The first step in diagnosing malnutrition is to undertake a nutritional assessment using a validated tool to identify those at risk of malnutrition. The second step is to apply the ESPEN criteria for those at risk.

Given the recency of the ESPEN definition and diagnostic criteria, there have thus far been few studies validating these criteria. One early study applied the definition and diagnostic criteria to describe the prevalence of malnutrition in four diverse populations: acutely ill middle-aged patients, geriatric outpatients, healthy old individuals and healthy young individuals.[245] The results found the criteria to be applicable to diverse population groups including for geriatric outpatients and healthy old and it is noteworthy that 13% of geriatric outpatients had an unintentional weight loss of more than 10% in an indefinite time frame or more than 5% in the past 3 months. That is, if not for the study, these people may not have been diagnosed with malnutrition, reflecting the invisibility and under-diagnosis of malnutrition in elderly people.[241,245]

Once an older person has lost weight or developed malnutrition, it is difficult to regain their prior health status; thus prevention, screening and early intervention are critical.[128] A malnourished older adult is more susceptible to an acute illness and is more likely to have an incomplete recovery due to poor nutritional and functional reserves, often triggering a cascade of worsening health and debility (see Fig. 17.4).

BOX 17.10 ESPEN diagnostic criteria for malnutrition

Option 1

BMI <18.5 kg/m^2

Option 2

Weight loss (unintentional) >10% indefinite of time, or >5% over the last 3 months combined with either
- BMI <20 kg/m^2 if <70 years of age or <22 km/m^2 if ≥70 years of age
  or
- Free-fat mass index (FFMI) <15 kg/m^2 and 17 kg/m^2 in women and men, respectively

Source: Cederholm T, Bosaeus I, Barazzoni R, et al. Diagnostic criteria for malnutrition: an ESPEN consensus statement. Clin Nutr 2015;34: 335–40.

Older adults are vulnerable to a diverse range of overlapping and compounding contributing risks for malnutrition. For example, chronic pain is a risk factor and it may lead to other risk factors including opioid use, which may lead to further risk factors such as dyspepsia, drowsiness, fatigue and constipation, all of which increase anorexia, reduce intake and exponentially increase the risk of malnutrition and the associated increased risk of morbidity and mortality. Contributing factors for malnutrition are outlined in Table 17.17.

Reduced protein intake is particularly problematic in older adults and may be due to an inability to afford meat and other animal protein sources, as well as difficulties in chewing and digesting protein owing to age-related physiological changes. Further, they may not be familiar with good plant-based protein sources or may experience undue digestive discomfort. Unlike cachexia, protein energy malnutrition can to varying degrees respond to dietary interventions.[103,121]

DISEASE-RELATED MALNUTRITION CATEGORIES

Malnutrition exists as a spectrum ranging from short-term mild 'simple starvation' to that associated with severe systemic disease and trauma.[103,249] Disease-related malnutrition may be sub-divided as follows, with the presence and degree of inflammation being a key determinant along with acuity of the disease.[118,249]

Starvation-related malnutrition (undernutrition)

The person is receiving care for a medical condition, there is no inflammation present and there is a significantly reduced energy intake. This may be through reduced oral intake, malabsorption or maldigestion. Starvation-related malnutrition is likely with a more than 25% reduction in kilojoules, a BMI of less than 20 kg/m^2, unintentional weight loss, no oral intake for more than a week, and reduced body fat and skin fold thickness. In elderly patients, this includes anorexia of ageing as well as malnutrition associated with depression, dysphagia or dementia.[118]

Chronic disease-related malnutrition

Chronic disease-related malnutrition is characterised by the presence of chronic disease that causes a subclinical, mild

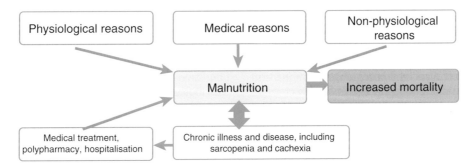

FIGURE 17.4 Risks and consequences of malnutrition

TABLE 17.17 Contributing factors to anorexia and malnutrition		
Physiological	**Non-physiological**	**Disease/medical-related**
• Reduced sense of taste and smell • Reduced sense of thirst (hypodipsia) • Diminished appetite • Changes in appetite-regulating peptides • Changes in GIT hormones • Delayed gastric emptying • Reduced neural sensitivity to GIT distension leading to early satiety, distension, slower gastric emptying and reduced intake • Reduced stomach acid, reduced gut motility • Xerostomia, or dry mouth, which impairs the ability to lubricate, chew and swallow food • Degeneration of brush border and reduced enzymes, increasing lactose and other intolerances.	• Physical and psychological abuse • <2 meals a day and inadequate snacks • Inadequate serving size • Limited income (reduced quality and quantity of food) • Reduced access to shopping • Physical disability or impaired motor performance affecting ability to prepare food • Disordered eating behaviours, food anxiety, fads • Cultural/religious values about appropriate diet • Reduced pleasure of eating • Inability to feed self • Living alone (especially males) • Social isolation • Bereavement (especially recent) • Institutionalised • Poor food knowledge • Cooking and food preparation techniques that reduce bioavailability of nutrients • Contemporary foods unfamiliar • Making change is difficult • Limited English skills/non–English speaking • From diverse cultures including Indigenous populations • Failure to cater to ethnic/religious food preferences in institutionalised settings.	• Medications, especially polypharmacy • Depression, anxiety • Cognitive decline, dementia, delirium • Disordered behaviour, psychosis and other mental health issues Comorbidities: GIT • Poor dental health (including cavities, gum disease, missing teeth and ill-fitting dentures) • Dysphagia and achalasia • Malabsorption syndromes • GIT disease (e.g. IBD) • Dyspepsia, GORD • *Helicobacter pylori* infection • Pernicious anaemia • Altered bowel flora and permeability • Constipation, diarrhoea Comorbidities: other • Hypermetabolic states (hyperthyroidism, infection) • Cardiovascular (especially heart failure), respiratory, renal disease • Diabetes, cancer, arthritis • Chronic and acute pain • Infection • Alcoholism.

Source: [121,241,246–248].

or moderate inflammation, the metabolic effects of which contribute to the malnutrition. Chronic inflammation, even at low levels, may alter nutrient requirements, body composition and metabolism and increase anorexia.[118] In addition to the risks identified in starvation-related malnutrition noted above (e.g. unintentional weight loss, no oral intake for a week), the patient with chronic disease-related malnutrition will have reduced muscle mass and signs of inflammatory activity such as elevated CRP or may be more specifically defined based on the disease, such as the American College of Rheumatology criteria.[118,250] In elderly patients, this is seen with common diseases such as heart failure, atherosclerosis, hypertension, inflammatory bowel disease, cancer and rheumatoid arthritis.

Acute disease or injury-related malnutrition

In this situation malnutrition is caused by an immense and potentially unmanageable protein catabolism associated with an acute inflammatory response during critical illness or injury. This is also referred to as stress metabolism.[118] Acute disease or injury-related malnutrition is defined by severe inflammation in response to a critical illness or major injury or trauma. It is typical of massive trauma, burns and sepsis. In the elderly patient, this may be associated with falls-induced fractures and closed-head injuries. Further, an older person with diminished reserves is less capable of responding to these insults and is more likely to have a poor clinical outcome.[118]

ASSESSMENT

Nutritional assessment is one aspect of a comprehensive health assessment and validated assessment tools exist for varying environments, including community-living, acute hospital and residential care facilities. The flowchart in Fig. 17.5 provides an overview of diagnosing disease-related malnutrition categories.

This information will help inform the development of naturopathic therapeutic goals and strategies, in particular for starvation-related malnutrition and chronic disease-related malnutrition. A naturopath is only likely to be involved in the care of patients who have had acute disease or injury-related malnutrition as part of their long-term recovery after what is typically a protracted hospital and rehabilitation in-patient admission, at which time they are more likely to be categorised as having chronic disease-related malnutrition as the intense catabolic state has resolved.

CACHEXIA

The term 'cachexia' is derived from the Greek words *kakòs* (bad) and *héxis* (condition), which aptly describe the condition[120]: cachexia is a complex inflammatory metabolic condition associated with an underlying disease that causes increased protein catabolism and severe loss of body weight, fat and muscle. It is different from non-inflammatory weight loss, malnutrition and sarcopenia. Indeed, while all patients with cachexia have weight loss and malnutrition not all malnourished and underweight people have cachexia.

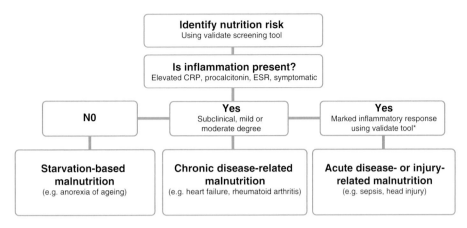

FIGURE 17.5 Assessment of disease-related malnutrition categories

Adapted from Valentini L, Volkert D, Schutz T, et al. Suggestions for terminology in clinical nutrition. ESPEN J 2014;9:e97–108. Jensen GL. Malnutrition and inflammation 'Burning down the house': inflammation as an adaptive physiologic response versus self-destruction. J Parenter Enteral Nutr 2015;39(1):56–62.

TABLE 17.18 Comparison of disease-related malnutrition and cachexia				
	Starvation-related malnutrition	**Chronic disease-related malnutrition**	**Acute disease or injury-related malnutrition**	**Cachexia**
Loss of fat?	Yes	Yes	Yes	Yes
Loss of muscle?	No, or minor compared with fat loss	Yes	Yes	Yes
Inflammation?	No	Low–moderate	Severe	Low–moderate
Can malnutrition be reversed by nutritional intervention?	Yes	Yes	Variable, possibly	No, or incomplete

Cachexia involves loss of lean muscle mass with or without loss of fat mass and is characterised by an increase in inflammatory cytokines (e.g. TNF, IL-1, IL-6, interferon-γ), weight loss, fatigue, weakness, muscle atrophy, metabolic alterations and reduced availability of nutrients, anorexia and insulin resistance.[102,120,122] Whereas to some degree non-inflammatory weight loss is considered a normal part of ageing, inflammatory cachexia is not, and it is associated with pathology such as heart failure, chronic renal failure, liver failure, rheumatoid arthritis, chronic obstructive pulmonary disease and cancer, though there are operational differences in the definition of cancer cachexia.[119,120,122] Cachexia is associated with increased morbidity and mortality, and there is a threshold in advanced cachexia past which there is little or no response to the available nutritional and pharmacological treatments and where death is inevitable.[102,120] There is significant overlap in the definitions of malnutrition and cachexia, with the main difference being that in cachexia the loss of body mass cannot be fully reversed with nutritional interventions (see Table 17.18).[102, 119]

ANOREXIA OF AGEING

Anorexia may be present by itself or concurrently with chronic illness, polypharmacy, sarcopenia, protein-energy malnutrition or cachexia, and it is a major contributing factor to malnutrition and adverse health outcomes.[251]

Anorexia and reduced energy intake are common with increasing age even in the absence of disease; the term 'anorexia of ageing' is used to denote this isolated anorexia in older adults and includes a reduced appetite as well as increased fullness and early satiation.[103,121] Anorexia of ageing is recognised as an independent predictor of morbidity and mortality.[103,251]

With increasing age the physiological processes that regulate body weight and the correlation of intake with metabolic requirements appear to lose their compensatory responsiveness to changes in energy requirements.[103] For example, a 2016 meta-analysis including 59 trials analysed the effect of ageing on appetite (hunger/fullness) and energy intake after overnight fasting and in a postprandial state.[252] Compared with younger adults (n = 4111, average 26 years), for the older adults (n = 3574, average 70 years) energy intake was 16–20% lower, hunger was 25% (after overnight fasting) to 39% (postprandial) lower, and fullness was 37% greater.

Weight loss associated with decreased intake affects young and old people differently through altered homeostatic mechanisms as we age.[121] In a landmark study, young and older men had marked calorie restriction of 750 calories (3138 kJ) per day for 21 days after which they could eat unrestricted. Following the period of underfeeding the young men exhibited hyperphagia and overfeeding followed by a period of hypophagia, after which they returned to their baseline body weight. The older men did not exhibit hyperphagia or the balancing hypophagia and did not regain the lost weight.[120] This highlights the risk of even a short period of reduced intake and has influenced more recent changes to preoperative preparation for bowel surgery. Whereas once patients had days of a clear fluid diet, fasting and extensive purgative bowel preparation in the belief it would reduce wound and peritoneal infection, it has been shown that this in fact increases the risk.[170,253] Fasting is associated with increased infection, slower return of bowel function, electrolyte imbalances, longer time to return of normal bowel function and extended length of hospital admission, and this effect is greatest in the elderly.[170,253] For example, having a carbohydrate drink preoperatively reduced the length of hospitalisation from 13 days for those who did not have the carbohydrate drink to a median of 7.5 days for those who did, and patients had their first bowel motion 2 days postoperatively compared to 5 days.[253]

Researchers have sought to identify key hormonal, adipokine and neuropeptide influences on the onset and severity of anorexia of ageing. It is believed that identifying these metabolic processes is most relevant in anorexia of ageing as no other overt disease or dysfunction has been identified as causative and this potentially would open an avenue for future treatment. To date, there is growing evidence for the role of GIT hormones (ghrelin, cholecystokinin and glucagon-like peptide) and adipokines but as yet animal studies on neuropeptide have not been convincingly repeated in humans.[103,121,246,254]

Older people have altered levels of gastrointestinal hormones, such as increased cholecystokinin (both basal and postprandial) and lower levels of and greater resistance to ghrelin, which normally increases hunger and appetite.[121,246,247] In addition to stimulating feeding, ghrelin releases growth hormone from the pituitary gland.[246,247] In older adults a high-fat diet increases the satiety signal from glucagon-like peptide 1 (GLP-1), which then decreases hunger through increasing insulin sensitivity in parts of the brain, including the hypothalamus, which in turn initiates anorexia.[246,247]

Regulation of appetite is also controlled by peptides. Animal studies show a decreased activity of endogenous opioid peptides, beta-endorphin, encephalin and dynorphin, which stimulate feeding behaviour and preferentially increase the ingestion of a high-fat diet through the κ receptor.[246] Human studies on neuropeptide-Y (NPY), a potent orexigenic agent whose effects are predominantly on carbohydrate-rich food, are also inconclusive, but there is evidence of decreased expression and numbers of receptors in animal studies.[103,121,246,255] Leptin is a hormone secreted by the adipose tissue that regulates fat storage. Leptin decreases the sensation of hunger and food intake, and adjusts energy expenditure; it is lower with age but may be affected by reduced testosterone in men.[121,246,255] Galanin is produced in the brain and peripherally and has an orexigenic activity; it is lowered in older women but not men.[121,246] Cocaine- and amphetamine-regulated transcript (CART) is a neuropeptide produced mainly in the hypothalamus and it suppresses appetite by the inhibition of NPY neurons but research on age-related changes is inconclusive.[121,246] Two orexins

(orexin-A and orexin-B, also named hypocretin-1 and hypocretin-2) increase the craving for food and their activity is inhibited by leptin (through the leptin receptor pathway) and activated by ghrelin and hypoglycaemia. No human studies are available but animal studies suggest that reduced neurons with ageing reduced the orexins.[121,246]

Adipose tissue was once believed to be an inert energy storage organ but is now recognised to be metabolically active and increasingly it is recognised as an endocrine organ in its own right.[224,254,256] Adipokines are a group of cytokines and proteins involved in cell-signalling, in particular in relation to inflammation and immune function, and include both pro-inflammatory actions (e.g. IL-6, TNF-α) and anti-inflammatory actions (e.g. adiponectin, which also has insulin-sensitising properties and is involved in fatty-acid breakdown). Adipocytes modulate energy status through eating behaviour, energy expenditure and insulin sensitivity.[256] Moreover, adipose tissue has become a central node for driving local and systemic sterile inflammation and adipokine dysregulation has a critical role in adiposity, insulin-resistance and metabolic syndrome.[256]

With progressive ageing the increased proportion of fat mass to lean muscle mass increases TNF-α and IL-6 and other pro-inflammatory cytokines, leading to anorexia.[103,121,247,255,256] This age-related increase in inflammation is compounded by the presence of physical stressors such as diseases (e.g. atherosclerosis) and infection as well as psychological stress.[121] Inflammatory cytokines are most elevated in acute disease- or injury-related malnutrition followed by cachexia.

CONSEQUENCES OF ANOREXIA OF AGEING AND MALNUTRITION

Anorexia, weight loss and malnutrition contribute to loss of lean muscle mass, reduced functioning, decreased function of respiratory muscles, impaired immune function with depressed antibody- and cell-mediated immune responses leading to increased susceptibility to infections, reduced gut function and increased bacterial translocation (of intestinal bacterial to extra-intestinal sites such as mesenteric nodes, bloodstream and organs).[248] Anorexia and reduced dietary intake lead to hypoalbuminaemia, increased synthesis of acute-phase proteins (e.g. CRP, alpha-1-acid glycoprotein and fibrinogen) and decreased coagulation capacity leading to increased oxidative stress and increased tissue damage, likely magnifying the underlying reasons for the anorexia (e.g. ill-health, depression).[155] Inflammation is thus both a cause and an effect of anorexia and malnutrition and is characteristic of cachexia and central to the pathogenesis of depression, cardiovascular disease, diabetes mellitus, autoimmune disease, infections, cancer and accelerated ageing.[224,257] The consequences of malnutrition and weight loss in an older adult are outlined in Table 17.19.

Malnutrition is a prognostic factor for increased morbidity and mortality, especially for those requiring hospitalisation where it is associated with:
- Increased rates of hospitalisation
- Functional decline while in hospital

TABLE 17.19 Consequences of weight loss and malnutrition in older adults

Consequences of weight loss and malnutrition for older people

↓ muscle mass, function, relaxation and strength; sarcopenia	Impaired immune function
↑ falls and resultant morbidity and mortality	↑ risk of infection
↓ bone density	↓ synthesis of T-cells
↑ risk of fractures	↓ synthesis IL-2
↓ functional status	↓ cytolytic cells activity
Anaemia	↓ immunoglobulin response to vaccination
Poor wound healing	↑ risk of pneumonia
↑ risk of pressure sores	↑ hospital admission and length of stay
Poor recovery from surgery and injury	↓ cardiac output
↑ risk of sepsis and delirium in hospital	↓ maximal breathing capacity
Fatigue	↓ circulating blood volume
↓ cognitive function	↑ frailty
↓ QOL	↑ morbidity and mortality.
↓ vitality.	

Source: Bernstein M, Munoz N, Academy of Nutrition and Dietetics. Position of the Academy of Nutrition and Dietetics: food and nutrition for older adults — promoting health and wellness. J Acad Nutr Diet 2012;112(8):1255–77. Johnson LE, Sullivan DH. Malnutrition in Older Adults. In: Fillit HM, Rockman K, Young J (eds). Brocklehurst's textbook of geriatric medicine and gerontology. 8th edn. Philadelphia: Elsevier; 2017, pp. 914–22. Soenen S, Chapman IM. Body weight, anorexia, and undernutrition in older people. J Am Med Dir Assoc 2013;14:642–8. van Asselt D, van Bokhorst DE, van der Schueren M, et al. Assessment and treatment of malnutrition in Dutch geriatric practice: consensus through a modified Delphi study. Age Ageing 2012;41:399–404.

- Delayed or reduced recovery of function upon discharge
- Increased risk of life-threatening complications (e.g. sepsis and delirium)
- Longer hospital admissions
- Increased risk of post-discharge readmission
- Poor QOL
- Increased in-hospital and later mortality.[243,245,258]

HYDRATION

Hydration presents a unique challenge for older people who may be negotiating a conflicting need for hydration with conditions such as arthritis and limited mobility, incontinence and heart failure. Dehydration increases the risk of falls, constipation and laxative use, poor recovery and rehabilitation, and postprandial orthostatic hypotension.[103] Risks for dehydration include medications (especially diuretics), dependency in ADLs including requiring assistance to get fluids and to eat and drink, cognitive decline and dementia, delirium, dismissed thirst drive and chronic disease. Further, hypodipsia is common with increasing age, especially in conjunction with chronic disease, and is estimated to be present in up to 30% of residents in nursing homes.[103]

Nutritional strategies

Nothing would be more tiresome than eating and drinking if God had not made them a pleasure as well as a necessity.
Voltaire

Malnutrition, inflammation and loss of lean muscle mass are key mechanisms for the development of geriatric syndromes, reduced QOL and increased morbidity and mortality in older adults, and nutritional interventions need to underpin any therapeutic plan. Further, those nutritional interventions need to be pleasurable.

ENERGY REQUIREMENTS

Lean muscle mass and physical activity are the main determinants of energy requirements and as both of these decline with age, so too does the required energy intake.[102] There are numerous formulas for calculating energy requirements and these vary across countries. In Australia, estimated nutrient and energy recommendations are provided by the National Health and Medical Research Council (NHMRC).[218] The calculations are based on a BMI of 22 kg/m² and in the example provided below the male is 1.8 m and the female is 1.7 m. Younger ages are provided to demonstrate the reduced energy requirements even when the BMI and perceived physical activity level are constant (see Table 17.20). For example, a male 19–30 years requires 13 000 kJ/day if he has moderate activity, whereas a man 70 years and older with the same activity requires only 10 700 kJ/day. Finally, as discussed above, the recommended BMI for an older person is closer to 25 kg/m², but how this may influence energy requirements depends more on body composition and the amount of lean muscle mass to fat mass.

PROTEIN

Older adults require additional protein to compensate for age-related changes in protein metabolism (including a declining anabolic response to consumed protein), and to counterbalance inflammation and catabolic processes associated with acute and chronic multi-morbidities increasingly common with progressive ageing.[259] The impact of increasing protein intake will vary according to the age and health of the individual but improvements can be found in most measures.

A Cochrane Review of 62 trials with 10 187 randomised participants aged 65–88 years who were inpatients in acute-care hospitals (71%) or living in aged care facilities (14%) or community-dwelling (15%) found a small but consistent increase in weight using energy and protein supplementation.[260] Mortality was only reduced for those who were over 75 years of age and undernourished. Further, the risk of complications such as development of pressure sores and surgical wound infections was reduced.

Another systematic review included 36 randomised controlled trials (*n* = 3790) of older people (mean age 74 years) using high-protein oral nutritional supplements, meaning that >20% of energy intake was from protein.[261] Outcomes included reduced complications (e.g. vomiting

Age	Energy requirements (MJ/day)					
	PAL 1.2 bed rest	PAL 1.4 very sedentary	PAL 1.6 light activity	PAL 1.8 moderate activity	PAL 2.0 heavy activity	PAL 2.2 vigorous activity
Male 1.8 m tall						
19–30 years	8.9	10.3	11.8	13.3	14.8	16.3
31–50 years	8.5	9.9	11.3	12.7	14.2	15.6
51–70 years	7.8	9.1	10.4	11.7	13.1	14.4
>70 years	7.1	8.3	9.5	10.7	11.9	13.1
Female 1.7 m tall						
19–30 years	7.2	8.4	9.6	10.8	12.0	13.2
31–50 years	6.8	8.0	9.1	10.3	11.4	12.5
51–70 years	6.5	7.6	8.7	9.8	10.7	12.0
>70 years	6.2	7.2	8.3	9.3	10.3	11.4

TABLE 17.20 NHMRC estimated energy requirements

Excludes pregnant or lactating women. PAL: physical activity level; 1 MJ (megajoule) = 1000 kJ.
Source: NHMRC. Dietary energy: nutrient reference values, 2014. [Cited 10 September 2016. Available from www.nrv.gov.au/dietary-energy.]

and nausea), reduced hospital length of stay and reduced readmissions to hospital. Functional improvements included significantly improved grip strength (a surrogate measure of muscle strength and sarcopenia) but there was no change to ADLs or mobility. Finally, supplementation increased energy intake (mean 314 calories [1314 kJ]) and protein intake (mean 22 g) without reducing regular food intake and the high-protein group increased their weight compared with the control group by an average of 1.7 kg.

In 2013 the European Union Geriatric Medicine Society and associated organisations formed the PROT-AGE Study Group to develop updated, evidence-based recommendations for optimal protein intake for adults aged 65 years and older.[259] The recommended protein intake to maintain and regain lean muscle mass and function was determined to be *at least* 1.0–1.2 g protein per kg of weight. Further, if the person is active and exercising the recommended amount is 1.2 g/kg and if they have acute or chronic disease it is further increased to 1.2–1.5 g/kg (with the caveat of conditions that require restricted protein, e.g. CKD).[259] The US Academy of Nutrition and Dietetics recommends 1.0–1.6 g/kg.[102] The NHMRC has increased protein requirements for older adults in alignment with other advisory and regulatory bodies and in recognition that protein requirements are approximately 25% higher in older adults than younger adults.[128,262] This increase still falls below the EU and US recommendations, but is above the British Nutrition Foundation recommendation, which does not make any increase for older adults.[263] The NHMRC is the only agency at this stage to make different recommendations for males and females. Most recommendations average 1.0–1.6 g/kg per day.[102] A comparison of the recommended daily intake (RDI) for protein for men and women over 70 years of age is provided in Table 17.21. The NHMRC recommendations for protein intake translate to 85.6 g for

EU Geriatric Medicine Society	US Academy of Nutrition and Dietetics	British Nutrition Foundation	Australian NHMRC
1.0–1.2 g/kg Increase to 1.2–1.5 g/kg exercising or ill	1.0–1.6 g/kg	0.75 g/kg	0.97 g/kg female 1.07 g/kg male

TABLE 17.21 Summary of protein recommendations

Source: Bernstein M, Munoz N, Academy of Nutrition and Dietetics. Position of the Academy of Nutrition and Dietetics: food and nutrition for older adults — promoting health and wellness. J Acad Nutr Diet 2012;112(8):1255–77. Jensen GL. Malnutrition and inflammation 'Burning down the house': inflammation as an adaptive physiologic response versus self-destruction. J Parenter Enteral Nutr 2015;39(1):56–62. NHMRC. Nutrients. In: Nutrient reference values, 2014. [Cited 10 November 2016. Available from www.nrv.gov.au/dietary-energy.] British Nutrition Foundation. Nutrient requirements, 2016. [Cited 10 September 2016. Available from www.nutrition.org.uk/healthyliving/resources/nutritionrequirements.html.]

males and 65.8 g for females aged over 70 years (with a BMI of 22 kg/m^2).

The maximal amount of protein that can be used for muscle synthesis (anabolic threshold) from one meal is 30 g and is higher in older adults than younger adults. Therefore, it is recommended to space protein intake over the day with meals providing a maximum of 25–30 g (containing about 2.5–2.8 g leucine) and for the remainder to be obtained through snacks.[102,259]

Strategies to increase protein intake include:
- Increase nutrient density by enriching with milk powder, whey powder, cheese, eggs and yoghurt. For example, add protein powder to pumpkin soup or mashed potatoes
- Use fortified foods as appropriate

- Include protein-enriched drinks, such as smoothies, shakes and juices
- Include protein sources for snacks, such as nuts with sliced apples, hummus and crackers or capsicum strips, boiled eggs, yoghurt and berries, small serve of baked beans, smoothies, cheese and pumpernickel
- Include protein in all meals, including plant-based protein. Deficiencies in B vitamins and zinc may affect the biological value of protein; conversely, large supplemental doses of nutrients can increase the metabolic demand for protein to metabolise the nutrients.[264]

PROTEIN SUPPLEMENTS

In younger adults protein is known to be the most satiating of the macronutrients but it is different in older adults. A study comparing the response of younger and older men found that appetite and energy intake were suppressed more in younger men than in older men, and the older men who added a protein drink had a greater increase in total energy and protein.[265]

Protein energy malnutrition and loss of lean muscle mass can be remediated through dietary changes and resistance exercises, and protein powders offer a convenient way of increasing protein intake. Research on whey protein in particular has found it to be more effective in increasing lean muscle mass than casein protein in older men and that adding whey protein to meals increased amino acid absorption and muscle protein synthesis, essential in avoiding or minimising sarcopenia and related disability and frailty.[266,267] Whey protein powder contains the essential amino acids, including branched chain amino acids which help conserve energy in exercise and prevent muscle loss, as well as alpha-lactalbumin, which is rich in tryptophan, a precursor of serotonin and niacin.[268] In addition, whey powder may have other features that would be helpful in an older population, including antimicrobial, antioxidant, hypolipidaemic, chelating, beneficial to gut microbiota such as *Bifidobacteria* and secondary immunity-enhancing properties.[268] A review of 17 studies of older adults (total participants 1287) reviewed the efficacy of protein supplements in sarcopenia and found them to be effective in improving muscle mass, especially when combined with exercise.[269]

ESSENTIAL FATTY ACIDS

The inclusion of healthy fats is an important part of a healthy diet for older adults. In particular, research has shown improvements in depression and cognitive performance with increased essential fatty acids. Of particular note is that essential fatty acids (especially omega-3 fatty acids) are anti-inflammatory and as such are an essential part of any approach to reduce the systemic inflammation that characterises ageing, multi-morbidities and geriatric syndromes. A brief summary of benefits from long-term consumption of fish as well as supplementing with omega-3 fatty acids that are of particular relevance for older adults includes:

- Improved memory and cognitive performance, including for those already with mild cognitive impairment, and reduced incidence of dementia[270–272]
- Reduced depression[51,273,274]
- Reduced CVD markers including hyperlipidaemia, platelet aggregation[271,275–277]
- Reduced hypertension, heart failure and arrhythmias[268,276,278]
- Reduced inflammation[271,276]
- Lower risk of hip fractures[279]
- Improved kidney function.[272]

For example, a 13-year study of 3294 older adults found improvements in self-reported cognitive difficulties with higher intake of omega-3 fatty acids.[270] Improvements in omega-3 fatty acid intake are observed in dietary inclusion of fatty and mixed fish as well as supplementation. If supplementing, care needs to be taken to ensure that there are no adverse interactions with the patient's medications.

FRUIT AND VEGETABLES

More than half of older Australians are consuming two serves of fruit per day but less than 15% consume the recommended five or more serves of vegetables.[105] Fruit and vegetables provide vitamins, minerals, fibre, antioxidants, carotenoids, anti-inflammatory phytonutrients and other constituents associated with core nutrient requirements, health and longevity.[102,280] Higher antioxidant consumption is associated with lower risk of degenerative diseases and increased maintenance of physiological function, vision and cognitive function in older adults.[102]

Confirming earlier findings, a Spanish study found that a lower level of fruit intake was associated with an increased risk of exhaustion, slow walking speed and low physical activity.[280] Similarly, a study of polyphenol intake found the highest polyphenol intake was associated with the lowest risk of frailty, exhaustion and slowness.[281] Further, a higher intake of vegetables was associated with a lower risk of exhaustion and unintentional weight loss, an important nutritional health marker with increasing age. Research from Brazil found that women who ate lower levels of vegetables had lower cognition scores.[282]

Phytonutrients, in particular polyphenols (flavonoids, flavones, flavonols, flavanones, anthocyanins and isoflavonoids, lignans, curcuminoids and tannins) and aromatic acids (phenolic acids, hydroxycinnamic acids and hydroxybenzoic acid) are associated with reduced cancer risk and reduced inflammation, including by inhibiting NF-κβ signalling.[283] Research on phytonutrients shows a broad range of benefits, including:

- Improvements in cognition from flavonoid-rich cocoa-based drink, grape juice, resveratrol[51]
- Reduced oxidative stress and promoted longevity from cocoa polyphenols[268]
- Reduced oxidative damage[284]
- Reduced sarcopenia from green tea catechins[285]
- Red wine (alcohol free) ingestion seemed to facilitate the swallowing reflex in elderly patients with dysphasia, a pathology associated with GIT dysfunction[51]
- Reduced incidence of degenerative disease[271]
- Curcuminoids have potent antioxidant, anti-inflammatory and anticancer properties[271]
- Reduced risk and progression of macular degeneration with lutein and zeaxanthin[286,287]

- Reduced cancer risk, especially for lycopene and prostate cancer[51,288]
- Lycopene may also lower HDL-associated inflammation, modulate T-lymphocyte activity and inhibit atherogenesis[289]
- Improve endothelial function and cerebral blood flow[290]
- Spermidine (citrus fruits and soybean) has positive effects on epigenetic modifications, autophagy and necrosis in preclinical trials.[271]

FIBRE, GRAINS AND LEGUMES

The NHMRC recommendation for fibre intake is 30 g for men and 25 g for women. Dietary fibre sources include fruit and vegetables, legumes, grains, nuts and seeds.[216] In addition to the other nutritional advantages of these foods, the fibre is particularly associated with reduced bowel cancer and obesity, provides food for beneficial microbiota, reduces inflammation and is valuable in regulating bowel movements and managing blood glucose and blood lipid levels.[51,56,291] Consistently, wholegrains are found to provide the most benefit as fibre and to gut microbiota.[51,291] In order to facilitate the inclusion of wholegrains, additional soaking and inclusion of acid (e.g. buttermilk, lemon juice) to the soaking water will improve their digestibility. The only caveats with increasing fibre in the diet are: ensure adequate hydration, increase fibre content gradually to reduce digestive disturbance, and be mindful of the satiating effect of fibre as generally the goal will be to increase intake, not decrease it.[102]

MICROBIOTA

As discussed earlier, in the absence of disease and antibiotics, the microbiota is stable until the ninth decade at which point it tends towards being pro-inflammatory. For an older adult, the likelihood of no acute or chronic disease and no antibiotic and pharmaceutical use is slim and thus actively promoting a healthy microbiota is recommended. A varied and complex diet provides the assorted substrates required for specific bacterial fermentation which confers health benefits such as production of short-chain fatty acids (anti-inflammatory, immune-modulating and cancer protective) and vitamins.[56] Interventions as short as 6 weeks with 60 g of combined brown rice and wholegrain barley have been found to positively alter the intestinal microbial composition, lower plasma IL-6 and peak postprandial glucose levels.[291]

The inclusion of fermented foods and drinks in the diet may be beneficial, including sauerkraut, kimchi, kefir and kombucha. Fermented dairy such as kefir and traditional yoghurt can enhance immune function (e.g. reduced respiratory tract infections and gastrointestinal infections with *Clostridium difficile*), has anti-inflammatory action and may decrease the mutagenicity of the digestive system.[51,292,293]

INFLAMMATION AND DIET

Discretionary foods and drinks (cakes, soft drink, alcohol, biscuits and so forth) can constitute a large part of the diet. In the older adult, quick, easy-to-prepare or snack foods may appeal if fatigue, a lack of mobility and dexterity, pain and food boredom are an issue. However, their inclusion is not only detrimental in and of themselves, but also often at the cost of including foods that confer health benefits. For example, a cross-sectional analysis of dietary intake data collected from participants of the 2007–2009 Blue Mountains Eye study ($n = 879$) found a significant inverse relationship with added sugar intake and protein, fibre and micronutrient intake, including vitamins A, B_6, B_{12}, C, E and D, and minerals including calcium, iron and magnesium.[294] The authors concluded that greater than 10% energy intake from sugar resulted in a deleterious dilution effect of nutrients.

Sugars, processed food and red meat in excess of recommended intake are associated with inflammation. Inflammation is recognised as the underlying pathophysiological process in key chronic disease such as cardiovascular disease, diabetes, obesity, depression, dementia and cancer.[295,296] Diets such as the DASH diet and the Mediterranean diet have been shown to improve cardiovascular risk and are associated with lower inflammatory markers, leading researchers to devise a dietary inflammatory index to quantify dietary impacts on inflammation.[296] Lower dietary-related inflammation (and thus markers such as hs-CRP, IL-1β, IL-6, TNF-α, IL-4 or IL-10) is correlated with higher intake of fruit and vegetables, legumes, nuts, olive oil, omega-3 fatty acids and dietary fibre.[295,296]

Inflammation and oxidation, as seen with obesity, diabetes and cardiovascular disease, are associated with telomere shortening and dysfunction, which is associated with ageing. Nutrients found to be supportive of telomere health include B vitamins (folate in particular), vitamins D, E and C and zinc.[257]

The Western diet is mainly characterised by high intake of processed foods, red meat, dairy, alcohol, high-energy saturated fat and refined sugar, and low intake of vegetables and fruit, fibre and complex carbohydrates, with a typical omega-6 (arachidonic acid) to omega-3 (DHA) fatty acid ratio found around an unhealthy 10–20:1.[290] The Western diet is associated with an increased risk of inflammation, oxidative damage and the development of chronic diseases such as obesity, type 2 diabetes, cardiovascular disease, dementia, stroke and cancer. Diets high in arachidonic acid increase triglycerides, which reduce leptin levels in the prefrontal cortex and hippocampus, and this is associated with impaired cognitive function.[290] Conversely, diets with a higher proportion of omega-3 fatty acids (including the Mediterranean diet) appear to have protective effects on the brain by lowering inflammation and oxidative stress, regulating neural membrane permeability, enhancing receptor function and neuroplasticity and dampening insulin resistance.[290]

The concept of the Mediterranean diet was originally based on traditional diets from Crete and Greece, and later included diets from Italy, Portugal and other countries. Unlike the Western diet, the Mediterranean diet is characterised by higher intake of vegetables, including legumes, and less meat. The Mediterranean 'diet pyramid' is as follows:

- Every meal: 1–2 serves of fruit, 2 or more serves of vegetable, olive oil, 1–2 serves of grains
- Every day: 2 serves of dairy, 1–2 serves of oils, nuts or seeds, herbs, spices, garlic and onion
- Weekly: 2 serves each of white meat and fish/seafood, 2–4 eggs, 2 or more serves of legumes, less than 2 serves of red meat, 1 or no serves of processed meat, 2 or fewer serves of sweets
- Wine in moderation, ample water and/or herbal infusions.[297]

In addition, the Mediterranean diet specifies engaging in regular physical activity, adequate rest, conviviality, biodiversity and seasonality, and local and eco-friendly products and culinary activities, thus it is more a philosophy or an approach to life than just a diet.[297] Numerous studies have sought to identify the health value of the Mediterranean diet by analysing the dietary components but importantly, the Mediterranean diet is not just about food, rather it includes the values of culture, tradition and community.[297–299] In 2013 UNESCO added the Mediterranean diet to the Representative List of the Intangible Cultural Heritage of Humanity of Italy, Morocco, Spain, Portugal, Greece, Cyprus and Croatia and describes the diet as follows:

The Mediterranean diet involves a set of skills, knowledge, rituals, symbols and traditions concerning crops, harvesting, fishing, animal husbandry, conservation, processing, cooking, and particularly the sharing and consumption of food. Eating together is the foundation of the cultural identity and continuity of communities throughout the Mediterranean basin. The Mediterranean diet emphasizes values of hospitality, neighbourliness, intercultural dialogue and creativity and plays a vital role in cultural spaces, festivals and celebrations, bringing together people of all ages, conditions and social classes.[299]

These intangibles, especially community and connection, may be missing from the lives of older adults, especially if they are isolated or widowed, and this influences their dietary choices as well as their emotional and psychological wellbeing. Depression, loneliness and isolation can reduce pleasure in eating and reduce intake.[240] While not all studies have shown the Mediterranean diet to be beneficial, the majority do. One concern about the diet is the level of wheat and gluten, but this can be substituted with wheat-free/gluten-free options. The diet is high in vegetables, fibre and wholegrains and has modest animal products; it is anti-inflammatory, rich in polyphenols and other phytonutrients and has been found to reduce cognitive impairment and dementia, and cerebrovascular and cardiovascular risk.[290] A recent meta-analysis of 22 studies on the Mediterranean diet found that it was consistently associated with reduced risk of leading causes of morbidity and mortality in older adults, that is stroke, depression, cognitive impairment and dementia.[300] A 2015 randomised control trial found all participants in the Mediterranean group showed cognitive improvement while those in the control group showed cognitive decline.[298]

STRATEGIES TO IMPROVE HYDRATION

Many older adults do not meet the recommended intake of fluids.[102] Refer to Box 17.11 for strategies to improve hydration where indicated.

STRATEGIES TO IMPROVE NUTRITIONAL STATUS – FOOD AND LIFESTYLE

The above information provides information on dietary components, such as ensuring adequate vegetable intake. Anorexia of ageing includes a reduced appetite as well as increased fullness and early satiation.[121] In addition, the energy intake may not need to be increased to the same degree as the nutrient intake, so the approach is to aim for nutritional density and eating enjoyment, even in the minority of times where weight loss is a goal. For all older adults, the goal is to maintain and ideally build lean muscle mass.[128] Refer to Box 17.12 for the components of the nutritional therapy plan.

To meet energy, protein and micronutrient requirements the first step is to conduct a dietary analysis to review intake as well as food preferences, beliefs and other factors. If there are deficiencies or malnutrition, identify and treat the probable causes and contributing factors as much as able. For example, the patient may

BOX 17.11 Strategies to improve hydration

- Ensure that the patient is not on restricted fluids due to heart failure or renal disease
- Prepare for high-risk situations (e.g. high ambient temperatures, acute illness)
- Evaluate swallowing ability, including use of a straw (refer to speech therapist if required)
- Offer fluid regularly
- Vary fluids – water, diluted juices, ice blocks, water-rich fruit (e.g. watermelon, grapes) and vegetables (e.g. tomatoes, lettuce, zucchini) and herbal tea
- Review timing and dosing of diuretics with doctor.

BOX 17.12 Components of the nutritional therapy plan

- Nutritional assessment
- Estimation of energy and nutrient requirements
- Specific and measureable nutrition goals (immediate and long term)
- Clear instructions (verbal and written), using other media as appropriate (e.g. food preparation videos)
- Monitoring and assessment schedule
- Supplements (with consideration of potential issues identified in the section on 'Pharmacotherapy')
- Anticipated duration of therapy.

Source: Adapted from Valentini L, Volkert D, Schutz T, et al. Suggestions for terminology in clinical nutrition. ESPENJ 2014;9: e97–108.

require dental work, medication adjustment, treatment for depression or may benefit from increased social interaction or home support with food preparation.[128] Working with the patient, consider removing any unnecessary dietary restrictions, provide advice and support in learning about new foods or cooking techniques and provide practical suggestions. Engage the support of family to cook and freeze meals and bulk cook to reduce preparation time. Home-delivered meals or home-delivered groceries may be helpful and home-care support services may also be able to attend shopping and food preparation tasks.

- Eat in company if possible
- If in a residential care facility, enhance the environment and have people eat together in a communal space
- Speech therapist review if swallowing difficulties experienced
- Occupational therapist input if dexterity, strength and coordination issues (e.g. after an injury or stroke)
- Consider home-delivered meals or have family/friends prepare nutritious meals
- Regularly monitor intake, body composition, weight and any concerns or difficulties the patient is experiencing with their diet
- Review polypharmacy, especially drugs with known impacts on nutrition; refer to prescribing doctor for review as required
- Review nutritional supplements and herbal medicine that may be contributing to anorexia or that may help improve appetite
- Review and optimise gastrointestinal function (especially dyspepsia, GORD, constipation and diarrhoea)
- Review depression and pain status as both reduce appetite and dietary intake
- Assess for hyperthyroidism, systemic inflammation, infection or other causes of weight loss and increased metabolism
- Seek to maintain a BMI of 22–27 kg/m²
- Aim for at least three meals and two snacks per day
- Aim for nutrient density
- If appropriate, try to increase what they already like and eat – it is more familiar, easier to incorporate and less likely to have significant extra cost
- Improve the quality of the foods the patient likes; for example, wholegrain or wholemeal bread instead of white bread, whole oats instead of instant oats
- Add flavour enhancers such as herbs and spices and sauces as desired and indicated
- If undernourished or malnourished, provide oral supplementation of 400–600 calories (1675–2510 kJ)/day (e.g. protein-enriched smoothie)[128]
- Aim for a protein intake of 1.0–1.6 g/kg
- Aim for rich dietary variety as it is most likely to provide nutrient diversity and complexity.

SUPPLEMENTATION

The nutritional requirements of older adults may be increased due to physiological changes that affect absorption and use of nutrients as well as acute and chronic illness and polypharmacy. Older adults tend to reduce their intake and

lose weight even when this is not desirable and a restrained diet risks inadequate intake of both macro- and micronutrients. Supplementing may be beneficial for older adults, especially for those who have increased needs that may be difficult to meet through diet alone (see Table 17.22).[102,268] Even when a deficiency is overt or suspected, and when supplementation is implemented, it is important to include good dietary sources of the nutrient where possible. Food sources provide greater nutrient complexity and synergies, are sustainable, provide less risk of nutrient–herb–drug interactions, are more enjoyable and are likely to be more cost-effective than supplements; ideally, food sources will be adequate once the patient is nutrient-replete from supplementing.[102]

Nutritional insufficiencies have been associated with cognitive impairment, fatigue, poor wound healing, anaemia, impaired immune function, neurological disorders, stroke, lower bone mineral density and some

TABLE 17.22 Possible supplementation for older adults	
Phytonutrients/ nutraceuticals	**Target disease/condition**
Calcium and vitamin D	Osteoporosis, cancer, diabetes, depression
Antioxidants (vitamin E, vitamin C, polyphenols, selenium)	Cancer, heart disease, neurodegenerative disease, systemic inflammation and oxidative damage, healing
B vitamins (especially B_3, folate, B_6, B_{12})	Heart disease, dyslipidaemia, hyperhomocysteinaemia, cognition, neurodegenerative disease
Omega-3 fatty acids (fish oil, DHA, EPA)	Inflammation, heart disease, stroke, depression
Phytosterols	Elevated cholesterol, cardiovascular disease
Glucosamine, chondroitin and collagen	Osteoarthritis
Lutein, zeaxanthin and lycopene	Macular degeneration
Epigallocatechin-3-gallate	Cancer
Fibre (soluble and insoluble)	Diabetes, constipation, cancer
Prebiotics and probiotics	Gastrointestinal health, immunity, inflammation, mental health
Coenzyme Q10	Inflammation, endothelial dysfunction
Zinc	Immunity, macular degeneration, mood disorders, diabetes, anorexia
Magnesium	Fatigue, myalgia and cramps, hypertension, diabetes
(Whey) protein	Sarcopenia

Source: [40,51,102,104,117,155,268,276].

SAMPLE DAILY DIET

Breakfast	Scrambled eggs with baked beans and avocado	Eggs combined with baked beans provide an affordable and nutritious source of protein. Approximately 1.2–1.6 g protein/kg/day is recommended to prevent sarcopenia in older adults. Baked beans also provide a source of fibre to help prevent constipation as ageing is associated with prolonged transit time in the colon. All foods are soft and moist for ease when swallowing.
Lunch	Local restaurant meal: slow-cooked lamb roast cooked with fresh herbs and garlic served with carrots, green beans, pumpkin, broccoli and Brussels sprouts	A decline in gustatory function due to ageing is associated with a gravitation towards more sweet and salty foods. Instead of refined foods, naturally sweet vegetables such as pumpkin, carrot and sweet potato should be encouraged. Foods should be cooked using plenty of herbs and spices to enhance taste. Lamb provides a source of zinc; zinc deficiency is a common cause of loss of taste in ageing adults.
Dinner	Salmon and sweet potato fish cakes with lemon, salad and vegetables containing bitter greens	High intake of omega-3 fatty acids has been shown to be beneficial for brain function in healthy older adults with visible improvements in executive functioning, MRI measures of grey matter atrophy, and white matter microstructural integrity seen in healthy older adults following supplementation with fish oil. Tinned salmon can be used in place of fresh if more affordable. A higher incidence of achlorhydria is seen in the ageing population, thus bitter foods should be encouraged to stimulate digestive juices.
Snacks	Blueberries Walnuts Oats	Ageing is associated with increasing susceptibility to chronic and debilitating brain diseases. Consumption of blueberries may help to reverse age-related neuronal deficits, due to their anti-inflammatory and antioxidant activity. PUFAs and polyphenols in walnuts reduce oxidant and inflammatory load on brain cells and may increase neurogenesis and enhance sequestration of insoluble toxic protein aggregates. Oats can be soaked to make a porridge and topped with fresh fruit and nuts. Texturally they are soft; they also provide fibre and may help to reduce possible comorbid conditions such as hyperlipidaemia and constipation.

Source: [314–320].

cancers. The most common micronutrient deficiencies are vitamin B_{12} and vitamin D.

Vitamin B_{12} and folate

It is estimated that 10–20% of older adults are at risk of clinically significant vitamin B_{12} deficiency,[301] with up to 11–90% of elderly vegetarians at risk of deficiency.[302] Vitamin B_{12} levels decline significantly with ageing, primarily due to atrophic gastritis and its associated impairment in protein-bound vitamin B_{12} absorption.[301] The prevalence of pernicious anaemia also increases with ageing and *Helicobacter pylori* infection is another important risk. Proton pump inhibitors and metformin are commonly used by older adults and may reduce B_{12} levels.[301] Consequences of vitamin B_{12} deficiency include megaloblastic anaemia; pancytopenia; demyelination of peripheral nerves, the posterior and lateral columns of spinal cord, and nerves within the brain; paraesthesia; ataxia; altered cognition and memory; depression, dementia and psychoses; and gastrointestinal

disturbances.[51,102,155,301] Vitamin B_{12} is also required with vitamin B_6 and folate for methylation and insufficiency may lead to hyperhomocysteinaemia and associated cardiovascular and neurological risks. Folic acid supplementation may mask vitamin B_{12} deficiency and expose the individual to the risk of irreversible neurological damage.[155] Folate insufficiency may be present due to low intake and impaired absorption and is associated with cognitive decline, megaloblastic anaemia, fatigue, irritability, depression and weight loss.[155]

Vitamin D

Vitamin D deficiency is influenced by reduced exposure and response to sunlight, reduced gastrointestinal absorption and altered renal and liver hydroxylation. It is estimated in Australia that approximately 30% of all adults have an inadequate vitamin D status, with those living in residential care, with chronic illness and of increasing age being at greater risk.[302] Vitamin D deficiency is associated with osteoporosis, cardiovascular disease, impaired immunity, cancer, insulin resistance and diabetes, sarcopenia, autoimmune diseases, cognitive decline, depression, neurological conditions and all-cause mortality.[302,303] For example, a 2012 review found that vitamin D levels below 50 nmol/L were associated with increased risk of myocardial infarction, fractured hip, cancer and death.[303]

Other nutrients

Calcium absorption decreases with age, possibly due to altered gastrointestinal physiology that is compounded by alterations in the metabolism of vitamin D. Low calcium can impact on bone mineral density as well as neuromuscular function.[155] A mild zinc deficiency is common in older adults and is associated with inflammageing due to dysregulation that causes an increased production of pro-inflammatory cytokines.[268,304] In addition, zinc deficiency is associated with impaired immune function and wound healing, anorexia and mood disorders.[155] Selenium is important for selenium-dependent enzyme actions and as an anti-inflammatory antioxidant. Low selenium is associated with immune dysfunction, impaired thyroid function, rheumatoid arthritis, altered CYP450 function and cancer.[155] Iron requirements do not increase but intake and absorption may decrease and anaemia of chronic illness and age may be present. Vitamin E is an antioxidant with a specific role in protecting membranous proteins and polyunsaturated fats and supplementing may be beneficial for cardiovascular and cerebrovascular health and there is a statistically significant inverse association with Alzheimer's disease, dementia and cognitive decline.[51,155]

Herbal medicines[199]

The diversity of conditions that an older person may have means that all but the reproductive herbal medicines could be applicable. Many herbs that the older adult might use primarily relate to defined or diagnosed conditions that are covered in other chapters; for example, *Crataegus monogyna* for cardiovascular diseases, *Serenoa repens* for benign prostatic hypertrophy or *Passiflora incarnata* for anxiety and depression. Further, there is no 'typical aged patient' and thus no formulaic response to their unique presentation and requirements.

Reflecting on the geriatric syndromes, key qualities include loss of stamina and energy, loss of muscle mass and appetite, depression and immunosenescence. These conditions are underpinned by oxidative and inflammatory damage, and together these characteristics will inform herbal medicine decisions for the patient. A brief review of the application of herbal medicines with older adults follows (note, not all actions, cautions and contraindications are covered).

Fatigue, low energy and lack of stamina may be addressed by adrenal herbs such as *Glycyrrhiza glabra* and *Rehmannia glutinosa* as well as adaptogens and tonics. *Withania somnifera* is perhaps a standout 'geriatric herb' as it is a tonic and adaptogen, has anti-degenerative and neuroprotective properties, and is anti-inflammatory, anti-anaemic and immune-modulating. Other options include *Eleutherococcus senticosus* and *Centella asiatica*, which has the added benefit of supporting microvascular circulation, or *Astragalus membranaceus*, which is also immunity-enhancing. Indeed,

one of the great benefits of herbal medicine is the multiple actions provided by one herb.

Depression may be supported by *Hypericum perforatum* or *Lavandula officinalis*. *Rhodiola rosea* may help with depressed mood, energy and cognition. If anxiety is present with digestive disturbances *Chamomilla recutita* would be ideal, or if anxiety is accompanied by palpitations *Leonurus cardiaca* may be appropriate. Appetite can be supported with bitters, and a herb such as *Gentiana luteum* may support pancreatic function and blood glucose control. Likewise, *Silybum marianum* is a useful hepatic but also helps with blood glucose control.

Preservation of cognitive function is a significant issue for many ageing adults and herbs such as *Ginkgo biloba*, *Bacopa monnieri* and *Rosmarinus officinalis* may be appropriate. Inflammation is acknowledged as impacting neurological decline and these herbs are also anti-inflammatory. It may also be indicated to include *Curcuma longa* or *Zingiber officinalis*, which also support the liver and circulation, respectively. Finally, *Vaccinium myrtillus* may be used for age-related macular degeneration and to strengthen capillary integrity.

The naturopath/herbalist is more likely to be prescribing in an environment of multiple morbidities and polypharmacy than for any other age group and particular care needs to be taken with interactions and contraindications. The ageing patient is likely to have some degree of reduced function and reserve in the major organs of metabolism and excretion, the liver and kidneys. This is particularly important for renally active and excreted herbal medicines such as some urinary antiseptics (e.g. *Juniperus communis*).

The issues covered in the sections on 'Polypharmacy' and 'Pharmacotherapy' apply to the use and prescribing of herbal medicine. Herbal medicine is not subsidised and long-term use is potentially costly, therefore prudent and creative prescribing may be needed. The aforementioned multiple actions of individual herbs helps in this regard, as does the ability to take herbal medicine as an herbal infusion, and indeed, potentially even grow your own herbs.

Lifestyle

In addition to improvements in nutrition and dietary intake, older adults are able to make meaningful improvements to health and overall QOL (see Table 17.23 for strategies).[12,305] Social isolation is recognised as a key determinant of health, especially in older adults. Isolation is associated with poor health and premature death, whereas social connectedness and good relationships are associated with better health status and longevity.[306,307] Maintaining social connectedness may require greater effort for older adults, especially if they have no family (at all, or nearby) and basic issues such as transport may prove a barrier. Involvement with community groups that can provide transport may help overcome this obstacle.

Research into healthy ageing, or ageing well, highlights areas such as planning for ageing physically, financially, socially, behaviourally and cognitively. Strategies include meditation and relaxation, exercising, actively working on maintaining relationships and having hobbies.[308] Maintaining a satisfying sex life can have its challenges

TABLE 17.23 Lifestyles strategies for older adults

Strategy	Area of potential benefit
Regular exercise	Sarcopenia, depression, neurodegenerative diseases (e.g. dementia), cardiovascular and cerebrovascular diseases, reduced falls, stress, quality of life, improved immunity.
Social connection	Depression, anorexia, isolation, stress, memory, malnutrition, cardiovascular disease, quality of life, longevity.
Mental activity and creativity	Cognitive function and engagement, depression, isolation, self-esteem. (Includes working and volunteering.)
Sexual activity	Self-esteem, enjoyment, depression, maintaining cognitive function.

Source: [12,305,306–313].

with age (both physical and psychological); however, sexuality is a basic component of human life and remains so in older age. While sex is usually taken to mean a physical function, sexuality has broader dimensions and also includes social and psychological aspects:

> *This human dimension encompasses self, interactions with others, and various stages of expression and affection throughout life ... Sexual needs in old age are similar to those in young age, with some variations, mainly in mode of expression.*[309]

Sex may also help maintain cognitive function. The English Longitudinal Study on Ageing (ELSA) analysed data from 6833 participants aged 50–89 years and found a significant association between sexual activity and memory/recall in men and women and with number sequencing in men.[310]

CASE STUDY 17.1: FRAIL AGED

OVERVIEW

FV is an 82-year-old woman who presents with increasing weakness and 'feeling her age'. Her daughter JC accompanies her and explains that up until her father's death 8 months ago her mother was vibrant, active and motivated. FV no longer attends her book club or does the volunteer work that she once loved as she 'doesn't have the energy' and it tires her too much. She lives alone and consequently her only contact is with her daughter JC and her grandchildren once or twice a week. She feels she has no muscle strength and has lost the confidence to go for a walk by herself.

PATHOLOGY AND INVESTIGATIONS

FV was reviewed by her GP recently and there was no overt pathology on EUC, FBC, hsCRP, lipid profile or TSH and

her vital signs are within normal limits. The GP conducted a geriatric depression assessment and noted she had some indication of depression but not enough to diagnose her as having major depression.

PAST HISTORY

FV has a fairly uncomplicated medical history given her age and currently takes no medication on a regular basis. She grew up in northern Europe and as a child experienced food shortages and other deprivations and trauma during WWII. FV married in her country of birth and migrated to Australia when she was in her early 20s. She had 6 pregnancies and 4 children (2 miscarriages). Her only surgery has been dilation and evacuation of remaining products of conception following her second miscarriage. She has full upper and lower dentures which have been a bit loose in recent months and she is using a gel to help with fit and discomfort.

CLINICAL EXAMINATION

FV is underweight at 47 kg (160 cm tall, BMI of 18.4); she has lost 8% of her body weight in the past 8 months. Her skin is moderately dry and pale as she has been an avid sun-avoider her whole life.

FV has a weak hand grip and relies on a single walking stick for balance (only for the past 4–5 months).

FV has some difficulty chewing tougher cuts of meat and hard foods such as nuts or hard biscuits and food sometimes 'catches' in her throat.

Cognitively FV performs well on the Mini Mental Assessment with 19/20 although she is a little slow in responding. She has a flat affect and appears withdrawn.

TREATMENT PLAN

The goals of treatment are to enhance FV's quality of life by improving muscle density, tone and strength, increasing weight, improving balance, avoiding falls, improving her nutritional status and avoiding issues associated with nutrient deficits, and help reduce depression. FV takes no medications and would like to avoid taking multiple supplements. Further, as she has difficulty swallowing tablets FV asks for alternatives such as drops.

REFERRALS

– Occupational therapist to review the home environment for safety risks and possible strategies to ease attending normal ADLs (e.g. may require grab rails, there may be uneven flooring and other trip hazards). The occupational therapist will also assess general physical strength and capability as well as cognitive function and memory
– Speech therapist to assess swallowing: dysphagia may indicate broader issues, including the risk of silent aspiration
– Grief counselling may also be helpful.

LIFESTYLE/EDUCATIONAL

– As her stamina improved, FV was encouraged to return to activities she previously enjoyed, including volunteer work. In addition, information was provided

- about other group activities (e.g. garden visits and film outings)
- JC was encouraged to make contact (even by phone or social media) with her mother more frequently as were her children. It became apparent that FV was interested in computer games and she connected with some of her grandchildren doing this. Eating alone can reduce interest and motivation so FV was encouraged to join her family as well as attend shared meals with her book club and other groups
- As safety allowed, FV returned to the garden to potter about and have some safe sun exposure.

NUTRITION

It was important that FV not lose any more weight or muscle bulk, so increasing her protein and energy intake was paramount.

- Whey protein powder was added to yoghurt, soups, stews, smoothies and baking
- Eggs were added to a breakfast of toast and as an occasional snack
- Fish-based meals were increased and other meats returned to the menu but in minced, stewed or poached forms so as to be easier to chew and swallow
- Re-introduction of foods that FV loved when younger: cheese, rye, fermented vegetables and pickles and occasional cured meats
- Anti-inflammatory and nutritive fats were increased including oily fish (especially herrings and sardines which FV enjoys), avocado, softened and ground nuts and seeds (either soaked and eaten soft and raw, or added to smoothies and porridge ground)
- FV was encouraged to have fresh fruit and vegetables where able, but also reminded about bulk cooking (with family help) and using snap-frozen vegetables if easier
- Eat three meals plus two snacks
- Make snacks higher in kilojoules and nutrients, e.g. nut butter on pumpernickel, a boiled egg with tomato and pickle, full-fat yoghurt
- A small gin and tonic as an aperitif if desired (20 mL gin).

SUPPLEMENTS

FV did not want to take multiple supplements and especially did not want tablets. For muscle, mood, energy and stamina the following were prescribed:

- B-complex powder or green powder (FV could use either depending on what she was eating that day and how she felt)
- B$_{12}$ spray or sublingual: 500 micrograms
- Liquid fish oil: 2.5 mL, 1.25 g EPA, 0.47 g DHA
- Zinc 30 mg: this was a smaller tablet and FV could swallow it or crush it and take with yoghurt or jam
- Vitamin D spray or drops: 2000 IU.

HERBAL MEDICINE

Herbal medicine was used to help lift mood, energy and stamina. FV has taken liquid herbs on and off since childhood and had no concerns about the taste or the small alcohol content.

Lavandula angustifolia (lavender) 1:2	2.5 mL per day
Hypericum perforatum (St John's wort) 1:2	4 mL per day
Eleutherococcus senticosus (Siberian ginseng) 1:2	2.5 mL per day
Withania somnifera (ashwagandha) 2:1	3 mL per day

Total: 12 mL taken as either 6 mL b.i.d. or 4 mL t.d.s.

REFERENCES

[1] World Health Organization. Nutrition for older persons. Available from: www.who.int/nutrition/topics/olderpersons/en. [Cited 20 August 2016].

[2] Rayner CK, Horowitz M. Physiology of the ageing gut. Curr Opin Clin Nutr Metab Care 2013;16(1):33–8.

[3] Australian Institute of Health and Welfare. Ageing. Available from: www.aihw.gov.au/ageing. [Cited 20 August 2016].

[4] Australian Bureau of Statistics. 4430.0.10.001. Disability, ageing and carers, Australia: first results; 2015. Available from: www.abs.gov.au/ausstats/abs@.nsf/mf/4430.0.10.001. [Cited 20 August 2016].

[5] Australian Bureau of Statistics. 2071.0. Reflecting a nation: stories from the 2011 census, 2012–2013. Available from: http://abs.gov.au/ausstats/abs@.nsf/Lookup/2071.0main+features602012-2013. [Cited 10 September 2016].

[6] Masoro EJ. Physiology of aging. In: Rockwood K, Woodhouse K, Brocklehurst JC, et al, editors. Brocklehurst's textbook of geriatric medicine and gerontology. 7th ed. Philadelphia: Saunders; 2010. p. 51–8.

[7] Browne W, Nair K. Geriatric medicine. In: Talley NJ, Frankhum B, Currow D, editors. Essentials of internal medicine. 3rd ed. Philadelphia: Churchill Livingstone; 2015. p. 777–90.

[8] Warner HR, Sierra F, Thompson LDV. Biology of aging. In: Rockwood K, Woodhouse K, Brocklehurst JC, et al, editors. Brocklehurst's textbook of geriatric medicine and gerontology. 7th ed. Philadelphia: Saunders; 2010.

[9] Fries JF. Aging, natural death, and compression of morbidity. N Engl J Med 1980;303(3):130–5.

[10] Vickery DM, Fries JF. Take care of yourself: a consumer's guide to medical care. Reading: Perseus Books Publishing Company; 2006.

[11] World Health Organization. World report on ageing and health. Geneva: WHO; 2015.

[12] Strandberg T. Healthy ageing: evidence that improvement is possible at every age. Eur Geriatr Med 2016;7(4):293–4.

[13] da Costa JP, Vitorino R, Silva GM, et al. A synopsis on aging: theories, mechanisms and future prospects. Ageing Res Rev 2016;29:90–112.

[14] Cronin H, Kenny RA. Biology and physiology of aging. In: Walsh D, Caraceni AT, Fainsinger R, et al, editors. Palliative medicine. Philadelphia: Saunders; 2009. p. 1123–9.

[15] Navaratnarajah A, Jackson S. The physiology of ageing. Medicine (Baltimore) 2013;41(1):5–8.

[16] Hevesi ZG, Hammel LL. Geriatric disorders. In: Hines LH, Marschall KE, editors. Stoelting's anesthesia and co-existing disease. 6th ed. Philadelphia: Saunders; 2012. p. 642–54.

[17] Swartz MH. The geriatric patient. In: Swartz MH, editor. Textbook of physical diagnosis. 7th ed. Philadelphia: Saunders; 2014. p. 743–57.

[18] Galvin JE. Neurological signs in older adults. In: Fillit HM, Rockwood K, Young J, editors. Brocklehurst's Textbook of geriatric medicine and gerontology. 8th ed. Philadelphia: Saunders; 2017. p. 105–9.

[19] Patel D, Lunn AD, Smith AD, et al. Cognitive decline in the elderly after surgery and anaesthesia: results from the Oxford Project to Investigate Memory and Ageing (OPTIMA) cohort. Anaesthesia 2016;71(10):1144–52.

[20] Plassman BL, Williams JW, Burke JR, et al. Systematic review: factors associated with risk for and possible prevention of cognitive decline in later life. Ann Intern Med 2010;153(3):182–93.

[21] MacDonald SWS, DeCarlo CA, Dixon RA. Linking biological and cognitive aging: toward improving characterizations of developmental time. J Gerontol B Psychol Sci Soc Sci 2011;66B(Suppl.I):I59–70.

[22] Cunnane SC, Courchesne-Loyer A, Vandenberghe C, et al. Can ketones help rescue brain fuel supply in later life? Implications for cognitive health during aging and the treatment of Alzheimer's disease. Front Mol Neurosci 2016;9(53):1–21.

[23] Hashimoto M, Hagie MA, Hara Y. Effect of green tea catechins on cognitive learning ability and dementia. In: Preedy VR, editor. Tea in health and disease prevention. Philadelphia: Saunders; 2012. p. 1363–71.

[24] World Health Organization. The top 10 causes of death. Available from: www.who.int/mediacentre/factsheets/fs310/en. [Cited 10 September 2016].

[25] Chaudhary KR, El-Sikhry H, Seubert JM. Mitochondria and the aging heart. J Geriatr Cardiol 2011;8:159–67.

[26] Georgakopoulou EA, Tsimaratou K, Evangelou K, et al. Specific lipofuscin staining as a novel biomarker to detect replicative and stress-induced senescence. A method applicable in cryo-preserved and archival tissues. Aging 2013;5(1):37–50.

[27] Birnbaumer DM. The elder patient. In: Marx JA, Hockberger RS, Walls RN, editors. Rosen's emergency medicine: concepts and clinical practice. 8th ed. Philadelphia: 2014. p. 2351–5.

[28] Maguire SL, Slater BM. Physiology of ageing. Anaesth Intensive Care Med 2010;11:310–12.

[29] Phelps K, Hassed C. Ageing. In: Phelps K, Hassed C, editors. General practice: the integrative approach. Sydney: Churchill Livingstone; 2011. p. 841–57.

[30] Conti S, Cassis P, Benigni A. Aging and the renin-angiotensin system. Hypertension 2012;60:878–83.

[31] Pacurari M, Kafoury R, Tchounwou P, et al. The renin-angiotensin-aldosterone system in vascular inflammation and remodeling. Int J Inflam 2014.

[32] Lalley PM. The aging respiratory system: pulmonary structure, function and neural control. Respir Physiol Neurobiol 2013;187(3):199–210.

[33] Davies GA, Bolton CE. Age-related changes in the respiratory system. In: Fillit HM, Rockwood K, Young J, editors. Brocklehurst's textbook of geriatric medicine and gerontology. 8th ed. Philadelphia: Saunders; 2017. p. 101–4.

[34] Lee SH, Yim SJ, Kim HC. Aging of the respiratory system. Kosin Med J 2016;31:11–18.

[35] Karam Z, Tuazon J. Anatomic and physiologic changes of the aging kidney. Clin Geriatr Med 2013;29:555–64.

[36] Weinstein JR, Anderson S. The aging kidney: physiological changes. Adv Chronic Kidney Dis 2010;17(4):302–7.

[37] Glassock RJ. Is the presence of microalbuminuria a relevant marker of kidney disease? Curr Hypertens Rep 2010;12(5):364–8.

[38] Choudhury D, Levi M. Aging and kidney disease. In: Skorecki K, Chertwo GM, Marsden PA, et al, editors. Brenner and Rector's the kidney. 10th ed. Philadelphia: Elsevier; 2016. p. 727–51.

[39] Masoro EJ. The physiology of aging. In: Boron WF, Boulpaep EL, editors. Medical physiology. 3rd ed. Philadelphia: Elsevier; 2017. p. 1235–47.

[40] Gallagher JC. Vitamin D and aging. Endocrinol Metab Clin North Am 2013;42(2):319–32.

[41] Griebling TL. Aging and geriatric urology. In: Wein AJ, Kavoussi LR, Partin AW, et al, editors. Campbell-Walsh urology. 11th ed. Philadelphia: Elsevier; 2012. p. 2083–102.

[42] Pilotto A, Maggi S, Noale M, et al. Association of upper gastrointestinal symptoms with functional and clinical characteristics in elderly. World J Gastroenterol 2011;17(25):3020–6.

[43] Luciano GL, Brennan MJ, Rothberg M. Postprandial hypotension. Am J Med 2010;123(3):281.

[44] Tarnawski AS, Ahluwalia A, Jones MK. Increased susceptibility of aging gastric mucosa to injury: the mechanisms and clinical implications. World J Gastroenterol 2014;20(16):4467–82.

[45] Slomiany BL, Slomiany A. Induction in gastric mucosal prostaglandin and nitric oxide by *Helicobacter pylori* is dependent on MAPK/ERK-mediated activation of IKK-β and cPLA 2: modulatory effect of ghrelin. Inflammopharmacology 2013;21(3):241–51.

[46] Andres E, Serraj K. Optimal management of pernicious anemia. J Blood Med 2012;3:97–103.

[47] Holzer P. Opioid receptors in the gastrointestinal tract. Regul Pept 2009;155(1–3):11–17.

[48] Mackowiak P, Giamarellos-Bourboulis E. Recycling Metchnikoff: probiotics, the intestinal microbiome and the quest for long life. Front Public Heal 2013;1(52).

[49] D'argenio V, Salvatore F. The role of the gut microbiome in the healthy adult status. Clin Chim Acta 2015;451:97–102.

[50] Lakshminarayanan B, Stanton C, O'Toole PW, et al. Compositional dynamics of the human intestinal microbiota with aging: implications for health. J Nutr Health Aging 2014;18(9):773–86.

[51] Rémond D, Shahar D, Gille D, et al. Understanding the gastrointestinal tract of the elderly to develop dietary solutions that prevent malnutrition. Oncotarget 2015;6(16):13858–83.

[52] Biagi E, Candela M, Franceschi C, et al. The aging gut microbiota: new perspectives. Ageing Res Rev 2011;10(4):428–9.

[53] Leung K, Thuret S. Gut microbiota: a modulator of brain plasticity and cognitive function in ageing. Healthcare (Basel) 2015;3(3):898–916.

[54] O'Toole PW, Jeffery IB. Gut microbiota and aging. Science 2015;350(6265):1214–15.

[55] David LA, Maurice CF, Carmody RN, et al. Diet rapidly and reproducibly alters the human gut microbiome. Nature 2014;505(7484):559–63.

[56] Graf D, Di Cagno R, Fåk F, et al. Contribution of diet to the composition of the human gut microbiota. Microb Ecol Health Dis 2015;26:26164.

[57] Saraswati S, Sitaraman R. Aging and the human gut microbiota: from correlation to causality. Front Microbiol 2015;5:1–4.

[58] Makivuokko H, Tiihonen K, Tynkkynen S, et al. The effect of age and non-steroidal anti-inflammatory drugs on human intestinal microbiota composition. Br J Nutr 2010;103(2):227–34.

[59] Claesson MJ, Cusack S, O'Sullivan O, et al. Composition, variability, and temporal stability of the intestinal microbiota of the elderly. Proc Natl Acad Sci USA 2011;108(Suppl. 1):4586–91.

[60] Biagi E, Nylund L, Candela M, et al. Through ageing, and beyond: gut microbiota and inflammatory status in seniors and centenarians. PLoS ONE 2010;5(5):1–13.

[61] Serste T, Bourgeois N. Ageing and the liver. Acta Gastroenterol Belg 2006;69(3):296–8.

[62] Pawelec G. Hallmarks of human 'immunosenescence': adaptation or dysregulation? Immun Ageing 2012;9(1):15.

[63] McDevitt MA. Aging and the blood. In: Fillit HM, Rockwood K, Young J, editors. Brocklehurst's textbook of geriatric medicine and gerontology. 8th ed. Philadelphia: Elsevier; 2017. p. 145–51.

[64] Vanasse GJ, Berliner N. Anemia in elderly patients: an emerging problem for the 21st century. Hematology Am Soc Hematol Educ Program 2010;2010(1):271–5.

[65] Yilmax MI, Solak Y, Covic A, et al. Renal anemia of inflammation: the name is self-explanatory. Blood Purif 2011;32(3):220–5.

[66] Turner JE. Is immunosenescence influenced by our lifetime dose of exercise? Biogerontology 2016;17:518–602.

[67] Ongrádi J, Kövesdi V. Factors that may impact on immunosenescence: an appraisal. Immun Ageing 2010;7:7.

[68] Shi Z, Araujo AB, Martin S, et al. Longitudinal changes in testosterone over five years in community-dwelling men. J Clin Endocrinol Metab 2013;98(8):3289–97.

[69] De Fina LF, Butwell Radford N, Leonard D, et al. Testosterone level in men is lower with increasing BMI and decreasing cardiorespiratory fitness but is not related to age. In: Endocrine Society's 96th Annual Meeting. Chicago: Endocrine Society; 2014.

[70] Morley JE, McKee A. Endocrinology of aging. In: Fillit HM, Rockwood K, Young J, editors. Brocklehurst's textbook of geriatric medicine and gerontology. 8th ed. Philadelphia: Elsevier; 2017. p. 138–44.

[71] Lamberts SWJ, Van Den Beld AW, Van Den Beld W. Endocrinology and aging. In: Melmed S, Polonsky KS, Reed LP, et al, editors. Williams textbook of endocrinology. 13th ed. Philadelphia: Saunders; 2016. p. 1234–51.

[72] Camacho EM, Huhtaniemi IT, O'Neill TW, et al. Age-associated changes in hypothalamic-pituitary-testicular function in middle-aged and older men are modified by weight change and lifestyle factors: longitudinal results from the European Male Ageing Study. Eur J Endocrinol 2013;168:445–55.

[73] Gardner MP, Lightman S, Sayer AA, et al. Dysregulation of the hypothalamic pituitary adrenal (HPA) axis and physical performance at older ages: an individual participant meta-analysis. Psychoneuroendocrinology 2013;38(1):40–9.

[74] Adam EK, Hawkley LC, Kudielka BM, et al. Day-to-day dynamics of experience: cortisol associations in a population-based sample of older adults. Proc Natl Acad Sci USA 2006;7(10345).

[75] Schoorlemmer RMM, Peeters GMEE, Van Schoor NM, et al. Relationships between cortisol level, mortality and chronic diseases in older persons. Clin Endocrinol (Oxf) 2009;71(6):779–86.

[76] Watts J, Abimanyi-Ochom J, Sanders KM. Osteoporosis costing all Australians: a new burden of disease analysis, 2012 to 2022. Sydney: Osteoporosis Australia; 2014.

[77] Australian Institute of Health and Welfare. Who gets ostoporosis. Available from: www.aihw.gov.au/osteoporosis/who-gets. [Cited 19 September 2016].

[78] Fabbri E, An Y, Schrack JA, et al. Energy metabolism and the burden of multimorbidity in older adults: results from the Baltimore Longitudinal Study of Aging. J Gerontol A Biol Sci Med Sci 2015;70(11):1297–303.

[79] Lu C-H, Chen Y-C, Chang Y-C, et al. Effect of age on febrile response in patients with healthcare-associated bloodstream infection. Geriatr Nurs 2013;34(5):366–72.

[80] Lapin A, Mueller E. Laboratory diagnosis and geriatrics: more than just reference intervals for older adults. In: Fillit HM, Rockwood K, Young J, editors. Brocklehurst's textbook of geriatric medicine and gerontology. 8th ed. Philadelphia: 2017. p. 220–5.

[81] Rubenstein LZ, Rubenstein LV. Multidimensional geriatric assessment. In: Fillit MH, Rockwood K, Young J, editors. Brocklehurst's textbook of geriatric medicine and gerontology. 8th ed. Philadelphia: Elsevier; 2017. p. 213–19.

[82] Janu MR, Creasey H, Grayson DA, et al. Laboratory results in the elderly: the Sydney Older Persons Study. Ann Clin Biochem 2003;40:274–9.

[83] Edvardsson M, Levander MS, Ernerudh J, et al. Clinical use of conventional reference intervals in the frail elderly. J Eval Clin Pract 2015;21(2):229–35.

[84] Phillips J, Pond D, Goode SM. Timely diagnosis of dementia: can we do better? Canberra: Alzheimer's Australia; 2011.

[85] Advance Care Planning. Advance care planning. Available from: http://advancecareplanning.org.au. [Cited 10 September 2016].

[86] National Advance Care Directives Working Group. A national framework for advance care directives. Canberra: Australian Health Ministers' Advisory Council; 2011.

[87] RACGP. Position Statement: advance care planning should be incorporated into routine general practice. East Melbourne: The Royal Australian College of General Practitioners; 2012.

[88] de Vries NM, Staal JB, van Ravensberg CD, et al. Outcome instruments to measure frailty: a systematic review. Ageing Res Rev 2011;10(1):104–14.

[89] Fernández-Ballesteros R, Santacreu Ivars M. Aging and quality of life. In: Stone JH, Blouin M, editors. International encyclopedia of rehabilitation. Buffalo: 2010. Available from: http://cirrie.buffalo.edu/encyclopedia/en/article/296.

[90] World Health Organization. World Health Organization Quality of Life Instruments (WHOQOL-BREF); 2011. Available from: http://depts.washington.edu/seaqol/WHOQOL-BREF.

[91] Ware JE, Gandek B. Overview of the SF-36 Health Survey and the International Quality of Life Assessment (IQOLA) project. J Clin Epidemiol 1998;51(11):903–12.

[92] Ware JE, Gandek B, Guyer R, et al. Standardizing disease-specific quality of life measures across multiple chronic conditions: development and initial evaluation of the QOL Disease Impact Scale (QDIS®). Health Qual Life Outcomes 2016;14:84.

[93] Creavin ST, Wisniewski S, Noel-Storr AH, et al. Mini-Mental State Examination (MMSE) for the detection of dementia in clinically unevaluated people aged 65 and over in community and primary care populations. Cochrane Database Syst Rev 2016;(1):CD011145.

[94] Radovanovic D, Seifert B, Urban P, et al. Validity of Charlson Comorbidity Index in patients hospitalised with acute coronary syndrome. Insights from the nationwide AMIS Plus registry 2002–2012. Heart 2013;100(4):288–94.

[95] Storey J, Rowland J, Basic D, et al. The Rowland Universal Dementia Assessment Scale (RUDAS): a multicultural cognitive assessment scale. Int Psychogeriatr 2004;16(1):13–31.

[96] Morley JE. Function assessment scales. In: Sinclair AJ, Morley JE, Vellas B, editors. Pathy's principles and practice of geriatric medicine. 5th ed. Oxford: Wiley-Blackwell; 2012. p. i–x.

[97] Grosmaitre P, Le Vavasseur O, Yachouh E, et al. Significance of atypical symptoms for the diagnosis and management of myocardial infarction in elderly patients admitted to emergency departments. Arch Cardiovasc Dis 2013;106:586–92.

[98] SouthernCare University. Atypical presentation of disease in the elderly; 2015. Available from: https://drohanlon.wordpress.com/2014/02/24/atypical-presentation-of-disease-in-older-people/.

[99] Garcia MB, Rosen S, Koretz B, et al. Presentation of disease in old age. In: Fillit HM, Rockwood K, Young J, editors. Brocklehurst's textbook of geriatric medicine and gerontology. 8th ed. Philadelphia: Elsevier; 2017.

[100] Limpawattana P, Phungoen P, Mitsungnern T, et al. Atypical presentations of older adults at the emergency department and associated factors. Arch Gerontol Geriatr 2016;62:97–102.

[101] Reuben DB. Geriatric assessment. In: Goldman L, Schafer AI, editors. Goldman-Cecil medicine. 25th ed. Philadelphia: Elsevier; 2016.

[102] Bernstein M, Munoz N, Academy of Nutrition and Dietetics. Position of the Academy of Nutrition and Dietetics: food and nutrition for older adults — promoting health and wellness. J Acad Nutr Diet 2012;112(8):1255–77.

[103] Johnson LE, Sullivan DH. Malnutrition in older adults. In: Fillit HM, Rockman K, Young J, editors. Brocklehurst's textbook of geriatric medicine and gerontology. 8th ed. Philadelphia: Elsevier; 2017. p. 914–22.

[104] Camina-Martín MA, De Mateo-Silleras B, Malafarina V, et al. Nutritional status assessment in geriatrics: consensus declaration by the Spanish Society of Geriatrics and Gerontology Nutrition Work Group. Maturitas 2015;81:414–19.

[105] Australian Bureau of Statistics. 4364.0.55.001. National health survey: first results, 2014–15; 2015. Available from: www.abs.gov.au/ausstats/abs@.nsf/Lookup/by Subject/4364.0.55.001˜2014-15˜Main Features˜Key findings˜1. [Cited 10 September 2016].

[106] Almeida OP, Khan KM, Hankey GJ, et al. 150 minutes of vigorous physical activity per week predicts survival and successful ageing: a population-based 11-year longitudinal study of 12 201 older Australian men. Br J Sports Med 2014;48(3):220–5.

[107] Hamirudin AH, Charlton K, Walton K. Outcomes related to nutrition screening in community living older adults: a systematic literature review. Arch Gerontol Geriatr 2016.

[108] Malnutrition Advisory Group. Malnutrition Universal Screening Tool. Available from: www.bapen.org.uk/pdfs/must/must_full.pdf. [Cited 10 September 2016].

[109] Nestlé. Mini Nutritional Assessment-Short Form (MNA-SF). Available from: www.mna-elderly.com/forms/mna_guide_english_sf.pdf.

[110] Skipper A, Ferguson M, Thompson K, et al. Nutrition screening tools: an analysis of the evidence. J Parenter Enteral Nutr 2012;36(3):292–8.

[111] Fight Malnutrition. SNAQ 65+. Available from: www.fightmalnutrition.eu/fileadmin/content/malnutrition/Screening_tools/Snaq_65__engels_final.pdf.

[112] Inouye SK, Studenski S, Tinetti ME, et al. Geriatric syndromes: clinical, research, and policy implications of a core geriatric concept. J Am Geriatr Soc 2007;55(5):780–91.

[113] Brown RT, Kiely DK, Bharel M, et al. Factors associated with geriatric syndromes in older homeless adults. J Health Care Poor Underserved 2013;24(3):456–68.

[114] Morley JE, Vellas B, Abellan van Kan G, et al. Frailty consensus: a call to action. J Am Med Dir Assoc 2013;14(6):392–7.

[115] Cesari M, Theou O. Frailty. In: Fillit HM, Rockwood K, Young J, editors. Brocklehurst's textbook of geriatric medicine and gerontology. 8th ed. Philadelphia: Elsevier; 2017.

[116] Rockwood K, Mitnitski A. Aging and deficit accumulation. In: Fillit HM, Rockwood K, Young J, editors. Brocklehurst's textbook of geriatric medicine and gerontology. 8th ed. Philadelphia: Elsevier; 2017.

[117] Smit E, Winters-Stone KM, Loprinzi PD, et al. Lower nutritional status and higher food insufficiency in frail older US adults. Br J Nutr 2013;110(1):172–8.

[118] Valentini L, Volkert D, Schutz T, et al. Suggestions for terminology in clinical nutrition. ESPENJ 2014;9:e97–108.

[119] Muscaritoli M, Anker SD, Argilés J, et al. Consensus definition of sarcopenia, cachexia and pre-cachexia: joint document elaborated by Special Interest Groups (SIG) 'cachexia-anorexia in chronic wasting diseases' and 'nutrition in geriatrics'. Clin Nutr 2010;29(2):154–9.

[120] Roberts SB, Fuss P, Heyman MB, et al. Control of food intake in older men. JAMA 1994;272(20):1601–6.

[121] Soenen S, Chapman IM. Body weight, anorexia, and undernutrition in older people. J Am Med Dir Assoc 2013;14:642–8.

[122] Landi F, Calvani R, Tosato M, et al. Anorexia of aging: risk factors, consequences, and potential treatments. Nutrients 2016;8(2):69.

[123] Walston JD. Sarcopenia in older adults. Curr Opin Rheumatol 2012;24(6):623–7.

[124] Studenski S, Van Swearingen J. Falls. In: Fillit HM, Rockwood K, Young J, editors. Brocklehurst's textbook of geriatric medicine and gerontology. 8th ed. Philadelphia: Elsevier; 2017.

[125] Australian Institute of Health and Welfare. Falls in older people; 2016. Available from: www.aihw.gov.au/injury/falls. [Cited 16 September 2016].

[126] Seyedi HR, Mahdian M, Mohammadzadeh M. Prediction of mortality in hip fracture patients: role of routine blood tests. Arch Bone Jt Surg 2015;3(1):51–5.

[127] Neyens J, Halfens R, Spreeuwenberg M, et al. Malnutrition is associated with an increased risk of falls and impaired activity in elderly patients in Dutch residential long-term care (LTC): a cross-sectional study. Arch Gerontol Geriatr 2013;56(1):265–9.

[128] Flanagan D, Fisher T, Murray M, et al. Managing undernutrition in the elderly. Aust Fam Physician 2012;41(9):695–9.

[129] Haralambous B, Lin X, Dow B, et al. Depression in older age: a scoping study. Melbourne: beyondblue; 2009. Available from: www.beyondblue.org.au/about-us/research-projects/research-projects/depression-in-older-age-a-scoping-study.

[130] Heflin MT, Cohen HJ. The aging patient. In: Benjamin IJ, Griggs RC, Wing EJ, et al, editors. Andreoli and Carpenter's Cecil essentials of medicine. Philadelphia: Elsevier; 2016.

[131] Gana K, Bailly N, Broc G, et al. The Geriatric Depression Scale: does it measure depressive mood, depressive affect, or both? Int J Geriatr Psychiatry 2016.

[132] Comijs HC, Nieuwesteeg J, Kok R, et al. The two-year course of late-life depression; results from the Netherlands study of depression in older persons. BMC Psychiatry 2015;15:20.

[133] Australian Bureau of Statistics. 3303.0. Causes of death, Australia; 2013. Available from: www.abs.gov.au/ausstats/abs@.nsf/Lookup/by Subject/3303.0~2013~Main Features~Suicide by Age~10010. [Cited 16 September 2016].

[134] Beyondblue. Signs and symptoms of anxiety and depression in older people. Beyondblue. Available from: www.beyondblue.org.au/who-does-it-affect/older-people/signs-and-symptoms-of-depression-in-older-people. [Cited 16 September 2016].

[135] Davis DH, Muniz Terrara G, Keage H, et al. Delirium is a strong risk factor for dementia in the oldest-old: a population-based cohort study. Brain 2012;135(Pt 9):2809–16.

[136] World Health Organization. A global response to elder abuse and neglect. Geneva: WHO; 2008. Available from: http://apps.who.int/iris/bitstream/10665/43869/1/9789241563581_eng.pdf.

[137] Tinker A, Biggs S, Manthorpe J. The mistreatment and neglect of frail older people. In: Fillit HM, Rockwood K, Young J, editors. Brocklehurst's textbook of geriatric medicine and gerontology. 8th ed. Philadelphia: Elsevier; 2017.

[138] Callaghan H. Australian longitudinal study on women's health: 1921–26 cohort. Summary 1996–2013. Newcastle: University of Newcastle; 2014.

[139] Johannesen M, LoGiudice D. Elder abuse: a systematic review of risk factors in community-dwelling elders. Age Ageing 2013;42:292–8.

[140] Seniors Rights Victoria. Your rights: elder abuse. Available from: https://seniorsrights.org.au. [Cited 20 September 2016].

[141] NPS MedicineWise. Anticipating the risks of polypharmcy; 2013. Available from: www.nps.org.au/topics/ages-life-stages/for-individuals/older-people-and-medicines/for-health-professionals/polypharmacy#references. [Cited 31 August 2016].

[142] Kantor ED, Rehm CD, Haas JS, et al. Trends in prescription drug use among adults in the United States from 1999–2012. JAMA 2015;314(7):1818–31.

[143] Duerden M, Avery T, Payne R. Polypharmacy and medicines optimisation: making it safe and sound. London: The King's Fund; 2013. Available from: www.kingsfund.org.uk.

[144] Guthrie B, Makubate B, Hernandez-Santiago V, et al. The rising tide of polypharmacy and drug–drug interactions:population database analysis 1995–2010. BMC Med 2015;13(74):1–10.

[145] Greene-Naples J, Handler SM, Maher RL, et al. Geriatric pharmacotherapy and polypharmacy. In: Fillit HM, Rockwood K, Young J, editors. Brocklehurst's textbook of geriatric medicine and gerontology. 8th ed. Philadelphia. 2017.

[146] European Medicines Agency. EMA Geriatric Medicines Strategy, 17 February 2011. Available from: https://www.ema.europa.eu/documents/other/geriatric-medicines-strategy_en.pdf.

[147] Hanlon JT, Handler SM, Maher RL, et al. Geriatric pharmacotherapy and polypharmacy. In: Fillit HM, Rockwood K, Woodhouse K, editors. Brocklehurst's textbook of geriatric medicine and gerontology. 7th ed. Philadelphia: Elsevier; 2010. p. 880–5.

[148] Beckett NS, Peters R, Fletcher AE, et al. Treatment of hypertension in patients 80 years of age or older. N Engl J Med 2008;358:1887–98.

[149] Beckett N, Peters R, Tuomilehot J, et al. Immediate and late benefits of treating very elderly people with hypertension: results from active treatment extension to hypertension in the very elderly randomised controlled trial. BMJ 2012;344(d7541):1–10.

[150] Musini VM, Tejani AM, Bassett K, et al. Pharmacotherapy for hypertension in the elderly. Cochrane Database Syst Rev 2009;(4):CD000028.

[151] Cepeda OA, Morley JE. Polypharmacy. In: Sinclair AJ, Morley JE, Vellas B, editors. Principles and practice of geriatric medicine. 5th ed. Chichester: John Wiley; 2012. p. 145–51.

[152] Huang Z, Ung T. Effect of alpha-1-acid glycoprotein binding on pharmacokinetics and pharmacodynamics. Curr Drug Metab 2013;14(2):226–38.

[153] Australian Institute of Health and Welfare. Chronic kidney disease; 2016. Available from: www.aihw.gov.au/chronic-kidney-disease. [Cited 16 September 2016].

[154] Chang Y-P, Huang S-K, Tao P, et al. A population-based study on the association between acute renal failure (ARF) and the duration of polypharmacy. BMC Nephrol 2012;13(96).

[155] Braun L, Cohen M. Herbs and natural supplements: an evidence-based guide. 4th ed. Sydney: Elsevier; 2015.

[156] Seripa D, Pilloto A, Panza F, et al. Pharmacogenetics of cytochrome P450 (CYP) in the elderly. Ageing Res Rev 2010;9(4):457–74.

[157] Amin ML. P-glycoprotein inhibition for optimal drug delivery. Drug Target Insights 2013;27–34.

[158] Van Assema D, Lubberink M, Boellaard R, et al. P-glycoprotein function at the blood–brain barrier: effects of age and gender. Mol Imaging Biol 2012;14:771–6.

[159] Welker KL, Mycyk MB. Pharmacology in the geriatric patient. Emerg Med Clin North Am 2016;34:4469–81.

[160] Jansen PAF, Brouwers JRBJ. Clinical pharmacology in old persons. Scientifica (Cairo) 2012;1–32.

[161] Gallagher P, Ryan C, Byrne S, et al. STOPP (Screening Tool of Older Person's Prescriptions) and START (Screening Tool to Alert Doctors to Right Treatment). Consensus validation. Int J Clin Pharmacol Ther 2008;46(2):72–83.

[162] Chang KL, Weitzel K, Schmidt S. Pharmacogenetics: using genetic information to guide drug therapy. Am Fam Physician 2015;92(7):588–94.

[163] US Food and Drug Administration. Table of pharmacogenomic biomarkers in drug labeling. US Food and Drug Administration; 2016. Available from: www.fda.gov/drugs/scienceresearch/researchareas/pharmacogenetics/ucm083378.htm. [Cited 15 September 2016].

[164] Stefanska B, Macewan DJ. Epigenetics and pharmacology. Br J Pharmacol 2015.

[165] Moore DS. The developing genome. Oxford: Oxford University Press; 2015.

[166] Seripa D, Paroni G, Lauriola M, et al. To translate pharmacogenenics in geriatrics: towards a personalized medicine. Geriatr Care 2015;1(5461):30–3.

[167] Compton RD. Polypharmacy concerns in the geriatric population. Osteopath Fam Physician 2013;5:147–52.

[168] Gnjidic D, Hilmer SN, Blyth FM, et al. Polypharmacy cutoff and outcomes: five or more medicines were used to identify community-dwelling older men at risk of different adverse outcomes. J Clin Epidemiol 2012;65:989–95.

[169] Smith CA, Chang E, Brownhill S, et al. Complementary medicine health literacy among a population of older Australians living in retirement villages: a mixed methods study. Evid Based Complement Alternat Med 2016;5672050:http://doi.org/10.1155/2016/5672050.

[170] Jamshed Siddiqui M, Sze Min C, Kumar Verma R, et al. Role of complementary and alternative medicine in geriatric care: a mini review. Pharmacogn Rev 2014;8(16):81–7.

[171] Sackett K, Carter M, Stanton M. Elders' use of folk medicine and complementary and alternative therapies: an integrative review with implications for case managers. Prof Case Manag 2014;3:113–23.

[172] Naja F, Alameddine M, Itani L, et al. The use of complementary and alternative medicine among Lebanese adults: results from a national survery. Evid Based Complement Alternat Med 2015;682397.

[173] Schnabel K, Binting S, Witt CM, et al. Use of complementary and alternative medicine by older adults: a cross-sectional survey. BMC Geriatr 2014;14:38. http://doi.org/10.1186/1471-2318-14-38.

[174] Ho T, Rowland-Seymour A, Frankel ES, et al. Generational differences in complementary and alternative medicine (CAM) use in the context of chronic diseases and pain: baby boomers versus the silent generation. J Am Board Fam Med 2014;27(4):465–73.

[175] Horowitz S. CAM and the aging population: trends and clinical implications. Altern Complement Ther 2012;18(6):314–18.

[176] Goh LY, Vitry AI, Semple SJ, et al. Self-medication with over-the-counter drugs and complementary medications in South Australia's elderly population. BMC Complement Altern Med 2009;9:42. http://doi.org/10.1186/1472-6882-9-42.

[177] Yen L, Jowsey T, McRae IS. Consultations with complementary and alternative medicine practitioners by older Australians: results from a national survey. BMC Complement Altern Med 2013;13:73. http://doi.org/10.1186/1472-6882-13-73.

[178] Gallagher P, Lang PO, Cherubini A, et al. Prevalence of potentially inappropriate prescribing in an acutely ill population of older patients admitted to six European hospitals. Eur J Clin Pharmacol 2011;67(11):1175–88.

[179] Zadak Z, Hyspler R, Ticha A, et al. Polypharmacy and malnutrition. Curr Opin Clin Nutr Metab Care 2013;16(1):50–5.

[180] Doan J, Zakrzewski-Jakubiak H, Roy J, et al. Prevalence and risk of potential cytochrome P450-mediated drug-drug interactions in older hospitalized patients with polypharmacy. Ann Pharmacother 2013;47(3):324–32.

[181] Catic AG. Identification and management of in-hospital drug-induced delirium in older patients. Drugs Aging 2011;28(9):737–48.

[182] The Australian Kidney Foundation. Chronic kidney disease (CDK) management in general practice. 3rd edn; 2015. Available from: http://kidney.org.au/health-professionals/prevent/chronic-kidney-disease-management-handbook.

[183] Richardson K, Bennett K, Kenny RA. Polypharmacy including falls risk-increasing medications and subsequent falls in community-dwelling middle-aged and older adults. Age Ageing 2015;44(1):90–6.

[184] Wong H, Heuberger R, Logomarsino J, et al. Associations between alcohol use, polypharmacy and falls in older adults. Nurs Older People 2016;28(1):30–6.

[185] Pan HH, Li CY, Chen TJ, et al. Association of polypharmacy with fall-related fractures in older Taiwanese people: age- and gender-specific analyses. BMJ Open 2014;4:e004428.

[186] Iihara N, Bando Y, Ohara M, et al. Polypharmacy of medications and fall-related fractures in older people in Japan: a comparison between driving-prohibited and driving-cautioned medications. J Clin Pharm Ther 2016;41(3):273–8.

[187] Meid AD, Quinzler R, Freigofas J, et al. Medication underuse in aging outpatients with cardiovascular disease: prevalence, determinants, and outcomes in a prospective cohort study. PLoS ONE 2015;10(8):e0136339.

[188] National Coordinating Council for Medication Error Reporting and Prevention. About medication errors; 2016. Available from: www.nccmerp.org/about-medication-errors. [Cited 28 August 2016].

[189] Al Hamid A, Ghaleb M, Aljadhey H, et al. A systematic review of hospitalization resulting from medicine-related problems in adult patients. Br J Clin Pharmacol 2014;78(2):202–17.

[190] Parameswaran NN, Chalmers L, Peterson GM, et al. Hospitalization in older patients due to adverse drug reactions: the need for a prediction tool. Clin Interv Aging 2016;11:497–505.

[191] Gurwitz JH, Field TS, Avorn J, et al. Incidence and preventability of adverse drug events in nursing homes. Am J Med 2000;109(2):87–94.

[192] Gurwitz JH, Field TS, Judge J, et al. The incidence of adverse drug events in two large academic long-term care facilities. Am J Med 2005;118(3):251–8.

[193] Kaufmann CP, Tremp R, Hersberger KE, et al. Inappropriate prescribing: a systematic overview of published assessment tools. Eur J Clin Pharmacol 2014;70(1):1–11.

[194] American Geriatrics Society 2015 Beers Criteria Update Expert Panel. American Geriatrics Society 2015 updated Beers criteria for potentially inappropriate medication use in older adults. J Am Geriatr Soc 2015;63(11):2227–46.

[195] O'Mahony D, O'Sullivan D, Byrne S, et al. STOPP/START criteria for potentially inappropriate prescribing in older people: version 2. Age Ageing 2015;44:213–18.

[196] Kara O, Arik G, Kızılarslanoglu MC, et al. Potentially inappropriate prescribing according to the STOPP/START criteria for older adults. Aging Clin Exp Res 2016;28:761–8.

[197] Price S, Holman CD, Emery JD. Are older Western Australians exposed to potentially inappropriate medications according to the Beers criteria? A 13-year prevalence study. Australas J Ageing 2014;33(3):E39–48.

[198] Curtain CM, Bindoff IK, Westbury JL, et al. A comparison of prescribing criteria when applied to older community-based patients. Drugs Aging 2013;30(11):935–43.

[199] Bone K, Mills S. Principles and practice of phytotherapy: modern herbal medicine. 2nd ed. Philadelphia: Churchill Livingstone; 2013.

[200] Patterson SM, Cadogan CA, Kerse N, et al. Interventions to improve the appropriate use of polypharmacy for older people. Cochrane Database Syst Rev 2014;(10):CD008165.

[201] Pretorius RW, Gataric G, Swedlund SK, et al. Reducing the risk of adverse drug events in older adults. Am Fam Physician 2013;87(5):331–6.

[202] Yu YM, Shin WG, Lee J-Y, et al. Patterns of adverse drug reactions in different age groups: analysis of spontaneous reports by community pharmacists. PLoS ONE 2015;10(7):e0132916. http://doi.org/10.1371/journal.pone.0132916.

[203] McLachlan AJ, Pont LG. Drug metabolism in older people: a key consideration in achieving optimal outcomes with medicines. J Gerontol A Biol Sci Med Sci 2012;67(2):175–80.

[204] Hubbard RE, O'Mahony MS, Calver BL, et al. Plasma esterases and inflammation in ageing and frailty. Eur J Clin Pharmacol 2008;64(9):895–900.

[205] Singh S, Bajorek B. Pharmacotherapy in the ageing patient: the impact of age per se (a review). Ageing Res Rev 2015;24:99–110.

[206] Therapeutic Goods Adminsitration. Medicines safety update. Aust Prescr 2012;35(3):168–711.

[207] Therapeutic Goods Adminsitration. Renal function assessment in prescribing. Aust Prescr 2012;35(3):100.

[208] Ungar A, Iacomelli I, Giordano A, et al. Evaluation of renal function in the elderly, not as easy as it seems: a review. Aging Clin Exp Res 2015;27(4):397–401.

[209] Karsch-Völk M, Schmid E, Wagenpfeil S, et al. Kidney function and clinical recommendations of drug dose adjustment in geriatric patients. BMC Geriatr 2013;13(92).

[210] Modig S, Lannering C, Ostgren CJ, et al. The assessment of renal function in relation to the use of drugs in elderly in nursing homes: a cohort study. BMC Geriatr 2011;11(1):1–19.

[211] Schaeffner ES, Ebert N, Delanaye P, et al. Two novel equations to estimate kidney function in persons aged 70 years or older. Ann Intern Med 2012;157(7):471–81.

[212] The Royal College of Pathologists of Australia. eGFR. In: RCPA manual; 2015. Available from: www.rcpa.edu.au/Library/Practising-Pathology/RCPA-Manual/Items/Pathology-Tests/E/eGFR. [Cited 18 August 2016].

[213] Best Practice Advocacy Centre New Zealand. Guide to drug dose adjustment in renal impairment. Dunedin: BPACNZ. Available from: www.bpac.org.nz/resources/other/guides/bpac_renal.pdf.

[214] Hudson JQ, Bean JR, Burger CF, et al. Estimated glomerular filtration rate leads to higher drug dose recommendations in the elderly compared with creatinine clearance. Int J Clin Pract 2015;69(3):313–20.

[215] NPS MedicineWise. Measuring and estimating GFR; 2016. Available from: www.nps.org.au/publications/health-professional/nps-radar/2012/december-2012/?a=59879. [Cited 10 September 2016].

[216] NPS MedicineWise. Ten principles for medicines use in older people; 2016. Available from: www.nps.org.au/topics/

ages-life-stages/for-individuals/older-people-and-medicines/
for-health-professionals/medicines-management/
prescribing-principles. [Cited 10 September 2016].

[217] NSW Government. Code of conduct for unregistered health professionals; 2012. Available from: www.austlii.edu.au/au/legis/nsw/consol_reg/phr2012217/sch3.html.

[218] NHMRC. Dietary energy: nutrient reference values; 2014. Available from: www.nrv.gov.au/dietary-energy. [Cited 10 September 2016].

[219] Illario M, Maione AS, Rusciano MR, et al. NutriLive: an integrated nutritional approach as a sustainable tool to prevent malnutrition in older people and promote active and healthy ageing — the EIP-AHA Nutrition Action Group. Adv Public Heal 2016;1–9.

[220] Australian Institute of Health and Welfare. Aged care; 2016. Available from: www.aihw.gov.au/aged-care. [Cited 10 September 2016].

[221] O'Keefe JH, Bhatti SK, Bajwa A, et al. Alcohol and cardiovascular health: the dose makes the poison or the remedy. Mayo Clin Proc 2014;89(3):382–93.

[222] Chiva-Blanch G, Arranz S, Lamuela-Raventos RM, et al. Effects of wine, alcohol and polyphenols on cardiovascular disease risk factors: evidence from human studies. Alcohol Alcohol 2013;48(3):270–7.

[223] Midlöv P, Calling S, Memon AA, et al. Women's health in the Lund area (WHILA): alcohol consumption and all-cause mortality among women — a 17-year-follow-up study. BMC Public Health 2016;16(22).

[224] Pérez LM, Pareja-Galeano H, Sanchis-Gomar F, et al. 'Adipaging': ageing and obesity share biological hallmarks related to a dysfunctional adipose tissue. J Physiol 2016;594(12):3187–207.

[225] Nepal B, Brown L. Projection of older Australians with a history of midlife obesity and overweight 2010–2050. Obesity (Silver Spring) 2013;21(12):2579–81.

[226] World Health Organization. Body mass index. Available from: www.euro.who.int/en/health-topics/disease-prevention/nutrition/a-healthy-lifestyle/body-mass-index-bmi. [Cited 10 September 2016].

[227] Zapatero A, Barba R, Ruiz J, et al. Malnutrition and obesity: influence in mortality and readmissions in chronic obstructive pulmonary disease patients. J Hum Nutr Diet 2013;26(Suppl. 1):16–22.

[228] Zunzunegui MV, Sanchez MT, Garcia A, et al. Body mass index and long-term mortality in an elderly Mediterranean population. J Aging Health 2012;24(1):29–47.

[229] Dahl AK, Fauth EB, Ernsth-Bravell M, et al. Body mass index, change in body mass index, and survival in old and very old persons. J Am Geriatr Soc 2013;61(4):512–18.

[230] Winter JE, Macinnis RJ, Wattanapenpaiboon N, et al. BMI and all-cause mortality in older adults: a meta-analysis 1–3. Am J Clin Nutr 2014;99:875–90.

[231] Cederholm T, Bosaeus I, Barazzoni R, et al. Diagnostic criteria for malnutrition: an ESPEN consensus statement. Clin Nutr 2015;34:335–40.

[232] Lee JS, Visser M, Tylavsky FA, et al. Weight loss and regain and effects on body composition: the Health, Aging, and Body Composition Study. J Gerontol A Biol Sci Med Sci 2010;65(1):78–83.

[233] Chmelo EA, Beavers DP, Lyles MF, et al. Legacy effects of short-term intentional weight loss on total body and thigh composition in overweight and obese older adults. Nutr Diabetes 2016;6(4):e206.

[234] Beavers KM, Lyles MF, Davis CC, et al. Is lost lean mass from intentional weight loss recovered during weight regain in postmenopausal women? Am J Clin Nutr 2011;94(3):767–74.

[235] Somes GW, Kritchevsky SB, Shorr RI, et al. Body mass index, weight change, and death in older adults: the systolic hypertension in the elderly program. Am J Epidemiol 2002;156(2):132–8.

[236] Newman A, Yanez D, Harris T, et al. Weight change in old age and its association with mortality. J Am Geriatr Soc 2001;49(10):1309–18.

[237] Karahalios A, Simpson JA, Baglietto L, et al. Change in body size and mortality: results from the Melbourne collaborative cohort study. PLoS ONE 2014;9(7):e99672.

[238] Pownall HJ, Bray GA, Wagenknecht LE, et al. Changes in body composition over eight years in a randomized trial of a lifestyle intervention: the Look AHEAD Study HHS Public Access. Obesity (Silver Spring) 2015;23(3):565–72.

[239] Santanasto AJ, Goodpaster BH, Kritchevsky SB, et al. Body composition remodeling and mortality: the Healthy Aging and Body Composition Study. J Gerontol A Biol Sci Med Sci 2017;72(4):513–19.

[240] Bailly N, Maitre I, Wymelbeke V. Relationships between nutritional status, depression and pleasure of eating in aging men and women. Arch Gerontol Geriat 2015;61(3):330–6.

[241] Konturek PC, Herrmann HJ, Schink K, et al. Malnutrition in hospitals: it was, is now, and must not remain a problem! Med Sci Monit 2015;21:2969–75.

[242] Meijers JM, van Bokhorst-de van der Schueren M, Schols J, et al. Defining malnutrition: mission or mission impossible? Nutrition 2010;6:432–40.

[243] van Asselt D, van Bokhorst DE, van der Schueren M, et al. Assessment and treatment of malnutrition in Dutch geriatric practice: consensus through a modified Delphi study. Age Ageing 2012;41:399–404.

[244] Sobokta L, Allison SP, Forbes A, et al, editors. Basics in clinical nutrition. 4th ed. Prague: Galen; 2011.

[245] Rojer AGM, Kruizenga HM, Trappenburg MC, et al. The prevalence of malnutrition according to the new ESPEN definition in four diverse populations. Clin Nutr 2016;35(3):758–62.

[246] Wysokinski A, Sobów T, Kloszewska I, et al. Mechanisms of the anorexia of aging: a review. Age (Dordr) 2015;37(4):81.

[247] Morley JE. Pathophysiology of the anorexia of aging. Curr Opin Clin Nutr Metab Care 2013;16(1):27–32.

[248] Martone AM, Onder G, Vetrano DL, et al. Anorexia of aging: a modifiable risk factor for frailty. Nutrients 2013;5(10):4126–33.

[249] Jensen GL. Malnutrition and inflammation 'Burning down the house': inflammation as an adaptive physiologic response versus self-destruction. J Parenter Enteral Nutr 2015;39(1):56–62.

[250] American College of Rheumatology. ACR-endorsed criteria for rheumatic diseases; 2010. Available from: www.rheumatology.org/Practice-Quality/Clinical-Support/Criteria/ACR-Endorsed-Criteria. [Cited 10 September 2016].

[251] Landi F, Calvani R, Tosato M, et al. Anorexia of aging: risk factors, consequences, and potential treatments. Nutrients 2016;8(2):69.

[252] Giezenaar C, Chapman I, Luscombe-Marsh N, et al. Ageing is associated with decreases in appetitie and energy intake: a meta-analysis in healthy adults. Nutrients 2016;7(8):28.

[253] Jones C, Badger SA, Hannon R. The role of carbohydrate drinks in pre-operative nutrition for elective colorectal surgery. Ann R Coll Surg Engl 2011;93(7):504–7.

[254] Galic S, Oakhill JS, Steinberg GR. Adipose tissue as an endocrine organ. Mol Cell Endocrinol 2010;316(2):129–39.

[255] Malafarina V, Uriz-Otano F, Gil-Guerrero L, et al. The anorexia of ageing: physiopathology, prevalence, associated comorbidity and mortality. A systematic review. Maturitas 2013;74(4):293–302.

[256] Kwon H, Pessin JE. Adipokines mediate inflammation and insulin resistance. Front Endocrinol (Lausanne) 2013;4(71).

[257] Boccardi V, Paolisso G, Mecocci P. Nutrition and lifestyle in healthy aging: the telomerase challenge. Aging 2016;8(1):12–15.

[258] Van Bokhorst DE, van der Schueren MA, Lonterman-Monasch S, et al. Prevalence and determinants for malnutrition in geriatric outpatients. Clin Nutr 2013;32:1007–11.

[259] Bauer J, Biolo G, Cederholm T, et al. Evidence-based recommendations for optimal dietary protein intake in older people: a position paper from the prot-age study group. J Am Med Dir Assoc 2013;14:542–59.

[260] Milne AC, Avenell A. Protein and energy supplementation in elderly people at risk from malnutrition. Cochrane Database Syst Rev 2009;(2):CD003288.

[261] Cawood AL, Elia M, Stratton RJ. Systematic review and meta-analysis of the effects of high protein nutrition supplements. Ageing Res Rev 2012;11(2):279–96.

[262] NHMRC. Nutrients 2014;Available from: www.nrv.gov.au/dietary-energy. [Cited 10 November 2016]. In: Nutrient reference values.

[263] British Nutrition Foundation. Nutrient requirements; 2016. Available from: www.nutrition.org.uk/healthyliving/resources/nutritionrequirements.html. [Cited 10 September 2016].

[264] Nowson C, O'Connell S. Protein requirements and recommendations for older people: a review. Nutrients 2015;7:6874–99.

[265] Giezenaar C, Trahair LG, Rigda R, et al. Lesser suppression of energy intake by orally ingested whey protein in healthy older men compared with young controls. Am J Physiol Regul Integr Comp Physiol 2015;309(8):R845–54.

[266] Pennings B, Groen B, de Lange A, et al. Amino acid absorption and subsequent muscle protein accretion following graded intake of whey protein in elderly men. Am J Physiol Endocrinol Metab 2012;302(8):E992–9.

[267] Pennings B, Boirie Y, Senden JM, et al. Whey protein stimulates postprandial muscle protein accretion more effectively than do casein and casein hydrolysate in older men. Am J Clin Nutr 2011;93(5):997–1005.

[268] Gupta C, Prakash D. Nutraceuticals for geriatrics. J Tradit Complement Med 2014;5(1):5–14.

[269] Malafarina V, Uriz-Otano F, Iniesta R, et al. Effectiveness of nutritional supplementation on muscle mass in treatment of sarcopenia in old age: a systematic review. J Am Med Dir Assoc 2013;14(1):10–17.

[270] Kesse-Guyot E, Péneau S, Ferry M, et al. Thirteen-year prospective study between fish consumption, long-chain n-3 fatty acid intake and cognitive function. J Nutr Health Aging 2011;15(2):115–20.

[271] Baierle M, Vencato P, Oldenburg L, et al. Fatty acid status and its relationship to cognitive decline and homocysteine levels in the elderly. Nutrients 2014;6(9):3624–40.

[272] Chrysohoou C, Pitsavos C, Panagiotakos D, et al. Long-term fish intake preserves kidney function in elderly individuals: the Ikaria study. J Ren Nutr 2013;23(4):e75–82.

[273] Pusceddu MM, Kelly P, Stanton C, et al. N-3 polyunsaturated fatty acids through the lifespan: implication for psychopathology. Int J Neuropsychopharmacol 2016;19(12):pyw078.

[274] Horikawa C, Otsuka R, Kato Y, et al. Cross-sectional association between serum concentrations of n-3 long-chain PUFA and depressive symptoms: results in Japanese community dwellers. Br J Nutr 2016;115(4):672–80.

[275] Mustafa R, Ahmed S, Gupta A, et al. A comprehensive review of hypertension in pregnancy. J Pregnancy 2012;105918.

[276] Molfino A, Gioia G, Fanelli FR, et al. The role for dietary omega-3 fatty acids supplementation in older adults. Nutrients 2014;6(10):4058–73.

[277] Panagiotakos DB, Zeimbekis A, Boutziouka V, et al. Long-term fish intake is associated with better lipid profile, arterial blood pressure, and blood glucose levels in elderly people from Mediterranean islands (MEDIS epidemiological study). Med Sci Monit 2007;13(7).

[278] Todoroki K, Ikeya Y, Fukui S, et al. Nutrition-dependent eicosapentaenoic acid deficiency in care house residents. Nutrition 2016;32(7–8):806–10.

[279] Fan F, Xue W-Q, Wu B-H, et al. Higher fish intake is associated with a lower risk of hip fractures in Chinese men and women: a matched case-control study. PLoS ONE 2013;8(2):e56849.

[280] García-Esquinas E, Rahi B, Peres K, et al. Consumption of fruit and vegetables and risk of frailty: a dose-response analysis of 3 prospective cohorts of community-dwelling older adults. Am J Clin Nutr 2016;104(1):132–42.

[281] Urpi-Sarda M, Andres-Lacueva C, Rabassa M, et al. The relationship between urinary total polyphenols and the frailty phenotype in a community-dwelling older population: the InCHIANTI Study. J Gerontol A Biol Sci Med Sci 2015;70(9):1141–7.

[282] França VF, Barbosa AR, D'Orsi E. Cognition and indicators of dietary habits in older adults from Southern Brazil. PLoS ONE 2016;11(2):e0147820.

[283] Salminen A, Kauppinen A, Kaarniranta K. Phytochemicals suppress nuclear factor-κB signaling: impact on health span and the aging process. Curr Opin Clin Nutr Metab Care 2012;15(1):23–8.

[284] González S, Cuervo A, Lasheras C. Polyphenol intake in elderly people is associated with lipid oxidative damage. J Am Coll Nutr 2013;32(6):384–90.

[285] Kim H, Suzuki T, Saito K, et al. Effects of exercise and tea catechins on muscle mass, strength and walking ability in community-dwelling elderly Japanese sarcopenic women: a randomized controlled trial. Geriatr Gerontol Int 2013;13(2):458–65.

[286] Ma L, Dou HL, Huang YM, et al. Improvement of retinal function in early age-related macular degeneration after lutein and zeaxanthin supplementation: a randomized, double-masked, placebo-controlled trial. Am J Ophthalmol 2012;154(4):625–34.

[287] Ma L, Dou H-L, Wu Y-Q, et al. Systematic review and meta-analysis of lutein and zeaxanthin intake and the risk of age-related macular degeneration: a systematic review and meta-analysis. Br J Nutr 2016;107:350–9.

[288] Chen P, Zhang W, Wang X, et al. Lycopene and risk of prostate cancer a systematic review and meta-analysis. Medicine (Baltimore) 2015;94(33):e1260.

[289] Thies F, Mills LM, Moir S, et al. Cardiovascular benefits of lycopene: fantasy or reality? Proc Nutr Soc 2016;1–8.

[290] Knight A, Bryan J, Murphy K. Is the Mediterranean diet a feasible approach to preserving cognitive function and reducing risk of dementia for older adults in Western countries? New insights and future directions. Ageing Res Rev 2016;25:85–101.

[291] Martínez I, Lattimer JM, Hubach KL, et al. Gut microbiome composition is linked to whole grain-induced immunological improvements. ISME J 2012;7(10):269–80.

[292] Fujita R, Iimuro S, Shinozaki T, et al. Decreased duration of acute upper respiratory tract infections with daily intake of fermented milk: a multicenter, double-blinded, randomized comparative study in users of day care facilities for the elderly population. Am J Infect Control 2013;41(12):1231–5.

[293] Lahtinen SJ, Forssten S, Aakko J, et al. Probiotic cheese containing *Lactobacillus rhamnosus* HN001 and *Lactobacillus acidophilus* NCFM modifies subpopulations of fecal lactobacilli and *Clostridium difficile* in the elderly. Age (Dordr) 2012;34:133–43.

[294] Moshtaghian H, Louie J, Charlton KE, et al. Added sugar intake that exceeds current recommendations is associated with nutrient dilution in older Australians. Nutrition 2016;32:937–42.

[295] García-Calzón S, Zalba G, Ruiz-Canela M, et al. Dietary inflammatory index and telomere length in subjects with a high cardiovascular disease risk from the PREDIMED-NAVARRA study: cross-sectional and longitudinal analyses over 5 y. Am J Clin Nutr 2015;102(4):897–904.

[296] Ruiz-Canela M, Bes-Rastrollo M, Martínez-González MA. The role of dietary inflammatory index in cardiovascular disease, metabolic syndrome and mortality. Int J Mol Sci 2016;17(8):e1265.

[297] Trichopoulou A, Martínez-González MA, Tong TY, et al. Definitions and potential health benefits of the Mediterranean diet: views from experts around the world. BMC Med 2014;12:112.

[298] Valls-Pedret C, Sala-Vila A, Serra-Mir M, et al. Mediterranean diet and age-related cognitive decline: a randomized clinical trial. JAMA Intern Med 2015;175(7):1094–103.

[299] UNESCO. Mediterranean diet; 2013. Available from: www.unesco.org/culture/ich/en/RL/mediterranean-diet-00884. [Cited 1 September 2016].

[300] Psaltopoulou T, Sergentanis TN, Panagiotakos DB, et al. Mediterranean diet, stroke, cognitive impairment, and depression: a meta-analysis. Ann Neurol 2013;74(4):580–91.

[301] Mason JB. Vitamins, trace minerals, and other micronutrients. In: Goldman L, Schafer A, editors. Goldman-Cecil medicine. 25th ed. Philadelphia: Elsevier; 2016.

[302] Nowson CA, McGrath JJ, Ebeling PR, et al. Vitamin D and health in adults in Australia and New Zealand. Med J Aust 2012;196(11):686–7.

[303] De Boer IH, Levin G, Robinson-Cohen C, et al. Serum 25-hydroxyvitamin D concentration and risk for major clinical disease events in a community-based population of older adults: a cohort study. Ann Intern Med 2012;156(9):627–34.

[304] Maywald M, Rink L. Zinc homeostasis and immunosenescence. J Trace Elem Med Biol 2015;29:24–30.

[305] Michel J-P, Dreux C, Vacheron A. Healthy ageing: evidence that improvement is possible at every age. Eur Geriatr Med 2016;7:298–305.

[306] Learmonth E, Taket A, Hanna L. Ways in which 'community' benefits frail older women's well-being: 'we are much happier when we feel we belong'. Australas J Ageing 2012;31(1):60–3.

[307] Rapacciuolo A, Perrone Filardi P, Cuomo R, et al. The impact of social and cultural engagement and dieting on well-being and resilience in a group of residents in the metropolitan area of Naples. J Aging Res 2016;4768420.

[308] Wilhelm K, Geerligs L, Peisah C. Successful transition to later life: strategies used by baby boomers. Australas J Ageing 2014;33:81–5.

[309] Dominguez LJ, Barbagallo M. Ageing and sexuality. Eur Geriatr Med 2016;7(6):512–18.

[310] Wright H, Jenks RA. Sex on the brain! Associations between sexual activity and cognitive function in older age. Age Ageing 2016;45:313–17.

[311] Grassi C, Landi F, Delogu G. Lifestyles and ageing: targeting key mechanisms to shift the balance from unhealthy to healthy ageing. Stud Health Technol Inform 2014;203:99–111.

[312] Giles LC, Anstey KJ, Walker RB, et al. Social networks and memory over 15 years of followup in a cohort of older Australians: results from the Australian longitudinal study of ageing. J Aging Res 2012.

[313] Turner JE. Is immunosenescence influenced by our lifetime dose of exercise? Biogerontology 2016;17.

[314] Lancha AH, Zanella R, Tanabe SG, et al. Dietary protein supplementation in the elderly for limiting muscle mass loss. Amino Acids 2016.

[315] Merchant HA, Liu F, Orlu Gul M, et al. Age-mediated changes in the gastrointestinal tract. Int J Pharm 2016;512(2):382–95. doi:10.1016/j.ijpharm.2016.04.024. [Epub 2016 Apr 13].

[316] Sergi G, Bano G, Pizzato S, et al. Taste loss in the elderly: possible implications for dietary habits. Crit Rev Food Sci Nutr 2017;57(17):3684–9.

[317] Imoscopi A, Inelmen EM, Sergi G, et al. Taste loss in the elderly: epidemiology, causes and consequences. Aging Clin Exp Res 2012;24(6):570–9. doi:10.3275/8520.

[318] Witte AV, Kerti L, Hermannstädter HM, et al. Long-chain omega-3 fatty acids improve brain function and structure in older adults. Cereb Cortex 2014;24(11):3059–68. doi:10.1093/cercor/bht163.

[319] Merchant HA, Liu F, Orlu Gul M, et al. Age-mediated changes in the gastrointestinal tract. Int J Pharm 2016;512(2):382–95. doi:10.1016/j.ijpharm.2016.04.024.

[320] Poulose SM, Miller MG, Shukitt-Hale B. Role of walnuts in maintaining brain health with age. J Nutr 2014;144(4 Suppl.): 561S–6S. doi:10.3945/jn.113.184838.

18

Autism spectrum disorder (ASD)

Helen Padarin

EPIDEMIOLOGY

Once classified into separate categories of autism and autism spectrum disorders (including autistic disorders, Asperger's disorder, Rett's syndrome, childhood disintegrative disorder and pervasive developmental disorder not otherwise specified), the 2013 release of the 5th edition of the *Diagnostic and Statistical Manual for Mental Disorders* (DSM-V)[1] now combines all categories under the banner of autism spectrum disorder (ASD). ASD is a pervasive developmental disorder (PDD). In 1980, autism was a rare disorder that few paediatricians saw. The incidence of autism was 2–5 per 10 000 people. Kanner, the psychiatrist who first diagnosed autism, saw an average of only eight patients per year in over 20 years of practice in a clinic dedicated to the specialty, and therefore attracting such patients from around the US. Through the Survey of Disability, Ageing and Carers (SDAC), the Australian Bureau of Statistics (ABS) reported a 79% increase in rates of ASD from 2009 to 2012 (the latest SDAC to date).[2] Thirty-one per cent of participants in the National Disability Insurance Scheme (NDIS) have ASD, according to its June 2015 report.[3] In 2012, Autism Aspergers Advocacy Australia (A4)[231] stated that the rate of ASD in Australian schools is 1 in 63 (children with a registered diagnosis who receive a carer allowance). Numbers are similar in other developed countries. In some areas, including the US, rates are 1 in 68.[4] Boys are more frequently affected than girls by a ratio of 4.5:1 (1 in 42), with several studies showing testosterone plays a role in autism severity.[4] Studies in Asia, Europe and North America have shown the prevalence of ASD to be between 1% and 2% of the population.[4] Between 18% and 29% of children with ASD are also affected by epilepsy.[5]

OVERVIEW

Genetics alone cannot be responsible for such a rapid rise in prevalence of autism. Better diagnosis also cannot account for the rapid rise.[6] DSM-V has more stringent diagnostic criteria, with individuals needing to meet more criteria than in DSM-IV. There is concern that as a result of this change in criteria, financial support for services for some individuals previously diagnosed under DSM-IV may be withdrawn if they no longer fit the new criteria. While

the cause of autism is not clear, an understanding of numerous contributing factors is growing. Growing evidence is showing that autism is not a psychological disorder; rather, it is a whole-body disorder with severe impact on neurological function. Numerous environmental, metabolic, immunological and digestive disorders have been found to be underlying contributory factors to the neurological symptoms of autism. These contributory factors go a long way to explaining the epidemic of ASD. See Table 18.1 in the article by Stigler et al. 2009[7] for studies on the immune factors involved with ASD.

CLASSIFICATION

Types of autism/ASD

As practitioners may be seeing patients diagnosed prior to the release of the DSM-V, it is worthwhile to be familiar with types of autism previously identified in DSM-IV. In infantile autism, typical neurological development never occurs. Some autistic symptoms are evident from birth, while others will become obvious as developmental milestones are not reached, particularly with speech. Regressive autism occurs when initial development is normal and healthy, and then at a point, often around 18 months of age, development starts to regress. First signs may be a loss of language skills and/or eye contact. High-functioning autism (HFA) is a condition where individuals display autistic characteristics, particularly with social impairment, but they are able to function close to a normal level in society. They are often very intelligent and sometimes gifted, with their symptoms only becoming obvious in social situations where they may be unable to predict or read other people's emotional responses to events, such as something that has been said. They may also appear somewhat disconnected or removed, particularly in situations where there is a lot of sensory stimulation. Asperger's syndrome (AS) is a PDD often referred to as a form of HFA. AS is often characterised by normal or above average intelligence, with poorly developed social skills and emotional and social development occurring later than normal. Some children previously diagnosed with autism may be re-diagnosed with AS if they show improvement. Children who do not clearly fit into any set diagnostic criteria are diagnosed

TABLE 18.1 Immune factors involved with ASD[7]		
Category	**Results**	**N**
Infections		
Singh et al. (2002)	Atypical MMR antibody in 60% of autistic sera vs 0% control sera	A = 125, C = 92
Singh and Jensen (2003)	Increased measles virus antibody levels in autistic sera vs sibling and control sera	A = 88, S = 15, C = 32
Vaccines		
Fombonne et al. (2006)	No relationship between PDD rates and trends in MMR vaccination use and two dose MMR vaccine schedule	
Richler et al. (2006)	No association of onset of autistic symptoms or regression to MMR vaccination	P = 351, C = 51
Neuroimmune		
Connolly et al. (1999)	Increased IgG and IgM binding to the temporal lobe in autistic subjects	A = 11, C = 71
Plioplys et al. (1994a)	Increased IgG and IgM antibodies to cerebellum; no reactivity to frontal cortex	A = 17, C (IgG) = 248, C (IgM) = 111
Singer et al. (2006)	Autistic subjects with more autoimmune complexes in basal ganglia and frontal lobe	P = 29, A = 22, S = 9, C = 13
Singh and Rivas (2004)	Autistic subjects with anti-caudate antibodies vs none in control group	A = 68, C = 30
Todd et al. (1988)	No difference in IgG antibody binding to frontal cortex among groups	A = 20, MR = 5, D = 5, C = 15
Immunogenetics		
Daniels et al. (1995)	Gene frequency of B44-SC30-DR-4 (contains null allele at C4B gene) greater in autistic subjects and their mothers vs controls	A = 45, PA = 78, C = 64
Einstrom et al. (2008)	Altered gene expression and function of NK cells in children with autism	A = 52, C = 27
Odell et al. (2005)	42.4% of autistic subjects carried at least one null allele (C4B) vs 14.5% of controls	A = 85, C = 69
Torres et al. (2006)	Autistic probands with increased frequency of HLA-A2 allele vs controls	A = 129, C = 265
Warren et al. (1992)	Gene frequency of B44-SC30-DR4 greater in autistic subjects and their mothers vs controls	A = 21, AP = 42, C = 21
Warren et al. (1996)	54% of autistic subjects with null allele (C4B) vs 20.2% of controls	A = 50, C = 79
Autoimmunity		
Coml et al. (1999)	Mean number of autoimmune diseases. Increased in families with autistic children vs control families.	AF = 61, CF = 46
Croen et al. (2005)	Maternal autoimmune disorders present in women around the time of pregnancy unlikely to contribute to autism risk; 2-fold risk of PDD for maternal asthma and allergy during 2nd trimester	AM = 407, CM = 2095
Micall et al. (2004)	No increase in number of autoimmune diseases in PDD family members vs control families	PF = 79, CF = 61
Sweeten et al. (2003)	Autoimmune disease reported more frequently in PDD family members vs families with autoimmune probands and control families	PF = 101, IF = 101, CF = 101
Immune Cells		
Denney et al. (1996)	Increased % of monocytes and decreased % of lymphocytes expressing bound IL-2 in autistic subjects vs controls	A = 10, C = 10.

with pervasive developmental disorder not otherwise specified (PDD-NOS). There are also subtypes of each category of PDD which depend on factors such as heredity, epigenetics, polymorphisms and immune tendencies.

CONTRIBUTING FACTORS

Environmental factors

As the increased rates of autism cannot be attributed to genetics alone, investigations into environmental impacts on risk of ASD have been undertaken. Environmental exposures can increase risk via a number of mechanisms – epigenetics, neurotoxicity, hormone disruption and immune disruption are some of the studied mechanisms of action. It is a challenging area to study as impacts of most chemicals and toxic compounds are studied in isolation, but real-life experience often means exposure to multiple compounds at once. Much of the time we do not know the effect of combined chemicals on health outcomes; however, studies on some toxins, such as heavy metals, show a synergistic effect of toxicity. This is worth bearing in mind when assessing environmental exposures in the person presenting to you in clinic.

Organophosphate pesticides affect gene expression and decrease expression of brain-derived neurotrophic factor (BDNF).

Pharmaceutical risk factors

Maternal use of valproic acid, a drug prescribed for epilepsy and some neuropsychological disorders, increases the risk of ASD in children.[8] Maternal use of selective serotonin reuptake inhibitors (SSRIs) also appears to increase risk of ASD; however, further research is required to clarify the effect of the medication versus the effect of the mother's condition, as well as effects of gestational window, specific medication and dosages.[9]

Both maternal use during the gestation period and early life use of paracetamol is associated with increased risk of ASD. Children with ASD may have a decreased sulfation activity. Sulfation is the primary route of paracetamol metabolism for children. When paracetamol requires metabolism through alternative routes, oxidative stress and immune dysregulation result, even at low doses.[10]

DIAGNOSIS

Diagnosis is now based on the 2013 DSM-V (see Box 18.1), and as such takes into account only psychiatric signs and symptoms, not physical signs or symptoms. For families to be able to receive financial support for autism services and treatments, a diagnosis must be made by a specialist paediatrician.

THE BIOMEDICAL APPROACH TO AUTISM AND ASD

The biomedical approach aims to address the underlying metabolic, digestive and immunological factors that contribute to the neurological symptoms of autism in order to reduce severity of symptoms as well as the impact on the lives of the individual, their family and carers. Complete recovery, rather than cure, is the goal, and success of this is becoming well documented. Doctors involved in the Autism Research Institute (ARI), The Walsh Research Institute, The Medical Academy of Paediatric Special Needs (MAPS), The Mindd Foundation (MINDD), the Pfeiffer Institute and the team of Dr Martha Herbert at Harvard Medical School are at the forefront of advances in biomedical autism research and treatment. Owing to the vast individuality and subtypes present in the ASD epidemic, prognosis varies greatly from child to child, but is clearly more positive the younger the child is when biomedical intervention begins and the greater the combination of interventions used.

There are several key principles to the biomedical approach to autism, ASD and attention deficit (hyperactivity) disorder (AD(H)D) including:

1. Dietary intervention
2. Digestive tract healing
3. Resolution of gut dysbiosis and parasitic infections
4. Nutritional medicine to balance biochemistry imbalances and deficiencies and to target oxidative stress and inflammation
5. Immune regulation – to address cytokine activity, inflammatory responses, autoimmunity, allergies, persistent viral infections (e.g. measles in gut pathologies)
6. Detoxification – promotion of methylation and sulfation as well as gentle chelation of heavy metals
7. Neurodevelopmental and behavioural therapies such as applied behavioural analysis (ABA), speech therapy, occupational therapy (OT), cognitive behavioural therapy (CBT) etc.
8. Reduction of oxidative stress
9. Mitochondrial support
10. Support for gene single nucleotide polymorphisms Medications may also be necessary for some children. See Fig. 18.1.

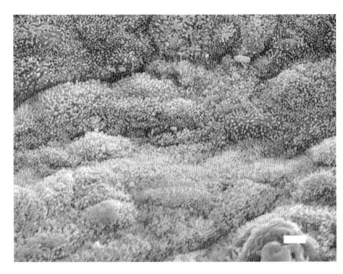

FIGURE 18.1 The gut microbiome–brain axis

http://link.springer.com/article/10.1007/s40474-016-0077-7

BOX 18.1 Autism spectrum disorder diagnostic criteria

Diagnostic criteria

A. Persistent deficits in social communication and social interaction across multiple contexts, as manifested by the following, currently or by history (examples are illustrative, not exhaustive):

1. Deficits in social–emotional reciprocity, ranging, for example, from abnormal social approach and failure of normal back-and-forth conversation; to reduced sharing of interests, emotions, or affect; to failure to initiate or respond to social interactions.

2. Deficits in nonverbal communicative behaviors used for social interaction, ranging, for example, from poorly integrated verbal and nonverbal communication; to abnormalities in eye contact and body language or deficits in understanding and use of gestures; to a total lack of facial expressions and nonverbal communication.

3. Deficits in developing, maintaining, and understanding relationships, ranging, for example, from difficulties adjusting behavior to suit various social contexts; to difficulties in sharing imaginative play or in making friends; to absence of interest in peers.

   Specify current severity:

   Severity is based on social communication impairments and restricted repetitive patterns of behavior (see Table 18.2).

B. Restricted, repetitive patterns of behavior, interests, or activities, as manifested by at least two of the following, currently or by history (examples are illustrative, not exhaustive):

1. Stereotyped or repetitive motor movements, use of objects, or speech (e.g., simple motor stereotypes, lining up toys or flipping objects, echolalia, idiosyncratic phrases).

2. Insistence on sameness, inflexible adherence to routines, or ritualized patterns of verbal nonverbal behavior (e.g., extreme distress at small changes, difficulties with transitions, rigid thinking patterns, greeting rituals, need to take same route or eat food every day).

3. Highly restricted, fixated interests that are abnormal in intensity or focus (e.g., strong attachment to or preoccupation with unusual objects, excessively circumscribed or perseverative interest).

4. Hyper- or hyporeactivity to sensory input or unusual interests in sensory aspects of the environment (e.g., apparent indifference to pain/temperature, adverse response to specific sounds or textures, excessive smelling or touching of objects, visual fascination with lights or movement).

   Specify current severity:

   Severity is based on social communication impairments and restricted, repetitive patterns of behavior (see Table 18.2).

C. Symptoms must be present in the early developmental period (but may not become fully manifest until social demands exceed limited capacities, or may be masked by learned strategies in later life).

D. Symptoms cause clinically significant impairment in social, occupational, or other important areas of current functioning.

E. These disturbances are not better explained by intellectual disability (intellectual developmental disorder) or global developmental delay. Intellectual disability and autism spectrum disorder frequently co-occur; to make comorbid diagnoses of autism spectrum disorder and intellectual disability, social communication should be below that expected for general developmental level.

   Note: Individuals with a well-established DSM-V diagnosis of autistic disorder, Asperger's disorder, or pervasive developmental disorder not otherwise specified should be given the diagnosis of autism spectrum disorder. Individuals who have marked deficits in social communication, but whose symptoms do not otherwise meet criteria for autism spectrum disorder, should be evaluated for social (pragmatic) communication disorder.

   Specify if:

   – *With or without accompanying intellectual impairment*

   – *With or without accompanying language impairment*

   – *Associated with a known medical or genetic condition or environmental factor*

   – (*Coding note:* Use additional code to identify the associated medical or genetic condition.)

   – Associated with another neurodevelopmental, mental, or behavioral disorder

   – (*Coding note:* Use additional code[s] to identify the associated neurodevelopmental, mental, or behavioral disorder[s].)

   – *With catatonia*

   – (*Coding note:* Use additional code 293.89 [F06.1] catatonia associated with autism spectrum disorder to indicate the presence of the comorbid catatonia.)

Source: *Diagnostic and Statistical Manual*, 5th edition, © 2013, American Psychiatric Association.

Working with diet offers a drug-free approach to the treatment of ASD and AD(H)D. It also builds the very important foundations on which medical treatment can be given in a safer, more effective manner.

The aim of dietary intervention is to help correct nutritional imbalances, resolve gut dysbiosis and heal the gut wall, enabling its function of digestion, absorption and elimination to work effectively. By doing this, the immune system is strengthened, resulting in fewer infections and an improved ability for the body to detoxify itself. Neurotransmitters that affect behaviours, concentration, mood, sleep and addictions are also balanced by resolving the nutritional deficiencies that create an imbalance of these critical brain chemicals.

While it is important that dietary modification be done concurrently with nutritional medicine, gut repair and

TABLE 18.2 Severity levels for autism spectrum disorder		
Severity level	Social communication	Restricted, repetitive behaviours
Level 1 'Requiring support'	Without supports in place, deficits in social communication cause noticeable impairments. Difficulty initiating social interactions, and clear examples of atypical or unsuccessful response to social overtures of others. May appear to have decreased interest in social interactions. For example, a person who is able to speak in full sentences and engages in communication but whose to-and-fro conversation with others fails, and whose attempts to make friends are odd and typically unsuccessful.	Inflexibility of behaviour causes significant interference with functioning in one or more contexts. Difficulty switching between activities. Problems of organisation and planning hamper independence.
Level 2 'Requiring substantial support'	Marked deficits in verbal and non-verbal social communication skills; social impairments apparent even with supports in place; limited initiation of social interactions; and reduced or abnormal responses to social overtures from others. For example, a person who speaks simple sentences, whose interaction is limited to narrow special interests, and who has markedly odd non-verbal communication.	Inflexibility of behaviour, difficulty coping with change or other restricted/repetitive behaviours appear frequently enough to be obvious to the casual observer and interfere with functioning in a variety of contexts. Distress and/or difficulty changing focus or action.
Level 3 'Requiring very substantial support'	Severe deficits in verbal and non-verbal social communication skills cause severe impairments in functioning, very limited initiation of social interactions, and minimal response to social overtures from others. For example, a person with few words of intelligible speech who rarely initiates interaction and, when he or she does, makes unusual approaches to meet needs only and responds to only very direct social approaches.	Inflexibility of behaviour, extreme difficulty coping with change, or other restricted/repetitive behaviours markedly interfere with functioning in all spheres. Great distress/difficulty changing focus or action.

detoxification for optimal results, treatments may also need to be staggered as children with ASD and AD(H)D are often hypersensitive to any treatment. Treatments are generally administered with the 'start low, go slow' approach.

Dietary intervention

Allergens and sensitivities need to be removed. They can be identified through IgE and IgG testing or from observation. Removing these reduces irritation to the gut wall, helping to minimise stress on an overburdened immune system. Many foods that initially cause sensitivity can often be reintroduced without any problem once gut dysbiosis is resolved and the gut wall is healed (this may take a couple of years for some foods). Some children may require a low-phenol/salicylate diet or a low-oxalate diet.

Most children (roughly 80%) benefit from the gluten- and casein-free (GFCF) diet. Gluten is the protein found in wheat, barley, oats, rye, spelt, triticale and kamut. Casein is the protein found in all animal milk and products made from milk. Eliminating these two proteins is an important first step to dietary intervention. Most children have significant improvement from eliminating gluten and casein. However, for others this has little effect, so then a premature conclusion is drawn that diet has no effect on autism. This has done a great disservice to the ASD community. Gluten and casein play only one part in a very big production of dysfunction.

THE GLUTEN EXORPHIN AND CASOMORPHIN FACTOR

The primary reason for removing gluten and casein from the diets of children with autism is that these two proteins break down into peptides called gluten exorphin and casomorphin respectively. These peptides have a very similar structure to opiates. Normally such peptides are not able to be absorbed through a healthy gut. In an inflamed gut, intestinal hyperpermeability results, allowing the peptides to be absorbed into the blood stream and cross the blood–brain barrier, where they attach to opiate receptor sites. This opiate response results in symptoms such as 'zoning out', repetitive behaviour, sleep disturbance, constipation and high pain tolerance – all very common autistic traits. This opiate response is also why many autistic children are very finicky eaters – their diet often completely consists of wheat- and dairy-based foods. In this sense, it is actually an addiction we are dealing with, a solid biochemical reason for demanding these foods. Many parents fear that their children will starve if they take gluten and casein out of the diet, but if the offending foods are removed in a calculated fashion, the child's palate tends to open up and they become willing to eat a much wider variety of foods.

As mentioned previously, removing gluten and casein is only one step of the dietary process and is not adequate as a therapeutic diet on its own. Other offending substances need to be removed and replaced with nutrient-dense foods that promote the colonisation of a healthy intestinal microbiota. Dysbiosis is common with autism and so becomes an important part of treatment.

Other substances that need to be eliminated from the diet are artificial colours, flavours, sweeteners, preservatives, other food additives and sugar. To address dysbiosis, certain carbohydrates, particularly di- and monosaccharides, will need to be eliminated for a period of time until intestinal microbiota are restored to a healthful state, basically heading towards a natural 'real food' diet.

Digestive tract healing

GASTROINTESTINAL PATHOLOGIES IN ASD AND AD(H)D

Gastrointestinal pathologies associated with autism and ASD include impaired activity of disaccharide enzymes,[11] impaired sulfation of ingested phenolic compounds,[12] intestinal dysbiosis with significant clostridial numbers,[13] intestinal hyperpermeability,[14] impaired gluten and casein digestion[15,16] and anatomical abnormalities at different sites including stomach, ileum, duodenum and colon.[17-19] A growing number of studies published in medical literature point to significant dysregulation of the Th1/Th2 immunity affecting mucosal integrity. Mucosal synthesis of pro-inflammatory cytokines IL-4, IL-5, IL-12, IL-6, IFN and TNF-α is often significantly increased, along with a deficiency in regulatory cytokine IL-10+.[20,21] These factors warrant treatments to balance Th1/Th2 regulation, reduce pro-inflammatory cytokines, repair integrity of gut mucosa, stimulate digestion, particularly of disaccharides and phenolics, and correct intestinal dysbiosis.

Dysbiosis in the gastrointestinal tract (GIT)

Several studies have shown that children with autism have a much higher rate of altered bacterial numbers in the bowel. Clinical observation of autistic children also strongly suggests a high correlation of dysbiosis – symptoms including marked abdominal distension, yeasty smelling breath, constipation and/or diarrhoea, asthma, allergies, eczema and recurrent infections, particularly otitis media. Opportunistic microbes often found in elevated numbers are: yeasts (particularly *Candida* spp.), *Clostridia*, *Prevotella*, *Streptococcus* and *Staphylococcus*. While *E. coli* can sometimes be elevated, it is common for children with autism to have little or no detectable *E. coli*. *Lactobacilli* and *Bifidobacteria* are elevated in some children with ASD and reduced in others.

The impact of opportunistic microbes

YEASTS

Yeasts, particularly *Candida* spp., are among the most common opportunistic microbes found in a dysbiotic gut. Without enough beneficial flora, yeasts are able to make contact with the mucous membrane of the digestive tract and implant themselves. Yeasts produce alcohol from any sugar or carbohydrate ingested, which can then have a devastating effect on an infant's neurological development. Yeast overgrowths can be a driver for fussy eating as they will often trigger cravings for sweet or starchy foods (the latter of which tends to be a staunch favourite among children with ASD). Yeast overgrowth symptoms can include silly giggly behaviour, laughing in the sleep, red ears and cheeks and a red ring around the anus.

CLOSTRIDIA

Clostridia spp. are found in the healthy human gut in small numbers. *Clostridia* are spore-forming Gram-negative bacteria found in soils everywhere in the world. Problems occur when there are not enough beneficial bacteria to keep *Clostridia* numbers in check. Exposure to these bacteria is guaranteed and constant.

Clostridia overgrowth is very common in children with ASD, especially in those with an aggressive ASD phenotype or those who had GI symptoms prior to the onset of ASD.[22]

Clostridium tetani produces one of the most powerful neurotoxins known to man as well as phenol, phenol alcohol and proprionic acid.[23] After *C. tetani* was injected into rat stomachs, the tetani neurotoxins were shown to travel up the vagus nerve and into the central nervous system (CNS). This resulted in stereotyped behaviour in rats that is very similar to stereotypical behaviour in children with autism: repetitious and intensive licking, sniffing, gnawing and repetitive movements. These symptoms were abated by the administration of lithium, diazepam, haloperidol, fenfluramine and valproic acid, all of which have been used to treat the behavioural symptoms of autism.[23] Children treated with antibiotics used to treat *Clostridia* were reported to experience significant improvements in hyperactivity, behaviour, eye contact, hypersensitivity, social interest and vocalisation for the duration of treatment, with a return of symptoms after treatment had ceased.[24] As *Clostridia* are spore forming, the spores are able to withstand antibiotic treatment and propagate once treatment has ceased. A biofilm treatment strategy is a warranted approach.

C. tetani neurotoxins are also used to cause epileptic activity in laboratory animals. Epileptic seizures are statistically very common in children with autism.[25-27] The subgroup of autistic children who are likely to have overgrowth of *C. tetani* will probably have symptoms such as history of chronic infection treated with antibiotics, elevated levels of phenolic metabolites present in urine and/or history of persistent loose bowel movements.[23]

Clostridia produce amines in the intestines,[28] so when *Clostridia* numbers are elevated, the increased amine production can contribute to amine sensitivity – a problem in a subset of children on the autism spectrum.

Proprionic acid is used as a food preservative and in agriculture. It is also produced by *Clostridia* and can impact on ASD severity as it is a potent mitochondrial toxin. Proprionic acid often complexes with L-carnitine, which may explain why a subset of children with ASD have low carnitine levels,[29,30] which in itself also affects mitochondrial function.

SULFATE-REDUCING BACTERIA (SRB)

This is a large group of bacteria including *Clostridia* spp., *Desulfomonas* and *Desulfovibrio*. SRB use sulfate as fuel, thereby depleting the host of sulfate and producing cytotoxic hydrogen sulfide as a byproduct. SRB have been implicated in the pathogenesis of inflammatory bowel disorders, periodontitis, appendicitis, rectal cancer and abdominal and brain abscesses.[31,32] Sulfate is essential for many enzymatic reactions in the body and plays a crucial role in detoxification – sulfation – in the liver. Without enough sulfate, the liver cannot properly break down or detoxify neurotransmitters, hormones, phenols (including salicylates and other phytochemicals in foods) and environmental toxins.[33] Recirculating 'used' neurotransmitters play havoc with neurological function.[34] Environmental toxins and heavy metals accumulate in cells throughout the body. Reduced sulfation has been associated with increased/reduced glutathione (i.e. oxidative stress) and increased prevalence of autism in several studies,[12,33,35] as has increased heavy metals, particularly mercury.[33,36–40] The correlation between high mercury and autism incidence may in part be due to reduced sulfation, ironically a pathway that mercury itself also impedes. Many children with autism have sensitivities to dietary phytochemicals such as salicylates, amines, oxalates and glutamates. This may also be due to reduced sulfation and/or increased mercury body burden. With sulfur being such an important part of detoxification of substances strongly implicated in the presentation of ASD, antimicrobial and reinoculation of healthy gastrointestinal microbes is warranted.

STREPTOCOCCUS AND PAEDIATRIC AUTOIMMUNE NEUROPSYCHIATRIC DISORDERS ASSOCIATED WITH STREPTOCOCCAL INFECTIONS (PANDAS)

Streptococcus spp., as well as anti-strep antibody titres, are often found to be elevated in the faeces and serum of children with autism, ASD, AD(H)D and OCD.[41,42] *Streptococcus* spp. produce a number of toxins that can contribute to the symptoms of these disorders. Streptokinase, an enzyme produced by *Streptococcus*, binds to the enzyme DPP-IV, also known as CD26 depending on the location and function it is involved in,[43] rendering it inactive. DPP-IV is a proline-specific enzyme responsible for breaking down peptides such as β-casomorphin and performs critical modulating of peptides such as neuropeptides, hormones, cytokines and chemokines.[44] This has important implications on autoimmunity, inflammation and neurological function. Disorders associated with lowered serum DPP-IV are many and include Crohn's disease,[45] depression and anxiety,[46–48] inflammatory bowel disease,[49] immunosuppression[50] and schizophrenia,[51] all of which have associations with autism, ASD and AD(H)D. Hence, overgrowth of *Streptococcus* in the gut can lead to streptokinase-induced DPP-IV deficiency. Other streptococcal toxins with implication in neurological disorders include neuraminidase, NAD-ase, glutathione peroxidase and streptococcal pyogenic toxins.[52] During treatment of streptococcal overgrowth, avoidance of D-lactic-acid-producing bacteria (and the foods that contain them) may be warranted as D-lactic acid is a food source for *Streptococcus* spp.

PANDAS is characterised by episodic, abrupt and sometimes explosive severity of symptoms, often following an overt group-A streptococcal infection such as a sore throat with fever.[53] Not all cases of PANDAS follow an overt infection, however, and so strep serology provides insights into the aetiology of symptoms. Symptoms of PANDAS include obsessive and compulsive behaviours, irritability, emotional liability, hyperactivity, tics, separation anxiety, oppositional defiance and major depression.[41,53] PANDAS is diagnosed in the clinical setting by using the following criteria:

1 presence of OCD and/or tic disorder, according to DSM-V criteria
2 onset occurring between 3 years of age and puberty
3 episodic course
4 temporal association of symptom exacerbations with group A beta-haemolytic streptococci infections
5 presence of abnormal results on neurological examination, in the absence of frank chorea.[53]

Although there are no laboratory tests to confirm a diagnosis, useful tests that can suggest the diagnosis include elevated anti-group-A strep antibodies and elevated faecal streptococcal count.

BIOFILM

Biofilm is a polysaccharide and mineral matrix produced by microbes in toxic environments. Emerging research is consistently showing a link between biofilm and chronic and/or recurrent infections.[54] Biofilm protocols pioneered by Dr Anju Usman and implemented in the past 15 years for children with ASD are showing promising outcomes for treatment of stubborn dysbiosis and recurrent infection of the ears, respiratory tract and, in particular, the GIT. The biofilm protocol consists of four steps, to be carried out each day, generally for a minimum of 3 months, and up to 1–2 years. The steps are:

1 lysis of biofilm using raw, unfiltered apple cider vinegar along with specific enzymes, on an empty stomach
2 antimicrobial herbal treatment 15–60 minutes after step 1
3 clean-up of dead microbes and their endotoxins roughly 2 hours later with the use of substances such as fractionated pectin, slippery elm, food-grade diatomaceous earth and charcoal
4 nourishing diet, repair of gut mucosa and reinoculation with deficient microbes.

The recommended diet for use during biofilm protocol is one or combination of: GAPS (gut and psychology syndrome diet)/SCD (specific carbohydrate diet)/BED (body ecology diet). Prebiotic and probiotic foods are also recommended, as is xylitol if streptococcal overgrowth is present.

Biomedically trained doctors may use sodium ethylenediaminetetraacetic acid as part of step one and pharmaceutical antibiotics or antifungals in step two. However, the naturopathic approach is always preferred. Biofilm treatment should be carried out under the strict supervision of a naturopath or doctor trained in biofilm and biomedical autism treatment as reactions, regressions and side effects may occur if individual pathophysiological/phenotypic needs of child are not taken into account.

Inflammatory and immune factors in ASD

MATERNAL TRANSFER

The role of inflammation in ASD may stem from time in utero. Autoantibodies against fetal neuronal tissue have been found in mothers of children with ASD.[55] The role of this autoantibody transfer is currently unclear; however, there does appear to be an association. Mothers of children with ASD are found to be four times more likely to carry antibodies against neural tissue than other women of childbearing age.[56] Epidemiological studies suggest that maternal exposure to infection resulting in maternal immune activation is associated with autism in the offspring, possibly due to microglial (macrophages of the CNS) priming.[57] Microglial priming is a process that results in the microglia multiplying and adopting an activated state, making the microglia more susceptible to secondary inflammatory stimuli, which can then trigger an exaggerated inflammatory response. Systemic illness with an inflammatory component can often provide the secondary stimulus,[58] as can exposure to environmental pollutants. Through a lung–brain axis (independent of the cytokine activity), a study showed that microglia in rats remained active 24 hours after exposure to ozone.[59] This increase in microglial production may be a contributing factor in increased head circumference commonly seen in children with ASD, as larger head circumference is significantly and positively associated with increased history of allergic and immune disorders in the patient as well as their immediate family.[60] This may also be a mechanism by which vaccines can affect some children with ASD.

CYTOKINES AND CHEMOKINES

Cytokines and chemokines are proteins that have multiple actions, not all of which are related to immune function. Cytokines are important at all stages of neural development. However, increased production or activation of cytokines in response to a stimuli, such as maternal infection or hypoxia, can adversely affect the neurodevelopment of the fetus.[61,62] It is well establish that cytokine activation can be triggered by mercury and other heavy metals, bacteria, amyloid and glutamate.[62] Systemic cytokines and/or local immune factors can activate astrocytes and microglia – the brain's immune system – resulting in elevated levels of reactive oxygen and nitrogen species, cytokines, arachidonic acid, cellular immune components and excitotoxins which can result in brain dysfunction. Proinflammatory chemokines (MCP-1 and TARC) are found to be elevated in brains of individuals with ASD.[63]

GABA, GLUTAMATE AND NEUROINFLAMMATION

GABA is the primary inhibitory neurotransmitter, while glutamate is the primary excitatory neurotransmitter, in the human brain. Elevated levels of glutamate, or an elevated glutamate to GABA ratio, is often seen in individuals with autism and is associated with increased risk of seizures, hyperactivity, aggression, difficulty concentrating and sleep disturbances.

ALLERGY, ALLERGY-LIKE SYMPTOMS AND MASTOCYTOSIS

Food allergies, rhinitis, allergic-type symptoms and atopic conditions such as eczema have a high prevalence in children with ASD.[64,65] Mast cells play a key role in inflammation, adaptive and innate immunity, autoimmunity and allergy.[66] They produce a variety of cytokines that disrupt the blood–brain barrier.[67] While mast cells are found in the brain and have been shown to have a direct effect on neuroinflammation[68] as well as microglia stimulation,[69] it has also been found that peripheral inflammation, outside of the CNS, can also activate microglia.[70] Mast cell activation due to allergy, environmental and/or stress triggers is hypothesised to be a contributing factor to the high rate of seizures in children with ASD by disrupting blood–brain barrier permeability.[71] Substances that inhibit mast cells and microglial activation and proliferation may have significant benefit to those with ASD with an inflammatory component. The flavonoid luteolin is one such compound that has this effect.[72] Mast cells are associated with perivascular oedema and may be an indicator of disrupted BBB function, which is a contributing factor in autism.[73,74]

AUTOIMMUNITY

Multiple studies have shown that autoimmune conditions are found significantly more frequently in children with ASD than in the neurotypical population, with type 1 diabetes and psoriasis being among the highest prevalence.[64,75] Family history of autoimmune diseases also increases the risk of ASD – children with ASD have a higher rate of first- and second-degree family members with autoimmune diseases.[76–80] For example, a 2015 population study demonstrated a greater risk of ASD in children of mothers who have systemic lupus erythematosus (SLE) than in matched controls.[81] Children with ASD have an increased risk of developing allergies and psoriasis,[64] which mirrored findings 10 years earlier that maternal allergies and psoriasis were associated with increased risk of ASD is offspring.[82] This may suggest genetic and/or environmental factors at play.

Many microbes – both pathogens and commensals – can induce brain autoantibodies (see Table 18.3). Treatment approaches that address the balance of the microbiota may be helpful in neuropsychiatric disorders via their effect on mediating autoimmunity.[83] The gut microbiota are likely at the foundation of the development of autoimmunity due to overproduction of Th17 cells when in a state of dysbiosis.[84] Furthermore, production of anti-neuronal antibodies, a common pathophysiology in children in autism, is correlated with family history of autoimmune illnesses.[77] Anti-neuronal antibodies cause cytotoxic neuronal damage and therefore lead to neuronal impairment and brain development abnormalities.[77]

TABLE 18.3 Microbes implicated in neuropsychiatric disorders		
Viruses	**Bacteria**	**Parasites**
Influenza virus HSV-1 and HSV-2 Epstein–Barr Virus Varicella zoster virus Cytomegalovirus Human herpesvirus-6 Rubella virus Measles Mumps Poliovirus HIV-1 and HIV-2 Endogenous retroviruses Bornavirus Parvovirus B19 and AAV-2 West Nile virus Enterovirus 71 Coxsackievirus B3 Polyomaviruses (JC virus and BK virus)	*Treponema pallidum* *Borrelia burgdorferi* Group A beta-haemolytic *Streptococcus pyogenes* *Chlamydiaceae* spp. *Mycoplasma* spp. Various gastrointestinal microflora	*Toxoplasma gondii* *Toxocara* spp.

Source: Hornig, M. The role of microbes and autoimmunity in the pathogenesis of neuropsychiatric illness. *Current Opinion in Rheumatology* 2013;25(4):488–795.

METHYLATION, DETOXIFICATION, OXIDATION, AUTOIMMUNITY AND EPIGENETICS

Methylation is a process of hundreds of reactions in the body involving the addition or removal of methyl groups to other compounds or elements. Methylation processes play critical roles in detoxification, particularly of environmental toxins, including heavy metals and pesticides, and phenols; DNA and RNA formation; neurotransmitter production; and the reading of genes. The rate of methylation therefore plays an important role in epigenetics (i.e. the effect that environment has on gene expression), and so abnormalities in rate of methylation have been linked to children with autism being more susceptible to environmental toxins and experiencing increased rates of oxidation. Methylation is also responsible for the formation of glutathione, a major antioxidant and detoxification compound in the body. Children with autism, ASD and AD(H)D have been shown to experience a great deal of oxidative stress as expressed by reduced levels of glutathione and superoxide dismutase,[77,85] caeruloplasmin and ferritin,[86] and increased levels of isoprostanes (a biomarker of oxidative stress and lipid peroxidation).[77,87] Nutrients essential in the methylation pathway are vitamins B_6, B_9 and B_{12}, zinc, magnesium, methionine and dimethylglycine (DMG)/ trimethylglycine (TMG).

High levels of oxidative stress are present in many autoimmune and neurological disorders. The brain has a

greater susceptibility than other body tissues to oxidative stress.[88] Oxidative stress leads to impaired methylation and damages polyunsaturated fatty acids in cell membranes, resulting in lipid peroxidation. Mostafa et al. showed significant association between markers of oxidative stress, autoimmunity and severity of autistic symptoms.[77]

PYRROLURIA/HPL

Pyrroles, or Mauve factor, recently more accurately identified as hydroxyhaemopyrrolin-2-one (HPL), are a byproduct of haemoglobin metabolism and have no known physiological function. Elevated HPL excretion via the urine is associated with emotional stress, which is in turn associated with oxidative stress.[89] Pyrroluria is a condition where elevated HPL is found in the urine. HPL binds to B_6 and zinc before all three are eliminated via the kidneys, rendering the B_6 and zinc unavailable for use in their many enzyme reactions. Early studies have shown that HPL is neurotoxic and affects the metabolism of haem, resulting in mitochondrial and neuronal decay.[89] Depressed haem results in increased oxidant release from mitochondria. Approximately 20% of children and adolescents with autism, ASD, AD(H)D and behavioural disorders have elevated HPL in their urine – an error of haemoglobin metabolism. This causes excessive losses and resultant deficiency in B_6 and zinc, often with elevated serum levels of copper. The cause of pyrroluria is epigenetic – a genetic susceptibility plus environmental factors such as stress, dysbiosis and heavy metal burden. Faulty fatty acid metabolism is another result of pyrroluria, with omega-3 fatty acids often aggravating symptoms of impulsiveness, aggression, depression, irritability, poor stress tolerance and anxiety. Treatment is usually very successful with the use of P5P, zinc (particularly zinc picolinate), magnesium, vitamins C and E, and omega-6 essential fatty acids such as those in evening primrose oil or blackcurrant oil.[90] Higher doses of these nutrients, particularly B_6, zinc and magnesium, during times of high emotional, psychosocial or physical stress may be useful in some individuals. Molybdenum can be used as an adjunct therapy in cases of copper excess (see Tables 18.4 and 18.5).

METALLOTHIONEIN

Metallothioneins (MTs) are intracellular low-molecular-weight, zinc- and cysteine-rich proteins with high metal-binding redox capabilities. Each MT protein contains seven molecules of zinc. They are found in high concentrations in the brain, liver, kidneys and GIT. MT plays vital roles in development of neurons, immune function, maturation of the GIT, free radical scavenging and metal transport, including the delivery of zinc into cells. MTs are involved in the homeostasis of metals in the body. MT has a protective effect against the adverse effects of zinc deficiency and zinc overload in the brain.[110] Other metals that MT binds to include copper, manganese, mercury, arsenic, aluminium and cadmium. MT is an important compound in the removal of heavy metals from the body. Individuals with under-functioning MT have a higher susceptibility to accumulation and toxic effects of

TABLE 18.4 Neurobehavioural disorders associated with elevated HPL

Diagnosis	Percentage high Mauve
AIP[91,92]	100
Latent AIP[93]	70
Down syndrome[94]	71
Schizophrenia, acute[95–98]	59–80
Schizophrenia, chronic[99–102]	40–50
Criminal behaviour: Adults, sudden deviance[103] Youths, violent offenders[104]	71 33
Manic depression[100,105]	47–50
Depression, non-schizophrenic[91,102,106]	12–46
Autism[106,107]	46–48
Epilepsy[106]	44
Learning disability/ADHD[102,106]	40–47
Neuroses[108]	20
Alcoholism[95,101,102,105,108,109]	20–84

AIP = acute intermittent porphyria
Source: McGinnis W, Audhya, T. *Discerning the Mauve Factor, part I*. [online] Walshinstitute.org; 2008.

TABLE 18.5 Signs, symptoms and traits clinicians report as more prevalent in high-Mauve patients*

Poor dream recall	Impotence
Nail spots	Eosinophilia
Stretch marks (striae)	B_6-responsive anaemia
Pale skin/poor tanning	Attention deficit/hyperactivity
Coarse eyebrows	Crime and delinquency
Knee and joint pain	Substance abuse
Acne	Alcoholism
Allergy	Stress intolerance
Cold hands or feet	Emotional lability
Abdominal tenderness	Explosive anger
Stitch in side	Anxiety
Constipation	Pessimism
Morning nausea	Dyslexia
Light/sound/odour intolerance	Familial or social withdrawal
Tremor/shaking/spasms	Depression
Hypoglycaemia/glucose intolerance	Paranoia
Obesity	Hallucinations
Migraine	Disordered perception
Delayed puberty	Bipolar disorder
Amenorrhoea/irregular periods	Autism

*The frequency of these features and their relationship to biochemical abnormalities associated with HPL are not well studied.
Source: https://nutripath.com.au/wp-content/uploads/2014/01/TestFlyerA4-MAUVE-FACTOR.pdf.

heavy metals as well as exposure to other environmental toxins. Zinc has been shown to be a potent stimulator of MT production. Low zinc results in low MT levels.

Due to the high concentration of cysteine in MT proteins, cysteine status may also impact on the body's ability to produce adequate MT. Studies at the Pfeiffer Treatment Center have found that children with autism, ASD and AD(H)D often have a high copper to zinc ratio, indicating malfunctioning MT.[111] Stimulation of MT production to promote detoxification, remove heavy metals, repair the intestinal mucosa, prevent oxidative damage and restore immune function is therefore utilised in the biomedical treatment of autism, ASD and AD(H)D. A study by Levin et al.[112] showed that malfunctioning/absent MT1 and MT2 resulted in decreased frontal dopamine levels when mice were exposed to mercury. Dopamine has a suspected protective mechanism against mercury exposure. Children with autism, ASD and AD(H)D are often found to have low dopamine levels. Dopamine is required for many functions including cognitive function, selective attention, motor function, reward mechanisms and neuroendocrine function. All are functions impaired in autism, ASD and AD(H)D, suggesting a possible link between metallothionein, zinc levels, mercury exposure and production of neurotransmitters.

HEAVY AND TOXIC METALS

Toxic metals attach to nutrient mineral binding sites on enzymes, inhibiting, overstimulating or otherwise destroying their function. Many of the symptoms of toxic metal burden mimic those of autism, ASD and AD(H)D, so it is important to determine whether toxicity is contributing to the neurological and immune issues presented in the individual. The toxicology of most metals has been studied independently of each other. More recent studies are showing that low levels of more than one toxic metal have a far greater toxic effect than each metal would have on its own. This raises big concerns in regards to children with ASD, autism and AD(H)D who have often been found to have increased levels of a number of toxic metals. The following metals described are only a few that are commonly raised in neurological disorders.

Lead

Lead is absorbed through GIT and lungs. More than 90% of the body burden of lead is found in bone;[113] however, toxic effects are found to target multiple organs and systems: liver, kidney, lung and immune and neurological systems.[114] Neurological symptoms of lead toxicity include: hyperactivity, restlessness, anxiety, irritability, fatigue, mood disorders, aggressiveness, reduced attention, inability to concentrate, reduced IQ, reduced memory, temper tantrums, fearfulness, insomnia and difficulties with reading, writing, language and visual and motor skills.

The accepted safe level of lead has decreased dramatically over the years. In the 1960s, acceptable blood levels of lead were 60 micrograms/dL. In 1985, that was reduced to 25 micrograms/dL, and then to 10 micrograms/dL in 1991. Studies have shown that neurodevelopmental effects of lead toxicity, including intellectual impairment, can occur at levels less than 10 micrograms/dL.[115,116]

Fetal exposure to maternal lead is of significant concern. Bone turnover increases during pregnancy and lactation, particularly if maternal calcium intake is inadequate. This causes mobilisation of lead, which is then easily able to cross the placenta and affect fetal development. Low-level exposure to lead during vulnerable periods of development has greater toxicological impacts than it would on a fully mature system. Fetal development, early childhood and adolescence are the most vulnerable developmental stages, and even minimal exposure during these times can cause significant cognitive impairment and immunotoxic effects.[117]

Exposure to lead causes a skewing of T cell function towards a Th2 dominance and Th1 impairment,[114,118,119] increasing the incidence of asthma, allergies, eczema and cancer, to name but a few. Studies have also demonstrated that lead exposure can increase autoantibody production, and, in doing so, bring about autoimmune illnesses.[120–122]

Perinatal and postnatal exposure to lead has now been clearly proven to be one cause of AD(H)D,[123,124] and has implications in the development of other neurological disorders such as ASD and autism. Many children with autism, ASD and AD(H)D have some degree of asthma, eczema and/or allergies, so it is possible that this is related to lead exposure.

Calcium and iron deficiency exacerbate symptoms of lead exposure. Lead competes with calcium for absorption, which can cause problems with calcium metabolism and affect neurotransmitter release via blockage of calcium channels. Calcium supplementation reduces the absorption of lead through the GIT.[125] During pregnancy and lactation, calcium supplementation can reduce the amount of lead mobilised from bone.[113,126,127] Sources of lead include crystal glassware, pottery, batteries, paint (in older homes), hair dyes and ammunitions.

Lead increases lipid peroxidation, causing oxidative damage to cells.[128,129] Several studies have demonstrated a protective effect of vitamin C and silymarin on hepatotoxicity of lead.[130–132] High levels of serum vitamin C are associated with low blood lead levels.[133] It is suspected that silymarin promotes the elimination of lead from the body via the bile.[134] Both silymarin and ascorbic acid provide antioxidant support and reduce lipid peroxidation.[129,135,136]

Arsenic

Not actually a metal, arsenic is a metalloid, and possibly is essential in minute amounts. Animal studies show that arsenic plays a role in the conversion of methionine to taurine and may be necessary for zinc metabolism.[137,138]

Sources of arsenic include drinking water (in some parts of the world), fish and seafood, pesticides, insecticides, herbicides and other agricultural chemicals, industrial pollution from mining smelting activities, computer chips and wood preservatives (used for children's playground equipment).[139]

Arsenic causes skin disorders, peripheral neuropathies and impairment of CNS function including impaired IQ, poor short- and long-term memory, impaired grip strength and hand–eye coordination, finger tapping and tremor.[139,140] Arsenic has also been shown to affect neurotransmitter production and function, particularly in regards to cholinergic, glutaminergic and monoaminergic systems. The dopaminergic system is the most profoundly disrupted. Studies have conflicting evidence of both upregulation and downregulation. However, this may depend on the type of arsenic and route of administration.

N-acetylcysteine is being studied for its possible role in treating arsenic-related liver damage.

Aluminium

Aluminium is ubiquitous in nature, the third most prevalent metal in the earth's crust, and yet it has no known requirement for human physiology. Sources of aluminium include water, food additives and utensils such as cookware and food containers. The largest dietary source is food additives. Different forms of aluminium are used in cake, bread, pancake and other baked goods flour mixes. It is used in processed cheeses, to clarify sugar and as an anticaking agent for salt, non-dairy creamers and other dry powdered products.[141] Aluminium is also used as a preservative in vaccines. Since the removal of thiomersal from many vaccines around 2001, aluminium-based preservatives in vaccines have been used instead.

Aluminium is a known potent neurotoxin, and maternal exposure to excess aluminium during pregnancy can cause skeletal and soft tissue abnormalities and growth retardation in the fetus.[141,142] Aluminium can potentiate reactive oxygen species in the presence of copper and iron,[143] causing oxidative damage to cells, and it can also cause inflammatory changes in neurons.[143]

Mercury

Mercury is particularly well absorbed by inhalation but also is absorbed via the GIT, and passes very easily into the brain. Body burden of mercury is concentrated in the nervous system, kidneys and liver. Mercury is well recognised as being cytotoxic and is one of the most potent neurotoxins known. Mercury causes oxidative damage, inflammation and disrupts the metabolism of minerals such as zinc and impairs the function of metallothioneins and methylation, which further impairs the ability to eliminate mercury. Mercury also decreases neurotransmitter production, testosterone and thyroid hormone.

Autoimmune reactions after mercury exposure have been considered a contributory factor to the pathogenesis of autism,[144] and children with autoimmune tendencies appear to be more susceptible to the negative effects of mercury in vaccines and other environmental sources.[145,146] Maternal exposure to mercury through flu vaccines and environmental exposure may put the developing fetus at risk of neurological and/or autoimmune disorders.

Symptoms of mercury toxicity include irritability, nervousness, anxiety, fatigue, memory loss, repetitive behaviour, social deficits, reduced attention, language/speech deficits, headache, dizziness, drowziness, emotional instability, depression and poor cognitive function. Sources of mercury include amalgam tooth fillings (during chewing, brushing and drinking hot drinks), some vaccines (including flu vaccine), seafood, pesticides, batteries, laxatives, paper and pulp manufacturing, drinking water and paint products.

MITOCHONDRIAL DYSFUNCTION

Dysfunctional mitochondrial activity is one of the most common findings in individuals with ASD, affecting a significant subset of children (some studies showing over 50%).[29] Organs and systems which are most affected by mitochondrial dysfunction are those with the biggest energy requirements and include the central and peripheral nervous system, the digestive system, the immune system and muscles. These are all systems in which problems commonly occur in ASD. Studies show the greater the mitochondrial dysfunction, the more significant the behavioural and cognitive symptoms are.[147] (See Box 18.2.) There is a strong correlation between mitochondrial dysfunction and GI symptoms. Mitochondrial dysfunction affects multiple organs of the system, including the liver and pancreas. Mitochondrial dysfunction also affects peristalsis of the intestines. As Frye and Rose and colleagues[22] outline, there are three possible mechanisms to this association, and they may occur singularly or in combination. The three mechanisms are first, that mitochondrial dysfunction itself can cause gastrointestinal symptoms. Secondly, many environmental stressors that are known to impact on ASD also impact on the mitochondria and the GI tract. Thirdly, there are

endogenous compounds from the GI tract such as lipopolysaccharides and metabolites from gut microbiota (such as proprionic acid from *Clostridia* spp.) that can affect mitochondrial and GI function.[22] (See 'The impact of opportunistic microbes' for further reading on *Clostridia*.)

The impacts on mitochondrial function of substances such as valproic acid, paracetamol, pesticides and mercury may partially explain the increased risk of ASD in those exposed to these substances.

In 2014 UC Davis researchers found that the mitochondria in granulocytes consumed less oxygen in children with ASD than in neurotypical children – a sign of diminished mitochondrial function. They also found that the level of response to fighting pathogens was lower and slower in the ASD population, leaving them more susceptible to infection. Mitochondria in children with ASD also produced more reactive oxygen species and had less capability to repair the damage, and therefore experienced more oxidative stress.[148]

Investigations

The following biochemical tests will help to determine contributory factors to ASD symptoms and to target interventions. The following tests are to determine abnormalities in metabolism (such as pyrroluria, impaired methylation or sulfation, and metallothionein activity). Stool tests provide invaluable insights into the microbial inhabitants of the large bowel and into possible digestive insufficiencies. Hair and urinary metal tests are used to evaluate heavy and toxic metal burden. Hair mineral analysis requires careful interpretation, as low levels do not necessarily indicate low body burden. Often retesting after a period of detoxifcation/chelation protocol will result in higher levels of toxic metals in hair. This is due to increased elimination. Re-testing will be required every 3–9 months until hair levels drop again, while still carrying out detoxification/chelation protocol. Urinary provocation test provides accurate indications of toxic metal burdens and is suitable in older, toilet-trained children with healthy kidney function.

FIRST-TIER TESTS

- Urinary HPL (pyrroles) – to determine if pyrroluria is present. Elevated HPL results in increased B$_6$ and zinc excretion and disrupted fatty acid metabolism.
- Plasma zinc (using Pfeiffer Center zinc collection protocol) and serum copper – often actual or relative plasma zinc is low and copper is elevated. This may be due to reduced absorption, pyrroluria, heavy metal burden, insufficient sulfation or impaired oxalate metabolism (due to either impaired sulfation or yeast overgrowth). Excess copper can lead to aggressive behaviours.
- Iron studies – low iron can be a result of inadequate intake, malabsorption due to gastrointestinal inflammation or lack of vitamin C or beneficial bacteria, or due to overgrowth of iron-loving bacteria.
- Full blood count.

> ## BOX 18.2 Symptoms of mitochondrial dysfunction
>
> - Developments delay
> - Aggression
> - Language impairment/speech delay
> - Social impairment
> - Intellectual disability
> - Neuropsychiatric symptoms typical of ADHD, anxiety, OCD and depression
> - Seizures
> - Headaches
> - Muscle weakness, poor posture
> - Small stature
> - Fatigue
> - GI symptoms

- Vitamin D – often low and may affect immune function and bone growth.
- Folate and B$_{12}$
- Serum creatinine
- Fasting homocysteine
- Whole blood histamine
- MTHFR and other SNPs relating to methylation
- HLA DQ2 and HLA DQ8
- Streptococcal serology (particularly if PANDAS is suspected)
- Lipid studies including breakdown
- hs-CRP
- ESR
- Complete faecal microbial analysis including parasitology, virology, bacteriology, worms and other.

SECOND-TIER TESTS

- Thyroid antibodies and thyroid receptor antibodies (common link between this and positive HLA DQ2 and HLA DQ8 gene).
- TSH, T3, T4 (dysregulated thyroid function can impact on multiple systems and/or organs, including effects on cognitive function).
- ANA and ENA if autoimmune activity suspected.
- 24 hr urinary creatinine clearance (will depend on toilet training/habits).
- Organic acids test (OAT) – very useful to give an overview of 55 urinary metabolites that shed light on mitochondrial function, adenosine triphosphate (ATP) production, neurotransmitter metabolism, dysbiosis markers and more.
- Live blood analysis (LBA) – gives a good overview of immune and digestive function and can give indications for further testing for allergies, heavy metals, mineral or hormonal imbalances. In combination with other investigations, helps to tailor treatment to child's specific needs.
- Bolan's clot retraction test (CRT) – a CRT will help determine which systems are being affected most by oxidative stress, a huge problem in children with ASD. Knowing what organ systems are being most affected will help to direct treatment appropriately. Results complement those of LBA and are of great benefit when both tests are done.

THIRD-TIER TESTS

- Urine toxic metal provocation test (in older children and adults and only if healthy kidney function is confirmed first). Not during acute inflamed periods.

Therapeutic considerations

CLINICAL DECISION MAKING AND RATIONALE

Decision making must be based strictly on the individual representation of symptoms and syndromes present in each child. It can be said that there are as many types of ASD as there individuals who have it. Before any significant therapeutic measures are carried out, a thorough case history must of course be taken, and it is advisable that the first tier of tests be carried out and results reviewed before introducing any specific supplements. Exceptions to that guideline may be cod liver oil and zinc if clinically indicated. Carefully considered probiotics may also be warranted at this time, such as in the case of chronic diarrhoea – *Saccharomyces boulardii* may be of great benefit. Additionally, if the patient is currently taking antibiotics, it may be of benefit to use a broad spectrum probiotic to help prevent antibiotic-associated GIT symptoms. Often it is best to wait until faecal microbial analysis has been completed before introducing probiotics. Probiotics and antibiotics/microbials need to be stopped for 2–4 weeks prior to faecal microbial analysis.

Therapeutic application

NATUROPATHIC PERSPECTIVE

The naturopathic perspective is to address the underlying immune, biochemical, metabolic and digestive disorders that are now clearly associated with the pathogenesis of ASD. Focus on these aspects often brings about improvements in neurological symptoms. The motto for treatment is 'low and slow' as the majority of children with ASD are hypersensitive and may react adversely to normal doses of certain nutrients and herbs. Only one new intervention should be introduced at a time. This is to make observations on effectiveness of individual interventions possible, to be able to tell what a child may be sensitive to and to avoid over-stimulating impaired metabolic pathways that may need to be addressed slowly in order not to cause distress, regression or a Jarisch–Herxheimer reaction.

NUTRITIONAL MEDICINE (DIETARY)

Dietary therapeutic objectives

Dietary intervention focuses on providing optimal delivery of nutrients required for growth, development and all physiological functions, gut healing, resolution of dysbiosis and reduction in inflammatory processes. Children with ASD are often very fussy eaters, which can pose a great challenge, particularly if changes are made too quickly. From clinical experience, it usually works best to introduce therapeutic foods first before trying to eliminate harmful foods. This is particularly true of the introduction of fermented vegetables – the sour tart taste helps to develop the palate, while the beneficial microbes in the fermented vegetables help to reduce cravings for starches and sugars by the effect they have on opportunistic microbes in the gut. Initially, these foods can be mixed into a child's favourite foods in order to get them ingested. The most important point is one step at a time. Wait until the first change has become habit before introducing the next change. ASD is a chronic disorder, so for treatment to be effective it must be maintainable over a long period of time.

Persuading children to become involved in food preparation where possible helps to pique their interest in eating and sets up good habits for later in life.

Specific dietary treatments

DIETARY INCLUSIONS

Fermented vegetables are usually the first dietary modification. They help to improve the child's willingness to try a wider variety of foods. Fermented vegetables are rich in enzymes, and the recognition of their sour/tart flavour by the tastebuds elicits the stimulation of production of hydrochloric acid in the stomach. Therefore, on both the acid and the enzyme front, the fermented vegetables can improve and support digestion. Fermented foods in general contain a wider array of microflora than probiotic supplements do, so they are a great way to get a broad spectrum of not only probiotics, but their beneficial byproducts including amino acids and vitamins B, K and biotin. They can help to reduce abdominal bloating and discomfort and may improve bowel habits. Many children actually tend to grow to love these foods and request them, much to their parents' disbelief! Any fermented food needs to be introduced in small amounts. The general recommendation is to start on ½–1 teaspoon of the juice of the fermented vegetables each day. This can be mixed into any food or drink that is not hot, or can be administered orally via syringe. After a week or so, a piece of solid vegetable can be introduced, and every week thereafter the amount of vegetable can be increased by ½–1 teaspoon until the child is consuming 1–2 dessert-spoonfuls with each meal.

Meat stocks/bone broths, for gastrointestinal healing and stimulation of digestion, can be given with each meal as a drink or used in cooking. These traditional foods are a rich source of proline and glycine-rich collagen as well as minerals, all of which aid in healing of connective tissue, including the GIT. Caution must be taken here for a very small subgroup of individuals who are sensitive to glutamates and who may deteriorate on bone broths/meat stock due to the high levels of glutamine. These individuals may experience more agitation, aggression or even seizures due to problems with glutamine, glutamate and GABA metabolism. This is rare, but noteworthy. For a small percentage of people, particularly those with histamine intolerance, it may be necessary to start with short-cooked broths of as little as half an hour, in small amounts (e.g. a shot diluted in a soup recipe, using filtered water instead of broth for the rest of the liquid), slowly increasing as gut flora begins to improve and liver function and metabolic pathways of detoxification are supported.

DIETARY EXCLUSIONS

The first items to be eliminated are added sugar (replace this with xylitol or green stevia) and artificial food additives – colours, flavours, preservatives, flavour enhancers and artificial sweeteners. Even natural or nature identical flavours need to be eliminated (the term natural is a loose one, and often still includes very synthetic compounds).

Xylitol can be particularly useful as a replacement sweetener if there is strep overgrowth, otitis media, dental plaque or PANDAS as xylitol has anti-strep activity.[149–151]

Any known allergens must be excluded.

Also exclude processed flour products – breads, pastas, cakes, biscuits and so on (unless homemade from grain-free flours).

Considering the extent of research now available demonstrating the effect of gluten on zonulin release and resultant increased intestinal and blood–brain barrier permeability,[152] any chronic condition that involves inflammation, the brain and/or the gut warrants at least a 3–6-month strict trial of gluten-free diet. ASD falls into this category. A 2013 dietary survey of children with ASD demonstrated that only 5% of children did not respond positively to a gluten-free diet. These 5% of children spent an average of 1 month on the diet, with 4.4% regressing on the diet (one would need to look at what other dietary influences were present). For all other children, the longer they spent on the diet, the greater their improvement. For example, 31 children who followed the diet for an average of 7 months experienced moderate improvements, 37 children who spent an average of 8 months had good improvement, 42 children who spent an average of 13 months on the diet had excellent improvements while 16 children who spent an average of 18 months on the diet experienced dramatic improvements. Age at start time of diet and length of time on diet were key predictors of outcome.[153]

Other dietary considerations

Depending on individual presentation, it may be necessary to consider implementing a low-phenol or low-oxalate diet. For children with painful IBS type symptoms, a low-FODMAP approach may help. If FODMAP-containing foods do result in IBS symptoms, this is a sign of gut dysbiosis. The low-FODMAP diet is meant to be short-term rather than long-term measure, utilised until gut healing and a better balance of gut microflora are restored.

A significant number of children often do not fare well on dairy foods for multiple reasons. One is the opiate-like effect of casomorphins which can create, among other things, fussy eating and a refusal to eat other food groups. For many, it also poses an allergy or sensitivity response. This is particularly true in children who have chronic catarrh conditions. Otitis media often clears remarkably quickly on a casein- and gluten-free diet. IBS symptoms also often significantly improve on removal of dairy and gluten.

The dairy- and gluten-free diet ideally needs to be soy free at the same time as soy proteins cross-react with gluten and casein and can keep inflammatory responses activating.

It is often a lot easier to notice the effect of certain food groups on reintroduction rather than elimination. Often, to notice a difference, multiple food triggers need to be eliminated at the same time. As a result, the easiest model to base dietary plans on is vegetables, fats, meats (from pasture-raised animals for healthy fatty acid and fat-soluble vitamin profiles), seafood and minimal fruit. This approach leaves out the most common triggers – grains, dairy and legumes – while including an abundance of nutrient-dense food groups. Once symptoms have reduced or cleared, after 3–6 months of trials, single foods can be reintroduced to see how the individual responds to each food. Food reintroductions need to be done one at a time and at least 4–7 days apart as food sensitivities can take up to 72 hours for symptoms to manifest.

Children with significant dysbiosis and/or *Candida*/yeast infections may need to eliminate all fruits and honey for a period of time until the microflora are returned to balance.

SAMPLE DAILY DIET

This diet is representative of what a child would be eating once they have completely adjusted to a BED (body ecology diet)/GAPS (gut and psychology syndrome)/paleolithic combined diet, which may take months.

BREAKFAST

Bone-broth-based soup or stew with a variety of tolerated vegetables.
Lamb chops or eggs (scrambled or fried in coconut oil) and fermented vegetables. 1 cup of meat stock.

LUNCH

Bone-broth-based chicken and vegetable soup (can make vegetables into noodles using a spiraliser to entice children).
Or homemade grain-, dairy- and soy-free chicken nuggets with veggie sticks and homemade guacamole.

DINNER

Meatballs and cooked vegetables, or GAPS/SCD (gut and psychology syndrome/specific carbohydrate diet) pizza and a cup of bone broth and teaspoon of fermented vegetables.

SNACKS

SCD banana pikelets; spicy nut cookies; gelatine gummies.
In the long term, think of food, rather than snack food; that is, have leftovers or smaller portions of regular meals. The aim is to slowly steer the palate away from sweet and starchy foods.

BEVERAGES

Herbal tea cordials: herbal teas such as peppermint, spearmint, lemon balm and/or hibiscus (for a great pink colour) sweetened with xylitol or stevia and cooled to room temperature.
Lemon twist – juice ½–1 lemon into 1 L of filtered or spring water and sweeten with xylitol or stevia.
Coconut water kefir diluted in water.
Pure water – filtered and remineralised.

NUTRITIONAL MEDICINE (SUPPLEMENTAL)

Nutritional medicine therapeutic objectives

- Balance biochemistry, address deficiencies – indicated by pathology results and clinical signs and symptoms
- Boost immunity

- Reduce inflammation
- Reduce oxidative damage
- Improve gastrointestinal integrity
- Provide nutrients for growth and development
- Support detoxifcation
- Support mitochondrial function
- Improve glutathione production
- Provide neurotrophic factors
- Support pathways of methylation and sulfation

Specific nutrients required

The range of beneficial nutrients can be diverse for children with ASD (see Table 18.6). The primary nutrients required include:

ZINC

Adequate zinc is required for immune responses, methylation, nucleic acid and protein synthesis, cell replication, tissue growth and repair neurotransmitter balance, including by controlling glutamate receptor activity. Zinc ions comprise the active centre of over 300 enzymes. Up to 85% of children with autism are low in zinc,[42] and zinc deficiency in early childhood is linked to ADHD – characteristics often seen in ASD. A study in 2013 of 1967 children with ASD aged between 0 and 15 found that 29.7% had low zinc levels, with almost half of the males aged 0–3 and over half of the females aged 0–3 being deficient.[155] This age group is likely the most significantly affected due to larger amounts of zinc per kilogram body weight being required at this time for growth and development.

Zinc deficiency is associated with poor wound healing, retarded growth, impaired immunity, depression, hyperactivity and neurodegenerative and neurodevelopmental disorders. Zinc supplementation affects the sense of taste and can make introduction of new foods easier as the child becomes more willing to try new flavours. Zinc stabilises sulfur, RNA and DNA,[42] and is required for the production of digestive acids and enzymes. Recent research demonstrates that zinc may

Mineral	Number of cases with deficiency	Rate (%) of deficiency
Zn	584	29.7
Mg	347	17.6
Ca	114	5.8
Co	40	2.0
Fe	17	0.9
Cr	12	0.6
Mn	4	0.2
Cu	4	0.2

TABLE 18.6 Prevalence of mineral deficiency in autistic children[154]

Source: http://www.mdpi.com/1660-4601/10/11/6027/htm (Table 3).

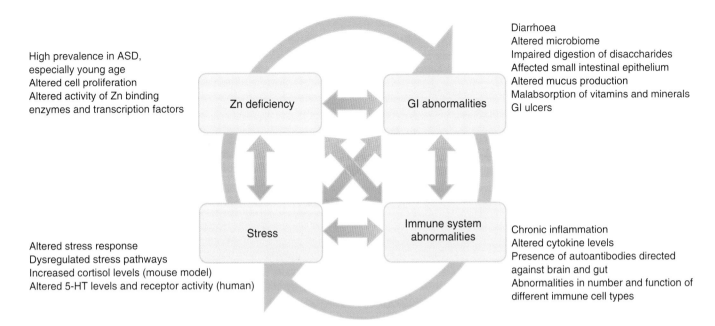

High prevalence in ASD,
especially young age
Altered cell proliferation
Altered activity of Zn binding
enzymes and transcription factors

Diarrhoea
Altered microbiome
Impaired digestion of disaccharides
Affected small intestinal epithelium
Altered mucus production
Malabsorption of vitamins and minerals
GI ulcers

Altered stress response
Dysregulated stress pathways
Increased cortisol levels (mouse model)
Altered 5-HT levels and receptor activity (human)

Chronic inflammation
Altered cytokine levels
Presence of autoantibodies directed
against brain and gut
Abnormalities in number and function of
different immune cell types

FIGURE 18.2 GI abnormalities, immune system dysfunction, stress and zinc deficiency may be highly linked processes contributing to the development of ASD

https://www.hindawi.com/journals/np/2015/972791/fig2/; https://www.hindawi.com/journals/np/2015/972791/#B3

reverse autism-related changes to the SHANK3 gene, improving neuronal communication that was previously weakened by changes to the gene.[156] This gene is associated with behavioural disorders and schizophrenia. The research of Yasuda and Tsutsui[155] also revealed an inverse relationship with zinc and toxic metals. Lower levels of zinc were found with increased levels of lead, aluminium and cadmium, indicating an association between toxic metal burden and zinc deficiency. Diarrhoea causes loss of zinc, and zinc deficiency results in morphological and functional changes of the intestinal epithelium and reduced activity of disaccharidases at the brush border[157] (see Fig. 18.2).

FOLATE

Folate is an important vitamin in ASD with epigenetic implications, being a key player in methylation reactions, the synthesis of nucleotides, metabolism of amino acids and production of neurotransmitters. The folate cycle is also required for the production of tetrahydrobiopterin (BH4), which is a cofactor for the synthesis of neurotransmitters such as serotonin and dopamine, the breakdown of phenylalanine and the production of nitric oxide.[158] BH4 has repetitively been found to be low in individuals with ASD. Prenatal deficiency of folate can increase autism risk as it influences maternal DNA methylation.[159] Cerebral folate deficiency is present in a significant subset of individuals with ASD, particularly infantile autism. The cerebral folate deficiency stems from a reduced ability to be able to transport folate to the brain (despite adequate systemic levels of folate). This appears to be due to the presence of autoantibodies to folate receptor alpha (FR-α) and low cerebral spinal fluid

methyl-tetrahydrofolate (5-MTHF). Using folinic acid or 5-MTHF (rather than folate or folic acid) supplementation bypasses several steps of folate metabolism and is better able to be transported across the blood–brain barrier. Ramaekers et al.[160] suggest starting at dosages of 0.5–1 mg/kg/day of folinic acid. If no therapeutic effect is seen at that dosage, then slow, gradual increments of dosage can be administered to achieve results. If genetic FR-α defects are present, dosages of 2–5 mg/kg/day may be required. Look for the natural L-stereoisomer rather than the synthetic DL form.

In a controlled study, 44 children with ASD and the FR-α autoantibody were treated with high doses of folinic acid (2 mg/kg/day in two divided doses, to a maximum of 50 mg/day). Four children discontinued due to adverse effects, three of whom were on risperidone and experienced increased irritability soon after starting the folinic acid. The fourth child experienced insomnia and gastro-oesophageal reflux after 6 weeks of treatment with folinic acid. In the 40 children remaining in the study, there were significant improvements over an average of 4 months in the areas of expressive and receptive language, verbal communication, attention and stereotypical behaviour.[161] Due to the adverse reactions in the three children taking resperidone, the authors suggested caution when using folinic acid in individuals already taking antipsychotic medications. An additional benefit of folinic acid supplementation is that it can increase glutathione metabolism as a treatment approach for oxidative stress. The L-stereoisomer of folinic acid has also been tested in adults with depression with positive outcomes for adults with SSRI-resistant depression.[162]

TABLE 18.7 Main clinical trials performed involving children on the effects of probiotics on neurological diseases		
Authors	**Study design**	**Main neurological results**
Parracho et al. 2010[165]	Randomised, double-blind, placebo-controlled study in children with ASD 3–16 years old treated with *L. plantarum* WCFS1 vs placebo for 3 weeks	Improvement of disruptive antisocial behaviours, anxiety and communication problems in probiotic arm
Kaluzna-Czaplinska et al. 2012[166]	Cohort study of children with ASD 4–10 years old treated with *L. acidophilus* strain Rosell-11 for 2 months	Improvement in their ability to concentrate and fulfil orders, with no impact on behavioural responses to other people's emotions or eye contact
Pärtty et al. 2015[167]	Randomised trial on infants followed for 13 years, giving *L. rhamnosus* GG vs placebo for the first 6 months of life	At the age of 13 years, 6 out of 35 (17.1%) children in the placebo group were diagnosed with ASD or attention deficit (hyperactivity) disorder, but none in the probiotic group were
Romeo et al. 2011[168]	Randomised trial in preterm infants treated with *L. reuteri* ATCC 55730 or *L. rhamnosus* ATCC 53103 or no supplementation for 6 weeks	Higher incidence of suboptimal neurological scores in the control group than in both the probiotic groups at 1 year of age

Source: Umbrello G, Esposito S. Microbiota and neurologic diseases: potential effects of probiotics. Journal of Translational Medicine 2016;14(1). doi: 10.1186/s12967-016-1058-7.

PROBIOTICS

Probiotics are defined as live microorganisms that upon digestion in specific and sufficient quantities confer health benefits to the host. Psychobiotics is a recently used term to describe a live microorganism that, when ingested in sufficient amounts, produces health benefits in patients with psychiatric illness.[163] Both probiotics and psychobiotics (referred to collectively from here as probiotics) are used to modulate immune and inflammatory responses via influences on Th1/Th2; to address gastrointestinal dysbiosis, diarrhoea and constipation; and to increase nutrient absorption.

Gut microbiota can elicit their effects on neurological function either directly via the bidirectional vagus nerve or by modulating pro- and anti-inflammatory cytokine production and activity. Metabolites produced by gut microbiota also have a significant influence on mitochondrial function, immune regulation and the gut–brain axis[164] (see Table 18.7).

Targeted probiotic therapy is advised in early stages of treatment rather than a broad spectrum approach. This is because overgrowths of commensal/beneficial bacteria may result in overproduction of metabolites that may adversely affect the host. For example, *Streptococcus* or *Lactobacilli* overgrowths may result in an excess production of D-lactic acid. With an inability to break down D-lactic acid due to dysbiosis, D-lactic acidosis can result, which can affect cognitive and mitochondrial function. In such a situation, D-lactate-free strains of probiotics, as well as those that aid in the breakdown of D-lactic acid, would make a wise choice. As such, a faecal microbial analysis and parasitology is advised prior to commencement of probiotic therapy. Failure to do this may result in either no benefit or a worsening of symptoms as a result of taking inappropriate probiotics.

Several studies on rats have showed some promise in the use of probiotics for neuropsychological symptoms. A study in 2011[169] demonstrated that *Lactobacillus rhamnosus* (JB-1) modulates GABA expression in the CNS and that the mode of action required an intact vagus nerve, indicating that neural transmission from the gut–brain axis was fundamental in producing the results. *L. rhamnosus* (JB-1) also reduced stress-induced corticosterone anxiety and depression-related behaviours. (See Fig. 18.3.)

Bacteroides fragilis (ATCC 9343) has been shown to correct intestinal permeability and correct tight junction alterations in tight junction and cytokine expression in maternal-immune-activated (MIA) offspring. It was also observed that *B. fragilis* ameliorated ASD-related behaviours including communicative, repetitive anxiety-like and sensorimotor behaviours. In addition, *B. fragilis* altered the metabolome, particularly in relation to two compounds that have potential relevance in the treatment of autism – indolepyruvate and 4-ethylphenylsulfate (4EPS, produced by some species of *Clostridia*, which is commonly elevated in children with autism and MIA offspring) – due to their effects on behaviour.[170]

A systematic review of 15 randomised controlled human trials and 25 animal trials showed that multiple strains of *Bifidobacterium* (*B. longum*, *B. breve* and *B. infantis*) and *Lactobacillus* (*L. helveticus* and *L. rhamnosus*) provided improvements in neuropsychiatric-disorder-related symptoms including memory abilities, anxiety, depression, ASD and obsessive compulsive disorder.[171]

A 2015 study indicated that maternal administration of *L. rhamnosus* GG from 4 weeks before expected delivery date, along with infant administration for the first 6 months of life, may reduce the risk of ASD and ADHD in offspring by mechanisms other than composition of the gut microbiota.[167]

B. longum NCC3001 demonstrated reversal of colitis-induced anxiety in mice,[172] while *B. breve* increased the fatty acid concentration of arachidonic acid and docosahexanoic acid in the brain, functions of which include neurodevelopment and protection from oxidative

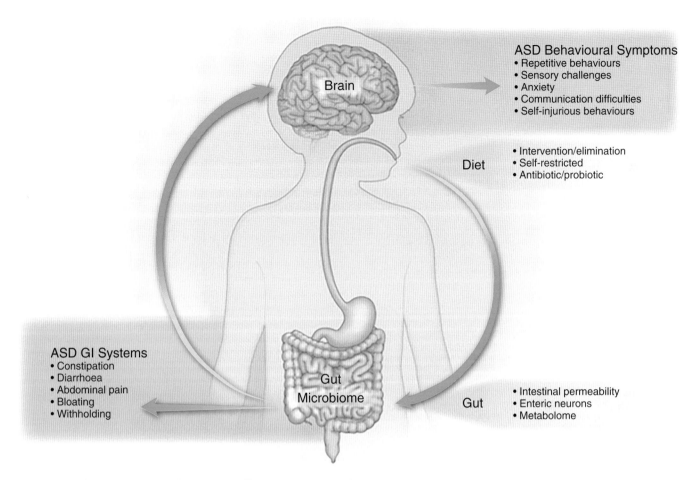

FIGURE 18.3 Mechanisms of probiotic effects on the central nervous system

stress, and deficiencies of which are known to influence depression, anxiety and memory.[173]

Saccharomyces boulardii is a helpful tool in the treatment of diarrhoea in individuals with ASD, and its inclusion in protocols against parasitic and *Clostridia* infections is very useful. *S. boulardii* can reduce the incidence of antibiotic-associated diarrhoea.[174,175]

VITAMIN A

Cod liver oil

Vitamin A is immune boosting and anti-infective, particularly against viruses. Some viral infections are associated with neurodegenerative and neurobehavioural disorders including ASD.[176,177] Vitamin-A-deficient mice exhibit major deficits in special learning and memory, so it will be interesting to see further research develop that can assess the benefit of vitamin A for cognitive function in ASD. Vitamin A also provides free radical scavenging benefits and reduces production of pro-inflammatory cytokines and chemokines by the microglia and astrocytes.[178,179] The vitamin A in cod liver oil occurs in a number of forms, increasing its stability when compared to the synthetic supplemental vitamin A. Vitamin D assists calcium absorption. Cod liver oil is excellent for general immune support, gut repair and prevention of recurrent infections such as otitis media. The fatty acids in cod liver

oil improve the flexibility of cell walls, improving nutrient supply and elimination of metabolic byproducts. DHA in particular is essential for normal neurological and visual development.

VITAMIN D

Being a neuroactive steroid, vitamin D affects brain development and function. Vitamin D is also protective against autoimmunity, involved in DNA repair, has anti-inflammatory function, stimulates antioxidant pathways and increases T regulatory cells.[180] In a 2015 meta-analysis of 11 studies including 870 ASD patients and 782 healthy controls, the ASD patients had significantly lower levels of vitamin D.[181] Poor maternal vitamin D, early childhood vitamin D deficiency, inadequate solar UVB exposure or perturbations of vitamin D enzyme activity can all result in a deficient vitamin D system and are risk factors in the development of ASD.

VITAMIN B$_6$

Pyridoxal-Phosphate (P5P)

Pyridoxal-5-phosphate (P5P) is the active form of pyridoxine hydrochloride (B$_6$) and is required for methylation and the folate cycle. It is involved in glucose regulation and the production of GABA, dopamine, serotonin, noradrenaline and melatonin[182] – all neurotransmitters or hormones that are often low or dysregulated in ASD populations. Even mild deficiency of B$_6$ can lead to downregulation of GABA and serotonin synthesis, resulting in disordered sleep.[182] Low levels of vitamin B$_6$ are inversely related to elevated levels of system markers of inflammation.[183] A large proportion of individuals with ASD have impaired ability to convert pyridoxine hydrochloride to P5P. Pyrroluria increases elimination of B$_6$, and supplementation with P5P and zinc often alleviates the symptoms of pyrroluria, such as depression, Jekyll and Hyde behaviour, emotional overwhelm, low stress tolerance and impulsivity.

METHYLATED B$_{12}$ (METHYLCOBALAMIN)

Processes of methylation and glutathione defence have been reported to be underfunctioning or low in children with ASD. As discussed previously, these deficits can result in children with ASD being more vulnerable to the effects of toxin exposure and stress of all kinds. As mentioned, there are several key nutrients required for the methylation process and adequate glutathione production to take place. These nutrients include vitamins B$_6$, B$_9$ and B$_{12}$. Zhang et al.[184] found low brain levels of vitamin B$_{12}$ in ASD (and schizophrenia and ageing). To compound this problem, for these B vitamins to be used in the methylation cycle, they themselves must be methylated into their active forms in order to be utilised. If methylation is underfunctioning, there can be insufficient conversion of these B vitamins into their active forms, further impeding the methylation process. Providing supplemental methylated B vitamins can help getting the methylation process going again, with the aim in the long term that the process will become self-regulated again. B$_{12}$ deficiency can also cause a functional folate deficiency.

A 2016 double-blind, placebo-controlled study of 50 children studied the impact of vitamin B$_{12}$ on autism symptoms and methylation capacity. Twenty-seven children received subcutaneous methyl B$_{12}$ injections, while 23 received subcutaneous saline injections. The subcutaneous route was chosen due to the opinion of physicians that this route was the most efficacious in their practices. Preliminary findings showed the methyl B$_{12}$ group had improved symptoms of ASD. These improvements were correlated with improvements in transmethylation metabolism. Those with the lowest baseline methionine status (i.e. the slowest methylators) showed the greatest improvements.[185]

VITAMIN C

Vitamin C neutralises free radicals, including hydroxyl radical, and regenerates vitamin E, which can then also be used to neutralise free radicals. It also elevates glutathione levels and is the most important antioxidant of all, and one that is commonly low in children with ASD. These antioxidant effects are exceptionally important as children with ASD have such high oxidative stress.[85,186–188] Vitamin C assists in the conversion of folic acid to the active form, folinic acid. It is a useful adjunct therapy when elevated HPL is present, and in high doses can be used to loosen stools and prevent faecal compaction.

CALCIUM

As most children undergoing biomedical treatment for ASD are on a casein-free diet, additional calcium supplementation may be required. In the study of 1967 children with autism by Yasuda and Tsutsui,[155] 5.8% were calcium deficient. Calcium is important for bone growth, cell signalling and hormone messenger systems.

MAGNESIUM

In the study of 1967 children with autism by Yasuda and Tsutsui,[155] 17.6% were magnesium deficient, making it the second most significant mineral deficiency in the ASD population (after zinc). Magnesium is essential for the conversion of methionine to SAM, the production of glutathione, and is an activator of phosphate and energy transfer enzymes, making it essential for energy production. It is involved in the methylation of serotonin to make melatonin, and so plays a role in sleep quality. Magnesium binds to GABA receptors, activating the receptors and increasing GABA activity. Improving GABA levels can improve symptoms such as insomnia, irritability, aggression, inattention, hyperactivity, nervousness and depression. Magnesium supports sulfation and is required to produce methylated adrenal hormones. Magnesium should be taken with B$_6$ to improve sulfation.[189]

POLYPHENOLS

Flavonoids (a subclass of polyphenols) hold potential for adjunctive treatment for ASD due to their anti-inflammatory and antioxidant activities. Luteolin, quercetin, rutin and epigallocatechin gallate (EGCG) are some such examples. Luteolin and quercetin inhibit the release of histamine, leukotrienes and inflammatory cytokines IL-8 and IL-6, as well as tumour necrosis factor (TNF). Luteolin is structurally related to 7,8-dihydroxyflavone, which has been shown to mimic brain-derived neurotrophic factor (BDNF), which may have a protective role in ASD.[190] BDNF regulates synaptic plasticity, neuronal differentiation and survival, and is often deleted in individuals with ASD and other neuropsychiatric and neurodegenerative disorders. Luteolin inhibits IL-6 release from activated microglia and is neuroprotective via its inhibition of microglial activation. In mouse brain models, luteolin protects against methylmercury-induced damage to mitochondria.[191]

Target of rapamycin (mTOR) regulates cell growth in response to nutrients, growth factors, cellular energy and stress. mTOR is upregulated to increase cell growth and energy when nutrients are abundant and stress is low. mTOR is important for cellular growth and energy, and also produces a lot of cellular waste, which is then mopped up via autophagy (the process of detoxification). Autophagy is initiated only once mTOR is downregulated, so detoxifcation cannot occur simultaneously with cell growth and increased energy production. Problems can occur when mTOR is continuously activated rather than cycled. When continuously activated, mTOR can result in neurodegeneration.[192] Dysregulated mTOR signalling is a phenotypic feature of some types of ASD and ASD-related syndromes, and inhibitors of mTOR are being investigated for the therapeutic potential in treating ASD.[193] Natural therapeutics shown to inhibit mTOR include epigallocatechin gallate (EGCG), resveratrol, curcumin and 3-diindolylmethane (DIM).[194] In a 2015 study, children with ASD were given a luteolin-containing supplement which resulted in reduced serum levels of TNF and IL-6 and correlated with improvements in ASD-related behaviours.[195]

N-ACETYLCYSTEINE (NAC)

N-acetylcysteine (NAC) is a form of the sulfur-containing amino acid cysteine, and is showing promise in a variety of areas of health, including that of ASD. A 2012 placebo-controlled study of 33 children aged 3.2–10.7 took NAC for 12 weeks (900 mg daily for 4 weeks, 900 mg twice daily for 4 weeks, then 900 mg 3 × daily or as tolerated for 4 weeks). The subjects had stable care and medications with no planned changes throughout the study period. Significant outcomes were observed in the treatment group of improvements on the Aberrant Behaviour Checklist (ABC) subscale for irritability. Reductions in hyperactivity, stereotypical and repetitive behaviours were also noted. Symptoms worsened in one patient.[196] In another similar-sized 2013 study, children had less irritability when on a combination of risperidone and NAC compared with risperidone alone or risperidone and placebo.[197] These effects may be due to glutamatergic effects of cysteine. Increasing extracellular cystine leads to lowering of the concentration of glutamate at the synapse. This may also be why NAC can be useful in diseases of addiction. NAC is also a powerful antioxidant and increases production of glutathione, which is regularly found to be low in populations with ASD. Improving glutathione levels may affect neurological function via its involvement in dopamine and glutamate regulation, neuroinflammation, neurogenesis and apoptosis, and mitochondrial function, as well as its antioxidant and immune-modulating activity.[198]

Use NAC with caution in individuals who have yeast/*Candida* overgrowth or infection as it may aggravate the condition.

DIMETHYLGLYCINE (DMG) AND TRIMETHYLGLYCINE (TMG)

Dimethylglycine and trimethylglycine act as methyl donors and can be useful for supporting methylation in some individuals. There is very limited research available. However, anecdotal evidence warrants a measured trial of these compounds (it is always best to start with low doses of anything that may upregulate methylation) in individuals with undermethylation and/or elevated homocysteine.

CARNITINE

Carnitine is an amino acid involved in energy production within the mitochondria and the conversion of fatty acids to ATP. A subset of individuals with autism have a gene variant that restricts the body's ability to produce carnitine. Problems can also occur with carnitine transport. Individuals with either of these dysfunctions in carnitine homeostasis may benefit from supplemental L-carnitine. Areas that commonly improve with L-carnitine

supplementation in these subsets of individuals include verbal and non-verbal communication, fatigue, using objects, fear and nervousness and interpersonal relationship skills. Delayed speech with low muscle tone appears to be a good indicator for potential responsiveness to carnitine (author's observations). A 2013 study of 213 children with ASD measured biomarkers of acquired mitochondrial dysfunction (which may be caused by the proprionic acid produced by enteric bacteria). In this study, 17% of the children demonstrated consistently abnormal acyl-carnitine abnormalities and glutathione metabolism abnormalities consistent with proprionic acid rat models.[29]

Dosage requirements

Use Clark's rule to determine dose, with adult doses listed below:
- Zinc: 30–100 mg per day, preferably towards the evening
- Cod liver oil: high vitamin varieties: ½–2 teaspoons per day. Regular strength: 1–4 teaspoons per day
- Vitamin C: 250–4000 mg per day, or to bowel tolerance for bowel cleanse
- Pyridoxal-5-phosphate (P5P): 50 mg per day, with food and preferably with some magnesium
- Magnesium: 100–400 mg per day
- Calcium: 600–900 mg per day.
- Folate: 200–800 micrograms:
  1 Folinic acid: starting at dosages of 0.5–1 mg/kg/day of folinic acid. If no therapeutic effect is seen at that dosage, then slow, gradual increments of dosage can be administered to achieve results. If genetic FR-α defects are present, dosages of 2–5 mg/kg/day may be required. Look for the natural L-stereoisomer rather than the synthetic DL form.
  2 L-5MTHF: 500 micrograms–15 mg/day. Always start low and gradually increase if need be. It is uncommon for more than 5 mg to be needed. Higher doses can be useful for depression and anxiety, but caution that high-dose B_9 does not cover B_{12} deficiency signs. L-5-MTHF requires lower dosages than D-5-MTHF.
- B_{12}: 500 micrograms–3 mg/day
NB Medical management required for higher dose prescriptions
- Vitamin D_3: 800–15 000 IU/day. Always provide with vitamins A and K (supplemental or grass-fed ghee and liver/cod liver oil). Only use high dosages when warranted, determined by 25-hydroxy-vitamin-D (25 OHD) blood test results.
- Polyphenols:
  1 Luteolin: 100 mg/10 kg.
  2 Quercetin: 12.5–25 mg/kg body weight per day (usually around 1100–2300 mg/day) if taken in isolation. Has synergistic effect when taken with other bioflavonoids.
  3 Rutin: 500–4000 mg/day
- NAC: 900–2700 mg/day
- TMG (betaine): 2500–6000 mg/day in divided dosages
- DMG: 125 mg 1–3 × daily
- Carnitine: 500–3000 mg/day
NB: Specific dosage for each child needs to be calculated based on their weight.

HERBAL MEDICINE

Herbal medicine therapeutic objectives

- Improve integrity of digestive lining
- Antimicrobials for gastrointestinal dysbiosis/candidiasis/parasitic infections
- Support liver function
- Stimulate digestion
- Improve immune function
- Treatment of acute infections
- Assist detoxification and elimination – lymphatic, liver, kidney, lung, dermal, bowels
- Reduce systemic inflammation
- Adrenal support
- Calm nervous system – promote parasympathetic function of autonomic nervous system
- Enhance cognition and learning abilities
- Neuroprotection
- Antioxidant support

Herbal medicine classes

Owing to the number of underlying syndromes present in ASD, virtually every herbal class may need to be employed at some stage during treatment – the whole materia medica comes into play. Immune modulators are required to address the many immunological dysfunctions present in children with ASD.[7] There may be underactive immunity in response to infections and a concomitant hyper-responsiveness to allergens. Vulneraries and mucous membrane trophorestoratives play a significant role in repair of gut wall and integrity of tissues in the inner ear, respiratory tract and urinary tract. Hepatostimulants and hepatorestoratives aid in liver function and help repair subclinical liver damage caused by toxic body burden. Depuratives and lymphatics aid in the detoxification process so crucial to the improvement and recovery of children with ASD. Bitters, cholagogues and digestive stimulants are required to promote proper digestion of foods, thereby reducing the load on an often already inflamed gastrointestinal tract and immune system. Anti-inflammatories are employed for any number of systems, depending on what syndromes the child is presenting with.

Specific herbal medicines

IMMUNE

Immune modulators used include Echinacea spp., Uncaria tomentosa, Bupleurum falcatum, Astragalus membranaceus (not during acute infections), Glycyrrhiza glabra, Scutellaria baicalensis (particularly when there are allergies) and Baptisia tinctoria.

Antimicrobial herbs are used frequently for gastrointestinal, respiratory, urinary and integumentary system infections, particularly *Calendula officinalis*, *Tabebuia avellanedae*, *Solidago virgaurea*, *Uncaria tomentosa*, *Echinacea* spp., *Arcostaphylos uva-ursi* and *Melissa officinalis*. *Berberis vulgaris* and *Hydrastis canadensis* are generally inadvisable for paediatric prescription. They are also unlikely to pass the GIT wall and are poorly effective for respiratory or urinary complaints. Parasite infections appear to be common in children with ASD, and considering the impact on immune function and increased inflammation that parasitic infections can elicit, resolving parasitic infections is very worthwhile, though not necessarily simple. Useful herbs to consider for parasite include pomegranate, walnut hulls, pumpkin seeds, wormwood, aniseed, garlic and clove. The seeds of papaya can be used fresh or dehydrated for a peppery-flavoured antiparasitic seasoning.

Whether for bacterial or yeast overgrowths of parasite infections, the biofilm protocol should be employed to help reduce likelihood of future recurrence. With restoring the microbiota, one must put therapeutic attention to changing the environment of the gut, as the environment plays a major role in the composition of gut flora. This means ensuring adequate digestive acid and enzyme production, addressing any gastrointestinal hyperacidosis, ensuring effective evacuation of bowels and a diet that supports growth of beneficial microbes.

HEPATOBILIARY

Liver support is often required, along with antioxidant support, making herbs such as *Silybum marianum* and *Rosmarinus officinalis* and *Curcuma longa* particularly useful. *Taraxacum officinale radix* is useful liver support when there is constipation present and *Bupleurum falcatum* is a useful hepatic herb to use when there is an acute infection. *Berberis vulgaris* is commonly used for liver support and for its berberine content, which is useful against overgrowth of organisms such as *Streptococcus* and *Clostridia* in the gut. *B. vulgaris* also stimulates digestion and bile production, resulting in a gastrointestinal environment that is more resistant to infection and inflammation. Other berberine-containing herbs such as *Hydrastis canadensis* are employed for the same reasons, as well as to dry up excessive mucus production and repair mucous membranes. *Calendula officinalis* is excellent for use in children and has many supportive actions in regards to immune and gastrointestinal integrity. *Calendula officinalis* is anti-inflammatory, antiseptic in the GIT, stimulates bile production and is vulnerary and astringent, helping to repair the gut wall and providing lymphatic support.

INFLAMMATION

Anti-inflammatory herbs include *Bupleurum falcatum* (particularly if there are signs of liver inflammation), *Calendula officinalis*, *Filipendula ulmaria* (meadowsweet), *Chamomilla recutita* and *Glycyrrhiza glabra*. They all provide anti-inflammatory support for the digestive tract. *Curcuma longa* provides excellent anti-inflammatory support and is also a hepatic and antioxidant herb, the latter action accentuating the anti-inflammatory effects. Herbs providing anti-inflammatory support for the urinary tract include *Agropyron repens* (couch grass), *Althaea officinalis* (marshmallow), *Plantago lanceolata* and *Solidago virgaurea* – the latter three also providing excellent anti-inflammatory support for the respiratory tract.

NEUROLOGICAL

Ginkgo biloba is an excellent herb for enhancing cognition (after 6 weeks of use) and provides powerful antioxidant support. The antioxidant *Rosmarinus officinalis* can also be used for enhancing cognitive function. *Bacopa monnieri* (bacopa) may be used for its adaptogenic, nervine, sedative and cognition-enhancing properties.

Adrenal and nervous system support are often required to dampen the sympathetic nervous system response and to enhance parasympathetic responses. Herbs used for this include *Withania somnifera*, *Astragalus membranaceus*, *Rehmannia glutinosa*, *Passiflora incarnata*, *Valeriana officinalis*, *Melissa officinalis*, *Scutellaria lateriflora* and *Lavandula officinalis*. Lion's mane (*Hericium erinaceus*) is showing promising anti-inflammatory and neuroprotective activity. It suppresses lipopolysaccharide-induced inflammation and protects against hydrogen peroxide oxidative stress.[199] This medicinal mushroom contains two types of compounds (hericenones and erinacines) known to stimulate nerve growth factor (NGF), and while more research needs to be done, there are promising indications for its use in a range of neurodegenerative disorders.[200] Erinacines are among the most powerful inducers of NGF in the natural world. *H. erinaceus* has been shown to improve cognitive function (including memory, attention and creativity), improve digestion, relieve gastritis and provide immunosupportive, anti-inflammatory and antioxidant functions, as well as modulating improvements in lipid profiles. All of these actions may support many of the underlying inflammatory, gastrointestinal, immunological and neurological features associated with ASD.

Lifestyle recommendations

Parents are usual overwhelmed by the amount of information covered in the initial consultation, and understandably so – there is a lot for them to take in. Therefore, lifestyle advice should remain very simple initially, focusing more on education in order for parents to solidify new information and fill in any gaps missed during the consultation. Send parents away with resources – websites and books on the basics of biomedical intervention as well as sources for recipes and meal ideas. The better informed and prepared the parent is, the easier it is for them to carry out biomedical intervention, as it does take considerable commitment.

EPSOM SALT BATHS

One simple lifestyle factor that may be suitable to start immediately is Epsom salt baths. Add 1 tablespoon–3 cups of Epsom salt to the child's warm bath. While there is very limited research available on the mechanism of action of Epsom salt baths, an unpublished study by Dr Waring at the University of Birmingham measured blood and urine sulfur and magnesium levels in 19 subjects before and after 12-minute Epsom salt baths, finding an increase in both after bathing in Epsom salts.[201] Both magnesium and sulfur aid in sulfation pathways, and magnesium is calming due to its role in GABA production. Epsom salt baths tend to be an effective adjunct treatment (in the author's clinical practice) for reducing histamine reactions. The reason for the wide dosage range is that some children react quite strongly to having the salts in the bath. It is

possible that in this scenario, sulfation/detoxifcation is being stimulated too quickly. In most of these children, starting off with a very small amount (e.g. 1 tablespoon) and slowly increasing appears to work well. For a very small subset of children, the salts tend to aggravate rather than help, no matter the dosage. The reason for this is not fully understood.

ESSENTIAL OILS

Baths are also a valuable time to employ therapeutic 100% essential oils if tolerated. Calming oils such as neroli (*Citrus aurantium*), chamomile (*Anthemis nobilis*), lavender (*Lavandula angustifolia*) and rose (*Rosa damascena* or *Rosa centifolia*) are very suitable for helping relaxation in children. Individuals with salicylate sensitivity may also be sensitive to essential oil components. Several studies (mostly animal studies) have shown that vetiver has both anxiolytic and nootropic effects and improves maintenance of attention during visual display tasks.[202–204] The ethanol extract of vetiver (*Chrysopogon zizanioides*) has also demonstrated anticonvulsant effects,[205] though no studies could be found as to whether the essential oil has the same effect.

ENEMAS

Enemas can be useful in helping to clear impacted faeces from the large intestine. They can also be used for stimulating detoxification, alkalising the bowel if there is acidosis present from overgrowth of D-lactic-acid-producing bacteria and delivering live probiotics to the area to improve the chances of colonisation. Enemas can be done with filtered water on its own, with added bicarb soda, apple cider vinegar or high-quality (ideally homemade) D-lactate-free coconut yoghurt. While not such a common modern therapeutic tool, anecdotal evidence shows safe and appropriately administered enemas can provide a very valuable tool in restoring gastrointestinal health and the gut microbiota and supporting detoxification. Caution of course needs to be exercised not to disrupt electrolyte levels. One case has been reported of a child with ASD receiving two water enemas (1 L each) daily over a period of months resulting in hypomagnesaemia presenting as tetany.[206]

OTHER THERAPIES

Patients may be using or benefiting from seeing practitioners of:
- occupational therapy (OT)
- speech therapy
- Tomatis Method – particularly useful for auditory processing problems
- The Son-Rise Program
- physical therapy
- art therapy
- applied behavioural analysis (ABA)
- hippotherapy (OT through horse riding)
- cognitive behavioural therapy (CBT)
- social skills training (for older children and adults).

CASE STUDY

OVERVIEW

TJ is a 4-year-and-3-month-old boy diagnosed with autism at 3.5 years of age. TJ was developing normally until 19 months of age, at which point he lost eye contact and stopped trying to use words and, in his mother's words, would regularly 'drift off to another place'. His parents cannot remember any significant responses to 18-month vaccinations except for a runny nose for a few weeks. In the past 8 months, he has had six bouts of otitis media with concomitant nasosinal congestion, requiring a course of antibiotics each time. He has been fed yoghurt in the belief that this will help protect against adverse effects of antibiotics. Since the second course of antibiotics, TJ has had wet, loose bowel motions 2–6 times daily. He has poor sleep, often waking two or three times per night and taking up to an hour to fall back to sleep.

TJ exhibits stimming behaviour of scribbling incessantly with pencils (fortunately on paper) and clapping his hands. He often stands, leaning over either parent's lap when they are sitting down.

TJ is described as being a fussy eater, his favourite foods being Vegemite on white toast, pasta with butter and salt and chicken nuggets.

TJ's father has a family history of rheumatoid arthritis; his mother has a history of vaginal thrush and IBS. His maternal aunt has asthma. TJ has no siblings yet, though his parents were planning for more children.

CLINICAL EXAMINATION

- Nails – white spots on 6 out of 10 finger nails
- Skin – dry, itchy, dermatographia, pale face, red ears, red cheeks
- Eyes – dark rings under eyes, puffiness under eyes, sideways glancing, poor eye contact
- Skinny with abdominal distension
- Fidgety, but looks tired
- Red ring around anus (described by mother)

TREATMENT PROTOCOL

INITIAL APPOINTMENT

- Education of parents of gut-immune-brain connection.
- Education on effects of artificial food additives.
- Explanation of T helper cell 1 (Th1) and T helper cell 2 (Th2) immunity in association with gut bacteria and eczema.
- Referrals for investigations – blood biochemistry (tier one), faecal microbial analysis.
- Explanation of benefits of fermented vegetables and instructions on how to make them.

HERBAL MEDICINE

Herbal formula for immune, digestive and nervous system support	
Echinacea spp. (1:2)	25 mL
Tabebuia avellanedae (1:2)	30 mL
Melissa officinale (1:2)	25 mL
Calendula officinalis (1:2)	20 mL
Total:	100 mL

Base on adult dose of 5 mL twice daily, calculate child dosage. (Twice daily is usually sufficient for infants and children.)

NUTRITIONAL MEDICINE

Dietary

- Introduction of fermented vegetables to reinoculate gut with beneficial bacteria.
- Introduction of bone broths to boost immunity and heal gut wall.
- Removal of artificial additives.
- Removal of any added sugars. Use xylitol instead (or stevia if xylitol aggravates loose bowels). Xylitol will help in the treatment of otitis media.[149]

Supplemental

- Each supplement was introduced one at a time, 4 days apart.
- Zinc picolinate: 60 mg at night time (start on 15 mg and increase by 15 mg once every 7 days until full dose is reached).
- High vitamin cod liver oil: 1 teaspoon per day for 1 week then 2 teaspoons daily for 1 week, and then back to 1 teaspoon daily.
- Probiotic providing 250 mg Saccharomyces boulardii, twice daily.

LIFESTYLE/EDUCATION

- Epsom salt baths every second night. Recommended reading:
- Gut and Psychology Syndrome by Dr Natasha Campbell-McBride
- Body Ecology Diet by Donna Gates Website site resources:
- www.mind.org
- www.autism.org Epsom salt baths every second night.

FOLLOW-UP

TJ came back 7 weeks later. He has been taking all his supplements (a little defiantly at first) and is on 1 teaspoon of fermented vegetables daily. He has not had any further bouts of otitis media and his bowels have slowed slightly to 2–3 bowel motions per day with a tendency to be soft. There is still obvious abdominal distension but it has reduced noticeably. He is slightly more settled and is waking less frequently during the night, although he still wakes once most nights. His parents are happy with progress so far, especially the absence of otitis media. No changes in autistic symptoms as yet.

The aim for this follow-up visit was to review all test results and implement the next stage of suitable diet changes, starting with the elimination of gluten and dairy. In light of test results, any significant deficiencies may be addressed with supplements, otherwise the focus will be on foods for the first few months to improve digestion and heal the gut so that all nutrients are better absorbed, and when specific supplements are required, that they are also absorbed.

Recommended reading

- *Gut and Psychology Syndrome* by Dr Natasha Campbell-McBride
- *Body Ecology Diet* by Donna Gates
- *Changing the Course of Autism* by Dr Bryan Jepsen
- *The Autism Revolution* by Martha Herbert MD
- *Nutrient Power: Health Your Biochemistry and Heal Your Brain* by William Walsh PhD
- *Mental and Elemental Nutrients: A Physician's Guide to Nutrition and Health Care* by Carl Pfeiffer

Website site resources

- www.mindd.org
- www.autism.org
- www.biobalance.org.au

ATTENTION DEFICIT (HYPERACTIVITY) DISORDER – AD(H)D

Epidemiology

Attention deficit (hyperactivity) disorder (AD(H)D) is estimated to affect between 3 and 20% of school-aged children, the average being 8–10%. AD(H)D is diagnosed using the DSM-V criteria (see Box 18.3).

Classification

AD(H)D is characterised by short or poor attention span and impulsivity, with or without hyperactivity. AD(H)D has academic, social and emotional ramifications,[207] and if untreated, it persists throughout adolescence and adulthood. Adolescents and adults with AD(H)D are more likely to suffer drug and alcohol addiction and have trouble maintaining employment.[208–210]

Aetiology

There are as many contributing factors to the epidemiology of AD(H)D as there are to ASD. As a result, many of the metabolic, immune and digestive factors discussed under ASD also apply here for ADHD. There is an element of heredity involved in AD(H)D, but twin studies confirm that genetics do not solely account for aetiology in AD(H)D.[211–213] Environmental factors play a significant role in pathogenicity.

FETAL EXPOSURE

Fetal lead, alcohol, marijuana and cigarette exposure are documented causes.[123,124,214–216] Immune discombobulation is common among children with AD(H)D, with a strong

---

BOX 18.3 DSM-5 criteria for ADHD

A. A persistent pattern of inattention and/or hyperactivity-impulsivity that interferes with functioning or development, as characterized by (1) and/or (2):

1. **Inattention:** Six (or more) of the following symptoms have persisted for at least 6 months to a degree that is inconsistent with developmental level and that negatively impacts directly on social and academic/occupational activities:

   Note: The symptoms are not solely a manifestation of oppositional behavior, defiance, hostility, or failure to understand tasks or instructions. For older adolescents and adults (age 17 and older), at least five symptoms are required.

   a) Often fails to give close attention to details or makes careless mistakes in schoolwork, at work, or during other activities (e.g., overlooks or misses details, work is inaccurate).

   b) Often has difficulty sustaining attention in tasks or play activities (e.g., has difficulty remaining focused during lectures, conversations, or lengthy reading).

   c) Often does not seem to listen when spoken to directly (e.g., mind seems elsewhere, even in the absence of any obvious distraction).

   d) Often does not follow through on instructions and fails to finish schoolwork, chores, or duties in the workplace (e.g., starts tasks but quickly loses focus and is easily side-tracked).

   e) Often has difficulty organizing tasks and activities (e.g., difficulty managing sequential tasks; difficulty keeping materials and belongings in order; messy, disorganized work; has poor time management; fails to meet deadlines).

   f) Often avoids, dislikes, or is reluctant to engage in tasks that require sustained mental effort (e.g., schoolwork or homework; for older adolescents and adults, preparing reports, completing forms, reviewing lengthy papers).

   g) Often loses things necessary for tasks or activities (e.g., school materials, pencils, books, tools, wallets, keys, paperwork, eyeglasses, mobile telephones).

   h) Is often easily distracted by extraneous stimuli (for older adolescents and adults, may include unrelated thoughts).

   i) Is often forgetful in daily activities (e.g., doing chores, running errands; for older adolescents and adults, returning calls, paying bills, keeping appointments).

2. **Hyperactivity and impulsivity:**

   a) Six (or more) of the following symptoms have persisted for at least 6 months to a degree that is inconsistent with developmental level and that negatively impacts directly on social and academic/occupational activities: Note: The symptoms are not solely a manifestation of

Continued

BOX 18.3 DSM-5 criteria for ADHD—cont'd

oppositional behaviour, defiance, hostility, or a failure to understand tasks or instructions. For older adolescents and adults (age 17 and older), at least five symptoms are required.

b) Often fidgets with or taps hands or feet or squirms in seat.

c) Often leaves seat in situations when remaining seated is expected (e.g., leaves his or her place in the classroom, in the office or other workplace, or in other situations that require remaining in place).

d) Often runs about or climbs in situations where it is inappropriate. (Note: In adolescents or adults, may be limited to feeling restless.)

e) Often unable to play or engage in leisure activities quietly.

f) Is often "on the go," acting as if "driven by a motor" (e.g., is unable to be or uncomfortable being still for extended time, as in restaurants, meetings; may be experienced by others as being restless or difficult to keep up with).

g) Often talks excessively.

h) Often blurts out an answer before a question has been completed (e.g., completes people's sentences; cannot wait for turn in conversation).

i) Often has difficulty waiting his or her turn (e.g., while waiting in line).

j) Often interrupts or intrudes on others (e.g., butts into conversations, games, or activities; may start using other people's things without asking or receiving permission; for adolescents and adults, may intrude into or take over what others are doing).

B. Several inattentive or hyperactive-impulsive symptoms were present prior to age 12 years.

C. Several inattentive or hyperactive-impulsive symptoms are present in two or more settings (e.g., at home, school, or work; with friends or relatives; in other activities).

D. There is clear evidence that the symptoms interfere with, or reduce the quality of, social, academic, or occupational functioning.

E. The symptoms do not occur exclusively during the course of schizophrenia or another psychotic disorder and are not better explained by another mental disorder (e.g., mood disorder, anxiety disorder, dissociative disorder, personality disorder, substance intoxication or withdrawal).

Specify whether:

314.01 (F90.2) Combined presentation: If both Criterion A1 (inattention) and Criterion A2 (hyperactivity-impulsivity) are met for the past 6 months.

314.00 (F90.0) Predominantly inattentive presentation: If Criterion A1 (inattention) is met but Criterion A2 (hyperactivity-impulsivity) is not met for the past 6 months.

314.01 (F90.1) Predominantly hyperactive/impulsive presentation: If Criterion A2 (hyperactivityimpulsivity) is met but Criterion A1 (inattention) is not met over the past 6 months.

Specify if:

In partial remission: When full criteria were previously met, fewer than the full criteria have been met for the past 6 months, and the symptoms still result in impairment in social, academic, or occupational functioning.

Specify current severity:

Mild: Few, if any, symptoms in excess of those required to make the diagnosis are present, and symptoms result in only minor functional impairments.

Moderate: Symptoms or functional impairment between "mild" and "severe" are present.

Severe: Many symptoms in excess of those required to make the diagnosis, or several symptoms that are particularly severe, are present, or the symptoms result in marked impairment in social or occupational functioning.

Source: https://images.pearsonclinical.com/images/assets/basc-3/basc3resources/DSM5_DiagnosticCriteria_ADHD.pdf.

---

tendency for Th2 dominance resulting in a high incidence of comorbidities such as asthma, eczema, allergies and food sensitivities. It is common for children with AD(H)D to have a history of recurrent otitis media, dark and puffy circles under the eyes, dyslexia, dyspraxia, obsessive or compulsive behaviours, dysbiosis, constipation and/or diarrhoea and cravings for certain foods – particularly sugary, carbohydrate and dairy foods (often driven by dysbiosis, intestinal hyperpermeability and poorly managed blood sugar levels).

AUTOIMMUNITY

Autoimmunity is associated with AD(H)D and other neurological disorders. Paediatric autoimmune neuropsychiatric disorder associated with streptococcus (PANDAS) is relatively common in children with AD(H)D. PANDAS results in transient exacerbations in symptoms such as obsessive compulsive behaviours, defiant behaviours and tics. The exacerbation of symptoms often, but not always, follows an overt group A streptococcal infection. There are no diagnostic tests to confirm PANDAS, though serum strep titres are often raised. Diagnosis of PANDAS is made on the following criteria:

1. presence of obsessive–compulsive disorder, AD(H)D symptoms and/or a tic disorder
2. paediatric onset of symptoms (age 3 years to puberty)
3. episodic course of symptom severity
4. association with group A beta-haemolytic streptococcal infection (a positive throat culture for strep or history of scarlet fever)
5. association with neurological abnormalities (motor hyperactivity, or adventitious movements, such as choreiform movements).

Investigations

Investigations in biochemistry are an excellent way of assessing nutritional and metabolic status and will alert of any problems, particularly with methylation, zinc and copper metabolism and iron absorption, all of which affect neurological development and neurotransmitter production, as well as immune status, which is often impaired or overactive.

FIRST-TIER TESTS

Urinary pyrroles

Signs of pyrroluria are very similar to those often attributed to AD(H)D, including impulsivity, lack of morning appetite, reading difficulties (e.g. dyslexia), mood swings and temper outbursts, explosive anger episodes, pale skin, stress intolerance, emotional sensitivity and anxiousness.

PCR stool test (parasitology)

This should be taken especially if allergy, inflammation or digestive factors are suspected to play a role and if allergy shiners (dark circles under the eyes) are present.

Blood tests

- Plasma zinc (using the Pfeiffer Center collection protocol)
- Serum copper
- Iron studies
- Full blood count
- Folate/B_{12}
- Vitamin D (25 OHD) Vitamin D_3 (25(OH)D_3)
- Blood glucose
- Insulin
- Streptococcal serology (especially if PANDAS is suspected)
- Serum creatinine (to assess kidney function, in case urinary toxic metal provocation test is indicated)
- hs-CRP
- ESR
- MTHFR and other SNPs
- Fasting homocysteine
- Faecal microbial analysis to assess gut flora composition and address gut–microbe–brain axis.

SECOND-TIER TESTS

- Hair mineral analysis or urinary toxic metals provocation test (the latter only in toilet trained children with confirmed healthy kidney function)
- Food allergy and sensitivity testing

Dietary factors

Diet, in particular sugars and synthetic food additives, has been proven to have a direct correlation with AD(H)D symptoms. Feingold first published his research in 1975 outlining the effects of additives on children with learning difficulties and hyperactivity.[217] It has now been confirmed that many synthetic food colours, flavours and preservatives are neurotoxic, although their use is still approved. Recent studies have shown that multiple food additives have a synergistic toxic effect far more pronounced than any of the individual additives on their own. This has been demonstrated with commonly occurring colour and preservative combinations[218] and with colours and flavourants.[219] In addition to this, many food additives contain heavy metals (lead, arsenic and mercury),[220] further adding to their neurotoxicity and possibly also adding to toxic synergistic effects with other food and environmental chemicals.

Clinically speaking, AD(H)D could be placed with asthma and eczema at the bottom end of the autism spectrum, meaning there are many common underlying metabolic, immune, digestive and neurological factors, the difference being the number of contributing factors and/or the severity of each factor. For further reading, please see the material on autism and ASD above.

Therapeutic considerations

CLINICAL DECISION MAKING AND RATIONALE

- Minimisation of medications:
  1. Support, in cooperation with a doctor, to reduce requirements for current medications
  2. Preventing the perceived need for medications
- Correction of nutritional deficiencies, particularly zinc, iron and B vitamins
- Normalisation of appetite
- Repair of digestive tract
- Restoration of healthy gut flora
- Support of methylation pathways if indicated
- Addressing urinary kryptopyrroles if indicated
- Rebalancing of immune function
- Cognitive support
- Parasympathetic nervous system support
- Heavy metal detoxification support
- Reduction in exposure to contributing environmental factors:
  1. Heavy metal exposure
  2. Artificial food additives
  3. Stress management and relaxation techniques
  4. Exposure to cigarette smoke
  5. Address allergies and sensitivities
  6. Screen time

Therapeutic application

NUTRITIONAL MEDICINE (DIETARY)

Specific dietary considerations

ADDITIVES

First and foremost, the removal of additives from the diet is called for. This simple step on its own often brings about drastic improvements – for some, this will resolve all symptoms of AD(H)D and no further specific treatment may be required.

SUGAR

Sugar cravings and high sugar intake are associated with hyperactivity, depression, moodiness and AD(H)D. Sugar cravings are an indication of a physiological dysfunction, so the aim should be the identification and resolution of the cause of the cravings rather than the abstinence approach, which usually fails. Chromium is often used to regulate blood sugar levels; however, this is rarely enough, or the ideal first approach. Sugar craving is a good indication of dysbiosis, which can be confirmed by a number of tests, predominantly faecal microbial analysis and/or comprehensive digestive stool analysis. The introduction of homemade lactofermented foods is a powerful way effectively to reduce sugar cravings and to develop the palate to a point where a wider range of flavours are enjoyed, or at least tolerated by previously fussy eaters.

BODY ECOLOGY DIET (BED), GUT AND PSYCHOLOGY SYNDROME DIET (GAPS) AND THE PALEO DIET

A low-glycaemic-load diet will help with blood sugar regulation and is also indicated if dysbiosis is suspected or confirmed. In the case of dysbiosis, a diet such as the body ecology diet (BED) and/or gut and psychology syndrome diet (GAPS) and/or a high plant-based paleo diet, all of which are low in starch and di- and polysaccharides, is indicated.

PHENOL/SALICYLATE/GLUTAMATE SENSITIVITY

Some children may need briefly to go on a low phenol, glutamate or oxalate diet. Often these children have heavy metal burden impacts on the detoxification pathways (e.g. sulfation and methylation) that phenols such as salicylates stimulate. Often addressing the underlying burden and promoting sulfation and methylation will resolve the phenol/salicylate sensitivity.

WHOLEFOOD PRINCIPLES

Eventually the diet needs to be focused on nutrient-dense wholefoods, with a focus on proteins and non-starchy vegetables, grains such as millet, quinoa, buckwheat and amaranth, legumes if tolerated and a limited amount of fruit (maximum of two pieces per day). Dietary changes should be made one step at a time, only introducing a new change when the previous has become habit. This ensures changes are manageable and sustainable, becoming part of the individual's, or the family's, lifestyle.

Dietary inclusions

- Fermented foods – fermented vegetables, water kefir, young coconut kefir, possibly milk kefir (depending on gut integrity)
- All fresh meats, no deli meats unless they are organic and free of all artificial food additives
- Bone broths as a drink with meals and/or in cooking
- All non-starchy vegetables
- Millet, quinoa, buckwheat, amaranth if tolerated (whole not puffed or flaked)
- Maximum two pieces of fruit per day (with exception of a greater quantity of organic berries allowed if tolerated – they are very high in antioxidant and anti-inflammatory activity while being low in sugar)

SAMPLE DAILY DIET

BREAKFAST

- Bone-broth-based soup or casserole with vegetables and chicken
  OR
- Soaked buckwheat pancakes
  OR
- Eggs any way or grain-free organic sausages with fermented vegetables and avocado
  OR
- Dinner leftovers

LUNCH

- Dinner leftovers
  OR
- Coconut flour crêpes with fillings
  OR
- Mini chicken satays and vegetables/salad
  OR
- Chicken salad

DINNER

- Stuffed capsicums (stuffed with savoury mince) and cooked green vegetables or salad drizzled with olive or flax oil and balsamic vinegar
  OR
- Meat cutlets and vegetables
  OR
- Baked crispy skin spiced chicken with salad
  OR
- Broth-based soup or casserole with meat and vegetables

SNACKS

- Vegetable sticks and additive-free hummus
- Soaked crunchy sea-salted nuts
- Apple and cinnamon muffin (made with almond flour)
- Tasty liver meatballs (do not tell them and they will never know there is liver in there!)
- Seaweed snacks
- Smaller serves of main meal options
- Avocado and/or olives to provide good fats

BEVERAGES

- Xylitol-sweetened herbal tea cordials such as:
  1. Lavender
  2. Peppermint and spearmint
  3. Lemon balm with a squeeze of fresh lemon
- Pure water
- Water kefir
- Coconut water kefir

Dietary exclusions

- Added sugar, soft drinks, etc.
- Artificial food additives
- Processed grain flour products – pasta, cakes, cookies, baked goods, puffed and flaked grains
- Shop-bought fruit juices, cordials, fruit drinks
- Chips and other junk foods
- Gluten, dairy and any known food sensitivities or allergies

NUTRITIONAL MEDICINE (SUPPLEMENTAL)

Nutrient supplementation will depend on the subclass or combination of aetiological factors. However, there are a few commonly featured nutrients in the treatment of AD(H)D. Also refer to 'Nutritional medicine' for information on folate, B_{12}, polyphenols, NAC, TMG and more, as there are many metabolic commonalities.

Zinc

The phrase 'no zinc no think' applies perfectly to children with AD(H)D. Zinc status is often deficient in children with AD(H)D.[221,222] Zinc plays essential roles in neurotransmitter, neurological, immune and digestive function. Zinc supplementation has been shown to reduce impulsivity and hyperactivity.[223] Zinc is the primary nutrient required for methylation, along with magnesium, B_6, DMG and folinic acid.

Iron

Low serum ferritin levels are associated with AD(H)D symptoms,[224] and symptoms have improved with supplementation, even in non-anaemic children.[225] Reduced ferritin levels may be due to impaired digestion as a result of zinc deficiency, mucosal immune inflammation or dysbiosis featuring an overgrowth of iron-consuming microbes such as *Streptococcus* and *Clostridia*.

Essential fatty acids

Essential fatty acids have been studied extensively and overall provided very positive results in addressing focus and concentration in AD(H)D.[226] Studies have confirmed that children with AD(H)D have lower levels than non-AD(H)D children of omega-3 fatty acids. Essential fatty acids provide anti-inflammatory support, and by increasing fluidity of cell membranes, they improve communication between cells and assist in efficient detoxification. Cod liver oil is the oil of choice. Not only does it contain EPA and DHA, it also has valuable vitamins D and A, both of which are often low in children with AD(H)D. Vitamins A and D play important roles in immune function, and so greatly help children with skewed immunology and recurrent infections. Children with pyrroluria may become more irritated on omega-3 fatty acids and benefit more from taking omega-6 fatty acids.

Magnesium

Magnesium is often low in children with hyperactivity, cognitive and mood disorders, and can result in tics, anxiety, depression, headaches and poor appetite. Magnesium plays a critical role in the pathways of methylation and sulfation and is therefore critical to the detoxification process often so important for children with AD(H)D. Deficiencies of magnesium, zinc and B vitamins, particularly B_6 and folate, result in reduced levels of dopamine, which is often low in children with AD(H)D. B_6 may need to be provided in its active form, P5P.

Vitamin B$_6$

P5P, or vitamin B6, is involved in metabolism of polyunsaturated fatty acids, haemoglobin synthesis and neurotransmission. It is a cofactor in the metabolism of dopamine, serotonin, glutamate and GABA, and as a result, deficiencies in this vitamin can have a negative influence on mood, behaviour and cognition.[227] Supplementing with B_6, often in its active form of P5P, can have positive outcomes in mood, hyperactivity, impulsivity and other symptoms associated with both ADHD and urinary kryptopyrroles.

Vitamin D

Data associating low vitamin D with ADHD is lacking. However, a 2014 study of 1331 children in Qatar indicated that there is a higher prevalence of vitamin D deficiency among children with ADHD compared to controls.[228] Vitamin D promotes normal brain development, enhances neuroprotection, modulates matrix metalloproteinases and anti-inflammatory mechanisms and boosts glutathione production in the brain. Animal studies have shown that vitamin D deficiency alters behaviours and locomotion, reflective of behaviours in children with ADHD. Vitamin D deficiency is common around the world, even in areas of the globe that are not sunshine limited. This is believed to be due to limited sun exposure due to extreme climate or lifestyle factors such as clothing type, increase in indoor activities and fewer outdoor activities, and fastidious use of sun-blocking agents. The 2014 study by Kamal et al.[228] indicated that vitamin D therapy via sunshine or supplementation may be warranted in children with ADHD and vitamin D deficiency.

L-theanine

L-theanine is a non-protein amino acid that readily crosses the blood–brain barrier. In 2011, a double-blind, placebo-controlled study was carried out to investigate L-theanine's effect on sleep in children with AD(H)D. Forty-six children between 8 and 12 years of age were given 400 mg of L-theanine daily (200 mg morning, 200 mg afternoon). Compared with the control group (47 children), there was no significant difference in sleep latency or total sleep time, but there was a significant improvement in sleep efficiency and a reduction in nocturnal activity.[229]

Aside from improvements in sleep quality, L-theanine has a number of actions, making it a useful tool in addressing the symptoms of ADHD. It has anti-anxiolytic effects due to upregulation of GABA and possible modulation of serotonin and dopamine. Brain-derived neurotrophic factor is increased with use of L-theanine, and studies show that it is neuroprotective. In both animal and human studies, L-theanine promotes improved cognition, including learning and memory. Interestingly, L-theanine produces selective alpha brain wave activity, much like meditation does, resulting in calmer and more focused behaviour.[230]

Probiotics

Probiotics are essential in virtually every child with AD(H)D. The high prevalence of digestive dysbiosis and immune imbalance indicates the need for beneficial bacteria to help restore digestive and immune function. Ideally, a stool test (faecal microbial analysis) is carried out to determine which beneficial microbes are missing, and which opportunistic or pathogenic microbes are overgrown, so that probiotic therapy can be targeted at specific needs.

Other

Antioxidant nutrients are often called for when there is evidence of neural, digestive or immune oxidative stress. Nutrients to consider include vitamin E, vitamin C, NAC, N-acetylcarnitine, CoQ10, B vitamins and polyphenols such as luteolin, pine bark extract and quercetin, which may be required for increased mitochondrial function and energy production. Vitamin C and vitamin A, magnesium and potassium support adrenal function, essential in a sympathetic dominant autonomic nervous system. For heavy metal detoxification, nutrients such as vitamin C, selenium, NAC, TMG, DMG, zinc and folate may also need to be considered.

Dosage requirements

Use Clark's rule to determine dose, with adult doses listed below:
Iron: 10–30 mg/day
Zinc: 30–100 mg/day
Magnesium: 100–400 mg/day
B6 (P5P): 10–50 mg/day
Vitamin D: 800–15 000 IU/day (calculate dose pending blood test results)
L-theanine: 200–600 mg/day (200–400 mg dose fine for children)

HERBAL MEDICINE

Herbal medicine therapeutic objectives

- Balance immune function
- Repair gastrointestinal integrity/hyperpermeability
- Resolve gastrointestinal dysbiosis
- Improve cognitive function
- Provide antioxidant and liver support
- Improve quality of sleep
- Improve energy levels while reducing hyperactivity
- Adrenal support
- Promoting parasympathetic nervous system response

Herbal medicine classes

Initial treatment often requires adrenal and parasympathetic nervous system support as well as digestive support. Nervines and adaptogens feature prominently. Sedative herbs may also be employed to improve sleep quality, and at lower doses may be used to promote calmness during the day. Use of mucous membrane trophorestoratives, vulneraries, digestive stimulants and antimicrobials addresses gastrointestinal pathologies involved in the pathogenesis of AD(H)D. Other primary classes of herbs are cognition enhancers, antioxidants and inflammatories.

Specific herbal medicines
NEUROLOGICAL

Excellent herbs shown to be effective for improving focus and concentration include *Ginkgo biloba* (ginkgo) and *Bacopa monnieri* (bacopa). *Rosmarinus officinalis* (rosemary) stimulates cognitive function and supports phase 2 liver detoxification, relevant for many AD(H)D children, though for some children rosemary may be too stimulating. *Hericium erinaceus* (lion's mane) improves cognitive function (including memory, attention and creativity). Adaptogens such as *Withania somnifera* (withania), *Astragalus membranaceus* (astragalus), *Glycyrrhiza glabra* (liquorice) and *Rehmannia glutinosa* (rehmannia) help increase tolerance to stress, build immune function and aid sleep. Nervines such as *Melissa officinalis* (lemon balm), *Matricaria recutita* (chamomile), *Valeriana officinalis* (valerian) and *Passiflora incarnata* (passionflower) help to dampen the sympathetic response, promoting calm behaviour and restful sleep.

DIGESTIVE

Herbs to consider for digestive repair and stimulation include *Hydrastis canadensis* (goldenseal), *Calendula officinalis* (calendula), *Berberis vulgaris* (barberry) and *Silybum marianum* (St Mary's thistle). The berberine in *Hydrastis canadensis*, *Berberis vulgaris* and *Arctostaphylos uva-ursi* is useful for addressing several intestinal microbial overgrowths, including *Clostridia* and *Streptococcus*. Antioxidant herbs such as *Silybum marianum*, *Rosmarinus officinalis*, *Curcuma longa* (turmeric), *Ginkgo biloba*, *Olea europa* (olive leaf) and pycnogenol can provide protection and repair from oxidative damage to liver, gastrointestinal tract and nervous system. Suitable immune herbs include *Echinacea* spp., *Uncaria tomentosa* (cat's claw), *Andrographis paniculata* (andrographis), *Glycyrrhiza glabra* and *Astragalus membranaceus* (do not use astragalus during acute infections). *Andrographis paniculata*, *Curcuma longa*, *Glycyrrhiza glabra* and *Astragalus membranaceus* also provide liver support and *Andrographis paniculata* stimulates secretion of digestive acids, improving digestion.

CASE STUDY

OVERVIEW

SB is a 12-year-old girl in her first year of high school. She is having trouble keeping up with school work as she struggles with dyslexia, nervousness and hyperactivity. She cannot complete homework without the constant assistance of her parents. Normally of a happy and affectionate temperament, she can become easily frustrated, has a low stress tolerance and can 'snap', becoming quickly upset or angry. Her family doctor has recommended commencing the use of Ritalin owing to concerns of academic struggle through high school. SB's parents are hesitant to start this treatment and would prefer to find an alternative approach.

SB has trouble falling asleep as she says she cannot stop thinking. It takes about an hour for her to fall asleep. Once asleep she sleeps through the night, but does not recall her dreams. She wakes feeling tired and has no appetite for breakfast, often skipping it or having only half a glass of full-strength shop-bought orange juice. At school she has trouble focusing and concentrating on the task at hand. She enjoys music lessons the most, particularly the practical aspect, sometimes struggling with theory.

SB has had mild to moderate eczema since she was 2 years old. Hydrocortisone cream is applied when the eczema flares up (use on average is for about 7 days in a row, once every 3–6 weeks). She also has verrucas growing on knuckles of both hands, which have been there for the past 3 years. In between skin is moisturised with sorbolene.

Bowel motions are on average once per day, although once or twice a week she will go a day without a bowel motion. They usually feel incomplete.

SB craves anything sweet, chocolate and salty chips.

Parents' primary concern is SB's ability to focus and concentrate. They are interested in treatments for eczema and warts, but not right now.

Relevant family history: younger brother has asthma and eczema. Mother has asthma.

CLINICAL EXAMINATION

- Pale skin
- Dark circles under eyes
- White spots on three finger nails
- Dry skin
- Underweight

TREATMENT PROTOCOL

INITIAL APPOINTMENT

Referral for investigations
- Urinary HPL (pyrroles)
- Blood tests
- Plasma zinc (Pfeiffer Center collection protocol)
- Serum copper
- Iron studies
- Full blood count
- Vitamin D
- B$_{12}$/folate

- Strep serology
- Serum creatinine
- Faecal microbial analysis

HERBAL MEDICINE

- Passiflora incarnata (1:2) 20 mL
- Withania somnifera (1:1) 40 mL
- Rosmarinus officinalis (1:2) 30 mL
- Taraxacum officinale radix (1:2) 40 mL
- Bacopa monnieri (1:2) 80 mL
- Dose: 5 mL twice daily
- Total 210 mL

NUTRITIONAL MEDICINE

Dietary

- Introduction of fermented vegetables
- Elimination of artificial food additives
- Elimination of sugar. Replace with xylitol
- Increase water to 6–8 glasses per day. Make herbal tea (e.g. lemon balm, peppermint and spearmint) or freshly squeezed lemon cordials using xylitol to sweeten.

Supplemental

- Zinc picolinate: 60 mg at night time – start as soon as urinary pyrrole test has been completed
- P5P: 50 mg per day, with a meal, preferably breakfast or lunch
- Magnesium: 150 mg daily
- High-vitamin-fermented cod liver oil: 1 teaspoon daily (or double for regular strength cod liver oil)

LIFESTYLE/EDUCATION

- Education about the gut–immune–brain connection, including Th1 and Th2 immune function and linking this to AD(H)D, warts and eczema
- Significance of biochemical investigations
- Significance of faecal microbial analysis (i.e. microbiota effects on neurotransmitter production and immune function)
- Recommended reading: *Gut and Psychology Syndrome* by Dr Natasha Campbell-McBride

FOLLOW-UP

6 weeks later.

SB is feeling calmer and more stable, a little less anxious, and is finding focus and concentration are beginning to improve, though she can still get frustrated, particularly with reading and writing. Sleep has improved significantly, only having trouble falling asleep if there is additional stress present. Dream recall has improved and SB now remembers her dreams most nights. Although a little better, she is still waking quite tired and struggles to get out of bed. Morning appetite has improved slightly and she now has either one egg for breakfast or a piece of toast with butter and peanut butter. She is now having roughly 3 teaspoons of fermented vegetables per day and has grown accustomed to the flavour and does not mind having it with any of her meals.

CASE STUDY CONTINUED

Plan: Review all test results. Parents have a much better idea of the gut–immune–brain connection and are eager to begin treatment in this direction.
Protocol:
- Add L-theanine: 200 mg capsule 30 minutes before bed to improve sleep quality
Further testing:
- Bioscreen faecal microbial analysis and parasitology (not previously completed, but now parents motivated to follow up)

REFERENCES

[1] American Psychiatric Association. Diagnostic and statistical manual of mental disorders. 5th ed. Arlington, VA: American Psychiatric Association; 2013.

[2] Australian Bureau of Statistics. 4428.0 – Autism in Australia, 2012; 2012. Available from: https://www.abs.gov.au/ausstats/abs@.nsf/Latestproducts/4428.0Main%20Features32012?opendocument&tabname=Summary&prodno=4428.0&issue=2012&num=&view=.

[3] National Disability Insurance Scheme. Report to COAG Disability Reform Council 30 June 2016 (Quarter 4, year 3). Available from: https://www.ndis.gov.au/about-us/publications/quarterly-reports.

[4] Christensen DL, Baio J, Van Naarden Braun K, et al. Prevalence and characteristics of autism spectrum disorder among children aged 8 years – Autism and Developmental Disabilities Monitoring Network, 11 sites, United States, 2012. MMWR Surveill Summ 2016;65(SS–3):1–23.

[5] Yates K, Le Couteur A. Diagnosing autism. Paediatr Child Health 2009;19(2):55–9.

[6] Jepson B, Johnson J. Changing the course of autism. Boulder, Colorado: Sentient Publications; 2007.

[7] Stigler KA, Sweeten TL, Posey DJ, et al. Autism and immune factors: a comprehensive review. Res Autism Spectr Disord 2009;3(4):840.60.

[8] Christensen J, Grønborg TK, Sørensen MJ, et al. Prenatal valproate exposure and risk of autism spectrum disorders and childhood autism. JAMA 2013;309(16):1696. doi:10.1001/jama.2013.2270.

[9] Boukhris T, Bérard A. Selective serotonin reuptake inhibitor use during pregnancy and the risk of autism spectrum disorders: a review. J Pediatr Genet 2015;4(2):84–93. doi:10.1055/s-0035-1556744.

[10] Bauer AZ, Kriebel D. Prenatal and perinatal analgesic exposure and autism: an ecological link. Environ Health 2013;12(1):doi:10.1186/1476-069x-12-41.

[11] Horvath K, Papadimitriou JC, Rabsztyn A, et al. Gastrointestinal abnormalities in children with autistic disorder. J Pediatr 1999;135:533–5.

[12] Alberti A, Pirrone P, Elia M, et al. Sulphation deficit in 'low-functioning' autistic children: a pilot study. Biol Psychiatry 1999;46:420–4.

[13] Finegold SM, Molitoris D, Song Y, et al. Gastrointestinal microflora studies in late-onset autism. Clin Infect Dis 2002;35(Suppl. 1):S6–16.

[14] D'Eufemia P, Celli M, Finocchiaro R, et al. Abnormal intestinal permeability in children with autism. Acta Paediatr 1996;85(9):1076–9.

[15] Knivsberg A, Reichelt K, Hoien T, et al. A randomized, controlled study of dietary intervention in autistic syndromes. Nutr Neurosci 2002;5:251–61.

[16] Knivsberg A, Reichelt K, Nodland M, et al. Autistic syndromes and diet: a follow-up study. Scand J Educ Res 1995;39:223–36.

[17] Ashwood P, Anthony A, Pellicer AA, et al. Intestinal lymphocyte populations in children with regressive autism: evidence for extensive mucosal immunopathology. J Clin Immunol 2003;23(6):504–17.

[18] Ashwood P, Anthony A, Torrente F, et al. Spontaneous mucosal lymphocyte cytokine profiles in children with autism and gastrointestinal symptoms: mucosal immune activation and reduced counter regulatory interleukin-10. J Clin Immunol 2004;24(6):666–73.

[19] Wakefield AJ, Ashwood P, Limb K, et al. The significance of ileo-colonic lymphoid nodular hyperplasia in children with autistic spectrum disorder. Eur J Gastroenterol Hepatol 2005;17(8):827–36.

[20] Ashwood P, Wakefield AJ. Immune activation of peripheral blood and mucosal CD3+ lymphocyte cytokine profiles in children with autism and gastrointestinal symptoms. J Neuroimmunol 2006;173(1–2):126–34.

[21] Wilner AN. Elevated TNF found in CSF of autistic children. CNS News 2007;9:4.

[22] Frye RE, Rose S, Slattery J, et al. Gastrointestinal dysfunction in autism spectrum disorder: the role of the mitochondria and the enteric microbiome. Microb Ecol Health Dis 2015;26:doi:10.3402/mehd.v26.27458.

[23] Bolte ER. Autism and Clostridium tetani. Med Hypotheses 1998;51(2):133–44.

[24] Shaw W, Chaves E. Experience with organic acid testing to evaluate abnormal microbial metabolites in the urine of children with autism. Proceedings of 1996 ASA Conference. Milwaukee, WI, July 13; 1996.

[25] Rapin I. Autistic children: diagnosis and clinical features. Pediatrics 1991;81(5 Pt 2):751–60.

[26] Gillberg C, Coleman M. The biology of the autistic syndromes. 2nd ed. New York: Cambridge University Press; 1992.

[27] Olsson I, Steffenburg S, Gillberg C. Epilepsy in autism and autistic-like conditions: a population-based study. Arch Neurol 1988;45(6):666–8.

[28] Smith EA, Macfarlane GT. Studies on amine production in the human colon: enumeration of amine forming bacteria and physiological effects of carbohydrate and pH. Anaerobe 1996;2:285–97.

[29] Frye R, Melnyk S, MacFabe D. Unique acyl-carnitine profiles are potential biomarkers for acquired mitochondrial disease in autism spectrum disorder. Transl Psychiatry 2013;3(1):e220.

[30] MacFabe D. Autism: metabolism, mitochondria, and the microbiome. Glob Adv Health Med 2013;2(6):52–66. doi:10.7453/gahmj.2013.089.

[31] Loubinoux J, Valente FMA, Pereira IAC, et al. Reclassification of the only species of the genus Desulfomonas, Desulfomonas pigra, as Desulfovibrio piger comb. nov. Int J Syst Evol Microbiol 2002;52:1305–8.

[32] Loubinoux J, Jaulhac B, Piemont Y, et al. Isolation of sulfate-reducing bacteria from human thoracoabdominal pus. J Clin Microbiol 2003;41(3):1304–6.

[33] Geier DA, Kern JK, Garver CR, et al. Biomarkers of environmental toxicity and susceptibility in autism. J Neurol Sci 2009;280(1–2):101–8.

[34] Campbell-McBride N. Gut and psychology syndrome. Cambridge: Medinform Publishing; 2004.

[35] Strous RD, Golubchik P, Maayan R, et al. Lowered DHEA-S plasma levels in adult individuals with autistic disorder. Eur Neuropsychopharmacol 2005;15:305–9.

[36] Adams JB, Romdalvik J, Levine KE, et al. Mercury in first-cut baby hair of children with autism vs. typically developing children. Toxicol Environ Chem 2008;90(4):739–53.

[37] Adams JB, Romdalvik J, Ramanujam VM, et al. Mercury, lead, and zinc in baby teeth of children with autism versus controls. J Toxicol Environ Health 2007;70(12):1046–51.

[38] Desoto MC, Hitlan RT. Blood levels of mercury are related to diagnosis of autism: a reanalysis of an important data set. J Child Neurol 2007;22:1308–11.

[39] Geier DA, Geier MR. A case series of children with apparent mercury toxic encephalopathies manifesting with clinical symptoms of regressive autistic disorders. J Toxicol Environ Health A 2007;70:837–51.

[40] Sajdel-Sulkowska EM, Lipinski B, Windom H, et al. Oxidative stress in autism: elevated cerebellar 3-nitrotyrosine levels. Am J Biochem Biotech 2008;4:73–84.

[41] Martino D, Defazio G, Giovannoni G. The PANDAS subgroup of tic disorders and childhood-onset obsessive–compulsive disorder. J Psychosom Res 2009;67(6):547–57.

[42] Pangborn J, MacDonald Baker S. Autism: effective biomedical treatments. San Diego, CA: Autism Research Institute; 2005.

[43] Boonacker E, Van Noorden C. The multifunctional or moonlighting protein CD26/DPPIV. Eur J Cell Biol 2003;82(2):53–73.

[44] Yaron A, Naider F. Proline-dependent structural and biological properties of peptides and proteins. Crit Rev Biochem Mol Biol 1993;28:31–81.

[45] Rose M, Hildebrandt M, Fliege H, et al. T-cell immune parameters and depression in patients with Crohn's disease. J Clin Gastroenterol 2002;34:40–8.

[46] Maes M, Bonaccorso S, Marino V, et al. Treatment with interferon-alpha (IFN-alpha) of hepatitis C patients induces lower serum dipeptidyl peptidase IV activity, which is related to IFN alpha-induced depressive and anxiety symptoms and immune activation. Mol Psychiatry 2001;6:475–80.

[47] Maes M, Capuron L, Ravaud A, et al. Lowered serum dipeptidyl peptidase IV activity is associated with depressive symptoms and cytokine production in cancer patients receiving interleukin-2-based immunotherapy. Neuropsychopharmacology 2001;24:130–40.

[48] Polgar L. Structural relationship between lipases and peptidases of the prolyl oligopeptidase family. FEBS Lett 1992;311:281–4.

[49] Hildebrandt M, Rose M, Ruter J, et al. Dipeptidyl peptidase IV (DP IV, CD26) in patients with inflammatory bowel disease. Scand J Gastroenterol 2001;36:1067–72.

[50] Schmitz T, Underwood R, Khiroya R, et al. Potentiation of the immune response in HIV-1 individuals. J Clin Invest 1996;97:1545–9.

[51] Maes M, De Meester I, Scharpe S, et al. Alterations in plasma dipeptidyl peptidase IV enzyme activity in depression and schizophrenia: effects of antidepressants and antipsychotic drugs. Acta Psychiatr Scand 1996;93:1–8.

[52] Fewtrell D. Lecture and notes from MINDD International Forum on Children, May 2009.

[53] Hoekstra PJ. PANDAS (pediatric autoimmune neuropsychiatric disorders associated with streptococcal infections) encyclopedia of neuroscience. Cambridge, MA: Academic Press; 2009. p. 415–20.

[54] Del Pozo JL. Biofilm-related disease. Expert Rev Anti Infect Ther 2017;16(1):51–65. doi:10.1080/14787210.2018.1417036.

[55] Young AMH, Chakrabarti B, Roberts D, et al. From molecules to neural morphology: understanding neuroinflammation in autism spectrum condition. Mol Autism 2016;7(1):doi:10.1186/s13229-016-0068-x.

[56] Brimberg L, Sadiq A, Gregersen PK, et al. Brain-reactive IgG correlates with autoimmunity in mothers of a child with an autism spectrum disorder. Mol Psychiatry 2013;18(11):1171–7. doi:10.1038/mp.2013.101.

[57] Knuesel I, Chicha L, Britschgi M, et al. Maternal immune activation and abnormal brain development across CNS disorders. Nat Rev Neurol 2014;10(11):643–60. doi:10.1038/nrneurol.2014.187.

[58] Perry VH, Holmes C. Microglial priming in neurodegenerative disease. Nat Rev Neurol 2014;10(4):217–24. doi:10.1038/nrneurol.2014.38.

[59] Mumaw CL, Levesque S, McGraw C, et al. Microglial priming through the lung–brain axis: the role of air pollution-induced circulating factors. FASEB J 2016;30(5):1880–91. doi:10.1096/fj.201500047.

[60] Sacco R, Militerni R, Frolli A, et al. Clinical, morphological, and biochemical correlates of head circumference in autism. Biol Psychiatry 2007;62(9):1038–47. doi:10.1016/j.biopsych.2007.04.039.

[61] Deverman BE, Patterson PH. Cytokines and CNS development. Neuron 2009;64(1):61–78. doi:10.1016/j.neuron.2009.09.002.

[62] El-Ansary A, Al-Ayadhi L. GABAergic/glutamatergic imbalance relative to excessive neuroinflammation in autism spectrum disorders. J Neuroinflammation 2014;11(1). doi:10.1186/s12974-014-0189-0.

[63] Al-Ayadhi LY, Mostafa GA. Elevated serum levels of macrophage-derived chemokine and thymus and activation-regulated chemokine in autistic children. J Neuroinflammation 2013;10(1):doi:10.1186/1742-2094-10-72.

[64] Zerbo O, Leong A, Barcellos L, et al. Immune mediated conditions in autism spectrum disorders. Brain Behav Immun 2015;46:232–6. doi:10.1016/j.bbi.2015.02.001.

[65] Chaidez V, Hansen RL, Hertz-Picciotto I. Gastrointestinal problems in children with autism, developmental delays or typical development. J Autism Dev Disord 2013;44(5):1117–27. doi:10.1007/s10803-013-1973-x.

[66] Theoharides TC, Valent P, Akin C. Mast cells, mastocytosis, and related disorders. N Engl J Med 2015;373(2):163–72. doi:10.1056/nejmra1409760.

[67] Ribatti D. The crucial role of mast cells in blood–brain barrier alterations. Exp Cell Res 2015;338(1):119–25. doi:10.1016/j.yexcr.2015.05.013.

[68] Nelissen S, Lemmens E, Geurts N, et al. The role of mast cells in neuroinflammation. Acta Neuropathol 2013;125(5):637–50. doi:10.1007/s00401-013-1092-y.

[69] Skaper SD, Facci L, Giusti P. Mast cells, glia and neuroinflammation: partners in crime? Immunology 2014;141(3):314–27. doi:10.1111/imm.12170.

[70] Hoogland ICM, Houbolt C, van Westerloo DJ, et al. Systemic inflammation and microglial activation: systematic review of animal experiments. J Neuroinflammation 2015;12(1):doi:10.1186/s12974-015-0332-6.

[71] Theoharides TC, Zhang B. Neuro-inflammation, blood-brain barrier, seizures and autism. J Neuroinflammation 2011;8(1):168. doi:10.1186/1742-2094-8-168.

[72] Theoharides TC, Asadi S, Patel AB. Focal brain inflammation and autism. J Neuroinflammation 2013;10(1):doi:10.1186/1742-2094-10-46.

[73] Theoharides TC, Stewart JM, Panagiotidou S, et al. Mast cells, brain inflammation and autism. Eur J Pharmacol 2016;778:96–102. doi:10.1016/j.ejphar.2015.03.086.

[74] Bradstreet JJ, Ruggiero M, Pacini S. Commentary: structural and functional features of central nervous system lymphatic vessels. Front Neurosci 2015;9. doi:10.3389/fnins.2015.00485.

[75] Kohane IS, McMurry A, Weber G, et al. The co-morbidity burden of children and young adults with autism spectrum disorders. PLoS ONE 2012;7(4):e33224. doi:10.1371/journal.pone.0033224.

[76] Di Marco B, Bonaccorso CM, Aloisi E, et al. Neuro-inflammatory mechanisms in developmental disorders associated with intellectual disability and autism spectrum disorder: a neuro-immune perspective. CNS Neurol Disord Drug Targets 2016;15(4):448–63.

[77] Mostafa GA, El-Hadidi ES, Hewedi DH, et al. Oxidative stress in Egyptian children with autism – relation to autoimmunity. J Neuroimmunol 2010;219(1–2):114–18.

[78] Mostafa GA, Kitchener N. Serum anti-nuclear antibodies as a marker of autoimmunity in Egyptian autistic children. Pediatr Neurol 2009;40:107–12.

[79] Sweeten TL, Bowyer SL, Posey DJ, et al. Increased prevalence of familial autoimmunity in probands with pervasive developmental disorders. Pediatrics 2003;112:420–4.

[80] Atladóttir HO, Pedersen MG, Thorsen P, et al. Association of family history of autoimmune diseases and autism spectrum disorders. Pediatrics 2009;12(2):687–94.

[81] Vinet É, Pineau CA, Clarke AE, et al. Increased risk of autism spectrum disorders in children born to women with systemic lupus erythematosus: results from a large population-based cohort. Arthritis Rheumatol 2015;67(12):3201–8. doi:10.1002/art.39320.

[82] Croen LA, Grether JK, Yoshida CK, et al. Maternal autoimmune diseases, asthma and allergies, and childhood autism spectrum disorders: a case-control study. Arch Pediatr Adolesc Med 2005;159:151–7.

[83] Hornig M. The role of microbes and autoimmunity in the pathogenesis of neuropsychiatric illness. Curr Opin Rheumatol 2013;25(4):488–795.

[84] McGeachy MJ, McSorley SJ. Microbial-induced Th17: superhero or supervillain? J Immunol 2012;189(7):3285–91. doi:10.4049/jimmunol.1201834.

[85] McGinnis WR. Oxidative stress in autism. Altern Ther Health Med 2004;10:22–36.

[86] Chauhan A, Chauhan V, Brown WT, et al. Oxidative stress in autism: increased lipid peroxidation and reduced serum levels of ceruloplasmin and transferrin – the antioxidant proteins. Life Sci 2004;75(21):2539–49.

[87] Basu S. F2-isoprostanes in human health and diseases: from molecular mechanisms to clinical implications. Antioxid Redox Signal 2008;10:1405–34.

[88] Ng F, Berk M, Dean O, et al. Oxidative stress in psychiatric disorders: evidence base and therapeutic implications. Int J Neuropsychopharmacol 2008;11:851–76.

[89] McGinnis W, Audhya T. Discerning the Mauve factor, part II. [online] Walshinstitute.org; 2008. Available from: https://www.walshinstitute.org/uploads/1/7/9/9/17997321/discerning-the-mauve-factor-part-ii-galley.pdf. [Accessed 3 October 2019].

[90] Walsh W, Glab LB, Haakenson ML. Reduced violent behavior following biochemical therapy. Physiol Behav 2004;82(5):835–9.

[91] Irvine DG, Ell D, Crichlow EC. Anticonvulsant and EEG activities of kryptopyrrole and a possible underlying neurochemical mechanism. Proceedings of the 4th International Meeting of the International Society for Neurochemistry. Tokyo; 1973:359.

[92] Jacobson SJ, Rapoport H, Ellman GL. The nonoccurence of hemo- and kryptopyrrole in the urine of schizophrenics. Biol Psychiatry 1975;10(1):91–3.

[93] Hoffer A. Megavitamin B3-therapy for schizophrenia. Can Psychiatr Assoc J 1971;16(6):499–504.

[94] Hoffer A. Malvaria and the law. Psychosomatics 1966;7(5):303–10.

[95] Hoffer A, Osmond H. Malvaria: a new psychiatric disease. Acta Psychiatr Scand 1963;39:335–66.

[96] Hoffer A, Osmond H. How to survive with schizophrenia. Secaucus, NJ: University Books; 1974.

[97] Walsh WJ, Glab LB, Haakenson ML. Reduced violent behavior following biochemical therapy. Physiol Behav 2004;82(5):835–9.

[98] Audhya T. Urinary EHHPL in neurobehavioral disorders: Think-tank presentation. Presented at: Defeat Autism Now! (DAN!) Conference. October 24–27, 2002; San Diego, CA.

[99] Wetterberg L. Pharmacological and toxic effects of kryptopyrrole in mice. Ups J Med Sci 1973;78(1):78–80.

[100] Brodie MJ, Graham DJM, Thompson GG, et al. The porphyrinogenic effects of kryptopyrrole in the rat and the occurrence of urinary kryptopyrrole in human hereditary hepatic porphyria. Clin Sci Mol Med 1976;50(5):431–4.

[101] Isaacson HR, Moran MM, Hall A, et al. Autism: a retrospective outcome study of nutrient therapy. J Appl Nutr 1996;110–18.

[102] Hoffer A. A program for the treatment of alcoholism: LSD, malvaria and nicotinic acid. In: Abramson HA, editor. The use of LSD in psychotherapy and alcoholism. Indianapolis: Howard W. Sams and Company, Inc.; 1967. p. 343–406.

[103] No authors listed. The 'mauve factor' in schizophrenia. Medical World News. 14 December 1973. p. 49.

[104] Pfeiffer CC, Maillous R, Forsythe L. The schizophrenias: ours to conquer. Wichita, Kansas: Bio-Communications Press; 1988.

[105] Cutler P. Pyridoxine and trace element therapy in selected clinical cases. J Orthomolec Psychiatr 1974;89–95.

[106] Jaffee R, Kruesi OR. The biochemical-immunology window: a molecular view of psychiatric case management. J Appl Nutr 1992;44:26–42.

[107] Pfeiffer CC, Audette L. Pyroluria-zinc and B6 deficiencies. Int Clin Nutr Rev 1988;8:107–9.

[108] Sohler A, Pfeiffer CC. Vitamin B6 nutritional status of a psychiatric outpatient population. J Orthomolec Psychiatr 1982;11:81–6.

[109] Hoffer A. The discovery of kryptopyrrole and its importance in diagnosis of biochemical imbalances in schizophrenia and in criminal behavior. J Orthomolec Med 1995;10:3–7.

[110] Kelly EJ, Quaife CJ, Froelick GJ, et al. Metallothionein I and II protect against zinc deficiency and zinc toxicity in mice. J Nutr 1996;126:1782–90.

[111] Walsh W, Usman A. Metal metabolism and autism. Presented at the American Psychiatric Association Annual Meeting, May 10, 2001. New Orleans, LA.

[112] Levin ED, Aschner M, Heberlein U, et al. Genetic aspects of behavioural neurotoxicology. Neurotoxicology 2009;30(5):741–53.

[113] Gulson BL, et al. Mobilization of lead from human bone tissue during pregnancy and lactation – a summary of long-term research. Sci Total Environ 2003;303(1–2):79–104.

[114] Dietert RR, Lee JE, Hussain I, et al. Developmental immunotoxicology of lead. Toxicol Appl Pharmacol 2004;198(2):86–94.

[115] Canfield RL, Henderson CRJ, Cory-Slechta DA, et al. Intellectual impairment in children with blood lead concentrations below 10 microgram per deciliter. N Engl J Med 2003;348:1517–26.

[116] Chiodo LM, Jacobson SW, Jacobson JL. Neurodevelopmental effects of postnatal lead exposure at very low levels. Neurotoxicol Teratol 2004;26:359–71.

[117] Holladay SD, Smialowicz RJ. Development of the murine and human immune system: differential effects of immunotoxicants depend on time of exposure. Environ Health Perspect 2000;108(Suppl. 3):463–73.

[118] Dietert RR, Lee JE, Bunn TL. Developmental immunotoxicology: emerging issues. Hum Exp Toxicol 2002;21:479–85.

[119] Snyder JE, Filipov NM, Parsons PJ, et al. The efficiency of maternal transfer of lead and its influence on plasma IgE and splenic cellularity of mice. Toxicol Sci 2000;57:87–94.

[120] Bunn TL, Marsh JA, Dietert RR. Gender differences in developmental immunotoxicity to lead in the chicken: analysis following a single early low-level exposure in ovo. J Toxicol Environ Health A 2000;61:677–93.

[121] Hudson CA, Cao L, Kasten-Joly J, et al. Susceptibility of lupus-prone NZM mouse strains to lead exacerbation of systemic lupus erythematous symptoms. J Toxicol Environ Health A 2003;66:895–918.

[122] McCabe MJ Jr, Singh KP, Reiners JJ Jr. Low level lead exposure in vitro stimulates the proliferation and expansion of alloantigen-reactive CD4 (high) T cells. Toxicol Appl Pharmacol 2001;177:219–31.

[123] Braun JM, Kahn RS, Froehlich T, et al. Exposure to environmental toxicants and ADHD in US children. Environ Health Perspect 2006;114:1904–9.

[124] Ha M, Kwon HJ, Lim MH, et al. Low blood levels of lead and mercury and symptoms of attention deficit hyperactivity in children – a report of the children's health and environment research (CHEER). Neurotoxicology 2008;30(1):31–6.

[125] Mahaffey KR. Absorption of lead by infants and young children. In: Schmidt EHF, Hildebrandt AG, editors. Health evaluation of heavy metals in infant formula and junior food. Berlin: Springer; 1983. p. 69–85.

[126] Hernandez-Avila M, Gonzalez-Cossio T, Palazuelos E, et al. Dietary and environmental determinants of blood and bone lead levels in lactating postpartum women living in Mexico City. Environ Health Perspect 1996;104:1076–82.

[127] Farias P, Borja-Aburto VH, Rios C, et al. Blood lead levels in pregnant women of high and low socioeconomic status in Mexico City. Environ Health Perspect 1996;104:1070–4.

[128] Ahamed M, Siddiqui MKJ. Low level lead exposure and oxidative stress – current opinions. Clin Chim Acta 2007;383(1–2):57–64.

[129] Upasani CD, Khera A, Balaraman R. Effect of lead with vitamins E, C, or spirulina on malondialdehyde: conjugated dienes and hydroperoxides in rats. Indian J Exp Biol 2001;39(1):70–4.

[130] Halim AB, El-Ahmady O, Hassab-Allah S, et al. Biochemical effect of antioxidants on lipids and liver function in experimentally induced liver damage. Ann Clin Biochem 1997;34(Pt 6):656–63.

[131] Schreiber M, Trojan S. Protective effect of flavonoids and tocopherol in high altitude hypoxia in the rat: comparison with ascorbic acid. Cesk Fysiol 1998;47(2):51–2.

[132] Zou CG, Agar NS, Jones GL. Oxidative insult to human red blood cells induced by free radical initiator AAPH and its inhibition by a commercial antioxidant mixture. Life Sci 2001;69(1):75–86.

[133] Simon JA, Hudes ES. Relationship of ascorbic acid to blood lead levels. JAMA 1999;281(24):2289–93.

[134] Shalan MG, Mostafa MS, Hassouna MM, et al. Amelioration of lead toxicity on rat liver with vitamin C and silymarin supplements. Toxicology 2005;206(1):115.

[135] Hsu PC, Guo YL. Antioxidant nutrients and lead toxicity. Toxicology 2002;180(1):33–44.

[136] Soto CP, Perez BL, Favari LP, et al. Prevention of alloxan-induced diabetes mellitus in the rat by silymarin. Comp Biochem Physiol Pharmacol Toxicol Endocrinol 1998;119(2):125–9.

[137] Nielsen FH. Nutritional requirements for boron, silicon, vanadium, nickel, and arsenic: current knowledge and speculation. FASEB J 1991;5:2661–7.

[138] Uthus EO. Effects of arsenic deprivation in hamsters. Magnes Trace Elem 1990;9:227–32.

[139] Rodriguez VM, Jiménez-Capdeville ME, Giordano M. The effects of arsenic exposure on the nervous system. Toxicol Lett 2003;145(1):1–18.

[140] Calderon J, Navarro ME, Jimenez-Capdeville ME, et al. Exposure to arsenic and lead and neuropsychological development in Mexican children. Environ Res 2001;85:69–76.

[141] Domingo JL. Aluminium, toxicology encyclopedia of food sciences and nutrition. Cambridge, MA: Academic Press; 2003. p. 160–6.

[142] Domingo JL. Reproductive and developmental toxicity of aluminum – a review. Neurotoxicol Teratol 1994;17(4):515–21.

[143] Bondy SC. Aluminum encyclopedia of neuroscience. Cambridge, MA: Academic Press; 2009. p. 253–7.

[144] Russo AJ. Anti-metallothionein IgG and levels of metallothionein in autistic children with GI disease. Drug Healthc Patient Saf 2009;1:1–8.

[145] Havarinasab S, Häggqvist B, Björn E, et al. Immunosuppressive and autoimmune effects of thiomersal in mice. Toxicol Appl Pharmacol 2005;15(204):109–21.

[146] Havarinasab S, Hultman P. Organic mercury compounds and autoimmunity. Autoimmun Rev 2005;4:270–5.

[147] Frye RE, Rossignol DA. Mitochondrial dysfunction can connect the diverse medical symptoms associated with autism spectrum disorders. Pediatr Res 2011;69(5 Pt 2):41R–7R. doi:10.1203/pdr.0b013e318212f16b.

[148] Napoli E, Wong S, Hertz-Picciotto I, et al. Deficits in bioenergetics and impaired immune response in granulocytes from children with autism. Pediatrics 2014;133(5):e1405–10. doi:10.1542/peds.2013-1545.

[149] Salli K, Lehtinen MJ, Tiihonen K, et al. Xylitol's health benefits beyond dental health: a comprehensive review. Nutrients 2019;11(8):1813. doi:10.3390/nu11081813.

[150] Kurola P, Tapiainen T, Kaijalainen T, et al. Xylitol and capsular gene expression in Streptococcus pneumoniae. J Med Microbiol 2009;58(11):1470–3. doi:10.1099/jmm.0.011700-0.

[151] Lee H-J, Kim SC, Kim J, et al. Synergistic inhibition of Streptococcal biofilm by ribose and xylitol. Arch Oral Biol 2015;60(2):304–12. doi:10.1016/j.archoralbio.2014.11.004.

[152] Fasano A. Zonulin and its regulation of intestinal barrier function: the biological door to inflammation, autoimmunity, and cancer. Physiol Rev 2011;91(1):151–75. doi:10.1152/physrev.00003.2008.

[153] Klaveness J, Bigam J, Reichelt K. The varied rate of response to dietary intervention in autistic children. Open J Psychiatr 2013;3:56–60. doi:10.4236/ojpsych.2013.32A009.

[154] Wisniewski S. Child nutrition, health problems, and school achievement in Sri Lanka. World Dev 2010;38(3):315–32.

[155] Yasuda H, Tsutsui T. Assessment of infantile mineral imbalances in autism spectrum disorders (ASDs). Int J Environ Res Public Health 2013;10(11):6027–43. doi:10.3390/ijerph10116027.

[156] Arons MH, Lee K, Thynne CJ, et al. Shank3 is part of a zinc-sensitive signaling system that regulates excitatory synaptic strength. J Neurosci 2016;36(35):9124–34. doi:10.1523/jneurosci.0116-16.2016.

[157] Vela G, Stark P, Socha M, et al. Zinc in gut-brain interaction in autism and neurological disorders. Neural Plast 2015;2015:1–15. doi:10.1155/2015/972791.

[158] Desai A, Sequeira JM, Quadros EV. The metabolic basis for developmental disorders due to defective folate transport. Biochimie 2016;126:31–42. doi:10.1016/j.biochi.2016.02.012.

[159] Guéant J-L, Namour F, Guéant-Rodriguez R-M, et al. Folate and fetal programming: a play in epigenomics? Trends Endocrinol Metab 2013;24(6):279–89. doi:10.1016/j.tem.2013.01.010.

[160] Ramaekers VT, Sequeira JM, Quadros EV. The basis for folinic acid treatment in neuro-psychiatric disorders. Biochimie 2016;126:79–90. doi:10.1016/j.biochi.2016.04.005.

[161] Frye RE, Sequeira JM, Quadros EV, et al. Cerebral folate receptor autoantibodies in autism spectrum disorder. Mol Psychiatry 2012;18(3):369–81. doi:10.1038/mp.2011.175.

[162] Papakostas GI, Shelton RC, Zajecka JM, et al. L-methylfolate as adjunctive therapy for SSRI-resistant major depression: results of two randomized, double-blind, parallel-sequential trials. Am J Psychiatry 2012;169(12):1267–74.

[163] Dinan TG, Stanton C, Cryan JF. Psychobiotics: a novel class of psychotropic. Biol Psychiatry 2013;74(10):720–6. doi:10.1016/j.biopsych.2013.05.001.

[164] Rogers GB, Keating DJ, Young RL, et al. From gut dysbiosis to altered brain function and mental illness: mechanisms and pathways. Mol Psychiatry 2016;21(6):738–48. doi:10.1038/mp.2016.50.

[165] Parracho HM, Gibson GR, Knott F, et al. A double-blind, placebo-controlled, crossover-designed probiotic feeding study in children diagnosed with autistic spectrum disorders. Int J Probiot Prebiot 2010;5:69–74.

[166] Kaluzna-Czaplinska J, Blaszczyk S. The level of arabinitol in autistic children after probiotic therapy. Nutrition 2012;28:124–6. doi:10.1016/j.nut.2011.08.002.

[167] Pärtty A, Kalliomäki M, Wacklin P, et al. A possible link between early probiotic intervention and the risk of neuropsychiatric disorders later in childhood: a randomized trial. Pediatr Res 2015;77:823–8. doi:10.1038/pr.2015.51.

[168] Romeo MG, Romeo DM, Trovato L, et al. Role of probiotics in the prevention of the enteric colonization by Candida in preterm newborns: incidence of late-onset sepsis and neurological outcome. J Perinatol 2011;31(1):63–9. doi:10.1038/jp.2010.57.

[169] Bravo JA, Forsythe P, Chew MV, et al. Ingestion of Lactobacillus strain regulates emotional behavior and central GABA receptor expression in a mouse via the vagus nerve. Proc Natl Acad Sci U S A 2011;108(38):16050–5. doi:10.1073/pnas.1102999108.

[170] Hsiao EY, McBride SW, Hsien S, et al. Microbiota modulate behavioral and physiological abnormalities associated with neurodevelopmental disorders. Cell 2013;155(7):1451–63. doi:10.1016/j.cell.2013.11.024.

[171] Wang H, Lee I-S, Braun C, et al. Effect of probiotics on central nervous system functions in animals and humans: a systematic review. J Neurogastroenterol Motil 2016;22(4):589–605. doi:10.5056/jnm16018.

[172] Bercik P, Park AJ, Sinclair D, et al. The anxiolytic effect of Bifidobacterium longum NCC3001 involves vagal pathways for gut-brain communication. Neurogastroenterol Motil 2011;23(12):1132–9. doi:10.1111/j.1365-2982.2011.01796.x.

[173] Luchtman DW, Song C. Cognitive enhancement by omega-3 fatty acids from childhood to old age: findings from animal and clinical studies. Neuropharmacology 2013;64:550–65. doi:10.1016/j.neuropharm.2012.07.019.

[174] Johnston BC, Goldenberg JZ, Parkin PC. Probiotics and the prevention of antibiotic-associated diarrhea in infants and children. JAMA 2016;316(14):1484. doi:10.1001/jama.2016.11838.

[175] McFarland LV, Ozen M, Dinleyici EC, et al. Comparison of pediatric and adult antibiotic-associated diarrhea and Clostridium difficile infections. World J Gastroenterol 2016;22(11):3078. doi:10.3748/wjg.v22.i11.3078.

[176] Karim S, Mirza Z, Kamal M, et al. The role of viruses in neurodegenerative and neurobehavioral diseases. CNS Neurol Disord Drug Targets 2014;13(7):1213–23.

[177] Kanduc D, Polito A. From viral infections to autistic neurodevelopmental disorders via cross-reactivity. J Psychiatry Brain Sci 2018;3(6):14.

[178] Sodhi R, Singh N. Retinoids as potential targets for Alzheimer's disease. Pharmacol Biochem Behav 2014;120:117–23.

[179] Ray S, Das B, Dasgupta S. Potential therapeutic roles of retinoids for prevention of neuroinflammation and neurodegeneration in Alzheimer's disease. Neural Regen Res 2019;14(11):1880.

[180] Neggers YH. Increasing prevalence, changes in diagnostic criteria, and nutritional risk factors for autism spectrum disorders. ISRN Nutr 2014;2014:https://doi.org/10.1155/2014/514026. Article ID 514026.

[181] Wang T, Shan L, Du L, et al. Serum concentration of 25-hydroxyvitamin D in autism spectrum disorder: a systematic review and meta-analysis. Eur Child Adolesc Psychiatry 2015;25(4):341–50. doi:10.1007/s00787-015-0786-1.

[182] Kennedy D. B vitamins and the brain: mechanisms, dose and efficacy – a review. Nutrients 2016;8(2):68. doi:10.3390/nu8020068.

[183] Sakakeeny L, Roubenoff R, Obin M, et al. Plasma pyridoxal-5-phosphate is inversely associated with systemic markers of inflammation in a population of U.S. adults. J Nutr 2012;142(7):1280–5.

[184] Zhang Y, Hodgson NW, Trivedi MS, et al. Decreased brain levels of vitamin B12 in aging, autism and schizophrenia. PLoS ONE 2016;11(1):e0146797. doi:10.1371/journal.pone.0146797.

[185] Hendren RL, James SJ, Widjaja F, et al. Randomized, placebo-controlled trial of methyl B12 for children with autism. J Child Adolesc Psychopharmacol 2016;26(9):774–83. doi:10.1089/cap.2015.0159.

[186] James SJ. Abnormal folate-dependant methionine and glutathione metabolism in children with autism: potential for increased sensitivity to thiomersal and other pro-oxidants. Spring DAN! Conference Proceedings, Washington DC; 2004. p. 59–63.

[187] Michelson AM. Pathology of oxygen. New York: Academic Press; 1982. p. 278–9.

[188] Pangborn J. Detection of metabolic disorders in people with autism. Proceedings, NSAC Annual Conference San Antonio Texas, International Autism Conference of the Americas 1984:3639.

[189] Rimland B. What is the right dosage for vitamin B, DMG and other nutrients in autism? Autism Res Rev Int 1997;11(4):3.

[190] Kasarpalkar NJ, Kothari ST, Dave UP. Brain-derived neurotrophic factor in children with autism spectrum disorder. Ann Neurosci 2014;21(4):doi:10.5214/ans.0972.7531.210403.

[191] Franco JL, Posser T, Missau F, et al. Structure–activity relationship of flavonoids derived from medicinal plants in preventing methylmercury-induced mitochondrial dysfunction. Environ Toxicol Pharmacol 2010;30(3):272–8. doi:10.1016/j.etap.2010.07.003.

[192] Laplante M, Sabatini DM. mTOR signaling in growth control and disease. Cell 2012;149(2):274–93. doi:10.1016/j.cell.2012.03.017.

[193] Sawicka K, Zukin RS. Dysregulation of mTOR signaling in neuropsychiatric disorders: therapeutic implications. Neuropsychopharmacology 2011;37(1):305–6. doi:10.1038/npp.2011.210.

[194] Zhou H, Luo Y, Huang S. Updates of mTOR inhibitors. Anticancer Agents Med Chem 2010;10(7):571–81. doi:10.2174/187152010793498663.

[195] Tsilioni I, Taliou A, Francis K, et al. Children with autism spectrum disorders, who improved with a luteolin-containing dietary formulation, show reduced serum levels of TNF and IL-6. Transl Psychiatry 2015;5(9):e647. doi:10.1038/tp.2015.142.

[196] Hardan AY, Fung LK, Libove RA, et al. A randomized controlled pilot trial of oral N-acetylcysteine in children with autism. Biol Psychiatry 2012;71:956–61. doi:10.1016/j.biopsych.2012.01.014.

[197] Ghanizadeh A, Moghimi-Sarani E. A randomized double blind placebo controlled clinical trial of N-acetylcysteine added to risperidone for treating autistic disorders. BMC Psychiatry 2013;13(1). doi:10.1186/1471-244x-13-196.

[198] Slattery J, Kumar N, et al. Clinical trials of N-acetylcysteine in psychiatry and neurology: a systematic review. Neurosci Biobehav Rev 2015;55:294–321. doi:10.1016/j.neubiorev.2015.04.015.

[199] Kushairi N, Phan CW, Sabaratnam V, et al. Lion's mane mushroom, Hericium erinaceus (Bull.: Fr.) Pers. suppresses H2O2-induced oxidative damage and LPS-induced inflammation in HT22 hippocampal neurons and BV2 microglia. Antioxidants (Basel) 2019;8(8):261. doi:10.3390/antiox8080261.

[200] Phan CW, David P, Naidu M, et al. Therapeutic potential of culinary-medicinal mushrooms for the management of neurodegenerative diseases: diversity, metabolite, and mechanism. Crit Rev Biotechnol 2014;35(3):355–68. doi:10.3109/07388551.2014.887649.

[201] Waring R. Absorption of magnesium sulfate. [online] Mgwater.com; n.d. Available from: https://www.mgwater.com/transdermal.shtml. [Accessed 9 October 2016].

[202] Matsubara E, Shimizu K, Fukagawa M, et al. Volatiles emitted from the roots of Vetiveria zizanioides suppress the decline in attention during a visual display terminal task. Biomed Res 2012;33(5):299–308.

[203] Nirwane A, Gupta P, Shet J, et al. Anxiolytic and nootropic activity of Vetiveria zizanioides roots in mice. J Ayurveda Integr Med 2015;6(3):158.

[204] Saiyudthong S, Pongmayteegul S, Marsden CA, et al. Anxiety-like behaviour and c-fos expression in rats that inhaled vetiver essential oil. Nat Prod Res 2015;2:1–4.

[205] Gupta R, Sharma KK, Afzal M, et al. Anticonvulsant activity of ethanol extracts of Vetiveria zizanioides roots in experimental mice. Pharm Biol 2013;51(12):1521–4.

[206] Foley D, Reid N, Neels A, et al. Profound hypomagnesaemia secondary to alternative therapy in a child with autism spectrum disorder. J Paediatr Child Health 2015;51(7):744–5. doi:10.1111/jpc.12946.

[207] Worley KA, Wolraich ML. Attention-deficit hyperactivity disorder. In: Wolraich ML, editor. Disorders of development and learning. 3rd ed. London: BC Decker; 2003.

[208] Faraone SV, Biederman J, Spencer T. Attention-deficit/hyperactivity disorder in adults: an overview. Biol Psychiatry 2000;48:9–20.

[209] Ingram S, Hechtman L, Morgenstern G. Outcome issues in ADHD: adolescent and adult long-term outcome. Ment Retard Dev Disabil Res Rev 1999;5:243–50.

[210] Spencer TJ, Biederman J, Wilens TE, et al. Overview and neurobiology of attention-deficit/hyperactivity disorder. J Clin Psychiatry 2002;63(Suppl.):3–9.

[211] Nadder TS, Silberg JL, Eaves LJ, et al. Genetic effects on ADHD symptomatology in 7- to 13-year-old twins: results from a telephone survey. Behav Genet 1998;28(2):83–100.

[212] Sharp WS, Gottesman RF, Greenstein DK, et al. Monozygotic twins discordant for attention-deficit/hyperactivity disorder: ascertainment and clinical characteristics. J Am Acad Child Adolesc Psychiatry 2003;42(1):93–7.

[213] Castellanos FX, Sharp WS, Gottesman RF, et al. Anatomic brain abnormalities in monozygotic twins discordant for attention deficit hyperactivity disorder. Am J Psychiatry 2003;160(9):1693–6.

[214] Neuman RJ, Lobos E, Reich W, et al. Prenatal smoking exposure and dopaminergic genotypes interact to cause a severe ADHD subtype. Biol Psychiatry 2007;61(12):1320–8.

[215] Stein J, Schettler T, Wallinga D, et al. In harm's way: toxic threats to child development. J Dev Behav Pediatr 2002;23(S1):S13–21.

[216] Goldschmidt L, Day NL, Richardson GA. Effects of prenatal marijuana exposure and child behavior problems at age 10. Neurotoxicol Teratol 2000;22(3):325–36.

[217] Feingold BF. Hyperkinesis and learning disabilities linked to artificial food flavors and colors. Am J Nurs 1975;75:797–803.

[218] Bateman B, Warner JO, Hutchinson E, et al. The effects of a double blind, placebo controlled, artificial food colourings and benzoate preservative challenge on hyperactivity in general population sample of preschool children. Arch Dis Child 2004;89(6):506–11.

[219] Lau KL, McLean WG, Williams DP, et al. Synergistic interactions between commonly used food additives in a developmental neurotoxicity test. Toxicol Sci 2006;90(1):178–87.

[220] United States Food and Drug Administration. Code of Federal Regulations 21 CFR 74. Available from: www.cfsan.fda.gov/~lrd/cfr74102.hmtl.

[221] Akhondzadeh S, Mohammadi MR, Khademi M. Zinc sulfate as an adjunct to methylphenidate for the treatment of attention deficit hyperactivity disorder in children: a double blind and randomized trial [ISRCTN64132371]. BMC Psychiatry 2004;4:9.

[222] Toren P, Elder S, Sela BA, et al. Zinc deficiency in attention-deficit hyperactivity disorder. Biol Psychiatry 1996;40(12):1308–10.

[223] Sinn N, Bryan J. Effect of supplementation with polyunsaturated fatty acids and micro nutrients on learning and behavior problems associated with child ADHD. J Dev Behav Pediatr 2007;28:82–91.

[224] Arnold LE, Bozzolo H, Hollway J, et al. Serum zinc correlates with parent- and teacher-rated inattention in children with attention-deficit/hyperactivity disorder. J Child Adolesc Psychopharmacol 2005;15:628–36.

[225] Konofal E, Lecendreux M, Arnulf I, et al. Iron deficiency in children with attention-deficit/hyperactivity disorder. Arch Pediatr Adolesc Med 2004;158:1113–15.

[226] Richardson AJ. Omega-3 fatty acids in ADHD and related neurodevelopmental disorders. Int Rev Psychiatry 2006;18:155–72.

[227] Esparham A, Evans R, Wagner L, et al. Pediatric integrative medicine approaches to attention deficit hyperactivity disorder (ADHD). Children 2014;1(2):186–207. doi:10.3390/children1020186.

[228] Kamal M, Bener A, Ehlayel MS. Is high prevalence of vitamin D deficiency a correlate for attention deficit hyperactivity disorder? Atten Defic Hyperact Disord 2014;6(2):73–8. doi:10.1007/s12402-014-0130-5.

[229] Lyon M, Kapoor M, Junejar L. The effects of L-theanine (Suntheanine®) on objective sleep quality in boys with attention deficit hyperactivity disorder (ADHD): a randomized, double-blind, placebo-controlled clinical trial. Altern Med Rev 2011;16(4):348–54.

[230] Lardner AL. Neurobiological effects of the green tea constituent theanine and its potential role in the treatment of psychiatric and neurodegenerative disorders. Nutr Neurosci 2013;17(4):145–55. doi:10.1179/1476830513y.0000000079.

[231] Autism Aspergers Advocacy Australia. Autism prevalence in Australia. Available from: http://a4.org.au/prevalence2015.

19

Down syndrome

Belinda Robson

INTRODUCTION

Down syndrome (trisomy 21) is the most common chromosomal cause of intellectual disability and affects 1 in 691 live births.[1] Down syndrome is classified as a developmental disability of chromosomal origin. Duplication of chromosome 21, resulting in three copies of this chromosome, influences protein encoding for immune meditators, kinases, proteases, protease inhibitors, methylation pathways, energy metabolism, transcription factors and many other regulatory pathways in the body.[2] Implications of this additional chromosome are broad, affecting many different body systems and resulting in a diverse range of comorbid health conditions and predispositions. Gene triplication affects expression of genes, not only in trisomic genes due to over-expression, but also in disomic genes, which may be under-expressed.[3] Downregulation of disomic genes, combined with upregulation of trisomic genes, contributes to the clinical phenotype observed in Down syndrome.[3] Furthermore, it has been demonstrated that in people with Down syndrome, global changes in gene expression occur throughout the entire genome.[4] This results in altered neurological development, cardiovascular malformations, dysfunctional tendencies and/or malformations of the musculoskeletal system and gastrointestinal system, metabolic disorders, nutritional deficiencies, altered immune function, endocrine disruption (hypothalamic-pituitary-thyroid axis) and intellectual impairment.[5] As this change is present from conception, malformations and developmental abnormalities begin in utero, and metabolic differences continue throughout the life span. Degenerative neurological disorders present earlier in people with Down syndrome than in the general population, and are a collective result of altered gene expression on neurological, metabolic, immunological and inflammatory processes.[5]

Discrimination is a significant issue for all people with disabilities. They face increased risk of abuse (emotional, sexual, verbal and physical), physical exclusion from community services and facilities due to inaccessible infrastructure, and literature that does not accommodate learning disabilities and sensory impairments. Attitudinal discrimination is also a persistent barrier to accessing health services. In general, people with intellectual and developmental disabilities experience significant health disparities, which is evidenced by lower life expectancy, poorer health status and lower access to preventive health initiatives and healthcare services.[6] Part of this disparity includes educational knowledge of general practitioners (GPs) to be able to communicate with, appropriately diagnose and treat people with disabilities. Trollor et al., in an audit of the disability education of medical practitioners, found that current medical school curricula contain on average only 2.55 hours of compulsory intellectual disability content.[7] Furthermore, they found that while the compulsory content included minimal information regarding sexual health and emergency medicine, issues such as human rights, teamwork between disciplines and preventive healthcare were largely neglected.[7] People with disabilities may present with signs and symptoms in unusual ways, lack the capacity to clearly understand questions or be able to express themselves in normative ways, may present by proxy and may have resistance or difficulty with examination procedures.[8] This directly affects healthcare outcomes, in that mainstream doctors have little training in how to best accommodate these additional challenges. Short appointment times and an overburdened public healthcare system may also reduce the likelihood of these appointments successfully identifying health problems. Without immediate improvement, current medical practitioner training is inadequate to address the disparities in health status of people with developmental disabilities.[7]

The Disability Inclusion Act 2014 acknowledges the human rights of people with disabilities and sets goals for promoting independence, enabling choice and control and improving access to mainstream services.[9] This includes naturopathic practitioners, and arguably the training of naturopaths is at least as inadequate as that of medical practitioners. Improving the knowledge, confidence and skill base of naturopaths will improve the quality and provision of services for people with Down syndrome and result in improved quality of care. It is easy in clinical practice to assume that another practitioner involved in the patient's care is keeping vigilance for deterioration in their condition. For many people with disabilities, however, this is seldom the case. The vigilance of a caring naturopath, who is able to look at health through a wider lens than speciality-specific medicine, and in more detail than the over-extended general practitioner, is a valuable asset to the care team for people with Down syndrome. Longer appointment times provided by naturopaths may help facilitate improved detection of health problems. The complexity of health conditions in people with Down syndrome necessitates multidisciplinary care and a high level of communication and coordination between service providers.

Pathogenesis of Down syndrome

For people with Down syndrome, their intellectual disability may be mild to moderate, with an intelligence quotient (IQ) ranging from 40 to 70.[5,10] Physical features characteristic of Down syndrome include:

- Flattened posterior head
- Flat facial profile
- Small low-set ears
- Low-set eyes with upward slant towards epicanthic folds
- Flat bridge of the nose
- Small mouth
- Large and protuberant tongue
- High arched palate
- Broad hands with a single crease
- Large space between first and second toes
- Low birth weight and poor weight gain in infancy
- Hypotonic muscles
- Joint hypermobility.[11]

Muscular hypotonia and joint hypermobility are present in most babies with Down syndrome at birth, resulting in a floppy-appearing infant.[12] Health complications throughout the life span include a higher incidence of comorbidities, including thyroid disease, coeliac disease, autism, congenital heart disease, sensory impairment, gastrointestinal malformations, seizures, obesity, leukaemia, diabetes mellitus, early menopause and earlier onset of age-related diseases.[13,14] Adults with Down syndrome with more severe health problems, resulting in frequent hospitalisation and GP visits, are less likely to be able to participate in a broad range of adult life experiences, including employment, community activities and leisure activities.[6,15] Diligent attendance to healthcare needs throughout childhood and adulthood to prevent disease and manage chronic conditions is therefore essential.[14]

Naturopathic support

The goals of naturopathic support for people with Down syndrome include:

- Optimise nutritional intake
- Support optimal growth and development
- Improve management of chronic health conditions, to prevent secondary complications and further disability
- Monitor for signs of health change or decline, and refer for further investigations when signs of ill-health are apparent
- Advocate for best health outcomes, including regular health screening

- Raise awareness of local support groups (including social media), community services and advocacy, where appropriate
- Ensure adequate support for parents and/or carers.

PERI-CONCEPTION SUPPLEMENTATION

Iron and folate supplementation within the first month of pregnancy has been shown to decrease the incidence of Down syndrome.[16] Significant risk reduction was observed with iron supplementation alone, and with folic acid supplementation above 6 mg per day.[16] While folic acid supplementation of 800 micrograms appears sufficient to decrease the incidence of neural tube defects, doses under 1 mg per day are insufficient to decrease Down syndrome risk.[16] With increased advanced maternal age in Western countries, this finding has substantial relevance for perinatal care.

METHYLATION

Inadequate methylation appears to play a role in the incidence of Down syndrome. Miscarriage is more common in mothers who have conceived a baby with Down syndrome than in those who have not, and 80% of Down syndrome pregnancies spontaneously miscarry.[17] Polymorphism in homocysteine-folate pathways results in DNA hypo-methylation and chromosomal aberrations during oogenesis.[18] The allele MTHFR C677T has been implicated in Down syndrome pathogenesis and impairs DNA methylation at the very first meiotic division.[18] Hypo-methylation also appears to be implicated in congenital heart disease associated with Down syndrome.[19,20] Studies to date are inconsistent about the relevance of MTHFR mutations on Down syndrome incidence, but increasingly research suggests that there is a link between Down syndrome risk and maternal gene mutations that impair methylation pathways. Nutritional variations may contribute to inconsistencies in existing research. The presence of the MTHFR C677T allele in the mother combined with no pre-conception supplementation of folic acid results in a two-fold increase in the incidence of congenital heart defects in children with Down syndrome.[21] The combined presence of two gene mutations (C677T and A1298C) in mothers has been observed to result in a 5.7-fold increase in Down syndrome risk.[22] A five-fold increase in risk of a subsequent neural tube defect during pregnancy has also been observed in mothers who already have a child with Down syndrome, supporting the importance of peri-conception supplementation in these women.[23]

Dietary modification or supplementation to include a therapeutic amount of folate and vitamin B_{12} has the potential to modify the impact of this polymorphism.[17] More detail is included in Chapter 7. Current prescribing patterns focus on methylated forms of folate that theoretically circumvent methylation issues associated with MTHFR polymorphisms; however, it is important to note that research linking folate and MTHFR polymorphisms to neural tube defects, Down syndrome and congenital heart defects is based on folic acid. Evidence-based prescribing therefore would suggest high-dose folic acid to reduce the risk of Down syndrome and congenital heart defects in mothers with increased risk. Further research into the clinical efficacy of methylated forms of folate (e.g. 5-methyl-tetrahydrofolate) is necessary to confirm the benefit of supplementing methylated forms instead of folic acid. Modification of this risk factor further highlights the importance of pre-conception care in mothers of all ages, but particularly those who are of advanced age (for more information, refer to Chapter 14). Other factors that negatively influence DNA methylation include poor diet, cigarette smoking, high alcohol intake and obesity.[18] Evidence to date suggests that perinatal care is of increasing importance in mothers with a personal or family history of miscarriage, neural tube defects, Down syndrome or MTHFR polymorphisms.

PRENATAL DIAGNOSIS

Prenatal screening for Down syndrome has advanced greatly within the last decade, and women now have access to testing that has 98.6% sensitivity for detection within the first trimester of pregnancy.[1] However, no test gives 100% sensitivity and specificity for Down syndrome detection. Previously, amniocentesis was the standard screening method, but it carries a risk of spontaneous abortion.[24] In the 1980s, amniocentesis was offered to all mothers over 35 years of age, though back then this group represented only 30% of babies born with Down syndrome.[25] This is largely due to the higher amount of babies born to younger mothers. More recently, less-invasive tests that combine maternal age, nuchal translucency and maternal serum markers (AFP, β-hCG, oestriol and inhibin) have been developed and they provide increased detection without risk to the fetus.[24] Late Down syndrome maternal serum marker screening has well demonstrated efficacy at 14–18 weeks gestation.[26] Many women, however, prefer earlier detection, so that decisions to terminate are less traumatic.

First-trimester combined screening measures the thickness of nuchal translucency and serological tests to provide detection at 85–90% sensitivity, with a 5% false positive rate, and is offered at 10–13 weeks gestation.[27] This test is most effective at 11–12 weeks gestation, with 92.3% sensitivity and a 5.7% false positive rate.[27] First-trimester screening combined with second-trimester screening yields 95% sensitivity with a 5% false positive rate.[27] Increased false positive rates have been observed in the pregnancies of mothers who follow a vegetarian diet and are linked to low serum vitamin B_{12} levels, which delays DNA synthesis resulting in elevated β-hCG.[28] Other screening methods will be more reliable for women who follow a vegetarian diet and should be used to reduce any unnecessary anxiety caused by a false positive reading. This anomaly in β-hCG readings does, however, highlight the need for vitamin B_{12} supplementation during pregnancy for women who are vegetarian. Improvements in non-invasive testing have limited the need for invasive tests, resulting in reduced iatrogenic miscarriages.[25] The most accurate non-invasive test available assesses free fetal DNA circulating in maternal plasma and has 98–99%

sensitivity and only a 1% false positive rate, and should be used in high-risk cases.[25,29]

Choice to screen

The ease of modern testing methods means Down syndrome screening has the potential to become part of routine pregnancy screening. Early testing with other routine pregnancy tests allows greater decision-making capacity for parents to choose to terminate or to choose to accept and nourish the pregnancy. A survey of health professionals found that they viewed informed consent for non-invasive Down syndrome screening less rigorously than invasive tests.[30] Some studies suggest that testing early in the first trimester, when there has been less opportunity for maternal bonding with the unborn child and there is less public knowledge of the pregnancy, gives mothers scope to make this decision with less societal pressure and feelings of judgment.[31] At this stage, Down syndrome screening is still an optional test, as opposed to routine pregnancy screening, and health professionals need to explain the consequences of the test in order to facilitate informed decision making.[30] Not all expectant mothers will have their babies screened for Down syndrome. Often this choice reflects the parents' ethics about termination and whether they would terminate if the baby had Down syndrome.[32] Lower child-related anxiety has been reported in mothers who decline Down syndrome screening; however, increased anxiety in mothers who accepted screening returned to normal after receiving a negative result.[33] Furthermore, maternal anxiety returns to baseline in the third trimester in women with a positive result.[33] This may reflect acceptance of the baby and the plans and preparations the family have made to accommodate the child's additional needs. Some women report concern that routine early testing may reduce acceptance of people with Down syndrome, and people with disabilities in general, and result in a shift towards people expecting to be able to choose the 'perfect baby'.[31] A caring, non-judgmental, supportive approach is required for these discussions with potential parents.

Impact of prenatal screening on the prevalence of Down syndrome

In the UK between 1998 and 2008 live births of babies with Down syndrome decreased by 1%, while the number of Down syndrome pregnancies increased by 71%.[25] This is not due to improved detection alone, but reflects the increasing average maternal age. It is suggested that without screening, Down syndrome birth rates would have increased by 48% over this time period.[25]

The rate of termination of a pregnancy once Down syndrome has been detected is 92% in the UK.[34,35] The rate is similar in Australia, with 94.7% of pregnancies terminated after Down syndrome has been detected.[36] Similarly, a 95% termination rate has been reported in the Netherlands,[37] while population studies from the US report variability across different states, with 61.4% reported in California and 93.3% in Maine.[38] Parents' decision to screen during pregnancy will depend on multiple factors, including their ethics about termination, social acceptance of disability, age and relative risk, ethnicity and religious beliefs. Termination rates of Down syndrome pregnancies are correlated with increased maternal age and with detection at an earlier gestational age.[38] Access to screening creates changes in the socioeconomic demographic trends of families that babies with Down syndrome are born into. Screening programs in the 1980s that offered screening to mothers over 35 years of age created an increase in the proportion of babies with Down syndrome born to younger mothers. While screening is now offered to mothers of all ages, it is more likely that older mothers will take up the option and less likely that mothers under 30 years will do so due to the lower risk. This difference in uptake of screening may also influence termination rates, in that mothers who choose to screen their pregnancies may also be more likely to terminate in the event of Down syndrome being detected.

In France it has been noted that mothers with greater social disparity are less likely to present to a medical professional during their pregnancy until the second and in some cases third trimester.[26] Similarly in China, higher proportions of late gestational detection of Down syndrome (>28 weeks) result in a higher birth rate of babies with Down syndrome born in rural areas.[32] Decreased potential for screening in these groups results in a shift towards a higher prevalence of Down syndrome in low socioeconomic populations. This is concerning, in that increased social disparity increases the likelihood of poor access to ongoing healthcare, poor health outcomes and greater propensity towards secondary disabilities.

The advent of prenatal screening and subsequent termination creates a disability ethics conundrum: reduced incidence of Down syndrome, through the prevention of life, at a time when terminating life is legal. Pro-life lobbyists increase the burden of guilt for parents who make this decision, and religious beliefs may also impact on how parents feel. Korenromp et al. reported that parental reasons for terminating a Down syndrome pregnancy include:

- Belief that the child would never function independently (92%)
- Concern that the abnormality would be too severe (90%)
- Burden for caring for a child with disabilities is too heavy (83%)
- Burden on siblings is too high (73%)
- Burden on relationship is too high (55%)
- Concern about the future for the child after the death of the parents (82%)
- Uncertainty about the consequences of disability (78%)
- Low societal respect for people with disability (45%)
- Fear of regretting having a child with disabilities (45%)
- Impact on potential for career (23%)
- Financial burden (6%).[37]

Furthermore, Korenromp et al. found that only 35% of parents were confident in their decision to terminate, 44% felt some level of doubt and 21% felt considerable doubt.[37] Doubts included conflict with feelings and/or religion, disagreement with partner about the decision, uncertainty about the severity and consequences of disability, and doubts about the accuracy of the diagnosis.[37]

Ultimately it is the parents' right to make this decision and they must be informed by the best possible medical information. Indeed, a court in Italy found in favour of parents who sued their gynaecologist and a hospital for failing to recommend available tests that would have identified fetal deformity in utero for their baby with severe disabilities.[39] Medical liability for 'wrongful life' or 'wrongful birth' is not pursuable in most countries, so the situation in Italy is somewhat unique.[39] This premise supports a woman's right to self-determination and reproductive freedoms, but is also a relic of the eugenics movement, which views life with severe disability as being without value.[39] In clinical practice, extreme care and sensitivity are needed to support parents with this decision.

Support groups for parents who make the decision to terminate and struggle with it are lacking. Middle and late termination carry with it both psychological and physical trauma, and parents may grieve heavily for the life and hopes they have let go. This grief may be more than for those who miscarry, in that the parents have taken an active role in deciding to terminate the pregnancy. Counselling and psychological support are a critical part of caring for these parents.

Parents who choose to continue with the pregnancy also require additional support, and while diagnosis often focuses on the negatives, parents report that this can be a positive experience and they have every right to celebrate and look forward to the birth of their child.[40]

DIAGNOSIS AT BIRTH: IMPACT ON PARENTS

Parents report that a postnatal diagnosis of Down syndrome leaves them feeling shocked, overwhelmed, devastated, stunned, helpless, sad, grief-stricken and angry.[40,41] Furthermore, doctors and medical students say that they are given little training about developmental disabilities, and no training on how to deliver this news.[40] Parents report that the diagnosis is often shared by nurses or lactation consultants, who assume that the parents have already been made aware.[40] Insensitive handling of their privacy and their child's diagnosis creates additional trauma for parents at this time. While research is being undertaken to study the ways parents receive this information, and how best to deliver it, improvements are yet to filter through to clinical practice. Gentleness, respectful dialogue and sensitivity on the part of the naturopath are necessary to avoid adding to this trauma.

The concept of post-traumatic growth has been explored over the last 15 years in relation to the way parents of children with a serious diagnosis respond over time.[42] Initially, the diagnosis of a disability is met by parents with complex and conflicting emotions. Grief, loss and disappointment for the future life they imagined compete with the initial joy and discovery of their new baby. Acceptance of their child is compounded by lack of surety about what the future holds for the child, the family and the parents as individuals with their own life aspirations. While it would be insensitive as a therapist to wax lyrical about the amazing journey of personal growth these parents have been granted, naturopaths are well placed to gently guide and support parents in ways that foster personal growth and lead to their own needs being better met.

The stresses of raising a child with a disability go well beyond normal parental stresses and typically require lifelong additional responsibility.[43] Interestingly, a study of parents with a child with Down syndrome reported that only 13% would pursue pregnancy screening for subsequent pregnancies and, of those, the majority stated reasons of improved pregnancy planning and early intervention care.[41] Furthermore, with the exception of fetal malformations that are able to be detected through ultrasound, testing does not predict the severity of intellectual disability or functional capacity. People with Down syndrome vary from very mild disability and borderline intellectual function to very severe disability and profound intellectual impairment. Despite being a more severe handicap, associated with many more coexisting health problems, parents of adolescents with Down syndrome report much less distress, better psychological wellbeing and greater feelings of bonding and affection than parents of adolescents with autism or fragile X syndrome.[44] This is likely to be due to having fewer behavioural challenges in children with Down syndrome, and greater social acceptance and support.[44] People with Down syndrome are now living longer, healthier and more independent lives, and health conditions that previously carried high mortality rates are better managed.[45]

IMPROVING COGNITIVE POTENTIAL THROUGH ENHANCED PREGNANCY CARE

To date there has been no research to guide enhanced pregnancy care for mothers who decide to continue with a known Down syndrome pregnancy. Arguably this is an opportune time to ensure high-quality care and ideal nutrition. While pregnancy metabolism enhances nutrient absorption and will prioritise the baby's development for most nutrients, hypo-methylation will continue to impair development unless nutritionally addressed. Guidelines proposed in Chapters 7 and 14 should be considered when guiding dietary and supplement choices for women with Down syndrome pregnancies. Research is needed to assess the extent to which enhanced pregnancy care through nutritional intervention may improve lifelong health outcomes.

Table 19.1 is intended as a suggested guide for women continuing with a known Down syndrome pregnancy to reduce the impact of pathological changes that occur in utero. Critical changes at this time of development have lifelong consequences, so any attempt at improving pregnancy nutrition is likely to be beneficial.

FAMILY

Having a child with Down syndrome adds stress to the family, though less than other intellectual and developmental disabilities.[74] Many variables contribute to this. Parents of children with Down syndrome tend to be older and therefore have greater financial security, while the children themselves have fewer behavioural challenges than children with autism or ADHD.[74] Studies of parental style and family impact often explore the teenage years, predominantly from a maternal perspective, with little exploration of the experience of fathers.[75] Mothers of children with Down syndrome are observed to display more open warmth and affection, their parenting style is more directive and they report less child-related stress and greater child acceptance.[74] In addition to dealing with the daily issues of providing high-needs care, parents worry about the health problems of their child, future dependence, impact on siblings, social isolation and career aspirations.[76] Included within the stressors of raising a child with Down syndrome is the prospect of premature death of the child, and the burden of comorbid health conditions.[75]

Parental confidence and wellbeing are associated with better outcomes for children with Down syndrome and positively correlated with access to social services and resources, the support of extended family, a harmonious marital relationship and community-based support groups.[76] A supportive cohesive family unit also increases access to other support and services that have positive implications on success through adulthood, including future employment. Supporting the parents of children with Down syndrome with stress management is an important role that naturopaths can play.

INFANT CARE

Initial assessment

Children with Down syndrome have an increased predisposition to a range of health problems, some of which should be screened for at birth. Congenital cardiac abnormalities occur in 50% of children with Down syndrome, and can be fatal if left untreated.[77] Comprehensive health screening should include:
- Hearing assessment
- Visual assessment
- Cardiac assessment
- Feeding assessment
- Reflexes
- Blood tests: full blood count, thyroid function test.

Infant survival to 12 months of age is lower in females (82% compared with 94% for non-gender specific), babies born with cardiac abnormalities (78%), low birthweight babies (75%) and in Australia, being Aboriginal (78%).[78] Lower survival in female babies is attributed to a higher incidence of congenital heart defects.[78] Higher mortality in Aboriginal babies with Down syndrome may be attributable to higher infant and child mortality observed in Indigenous populations and higher incidence of low

TABLE 19.1 Suggested nutrition guide for women continuing with a Down syndrome pregnancy

Nutrient	Rationale	Dose and timing
Antioxidants	Reduce the impact of oxidative stress	Include abundant and varied sources in the diet throughout the pregnancy.
Calcium	Healthy fetal bone development is dependent on adequate maternal calcium intake. Fetal calcium deposition is greatest during the third trimester. Supplementation of calcium during the third trimester is also associated with decreased maternal bone resorption.[46]	Supplementation should be guided by existing sources of calcium in a woman's diet. Where appropriate, it is reasonable to achieve recommended daily intake through diet alone. When food restrictions limit calcium intake, supplement additional calcium to achieve a combined total of 1000 mg per day.
Folate	Hypo-methylation is implicated in congenital heart defects in Down syndrome. While folinic acid or L-5-methyl tetrahydrofolate is likely to be a more clinically appropriate form of folate to supplement when MTHFR mutations are involved, current research demonstrating a clinical benefit is based on folic acid supplementation. The benefit of folate supplementation appears to be highest within the first 6 weeks of pregnancy, which is earlier than detection of Down syndrome for most women.[47] Current evidence regarding increased incidence of allergic disease with supplementation of folate in the latter half of pregnancy is inconclusive and warrants further investigation.[48]	4–5 mg/day in first trimester.[49] Also include abundant sources of natural folate through dietary sources (e.g. leafy green vegetables).
Iodine	Iodine deficiency and insufficiency in pregnancy are prevalent in many countries and result in intellectual impairment, hearing loss, short stature and neurological impairment.[50] Iodine deficiency also increases the risk of thyroid disease in both the mother and the fetus.[51]	Caution is warranted with iodine supplementation, as high doses may stimulate iodine-induced hyperthyroidism and autoimmune thyroid disease in vulnerable populations.[52] 200 micrograms per day in addition to iodised salt through the diet.[51]
Iron	Iron is critical to fetal development. Deficiency in pregnancy is associated with cognitive impairment[53] and increased thyroid autoimmunity.[54] However, excessive iron is toxic and is associated with increased oxidative stress.[53] Iron excess is also associated with a higher incidence of gestational diabetes.[55] Iron levels should be regularly checked during pregnancy (weeks 12, 24 and 36) to assess additional needs. More frequent testing is necessary while supplementing to monitor changes in iron levels and adjust supplementation as necessary.	The recommended daily intake of iron in pregnancy is 27 mg per day. Supplementation should be guided by blood levels: • Severe deficiency (ferritin <15 micrograms/L): 100 mg/day • Moderate deficiency (ferritin 16–30 micrograms/L): 60–80 mg/day • Mild deficiency (ferritin 31–70 micrograms/L): 40 mg daily • Iron replete (ferritin >70 micrograms/L): no supplementation.[56] Choose well-absorbed forms of iron such as iron amino acid chelate or iron bisglycinate.
Magnesium	Magnesium deficiency and subclinical deficiency are common in women in both developed and developing countries and are implicated in preeclampsia pathogenesis, gestational diabetes and interuterine growth restriction.[57] Magnesium is also involved in bone formation, neurological development and function, muscular contraction, blood sugar regulation, vascular tone and cardiac excitability.[54]	100–350 mg of elemental magnesium per day, in divided doses, with food.[54] Choose a well-absorbed form of magnesium such as magnesium citrate or magnesium amino acid chelate.
Methylated B vitamins	Association between Down syndrome and MTHFR polymorphisms highlights the need for supplementation of methylated B vitamins in Down syndrome pregnancies. While research to validate this is currently lacking, the implications of inadequate methylation on neural development are well documented.	A high-quality methylated B-complex is likely to be more beneficial than isolated B vitamins.

TABLE 19.1 Suggested nutrition guide for women continuing with a Down syndrome pregnancy—cont'd

Nutrient	Rationale	Dose and timing
Omega-3 fatty acids	Omega-3 fatty acids are involved in neurological development and prostaglandin pathways. Supplementation with omega-3 fatty acids has been shown to reduce inflammation and oxidative stress in gestational diabetes.[58] Inconsistency exists within the literature as to the benefits of omega-3 supplementation in pregnancy, but supplementation has been shown to decrease neonatal mortality and hospitalisations.[59] Given the safety profile of omega-3 fatty acids, and that Down syndrome neurological impairment begins in utero, omega-3 supplementation is likely to be beneficial.	3000–5000 mg of high-quality molecularly distilled fish oil concentrate. Consider dietary intake when recommending omega-3 supplementation.
Prebiotics: fructooligosaccharides (FOS), galactooligosaccharides (GOS), lactulose	Prebiotics selectively feed specific types of beneficial bacteria in the colon and increase the growth of both endogenous and supplemented lactobacilli and bifidobacteria.[60] Prebiotic supplementation has been shown to have immunomodulatory benefits, reduce pro-inflammatory mediators and improve mineral absorption.[60] While there are no clinical data to verify the benefits of prebiotic supplementation in Down syndrome pregnancies, improving gastrointestinal health will alter the inflammatory mediators the unborn baby is exposed to.	Bloating and discomfort may occur with moderate to large doses. Start with a small dose and increase gradually: • FOS: 4–10 g/day • GOS: 2.5–10 g/day • Lactulose: 3–15 g/day.
Probiotics: lactobacillus rhamnosus (LGG)	Probiotic supplementation has been shown to have a beneficial effect on the production of anti-inflammatory, mediatory, immunomodulatory compounds and strengthens the intestinal barrier, thereby reducing intestinal permeability.[61] When taken during pregnancy, LGG has been shown to reduce the incidence of atopic eczema, due to reduced transportation of antigens through the intestinal lumen.[61]	$>10^9$ bacteria/dose.[61]
Selenium	Selenium deficiency in pregnancy exacerbates the effect of insufficient iodine on the fetus and the mother and is associated with poorer childhood outcomes including language and psychomotor development.[62] Selenium is also involved in immune system function and is a potent antioxidant.[63]	100–200 micrograms per day.
Vitamin C	Vitamin C is a potent antioxidant, involved in recycling other antioxidants, and plays a critical role in the immune system. Vitamin C deficiency in pregnancy is associated with increased blood pressure, preeclampsia, anaemia and low birthweight babies.[64] Studies to date have failed to demonstrate benefit, though vitamin C supplementation has been shown to decrease the risk of placental abruption and premature rupture of the membranes.[64] Given the high antioxidant load in Down syndrome pregnancies, vitamin C may be beneficial, though clinical studies are needed to confirm this.	500–1000 mg per day.
Vitamin D	Vitamin D influences maternal gene expression, neonatal lung maturation and the likelihood of allergic disease in the child.[65] Vitamin D is also involved in calcium regulation, cellular proliferation and differentiation, and is a common deficiency in pregnant mothers.[66] Vitamin D supplementation in pregnancy has been shown to decrease the incidence of allergic sensitisation in children[67] as well as the incidence of upper and lower respiratory tract infections in neonates.[68]	Supplement 5000–6400 IU per day in sunlight-deprived populations. Ideal blood levels of vitamin D should be 100–150 nmol/L. Supplementation with 4000–6400 IU per day has been shown to be safe in pregnancy to achieve this.[69]
Vitamin E	Lower vitamin E intake in pregnancy is associated with increased risk of hyperglycaemia and insulin resistance.[70] Yet there is little clinical evidence to support vitamin E supplementation in pregnancy. Some research suggests that vitamins E and C supplementation may be associated with an increased risk of preeclampsia, hypertension and premature rupture of the membranes.[71]	Include abundant sources of vitamin E through the diet, including nuts, seeds, avocados and fresh green leafy vegetables.
Zinc	Poor zinc status in pregnancy has negative outcomes for mother and baby, including increased risk of spontaneous abortion, preterm labour, congenital malformations, interuterine growth retardation and preeclampsia.[72]	30 mg of elemental zinc per day, both in isolation and in combination with a multivitamin, has been shown to improve neonatal pregnancy outcomes.[73]

birthweight babies,[78] and reflects the persistent health disparity between Indigenous and non-Indigenous Australians. Slower growth is observed during infancy in babies with Down syndrome, as babies have difficulty gaining weight.[12]

Neonates with Down syndrome tend to spend longer in hospital than age-matched peers without Down syndrome, require longer times on oxygen, longer stays in intensive care units and are often discharged home while still needing oxygen.[79] Hospital admissions also occur more frequently in babies of lower birthweight.[79]

Breastfeeding

The importance of breastfeeding any infant cannot be overstated – and within a culture that has adopted artificial formula as the norm since the 1950s, much support and encouragement are needed for mothers to successfully initiate and continue to breastfeed their children. The World Health Organization recommends breastfeeding exclusively for the first 6 months, with continued breastfeeding alongside appropriate foods for 2 years and beyond, for as long as mutually agreeable between mother and baby.[80] Breastmilk contains compounds that continue maturation of the gastrointestinal tract, immune system, neurological system and microbiota, among many other benefits (for more detail, see Chapter 15). Additionally, skin-to-skin contact inherent with breastfeeding further enhances the baby's skin flora. The additional risks of comorbid conditions, gastrointestinal dysfunction, autoimmune predisposition and developmental delay in children with Down syndrome increase the importance of successful breastfeeding. Breastfeeding provides protection from gastrointestinal and respiratory infections, which are more common in babies with Down syndrome.[81,82] Breastfeeding also helps decrease the incidence of allergic diseases (including asthma and allergic rhinitis), autoimmune disease and obesity.[83] Additional hospital visits and hospital stays expose babies with Down syndrome to a greater number of more virulent pathogens, which their immune systems are poorly equipped to deflect. Breastfeeding mothers who accompany their babies during these hospital stays will also encounter these pathogens and produce antibodies in response, which the baby will receive through the breastmilk. In this respect, breastmilk may certainly be thought of as 'food as medicine' and provides the means for critical immune protection and development.

Children with Down syndrome may have increased difficulty with attachment to the breast, due to anatomical differences of the palate and tongue, and poor muscle tone. However, breastfeeding stimulates all of a baby's senses, through touch, smell, intimacy with the mother and feeding, and helps strengthen and coordinate the muscles of the tongue, lips and palate.[81,82] Babies with Down syndrome may tire quickly at the breast and need more guidance with attachment, but will breastfeed more effectively as they grow and become stronger. Patience and persistence are needed to establish effective feeding. Early development of these muscles is important groundwork

for eating solids, speech acquisition and orofacial development.

Maternal stress around diagnosis and prognosis of the child may impede establishment of milk supply. Initial diagnosis at birth can leave families in a state of 'disenfranchised joy' with hesitant congratulations from friends and loved ones, awkward interactions with health professionals and bonding interrupted by grief, shock and uncertainty. Supporting mothers to breastfeed at this time gives a sense of normalcy and facilitates bonding between mother and baby. Hormones produced during breastfeeding help with maternal coping skills, reduce the risk of postnatal depression and contribute towards acceptance of the child. Including fathers in the cuddles and intimacy of learning to breastfeed will assist with paternal bonding, acceptance and coping, and may lay the early groundwork for the couple to progress through this challenge together. Support of a skilled, understanding, well-trained lactation consultant is needed to help guide parents to establish bonding and breastfeeding, and make well-educated decisions about infant nutrition.

Early intervention and environmental enrichment

'Early intervention' refers to therapeutic strategies implemented within the first 6 years of life.[84] Little clinical or experimental data currently exist to guide policy on early intervention for children with Down syndrome.[85] Capone asserts that while improvements have been observed in adaptive behaviours, progress in cognitive function as measured by IQ is temporary.[86] Capone argues that defective 'hardware' is responsible for this lack of progress – Down syndrome children lack the neurological organisation to use early intervention education.[86] This kind of opinion when carried by health professionals, child educators and parents creates low expectations of development and performance, which in turn reduces attentiveness to stimulating the child's intellect.[76] This is disempowering for parents and detrimental to the child, and is reflective of attitudinal discrimination.

Recent studies present a more positive perspective. Early intervention beginning at birth improves parental confidence and provides positive goals to work towards at a time when parents may be overwhelmed by the diagnosis.[76] The concept of 'environmental enrichment' builds on the work of Skeels and Dye, who demonstrated that a loving and intellectually stimulating environment can greatly enhance IQ and cognitive function, whereas depriving children of this environment is detrimental.[87] This research was the first study to demonstrate that cognitive potential is not predetermined by genetics and that early developmental conditioning, exposure and environment have great scope to influence lifelong outcomes. Environmental enrichment can be used to increase sensory and motor neuron stimulation. Infant massage as a form of environmental enrichment has been shown to significantly improve visual acuity in infants with Down syndrome when performed from birth to 6 months of age.[85] Purpura et al. highlight the importance of this finding – that not only is the neonatal period highly neuroplastic, but also visual function is integral to other learning, social, communication and neurodevelopmental outcomes.[85]

Environmental enrichment also occurs through providing a stimulating environment in the home, developmentally appropriate toys and contact with other children and adults.[76] People with Down syndrome continue to improve non-verbal cognitive skills through adolescence and adulthood.[88]

Developmental milestones

Parents often enquire about expected developmental milestones in children with Down syndrome, which occur later than in children within the general population. Delayed development of motor skills limits the experiences the child can have in exploring the world around them, which will further delay cognitive and motor development.[89] Early gross motor performance in infants is predictive of motor skill performance at 2 years of age.[89] Early gross motor movements include head holding, head stability, posture, kicking and visual tracking. Active engagement of the child and physiotherapy exercises to build muscle strength and coordination are necessary to improve motor skill development.[89] The following can be used to guide parents and clinicians to understand the range of normal development for children with Down syndrome:

– Anterior fontanel closure: around 2 years of age[12]
– Holds own head independently: 1–18 weeks (average: 3.95 weeks)[90]
– Smiling 1.5–4 months (average: 2 months)[91]
– Rolling over: 1–60 months (average: 6.38 months)[90]
– Sits unsupported: 5–72 months (average: 11.14 months in girls, 12.52 months in boys)[90]
– Creeping: 4–24 months (average: 12 months)
– Talking, words: 6–84 months (average: 21.82 months in girls, 26.59 months in boys)[90]
– Talking, sentences/phrases: 12–132 months (average: 41.82 months for phrases, 52 months for sentences)[90]
– Standing: 11–42 months (average: 20 months)[91]
– Teeth: often do not start to erupt until after 1 year old[12]
– Walking: 12–65 months (average 24 months)[91]
– Eating finger foods: 8–28 months (average 12 months)[91]
– Eating with spoon: 28–72 months[92]
– Eating with a fork: 28–90 months[92]
– Toilet training, bladder: 20–95 months (average: 48 months)[91]
– Toilet training, bowel: 28–90 months (average: 42 months)[91]
– Undressing: 29–72 months (average: 40 months)[91]
– Dressing: 38–98 months (average: 58 months)[91]

– Puberty: appears early, but with slower growth during adolescence than typically developing peers, and there is a tendency towards obesity.[12]

CHILDHOOD–SCHOOL-AGE YEARS

Cognitive capacity

Children with Down syndrome present with a wide variation in cognitive ability, from mild (IQ: 55–69) to moderate (IQ: 40–54) to severe (IQ: 20–39) intellectual disability.[93] Lower IQ is associated with lower adaptive functioning, reduced capacity for reasoning and increased need for support with activities of daily living.[94] Reduced brain volume and brachycephaly (flattening of the back of the skull) is observed on autopsy and magnetic resonance imaging (MRI) studies in people with Down syndrome, with disproportionately reduced size of the frontal cortex, temporal cortex, uncus, hippocampus and cerebellum.[95] In contrast, the parahippocampal gyrus appears larger on MRI and other areas of the brain appear to be of normal size.[95] These differences in brain structure have a profound impact on short- and long-term memory and capacity to use old strategies or experiences to understand and respond to new situations.[95] Slower memory recall and responsiveness, and reduced behavioural flexibility, also result from these neurological differences.[95]

Cognitive deficits in people with Down syndrome have negative consequences for learning, memory, language acquisition and capacity for executive function.[95] 'Executive function' refers to the ability to coordinate cognitive functions and behaviours in order to plan, negotiate, access working memory and respond to stimuli.[96] Executive function requires complex organisation of multiple areas of the brain, drawing on memories and stored knowledge, decision making, rationalisation of the situation, and action. Cognitive deficits result in multiple opportunities for this process to be unsuccessful, resulting in poor learning outcomes. This also has negative implications for task performance and perceptual capabilities.[97]

Cognitive capacity is correlated with expressive language, though this may be difficult to assess due to oro-muscular impacts on speech intelligibility.[93] Difficulty in physically forming words increases the complexity of assessing IQ. Listening comprehension is typically poorer than literacy and reading comprehension,[98] which may be related to slower processing time. Slower auditory processing results in differences in task performance, and auditory tasks being more challenging than visual tasks.[97] Literacy is improved when drawings are used alongside text to give meaning and relevance to written prose.[99] Pictures that directly represent written text are highly effective in improving comprehension and recall of text, not just in children with Down syndrome, but also in children with reading difficulties and other causes of intellectual impairment.[99] A reciprocal relationship exists between memory and reading, by which memory is enriched by reading tasks, and reading and comprehension are enhanced by improved memory capacity.[99] Memory training in children with Down syndrome has been shown to improve not only memory skills, but also the cognitive mechanisms involved with verbal memory span.[100]

Adaptive functioning

Children and adolescents with Down syndrome require greater assistance from carers with household and self-care tasks, and have lower levels of independence than typically developing children.[101] Difficulties with household tasks can be due to a combination of physical limitations (e.g. balance, coordination, short stature, low muscle tone) and cognitive capacity, which involves memory of where things are kept, and task sequencing.[101] Tasks of daily living require additional support from family members and carers. Researchers in the Netherlands found that only 60% of older teenagers with Down syndrome were able to maintain adequate personal hygiene, 55–60% were able to prepare and eat their own breakfast without assistance, 7% were able to cook a simple meal without assistance, and 12% were able to pay for goods in a store unassisted.[102] Ability to tell the time, make phone calls or make short journeys on foot around the neighbourhood, or having sufficient self-competence to be left at home unsupervised for short periods, is lacking in most teenagers with Down syndrome.[102] Parents report that they place less importance on life skills than academic progress, thus this is often overlooked.[103] Furthermore, Bouck reports that in children with intellectual disability, being taught life skills was not associated with level of intellectual impairment.[103] While assumptions of capability might be made for those with very severe intellectual disabilities, this suggests that even more capable children are not receiving life skills training.

Children and adolescents with Down syndrome can be taught a range of tasks in the home that will help prepare them for greater independence throughout adulthood, by breaking down tasks into individual steps, and with supported participation. Parents of children with Down syndrome often tailor their expectations of household contributions to their child's individual abilities.[101] While this is positive in that it sets the child up to succeed at the task, it does not help them to expand their skill set or foster greater independence. Learning life skills throughout the teenage years is essential for successful transitioning from life as a student to life within the adult world.[103] Encouraging parents to expand the range of tasks they engage their child in will enhance long-term independence and has long-term implications for health and satisfaction with life. Resources are available to help parents teach life skills to their teenagers with Down syndrome and can be found through local disability support services. Disability Services Australia (www.dsa.org.au) covers a comprehensive range of essential life skills and considerations for independent living: transport, career planning, budgeting and money management, living arrangements, adult rights and responsibilities, emotional and physical health, transition to work programs and guardianship.

School choices and impact on cognitive development and health

Expectations of low achievement contribute to poor educational outcomes for children with Down syndrome in both integrated and segregated schools.[104] Higher levels of cognitive and adaptive function increase the success of employment as adults, so every opportunity to develop to potential during school years should be taken.[105] A 2006 comparison of integrated and segregated schools found no difference between the two settings for daily living skills, play and leisure activities or social coping skills.[104] Relationship development was more advanced in segregated education, which may be due to greater opportunities to develop friendships with peers of similar ability.[104] Communication and expressive language, however, were more advanced in integrated schools, due to the increased demands of communicating with peers who do not have disabilities.[104] Communication skills are essential for independence in adult life. Social skills are also of importance in workplace settings. Thus it is imperative that regardless of the type of school, social and communication skills are well attended to.

ADOLESCENCE

Behaviour

A study in the Netherlands reported a higher incidence of problem behaviour in older teenagers with Down syndrome than in teenagers without Down syndrome: 51% of children with Down syndrome were found to have clinical or borderline behaviour problems, and 50% were found to have social problems.[106] Severity of social and behavioural problems was found to correlate with severity of intellectual disability, with those with mild disability showing the least problems, and those with severe disability showing more severe social and behavioural problems.[106] Behaviours included mood swings (43%), persistent disobedience (33%) and anger (33%).[102] In general, boys showed less skill acquisition and language mastery than girls, though no significant difference was observed with social abilities.[102] Reasons for this may be multifactorial and include difficulties that arise through sexual maturation, challenges of relating to age-equivalent peers and conflict between teenager expectations and parental limitations to activities.

Expectations

Some studies have found that as teenagers with Down syndrome get older, social activity becomes more focused on formal activities (structured or organised activities such as music lessons, skill-building classes, sports, youth groups) and less informal activities (more spontaneous activities, such as phone calls to friends, reading, board games).[107] While formal activities encourage friendship development with peers, particularly those who also have disabilities and can relate to the challenges young people with Down syndrome face, encouraging informal activities is also important to reduce tendencies towards sedentary behaviour and improve community acceptance and engagement.[107]

Developing life skills

Acquiring functional life skills, or skills of daily living, is essential for successful transitioning from school expectations to adult life and employment.[103] These skills include money handling, self-care, cooking, house-keeping, negotiating public transport, relationship skills and time management. Life skill focus is often lacking in school curricula, where academic achievement is prioritised.[103] Furthermore, a 2010 study found that parents prioritise academic achievement above life skill development, and that low numbers of people with intellectual disability receive life skills training after high school.[103] Engagement in life skill programs has been positively correlated with satisfaction with life, successful employment and higher wages.[103] If absent at school, life skill training needs to be attained through other training or therapy-based programs.

ADULTHOOD

Access to services and opportunities

Community engagement is a strong predictor of quality of life and functional capacity in people with Down syndrome. Bertoli et al. reported that only 30–40% of people with Down syndrome were involved in some kind of work or educational activity past the age of 20 years and that this correlated with sedentary leisure time and deterioration of mental function and capacity.[108] While school provides an ongoing source of intellectual stimulation and social opportunities, vulnerability exists for people with Down syndrome entering adult life without further meaningful activity to pursue. Barriers to community and social participation can be attitudinal, environmental, financial and logistical. Attitudinal barriers can be through negative attitudes of friends or strangers, unwillingness of people to associate with a person with a disability or involve low expectations of what a person with Down syndrome is capable of or can achieve.[109] The physical environment, and how accessible it is, remains a persistent barrier that is more resistant to change, because it involves the physical infrastructure of the towns and cities we live in.[109] Building legislation in most developed countries now requires disability access to be designed into new buildings, but this does not change the inaccessibility of buildings that already exist. Logistical challenges are a barrier for people with Down syndrome when needing family or paid carers to assist with transport to and from places, or to organise membership or application forms for community events. Consideration of a broad range of factors is needed when recommending activities or programs for people with Down syndrome, to ensure that they are physically and logistically able to participate, and have the support they need to attend.

Independent or supported living

People with Down syndrome often remain living with their parents into adulthood and continue to need support with activities of daily living.[109] This has implications for the family in terms of finance and maintaining an ongoing carer relationship, while also limiting independence and socialisation for the person with Down syndrome.[109] Community integration has benefits for people with disabilities and the community. This is through increased awareness of disability, enhanced socialisation and relationship development, life skill development and fostering appreciation of people with disabilities as valued members of the community.[110]

Supported employment transition

Participation of people with disabilities including Down syndrome in employment is relatively low.[111] People with intellectual disabilities are three to four times more likely to be unemployed than people without an intellectual disability.[110] Teenagers benefit from training focused on presenting themselves to employers, resume writing, casual work and volunteer work experience while still at school.[112] Teenagers with disabilities also need specific training about disability discrimination, their rights within the workplace and how to discuss their disability and capabilities with an employer.[112]

Transition into the workforce after school is an important goal for all school leavers, but is particularly difficult for people with disabilities.[113] Transition to work (TTW) programs can be an effective way of bridging the gap between school and employment. TTW programs involve a disability worker helping to secure a job placement and providing ongoing support, and are an effective means of facilitating employment.[105,114] Furthermore, people who have received a supported employment position are more likely to remain employed and have reduced dependence on social security benefits.[114]

Workplace participation of people with Down syndrome fosters appreciation of people with disabilities, fills a valuable role within workplaces and improves acceptance of diversity within communities. It also improves quality of life outcomes, provides the opportunity for greater socialisation and relationship development and improves family life. Greater involvement in decision making and planning for transition into the workforce by the person with Down syndrome is correlated with greater success.[15] This impact is independent of other factors such as family income, age, gender, health conditions, behaviour and functional capacity.[15]

Support needs

Most young people with Down syndrome require assistance with communication, more complex cognitive functions and complex self-care tasks.[115] Mobility is in general more independent, though most will require assistance with transport, with one study reporting that only 17% of young adults with Down syndrome were able to use public transport independently.[115] Travel training is manageable for most people with Down syndrome, is an effective means to improve day-to-day independence (e.g. to and from employment/school) and helps reduce additional long-term duties for family/paid carers.[116]

Friendships and social opportunities tend to decline once young people with Down syndrome finish school and may contribute to loneliness, isolation and depression.[15] Planning for the next phase of life is important to prevent or lessen the impact of this reduction in daily activity and social engagement. Moving into employment is not guaranteed and may take time. Encouraging families to access support services that facilitate transition to work or supported employment opportunities, as well as community activities that enable social engagement and recreation, is one way natural therapists can help mitigate this risk. Participation in supported employment is associated with improved psychological wellbeing, quality of life, self-knowledge, self-confidence and feelings of adequacy.[15] For those who are unable to work, due to inadequate opportunities or severity of disability, many day services exist within disability support and mainstream services. Engagement in these services does not provide all of the same benefits of employment, but will help with social engagement and intellectual stimulation, and may result in further opportunities arising.

Supporting carers

Carers of people with Down syndrome are more often than not ageing parents or siblings who have taken over responsibility after their parents have passed away or are no longer able to fill this role. Family carers report a sense of sadness and emotional strain with the onset of dementia symptoms that occur at a younger age in people with Down syndrome.[117] Family carers also report:

- Grief at watching their family member decline
- Dementia symptoms that are abusive or aggressive are emotionally difficult
- Night-time disruptions reduce capacity to cope during the day and stay patient and loving
- Lack of knowledge about disease progression and support services creates anxiety and fearfulness about the future, and whether they can continue to provide care
- Having very little time to themselves.[117]

The commitment and responsibility taken on by family members is through dedication and love, and requires additional support. Family carers are often on-call throughout the day and night, and may have little in the way of respite care. Physical and emotional exhaustion are common. It is important to gently enquire as to how well they are coping. Naturopaths can gently guide carers towards better self-care to support them to continue caring. This may be through herbal medicines, ensuring nutritional (and other) needs are met, massage and referral for psychological support.

END-OF-LIFE CARE

Death is a very uncomfortable subject in most Western societies. Children and people with disabilities are particularly sheltered from it, though children do get some exposure through stories in children's picture books. Stories are one of the ways we teach children about death and the impermanence of life and grief, and can also be used to help people with intellectual impairment to learn about these topics. Traditions in other parts of the world like Day of the Dead celebrations hold space for death, for remembering those who are no longer with us and for accepting death as an inevitability for all of us.

People with disabilities often experience a 'disenfranchised death', in which they are protected from being taught about death and understanding illness or accidents that may result in death.[118] Lack of understanding of causality, ageing and cessation of life leaves people with intellectual disabilities vulnerable to misinterpretation, fear and anxiety for themselves and loved ones, confusion and irrational thinking.[119] This may extend to maladaptive responses to grief, separation anxiety, feelings of misplaced guilt and insecurities about friends or loved ones.[119] This results in having even more limited capacity to understand the death of a loved one or their own impending death, to make choices regarding treatment and funeral services, to say goodbyes and engage in particular activities they would like to do before they die. This misplaced protection denies people with disabilities the respect and dignity required to make autonomous decisions.[118] People with Down syndrome with a higher level of intellectual capacity will have greater ability to understand concepts around death and dying than people with more severe impairment. In naturopathic care, it is important that we make no assumptions about what people may or may not know, and sensitively enquire about their knowledge when death and dying are pertinent to their own situation or that of close friends or loved ones. While it is outside the scope of naturopathic medicine to counsel patients about end-of-life education, naturopaths are well placed to identify this as a topic that needs further exploration and guidance.

SPECIFIC HEALTH CONCERNS

Many diseases occur in increased frequency in people with Down syndrome due to the duplication of chromosome 21. The additional copy of this gene increases the likelihood of gene expression of oncogenes, resulting in increased leukaemia and other cancer risk.[120] Other comorbidities that occur with increased frequency in people with Down syndrome are explored in Table 19.2.

Cardiac complications

Congenital heart defects (CHD) occur in up to 50% of babies born with Down syndrome.[122–125] While maternal age increases the risk of a Down syndrome pregnancy, increased maternal age is associated with lower risk of CHD – a 1% reduction in risk per year of maternal age.[126] This may be due to increased preconception and perinatal

TABLE 19.2 Common health conditions that occur more frequently in people with Down syndrome

System	Specific health conditions
Cardiac	Congenital cardiac malformations (approximately 50%) Cor pulmonale Pulmonary hypertension Valvular dysfunction Mitral valve prolapse (adults, 50%) and aortic regurgitation (young adults and adolescents)
Dental	Delayed and abnormal dentition Over-crowding of teeth due to smaller oral cavity
Dermatological	Alopecia Dry skin Eczema Folliculitis Hyperkeratosis Seborrhoeic dermatitis Vitiligo
Developmental	Developmental delay Learning difficulties (100%) Intellectual impairment (100%) Short stature Early-onset dementia and cognitive decline
Ear, nose and throat, and other respiratory disorders	Asthma Chronic catarrh Eustachian tube dysfunction Hearing loss (conductive or sensorineural) (75%) Recurrent and chronic otitis media, and serous otitis media Sleep-related breathing disorders, including sleep apnoea Stenotic (narrow) ear canals
Endocrine	Diabetes mellitus (type 1) Hyper- and hypothyroidism (15%)
Gastrointestinal	Coeliac disease (4–17%) Congenital malformations to digestive tract (12%) Constipation Dietary intolerances and allergies Feeding difficulties, including forward thrust tongue, dysphagia and poor latch (infant) Gastro-oesophageal reflux Hirschsprung's disease
Haematological	Leukaemia Neonatal polycythaemia Neonatal thrombocytopenia Polycythaemia, macrocytosis, leukopenia Transient myeloproliferative states Transient neonatal myeloproliferative states
Neuropsychiatric	Autistic spectrum disorder Dementia (adults) Depressive illness Epilepsy Infantile spasms and other myoclonic epilepsies
Metabolic	Obesity
Ophthalmic	Blepharitis (eyelid inflammation) Cataracts: congenital (3%) and acquired (50%) Glaucoma Keratoconus (degenerative thinning of cornea to cone shape) Nasolacrimal obstruction Nystagmus (20%) Refractive errors (50%) Strabismus (squint) (44%)

Continued

TABLE 19.2 Common health conditions that occur more frequently in people with Down syndrome—cont'd

System	Specific health conditions
Orthopaedic	Atlanto-occipital instability (14%) Cervical spine disorders Hip subluxation/dislocation (6%) Hypotonia Joint hypermobility Patella instability Metatarsus varus (also called intoe, toeing in or 'pigeon toed') Osteoporosis Pes planus (flat foot) Scoliosis
Reproductive	Early-onset menopause in women Infertility and subfertility in males Hypogenitalia in males High rate of Down syndrome in offspring (in females, 50%) Undescended testes Testicular microlithiasis Testicular cancer

Source: [1, 34, 121]

care, as later pregnancies may be more likely to be planned and more likely to entail a higher degree of medical supervision. In Brazil, the rate of CHD in Down syndrome babies has been found to be as high as 70%, which may reflect differences in prenatal care and screening, or greater accuracy in neonatal cardiac screening.[127] Maternal obesity and smoking have been shown to increase the risk of CHD, while diabetes and hypertension have no significant effect on CHD in Down syndrome.[126]

Between 1992 and 2012 in Sweden, complex malformations in babies with Down syndrome fell by 40%, though the rate of CHD developing later in life remained high.[126] This rate may reflect neonatal screening practices in Sweden, where early second-trimester ultrasound may detect complex cardiac malformations, leading to further testing and termination of the pregnancy.[126] Gender discrepancy has been observed in some studies, in which 38% of male babies with Down syndrome and 49% of female babies with Down syndrome were born with a congenital cardiac abnormality.[78,126] This gender disparity continues throughout the life span.

Physical examination by a cardiologist detects the majority of cases of CHD in Down syndrome, but many cases are missed, with 34% remaining undiagnosed at 6 weeks and 25% remaining undiagnosed at 12 weeks.[128] Physical examination relies on the presence of signs and symptoms of cardiac abnormalities and will therefore not necessarily detect cases that are asymptomatic.[128] Assessment by an echocardiogram is recommended for all babies born with Down syndrome by 6 weeks of age[34] and to date is the most sensitive method for assessing cardiac abnormalities in babies.[128] Surgical correction of cardiac malformations is usually performed by 6 months of age, with a 1-year survival rate of 95%.[34] Surgery is performed as early as is safe to do so, usually within the first 6 months of life, and in some hospitals as early as 3–4

months.[124] Early surgery reduces the overall impact of CHD on growth, development and secondary complications including abnormal heart and lung development, pulmonary hypertension, ischaemia, embolic events and heart failure, but must be balanced against the risk of surgery in babies so young.[128,129] CHD also has implications for language development delay[130] and gross motor development.[131] Pulmonary infections including pneumonia and sepsis are more common in babies with Down syndrome and CHD, which has implications for mortality and timing of corrective cardiac surgery.[127]

In recent times, infants and young children have been denied access to corrective cardiac surgery, due to perceived lower quality of life and reduced life expectancy, resulting in increased fatality.[132] Discrimination on the basis of disability is not acceptable under internationally accepted human rights conventions. Improvements in cardiac surgery have contributed dramatically to the increased life expectancy now observed in people with Down syndrome, though it is still around 20 years less than the general population.[132] Proactive surgical intervention for babies with CHD and Down syndrome has resulted in a 10-fold improvement in life expectancy, and should occur as early as is safe to do so.[124]

Weight and height impairment occurs from birth in babies with CHD, more so than for babies with Down syndrome and CHD than babies with Down syndrome but not CHD, or babies with CHD alone.[123] Postoperative recovery takes longer in babies with Down syndrome than babies without Down syndrome.[123] Neurological development remains poorer in children with Down syndrome and cardiac abnormalities after corrective surgery, but little difference is seen between these children and age-matched peers with Down syndrome by the time they reach school age.[129] Risk of pulmonary hypertension and other cardiac dysfunction is not completely eliminated by surgery, so regular monitoring by a cardiologist over time will be necessary to detect and appropriately manage cardiac conditions as they arise.[124] Surgical practices have improved greatly over the last two decades, and congenital heart surgery now confers less mortality risk in babies with Down syndrome.[133] Mortality for cardiac surgery is not significantly different between babies with CHD with and without Down syndrome, though morbidity, length of hospital stay and complications remain higher in babies with Down syndrome.[133] Predisposition to infections, upper airway obstruction, increased respiratory secretions and gastro-oesophageal reflux increase complications and result in increased length of time spent in neonatal intensive care units pre- and postoperatively.[133]

Cardiovascular disease, however, seems to be low in people with Down syndrome, despite a predisposition to CHD, obesity and sedentary lifestyles.[134] Atherosclerosis is lower in people with Down syndrome than in the general population and does not appear to be a significant risk for cardiovascular health.[135] Hospitalisation rates are higher in adults with Down syndrome, though the number of hospitalisations due to CHD in adults with Down syndrome has decreased due to improved surgical correction of congenital cardiac malformations.[136] Despite this, death following hospitalisation is higher in adults with Down syndrome than in the general population, as is relative risk of heart failure, pulmonary hypertension and cyanosis.[136] Death during a hospital stay is twice as likely for adults with Down syndrome and CHD compared with adults without Down syndrome with CHD.[136] This may reflect attitudinal discrimination in the types of treatments and care that are offered to people with Down syndrome, or concern about perceived elevated surgical risk, or may be secondary to other comorbid health conditions.[136] Surgical cardiac procedures for CHD have been reported to be 70% less likely to be performed in adults with Down syndrome than in adults with CHD without Down syndrome.[136] Women with Down syndrome are more likely than men with Down syndrome to present to hospital due to CHD, and have higher mortality secondary to CHD.[136]

Dental problems

Dental problems are more prevalent in people with Down syndrome due to a small oral cavity, enlarged tongue, overcrowding of teeth and dental malocclusion.[34] Development of teeth is typically delayed.[34] Rapid maxillary expansion (RME) is an orthodontic procedure offered to some children with Down syndrome and is used to correct craniofacial abnormalities. RME creates extra space for overcrowded teeth and reduces the incidence of upper respiratory infections by 60% and mouth breathing by 87%, and improves nasal patency in up to 91% of patients.[137] Other improvements with RME include improved upper airway airflow, reduced tongue protrusion and reduced dribbling.[137] Regular dental assessment and good oral hygiene are particularly important for children and adults with Down syndrome to

prevent further complications of oral and craniofacial abnormalities.

Dermatological conditions

Alopecia, dry skin, eczema, folliculitis, hyperkeratosis, seborrhoeic dermatitis and vitiligo are more common in people with Down syndrome than in the general population, and may be more persistent due to atopic and autoimmune tendencies. Alopecia areata is of autoimmune origin and is discussed in the autoimmune section of this chapter. Xerosis (dry skin) may occur secondary to low thyroid function or poor hydration, or may be due to poor gastrointestinal absorption of essential fatty acids and other nutrients essential to maintaining skin integrity. Xerosis occurs in 75% of children with Down syndrome over 5 years old, and increases to 85% in patients aged 12–48 years, with patchy lichenification occurring in some.[138] Eczema (atopic dermatitis) occurs as an allergic response to dietary or environmental triggers and occurs in approximately 20% of children with Down syndrome.[138] Treatment of eczema in children and adults with Down syndrome is the same as for the general population, with a strong emphasis on maintaining gastrointestinal integrity and soothing topical applications.

Seborrhoeic dermatitis occurs in 30–36% of people with Down syndrome, compared with 2–5% of the general population, and is related to being immunocompromised.[138] Seborrhoeic dermatitis resembles cradle cap in babies and younger children, and typically involves erythema, with yellow-brown scales, which may or may not weep serous fluid. It occurs most often on the scalp and face, particularly around the sides of the nose, eyelashes and eyebrows, and may also occur in or around the ears.[138] Cheilitis (cracking, scaling and fissuring of the lips) occurs in approximately 6% of people with Down syndrome and is more common in males.[138] Cheilitis may present more frequently due to chronic mouth breathing, secondary to an oversized tongue and small oral cavity, or chronic sinus congestion.

Folliculitis occurs in 10% of people with Down syndrome and involves inflammation of a hair follicle, usually occurring on the upper back, chest or shoulders, and often results in infection.[138] Folliculitis occurs in Down syndrome secondary to immunological deficit.[138] Anetoderma may occur secondary to folliculitis, in which the skin loses elastic fibres, resulting in patches of flaccid skin, often with herniation of adipose tissue.[138]

Persistent furunculosis (boils) is also common in people with Down syndrome, and similarly occurs due to immune deficit. Staphylococcal or streptococcal infection is usually involved, resulting in pain and scarring.[138] In patients with Down syndrome, this typically occurs on the thighs or trunk, and may cause pain with walking and sitting. Naturopathic treatment of both folliculitis and furunculosis involves internal immune stimulants, with topical applications that combine antimicrobial essential oils with vulnerary and anti-inflammatory herbs.

CASE STUDY 19.1

OVERVIEW

A 17-year-old male with Down syndrome presented with a 3-month history of frequent boils on his buttocks, inner thighs and groin area. Boils were up to 3 cm in diameter and caused pain and discomfort when walking or sitting. The first boil appeared 3 months ago and he had six active boils. The boils were limiting physical exercise, as friction and sweating at the gym exacerbate pain and itching, and he was embarrassed by them at the swimming pool. He is mildly overweight, eats a dairy-free but otherwise well-balanced wholefood diet and lives at home with both parents and two siblings. Previous home-based treatment involved salt-water baths and topical application of Dettol, which provided some relief but had not resolved the problem.

TREATMENT

Initial treatment included a herbal tincture, aimed at stimulating the immune system, lymphatics, general circulation and excretory pathways. No attempt was made with this mixture to improve taste, as he has a long history of herb taking and is very compliant. Topical cream combines demulcent herbs with analgesia and strong antimicrobial essential oils. Essential oils were chosen due to their capacity to penetrate through the skin to address deeper infection. Herbal sitz baths with strong oregano and calendula tea were also recommended.

HERBAL TINCTURE

Echinacea spp. 95 mL
Piper longum 20 mL
Zanthoxylum americanum 40 mL
Phytolacca decandra 5 mL
Rumex crispus 40 mL
Dose: 5 mL three times daily.

TOPICAL CREAM

Plantago lanceolata 10%
Syzygium aromaticum tincture 5%
Origanum vulgare essential oil 2%
Lavandula angustifolia essential oil 5%
Backhousia citriodora essential oil 2%
Zinc oxide 10%
Base: 1 part beeswax, 4 parts organic olive oil
Apply topically 3–4 times daily

NUTRITIONAL INTERVENTION

Vitamin D: 5000 IU per day
Zinc: 30 mg per day

FOLLOW-UP (2 WEEKS)

Boils had reduced in size and pain significantly; four had resolved completely and two remained. His mother reported that he was enjoying the sitz baths, but found the cream messy. They had been applying the cream only twice daily, under large plasters to keep it contained. Mild topical irritation was occurring secondary to the adhesive plasters. He continued with the baths, topical treatment and herbal

tincture for a further 2 weeks, by which stage the boils had resolved completely. The family now keep the tincture and cream at home to use at the first sign of boils recurring. Nutritional supplements are ongoing.

Other dermatological manifestations occur more frequently in people with Down syndrome due to a higher propensity towards autoimmune disease, malabsorption and lowed immune function. These include, but are not limited to, vitiligo, geographic tongue, fissured tongue, scabies, onychomycosis (fungal infection of the nails) and tinea.[138] Bates reported fissured tongue in 28% of patients with Down syndrome aged 3–20 years, and hypertrophy of the tongue papillae in 22% of children with Down syndrome.[139] Scabies may occur due to decreased immune defences combined with absence of itching, resulting in decreased manual removal of mites, and delayed detection and treatment.[140,141] Incidence of scabies is more common in institutionalised settings, and in some studies does not present as a Down syndrome–specific problem at all where participants are living at home with their parents and are well cared for.[140] Similarly, onychomycosis and tinea are opportunistic conditions and are less likely to persist when adequate nutrition and personal care are provided.

ACCELERATED AGEING

People with Down syndrome experience accelerated ageing of the skin, with wrinkles appearing at an earlier age and greater effects from sun damage.[138] Accelerated wrinkling occurs due to loss of skin elasticity, increased oxidative stress and poor wound healing. Other non-dermatological effects such as alopecia, loss of hair pigmentation, early-onset dementia, premature menopause, osteoarthritis and osteoporosis contribute to a visual and actual experience of premature ageing.[138,140] Loss of hair pigmentation, or premature greying, can happen quite young and has been reported in as many as 55% of young adults with Down syndrome aged 16–20 years, 12% aged 11–15 years and 9% aged 6–10 years.[142] Gender discrepancy was found, with males showing a slightly higher incidence of premature greying in all three age groups.[142]

Respiratory illness

Respiratory illness is particularly prevalent in children with Down syndrome and contributes considerably to increased mortality. In neonates with Down syndrome, lung or airway disease accounts for 42% of hospital admissions, while in children respiratory infections contribute to 80% of hospital admissions and 78% of intensive care admissions.[143] Wheeze is reported more frequently in children with Down syndrome (18.5%) compared with their siblings without Down syndrome (6.6%).[144] Persistent rhinitis is also common in children with Down syndrome, while asthma, respiratory allergies and fever are less common.[144] Impaired immune system responsiveness contributes to increased severity of respiratory infections, resulting in higher rates of pneumonia and other complications. Furthermore, anatomical abnormalities of the airways may cause chronic respiratory aspiration, resulting in chronic wheeze, pneumonia, persistent coughing, interstitial inflammation and bronchiectasis.[143]

Pulmonary hypertension may present in children with Down syndrome due to cardiac abnormalities, but occurs in higher frequency in children with Down syndrome without congenital heart defects than in the general population.[143] Structural and vascular abnormalities of the lungs in children and babies with Down syndrome contribute to pulmonary resistance, resulting in increased rates of pulmonary oedema and pulmonary haemorrhage.[143] Children with Down syndrome also have increased prevalence of parenchymal lung disease, subpleural cysts, tracheobronchomalacia, subglottic stenosis, tracheal stenosis, sleep-disordered breathing and upper airway obstruction due to adenoid or tonsillar hypertrophy.[143]

Asthma is not statistically more prevalent in children with Down syndrome, though it is often suspected due to wheeze, stridor and other breathing difficulties. Feasibility of testing children with Down syndrome for asthma is limited by low muscle tone and coordination, and reduced cognitive capacity to understand how to perform the test.[144] Thorough assessment by a skilled paediatric pulmonologist is necessary to diagnose and assess risk in children with Down syndrome presenting with respiratory symptoms.

Hospitalisation for respiratory syncytial virus (RSV) occurs six times more frequently in children with Down syndrome than in age-matched peers within the first 2 years of life and presents as more severe illness.[145] This greater severity of RSV in children with Down syndrome is due to inherent immune system deficiencies, poor upper airway tone, abnormal lung development and cardiopulmonary abnormalities.[146] RSV lower respiratory tract infections in children with Down syndrome are more likely to progress to pneumonia and bronchiolitis and may be complicated by a secondary or concomitant bacterial infection.[145] Congenital heart disease, chronic lung disease, prematurity, low birthweight and neuromuscular impairment predispose children with Down syndrome to increased incidence and severity of RSV, though Down syndrome in itself has been recognised as an independent risk factor.[145]

ATOPY

Dietary and airborne allergies may contribute to respiratory difficulties in children with Down syndrome. However, current medical evidence suggests there is a lesser rate of sensitisation to airborne allergens in children with Down syndrome than in the general population.[147] Mannan et al. reported that 77% of children with Down syndrome have a family history of atopy, defined as having at least one family member with asthma, allergic rhinitis or atopic dermatitis, but only 18% of children themselves had respiratory sensitivities identified.[147] This may be due to differences in the production of immune mediators, and

suggests that other physiological and anatomical abnormalities contribute more to respiratory disease in people with Down syndrome.[147]

EAR, NOSE AND THROAT (ENT) HEALTH

Persistent otitis media (middle ear infection) occurs secondary to stenotic (narrow) ear canals, persistent/ chronic catarrh and lowered immune function. Narrowness of the ear canals can make viewing the tympanic membrane with an otoscope difficult.[1] Regular examination by an otolaryngologist with a specialised microscopic otoscope attachment is recommended.[83] Effective management of ear infections is necessary to prevent hearing loss, which has important implications for language acquisition, social development, cognitive development and learning outcomes. Close monitoring of ENT health is necessary to detect, manage and appropriately treat ear infections in children with Down syndrome. Fortunately this is an area that can be managed well by the natural therapist. Competence in physical examination is necessary to monitor ear health.

CASE STUDY 19.2

The patient is an 8-year-old girl with Down syndrome presenting with recurrent otitis media.

Goals of naturopathic treatment:
- Relieve pain
- Resolve infection
- Stimulate immune function
- Decongest
- Prevent further complications:
  - Mastoiditis
  - Bacterial meningitis
  - Recurrent middle ear inflammation
  - Recurrent scarring of tympanic membrane
  - Hearing loss.

Topical treatment: herbal ear oil:
- *Calendula officinalis* (flower) infused in olive oil (28%)
- *Hypericum perforatum* (aerial parts) infused in olive oil (30%)
- *Verbascum thapsus* (flower) infused in olive oil (25%)
- *Allium sativum* (in 0.05% in olive oil [10%])
- *Lavandula officinalis* essential oil (5%)
- Tocopherol acetate oil (2%).

This mixture has been clinically trialled in children with otitis media and was found to be more effective than topical antibiotic combined with a topical anaesthetic, for both pain relief and resolution of infection. Reduction of pain occurs in less than 30 minutes.[120] Apply warmed (place bottle in a hot water bath) to both ears four to five times daily. Continue with treatment for 48 hours after symptoms have resolved to ensure complete resolution of infection.

Internal treatment: herbal tincture
- *Echinacea* spp. 20%
- *Echinacea* spp. glycetract 20%
- *Glycyrrhiza glabra* 20%
- *Thymus vulgaris* 10%
- *Mentha × piperita* 5%
- *Sanguinaria canadensis* 5%
- *Hyssopus officinalis* 20%

Mucolytic properties of echinacea, bloodroot and liquorice help break up or thin congested catarrh, making it easier to pass. Liquorice is also anti-inflammatory and soothing to respiratory mucosa. Peppermint is useful as a pleasant-tasting decongestant and masks the flavour of thyme (antimicrobial) reasonably well. Hyssop is included for its anti-catarrhal properties and pleasant taste and is a gentle relaxing nervine. The combination of echinacea glycetract and liquorice improves taste compliance with this mixture.

Dosage:

Adjust dose according to body weight using Clark's rule:
    child's weight ÷ adult's weight (70 kg) × adult dose
Example: 35 kg child ÷ 70 kg × 15 mL/day = 7.5 mL/day = 2.5 mL three times daily.

Note: for acute prescribing, in adults it is reasonable to use 20–30 mL per day short term. In this case, dosing becomes 3 mL five times per day.

Therapeutic considerations:

- Consider dairy allergy in children with chronic catarrh and recurrent otitis media. Dairy exclusion for 4–6 weeks followed by dairy challenge is an effective means to identify whether dairy allergy is contributing to the frequency of infections. Ensure calcium needs are met through other sources in the diet.
- Possible nutritional deficiencies due to poor dietary intake or gastrointestinal abnormalities.
- Immune system dysfunction.
- Healthy home environment: ideal home temperature for respiratory health is >18°C. Living temperatures below 16°C impair normal respiratory function, resulting in increased frequency of infections, asthmatic episodes and hospitalisations, and mortality.[121]
- Herbal dosing considerations: adjust dose appropriate to child's weight and individual sensitivity to herbs. Effective treatment is important to prevent further complications and sequelae. Dosage needs to be high enough for medicine to be effective, but not so high as to give child adverse effects (e.g. vomiting).

TONSILS AND ADENOIDS

Enlarged tonsils occur in up to 90% of children with Down syndrome and may obstruct 50–75% of the pharyngeal space.[148] Parents of children with Down syndrome who have undergone tonsillectomy report fewer problems with mouth breathing and sleep apnoea.[148] Adeno-tonsillectomy is very common, with one study reporting that by school age 79% of children with Down syndrome had either undergone adeno-tonsillectomy or suffered ongoing obstructive breathing problems due to hypertrophic glandular tissue in the tonsils and adenoids.[149]

Otitis media with effusion (OME, commonly known as glue ear) is a frequent problem for children with Down syndrome. Incidence across different age groups varies; the highest incidence has been found in a study in Glasgow in which 93% of one-year-olds were found to have OME, though not all were symptomatic.[149] This is concerning, in that children who are not symptomatic will seldom receive treatment for OME, which has long-term implications for hearing, language, social development and cognition. Grommets (ventilation tubes) are the standard treatment for OME. A review of the available published literature reveals that insertion of grommets in children with Down syndrome is efficacious in serous otitis media, but not recurrent acute otitis media.[150] In cases where grommets are effective, significant improvement in quality of life is experienced.[150] By school age, the incidence of OME falls to 68%, which is still significantly higher than in the general population and poses a major risk for ongoing hearing difficulties.[149] Declining trends in OME have been observed in children with Down syndrome after 8 years of age, which may reflect surgical intervention, improvements in health management and maturation of the immune system.[151] A Cochrane Collaboration Review of antibiotic treatment for OME in children revealed moderate evidence of resolution of infection; however, there are currently no data on long-term effects such as impact on rates of grommet insertion, speech, language development, cognitive development or quality of life.[152]

Chronic rhinosinusitis is common in children with Down syndrome, and occurs due to a number of factors.[153] Adenoid hypertrophy reduces the respiratory airflow, and unaddressed allergies may contribute to excessive mucus production.[153] Immune system immaturity and dysfunction predispose children with Down syndrome to infections and chronic allergies. Reducing irritants in the living environment can be of benefit, as mucous membranes that are already inflamed will be more susceptible to non-allergen irritants present in the environment. Chronic mucus production, combined with stenotic passages, lowered immune function and inflammation, contributes to ongoing sinus congestion and predisposes children with Down syndrome to recurrent upper respiratory infections. Herbal medicines that reduce congestion, reduce inflammation and have anti-allergy and immune-enhancing effects can be helpful to manage upper airway health and reduce secondary complications of otitis media and OME.

Compliance with hearing aids can be difficult due to sensitivity to noise.[1] Hearing aids are also often impractical in children with Down syndrome, due to the narrowness of the ear canals, difficulties with compliance, wax accumulation and auditory feedback.[153] Appropriate management of wax accumulation and ear infections is essential to improve compliance outcomes, where hearing aids are necessary. For children who are struggling with hearing, simplified sign language (Key Sign) can be a useful way of continuing to engage in active communication while the hearing difficulties are addressed. Any period of hearing loss has negative implications on language, social and intellectual development. Sign language in children who are deaf has been shown to have a protective effect on both cognitive and psychosocial development, which likely occurs through improving the capacity to interact with peers, carers and teachers.[154] Parents may be reluctant, due to a stigma of signing in public or the perception that no-one else will be able to sign with their child. Children, however, pick up new languages easily and will often pick up signs to be able to better communicate with their peers. The simplified signs of Key Sign provide the basics so that communication is easily re-established, and easily learned by adults. Improved capacity to communicate with the child is important not only to maintain development, but also as a safety consideration.

Endocrine disorders

Thyroid disorders are the most common endocrine disorders observed in people with Down syndrome.[155] Hypothyroidism occurs more frequently in people with Down syndrome than in the general population, and it has been suggested that impaired subclinical thyroid dysfunction may be present at birth and continue to persist throughout life.[156] Decreased selenium levels are observed in people with Down syndrome; selenium plays a critical antioxidant role for thyrocytes and is involved in the conversion of thyroid hormones.[156] The clinical metabolic presentation in patients with Down syndrome has overlapping features with hypothyroidism, and may result in diagnostic overshadowing and thyroid dysfunction remaining undetected. As most thyroid disease in people with Down syndrome is of autoimmune origin, more detail is covered in the autoimmune section of this chapter.

Differences in sex hormone production are also observed in people with Down syndrome. In women, plasma levels of oestradiol and progesterone are lower than in age-matched menstruating women, with higher propensity for anovulatory cycles, suggesting impaired follicular and luteal phase function.[157] In men, low testosterone and elevated luteinising hormone (LH) and follicle-stimulating hormone (FSH) levels have been observed.[158] More detail as to the health implications of these hormonal differences is covered in the sexual health section of this chapter.

Epilepsy

In people with Down syndrome, seizure presentation occurs most frequently either as infantile spasms (40%) under the age of 1 year or late-onset epilepsy after 50 years of age (46%).[2] In the general population, infantile spasms are associated with profound developmental delay in 80–90% of cases, with worse prognosis associated with earlier onset of seizures.[27] Infantile spasms are less persistent in children with Down syndrome than in the general population, with 19–28% of children with Down syndrome and infantile spasms progressing to develop epilepsy, compared with 35–60% in the general population.[159] Epileptic spasms typically occur in clusters and affect the axial muscles, resulting in flexion or extension of limbs.[160] Febrile seizures may also occur in children with Down syndrome, though this appears to be less common than in the general population.[161] Immune system dysfunction in children with Down syndrome reduces the potential to produce a fever in response to illness, so febrile seizures when they occur in children with Down syndrome typically occur at <38°C.[161]

Poor neurodevelopment and autistic-like symptoms are more common in children with infantile spasms.[162]

Aggressive early-onset treatment of seizures in infants is associated with better responsiveness to treatment and improved psychomotor development.[159] Anti-epileptic medications include vigabatrin and topiramate, though success rates for remission of infantile spasms are variable, 1–60% and 20–30% respectively.[163] Adrenocorticotropic hormone (ACTH) is used in combination with vigabatrin, which improves seizure management to 76%.[163] However, these medications appear to have lower efficacy in infants with Down syndrome, with one study reporting that seizure control was eventually achieved in 88% of patients, but the time taken to achieve control varied between 3 and 13 months.[160] It is possible that with this time frame, some children outgrow their infantile spasms rather than finally achieving seizure control with medications. Other medications used for seizures in children with Down syndrome include pyridoxine, hydrocortisone, phenobarbitone (phenobarbital), phenytoin, diazepam and primidone, though their safety and efficacy have not been demonstrated specifically for children with Down syndrome.[164] Unique differences to neuronal structure, abnormal neurotransmission inhibitors and hyperexcitable membranes in children with Down syndrome increase the likelihood of developing seizures,[160] and may also influence predisposition to treatment resistance. Other structural abnormalities that may predispose patients with Down syndrome to seizures include decreased neural density, abnormal lamination of the neural cortex, and lowered volume of the hippocampus and cerebellum, though exact mechanisms are not known.[164] Few data exist specifically for effective medical intervention for infantile spasms in infants with Down syndrome. Medication trials in children with infantile spasms are typically small and limited to retrospective studies, due to ethical issues regarding blind placebo trials in a serious condition in infants with long-term consequences. It is common practice to combine multiple medications to achieve seizure control, with reports that only 32% of patients become seizure-free with the first anti-epileptic medication prescribed and only 54% achieving long-term seizure-free status (>2 years).[163]

The ketogenic diet has been found to be effective for treating seizures in 70% of children with intractable infantile spasms.[163] Mechanism of action is poorly understood; it is theorised that increased short-chain fatty acid production may exhibit protective effects within brain tissue and promote inhibitory pathways that improve seizure control.[165] A 2006 meta-analysis of the ketogenic diet in epilepsy found that 24% of patients achieved complete seizure control and a further 52% experienced at least 90% seizure reduction.[166] Similar results have been found in more recent studies,[167–171] though one study reported poorer results.[172] Variation in success may be due to compliance or, more importantly, the level of guidance and education given to parents or patients as to successfully implementing the diet. The ketogenic diet has been researched in children ranging in age, with reasonable success in either decreasing seizures or achieving complete seizure control.[173] However, the drop-out rate is high and side effects include constipation (14%), weight loss, lack of appetite or growth retardation

(13%), nausea and vomiting (5%), irritability or behavioural difficulties (4%), increased cholesterol and triglycerides (4%), lethargy (4%), hypercalciuria (2.5%), raised liver enzymes (2.4%), renal stones (1.9%), diarrhoea (1.6%) and hypoglycaemia (1.3%).

Current studies suggest that most children respond with seizure reduction within 2 weeks on the ketogenic diet, with a recommendation to persist with the diet for 3 months even if initially ineffective.[173] The ketogenic diet is generally discontinued after 1–2 years, as it is difficult to maintain long term, and apparent remission of epilepsy symptoms may precipitate the decision to try a normal diet again.[166] Caraballo et al. found that after discontinuation of the diet seizure recurrence occurred in 25% of patients who were seizure-free (75% remained seizure-free) and, of those with reduced seizures on the diet, 75% remained at the same frequency of seizures.[173] Careful planning and supervision are necessary to ensure that dietary intake is sufficient to meet growth and development needs.

Epilepsy is associated with more severe intellectual disability in children with Down syndrome, and delays in achieving effective seizure control worsen developmental and intellectual outcomes.[174] Children with effective seizure management appear to have slight improvement in cognitive and language skills.[17] However, topiramate may also increase cognitive impairment in some patients.[164] Clinical practice preference in most studies is to attempt single medication treatment first, followed by combined medications if unsuccessful; different combinations of medications if still unsuccessful; and the ketogenic diet in treatment-resistant or intractable cases. Given the severity of side effects of anti-epileptic medications compared with the side effects and compliance difficulty with the ketogenic diet, it may be advisable to attempt the ketogenic diet earlier in children whose first-line treatment is ineffective.

Medical cannabis is currently receiving much attention as a possible treatment for seizures. Cannabinoids appear to be involved in the therapeutic effect, as distinct from tetrahydrocannabinol (THC), which can have pro-convulsant effects in epilepsy-prone neural tissue.[175] Studies mostly use isolated cannabidiol, though other cannabinoids (of which there are over 80 present in cannabis) may also exert therapeutic benefit.[175] A Canadian survey of patients with epilepsy found that 24% reported that cannabis was effective at controlling their seizures, and 84% of parents of children with epilepsy reported seizure reduction using cannabidiol-enriched cannabis.[176] Other benefits reported by parents included improved sleep outcomes, mood and daytime alertness.[175,176] Efficacy so far appears better than the standard medications used in epilepsy management, with a lesser side effect profile.[177] Anticonvulsant effects have been well demonstrated in animal models and further investigation in humans is warranted.[178] The mechanism of action appears to be via the cannabinoid receptors (CB1 and CB2), expressed at presynaptic neuronal sites, reducing neuronal excitability, while also ameliorating muscle spasm, spasticity and tremors.[179] In animal studies, cannabinoid treatment appears to reduce the spread of seizure activity in the brain, irrespective of the focal origin of the seizure.[178] Decreased propagation of seizure activity has the potential to reduce the severity of seizures and possibly reduce some of the cognitive damage associated with sustained seizures.

Negative stigma remains evident within medical literature and social discussion of cannabis as a potential medicine. Current trials have increased public and medical discourse about medical cannabis; however, at the time of writing, most patients in Australia have to obtain cannabis by illegal means to use it therapeutically in seizure management. This has obvious implications for the consistency of quality, adulteration, variation in THC content and legal risk. This is challenging, particularly for parents of children with treatment-resistant seizures or who find that the medication side effects negate adequate quality of life. Some parents report that side effects of anti-epileptic medications impair quality of life for their children just as severely as the seizures do.[175] Furthermore, increasing reports are emerging of parents being able to wean their children off their antiepileptic medications due to the seizure control achieved with cannabidiol-enriched cannabis, further improving quality of life by eliminating negative medication side effects.[175] Some medical investigators suggest that whole plant cannabis extract could be considered 'ethically reasonable' when all other therapeutic interventions have failed.[180] This is reflective of attitudinal bias towards therapeutic interventions that are pharmaceutical and therefore legitimate, as opposed to one that has a less socially acceptable history of use, regardless of differences in therapeutic benefit, safety and side effect profiles. Maa and Figi state: 'Growers and regulators must satisfy concerns about consistency, quality, and safety before medical cannabis will ever gain legitimacy as a mainstream therapeutic option.'[181] Calm, objective and non-sensationalist investigation of the potential therapeutic outcomes of this herb, and the ways in which it can be grown and regulated to assure quality, while not increasing risk of abuse, is needed.

Other potential supportive nutritional interventions for improving epilepsy management in Down syndrome are lacking research and must be extrapolated from mainstream epilepsy research, which is also limited in scope. A brief summary of potential therapies is included in Table 19.3.

LATE-ONSET EPILEPSY

Late-onset epilepsy typically presents with myoclonic seizures, early morning myoclonic jerks and photosensitivity.[216] Cognitive deterioration typically occurs at the same time, presenting clinically as a loss of interest in social interactions, forgetfulness, confusion about space and time, and behavioural changes.[217] Loss of independent living skills, reduced engagement in activities of daily living and reduced coordination occur as the condition progresses.[216] Development of late-onset epilepsy may be related to synaptic degeneration and abnormal synchronisation of neurons secondary to accumulation of amyloid peptides, and in people with Down syndrome is

TABLE 19.3 Evidence for herbal and nutritional supplementation in the treatment of epilepsy

Supplement	Clinical findings
Curcumin	Curcumin (100–300 mg/kg) demonstrated dose-dependent anticonvulsant effects in animal models. Antioxidant effects reduce oxidative stress and cognitive impairment. Ability to cross the blood–brain barrier enables potential for reducing oxidative stress in neural tissue.[182]
Fish oil	1080 mg EPA + DHA daily was associated with 33.6% reduction in seizure frequency, 25% response rate and 10% seizure-free rate.[183] 700 mg DHA + 300 mg EPA daily supplementation for 6 months was associated with improved serum levels of DHA and 50% reduction in seizure frequency.[184] 1200 mg fish oil (240 mg DHA + 360 mg EPA) given daily to children aged 4–12 years for 3 months resulted in reduced frequency but not severity of seizures in 91% of children; 57.1% of children became seizure-free within 3 months of supplementation, 28.6% reduced seizure frequency to 1–3 per months and 8.6% remained having >30 seizures per month.[185] 5 g omega-3 polyunsaturated fat-enhanced dietary spread (2300 mg DHA, 900 mg EPA) daily for 6 months: 16 out of 21 patients refused to eat the spread; the 5 remaining experienced significant reduction in the severity and frequency of seizure symptoms. Participant numbers are too small to extrapolate much; however, this result is consistent with other research. This study highlights the need for palatable dosing methods.[186]
Magnesium	Magnesium deficiency is correlated with seizure occurrence. There is a sparsity of research examining the benefits of magnesium in seizures or epilepsy; however, evidence from human clinical trials and case studies has found that magnesium supplementation increases the seizure threshold in eclampsia and seizures resulting from *TRPM6* gene mutations. Further research is needed to explore potential therapeutic benefits of magnesium in patients with Down syndrome and epilepsy.[187] Magnesium deficiency or hypomagnesia has been reported in case studies of infants and adults with seizures. Small studies have demonstrated lower magnesium levels in patients with epilepsy. Pilot studies have found magnesium supplementation improves responsiveness to anti-epileptic medications.[188]
Calcium	Calcium plays a critical role in normal functioning of neurons. Increased intracellular calcium contributes to acute neuronal injury under conditions of excessive stimulation during a seizure. Low serum calcium is observed in patients with epilepsy, with rapid accumulation of calcium in the brain during a seizure, producing increased neuronal hyper-excitability.[189]
Calcium and vitamin D	Calcium and vitamin D supplementation in patients taking anti-epileptic medications resulted in lower rates of bone fractures in patients with epilepsy.[190] Similar results have been reported in babies born with rickets and vitamin D deficiency. These cases highlight the need for improved pregnancy care. Supplementation with calcium and vitamin D effectively eliminated seizures and was discontinued after 2 months.[191] Case report of afebrile seizures in an exclusively breastfed infant, born to a mother with severe vitamin D deficiency secondary to veiling as part of religious practice. This case highlights the need to supplement vitamin D in at-risk populations.[192]
Selenium	Selenoproteins are involved in antioxidant activities that promote neuron cell survival. Case reports have indicated reduction in seizures with selenium supplementation in medication-resistant epilepsy.[193] Some anti-epileptic medications (e.g. valproic acid) deplete selenium and reduce selenium-dependent glutathione peroxidase (GSH-Px) activity. Selenium deficiency is implicated in the pathogenesis of epilepsy and contributes to calcium dysregulation, oxidative stress and neurotoxic sequelae.[194] Decreased serum zinc and selenium observed in patients with idiopathic intractable epilepsy, compared with age-matched peers.[195] The role of selenium in brain function is greater than just its antioxidant action; it has a significant role in neurotransmission, inflammation, protein phosphorylation, calcium homeostasis and brain cholesterol metabolism.[196] Selenium found to reduce seizure genesis and oxidative stress, and reduce the toxicity of topiramate.[197]
Caffeine	Case report of a tonic-clonic seizure following high consumption of caffeinated energy drinks (4–6 cans per day for 5 months). No other seizures were reported after discontinuing use of energy drinks.[198] Case report of increased seizure frequency associated with increased consumption of caffeinated beverages.[199] Retrospective study of 145 people with epilepsy found no difference in seizure incidence with short-term increase or decrease in caffeine intake. Avoidance of caffeine in caffeine-naïve individuals is recommended to avoid sleep disruption, which has a demonstrated negative effect on seizure incidence.[199]

Continued

TABLE 19.3 Evidence for herbal and nutritional supplementation in the treatment of epilepsy—cont'd

Supplement	Clinical findings
Folic acid	Scarcity of evidence (mostly case reports) suggesting seizure-provoking effect of folic acid. Anti-epileptic medications deplete folate. Folic acid supplementation through food fortification is common practice. Involvement in methylation pathways highlights the importance of folate in neurological function.[200] Folic acid deficiency is associated with neurological impairment and is common in people taking anti-epileptic medications.[201]
Vitamin B_6	Case report in a newborn: epilepsy identified 8 hours after birth and treated with vitamin B_6 injection. Continuous treatment throughout life resulted in reasonable seizure management, with occasional breakthrough seizures during illness or attempts to withdraw supplementation. Patient was seizure-free from age 9 to 31 years on a dose of 50 mg twice daily.[202] Neonatal seizures secondary to vitamin B_6 deficiency occur within hours to days of birth. Intravenous doses between 1 and 680 mg of pyridoxine have been given to control seizures in neonates. Familial tendency has been observed.[203] Case report in an adult demonstrating seizures secondary to vitamin B_6 deficiency, which resolved after normalisation of vitamin B_6 levels.[204] Review article: vitamin B_6 in infants and children (age 3 months to 5 years) has a dose-dependent effect on seizures associated with vitamin B_6 deficiency. Little clinical effect is observed with low doses of 10–40 mg, increased clinical effect is observed at doses of 30–50 mg and dramatic clinical improvement is observed at higher doses of 100–400 mg.[205] Vitamin B_6 supplementation in pyridoxine-deficient or pyridoxine-dependent seizures may have a positive effect on cognitive development in infants with seizures.[206] Vitamin B_6 (100 mg per day) administration during pregnancy in mothers with a familial risk of vitamin B_6 dependent seizure may reduce the incidence of infantile seizures after birth. Mothers who already have one child with vitamin B_6 dependent seizures have a 25% recurrence risk for subsequent pregnancies. Long-term dosage of up to 200 mg per day in infants, or 500 mg in adults, is safe and efficacious for seizure management.[207]
Vitamin B_{12}	Epileptic seizures in infants can be secondary to vitamin B_{12} deficiency and are most likely to occur in babies born to vegetarian or vegan mothers. Vitamin B_{12} deficiency presents within 1–2 months in infants, as infant hepatic reserves are minimal.[208]
Vitamin C	Vitamin C has been demonstrated to increase the latency of induced seizures in animal models and may have a protective antioxidant effect in seizure genesis.[209] Vitamin C reduced oxidative stress and lipid peroxidation in induced seizures in animal models.[210]
Vitamin D	Hypocalcaemia secondary to severe vitamin D deficiency has been identified in some case studies as a cause of rickets, seizures and myopathies in children. Hypercalcaemic seizures are more likely to present in early childhood and adolescence due to increased demands of growth and have a higher prevalence in boys; 24% of patients with this presentation were <1 month old. Vitamin D supplementation during pregnancy is advisable to prevent vitamin D deficiency in neonates and secondary implications for bone and neural development.[211] Correction of vitamin D deficiency in treatment-resistant patients with epilepsy resulted in an average drop in seizures of 40% over 3 months following vitamin D supplementation.[212] Low vitamin D levels are common in patients with seizures. Screening for and correction of vitamin D deficiency in people with seizures should be part of routine management.[213]
Vitamin E	Co-administration of vitamin E (400 IU per day for 6 months) with anti-epileptic medications reduces oxidative stress and improves seizure control.[214]
Zinc	Zinc is involved in a wide range of bodily processes, including post-synaptic excitability and immune system regulation. Zinc may play a role in seizure genesis, though mechanisms and therapeutic potential need further research.[215] Increased copper and decreased zinc and chromium have been observed in children with epilepsy, with additional decreased iron in girls, compared with age-matched peers.[197]

usually comorbid with dementia.[216] Progressive deterioration over 2–4 years is generally observed, with the highest intensity of seizures being experienced in the earlier part of the disease.[216] Medications used for seizure control include levetiracetam, which has a small number of positive case reports to support its use in older adults with Down syndrome and myoclonic seizures; however, seizure control does not appear to reduce cognitive decline in these patients.[217,218] Sudden unexpected death in epilepsy can occur in people with Down syndrome, though to date little knowledge exists for predicting or preventing this.[219] Sudden unexpected death is more likely in poorly controlled epilepsy with tonic-clonic seizures, longer duration of epilepsy, use of multiple medications, cardiac arrhythmias and poor electrolyte balance.[164] Avoidable causes of death are also possible when seizures occur while unattended in a bath or precipitate a serious fall. Care plans for people with Down syndrome and epilepsy or seizures need to accommodate these risks and include measures to avoid them.

OTHER THERAPEUTIC CONSIDERATIONS FOR SEIZURES OR EPILEPSY IN DOWN SYNDROME

Electrolyte disturbances can trigger seizures or result from chronic or severe seizures, and if overlooked can result in severe and life-threatening complications.[220] Electrolyte disturbances may occur due to medication side effects, excessive water intake, excessive fluid loss (vomiting, diarrhoea, laxative abuse, sodium overload, extreme exercise), hyperparathyroidism or severe vitamin D deficiency.[220] Electrolytes have a critical role in neuronal excitability, excitotoxicity, mitochondrial dysfunction and protein aggregation, which influences the potential for seizures to occur.[189] Identifying potential causes of electrolyte disruption in individual patients and correcting the imbalance may help prevent seizure occurrence and other more critical sequelae.

Gastrointestinal tract abnormalities

Gastrointestinal tract abnormalities are present in 12% of children with Down syndrome.[221] These include an increased predisposition towards oral cavity defects, including dental malocclusion, delayed and atypical tooth eruptions, congenital absence of teeth, periodontal disease and dental caries.[221] Chewing and swallowing may also be complicated by low muscle tone and poor muscle coordination, leading to a preference towards foods that are softer and easier to swallow.[221] Coeliac disease occurs more frequently, especially in people with Down syndrome with a history of other autoimmune diseases or leukaemia, and is discussed further in the autoimmune section of this chapter. Inflammatory bowel disease (IBD) has been described in case reports of adults with Down syndrome, though it appears to occur relatively infrequently and is of similar incidence to the general population.[222] Chronic constipation is reported by around 34% of patients with Down syndrome, and may occur alongside other related symptoms including abdominal cramps, bloating, flatulence and behavioural difficulties.[40] Chronic constipation may occur more frequently due to hypotonic muscles or low dietary fibre intake or may be due to other comorbid conditions such as coeliac disease, hypothyroidism and tethered spinal cord.[40]

CASE STUDY 19.3

OVERVIEW

The patient is a 16-year-old male with Down syndrome who has always experienced constipation but it has become progressively worse over the last 6 months. Stools are large, dry and hard, and without pharmaceutical laxatives bowel

movements occur once every 10–14 days. Recent x-ray revealed severe faecal impaction, which was manually evacuated. Parents comment that his breath has become quite foul recently. Appetite is good, though he tends not to chew foods, due to a large tongue and poor oral motor control. Diet consists mostly of steamed vegetables, tinned tuna, milk shakes and three serves per day of breakfast cereals.

Other pertinent health history and concerns:
- No history of asthma, but appears to be wheezing and coughs regularly through night
- Adenoidectomy and tonsillectomy at 3 years old
- Negative thyroid and coeliac screen
- Frequent antibiotic use due to frequent upper respiratory tract infections
- Surgical correction of cardiac defect at 6 months old
- Limited exercise due to hip instability
- Mild central obesity.

INITIAL PLAN

- Smoothies for breakfast, including:
  - Vaalia yoghurt (probiotic yoghurt containing *Lactobacillus rhamnosus* LGG, *Lactobacillus acidophilus* LA5, *Bifidobacterium lactis* Bb12): minimum ½ cup
  - Partially hydrolysed guar gum (PHGG): 5 g
  - Banana
  - Blueberries: ½ cup
  - Flaxseed oil: 20 mL
  - Cashews soaked overnight
  - Milk
- Increase water intake to 1.5–2 L per day
- Lactulose: 30 mL diluted in water before bed
- Gentle exercise daily.

FIRST FOLLOW-UP (2 WEEKS LATER)

Bowel movements occurring every morning, with some urgency. Breath improved significantly. Patient was feeling happier and more energetic, and parents reported he seemed less fidgety and less moody. Smoothies were well accepted and resulted in less cereal consumption through the day.

FURTHER TREATMENT

- Continue with smoothies (with PHGG, Vaalia yoghurt, flaxseed oil and berries) long term
- Reduce lactulose to 10 mL in the evening, and monitor bowel frequency. Increase dose to 20 mL if needed to ensure daily bowel movement
- Increase vegetable sources of protein in the diet: legumes, lentils, nuts (soaked or blended), seeds (soaked or blended).

SECOND FOLLOW-UP (4 WEEKS LATER)

Family and patient happy with treatment and exploring vegetarian cooking that includes legumes, brown rice, quinoa and more vegetables than in previous diet. Water intake is a persistent issue, but otherwise compliant with everything else. Currently taking 10 mL lactulose every night before bed. Bowel movements daily, without straining.

Future planning:
- Refer for assessment for potential sleep apnoea
- Refer to physiotherapist or hydrotherapy for hip instability
- Increase social activities outside of school, skill-building and community engagement
- Increase engagement in cooking meals with parents.

ACHALASIA

Achalasia is a rare presentation in the general population that appears to be more common in children with Down syndrome and should be investigated in any child with Down syndrome who presents with frequent choking or vomiting of food.[223] Achalasia involves motor dysfunction of the oesophagus, creating functional obstruction of the oesophago-gastric junction.[223] Aetiology is unknown; achalasia results from loss of myenteric neurons in the oesophagus and lower oesophageal sphincter, which may occur via genetic, infectious or autoimmune processes.[223] Treatment involves surgical correction, either by pneumatic dilation (effective in 50%) or oesophagomyotomy, which is more effective but also more invasive.[223] Postoperative GORD occurs in 3.8% of successfully operated cases.[223] Nutritional intake needs to be guided to prevent nutritional deficiencies and low fibre intake, while working within the oral competencies of the child.

Haematology

Neonates with Down syndrome have been observed to have higher haemoglobin concentrations, increased circulating erythroblasts, abnormal red cell morphology, thrombocytopenia and abnormal platelet morphology.[224] Total lymphocyte count is lower in neonates and children with Down syndrome, particularly B lymphocytes, which is reflective of deficient production in the bone marrow.[224] Leukaemia is substantially more common in children with Down syndrome than in the general population; this is discussed further in the immunology section of this chapter.

Neurological conditions

Delayed maturation of the cerebellum and the smaller relative size of the cerebellum and brainstem contribute to poor balance and coordination and disordered proprioception in people with Down syndrome.[225] This results in perceived clumsiness and greater propensity towards tripping, falling and other accidents. Dysfunctional sensory integration processes, muscle hypotonia, cartilage hypoplasia and inadequate muscular co-contraction also contribute to clumsiness and poor balance.[226] Motor coordination is closely related to proprioception and balance, which are better developed in children with more

advanced motor development.[226] Physical conditioning is necessary in children and adults with Down syndrome to improve muscular strength and sensory perception, thereby reducing the incidence of falls and degenerative processes over time.[227] Attention to developing motor skills should occur from birth, as motor skill development sets the basis for learning about the world and other people from birth, and is strongly correlated with social, cognitive and language development.[226]

Neurological response to pain is abnormal in people with Down syndrome. Children with Down syndrome are less likely to be able to explain a situation that has led to a painful event and present with a more emotional response than similar-aged peers.[228] This is likely to be due to decreased cognitive ability to understand what has happened and slower processing of how to manage the situation.[228] Delayed peripheral conduction and cerebral processing also slow the response to pain and may reduce comprehension of events leading up to a painful sensation.[229] Limited verbal and behavioural capacity to express a reaction to pain contributes to difficulty in assessing traumatic events in children with Down syndrome.[230] Pain studies demonstrate that children with Down syndrome are also less precise in their ability to localise the source of stimuli and have a higher sensory threshold.[231] Children with Down syndrome show reduced capacity to differentiate between blunt and sharp sensations, which may also contribute towards difficulty in describing events and sensations.[229] Parents express uncertainty in assessing and responding to pain, because the child may present in unusual ways, may lack the ability to show where the pain is or be unable to explain what happened.[228] Response to pain is often similar to the emotional response of a much younger child and may not indicate the severity of the injury.[228] Extra care is needed to assess children with Down syndrome, as injuries can be disproportionate to the level of discomfort expressed and be poorly identified by parents, carers and the child themselves. Coping strategies for pain in children with Down syndrome are less sophisticated than similar-aged peers and reflective of cognitive age equivalent.[229] Parents often use distraction strategies, as used in much younger children, such as ball squeezing, music, stories or bubble blowing.[229] Adequate strategies for coping with pain are needed, particularly for surgery and other medical procedures, immunisations, dental procedures and chronic illness.

Neuropsychology

With the exception of research into the psychosocial manifestations of Alzheimer's disease in older people with Down syndrome, little research attention has been directed to mental health parameters in children and adults with Down syndrome.[232] In younger children, challenging behaviours and emotional difficulties are less common in children with Down syndrome than in children with other causes of developmental delay, and tend to reduce over time.[232] Adolescence appears to be more problematic for some young people with Down syndrome, with 'young adult disintegrative syndrome' (YADS) observed in some, presenting with aggression, withdrawal, depression and regression of social, cognitive, language and motor skills.[233] This disorder shares some characteristics observed in dementia-related cognitive decline, without meeting complete diagnostic criteria.[233] Some improvement is observed with antidepressant medication in these cases, but loss of cognitive, behavioural and social skills does not appear to ameliorate.[233] Case studies attribute potential triggers for regression as being loss of routines, such as finishing high school, 'identity rupture' on becoming more aware of their disability and impairments, or onset of severe depression.[234]

In post-school young adults with Down syndrome, behaviour and psychological health is significantly better in those who are able to find meaningful employment, compared with those who remain in other day activities.[15] Late teens through to late 20s appears to be a vulnerable age for people with Down syndrome adjusting into the adult world, comparing their lives and expectations to siblings and peers, coping with adversity, and grappling with self-acceptance. Nurturing self-esteem throughout childhood and early adulthood, with a focus on capabilities, skill-building and independence, may help prevent identity crises that may precipitate regression.[234]

Psychiatric disorders that occur in the general population also occur in people with Down syndrome, including anxiety, depression, bipolar, psychosis, mood dysphoria and impulse control disorders,[232] though prevalence appears to be lower.[235] Psychosis, delusions and hallucinations are more common in older people with Down syndrome and may be associated with dementia and cognitive decline.[232] In younger people, delusions or hallucinations may be reflective of behaviours consistent with cognitive impairment and age-matched development, and include fantasies, having imaginary friends or engaging in magical thinking.[232] Self-talk is also very common in people with Down syndrome, and rather than being indicative of psychiatric disorder, serves as a way of processing previous conversations or situations.[232]

Depression may be more difficult to detect in patients with Down syndrome, due to intellectual impairment, poor communication and secondary impacts of comorbid health complaints, including hypothyroidism, sleep apnoea, digestive disorders and sensory impairments.[234] Questioning of carers may reveal loss of friendliness, withdrawal and reduced pleasure in activities they have previously enjoyed.[235] Vulnerability to developing depression occurs due to increased likelihood of adverse life events (discrimination, poor health, dislocation following death of carer), lower IQ, deficits in language and working memory, and other somatic disorders.[236] Symptoms of depression are similar to those observed in the general population, but in people with Down syndrome require information gathering from family or carers; see Table 19.4.[234]

As for disintegrative disorders, poor prognosis has been observed in people with Down syndrome and depression.[234] A multifaceted approach is needed to effectively treat depression in people with Down syndrome, that may include:

TABLE 19.4 Symptoms of depression in people with Down syndrome

Symptoms reported by individual	Symptoms reported by carers or family
Sadness	Slowing of activities
Apathy	Appetite loss
Feeling useless	Loss of memory and skills
Tired of life	Reduced cognitive capacity
Poor sleep	Tendency to disconnect or withdraw from social engagement
	Mood swings
	Passivity
	Weeping

Source: [234]

- Removal of stressors:
  - Work demands that exceed their cognitive or physical capacity
  - Insufficient support for activities of daily living or community participation
  - Condescending, derogatory or demeaning treatment from others
- Antidepressant medication: pharmacological or complementary medicines
- Psychotherapy or counselling to:
  - Address personal difficulties, self-acceptance and build coping skills
  - Improve mental health and biopsychosocial well being
- Leisure, sporting, vocational and occupational activities that include relationships with other people and meaningful activity:
  - Friendships and social outings outside the family home
  - Opportunities to develop social, interpersonal and communication skills
  - Opportunities for personal growth and self-esteem building
  - Meaningful employment
  - Physical activity suited to physical limitations.[234]

Applying these same strategies to circumvent the development of depression should be part of routine planning for all people with Down syndrome. Prevention of depression occurs through promotion of an active, healthy engaged lifestyle, fostering acceptance and promoting a positive self-image.[234] Physical fitness, through regular exercise, is also a vital part of maintaining healthy emotional wellbeing.[234] Cognitive behavioural therapies can be adapted to meet the needs of people with Down syndrome with mild intellectual disability and can be an effective treatment option.[236] Herbal and nutritional interventions used for people in the general population who are suffering depression are likely to also be of benefit for people with Down syndrome, though further research in this area is needed.

Anxiety and fears have been studied in typically developing children, but little research exists to understand fears and phobias in children with Down syndrome. In children with Down syndrome, fearfulness has been found to be negatively correlated with impulsiveness and hyperactivity[237] and positively correlated with increased expression of pain.[228] Overall, children with Down syndrome appear to be less fearful than children with autism spectrum disorder, and also less fearful than age-matched and development-matched peers.[237] Fearfulness does not appear to be part of the phenotypical presentation in Down syndrome, though it may occur depending on environmental, social and situational experiences. However, clinical attention should be given to any presentation that causes the child significant distress or results in changes in social, cognitive or emotional development.[237]

Repetitive and compulsive behaviours have been observed in some children and adults with Down syndrome, and appears to be an adaptive response to cognitive limitations, as opposed to pathology.[238] It is suggested that routines, preference for sameness and control assist people with intellectual disability, who otherwise have difficulty with quick thinking and flexibility, and reduce difficulty in making sense of the world around them.[238] Similarly, repetitive or compulsive behaviours may be an adaptive response in children and adults who otherwise have difficulty remembering to do things.[238] Rigidity and insistence on sameness early in life appear to be adaptive, but later in life may become maladaptive and negatively reinforce fears and anxiety.[239] Behaviours that appear to be causing emotional distress should be clinically evaluated by a psychotherapist who has experience meeting the needs of people with developmental and intellectual disabilities.

Autism spectrum disorder (ASD) occurs more frequently in people with Down syndrome, and should be screened for by a clinical psychologist.[40] Behavioural difficulties that arise in children with Down syndrome are related to frustrations with expressive language, which may be mitigated by additional speech therapy.[40] Where dual diagnosis with ASD occurs, referral to an occupational therapist who specialises in children with developmental disorders may be helpful to identify therapeutic interventions that facilitate learning and development in a manner that is best suited to the child's individual needs.

Metabolic conditions

At birth, children with Down syndrome are typically smaller than children without Down syndrome, and while short stature remains a prominent feature throughout life, 30% of children with Down syndrome are overweight by 3 years of age.[240] Decreased resting metabolic rate, which may be related to muscular hypotonia, contributes to weight accumulation in children with Down syndrome.[240]

OBESITY RISK

Obesity risk is higher in children and adults with Down syndrome, due to the genetic phenotype specific to Down syndrome, but is also compounded by diet and exercise.

Esposito et al. found that 45.5% of the children with Down syndrome they observed were overweight or obese, and very few were engaged in vigorous physical exercise of more than 60 minutes per day.[241] Hours of sedentary activity were high, although this was consistent with sedentary behaviours of age-matched peers without Down syndrome.[241] Activity levels were reported to be highest in the 10–11-year-old age group, and declined throughout the teenage years to be lowest at 15–16 years of age.[241] Tendency to accumulate weight is also likely to be influenced by subclinical or clinical hypothyroidism, which is common in children and adults with Down syndrome.

Obesity correlates negatively with motor performance and has a negative impact on participation in social activities that would promote opportunities for social development.[240] This is important in that children with Down syndrome are already likely to experience social exclusion. Obesity also has a negative impact on social inclusion, which is compounded by self-exclusion due to not feeling physically fit enough to participate.

DIABETES RISK

Diabetes risk in people with Down syndrome is largely due to autoimmune processes and is discussed further within the autoimmune section of this chapter. Type 2 diabetes seldom occurs in people with Down syndrome, despite a tendency towards obesity.[242] Two cases have been reported within the medical literature of diabetes presenting in adults with Down syndrome, one in a 28-year-old man, the other in a 26-year-old woman.[242] Genetic predisposition is likely to be implicated in the pathogenesis of these cases.[242] Management of diabetes in people with Down syndrome follows the same protocols as for the general population.

WEIGHT MANAGEMENT

Obesity is a significant problem for people with Down syndrome and begins very early in life. A tailored exercise and dietary plan, with consideration of physical limitations and requirements for support, can help manage body weight throughout the younger years and may help establish life-long healthy eating and lifestyle habits. A study investigating the importance of parental involvement found improved weight management outcomes with a 16-session weekly education and training program aimed at parents to be implemented in the home with their teenager with Down syndrome.[243] Parent feedback suggested that longer gaps between appointments would allow better time to implement each week's strategies, and that they would have liked more support to accommodate the restricted eating program.[243] Small trial sizes and a dearth of controlled trials highlights the need for more research into effective weight loss strategies for people with Down syndrome.[244]

Evidence from mainstream practice suggests that weight management is more effective when multi-component interventions are implemented, which include physical exercise, dietary modification and behavioural therapy.[245] Individualising intervention programs to suit the person's needs and level of risk, combined with positive reinforcement from the therapist, improves outcomes in weight management.[245]

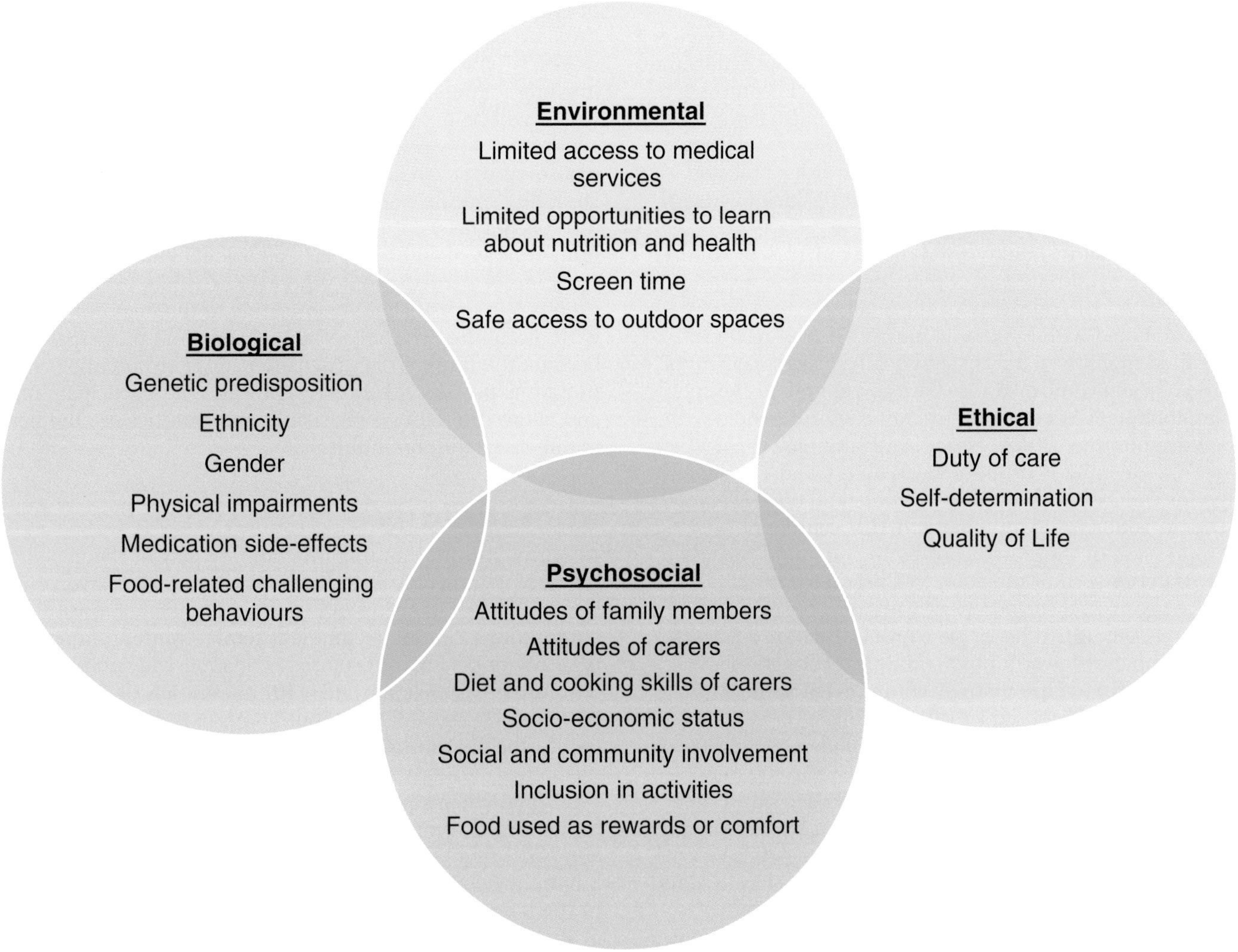

FIGURE 19.1 Environmental, psychosocial and ethical factors that influence weight management for people with developmental disabilities

[247–249]

Multi-component weight loss strategies have also been found to be effective in people with intellectual disability: Melville reported that while there was no significant change to intense or vigorous exercise in his study cohort, a multi-component weight loss program was successful at decreasing sedentary behaviours and increasing light physical exercise.[246] Decreasing sedentary behaviours has the potential to support longer term change, through changes to habitual activity patterns. Ongoing follow-up with a health professional who is providing weight management support is also predictive of longer term success in mainstream studies[245] and should be incorporated into weight management care for people with Down syndrome.

Multiple factors influence the predisposition towards obesity in people with Down syndrome, not least of all genetics. Other factors that more broadly influence tendency towards obesity are explored in Fig. 19.1. These factors should be taken into consideration when creating individualised plans for children, adolescents and adults with Down syndrome.

Orthopaedic conditions

Hypermobility of the joints has implications for posture, joint injuries, gait and long-term structural stability. Combined with low muscle tone, joint hypermobility produces alterations of gait that affect pelvic tilt, hip flexion, knee and ankle joints.[250] Compensatory strategies to maintain balance and centre of gravity reduce propulsion in walking movements, resulting in a cautious and unusual gait pattern.[250] Poor postural control also results in generalised clumsiness, slower reaction time and a greater risk of falls due to reduced ability to self-correct body positioning.[251] Somatosensory input also influences gait and postural control, and is poorer in younger children (under 6 years old) than in older children or adults.[252] Sensory deficits (hearing or visual) should be monitored, as these will influence capacity to predict changes in the physical environment.[252] Physical exercise training in children and adolescents with Down syndrome improves static balance and voluntary muscle control.[251] Physiotherapy programs that strengthen musculature without creating overt impacts or risks to joint stability are advisable to ensure mobility, reduce the risk of falls or other accidents and maintain sufficient balance to engage in social and functional activities.

Atlantoaxial instability (AAI) occurs in 15% of children with Down syndrome and is potentially dangerous.[253] It is characterised by instability of the atlas and axial bones, and combined with hypotonic muscles it may result in impaired mobility, paralysis and death.[11] The majority of radiologically confirmed cases are asymptomatic, with symptomatic AAI occurring in only 1–2% of people with Down syndrome.[253] AAI is not static and may occur at any age.[253] Screening is recommended at 3, 5 and 12 years of age for children with Down syndrome and once every 10 years in adults.[253] Symptomatic AAI is caused by compression of the spinal cord by the odontoid process or the posterior arch of the atlas.[254] Clinical signs of symptomatic AAI include neck pain, new onset of impaired gait, torticollis or new onset of motor difficulties in the upper or lower limbs.[255] Surgical correction is imperative for symptomatic AAI to prevent spinal cord compression and subsequent immobility.[253]

Hypermobility allows for unusual body positioning for sleep and sitting. Children with Down syndrome may be found to sleep with the head resting between or on their legs.[12] Hip flexibility also enables them to sit comfortably in a 'W' or reverse tailor position.[12] Orthopaedic concerns with this position include potential for hip dislocation and inhibition of other movement patterns due to limited capacity to rotate the trunk, reach for objects or move the body forwards, as well as poor gluteal development and delayed maturation of gait.[256] Encouraging a range of body positions and physical activity is advisable to accommodate joint hypermobility.

Pes planus (otherwise known as flat feet or fallen arches) is found in 60–75% of children with Down syndrome and occurs due to ligament laxity and hypotonic musculature.[257] Referral to a physiotherapist to design a program to strengthen the musculature of the feet and improve arch strength should be undertaken as early as possible to counteract hypertonia and prevent further loss of arch height.[257] Weight management is also helpful, as increased weight exacerbates changes to foot architecture.[257] Assessment of the structural integrity of the feet by a paediatric podiatrist is also advisable, and may result in individually designed orthotics that support healthy development of foot arches.

MUSCULAR STRENGTH

Muscle strengthening exercise programs improve many outcomes for people with Down syndrome, including issues associated with muscular hypotonia and joint hypermobility. Physical training regimens can be used to improve balance and coordination, and also provide social and recreational opportunities.[225] Three sessions per week

of a physical training program have been shown to improve balance and coordination outcomes over 12 weeks.[225] Obviously physical exercise needs to be part of life-long maintenance of health, so while more than 12 weeks will be necessary for all people with Down syndrome, it is encouraging that vast improvements can be measured over a relatively short period of time. Disability-specific exercise programs may cater better for the specific needs of people with Down syndrome, but are limited in availability and lack additional benefits of community participation. Wherever possible, community exercise programs should be flexible to the needs of people with disabilities, so that social inclusion and participation become the norm. This widens the scope of potential programs people with Down syndrome can participate in, and allows the same choices and opportunities as all other members of the community.

Immunology

Abnormalities in immune function are part of the genetic phenotype in people with Down syndrome and have bearing on resistance to infection and tendency towards autoimmune conditions and leukaemia. Immune function typically undergoes substantial activation and proliferation within the first years of life, with maturation of T and B lymphocytes secondary to continuous exposure to antigens within the environment[258] and in response to immune mediators in breast milk. In children with Down syndrome, the adaptive response of the immune system is limited.[258] B- and T-lymphocyte production is low, due to abnormal thymus gland development and function. B-lymphocyte development is irregular from genesis stage in the bone marrow, which produces only half the number of B lymphocytes generated in chromosome typical children.[259] Decreased maturation of B lymphocytes and possibly increased apoptosis results in B lymphocytopenia in people with Down syndrome.[258] Immune system irregularities also favour production of inflammatory mediators, which influences progression towards chronic inflammatory comorbidities.[260] The thymus gland is typically smaller in people with Down syndrome, with marked thymocyte depletion.[261] Decreased switched memory B-cells are produced, resulting in poor immune antigen memory and increased susceptibility to respiratory and other infections including sepsis.[259] Increased immunological capacity to differentiate cells into antibody-producing cells has been demonstrated in people with Down syndrome.[259] Some authors postulate that T-lymphocyte abnormalities observed in people with Down syndrome represent intrinsic immunodeficiency, with gradual deterioration of the immune system resulting in reduced response of immune memory.[262] Intrinsic immunodeficiency results in lower immune surveillance, higher susceptibility to infections, malignancies and autoimmunity.[263] Altered lymphocyte production, differentiation and maturation are observed in people with Down syndrome from birth.[263] Poor lymphocyte production and function impair adaptive immune cell response and reduce vaccine responsiveness to new vaccinations and boosters.[259,263] B-cell memory in children with Down syndrome improves by age 7–17 years, resulting in a lower susceptibility to infection than in children 0–5 years, but is still markedly lower than age-matched peers in the general population.[264]

INFECTION SUSCEPTIBILITY

Mortality from infections is 12 times higher in people with Down syndrome than in the general population.[120] Increased susceptibility to respiratory infections occurs in people with Down syndrome, including chronic rhinitis, tonsillitis, tonsillar hypertrophy, middle and outer ear infections, influenza, bronchitis and pneumonia.[262] Poor retention of immunological memory results in slower response time to infections and greater proliferation of pathogens before the immune defences are engaged.[262] This, combined with lower overall numbers of lymphocytes, results in greater severity and duration of infections. People with Down syndrome also have lower capacity to produce a fever, which is a critical immune response to infection.

LEUKAEMIA

Malignancies in people with Down syndrome are typically haematological.[263] Down syndrome is associated with a marked increased risk of childhood leukaemia, which includes a 150-fold increased risk of acute megakaryocyte-erythroid leukaemia (AMKL) and a 10–20-fold increased risk of acute lymphoblastic leukaemia (ALL).[224] AMKL is a subtype of acute myeloid leukaemia (AML), referred to as myeloid leukaemia of Down syndrome (ML-DS) when occurring in children with Down syndrome.[224] The highest incidence of leukaemia occurs in children with Down syndrome aged 1–4 years old,[120] with over 95% of cases of ML-DS diagnosed by 4 years of age.[224] Mutations in the gene encoding for megakaryocyte-erythroid transcription factor GATA1 occur in up to 28% of fetuses and newborns with Down syndrome, which may be clinically silent or may precipitate a pre-leukaemia disorder of impaired myelopoiesis and lymphopoieses.[224] Transient leukaemia occurs in approximately 10% of newborns with Down syndrome and is clinically indistinguishable from AMKL.[265] Transient leukaemia is often uncomplicated, may be asymptomatic and remain undetected, and usually resolves spontaneously within the first 3 months of life.[265] In 15% of cases, however, transient leukaemia causes life-threatening complications, caused by leukaemic blasts infiltrating other organs (liver, heart, skin), resulting in fibrosis and failure of affected organs.[265] AMKL develops later in life in 20–25% of children with a history of transient leukaemia.[265]

Close monitoring of children with Down syndrome is warranted to detect early signs of myelodysplasia, which includes progressive anaemia and thrombocytopenia, and results in profuse and excessive bruising. Regular blood tests that include iron studies and a full blood count can help detect leukaemia in the early phases, prior to clinical symptoms manifesting.[224] Improvements to treatment regimens for children with Down syndrome and leukaemia have been made, though medication toxicity is higher in children with Down syndrome and contributes to medication-induced deaths.[266] Relapse rates are higher in children with Down syndrome than in children without Down syndrome (31.6% and 23.5%, respectively), and death during induction and remission is significantly higher in children with Down syndrome.[266] Poorer outcomes in children with Down syndrome may be due to differences in medication regimens, due to increased toxicity and adverse effects, and increased immunological deficiency resulting in more severe infections.[266] Better treatment outcomes are reported in ML-DS than ALL, due to sensitivity of myeloid leukaemic blasts to chemotherapy, resulting in a survival probability of 70–90%.[265] Survival rates in ALL are substantially lower, ranging from 19% to 49%.[266,267]

Development of autoimmune conditions is associated with leukaemia in children with Down syndrome.[268] Transient diabetes mellitus is diagnosed in approximately 10% of children with ALL, either concurrently or after leukaemia diagnosis, while chronic diabetes and hypothyroidism occur more frequently in ALL survivors.[268] Furthermore, developmental outcomes for leukaemia survivors are slightly poorer for children with Down syndrome, but otherwise follow similar patterns to children with Down syndrome who have not had leukaemia.[269] Children treated for AML appear to have worsening of verbal intelligence and receptive vocabulary, while children treated for ALL are more globally affected, with significant reductions in adaptive function, visual-motor skills, verbal intelligence, vocabulary and spelling.[269] Treatment for ALL typically requires longer duration of chemotherapy that is directed at the central nervous system, with medications that have greater toxicity, resulting in detrimental changes to neuropsychological function.[269] It has also been suggested that the longer duration of treatment for ALL results in prolonged changes to parenting style, with less focus on intellectually stimulating activities, resulting in stalled intellectual development.[269]

Naturopathic support during treatment of leukaemia for children with Down syndrome should include therapies that improve clinical outcomes and reduce the toxic effects of medications. There is, however, no clinical evidence for the use of natural therapies for children with leukaemia and Down syndrome. Vitamin D status in paediatric leukaemia patients in the general population varies, though there may be a higher prevalence of vitamin D deficiency and insufficiency in this population, consistent with deficiency observed in other types of malignancies.[270] Some caution has been suggested with high-dose vitamin D supplementation, secondary to in vitro research demonstrating the role of vitamin D in leukaemia cell differentiation and proliferation.[271] However, low vitamin D levels have consistently been associated with poorer survival rates in a range of types of leukaemia, across a broad range of age groups.[272,273] While vitamin D supplementation does not improve survival rates as a monotherapy, in conjunction with standard medical treatment for leukaemia, higher vitamin D levels are associated with fewer episodes of febrile neutropenia, shorter hospitalisations and reduced infectious complications.[273] Vitamin D testing should occur in all leukaemia patients, and where deficient, appropriate supplementation should be given to achieve optimal levels.

Other supportive natural therapies have potential use for patients with Down syndrome and paediatric leukaemia. Due to the sparsity of research in this area, sensible clinical judgment is required to support patients in maintaining body weight and nutritional status and managing medication side effects. Therapeutic guidelines in Chapters 21 and 22 may be used to guide clinical prescribing.

AUTOIMMUNITY

An increased risk of autoimmune disease affecting the thyroid, gastrointestinal tract and pancreatic islet cells has been observed in people with Down syndrome.[274] Absence of tolerance to self-antigens is required for autoimmunity to develop, though the processes of how this happens are poorly understood.[275] In patients with Down syndrome, dysregulation of genes involved with autoimmune pathogenesis, and failure of immunological development in the thymus gland to establish self-tolerance, results in increased incidence of autoimmune disease.[262,275]

THYROID DISORDERS

Hypothyroidism, and to a lesser extent hyperthyroidism of autoimmune origin, is more common in people with Down syndrome than in the general population.[276] Antithyroid antibodies have been measured in 30% of patients with Down syndrome, with up to 88% of people with Down syndrome expressing some sort of thyroid dysfunction.[276] This includes congenital hypothyroidism, Graves' disease, Hashimoto's thyroiditis, non-autoimmune hypothyroidism and sub-clinical hypothyroidism.

Congenital hypothyroidism

Congenital hypothyroidism occurs in 1 : 141 neonates with Down syndrome[277] compared with 1 : 2000–1 : 3000 in the general population.[278]

Graves' disease

Graves' disease occurs in about 6.5 : 1000 people with Down syndrome. It typically presents at a younger age than in the general population and demonstrates a female gender dominance of 6.7 : 1.[279] Patients with Graves' disease and Down syndrome show a similar clinical picture to patients with Graves' disease without Down syndrome, but a few key differences have been described in medical literature. Firstly, with earlier presentation during childhood or adolescence, accelerated growth in Graves' disease may accelerate maturation of epiphyseal plates and exacerbate the shorter stature observed in people with Down syndrome.[276] The effect of this is minimal with early identification and initiation of treatment, though little is known about the effects of Graves' disease when it presents at puberty.[276] Secondly, the clinical course of Graves' disease in Down syndrome is significantly less severe, with higher remission rates and lower rates of relapse.[280] Communication difficulties may impede early detection of Graves' disease in children and adolescents with Down syndrome, which may initially be mistaken for behavioural difficulties or a growth spurt. However, the abruptness of presentation with Graves' disease makes this easier to identify than hypothyroidism. Thirdly, people with Down syndrome experience a high rate of other autoimmune diseases and a higher overall burden of comorbid health conditions.[276,279,280] Some studies have reported a lower incidence of exophthalmos (16% compared with 25% for people with Graves' disease and not Down syndrome),[276] while other studies have reported similar rates to the general population with Graves' disease.[280] Other symptoms patients describe at the time of diagnosis include irritability, weight loss, palpitations, insomnia, distal tremor, increased bowel frequency and painful eyes.[279]

Medical intervention for Graves' disease in Down syndrome is similar to that for the general population and includes carbimazole, radioactive iodine or surgical removal of the thyroid.[276] Surgical intervention is complicated in patients with Down syndrome, due to craniofacial abnormalities, shorter neck and higher incidence of obstructive airway conditions, so medication-based treatments are usually preferred and are less invasive for the patient.[276]

Hashimoto's thyroiditis

Hashimoto's thyroiditis is the most prevalent thyroid disorder in people with Down syndrome, with onset usually occurring from school age onwards.[281] Phenotypical overlap with Down syndrome traits often obscures detection of Hashimoto's thyroiditis, so regular screening is recommended to ensure this is not overlooked. Growth retardation may occur in very young children with Hashimoto's thyroiditis, particularly if it is slow to be detected and treated. Key differences in the presentation of Hashimoto's thyroiditis in people with Down syndrome compared with the general population are the lack of gender preponderance and lack of goitre due to atrophic thyroiditis. Diagnostic overshadowing often delays diagnosis, thus most cases are identified during screening, not due to presentation of symptoms.[281]

Non-autoimmune hypothyroidism

Non-autoimmune hypothyroidism may also occur in people with Down syndrome, though the majority of cases of thyroid disease are of autoimmune origin.

Subclinical hypothyroidism

Subclinical hypothyroidism is noted by elevated TSH levels, with normal plasma T4 and T3, and occurs in 25–60% of children with Down syndrome.[282] Children with subclinical hypothyroidism may present with no symptoms, or with some symptoms of hypothyroidism, though these are often clinically indistinguishable from Down syndrome characteristics.[277] Detection of subclinical hypothyroidism usually occurs during routine screening. Progression to clinical hypothyroidism occurs in less than 50% of cases and is dependent on other factors, such as the presence of thyroid antibodies, goitre and thyroid hypoplasia.[277] Subclinical hypothyroidism may have profound effects on quality of life and may exacerbate already existing characteristics of Down syndrome. These effects include moderate to severe hypotonia and normocytic anaemia resulting in fatigue.[283] Other potential effects of low thyroid function, including reduced cognitive and motor function, and constipation, have not been clinically demonstrated to date.[283] T4 levels decline with age, and should be monitored regularly.[283]

Nutritional and herbal recommendations for treating thyroid conditions follow the same recommendations as for Graves' disease and Hashimoto's thyroiditis in the general population, though antioxidant needs are probably higher due to increased oxidative stress inherent in Down syndrome.

COELIAC DISEASE

The incidence of coeliac disease varies globally, but is consistently higher in people with Down syndrome than in the general population when compared with others in the same region.[284] Coeliac disease is an autoimmune response to gluten that results in inflammation of the duodenal mucosa, reduced intestinal villi length and hyperplastic crypta, and may result in complete atrophy of the small intestinal villi.[285] Prevalence in people with Down syndrome in developed countries is estimated at 4–17%,[286-291] with a male to female ratio of 2 : 1.[289] This is approximately 7–10 times higher than in the general population in developed countries, which is generally between 1% and 2%.[291,292] As within the general population, age at diagnosis varies and is likely to be related to disease severity. Symptomatic presentation of coeliac disease is 8–10 times more likely to be detected than silent or asymptomatic presentation.[289] Growth failure in children with Down syndrome is more likely with comorbid coeliac disease, but due to other gastrointestinal abnormalities children with Down syndrome without coeliac disease may also present with growth failure. Early detection of coeliac disease in children with Down syndrome improves clinical outcomes and gives opportunity for reversing small intestinal damage.[293] Treatment involves strict adherence to a gluten-free diet, which in most cases leads to resolution of symptoms. However, in patients with complete small intestinal villi atrophy, malabsorption syndromes may persist.[285]

Serological screening for coeliac disease needs to occur multiple times throughout the life span, as development of coeliac disease can occur at any age.[293] Screening should begin early in life to reduce long-term complications. In clinical practice, children who have gastrointestinal symptoms or growth failure are obvious candidates for referral for coeliac screening,[294] but given the increased prevalence, it would be prudent to include coeliac screening with routine screens for other autoimmune diseases and health assessments. The method of screening should include anti-endomysium antibodies (EMA), IgA anti-tissue transglutaminase antibodies (IgA tTG) and IgG anti-tissue transglutaminase antibodies (IgG tTG). Small bowel biopsy is the definitive way of diagnosing coeliac disease, but this is not always practical or advisable in

children with Down syndrome[295] due to poorer recovery from medical procedures and increased risk of complications. IgA production is immature in children under 2 years old and may give false negative results.[296] Furthermore, IgA deficiency in patients with coeliac disease is estimated to be 5%.[297] Older testing methods using antigliadin antibodies (IgA AGA and IgG AGA) are less reliable, as they have poorer sensitivity and specificity.[296] Altered immunoglobulin levels in Down syndrome result in up to 80% of patients showing a positive result for IgA AGA, rendering this less reliable as a test of coeliac disease in patients with Down syndrome.[297] A positive result for coeliac disease is also higher in mothers of children with coeliac disease (4.2%) than in mothers of children without coeliac disease (0.3%).[292]

Patients with untreated coeliac disease have an increased probability of developing other autoimmune diseases, including hypothyroidism and type 1 diabetes, so early detection is preferable, regardless of whether the presentation is silent or symptomatic.[295] Other complications include an increased risk of lymphoma and increased overall mortality.[292] Tissue typing (HLA DQ2, HLA DQ8) may also be of benefit in patients already on a gluten-free diet who have either growth failure or digestive symptoms. It is particularly prudent when adherence to the diet is inconsistent, due to perceived 'tolerance' of small amounts of gluten. While a positive HLA result does not specifically indicate coeliac disease, a negative result eliminates the need for repeated coeliac screening throughout the life span.[291,296]

Non-coeliac gluten sensitivity may also occur and is more elusive to diagnose than coeliac disease. Typical presentation involves gastrointestinal or extra-intestinal symptoms that are present on a gluten-inclusive diet and resolve with strict exclusion of gluten.[285] To date, no serological markers have been identified to diagnose non-coeliac gluten sensitivity.[285] Diagnosis involves strict exclusion of gluten for a period of time long enough to elicit resolution of symptoms (2–3 months), followed by return of symptoms with a one-off reintroduction (gluten challenge or gluten binge) of gluten-containing foods.

OTHER MALABSORPTION SYNDROMES

Other autoimmune enteropathic conditions have been reported in people with Down syndrome, resulting from immune system dysregulation.[298] Non-coeliac autoimmune enteropathy may or may not respond to a gluten-free diet and is histologically distinct from other autoimmune pathology of the bowel, such as Crohn's disease and ulcerative colitis.[298]

INSULIN-DEPENDENT DIABETES MELLITUS

Increased production of autoantibodies that attack the pancreatic islet cells contributes to over-representation of insulin-dependent diabetes mellitus (IDDM) in people with Down syndrome.[299] Early-onset autoimmune diabetes has been observed in infants within the first 6 months of life and is not aetiologically distinct from autoimmune pathogenesis of IDDM in the general population.[274] IDDM presents in 22% of children with Down syndrome under the age of 2 years and is associated with increased predisposition towards other autoimmune presentations.[274] Islet autoantibodies have been detected in 72% of children with IDDM, and 10 years after diagnosis, one study reported 80% also had other types of autoantibodies detected.[274] Biphasic presentation occurs, with a second peak onset occurring around adolescence.[274] Overall, IDDM occurs up to six times more frequently in children with Down syndrome than in the general population, typically presenting before the age of 20 years.[300] Management of IDDM in people with Down syndrome follows the same guidelines as for the general population. Additional herbal and nutritional support for moderating the immune system response could also be of benefit.

ALOPECIA AREATA

Alopecia areata is of autoimmune origin and presents as episodic circular patches of hair loss 2–5 cm in diameter, with coalesced patches occurring in severe cases, and may affect other hair-producing areas of the body.[301] Alopecia areata produces non-scarring hair loss[302] and is estimated to occur in 1.3–11% of people with Down syndrome, with familial tendency observed in 10–25% of cases.[301] Episodes vary in length, ranging from 20 weeks to 2.4 years, with remission between episodes for some and persistence of patches for others.[301] Sources of emotional or physiological stress, such as a change of classroom teacher for children, a change of residence, death of a loved one, family conflict, puberty or illness may trigger an episode.[301] Medical management includes topical corticosteroid creams combined with internal immunosuppressant medications.[302] Phototherapy and photochemotherapy are generally not recommended, due to low response rates.[302] An evidence base for naturopathic treatment of alopecia areata in Down syndrome is lacking. Potential treatment regimens should focus on topical and internal treatments that support optimal function of the immune system, improve nutritional status, reduce oxidative stress and improve stress management.

ARTHROPATHY

Articular complaints are common in children with Down syndrome and may include typical rheumatoid arthritis or be a unique arthopathy specific to Down syndrome.[303] Rheumatoid factor is observed in 28% of people with Down syndrome, but is not correlated with presentation of rheumatoid arthritis.[303] Arthropathy similar to juvenile rheumatoid arthritis occurs in 1–2% of children and adolescents with Down syndrome, with an average age of onset of 3.3 years[304] and a range of onset age of 20 months to 12 years.[305] Delays in the treatment of inflammatory arthritis in children with Down syndrome result in ongoing pain, delayed motor development, irreversible damage to joints and functional limitations.[305] Iritis and other complications typically associated with juvenile rheumatoid arthritis do not seem to occur in arthropathy associated with Down syndrome.[305] Serum markers of inflammation are not sufficient for diagnosis, as few inflammatory markers aside from ESR reliably

present in children with Down syndrome and arthopathy.[305] Screening for autoimmune arthropathy in children with Down syndrome is not currently part of standard health screening, but needs to be to prevent degeneration of joints, pain and limitations to function and movement.[305]

Speech and language acquisition

Children with Down syndrome have multiple difficulties that compound their ability to speak. Hypotonia, midface hyperplasia, an enlarged tongue and difficulty coordinating the oral muscles involved in forming sounds contribute to verbal apraxia.[12,148] Speech difficulties remain a persistent problem throughout the teenage years, with one study reporting that only 44% of older teenagers could be understood by others, 29% could be understood by people they knew and 20% by close carers.[102] Many children with Down syndrome communicate with a combination of spoken words and manual signs.[148] While spoken language is preferred socially, children have a preference for expressive language that is most achievable for them and is effective in meeting their needs. A small study of children with Down syndrome undergoing partial plate therapy found that 40% preferred spoken language, 30% used a mixture of spoken and signed language and 30% preferred manual signs.[148]

Expressive language is generally much poorer than receptive language, suggesting that children with Down syndrome understand more of what is said to them than they are capable of articulating.[12] However, phonological skills are limited in children with Down syndrome compared with children of the same intellectual age equivalent.[115] Grammar and tense, rhyme awareness and vocabulary development are limited, which may be attributable to limited cognitive function.[306]

Facial expression, an important component of non-verbal expression, is also delayed in children with Down syndrome due to slower motor skill development, poor muscular coordination and hypotonic orofacial muscles.[148] Language development is significantly delayed with any disruption to hearing, which is more common in children with Down syndrome due to deformities of the inner and middle ear structures, poor immune function and persistent ear infections. This may also compromise literacy development.[307] Speech therapy should be provided to any child with ongoing hearing difficulties.[307]

Medical therapeutic interventions to improve speech development in children with Down syndrome include partial plate therapy, which reduces tongue protrusion, improves articulation of words and improves facial expression.[148] Tonsillectomy may also improve the capacity to form words and therefore improve the intelligibility of speech.[148]

Hearing

Hearing appears to be about 15 decibels lower than the average for the general population in 38–78% of people with Down syndrome, compared with 2.5% of the general population and 9% of people with intellectual disabilities other than Down syndrome.[308] In children with Down syndrome, the pinna (ear lobe) is about two standard deviations smaller than in the general population, resulting in decreased sound localisation and concentration.[153] Stenosis (narrowing) of the ear canal also contributes to poor sound conduction.[153] Predisposition to cerumen (wax) impaction further impedes sound conduction.[153] Specialist ear assessment is recommended once every 3 months until children are 3 years old to avoid missed diagnosis of ear effusions.[153] Conductive hearing loss occurs in up to 80% of children with Down syndrome secondary to OME. Improved management of OME, upper respiratory inflammation and congestion is essential to preventing long-term hearing loss.

Sensorineural hearing loss also occurs in children with Down syndrome, though this is less well defined than conductive hearing loss, and may occur due to internal auditory canal hypoplasia, enlarged vestibular aqueducts or cochlear nerve hypoplasia.[153] Inner ear dysplasia may also present as decreased size of cochlear spiral, vestibular apparatus and labyrinth.[309] These abnormalities may contribute to sensorineural hearing deficits.[309] Sensorineural hearing loss has been found in 26% of neonates and up to 55% of children with Down syndrome.[310]

Sleep

Sleep apnoea may contribute to chronic sleep disruption, which may in turn have implications for behaviour, learning, attentiveness and concentration,[149] pulmonary hypertension and failure to thrive.[153] Continuous positive airway pressure (CPAP) is used as a measure in adults, but is poorly tolerated in children and may be less effective in children with Down syndrome due to the obstructive tendencies of airway abnormalities.[153] At this stage, adeno-tonsillectomy remains the first-line treatment and is effective for children with Down syndrome to reduce airway obstruction and reduce obstructive sleep apnoea.[153] Any surgery in children with Down syndrome requires extra follow-up care to prevent and monitor for complications. Children with Down syndrome have a five-fold increase in complications following surgery, require longer hospital stays, usually require increased intravenous fluids and have a 50% chance of obstruction persisting after surgery.[153] Postoperative naturopathic care to support wound healing, reduce inflammation, prevent opportunistic infections and enhance recovery could be beneficial in these children.

Medications

Adolescents and teenagers with Down syndrome (age 12–21 years) are more likely to be on medication than younger children (age 5–11 years).[311] Classes of medications commonly used include:
- Central nervous system stimulants: used for the treatment of attention deficit-hyperactivity disorder (ADHD) symptoms. Most commonly used for children with Down syndrome aged 5–11 years.[311] Frequency increases by 1.37 times for every year of life from age 5 to 11.[311]

- Selective serotonin reuptake inhibitors (SSRIs): higher use has been observed for teenagers than for younger children with Down syndrome.[311]
- Atypical antipsychotics (AAPs): often prescribed off-label for the management of behavioural problems, such as irritability, aggression and disruptive behaviours.[311] Use of AAPs is highest for children with Down syndrome aged 11–14 years, and four times higher for children with public funding compared with those with private medical insurance.[311]

Prescribing of psychotropic medications for children with Down syndrome is based on data from trials conducted in the general population, as there is very little evidence on people with developmental disabilities for these medications, or more specifically Down syndrome. Close monitoring of children and adolescents with Down syndrome taking pharmacological medications is required, as response rates to these medications appears to be lower than in the general population, while side effects and adverse effects are higher.[311] This may be due to methylation factors, differences in expression of serotonin and dopamine, or other neurotransmitter and neurological anomalies specific to Down syndrome.[311] Historically AAPs have been used in large institutions for people with intellectual disabilities to make them more pliable, or easier to manage. This practice is now considered unethical from a disability perspective, although prescription of psychotropic medications still occurs for individuals with Down syndrome and significant behavioural challenges, particularly children.

Medication use for other conditions that arise with Down syndrome is specific to the comorbid conditions in the individual, as opposed to any one medication being specific to treat the syndrome. Few medications have specific research relating to people with Down syndrome, so prescribing is based on applications for comorbidities within the general population. For children with Down syndrome, medication prescription is largely to manage cardiac abnormalities in infants or psychological medications in children. Medications used for psychological or behavioural interventions in children and young adults are included in Table 19.5 and in adults in Table 19.6.

TABLE 19.5 Psychotropic medication use in children and young adults with Down syndrome

Medication type	5–11 years old	12–21 years old
Central nervous system stimulant	52%	28%
Selective serotonin reuptake inhibitor (SSRI)	22%	54%
Atypical antipsychotic (AAP)	19%	33%
Alpha-adrenergic agonist (AAG)	38%	35%
Any psychotropic medication	92%	92%

Source: [311]

TABLE 19.6 Psychotropic medication use in adults with Down syndrome

Medication type	<50 years old	>50 years old
Anti-anxiety	16%	16%
Anticonvulsant	16%	38%
Anti-depressant	25%	14%
Anti-hypertension	4%	19%
Antipsychotic	9%	19%
Antispasmodic	1%	5%
Cholesterol-lowering agent	9%	11%
Cholinesterase inhibitor	12%	8%
Fosamax	21%	23%
GORD-related medication	18%	22%
Hormones	13%	14%
Hypothyroid medication	35%	38%
Respiratory medication	26%	28%
Vitamin A	1%	0%
Vitamin B$_{12}$	3%	8%
Vitamin C	4%	6%
Vitamin E	51%	55%
Calcium	30%	30%
Folic acid	1%	5%
Iron	1%	0%
Multivitamin	30%	38%
Other medication	34%	47%

Source: [312]

Sexual health and relationships

The World Association for Sexual Health asserts that sexual health education needs to be broader than just the physical act of sex.[313] When thinking about people with disabilities, sexuality is often left out, under the assumption that sex is not something they should think about or would be inappropriate for them. The persistence of the 'eternal child' way of thinking about people with Down syndrome often denies them access to sex education, which in turn leaves them vulnerable to sexual abuse, sexually transmitted infections, inappropriate displays of affection and not knowing how to express their feelings and desires.[314] Discrimination and marginalisation of people with disabilities carry through into sexual health and sexual freedoms and are the basis for paternalistic attitudes towards sex and sexuality that persist within communities with regards to people with disabilities wanting to live full and unencumbered lives.[315] In very recent history, this included sterilisation of girls and young women without their consent.[316] While in most developed

countries legislation is now in place to prevent this happening, the idea that a person can be denied the right to choose their own reproductive future still persists, but involuntary or coerced sterilisation is viewed as a violation of human rights.[317]

Fear of sexual deviance is another reason that sex education is often withheld from young people with disabilities. Sexually deviant behaviour may occur in people with disabilities, just as it does in the general population, and is often termed 'counterfeit deviance'. Counterfeit deviance refers to inappropriate sexual behaviour that occurs 'due to low socio-sexual knowledge, poor social skills, sexual naivety, limited opportunities and unmet sexual needs'.[318] These behaviours may be benign, offensive or hypersexualised.[319] Inappropriate sexual expression may be due to not understanding norms, expectations or feelings of sexual oppression. Parents often withhold sex education for fear of their children embarrassing themselves, but ironically this predisposes them to social errors that are misinterpreted by others. Sexual health education for people with Down syndrome must consider their needs for sexual intimacy, pleasure and human connectedness, and that these needs are integral to human happiness and wellbeing. It is critical that sex education encompasses broader concepts of sexual health, so it should be more than physical coitus and absence of disease[320] and include the basics of human physiology and anatomy, menstruation, reproduction, masturbation, feelings, intimacy, rights and appropriate expression, diversity of sexual experiences (same-sex and heterosexual couplings), STIs and HIV. Furthermore, informal and formal sexual education is needed that includes discussion of the need to provide privacy, opportunities for relationship development and scope for sexual expression. Sexual health education programs need to be adapted to meet the learning needs of people with Down syndrome, which includes simpler language, and may need to be adapted based on sensory impairments and level of literacy.

Rates of sexual abuse in children and adults with intellectual disability are higher than in the general population. A number of factors contribute towards this. Lack of self-esteem and poor social and communication competence increase the likelihood of being taken advantage of by others.[321] Low respect for people with disabilities in our communities increases the likelihood that negative attitudes exist about people with disabilities and their right to the same human rights as the rest of the community.[322] Poor sexual health education may also result in limited knowledge about safe sex practices, sexual expectations, consent and pregnancy as a potential result of sexual encounters.[321] Disclosure of sexual abuse may be limited in people with Down syndrome due to communication difficulties, and may be expressed instead through increased behavioural difficulties, withdrawal, low self-esteem, depression, regression of skills, self-injury, sleep disturbance or substance abuse.[323] Embarrassment, shame and fear of retribution from the perpetrator may also limit disclosure of abuse.[323] As primary healthcare practitioners, naturopaths need to be aware that sexual and reproductive health is just as important for people with

Down syndrome and other disabilities as it is for the general population. Case taking must include sensitive assessment of reproductive and sexual health, and may uncover a history of sexual abuse or exploitation. Adequate referral for counselling and sexual health screening is necessary in these cases.

SEXUAL DEVELOPMENT AND MALE SEXUAL HEALTH

Hypogonadism, cryptorchidism (undescended testes), a small penis and small testicular size occur frequently in males of all ages with Down syndrome and are associated with low testosterone levels.[158] Hypogonadism may occur in as many as 48% of men with Down syndrome.[324] Luteinising hormone (LH) and follicle-stimulating hormone (FSH) levels have been found to be elevated, which may have a negative impact on testicular development.[158,324] Infertility and subfertility are observed in adults with Down syndrome, more so in males than females. Men with Down syndrome are generally considered to be infertile, with only three pregnancies fathered by two men with Down syndrome recorded in the medical literature.[325-327] Multiple factors contribute to high rates of infertility in men with Down syndrome, including low testosterone. Low testosterone levels may also reduce libido and lean muscle mass and increase the likelihood of osteoporosis. Cryptorchidism occurs more frequently in boys with Down syndrome than in boys without Down syndrome, and also contributes to infertility. Clinical studies vary in reports of incidence from 6.52% to 27%.[328] Testicular cancer has a fifty-fold increased incidence in men with Down syndrome, which may be related to increased incidence of cryptorchid testes, combined with immunological abnormalities.[329]

Genital hygiene tends to be poor in men and boys with intellectual disability, resulting in increased risk of paraphimosis, urinary tract infections, thrush and penile cancer.[330] In some this is due to poor coordination or other limitations to being physically capable of washing the genital area, including cleaning under the foreskin. In others it is due to poor cognition and remembering to wash this area, and why it is important to do so. Baths as opposed to showers may improve successful hygiene, in that self-exploration in the bath will result in adequate flushing and irrigation of the foreskin. Genital hygiene continues to be an issue into adulthood, due to dependence on others for personal care. Personal care may be performed by family members or support staff, who may find the intimacy of such care confronting or be concerned about being accused of sexual misconduct.[330] However, inadequate personal hygiene has long-term implications and good hygiene is necessary to avoid infections and detect problems such as paraphimosis and testicular cancer as early as possible.

Testicular microlithiasis occurs in 22.8% of boys with Down syndrome under 18 years of age, compared with 4.2% of boys in the general population.[331] Testicular microlithiasis involves small clusters of calcium accumulating in the testicles and is associated with increased risk of testicular cancer.[332] Testicular

microlithiasis is more common in boys with Down syndrome and undescended testes (50%) than in boys with Down syndrome and descended testes (16%).[331] It is also associated with germ cell testicular cancer in 40–50% of testicular cancer cases, so close surveillance is advisable when testicular microlithiasis is detected.[333] It is recommended that all adolescents and young men engage in regular testicular self-examination, though this may be poorly adhered to by men with Down syndrome due to intellectual impairment.[331] Some authors recommend annual testicular ultrasound for all males with Down syndrome over 15 years of age, especially those with increased risk of malignancy, as indicated by testicular pain, history of germ cell tumour, testicular microlithiasis or undescended testes.[331] Resources are available to assist men with intellectual disability to learn how to perform self-examination, why it is important and what to do if they do find an abnormality (see Appendices 19.1 and 19.2).

In general, there is a paucity of research regarding sexual health in men with Down syndrome. Marginally more research exists for men with intellectual disability, of which men with Down syndrome represent a considerable portion, but this is scant to draw conclusions from regarding typical health problems that occur or best evidence-based practice. While inappropriate sexual behaviours are over-represented in clinical literature, little exists to guide clinical practice with regards to supporting men with Down syndrome with healthy sexuality.

SEXUAL DEVELOPMENT AND FEMALE SEXUAL HEALTH

Menarche, menstruation and premenstrual mood dysphoria show similar patterns in teenagers with Down syndrome and the general population.[334] Girls who are given inadequate reproductive health education are often unprepared for the onset of menstruation, and are shocked or frightened when it occurs.[335] In contrast, girls who are well prepared seem to experience less difficulty and greater acceptance, and some report looking forward to menstruation as part of becoming a woman.[335] This is consistent within the general population and for girls with Down syndrome. Understanding of menstruation varies widely among teenagers with Down syndrome and is influenced by severity of intellectual disability and capacity to comprehend concepts, the comfort of parents (particularly mothers) discussing sex education with their daughters, and inclusiveness of sex education programs in schools.[335] Some mothers report that they too were underprepared and that they expected menarche would occur later, as with most other developmental milestones in people with Down syndrome.[335] Timing of menarche, however, is not significantly different in girls with Down syndrome than in the general population, and is influenced more predictively by body weight and adiposity.[334]

Menorrhagia, dysmenorrhoea, irregular bleeding and hygiene issues are the most commonly reported gynaecological complaints in adolescents with Down syndrome. Mason and Cunningham, in a survey of teenage girls with Down syndrome, reported that independent self-care during menses was achievable for about 30%, a further 30% were able to self-care with reminders, while the remaining 40% required a greater level of support to manage their periods.[335] Cognitive difficulty and fine motor skills may limit capacity to manage sanitary pads, remember how often to change them and practise discretion in disclosure about their menses. Mothers report that creating routines and involving their daughters in recording their menstrual cycle improve engagement in self-care and acceptance of menstrual hygiene practices.[335]

Women with intellectual disabilities are often not given access to the same range of contraceptive choices as women within the general population. In recent history, hysterectomy was viewed as an appropriate method for preventing reproduction and mitigating the need for managing menstruation in adolescents and women with disabilities.[336] This is no longer considered acceptable practice within international human rights conventions. Long-acting contraceptives, including intra-uterine devices (hormonal or copper), subdermal implants (Implanon) and intra-muscular injections (e.g. depot medroxyprogesterone acetate), are commonly prescribed for women with Down syndrome to prevent unwanted pregnancies but enable greater choice.[336] These choices negate the potential for error involved with taking the oral contraceptive pill daily, inserting a diaphragm or correctly putting on a condom. However, for most women with disabilities, this decision is still made for them, or made with little education about options, side effects or limitations.[336] In many cases, decisions are made with assumed consent or consent that falls considerably short of informed consent. [336] The importance of education about condom use for the prevention of HIV and other sexually transmitted infections is needed for women regardless of whether they are using long-acting contraceptives and are sexually active.

Consistent with other areas of healthcare, gynaecological and breast screening are poorly accessed by women with disabilities. Regular Pap smears and breast examination are recommended for all women with Down syndrome. In the general population breast cancer is the most common type of cancer in women and second only to lung cancer for cause of death from cancer in women.[337] However, the incidence of breast cancer in women with Down syndrome is lower than in the general population. People with Down syndrome are 50% less likely to develop solid tumours, and of those, mortality from breast cancer is 10–25-fold less than in the general population.[338] While increased incidence of other conditions may be explained by over-expression of genes found on chromosome 21, it is hypothesised that one or more tumour suppressor genes are also located on chromosome 21, thus providing a protective effect.[338] It is known that the effects of ionising radiation involved with mammography increase the risk of breast cancer in women, a risk that is outweighed by the benefits of early detection within the general population.[339] Psychological trauma associated with mammography is higher in women with Down syndrome, who may lack the capacity to understand the procedure.[339] Further investigations including biopsy in women with Down syndrome often require general anaesthesia, which is associated with increased complications.[339] Some research suggests that regular mammography should be re-evaluated in women with Down syndrome, in terms of cost-effectiveness, time and psychological trauma, and potential harm caused by unwarranted exposure to radiation.[339] Supporting women to make well-informed decisions about breast screening is essential and may include exploring less traumatic methods of breast screening such as physical examination and ultrasound.[340]

Age at menopause is generally 4–5 years earlier in women with Down syndrome than in women without Down syndrome, occurring on average at 45.8 years of age.[341] Reduced cognitive function and increased incidence of Alzheimer's disease are associated with earlier menopause (<40 years of age) experienced by women with Down syndrome.[342] Post-menopausal health initiatives that include strategies for maintaining bone mineral density, lean muscle mass, weight management and cognitive health should be implemented in post-menopausal women with Down syndrome.

A summary of sexual health education resources for adolescents and adults with intellectual disabilities is included in Appendices 19.1 and 19.2.

Health literacy

Increased predisposition to multiple health problems necessitates life-long attention to health screening and management of acute and chronic health conditions as they arise. Health literacy has been found to be poor in adolescents with Down syndrome.[343] Specific areas of vulnerability include:

- Personal hygiene
- Choice of healthy foods
- Regular exercise
- Regular health screening
- Sedentary behaviours.

Vulnerability in these areas necessitates additional support. Competence with daily hygiene practices is achievable for the majority of adolescents with Down syndrome, though few will be able to maintain this completely independently. Understanding of food hygiene, contamination and possibility of illness resulting from inadequate cleaning has been found to be particularly poor in people with intellectual disabilities.[343] Similarly, understanding of taking medications and supplements including vitamins and minerals is poor. Health literacy will be limited by cognitive capacity. Jobling and Cuskelly report that in adolescents with Down syndrome food selection was more likely to be based on foods they liked, rather than foods that were good for them, and that food preference tended to favour high-fat and high-sugar choices.[343] While this is unlikely to be considerably different from the choices made by other adolescents, it is particularly relevant to people with Down syndrome due to an increased risk of obesity, constipation and other health conditions that is exacerbated by poor dietary choices.

Health literacy will also be influenced by the health literacy of family members and carers. Treats are often used as part of a reward system for children and adults with intellectual disabilities and may result in a poor awareness of the contribution these foods make to weight gain.[343] While these strategies are effective in motivating children with tasks and learning activities, careful attention needs to be given to ensure healthier food choices constitute the bulk of the diet. Recipe books are available to teach people with intellectual disabilities healthy cooking skills and food hygiene practices. These books are printed in large print, with simplified language and steps broken down into smaller components to allow easier comprehension. Facilitating acquisition of healthy eating skills is a necessary part of long-term healthy eating habits. A range of cookbooks suitable to meet the learning needs of adolescents and adults with Down syndrome are available from Independent Living Skills Resources (https://www.easycookbook.org). Each book has easy-to-clean laminated pages including step-by-step instructions with photographs for a range of easy-to-prepare, nutritious, visually attractive meals, salads and desserts. Each recipe includes a list of ingredients and utensils, in both picture format and written list. Shopping cards are also available, with pictorial and written shopping lists.

Adults with an intellectual disability who live in dispersed housing are at increased risk of developing health problems resulting from inadequate screening and problematic lifestyle and dietary choices, compared with those who live in clustered or institutionalised settings.[344–346] This is due to a higher level of choice of what to eat and when to eat, combined with a lack of understanding about health needs and how to access services.[344] Routine health screening and monitoring that occurs in more controlled facilities is often absent in independent settings. This increased risk can be mitigated by ensuring that service providers encourage healthy eating practices and regular physical exercise, and are observant for changes in people's mental and physical wellbeing. Annual health check-ups also facilitate screening processes for early detection of problems. Changes in body weight, mood and activity levels should be observed, as well as medication and supplement compliance, and changes to control of existing health conditions.

Oxidative stress

Glyco-oxidation damage occurs from birth in people with Down syndrome and contributes to accelerated ageing.[347] High oxidative stress through elevated reactive oxygen species (ROS) has been measured in children and teenagers with Down syndrome and contributes to antioxidant depletion.[348,349] Glutathione depletion occurs in response to high oxidant load and limits availability for other processes glutathione is used in, including recycling of other antioxidants (vitamins E and C), amino acid transport, immunological functions and cellular signalling.[348] Supplementation with vitamins E and C has been shown to reduce oxidative stress in

people with Down syndrome when supplemented over 6 months.[348]

ROS are highly toxic to cells and contribute to further generation of free radicals.[156] Increased ROS generation interacts with proteins, lipids and DNA, and contributes to increased cellular death.[350] These interactions, particularly where DNA, mitochondrial-DNA and RNA are involved, contribute to comorbidities and earlier disease progression observed in people with Down syndrome.[350]

While oxidative stress contributes to advanced pathological development in Down syndrome throughout the life span, it should be noted that increased oxidative stress is a feature of Down syndrome in utero and contributes to neurological and developmental impairment.[351] Duplication of chromosome 21 predisposes patients to degenerative oxidative processes, which is evidenced by studies of amniotic fluid, and begins early in gestation.[351] Amniotic fluid in Down syndrome pregnancies has been found to be nine times higher in isoprostane (IP), a marker of lipid peroxidation.[351] While very few known Down syndrome pregnancies progress to birth, there is scant research agenda for improving pregnancy and life-long outcomes. However, it is plausible that increasing the dietary intake and supplementation of antioxidants during known Down syndrome pregnancies may have a beneficial effect on the oxidative environment in utero. This should also include supporting methylation pathways.

Bone mineral density

Osteoporosis and low bone mineral density (BMD) are more common in people with Down syndrome of all ages than in the general population.[352–354] Low BMD appears to begin very early in life and is observed in children and adolescents with Down syndrome,[355,356] even in children as young as 2–5 years old.[357] Some studies have found low BMD to be more common in men with Down syndrome than women with Down syndrome, particularly compared with the general population in which low BMD is more common in women.[358] Men with Down syndrome have also been found to have lower BMD than men within the general population and men with intellectual disability but not Down syndrome.[359,360] While low levels of physical activity are a persistent problem for people with intellectual disability, including people with Down syndrome, this finding suggests that other factors specific to Down syndrome further compound lifestyle influences on BMD.[353]

Low muscle tone in Down syndrome may account for this difference, due to inferior muscular stress being placed on bones, to stimulate bone mineralisation.[359] BMD is affected by gravitational force and muscular contraction, which shapes the distribution of bone mineralisation and stimulates functional remodelling.[360] Joint instability and a tendency towards not only less exercise but also low-impact exercise to reduce impact on joints may also impact on muscular engagement and bone strength, more so for people with Down syndrome than people with intellectual disability of other causes. Low testosterone levels associated with hypogonadism observed in men with Down syndrome may also influence this, as will other endocrine abnormalities such as hypothyroidism.[352] Low osteoblast activity and bone mineralisation have been observed in people with Down syndrome, but not increased osteoclast or bone mineral resorption activity.[361] This suggests that anti-resorptive medications may be less effective than therapies that encourage increased osteoblast activity.

Poor BMD in people with Down syndrome increases the risk of developing osteoporosis. Higher fracture risk is observed in people with Down syndrome, due to increased bending and torsion stresses with increased weight, low BMD and low muscle tone.[362] Slower muscle response rates also result in slower self-correction and increased severity of falls, increasing the importance of attending to this area of preventive care in people with Down syndrome.

Screening for osteoporosis and low BMD is lower in people with intellectual disabilities than in the general population.[363] This may reflect deficiencies in preventive care services provided to people with disabilities. Dreyfus et al. reported that people living in residential facilities with care 24 hours per day were more likely to receive preventive care services than those living in other settings, but that this care was more likely to be procedures that are considered easy such as the influenza vaccine, and less likely to include clinical assessments such as BMD.[363]

BMD is highly responsive to changes in physical training and activity, and is an important consideration not only for preventing osteoporosis, but also for life-long health. Increased levels of physical exercise in adolescents with Down syndrome are correlated with improved long-term health outcomes and decreased fracture risk.[364] Peak bone mass occurs by around the age of 20 as a result of hormonal changes during adolescence.[358] Multiple studies have demonstrated that improvements in BMD in people with Down syndrome can occur secondary to improvements in physical activity, which is of particular importance during adolescence. Improved bone mineralisation has been demonstrated in teenagers with Down syndrome undergoing a 12-month physical training program for 60 minutes twice per week, in addition to their normal daily activities.[365] Motor skill improvement was also reported in this study. Furthermore, improvements have been found in a 21-week study of a physical training program in teenagers with Down syndrome consisting of a 25-minute program twice per week.[355]

Exercise regimens vary throughout studies, but consistently demonstrate that doing any exercise is better than doing no exercise, and that regularity of exercise is of key importance. Regular physical activity will also improve muscle coordination, balance, confidence and muscle control, which have implications for decreasing fracture risk. Furthermore, combining adequate calcium intake, through either diet or supplementation, improves BMD achieved with increased physical exercise.[366] Testosterone treatment in men with low testosterone in the general population has been shown to improve BMD,[367] but specific research in men with Down syndrome and testosterone deficiency is needed to confirm whether this has therapeutic efficacy in this group. Guidelines for promoting adequate BMD are included in Table 19.7.

Life expectancy and quality of life

There have been substantial advances in life expectancy for people with Down syndrome over the last two decades, largely due to improvements in healthcare. Higher detection of health problems with routine screening in childhood enables congenital health problems to be more effectively managed and so they are less likely to lead to secondary disabilities or increased mortality.[134] Health-related quality of life is a measure that takes into account physical and mental health and the impact this has on satisfaction with life.[379] Increased incidence of health problems in people with Down syndrome impacts on quality of life and wellbeing. Quality of life for older people with Down syndrome seems strongly related to level of community participation, socialisation and self-determination.[379]

Premature ageing: dementia, cognitive decline and Alzheimer's disease

Increased life expectancy for people with Down syndrome, through improvements in healthcare, has necessitated advancements in research into differences in ageing in this population. Premature ageing is common in people with Down syndrome and includes earlier onset of cognitive decline, cataracts, dementia and musculoskeletal disorders.[134] Loss of social and conceptual skills has stronger association with age-related decline than adaptive skill loss in Down syndrome.[380] This would suggest that with appropriate support, people with Down syndrome can be encouraged to maintain autonomy and activity into their later years.[380] However, other studies report that older people with Down syndrome may also lose practical skills associated with activities of daily living, as well as communication and memory decline.[381]

Neuro-inflammation is implicated in the pathogenesis of Alzheimer's disease and is more prevalent in people with Down syndrome due to over-expression of genes involved in pro-inflammatory processes.[382] Specifically, increases in amyloid plaques, higher levels of inflammation and increased neurofibrillary tangles are observed in people with Down syndrome from the age of 40 onwards.[383] The incidence of Alzheimer's disease in people with Down syndrome is approximately 10–15% in those aged 40–50 and up to 50% in people over 50.[384] Comparatively, the rate of Alzheimer's disease in the general population is 9% in people over 65.[385] Screening for Alzheimer's disease should occur once every 2 years for people with Down syndrome from the age of 40 onwards, and annually after 50 years of age. While there is no cure for Alzheimer's disease, detection in this population will help identify changes to the level of support needed and

TABLE 19.7 Guidelines for promoting adequate bone mineral density					
	Infants	**Children**	**Adolescents**	**Adults**	**Older adults**
Calcium	—	1–3 years: 500 mg 4–8 years: 700 mg	9–11 years: 1000 mg 12–13 years: 1300 mg 14–18 years: 1300 mg	♀19–70 years: 1000 mg Pregnancy: 1000 mg Lactation: 1000 mg ♂19–50 years: 1300 mg	♀ >50 years: 1300 mg ♂ >70 years: 300 mg
Magnesium	Normally received in breast milk: 0–6 months: 30 mg 7–12 months: 75 mg	1–3 years: 80 mg 4–8 years: 130 mg	9–13 years: 240 mg ♀14–18 years: 360 mg ♂14–18 years: 410 mg	♀19–30 years: 310 mg ♀31–70 years: 320 mg Pregnancy: 350–400 mg Lactation: 310–360 mg ♂19–30 years: 400 mg ♂31–70 years: 420 mg	♀ >50 years: 320 mg ♂ >70 years: 420 mg
Zinc	0–6 months: 2 mg (UL: 4 mg) 7–12 months: 3 mg (UL: 5 mg)	1–3 years: 3 mg (UL: 7 mg) 4–8 years: 4 mg (UL: 12 mg)	9–13 years: 6 mg (UL: 25 mg) ♀14–18 years: 7 mg ♂14–18 years: 10 mg (UL: 35 mg)	♀19–70 years: 8 mg Pregnancy: 11 mg Lactation: 12 mg ♂19–70 years: 14 mg (UL: 40 mg)	♀ >70 years: 8 mg ♂ >70 years: 14 mg (UL: 40 mg)
Boron* (estimated average daily intake)	Estimated amount received in breast milk: 0.21 mg/day	1–6 years: 0.27 mg (UL 1–3 years: 3 mg) 6–8 years: 0.85 mg (UL: 4–8 years: 6 mg)	9–13 years: 0.92 mg (UL: 11 mg) 14–18 years: 1.06 mg (UL: 17 mg)	1.0–1.5 mg (UL: 20 mg)	1.0–1.5 mg
Vitamin D	Current RDI and EAR are inadequate to maintain or increase serum vitamin D levels in sunshine-limited or deprived populations. Higher serum vitamin D is necessary for managing increased prevalence of autoimmune conditions, infections and oxidative stress. Aim to build serum levels to 100–200 nmol/L. Dosing of children and adolescents: 1000 IU/14 kg body weight per day for maintenance; upper limit for building vitamin D levels is 2000 IU/14 kg body weight.			5000 IU per day in sunlight-deprived populations and pregnancy. 6400 IU/day is the highest daily dose that has been demonstrated to be safe in pregnancy. 7000 IU per day required in lactation.	5000 IU per day in sunlight-deprived populations.
Vitamin K	2.5 micrograms derived from breast milk	1–3 years: 25 micrograms 4–8 years: 35 micrograms	9–13 years: 45 micrograms 14–18 years: 55 micrograms	♀19–70 years: 60 micrograms ♂19–70 years: 70 micrograms	♀19–70 years: 60 micrograms ♂19–70 years: 70 micrograms
Exercise	0–1 year: encourage floor-based play in safe environment.	1–5 years: encourage active play. Young children should be active for at least 3 hours every day, spread out throughout the day. 5–17 years: at least 60 minutes of moderate to vigorous intensity exercise daily, including aerobic and strengthening exercises.		18–64 years: at least 150 minutes of moderate to vigorous intensity exercise per week, with additional health benefits achieved at 300 minutes per week. Muscle strengthening exercises should be done at least twice per week. 65+ years: in older adults, physical activity includes activities of daily living, leisure activities, incidental exercise, sports and planned activities. A minimum of 150 minutes per week is recommended, with additional health benefits achieved with 300 minutes per week and aerobic bursts of at least 10 minutes. Physical activity should include balance-promoting activities 3 days per week, and muscle strengthening activities at least 2 days per week. Adjust activities to level of ability.	

*No standard recommendations exist for supplementing boron. Boron requirements are easily fulfilled through a healthy well-balanced diet.[378]
Source: Adapted from [368–377]

precipitate planning of ongoing care. Awareness of carers and family members to be observant of changes in behaviour and cognitive function facilitates the detection of onset of decline, which may be difficult for the individual to express due to communication deficits.[386] It is generally recommended that people with Down syndrome are supported to remain living in their own home with additional support as needed, as this is associated with better quality of life outcomes.[387] People with Down syndrome are more likely than people with other intellectual disabilities to remain living with family members as they age.[387] Early-onset Alzheimer's disease creates additional challenges for family carers, who may be ageing themselves. Alzheimer's disease changes include behavioural changes (e.g. wandering), cognitive decline, personality changes (e.g. aggression), incontinence and reduced capacity for self-care and activities of daily living.[387] These changes may precipitate carers seeking additional support, though most families prefer to keep their loved one at home rather than admitting them to an aged care facility.[387]

Changes may be gradual, or quite sudden. The Plymouth dementia screening checklist (see Appendix 19.3) is an effective tool for assessing the need for referral for dementia assessment.[388] The checklist can easily be filled out by family or paid carers. In the general population, a score of three or above indicates the need for dementia assessment.[388] In a clinical trial, the checklist had a 72% sensitivity in the general population, though it was found that the majority of false negatives occurred in people with Down syndrome.[388] The study authors recommend that people with Down syndrome scoring one or two on the checklist should be referred for dementia assessment.[388] Whitwham et al. report that false positives with this screening were 12.5%, though a quarter of these patients were diagnosed with dementia within the following year and a further quarter were undergoing dementia investigations within the following year.[388] This may suggest that the screening checklist is also effective at indicating early pre-clinical signs of dementia and is thus a very useful low-cost method of tracking decline over time.

Medical therapies used in the treatment of Alzheimer's disease in the general population are not necessarily effective for people with Down syndrome. A recent study of memantine in people with Down syndrome showed no significant difference in cognitive decline, challenging behaviours, independent ability or global outcomes.[389] People with Down syndrome and cognitive decline are generally much younger than people with Alzheimer's disease in the general population, and show distinct differences in neurological function, myelination and amyloid clearance.[389]

Supporting healthy ageing in people with Down syndrome is imperative to improving quality of life outcomes and must begin earlier than in the general population due to earlier onset of age-associated decline. Recommendations as stipulated in the NHMRC 2013 Australian Dietary Guidelines include a plant food-based diet rich in fresh vegetables, fruit, wholegrains and legumes, with moderate intake of dairy products (if tolerated) or other calcium-enriched alternatives, lean meat, poultry, fish, eggs and plenty of water.[390]

Early onset of ageing is correlated with lack of activity and engagement in activities of daily living in early adulthood in people with Down syndrome.[391] To an extent this may reflect differences in severity of disability and functional abilities. Sedentary lifestyles are, however, a significant problem for many people with disabilities and in Down syndrome appear to hasten age-related decline. This is not limited to cognitive decline, but also includes frailty, sensory loss (vision and hearing), sleep disturbance and loss of language skills.[391] Encouraging community participation, daily exercise and engagement in activities of self-care and daily living is therefore essential throughout the entire life span for people with Down syndrome.

Inflammation and oxidative stress play a significant role in age-related cognitive decline, neurodegeneration and Alzheimer's disease pathological processes in the brain.[392] While there is little evidence for the use of natural medicines in people with cognitive decline and Down syndrome, supplements and herbal medicines that are neuroprotective and enhance cognition have the potential to improve quality of life outcomes for these patients. To date, clinical trials in people with Down syndrome and dementia have demonstrated that supplementation improves blood antioxidant levels but does not improve clinical outcomes.[393,394] Treatment resistance in older people with Down syndrome may result from the complex nature of neurofibrillary tangles and plaque deposition, which begin very early in life. It is possible that antioxidant therapy in Down syndrome needs to occur earlier in the life span to reduce degenerative changes, and that by the time dementia or pre-dementia symptoms present, neurodegeneration is too advanced for antioxidant therapy to produce a measureable effect. Thiel and Fowkes suggest that nutrients such as vitamins B_6, C and E, selenium, zinc, alpha-lipoic acid and carnitine that have a role in free radical scavenging and reducing the accumulation of glycation end products may have a slowing effect on neurodegeneration and age-associated decline in people with Down syndrome.[347] Long-term cohort studies are necessary to confirm or dismiss this theory. However, given the tolerability of antioxidants, and that oxidative stress plays a significant role in many of the pathologies present in patients with Down syndrome, it is reasonable that antioxidant supplementation is an appropriate recommendation. Emphasis on a broad and antioxidant-rich diet should be part of routine care for people of all ages with Down syndrome. Additional supplementation with key antioxidants and minerals may have a role in decelerating cognitive decline and neurodegeneration when started at younger ages.

THERAPEUTIC CONSIDERATIONS

Health surveillance and timely intervention are of great importance for the multitude of health problems people with Down syndrome face throughout their lives. Naturopaths and herbalists perform a key role in

TABLE 19.8 Clinical examination procedures for health surveillance in people with Down syndrome

Examination or investigation	Rationale
Blood pressure	Cardiovascular risk
BMI	High risk of obesity and metabolic syndrome
Lung auscultation	Increased frequency and severity of respiratory tract infections
Random blood glucose	Diabetes risk
Temperature	Thyroid risk
Urinalysis	Detect urinary tract infections, early signs of kidney and liver disease, blood sugar control
Waist circumference	High risk of obesity and metabolic syndrome

TABLE 19.9 Health screening by the patient's GP or specialist for people with Down syndrome

Investigation	Frequency
Cardiac assessment	Cardiac assessment by a cardiologist by 6 weeks of age. Auscultate for signs of acquired heart disease at every health assessment.
Coeliac screen	Annually from 12 months.
ESR & CRP	At birth and annually from 12 months.
Full blood count	At birth and annually from 12 months.
Hearing assessment	Newborn hearing screen. Comprehensive hearing assessment by 10 months of age. Annual hearing assessment prior to school age. Hearing assessment once every 2 years from school age onwards.
Iron studies	Annually from 12 months.
Sleep-related breathing	Enquire about breathing at every health assessment.
Thyroid studies	At birth and annually from 12 months, including TSH, T4 and thyroid antibodies.
Vision assessment	Newborn assessment. Formal eye and vision assessment at 18–24 months. Vision assessment once every 2 years thereafter, unless more frequently recommended by an optometrist or ophthalmologist.
Vitamin D	Annually.

Source: [395]

comprehensive healthcare. Longer appointment times allow sufficient scope to assess changes in health status over time, progress with therapies and planning for long-term health maintenance. It is insufficient to assume that another health professional is responsible for health surveillance: holistic care entails a broad overview of the patient's health, alongside keen attention to detail to ensure health issues are not overlooked. Good communication with other health practitioners who are also involved in the patient's care is essential to coordinate and better inform clinical practice.

THERAPEUTIC APPLICATION

Clinical examination and investigations

Good clinical observation, sound case-taking skills and competence in physical examination are necessary to detect, manage and, where appropriate, refer patients with Down syndrome. Essential clinical examination procedures are included in Table 19.8.

More specialised assessment is also necessary on a regular basis to detect changes in health status early and allow for more timely intervention. Screening tests and investigations recommended for routine health assessment are included in Table 19.9.

Nutritional medicine (dietary)

Oral motor difficulties result in parents reporting that some children with Down syndrome swallow food without chewing and that meal choices reflect concerns about choking risk and soft textures to enable easier consumption.[396] These difficulties may persist through to adolescence, and for some people oral difficulties remain in adulthood.[74] Obesity risk in people of all ages with

Down syndrome is high, due to lower metabolic rate, low muscle tone and a tendency towards a sedentary lifestyle. Prevalence for obesity necessitates adherence to a healthy, well-balanced, antioxidant-rich, low glycaemic index diet. Naturopaths are well-placed to guide dietary interventions to improve nutrient intake and health outcomes. Key considerations in tailoring nutritional interventions are included in Table 19.10.

A gluten-free diet is advocated due to a higher incidence of autoimmune disease including coeliac disease and thyroiditis being reported in individuals with Down syndrome. Implementation of a gluten-free diet is associated with a number of benefits including improved behaviour with less irritability.[397] Individuals with Down syndrome have higher rates of overweight and obesity than those without Down syndrome, in part due to unfavourable diet, decreased metabolic rate and a tendency towards sedentary behaviours. Higher incidence of hypothyroidism also contributes towards weight gain, and may be clinical or subclinical. Meal planning should take

TABLE 19.10 Key nutritional considerations for people with Down syndrome	
Food or food components	**Considerations and recommendations**
Fruit	Adequate intake of a range of fresh fruit. Include berries regularly to improve antioxidant intake, and polyphenols to improve gastrointestinal microbiota.
Vegetables	Vegetable intake should include a broad range of types and colours, including green leafy vegetables, brassicas, root vegetables, legumes and curbits. A range of cooked and raw vegetables should be encouraged, including salads.
Protein	Protein may include a range of animal and non-animal sources, such as lean meat, fish, eggs, nuts, legumes, dairy and soy products. Encouraging people with Down syndrome to increase the proportion of vegetarian sources of protein will also serve to increase fibre intake and have beneficial effects on gastrointestinal flora.
Fibre	A range of soluble and insoluble fibre should be consumed daily to optimise gastrointestinal flora and reduce tendency towards constipation. This should include vegetables (including skins where reasonable), fruit, legumes, nuts, seeds and wholegrains.
Carbohydrate	A low glycaemic index diet should be encouraged. Carbohydrates should be from wholegrain sources wherever possible to improve fibre and nutrient intake.
Antioxidants	Diet should contain a range of antioxidant-rich foods daily. This includes brightly coloured fruits (including berries), vegetables and herbs. Fresh and dried herbs that contain substantial antioxidants include turmeric, rosemary, basil, oregano and parsley.
Fat	Foods rich in beneficial fats should be included in the diet, such as olive oil, avocados, nuts, seeds and fish. Saturated fats and trans fats should be limited, by choosing low-fat meats and avoiding processed foods.
Supplementation	Supplementation should be considered for any at-risk nutrients and will vary depending on individual dietary allergies or intolerances.
Vitamin D	Vitamin D is a growing concern, due to indoor lifestyles and sedentary behaviours. Consider risk factors including geographic location, regularity of unprotected time in the sun, premature skin ageing and skin pigmentation. Serum vitamin D testing is advisable for individuals who meet one or more risk factors.

this into account. Earlier onset and higher incidence of dementia, Alzheimer's disease and cognitive decline should also be considered in meal planning. While research currently offers no solutions once cognitive decline has been noted, improved dietary practices in earlier life are advisable. Though no research exists as yet, it is proposed that a Mediterranean-style diet rich in omega-3 fatty acids, anti-inflammatory constituents and antioxidants has been linked to lower rates of dementia in other groups and may be useful for individuals with Down syndrome to reduce cognitive and memory decline.

By necessity the naturopathic consultation involves a certain amount of trouble-shooting, solution finding and strategising with patients with Down syndrome and their families or carers. Each situation will be unique and entail case-specific challenges. Working with patients and their families to explore obstacles to sound nutrition and dietary intake is part of the process. Some challenges will be due to oral motor and physiological difficulties, others may be psychological, social or financial or due to time constraints. Patient autonomy and self-determination must be respected at all times, while also guiding, educating and supporting patients to understand the importance of nutrition to their overall health and wellbeing. Improving nutritional intake will have a positive impact on all other areas of the patient's health, and is thus an essential part of their care.

DIETARY INCLUSIONS

Include:
- Calcium-rich foods
- High-fibre foods such as fruit and vegetables, legumes, nuts and seeds, wholegrains
- Low glycaemic index meals; high glycaemic index foods should be balanced within meal planning with foods that lower the overall glycaemic impact – this includes sources of beneficial fats and protein
- Antioxidants from multiple sources.

DIETARY EXCLUSIONS

Consider a gluten-free diet due to the higher incidence of coeliac disease in this population. While regular testing is pertinent as a screening tool, it will not detect non-coeliac gluten enteropathy. A strict 8-week gluten exclusion followed by a gluten challenge for any patient who appears to have unresolved gastrointestinal upset, which may or may not be related to gluten, is a practical way of assessing the patient's symptomatic response where pathological testing is inconclusive.

Dairy exclusion may also be warranted for patients who appear to have a dairy protein allergy. This may present as chronic catarrh or eczema. A strict dairy exclusion for 8 weeks followed by reintroduction is a viable means of assessing this.

SAMPLE DAILY DIET

BREAKFAST

Smoothie: berries, banana, flaxseed oil, live yoghurt and mixed crushed nuts (including 2–4 Brazil nuts).	A smoothie provides an antioxidant-rich breakfast, which may help counter the impact of oxidative stress. Additionally, it is easy to digest given the higher incidence of dysphagia as a result of structural and anatomical issues in this population. Brazil nuts provide selenium, which is essential for thyroid function, an important consideration for people with Down syndrome due to the higher incidence of autoimmune thyroid disease.

LUNCH

Gluten-free wrap with hummus, boiled egg, tomato, cucumber, mixed lettuce or baby spinach, nori or wakame flakes, and avocado.	Including a source of high-quality protein (e.g. lean meat, eggs, tofu, lentils and legumes) will reduce the overall glycaemic index of the meal. The addition of nori or wakame provides minerals, in particular iodine, for healthy thyroid function.

DINNER

Baked or grilled fresh fish with steamed sweet potato or baby potatoes and a fresh green salad (e.g. mixed green lettuce and baby spinach, sautéed mushrooms, cashews/almonds/pepitas/pine nuts, thinly sliced fresh beetroot, carrot, radish, tamarillo/blackcurrants/tomato).	Though no research exists as yet, it is proposed that a Mediterranean-style diet may be useful for individuals with Down syndrome to reduce cognitive and memory decline. The addition of a salad dressing using both olive oil and apple cider vinegar will slow the blood sugar rise after the meal and is a valuable source of antioxidants and beneficial fats.

SNACKS

At least two pieces of fruit, as seasonally appropriate. Other low glycaemic index, nutrient-dense, lower-kilojoule snack options include:
    Cherry tomatoes, vegetable sticks (cucumber, carrot, beetroot, celery) and hummus
    Rice cakes with mixed nut spread or avocado and tomato
    Trail mix made with raw nuts and seeds
    Homemade gluten-free cake or slice. Improve nutrient density by supplementing gluten-free flour with buckwheat flour, almond or coconut flour, and ground sesame seeds.
	Fresh fruit is rich in vitamin C to help counter the increased risk of periodontal disease seen in people with Down syndrome.

BEVERAGES

1.5–2 L water per day.	Avoid soft drinks and pre-packaged juices, as these contribute significantly to sugar intake, blood sugar spikes and kilojoule intake. Green tea and other enjoyable herbal teas contribute to antioxidant and fluid intake.

Source: Nisihara RM, Bonacin M, da Silva Kotze LM, et al. Monitoring gluten-free diet in coeliac patients with Down's syndrome. J Hum Nutr Diet 2014;27(Suppl 2):1–3. doi:10.1111/jhn.12137; Zigman WB. Atypical aging in Down syndrome. Dev Disabil Res Rev 2013;18(1):1–67; Rafii MS. Improving memory and cognition in individuals with Down syndrome. CNS Drugs 2016;30(7):567–73. doi:10.1007/s40263-016-0353-4; Petersson SD, Philippou E. Mediterranean diet, cognitive function, and dementia: a systematic review of the evidence. Adv Nutr 2016;7(5):889–904. doi:10.3945/an.116.012138.

Nutritional medicine (supplemental)

Supplementation will vary on a case-by-case basis, depending on the health status of the patient, dietary intake and the health issues they present with. It is important that the practitioner is aware they are not treating Down syndrome but a subset of the population with a greater predisposition to a range of health conditions, poorer access to healthcare and greater need for health surveillance. Evidence for nutrient supplementation specifically for people with Down syndrome is provided in Table 19.11.

Zinc is involved in over 300 enzyme processes within the human body and is a catalytic metal in many other

TABLE 19.11 Therapeutically beneficial supplementation for people with Down syndrome

Nutrient	Supportive research
Alpha-lipoic acid and L-cysteine	30-day treatment with alpha-lipoic acid and L-cysteine followed by 30 days washout resulted in significantly improved antioxidant serum concentrations. Assessing a clinically relevant effect was outside the scope of this trial.[398]
Coenzyme Q10 (CoQ10)	10 mg/kg/day in children with Down syndrome for 4 weeks was well tolerated, though dosing needs to consider palatability. Improved plasma levels of CoQ10 were observed with divided dosing.[399] 10 mg/kg/day CoQ10 in children with Down syndrome for 4 weeks normalised antioxidant:oxidant imbalance.[400] 4 mg/kg/day CoQ10 for 20 months in children aged 5–17 years with Down syndrome produced a significant rise in plasma CoQ10.[401]
Epigallocatechin gallate (EGCG): mouse models	Improvement of skeletal parameters, including bone mineral density.[402] Inhibition of *DYRK1A* gene (involved in brain morphogenesis, learning impairments), resulting in reduced brain morphogenesis defects.[403] Improvement in synaptic pathways and methylation activity.[404] 2 weeks of EGCG treatment in mouse pups from 3 days old induced restoration of neurogenesis, and improved hippocampal granule cell numbers and synaptic proteins in the hippocanthus and neural cortex, but none of these effects was maintained 30 days after cessation of treatment.[405] Resveratrol and EGCG demonstrated improvements in mitochondrial dysfunction in hippocampal progenitor cells.[406]
EGCG: human trials	9 mg/kg/day EGCG combined with cognitive training for 12 months was more effective than cognitive training and placebo for improving memory, inhibition control and adaptive skills in young adults with Down syndrome.[407]
Multivitamin and minerals	Multivitamin preparation (high dose of 11 vitamins, low dose of 8 minerals) or placebo was given to 20 children with Down syndrome for 8 months. No significant difference was observed in IQ, behaviour, speech and language development, school achievement, growth or health.[408]
Vitamin B$_6$	Supplementation with vitamin B$_6$ from infancy (under 8 weeks old) for 3 years in a double-blind study in 19 children (25 mg/kg/day for the first 6 months, 35 mg/kg/day thereafter, or placebo) and an open trial of 400 older children (15–65 mg/kg/day) for up to 8 years. No change in psychological testing at 3 years old, but significantly better social development in the treatment group at 6 years old. The open trial revealed tolerance issues, including photosensitivity, sun blisters, vomiting and peripheral neuropathy.[409] Supplementation with vitamin B$_6$ from infancy (under 8 weeks old) for 3 years in a double-blind study in 19 children (25 mg/kg/day for the first 6 months, 35 mg/kg/day thereafter, or placebo). Significant improvement in cortical auditory evoked potentials at 3 years old but not 1 year old.[410]
Vitamin D	Vitamin D deficiency is common in people with Down syndrome and increases predisposition to developing autoimmune disease. Obesity, sedentary lifestyles and already existing autoimmune disease increase vitamin D deficiency.[411] In recent history, people with Down syndrome were at risk of vitamin D deficiency due to institutionalisation. While institutionalisation of people with intellectual disabilities is being phased out in most developed countries globally, vitamin D deficiency is still prevalent due to sedentary lifestyle patterns.[412]
Vitamin E	400 IU/day significantly reduced oxidative stress in children with Down syndrome. No negative effects were reported.[413] 100 micrograms vitamin E/day reduced chromosomal and lymphocyte damage secondary to increased oxidative stress.[414] 1000 IU vitamin E orally twice daily or placebo, given for 3 years, to 337 people with Down syndrome over 50 years of age did not slow the onset of ageing or have a clinically significant effect on cognition, functionality or behaviour. No markers of antioxidant status were measured.[394]
Vitamins E and C	500 mg/day vitamin C and 400 mg/day vitamin E over 6 months produced measureable reduction in oxidative stress, increased plasma concentration of vitamin E and restored glutathione blood levels in children with Down syndrome.[415] 500 mg/day vitamin C and 400 mg/day vitamin E over 6 months persistently attenuated oxidative stress 6 months after cessation of supplementation in children with Down syndrome.[416]
Vitamins E and C and alpha-lipoic acid	Treatment group was given 900 IU alpha tocopherol, 200 mg ascorbic acid and 600 mg alpha-lipoic acid twice daily and a multivitamin supplement once daily, plus standard dementia medication (acetylcholinesterase inhibitor) for 2 years. Participants were patients with Down syndrome and pre-dementia diagnosis. Increased blood levels of vitamin E were measured, but no clinically discernible therapeutic effect was observed. No adverse events or safety issues were reported.[393]

TABLE 19.11 Therapeutically beneficial supplementation for people with Down syndrome—cont'd	
Nutrient	**Supportive research**
Zinc	Zinc supplementation (1 mg elemental zinc (sulfate)/kg bodyweight per day for 4 months) in children with Down syndrome accelerated the rate of DNA repair to a level that was similar to control participants.[417]
	Zinc supplementation (1 mg elemental zinc (sulfate)/kg bodyweight per day for 4 months) in boys with Down syndrome reduced the number of infective episodes and the number of days with an elevated body temperature. Girls in this study had a lower baseline of infections, which remained low after zinc supplementation.[418]
	Zinc supplementation in children (25 mg per day for children aged 1–9 years; 50 mg per day for children aged 10–19 years) for 3 months produced lower incidence of cough and fever, but did not alter other clinically relevant variables.[419]
	Surveyed dietary intake for zinc is similar to age-matched peers, but lower levels of serum zinc suggest altered metabolism. Zinc supplementation (30 mg zinc daily for 4 weeks) in adolescents with Down syndrome (aged 10–19 years) was effective in improving plasma and erythrocyte concentrations of zinc, but had no influence on thyroid hormone metabolism.[420]
	Level of zinc deficiency in people with Down syndrome was not found to be correlated with particular comorbidities, including growth hormone dysfunction and immune system irregularities, or predisposition to coeliac disease or hypothyroidism.[421]
	Oral administration of zinc sulfate (20 mg/kg/day for 2 months) resulted in increased DNA synthesis and improved lymphocyte proliferative response.[422]

metabolic functions.[423] Multiple studies have found zinc to be lower in people with Down syndrome across a range of age groups.[418,422,424,425] Stabile et al. found that only some children with Down syndrome were zinc deficient (20%) and that the effect of zinc on the immune system was transitory. Increased lymphocyte proliferation, however, was demonstrated with zinc supplementation.[422] While nutritional intake in adolescents with Down syndrome is not significantly different from that of the general population, zinc status has been found to be lower, as measured by plasma and urine concentrations, and is elevated in erythrocytes.[420] Romano et al. conducted a study of the levels of zinc deficiency in people with Down syndrome and found that severity of zinc deficiency was not correlated with particular comorbidities, including growth hormone dysfunction, immune system irregularities, predisposition to coeliac disease or hypothyroidism.[421] It is likely that more than one factor is involved in the incidence of these disorders and so it is unsurprising that this study did not find a direct correlation. While zinc deficiency in isolation will not cause these conditions, it is likely that it may contribute to disease progression. Zinc absorption is also lower in older people. Maintaining adequate zinc status is important for cellular proliferation and differentiation, growth factors, cell growth arrest, apoptosis, oncogene expression, chemokines and hormone function.[423] Zinc plays a critical role in immune function through both cellular maturation and migration of immune cells.[423] It is also implicated in inflammatory processes, through cytokine production, and is involved in DNA-repair during accelerated oxidative stress associated with ageing.[423] Current studies on zinc supplementation in Down syndrome are sparse but, as a critical nutrient that is well-tolerated and has been found to be deficient in both ageing populations and people with Down syndrome throughout the life span, zinc supplementation is worth considering.

Carnosine has a potential role in Down syndrome, as it is involved in free radical scavenging and has been shown to have anti-inflammatory properties.[347] Potential for reducing cognitive impairment and cognitive decline has been proposed by some authors,[347] though as yet no clinical trials have been conducted to assess the benefits of supplementation.

Acetyl-L-carnitine has been found to be lower in children with Down syndrome than in age-matched peers.[426] Acetyl-L-carnitine has been clinically trialled in an elderly population and found to reduce physical and mental fatigue, and improve exercise tolerance and cognitive status.[427] This has potential application for people with Down syndrome. One small study ($n = 40$) of men with Down syndrome found no significant improvement with a dose of 10–30 mg/kg/day acetyl-L-carnitine on neurological, cognitive, behavioural or social functions.[428] Higher doses may be needed to achieve a clinically significant result, though further research is needed to support this.

Cysteine has been observed to be elevated in people with Down syndrome, possibly due to over-expression of genes involved in enzyme production that convert homocysteine to cysteine.[347] N-acetyl-cysteine is an anti-glycation agent and has been proposed for use in people with Down syndrome; however, there is limited evidence that it may induce seizures in susceptible individuals and no direct evidence of beneficial effects.[347]

Resveratrol, present in red wine, is a potent antioxidant able to penetrate the blood–brain barrier and is associated with lower incidence of Alzheimer's disease.[429] Other benefits in patients with Alzheimer's disease include weight loss, fat loss and enhanced mitochondrial biogenesis.[429] To date, research on resveratrol is limited, with only a single animal trial conducted in Down syndrome, with positive effects.[406] Preliminary research suggests that resveratrol is well-tolerated and may help reduce the premature neurological ageing that occurs in Down syndrome, though further research is needed to confirm this.

While human clinical trials on people with Down syndrome for herbal, nutritional and supplemental therapies are scarce, often inconsistent or based on inadequate dosing regimens, many of the above nutrients and antioxidants can be sourced through a varied and well-balanced diet. Common sense and sound knowledge of nutritional and herbal medicine should guide therapeutic interventions in the management of the many health complaints that arise in people with Down

syndrome. Nutrients to consider supplementing for specific health presentations are included in Table 19.12.

Herbal medicine

Therapeutic objectives for people with Down syndrome are focused on improving access to quality healthcare, health surveillance and improving the management of acute and chronic health conditions and comorbidities. Herbal medicines used will vary depending on the specific health problems individual patients present with. Herbs that exhibit strong antioxidant activity are of particular

Condition	Nutrients to consider supplementing	Adult dosage	Child dosage	
Anxiety and depression	Antioxidants Curcumin	Include a range of antioxidants from dietary sources. Dose will vary depending on body size. Ensure supplement includes piperine, quercetin or a phospholipid to improve absorption. Inclusion of curcumin in the diet may be preferable in very young children.		
	Magnesium	150–600 mg/day	3–8 years: 80–150 mg/day 9–15 years: 240–360 mg/day 15+ years: dose as for adults depending on child's size	
	Methylated B vitamins, including folic acid	While epidemiological research suggests a link between depression and low B vitamin intake, particularly B_{12} and folate, current evidence for supplementing B vitamins is inconsistent. Given the methylation issues inherent in people with Down syndrome, supplementation is likely to be beneficial and warrants further research. Supplementation with a high-quality methylated B complex is likely to be more beneficial than isolated B vitamins.		
	Omega-3 fatty acids Vitamin D	>3000 mg/day 2000–5000 IU per day	1000–5000 mg/day 1000 IU per 14 kg body weight for maintenance or 2000 IU per 14 kg body weight for building vitamin D levels	
	Zinc	15–30 mg/day	1–3 years: 3–5 mg 4–8 years: 4–10 mg 9–13 years: 10–20 mg 14–18 years: 15–30 mg	
Arthropathy	Antioxidants Curcumin	Include a range of antioxidants from dietary sources. Dose will vary depending on body size. Ensure supplement includes piperine, quercetin or a phospholipid to improve absorption. Inclusion of curcumin in the diet may be preferable in very young children.		
	Omega-3 fatty acids	6000–16 000 mg/day	1000–5000 mg/day	
Chronic constipation	Ground flaxseeds Lactulose	1–2 tablespoons daily 20–30 mL acute dose 5–15 mL maintenance dose	½–1 tablespoon daily Acute dose: 1–6 years: 10 mL 7–14 years: 15 mL	Maintenance dose: <1 year: 2.5 mL 1–5 years: 5 mL 7–14 years: 5–10 mL
	Partially hydrolysed guar gum Probiotics: *Lactobacillus acidophilus* La-14 *Bifidobacterium longum* Bl-05 *Lactobacillus plantarum* Lp-115	5 g daily 10^9–10^{11} organisms per strain	5 g daily 10^9–10^{11} organisms per strain	

TABLE 19.12 Nutrients to consider supplementing for health conditions arising in people with Down syndrome

TABLE 19.12 Nutrients to consider supplementing for health conditions arising in people with Down syndrome—cont'd

Condition	Nutrients to consider supplementing	Adult dosage	Child dosage
Coeliac disease	Glutamine	10–20 mg/day	0.3–0.5 g/kg body weight
	Iron (if deficiency confirmed)	30–50 mg daily for 3 months, then re-test	1 mg/kg/day for 3 months, then re-test
	Multivitamin and minerals	Clinical decision will vary depending on the needs of the patient, quality of dietary intake and patient budget.	High-quality paediatric multivitamin and mineral powder.
	Omega-3 fatty acids	>3000 mg/day	1000–5000 mg/day
	Probiotics: *Lactobacillus rhamnosus* LGG *Saccharomyces cerevisiae var boulardii* (biocodex strain)	10^9–10^{11} organisms per strain	10^9–10^{11} organisms per strain
	Protein powder	Protein supplement may be useful for patients with dysphagia or other oral motor difficulties. Preference food sources of protein and supplement additional protein as needed on a case-by-case basis.	
	Zinc	15–30 mg/day	1–3 years: 3–5 mg 4–8 years: 4–10 mg 9–13 years: 10–20 mg 14–18 years: 15–30 mg
Diabetes and metabolic syndrome	Chromium	200–600 micrograms/day	
	L-carnitine	2–4 g/day	
	Magnesium	150–600 mg/day	3–8 years: 80–150 mg/day 9–15 years: 240–360 mg/day 15+ years: dose as for adults depending on child's size
	Zinc	15–30 mg/day	1–3 years: 3–5 mg 4–8 years: 4–10 mg 9–13 years: 10–20 mg 14–18 years: 15–30 mg
Eczema	Antioxidants	Include a range of antioxidants from dietary sources.	
	Omega-3 fatty acids	>3000 mg/day	1000–5000 mg/day
	Prebiotics: Fructooligosaccharides	3–10 g daily	3–10 g daily
	Probiotics: *Lactobacillus rhamnosus* LGG *Lactobacillus reuteri* MM53	10^9–10^{11} organisms per strain	10^9–10^{11} organisms per strain
	Selenium	100–200 micrograms/day	25–100 micrograms/day
	Vitamin C	1000–3000 mg/day	500–2000 mg/day
	Vitamin D	5000 IU per day in sunlight-deprived populations.	1000 IU per 14 kg bodyweight for maintenance or 2000 IU per 14 kg body weight for building vitamin D levels
	Zinc	15–30 mg/day	1–3 years: 3–5 mg 4–8 years: 4–10 mg 9–13 years: 10–20 mg 14–18 years: 15–30 mg
Growth failure and/or developmental delay	Glutamine	N/A	0.3–0.5 g/kg
	Multivitamin and minerals	N/A	High-quality paediatric multivitamin and mineral powder
	Omega-3 fatty acids	N/A	1000–3000 mg/day
	Protein powder	N/A	Case-dependent
	Vitamin D	N/A	1000 IU per 14 kg bodyweight for maintenance, or 2000 IU per 14 kg body weight for building vitamin D levels
	Zinc	N/A	1–3 years: 3–5 mg 4–8 years: 4–10 mg 9–13 years: 10–20 mg 14–18 years: 15–30 mg

Continued

TABLE 19.12 Nutrients to consider supplementing for health conditions arising in people with Down syndrome—cont'd			
Condition	**Nutrients to consider supplementing**	**Adult dosage**	**Child dosage**
Hyper-thyroidism	Antioxidants	Include a range of antioxidants from dietary sources.	
	Selenium Zinc	200 micrograms/day 15–30 mg/day	25–100 micrograms/day 1–3 years: 3–5 mg 4–8 years: 4–10 mg 9–13 years: 10–20 mg 14–18 years: 15–30 mg
Hypo-thyroidism	Antioxidants Iodine	Include a range of antioxidants from dietary sources. 150–290 micrograms/day	 <12 months: 110–130 micrograms/day 1–8 years: 90 micrograms/day 9–13 years: 13 micrograms/day >14 years: 150 micrograms/day
	Selenium Zinc	200 micrograms/day 15–30 mg/day	25–100 micrograms/day 1–3 years: 3–5 mg 4–8 years: 4–10 mg 9–13 years: 10–20 mg 14–18 years: 15–30 mg
Leukaemia		Supplements for patients with leukaemia need to be considered within the context of medications and other concomitant therapies. Supportive therapies for people with Down syndrome follow the same guidelines as for the general population.	
Osteoporosis And osteopenia	Boron	0.2–1 mg/day estimated daily intake	2 mg per day
	Calcium	1000–1300 mg/day	1–3 years: 500 mg 4–8 years: 700 mg 9–11 years: 1000 mg 12–18 years: 1300 mg
	Magnesium	150–600 mg/day	3–8 years: 80–150 mg/day 9–15 years: 240–360 mg/day 15+ years: dose as for adults depending on child's size
	Vitamin D	5000 IU per day in sunlight-deprived populations	1000 IU per 14 kg body weight for maintenance or 2000 IU per 14 kg body weight for building vitamin D levels
	Vitamin K	60–70 micrograms	1–3 years: 25 micrograms 4–8 years: 35 micrograms 9–13 years: 45 micrograms 14–18 years: 55 micrograms
	Zinc	15–30 mg/day	1–3 years: 3–5 mg 4–8 years: 4–10 mg 9–13 years: 10–20 mg 14–18 years: 15–30 mg
Oxidative stress and premature ageing	Alpha-lipoic acid	600–1200 mg/day	Doses have not been established for children.
	Antioxidants	Include a range of antioxidants from dietary sources.	
	Co-enzyme Q10 Epigallocatechin gallate (EGCG)	150–300 mg 9 mg/kg	4–10 mg/kg/day CoQ10 Older adolescents: 9 mg/kg
	Multivitamin and minerals	Clinical decision will vary depending on the needs of the patient, quality of dietary intake and patient budget.	
	Vitamin C Vitamin D	1000–3000 mg/day 5000 IU per day in sunlight-deprived populations	500–2000 mg/day 1000 IU per 14 kg body weight for maintenance or 2000 IU per 14 kg body weight for building vitamin D levels
	Vitamin E Zinc	500 IU/day 15–30 mg/day	100 IU/day 1–3 years: 3–5 mg 4–8 years: 4–10 mg 9–13 years: 10–20 mg 14–18 years: 15–30 mg

TABLE 19.12 Nutrients to consider supplementing for health conditions arising in people with Down syndrome—cont'd

Condition	Nutrients to consider supplementing	Adult dosage	Child dosage
Persistent infections and poor immune function	Antioxidants	Include a range of antioxidants from dietary sources.	
	Prebiotic: Fructooligosaccharides	3–10 g/day	3–10 g/day
	Lactulose	5–15 mL/day	2.5–10 mL/day
	Probiotic: *Lactobacillus rhamnosus* LGG	10^9 organisms	10^9 organisms
	Vitamin A	3000–5000 IU/day	1000–2000 IU/day
	Vitamin C	2000–3000 mg/day	500–2000 mg/day
	Vitamin D	5000 IU per day in sunlight-deprived populations	1000 IU per 14 kg body weight for maintenance or 2000 IU per 14 kg body weight for building vitamin D levels
	Zinc	15–30 mg/day	1–3 years: 3–5 mg 4–8 years: 4–10 mg 9–13 years: 10–20 mg 14–18 years: 15–30 mg
Post-surgery	Glutamine	10–20 g/day	
	Multivitamin and minerals	Clinical decision will vary depending on the needs of the patient, quality of dietary intake and patient budget.	High-quality paediatric multivitamin and mineral powder.
	Omega-3 fatty acids	>3000 mg/day	1000–5000 mg/day
	Protein powder	Protein supplement may be useful for patients with dysphagia or other oral motor difficulties. Preference food sources of protein and supplement additional protein as needed on a case-by-case basis.	
	Zinc	15–30 mg/day	1–3 years: 3–5 mg 4–8 years: 4–10 mg 9–13 years: 10–20 mg 14–18 years: 15–30 mg
Seizures and epilepsy	Antioxidants	Include a range of antioxidants from dietary sources.	
	Calcium	1000–1300 mg/day	1–3 years: 500 mg 4–8 years: 700 mg 9–11 years: 1000 mg 12–18 years: 1300 mg
	Curcumin	Dose will vary depending on body size. Ensure supplement includes piperine, quercetin or a phospholipid to improve absorption. Inclusion of curcumin in the diet may be preferable in very young children.	
	Electrolytes	Dose as needed in 500 mL–1 L of water.	
	Magnesium	150–600 mg/day	3–8 years: 80–150 mg/day 9–15 years: 240–360 mg/day 15+ years: dose as for adults depending on child's size.
	Methylated B vitamins, including folic acid	Supplementation with a high-quality methylated B complex is likely to be more beneficial than isolated B vitamins.	
	Omega-3 fatty acids	>3000 mg/day	1000–5000 mg/day
	Selenium	200 micrograms/day	25–100 micrograms/day
	Vitamin C	1000–3000 mg/day	500–2000 mg/day
	Vitamin D	5000 IU per day in sunlight-deprived populations	1000 IU per 14 kg body weight for maintenance or 2000 IU per 14 kg body weight for building vitamin D levels
	Zinc	15–30 mg/day	1–3 years: 3–5 mg 4–8 years: 4–10 mg 9–13 years: 10–20 mg 14–18 years: 15–30 mg

Source: [430]

importance for people with Down syndrome. Curcumin, the active component in *Curcuma longa* (turmeric), is a potent anti-inflammatory and antioxidant and demonstrates neuroprotective effects through free radical scavenging.[350] *Ginkgo biloba* is known for its antioxidant properties and has been shown to improve cognitive function in patients with Alzheimer's disease.[350] Other strongly antioxidant herbs, particularly those with evidence of a history of use for cognitive support, should be considered. These include, but are not limited to, *Pinus pinaster* (maritime pine), *Rosmarinus officinalis* (rosemary), *Salvia officinalis* (sage), *Melissa officinalis* (lemon balm), *Ocimum tenuiflorum* (Krishna tulsi) and *Panax ginseng* (Korean ginseng). Table 19.13 includes a range of herbs that may be useful in the management of health conditions experienced by people with Down syndrome. Consider potential herb–drug interactions in the choice of herbal medicines when patients are taking prescribed medications.

Green tea contains multiple antioxidant compounds including EGCG, which has demonstrated anti-cancer and antioxidant properties and may reduce neurodegenerative processes.[350] To date, most research on EGCG in Down syndrome has been conducted in mouse models. While one cannot directly extrapolate benefit in humans from these studies, they do demonstrate potential therapeutic benefits, including improved bone mineral density, neurotransmitter and synaptic enhancement and reduced maladaptive neurogenesis (see Table 19.11). To date only one study has investigated EGCG in humans as well as mice: de la Torre et al. demonstrated improvements in visual memory recognition, spatial working memory, social functioning and quality of life in adolescents with Down syndrome.[407] Further research is needed to explore the therapeutic potential of EGCG in young and older people with Down syndrome.

TABLE 19.13 Potential herbal medicines to consider in the treatment of health complaints experienced by people with Down syndrome

System	Therapeutic objective	Herbal medicine
Cardiac	Cardiotonic and cardioprotective	*Crataegus oxycanthus* (hawthorn) *Leonuris cardiaca* (motherwort) *Terminalia arjuna* (arjuna)
	Hypotensive	*Allium sativum* (garlic) *Leonuris cardiaca* (motherwort) *Olea europaea* (olive leaf) *Tilia europaea* (linden, or lime blossom) *Viscum album* (mistletoe)
Dental	Improve oral flora	*Camellia sinensis* (green tea)
Dermatological	Anti-inflammatory	*Calendula officinalis* (calendula) *Glycyrrhiza glabra* (liquorice) *Hypericum perforatum* (St John's wort) *Lavandula officinalis* (lavender) *Matricaria recutita* (chamomile) *Plantago lanceolata* (ribwort)
	Antimicrobial	*Allium sativum* (garlic) *Camellia sinensis* (green tea) *Hydrastis canadensis* (golden seal) *Melaleuca alternifolia* (tea tree) *Ocimum tenuiflorum* (Krishna tulsi) *Origanum vulgare* (oregano) *Rosmarinus officinalis* (rosemary) *Salvia officinalis* (sage) *Thymus vulgaris* (thyme)
	Vulnerary	Topical: *Aloe barbadensis* (aloe vera) *Plantago lanceolata* (ribwort) *Vitellaria paradoxa*, formerly known as *Butyrospermum parkii* (shea butter)
Developmental delay and learning difficulties	Cognitive enhancer/brain tonic	*Bacopa monnieri* (brahmi) *Camellia sinensis* (green tea) *Ginkgo biloba* (ginkgo) *Rosmarinus officinalis* (rosemary) *Salvia officinalis* (sage) *Melissa officinalis* (lemon balm) *Panax ginseng* (Korean ginseng)

TABLE 19.13 Potential herbal medicines to consider in the treatment of health complaints experienced by people with Down syndrome—cont'd

System	Therapeutic objective	Herbal medicine
ENT and other respiratory disorders	Antimicrobial	*Allium sativum* (garlic) *Camellia sinensis* (green tea) *Hydrastis canadensis* (golden seal) *Ocimum tenuiflorum* (Krishna tulsi) *Origanum vulgare* (oregano) Propolis *Commiphora myrrha* (myrrh) *Salvia officinalis* (sage) *Thymus vulgaris* (thyme)
	Anti-spasmodic	*Pimpinella anisum* (aniseed) *Thymus vulgaris* (thyme) *Adhatoda vasica* (adhatoda)
	Decongestant	*Eucalyptus globulus* (southern blue gum) *Mentha x piperita* (peppermint)
	Demulcent	*Codonopsis pilosula* (codonopsis) *Glycyrrhiza glabra* (liquorice) *Plantago lanceolata* (ribwort) *Verbascum thapsus* (mullein)
	Expectorant	*Marrubium vulgare* (white horehound) *Origanum vulgare* (oregano) *Polygala tenuifolia* (polygala) *Thymus vulgaris* (thyme) *Verbascum thapsus* (mullein)
	Febrifuge	*Achillea millefolium* (yarrow) *Eupatorium perfoliatum* (boneset)
	Immune stimulant	*Andrographis paniculata* (andrographis) *Uncaria tomentosa* (cat's claw) *Echinacea* spp. (echinacea) *Eleutherococcus senticosus* (Siberian ginseng) *Panax ginseng* (Korean ginseng) *Panax quinquefolius* (American ginseng)
	Immune tonic	*Astragalus membranaceus* (astragalus) *Codonopsis pilosula* (codonopsis) *Eleutherococcus senticosus* (Siberian ginseng) *Panax ginseng* (Korean ginseng) *Panax quinquefolius* (American ginseng) *Sutherlandia frutescens* (Sutherlandia) *Withania somnifera* (ashwagandha)
	Lung tonic	*Inula helenium* (elecampane) *Panax quinquefolius* (American ginseng) *Verbascum thapsus* (mullein)
	Lymphatic	*Calendula officinalis* (calendula) *Galium aparine* (clivers) *Phytolacca decandra* (poke root)
	Mucolytic	*Glycyrrhiza glabra* (liquorice) *Polygala tenuifolia* (polygala) *Sanguinaria canadensis* (bloodroot)
	Sinus tonic	*Hydrastis canadensis* (golden seal) *Hyssopus officinalis* (hyssop) *Solidago canadensis* (golden rod)
Endocrine	Hypoglycaemic	*Cinnamomum zeylanicum* (true cinnamon) *Galega officinalis* (goat's rue) *Gymnema sylvestre* (gymnema) *Momordica charantia* (bitter melon) *Trigonella foenum-graecum* (fenugreek)
	Thyroid stimulant	*Coleus forskohlii* (coleus) *Fucus vesiculosus* (bladderwrack)
	Thyroid suppressant	*Lycopus virginicus* (bugleweed)

Continued

TABLE 19.13 Potential herbal medicines to consider in the treatment of health complaints experienced by people with Down syndrome—cont'd

System	Therapeutic objective	Herbal medicine
Gastrointestinal	Alleviate constipation	*Linum usitatissimum* (flaxseed) *Rhamnus purshiana* (cascara sagrada) *Rheum palmatum* (rhubarb) *Rumex crispus* (yellow dock) *Ulmus rubra* (slippery elm)
	Carminative	*Angelica archangelica* (angelica) *Anethum graveolens* (dill) *Carum carvi* (caraway) *Cinnamomum zeylanicum* (true cinnamon) *Foeniculum vulgare* (fennel) *Hyssopus officinalis* (hyssop) *Lavandula officinalis* (lavender) *Matricaria recutita* (chamomile) *Melissa officinalis* (lemon balm) *Mentha × piperita* (peppermint) *Nepeta cataria* (catnip) *Pimpinella anisum* (aniseed) *Zingiber officinale* (ginger)
	Emollients	*Althaea officinalis* (marshmallow) *Plantago lanceolata* (ribwort) *Ulmus rubra* (slippery elm)
	Manage gastro-oesophageal reflux	*Althaea officinalis* (marshmallow) *Filipendula ulmaria* (meadowsweet) *Ulmus rubra* (slippery elm)
Haematological	Nutritive/blood building	*Codonopsis pilosula* (codonopsis) *Eleutherococcus senticosus* (Siberian ginseng) *Panax ginseng* (Korean ginseng) *Panax quinquefolius* (American ginseng) *Urtica dioca* (nettle) *Withania somnifera* (ashwagandha)
Neuropsychiatric	Adaptogens	*Codonopsis pilosula* (codonopsis) *Eleutherococcus senticosus* (Siberian ginseng) *Panax ginseng* (Korean ginseng) *Panax quinquefolius* (American ginseng) *Rhodiola rosea* (Arctic rose) *Withania somnifera* (ashwagandha)
	Anti-depressant	*Avena sativa* (green oats) *Crocus sativus* (saffron) *Hypericum perforatum* (St John's wort) *Lavandula officinalis* (lavender) *Leonurus cardiaca* (motherwort) *Melissa officinalis* (lemon balm) *Sceletium tortuosum* (sceletium) *Verbena officinalis* (vervain)
	Enhance cognitive function	*Bacopa monnieri* (brahmi) *Melissa officinalis* (lemon balm) *Ocimum tenuiflorum* (Krishna tulsi) *Rosmarinus officinalis* (rosemary) *Salvia officinalis* (sage)
	Neuroprotective	*Centella asiatica* (gotu kola) *Curcuma longa* (turmeric)

TABLE 19.13 Potential herbal medicines to consider in the treatment of health complaints experienced by people with Down syndrome—cont'd

System	Therapeutic objective	Herbal medicine
Neuropsychiatric (cont'd)	Reduce anxiety	*Avena sativa* (green oats) *Crocus sativus* (saffron) *Eschscholzia californica* (Californian poppy) *Hypericum perforatum* (St John's wort) *Lavandula officinalis* (lavender) *Leonurus cardiaca* (motherwort) *Matricaria chamomilla* (chamomile) *Melissa officinalis* (lemon balm) *Passiflora incarnata* (passionflower) *Piper methysticum* (kava) *Sceletium tortuosum* (sceletium) *Scutellaria lateriflora* (skullcap) *Valeriana officinalis* (valerian) *Verbena officinalis* (vervain)
	Sedative	*Eschscholzia californica* (Californian poppy) *Lavandula officinalis* (lavender) *Passiflora incarnata* (passionflower) *Piper methysticum* (kava) *Valeriana officinalis* (valerian) *Zizyphus spinosa* (zizyphus)
Metabolic	Metabolic stimulant	*Camellia sinensis* (green tea) *Coleus forskohlii* (coleus) *Eleutherococcus senticosus* (Siberian ginseng) *Panax ginseng* (Korean ginseng) *Panax quinquefolius* (American ginseng)
Ophthalmic	Anti-inflammatory Microvascular tonic	Topical: *Plantago lanceolata* (ribwort) (dilute in saline) *Pinus pinaster* (maritime pine) *Vaccinium myrtillus* (bilberry) *Vitis vinifera* (grape: skin and seed)
Orthopaedic	Anti-rheumatic/anti-inflammatory Spasmolytic	*Apium graveolens* (celery seed) *Boswellia serrata* (boswellia) *Curcuma longa* (turmeric) *Harpagophytum procumbens* (devil's claw) *Salix alba* (willow bark) *Urtica dioca* (nettle) *Corydalis ambigua* (corydalis) *Piper methysticum* (kava) *Valeriana officinalis* (valerian) *Viburnum opulus* (cramp bark)
Sexual and reproductive health: female	Anodyne Luteal phase tonic Ovulatory tonic Uterine tonic	*Corydalis ambigua* (corydalis) *Matricaria chamomilla* (chamomile) *Piscidia piscipula* (Jamaican dogwood) *Viburnum opulus* (cramp bark) *Viburnum prunifolium* (black haw) *Vitex agnus-castus* (chaste tree) *Paeonia lactiflora* (peony) *Alchemilla vulgaris* (lady's mantle) *Rubus idaeus* (raspberry leaf) *Viburnum prunifolium* (black haw)
Sexual and reproductive health: male	Tonic	*Panax ginseng* (Korean ginseng) *Serenoa repens* (saw palmetto) *Smilax ornata* (sarsaparilla) *Turnera diffusa* (damiana) *Withania somnifera* (ashwagandha)

Lifestyle: exercise

Exercise requirements follow the same guidelines as for the general population and should be adapted to the physical capabilities of the patient. While physical impairments may limit some types of exercise, more often than not activities are possible with a greater degree of support. For babies aged 0–1 year old, encourage floor-based play in safe environments.[374] Floor-based play not only is a valuable form of exercise, but also facilitates interaction with objects and the environment, family members and carers, and provides great scope for environmental enrichment. Children aged 1–5 years should be encouraged to engage in active play. Young children should be active for at least 3 hours every day, spread out throughout the day.[374] This should include a broad range of activities that encourage muscular development, balance, proprioception and intellectual stimulation. School-aged children (aged 5–17 years) should engage in at least 1 hour of moderate to vigorous intensity exercise daily, including aerobic and strengthening exercises.[375] Healthy exercise practices established during childhood may reduce the tendency towards sedentary activity and may help establish a lifelong habitual exercise.

In adults, physical activity includes activities of daily living, leisure activities, incidental exercise, sports and planned activities. A minimum of 150 minutes per week is recommended, with additional health benefits achieved with 300 minutes per week, including aerobic bursts of at least 10 minutes. In older adults (50–70 years), physical activity should include balance-promoting activities 3 days per week, and muscle strengthening activities at least 2 days per week. The type of activities enjoyed will need to be adjusted to accommodate the individual's physical abilities.[377]

CASE STUDY 19.4

OVERVIEW

Wendy, a 42-year-old woman with Down syndrome, presents with a recent history of irregular menses, mood swings, night sweats and irritability. Her menstrual history is unremarkable and her periods were regular and non-painful until 6 months ago. She lives in a group home with two other women with intellectual disabilities. Wendy and her housemates have support workers who assist them with evening meal preparation and domestic duties. The household food budget is shared; the three women eat together most nights and organise other meals independently of each other. Wendy is assertive with her ideas and is frustrated when people don't take the time to understand what she has to say. Her speech is intelligible, but words are often poorly formed due to oral motor difficulties and an oversized tongue. Wendy was accompanied by her carer for the initial appointment.

RELEVANT HEALTH HISTORY

Wendy was born at 41 weeks' gestation via normal vaginal delivery and was breastfed for 14 months. She has no history of congenital heart disease. Wendy suffered frequent respiratory tract infections as a child, including recurrent middle ear infections, croup and pneumonia, resulting in frequent antibiotic use and many hospitalisations. Adenoidectomy and tonsillectomy were performed at 4 years old. Wendy works 4 days per week at a local disability support agency. She reports that she is not stressed, though on further questioning she reveals she has frequent disagreements with one of her housemates. Wendy has lived in the group home for 8 months following the death of her father and her mother moving into an aged care facility. Prior to this she lived in the family home with her ageing parents. Her mother has multiple autoimmune conditions, has become increasingly frail over the last decade and decided she could no longer care for herself or Wendy following her husband's death. Wendy has dinner with her mother once a week, which she tearfully says is not enough. She has one sister and three nephews, who she has little contact with, even though they live within 10 km of Wendy. Wendy does not drive and feels her sister makes little effort to include her in their lives. She misses living with her family and sometimes cries herself to sleep. Her carer reports that she tends to be withdrawn in the evenings and that her boss has expressed concern that she is listless and less focused at work. Wendy has received no counselling, and has little understanding of death.

Wendy says she gets very tired and wants to take a nap at work, but is not allowed. She has gained 6 kg over the last 8 months. She has had no other contact with health professionals in the last 2 years. Wendy is not currently taking any supplements or pharmaceutical medications.

CLINICAL EXAMINATION

Height: 148 cm	Weight: 71 kg	BMI: 32 (obese)
Waist circumference: 88 cm	Blood pressure: 134/77 mmHg	Pulse: 77 bpm
Breathing: 24 breaths per minute	Temperature 35.9°C (per axilla)	Blood glucose: 7.8 mmol/L (fruitcake and coffee 30 minutes prior to appointment)
Urinalysis: Specific gravity: 1.030 pH: 5.0 Otherwise NAD	Physical appearance: Wendy appears flushed and out of breath. She is visibly obese, with central obesity. She has mild vertical ridging on her nails, some white flecks and 3-second capillary refill. She is a little bashful when she talks about eating fruitcake prior to her appointment.	

TREATMENT PROTOCOL

INITIAL APPOINTMENT

Treatment considerations:
- Menstrual irregularities consistent with early menopause
- Unexplained weight gain

- Possible depression
- Inadequate bereavement support
- Dislocation and isolation from family
- Inadequate health surveillance

Prescription		Rationale
Herbal medicine	200 mL herbal tincture	
	Leonurus cardiaca 80	Thymoleptic Anti-depressant
	Crocus sativum 40	
	Actaea racemosa 30	Clinically shown to reduce hot flushes
	Salvia officinalis 50	Cooling, cognition enhancer
	Dose: take 7.5 mL in a little water twice daily	
Nutritional medicine	Vitamin D: 5000 IU per day from March to November	Wendy lives in a region where vitamin D deficiency is endemic; vitamin D deficiency contributes to depression
	Activated B complex	MTHFR implicated in Down syndrome and depression
Dietary	Increase green leafy vegetables Berries: ¼–½ cup daily Therapeutically active yoghurt Increase water intake	Inadequate dietary intake of vegetables, water and antioxidants
Further investigations	Iron studies Thyroid function test Full blood count ESR/CRP Fasting blood glucose	Heavy menstrual loss Unexplained fatigue
Referral	Bereavement counselling	Inadequate support following loss of father, dislocation from family

FOLLOW-UP

Wendy was feeling significantly better at her second appointment. She had been to see her GP, who ordered multiple blood tests. Her iron stores were low, but no other abnormalities were detected. She had also had her first appointment with a counsellor, who she seemed happy with. Wendy discussed having a better understanding about where her father had 'gone' and though she still felt sad, she felt more at peace with his passing. She had been compliant with the herbs and did not mind that they tasted 'yucky' because they made her feel happier. Her carer reported she was arguing less with her housemate and was motivated to help more with the evening cooking. This consultation focused on educating Wendy about menopause, the changes that were happening in her body, and encouraging further improvements to her dietary intake.

Prescription		Rationale
Herbal medicine	Continue with herbal tincture	
Nutritional medicine	Continue with vitamin D and activated B complex	
	25 mg iron bisglycinate for 3 months, then re-test	Low iron stores
Dietary	Low glycaemic index diet	Central obesity, possible insulin resistance
	Increase fresh fruit and vegetables	Improve nutritional intake
	Increase wholegrains	Increase fibre intake
Educational resources	Life Without Barriers (http://www.lwb.org.au)	Support services for people of all ages with disabilities
	Lifestyle Easy Cookbooks (https://www.easycookbook.org/home)	Easy-to-prepare, simple nutritious meals designed for people with intellectual disabilities; laminated for easy cleaning
Lifestyle	Encourage participation in local Down syndrome support group	Increase community participation
	Increase exercise: 30–45 minutes of walking daily	Exercise is associated with many health benefits, including improved mood, weight management and easier menopause transition
	Organise travel training through support workers	Greater transport independence would allow Wendy more freedom to visit her mother and sister
Referral	Continue with bereavement counselling	Bereavement support for people with intellectual disabilities is typically lacking and can lead to pathological grieving processes

ONGOING SUPPORT

Wendy intends to continue seeing her counsellor and her naturopath as needed for further support. She is enjoying having greater control over what she eats, and at follow up 2 months later had lost 3 kg. She has taken up table tennis through her local Down syndrome support group and has joined a local choir. She has started travel training and is learning the bus routes to various services in her community. Wendy is happier, healthier and enjoying making new friends.

REFERENCES

[1] Hickey F, Hickey E, Summar KL. Medical update for children with Down syndrome for the pediatrician and family practitioner. Adv Pediatr 2012;59(1):137–57.

[2] Araujo BH, Torres LB, Guilhoto LM. Cerebal overinhibition could be the basis for the high prevalence of epilepsy in persons with Down syndrome. Epilepsy Behav 2015;53:120–5.

[3] Hibaoui Y, Grad I, Letourneau A, et al. Modelling and rescuing neurodevelopmental defect of Down syndrome using induced pluripotent stem cells from monozygotic twins discordant for trisomy 21. EMBO Mol Med 2014;6(2):259–77.

[4] Rachidi M, Lopes C. Mental retardation in Down syndrome: from gene dosage imbalance to molecular and cellular mechanisms. Neurosci Res 2007;59(4):349–69.

[5] Mazurek DWJ. Down syndrome: genetic and nutritional aspects of accompanying disorders. Rocz Panstw Zakl Hig 2015;66(3):189–94.

[6] Durvasula S, Beange H. Health inequalities in people with intellectual disability: strategies for improvement. Health Promotion J Austr 2001;11(1):27–31.

[7] Trollor J, Ruffell B, Tracy J, et al. Intellectual disability health content within medical curriculum: an audit of what our future doctors are taught. BMC Med Educ 2016;16(105):1–9.

[8] Wallace RA, Beange H. On the need for a specialist service within the generic hospital setting for the adult patient with intellectual disability and physical health problems. J Intellect Dev Disabil 2008;33(4):354–61.

[9] NSW Disability Inclusion Act 2014. Available from: www.legislation.nsw.gov.au.

[10] Daunhauer LA, Fidler DJ, Will E. School function in students with Down syndrome. Am J Occup Ther 2014;68(2):167–76.

[11] Herron-Foster BJ, Bustos JJ. Special needs: caring for the older adult with Down syndrome. Medsurg Nurs 2014;23(225):2014.

[12] Baum RA, Nash PL, Foster JE, et al. Primary care of children and adolescents with Down syndrome: an update. Curr Probl Pediatr Adolesc Health Care 2008;38(8):241–61.

[13] Pikora TJ, Bourke J, Bathgate K, et al. Health conditions and their impact among adolescents and young adults with Down syndrome. PLoS ONE 2014;9(5):e96868.

[14] Ross WT, Olsen M. Care of the adult patient with Down syndrome. South Med J 2014;107(11):715–21.

[15] Foley KR, Jacoby P, Girdler S, et al. Functioning and post-school transition outcomes for young people with Down syndrome. Child Care Health Dev 2013;39(6):789–800.

[16] Czeizel AE, Puho E. Maternal use of nutritional supplements during the first month of pregnancy and decreased risk of Down's syndrome: case-control study. Nutrition 2005;21(6):698–704, discussion 74.

[17] Sukla KK, Jaiswal SK, Rai AK, et al. Role of folate-homocysteine pathway gene polymorphisms and nutritional cofactors in Down syndrome: a triad study. Hum Reprod 2015;30(8):1982–93.

[18] Bozovic IB, Stankovic A, Zivkovic M, et al. Altered LINE-1 methylation in mothers of children with Down syndrome. PLoS ONE 2015;10(5):e0127423.

[19] Locke AE, Dooley KJ, Tinker SW, et al. Variation in folate pathway genes contributes to risk of congenital heart defects among individuals with Down syndrome. Genet Epidemiol 2010;34(6):613–23.

[20] van Driel LMJW, de Jonge R, Helbing WA, et al. Maternal global methylation status and risk of congenital heart diseases. Obst Gynecol 2008;112(2):277–83.

[21] Brandalize AP, Bandinelli E, dos Santos PA, et al. Evaluation of C677T and A1298C polymorphisms of the MTHFR gene as maternal risk factors for Down syndrome and congenital heart defects. Am J Med Genet A 2009;149A(10):2080–7.

[22] Acacio GL, Barini R, Bertuzzo CS, et al. Methylenetetrahydrofolate reductase gene polymorphisms and their association with trisomy 21. Prenat Diagn 2005;25(13):1196–9.

[23] Barkai G, Arbuzova S, Berkenstadt M, et al. Frequency of Down's syndrome and neural-tube defects in the same family. Lancet 2003;361:1331–5.

[24] Martin I, Gibert MJ, Aulesa C, et al. Bauca JM. Comparing outcomes and costs between contingent and combined first-trimester screening strategies for Down's syndrome. Eur J Obstet Gynecol Reprod Biol 2015;189:13–18.

[25] McEwan A, Godfrey A, Wilkins J. Screening for Down syndrome. Obst Gynaecol Reprod Med 2012;22(3):70–5.

[26] Dreux S, Nguyen C, Czerkiewicz I, et al. Down syndrome maternal serum marker screening after 18 weeks of gestation: a countrywide study. Am J Obstet Gynecol 2013;208(5):e1–5.

[27] Lee FK, Chen LC, Cheong ML, et al. First trimester combined test for Down syndrome screening in unselected pregnancies: a report of a 13-year experience. Taiwan Province of China J Obstet Gynecol 2013;52(4):523–6.

[28] Cheng P-J, Chu D-C, Chueh H-Y, et al. Elevated maternal midtrimester serum free b-human chorionic gonadotropin levels in vegetarian pregnancies that cause increased false-positive Down syndrome screening results. Am J Obst Gynecol 2004;190:442–7.

[29] Porreco RP, Garite TJ, Maurel K, et al; the Obstetrix Collaborative Research. Noninvasive prenatal screening for fetal trisomies 21, 18, 13 and the common sex chromosome aneuploidies from maternal blood using massively parallel genomic sequencing of DNA. Am J Obstet Gynecol 2014;211(4):e1–12.

[30] van den Heuvel A, Chitty L, Dormandy E, et al. Will the introduction of non-invasive prenatal diagnostic testing erode informed choices? An experimental study of health care professionals. Patient Educ Couns 2010;78(1):24–8.

[31] Lewis C, Silcock C, Chitty LS. Non-invasive prenatal testing for Down's syndrome: pregnant women's views and likely uptake. Public Health Genomics 2013;16(5):223–32.

[32] Deng C, Yi L, Mu Y, et al. Recent trends in the birth prevalence of Down syndrome in China: impact of prenatal diagnosis and subsequent terminations. Prenat Diagn 2015;35(4):311–18.

[33] Lou S, Mikkelsen L, Hvidman L, et al. Does screening for Down's syndrome cause anxiety in pregnant women? A systematic review. Acta Obstet Gynecol Scand 2015;94(1):15–27.

[34] Charleton PM, Dennis J, Marder E. Medical management of children with Down syndrome. Paediatr Child Health 2010;20(7):331–7.

[35] Mansfield C, Hopfer S, Marteau TM. Termination rates after prenatal diagnosis of Down syndrome, spina bifida, anencephaly, and Turner and Klinefelter syndromes: a systematic literature review. Prenat Diagn 1999;19:808–12.

[36] Collins VR, Muggli EE, Riley M, et al. Is Down syndrome a disappearing birth defect? J Pediatr 2008;152(1):20–4.

[37] Korenromp MJ, Page-Christiaens GC, van den Bout J, et al. Maternal decision to terminate pregnancy in case of Down syndrome. Am J Obstet Gynecol 2007;196(2):e1–11.

[38] Natoli JL, Ackerman DL, McDermott S, et al. Prenatal diagnosis of Down syndrome: a systematic review of termination rates (1995–2011). Prenat Diagn 2012;32(2):142–53.

[39] Frati P, Gulino M, Turillazzi E, et al. The physician's breach of the duty to inform the parent of deformities and abnormalities in the foetus: 'wrongful life' actions, a new frontier of medical responsibility. J Matern Fetal Neonatal Med 2014;27(11):1113–17.

[40] Skotko BG, Davidson EJ, Weintraub GS. Contributions of a specialty clinic for children and adolescents with Down syndrome. Am J Med Genet A 2013;161A(3):430–7.

[41] Nelson Goff BS, Springer N, Foote LC, et al. Receiving the initial Down syndrome diagnosis: a comparison of prenatal and postnatal parent group experiences. Intellect Dev Disabil 2013;51(6):446–57.

[42] Strecker S, Hazelwood ZJ, Shakespeare-Finch J. Postdiagnosis personal growth in an Australian population of parents raising children with developmental disability. J Intellect Dev Disabil 2013;39(1):1–9.

[43] Raina P, O'Donnell M, Schwellnus H, et al. Caregiving process and caregiver burden: conceptual models to guide research and practice. BMC Pediatr 2004;4(1):1–13.

[44] Abbeduto L, Mallick Seltzer M, Shattuck P. Psychological Well-being and coping in mothers of youths with autism, Down syndrome, or fragile X syndrome. Am J Ment Retard 2004;109(3):237–54.

[45] Thomas GM. An elephant in the consultation room? Configuring Down syndrome in British antenatal care. Med Anthropol Q 2016;30(2):238–58.

[46] Thomas M, Weisman SM. Calcium supplementation during pregnancy and lactation: effects on the mother and the fetus. Am J Obstet Gynecol 2006;194(4):937–45.

[47] Gomes S, Lopes C, Pinto E. Folate and folic acid in the periconceptional period: recommendations from official health organizations in thirty-six countries worldwide and WHO. Public Health Nutr 2016;19(1):176–89.

[48] Wang T, Zhang HP, Zhang X, et al. Is folate status a risk factor for asthma or other allergic diseases? Allergy Asthma Immunol Res 2015;7(6):538–46.

[49] Cavalli P. Prevention of neural tube defects and proper folate periconceptional supplementation. J Prenatal Med 2008;2(4):40–1.

[50] Charoenratana C, Leelapat P, Traisrisilp K, et al. Maternal iodine insufficiency and adverse pregnancy outcomes. Matern Child Nutr 2016;12(4):680–7.

[51] Berbel P, Obregon MJ, Bernal J, et al. Iodine supplementation during pregnancy: a public health challenge. Trends Endocrinol Metab 2007;18(9):338–43.

[52] Shi X, Han C, Li C, et al. Optimal and safe upper limits of iodine intake for early pregnancy in iodine-sufficient regions: a cross-sectional study of 7190 pregnant women in China. J Clin Endocrinol Metab 2015;100(4):1630–8.

[53] Best CM, Pressman EK, Cao C, et al. Maternal iron status during pregnancy compared with neonatal iron status better predicts placental iron transporter expression in humans. FASEBJ 2016;30(10):3541–50.

[54] Veltri F, Decaillet S, Kleynen P, et al. Prevalence of thyroid autoimmunity and dysfunction in women with iron deficiency during early pregnancy: is it altered? Eur J Endocrinol 2016;175(3):191–9.

[55] Khambalia AZ, Aimone A, Nagubandi P, et al. High maternal iron status, dietary iron intake and iron supplement use in pregnancy and risk of gestational diabetes mellitus: a prospective study and systematic review. Diabet Med 2016;33(9):1211–21.

[56] Milman N. Iron in pregnancy: how do we secure an appropriate iron status in the mother and child? Ann Nutr Metab 2011;59(1):50–4.

[57] Dalton LM, Ni Fhloinn DM, Gaydadzhieva GT, et al. Magnesium in pregnancy. Nutr Rev 2016;74(9):549–57.

[58] Jamilian M, Samimi M, Kolahdooz F, et al. Omega-3 fatty acid supplementation affects pregnancy outcomes in gestational diabetes: a randomized, double-blind, placebo-controlled trial. J Matern Fetal Neonatal Med 2016;29(4):669–75.

[59] Saccone G, Saccone I, Berghella V. Omega-3 long-chain polyunsaturated fatty acids and fish oil supplementation during pregnancy: which evidence? J Matern Fetal Neonatal Med 2016;29(15):2389–97.

[60] Hawrelak J. Prebiotics. In: Braun L, Cohen M, editors. Herbs and natural supplements. 4th ed. Sydney: Elsevier; 2015. p. 760–70.

[61] Hawrelak J. Probiotics. In: Braun L, Cohen M, editors. Herbs and natural supplements. 4th ed. Sydney: Elsevier; 2015. p. 979–94.

[62] Skroder HM, Hamadani JD, Tofail F, et al. Selenium status in pregnancy influences children's cognitive function at 1.5 years of age. Clin Nutr 2015;34(5):923–30.

[63] Pieczynska J, Grajeta H. The role of selenium in human conception and pregnancy. J Trace Elem Med Biol 2015;29:31–8.

[64] Rumbold A, Ota E, Nagata C, et al. Vitamin C supplementation in pregnancy. Cochrane Database Syst Rev 2015;(9):CD004072.

[65] Al-Garawi A, Carey VJ, Chhabra D, et al. The role of vitamin D in the transcriptional program of human pregnancy. PLoS ONE 2016;11(10):e0163832.

[66] Awker AL, Herbranson AT, Rhee TG, et al. Impact of a vitamin D protocol in pregnancy at an urban women's health clinic. Ann Pharmacother 2016;50(11):935–41.

[67] Grant CC, Crane J, Mitchell EA, et al. Vitamin D supplementation during pregnancy and infancy reduces aeroallergen sensitization: a randomized controlled trial. Allergy 2016;71(9):1325–34.

[68] Morris SK, Pell LG, Rahman MZ, et al. Maternal vitamin D supplementation during pregnancy and lactation to prevent acute respiratory infections in infancy in Dhaka, Bangladesh (MDARI trial): protocol for a prospective cohort study nested within a randomized controlled trial. BMC Pregnancy Childbirth 2016;16(1):309.

[69] Pludowski P, Holick MF, Pilz S, et al. Vitamin D effects on musculoskeletal health, immunity, autoimmunity, cardiovascular disease, cancer, fertility, pregnancy, dementia and mortality: a review of recent evidence. Autoimmun Rev 2013;12(10):976–89.

[70] Ley SH, Hanley AJ, Sermer M, et al. Lower dietary vitamin E intake during the second trimester is associated with insulin resistance and hyperglycemia later in pregnancy. Eur J Clin Nutr 2013;67(11):1154–6.

[71] Conde-Agudelo A, Romero R, Kusanovic JP, et al. Supplementation with vitamins C and E during pregnancy for the prevention of preeclampsia and other adverse maternal and perinatal outcomes: a systematic review and metaanalysis. Am J Obstet Gynecol 2011;204(6):503.e1–e12.

[72] Zahiri Sorouri Z, Sadeghi H, Pourmarzi D. The effect of zinc supplementation on pregnancy outcome: a randomized controlled trial. J Matern Fetal Neonatal Med 2016;29(13):2194–8.

[73] Nossier SA, Naeim NE, El-Sayed NA, et al. The effect of zinc supplementation on pregnancy outcomes: a double-blind, randomised controlled trial, Egypt. Br J Nutr 2015;114(2):274–85.

[74] Smith CH, Teo Y, Simpson S. An observational study of adults with Down syndrome eating independently. Dysphagia 2014;29(1):52–60.

[75] Reilly D, Huws J, Hastings R, et al. Life and death of a child with Down syndrome and a congenital heart condition: experiences of six couples. Intellect Dev Disabil 2010;48(6):403–16.

[76] van Hooste A, Maes B. Family factors in the early development of children with Down syndrome. J Early Intervention 2003;25(4):296–309.

[77] Bunt CW, Bunt SK. Role of the family physician in the care of children with Down syndrome. Am Fam Phys 2014;90(12):851–8.

[78] Leonard S, Beaver C, Petterson B, et al. Survival of infants born with Down's syndrome: 1980–96. Paediatr Perinatal Epidemiol 2000;14:163–71.

[79] Mann JP, Statnikov E, Modi N, et al. Management and outcomes of neonates with Down syndrome admitted to neonatal units. Birth Defects Res A Clin Mol Teratol 2016;106:468–74.

[80] World Health Organization. Breastfeeding; 2016. Available from: https://www.who.int/nutrition/topics/exclusive_breastfeeding/en/.

[81] Australian Breastfeeding Association. Breastfeeding your baby with Down syndrome; 2015. Available from: https://www.breastfeeding.asn.au/bf-info/down.

[82] La Leche League International. Is it possible to breastfeed my baby who was born with Down syndrome? 2016.

[83] Canadian Down Syndrome Society. Breastfeeding a baby with Down syndrome; 2016. Available from: https://www.ndsccenter.org/wp-content/uploads/CDSS_breastfeeding_brochure.pdf.

[84] Buzunariz Martinez N, Martinez Garcia M. Psychomotor development in children with Down syndrome and physiotherapy in early intervention. Int Med J Down Syndrome 2008;12(2):28–32.

[85] Purpura G, Tinelli F, Bargagna S, et al. Effect of early multisensory massage intervention on visual functions in infants with Down syndrome. Early Hum Dev 2014;90(12):809–13.

[86] Capone GT. Down syndrome: genetic insights and thoughts of early intervention. Infant Young Child 2004;17(1):45–8.

[87] Skeels HM, Dyer HB. A study of the effects of differential stimulation on mentally retarded children. Proc Am Assoc Mental Deficiency 1939;44(1):114–36. (Republished in Blacher J, Baker BL (eds). The best of AAMR. Families and mental retardation: a collection of notable AAMR journal articles across the 20th century. Washington DC: American Association on Mental Retardation; 2002, p. 19–33.)

[88] Channell MM, Thurman AJ, Kover ST, et al. Patterns of change in nonverbal cognition in adolescents with Down syndrome. Res Dev Disabil 2014;35(11):2933–41.

[89] Cardoso AC, Campos AC, Santos MM, et al. Motor performance of children with Down syndrome and typical development at 2 to 4 and 26 months. Pediatr Phys Ther 2015;27(2):135–41.

[90] Melyn MA, White DT. Mental and developmental milestones of noninstitutionalized Down's syndrome children. Pediatrics 1973;52(4):542–5.

[91] Pueschel SM. As cited in: Cohen WI. Down syndrome: care of the child and family. In: Levine MD, Carey WB, Crocker AC, editors. Developmental-behavioral pediatrics. 3rd ed. Philadelphia: WB Saunders; 1978. p. 241–8.

[92] Frank K, Esbensen AJ. Fine motor and self-care milestones for individuals with Down syndrome using a retrospective chart review. J Intellect Disabil Res 2015;59(8):719–29.

[93] Cleland J, Wood S, Hardcastle W, et al. Relationship between speech, oromotor, language and cognitive abilities in children with Down's syndrome. Int J Lang Commun Disord 2010;45(1):83–95.

[94] Koriakin TA, McCurdy MD, Papazoglou A, et al. Classification of intellectual disability using the Wechsler Intelligence Scale for Children: full scale IQ or general abilities index? Dev Med Child Neurol 2013;55(9):840–5.

[95] Lott IT, Dierssen M. Cognitive deficits and associated neurological complications in individuals with Down's syndrome. Lancet Neurol 2010;9(6):623–33.

[96] Costanzo F, Varuzza C, Menghini D, et al. Executive functions in intellectual disabilities: a comparison between Williams syndrome and Down syndrome. Res Dev Disabil 2013;34(5):1770–80.

[97] Trezise KL, Gray KM, Sheppard DM. Attention and vigilance in children with Down syndrome. J App Research Intellect Disabil 2008;21(6):502–8.

[98] Roch M, Florit E, Levorato C. Follow-up study on reading comprehension in Down's syndrome: the role of reading skills and listening comprehension. Int J Lang Commun Disord 2011;46(2):231–42.

[99] de la Iglesia CJF, Buceta JM, Campos A. Prose learning in children and adults with Down syndrome: the use of visual and mental image strategies to improve recall. J Intellect Dev Disabil 2005;30(4):199–206.

[100] Conners FA, Rosenquist CJ, Arnett L, et al. Improving memory span in children with Down syndrome. J Intellect Disabil Res 2008;52(Pt 3):244–55.

[101] Amaral MF, Drummond Ade F, Coster WJ, et al. Household task participation of children and adolescents with cerebral palsy, Down syndrome and typical development. Res Dev Disabil 2014;35(2):414–22.

[102] Van Gameren-Oosterom HB, Fekkes M, Reijneveld SA, et al. Practical and social skills of 16–19-year-olds with Down syndrome: independence still far away. Res Dev Disabil 2013;34(12):4599–607.

[103] Bouck EC. Reports of life skills training for students with intellectual disabilities in and out of school. J Intellect Disabil Res 2010;54(12):1093–103.

[104] Buckley S, Bird G, Sacks B, et al. A comparison of mainstream and special education for teenagers with Down syndrome. Down Syndrome Res Pract 2006;9(3):54–67.

[105] Su CY, Lin YH, Wu YY, et al. The role of cognition and adaptive behavior in employment of people with mental retardation. Res Dev Disabil 2008;29(1):83–95.

[106] van Gameren-Oosterom HB, Fekkes M, van Wouwe JP, et al. Problem behavior of individuals with Down syndrome in a nationwide cohort assessed in late adolescence. J Pediatr 2013;163(5):1396–401.

[107] Wuang Y, Su CY. Patterns of participation and enjoyment in adolescents with Down syndrome. Res Dev Disabil 2012;33(3):841–8.

[108] Bertoli M, Biasini G, Calignano MT, et al. Needs and challenges of daily life for people with Down syndrome residing in the city of Rome, Italy. J Intellect Disabil Res 2011;55(8):801–20.

[109] Foley KR, Girdler S, Bouck J, et al. Influence of the environment on participation in social roles for young adults with Down syndrome. PLoS ONE 2014;9(9):e108413.

[110] Verdonschot MM, de Witte LP, Reichrath E, et al. Community participation of people with an intellectual disability: a review of empirical findings. J Intellect Disabil Res 2009;53(4):303–18.

[111] Holwerda A, van der Klink JJ, de Boer MR, et al. Predictors of work participation of young adults with mild intellectual disabilities. Res Dev Disabil 2013;34(6):1982–90.

[112] Feldman DC. The role of physical disabilities in early career: vocational choice, the school-to-work transition, and becoming established. Hum Res Manag Rev 2004;14(3):247–74.

[113] Sabbatino ED, Macrine SL. Start on success: a model transition program for high school students with disabilities. Preventing School Failure 2007;52(1):33–9.

[114] Wehman P, Chan F, Ditchman N, et al. Effect of supported employment on vocational rehabilitation outcomes of transition-age youth with intellectual and developmental

[115] disabilities: a case control study. Intellect Dev Disabil 2014;52(4):296–310.

[115] Danielsson H, Henry L, Messer D, et al. Developmental delays in phonological recoding among children and adolescents with Down syndrome and Williams syndrome. Res Dev Disabil 2016;55:64–76.

[116] Haveman M, Tillman V, Stoppler R, et al. Mobility and public transport use abilities of children and young adults with intellectual disabilities: results from the 3-year Nordhorn Public Transportation Intervention Study. J Pol Pract Intellect Disabil 2013;10(4):289–99.

[117] Furniss KA, Loverseed A, Lippold T, et al. The views of people who care for adults with Down's syndrome and dementia: a service evaluation. Br J Learn Disabil 2012;40(4):318–27.

[118] Read S, Morris H. Living and dying with dignity. The best practice guide to end-of-life care for people with a learning disability. London: Mecap, The Voice of Learning Disability; 2008.

[119] McEvoy J, MacHale R, Tierney E. Concept of death and perceptions of bereavement in adults with intellectual disabilities. J Intellect Disabil Res 2012;56(2):191–203.

[120] Hill DA, Gridley G, Cnattingus S, et al. Mortality and cancer incidence among people with Down syndrome. Arch Int Med 2003;13:705–11.

[121] Tracy J. Australians with Down syndrome: health matters. Aus Fam Phys 2011;40(4):202.

[122] Akinci O, Mihci E, Tacoy S, et al. Neutrophil oxidative metabolism in Down syndrome patients with congenital heart defects. Environ Mol Mutagen 2010;51(1):57–63.

[123] Bravo-Valenzuela N, Passarelli MLB, Coates MV, et al. Weight and height recovery in children with Down syndrome and congenital heart disease. Rev Bras Cir Cardiovasc 2011;26(1):61–8.

[124] Dimopoulos K. Kempny A. Patients with Down syndrome and congenital heart disease: survival is improving, but challenges remain. Heart 2016;102(19):1515–17.

[125] Espinola-Zavaleta N, Soto ME, Romero-Gonzalez A, et al. Prevalence of congenital heart disease and pulmonary hypertension in Down's syndrome: an echocardiographic study. J Cardiovasc Ultrasound 2015;23(2):72–7.

[126] Bergstrom S, Carr H, Petersson G, et al. Trends in congenital heart defects in infants with Down syndrome. Pediatrics 2016;138(1).

[127] Faria PF, Nicolau JAZ, Melek M, et al. Association between congenital heart defects and severe infections in children with Down syndrome. Revista Portuguesa de Cardiologia (English Edition) 2014;33(1):15–18.

[128] Flanders L, Tulloh R. Cardiac problems in Down syndrome. Paediatr Child Health 2011;21(1):25–31.

[129] Alsaied T, Marino BS, Esbensen AJ, et al. Does congenital heart disease affect neurodevelopmental outcomes in children with Down syndrome? Congen Heart Dis 2016;11(1):26–33.

[130] Visootsak J, Hess B, Bakeman R, et al. Effect of congenital heart defects on language development in toddlers with Down syndrome. J Intellect Disabil Res 2013;57(9):887–92.

[131] Visootsak J, Mahle WT, Kirshbom PM, et al. Neurodevelopmental outcomes in children with Down syndrome and congenital heart defects. Am J Med Genet A 2011;155A(11):2688–91.

[132] Roussot MA, Lawrenson JB, Hewitson J, et al. Is cardiac surgery warranted in children with Down syndrome? S Afr Med J 2006;96(9):924–30.

[133] Fudge JC Jr, Li S, Jaggers J, et al. Congenital heart surgery outcomes in Down syndrome: analysis of a national clinical database. Pediatrics 2010;126(2):315–22.

[134] Real de Asua D, Quero M, Moldenhauer F, et al. Clinical profile and main comorbidities of Spanish adults with Down syndrome. Eur J Intern Med 2015;26(6):385–91.

[135] Goi G, Baquero-Herrera C, Licastro F, et al. Advanced oxidation protein products (AOPP) and high-sensitive C-reactive protein (hs-CRP) in an 'atheroma-free model': Down's syndrome. Int J Cardiol 2006;113(3):427–9.

[136] Baraona F, Gurvitz M, Landzberg MJ, et al. Hospitalizations and mortality in the United States for adults with Down syndrome and congenital heart disease. Am J Cardiol 2013;111(7):1046–51.

[137] de Moura CP, Andrade D, Cunha LM, et al. Down syndrome: otolaryngological effects of rapid maxillary expansion. J Laryngol Otol 2008;122(12):1318–24.

[138] Barankin B, Guenther L. Dermatological manifestations of Down's syndrome. J Cutan Med Surg 2001;5(4):289–93.

[139] Bates B. Skin and mucosal conditions prevalent in Down syndrome (Clinical Rounds). Skin Allergy News 2005;36(4).

[140] Madan V, Williams J, Lear JT. Dermatological manifestations of Down's syndrome. Clin Exp Dermatol 2006;31(5):623–9.

[141] Schepis C, Barone C, Siragusa M, et al. An updated survey on skin conditions in Down syndrome. Dermatology 2002;205(3):234–8.

[142] Daneshpazhooh M, Nazemi TM, Bigdeloo L, et al. Mucocutaneous findings in 100 children with Down syndrome. Pediatr Dermatol 2007;24(3):317–20.

[143] McDowell KM, Craven DI. Pulmonary complications of Down syndrome during childhood. J Pediatr 2011;158(2):319–25.

[144] Weijerman ME, Brand PL, van Furth MA, et al. Recurrent wheeze in children with Down syndrome: is it asthma? Acta Paediatr 2011;100(11):e194–7.

[145] Zachariah P, Ruttenber M, Simoes EA. Down syndrome and hospitalizations due to respiratory syncytial virus: a population-based study. J Pediatr 2012;160(5):827–31, e1.

[146] Stagliano DR, Nylund CM, Eide MB, et al. Children with Down syndrome are high-risk for severe respiratory syncytial virus disease. J Pediatr 2015;166(3):703–9, e2.

[147] Mannan SE, Yousef E, Hossain J. Prevalence of positive skin prick test results in children with Down syndrome: a case-control study. Ann Allergy Asthma Immunol 2009;102(3):205–9.

[148] Carlstedt K, Henningsson G, Dahllöf G. A four-year longitudinal study of palatal plate therapy in children with Down syndrome: effects on oral motor function, articulation and communication preferences. Acta Odontol Scand 2009;61(1):39–46.

[149] Barr E, Dungworth J, Hunter K, et al. The prevalence of ear, nose and throat disorders in preschool children with Down's syndrome in Glasgow. Scott Med J 2011;56(2):98–103.

[150] Hellstrom S, Groth A, Jorgensen F, et al. Ventilation tube treatment: a systematic review of the literature. Otolaryngol Head Neck Surg 2011;145(3):383–95.

[151] Maris M, Verhulst S, Wojciechowski M, et al. Sleep problems and obstructive sleep apnea in children with Down syndrome, an overview. Int J Pediatr Otorhinolaryngol 2016;82:12–15.

[152] Venekamp RP, Hearne BJ, Chandrasekharan D, et al. Tonsillectomy or adenotonsillectomy versus non-surgical management for obstructive sleep-disordered breathing in children. Cochrane Database Syst Rev 2015;(10):CD011165.

[153] Chin CJ, Khami MM, Husein M. A general review of the otolaryngologic manifestations of Down syndrome. Int J Pediatr Otorhinolaryngol 2014;78(6):899–904.

[154] Kiani R, Miller H. Sensory impairment and intellectual disability. Adv Psychiatric Treat 2010;16(3):228–35.

[155] Musat MD, Zah L, Danciulescu R, et al. The endocrine and metabolic profile in adult patients with Down syndrome. The Endocrine Society's 93rd Annual Meeting & Expo, 4–7 June 2011, Boston.

[156] Campos C, Guzman R, Lopez-Fernandez E, et al. Evaluation of urinary biomarkers of oxidative/nitrosative stress in adolescents and adults with Down syndrome. Biochim Biophys Acta 2011;1812(7):760–8.

[157] Cento RM, Raqusa L, Proto C, et al. Basal body temperature curves and endocrine pattern of menstrual cycles in Down syndrome. Gynecol Endocrinol 1996;10(2):133–7.

[158] Suzuki K, Nakajima K, Kamimura S, et al. Eight case reports on sex-hormone profiles in sexually mature male Down syndrome. Int J Urol 2010;17(12):1008–10.

[159] Eisermann MM, DeLaRaillère A, Dellatolas G, et al. Infantile spasms in Down syndrome: effects of delayed anticonvulsive treatment. Epilepsy Res 2003;55:1–2.

[160] Meeus M, Kenis S, Wojciechowski M, et al. Epilepsy in children with Down syndrome: not so benign as generally accepted. Acta Neurol Belgica 2015;115(4):569–73.

[161] Shimakawa S, Tanabe T, Ono M, et al. Incidence of febrile seizure in patients with Down syndrome. Pediatr Int 2015;57(4):670–2.

[162] Goldberg-Stern H, Strawsberg RH, Peatterson B, et al. Seizure frequency and characteristics in children with Down syndrome. Brain Dev 2001;23(6):375–8.

[163] Lee J, Lee JH, Yu HJ, et al. Prognostic factors of infantile spasms: role of treatment options including a ketogenic diet. Brain Dev 2013;35(8):821–6.

[164] Ulate-Campos A, Nascimento A, Ortez C. Down's syndrome and epilepsy. International Medical Review on Down Syndrome 2014;18(1):3–8.

[165] Chang P, Zuckermann AM, Williams S, et al. Seizure control by derivatives of medium chain fatty acids associated with the ketogenic diet show novel branching-point structure for enhanced potency. J Pharmacol Exp Ther 2015;352(1):43–52.

[166] Henderson CB, Filloux FM, Alder SC, et al. Efficacy of the ketogenic diet as a treatment option for epilepsy: meta-analysis. J Child Neurol 2006;21(3):193–8.

[167] Hong AM, Turner Z, Hamdy RF, et al. Infantile spasms treated with the ketogenic diet: prospective single-center experience in 104 consecutive infants. Epilepsia 2010;51(8):1403–7.

[168] Kang HC, Lee YJ, Lee JS, et al. Comparison of short- versus long-term ketogenic diet for intractable infantile spasms. Epilepsia 2011;52(4):781–7.

[169] Kayyali HR, Gustafson M, Myers T, et al. Ketogenic diet efficacy in the treatment of intractable epileptic spasms. Pediatr Neurol 2014;50(3):224–7.

[170] Kossoff EH, Hedderick EF, Turner Z, et al. A case-control evaluation of the ketogenic diet versus ACTH for new-onset infantile spasms. Epilepsia 2008;49(9):1504–9.

[171] Pires ME, Ilea A, Bourel E, et al. Ketogenic diet for infantile spasms refractory to first-line treatments: an open prospective study. Epilepsy Res 2013;105(1–2):189–94.

[172] Hussain SA, Shin JH, Shih EJ, et al. Limited efficacy of the ketogenic diet in the treatment of highly refractory epileptic spasms. Seizure 2016;35:59–64.

[173] Caraballo R, Vaccarezza M, Cersosimo R, et al. Long-term follow-up of the ketogenic diet for refractory epilepsy: multicenter Argentinean experience in 216 pediatric patients. Seizure 2011;20(8):640–5.

[174] Barca D, Tarta-Asene O, Dica A, et al. Intellectual disability and epilepsy in Down syndrome. Maedica 2014;9(4):344.

[175] Porter BE, Jacobson C. Report of a parent survey of cannabidiol-enriched cannabis use in pediatric treatment-resistant epilepsy. Epilepsy Behav 2013;29(3):574–7.

[176] Detyniecki K, Hirsch L. Marijuana use in epilepsy: the myth and the reality. Curr Neurol Neurosci Rep 2015;15(10):65.

[177] Gross DW, Hamm J, Ashworth NL, et al. Marijuana use and epilepsy: prevalence in patients of a tertiary care epilepsy center. Neurology 2004;62(11):2095–7.

[178] Jones NA, Glyn SE, Akiyama S, et al. Cannabidiol exerts anti-convulsant effects in animal models of temporal lobe and partial seizures. Seizure 2012;21(5):344–52.

[179] Kolikonda MK, Srinivasan K, Manasa E, et al. Medical marijuana for epilepsy? Innov Clin Neurosci 2015;13.

[180] Rosemergy I, Adler J, Psirides A. Cannabidiol oil in the treatment of super refractory status epilepticus. A case report. Seizure 2016;35:56–8.

[181] Maa E, Figi P. The case for medical marijuana in epilepsy. Epilepsia 2014;55(6):783–6.

[182] Mehla J, Reeta KH, Gupta P, et al. Protective effect of curcumin against seizures and cognitive impairment in a pentylenetetrazole-kindled epileptic rat model. Life Sci 2010;87(19–22):596–603.

[183] DeGiorgio CM, Miller PR, Harper R, et al. Fish oil (n-3 fatty acids) in drug resistant epilepsy: a randomised placebo-controlled crossover study. J Neurol Neurosurg Psychiatry 2015;86(1):65–70.

[184] Khayat H, Awadalla M, Waked A. Marzook Z. Polyunsaturated fatty acids in children with idiopathic intractable epilepsy serum levels and therapeutic response. J Pediatr Neurol 2010;8:175–8.

[185] Reda DM, Abd-El-Fatah NK, Omar Tel S, et al. Fish oil intake and seizure control in children with medically resistant epilepsy. N Am J Med Sci 2015;7(7):317–21.

[186] Schlanger S, Shinitzky M, Yam D. Diet enriched with omega-3 fatty acids alleviates convulsion symptoms in epilepsy patients. Epilepsia 2002;43(2):103–4.

[187] Osborn KE, Shytle RD, Frontera AT, et al. Addressing potential role of magnesium dyshomeostasis to improve treatment efficacy for epilepsy: a reexamination of the literature. J Clin Pharmacol 2016;56(3):260–5.

[188] Yuen AW, Sander JW. Can magnesium supplementation reduce seizures in people with epilepsy? A hypothesis. Epilepsy Res 2012;100(1–2):152–6.

[189] Prasad DK, Shaheen U, Satyanarayana U, et al. Association of serum trace elements and minerals with genetic generalized epilepsy and idiopathic intractable epilepsy. Neurochem Res 2014;39(12):2370–6.

[190] Espinosa PS, Perez DL, Abner E, et al. Association of antiepileptic drugs, vitamin D, and calcium supplementation with bone fracture occurrence in epilepsy patients. Clin Neurol Neurosurg 2011;113(7):548–51.

[191] Jo BW, Shim YJ, Choi JH, et al. Formula fed twin infants with recurrent hypocalcemic seizures with vitamin D deficient rickets and hyperphosphatemia. Ann Pediatr Endocrinol Metab 2015;20(2):102–5.

[192] Mantadakis E, Deftereos S, Tsouvala E, et al. Seizures as initial manifestation of vitamin D-deficiency rickets in a 5-month-old exclusively breastfed infant. Pediatr Neonatol 2012;53(6):384–6.

[193] Ashrafi MR, Shabanian R, Abbaskhanian A, et al. Selenium and intractable epilepsy: is there any correlation? Pediatr Neurol 2007;36(1):25–9.

[194] Naziroglu M. Role of selenium on calcium signaling and oxidative stress-induced molecular pathways in epilepsy. Neurochem Res 2009;34(12):2181–91.

[195] Seven M, Basaran SY, Cengiz M, et al. Deficiency of selenium and zinc as a causative factor for idiopathic intractable epilepsy. Epilepsy Res 2013;104(1–2):35–9.

[196] Solovyev ND. Importance of selenium and selenoprotein for brain function: from antioxidant protection to neuronal signalling. J Inorg Biochem 2015;153:1–12.

[197] Wojciak RW, Mojs E, Stanislawska-Kubiak M, et al. The serum zinc, copper, iron, and chromium concentrations in epileptic children. Epilepsy Res 2013;104(1–2):40–4.

[198] Calabro RS, Italiano D, Gervasi G, et al. Single tonic-clonic seizure after energy drink abuse. Epilepsy Behav 2012;23(3):384–5.

[199] Kaufman KR, Sacdeo RC. Caffeinated beverages and decreased seizure control. Seizure 2003;12(7):519–21.

[200] Moore JL. The significance of folic acid for epilepsy patients. Epilepsy Behav 2005;7(2):172–81.

[201] Morrell MJ. Folic acid and epilepsy. Epilepsy Curr 2002;2:31–4.

[202] Baynes K, Tomaszewski Farias S, Gospe S. Pyridoxine-dependent seizures and cognition in adulthood. Devel Med Child Neurol 2003;45(11):782–5.

[203] Gospe SM. Current perspectives on pyridoxine-dependent seizures. J Pediatr 1998;132(6):919–23.

[204] Lee D, Lee YJ, Shin H, et al. Seizures related to vitamin B6 deficiency in adults. J Epilepsy Res 2015;5:23–4.

[205] Ohtahara S, Yamatogi Y, Ohtsuka Y, et al. Vitamin B6 treatment of intractable seizures. Brain Dev 2011;33(9):783–9.

[206] Ohtsuka Y, Ogino T, Asano T, et al. Long-term follow-up of vitamin B6-responsive West syndrome. Pediatr Neurol 2000;23(3):202–6.

[207] Stockler S, Plecko B, Gospe SM Jr, et al. Pyridoxine dependent epilepsy and antiquitin deficiency: clinical and molecular characteristics and recommendations for diagnosis, treatment and follow-up. Mol Genet Metab 2011;104(1–2):48–60.

[208] Benbir G, Uysal S, Saltik S, et al. Seizures during treatment of vitamin B12 deficiency. Seizure 2007;16(1):69–73.

[209] Gonzalez-Ramirez M, Razo-Juarez LI, Sauer-Ramirez JL, et al. Anticonvulsive effect of vitamin C on pentylenetetrazol-induced seizures in immature rats. Pharmacol Biochem Behav 2010;97(2):267–72.

[210] Santos LF, Freitas RL, Xavier SM, et al. Neuroprotective actions of vitamin C related to decreased lipid peroxidation and increased catalase activity in adult rats after pilocarpine-induced seizures. Pharmacol Biochem Behav 2008;89(1):1–5.

[211] Basatemur E, Sutcliffe A. Incidence of hypocalcemic seizures due to vitamin D deficiency in children in the United Kingdom and Ireland. J Clin Endocrinol Metab 2015;100(1):E91–5.

[212] Hollo A, Clemens Z, Kamondi A, et al. Correction of vitamin D deficiency improves seizure control in epilepsy: a pilot study. Epilepsy Behav 2012;24(1):131–3.

[213] Teagarden DL, Meador KJ, Loring DW. Low vitamin D levels are common in patients with epilepsy. Epilepsy Res 2014;108(8):1352–6.

[214] Mehvari J, Motlagh FG, Najafi M, et al. Effects of vitamin E on seizure frequency, electroencephalogram findings, and oxidative stress status of refractory epileptic patients. Adv Biomed Res 2016;5:36.

[215] Saghazadeh A, Mahmoudi M, Meysamie A, et al. Possible role of trace elements in epilepsy and febrile seizures: a meta-analysis. Nutr Rev 2015;73(11):760–79.

[216] d'Orsi G, Specchio LM. Apulian Study Group on Senile Myoclonic E. Progressive myoclonus epilepsy in Down syndrome patients with dementia. J Neurol 2014;261(8):1584–97.

[217] De Simone R, Puig XS, Gelisse P, et al. Senile myoclonic epilepsy: delineation of a common condition associated with Alzheimer's disease in Down syndrome. Seizure 2010;19(7):383–9.

[218] Sangani M, Shahid A, Amina S, et al. Improvement of myoclonic epilepsy in Down syndrome treated with levetiracetam. Epileptic Disord 2010;12(2):151–4.

[219] Scorza CA, Scorza FA, Arida RM, et al. Sudden unexpected death in people with Down syndrome and epilepsy. Clinics 2011;66(5):719–20.

[220] Nardone R, Brigo F, Trinka E. Acute symptomatic seizures caused by electrolyte disturbances. J Clin Neurol 2016;12(1):21–33.

[221] Mazurek D, Wyka J. Down syndrome-genetic and nutritional aspects of accompanying disorders. Roczniki Państwowego Zakl Hig 2015;66(3).

[222] Souto-Rodríguez R, Barreiro-de-Acosta M, Domínguez-Muñoz JE. Down's syndrome and inflammatory bowel disease: is there a real link. Rev Esp Enferm Dig 2014;106:220–2.

[223] Viegelmann G, Low Y, Sriram B, et al. Achalasia and Down syndrome: a unique association not to be missed. Singapore Med J 2014;55(7):e107–8.

[224] Maloney KW, Taub JW, Ravindranath Y, et al. Down syndrome preleukemia and leukemia. Pediatr Clin North Am 2015;62(1):121–37.

[225] Tsimaras VK, Fotiadou EG. Effect of training on the muscle strength and dynamic balance ability of adults with Down syndrome. J Strength Cond Res 2004;18(2):343–7.

[226] Malak R, Kotwicka M, Krawczyk-Wasielewska A, et al. Motor skills, cognitive development and balance functions of children with Down syndrome. Ann Agricul Environ Med 2013;20(4):803–6.

[227] Cabeza-Ruiz R, Garcia-Masso X, Centeno-Prada RA, et al. Time and frequency analysis of the static balance in young adults with Down syndrome. Gait Posture 2011;33(1):23–8.

[228] Davies RB. Pain in children with Down syndrome: assessment and intervention by parents. Pain Manag Nurs 2010;11(4):259–67.

[229] Valkenburg AJ, Tibboel D, van Dijk M. Pain sensitivity of children with Down syndrome and their siblings: quantitative sensory testing versus parental reports. Dev Med Child Neurol 2015;57(11):1049–55.

[230] Mafrica F, Schifilliti D, Fodale V. Pain in Down's syndrome. Sci World J 2006;6:140–7.

[231] Hennequin M, Morin C, Feine JS. Pain expression and stimulus localisation in individuals with Down's syndrome. Lancet 2000;356(9245):1882–7.

[232] Dykens E, Shah B, Davis B, et al. Psychiatric disorders in adolescents and young adults with Down syndrome and other intellectual disabilities. J Neurodev Dis 2015;7(1).

[233] Prasher V. Disintegrative syndrome in young adults. Irish J Psychol Med 2014;19(03):101.

[234] Garvia B, Benejam B. Regression in young adults with Down's syndrome. A three cases review. Int Med Rev Down Syndrome 2014;18(3):43–6.

[235] Myers B, Pueschel SM. Major depression in a small group of adults with Down syndrome. Res Dev Disabil 1995;16(4):285–99.

[236] Walker JC, Dosen A, Buitelaar JK, et al. Depression in Down syndrome: a review of the literature. Res Dev Disabil 2011;32(5):1432–40.

[237] Evans DW, Canavera K, Kleinpeter FL, et al. The fears, phobias and anxieties of children with autism spectrum disorders and Down

syndrome: comparisons with developmentally and chronologically age matched children. Child Psychiatry Hum Dev 2005;36(1):3–26.

[238] Glenn S, Cunningham C, Nananidou A, et al. Routinised and compulsive-like behaviours in individuals with Down syndrome. J Intellect Disabil Res 2015;59(11):1061–70.

[239] Uljarevic M, Evans DW. Relationship between repetitive behaviour and fear across normative development, autism spectrum disorder, and down syndrome. Autism Res 2016.

[240] Luke A, Roizen NJ, Sutton M, et al. Energy expenditure in children with Down syndrome: correcting metabolic rate for movement. J Pediatr 1994;125(5):829–38.

[241] Esposito PE, MacDonald M, Hornyak JE, et al. Physical activity patterns of youth with Down syndrome. Intellect Dev Disabil 2012;50(2):109–19.

[242] Kota SK, Tripathy PR, Kota SK, et al. Type 2 diabetes mellitus: an unusual association with Down's syndrome. Indian J Hum Genet 2013;19(3):358–9.

[243] Curtin C, Bandini LG, Must A, et al. Parent support improves weight loss in adolescents and young adults with Down syndrome. J Pediatr 2013;163(5):1402–8.e1.

[244] Jinks A, Cotton A, Rylance R. Obesity interventions for people with a learning disability: an integrative literature review. J Adv Nurs 2011;67(3):460–71.

[245] Kirk SF, Penney TL, McHugh TL, et al. Effective weight management practice: a review of the lifestyle intervention evidence. Int J Obes (Lond) 2012;36(2):178–85.

[246] Melville CA, Boyle S, Miller S, et al. An open study of the effectiveness of a multi-component weight-loss intervention for adults with intellectual disabilities and obesity. Br J Nutr 2011;105(10):1553–62.

[247] Johnson C, Hobson S, Garcia AC, et al. Nutrition and food skills education: for adults with developmental disabilities. Canadian J Diet Prac Res 2011;72(1):7–13.

[248] Robinson KT, Butler J. Understanding the causal factors of obesity using the International Classification of Functioning, Disability and Health. Disabil Rehabil 2011;33(8):643–51.

[249] Slevin E, Northway R. Health promotion for people with intellectual and developmental disabilities. Berks, UK: Open University Press/McGraw-Hill Education; 2014.

[250] Rigoldi C, Galli M, Albertini G. Gait development during lifespan in subjects with Down syndrome. Res Dev Disabil 2011;32(1):158–63.

[251] Wang HY, Long IM, Liu MF. Relationships between task-oriented postural control and motor ability in children and adolescents with Down syndrome. Res Dev Disabil 2012;33(6):1792–8.

[252] Villarroya MA, Gonzalez-Aguero A, Moros-Garcia T, et al. Static standing balance in adolescents with Down syndrome. Res Dev Disabil 2012;33(4):1294–300.

[253] Dedlow ER, Siddiqi S, Fillipps DJ, et al. Symptomatic atlantoaxial instability in an adolescent with trisomy 21 (Down's syndrome). Clin Pediatr 2013;52(7):633–8.

[254] Leas D. Atlantoaxial instability. Medscape; 2015. Available from: http://emedicine.medscape.com/article/1265682-overview#a3.

[255] Alvarez N. Atlantoaxial instability in Down syndrome. Medscape; 2016. Available from: http://emedicine.medscape.com/article/1180354-overview#a6.

[256] Goelz T, Butler M, Lee PDK, et al. Motor developmental interventions. In: Butler M, Lee PDK, Whitman BY, editors. Management of Prader-Willi syndrome. USA: Springer; 2006.

[257] Pau M, Galli M, Crivellini M, et al. Foot-ground interaction during upright standing in children with Down syndrome. Res Dev Disabil 2012;33(6):1881–7.

[258] de Hingh YC, van der Vossen PW, Gemen EF, et al. Intrinsic abnormalities of lymphocyte counts in children with Down syndrome. J Pediatr 2005;147(6):744–7.

[259] Carsetti R, Valentini D, Marcellini V, et al. Reduced numbers of switched memory B cells with high terminal differentiation potential in Down syndrome. Europ J Immunol 2015;45(3):903–14.

[260] Bloemers BLP, van Bleek GM, Kimpen JLL, et al. Distinct abnormalities in the innate immune system of children with Down syndrome. J Pediatr 2005;156(5).

[261] Ugazio AG, Maccario R, Notarangelo LD, et al. Immunology of Down syndrome: a review. Am J Med Genet 1990;37(S7):204–12.

[262] Jakubiuk-Tomaszuk A, Sobaniec W, Rusak M, et al. Decrease of interleukin (IL)17A gene expression in leucocytes and in the amount of IL-17A protein in CD4+ T cells in children with Down syndrome. Pharmacol Rep 2015;67(6):1130–4.

[263] Kusters MAA, Verstegen RHJ, de Vries E. Down syndrome: is it really characterized by precocious immunosenescence? Aging Dis 2014;2(6):538–45.

[264] Verstegen RH, Driessen GJ, Bartol SJ, et al. Defective B-cell memory in patients with Down syndrome. J Allergy Clin Immunol 2014;134(6):1346–53.e9.

[265] Hitzler JK. Acute megakaryoblastic leukemia in Down syndrome. Pediatr Blood Cancer 2007;49(S7):1066–9.

[266] Arico M, Ziino O, Valsecchi MG, et al. Acute lymphoblastic leukemia and Down syndrome: presenting features and treatment outcome in the experience of the Italian Association of Pediatric Hematology and Oncology (AIEOP). Cancer 2008;113(3):515–21.

[267] Goto H, Kaneko T, Shioda Y, et al. Hematopoietic stem cell transplantation for patients with acute lymphoblastic leukemia and Down syndrome. Pediatr Blood Cancer 2015;62(1):148–52.

[268] Linabery AM, Li W, Roesler MA, et al. Immune-related conditions and acute leukemia in children with Down syndrome: a Children's Oncology Group report. Cancer Epidemiol Biomarkers Prev 2015;24(2):454–8.

[269] Roncadin C, Hitzler J, Downie A, et al. Neuropsychological late effects of treatment for acute leukemia in children with Down syndrome. Pediatr Blood Cancer 2015;62(5):854–8.

[270] Revuelta Iniesta R, Rush R, Paciarotti I, et al. Systematic review and meta-analysis: prevalence and possible causes of vitamin D deficiency and insufficiency in pediatric cancer patients. Clin Nutr 2016;35(1):95–108.

[271] Al-Nawakil C, Park S, Chapuis N, et al. Salvage therapy of autoimmune thrombocytopenic purpura revealing non-Hodgkin lymphoma by the thrombopoietin receptor agonist romiplostim. Br J Haematol 2012;156(1):145–7.

[272] Lee HJ, Muindi JR, Tan W, et al. Low 25(OH) vitamin D3 levels are associated with adverse outcome in newly diagnosed, intensively treated adult acute myeloid leukemia. Cancer 2014;120(4):521–9.

[273] Radujkovic A, Schnitzler P, Ho AD, et al. Low serum vitamin D levels are associated with shorter survival after first-line azacitidine treatment in patients with myelodysplastic syndrome and secondary oligoblastic acute myeloid leukemia. Clin Nutr 2016.

[274] Aitken RJ, Mehers KL, Williams AJ, et al. Early-onset, coexisting autoimmunity and decreased HLA-mediated susceptibility are the characteristics of diabetes in Down syndrome. Diabetes Care 2013;36(5):1181–5.

[275] Gimenez-Barcons M, Casteras A, Armengol M, et al. Autoimmune predisposition in Down syndrome may result from a partial central tolerance failure due to insufficient intrathymic expression of AIRE and peripheral antigens. J Immunol 2014;193(8):3872–9.

[276] Claret-Torrents C, Goday-Arno A, Cerda-Esteve M, et al. Hyperthyroidism in Down syndrome. Int Med J Down Syndrome 2009;13(1):2–8.

[277] Kariyawasam D, Carre A, Luton D, et al. Down syndrome and nonautoimmune hypothyroidisms in neonates and infants. Horm Res Paediatr 2015;83(2):126–31.

[278] Leger J, Olivieri A, Donaldson M, et al. European Society for Paediatric Endocrinology consensus guidelines on screening, diagnosis, and management of congenital hypothyroidism. J Clin Endocrinol Metab 2014;99(2):363–84.

[279] Goday-Arno A, Cerda-Esteva M, Flores-Le-Roux JA, et al. Hyperthyroidism in a population with Down syndrome (DS). Clin Endocrinol 2009;71(1):110–14.

[280] De Luca F, Corrias A, Salerno M, et al. Peculiarities of Graves' disease in children and adolescents with Down's syndrome. Eur J Endocrinol 2010;162(3):591–5.

[281] Popova G, Paterson WF, Brown A, et al. Hashimoto's thyroiditis in Down's syndrome: clinical presentation and evolution. Horm Res 2008;70(5):278–84.

[282] King K, O'Gorman C, Gallagher S. Thyroid dysfunction in children with Down syndrome: a literature review. Ir J Med Sci 2014;183(1):1–6.

[283] Tenenbaum A, Lebel E, Malkiel S, et al. Euthyroid submedian free T4 and subclinical hypothyroidism may have a detrimental clinical effect in Down syndrome. Horm Res Paediatr 2012;78(2):113–18.

[284] Bhat AS, Chaturvedi MK, Saini S, et al. Prevalence of celiac disease in Indian children with Down syndrome and its clinical and laboratory predictors. Indian J Pediatr 2013;80(2):114–17.

[285] Tonutti E, Bizzaro N. Diagnosis and classification of celiac disease and gluten sensitivity. Autoimmun Rev 2014;13(4–5):472–6.

[286] Carlsson A, Axelsson I, Bourulf S, et al. Prevalence of IgA-antigliadin antibodies and IgA-antiendomysium antibodies related to celiac disease in children with Down syndrome. Pediatrics 1998;101(2):272–5.

[287] Costa Gomes R, Cerqueira Maia J, Fernando Arrais R, et al. The celiac iceberg: from the clinical spectrum to serology and histopathology in children and adolescents with type 1 diabetes mellitus and Down syndrome. Scand J Gastroenterol 2016;51(2):178–85.

[288] George EK, Mearin ML, Bouquet J, et al. High frequency of celiac disease in Down syndrome. J Pediatr 1996;128:4.

[289] Martinez AR, Jaime BE, Lopez AG, et al. Coeliac disease profile in Down syndrome patients. Int Med Rev Down Syndrome 2010;14(1):3–9.

[290] Szaflarska-Poplawska A, Soroczynska-Wrzyszcz A, Barg E, et al. Assessment of coeliac disease prevalence in patients with Down syndrome in Poland: a multi-centre study. Prz Gastroenterol 2016;11(1):41–6.

[291] Wouters J, Weijerman ME, Van Furth MA, et al. Prospective human leukocyte antigen, endomysium immunoglobulin A antibodies, and transglutaminase antibodies testing for celiac disease in children with Down syndrome. J Pediatr 2009;154(2):239–42.

[292] Mårild K, Stephansson O, Grahnquist L, et al. Down syndrome is associated with elevated risk of celiac disease: a nationwide case-control study. J Pediatr 2013;163(1):237–42.

[293] Csizmadia CG, Mearin ML, Oren A, et al. Accuracy and cost-effectiveness of a new strategy to screen for celiac disease in children with Down syndrome. J Pediatr 2000;137(6):756–61.

[294] Cogulu O, Ozikinay F, Gunduz C, et al. Celiac disease in children with Down syndrome: importance of follow-up and serologic screening. Pediatr Int 2003;45(4):395–9.

[295] Hansson T, Dahlbom I, Rogberg S, et al. Antitissue transglutaminase and antithyroid autoantibodies in children with Down syndrome and celiac disease. J Pediatr Gastroenterol Nutr 2005;40(2):170–4.

[296] Langguth D. Coeliac disease testing recommendations. Sullivan Nicolaides; 2012. Available from: www.snp.com.au/media/274287/coeliac_disease_testing_recommendations.pdf.

[297] Shamaly H, Hartman C, Pollack S, et al. Tissue transglutaminase antibodies are a useful serological marker for the diagnosis of celiac disease in patients with Down syndrome. J Pediatr Gastroenterol Nutr 2007;44(5):583–6.

[298] Depince-Berger A, Cremilieux C, Rinaudo-Gaujous M, et al. A difficult and rare diagnosis of autoimmune enteropathy in a patient affected by Down syndrome. J Clin Immunol 2016;36(5).

[299] Soderbergh A, Gustafsson J, Ekwall O, et al. Autoantibodies linked to autoimmune polyendocrine syndrome type I are prevalent in Down syndrome. Acta Paediatr 2006;95(12):1657–60.

[300] Gillespie KM, Dix RJ, Williams AJK, et al. Islet autoimmunity in children with Down's syndrome. Diabetes 2006;55(11):3185–8.

[301] Estefan J, Queriroz M, Costa F, et al. Clinical characteristics of alopecia areata in Down syndrome. Acta Dermatovenerol Croat 2014;21(4):253–8.

[302] Alves R, Ferrando J. Alopecia areata in Down's syndrome. Int Med Rev Down Syndrome 2011;15(3):34–6.

[303] da Rosa Utiyama S, Nisihara R, Nass FR, et al. Autoantibodies in patients with Down syndrome: early senescence of the immune system or precocious markers for immunological diseases? J Paediatr Child Health 2008;44(4):182–6.

[304] Roizen N, Patterson D. Down's syndrome. Lancet 2003;361:1281–9.

[305] Juj H, Emery H. The arthropathy of Down syndrome: an underdiagnosed and under-recognized condition. J Paediatr 2009;154(2):234–8.

[306] Naess KA. Development of phonological awareness in Down syndrome: a meta-analysis and empirical study. Dev Psychol 2016;52(2):177–90.

[307] Laws G, Hall A. Early hearing loss and language abilities in children with Down syndrome: early hearing loss and language abilities in children with DS. Int J Lang Commun Disord 2014;49(3):333–42.

[308] Diaz F. Zurron M. Auditory evoked potentials in Down's syndrome. Electroencephalogr Clin Neurophysiol 1995;96:526–37.

[309] Blaser S, Propst EJ, Martin D, et al. Inner ear dysplasia is common in children with Down syndrome (trisomy 21). Laryngoscope 2006;116(12):2113–19.

[310] Park AH, Wilson MA, Stevens PT, et al. Identification of hearing loss in pediatric patients with Down syndrome. Otolaryngol Head Neck Surg 2012;146(1):135–40.

[311] Downes A, Anixt JS, Esbensen AJ, et al. Psychotropic medication use in children and adolescents with Down syndrome. J Devel Behav Pediatr 2015;36(8):613–19.

[312] Kerins G, Petrovic K, Bruder M, et al. Medical conditions and medication use in adults with Down syndrome: a descriptive analysis. Down Syndrome Res Pract 2008;12(2):141–7.

[313] Maticka-Tyndale E. Sexual Health for the millennium. A declaration and technical document. Int J Sexual Health 2008;20:1.

[314] Hollomotz A. 'May we please have sex tonight?' People with learning difficulties pursuing privacy in residential group settings. Br J Learn Disabil 2009;37(2):91–7.

[315] Young R, Gore N, McCarthy M. Staff attitudes towards sexuality in relation to gender of people with intellectual disability: a qualitative study. J Intellect Dev Disabil 2012;37(4):343–7.

[316] Diekema DS. Involuntary sterilization of persons with mental retardation: an ethical analysis. Ment Retard Dev Disabil Res Rev 2003;9(1):21–6.

[317] Senate Community Affairs Committee Secretariat, Holland I, McInally G, et al. Involuntary or coerced sterilisation of people with disabilities in Australia. Canberra, ACT: Commonwealth of Australia; 2013.

[318] Lockhart K, Guerin S, Shanahan S, et al. Expanding the test of counterfeit deviance: are sexual knowledge, experience and needs a factor in the sexualised challenging behaviour of adults with intellectual disability? Res Dev Disabil 2010;31(1):117–30.

[319] Griffiths D, Hingsburger D, Hoath J, et al. 'Counterfeit deviance' revisited. J Appl Res Intell Disabil 2013;26(5):471–80.

[320] World Health Organization (WHO). Promoting sexual and reproductive health for persons with disabilities: WHO/UNFPA guidance note. Geneva: WHO; 2009.

[321] Eastgate G, Schreermeyer E, van Driel ML, et al. Intellectual disability, sexuality and sexual abuse prevention: a study of family members and support workers. Aus Fam Phys 2012;41(3):135.

[322] Gill M. Rethinking sexual abuse, questions of consent, and intellectual disability. Sex Res Soc Policy 2010;7(3):201–13.

[323] Burke L, Bedard C, Ludwig S. Dealing with sexual abuse of adults with a developmental disability who also have impaired communication: supportive procedures for detection, disclosure and follow up. Can J Human Sexual 1998;7(1):79–91.

[324] McElduff A, Center J, Beange H. Hypogonadism in men with intellectual disabilities: a population study. J Intellect Dev Disabil 2003;28(2):163–70.

[325] Bobrow M, Barby T, Hajianpour A, et al. Fertility in a male with trisomy 21. J Med Genet 1992;29(2):141.

[326] Sheridan R, Llerena J, Matkins S, et al. Fertility in a male with trisomy 21. J Med Genet 1989;26(5):294–8.

[327] Zühlke C, Thies U, Braulke I, et al. Down syndrome and male fertility: PCR-derived fingerprinting, serological and andrological investigations. Clin Genet 1994;46(4):324–6.

[328] Chew G, Hutson JM. Incidence of cryptorchidism and ascending testes in trisomy 21: a 10-year retrospective review. Pediatr Surg Int 2004;20(10):744–7.

[329] Dada R, Kumar R, Kucheria K. A 2-year-old baby with Down syndrome, cryptorchidism and testicular tumour. Eur J Med Genet 2006;49(3):265–8.

[330] Wilson NJ, Cumella S, Parmenter TR, et al. Penile hygiene: puberty, paraphimosis and personal care for men and boys with an intellectual disability. J Intellect Disabil Res 2009;53(2):106–14.

[331] Goede J, Weijerman ME, Broers CJ, et al. Testicular volume and testicular microlithiasis in boys with Down syndrome. J Urol 2012;187(3):1012–17.

[332] Costabile RA. How worrisome is testicular microlithiasis? Curr Opin Urol 2007;17(6):419–23.

[333] Vachon L, Fareau GE, Wilson MG, et al. Testicular microlithiasis in patients with Down syndrome. J Pediatr 2006;149(2):233–6.

[334] Goldstein H. Menarche, menstruation, sexual relations and contraception of adolescent females with Down syndrome. Eur J Obstet Gynecol Reprod Biol 1988;27(4):343–9.

[335] Mason L, Cunningham C. An exploration of issues around menstruation for women with Down syndrome and their carers. J Appl Res Intell Disabil 2008;21(3):257–67.

[336] Stinson J, Christian L, Dotson LA. Overcoming barriers to the sexual expression of women with developmental disabilities. Res Pract Persons Severe Disabil 2002;27(1):18–26.

[337] Cancer Council Australia. Breast cancer; 2016. Available from: www.cancer.org.au/about-cancer/types-of-cancer/breast-cancer.html.

[338] Kwak HI, Gustafson T, Metz RP, et al. Inhibition of breast cancer growth and invasion by single-minded 2s. Carcinogenesis 2007;28(2):259–66.

[339] Chicoine B, Roth M, Chicoine L, et al. Breast cancer screening for women with Down syndrome: lessons learned. Intellect Dev Disabil 2015;53(2):91–9.

[340] Willis D. Breast screening: participation of women with intellectual disabilities: Diane Willis discusses how overdiagnosis of cancer can influence service users' decisions to take part in screening programmes. Learn Disabil Prac 2012;16(4):24–6.

[341] Seltzer GB, Schupf N, Wu H-S. A prospective study of menopause in women with Down's syndrome. J Intellect Disabil Res 2001;45(1):1–7.

[342] Ejskjaer K, Uldbjerg N, Goldstein H. Menstrual profile and early menopause in women with Down syndrome aged 26–40 years. J Intellect Disabil Res 2006;31(3):166–71.

[343] Jobling A, Cuskelly M. Young people with Down syndrome: a preliminary investigation of health knowledge and associated behaviours. J Intellect Dev Disabil 2006;31(4):210–18.

[344] Havercamp SM, Scott HM. National health surveillance of adults with disabilities, adults with intellectual and developmental disabilities, and adults with no disabilities. Disabil Health J 2015;8(2):165–72.

[345] Mansell J, Beadle-Brown J. Dispersed or clustered housing for disabled adults: a systematic review. Dublin: National Disability Authority; 2009.

[346] Sutherland G, Couch MA, Iacono T. Health issues for adults with developmental disability. Res Develop Disabil 2002;23(6):422–45.

[347] Thiel R, Fowkes SW. Can cognitive deterioration associated with Down syndrome be reduced? Med Hypotheses 2005;64(3):524–32.

[348] Garlet TR, Parisotto EB, de Medeiros G, et al. Systemic oxidative stress in children and teenagers with Down syndrome. Life Sci 2013;93(16):558–63.

[349] Ko JW, Lim SY, Chung KC, et al. Reactive oxygen species mediate IL-8 expression in Down syndrome candidate region-1-overexpressed cells. Int J Biochem Cell Biol 2014;55:164–70.

[350] Zana M, Janka Z, Kalman J. Oxidative stress: a bridge between Down's syndrome and Alzheimer's disease. Neurobiol Aging 2007;28(5):648–76.

[351] Perrone S, Longini M, Bellieni CV, et al. Early oxidative stress in amniotic fluid of pregnancies with Down syndrome. Clin Biochem 2007;40(3–4):177–80.

[352] Baptista F, Varela A, Sardinha LB. Bone mineral mass in males and females with and without Down syndrome. Osteoporos Int 2005;16(4):380–8.

[353] Geijer JR, Stanish HI, Draheim CC, et al. Bone mineral density in adults with Down syndrome, intellectual disability, and nondisabled adults. Am J Intellect Dev Disabil 2014;119(2):107–14.

[354] Guijarro M, Valero C, Paule B, et al. Bone mass in young adults with Down syndrome. J Intellect Disabil Res 2008;52(Pt 3):182–9.

[355] Gonzalez-Aguero A, Vicente-Rodriguez G, Moreno LA, et al. Bone mass in male and female children and adolescents with Down syndrome. Osteoporos Int 2011;22(7):2151–7.

[356] Wu J. Bone mass and density in preadolescent boys with and without Down syndrome. Osteoporos Int 2013;24(11):2847–54.

[357] Jasien J, Daimon CM, Maudsley S, et al. Aging and bone health in individuals with developmental disabilities. Int J Endocrinol 2012;469235.

[358] Angelopoulou N, Souftas V, Sakadamis A, et al. Bone mineral density in adults with Down's syndrome. Eur Radiol 1999;9:648–51.

[359] Angelopoulou N, Matziari C, Tsimaras V, et al. Bone mineral density and muscle strength in young men with mental retardation (with and without Down syndrome). Calcif Tissue Int 2000;66(3):176–80.

[360] da Silva VZ, de Franca Barros J, de Azevedo M, et al. Bone mineral density and respiratory muscle strength in male individuals with mental retardation (with and without Down Syndrome). Res Dev Disabil 2010;31(6):1585–9.

[361] McKelvey KD, Fowler TW, Akel NS, et al. Low bone turnover and low bone density in a cohort of adults with Down syndrome. Osteoporos Int 2013;24(4):1333–8.

[362] Gonzalez-Aguero A, Vicente-Rodriguez G, Gomez-Cabello A, et al. Cortical and trabecular bone at the radius and tibia in male and female adolescents with Down syndrome: a peripheral quantitative computed tomography (pQCT) study. Osteoporos Int 2013;24(3):1035–44.

[363] Dreyfus D, Lauer E, Wilkinson J. Characteristics associated with bone mineral density screening in adults with intellectual disabilities. J Am Board Fam Med 2014;27(1):104–14.

[364] Matute-Llorente Á, González-Agüero A, Gómez-Cabello A, et al. Decreased levels of physical activity in adolescents with Down syndrome are related with low bone mineral density: a cross-sectional study. BMC Endocr Disord 2013;13(1):22.

[365] Ferry B, Gavris M, Tifrea C, et al. The bone tissue of children and adolescents with Down syndrome is sensitive to mechanical stress in certain skeletal locations: a 1-year physical training program study. Res Dev Disabil 2014;35(9):2077–84.

[366] Reza SM, Rasool H, Mansour S, et al. Effects of calcium and training on the development of bone density in children with Down syndrome. Res Dev Disabil 2013;34(12):4304–9.

[367] Torr J, Strydom A, Patti P, et al. Aging in Down syndrome: morbidity and mortality. J Pol Pract Intellect Disabil 2010;7:70–81.

[368] Department of Health and Aging. New Zealand Ministry of Health. Nutrient reference values for Australia and New Zealand. National Health and Medical Research Council; 2005.

[369] Cannell JJ, Hollis BW. Use of vitamin D in clinical practice. Alt Med Rev 2008;13(1):6.

[370] Hollis BW. Vitamin D requirement during pregnancy and lactation. J Bone Min Res 2007;22(S2):V39–44.

[371] Holick MF, Binkley NC, Bischoff-Ferrari HA, et al. Evaluation, treatment, and prevention of vitamin D deficiency: an Endocrine Society clinical practice guideline. J Clin Endocrinol Metab 2011;96(7):1911–30.

[372] Vitamin D Council. How do I get the vitamin D my body needs? Available from: www.vitamindcouncil.org/about-vitamin-d/how-do-i-get-the-vitamin-d-my-body-needs.

[373] Dawodu A, Wagner CL. Mother–child vitamin D deficiency: an international perspective. Arch Dis Childhood 2007;92(9):737–40.

[374] Department of Health. Move and play every day. National physical activity recommendations for children 0–5 years; 2014. Available from: www.health.gov.au/internet/main/publishing.nsf/content/F01F92328EDADA5BCA257BF0001E720D/$File/Move%20and%20play%20every%20day%200-5 years.PDF.

[375] World Health Organization. Global recommendations on physical activity for health, 5–17 years old; 2011. Available from: www.who.int/dietphysicalactivity/factsheet_young_people/en.

[376] World Health Organization. Global recommendations on physical activity for health, 18–64 years; 2011. Available from: www.who.int/dietphysicalactivity/physical-activity-recommendations-18-64years.pdf?ua=1.

[377] World Health Organization. Global recommendations on physical activity for health, 65 years and above; 2011. Available from: www.who.int/dietphysicalactivity/physical-activity-recommendations-65years.pdf?ua=1.

[378] Institute of Medicine (US). Panel on Micronutrients. Dietary reference intakes for vitamin A, vitamin K, arsenic, boron, chromium, copper, iodine, iron, manganese, molybdenum, nickel, silicon, vanadium, and zinc. Washington, DC: National Academies Press; 2002.

[379] Graves RJ, Graff JC, Esbensen AJ, et al. Measuring health-related quality of life of adults with Down syndrome. Am J Intellect Dev Disabil 2016;121(4):312–26.

[380] Makary AT, Testa R, Tonge BJ, et al. Association between adaptive behaviour and age in adults with Down syndrome without

dementia: examining the range and severity of adaptive behaviour problems. J Intellect Disabil Res 2015;59(8):689–702.

[381] McLaughlin K, Jones DA. 'It's all changed': carers' experiences of caring for adults who have Down's syndrome and dementia. Br J Learn Disabil 2010.

[382] Wilcock DM, Hurban J, Helman AM, et al. Down syndrome individuals with Alzheimer's disease have a distinct neuroinflammatory phenotype compared to sporadic Alzheimer's disease. Neurobiol Aging 2015;36(9):2468–74.

[383] Dekker AD, Strydom A, Coppus AM, et al. Behavioural and psychological symptoms of dementia in Down syndrome: early indicators of clinical Alzheimer's disease? Cortex 2015;73: 36–61.

[384] McBrien J. Screening adults with Down's syndrome for early signs of dementia. J Integrat Care 2009;17(3):3–7.

[385] Laver K, Cumming RG, Dyer SM, et al. Clinical practice guidelines for dementia in Australia. Med J Aust 2016;204(5):191–3.

[386] Bishop KM, Hogan M, Janicki MP, et al. Guidelines for dementia-related health advocacy for adults with intellectual disability and dementia: National Task Group on Intellectual Disabilities and Dementia Practices. Intellect Dev Disabil 2015;53(1):2–29.

[387] Janicki MP, Zendell A, DeHaven K. Coping with dementia and older families of adults with Down syndrome. Dementia 2010;9(3):391–407.

[388] Whitwham S, McBrien J, Broom W. Should we refer for a dementia assessment? Br J Learn Disabil 2010;39(1):17–21.

[389] Hanney M, Prasher V, Williams N, et al. Memantine for dementia in adults older than 40 years with Down's syndrome (MEADOWS): a randomised, double-blind, placebo-controlled trial. Lancet 2012;379(9815):528–36.

[390] Brownie S, Muggleston H, Oliver C. The 2013 Australian dietary guidelines and recommendations for older Australians. Aus Fam Phys 2013;44(5):311.

[391] Lin JD, Lin LP, Hsu SW, et al. Are early onset aging conditions correlated to daily activity functions in youth and adults with Down syndrome? Res Dev Disabil 2014;36C:532–6.

[392] Kamer AR, Fortea JO, Videla S, et al. Periodontal disease's contribution to Alzheimer's disease progression in Down syndrome. Alzheimers Dement 2016;2:49–57.

[393] Lott IT, Doran E, Nguyen VQ, et al. Down syndrome and dementia: a randomized, controlled trial of antioxidant supplementation. Am J Med Genet 2011;155A(8):1939–48.

[394] Sano M, Aisen P, Andrews HF, et al. Vitamin E in aging persons with Down syndrome: a randomized, placebo-controlled clinical trial. Neurology 2016;86(22):2071–6.

[395] Charleton PM, Dennis J, Marder E. Medical management of children with Down syndrome. Paediatr Child Health 2014;24(8):362–9.

[396] Collins MSR, Kyle R, Smith S, et al. Coping with the usual family diet eating behaviour and food choices of children with Down's syndrome, autistic spectrum disorders or cri du chat syndrome and comparison groups of siblings. J Learn Disabil 2003;7(2):137–55.

[397] Nisihara R, Bonacin M, da Silva Kotze L, et al. Monitoring gluten-free diet in coeliac patients with Down's syndrome. J Hum Nutr Dietet 2013;27(2):1–3.

[398] Gualandri W, Gualandri L, Demartini G, et al. Redox balance in patients with Down's syndrome before and after dietary supplementation with alpha-lipoic acid and L-cysteine. Int J Clin Pharmacol Res 2003;23(1):23–30.

[399] Miles MV, Patterson BJ, Schapiro MB, et al. Coenzyme Q10 absorption and tolerance in children with Down syndrome: a dose-ranging trial. Pediatr Neurol 2006;35(1):30–7.

[400] Miles MV, Patterson BJ, Chalfonte-Evans ML, et al. Coenzyme Q10 (ubiquinol-10) supplementation improves oxidative imbalance in children with trisomy 21. Pediatr Neurol 2007;37(6): 398–403.

[401] Tiano L, Padella L, Santoro L, et al. Prolonged coenzyme Q10 treatment in Down syndrome patients: effect on DNA oxidation. Neurobiol Aging 2012;33(3):626.e1–e8.

[402] Abeysekera I, Thomas J, Georgiadis TM, et al. Differential effects of epigallocatechin-3-gallate containing supplements on correcting skeletal defects in a Down syndrome mouse model. Mol Nutr Food Res 2016;60(4):717–26.

[403] Guedj F, Sebrie C, Rivals I, et al. Green tea polyphenols rescue of brain defects induced by overexpression of DYRK1A. PLoS ONE 2009;4(2):e4606.

[404] Ramakrishna N, Meeker HC, Brown WT. Novel epigenetic regulation of alpha-synuclein expression in Down syndrome. Mol Neurobiol 2016;53(1):155–62.

[405] Stagni F, Giacomini A, Emili M, et al. Short- and long-term effects of neonatal pharmacotherapy with epigallocatechin-3-gallate on hippocampal development in the Ts65Dn mouse model of Down syndrome. Neuroscience 2016;333:277–301.

[406] Valenti D, de Bari L, de Rasmo D, et al. The polyphenols resveratrol and epigallocatechin-3-gallate restore the severe impairment of mitochondria in hippocampal progenitor cells from a Down syndrome mouse model. Biochim Biophys Acta 2016;1862(6):1093–104.

[407] de la Torre R, de Sola S, Hernandez G, et al. Safety and efficacy of cognitive training plus epigallocatechin-3-gallate in young adults with Down's syndrome (TESDAD): a double-blind, randomised, placebo-controlled, phase 2 trial. Lancet Neurol 2016;15(8): 801–10.

[408] Bennett FC, McClelland S, Kriegsmann EA, et al. Vitamin and mineral supplementation in Down's syndrome. Pediatrics 1983;72(5):707–13.

[409] Coleman M, Sobel S, Bhagavan HN, et al. A double blind study of vitamin B6 in Down's syndrome infants. Part 1: clinical and biochemical results. J Ment Defic Res 1985;29(Pt 3): 233–40.

[410] Frager J, Barnet A, Weiss I, et al. A double blind study of vitamin B6 in Down's syndrome infants. Part 2: cortical auditory evoked potentials. J Ment Defic Res 1985;29(Pt 3):241–6.

[411] Stagi S, Lapi E, Romano S, et al. Determinants of vitamin D levels in children and adolescents with Down syndrome. Int J Endocrinol 2015;896758.

[412] Zubillaga P, Garrido A, Mugica I, et al. Effect of vitamin D and calcium supplementation on bone turnover in institutionalized adults with Down's syndrome. Eur J Clin Nutr 2006;60(5): 605–9.

[413] Mustafa Nachvak S, Reza Neyestani T, Ali Mahboob S, et al. Alpha-tocopherol supplementation reduces biomarkers of oxidative stress in children with Down syndrome: a randomized controlled trial. Eur J Clin Nutr 2014;68(10):1119–23.

[414] Pincheira J, Navarrete MH, de la Torre C, et al. Effect of vitamin E on chromosomal aberrations in lymphocytes from patients with Down's syndrome. Clin Genet 1999;55:192–7.

[415] Parisotto EB, Garlet TR, Cavalli VL, et al. Antioxidant intervention attenuates oxidative stress in children and teenagers with Down syndrome. Res Dev Disabil 2014;35(6):1228–36.

[416] Parisotto EB, Giaretta AG, Zamoner A, et al. Persistence of the benefit of an antioxidant therapy in children and teenagers with Down syndrome. Res Dev Disabil 2015;45-46:14–20.

[417] Chiricolo M, Musa AR, Monti D, et al. Enhanced DNA repair in lymphocytes of Down syndrome patients: the influence of zinc nutritional supplementation. Mutat Res 1993;295(3): 105–11.

[418] Licastro F, Chiricolo M, Mocchegiani E, et al. Oral zinc supplementation in Down's syndrome subjects decreased infections and normalized some humoral and cellular immune parameters. J Intellect Disabil Res 1994;38(2):149–62.

[419] Lockitch G, Puteman M, Godolphin W, et al. Infection and immunity in Down syndrome: a trial of long-term low oral doses of zinc. J Pediatr 1989;114(5):781–7.

[420] Marreiro DN, de Sousa AF, Nogueira N, et al. Effect of zinc supplementation on thyroid hormone metabolism of adolescents with Down syndrome. Biol Trace Elem Res 2009;129(1–3): 20–7.

[421] Romano C, Pettinato R, Ragusa L, et al. Is there a relationship between zinc and the peculiar comorbidities of Down syndrome? Down Syndrome Res Pract 2002;8(1):25–8.

[422] Stabile A, Pesaresi MA, Stabile AM, et al. Immunodeciency and plasma zinc levels in children with Down's syndrome: a long-term follow up of oral zinc supplementation. Clin Immunol Immunopathol 1991;58:207–16.

[423] Mocchegiani E, Costarelli L, Giacconi R, et al. Micronutrient (Zn, Cu, Fe)-gene interactions in ageing and inflammatory age-related

diseases: implications for treatments. Ageing Res Rev 2012;11(2):297–319.

[424] Lima AS, Cardoso BR, Cozzolino SF. Nutritional status of zinc in children with Down syndrome. Biol Trace Elem Res 2010;133(1):20–8.

[425] Marques RC, de Sousa AF, do Monte SJ, et al. Zinc nutritional status in adolescents with Down syndrome. Biol Trace Elem Res 2007;120(1–3):11–18.

[426] Seven M, Cengiz M, Tüzgen S, et al. Plasma carnitine levels in children with Down syndrome. Am J Hum Biol 2001;13(6):721–5.

[427] Malaguarnera M, Gargante MP, Cristaldi E, et al. Acetyl L-carnitine (ALC) treatment in elderly patients with fatigue. Arch Gerontol Geriatr 2008;46(2):181–90.

[428] Pueschel SM. The effect of acetyl-L-carnitine administration on persons with Down syndrome. Res Dev Disabil 2006;27(6):599–604.

[429] Turner RS, Thomas RG, Craft S, et al. A randomized, double-blind, placebo-controlled trial of resveratrol for Alzheimer disease. Neurology 2015;85(16):1383–91.

[430] Hawrelak J. Probiotics. In: Murray M, Pizzorno J, editors. Textbook of natural medicine. St Louis: Churchill Livingstone; 2013. p. 966–78.

[431] Anderson J, Hasler K, Yates R, et al. Sexual health and relationships: a review of resources for people with learning disabilities. Glasgow: NHS Health Scotland; 2008.

APPENDIX 19.1

Sexual health resources for parents, carers and health professionals working with people with Down syndrome and other learning disabilities

Resource	Topics included
Hart P, Douglas-Scott S. *Batteries not included: a sexuality resource pack for working with people with complex communication support needs.* Common Knowledge; 2005.	Masturbation Moral issues Policy issues Relationships Rights and responsibilities Same-sex relationships Sex aids/sex toys Sex and the law
Cooper E. *Becoming a woman: a teaching pack on menstruation for women with learning disabilities.* Pavilion Publishing; 1999.	Anatomy of sexual organs Body changes Intimate care Menstruation Mood swings Personal hygiene and grooming Puberty
Body board (variety of packs available) Headon Productions; 1999.	Communication skills Drugs Emotions, pregnancy, contraception, love, hygiene Flirting and body language Human reproduction Masturbation Organs of the body Sex and relationships education Sexual intercourse/penetration (Only includes heterosexual sex)
Dixon H. *Chance to choose: sexuality and relationships education for people with learning difficulties.* LDA; 2005.	Appropriate behaviour Assertiveness Body image Communication skills Contraception Group work Masturbation Menstruation Puberty Relationships Self-esteem STIs — symptoms and consequences

Continued

Resource	Topics included
Sherlin M, McCormick G. *Exploring sexuality and disability: walk your talk.* FPA; 1997.	Assertiveness Attitudes or attitudinal change Avoiding risky situations Choices, making informed decisions Condoms Disability politics/rights/issues Emergency contraception Heterosexuality Learning disabilities Love Options if pregnant Other disabilities Personal hygiene and grooming Preventing pregnancy Safer sex Sexual health and sexual health services STIs — symptoms and consequences Staff values
Drury J, Hutchinson L, Wright J. *Holding on, letting go: sex, sexuality and people with learning disabilities.* Souvenir Press; 2000.	Disability politics/rights/issues Parenting Relationships Rights and responsibilities Sexual abuse or coercion Sexual health services Sexuality
How it is: an image vocabulary for children about feelings, rights and safety, personal care and sexuality. NSPCC; 2002.	Sexual organs Body changes Communication skills Emotions/feelings Friendships Heterosexuality Intimate care Masturbation Rights and responsibilities Sexual language Sexually explicit material
Atkinson D, Gingell A, Martin J. *I have the right to know: how to run a course on sexuality and personal relationships for people with learning disabilities.* BILD; 1997.	Abortion/termination of pregnancy Anatomy of sexual organs Assertiveness Bisexuality Body changes Contraception Gender differences Homosexuality Masturbation Personal hygiene and grooming Policy issues Pregnancy and parenthood Relationships Reproductive health Rights and responsibilities Self-esteem Sexual behaviour Sexual language STIs — symptoms and consequences

Resource	Topics included
Meinertzhagen K, Kennard M, Hall L. *It's my life* (picture signed for people working with individuals with hearing impairment or deafness). SIGNALONG Group; 2000.	Anal sex Anatomy of sexual organs Bisexuality Bullying Circumcision Communication skills Confidentiality Contraception Emotions/feelings Gender issues Heterosexuality Homosexuality Masturbation Medical examinations Menstruation Options if pregnant Oral sex Pregnancy Puberty Relationships Sexual abuse or coercion Sexual language STIs — symptoms and consequences Transgender issues
Queens Road Sexual Health Team. *It's only natural: for parents, carers and others involved in the lives of young people with learning disabilities — a resource which looks at issues of sexuality and sexual health*. Barnardos; 1996.	Confidentiality Parents Relationships Rights and responsibilities Self-esteem Sex and relationships education (SRE) SRE program development STIs — symptoms and consequences
Hingsburger D. *Just say know! Understanding and reducing the risk of sexual victimisation of people with developmental disabilities*. Diverse City Press; 1995.	Attitudes/attitudinal change Disability politics/rights/issues Gender issues Learning disabilities Parents Power issues in relationships Rights and responsibilities Self-esteem Sex and relationships education Sexual abuse or coercion Staff values
Frawley P, Johnson K, Hillier L, Harrison L. *Living safer sexual lives: a training and resource pack for people with learning disabilities and those who support them*. Pavilion Publishing; 2000.	Attitudes/attitudinal change Emotions/feelings Friendships Gay men Heterosexuality and homosexuality Learning disabilities Lesbians Love Media Men who have sex with men Parenthood and parents Policy issues Power issues in relationships Relationships rights and responsibilities Same-sex partnerships Self-esteem Sexual abuse or coercion Sexuality Staff values

Continued

Resource	Topics included
Making choices, keeping safe. Interagency Guideline for Lothian. Issue 1. Author: NHS Lothian; 2004.	Abortion/termination of pregnancy Bisexuality Choices, making informed decisions Condoms Consent Contraception Emergency contraception Heterosexuality HIV infection/AIDS Homosexuality Intimate care Masturbation Parenthood Preventing pregnancy Privacy Same-sex partnerships Sex and the law Sexual health services Sexually explicit material
McCarthy M, Thompson D. *Sex and the 3Rs – rights, responsibilities and risks:a sex education package for working with people with learning difficulties*. Pavilion Publishing; 1998 (rev edn).	Anal sex Appropriate touch Contraception Gender differences Heterosexuality Homosexuality Oral sex Pregnancy Saying no to sex Sexual abuse and coercion STIs — symptoms and consequences
Adcock K, Stanley G. *Sexual health education and children and young people with learning disabilities: a practical way of working for professionals, parents and carers*. BILD/Barnados; 1996.	Group work Sex and relationships education
Scott L, Kerr-Edwards L. *Talking together … about growing up*. FPA; 1999.	Behaviour Body changes Body image Choices, making informed decisions Emotions/feelings Masturbation Menstruation Public/private Relationships Sex and relationships Sexual language
Couwenhoven T. *Teaching children with Down syndrome about their bodies, boundaries, and sexuality: a guide for parents and professionals*. Woodbine House; 2007.	Anticipating and understanding puberty Dealing with periods, bras for girls Experiencing erections, wet dreams for boys Explaining sexual relationships Identifying and expressing emotions Labelling and explaining private body parts Preventing sexual abuse Relating to the opposite sex Respecting personal space Sharing parental values about sexuality Showing appropriate levels of affection Teaching self-care and hygiene Understanding gender identity Understanding how Down syndrome affects puberty and fertility rates Understanding norms of privacy

Source: Anderson J, Hasler K, Yates R, et al. Sexual health and relationships: a review of resources for people with learning disabilities. Glasgow: NHS Health Scotland; 2008.

APPENDIX 19.2

Sexual health resources for people with Down syndrome and other learning disabilities, with the support of carers or family members

Resource	Topics included
Hollins S, Sinason V. *Bob tells all* (books beyond words). Gaskell/Royal College of Psychiatrists; 1992.	Appropriate sexual and non-sexual behaviour Sexual abuse or coercion
Fraser J (ed.). *Building friendships: a resource pack to help young people make friendships and develop relationships*. Brook Publications; 1994.	Avoiding risky situations Communication skills Friendships and relationships Icebreakers Social skills Building friendships Helping others get to know you
Cathy has thrush. Women's Health; 2001.	Intimate care Medical examinations Personal hygiene and grooming Sexual health services Thrush
Poynor L et al. *Cervical screening: a teaching pack for women with learning disabilities and those who work with them*. Surrey Oaklands NHS Trust; 2004.	Anatomy of sexual organs Body changes Cervical cancer Cervical screening Choices and making informed consent Medical examinations Sexual health services Smear tests
Hollins S. *Falling in love* (books beyond words). Gaskell/Royal College of Psychiatrists; 1999.	Communication skills Emotions/feelings Love Parents Privacy Relationships
Feeling grown up. Shepherd School; 1999.	Appropriate behaviour Masturbation Menstruation Personal hygiene and grooming Public/private Wet dreams
Hollins S, Flynn M, Russell P. *George gets smart* (books beyond words). Gaskell/Royal College of Psychiatrists; 2001.	Friendships Personal hygiene and grooming
FAIR/NHS Health Scotland. *A guide to examining your breasts*. NHS Health Scotland; 2002.	Breast awareness and screening Choices, making informed decisions Medical examinations Self-examination (breasts)
FAIR/NHS Health Scotland. *A guide to examining your testicles*. NHS Health Scotland; 2002.	Choices, making informed decisions Self-examination (testicles) Sexual health services Testicular examination
FAIR/NHS Health Scotland. *A guide to having a period*. NHS Health Scotland; 2003.	Anatomy of sexual organs Emotions/feelings Intimate care Menstruation Mood swings Personal hygiene and grooming Puberty Sexual health services

Continued

Resource	Topics included
FAIR/NHS Lothian. *A guide to having a smear test.* FAIR Multimedia/NHS Lothian; 2004.	Anatomy of sexual organs Cervical cancer Cervical screening Medical examinations Smear tests
Hollins S, Roth T. *Hug me touch me.* Gaskell/Royal College of Psychiatrists; 1994.	Appropriate behaviour Friendships and relationships Touch
I want to be a good parent. The BILD parenting series. BILD; 1994 (reprinted 1998).	Child development Child needs: health, hygiene, warmth, safety, love Feeding children healthy food Parenthood Realities of becoming a parent
Hollins S, Sinason V. *Jenny speaks out* (books beyond words). Gaskell/Royal College of Psychiatrists; 2005.	Communication skills Sexual abuse or coercion
Hollins S, Downer J. *Keeping healthy down below* (books beyond words). Gaskell/Royal College of Psychiatrists; 2000.	Cervical screening Choices, making informed decisions Medical examinations Menstruation Sexual health services Smear tests
Johns R, Scott L, Bliss J. *Let's do it: creative activities for sex education for young people with learning disabilities* (3rd edn). Image in Action; 2002.	Anatomy of sexual organs Assertiveness Body changes Body image Condoms Emotions /feelings Gender differences Group work HIV infection/AIDs Masturbation Public/private Relationships Self-esteem Sexual arousal Sexual health services Sexual intercourse/penetration
Marsden L. *Let's talk about puberty: a booklet about growing up for young people who have a learning disability.* Down's Syndrome Scotland; 2004.	Body changes Body images Choices, making informed decisions Emotions/feelings Masturbation Menstruation Mood swings Personal hygiene and grooming Puberty Self-esteem Sexual arousal
Hollins S, Wilson J. *Looking after my balls* (books beyond words). Gaskell/Royal College of Psychiatrists; 2004.	Medical examinations Self-examination (testicles) Sexual health services Testicular cancer
Hollins S, Perez W. *Looking after my breasts* (books beyond words). Gaskell/Royal College of Psychiatrists; 2000.	Breast awareness and screening Mammograms Self-examination (breasts)
Hollins S, Roth T. *Making friends* (books beyond words). Gaskell/Royal College of Psychiatrists; 1995.	Appropriate touch Behaviour Emotions/feelings Friendships

Resource	Topics included
FAIR/NHS Health Scotland. *A man's guide to keeping clean*. NHS Health Scotland; 2003.	Anatomy of sexual organs Body image Intimate care Personal hygiene and grooming
FAIR/NHS Health Scotland. Shaving card. NHS Health Scotland; 2003.	Laminated card for men with intellectual disabilities with step-by-step guide to wet and dry shaving
Hollins S, Sinason V. *Susan's growing up*. Gaskell/Royal College of Psychiatrists; 2001.	Menstruation Personal hygiene and grooming
Thinking about sex? How to use condoms. Caledonia Youth; 1999 (reprinted 2003).	Anatomy of sexual organs Condoms Heterosexuality Preventing pregnancy Safer sex (Note: only contains heterosexual images)
FAIR/NHS Health Scotland. *A woman's guide to keeping clean*. NHS Health Scotland; 2003.	Body image Intimate care Personal hygiene and grooming

Source: Anderson J, Hasler K, Yates R, et al. Sexual health and relationships: a review of resources for people with learning disabilities. Glasgow: NHS Health Scotland; 2008.

APPENDIX 19.3

Plymouth dementia screening checklist

Plymouth Dementia Screening Checklist

1. **Has there been a <u>negative change</u> in memory functioning over the past 12 months?**

   For example: *Short-term memory problems? Repetitive in conversation? Needs frequent reminding/prompting? Concentration problems?*

   No change ⟷ Extensive change

   Point =   ☐ 0   ☐ 1   ☐ 2   ☐ 3   Total /3

2. **Has there been a <u>negative change</u> in mood over the past 12 months?**

   For example: *Low in mood? Withdrawn? Mood swings?*

   No change ⟷ Extensive change

   Point =   ☐ 0   ☐ 1   ☐ 2   ☐ 3   Total /3

3. **Has there been a <u>negative change</u> in behaviour over the past 12 months?**

   For example: *Difficult behaviours? Night wandering? Inappropriate behaviour? Aggression? Incontinence? Losing skills?*

   No change ⟷ Extensive change

   Point =   ☐ 0   ☐ 1   ☐ 2   ☐ 3   Total /3

   Total /9

   Have any other changes been noticed?
   Please consider: Language and communication skills? Self-help skills? Activities of daily living?

   ....

   ....

   ....

   ....

   ....

20

The endocannabinoid system and cannabis

Justin S Sinclair

INTRODUCTION

The endocannabinoid system (ECS) is a relatively recent scientific discovery, with its unearthing owed largely to the research conducted on the *Cannabis* genus and its unique pharmacological effects. This ubiquitous neuromodulatory system exhibits key functions across many different organ systems, tissues, cells and physiological settings[1,2] and comprises specific endocannabinoid receptors, the endogenous ligands that bind with these receptors and the enzymes that are responsible for ligand synthesis and degradation. Despite being researched for more than 30 years, there is sparse representation of the endocannabinoid system in current tertiary medicine, nursing and allied health curriculums. This is potentially contributing to a delay in access to *Cannabis* spp. and cannabinoid-based medicines for certain patient populations in Australia and New Zealand, while also slowing research into our understanding of the aetiological basis behind numerous medical conditions.

EVOLUTION OF THE ENDOCANNABINOID SYSTEM

The evolutionary development of the ECS has taken place over millions of years across diverse biological organisms, with evidence of cannabinoid receptor genes being found in the Deuterostomian invertebrate *Ciona intestinalis* (sea squirt), suggesting that the receptors developed in this class some 500 million years ago.[3] Recent research has highlighted that genes for these receptors and their related endocannabinoid ligands need to coevolve in order to maintain binding affinities and coordinated gene expression.[4] Further investigation has uncovered that cannabinoid receptors are also distributed widely throughout the vertebrates and have been documented in fish, amphibians, sea urchins, molluscs, leeches and mammals.[5–7]

Research into how the phytochemicals in *Cannabis* spp. interacted with human physiology was a slow evolution also, taking place in three distinct phases. Academic investigation has been impeded largely by inconsistent *Cannabis* spp. plant samples, prohibitive laws hampering its availability in academic research[2] and a poor understanding of the chemical structure of the plant cannabinoids. With more than 100 phytocannabinoids[8–10] in various *Cannabis* spp. and strains, many being artefacts of analysis, this made isolation difficult due to similarities in structure and physical properties.[2] Advances in modern analytical separation techniques finally elucidated the main psychoactive principle, the phytocannabinoid known as Δ^9-tetrahydrocannabinol (THC), in 1964,[11] which led to its chemical synthesis 3 years later.[12] It thus became more readily available for scientific research, allowing for the investigation of its physiological mechanism of action.[13]

The first phase in our understanding of the ECS came almost 20 years later in the mid-1980s,[13] when research teams began closing in on potential receptors with which THC interacted. Studies in 1984 elucidated that cannabimimetic agents inhibited cAMP accumulation in neuronal cells via a receptor-mediated cellular response,[14] and in 1988 research undertaken by Mechoulam and colleagues demonstrated that THC was stereospecific, suggesting that it required a specific site of action for binding.[13,15] Later that same year a specific cannabinoid receptor was discovered,[16] with structural expression of this receptor being defined in 1990.[17] This cannabinoid receptor became known as the CB_1 receptor and THC binds with relatively high affinity to it within the central nervous system (CNS). Just 3 years later, a second receptor, known as the CB_2 receptor, was discovered[18] and it is believed to exist mainly in the peripheral nervous system and tissues.

The endogenous ligands that interact with the CB_1 and CB_2 receptors represent the second phase and were the next piece of the anatomical and physiological puzzle of the ECS. Based on the highly lipophilic structure of the terpenophenolic THC,[10] it was hypothesised that the endogenous ligands would also be lipid derived.[2,13] This hypothesis was later proven correct, with the endocannabinoids being shown to be derivatives of arachidonic acid, which is a progenitor compound to other endogenous molecules such as leukotrienes, thromboxanes, prostacyclins and prostaglandins.[13] Using lipid separation techniques, in 1992 Devane and colleagues[19] isolated anandamide (AEA; N-arachidonoylethanolamine), with a second endocannabinoid known as 2-AG (2-arachidonoylglycerol) being identified in 1995.[20,21] These endocannabinoids are chemically derived from long-chain polyunsaturated fatty acids as amides, esters and even ethers and bind with varying affinity to the CB_1 and CB_2 receptors.[5,22] While anandamide and 2-AG are the most studied endocannabinoids currently, others have been identified such as 2-arachidonylglyceryl ether (noladin ether), O-arachidonoyl-ethanolamine (virodhamine) and N-arachidonoyl-dopamine (NADA),[5] but their physiological importance is as yet largely undetermined.[23]

Lastly, the third phase includes the enzymes involved in the synthesis and degradation of the endocannabinoids have been described[13] and are continuing to be researched. Various enzymes, such as N-acyltransferase, N-acyl-phosphatidylethanolamine phospholipase D (NAPE-PLD), phospholipase C (PLC) and diacylglycerol lipase (DAGL) are involved in endocannabinoid synthesis, whereas fatty acid amide hydrolase (FAAH) and monoacylglycerol lipase are specific for degradation pathways.[24]

All of these components comprising the ECS represent perhaps one of the most significant anatomical and physiological discoveries in the fields of biology, pharmacology and medicine in the last 100 years and open up an entirely new chapter in our understanding of homeostatic mechanisms and regulation within the human organism. The potential of this understanding to enrich our current knowledge base and treatment of numerous idiopathic diseases, disorders and conditions has far-reaching implications, and was made possible by initial research into the cannabis plant and how it impacted human physiology.

ANATOMY OF THE ENDOCANNABINOID SYSTEM

The ECS represents a vital and integral neuromodulatory system involved in the regulation of many facets of homeostasis, with cannabinoid receptors widely expressed in many cells and tissues of the body.[23] Essentially, the ECS is comprised of three major components:

– Cannabinoid receptors (i.e. CB_1 and CB_2),[25] which are distributed throughout the various organs and tissues
– Endogenous ligands (i.e. endocannabinoids), which interact with these receptors
– Enzymes that are involved in synthesis or degradation of the ligands.[3,26–29]

Of key clinical interest here is that any individual variability or genetic polymorphic modifications to any one of these components may potentially modify the normal functioning of the entire ECS and the body systems it regulates. This invariably highlights not only the complexity of cannabis pharmacotherapy in clinical application, but also the need for discussion about the concept of a precision-medicine initiative around the medicinal cannabis debate, optimised for individual patients and their physiological expression.

Receptors

The CB_1 and CB_2 cannabinoid receptors belong to the family of 7-transmembrane (comprised of α-helices, a glycosylated amino terminus and an intracellular carboxyl terminus)[25] $G_{i/o}$ protein-coupled receptors (GPCRs),[13,22,28,30–33] being expressed in abundance in the CNS where it far exceeds those present for the neurotransmitters it modulates.[27] Widespread tissue distribution of cannabinoid receptor 1 and 2 subtypes is suggestive that they have a broad scope and variance in physiological roles around the body. Recent research has also identified other targets for endocannabinoids, with the G protein-coupled receptor 55 (GPR55)[34] and G protein-coupled receptor 119 (GRP119) being postulated as new members of the cannabinoid receptor family.[25,35] Further research suggests that the transient receptor potential vanilloid 1 (TRPV1) and the peroxisome proliferator-activated receptor (PPAR) α and γ subtypes are also a target for endocannabinoid binding.[13,36,37]

The CB_1 and CB_2 receptors, coupled to $G_{i/o}$ proteins, demonstrate physiological effects by inhibiting adenylate cyclases (thus inhibiting the conversion of ATP to cyclic AMP),[5,38] stimulating mitogen-activated protein kinases (MAPK) and modulating the activity of K^+ and Ca^{2+} ion channels assisting in transducing the binding of agonists.[39] This latter protein-mediated modulation of ion channels includes activating inwardly rectifying A-type K^+ channels or inhibiting L-, N- and P/Q-type voltage gated Ca^{2+} channels,[40,41] thus modulating neurotransmitter release such as inhibiting central neurotransmitter release with noradrenaline, acetylcholine and glutamate.[25,29,42]

CB_1 receptors, which have CB_{1A} and CB_{1B} subtypes,[43,44] are encoded by the *CNR1* gene[45] and are the most widely expressed GPCRs in the brain and spinal cord, with high density present on presynaptic terminals, particularly of GABAergic and glutamatergic neurons.[23,46–48] CB_1 activation inhibits the specific neurotransmitter release of GABA, glutamate, dopamine, serotonin, acetylcholine, D-aspartate and noradrenaline[49–51] of both excitatory and inhibitory synapses. Thus CB_1 receptors are primarily involved in modulation of neurotransmitter release centrally, but also have roles in causing coronary and cerebral dilation, neuroprotective signalling, relief of pain and promoting neural stem cell differentiation.[52–55]

Receptor locations within the CNS include numerous regions within the cortex (see Box 20.1).[2,3,39] Interestingly, there is a paucity of CB_1 receptors in the brainstem (specifically the cardiopulmonary centres), which may explain the lack of respiratory depression in *Cannabis* spp. overuse compared to that observed in opiate medication overdose, despite CB_1 receptors being ten times more common than mu-opioid receptors in the brain.[3] Furthermore, cannabinoid receptors have been shown to co-localise with opioid receptors and may amplify analgesic effects via potential pharmacodynamic activity.[3]

The CB_1 receptor subtype was originally believed to be expressed mainly in the CNS[2]; however, recent research has demonstrated that it is also expressed in peripheral neurons presynaptically and other extra-neural tissues and organs such as adipocytes, myocytes, hepatocytes, epithelial cells, the digestive system, male (e.g. testis) and female reproductive organs, eyes, vascular endothelium, heart, lungs and kidneys and the pituitary, adrenal and thyroid glands,[39,45,56,57] albeit with lower receptor expression levels

BOX 20.1 CNS distribution of CB₁ receptors

Amygdala
Basal ganglia*
Cerebellum*
Cerebral cortex*
  – Frontal lobe
  – Olfactory cortex
  – Entorhinal cortex
  – Somatosensory cortex
Globus pallidus
Hippocampus*
Periaqueductal grey matter
Rostroventrolateral medulla (RVM)
Spinal interneurons
Substantia gelatinosa (spinal cord)
Substantia nigra
*Highest receptor concentration

than observed in the CNS. CB_1 is also highly expressed in the enteric nervous system throughout all neuronal types except for inhibitory motor neurons.[58,59]

The CB_1 receptor is encoded by the *CNR1* gene located at chromosome 6q 14-15,[60] for which multiple single-nucleotide polymorphisms (SNPs) have been documented. Due to such widespread distribution in the CNS, CB_1 receptors are thought to be important for motivation, cognition,[2] sedation, pain, appetite regulation and muscle relaxation, and are the predominant targets involved for the psychotropic activity of *Cannabis* spp. rich in THC or other exogenous cannabinoids.

Conversely, CB_2 receptors were thought to exist mainly in the periphery and immune cells with little, if any, CNS distribution. However, in 2006 researchers discovered the functional expression of this receptor subtype within the brain,[28,61–63] particularly in microglial cells and more recently neural stem cells.[64] More commonly, CB_2 receptors are widely expressed throughout peripheral tissues within the immune system, including the spleen, thymus, tonsils, mast cells and gastrointestinal tract (GIT).[45] Specific immune cells with high levels of CB_2 expression include CD4+ T cells, CD8+ T cells, B-cells, natural killer (NK) cells, macrophages, monocytes and neutrophils.[48,65] The *CNR2* gene encodes for the CB_2 receptor, with both CB_1 and CB_2 receptors demonstrating 44% similarity in their amino acid sequences.[45]

CB_2 receptor expression in peripheral immune cells and tissues is currently considered responsible for the effects that cannabinoids have on immunomodulatory activity,[66] thought largely to be due to the CB_2 signalling pathway playing a critical role in regulating microglial activities within the CNS.[67] CB_2 receptors do not cause any noted psychoactive activity but they do contribute to local analgesic effects.[3] Furthermore, CB_2 receptors demonstrate important neuroprotective and anti-inflammatory activities, with CB_2 expression being enhanced by inflammation, which suggests that this receptor subtype may be involved in the endogenous response to injury.[55,68–70] Recent

evidence has demonstrated the role of CB_2 activation in analgesia in acute and neuropathic models of pain.[71]

It has been posited that the CB_2 receptor is part of an integral protective system within the body,[2] with Pacher and Mechoulam speculating that:

> The mammalian body has a highly developed immune system which guards against continuous invading protein attacks and aims at preventing, attenuating or repairing the inflicted damage. It is conceivable that through evolution, analogous biological protective systems have evolved against nonprotein attacks. There is emerging evidence that lipid endocannabinoid signaling through CB_2 receptors may represent an example/part of such a protective system.[72]

It should be noted that non-CB_1/CB_2 receptor effects have been reported in the scientific literature, with examples of certain cannabinoid ligands being mediated by α-7-nicotinic acetylcholine receptors, serotonin type 3 receptors, peroxisome proliferator-activated receptor-α, peroxisome proliferator-activated receptor-γ[37,73] and transient receptor potential vanilloid type 1 (TRPV1) receptors.[25,36,74–76] Interestingly, cannabinoid effects have been noted independent of any currently known receptor types, suggesting the possibility of either as yet unidentified cannabinoid receptor subtypes or the ability of the endocannabinoids to diffuse directly through the cellular phospholipid bilayer.[25,77]

The discovery of the cannabinoid receptors and an evolving understanding of the regulatory mechanisms of the ECS, with its subsequent role in the aetiology and pathogenesis of multiple diseases and conditions, has seen the pharmacological development of many synthetic substances that are agonists and antagonists to CB_1/CB_2 receptors. Examples of CB_1 synthetic inverse agonists or antagonists include SR141716A (Rimonabant), AM251 and AM281, while SR144528 and AM630 are selective for CB_2 receptors.[25,78] These synthetic derivatives can express very high levels of specificity and affinity for the various cannabinoid receptors, but are not without risks. For example, Rimonabant (Acomplia, Zimulti) was marketed as an anti-obesity drug, but it has been withdrawn from the US market due to serious adverse effects such as suicidality and depression, with a 2006 Cochrane Review suggesting that more rigorous studies are required to examine the safety and efficacy to evaluate the benefit/risk ratio in more detail.[79]

Apart from endogenous ligands and synthetically manufactured agonists and antagonists, the CB_1 and CB_2 receptors can also interact with phytocannabinoids (i.e. secondary plant metabolites of terpenophenolic origin) such as THC and synthetically derived cannabinoids, all with varying receptor affinities and physiological outcomes. This is discussed later under the phytochemistry of the *Cannabis* genus.

Endogenous ligands (endocannabinoids)

Being derivatives of polyunsaturated fatty acids, the endocannabinoids differ structurally from the

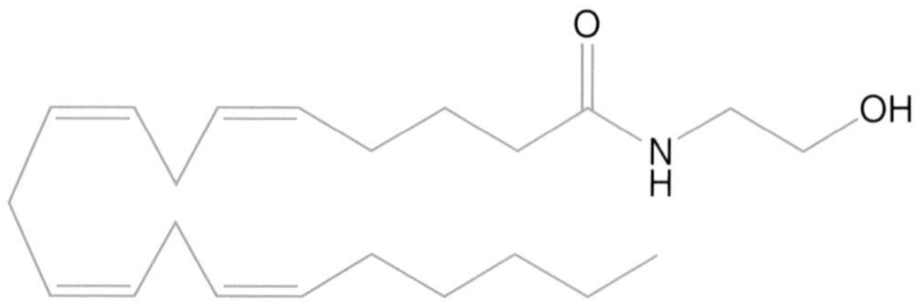

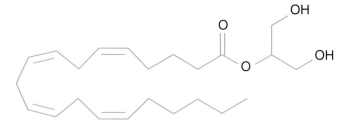

FIGURE 20.1 Chemical structure of anandamide

FIGURE 20.2 Chemical structure of 2-AG

phytocannabinoids produced in the *Cannabis* genus or other synthetically derived exocannabinoids.[5] Currently, two main endocannabinoids have emerged in the research as prevalent regulators of synaptic function, anandamide[80] and 2-AG,[20,21] but others have been highlighted in the literature – for example, non-amide derivatives such as virodhamine[81] and ether derivatives such as noladin ether.[25,76,82,83] The latter, which is generally quite stable in vivo unlike anandamide or 2-AG, is of particular interest in drug development.[84] Furthermore, *N*-palmitoylethanolamine (PEA), *N*-oleoylethanolamine (OEA) and *N*-stearoylethanolamine (SEA) have been described as 'endocannabinoid-like' compounds found in rat, mouse and human brain tissue,[84,85] but research on their physiological significance is still ongoing.

ANANDAMIDE

Anandamide was the first endocannabinoid isolated in 1992 and it was named after the Sanskrit word *ananda* meaning 'supreme joy' or 'bliss'[2] due to its cannabimimetic activity, pertaining to its ability to interact with cannabinoid receptors and mimic the psychotropic effect of THC from *Cannabis* spp.[84,86] Of all the posited endocannabinoids, anandamide is the most studied in the literature at this time[87] (see Fig. 20.1).

Interestingly, anandamide binds to cannabinoid receptors with higher affinity (it binds with modestly higher affinity at CB_1 receptors in comparison to CB_2) than 2-AG[88] but exhibits only partial agonistic activity at both cannabinoid receptor types. It is, however, a full agonist for the TRPV1 receptor, with research suggesting that anandamide activation of cannabinoid receptors regulates TRPV1 responsiveness and that TRPV1 activation regulates anandamide synthesis postsynaptically.[89]

2-AG

Conversely, 2-AG is the most abundant of the currently studied endocannabinoids[55,90] and is considered a fast retrograde synaptic messenger, with recent evidence indicative that it is the most efficacious endogenous ligand for the cannabinoid receptors and the key endocannabinoid involved in retrograde signalling within the brain.[91–93] It is a full agonist of both CB_1 and CB_2 receptors,[91,94] unlike the only partial agonistic activity of anandamide (see Fig. 20.2).

Within the nervous system, endocannabinoids are currently believed to be synthesised on demand (i.e. in response to injury, ischaemia or stress)[13,55] in an activity-dependent manner by the catabolism of

phospholipid membrane components located within the postsynaptic neuron.[2,25,58,95] Once manufactured, the endocannabinoids exert physiological effects by travelling back across the synaptic cleft and binding to cannabinoid receptors on presynaptic neurons, inhibiting either inhibitory or excitatory neurotransmitters. This action is known as retrograde synaptic flow.

Enzymes

The endocannabinoid system also incorporates a variety of different enzymes that are responsible for the biosynthesis and catabolism of the endogenous lipid-based ligands. The various endocannabinoids, whether anandamide or 2-AG, are manufactured in an activity-dependent manner (i.e. on demand) in a process that is not yet fully understood but seems to be a response to various pathophysiological stimuli.[13,25,84] While this is believed to be the canonical view currently held in the literature, recent research posits that endocannabinoid production and metabolic control may be complemented by intracellular trafficking and storage in specific reservoirs.[96]

Anandamide is synthesised from membrane phospholipid precursors such as N-arachidonoyl phosphatidylethanolamine (NAPE), which is formed by the transfer of arachidonic acid from the *sn*-1 position of a donor phospholipid to phospatidylethanolamine by the calcium-dependent enzyme *N*-acyltransferase (see Fig. 20.3).[13,58] Biosynthesis continues with the hydrolysis of NAPE by the enzyme NAPE-PLD,[97] which produces anandamide.[23,98,99] While this is considered one of the main biosynthetic pathways of anandamide, other alternative biochemical pathways for synthesis have been described in the literature,[100] including enzymes such as α/β-hydrolase domain 4 (ABHD4), protein tyrosine phosphatase, non-receptor type 22 (PTPN22) and glycerophosphodiester phosphodiesterase (GDE1).[13]

The catabolism (i.e. hydrolysis) of anandamide is primarily mediated by the enzyme FAAH,[23,101] which degrades anandamide to arachidonic acid and ethanolamine. Alternatively, anandamide can be oxidised by N-acylethanolamine-hydrolysing acid amidase (NAAA), cytochrome P450 enzymes, lipoxygenases and cyclooxygenase-2.[13]

The more prevalent endocannabinoid, 2-AG, is similarly synthesised from membrane phospholipid precursors (see Fig. 20.4). In contrast, the progenitor compound phosphatidylinositol is degraded to diacylglycerol by the enzyme phospholipase C (PLC) and then to 2-AG by either

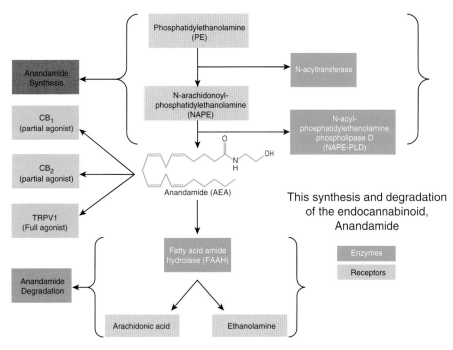

FIGURE 20.3 Anandamide synthesis and degradation

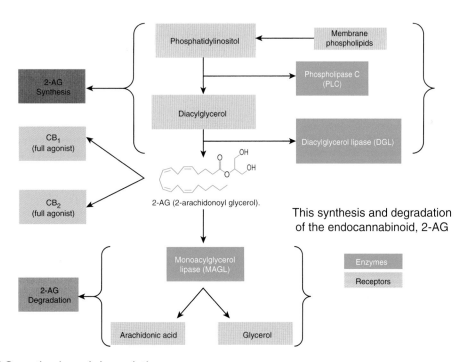

FIGURE 20.4 2-AG synthesis and degradation

diacylglycerol lipase α (DAGL α) or diacylglycerol lipase β (DAGL β).[13]

The catabolism of 2-AG mimics that of anandamide via oxidative processes of the cytochrome P450 enzymes, lipoxygenases and cyclooxygenase-2; however, the specific degrading enzymes are monoacylglycerol lipase (MAGL) and the membrane-associated α/β-hydrolase domain 6 (ABHD6) and α/β-hydrolase domain 12 (ABHD12)

enzymes.[13] End products of enzymatic degradation of 2-AG include arachidonic acid and glycerol.

The diverse and complex enzymatic mechanisms involved in endocannabinoid biological metabolism in vivo are important in maintaining the resting 'tone' of this entire neuromodulatory system.[13,102] This diversity also highlights that the inherent abundance or deficiency of these enzymes in the individual can have dramatic influence over ECS functioning. As such, if the enzymes responsible for endocannabinoid degradation are suppressed experimentally, a prolonged therapeutic activity of the endocannabinoids is achieved, demonstrating another promising target for cannabinoid pharmacotherapy.[2,26]

PHYSIOLOGY OF THE ENDOCANNABINOID SYSTEM

Fundamentally, the ECS is largely responsible for homeostatic regulation and physiological balance. Due to the anatomical distribution of the ECS throughout the brain, spinal cord, enteric and peripheral nervous systems,[2] it plays a pivotal role in regulating a broad list of physiological homeostatic processes including the regulation of stress and emotions, digestion, nociception (i.e. pain),[103] cardiovascular[104] and respiratory function,[105] immune function, neural development, synaptic plasticity and learning, memory, movement, metabolism, energy expenditure and balance, inflammation, appetite regulation, sleep/wake cycles, thermogenesis and psychomotor behaviour.[49,50,106–108] Ongoing research into the scope and influence of the ECS in organ system dysfunction and disease should be a priority, as an evolving evidence base is showing that dysfunction or modulation of this system may be where future breakthroughs in understanding disease aetiology, pathogenesis and treatment reside.

Neurological system

With its ubiquitous distribution throughout the central and peripheral nervous systems, the ECS may play a meaningful role in various neurological pathophysiologies, such as epilepsy. Early studies have demonstrated defects within the ECS in epilepsy patients, with one study showing patients with newly diagnosed temporal lobe epilepsy exhibiting significantly lower levels of anandamide in their cerebrospinal fluid (CSF) in contrast to healthy controls.[40,109] Further supporting the hypothesis that the ECS may play a role in seizure inhibition in epilepsy was a study on resected tissue following surgery for epilepsy, whereby epilepsy patients demonstrated lower levels of CB_1 receptor mRNA expression in the glutamatergic terminals of the dentate gyrus in contrast to postmortem controls of non-epileptic subjects.[40] Interestingly, reduced expression of DAGL α was also found in epilepsy patients, which is the enzyme responsible for 2-AG synthesis postsynaptically.[110]

Reduced levels of anandamide have also been identified in the CSF of patients with chronic migraine,[3,111] with subsequent studies showing the gene encoding for the CB_1 receptor, CNR1, being linked to a chromosomal region linked with migraine,[112] and variations in CNR1 gene expression showing predisposition to higher risk of migraine development.[113] Not surprisingly, a clinical endocannabinoid deficiency (CECD) has been posited[114] as being potentially critical in our pathophysiological understanding of migraine and numerous functional pain conditions, such as irritable bowel syndrome (IBS) and fibromyalgia.[3,114] Conversely, elevated levels of endocannabinoids have been noted within normal and abnormal ECS functioning. Increased anandamide plasma levels (but not 2-AG) have been observed after moderate intensity aerobic activity in healthy individuals,[87,115] changing our previous physiological understanding of the association between 'runner's high' and reward-seeking behaviours.[116]

Additionally, schizophrenia and dysfunction in ECS anatomy and physiology have been observed in the literature. Recent evidence of potential anandamidergic dysfunction has shown markedly increased levels of anandamide in patients with schizophrenia, not only in CSF, but also in plasma, in contrast to healthy controls.[117] Significantly elevated plasma levels of anandamide have been reported in the acute phase of schizophrenia relative to the control group.[118] Moreover, research into the CNR1 gene, which is located on chromosome 6q 14-15, has suggested it may be a susceptibility locus for schizophrenia.[119] SNPs have also been described for the CNR2 gene, which codes for the CB_2 receptor, with researchers suggesting that susceptibility for schizophrenia may be increased by a genetically predetermined decrease in functioning of CB_2 receptors.[117,120]

Other neurological conditions demonstrate a strong coexistent link between neurodegeneration and inflammation, for which the ECS is being implicated in potential treatment options. Conditions such as HIV-associated dementia and multiple sclerosis (MS) represent inflammatory conditions that lead to wide-ranging neuronal damage, while diseases such as amyotrophic lateral sclerosis ALS [MND – motor neuron disease], Parkinson's disease and Alzheimer's disease are classic neurodegenerative diseases with concurrent tissue inflammation.[121] Marsicano and colleagues posit that neuronal injury and the subsequent release of endocannabinoids may be a protective mechanism,[122] with endocannabinoids, various phytocannabinoids and other exogenous cannabinoids demonstrating neuroprotective activity.[25,54,123] Centonze and colleagues describe a multitude of mechanisms that may be at work in achieving this neuroprotective activity, including:

1. The prevention of excitotoxicity by CB_1-receptor-mediated inhibition of glutamate-mediated transmission via the closing of N- and P/Q-type Ca2+ channels
2. A reduction of Ca2+ influx at both the pre- and postsynaptic level, followed by inhibition of subsequent noxious cascades
3. Antioxidant activity (owing to the phenol group present on certain resorcinol-type cannabinoids)
4. Suppression of the production of tumour necrosis factor-α (TNF-α)
5. Activation of protein B pathway and phosphatidylinositol 3-kinase
6. The induction of the expression of transcription factors and neurotrophins.[121]

Both CB_1 and CB_2 receptors have been found to play an important role in neuroprotection and immunomodulation, respectively,[69,124–127] with ongoing research being conducted internationally, particularly in identifying other cannabinoid receptors within the ECS.

Cardiovascular system

With CB_1, CB_2, endocannabinoids and the associated synthetic and degrading enzymes being present in cardiovascular system (CVS) tissue, the ECS can play an important regulatory role in CVS physiology and the development or progression of common CVS disorders.[13,56,57,128] Studies have demonstrated that in cases of heart failure endocannabinoids are produced by activated monocytes, which in turn contribute to the development of hypotension and negative inotropic activity.[56] Further research shows that under pathophysiological conditions, cardiac myocytes and vascular smooth muscle cells can generate endocannabinoids. These can then interact with CB_1 receptors and cause reactive oxygen species and advanced glycation end product accumulation, which, among other physiological mechanisms, can contribute to cell death and injury.[129,130] Interestingly, upregulation of CB_1 receptors and an increase in endocannabinoid expression were noted in the myocardium in these experimental models.[13]

Furthermore, this pro-inflammatory effect of CB_1 receptors in the CVS has been confirmed in knockout (i.e. of the enzyme FAAH) animal testing and using inhibitors in models of cardiomyopathy and atherosclerosis.[13,130] This CB_1 interactivity may pose safety risks, with several case reports showing young adults using cannabis recreationally presenting with CVS problems, but more research is needed to understand the underlying potential risk, the strains of cannabis that may have been used and the potential physiological mechanisms being exploited.[131]

Conversely, CB_2 receptor involvement in the CVS appears to be protective, with activation decreasing pro-inflammatory and fibrotic responses and initiating protective effects in cardiac myocytes.[13,128] CB_2 activation reduces immune cell chemotaxis, inflammatory cell adhesion and cellular activation, which appears to be behind the protective effects in preclinical models of myocardial infarction, stroke, restenosis and atherosclerosis.[128]

While a great deal more research into the influence of the ECS over CVS function and pathophysiology is required, it is clear that ECS dysfunction is present (particularly CB_1 overactivity) in various CVS diseases and that CB_1 antagonists and CB_2 agonists are of great clinical interest in pharmacotherapy for specific CVS disorders and conditions.[13]

Gastrointestinal tract

As previously mentioned, both CB_1 and CB_2 receptors are widely distributed throughout the GIT, being highly expressed on enteric nerves and intestinal mucosa. CB_1 receptors are specifically present on enteroendocrine cells, immune cells and enterocytes, whereas CB_2 expression is mostly observed on immune cells and enterocytes.[13] Recent research has highlighted a novel mechanism of ECS regulation within the GIT involving the endocannabinoids, primarily 2-AG. While 2-AG is a fast retrograde messenger in neuronal tissue of the brain, within the enteric nervous system it undertakes a previously unknown form of synaptic control involving 2-AG and a purine nucleotide,

which work in opposite directions to control synaptic strength[13] and tone. This system has been described as metaplasticity[132] and has reinforced our understanding of the relationship between the GIT and the CNS, showing that virtually all GIT function is regulated by the ECS and that this may lay the foundation for the neuromodulatory control of metabolic and homeostatic functions of the body.[13]

Primarily, the ECS is involved in the regulation of nausea, vomiting, food intake and energy,[133] hunger,[134] gastric secretions and gastroprotection, GI motility,[135,136] visceral sensation, ion transport, intestinal inflammation,[137,138] intestinal barrier protection[139] and normal cellular proliferation in the GIT.[140] Most endocannabinoid activity in the GIT is mediated by CB_1 receptors under normal physiological conditions, with mesenteric vasodilation, acid suppression, motility stimulation and fluid secretion being examples.[140] With a growing research base demonstrating the connection between a balanced intestinal microbiota and normalised immune, GIT and neurological functioning, it may not surprise many in the naturopathic or herbal fields to read that CB_1 expression on enterocytes is regulated by the enteric microbiota, with CB_1 activation increasing epithelial permeability by reduced expression of tight gap junction proteins, permitting bacterial translocation and potential metabolic endotoxaemia[13,139] as sequelae. Blocking CB_1 expression therefore may help normalise intestinal barrier function and has also been investigated for reducing obesity.[13] Conversely, CB_2 activation within the GIT can exert a normalising activity in instances of increased gastric motility observed in specific GIT conditions.[136]

While an accessory organ of digestion, the liver is also firmly enmeshed in ECS physiology. Both CB_1 and CB_2 receptors are found in the liver. CB_1 receptors are located primarily in stellate cells, hepatocytes and vascular endothelial cells, whereas CB_2 receptors are expressed on immune cells, Kupffer cells and myofibroblasts.[13]

Activation of the CB_1 receptor in the liver promotes vasodilation, which can lead to the development of ascites and increases fat accumulation (fatty liver), insulin resistance[141] and fibrosis.[13] CB_2 opposes such changes, reduces cytokine production, is anti-inflammatory (via induction of haemoxygenase-1 switching Kupffer cells from a pro-inflammatory M1 phenotype to an anti-inflammatory M2 phenotype), minimises reperfusion injury,[142] is antifibrotic [143,144] and reduces fatty deposition in the liver.[13]

This growing understanding of the neuromodulatory role of the ECS and the GIT paves the way to a new perception of gut-specific pathology. Conditions such as IBS,[8] coeliac disease[145] and inflammatory bowel diseases show patterns of ECS dysfunction or alteration.[146] With CB_1 and CB_2 receptors and endocannabinoids distributed throughout the enteric nervous system and GIT, and physiological actions that regulate gastric hormone and enteric neurotransmitter release, suppress immune activation and regulate intestinal permeability,[13] the likelihood that continuing research in this field will unearth new understandings of GIT disease aetiology and pathogenesis is highly plausible.

Immune system

As has been demonstrated, CB_2 expression predominates in immune cells, particularly CD4+ T-cells, CD8+ T-cells, B-cells, NK cells, macrophages, monocytes and neutrophils. A growing research base shows that anandamide may inhibit immune function by reducing the production of pro-inflammatory cytokines, whereas 2-AG acting through CB_2 receptors may inhibit the migratory activities of certain immune cells by modulating various pathways.[13,147] Of particular interest is that studies have shown anandamide reduced IL-6 and IL-8 in human monocytes while also suppressing the release of IL-2, TNF-α and IFN-γ from activated T lymphocytes, the latter via CB_2 receptors.[13,148,149] While more focused human research is needed, a growing body of case study reports in the US suggests that cannabinoid-based therapies may be of benefit in autoimmune, neurodegenerative and neuroinflammatory disorders.

While the main focus of this physiological review of the ECS has targeted the larger regulatory systems, evidence exists to show the ECS functioning in a modulatory or regulatory capacity in the skin, muscles, bone and respiratory and reproductive systems. Maccarrone and colleagues provide an excellent review of these systems and ECS involvement.[13,85]

THE ECS AND CLINICAL CHALLENGES

There are various clinical challenges in using cannabinoid-based pharmacotherapy for ECS modulation. While certainly not insurmountable, they may require a deviation away from the 'one size fits all' pharmaceutical and clinical medical model, to rather embrace a more holistic focus on personalised medicine for the individual. Such deviation can use the latest technological advancements in genetic and biochemical testing to identify mutations and imbalances, respectively, in the individual and therefore allow for accurate dosage titration and even specific cannabis strain or extract selection to develop a patient-centred, customised and highly personalised focus to disease and symptom management.

Clinical endocannabinoid deficiency

As already noted, research evidence, along with expert academic and clinical opinion, suggests that a CECD may be a plausible aetiology behind various medical conditions and diseases.[150] In 2008, Russo posited that conditions such as migraine, fibromyalgia and IBS could be due to a CECD.[150] While this is in itself of clinical importance in order to elicit greater understanding of disease aetiology, pathophysiology and potential treatment options for many conditions of unknown cause, perhaps just as important is that it highlights that certain individual differences in endocannabinoid expression may be an important consideration in treatment. The plasma or CSF levels of the various endocannabinoids can be measured to potentially identify ECS involvement and allow for modification or inclusion of various cannabinoid-based therapies, particularly for conditions where current treatment options are resistant.

Receptor expression and genetic polymorphisms

Not only can individuals express endocannabinoids at differing levels, but also the receptors they bind to are an important clinical consideration. *CNR1* and *CNR2* SNPs have been identified, potentially affecting individual receptor expression (up-regulation or down-regulation). Of particular interest is CB_1 receptor gene SNPs and various halotypes. While their importance is still a matter of debate, suggestions that such modifications could increase susceptibility to neuropsychiatric conditions could be plausible.[2,60] Such individual expression could therefore affect both the functional tone of the ECS and how cannabinoid-based therapeutics affect the individual.

ECS enzyme variability

While individual receptor expression and endocannabinoid levels are certainly well-established variables that could impact ECS tone and function, so too is any ECS-specific enzyme abundance or deficiency. Endocannabinoids may be affected by innate genetic aberrations or a lack of nutritional components required for their biosynthesis or degradation. Their synthesis and degradation are enzymatically controlled by enzymes such as FAAH, PLC, NAPE and MAGL, identifying yet another potential variable that could impact functional ECS tone and alter cannabinoid-based pharmacotherapy.

As can be seen, key to understanding the ECS and its role in homeostatic regulatory mechanisms is that every individual expresses this neuromodulatory system with slight differences. Other variables that need to be considered are age-related changes to organ function as well as individual expression of cytochrome P450 enzymes and pharmacokinetic metabolic biotransformation of key therapeutic constituents of cannabinoid-based pharmacotherapy. The latter aspect is discussed in greater detail later in the chapter.

> *All truth passes through three stages.*
> *First, it is ridiculed.*
> *Second, it is violently opposed.*
> *Third, it is accepted as being self-evident.*
> *Arthur Schopenhauer (1788–1860)*

THE GENUS *CANNABIS*

The Cannabaceae family (order Rosales) is a relatively small family of flowering plants encompassing around 11 genera and 170 different species.[151] The *Cannabis* genus encompasses several species that have been highly prized since ancient times for use as a medicine[152] or foodstuff[153] and in textile and cordage production.[154–157] The psychoactive effects of the plant have also seen it used in various spiritual and shamanistic practices and rituals throughout the ages.[158,159]

History of use

The inflorescences, seeds, leaves, stems, glandular trichomes and roots of the cannabis plant have been a valuable commodity and medicine to humans for millennia. The plant is believed to have originated in central Asia,[160,161] with 20th-century scholars placing the centre of *Cannabis* genus diversity in a region extending from the Pamir plain of Tajikistan and bordering Afghanistan, Kyrgyzstan and the Xinjiang region of Western China.[162] However, more recent ethnobotanical modelling suggests it originated in the Himalayan mountains from Kashmir to Nepal and into Bhutan and Burma,[161,163,164] and probably spread from there through human use and trade. Specific psychoactive strains, most likely the broadleaf drug variety *Cannabis indica* subspp. *afghanica*, which is rich in THC, originated in the latter region, spreading through China, India, the Middle East and regions of Northern Africa via established trade routes. The seeds of this subspecies and others would have been highly valued for their medicinal qualities and enabled the spread and cultivation of the plant, as well as its own hybridisation and evolution, across the ancient world. A more detailed review of the ethnobotany of the *Cannabis* genus and its evolution is provided in Clarke and Merlin, for example.[161]

Determining the exact time that our hominoid ancestors started using *Cannabis* spp. is difficult to quantify due to the fact that its cultivation, use and consumption most probably predated currently accepted archaeological timelines for the appearance of writing in human evolution.[160] Some of the earliest evidence of human usage of *Cannabis* spp. is as a fibre in a net made by the Gravettians, an Upper Palaeolithic industrial culture situated throughout Europe.[165] Primarily hunters and gatherers, hunting nets made from cannabis fibre used by these people have been dated between 24 980 and 22 870 BCE.[166] Ethnobotanical evidence from Taiwan Province of China posits that cannabis was used as a fibre some 10 000 years ago.[167] More recent archaeological evidence suggests that various *Cannabis* spp. have been used since the late Neolithic period (4000–2000 BCE) throughout Asia as a medicine, fibre crop, food and entheogen,[159,168,169] while several respected scholars believe it has been used for at least 10 millennia or possibly longer as a medicine.[155,161,168]

Cannabis was a valuable medicine in many cultures in the ancient world. The use of cannabis as a medicine in China was first attributed to the Chinese Emperor Shen Nung (ca. 2700 BCE),[157,160,170] based on the *Shen-nung Pen-tsao Ching* (Divine Husbandman's *Materia Medica*). Similar evidence has been found in the written histories of India, the *Atharvaveda* (1500 BCE) and *Sushruta Samhita* (800–300 BCE).[171,172] Confirmation of the therapeutic use of cannabis also exists from Persia (600 BCE), found in the *Zend-Avesta*,[172] and Egypt from written evidence[173] encoded within stone in the *Pyramid Texts* from Memphis (2350 BCE)[162] and later in the *Papyrus Ramesseum III* (1799 BCE), *Hearst Papyrus* (ca. 1550 BCE), *Ebers Papyrus* (ca. 1550 BCE) and *Berlin Papyrus* (1300 BCE).[162] Because of established trade routes within Asia and the Middle East, this knowledge spread throughout the Mediterranean

too, with the Greek historian Herodotus (ca. 484–425 BCE) writing of cannabis use by the Scythians in the 5th century BCE.[167] The classic Greek herbalists Dioscorides, Galen and Pliny[153] wrote of the medicinal virtues of this plant in detail, with Dioscorides describing the plant in his magnum opus, *De Materia Medica*, which was used throughout the world as a foundational medicinal text for almost 1500 years.

Numerous Arabic physicians wrote about cannabis in managing various pathologies, including Ibn al-Baytar, Ishaq Ibn Sulayman[162] and the famous Avicenna, Ibn Sina, who wrote of it in the *Canon of Medicine* (ca. 1025 CE). While deemed an inebriant and forbidden under Islam recreationally, cannabis was nonetheless still revered as a medicine. With the Muslim conquest of the Iberian peninsula (i.e. Spain and Portugal) in the 7th century, and later parts of North Africa, *Cannabis* spp. probably spread to places such as Northern Morocco,[174] where it currently inhabits large regions such as the Rif Mountains. From here it could have spread through Western Europe.

Credited with bringing *Cannabis* spp. into Western medicine, the Irish doctor William B. O'Shaughnessy (1809–1889) was an assistant surgeon contracted to the East India Company. He became fascinated with the therapeutic benefits of the *Cannabis* genus while in India, identifying antiemetic, appetite stimulant, analgesic, muscle relaxant and anticonvulsant actions.[160] He took this information back to London and was elected into the Royal Society as a Fellow for his contributions to science.

Following this, cannabis swept through European dispensaries, being used in patent medicines and as a 'simple', and included in the United States Dispensatory in 1854.[175] This continued throughout most of the developed world until problems with lack of standardisation, quality assurance and an inability to accurately titrate dose hampered its use in a growing scientific evidence-based medical profession in the early to mid-20th century.[162] In 1937 the passing of the Marijuana Tax Act (US) effectively made cannabis use illegal, even though this was opposed by the American Medical Association at the time. This eventually led to *Cannabis* spp. being classified as a Schedule 1 drug of addiction in accordance with the Controlled Substances Act (US), and international laws prohibited its trade and use soon after. It is only now, in certain international jurisdictions, and after isolating many of the key phytochemicals within the various *Cannabis* species, that this herbal medicine is being reintroduced to the medical armamentarium and is gaining acceptance once more.

Botany and morphology

Cannabis and its relevant species (*Cannabis indica*, *Cannabis sativa*, *Cannabis ruderalis*) and subspecies of medicinal interest are annual, herbaceous (i.e. green-stemmed), dicotyledonous (i.e. possesses a taproot), dioecious (i.e. female and male reproductive parts occur on separate plants) flowering plants (angiosperms) (see Fig. 20.5).[10,161,176] Rarely, *Cannabis* spp. may exhibit monoecious characteristics (i.e. male and female reproductive parts occur on the same plant), but true hermaphrodism is uncommon.

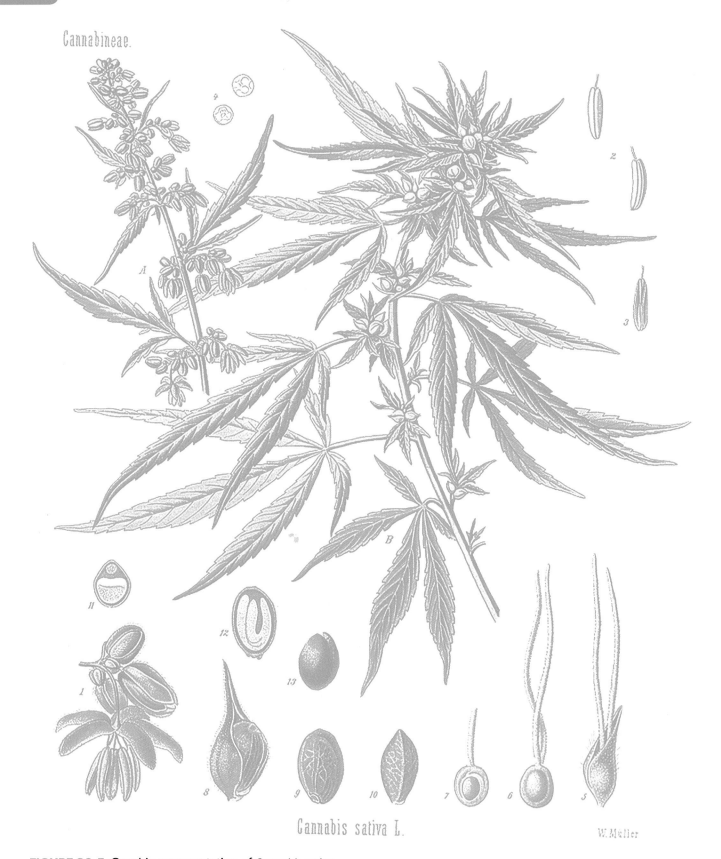

FIGURE 20.5 Graphic representation of *Cannabis sativa*

Franz Eugen Köhler's Medizinal-Pflantzen. Published and copyrighted by Gera-Untermhaus, FE Köhler in 1887 (1883–1914). Obtained from http://caliban. mpiz-koeln.mpg.de/~stueber/koehler.

Morphologically, *Cannabis* spp. exhibit a strong taproot (dependent on plant size and genetics) between 120 and 240 mm deep, with a strong erect stem, which is roughly round to hexagonal in cross-section.[10] The stem is usually 1–3 m tall and often hollow, with male plants typically being less tall and robust than female plants.[10] Leaves exhibit opposite or alternate petiolate attachment with the characteristic palmately compound leaf arrangement comprising 5–11 leaflets, they are typically lanceolate to linear in shape and the leaf margin is serrate, terminating in an acuminate apex.[10] The part of medicinal interest is the unfertilised female inflorescence, which is typically green (occasionally red or purple depending on genetics) and sessile. Proximal surfaces of the bract are covered in capitate glandular trichomes.[10] The bracteole is covered with resinous glandular trichomes and the calyx measures 2–6 mm in length and contains the ovary which produces the fruit (seed),[161] which is an achene.[10] A full botanical and morphological description of the *Cannabis* genus is beyond the scope of this textbook. For further information, the American Herbal Pharmacopoeia monograph on *Cannabis inflorescence*[10] is highly recommended as being authoritative on the subject.

Taxonomy and nomenclature

The taxonomic classification of the *Cannabis* genus has undergone considerable and rigorous academic and legal debate over the last 100 years[177] based on the necessity to provide a scientifically acceptable statement not only to confirm the orientation and hierarchy of the *Cannabis* genus taxonomically, but also to potentially identify lawful versus illicit species for legal commercial use.[165] Emerging scientific fields such as plant genetics and chemotaxonomy have been added to the arsenal of traditional botanical studies of taxonomy and morphology, enabling detailed analysis of the plant. The evolution of this contentious taxonomic debate has up until recently embraced two major models for the *Cannabis* genus, believing that it exhibits either monotypic (single species) or polytypic (multiple species) characteristics.[10,153,155]

Cannabis sativa was first described by Carl Linnaeus in 1753,[10,165] setting up a single species orientation for the genus. Some 32 years later, French biologist Jean Lamarck challenged the single species convention by describing *Cannabis indica*, which exhibited very different morphological characteristics from *C. sativa*, such as poor bast fibre (phloem), smaller leaves, narrower leaflets, shorter habit and greater use as an inebriant (i.e. psychoactivity).[10] By 1849, Delile had described a new species from China named *Cannabis chinensis* and later in 1851 described another species *Cannabis gigantea*.[165,178] Russian botanist Dmitri Janischewsky described a new species named *Cannabis ruderalis* in 1924, and later in 1929 Vavilov and Bukinich named a new variety of *Cannabis indica var kafiristanica*.[10,165]

With a growing body of botanical evidence, between 1974 and 1980 Schultes[155,179] and Anderson[180] undertook reviews finding evidence supporting the polytypic model, yet Small and Cronquist[181] analysed 350 worldwide accessions in a common garden experiment in 1976

positing that only one polymorphic species, *C. sativa*, existed. Finally, in 2005 genetic and phytochemical evidence was brought to bear in this growing taxonomic argument by Hillig[182] using cannabinoid[183] and terpene profiles[184] as well as host–parasite data.[10] Findings included the recognition of a *sativa* gene pool inclusive of seed- and fibre-rich landraces located in Central Asia and Europe, an *indica* gene pool rich in cannabinoids originating from Pakistan, Afghanistan, South America, Southern Asia and Africa, and a third *ruderal* gene pool from ruderal accessions in Central Asia.[10] This has been further expanded by Clarke and Merlin,[161] based on the work by Hillig, classifying the various *Cannabis* spp. into different biotypes, as shown in Table 20.1.

McPartland[185] has since proposed a revised nomenclature at the 2014 meeting of the International Cannabinoid Research Society. The extensive crossbreeding practices by breeders and natural cross-pollination[10] make accurate botanical identification difficult, and while the introduction of genetics into the taxonomic discussion has certainly increased knowledge, this new nomenclature is not yet universally accepted academically. The International Code of Nomenclature for Cultivated Plants has suggested that a cultonomic, rather than purely botanical, differentiation of nomenclature may be more appropriate in modern applications, as it is based on economically or medicinally important characteristics such as a THC drug group, the cannabidiol (CBD) drug group or fibre-hemp groups.[10]

Less contentious are the common names associated with *Cannabis* spp. and its products, including ganja, hemp, kif, marijuana, bhang, weed, hashish (i.e. pure

TABLE 20.1 Different *Cannabis* spp. gene pools (biotypes)

Biotype	Latin binomial	Range	Uses
PA	*Cannabis ruderalis*	North Central Asia	Seed and fibre
NLHA	*C. sativa* subspp. *spontanea*	Eastern Europe and Central Asia	Seed and fibre
NLH	*C. sativa* subspp. *sativa*	Europe	Seed and fibre
BLH	*C. indica* subspp. *chinensis*	China, Korea, Japan, Southeast Asia	Seed and fibre
NLDA	*C. indica* subspp. *kafiristanica*	Himalayan foothills	Drug/hashish
NLD	*C. indica* subspp. *indica*	Southeast Asia, Middle East	Drug/hashish/seed and fibre
BLD	*C. indica* subspp. *afghanica*	Afghanistan and Pakistan	Drug/hashish

PA, putative ancestor; NLHA, narrow-leaf hemp ancestor; NLH, narrow-leaf hemp; BLH, broad-leaf hemp; NLDA, narrow-leaf drug ancestor; NLD, narrow-leaf drug; BLD, broad-leaf drug.
Source: Adapted from Clarke R, Merlin MD. Cannabis evolution and ethnobotany. Berkeley, CA: University of California Press; 2013

glandular trichomes), pot, grass, dagga, charas and sinsemilla (i.e. female, unfertilised inflorescence only).[10,161]

Cultivation and growth cycle

Cannabis sativa and *Cannabis indica* are known to be affected by photoperiodism, which is defined as the developmental response or physiological reaction of a plant to the relative length of the daylight cycle. The growth cycle of *Cannabis* spp. is quite unique. During spring and summer months, when sunlight exposure is approximately 15–18 hours per day (depending on geographical location), the plants undertake vegetative growth. During this phase, they maximise growth of the leaves to produce carbohydrates through photosynthesis, which provides the fuel to increase the growth and vitality of the plant. As the sunlight wanes and reduces in length in autumn and winter, dropping down to 10–12 hours per day,[161] this initiates the process of flowering, which is the main morphological structure of interest medicinally. Conversely, *Cannabis ruderalis* produces inflorescences based on its age, not light exposure – a flowering process known as autoflowering.[165] As such, this species is favoured among certain social growers who know little about the select needs of the plant. The time from seedling to harvest is typically 75 days. Of particular interest is that *Cannabis ruderalis* is seen as being the species exhibiting the lowest profile of phytochemicals of specific medicinal interest, and is seen as inferior to *Cannabis indica* and *Cannabis sativa* and associated hybrids/phenotypes.

This understanding of photoperiodism and the regulation of light has enabled cannabis to be grown indoors, a popular method of cultivation in jurisdictions where medicinal and social cannabis use is legal and consistent sunlight is difficult to obtain. Indoor cultivation also enables the tight regulation of factors such as humidity and temperature that optimise phytocannabinoid and terpene production. Growers also use technology that is designed to replicate the sun's UV spectrum by using lights that emit high photosynthetic photon flux density (PPFD). Through the specific use of fluorescent, metal halide, high-pressure sodium and light-emitting diode technology,[165] plants can grow quickly, but whether these forms of technology can ever truly replicate the broad spectrum of photons available, for free, from the sun is currently a matter of scientific investigation and debate. Indoor operations use large amounts of energy to power the lighting and cooling systems, which increases costs and contributes to greenhouse gas emissions, therefore making outdoor cultivation or the use of greenhouses with supplemental lighting a more environmentally sustainable and cost-effective option to optimise net clinical and economic benefit.

In modern cannabis cultivation, unfertilised female inflorescences (florets) are considered to have the highest concentration of tetrahydocannabinolic acid (THCA), which can be converted into the psychoactive and medicinally potent THC and its derivatives through the use of heat, drying and curing.[10] Numerous other cannabinoids and terpenes are located within the glandular trichomes of the inflorescence.[8] As such, it is common horticultural practice to use female clones[165] from a mother plant, which will be phytochemically and genetically identical if growing conditions are optimally stable. Male plants, once identified after a relatively short period of propagation from seed, are removed early so that they cannot release pollen, which would send female flowers in the surrounding environment to seed and thus reduce the phytochemical concentration of medicinally active constituents.

Cannabis phytochemistry

The various species and strains of the *Cannabis* genus exhibit complex secondary metabolites that can be used as therapeutic agents. Currently researchers have identified more than 750 different phytochemical constituents[10] from *Cannabis* spp., many of which are located within the specialised glandular trichomes found on the inflorescence of the plant. ElSohly describes a broad spectrum of phytochemical constituents within the plant, including phytocannabinoids (i.e. plant-derived cannabinoids),[5] terpenes, flavonoids, nitrogenous compounds (i.e. alkaloids), amino acids, glycoproteins, enzymes, hydrocarbons, alcohols, aldehydes, ketones, fatty acids, steroids, phenols (non-cannabinoid) and vitamins.[186]

Of greatest clinical interest since phytochemical research has been undertaken on the plant are the cannabinoids. Cannabinoid concentration within the plant depends largely on the genetics (genotype), sex and senescence of the plant, but many environmental variables such as light exposure, light intensity, temperature, elevation, soil pH and soil mineral concentration play an important role.[10,176,187,188] To date, more than 66 cannabinoids[5,186,189–193] have been identified, belonging to several subclasses, of which the cannabigerol (CBG) type, cannabichromene (CBC) type, THC type, CBD type, Δ^8-tetrahydrocannabinol (delta-8-THC) type, cannabinol (CBN) type and cannabinidiol (CBDL) type exist.[5,186,194] The CBN and CBDL types are viewed as being artefacts of oxidation of the parent compounds THC and CBD, respectively.[186,195] All cannabinoids, along with the terpene class, undergo biosynthesis and storage within the glandular trichomes of the plant.[10]

Structurally, the cannabinoids are terpeno-phenolic compounds derived from the enzymatic condensation of both a terpene moiety (i.e. geranyl pyrophosphate) and a phenolic moiety (i.e. generally olivetolic or diverinic acid).[196] This is catalysed by the enzyme geranylpyro-phosphate:olivetolate geranyltransferase (GOT) and produces the progenitor compound cannabigerolic acid (CBGA), from which the major cannabinoid acids are derived.[197] Cannabidiolic acid (CBDA), Δ^9-tetrahydrocannabinolic acid (THCA) and cannabichromenic acid (CBCA) are the main acidic cannabinoids produced from the oxidocyclisation of CBGA by the independent enzymes, CBDA-synthase, THCA-synthase and CBCA-synthase, respectively.[10,196] See Fig. 20.6.

Cannabinoids have certain chemical characteristics that are considered pharmacologically important. Of primary interest is that the cannabinoids are stored in a carboxylated (i.e. COOH) form within the plant, making them cannabinoid acids and devoid of any psychoactive pharmacological effects.[196] This carboxylic acid group is

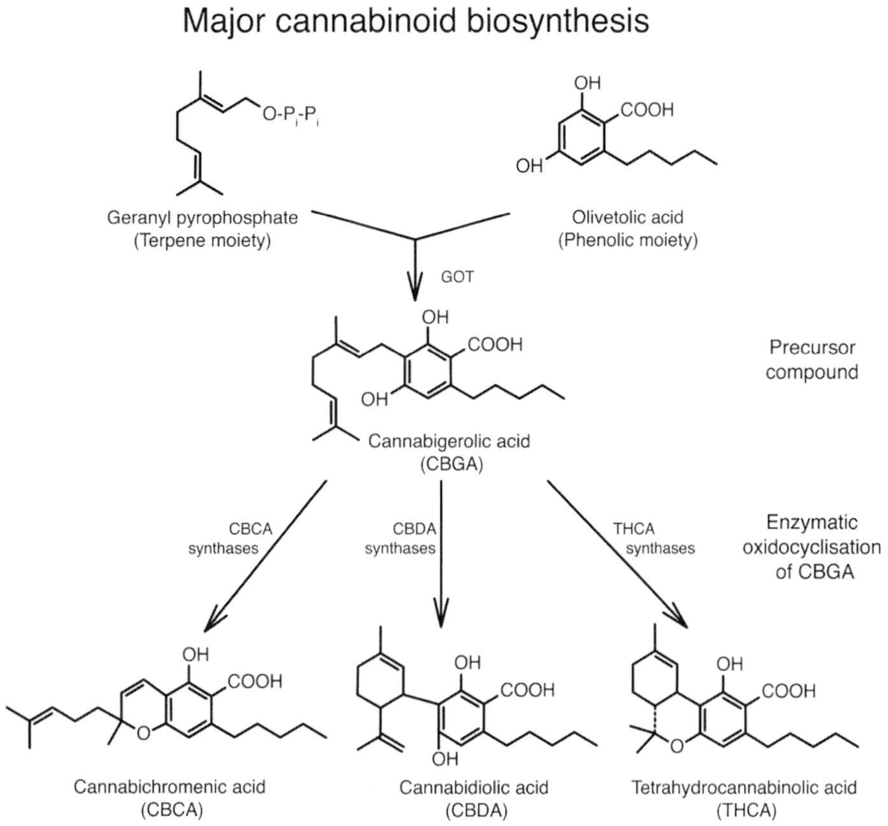

Major cannabinoid biosynthesis

FIGURE 20.6 Cannabinoid biosynthesis

Adapted from Giacoppo S, Mandolino G, Galuppo M, et al. Cannabinoids: new promising agents in the treatment of neurological diseases. Molecules 2014;19(11):18781–816.

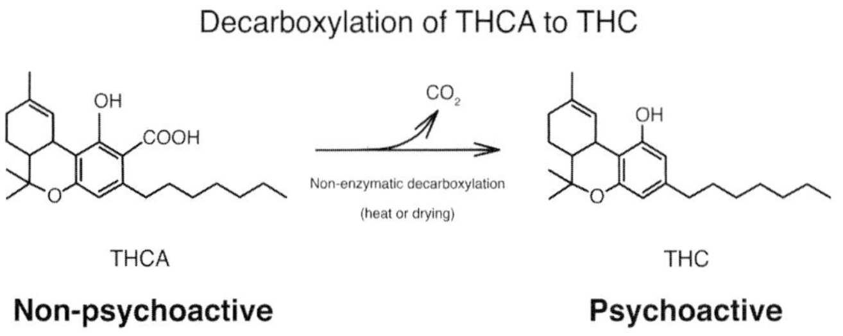

FIGURE 20.7 The decarboxylation process

Adapted from Giacoppo S, Mandolino G, Galuppo M, et al. Cannabinoids: new promising agents in the treatment of neurological diseases. Molecules 2014;19(11):18781–816.

attached to the phenolic ring of the cannabinoid acid structure[196] and stops the phytochemical from binding to cannabinoid receptors. It is only through exposure to drying or heat that decarboxylation takes place[10,196] and the various cannabinoid acids are converted into their active forms and can thus interact with receptors (see Fig. 20.7).

Secondly, the alkyl group positioned at the third carbon atom is deemed an important site for substrate/receptor interactions.[10] In the case of major cannabinoids such as THC, CBG, CBD and CBN, this is typically a pentyl group (C5), but it can also extend to being a propyl group

(C3).[198] In such cases, the suffix 'varin' is added to the original pentylated analogue,[10] for example cannabivarin (CBV), cannabigerovarin (CBGV), cannabidivarin (CBDV) and tetrahydrocannabivarin (THCV), each of which exerts its own pharmacological activity (see Fig. 20.8),[199,200] but these are much less researched than the major cannabinoids.

Based on their unique structure, cannabinoids are highly lipophilic, which enables them to both cross the blood–brain barrier and penetrate cellular membranes,[10] allowing many different phytochemical dosage forms to be used in clinical practice. The various major cannabinoids and other phytochemical classes are discussed in more detail below.

DELTA-9-THC

Having been first discovered in 1964, it is not surprising that there is a large amount of research on this cannabinoid in the literature. Once THCA undergoes decarboxylation, it produces the active compound THC (see Fig. 20.9). Interestingly, THCA is not just a simple progenitor compound, but has been shown to be a TRPA1 partial agonist and a TRPM8 antagonist, both potentially suggestive of a role in analgesia.[201]

THC is a partial agonist[200,202] at both the CB$_1$ and the CB$_2$ receptors with relatively high affinity, expressing similarity to the endogenous cannabinoid

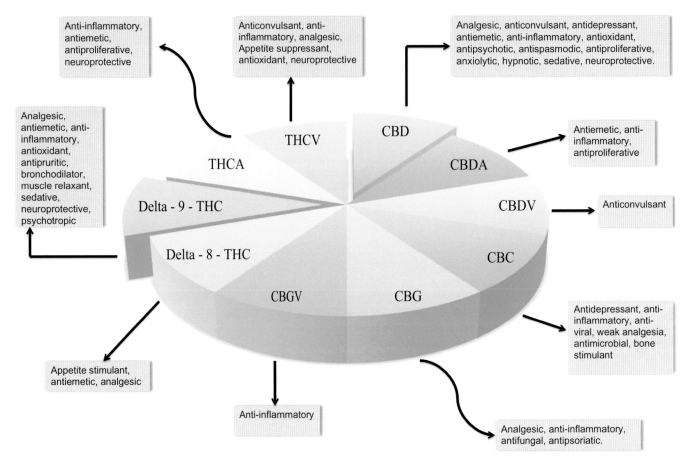

FIGURE 20.8 List of actions associated with the cannabinoids.

Russo EB. Taming THC: potential cannabis synergy and phytocannabinoid-terpenoid entourage effects. Br J Pharmacol 2011;163(7):1344–64. Upton R, ElSohly M, Romm A, et al (eds). Cannabis inflorescence. Scotts Valley, CA: American Herbal Pharmacopoeia; 2013. Elsohly MA, Slade D. Chemical constituents of marijuana: the complex mixture of natural cannabinoids. Life Sci 2005;78(5):539–48. Howard P, Twycross R, Shuster J, et al. Cannabinoids. J Pain Symptom Manage 2013;46(1):142–9.

FIGURE 20.9 THC structure

anandamide.[8,10,203,204] Interacting with the CB_1 receptor, THC is the main psychoactive phytochemical contained within drug varieties of *Cannabis* spp.; however, its main active metabolite after absorption is 11-OH-THC (11-hydroxy-THC), which is more potent therapeutically[5,200] and has higher permeability for the blood–brain barrier. Of interest is that 11-OH-THC is found in higher amounts after oral ingestion due to liver biotransformation than for inhalant methods of administration.

A wide range of therapeutic activity has been described for THC in the literature, including analgesic,[106,205] anti-inflammatory, antioxidant, neuroprotective,[206] muscle relaxant,[207] bronchodilatory,[208] antipruritic,[209] anticancer,[210–216] appetite stimulant and antiemetic actions.[8,217] Such pharmacological activity makes it clinically useful for many different indications, including neuropathic pain,[218,219] migraine,[3] cancer pain,[220,221] chemotherapy-induced nausea and vomiting,[222] chronic pain,[223] weight loss in cancer and AIDS patients (i.e. as an appetite-promoting agent),[224] spinal cord injury,[225] postsurgical pain and phantom limb pain.[10] It also holds value for the management of various neurological disorders such as multiple sclerosis (i.e. muscle spasticity)[226] and Alzheimer's disease,[227] and can lower intraocular pressure in glaucoma.[228] THC exhibits significant anti-inflammatory activity, which may be a mechanism of action of great therapeutic interest, particularly in neurological degenerative disorders (and when combined with other cannabinoids such as CBD),[196] with studies suggesting that THC has 20 times the anti-inflammatory power of aspirin and twice the strength of hydrocortisone.[8,229]

THC is not without adverse effects, however. In numerous clinical studies it has been shown to produce central effects such as anxiety, restlessness and dysphoria

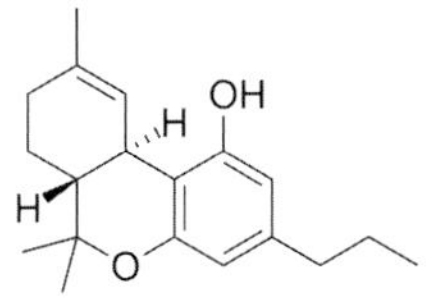

FIGURE 20.10 THCV structure

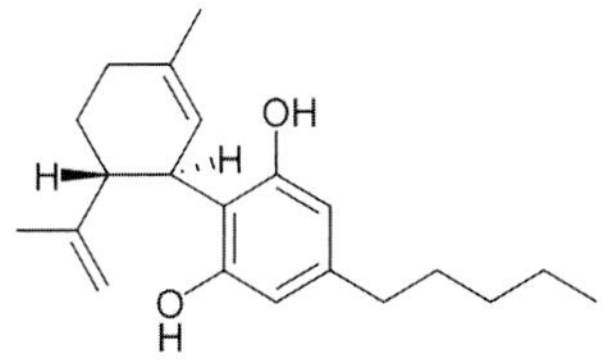

FIGURE 20.11 CBD structure

in certain individuals or at high dose. Interestingly, when administered with other cannabinoids, particularly CBD, this can be mitigated.

THCV

Belonging to the THC cannabinoid type subclass, THCV is the propyl (CH_2—CH_2—CH_3) homologue of THC,[10] but lacks major psychoactive effects. Unlike THC, which is derived from CBGA, THCV is derived when geranyl pyrophosphate binds with divarinolic acid to produce cannabigerovarin acid (CBGVA). Divarinolic acid has two fewer carbon atoms and therefore makes THCV propyl instead of pentyl like THC, CBD, CBG and CBN.[10] CBGVA is then broken down via THCV synthase to tetrahydrocannabivarin carboxylic acid, and in a similar decarboxylation process to CBD and THC via exposure to heat or drying, degrades to THCV (see Fig. 20.10).

Generally, THCV occurs in cannabis in small concentrations, although plant breeding projects are aiming to soon correct this. THCV is a CB_1 antagonist at low doses,[230] but with high doses it can act as an agonist at both the CB_1 and the CB_2 receptors.[10,231] Research is currently being conducted into its potential appetite suppressant action, with preliminary data suggesting that it can produce weight loss and decreased body fat in animal models.[232] Research has shown anticonvulsant, euphoric, anti-inflammatory and analgesic properties for THCV, as well as antioxidant and neuroprotective effects.[10,231]

CBD

CBD is a non-psychoactive cannabinoid with a well-established safety profile[201] that is derived from CBDA once decarboxylation has taken place. Next to THC, it is the most extensively studied cannabinoid, particularly in recent times in the field of epilepsy and other neurological conditions. Intriguingly, CBD displays very little affinity for cannabinoid receptors, which probably contributes to its lack of psychotropic activity.[233] As such, emphasis has focused on non-cannabinoid receptor interactivity for CBD, with research demonstrating that it is an agonist at serotonin ($5\text{-}HT_{1A}$) receptors and TRPV1 and TRPV2 receptors,[233–235] while also enhancing the activity of $\alpha 1$ and $\alpha 3$ glycine receptors, the transient receptor potential of ankyrin type 1 (TRPA1) channel and PPAR-γ (i.e. at a higher concentration). CBD has been found to be a blocker of the equilibrative nucleoside transporter (ENT) GPR55[236] and the transient receptor potential of melastatin type 8 (TRPM8) channel.[233] This diversity and complexity, along with its unique polyphenolic structure (see Fig. 20.11), makes it both a potent antioxidant and a truly unique multi-target phytochemical.[233]

CBD is an antagonist of cannabinoid receptors agonists and has been found to reduce the psychoactivity of THC when co-administered, reducing symptoms such as paranoia, dysphoria and anxiety,[237–242] while also potentiating THC's beneficial effects to enhance its tolerability and broaden its therapeutic scope.[233,243] This phytochemical synergy is discussed later in more detail and is what researchers are terming the 'entourage effect'. It provides a theory as to why full-spectrum extracts maximising various cannabinoids (and other phytochemicals such as terpenes) may be more effective therapeutically than single active synthetic or naturally derived isolates.

With a broad array of interactivity at various receptors, CBD has an equally wide scope therapeutically. CBD has well-researched anti-inflammatory activity, and it has been suggested that it can enhance adenosine signalling by inhibiting adenosine inactivation.[236] Adenosine A_{2A} receptors can down-regulate immune cell over-reactivity, which can protect from inflammatory damage and pain. While CBD is a potent anti-inflammatory,[244] it also exhibits significant neuroprotective,[25] antioxidant,[245] immunomodulatory,[25] anticonvulsive,[246] antipsychotic,[10,247–249] anxiolytic,[250] antidepressant,[192] hypnotic, sedative, anticancer,[251–256] analgesic and antiemetic activity.[10]

Due to a well-established safety and tolerability profile, along with absent psychoactivity, CBD is an incredibly promising agent in a number of medical conditions, particularly neurological conditions. Evidence and research are supportive of the application of CBD therapeutically in conditions such as multiple sclerosis,[25,257] epilepsy,[233,246,258–260] psychosis/schizophrenia,[249,261,262] Huntington's disease, Parkinson's disease, amyotrophic lateral sclerosis[263] and neurodegenerative diseases such as Alzheimer's disease,[264] although more research needs to be conducted across many of these conditions to fully understand the mechanisms of action and CBD's therapeutic potential. Interestingly, the propyl analogue of CBD, CBDV, may share a synergistic activity with CBD as it also demonstrates a noted anticonvulsant activity in animal models.[8,265,266]

CBG

CBG (see Fig. 20.12) is found in small concentrations in THC-rich strains, but in much higher concentrations in hemp strains commonly grown for fibre or seeds. Viewed as a minor therapeutic cannabinoid, a growing pool of research is making scientists look at this cannabinoid with more clinical interest.

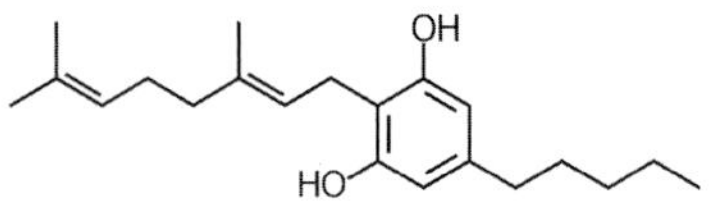

FIGURE 20.12 CBG structure

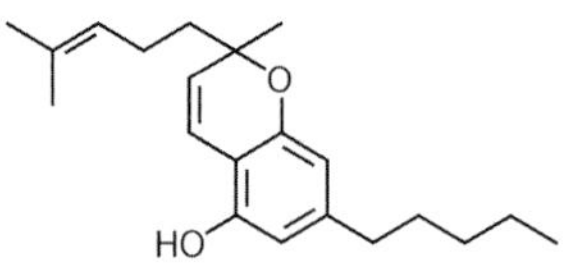

FIGURE 20.13 CBC structure

CBG is a non-psychoactive cannabinoid, with studies demonstrating it exhibits activity such as being a GABA uptake inhibitor,[267] an antagonist to TRPM8[268] and an alpha-2-adrenocorticotropic receptor agonist[269] and shows potential uptake inhibitory activity at $5HT_{1A}$ receptors.[10,267] Key areas of clinical interest for this cannabinoid are as an antimicrobial agent,[270] in psoriasis due to its ability to inhibit the proliferation of keratinocytes, as a potential anticancer agent[251] and as a potent analgesic exhibiting superiority over THC.[10,229]

CBC

Derived from CBGA, CBC (see Fig. 20.13) interacts with TRPV1 with strong affinity and is also a TRPA1 agonist[271] that can inhibit endocannabinoid inactivation, which could explain its anti-inflammatory effect.[10,193] Interestingly, it exhibits poor affinity for the CB1 receptor. Weak anandamide inhibition has also been noted in the literature.[251] Research on CBC is scarce, but demonstrates that this cannabinoid exhibits strong antibacterial activity and mild-to-moderate antifungal activity[272] and is a weak analgesic.[193]

DELTA-8-THC

Defined as a lesser cannabinoid, not a great deal of research interest has been expressed in delta-8-THC. While not completely non-psychotropic, it exhibits less psychotropic activity than THC and therefore may be more clinically appropriate. It has been shown to stimulate the appetite,[273] and also possesses antiemetic and analgesic actions.

Terpenes

The terpene class can be thought of as the essential oil phytochemical class contained within the glandular trichomes of *Cannabis* spp., and undergoes synthesis via the terpene moiety geranyl pyrophosphate. This class is responsible for the different aromas and tastes throughout the various strains of the *Cannabis* genus and is based chemically off the isoprene unit, a 5-carbon structure (see Fig. 20.14).[274] Terpenes found in the *Cannabis* genus are mainly of monoterpene ($C_{10}H_{16}$) and sesquiterpene ($C_{15}H_{24}$) derivation[10]; diterpenes ($C_{20}H_{32}$) and triterpenes ($C_{30}H_{48}$) are also observed, but in lesser amounts.[10]

To date, more than 200 terpenes[275,276] have been identified in the various *Cannabis* spp., but none of unique

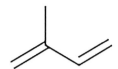

FIGURE 20.14 Isoprene (C5) structure

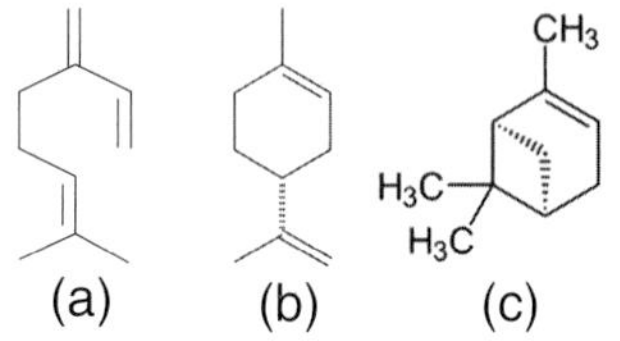

FIGURE 20.15 Structural representation of various monoterpenoids
(a) β-myrcene (b) limonene (c) α-pinene

presentation within the genus that have not been identified in other flora. While terpene composition within the plant is under genetic control,[277] environmental variables such as light exposure and decreased nitrogen can produce higher terpene yields prior to harvest.[8]

Terpenes exhibit their own potent and diverse pharmacology, are highly lipophilic (like the cannabinoids) and have the potential to interact with cell membranes, enzymes, second messenger systems, neurotransmitter receptors and neuronal ion channels.[8]

MONOTERPENES ($C_{10}H_{16}$)

The monoterpene class usually predominates distribution throughout the various *Cannabis* spp., with 47–92% of volatile oil extracted from the inflorescence coming from this class alone.[276] Examples of note are β-myrcene, pinene and limonene (see Fig. 20.15), with α-pinene and limonene acting as biological insect repellents to protect the plant.[8] Due to their structure, monoterpenes are incredibly volatile and heat-sensitive. They are also prone to loss during storage and drying procedures, so handling crude herb after harvest and appropriate manufacturing procedures are critical to maintaining phytochemical integrity.

β-myrcene

With noted sedative, muscle relaxant, analgesic[278] and anti-inflammatory properties,[279] β-myrcene is a very useful therapeutic phytochemical. Evidence suggests that it can block hepatic carcinogenesis by aflotoxin in vitro,[280] although most of its pharmacological actions show prominence in the area of pain management. The anti-inflammatory action has been shown to be due to prostaglandin-E_2 (PGE-2),[281] whereas the muscle relaxant action has been shown to potentiate barbiturate sleep time in an animal model.[8] Working by different mechanisms of action to the sedating and analgesic THC, a useful synergy may be therapeutically useful for intractable pain conditions.

α-pinene

α-pinene, a bicyclic monoterpene, is one of two isomers of pinene that is ubiquitously distributed throughout the plant kingdom.[8,282] It is responsible for the characteristic pine fragrance encountered in the division coniperophyta (i.e. conifers: fir, pine, redwood, spruce, yew, cypress), where it exists as an insect repellent secondary metabolite.[8] Like β-myrcene, it exhibits anti-inflammatory activity but via PGE-1, while uniquely exhibiting bronchodilatory activity via inhalation, and has demonstrated acetylcholinesterase inhibitory activity.[283]

Limonene

Being the second most distributed terpene in nature,[282] D-limonene is commonly found in members of the *Citrus* genus (family Rutaceae). D-limonene is the most common isomer that is used commercially in food and cosmetic production, and like α-pinene it is produced as a secondary metabolite as an antifeedant and insect repellent. D-limonene exhibits a powerful and diverse pharmacology, with antidepressant,[284] anxiolytic,[285] anticancer[286] and immunostimulant actions, the last via inhalation.[8,284] Further research has posited that the anxiolytic action is mediated by increasing serotonin in the pre-frontal cortex mediated by 5-HT$_{1A}$ in animal studies,[287] and later human clinical studies demonstrated normalised Hamilton depression (HAM-D) scores via citrus essential oil aerosol dispersal.[284]

SESQUITERPENES (C$_{15}$H$_{24}$)

Comprised of three isoprene units, the sesquiterpene class is expressed less than the monoterpenes in most cannabis samples. Surprisingly, over time the levels of sesquiterpenes in plant samples may actually increase due to the evaporation of the more volatile monoterpene class.[276] Representative examples of this class include β-caryophyllene, caryophyllene oxide, α-humulene, farnesene, elemene, trans-nerolidol and bergamotene.[10,184,276,288]

β-caryophyllene

Commonly distributed throughout plants such as *Piper nigrum* (black pepper) and *Syzygium aromaticum* (clove), β-caryophyllene is a secondary metabolite involved as an insect repellent.[277] Therapeutically it exhibits anti-inflammatory activity via PGE-1, along with antimalarial and gastric cytoprotective activity.[8,289] β-caryophyllene has also been shown to be a selective CB$_2$ receptor agonist, directly interacting with the ECS.

Caryophyllene oxide

Found also in *Melissa officinalis* (lemon balm), this non-toxic and non-sensitising sesquiterpene is ubiquitously distributed throughout the *Cannabis* genus, and for this reason it is generally considered to be the substance responsible for cannabis detection by canine drug units.[8] The plant produces this terpenoid as an antifeedant and insecticide, but it also has potent antifungal activity that is required in plant protection.[8] The latter action has also been demonstrated in an in vitro experimental model for onychomycosis, where it was found to be comparable to ciclopiroxolamine and sulconazole in an 8% preparation that achieved resolution (fungal eradication) within 15 days.[8,290]

For a summary of the actions of the major terpenoids within the *Cannabis* genus, see Fig. 20.16.

Flavonoids

As of 2013, 29 flavonoids had been characterised within the *Cannabis* genus, belonging to mainly the flavonol and flavone classes.[291] Many of the flavones and flavonols found in *Cannabis* spp. are found in numerous other medicinal plants, with specific flavone distribution including luteolin, orientin, vitexin, isovitexin and apigenin, and flavonol-specific examples including kaempferol and quercetin.[10,186] Flavonoids generally exhibit anti-inflammatory activity, with specific flavones such as apigenin expressing phyto-oestrogenic activity. The *Cannabis* genus, particularly the drug varieties such as *Cannabis indica*, produce unique flavanones known as cannflavins A, B and C.[10] These flavanones are prenylated aglycones that have been found to inhibit prostaglandin E$_2$ production as well as cyclooxygenase enzymes.[292]

Alkaloids

Two alkaloids belonging to the spermidine class (C-21 alkaloids), cannabisativine (C$_{21}$H$_{39}$N$_3$O$_3$) and anhydrocannabisativine, have been identified in *Cannabis* spp. samples.[293] Research is ongoing as to whether they have any specific therapeutically important actions.

Other pharmacological classes

Numerous other phytochemical classes are distributed throughout the *Cannabis* genus, but are beyond the scope of this textbook. While the focus of this chapter is on the *Cannabis* genus, other herbal medicines also interact with the ECS in meaningful ways.

- *Piper methysticum* (kava-kava) is a social and ritualistic beverage commonly enjoyed throughout Fiji and the Polynesian archipelago. Most studies of standardised extracts of kava lactones have focused on GABA$_B$ receptor activity, which modifies muscle tone and anxiety states. However, recently yangonin has been shown to exhibit significant CB$_1$ binding activity, but whether it possesses agonistic or antagonistic activity is still being researched[27]
- Known as Japanese liverwort, *Radula perrottetii* contains a structural THC analogue known as perrottetinene, but no clinical research has been conducted on its potential cannabimimetic activity.[27] New Zealand liverwort, *Radula marginata*, possesses perrottetinenic acid,[294] with research indicative that it is a CB$_1$ agonist. The clinical applications of both plants is currently unknown
- Whole plant extracts of *Salvia divinorum* have tested positive for CB$_1$ activity and the humble *Daucus carota* (Queen Anne's lace), which contains falcarinol, has been found to covalently bind CB$_1$ receptors acting as an inverse agonist[27]
- The purple cone flower (*Echinacea* spp.) contains alkylamides that have been shown to resemble the structures of anandamide and 2-AG and modulate

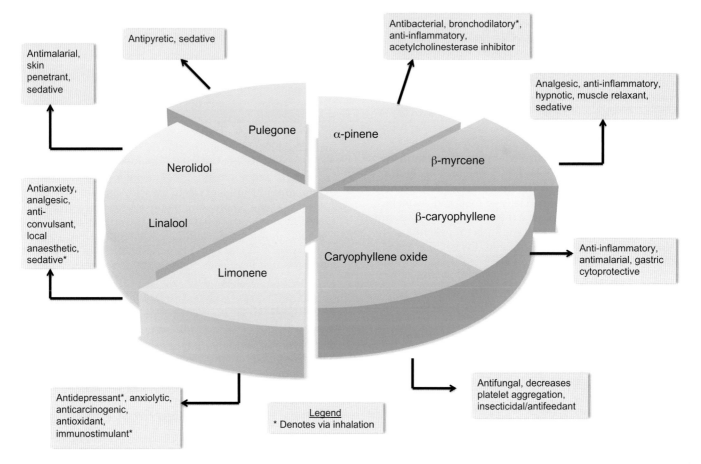

FIGURE 20.16 List of actions associated with the terpene class

Russo EB. Taming THC: potential cannabis synergy and phytocannabinoid-terpenoid entourage effects. Br J Pharmacol 2011;163(7):1344–64. Upton R, ElSohly M, Romm A, et al (eds). Cannabis inflorescence. Scotts Valley, CA: American Herbal Pharmacopoeia; 2013. Noma Y, Asakawa Y. Biotransformation of monoterpenoids by microorganisms, insects, and mammals. In: Baser K, Buchbauer, G (eds). Handbook of essential oils: science, technology, and applications. Boca Raton, FL: CRC Press; 2010.

TNF-α gene expression via the CB_2 receptor.[295] CB_2 receptor agonism has also been demonstrated along with modulation of cAMP, the ability to inhibit anandamide in vitro, and partial inverse agonist activity at the CB_1 receptor.[27,296,297] It is anticipated that with new understanding of the influence and physiological mechanisms of the ECS, more research will be undertaken into herbal medicines and other natural compounds that may interact with it and exert clinical application.

Phytochemical synergy (entourage effect)

The concept of multiple phytochemicals interacting in dynamic and meaningful ways to augment or support each other's absorption, reduce side effects or increase therapeutic potency is not a new concept to naturopathic or herbal practitioners, with examples of synergy being discussed in pharmacopoeias and formulary since ancient times.[298] Multiple herbal medicines, or indeed phytochemicals within the same plant, can have supportive and augmenting effects and complex interactivity. Science is now validating this concept, with Wagner and Ulrich-Merzenich identifying several synergistic mechanisms by which this can occur, including:

- Multi-target effects (i.e. targeting multiple receptors or organ systems at one time)
- Pharmacokinetic effects (i.e. modifying absorption, distribution, metabolism, excretion [ADME], improving bioavailability or improving solubility)
- Modulation of adverse events (i.e. reducing side effects).[299]

While studying the interactivity of endogenous fatty acid glycerol esters enhancing 2-AG activity, Ben-Shabat and Mechoulam[300,301] coined the term 'entourage effect' to describe this synergy. Since then, research into cannabinoids and terpenes has highlighted that this synergistic phenomenon also occurs between active constituents within the cannabis plant. Several examples of phytochemical synergy have been posited. CBD has been shown to reduce the severity of the psychotropic activity of THC when used in combination,[8] which

TABLE 20.2 Summary of cannabis-based dosage forms

Dosage form	Advantages	Disadvantages
Smoking	Quick onset of effect; cheap; easy to adjust dosing	Smoke can irritate the lungs; concurrent pulmonary disease may decrease absorption and effects
Vaporising	Quick onset of effect; better for lung health than smoking due to less combustible material	Vaporising units can be expensive.
Edibles (oral ingestion)	Long-lasting duration of effect; option for those who do not smoke or are health conscious	Delayed onset of effect due to slower absorption and liver metabolism
Juicing (of fresh plant/ no heat)	Rich in THCA; non-psychoactive	Not a great deal of evidence to support this dosage form currently
Tinctures/oils	Easy to control dosage; palatable; good for children; longer duration of effect	Delayed onset of effect due to slower absorption and liver metabolism
Capsules	Long-lasting effect; easy to control dosage; option for those who do not smoke	Delayed onset of effect due to slower absorption and liver metabolism; excipient ingestion
Suppositories	Absorbed relatively quickly; long-lasting effect	Difficult to administer; needs refrigeration
Topical	Can be used for local skin conditions; non-psychoactive	Not a great deal of evidence to support this dosage form currently

highlights the benefits of both THC and CBD being included at varying ratios in plant and full spectrum extracts to modify therapeutic outcomes.

More interesting is the synergistic potential between cannabinoids and terpenes. β-myrcene, a monoterpene found in *Humulus lupulus* (common hops) and various other herbal medicines such as cannabis, has muscle relaxant, hypnotic, anti-inflammatory and sedative actions associated with its clinical use, so when combined with cannabinoids such as THC or CBD which share similar pharmacological activity, albeit via different mechanisms of action, it may produce a potentiated pharmacodynamic activity and increase therapeutic efficacy. Factor into this pharmacodynamic interaction other anti-inflammatory classes such as the flavonoids or cannflavins, and it is possible to understand the potential for cannabis-based therapy using broad-spectrum phytochemical extracts. This level of phytochemical understanding enables plant breeders to select for certain chemotypes to maximise both cannabinoid and terpene profiles for specific medical conditions. This level of 'phytochemical optimisation' could represent a new paradigm in not only individual patient care and disease management, but also cannabis extract manufacturing procedures.

Cannabis dosage forms

Due to the pronounced lipophilic nature of cannabinoids and terpenes, the dosage form used in therapeutic delivery is a key consideration. Once a specific cannabis strain or single phytochemical has been selected for a certain symptom or condition, the application in an appropriate dosage form is a critical variable that can be the difference between treatment success or failure. Table 20.2 summarises the various advantages and disadvantages facing the application of different cannabis dosage forms.

Cannabis pharmacokinetic interactions

Limited research has been undertaken into potential interactions between *Cannabis* spp. and pharmaceutical medicines, but it is an emerging field now that more is known about the mechanisms of action and receptor activity of cannabinoids and other phytochemical classes.

Pharmacokinetics is defined as the quantitative study of the absorption, distribution, metabolism and excretion of a substance/medicine by the body.[302–304] In relation to cannabis and its derived extracts, any significant modification to bioavailability or clearance mechanisms can be potentially clinically meaningful in causing either positive or negative patient outcomes.[302]

ABSORPTION

Absorption is of great significance in impacting the bioavailability of orally ingested cannabis dosage forms. Any changes in factors such as gastric pH, gastric output, bile acid concentration, gastrointestinal motility, age-related changes to organ function, local organ (i.e. stomach, small intestine) blood supply or concurrent gastrointestinal pathology can impact on absorption rates.[302] Topical absorption is also worthy of consideration: age-related changes to the skin may modify absorption rates for cannabinoid-based products using transdermal liposomal or ethosomal delivery systems.[305–307]

METABOLISM

While genetic polymorphisms and individual variability within the ECS has been highlighted as potential challenges in navigating cannabis pharmacotherapy, so too can genetic variability impact on the metabolism of cannabinoids within the body.

Distributed in greatest concentrations within the liver,[308] but also in the intestines, skin, kidneys and lungs,[303] the cytochrome P450 (CYP450) enzyme system is a primary site for exogenous pharmaceutical medication and endogenous compound metabolism. The CYP1A2, 2C9, 2C19, 2D6 and 3A4 isoforms are metabolically involved in the processing of more than 50% of pharmaceutical medications.[302,308–310] Induction or inhibition of certain CYP450 enzymes can have serious clinical consequences, particularly when drugs of narrow therapeutic index (NTI) are involved. In such instances, induction of specific isoenzymes can hyper-metabolise medication serum levels and thus reduce therapeutic coverage, whereas inhibition can reduce clearance of medication levels which, after further dosing, can increase circulating levels in the blood and increase risks of toxicity or adverse effects. Both interaction types have potentially serious clinical implications.[302]

Individual expression of CYP450 enzymes and their relative concentration and distribution throughout the body is under genetic control.[311] Therefore, not only can certain exogenous substances induce or inhibit normal CYP450 function, but inbuilt genetic polymorphisms need to be considered for clinical cannabinoid optimisation for the individual patient. Individuals classified as poor metabolisers are at higher risk of side effects from drugs, whereas rapid metabolisers may have sub-therapeutic plasma concentrations and tissue distribution causing treatment failure due to hyper-metabolism.[302,309,312] This obviously has ramifications for the ingestion of cannabis-based extracts, as well as all xenobiotic drugs.

Orally administered cannabis dosage forms are typically absorbed primarily in the small intestine and are subsequently transported to the liver for biotransformation. The enzymes involved in this process are mainly the CYP2C and CYP3A families, where cannabinoids such as THC are transformed into 11-OH-THC, a more potent and therapeutically active form of THC. This is why edible or orally ingested forms are favoured by pain sufferers – they have a longer duration of effect and higher potency than smoked forms. Another clinically relevant cannabinoid, CBD, also undergoes biotransformation by these enzymes to 7-OH-CBD and 6-OH-CBD, but little research has been conducted on these metabolites to date. Worthy of consideration also are age-related changes[313] to liver function or the presence of concurrent hepatic pathology, which could detrimentally impact therapeutic outcomes.

Specific *Cannabis* spp. interactions are attracting more research interest with the increased therapeutic use of cannabis worldwide. Currently, research has demonstrated that CBD is metabolised by CYP1A1, 1A2, 2C9, 2C19, 2D6, 3A4 and 3A5 isoenzymes in human liver microsomes,[314] with another paper showing that CBD can potently inhibit CYP3A4 and CYP3A5 isoenzymes.[315] This has obvious clinical implications for medications metabolised by these specific enzyme pathways. Furthermore, CYP2C9 inhibition was demonstrated in vitro for multiple cannabinoids contained within cannabis smoke, including THC, CBN and CBD,[315–317] with the last also exhibiting strong CYP2D6 inhibition.[316] Of all the cannabinoids, it appears that CBD is the most potent deactivator of the CYP450 enzyme system, and may actually act as a competitive inhibitor.[318]

THC is specifically metabolised by CYP2C9 and CYP3A4 and therefore individuals who are poor metabolisers at these specific isoenzyme sites could potentially exhibit a three-fold higher concentration of THC than rapid metabolisers,[319] greatly increasing their risk of adverse effects such as anxiety, dysphoria and paranoia. Conversely, substances that could inhibit these enzymes are also worthy of clinical consideration, such as cimetidine, metronidazole, fluconazole, amiodarone, phenytoin, valproic acid, clopidogrel and fluoxetine.

Such individual genetic variability, coupled with knowledge of current inducers or inhibitors of certain enzyme pathways, could dramatically impact how well tolerated and efficacious cannabis is as a therapeutic substance. Clinically authorised prescribers of cannabis must pay close attention to such herb–drug interactions, and also consider that treatment failure or adverse effect presentation could actually be based on individual metabolic genetic polymorphisms. With technology in the area of genetic testing advancing rapidly, this is something that could potentially be tested for in patients to optimise therapeutic outcomes and avoid adverse effects.

Cannabis pharmacodynamic interactions

While generally easier to predict than pharmacokinetic interactions,[302] numerous pharmacodynamic interactions have been posited for cannabis. Not surprisingly, animal experiments have demonstrated that cannabis may increase the depressant action of pharmaceutical barbiturates and other drug classes such as opiates and benzodiazepines. This is largely due to the presence of the psychoactive constituent THC, which may also potentiate other psychoactive medications in an additive way. While not pharmaceutical, alcohol should also be considered as a CNS depressant and as an important questioning point for patients seeking to use medicinal cannabis. Although evidence is sparse and case studies are lacking, clinicians need to familiarise themselves with the multitude of pharmacological actions of cannabis and cross-check proposed mechanisms with prescription medications.

Interestingly, such herb–drug interactions should not always be seen in a negative light, as many positive interactions may be possible from modified (mostly augmented) pharmacodynamic effects that could potentially enable a decrease in drug dosage or lead to a reduction in side effects of the prescribed pharmaceuticals.

Cannabis controversies

Cannabis is not without its controversies and a great deal of research has been conducted on its illicit use over the last 50 years. This needs to be kept in mind, as the plant material grown for illicit use – which is what this research has been based on – is certainly not to be misconstrued as the medicinal-grade cannabis available today, regardless whether it has been used for symptomatic amelioration by patients or not. Large variances in quality, adulteration, pesticide residues, heavy metal contamination and the use of various growth hormones may affect the finished plant product. Most illicit strains are grown to maximise THC levels, with little other cannabinoid representation present to potentially reduce side effects due to entourage-like effects, or achieve optimised medical benefit. The data on illicit use collected over the last 50 years can skew the results of perceived adverse effects associated with cannabis, have certainly tainted the opinion of doctors in accepting cannabis back into medical use and must therefore be considered when pondering the previously published harm or risk/benefit analysis for the plant.

It has long been espoused that cannabis use can lower intelligence quotient (IQ) results in recreational users. While increased consumption of cannabis can certainly cause a decreased functioning of short-term memory in some people, these changes are not permanent and resolve with cessation. Long-term damage or permanent IQ deterioration is unlikely: a longitudinal twin study published in the Proceedings of the National Academy of Sciences in 2016 found that cannabis-using twins failed to show significantly greater IQ decline relative to their abstinent siblings, suggesting that observed declines in IQ are more attributable to familial or other factors.[320] Notwithstanding this, the impact of cannabis on the young developing brain is less certain and more research is needed to determine its safety.

The links with cannabis causing psychosis or schizophrenia have been a focus for addiction specialists and researchers for decades, with papers suggesting that cannabis increases the risk of both the incidence of psychosis in previously healthy people and a poor prognosis for those with established vulnerability to psychotic disorders.[321] This relationship is often used as an argument against the use of medicinal cannabis, but let us not forget that the mechanisms underlying this association have not been fully elucidated,[322] and our understanding of this mental illness is at best rudimentary.

Interestingly, recent research suggests that cannabis in itself does not cause psychosis, but rather that both early use and heavy use of cannabis are more likely in people with a vulnerability to psychosis.[323] Furthermore, Hickman and colleagues have sought to estimate how many cannabis users would need to be prevented from using in order to stop one case of schizophrenia or psychosis, with statistics suggesting that the annual mean number needed to prevent heavy cannabis use and schizophrenia in men ranged from 2800 in those aged 20–24 years to 4700 in those aged 35–39 years.[324] While more research on this relationship needs to be undertaken, it must be reiterated that illicit and medicinal cannabis strains are not synonymous, and that using this as an argument to prohibit the use of medicinal cannabis is laughing in the face of a risk/benefit analysis for those for whom no medical treatment can provide relief.

Another well-known controversy surrounding cannabis is its ability to cause dependence. Once again, this is touted as an argument against a compassionate medicinal cannabis access scheme. Anthony and colleagues conducted a study of 8000 people between the ages of 15

and 54 years as part of the National Comorbidity Survey in the US.[325] While it was found that cannabis can indeed cause dependency, it had an estimated prevalence of 4%. Conversely, 24% of participants surveyed had a history of dependence on tobacco (1 in 4) while 14% (1 in 7) had a dependence on alcohol.[325] These are both substances that are licit and legally obtainable and create a huge burden on the Australian healthcare system. According to the Australian government's Quitline, more than 50 Australians die of tobacco-related disease every day, with more than 19 000 deaths in 1998 alone. In 2010, 5500 deaths were attributed to alcohol, with an additional 157 000 hospitalisations that same year.[326] With such overwhelming statistics showing the harm and cost of these legal substances, in terms of both human suffering and costs to the public purse, hopefully balance can be brought to bear when considering the use of high-quality, expertly cultivated medicinal cannabis for patients requiring compassionate relief from suffering.

As Australia, New Zealand and many other countries are engaging in the process to re-introduce medicinal cannabis to the medical armamentarium of approved treatments, it allows for a pensive reflection to see that common sense and the traditional medical use and faith that hundreds of generations have placed in this plant has come full circle and cannabis is being returned to its rightful place. The evidence is not only encouraging, but also in many different areas of medicine it is overwhelming. To state that the evidence associated with cannabis is only anecdotal, as many still do, represents a wilful ignorance of the amassing evidence base of this diverse herbal medicine. It also draws attention to the broadening divide between hard science and the current evidence-based paradigm of clinical medicine, and the compassionate alleviation of suffering for patients for whom medicine has no answers or treatment.

In countries and states where medicinal cannabis has been implemented we can already see evidence of benefit across many different levels. In 2014, Bachhuber and colleagues noted that in 1999–2010 in states where medicinal cannabis was legal, there was a 24.8% lower mean opioid mortality rate compared with states without state medicinal cannabis laws in place.[327] Furthermore, this lowered rate strengthened over time to 33.3% after 6 years of implementation.[327] Such evidence is suggestive that medicinal cannabis may be an exit drug, rather than a gateway drug, which has been the line touted for the last 40 years by addiction specialists. Considering that the Australian Medical Association has issued a statement noting that prescription medicine abuse is a national emergency, such evidence from overseas should be comforting to authorised prescribers of medicinal cannabis moving forwards towards implementation.

In US states where medicinal cannabis is used, statistics show a 12% lower rate of Medicare pain relief prescriptions in patients over the age of 65 and 8–13% lower rates of prescription medications used for depression, anxiety, nausea, psychosis and sleep disorders.[328] Considering that severe pain is the single greatest qualifying condition for medicinal cannabis use in patients, and Australia and New Zealand are experiencing a burgeoning ageing population,[329] over the next few years medicinal cannabis could have serious economic benefits that can take some strain off the already struggling healthcare system.

Lastly, and perhaps most importantly, patients in palliative care and those suffering from intractable cases of epilepsy or pain may finally have another medical option to provide hope and symptomatic amelioration. Medicinal cannabis may well be the hope that many patients and doctors have been waiting for, and while this author understands that medicinal cannabis is certainly not the panacea that many proclaim it to be, and it will not help all people, it does beg the question that with science's blinkered focus on finding cure, are we losing our ability to act with compassion?

REFERENCES

[1] Mallat A, Teixeira-Clerc F, Lotersztajn S. Cannabinoid signaling and liver therapeutics. J Hepatol 2013;59(4):891–6.

[2] Mechoulam R, Parker LA. The endocannabinoid system and the brain. Annu Rev Psychol 2013;64:21–47.

[3] McGeeney BE. Cannabinoids and hallucinogens for headache. Headache 2013;53(3):447–58.

[4] McPartland JM, Norris RW, Kilpatrick CW. Coevolution between cannabinoid receptors and endocannabinoid ligands. Gene 2007;397(1–2):126–35.

[5] Grotenhermen F. Cannabinoids and the endocannabinoid system. Cannabinoids 2006;1(1):10–14.

[6] McPartland JM, Matias I, Di Marzo V, et al. Evolutionary origins of the endocannabinoid system. Gene 2006;370:64–74.

[7] Elphick MR, Satou Y, Satoh N. The invertebrate ancestry of endocannabinoid signalling: an orthologue of vertebrate cannabinoid receptors in the urochordate Ciona intestinalis. Gene 2003;302(1–2):95–101.

[8] Russo EB. Taming THC: potential cannabis synergy and phytocannabinoid-terpenoid entourage effects. Br J Pharmacol 2011;163(7):1344–64.

[9] Mehmedic Z, Chandra S, Slade D, et al. Potency trends of Delta9-THC and other cannabinoids in confiscated cannabis preparations from 1993 to 2008. J Forensic Sci 2010;55(5):1209–17.

[10] Upton R, ElSohly M, Romm A, et al, editors. Cannabis inflorescence. Scotts Valley, CA: American Herbal Pharmacopoeia; 2013.

[11] Gaoni Y, Mechoulam R. Isolation, structure and partial synthesis of an active constituent of hashish. J Am Chem Soc 1964;86:1646–7.

[12] Mechoulam R, Braun P, Gaoni Y. A stereospecific synthesis of (−)-delta 1- and (−)-delta 6- tetrahydrocannabinols. J Am Chem Soc 1967;89:4552–4.

[13] Maccarrone M, Bab I, Biro T, et al. Endocannabinoid signaling at the periphery: 50 years after THC. Trends Pharmacol Sci 2015;36(5):277–96.

[14] Howlett AC, Fleming RM. Cannabinoid inhibition of adenylate cyclase. Pharmacology of the response in neuroblastoma cell membranes. Mol Pharmacol 1984;26(3):532–8.

[15] Mechoulam R, Feigenbaum JJ, Lander N, et al. Enantiomeric cannabinoids: stereospecificity of psychotropic activity. Experientia 1988;44(9):762–4.

[16] Devane WA, Dysarz FA 3rd, Johnson MR, et al. Determination and characterization of a cannabinoid receptor in rat brain. Mol Pharmacol 1988;34(5):605–13.

[17] Matsuda LA, Lolait SJ, Brownstein MJ, et al. Structure of a cannabinoid receptor and functional expression of the cloned cDNA. Nature 1990;346(6284):561–4.

[18] Munro S, Thomas KL, Abu-Shaar M. Molecular characterization of a peripheral receptor for cannabinoids. Nature 1993;365(6441):61–5.

[19] Devane WA, Hanus L, Breuer A, et al. Isolation and structure of a brain constituent that binds to the cannabinoid receptor. Science 1992;258(5090):1946–9.

[20] Mechoulam R, Ben-Shabat S, Hanus L, et al. Identification of an endogenous 2-monoglyceride, present in canine gut, that binds to cannabinoid receptors. Biochem Pharmacol 1995;50(1):83–90.

[21] Sugiura T, Kondo S, Sukagawa A, et al. 2-arachidonoylglycerol: a possible endogenous cannabinoid receptor ligand in brain. Biochem Biophys Res Commun 1995;215(1):89–97.

[22] Di Marzo V, Bifulco M, De Petrocellis L. The endocannabinoid system and its therapeutic exploitation. Nat Rev Drug Discov 2004;3(Sept):771–84.

[23] Henry RJ, Kerr DM, Finn DP, et al. For whom the endocannabinoid tolls: modulation of innate immune function and implications for psychiatric disorders. Prog Neuropsychopharmacol Biol Psychiatry 2016;64:167–80.

[24] Blankman JL, Simon GM, Cravatt BF. A comprehensive profile of brain enzymes that hydrolyze the endocannabinoid 2-arachidonoylglycerol. Chem Biol 2007;14(12):1347–56.

[25] Sanchez AJ, Garcia-Merino A. Neuroprotective agents: cannabinoids. Clin Immunol 2012;142(1):57–67.

[26] Vemuri VK, Makriyannis A. Medicinal chemistry of cannabinoids. Clin Pharmacol Ther 2015;97(6):553–8.

[27] Russo EB. Beyond cannabis: plants and the endocannabinoid system. Trends Pharmacol Sci 2016;37(7):594–605.

[28] Castillo PE, Younts TJ, Chavez AE, et al. Endocannabinoid signaling and synaptic function. Neuron 2012;76(1):70–81.

[29] Cristino L, Becker T, Di Marzo V. Endocannabinoids and energy homeostasis: an update. Biofactors 2014;40(4):389–97.

[30] Maccarrone M, Guzman M, Mackie K, et al. Programming of neural cells by (endo)cannabinoids: from physiological rules to emerging therapies. Nat Rev Neurosci 2014;15(12):786–801.

[31] DiPatrizio NV, Piomelli D. The thrifty lipids: endocannabinoids and the neural control of energy conservation. Trends Neurosci 2012;35(7):403–11.

[32] Galve-Roperh I, Chiurchiu V, Diaz-Alonso J, et al. Cannabinoid receptor signaling in progenitor/stem cell proliferation and differentiation. Prog Lipid Res 2013;52(4):633–50.

[33] Glass M, Dragunow M, Faull RL. Cannabinoid receptors in the human brain: a detailed anatomical and quantitative autoradiographic study in the fetal, neonatal and adult human brain. Neuroscience 1997;77(2):299–318.

[34] Ross RA. The enigmatic pharmacology of GPR55. Trends Pharmacol Sci 2009;30(3):156–63.

[35] Baker D, Pryce G, Davies WL, et al. In silico patent searching reveals a new cannabinoid receptor. Trends Pharmacol Sci 2006;27(1):1–4.

[36] Di Marzo V, De Petrocellis L. Endocannabinoids as regulators of transient receptor potential (TRP) channels: a further opportunity to develop new endocannabinoid-based therapeutic drugs. Curr Med Chem 2010;17:1430–49.

[37] Pistis M, Melis M. From surface to nuclear receptors: the endocannabinoid family extends its assets. Curr Med Chem 2010;17(14):1450–67.

[38] Heifets BD, Castillo PE. Endocannabinoid signaling and long-term synaptic plasticity. Annu Rev Physiol 2009;71:283–306.

[39] De Petrocellis L, Bifulco M, Ligresti A, et al. Potential use of cannabimimetics in the treatment of cancer. In: Mechoulam R, Gaoni Y, editors. Cannabinoids as therapeutics. Basel: Birkhauser; 2005. p. 165–82.

[40] Friedman D, Devinsky O. Cannabinoids in the treatment of epilepsy. N Engl J Med 2015;373(11):1048–58.

[41] Kano M. Control of synaptic function by endocannabinoid-mediated retrograde signaling. Proc Jpn Acad Ser B Phys Biol Sci 2014;90(7):235–50.

[42] Mackie K, Lai Y, Westenbroek R, et al. Cannabinoids activate an inwardly rectifying potassium conductance and inhibit Q-type calcium currents in AtT20 cells transfected with rat brain cannabinoid receptor. J Neurosci 1995;15(10):6552–61.

[43] Shire D, Carillon C, Kaghad M, et al. An amino-terminal variant of the central cannabinoid receptor resulting from alternative splicing. J Biol Chem 1995;270(8):3726–31.

[44] Ryberg E, Vu HK, Larsson N, et al. Identification and characterisation of a novel splice variant of the human CB1 receptor. FEBS Lett 2005;579(1):259–64.

[45] Husni AS, McCurdy CR, Radwan MM, et al. Evaluation of phytocannabinoids from high potency using bioassays to

determine structure-activity relationships for cannabinoid receptor 1 and cannabinoid receptor 2. Med Chem Res 2014;23(9):4295–300.

[46] Herkenham M, Lynn AB, Johnson MR, et al. Characterization and localization of cannabinoid receptors in rat brain: a quantitative in vitro autoradiographic study. J Neurosci 1991;11(2):563–83.

[47] Mackie K. Cannabinoid receptors: where they are and what they do. J Neuroendocrinol 2008;20(Suppl. 1):10–14.

[48] Howlett AC, Barth F, Bonner TI, et al. International Union of Pharmacology. XXVII. Classification of cannabinoid receptors. Pharmacol Rev 2002;54(2):161–202.

[49] Baron EP. Comprehensive review of medicinal marijuana, cannabinoids, and therapeutic implications in medicine and headache: what a long strange trip it's been. Headache 2015;55(6):885–916.

[50] Serrano A, Parsons LH. Endocannabinoid influence in drug reinforcement, dependence and addiction-related behaviors. Pharmacol Ther 2011;132(3):215–41.

[51] Katona I, Freund TF. Endocannabinoid signaling as a synaptic circuit breaker in neurological disease. Nat Med 2008;14(9):923–30.

[52] Pacher P, Hasko G. Endocannabinoids and cannabinoid receptors in ischaemia-reperfusion injury and preconditioning. Br J Pharmacol 2008;153(2):252–62.

[53] Aguado T, Romero E, Monory K, et al. The CB1 cannabinoid receptor mediates excitotoxicity-induced neural progenitor proliferation and neurogenesis. J Biol Chem 2007;282(33):23892–8.

[54] van der Stelt M, Di Marzo V. Cannabinoid receptors and their role in neuroprotection. Neuromolecular Med 2005;7(1–2):37–50.

[55] Latorre JG, Schmidt EB. Cannabis, cannabinoids, and cerebral metabolism: potential applications in stroke and disorders of the central nervous system. Curr Cardiol Rep 2015;17(9):627.

[56] Pacher P, Batkai S, Kunos G. The endocannabinoid system as an emerging target of pharmacotherapy. Pharmacol Rev 2006;58(3):389–462.

[57] Steffens S, Pacher P. The activated endocannabinoid system in atherosclerosis: driving force or protective mechanism? Curr Drug Targets 2015;16(4):334–41.

[58] Sharkey KA, Wiley JW. Getting into the weed: the role of the endocannabinoid system in the brain–gut axis. Gastroenterology 2016;151(2):252–66.

[59] Trautmann SM, Sharkey KA. The endocannabinoid system and its role in regulating the intrinsic neural circuitry of the gastrointestinal tract. Int Rev Neurobiol 2015;125:85–126.

[60] Zhang PW, Ishiguro H, Ohtsuki T, et al. Human cannabinoid receptor 1: 5′ exons, candidate regulatory regions, polymorphisms, haplotypes and association with polysubstance abuse. Mol Psychiatry 2004;9(10):916–31.

[61] Onaivi ES, Ishiguro H, Gong JP, et al. Discovery of the presence and functional expression of cannabinoid CB2 receptors in brain. Ann N Y Acad Sci 2006;1074:514–36.

[62] Onaivi ES, Ishiguro H, Gong JP, et al. Functional expression of brain neuronal CB2 cannabinoid receptors are involved in the effects of drugs of abuse and in depression. Ann N Y Acad Sci 2008;1139:434–49.

[63] Samson MT, Small-Howard A, Shimoda LM, et al. Differential roles of CB1 and CB2 cannabinoid receptors in mast cells. J Immunol 2003;170(10):4953–62.

[64] Nunez E, Benito C, Pazos MR, et al. Cannabinoid CB2 receptors are expressed by perivascular microglial cells in the human brain: an immunohistochemical study. Synapse 2004;53(4):208–13.

[65] Dittel BN. Direct suppression of autoreactive lymphocytes in the central nervous system via the CB2 receptor. Br J Pharmacol 2008;153(2):271–6.

[66] Howlett AC. The cannabinoid receptors. Prostaglandins Other Lipid Mediat 2002;68–69:619–31.

[67] Tao Y, Li L, Jiang B, et al. Cannabinoid receptor-2 stimulation suppresses neuroinflammation by regulating microglial M1/M2 polarization through the cAMP/PKA pathway in an experimental GMH rat model. Brain Behav Immun 2016;58:118–29.

[68] Atwood BK, Mackie K. CB2: a cannabinoid receptor with an identity crisis. Br J Pharmacol 2010;160(3):467–79.

[69] Benito C, Tolon RM, Pazos MR, et al. Cannabinoid CB2 receptors in human brain inflammation. Br J Pharmacol 2008;153(2):277–85.

[70] Klein TW. Cannabinoid-based drugs as anti-inflammatory therapeutics. Nat Rev Immunol 2005;5(5):400–11.

[71] Anand P, Whiteside G, Fowler CJ, et al. Targeting CB2 receptors and the endocannabinoid system for the treatment of pain. Brain Res Rev 2009;60(1):255–66.

[72] Pacher P, Mechoulam R. Is lipid signaling through cannabinoid 2 receptors part of a protective system? Prog Lipid Res 2011;50(2):193–211.

[73] Chakrabarti B, Persico A, Battista N, et al. Endocannabinoid signaling in autism. Neurother 2015;12(4):837–47.

[74] Oz M, Zhang L, Ravindran A, et al. Differential effects of endogenous and synthetic cannabinoids on alpha7-nicotinic acetylcholine receptor-mediated responses in Xenopus oocytes. J Pharmacol Exp Ther 2004;310(3):1152–60.

[75] Zygmunt PM, Petersson J, Andersson DA, et al. Vanilloid receptors on sensory nerves mediate the vasodilator action of anandamide. Nature 1999;400(6743):452–7.

[76] De Petrocellis L, Di Marzo V. Non-CB1, non-CB2 receptors for endocannabinoids, plant cannabinoids, and synthetic cannabimimetics: focus on G-protein-coupled receptors and transient receptor potential channels. J Neuroimmune Pharmacol 2010;5(1):103–21.

[77] Mackie K, Stella N. Cannabinoid receptors and endocannabinoids: evidence for new players. AAPS J 2006;8(2):E298–306.

[78] Pertwee R. Receptors and channels targeted by synthetic cannabinoid receptor agonists and antagonists. Curr Med Chem 2010;17:1360–81.

[79] Curioni C, Andre C. Rimonabant for overweight or obesity. Cochrane Database Syst Rev 2006;(4):CD006162.

[80] Devane W, Hanus L, Breuer A, et al. Isolation and structure of a brain constituent that binds to the cannabinoid receptor. Science 1992;258:1946–9.

[81] Porter A, Sauer J, Knierman M, et al. Characterization of a novel endocannabinoid, virodhamine, with antagonist activity at the CB1 receptor. J Pharmacol Exp Ther 2002;301:1020–4.

[82] Hanus L, Abu-Lafi S, Fride E, et al. 2-arachidonyl glyceryl ether, an endogenous agonist of the cannabinoid CB1 receptor. Proc Natl Acad Sci USA 2001;98:3662–5.

[83] Di Marzo V, Petrosino S. Endocannabinoids and the regulation of their levels in health and disease. Curr Opin Lipidol 2007;18:129–40.

[84] Maccarone M, Finazzi-Agro A. The endocannabinoid system, anandamide and the regulation of mammalian cell apoptosis. Cell Death Differ 2003;10(9):946–55.

[85] Maccarone M, Finazzi-Agro A. Endocannabinoids and their actions. Vitam Horm 2002;65:225–55.

[86] Mechoulam R, Panikashvili D, Shohami E. Cannabinoids and brain injury: therapeutic implications. Trends Mol Med 2002;8(2):58–61.

[87] Justinova Z, Yasar S, Redhi GH, et al. The endogenous cannabinoid 2-arachidonoylglycerol is intravenously self-administered by squirrel monkeys. J Neurosci 2011;31(19):7043–8.

[88] Mackie K, Devane WA, Hille B. Anandamide, an endogenous cannabinoid, inhibits calcium currents as a partial agonist in N18 neuroblastoma cells. Mol Pharmacol 1993;44(3):498–503.

[89] Toth A, Blumberg PM, Boczan J. Anandamide and the vanilloid receptor (TRPV1). Vitam Horm 2009;81:389–419.

[90] Murataeva N, Straiker A, Mackie K. Parsing the players: 2-arachidonoylglycerol synthesis and degradation in the CNS. Br J Pharmacol 2014;171(6):1379–91.

[91] Sugiura T, Kobayashi Y, Oka S, et al. Biosynthesis and degradation of anandamide and 2-arachidonoylglycerol and their possible physiological significance. Prostaglandins Leukot Essent Fatty Acids 2002;66(2–3):173–92.

[92] Sugiura T, Kishimoto S, Oka S. Gokoh M. Biochemistry, pharmacology and physiology of 2-arachidonoylglycerol, an endogenous cannabinoid receptor ligand. Prog Lipid Res 2006;45(5):405–46.

[93] Tanimura A, Yamazaki M, Hashimotodani Y, et al. The endocannabinoid 2-arachidonoylglycerol produced by diacylglycerol lipase alpha mediates retrograde suppression of synaptic transmission. Neuron 2010;65(3):320–7.

[94] Gonsiorek W, Lunn C, Fan X, et al. Endocannabinoid 2-arachidonyl glycerol is a full agonist through human type 2 cannabinoid receptor: antagonism by anandamide. Mol Pharmacol 2000;57(5):1045–50.

[95] Katona I, Freund TF. Multiple functions of endocannabinoid signaling in the brain. Annu Rev Neurosci 2012;35:529–58.

[96] Maccarrone M, Dainese E, Oddi S. Intracellular trafficking of anandamide: new concepts for signaling. Trends Biochem Sci 2010;35(11):601–8.

[97] Rahman IA, Tsuboi K, Uyama T, et al. New players in the fatty acyl ethanolamide metabolism. Pharmacol Res 2014;86:1–10.

[98] Di Marzo V, Fontana A, Cadas H, et al. Formation and inactivation of endogenous cannabinoid anandamide in central neurons. Nature 1994;372(6507):686–91.

[99] Sugiura T, Kondo S, Sukagawa A, et al. Transacylase-mediated and phosphodiesterase-mediated synthesis of N-arachidonoylethanolamine, an endogenous cannabinoid-receptor ligand, in rat brain microsomes. Comparison with synthesis from free arachidonic acid and ethanolamine. Eur J Biochem 1996;240(1):53–62.

[100] Blankman JL, Cravatt BF. Chemical probes of endocannabinoid metabolism. Pharmacol Rev 2013;65(2):849–71.

[101] Walker JM, Krey JF, Chu CJ, et al. Endocannabinoids and related fatty acid derivatives in pain modulation. Chem Phys Lipids 2002;121(1–2):159–72.

[102] Di Marzo V, Maccarrone M. FAAH and anandamide: is 2-AG really the odd one out? Trends Pharmacol Sci 2008;29(5):229–33.

[103] Iversen L, Chapman V. Cannabinoids: a real prospect for pain relief? Curr Opin Pharmacol 2002;2(1):50–5.

[104] Randall MD, Harris D, Kendall DA, et al. Cardiovascular effects of cannabinoids. Pharmacol Ther 2002;95(2):191–202.

[105] Schmid K, Niederhoffer N, Szabo B. Analysis of the respiratory effects of cannabinoids in rats. Naunyn Schmiedebergs Arch Pharmacol 2003;368(4):301–8.

[106] Aggarwal SK. Cannabinergic pain medicine: a concise clinical primer and survey of randomized-controlled trial results. Clin J Pain 2013;29(2):162–71.

[107] Greco R, Gasperi V, Maccarrone M, et al. The endocannabinoid system and migraine. Exp Neurol 2010;224(1):85–91.

[108] Maccarrone M, Gasperi V, Catani MV, et al. The endocannabinoid system and its relevance for nutrition. Annu Rev Nutr 2010;30:423–40.

[109] Romigi A, Bari M, Placidi F, et al. Cerebrospinal fluid levels of the endocannabinoid anandamide are reduced in patients with untreated newly diagnosed temporal lobe epilepsy. Epilepsia 2010;51(5):768–72.

[110] Ludanyi A, Eross L, Czirjak S, et al. Downregulation of the CB1 cannabinoid receptor and related molecular elements of the endocannabinoid system in epileptic human hippocampus. J Neurosci 2008;28(12):2976–90.

[111] Sarchielli P, Pini LA, Coppola F, et al. Endocannabinoids in chronic migraine: CSF findings suggest a system failure. Neuropsychopharmacology 2007;32(6):1384–90.

[112] Nyholt DR, Morley KI, Ferreira MA, et al. Genomewide significant linkage to migrainous headache on chromosome 5q21. Am J Hum Genet 2005;77(3):500–12.

[113] Juhasz G, Lazary J, Chase D, et al. Variations in the cannabinoid receptor 1 gene predispose to migraine. Neurosci Lett 2009;461(2):116–20.

[114] Russo EB. Clinical endocannabinoid deficiency (CECD): can this concept explain therapeutic benefits of cannabis in migraine, fibromyalgia, irritable bowel syndrome and other treatment-resistant conditions? Neuro Endocrinol Lett 2004;25(1–2):31–9.

[115] Sparling PB, Giuffrida A, Piomelli D, et al. Exercise activates the endocannabinoid system. Neuroreport 2003;14(17):2209–11.

[116] Raichlen DA, Foster AD, Gerdeman GL, et al. Wired to run: exercise-induced endocannabinoid signaling in humans and cursorial mammals with implications for the 'runner's high'. J Exp Biol 2012;215(8):1331–6.

[117] Desfosses J, Stip E, Bentaleb LA, et al. Endocannabinoids and schizophrenia. Pharmaceuticals 2010;3:3103–26.

[118] De Marchi N, De Petrocellis L, Orlando P, et al. Endocannabinoid signalling in the blood of patients with schizophrenia. Lipids Health Dis 2003;2:5.

[119] Cao Q, Martinez M, Zhang J, et al. Suggestive evidence for a schizophrenia susceptibility locus on chromosome 6q and a

[120] Ishiguro H, Horiuchi Y, Ishikawa M, et al. Brain cannabinoid CB2 receptor in schizophrenia. Biol Psychiatry 2010;67(10):974–82.

[121] Centonze D, Finazzi-Agro A, Bernardi G, et al. The endocannabinoid system in targeting inflammatory neurodegenerative diseases. Trends Pharmacol Sci 2007;28(4):180–7.

[122] Marsicano G, Goodenough S, Monory K, et al. CB1 cannabinoid receptors and on-demand defense against excitotoxicity. Science 2003;302(5642):84–8.

[123] Sarne Y, Mechoulam R. Cannabinoids: between neuroprotection and neurotoxicity. Curr Drug Targets CNS Neurol Disord 2005;4(6):677–84.

[124] Mechoulam R, Lichtman AH. Neuroscience. Stout guards of the central nervous system. Science 2003;302(5642):65–7.

[125] Croxford JL, Pryce G, Jackson SJ, et al. Cannabinoid-mediated neuroprotection, not immunosuppression, may be more relevant to multiple sclerosis. J Neuroimmunol 2008;193(1–2):120–9.

[126] Jackson SJ, Pryce G, Diemel LT, et al. Cannabinoid-receptor 1 null mice are susceptible to neurofilament damage and caspase 3 activation. Neuroscience 2005;134(1):261–8.

[127] Fernandez-Ruiz J, Pazos MR, Garcia-Arencibia M, et al. Role of CB2 receptors in neuroprotective effects of cannabinoids. Mol Cell Endocrinol 2008;286(1–2, Suppl. 1):S91–6.

[128] Steffens S, Pacher P. Targeting cannabinoid receptor CB(2) in cardiovascular disorders: promises and controversies. Br J Pharmacol 2012;167(2):313–23.

[129] Rajesh M, Batkai S, Kechrid M, et al. Cannabinoid 1 receptor promotes cardiac dysfunction, oxidative stress, inflammation, and fibrosis in diabetic cardiomyopathy. Diabetes 2012;61(3):716–27.

[130] Pacher P, Kunos G. Modulating the endocannabinoid system in human health and disease: successes and failures. FEBS J 2013;280(9):1918–43.

[131] Jouanjus E, Lapeyre-Mestre M, Micallef J. French Association of the Regional Abuse and Dependence Monitoring Centres Working Group on Cannabis Complications. Cannabis use: signal of increasing risk of serious cardiovascular disorders. J Am Heart Assoc 2014;3(2):e000638.

[132] Hons IM, Storr MA, Mackie K, et al. Plasticity of mouse enteric synapses mediated through endocannabinoid and purinergic signaling. Neurogastroenterol Motil 2012;24(3):e113–24.

[133] Piomelli D. A fatty gut feeling. Trends Endocrinol Metab 2013;24(7):332–41.

[134] Sykaras AG, Demenis C, Case RM, et al. Duodenal enteroendocrine I-cells contain mRNA transcripts encoding key endocannabinoid and fatty acid receptors. PLoS ONE 2012;7(8):e42373.

[135] Wright KL, Duncan M, Sharkey KA. Cannabinoid CB2 receptors in the gastrointestinal tract: a regulatory system in states of inflammation. Br J Pharmacol 2008;153(2):263–70.

[136] Duncan M, Mouihate A, Mackie K, et al. Cannabinoid CB2 receptors in the enteric nervous system modulate gastrointestinal contractility in lipopolysaccharide-treated rats. Am J Physiol Gastrointest Liver Physiol 2008;295(1):G78–87.

[137] Fichna J, Bawa M, Thakur GA, et al. Cannabinoids alleviate experimentally induced intestinal inflammation by acting at central and peripheral receptors. PLoS ONE 2014;9(10):e109115.

[138] Kinsey SG, Nomura DK, O'Neal ST, et al. Inhibition of monoacylglycerol lipase attenuates nonsteroidal anti-inflammatory drug-induced gastric hemorrhages in mice. J Pharmacol Exp Ther 2011;338(3):795–802.

[139] Muccioli GG, Naslain D, Backhed F, et al. The endocannabinoid system links gut microbiota to adipogenesis. Mol Syst Biol 2010;6:392.

[140] Izzo AA, Sharkey KA. Cannabinoids and the gut: new developments and emerging concepts. Pharmacol Ther 2010;126(1):21–38.

[141] Liu J, Zhou L, Xiong K, et al. Hepatic cannabinoid receptor-1 mediates diet-induced insulin resistance via inhibition of insulin signaling and clearance in mice. Gastroenterology 2012;142(5):1218–28.

[142] Batkai S, Osei-Hyiaman D, Pan H, et al. Cannabinoid-2 receptor mediates protection against hepatic ischemia/reperfusion injury. FASEB J 2007;21(8):1788–800.

confirmation in an independent series of pedigrees. Genomics 1997;43(1):1–8.

[143] Guillot A, Hamdaoui N, Bizy A, et al. Cannabinoid receptor 2 counteracts interleukin-17-induced immune and fibrogenic responses in mouse liver. Hepatology 2014;59(1):296–306.

[144] Julien B, Grenard P, Teixeira-Clerc F, et al. Antifibrogenic role of the cannabinoid receptor CB2 in the liver. Gastroenterology 2005;128(3):742–55.

[145] Battista N, Di Sabatino A, Di Tommaso M, et al. Altered expression of type-1 and type-2 cannabinoid receptors in celiac disease. PLoS ONE 2013;8(4):e62078.

[146] D'Argenio G, Valenti M, Scaglione G, et al. Up-regulation of anandamide levels as an endogenous mechanism and a pharmacological strategy to limit colon inflammation. FASEB J 2006;20(3):568–70.

[147] Liu YJ, Fan HB, Jin Y, et al. Cannabinoid receptor 2 suppresses leukocyte inflammatory migration by modulating the JNK/c-Jun/Alox5 pathway. J Biol Chem 2013;288(19):13551–62.

[148] Berdyshev EV, Boichot E, Germain N, et al. Influence of fatty acid ethanolamides and delta9-tetrahydrocannabinol on cytokine and arachidonate release by mononuclear cells. Eur J Pharmacol 1997;330(2–3):231–40.

[149] Cencioni MT, Chiurchiu V, Catanzaro G, et al. Anandamide suppresses proliferation and cytokine release from primary human T-lymphocytes mainly via CB2 receptors. PLoS ONE 2010;5(1):e8688.

[150] Russo EB. Clinical endocannabinoid deficiency (CECD): can this concept explain therapeutic benefits of cannabis in migraine, fibromyalgia, irritable bowel syndrome and other treatment-resistant conditions? Neuro Endocrinol Lett 2008;29(2):192–200.

[151] Cannabaceae. Encyclopaedia Britannica. London: Encyclopaedia Britannica; 2016.

[152] Hosking RD, Zajicek JP. Therapeutic potential of cannabis in pain medicine. Br J Anaesth 2008;101(1):59–68.

[153] Russo E. History of cannabis as a medicine. In: Guy G, Whittle BA, Robson P, editors. The medicinal uses of cannabis and cannabinoids. London: Pharmaceutical Press; 2004. p. 1–16.

[154] Kalant H. Medicinal use of cannabis: history and current status. Pain Res Manag 2001;6(2):80–91.

[155] Schultes R. Random thoughts and queries on the botany of cannabis. In: Joyce C, Curry SH, editors. The botany and chemistry of cannabis. London: J&A Churchill; 1970. p. 11–38.

[156] McKim W. Drugs and behavior: an introduction to behavioral pharmacology. 4th ed. Saddle River, NJ: Prentice Hall; 2000.

[157] Li H. An archaeological and historical account of cannabis in China. Econ Bot 1974;28:437–48.

[158] Russo EB, Jiang HE, Li X, et al. Phytochemical and genetic analyses of ancient cannabis from Central Asia. J Exp Bot 2008;59(15):4171–82.

[159] Jiang HE, Li X, Zhao YX, et al. A new insight into Cannabis sativa (Cannabaceae) utilization from 2500-year-old Yanghai Tombs, Xinjiang, China. J Ethnopharmacol 2006;108(3):414–22.

[160] Ben Amar M. Cannabinoids in medicine: a review of their therapeutic potential. J Ethnopharmacol 2006;105(1–2):1–25.

[161] Clarke R, Merlin MD. Cannabis evolution and ethnobotany. Berkeley, CA: University of California Press; 2013.

[162] Russo EB. History of cannabis and its preparations in saga, science, and sobriquet. Chem Biodivers 2007;4(8):1614–48.

[163] Sharma G. Ethnobotany and its significance for cannabis studies in the Himalayas. J Psychedelic Drugs 1977;9(4):337–9.

[164] Sharma G. A botanical survey of cannabis in the Himalayas. J Bomb Nat Hist So 1980;76:17–20.

[165] Green G. The cannabis grow bible. San Francisco: Green Candy Press; 2010.

[166] Pringle H. Ice age communities may be earliest known net hunters. Science 1997;277(5330):1203–4.

[167] Abel E. Marihuana: the first twelve thousand years. New York: Plenum Publishers; 1980.

[168] Merlin M. Archaeological evidence for the tradition of psychoactive plant use in the old world. Econ Bot 2003;57:295–323.

[169] Merlin M. Man and marijuana: some aspects of their ancient relationship. Rutherford, NJ: Fairleigh Dickinson University Press; 1972.

[170] Maule WJ. Medical uses of marijuana (Cannabis sativa): fact or fallacy? Br J Biomed Sci 2015;72(2):85–91.

[171] Grierson G. The hemp plant in Sanskrit and Hindi literature. Indian Antiq 1894;Sept:260–2.

[172] Russo E. Cannabis in India: ancient lore and modern medicine. In: Mechoulam R, editor. Cannabinoids as therapeutics. Switzerland: Birkauser Verlag; 2005.

[173] Aboelsoud N. Herbal medicine in ancient Egypt. J Med Plant Res 2010;4(2):82–6.

[174] Merzouki A, Mesa JM. Concerning kif, a Cannabis sativa L. preparation smoked in the Rif mountains of northern Morocco. J Ethnopharmacol 2002;81(3):403–6.

[175] Robson P. Therapeutic aspects of cannabis and cannabinoids. Br J Psychiatry 2001;178:107–15.

[176] Clarke R. Marijuana botany: an advanced study of the propogation and breeding of distinctive cannabis. Oakland, CA: Ronin Publishing; 1981.

[177] Small E. On toadstool soup and legal species of marihuana. Plant Science Bulletin 1975;21:34–9.

[178] Dewey L. Yearbook of the United States Department of Agriculture: hemp. Bureau of Plant Industry; 1913.

[179] Schultes R, Klein WM, Plowman T, et al. Cannabis: an example of taxonomic neglect. Harv Univ Bot Mus Leafl 1974;23:337–67.

[180] Anderson L. Leaf variation among cannabis species from a controlled garden. Harv Univ Bot Mus Leafl 1980;28:10.

[181] Small E, Cronquist A. A practical and natural taxonomy for cannabis. Taxon 1976;25:405–35.

[182] Hillig KW. Genetic evidence for speciation in cannabis (Cannabaceae). Genet Resour Crop Evol 2005;52:161–80.

[183] Hillig KW, Mahlberg PG. A chemotaxonomic analysis of cannabinoid variation in cannabis (Cannabaceae). Am J Bot 2004;91(6):966–75.

[184] Hillig KW. A chemotaxonomic analysis of terpenoid variation in cannabis. Biochem Syst Ecol 2004;32:875–91.

[185] McPartland JM. Correct(ed) vernacular nomenclature. O'Shaughnessy's J Cannabis Clin Pract 2015;19.

[186] ElSohly M. Chemical constituents of cannabis. In: Grotenherman F, Russo E, editors. Cannabis and cannabinoids: pharmacology, toxicology and therapeutic potential. New York: Haworth Press Inc; 2002.

[187] Chandra S, Lata H, Khan IA, et al. Photosynthetic response of Cannabis sativa L. to variations in photosynthetic photon flux densities, temperature and CO2 conditions. Physiol Mol Biol Plants 2008;14(4):299–306.

[188] Valle J, Vieira JE, Aucelio JG, et al. Influence of photoperiodism on cannabinoid content of Cannabis sativa L. Bull Narc 1978;30:67–8.

[189] Kluger B, Triolo P, Jones W, et al. The therapeutic potential of cannabinoids for movement disorders. Mov Disord 2015;30(3):313–27.

[190] Demuth DG, Molleman A. Cannabinoid signalling. Life Sci 2006;78(6):549–63.

[191] Ashton CH. Pharmacology and effects of cannabis: a brief review. Br J Psychiatry 2001;178:101–6.

[192] Zanelati TV, Biojone C, Moreira FA, et al. Antidepressant-like effects of cannabidiol in mice: possible involvement of 5-HT1A receptors. Br J Pharmacol 2010;159(1):122–8.

[193] Turner CE, ElSohly MA, Boeren EG. Constituents of Cannabis sativa L. XVII. A review of the natural constituents. J Nat Prod 1980;43(2):169–234.

[194] Hanus L, Mechoulam R. Cannabinoid chemistry: an overview. In: Mechoulam R, editor. Cannabinoids as therapeutics. Switzerland: Birkhauser Verlag; 2005.

[195] ElSohly M, Slade D. Chemical constituents of marijuana: the complex mixture of natural cannabinoids. Life Sci 2005;78:539–48.

[196] Giacoppo S, Mandolino G, Galuppo M, et al. Cannabinoids: new promising agents in the treatment of neurological diseases. Molecules 2014;19(11):18781–816.

[197] Fellermeier M, Zenk MH. Prenylation of olivetolate by a hemp transferase yields cannabigerolic acid, the precursor of tetrahydrocannabinol. FEBS Lett 1998;427(2):283–5.

[198] de Zeeuw RA, Wijsbeek J, Breimer DD, et al. Cannabinoids with a propyl side chain in cannabis: occurrence and chromatographic behavior. Science 1972;175(4023):778–9.

[199] ElSohly MA, Slade D. Chemical constituents of marijuana: the complex mixture of natural cannabinoids. Life Sci 2005;78(5):539–48.

[200] Howard P, Twycross R, Shuster J, et al. Cannabinoids. J Pain Symptom Manage 2013;46(1):142–9.

[201] Izzo AA, Borrelli F, Capasso R, et al. Non-psychotropic plant cannabinoids: new therapeutic opportunities from an ancient herb. Trends Pharmacol Sci 2009;30(10):515–27.

[202] Gaoni Y, Mechoulam R. The isolation and structure of delta-1-tetrahydrocannabinol and other neutral cannabinoids from hashish. J Am Chem Soc 1971;93(1):217–24.

[203] Pertwee RG. The diverse CB1 and CB2 receptor pharmacology of three plant cannabinoids: delta9-tetrahydrocannabinol, cannabidiol and delta9-tetrahydrocannabivarin. Br J Pharmacol 2008;153(2):199–215.

[204] Howlett AC, Blume LC, Dalton GD. CB(1) cannabinoid receptors and their associated proteins. Curr Med Chem 2010;17(14):1382–93.

[205] Rahn EJ, Hohmann AG. Cannabinoids as pharmacotherapies for neuropathic pain: from the bench to the bedside. Neurother 2009;6(4):713–37.

[206] Hampson AJ, Grimaldi M, Axelrod J, et al. Cannabidiol and (-) delta9-tetrahydrocannabinol are neuroprotective antioxidants. Proc Natl Acad Sci USA 1998;95(14):8268–73.

[207] Kavia RB, De Ridder D, Constantinescu CS, et al. Randomized controlled trial of Sativex to treat detrusor overactivity in multiple sclerosis. Mult Scler 2010;16(11):1349–59.

[208] Williams SJ, Hartley JP, Graham JD. Bronchodilator effect of delta1-tetrahydrocannabinol administered by aerosol of asthmatic patients. Thorax 1976;31(6):720–3.

[209] Neff GW, O'Brien CB, Reddy KR, et al. Preliminary observation with dronabinol in patients with intractable pruritus secondary to cholestatic liver disease. Am J Gastroenterol 2002;97(8):2117–19.

[210] Munson AE, Harris LS, Friedman MA, et al. Antineoplastic activity of cannabinoids. J Natl Cancer Inst 1975;55(3):597–602.

[211] Sanchez C, Galve-Roperh I, Canova C, et al. Delta9-tetrahydrocannabinol induces apoptosis in C6 glioma cells. FEBS Lett 1998;436(1):6–10.

[212] Blazquez C, Salazar M, Carracedo A, et al. Cannabinoids inhibit glioma cell invasion by down-regulating matrix metalloproteinase-2 expression. Cancer Res 2008;68(6):1945–52.

[213] Carracedo A, Gironella M, Lorente M, et al. Cannabinoids induce apoptosis of pancreatic tumor cells via endoplasmic reticulum stress-related genes. Cancer Res 2006;66(13):6748–55.

[214] Ruiz L, Miguel A, Diaz-Laviada I. Delta9-tetrahydrocannabinol induces apoptosis in human prostate PC-3 cells via a receptor-independent mechanism. FEBS Lett 1999;458(3):400–4.

[215] Leelawat S, Leelawat K, Narong S, et al. The dual effects of delta(9)-tetrahydrocannabinol on cholangiocarcinoma cells: anti-invasion activity at low concentration and apoptosis induction at high concentration. Cancer Invest 2010;28(4):357–63.

[216] Whyte DA, Al-Hammadi S, Balhaj G, et al. Cannabinoids inhibit cellular respiration of human oral cancer cells. Pharmacology 2010;85(6):328–35.

[217] Machado Rocha FC, Stefano SC, De Cassia Haiek R, et al. Therapeutic use of Cannabis sativa on chemotherapy-induced nausea and vomiting among cancer patients: systematic review and meta-analysis. Eur J Cancer Care (Engl) 2008;17(5):431–43.

[218] Berman JS, Symonds C, Birch R. Efficacy of two cannabis-based medicinal extracts for relief of central neuropathic pain from brachial plexus avulsion: results of a randomised controlled trial. Pain 2004;112(3):299–306.

[219] Karst M, Salim K, Burstein S, et al. Analgesic effect of the synthetic cannabinoid CT-3 on chronic neuropathic pain: a randomized controlled trial. JAMA 2003;290(13):1757–62.

[220] Noyes R Jr, Brunk SF, Avery DA, et al. The analgesic properties of delta-9-tetrahydrocannabinol and codeine. Clin Pharmacol Ther 1975;18(1):84–9.

[221] Noyes R Jr, Brunk SF, Baram DA, et al. Analgesic effect of delta-9-tetrahydrocannabinol. J Clin Pharmacol 1975;15(2–3):139–43.

[222] McCabe M, Smith FP, Macdonald JS, et al. Efficacy of tetrahydrocannabinol in patients refractory to standard antiemetic therapy. Invest New Drugs 1988;6(3):243–6.

[223] Notcutt W, Price M, Miller R, et al. Initial experiences with medicinal extracts of cannabis for chronic pain: results from 34 'N of 1' studies. Anaesthesia 2004;59(5):440–52.

[224] Abrams DI, Hilton JF, Leiser RJ, et al. Short-term effects of cannabinoids in patients with HIV-1 infection: a randomized, placebo-controlled clinical trial. Ann Intern Med 2003;139(4):258–66.

[225] Wade DT, Robson P, House H, et al. A preliminary controlled study to determine whether whole-plant cannabis extracts can improve intractable neurogenic symptoms. Clin Rehabil 2003;17(1):21–9.

[226] Wade DT, Makela P, Robson P, et al. Do cannabis-based medicinal extracts have general or specific effects on symptoms in multiple sclerosis? A double-blind, randomized, placebo-controlled study on 160 patients. Mult Scler 2004;10(4):434–41.

[227] Currais A, et al. Amyloid proteotoxicity initiates an inflammatory response blocked by cannabinoids. NPJ Aging Mech Dis 2016;2.

[228] Merritt JC, Crawford WJ, Alexander PC, et al. Effect of marihuana on intraocular and blood pressure in glaucoma. Ophthalmology 1980;87(3):222–8.

[229] Evans FJ. Cannabinoids: the separation of central from peripheral effects on a structural basis. Planta Med 1991;57(7):S60–7.

[230] Thomas A, Stevenson LA, Wease KN, et al. Evidence that the plant cannabinoid delta9-tetrahydrocannabivarin is a cannabinoid CB1 and CB2 receptor antagonist. Br J Pharmacol 2005;146(7):917–26.

[231] Bolognini D, Costa B, Maione S, et al. The plant cannabinoid delta9-tetrahydrocannabivarin can decrease signs of inflammation and inflammatory pain in mice. Br J Pharmacol 2010;160(3):677–87.

[232] Riedel G, Fadda P, McKillop-Smith S, et al. Synthetic and plant-derived cannabinoid receptor antagonists show hypophagic properties in fasted and non-fasted mice. Br J Pharmacol 2009;156(7):1154–66.

[233] Devinsky O, Cilio MR, Cross H, et al. Cannabidiol: pharmacology and potential therapeutic role in epilepsy and other neuropsychiatric disorders. Epilepsia 2014;55(6):791–802.

[234] Bisogno T, Hanus L, De Petrocellis L, et al. Molecular targets for cannabidiol and its synthetic analogues: effect on vanilloid VR1 receptors and on the cellular uptake and enzymatic hydrolysis of anandamide. Br J Pharmacol 2001;134(4):845–52.

[235] Russo EB, Burnett A, Hall B, et al. Agonistic properties of cannabidiol at 5-HT1a receptors. Neurochem Res 2005;30(8):1037–43.

[236] Burstein S. Cannabidiol (CBD) and its analogs: a review of their effects on inflammation. Bioorg Med Chem 2015;23(7):1377–85.

[237] Karniol IG, Shirakawa I, Kasinski N, et al. Cannabidiol interferes with the effects of delta 9-tetrahydrocannabinol in man. Eur J Pharmacol 1974;28(1):172–7.

[238] Dalton WS, Martz R, Lemberger L, et al. Influence of cannabidiol on delta-9-tetrahydrocannabinol effects. Clin Pharmacol Ther 1976;19(3):300–9.

[239] Bhattacharyya S, Morrison PD, Fusar-Poli P, et al. Opposite effects of delta-9-tetrahydrocannabinol and cannabidiol on human brain function and psychopathology. Neuropsychopharmacology 2010;35(3):764–74.

[240] Englund A, Morrison PD, Nottage J, et al. Cannabidiol inhibits THC-elicited paranoid symptoms and hippocampal-dependent memory impairment. J Psychopharmacol 2013;27(1):19–27.

[241] Demirakca T, Sartorius A, Ende G, et al. Diminished gray matter in the hippocampus of cannabis users: possible protective effects of cannabidiol. Drug Alcohol Depend 2011;114(2–3):242–5.

[242] Zuardi AW, Shirakawa I, Finkelfarb E, et al. Action of cannabidiol on the anxiety and other effects produced by delta 9-THC in normal subjects. Psychopharmacol 1982;76(3):245–50.

[243] Karniol IG, Carlini EA. Pharmacological interaction between cannabidiol and delta 9-tetrahydrocannabinol. Psychopharmacologia 1973;33(1):53–70.

[244] Mukhopadhyay P, Rajesh M, Horvath B, et al. Cannabidiol protects against hepatic ischemia/reperfusion injury by attenuating inflammatory signaling and response, oxidative/nitrative stress, and cell death. Free Radic Biol Med 2011;50(10):1368–81.

[245] Castillo A, Tolon MR, Fernandez-Ruiz J, et al. The neuroprotective effect of cannabidiol in an in vitro model of newborn hypoxic-ischemic brain damage in mice is mediated by CB(2) and adenosine receptors. Neurobiol Dis 2010;37(2):434–40.

[246] Jones NA, Hill AJ, Smith I, et al. Cannabidiol displays antiepileptiform and antiseizure properties in vitro and in vivo. J Pharmacol Exp Ther 2010;332(2):569–77.

[247] Zuardi AW, Hallak JE, Dursun SM, et al. Cannabidiol monotherapy for treatment-resistant schizophrenia. J Psychopharmacol 2006;20(5):683–6.

[248] Morgan CJ, Curran HV. Effects of cannabidiol on schizophrenia-like symptoms in people who use cannabis. Br J Psychiatry 2008;192(4):306–7.

[249] Leweke FM, Piomelli D, Pahlisch F, et al. Cannabidiol enhances anandamide signaling and alleviates psychotic symptoms of schizophrenia. Transl Psychiatry 2012;2:e94.

[250] Bergamaschi MM, Queiroz RH, Chagas MH, et al. Cannabidiol reduces the anxiety induced by simulated public speaking in treatment-naive social phobia patients. Neuropsychopharmacology 2011;36(6):1219–26.

[251] Ligresti A, Moriello AS, Starowicz K, et al. Antitumor activity of plant cannabinoids with emphasis on the effect of cannabidiol on human breast carcinoma. J Pharmacol Exp Ther 2006;318(3):1375–87.

[252] Solinas M, Massi P, Cantelmo AR, et al. Cannabidiol inhibits angiogenesis by multiple mechanisms. Br J Pharmacol 2012;167(6):1218–31.

[253] Vaccani A, Massi P, Colombo A, et al. Cannabidiol inhibits human glioma cell migration through a cannabinoid receptor-independent mechanism. Br J Pharmacol 2005;144(8):1032–6.

[254] Shrivastava A, Kuzontkoski PM, Groopman JE, et al. Cannabidiol induces programmed cell death in breast cancer cells by coordinating the cross-talk between apoptosis and autophagy. Mol Cancer Ther 2011;10(7):1161–72.

[255] McKallip RJ, Jia W, Schlomer J, et al. Cannabidiol-induced apoptosis in human leukemia cells: a novel role of cannabidiol in the regulation of p22phox and nox4 expression. Mol Pharmacol 2006;70(3):897–908.

[256] Brown I, Cascio MG, Rotondo D, et al. Cannabinoids and omega-3/6 endocannabinoids as cell death and anticancer modulators. Prog Lipid Res 2013;52(1):80–109.

[257] Mecha M, Feliu A, Inigo PM, et al. Cannabidiol provides long-lasting protection against the deleterious effects of inflammation in a viral model of multiple sclerosis: a role for A2A receptors. Neurobiol Dis 2013;59:141–50.

[258] Cunha JM, Carlini EA, Pereira AE, et al. Chronic administration of cannabidiol to healthy volunteers and epileptic patients. Pharmacology 1980;21(3):175–85.

[259] Hofmann ME, Frazier CJ. Marijuana, endocannabinoids, and epilepsy: potential and challenges for improved therapeutic intervention. Exp Neurol 2013;244:43–50.

[260] Devinsky O, Marsh E, Friedman D, et al. Cannabidiol in patients with treatment-resistant epilepsy: an open-label interventional trial. Lancet Neurol 2016;15(3):270–8.

[261] Schubart CD, Sommer IE, Fusar-Poli P, et al. Cannabidiol as a potential treatment for psychosis. Eur Neuropsychopharmacol 2014;24(1):51–64.

[262] Gomes FV, Llorente R, Del Bel EA, et al. Decreased glial reactivity could be involved in the antipsychotic-like effect of cannabidiol. Schizophr Res 2015;164(1–3):155–63.

[263] de Lago E, Fernandez-Ruiz J. Cannabinoids and neuroprotection in motor-related disorders. CNS Neurol Disord Drug Targets 2007;6(6):377–87.

[264] Martin-Moreno AM, Reigada D, Ramirez BG, et al. Cannabidiol and other cannabinoids reduce microglial activation in vitro and in vivo: relevance to Alzheimer's disease. Mol Pharmacol 2011;79(6):964–73.

[265] Hill AJ, Mercier MS, Hill TD, et al. Cannabidivarin is anticonvulsant in mouse and rat. Br J Pharmacol 2012;167(8):1629–42.

[266] Hill AJ, Weston SE, Jones NA, et al. Delta(9)-tetrahydrocannabivarin suppresses in vitro epileptiform and in vivo seizure activity in adult rats. Epilepsia 2010;51(8):1522–32.

[267] Banerjee SP, Snyder SH, Mechoulam R. Cannabinoids: influence on neurotransmitter uptake in rat brain synaptosomes. J Pharmacol Exp Ther 1975;194(1):74–81.

[268] De Petrocellis L, Vellani V, Schiano-Moriello A, et al. Plant-derived cannabinoids modulate the activity of transient receptor potential channels of ankyrin type-1 and melastatin type-8. J Pharmacol Exp Ther 2008;325(3):1007–15.

[269] Cascio MG, Gauson LA, Stevenson LA, et al. Evidence that the plant cannabinoid cannabigerol is a highly potent alpha2-adrenoceptor agonist and moderately potent 5HT1A receptor antagonist. Br J Pharmacol 2010;159(1):129–41.

[270] Appendino G, Gibbons S, Giana A, et al. Antibacterial cannabinoids from Cannabis sativa: a structure-activity study. J Nat Prod 2008;71(8):1427–30.

[271] Romano B, Borrelli F, Fasolino I, et al. The cannabinoid TRPA1 agonist cannabichromene inhibits nitric oxide production in macrophages and ameliorates murine colitis. Br J Pharmacol 2013;169(1):213–29.

[272] Turner CE, ElSohly MA. Biological activity of cannabichromene, its homologs and isomers. J Clin Pharmacol 1981;21(8–9 Suppl.):283S–91S.

[273] Avraham Y, Ben-Shushan D, Breuer A, et al. Very low doses of delta 8-THC increase food consumption and alter neurotransmitter levels following weight loss. Pharmacol Biochem Behav 2004;77(4):675–84.

[274] Pengelly A. The constituents of medicinal plants: an introduction to the chemistry and therapeutics of herbal medicine. 2nd ed. Sydney: Allen & Unwin; 2004.

[275] Brenneisen R. Chemistry and analysis of phytocannabinoids and other cannabis constituents. In: ElSohly M, editor. Marijuana and the cannabinoids. New York: Humana Press; 2007. p. 17–49.

[276] Ross SA, ElSohly MA. The volatile oil composition of fresh and air-dried buds of Cannabis sativa. J Nat Prod 1996;59(1):49–51.

[277] Langenheim JH. Higher plant terpenoids: a phytocentric overview of their ecological roles. J Chem Ecol 1994;20(6):1223–80.

[278] Rao VS, Menezes AM, Viana GS. Effect of myrcene on nociception in mice. J Pharm Pharmacol 1990;42(12):877–8.

[279] do Vale TG, Furtado EC, Santos JG Jr, et al. Central effects of citral, myrcene and limonene, constituents of essential oil chemotypes from Lippia alba (Mill.) n.e. Brown. Phytomedicine 2002;9(8):709–14.

[280] De-Oliveira AC, Ribeiro-Pinto LF, Paumgartten JR. In vitro inhibition of CYP2B1 monooxygenase by beta-myrcene and other monoterpenoid compounds. Toxicol Lett 1997;92(1):39–46.

[281] Lorenzetti BB, Souza GE, Sarti SJ, et al. Myrcene mimics the peripheral analgesic activity of lemongrass tea. J Ethnopharmacol 1991;34(1):43–8.

[282] Noma Y, Asakawa Y. Biotransformation of monoterpenoids by microorganisms, insects, and mammals. In: Baser K, Buchbauer G, editors. Handbook of essential oils: science, technology, and applications. Boca Raton, FL: CRC Press; 2010.

[283] Perry NS, Houghton PJ, Theobald A, et al. In-vitro inhibition of human erythrocyte acetylcholinesterase by salvia lavandulaefolia essential oil and constituent terpenes. J Pharm Pharmacol 2000;52(7):895–902.

[284] Komori T, Fujiwara R, Tanida M, et al. Effects of citrus fragrance on immune function and depressive states. Neuroimmunomodulation 1995;2(3):174–80.

[285] Carvalho-Freitas MI, Costa M. Anxiolytic and sedative effects of extracts and essential oil from Citrus aurantium L. Biol Pharm Bull 2002;25(12):1629–33.

[286] Vigushin DM, Poon GK, Boddy A, et al. Phase I and pharmacokinetic study of D-limonene in patients with advanced cancer. Cancer Research Campaign Phase I/II Clinical Trials Committee. Cancer Chemother Pharmacol 1998;42(2):111–17.

[287] Komiya M, Takeuchi T, Harada E. Lemon oil vapor causes an anti-stress effect via modulating the 5-HT and DA activities in mice. Behav Brain Res 2006;172(2):240–9.

[288] Fischedick JT, Hazekamp A, Erkelens T, et al. Metabolic fingerprinting of Cannabis sativa L., cannabinoids and terpenoids for chemotaxonomic and drug standardization purposes. Phytochemistry 2010;71(17–18):2058–73.

[289] Basile AC, Sertie JA, Freitas PC, et al. Anti-inflammatory activity of oleoresin from Brazilian Copaifera. J Ethnopharmacol 1988;22(1):101–9.

[290] Yang D, Michel L, Chaumont JP, et al. Use of caryophyllene oxide as an antifungal agent in an in vitro experimental model of onychomycosis. Mycopathologia 1999;148(2):79–82.

[291] Vanhoenacker G, Van Rompaey P, De Keukeleire D, et al. Chemotaxonomic features associated with flavonoids of cannabinoid-free cannabis (Cannabis sativa subsp. sativa L.) in relation to hops (Humulus lupulus L). Nat Prod Lett 2002;16(1):57–63.

[292] Barrett ML, Gordon D, Evans FJ. Isolation from *Cannabis sativa* L. of cannflavin: a novel inhibitor of prostaglandin production. Biochem Pharmacol 1985;34(11):2019–24.

[293] ElSohly MA, Turner CE, Phoebe CH Jr, et al. Anhydrocannabisativine, a new alkaloid from *Cannabis sativa* L. J Pharm Sci 1978;67(1):124.

[294] Toyota M, Shimamura T, Ishii H, et al. New bibenzyl cannabinoid from the New Zealand liverwort *Radula marginata*. Chem Pharm Bull (Tokyo) 2002;50(10):1390–2.

[295] Gertsch J, Schoop R, Kuenzle U, et al. Echinacea alkylamides modulate TNF-alpha gene expression via cannabinoid receptor CB2 and multiple signal transduction pathways. FEBS Lett 2004;577(3):563–9.

[296] Raduner S, Majewska A, Chen JZ, et al. Alkylamides from echinacea are a new class of cannabinomimetics. Cannabinoid type 2 receptor-dependent and independent immunomodulatory effects. J Biol Chem 2006;281(20):14192–206.

[297] Hohmann J, Redei D, Forgo P, et al. Alkamides and a neolignan from *Echinacea purpurea* roots and the interaction of alkamides with G-protein-coupled cannabinoid receptors. Phytochemistry 2011;72(14–15):1848–53.

[298] Bone K. A clinical guide to blending liquid herbs: herbal formulations for the individual patient. St Louis, MI: Churchill Livingstone; 2003.

[299] Wagner H, Ulrich-Merzenich G. Synergy research: approaching a new generation of phytopharmaceuticals. Phytomedicine 2009;16(2–3):97–110.

[300] Ben-Shabat S, Fride E, Sheskin T, et al. An entourage effect: inactive endogenous fatty acid glycerol esters enhance 2-arachidonoyl-glycerol cannabinoid activity. Eur J Pharmacol 1998;353(1):23–31.

[301] Mechoulam R, Ben-Shabat S. From gan-zi-gun-nu to anandamide and 2-arachidonoylglycerol: the ongoing story of cannabis. Nat Prod Rep 1999;16(2):131–43.

[302] Sinclair J, Sinclair C. Integrative medicine: polypharmacy. In: Sarris J, editor. Clinical naturopathy: an evidence-based guide to practice. 2nd ed. Sydney: Elsevier; 2014.

[303] Braun L, Cohen M. Herbs and natural supplements: an evidence-based guide. 2nd ed. Sydney: Elsevier; 2007.

[304] Mills S, Bone K. The essential guide to herbal safety. St Louis, MI: Churchill Livingstone; 2005.

[305] Touitou E, Godin B, Dayan N, et al. Intracellular delivery mediated by an ethosomal carrier. Biomaterials 2001;22(22):3053–9.

[306] Touitou E, Dayan N, Bergelson L, et al. Ethosomes — novel vesicular carriers for enhanced delivery: characterization and skin penetration properties. J Control Release 2000;65(3):403–18.

[307] Lodzki M, Godin B, Rakou L, et al. Cannabidiol-transdermal delivery and anti-inflammatory effect in a murine model. J Control Release 2003;93(3):377–87.

[308] Watkins PB. Drug metabolism by cytochromes P450 in the liver and small bowel. Gastroenterol Clin North Am 1992;21(3):511–26.

[309] Shimada T, Yamazaki H, Mimura M, et al. Interindividual variations in human liver cytochrome P-450 enzymes involved in the oxidation of drugs, carcinogens and toxic chemicals: studies with liver microsomes of 30 Japanese and 30 Caucasians. J Pharmacol Exp Ther 1994;270(1):414–23.

[310] Guengerich FP. Cytochrome P450 enzymes. In: McQueen CA, editor. Comprehensive toxicology. 4th ed. Elsevier; 2010. p. 41–76.

[311] Pirmohamed M, Park BK. Cytochrome P450 enzyme polymorphisms and adverse drug reactions. Toxicology 2003;192(1):23–32.

[312] Shapiro LE, Shear NH. Drug interactions: proteins, pumps, and P-450s. J Am Acad Dermatol 2002;47(4):467–88.

[313] Klotz U. Effect of age on pharmacokinetics and pharmacodynamics in man. Int J Clin Pharmacol Ther 1998;36(11):581–5.

[314] Jiang R, Yamaori S, Takeda S, et al. Identification of cytochrome P450 enzymes responsible for metabolism of cannabidiol by human liver microsomes. Life Sci 2011;89(5–6):165–70.

[315] Yamaori S, Koeda K, Kushihara M, et al. Comparison in the in vitro inhibitory effects of major phytocannabinoids and polycyclic aromatic hydrocarbons contained in marijuana smoke on cytochrome P450 2C9 activity. Drug Metab Pharmacokinet 2012;27(3):294–300.

[316] Yamaori S, Okamoto Y, Yamamoto I, et al. Cannabidiol, a major phytocannabinoid, as a potent atypical inhibitor for CYP2D6. Drug Metab Dispos 2011;39(11):2049–56.

[317] Watanabe K, Yamaori S, Funahashi T, et al. Cytochrome P450 enzymes involved in the metabolism of tetrahydrocannabinols and cannabinol by human hepatic microsomes. Life Sci 2007;80(15):1415–19.

[318] Devitt-Lee A. CBD–drug interactions: the role of Cytochrome p450. O'Shaughnessy's J Cannabis Clin Pract 2015/16:10.

[319] Sachse-Seeboth C, Pfeil J, Sehrt D, et al. Interindividual variation in the pharmacokinetics of delta9-tetrahydrocannabinol as related to genetic polymorphisms in CYP2C9. Clin Pharmacol Ther 2009;85(3):273–6.

[320] Jackson NJ, Isen JD, Khoddam R, et al. Impact of adolescent marijuana use on intelligence: results from two longitudinal twin studies. Proc Natl Acad Sci USA 2016;113(5):E500–8.

[321] van Os J, Bak M, Hanssen M, et al. Cannabis use and psychosis: a longitudinal population-based study. Am J Epidemiol 2002;156(4):319–27.

[322] Thornicroft G. Cannabis and psychosis. Is there epidemiological evidence for an association? Br J Psychiatry 1990;157:25–33.

[323] Ksir C, Hart CL. Cannabis and Psychosis: a Critical Overview of the Relationship. Curr Psychiatry Rep 2016;18(2):12.

[324] Hickman M, Vickerman P, Macleod J, et al. If cannabis caused schizophrenia, how many cannabis users may need to be prevented in order to prevent one case of schizophrenia? England and Wales calculations. Addiction 2009;104(11):1856–61.

[325] Anthony J, Warner LA, Kessler RC. Comparative epidemiology of dependence on tobacco, alcohol, controlled substances, and inhalants: basic findings from the national comorbidity survey. Exp Clin Psychopharmacol 1994;2(3):244–68.

[326] Gao C, Ogeil R, Lloyd B. Alcohol's burden of disease in Australia. Canberra: FARE and VicHealth in collaboration with Turning Point; 2014.

[327] Bachhuber MA, Saloner B, Cunningham CO, et al. Medical cannabis laws and opioid analgesic overdose mortality in the United States, 1999–2010. JAMA Intern Med 2014;174(10):1668–73.

[328] Bradford AC, Bradford WD. Medical marijuana laws reduce prescription medication use in Medicare, part D. Health Aff (Millwood) 2016;35(7):1230–6.

[329] May J. The new age of old age. Sydney Morning Herald, 1 May 2012.

21

Cancer – Advanced I

Dr Janet Schloss

CANCER PATHOGENESIS AND TREATMENT

Cancer as a disease is a complex system that consists of various theories on pathogenesis. As scientists unravel the pathogenesis of cancer, it has helped not only the understanding of how a cell can transform into a tumour, but also the development of molecular testing that can now diagnose tumour development and provide prognosis for a variety of cancers. The following sections look at cancer pathogenesis understanding and how treatment options are now being developed to combat this insidious disease.

Scientific theories on cancer pathogenesis

The development and growth of scientific understanding of cancer has progressed tremendously over the past decade. There are, however, other alternative theories of carcinogenesis, but these theories lack substance and scientific evidence. The five basic theories of cancer pathogenesis are:

1 *Mutational theory.* The mutation theory of carcinogenesis has been the dominant force behind cancer research and the most prevalent theory for the past century. The basis behind this theory is that cancer is a clonal, cell-based disease and that successive DNA mutations in a cell can cause cancer. Therefore, this means that: 1) cancer is a defect of the control of cell proliferation; and 2) the default state of metazoan cells is quiescence.[1]

2 *Genome instability theory.* The genetic instability has been hypothesised as the cardinal feature of cancer development. Genetic alterations in all tumours have now been well established, including subtle changes in DNA sequence, in addition to cytogenetically visible changes such as chromosomal losses, gains and translocation. This theory posits that the genetic instability drives tumour progression by generating mutations in oncogenes and tumour-suppressor genes, thereby providing cancer cells with a selective growth advantage.[2]

3 *Non-genotoxic theory.* The non-genotoxic (epigenetic) theory of carcinogenesis is based on the thought that to induce tumour formation, disturbance of the balance between cell growth and cell death needs to occur. The posit of this theory is that there is a diverse group of chemicals that can induce tumour formation by mechanisms other than direct DNA damage. It believes that repeated exposure to cytotoxicants can result in chronic cell injury, compensatory cell proliferation, hyperplasia and, ultimately, tumour development. In addition, another class of epigenetic carcinogens can interfere with signal transduction mechanisms and gene expression involved in the regulation of cell growth, cell death and differentiation as well as disturbance of hormonal balance, immunosuppression and chronic inflammation.[3]

4 *Darwinian theory.* Since the mid 1970s, cancer development has been described as the process of Darwinian evolution. This states that somatic cellular selection and evolution is the fundamental process leading to malignancy and its many manifestations such as neoangiogenesis, evasion of the immune system, metastasis and resistance to therapies. The basis behind this theory is that cancer is a disease of opportunity.[4]

5 *Tissue organisation theory.* The tissue organisation theory posits that cancer is a tissue-based disease and that proliferation is the default state of all cells based on epistemological and experimental evidence. The premise behind this theory is that carcinogenesis occurs at the tissue level of biological organisation. This implies that chronic abnormal interactions between the mesenchyme/stroma and the parenchyma of a tissue are responsible for the appearance of a tumour, and the default state of all cells is proliferation. In addition, this theory believes that carcinogenesis is a reversible process, as normal tissue in contact with neoplastic tissues may normalise the latter.[5]

Understanding new molecular pathogenesis and prognostics of cancer

SYSTEMIC EVOLUTIONARY THEORY OF CANCER PATHOGENESIS

This new theory posits that cancer is generated by the demergence of the eukaryotic cell system and then the re-emergence of its archaea (genetic material and cytoplasm) and prokaryotic (mitochondria) subsystems. This re-emergence has uncoordinated behaviour and decreased coordination caused by the change in the organisation of the cell environment, which is mainly due to chronic inflammation, damage to mitochondrial DNA and/or its membrane composition by various agents (e.g. viruses, chemicals, hydrogenated fatty acids) and/or by damage to the nuclear DNA that controls mitochondrial energy production. This in turn can affect metabolic pathways including glycolysis within the tumour cell.[6]

PROGNOSTICS OF CANCER

Prognostics of cancer relates to the chances of survival for a person who has cancer. It relates to the estimate of how the disease will go or unravel for that person. The main factors that influence the prognosis include:

- type of cancer and where it is located in the body
- the stage of cancer (i.e. the size of tumour and if it has spread to other parts of the body)
- the grade of the cancer (i.e. how abnormal the cancer cells look under a microscope)
- what traits the cancer cells possess
- the person's age and how healthy they are prior to cancer diagnosis
- response to treatment options.

Currently, doctors estimate prognosis by using statistics that researchers have collected and collated over many years. The most commonly used statistics include:[7]

- *Cancer-specific survival* – the percentage of patients with a specific type and stage of cancer who have not died from their cancer during a certain period of time post diagnosis.
- *Relative survival* – the percentage of cancer patients who have survived for a certain period of time after diagnosis compared to people who do not have cancer.
- *Overall survival* – the percentage of people with a specific type and stage of cancer who have not died from any cause during a certain period of time post diagnosis.
- *Disease-free survival* – the percentage of patients who have no signs of cancer during a certain period of time post treatment.

In addition to the normal statistics used for prognosis, scientists are trying to develop new and progressive models to assist doctors to be more specific for cancer prognosis. Some of the new developments in prognostic tools include:

- *Isolation and characterisation of extracellular vesicles.* Extracellular vesicles contain a substantial amount of genetic information that can be transferred to other cells, thereby promoting the progression of metastatic cancer in patients. To date, several methods are being developed to isolate and analyse these vesicles. However, further work is needed to combat certain issues. Nevertheless, extracellular vesicles are emerging as an important biomarker for cancer diagnosis and prognosis.[8]
- *Single cell protein analysis.* The area of proteomics is an emerging scientific stream that can assist many aspects of health. The single cell protein analysis is a method by which two protein assays demonstrate that T cells communicate with each other and enhance their cytokine release upon contact. This technique is only new as it was developed through a recent PhD project, and further testing to confirm cancer prognosis technique is warranted.[9]
- *Epigenetic biomarkers.* The development and identification of epigenetic biomarkers is an exciting new area with potential to assist the prognostic ability of doctors. To date, prognostic values of the separate biomarkers are ambiguous with no established standards. However, epigenetic biomarkers still seem to have potential, with further research required.[10]
- *Multi-omics Data.* Currently, there have been individual types of omics data used to separately construct predictive models of a 10-year survival rate for breast cancer patients. The predictive model now constructed with proteome data achieved a better predictivity, and was found to out-perform other models. Future development of data-driven and domain-knowledge-based data fusion methods has the ability to lead to improved predictive ability in biomedicine.[11]
- *DNA methylation.* One of the epigenetic mechanisms of regulating gene expression is cytosine methylation in DNA. This plays an important role in cell differentiation or proliferation. Techniques or methods to determine methylation status of specific DNA are being developed to assist in the prognosis of cancer. Two of these techniques include MA-HRM (methylation-specific high-resolution melting) and electrochemistry. These techniques have shown great promise as both were tested successfully, which may lead to more precise diagnostic and prognostics of cancer.[12]

Medicinal cannabis

Studies examining the medicinal properties of *Cannabis sativa* have been increasingly conducted around the world, largely in line with the legalisation of medicinal cannabis occurring in certain states and countries. The medicinal properties identified in these studies include inhibition of chemotherapy-induced nausea and vomiting, appetite stimulation, pain reduction and decreased inflammation, cell proliferation and cell survival.[13] Based on these medicinal properties, the medical conditions identified for the potential benefits of medicinal cannabis properties include chronic pain, respiratory system disorders, glaucoma, multiple sclerosis, HIV/AIDS, muscle spasms, seizures, severe nausea and cachexia or dramatic weight loss.[14]

Cannabis sativa has been found to consist of approximately 60 unique compounds known as cannabinoids. Delta-9-tetrahydrocannabinol (THC) is the most widely studied constituent due to its high potency and abundance in cannabis.[15] Medicinally, THC consists of the main psychoactive component found in cannabis. The other main cannabinoid compound identified for potential beneficial properties is cannabidiol (CBD).[16]

Cannabinoid's pharmacological effects are exerted primarily through two specific plasma membrane G-protein-coupled receptors: cannabinoid receptor 1 (CB1) receptors (most commonly located in the hippocampus, basal ganglia and cerebellum) and cannabinoid receptor 2 (CB2) receptors located in peripheral tissues.[13,16] The anti-cancer properties of cannabinoids were recognised in 1975, with Munson et al.[17] showing in vitro and in vivo data on medicinal cannabis Lewis lung adenocarcinoma growth in mice. The cannabinoids delta-9-THC, delta 8-THC and cannabinol (CBN) but not CBD reduced the primary cancer growth.[17] In addition, in vitro work has identified that cannabinoids can limit inflammation, cell proliferation and cell survival via CB1 and CB2 receptors. This is through a variety of intracellular signal-transducing effects such as inhibition of adenylate cyclase (AC), activation of mitogen-activated protein kinase, regulation of calcium and potassium channels (CB1 only) and other signal transduction pathways.

Further information pertaining to the medicinal cannabis and the endocannabinoids can be found in Chapter 20: Endocannabinoid System.

Outline of treatment options available to people with cancer

In addition to traditional medical treatment for cancer and supportive therapies, there are several options available to people with cancer to assist their treatment or options that are considered to be an 'alternative' treatment. Each country enforces its own laws and regulations in regard to treatment options for cancer, with the World Health Organization setting its own guidelines.[18] Therefore, some of the treatments listed below may be illegal in certain countries but legal in others. There are many alternative therapies available to people – a number of treatments are outlined in Table 21.1.

People who have cancer and those who are assisting people with cancer all want the best for the person, and a 'cure' if possible. However, it is important to note that not all natural therapies are safe, and each case needs to be considered carefully to find what is best for the individual and the stage they are currently at. Some controversial alternative treatment options that are available and have claimed to 'cure' cancer can be seen in Table 21.2. Some of these options may be seen or are classified in certain countries as potentially dangerous. This list is not conclusive as there are quite a number of unsubstantiated alternative treatments for cancer.

MYTHS OF CANCER

Acid/alkaline diet

The human body is regulated by homeostasis, with certain areas requiring acidic environments and others requiring alkaline. The pH of individual cells is highly regulated and the extracellular matrix surrounding cells, although slightly less regulated, is the result of a delicate balance between metabolic processes, proton production and transportation, chemical buffering and vascular removal of waste products.[46] Malignant aggressive cells from a solid tumour are different in that they show a pronounced increase in metabolic processes. Aerobic glycolysis is one of the hallmarks of cancer metabolism and results in an increase

of protons which, if they stayed within the cell, would cause acidosis and cellular death.[46]

Therefore, malignant cancer cells aim to keep intracellular pH consistently alkaline to solve this problem by increasing proton transportation which expels the excess acidity. The accumulation in the extracellular matrix creates a hypoxic and acidic environment around the tumour. It is important to remember that not all cancer cells express or overexpress the same combination of proton transporters and there are important differences among various tumours – in particular, the slower or less aggressive malignant mitochondrial-based tumours.[46,47]

A systematic review on the association between dietary acid load, alkaline water and cancer was conducted and published in 2016.[48] The review evaluated the evidence for a causal relationship between the dietary acid/alkaline and alkaline water for the aetiology and treatment of cancer. Of the 8278 citations, only one study met the inclusion criteria, and no randomised trials were located. The only study found was a cohort study and it revealed no association between the diet acid load and bladder cancer, and no association was found among long-term smokers.[49] Therefore, despite the worldwide promotion of the alkaline diet and water by the internet, media and natural practitioners, there is no actual research to support or disprove this theory. Hence, as a cancer treatment, it is not justified.[48]

The acid/alkaline diet, although not proven for cancer prevention or as a treatment, can have benefits because people who follow this diet generally increase their intake of fresh fruits and vegetables and decrease the intake of highly fried and processed foods and red meat. This provides the body with good nutrients and can be beneficial for cancer prevention. High intake of red meat has been found to be associated with a higher risk of all-cause cancer and cardiovascular mortality, while the increase of fruits and vegetables has been found to decrease the risk.[50]

Sugar feeds cancer

The notion that sugar feeds cancer or cancer cells is touted throughout the internet, controversial anti-cancer sites, books and seminars, in addition to clinician/practitioner seminars. This notion is a very oversimplified and unhelpful assumption based on a highly complex area that science is still unravelling. While it is very sensible to limit sugary food or processed foods high in sugar as part of a healthy diet, the thought that sugar actually feeds cancer cells is incorrect. Researchers are investigating the connection, but this notion remains a source of anxiety-inducing speculation and misinformation from media, the internet and so-called 'experts'.

The main metabolic process of tumours varies depending on the tumour type, aggressiveness and requirements of those particular cells. In essence, blood glucose is the main energy source for all cells, and even without carbohydrate intake, the body can make blood glucose from other sources such as amino acids and fat. The theory that sugar feeds cancer is based on the fact that some solid tumours use aerobic glycolysis as their main

	TABLE 21.1 Alternative treatments for cancer
Treatment	**Description**
Artemisia	The most common form of this herb, which is touted to treat cancer, is *Artemisia annua*. This is a common type of wormwood and is native to Asia. Animal studies and in vitro studies have indicated potential anti-invasion and anti-metastatic capabilities by participating partially in the inhibition of the cancer cell adhesion to endothelial cells via suppression of vascular cell adhesion molecule-1 and suppression of epithelial-mesenchymal transition (EMT).[19–21] However, there are no human studies that have been conducted to date, so further research is required to validate potential anti-cancer activity.
Budwig protocol	This protocol primarily involves flaxseed oil with cottage cheese or quark. It was started by Dr Johanna Budwig in 1952, who developed a specific diet to counteract the 'cancer-causing' process. The basis of the diet is replacing processed fats with beneficial fats. For further information see the Budwig diet in Chapter 12 of CNM – The Immune System, Part C – Cancer.
Frankincense and/ or sandalwood essential oil therapy	Essential oils such as Frankincense (*Boswellia carterii* or *Ru Xiang*) and Sandalwood (*Santalum album* or *Tan Xiang*) have been said in Chinese medicine to have cancer preventive and therapeutic anti-cancer properties.[22] Currently, only in vitro studies have been conducted on these essential oils, with positive results indicating induction of apoptosis in cancer cell lines, but further human clinical trials are required.[22–24]
Hyperthermia	Hyperthermia treatment, which is predominantly used in Europe for cancer, is an emerging cancer treatment worldwide that involves applying heat to a malignant tumour or the whole body of a person with cancer. The heating process can be delivered by using electromagnetic (EM) energy or radiofrequency (RF) or microwave range.[25] Currently, there are clinical trials confirming the use of hyperthermia in conjunction with radiotherapy to help improve the therapeutic outcomes in various tumours. Clinical trials with chemotherapy and hyperthermia are also being conducted.[26] Accurate patient-specific hyperthermia treatment planning is an essential component for effective and safe treatments. Hyperthermia treatment has been found to be a good adjunct to cancer treatment.
Iscador (mistletoe)	Iscador, or mistletoe (*Viscum album*), is a common complementary medicine used in Europe and has been an essential part of herbal medicine for thousands of years. It has also been used as an adjuvant cancer therapy for almost a century in Europe. There are a number of published papers and clinical trials conducted on iscador during and post chemotherapy. It is considered a safe and effective adjunctive treatment for cancer that assists in reducing chemotherapy-related toxicity.[27,28]
Oxygen therapy and hyperbaric chambers	Limited studies have been published on oxygen therapy and hyperbaric chambers as a possible treatment for cancer, but it is promoted as a treatment for cancer. The main peer-reviewed publication on hyperbaric therapy and oxygen therapy as a treatment for cancer was published in 1975 and was a mice study.[29] Hyperbaric oxygen therapy has been stated as treatment for cancer due to the fact that hypoxia is a hallmark of solid tumours and is involved in cell survival, angiogenesis, glycolytic metabolism and metastasis. It has been assumed that increasing oxygenation creates an environment in which cancer cells cannot survive. However, a review conducted in 2012 on hyperbaric oxygen therapy and cancer found that there is no evidence that it has tumour-inhibitory effects.[30] Liquid oxygen is also suggested for cancer patients under the same thought process, but again, there is no literature to support this theory, and to date oxygenation has not been proven to be an effective treatment for cancer, but it may assist with side effects from treatment such as radiation.
Proteolytic enzyme therapy	The theory of enzyme therapy for cancer was initially published in 1911 by John Beard,[31] an English embryologist whose work was forgotten until the 1950s when Max Wolf and Helene Benitez adopted the concept of systemic enzyme therapy for oncology.[32] The basis of the theory is that oral proteolytic enzymes, when no food is being absorbed, are absorbed and distributed systemically. The initial animal studies showed that the growth of tumours was reduced when exposed to these enzymes. Both in vitro and in vivo studies have been conducted and have demonstrated that it may assist in decreasing tumour-induced and therapy-induced side effects and complaints in oncology. These include nausea, gastrointestinal complaints, fatigue, weight loss, restlessness and quality of life. In addition, it was found to increase the response rate of medical treatment, the duration of remissions and the overall survival times.[33] It is still to be proven as an effective alternative therapy for decreasing tumour size, but has promise as an adjunctive cancer treatment.
Vitamin C infusions	Vitamin C has been long connected with assisting people with cancer; however, confusion regarding the understanding and clinical application of the differences between oral and intravenous use has occurred. Early clinical studies by Linus Pauling[34] showed that high-dose vitamin C given intravenously and orally may improve symptoms and prolong life in patients with terminal cancer. Further scientific studies have now confirmed that oral vitamin C therapy has no benefit against cancer cells.[35] Only intravenous vitamin C can reach the plasma concentration necessary to cause toxicity against cancer cells. It is estimated that between 50 and 100 g of intravenous vitamin C, depending on the weight of a person, can reach the level of above 1000 micromol/L required to cause toxicity for cancer cells. Case studies and a few clinical trials have been conducted to date;[36,37] however, the main issue is that there is still no protocol for intravenous vitamin C, or algorithm for administration. Intravenous vitamin C has potential as an individual treatment as well as an adjunct treatment, but further research is required.

TABLE 21.2 Controversial cancer treatments	
Treatment	**Description**
Baking soda and black strap molasses	The Trojan horse remedy of mixing baking soda and black strap molasses is a remedy that is supposed to increase the pH immediately in the blood, increase energy levels and the ability of cells to intake oxygen. This treatment has no peer-reviewed evidence to support the theory and there is no evidence that increasing the pH or oxygenation can reduce tumours. However, there are no unforeseen dangers of undertaking this remedy if so desired.
Bicarbonate soda	Consuming bicarbonate soda daily is based on the theory of alkalising the body. This theory is a cancer myth as the body cannot be alkalised by diet or by taking foods or beverages that are considered alkaline. The body regulates this, not intake. By ingesting bicarbonate soda, stomach acid is decreased, which is good for reflux, but not good before meals. There is no danger if patients want to consume bicarbonate soda on a daily basis, but it must be consumed at least 1 hour post eating.
Black salve (cansema)	Black salve, or cansema, is a corrosive agent that consists of a combination of herbs including *Sanguinaria canadensis* (bloodroot) and zinc chloride. Black salve products have been advertised and promoted as a natural remedy for many different types of cancer, but primarily for skin cancers such as melanoma. Both topical and internal use has been suggested. A review conducted in 2014 examined the current literature as this treatment can be dangerous with or without medical supervision.[38] It found that the widespread use of internet non-peer-reviewed information has allowed anecdotal reports of alternative treatments being used for cancer. Laboratory evidence has documented anticarcinogenic and corrosive effects by black salve. Nine case studies have been published and no clinical trials on efficacy and safety have been documented.[38] Therefore, the concept of black salve as a cancer treatment is not unfounded. However, the side effects of the treatment are not well communicated or known and vary from significant cosmetic defects and scarring to unconfirmed clearance of all cancer cells to cancer recurrence or spread, and there has also been one case documented of death.[38] There are many dangers associated with its use and until clinical trials are conducted to prove safety and efficacy, this treatment is not recommended. Despite the numerous side effects, extreme pain and lack of predictable response or evidence that it works, individuals continue to choose this self-treatment over surgery or medical treatment. A survey of 340 adults regarding their perception of the use of black salve found that 17 of the 23 black salve users were unaware of the potential side effects, and 70% did not visit a dermatologist or doctor before treatment with black salve, but rather relied on personal experience of friends and family.[39]
Hydrogen peroxide treatment	Hydrogen peroxide treatment is one of the best known 'alternative cures' for cancer. It is promoted as being 'safe, readily available and dirt cheap'. It is promoted by controversial programs and publications such as the 'Truth about Cancer' and involves the ingestion of hydrogen peroxide water. However, to date, no case studies or clinical trials have been published on this treatment. Use of hydrogen peroxide internally, such as intravenous vitamin C, has been documented and found safe, and laboratory investigations of hydrogen peroxide on cells have also found it can induce cancer cell death.[40] Hydrogen peroxide is most commonly used as an oxidising agent. Medically, it has been used for wound irrigation at a concentration of 3%; however, its toxic effects preclude its routine use. Ingestion of hydrogen peroxide is a well-known poison. A 39-year-old man who accidentally ingested 250 mL of unlabelled 35% hydrogen peroxide, thinking it was water, suffered grade 2 diffuse oral, oropharynx and epigastric damage, and was admitted to hospital. He was considered 'lucky' because he realised as soon as he had ingested it that it was caustic, so consumed 500 mL of water and induced vomiting.[41] The patient told emergency staff that the substance was in a friend's fridge and was intended for natural health purposes. He mistook the unlabelled container for water. In conclusion, hydrogen peroxide diluted in water is caustic and is not considered a safe practice or treatment for cancer.
Laetrile (vitamin B$_{17}$ or amygdalin)	Laetrile, vitamin B$_{17}$, apricot kernels and amygdalin are all names given to the same substance. Laetrile is considered the best known 'cure for cancer'. The laetrile is used to describe a purified form of the chemical amygdalin, a cyanogenic glycoside found in the pits of many fruits, raw nuts, lima beans, clover and sorghum. In the body, the hydrogen cyanide dissolves to form the cyanide anion. The term vitamin B$_{17}$ was given to laetrile by E.T. Krebs Jr. It gained popularity in the 1970s as an anti-cancer agent.[42] Laetrile is not approved for use in any country. The studies to date have shown very little anti-cancer activity in animals and no anti-cancer activity in human clinical trials. The side effects associated with laetrile toxicity are very similar to cyanide poisoning. These include liver damage, difficulty walking due to nerve damage, fever, coma and death. The internet as an unpoliced source of information has promoted inappropriate advertising of laetrile, and investigations, charges and convictions of distributors have occurred in a number of countries including the US and Australia.[42] A Cochrane review conducted in 2015 found that claims that laetrile or amygdalin have beneficial effects for cancer patients are not currently supported by sound clinical data. Moreover, there is a considerable risk of serious adverse effects from cyanide poisoning after laetrile or amygdalin ingestion. The authors concluded that laetrile as a treatment for cancer is unambiguously negative and is not recommended for use.[43]

Continued

Treatment	Description
Machines (e.g. Rife machine)	There are a number of different types of machines that are used as an anti-cancer treatment. Probably the best known is the Rife machine, which was developed by Royal Raymond Rife in 1920. This machine produces electromagnetic energy in the form of electrical impulses which travel in waves. The theory behind these machines is that all parts of the body emit electrical impulses with different frequencies that may vary depending on health or disease, illnesses could be diagnosed by 'tuning in' on patients' blood or handwriting samples, and these diseases could be treated by feeding proper vibrations into the body with these devices. There are several websites claiming that the Rife machine can be used to treat a number of conditions including cancer. New devices, machines or diagnostic or treatment tools are required to undergo a long process of development and clinical trials to prove or disprove if they cause harm or benefit. The Rife machine and similar machines have not been through this process of scientific testing and there is no evidence to indicate that the Rife machine does what its supporters say, nor is there evidence of harm.[44] Therefore, this treatment had no scientific evidence of benefit and harm has not been formally excluded.
Urine therapy	Urine therapy is based on drinking one's own urine or, in India, drinking cow's urine, as an alternative therapy to treat cancer. There is no scientific evidence for drinking one's own urine as a treatment for cancer to date. India has published studies on cow's urine therapy on various cancer patients.[45] The theory behind the use of cow's urine in India is that cow's blood has life force (pran Shakti), and cow's urine is cow's blood that has been filtered by the kidney. One paper evaluated cow's urine therapy on cancer patients in an 8-day camp. A total of 68 cancer patients completed the survey. Of the 68 patients, five withdrew from the treatment. According to the results of the survey, the symptoms (pain, inflammation, burning sensation, difficulty swallowing, irritation etc.) were decreased in patients undergoing cow's urine therapy.[45] Urine therapy overall, has limited scientific benefit for cancer. It is not recommended but also does no harm.

TABLE 21.2 Controversial cancer treatments—cont'd

metabolic system to produce ATP or energy. This increased uptake of blood glucose has been misconstrued into the notion that consumption of sugar feeds cancer cells. The idea that consumption of sugar and carbohydrates feeds cancer cells has influenced people with cancer to avoid *all* carbohydrate-containing foods. This avoidance is counterproductive in most cases. Moreover, this fear-based approached creates stress and anxiety for the person, which in turn stimulates the fight and flight mechanism, producing hormones that raise blood glucose levels and suppress the immune system.

The science behind some cancer cells does include the upregulation of aerobic glycolysis and is often stimulated by oncogenes. In in vivo studies, researchers have now found that glucose-derived pyruvate can be diverted into the mitochondrial tricarboxylic acid cycle (which all cancer cells still contain) to produce additional energy or intermediates for the synthesis of fatty acids or amino acids such as glutamine.[51,52] Cancer cells can use blood glucose, amino acids or fats as their energy source. Hence, consuming carbohydrates does not 'feed' cancer cells as carbohydrates are only one of the cells' energy sources and restricting them cannot 'starve' the tumour.

MODERN MAINSTREAM TREATMENT, RECENT DEVELOPMENTS IN GENOMICS/ PROFILING/THERAPIES

New developments in immunotherapies and targeted cancer treatments

The medical treatment of cancer has been increasingly focused on new, more direct interventions. The development of immunotherapy and targeted cancer treatments has changed the way cancer is treated, developed patient- or mutation-centred care and enhanced the patients' experience, mortality and quality of life. The mechanism of cancer immunotherapy is the use of specific aspects of the immune system to treat cancer.[53] Some of the new therapies involve antibodies that block the immune checkpoints, cytotoxic T-lymphocyte-associated protein 4 (CTLA-4) and programmed cell-death protein 1 (PD-1 or PD-L1). These new innovations have specially assisted poor response cancers such as melanoma, renal cell carcinoma, bladder cancer, brain tumours and non-small-cell lung cancer.[54]

Targeted cancer therapies are different from immunotherapies. These therapies are linked to specific genetic lesions such as epidermal growth factor receptor mutations and inhibitors. Targeted cancer therapy has progressed cancer treatment from the non-selective, chemotherapy cytotoxic agents that have numerous side effects to a revolutionary molecularly targeted therapy.[55] An example of a targeted cancer treatment is Tarceva (erlotinib) for metastatic non-small-cell lung cancer.

Genomics and impact on treatment

The mapping of the human genome has accelerated the discovery and development of various cancer treatments. The implantation of tumour profiling has already entered the clinic setting and enhanced current treatment options. Understanding the differences in genomic results between different tumour profiling is becoming increasingly important for both patients and oncologists, but enhancing clinician literacy to applied cancer genomics is still required.[56]

Genomic profiling involves scientific assays targeting sequencing panels which may contain between 200 and 500 genes (or, extreme, $n = 20\,000$ genes) that can be implicated in cancer biology or clinical management of cancer. In addition, panel sequencing may emphasise rapid turnaround time by only profiling small gene sets ($n = $ 15–48 genes). These types of genetic profiling may assist clinicians in predicting mutational load for immunotherapy response or predict DNA mismatch repair protein-deficient tumours through mutational load.[56]

Genomic profiling is still a new development and a variety of studies are still being conducted. The use of genomic profiling with the combination of immunotherapy and targeted therapy to enhance the clinical outcome for the patient is a very positive step in cancer treatment.

Profiling and staging options now available

The tumour/node/metastasis staging system has been in use since the 1940s and has several limitations, including not actually reflecting the status of the solid or haematological cancer to predict prognosis. To resolve this issue, new methods of profiling and staging have been investigated. One of the innovations for profiling is the immunokine profiling for cancer staging.[57] This new form is based on the cytokine levels in tumour-bearing human patients. It has demonstrated that cytokine profiling is differential for local or systemic cancers and provides a better predictive tool for oncologists.[57]

Precision medicine

Precision medicine is used to describe how genetic information about a person's disease or cancer is used to assist in diagnosis or treatment.[58] As cancer is a disease of the genome, understanding the genetic changes that occur in cancer cells assists researchers to find more effective treatment strategies that can tailor the cancer treatment to a person's cancer from their genetic profile.[58]

An example of a new cancer treatment that exemplifies precision medicine is the drug imatinib (Gleevec), which was designed to inhibit the altered enzyme produced by a fused version of two genes found in chronic myelogenous leukaemia.[59] Another precision medicine drug that is well known due to its role in breast cancer is trastuzumab (Herceptin), which works only on women whose tumours have a particular genetic prolife called HER-2 positive.[60] There are quite a number of these types of drugs now available to patients, which has taken treatment and survival for patients with cancer to the next level.

Targeted chemotherapy and new radiation therapies

Chemotherapy, for many cancers and people, is an aggressive but effective treatment, but for most patients, the nasty side effects almost outweigh the benefits. Due to the side effects from systemic exposure to the chemotherapy drugs, scientists are now looking for more effective and less toxic ways of delivering these chemotherapy drugs. This includes the development of targeted chemotherapy and new radiation therapies.

One of the new techniques, particularly for liver cancer, is transarterial chemoembolisation.[61] This involves infusing chemotherapy directly into the hepatic artery, as hepatocellular and hepatoma carcinomas get their blood exclusively from this artery. This technique can also be used for metastatic cancers in the liver for similar reasons. This delivers the chemotherapy directly into the liver and to the tumours. There are still side effects from this technique, but they are not as severe as from systemic chemotherapy. In addition to transarterial chemotherapy, there is also intra-arterial chemotherapy, which is used for cancers such as local invasive bladder cancer.[62]

Intratumoural chemotherapy is also an innovative technique for cancers such as non-small-cell lung cancer.[63] This is still going through clinical trials but it involves a computed tomography (CT)-guided intratumoural injection into lesion. To date, it has been found to be safe, effective, aggressive (as it creates a high drug concentration in the tumour) and cost effective.[63] In addition to intratumoural chemotherapy, there is now intraperitoneal chemotherapy, whereby a catheter is inserted via laparoscopy for colorectal and ovarian cancer. This catheter sits just under the skin and connects to a large vein in the peritoneum. Chemotherapy drugs are injected through the catheter, directly targeting the cancer cells in the abdomen.[64]

New ways of delivering radiation have also been developed to assist in making it safer and more effective. Nanomedicine is one of these developments that has stepped into the spotlight. Nanoparticles have been found to potentiate radiotherapy by specifically delivering radionuclides or radiosensitisers into tumours, which enhances the efficacy and reduces the toxicity of radiation.[65] There are now a number of different types of nanoparticle radiosensitisation available to patients including gold nanoparticle dose-enhanced radiation therapy (GNPT)[66] and other metal-based nanoparticle radiosensitisation.[67]

Other new developments in radiotherapy include selective internal radiation therapy (SIRT), which has been used for liver metastasis.[68] This technique delivers millions of tiny radioactive microspheres or beads called SIR-Spheres® directly to the liver tumours.

Radioprotectors and mitigators of radiation-induced normal tissue injury are also another innovation to try to minimise the damage from radiation. Some of the technology used to reduce the toxicity to normal tissue include conformal radiotherapy, intensity-modulated radiotherapy, image-guided radiotherapy and proton radiotherapy.[69]

SCOPE OF PRACTICE FOR THE NATURAL HEALTHCARE PROVIDER

Role of a natural healthcare practitioner in assisting people who have cancer

The role of natural healthcare practitioners in assisting people with cancer will vary. Rarely will a natural healthcare practitioner be the primary health professional unless the patient has declined all or certain medical treatment and is relying totally on natural therapy support or treatment. In most situations, the role of the natural healthcare practitioner will be one of integration, complementary collaboration and/or support using complementary medicine.

To clarify the difference, complementary medicine is defined as complementary therapies used together with conventional medicine; alternative medicine is where natural therapies are used in place of conventional medical treatment; and integrative or collaborative medicine is the practice of medicine that reaffirms the importance of the relationship between a practitioner and patient and utilises all appropriate therapeutic approaches, healthcare professionals and disciplines to achieve optimal health and healing.

Therefore, the natural healthcare professional's role may be one of the following:

* *Primary healthcare practitioner* – if the patient declines traditional medical treatment. This role may use alternative medicine techniques.
* *Complementary healthcare practitioner* – supporting the patient by using natural health products, lifestyle advice or techniques to assist them through medical treatment and post treatment.
* *Integrative practitioner* – part of a team of health professionals assisting the patient with their scope of practice to achieve the best health and healing possible.

Natural healthcare practitioners may find themselves rotating between these roles between patients, and even for the same patient. What is important is being aware of where you stand when assisting that person.

Language and communication

Language, communication and practitioner interaction/relationships with patients is crucial in the wellbeing, health, compliance and mental health of people with cancer. Communication is a multidimensional concept, particularly with people who have or had cancer, as that can be particularly challenging. Unfortunately, it is one of the areas that is less focused on, but it can have the largest impact. Effective treatment and words practitioners use are the basic foundation for responsiveness to treatment, decisions made, positive health outcomes, patient-driven compliance and overall high quality of care.[70]

One of the most important aspects is compassion from the practitioner and patient-centred care, which means the interaction is about the patient being heard and listened to, and the words chosen and treatment suggestions are tailored to that person. It is really important to consider the needs of the patients, their perspectives and experiences. Also, provide opportunities for patients to participate in their own care and take note of how to best interact with the patient.

The current literature of practitioner–patient communication is that the communication must vary depending on which phase patients are in, and that it should be tailored to their evolving needs, preferences and state. Non-verbal communication, from both the patient and the practitioner, is vital. It is important that the practitioner identifies non-verbal as well as verbal cues from the patient and responds accordingly. Additionally,

the non-verbal expressions and language from the practitioner can influence the patient just as much as the verbal language used. Compassion and empathy are very important traits of practitioners, but patients generally do not like sympathy or being patronised.[71]

Scope of practice within and outside the medical system

In addition to language and communication, it is also important to acknowledge your scope of practice with the care of the person with cancer. As with all conditions and people, you should never practise outside your scope of practice. Where needed, refer to professionals if other modalities or assistance are required outside your scope of practice. Within the medical system, the scope of practice of a natural healthcare practitioner is one of support. A patient should never be put in a situation where they are made to choose between the medical fraternity and a natural healthcare practitioner. If a natural healthcare practitioner does not want to collaborate or work with patients who are under care of a medical practitioner, they should state that clearly so the patient is not put into an inappropriate situation.

When patients decline medical treatment

If patients decline medical treatment and choose natural alternatives, communication, ethical and legal considerations and outlining very clearly the scope of practice are imperative. Legally and ethically, natural healthcare professionals cannot state that they can 'cure' cancer. It is important still to promote hope as well as using evidence-based treatment options. The patient should at all stages know there are no guarantees but that the practitioner will do their best to assist them to achieve their goals.

Legality of treating people with cancer

Cancer is considered a 'red flag' disease and, as such, legal and ethical considerations are very crucial. In particular, the legality of treating people needs to be understood and adhered to as the risk of legal action against the practitioner is considered to be higher than for other conditions.

The general legal principles include:
* Every adult of sound mind has the right to determine what happens or is done to their body.
* Any healthcare treatment provided without consent is a trespass.
* Consent to treatment is distinct from the duty to warn about potential risks of treatment.
* A patient has the right to decline treatment.

In general, medical practitioners are ethically and legally obliged to provide patients with enough information to assist them in making adequately informed healthcare decisions. With the growth of complementary or natural therapy medicine, there has been a blurring of distinctions between complementary medicine and conventional medicine. This is particularly important in countries where natural health modalities are not registered. In natural healthcare modalities that are registered, legal and ethical issues are clearly outlined, whereas in the modalities that are not, there are no clear legal or ethical guidelines. However, all natural healthcare professionals are liable and can be made accountable via the legal system in their country.[72]

Understanding your scope of practice and working within that, taking detailed notes and practising within the legal requirements of the country are imperative. This is the same for treating all health conditions, but is emphasised more in 'red flag' conditions such as cancer.

Understanding of the oncological system and the options/approaches for engagement

OVERVIEW OF THE ONCOLOGY/MEDICAL SYSTEM

Oncology incorporates all aspect of cancer care. This includes prevention, diagnosis and treatment of cancer. The main medical staff involved in oncology include the surgeons, medical oncologists, radiation oncologists, haematology oncologists, cancer care nurses, oncology pharmacists and supportive and oncology palliative care doctors and nurses. In addition, all allied health professionals in oncology are classified under the oncology banner.

Primarily, the patients with or who have had cancer will be under a surgeon and/or a medical oncologist and/or a radiation oncologist. All or a combination of these will be the patient's primary carer.

COLLABORATION

Interaction between natural health practitioners and oncology medical staff will vary depending on the primary carer's beliefs regarding natural health. The best interaction a natural health practitioner can have with medical oncology staff is one of professionalism, similar to their interactions with other medical healthcare professionals. This includes written letters given to the patient for the oncologist or contact with the medical oncologist through email. Treating each professional associated with the person with cancer with respect and collaborating is an important aspect of care. The patient then feels that they are not torn between two different worlds of thought and that they are not having to hide something from either the medical or the natural health practitioners. The idea is to all collaborate professionally to achieve the best practice for the patient.

If a natural health professional finds that an oncologist does not want the patient to take any natural supplements throughout treatment, it is recommended that the natural health professional respect the oncologist's decision. The natural health professional may not agree with the statement; however, it is more important that no conflict or confusion for the patient is created. Being diagnosed

with cancer and undergoing medical treatment can be stressful enough without extra stress on the patient.

Alternatively, if a patient really wants to take natural supplements throughout their treatment, it is important to do everything possible to work collaboratively with the medical staff to assist this process and make it as easy and stress free as possible for the patient.

Support through surgery, radiation and chemotherapy – concurrent care

SUPPORT THROUGH SURGERY

Supporting patients through surgery for cancer can pose difficulties. Current practice has shown that patients diagnosed with cancer that can be surgically removed undergo surgery within weeks of diagnosis. There are many reasons for this urgency, but the main reason is that overall survival can be assessed from time of diagnosis to time of surgery. It has been found that the shorter the time interval, the better statistics for survival. In addition to the stress for the person being diagnosed, beginning treatment is crucial for them to feel that something is being done to eradicate the tumour(s). Surgery may not always be at the start of the cancer treatment. If a tumour is a significant size, chemotherapy and/or radiation may be commenced before surgical removal. Also, if the surgeon did not get clear margins, a second or third surgery may be required.

All of these factors need to be taken into consideration when supporting a patient during surgery for cancer. Cessation of natural ingestive products is recommended approximately 1–2 weeks prior to surgery, so the patient may not have time to commence certain supplements prior to surgery. Therefore, support for patients is mostly post surgery. Post-surgery support for tumour removal should focus on:
- wound healing (e.g. zinc, vitamin C, vitamin E, bromelain, wound healing herbs such as *Calendula officinalis*, *Hydrastis canadensis*)
- increasing immune function/system (e.g. *Echinacea purpurea*, *Uncaria tomentosa*, medicinal mushrooms, *Astragulus membranaceus*, zinc, vitamin C)
- restoring nutritional deficiencies (e.g. iron, zinc)
- reducing any risk of circulating tumour cells (e.g. *Uncaria tomentosa*, turmeric)
- rebuilding the body to a healthy state prior to the start of further cancer treatment (e.g. adaptogenic herbal medicines such as *Eleutherococcus senticosus*, *Panax ginseng*, *Withania somnifera*, *Rhodiola rosea*, *Centella asiatica*)

SUPPORT THROUGH RADIATION

Radiotherapy uses high-energy radiation to shrink tumours or kill potential cells. It works by damaging the DNA and creating charged particles (free radicals) within the cells that in turn can damage the DNA. Therefore, use of natural therapies during cancer radiation treatment needs to be evidence-based so no interference with the treatment occurs.

Vitamin D₃

Vitamin D₃ has attracted a lot of attention during cancer. In particular, a deficiency in vitamin D₃ has been found to increase the severity of side effects from treatment and increase the risk of osteoporosis. An overview of some of the studies on a vitamin D deficiency and radiation can be seen in Table 21.3. Overall, it is recommended that patients undergoing radiotherapy for cancer treatment should take a vitamin D₃ oral supplement.

Probiotics

Probiotics in general have been found to help strengthen homeostasis and reduce side effects associated with cancer treatment. To date, current evidence supporting the use of probiotics as an adjunctive therapy to cancer treatment is limited. However, there is some evidence to show benefit during radiotherapy.[76] A list of studies on probiotics and radiotherapy is listed in Table 21.4.

Glutamine

Glutamine as an amino acid has been used for side effects for both chemotherapy and radiation. In a recent meta-analysis on glutamine for radiation-induced severe oral mucositis in head and neck patients,[83] glutamine was found to significantly reduce the risk and the severity of oral mucositis during radiotherapy from the five clinical studies included in the review.

Melatonin

Melatonin is well known for its mechanism of action for insomnia and sleep disturbances. However, melatonin has also been found to have other beneficial activities in relation to radiation. In a phase II, prospective, double-blind randomised trial, patients with radiation-induced dermatitis were treated with a melatonin-containing emulsion which was found to significantly reduce the dermatitis compared to placebo.[84]

TABLE 21.3 Vitamin D₃ deficiency and cancer radiotherapy

Authors	Explanation of study	Dose
Ghorbanzadeh-Moghaddam A, Gholamrezaei A, Hemati S. *Int J Radiat Oncol Biol Phys* 2015[73]	Prospective observational study on cancer patients receiving pelvic radiation (*n* = 98)	Vitamin D deficiency was associated with increased severity of radiation-induced acute proctitis
Akinci MB, Sendur MA, Aksoy S et al. *Asian Pac J Cancer Prev* 2014[74]	A total of 113 colorectal cancer survivors treated with surgery and/or chemotherapy ± radiation were recruited	Results found 96.5% of patients were vitamin D₃ deficient and 66.4% had osteopenia/osteoporosis. Authors stated they were not related
Alco G, Igdem S, Dincer M, et al. *Asian Pac J Cancer Prev* 2014[75]	186 patients with breast cancer undergoing chemotherapy and radiation had their vitamin D₃ status measured	High prevalence of vitamin D₃ (25-OHD) deficiency/insufficiency (70%). Supplementation during is recommended

TABLE 21.4 Probiotic use and cancer radiotherapy

Authors	Explanation of study	Dose
Frazzoni L, Marca M, Guido A et al. 2015[77]	Radiotherapy is frequently employed for pelvic cancers. Despite recent advances in irradiation techniques, acute and late-onset radiation-induced gastrointestinal tract toxicity is frequently reported. Review on treatments	*Lactobacillus rhamnosus* can be administered orally 1.5 g three times a day for a week safely
Mansouri-Tehrani HA, Rabbani-Khorasgani M, Hosseini SM, et al. 2015[78]	67 pelvic cancer patients were randomised to: 1. probiotic capsules (*L. casei, L. acidophilus, L. rhamnosus, L. bulgaricus, Bifidobacterium breve, B. longum, Streptococcus thermophilus*) 2. probiotic caps plus honey 3. placebo capsules	Results were not significant. However, a trend was seen in favour of probiotics in patients receiving pelvic radiotherapy
Kumar M et al. 2013[79]	Probiotics during radiotherapy may reduce risk of heart disease	Rat study, no dose given
Sharma S et al. 2012[80]	*Enterococcus lactis* protects against acetaminophen- (paracetamol-) induced hepatotoxicity	Rat study, no dose given
Ki Y, Kim W, Nam J, et al. 2013[81]	*L. acidophilus* reduced percentage of volume change of the rectum during prostate cancer radiation	Probiotic capsule containing 1.0×10^8 colony-forming units of *L. acidophilus*
Demers M, Dagnault A, Desjardins J 2014[82]	Probiotics found to reduce radiation-induced diarrhoea (grade 204) at the end of treatment for pelvic cancer	Bifilact® probiotics (*L. acidophilus* LAC-361 and *B. longum* BB-536): a standard dose twice a day (1.3 billion CFU) or a high dose three times a day (10 billion CFU)

In addition, melatonin has also been found to be a potent stimulus for enhancing the efficacy of laser radiation on induction of apoptosis in tumour cells for ovarian cancer.[85]

A literature review has found that melatonin can effectively protect animals against injury to healthy tissues from ionising radiation, but no studies have been conducted on humans to date.[86] If human studies focus on healthy tissue protection from melatonin document similar protective effects, melatonin could provide a great adjunct in protection against radiation-induced side effects.

Deglycyrrhizinated liquorice

Studies examining the protective effects of liquorice for radiotherapy-induced side effects are limited. However, it is worth noting for its mucosal healing properties. One of the most common side effects of head and neck radiation is mucositis. One trial on *Glycyrrhiza glabra* protection for head and neck cancers found that the severity of radiation-induced mucositis for head and neck was reduced by a great extent. Therefore it was found beneficial for the prevention and treatment of radiation-induced mucositis, working in two ways: 1) there were no interruptions in the treatment; and 2) food intake was not severely affected, leading to maintenance of nutritional status and weight of patients.[87]

Calendula

Calendula officinalis is well known as a topical agent for skin conditions. It has been noted to increase skin healing and has been tested for oral mucositis as a mouthwash in hamsters[88] with positive effects. Similarly, in a randomised trial on 40 head and neck cancer patients receiving radiotherapy, those who were given the calendula mouthwash had a significantly lower intensity of oropharyngeal mucositis compared to placebo.[89] Calendula has also been assessed for the treatment of radiation-induced skin conditions such as radiation-induced dermatitis. A review examining calendula as a topical treatment and preventive agent of radiation-induced skin toxicity found that it was safe; however, the evidence for benefit remains weak.[90]

SUPPORT THROUGH CHEMOTHERAPY

The aim of using natural therapies during chemotherapy is to:
- reduce side effects, in particular long term
- increase efficacy of medical treatment
- increase the quality of life of the patient.

There is a risk of interference or interaction with chemotherapy drugs during treatment with natural supplements. An overview of potential interactions from ingestive complementary medicines can be seen in Table 21.5.

In regards to introducing natural ingestive medicines or supplements during chemotherapy, there are some essential points that need to be taken into consideration. Some of the general principles include stopping the ingestive complementary medicine 1–2 days prior to

TABLE 21.5 Ingestive complementary medicine interaction with chemotherapy

Action	Complementary ingestive medicine	Suggestions
Inhibit or induce cytochrome P450 enzymes	St John's wort[91,92] *Ginkgo biloba*[92,93] Kava[92,94] Black cohosh[94] *Panax ginseng*[95] *Echinacea purpurea*[96] Milk thistle[95] Evening primrose oil[92]	Avoid during chemotherapy treatment
Affect cellular protein P-glycoprotein	Curcumin[97,98] Ginseng[99] Piperine[98] Ginger[98] Capsaicin[98] Resveratrol[98] Green tea catechins[98] Quercetin[98] Silymarin[100]	A majority of these natural components have chemo-sensitising ability, especially for multi-drug resistant tumours

chemotherapy administration and then recommencing 2–3 days post administration. This may vary depending on the half-life of the chemotherapy drugs, but this is a general rule to follow. Some natural vitamin supplements may be safe and efficacious to take through the chemotherapy cycle, but it may be easier for the patient to keep all supplements away from chemotherapy for ease of taking and remembering to take them and so they do not become confused.

In addition, polypharmacy in cancer treatment is common, and precautions when adding ingestive complementary medicine is warranted. One of the major challenges for medical health professionals is the lack of awareness or understanding of natural health products. They may not have the time to research these products or may not have had heard of them. Therefore, it is important to consider dose, frequency, time of use and the administration of use. If a practitioner is in doubt about an ingestive supplement, do not prescribe it.

Diet

Diet or what people eat will vary greatly depending on the chemotherapy combination they are undertaking and which stage they are at. Diet in general, or what people eat, is often a controversial and hotly debated topic. Medical professionals may recommend that they eat what they want or continue their normal diet; dietitians may recommend certain foods or breakdown of foods to keep on weight; natural health professionals debate among themselves about certain types or styles of diets. All of this can be very confusing for patients to know what is best for them.

A general rule for people undergoing chemotherapy is to try to keep their diet as healthy as possible, limit highly processed foods, avoid delicatessen foods and ensure all foods are fully cooked (e.g. no raw eggs or fish, no leftovers that have been kept in the fridge for more than 1 day or any foods that are in a bain-marie). This is due to low neutrophils and the body's inability to fight normal bacteria and viruses.

In addition, many patients undergoing chemotherapy experience taste and smell changes and have malaise, nausea and either of, or a combination of, constipation and diarrhoea. Some general rules for people undergoing chemotherapy include:

- If something does not taste or smell good, and makes them feel sick, even though they know it is good for them, it is best not to eat or drink it, the reason being that there is a memory that is triggered, and if they eat it and it makes them sick, when they try to eat it after the treatment is finished, they will find it difficult to eat. Chemotherapy is only for a short time in general, so it is better to keep good foods for later when they can eat them for maintenance.
- Freeze foods and bring them out when needed. Having a range of frozen meals assists when they are not sure what they feel like, if they are served foods and then cannot eat them, and because of the fatigue they generally do not have energy at the end of the day, so this is a good way to ensure good nutrient intake. Note: do not freeze rice as it may harbour bacteria.
- Include complex carbohydrates. Due to chemotherapy's effect on blood glucose, the malaise and the nausea, consuming complex carbohydrates with protein gives the person slow-release energy, which helps them feel better.
- If the person is suffering from constipation, try pear juice or prune juice.
- If the person has diarrhoea, try grated apple that needs to be eaten only when the apple flesh goes brown.
- For nausea, eat every 2 hours and have crackers available if needed. Hot chips (oven baked if possible) have been found to help a lot of people with chemotherapy nausea.

There are many different dietary techniques that can assist people, but each person is different. Tailor the person's diet accordingly and be gentle with them as it is a very hard experience and they need assistance and compassion to get through it.

Exercise

Exercise during chemotherapy and post cancer treatment has received a lot of attention within the past 5 years. Exercise during treatment and after treatment is highly recommended. There are many benefits that have been found. The term used now is 'activity' rather than exercise during chemotherapy treatment to assist people to understand that because of the fatigue and other side effects, they may not be able to participate in an organised exercise regimen, but can still do moderate activity.

Exercise or activity has been found to mitigate several symptoms associated with chemotherapy treatment. This is because it influences biological pathways such as the inflammatory immune response, metabolic and neuroendocrine adaptations and genetic and epigenetic influences.[101] Moreover, a higher resting level of certain sympathetic hormones has been linked to fatigue,

depression and pain, which exercise can decrease.[101] Thus, exercise has been found to positively influence immune, metabolic, neuroendocrine, genetic and epigenetic functions in individuals without cancer, and now with cancer.[101]

Some specific studies addressing side effects of chemotherapy and exercise are listed below:
- Tai chi during chemotherapy has been found to be very beneficial. A randomised clinical trial assessing tai chi for lung cancer patients during chemotherapy found that it was an effective intervention for managing cancer-related fatigue.[102]
- A study conducted on 417 older patients (>65 years) during and after cancer treatment found that almost half of the older and oldest cancer patients reported that using exercise (activity) during and post treatment assisted in reducing their side effects, including sleep and skin problems.[103]
- A meta-analysis of randomised controlled trials on aerobic exercise for cancer-related fatigue found that it was very effective for the management of fatigue for patients who completed adjuvant chemotherapy treatment.[104]
- Chemotherapy-induced peripheral neuropathy (CIPN) is a debilitating side effect of a number of chemotherapy agents. The Pathways study found that patients who engaged in more than 5 hours per week of moderate-to-vigorous physical activity had less CIPN.[105]

Therefore, some basic advice for patients undergoing chemotherapy regarding exercise is:
- Adjust exercise depending on mobility and level of fatigue.
- Exercise at least three times a week to their ability.
- Walking in most cases is suggested as it is low cost, safe and can be conducted at their own pace.
- Tai chi and Qigong have been found to be beneficial for sleep and fatigue.
- Avoid public swimming pools due to risk of infection.
- Consult an exercise physiologist if required.

Meditation

The diagnosis and treatment of cancer is considered to be a major life stress. Implementing ways of managing this stress has been found to be highly beneficial for patients. Meditation, brief psychological interventions, mindfulness and gratitude have been found to assist patients psychologically.[106] Mindfulness, sitting meditation in particular, has been found to be extremely beneficial for patients who have higher symptoms of distress.[107]

Sleep

Insomnia is a common problem for patients undergoing chemotherapy, especially due to steroid use. A number of options have been trialled that showed possible benefit. These include melatonin, cognitive behaviour therapy, Qigong/tai chi and acupuncture. One study in particular was a double-blind, placebo-controlled randomised controlled trial (RCT) which assessed 50 patients (aged 20–65 years old) who had primary insomnia during cancer treatment. The intervention was 3 mg of melatonin or

TABLE 21.6 Natural therapies trialled for cisplatin

Complementary agent	Main mechanism of action	Dose
Vitamin E – alpha-tocopherol[112–115]	Decrease ototoxicity and CIPN	400 mg per day (300–600 mg/day)
Vitamin B₆[116]	Prevented CIPN, but affected dose response	Dose in the trial was 300 mg daily. Lower dose is recommended
Alpha-lipoic acid[117]	Sensitises cells to chemotherapy	Cell work, no dose given. Recommended 600–800 mg daily
Quercetin[118,119]	In animal studies, reduces renal and hepatic toxicity	No dose given. Recommended 500 mg administered orally twice a day
Melatonin[120,121]	Rat study showed protection against ototoxicity and fertility through decreased follicle loss	No dose given. Recommended 5 mg at night 2 hours before bed.

TABLE 21.7 Colorectal cancer regimens

Chemotherapy regimen	Chemotherapy agents
FOLFOX Every 2 weeks for 12 cycles	Oxaliplatin Leucovorin (folinic acid) Fluorouracil (5FU)
FOLFIRI Every 2 weeks for 12 cycles	Leucovorin (folinic acid) Irinotecan
CapeOX Every 2 weeks for 12 cycles	Capecitabine (Xeloda) Oxaliplatin
FOLFOXIRI Every 2 weeks for 12 cycles	Leucovorin (folinic acid) Oxaliplatin Irinotecan

TABLE 21.8 Supportive therapy for colorectal cancer

Complementary agent	Main mechanism of action	Dose
Alpha-lipoic acid[122,123]	Reduced severity of CIPN	800 mg daily
Vitamin B₆[124]	Possible reduction in CIPN	60 mg daily
PSK (Coriolus versicolor)[125,126]	Immune modulation during treatment and increased survival rate	3 g per day away from food

placebo 2 hours before bed for 14 days. It was found that the daily intake of the melatonin improved sleep induction and quality of sleep for the cancer patients.[108]

General support during chemotherapy

As mentioned, undertaking chemotherapy treatment for cancer can be very stressful. Being prepared and understanding the chemotherapy regimen may help lessen some of the stress associated with the treatment. As there are many different types of chemotherapy or anti-cancer drugs, a general list of some combinations for more common cancers and natural therapies that have been trialled are listed below. Some general tips for chemotherapy include:
- ginger for acute nausea and vomiting[109]
- vitamin D₃ for all patients[110]
- probiotics for chemotherapy-induced diarrhoea.[111]

Specific chemotherapy and combination regimens

Cisplatin is a platinum compound that is used to treat a number of cancers, including testicular, ovarian, breast, lung, bladder, oesophageal, brain, head and neck and cervical cancer, as well as mesothelioma and neuroblastoma. Natural therapies trialled for cisplatin can be seen in Table 21.6.

Please review Tables 21.7–21.15 for specific medication regimens for specific cancers.

TABLE 21.9 Breast cancer regimens

Chemotherapy regimen	Chemotherapy agents and cycles
AC – T(H)	Adriamycin, cyclophosphamide: every 3 weeks for 3–4 cycles Then paclitaxel weekly for 9–12 weeks If HER 2+, Herceptin and possibly pertuzumab (Perjeta) every 3 weeks
FEC – D(H)	5-fluorouracil, epirubicin, cyclophosphamide than docetaxel for 3 or 4 rounds, then docetaxel 3 or 4 rounds every 3 weeks
FEC – T(H)	5-fluorouracil, epirubicin, cyclophosphamide every 3 weeks for 3 or 4 cycles, then paclitaxel weekly for 9–12 weeks
TAC	Docetaxel, Adriamycin, cyclophosphamide every 3 weeks for 6 cycles
TC(H)	Docetaxel, cyclophosphamide plus Herceptin every 3 weeks for 4–6 cycles
CMF	Cyclophosphamide, methotrexate, 5-fluorouracil every 3 weeks for 6 cycles

TABLE 21.10 Supportive therapies for breast cancer

Complementary agent	Main mechanism of action	Dose
Omega-3 fatty acids[127]	Reduces CIPN	640 mg t.d.s.
Vitamin B$_{12}$[128,129]	Reduces CIPN	1000 micrograms daily
PSK[130]	Increases the prognosis of operable breast cancer with vascular invasion and patients positive for HLA-B40	3 g per day away from food
Lipoic acid[117]	Sensitises cells to chemotherapy agent	No dose given – cell culture Recommended 600–800 mg/day
Biobran (Ribraxx)[131]	Increases chemotherapy into cells, reduces drug resistance, increases natural killer cells, protects Peyer's patches in digestive tract	1 sachet per 30 kg of body weight
Withania somnifera[132]	Has potential for assisting against cancer-related fatigue. Tested in an open-label non-RCT on 100 breast cancer patients undergoing chemo with Taxotere, Adriamycin, cyclophosphamide, 5FU and epirubicin	2 g every 8 hours throughout course of chemotherapy treatment
Melatonin[133]	Melatonin prevents mitochondrial damage induced by doxorubicin in mouse fibroblasts	No dose given due to mice/rat study 2–5 mg 2 hours before bed

TABLE 21.11 Prostate cancer

Chemotherapy agent	Trial
Now treated with docetaxel (Taxotere)	Mainsail trial[134] Multi-national trial, RCT, phase III study 1059 patients received docetaxel, prednisone and lenalidomide or docetaxel, prednisone or placebo Authors looked at optimal number of docetaxel cycles Results: 8 or more cycles increased survival benefit
Same treatment support as breast cancer	

TABLE 21.12 Lymphoma regimens

Chemotherapy regimen	Chemotherapy agents
R-CHOP or CHOP Every 2–3 weeks for 6–8 cycles	Cyclophosphamide Doxorubicin Vincristine Prednisolone Rituximab (MabThera)
CVP (R) Every 2–3 weeks for 4–8 cycles May have rituximab or doxorubicin added	Cyclophosphamide Vincristine Prednisolone
Hyper-CVAD Schedule A (cycles 1, 3, 5, 7) Schedule B (cycles 2, 4, 6, 8)	Part A: Cyclophosphamide Vincristine Doxorubicin Dexamethasone Part B: Methotrexate Cytarabine

TABLE 21.13 Supportive therapy for lymphoma

Complementary agent	Main mechanism of action	Dose
CoQ10[135]	Used in conjunction with Adriamycin or doxorubicin. Non-toxic, did not affect anti-tumour activity, decreased cardiac dysfunction, decreased cardiotoxicity	200 and 350 mg/m^2. Continued daily dose of at least 50 mg of CoQ10
Lipoic acid[136]	Decreases cardiotoxicity associated with cyclophosphamide. Mice study, but reversed abnormal biochemical changes to near normalcy. Protective role	No dose given due to mice study. Recommended 600–800 mg a day
Melatonin[133,137]	Melatonin prevents mitochondrial damage induced by doxorubicin in mouse fibroblasts	No dose given due to mice/rat study. Recommended 2–5 mg 2 hours before bed
EPA/DHA[138,139]	Distribution of plasma fatty acids has been associated with patients' response to chemotherapy for non-Hodgkin's lymphoma. Poor response (not finishing due to death or toxicity) had significantly lower EPA/DHA, palmitoleic, linoleic acid, omega-3, omega-6. Cell lines showed omega-3 fatty acids to promote chemo-sensitivity for chemo for chronic lymphocytic leukaemia (vincristine, doxorubicin, fludarabine)	No dose given. Recommended 3–4 g of EPA/DHA
Withania somnifera[140]	Animal study showed Withania somnifera to protect against cyclophosphamide-induced urotoxicity	No dose given. Recommended 2 g per day

| TABLE 21.14 Lung cancer chemotherapy agents ||
Chemotherapy agent – a combination of these can be utilised	Chemotherapy agent – a combination of these can be utilised
Cisplatin	Vinorelbine
Carboplatin	Irinotecan
Paclitaxel/Abraxane	Etoposide
Docetaxel	Vinblastine or vincristine
Gemcitabine	Pemetrexed (Alimta)

| TABLE 21.15 Supportive therapy for lung cancer ||||
Complementary agent	Main mechanism of action	Dose
Lipoic acid[117]	Sensitises cells to chemotherapy agent	No dose given – cell culture Recommended 600–800 mg/day
Omega-3 fatty acids[127]	Reduces CIPN	640 mg t.d.s.
Vitamin B$_{12}$[128,129]	Reduces CIPN	1000 micrograms daily
PSK[141]	Found to improve immune function, reduce tumour-associated symptoms, extend survival in lung cancer patients	3 g per day away from food
Melatonin[142]	Melatonin in reduction of chemotherapy-induced toxicity trial was a double-blind, placebo-controlled RCT. Was found that it did not affect survival, did not interfere with chemotherapy, had no adverse events but helped quality of life for patients	10–20 mg 2 hours before bed
Biobran (Ribraxx)[131]	Increases chemotherapy into cells, reduces drug resistance, increases natural killer cells, protects Peyer's patches in digestive tract	1 sachet per 30 kg of body weight

DISCUSSION ON FASTING AND EVIDENCE

A new, novel way to assist people with cancer or who have had cancer is fasting overnight. A multi-site randomised trial on patients with breast cancer conducted a women's healthy eating and living study.[143] Data was collected from 2413 women with breast cancer, but without diabetes mellitus, aged 27–70 years at diagnosis. A dietary analysis was conducted at baseline, 1 year post and then 4 years. The major outcomes found that prolonged nightly fasting (13 hours or more) reduced the risk of breast cancer recurrence, reducing inflammation (lower C reactive protein), improved gluco-regulation (lower HbA$_{1c}$) and assisted sleep.[143]

Although this study was conducted on women who had breast cancer, it can be extrapolated for all cancers. The recommendation is no food consumption (including milk) after 8 pm, and fasting for at least 13 hours overnight. Water and herbal teas can still be consumed, but no food substance. This means that if the person finished their dinner around 7.30 pm, they do not eat again until 8.30 am the next day.

This is an easy-to-incorporate approach to assist in decreasing the risk of cancer, decreasing systemic inflammation, managing blood glucose control, assisting sleep and decreasing the risk of recurrence. Moreover, it is a non-pharmaceutical approach anyone can incorporate.

CASE STUDIES OF MOST COMMON TYPES OF CANCER TO HIGHLIGHT APPROACH

CASE STUDY 1
Breast cancer

OVERVIEW

RA is a 42 year-old-woman who was diagnosed with breast cancer 3 weeks ago (2 weeks before Christmas). Biopsy indicated invasive ductal carcinoma HER2 negative, oestrogen and progesterone positive with three possible axillary lymph node involvement. Due to the time of year and size, commenced chemotherapy 14 days post diagnosis before surgery and 1 week before presentation to the clinic consultation. The chemotherapy regimen is AC – Adriamyocin and cyclophosphamide 4 cycles, every 3 weeks. A scan will be conducted post 4th cycle and a decision will be made to either have surgery then or continue 9 weeks of paclitaxel weekly before surgery. Side effects of the first round of chemotherapy were constipation, nausea, increased smell sensation and body fatigue, or 'heaviness'.

Only known allergy was penicillin. She had just commenced a ketogenic diet prior to diagnosis and was unsure what she should do diet-wise throughout treatment, and wanted to work together to assist treatment. She is married with one child who is 2 years old.

CLINICAL EXAMINATION

- Weight 80.7 kg, height 1.62 m
- Temperature: 36.2°C
- Emotionally stable but stressed with the diagnosis

INVESTIGATIONS

Blood testing that precipitated medication prescription included:

Test	Result
Haemoglobin	122 (115–160)
Platelet count	198
White cell count	5.2 (4.0–11.0)
Neutrophils	4.1 (2.0–7.5)
Lymphocytes	1.9 (1.1–4.0)
Monocytes	0.4 (0.2–1.0)
Mean cell volume	85 (80–98)
Mean cell haemoglobin	29 (27–35)

TREATMENT PROTOCOL

The treatment focused on assisting RA through this stage of treatment until she knew if she was going to have surgery first or further chemotherapy. The aim was to minimise side effects and provide a dietary plan that would work for her and her family during this first period of time.

HERBAL MEDICINE

Due to her stress, a capsule formula of *Withania somnifera*, *Eletherococcus senticosis* and *Rhodiola rosea* was prescribed – two capsules a day but not on the day of and 2 days after chemotherapy administration. A majority of patients cannot tolerate liquid herbal mixtures due to smell and taste changes associated with chemotherapy administration. Capsules or tablets have a better compliance response in most cases.

NUTRITIONAL MEDICINE

Dietary

Dietary suggestions were given in accordance with what the patient would consume and the chemotherapy regimen she is undergoing currently. This regimen generally makes the patient feel sick in the morning and fatigued in the evening. Constipation occurs within the first week after chemotherapy administration. Water also tastes terrible and can leave a metallic taste in the mouth. Mouth ulcers are very common and taste changes occur after the first round of chemotherapy in most people. The following suggestions were given:

- Breakfast options may include:
  - Light rye or spelt toast with butter with Vegemite (can add avocado)
  - Cooked potatoes or hash browns
  - If she feels like it, scrambled eggs
- Largest meal should be lunch in the middle of the day and consist of either salad or cooked vegetables with some form of protein:
  - Salmon patties
  - Lentil patties
  - Chicken/turkey
  - Eggs – quiche, scrambled, omelette
  - Pork rissoles homemade
- For dinner, more cooked vegetables rather than raw due to fatigue and poor digestive ability (e.g. yellow Thai curry with small amount of basmati rice, slow-cooked meals)
  - *Avoid* – high tomato-based foods or creamy based sauces, no delicatessen foods, no grapefruit, no citrus fruits, chilli or hot, spicy foods
  - If feeling nauseous, eat every 2–3 hours, have crackers if needed; hot oven-baked chips can help manage and decrease the nausea
  - Consume a small cup of bone broth daily
  - Consume fresh ginger and/or peppermint tea
  - In water (drink cold) – put small amount of grated ginger, fresh mint, cut up apple or small amount of pomegranate or cranberry juice to change taste of water
  - Snacks if required: cut up vegetables such as carrot or celery with hummus

Supplemental

Nutrient	Dose	Justification
Vitamin D₃	1000 IU (1 capsule) after food	To maintain or increase vitamin D levels to decrease risk of osteoporosis, fatigue and aches and pains
Coriolus (medicinal mushrooms)	2 capsules twice a day	To support the immune system
Liposomal vitamin C	1 sachet per day	To assist immune system and healing

Note: Not to be administered on chemotherapy day and 2 days post chemotherapy administration.

Lifestyle/education

Emphasis was placed on listening to herself and her body. Rest when needed, manage stress, refer to an exercise physiologist for correct exercise advice, ensure good sleep habits, engage in activities she enjoys and socialise and have fun with her daughter and husband. Avoid large areas of people from days 8 to 14 post chemotherapy administration as she will be at higher risk of infection. Take her temperature daily, and if over 38°C, go to the hospital. Conduct good hygiene, particularly 48 hours post chemotherapy administration, as a majority is excreted through urine.

CASE STUDY 2
Lymphoma

OVERVIEW

KB is a 56-year-old woman who has been diagnosed with follicular B cell lymphoma grade 3, stage 3. History includes atrial fibrillation, haemorrhoids and anal fissure, two bowel prolapse surgeries, hysterectomy (ovaries not taken), bone marrow and tumour biopsies. Medication includes Noten, Tambocor, rectogesic for the anal fissure, antibiotic (Bactrum) twice a week, and has currently just completed chemotherapy treatment, R-CHOP six cycles every 2 weeks, 3 weeks ago at time of consultation. Currently taking magnesium capsules and has just taken Macu-Vision for her sight. She is walking briskly for about 3–4 km most days. Diet is very good, with a protein shake for breakfast (blueberries, pea protein powder, vital greens, almond milk, coconut yoghurt, spinach leaves, cinnamon, ginger and turmeric), lunch is a salad with spinach, tomato, avocado, olives with salmon. Dinner consists of cooked fish with cooked vegetables. Snacks include fruit, nuts, hummus with gluten-free crackers or falafel chips. She consumes water, herbal teas and, occasionally, almond decaf coffee. She is married with two children.

Current status, she is due for a PET/CT in a month's time to see progress of tumours. Last tumour showed main tumours had reduced in size. Had been administered Xarelto but had ceased use 1 month ago. Currently, she is experiencing CIPN grade 2 (currently not painful but had been), eyes and eyesight affected – tear ducts blocked, dry and inflamed, and extreme fatigue, particularly in the legs, has dizzy spells, headaches, ectopic heart beats, sore mouth (had oral thrush and was prescribed oral Nilstat), tongue sore and persistent stinging sensation around mouth, bowels are currently working 'OK' and is taking a laxative daily due to anal fissure.

CLINICAL EXAMINATION

Weight 63 kg, height 1.56 m

TREATMENT PROTOCOL

The treatment focused on decreasing the side effects from treatment. The CIPN, leg fatigue and nerve stinging sensations near the mouth are all from vincristine administration. The eye reactions are from the steroids, and the rest are from the chemotherapy combination. As she has only just finished her chemotherapy regimen, she is still experiencing acute and chronic side effects.

HERBAL MEDICINE

A tablet of *Ginkgo biloba* was prescribed, two tablets a day (120 mg twice a day). This is to assist in reducing CIPN pain and in restoring nerve fibre damage. Also may assist with chemo brain symptoms.

For fatigue, an American ginseng tablet 1000 mg a day was prescribed to be taken in the morning.

NUTRITIONAL MEDICINE
Dietary

Minimal dietary suggestions were given due to her diet, which she has worked on with an integrative doctor.
- Increase protein for lunch such as salmon, small amounts of organic chicken (no skin), organic lamb or beef, egg or sheep's cheese (haloumi) or goat's fetta

Supplemental

Nutrient	Dose	Justification
Acetyl-L-carnitine	2000 g a day on an empty stomach	To restore nerve damage (CIPN) and assist with fatigue and chemotherapy brain
Vitamin B$_{12}$	1000 micrograms of methylcobalamin daily	To assist in reversing CIPN
Sublingual CoQ10 lozenges	1–2 lozenges sucked daily	To assist in healing the mouth and help with fatigue and heart complications

Lifestyle/education

For her mouth, try rubbing coconut oil around her mouth and tongue daily. For her eyes, try putting wet tea bags on them daily, or an eye bath of Eyebright. Continue exercise and rest when needed.

CASE STUDY 3
Metastatic colorectal cancer

OVERVIEW

JL is a 73-year-old woman who has been diagnosed with metastatic colorectal cancer and adenocarcinoma. Six months prior to her first consultation, she thought she had a urinary tract infection, and went to an osteopath who thought it might be appendicitis, so sent her to the doctor. Upon seeing her general practitioner, she was sent straight to hospital where she was operated on immediately, and 27 cm of her large bowel was removed. She had 26 nodes removed, eight positive for cancer ($n = 8/26$). Staged T4a N2b, **carcinoembryonic antigen (CEA)** levels were 400, and received a PET scan a few days post surgery which identified lymphatic involvement. Was diagnosed stage 4 colorectal cancer and declined chemotherapy. History includes pleuroparenchymal scarring on both lungs, cysts on the liver, hay fever and haemochromatosis. Currently her CEA is 17.1. Allergies include intravenous dye and valerian. Currently, only medication is melatonin 3 mg per night. Complementary medicines include:
- Five-mushroom extract 20 drops three times day
- Citrus pectin 1 teaspoon three times a day

- Vitamin C 1000 mg three times a day
- Zinc 30 mg a day
- Magnesium 400 mg a day
- Vital greens
- CoQ10 150 mg daily
- Fish oil – two capsules daily
- Curcumin – two capsules daily
- Green-lipped muscle extract three capsules daily
- Gelatine
- Silica
- Fibergy
- Olive leaf extract.
  Diet consisted of:
  Breakfast: chia seeds soaked with almonds, magnesium powder, vital greens, Fibergy, silica, kefir yoghurt, goji berries, cranberries and ½ banana
  Lunch: greens from garden (home grown), lettuce, garlic chives, kale, steamed beetroot, sundried tomatoes, avocado, apple cider vinegar, boiled egg (from her own chickens), cashew cheese and 1 dessertspoon of sauerkraut
  Dinner: fish/chicken, vegetable burger patties (homemade) or egg-omelette with steamed vegetables
  Snacks: brazil nuts
  Beverages: 4 cups of water with apple cider vinegar in all of it, herbal teas – Jason Winters (3 cups a day), green tea (1–2 cups), ginger and lemon

CLINICAL EXAMINATION

Weight: 60 kg, height: 1.65 m

TREATMENT PROTOCOL

The treatment focused on working with her diet, improving her immune system, decreasing her diarrhoea, and trying to prevent further metastasis and reduce or stabilise cancer growth.

HERBAL MEDICINE

A liquid herbal mixture was prescribed:

Herb	Amount
Cat's claw (*Uncaria tomentosa*)	80 mL
Astragalus membranaceus	60 mL
Artemisia annua	20 mL
Withania somnifera	40 mL
TOTAL	200 mL

Dose: 8 mL to be taken twice daily.

NUTRITIONAL MEDICINE

Dietary

- Remove magnesium powder from the shake and take at night time before bed
- Consume plain filtered water with no apple cider vinegar in it
- Continue diet ensuring 2 cups of cooked vegetables at night

- Consume only 2 serves of fruit a day
- Consume lamb once a fortnight in a slow cooker
- Organic cheese in small amounts

Supplemental

Change vitamin C oral to liposomal vitamin C.

Nutrient	Dose	Justification
PSK	2 capsules three times a day away from food	To assist with immune system
Liposomal vitamin C	1 sachet twice a day	To support the immune system, act as an anti-cancer agent
Biobran (Ribraxx)	1 sachet twice a day	To assist immune system, healing, increase natural killer cells

Lifestyle/education

Emphasis was placed on listening to herself and her body. Recommended she try tai chi as an exercise, engage in activities she enjoys particularly gardening and bridge, and develop good sleep hygiene habits.

REFERENCES

[1] Sonnenschein C, Soto AM. Somatic mutation theory of carcinogenesis: why it should be dropped and replaced. Mol Carcinog 2000;29:205–11.

[2] Cahill DP, Kinzler KW, Vogelstein B, et al. Genetic instability and darwinian selection in tumours. Trends Cell Biol 1999;9(12):M57–60.

[3] Mally A, Chipman JK. Non-genotoxic carcinogens: early effects on gap junctions, cell proliferation and apoptosis in the rat. Toxicology 2002;180:233–48.

[4] Thomas F, Fisher D, Fort P, et al. Applying ecological and evolutionary theory to cancer: a long and winding road. Evol Appl 2012;6:1–10.

[5] Soto AM, Sonnenschein C. The tissue organization field theory of cancer: a testable replacement for the somatic mutation theory. Bioessays 2011;33(5):332–40.

[6] Mazzocca A, Ferraro G, Miciagna G, et al. A systemic evolutionary approach to cancer: hepatocarcinogenesis as a paradigm. Med Hypotheses 2016;93:132–7.

[7] National Cancer Institute. Understanding cancer prognosis; 2016. Available from https://www.cancer.gov/about-cancer/diagnosis-staging/prognosis.

[8] Sunkara V, Woo H, Cho YK. Emerging techniques in the isolation and characterization of extracellular vesicles and their role in cancer diagnostics and prognostics. Analyst 2016;141:371.

[9] Sutherland AM. Technology for single cell protein analysis in immunology and cancer prognosis. PhD dissertation; 2016. California Institute of Technology.

[10] Juodzbalys G, Kasradze D, Cicciu M, et al. Modern molecular biomarkers of head and neck cancer. Part 1. Epigenetic diagnostics and prognostics: systematic review. Cancer Biomark 2016;17(4):487–502.

[11] Ma S, Ren J, Fenyo D. Breast cancer prognostics using multi-omics data. AMIA Jt Summits Transl Sci Proc 2016;2016:52–9.

[12] Bartošik M, Ondroušková E. Novel approaches in DNA methylation studies – MS-HRM analysis and electrochemistry. Klin Onkol 2016;29(Suppl. 4):64–71.

[13] Zogopoulos P, Korkolopoulous P, Patsouris E, et al. The antitumour action of cannabinoids on glioma tumorigenesis. Histol Histopathol 2015;30:629–45.

[14] Pinkas J, Jablonski P, Kidawa M, et al. Use of marijuana for medical purposes. Ann Agric Environ Med 2016;23(3):525–8.

[15] Velasco G, Galve-Roperh I, Sánchez C, et al. Hypothesis: cannabinoid therapy for the treatment of gliomas? Neuropharmacology 2004;47:315–23.

[16] Shelef A, Barak Y, Berger U, et al. Safety and efficacy of medical cannabis oil for behavioural and psychological symptoms of dementia: an open label, add-on, pilot study. J Alzheimers Dis 2016;51:15–19.

[17] Munson AE, Harris LS, Friedman MA, et al. Antineoplastic activity of cannabinoids. J Natl Cancer Inst 1975;55(3):597–602.

[18] Various. World Health Organization Cancer Guideline publications; 2016. Available from http://www.who.int/cancer/publications/en/.

[19] Ko YS, Lee W, Panchanathan R, et al. Polyphenols from Artemisia annua L inhibit adhesion and EMT of highly metastatic breast cancer cells MDA-MB-231. Phytother Res 2016;30(7):1180–8.

[20] Yuan H, Lu X, Ma Q, et al. Flavonoids from Artemisia sacrorum Ledeb. and their cytotoxic activities against human cancer cell lines. Exp Ther Med 2016;12(3):1873–8.

[21] Michaelsen FW, Saeed M, Schwarzkopf J, et al. Activity of Artemisia annua and artemisinin derivatives, in prostate carcinoma. Phytomedicine 2015;22(14):1223–31.

[22] Dozmorov MG, Yang Q, Wu W, et al. Differential effects of selective frankincense (Ru Xiang) essential oil versus non-selective sandalwood (Tan Xiang) essential oil on cultured bladder cancer cells: a microarray and bioinformatics study. Chin Med 2014; 9:18.

[23] Ni X, Suhail M, Yang Q, et al. Frankincense essential oil prepared from hydrodistillation of Boswellia sacra gum resins induces human pancreatic cancer cell death in cultures and in a xenograft murine model. BMC Complement Altern Med 2012;12:253.

[24] Suhail MM, Wu W, Cao A, et al. Boswellia sacra essential oil induces tumor cell-specific apoptosis and suppresses tumor aggressiveness in cultured human breast cancer cells. BMC Complement Altern Med 2011;11:129.

[25] Cappiello G, McGinley B, Elahi MA, et al. Differential evolution optimization of the SAR distribution for head and neck hyperthermia. IEEE Trans Biomed Eng 2016;64(8):1875–85.

[26] Datta NR, Krishnan S, Speiser DE, et al. Magnetic nanoparticle-induced hyperthermia with appropriate payloads: Paul Ehrlich's 'magic (nano)bullet' for cancer theranostics? Cancer Treat Rev 2016;50:217–27.

[27] Bar-Sela G, Wollner M, Hammer L, et al. Mistletoe as complementary treatment in patients with advanced non-small-cell lung cancer treated with carboplatin-based combinations: a randomised phase II study. Eur J Cancer 2013;49(5):1058–64.

[28] Büssing A, Raak C, Ostermann T. Quality of life and related dimensions in cancer patients treated with mistletoe extract (iscador): a meta-analysis. Evid Based Complement Alternat Med 2012;2012:219402.

[29] Dole M, Wilson F, Fife WP. Hyperbaric hydrogen therapy: a possible treatment for cancer. Science 1975;190(4210):152–4.

[30] Moen I, Stuhr L. Hyperbaric oxygen therapy and cancer – a review. Targ Oncol 2012;7:233–42.

[31] Beard J. The enzyme treatment of cancer and its scientific basis. London, UK: Chatto & Windus; 1911.

[32] Leipner J, Saller R. Systematic enzyme therapy in oncology: effect and mode of action. Drugs 2000;59:769–80.

[33] Beuth J. Proteolytic Enzyme therapy in evidence-based complementary oncology: fact or fiction? Integr Cancer Ther 2008;7(4):311–16.

[34] Pauling L. Effect of ascorbic acid on incidence of spontaneous mammary tumors and UV-light-induced skin tumors in mice. Am J Clin Nutr 1991;54(6 Suppl.):1252S–1255S.

[35] Creagan ET, Moertel C, O'Fallon JR, et al. Failure of high-dose vitamin C (ascorbic acid) therapy to benefit patients with advanced cancer – a controlled trial. N Engl J Med 1979;301: 687–90.

[36] Padayatty SJ, Riordan H, Hewitt SM, et al. Intravenously administered vitamin C as cancer therapy: three cases. Research 2006;174(7):937–42.

[37] Riordan HD, Casciari J, González MJ, et al. A pilot clinical study of continuous intravenous ascorbate in terminal cancer patients. P R Health Sci J 2005;24(4):269–76.

[38] Eastman KL, McFarland L, Raugi GJ. A review of topical corrosive black salve. J Altern Complement Med 2014;20(4):284–9.

[39] Clark JJ, Woodcock A, Cipriano SD, et al. Community perceptions about the use of black salve. J Am Acad Dermatol 2016;74(5):1021–3.

[40] López-Lázaro M. Dual role of hydrogen peroxide in cancer: possible relevance to cancer chemoprevention and therapy. Cancer Lett 2007;252(1):1–8.

[41] Pritchett S, Green D, Rossos P. Accidental ingestion of 35% hydrogen peroxide. Can J Gastroenterol 2007;21(10):665–7.

[42] PDQ Integrative. Alternative, and complementary therapies editorial board. Laetrile/Amygdalin (PDQ®): health professional version. Bethesda, MD: National Cancer Institute; 2017.

[43] Milazzo S, Horneber M. Laetrile treatment for cancer. Cochrane Database Syst Rev 2015;(4):CD005476.

[44] Cancer Research UK. Rife machine and cancer; 2016. Available from http://www.cancerresearchuk.org/about-cancer/cancers-in-general/cancer-questions/rife-machine-and-cancer.

[45] Jain NK, Gupta VB, Garg R, et al. Efficacy of cow urine therapy on various cancer patients in Mandsaur District, India – a survey. Int J Green Pharm 2010;4(1).

[46] Koltai T. Cancer: fundamentals behind pH targeting and the double-edged approach. Onco Targets Ther 2016;9:6343–60.

[47] Pavlova NN, Thompson C. The emerging hallmarks of cancer metabolism. Cell Metab 2016;23(1):27–47.

[48] Fenton TR, Huang T. Systematic review of the association between dietary acid load, alkaline water and cancer. BMJ Open 2016;6(6):e010438.

[49] Wright ME, Michaud D, Pietinen P, et al. Estimated urine pH and bladder cancer risk in a cohort of male smokers (Finland). Cancer Causes Control 2005;16(9):1117–23.

[50] Bellavia A, Stilling F, Wolk A. High red meat intake and all-cause cardiovascular and cancer mortality: is the risk modified by fruit and vegetable intake? Am J Clin Nutr 2016;10(4):1137–43.

[51] Marin-Valencia I, Yang C, Mashimo T, et al. Analysis of tumor metabolism reveals mitochondrial glucose oxidation in genetically diverse human glioblastomas in the mouse brain in vivo. Cell Metab 2012;15:827–37.

[52] Maher EA, Marin-Valencia I, Bachoo RM. Metabolism of [U-13 C] glucose in human brain tumors in vivo. NMR Biomed 2012;25:1234–44.

[53] Altmann DM. A Nobel prize-worthy pursuit: cancer immunology and harnessing immunity to tumour neoantigens. Immunology 2018;155(3):283–4.

[54] Voena C, Chiarle R. Advances in cancer immunology and cancer immunotherapy. Discov Med 2016;21(114):125–33.

[55] Schmitt MW, Loeb L, Salk JJ. The influence of subclonal resistance mutations on targeted cancer therapy. Nat Rev Clin Oncol 2016;13(6):335–47.

[56] Garofalo A, Sholl L, Reardon B, et al. The impact of tumor profiling approaches and genomic data strategies for cancer precision medicine. Genome Med 2016;8:79.

[57] Park P, Dhupal M, Kim CS, et al. Implication of immunokine profiling for cancer staging. Med Hypotheses 2016;88:46–8.

[58] The Cancer Institute. Impact of cancer genomics on precision medicine for the treatment of cancer. The Cancer Cengome Atlas; 2016. Available from https://cancergenome.nih.gov/cancergenomics/impact.

[59] Teitelbaum A, Spencer D, Bollu VK, et al. Monitoring response and treatment outcome in patients with chronic phase chronic myeloid leukemia (CML) treated with imatinib. J Clin Oncol 2011;29(15_Suppl.):e16612.

[60] Olson EM, Najita J, Sohl J, et al. Predictors of survival in patients with HER2+ metastatic breast cancer (MBC) treated with trastuzumab. J Clin Oncol 2016;29(15_Suppl.):e11100.

[61] Wanebo HJ, Sanikommu S, Taneja C, et al. Hepatic artery infusion for recurrent or chemotherapy-resistant hepatic malignancy. J Clin Oncol 2016;29(15_Suppl.):e14151.

[62] Hongo F, Mikami K, Nakanouchi T, et al. Intra-arterial chemotherapy for local invasive bladder cancer. J Clin Oncol 2016;29(15_Suppl.):e15063.

[63] Yu B, Ma Z, Guan C, et al. Clinical introtumoral chemoimmunotherapy for late stages of lung cancer. J Clin Oncol 2016;29(15_Suppl.):e21001.

[64] Maciver AH, Lee N, Skitzki JJ, et al. Cytoreduction and hyperthermic intraperitoneal chemotherapy (CS/HIPEC) in colorectal cancer: evidence-based review of patient selection and treatment algorithms. Eur J Surg Oncol 2017;43(6):1028–39.

[65] Zhao J, Zhou M, Li C. Synthetic nanoparticles for delivery of radioisotopes and radiosensitizers in cancer therapy. Cancer Nanotechnol 2016;7(1):9.

[66] Martinov MP, Thomson R. Heterogeneous multiscale Monte Carlo simulations for gold nanoparticle radiosensitization. Med Phys 2017;44(2):644–53.

[67] Su XX, Liu P, Hao W, et al. Enhancement of radiosensitization by metal-based nanoparticles in cancer radiation therapy. Cancer Biol Med 2014;11(2):86–91.

[68] Van de Wiele C, Maes A, Brugman E, et al. SIRT of liver metastases: physiological and pathophysiological considerations. Eur J Nucl Med Mol Imaging 2012;39(10):1646–55.

[69] Citrin D, Cotrim A, Hyodo F, et al. Radioprotectors and mitigators of radiation-induced normal tissue injury. Oncologist 2010;15(4):360–71.

[70] Hasan I, Rashid T. Clinical communication, cancer patients & considerations to minimize the challenges. J Cancer Ther 2016;7:107–13.

[71] Shim E-J, Park JE, Yi M, et al. Tailoring communications to the evolving needs of patients throughout the cancer care trajectory: a qualitative exploration with breast cancer patients. BMC Womens Health 2016;16:65.

[72] Kerridge IH, McPhee J. Ethical and legal issues at the interface of complementary and conventional medicine. Med J Aust 2004;181(3):164–6.

[73] Ghorbanzadeh-Moghaddam A, Gholamrezaei A, Hemati S. Vitamin D deficiency is associated with the severity of radiation-induced proctitis in cancer patients. Int J Radiat Oncol Biol Phys 2015;92(3):613–18.

[74] Akinci MB, Sendur MA, Aksoy S, et al. Serum 25-hydroxy vitamin D status is not related to osteopenia/osteoporosis risk in colorectal cancer survivors. Asian Pac J Cancer Prev 2014;15(8):3377–81.

[75] Alco G, Igdem S, Dincer M, et al. Vitamin D levels in patients with breast cancer: importance of dressing style. Asian Pac J Cancer Prev 2014;15(3):1357–62.

[76] Mego M, et al. Probiotic bacteria in cancer patients undergoing chemotherapy and radiation therapy. Complement Ther Med 2013;21(6):712–23.

[77] Frazzoni L, Marca M, Guido A, et al. Pelvic radiation disease: updates on treatment options. World J Clin Oncol 2015;6(6):272–80.

[78] Mansouri-Tehrani HA, Rabbani-Khorasgani M, Hosseini SM, et al. Effect of supplements: probiotics and probiotic plus honey on blood cell counts and serum IgA in patients receiving pelvic radiotherapy. J Res Med Sci 2015;20(7):679–83.

[79] Kumar M, et al. Probiotic Lactobacillus rhamnosus GG and Aloe vera gel improve lipid profiles in hypercholesterolemic rats. Nutrition 2013;29(3):574–9.

[80] Sharma S, et al. Probiotic Enterococcus lactis IITRHR1 protects against acetaminophen-induced hepatotoxicity. Nutrition 2012;28(2):173–81.

[81] Ki Y, Kim W, Nam J, et al. Probiotics for rectal volume variation during radiation therapy for prostate cancer. Int J Radiat Oncol 2013;87(4):646–50.

[82] Demers M, Dagnault A, Desjardins J. A randomized double-blind controlled trial: impact of probiotics on diarrhea in patients treated with pelvic radiation. Clin Nutr 2014;33(5):761–7.

[83] Leung HW, Chan AL. Glutamine in alleviation of radiation-induced severe oral mucositis: a meta-analysis. Nutr Cancer 2016;68(5):734–42.

[84] Ben-David MA, et al. Melatonin for prevention of breast radiation dermatitis: a phase II, prospective, double-blind randomized trial. Isr Med Assoc J 2016;18(3–4):188–92.

[85] Akbarzadeh M, et al. Effects of combination of melatonin and laser irradiation on ovarian cancer cells and endothelial lineage viability. Lasers Med Sci 2016;31(8):1565–72.

[86] Zetner D, Andersen LP, Rosenberg J. Melatonin as protection against radiation injury: a systematic review. Drug Res (Stuttg) 2016;66(6):281–96.

[87] Das D, Agarwal SK, Chandola HM. Protective effect of Yashtimadhu (Glycyrrhiza glabra) against side effects of radiation/chemotherapy in head and neck malignancies. Ayu 2011;32(2):196–9.

[88] Tanideh N, et al. Healing acceleration in hamsters of oral mucositis induced by 5-fluorouracil with topical Calendula officinalis. Oral Surg Oral Med Oral Pathol Oral Radiol 2013;115(3):332–8.

[89] Babaee N, et al. Antioxidant capacity of Calendula officinalis flowers extract and prevention of radiation induced oropharyngeal mucositis in patients with head and neck cancers: a randomized controlled clinical study. Daru 2013;21(1):18.

[90] Kodiyan J, Amber K. A review of the use of topical calendula in the prevention and treatment of radiotherapy-induced skin reactions. Antioxidants (Basel) 2015;4(2):293–303.

[91] Goey AK, et al. The effect of St John's wort on the pharmacokinetics of docetaxel. Clin Pharmacokinet 2014;53(1):103–10.

[92] Zou L, Harkey MR, Henderson GL. Effects of herbal components on cDNA-expressed cytochrome P450 enzyme catalytic activity. Life Sci 2002;71(13):1579–89.

[93] Naccarato M, Yoong D, Gough K. A potential drug-herbal interaction between Ginkgo biloba and efavirenz. J Int Assoc Physicians AIDS Care (Chic) 2012;11(2):98–100.

[94] Gurley BJ, et al. In vivo effects of goldenseal, kava kava, black cohosh, and valerian on human cytochrome P450 1A2, 2D6, 2E1, and 3A4/5 phenotypes. Clin Pharmacol Ther 2005;77(5):415–26.

[95] Goey AK, et al. Relevance of in vitro and clinical data for predicting CYP3A4-mediated herb-drug interactions in cancer patients. Cancer Treat Rev 2013;39(7):773–83.

[96] Gorski JC, et al. The effect of echinacea (Echinacea purpurea root) on cytochrome P450 activity in vivo. Clin Pharmacol Ther 2004;75(1):89–100.

[97] Ooko E, et al. Modulation of P-glycoprotein activity by novel synthetic curcumin derivatives in sensitive and multidrug-resistant T-cell acute lymphoblastic leukemia cell lines. Toxicol Appl Pharmacol 2016;305:216–33.

[98] Khan M, et al. Enhancing activity of anticancer drugs in multidrug resistant tumors by modulating P-glycoprotein through dietary nutraceuticals. Asian Pac J Cancer Prev 2015;16(16):6831–9.

[99] Jia W, et al. Aglycone Protopanaxadiol, a ginseng saponin inhibits P-glycoprotein and sensitizes chemotherapy drugs on multidrug resistant cancer cells. J Clin Oncol 2004;22(14_Suppl.):9663.

[100] Park JH, et al. Effects of silymarin and formulation on the oral bioavailability of paclitaxel in rats. Eur J Pharm Sci 2012;45(3):296–301.

[101] Mustian KM, Cole C, Lin PJ, et al. Exercise recommendations for the management of symptoms clusters resulting from cancer and cancer treatment. Semin Oncol Nurs 2016;32(4):383–93.

[102] Zhang LL, Wang S, Chen HL, et al. Tai chi exercise for cancer-related fatigue in patients with lung cancer undergoing chemotherapy: a randomized controlled trial. J Pain Symptom Manage 2016;51(3):504–11.

[103] Sprod L, et al. Exercise and side effects among 417 older patients with cancer during and after cancer treatment: a URCC CCOP study. J Clin Oncol 2011;29(15_Suppl.):9036.

[104] Tian L, et al. Effects of aerobic exercise on cancer-related fatigue: a meta-analysis of randomized controlled trials. Support Care Cancer 2016;24(2):969–83.

[105] Leon-Ferre R, Ruddy K, Staff NP, et al. Fit for chemo: nerves may thank you. J Natl Cancer Inst 2016;109(2).

[106] Rush SE, Sharma M. Mindfulness-based stress reduction as a stress management intervention for cancer care: a systematic review. J Evid Based Complementary Altern Med 2017;22(2):348–60.

[107] Liu S, Qiu G, Louie W. Use of mindfulness sitting meditation in Chinese American women in treatment of cancer. Integr Cancer Ther 2017;16(1):110–17.

[108] Kurdi MS, Muthukalai SP. The efficacy of oral melatonin in improving sleep in cancer patients with insomnia: a randomized double-blind placebo-controlled study. Indian J Palliat Care 2016;22(3):295–300.

[109] Marx W, et al. Ginger – mechanism of action in chemotherapy-induced nausea and vomiting: a review. Crit Rev Food Sci Nutr 2017;57(1):141–6.

[110] Trivanovic D, et al. An open-label randomized phase II trial of oral vitamin D3 supplementation in combination with standard chemotherapy or best supportive care compared with standard chemotherapy and best supportive care in patients with advanced solid tumors. J Clin Oncol 2011;29(15_Suppl.):e19566.

[111] Abd El-Atti S, et al. Use of probiotics in the management of chemotherapy-induced diarrhea: a case study. JPEN J Parenter Enteral Nutr 2009;33(5):569–70.

[112] Argyriou AA, et al. Preventing paclitaxel-induced peripheral neuropathy: a phase II trial of vitamin E supplementation. J Pain Symptom Manage 2006;32(3):237–44.

[113] Argyriou AA, et al. Vitamin E for prophylaxis against chemotherapy-induced neuropathy: a randomized controlled trial. Neurology 2005;64(1):26–31.

[114] Villani V, et al. Vitamin E neuroprotection against cisplatin ototoxicity: preliminary results from a randomized, placebo-controlled trial. Head Neck 2016;38(Suppl. 1):E2118–21.

[115] Pace A, Bove L, Jandolo B. Vitamin E for prophylaxis against chemotherapy-induced neuropathy: a randomized controlled trial. Neurology 2005;65(3):501–2.

[116] Wiernik PH, et al. Hexamethylmelamine and low or moderate dose cisplatin with or without pyridoxine for treatment of advanced ovarian carcinoma: a study of the Eastern Cooperative Oncology Group. Cancer Invest 1992;10(1):1–9.

[117] Puchsaka P, Chaotham C, Chanvorachote P. Alpha-lipoic acid sensitizes lung cancer cells to chemotherapeutic agents and anoikis via integrin beta1/beta3 downregulation. Int J Oncol 2016;49(4):1445–56.

[118] Dora CL, et al. Oral delivery of a high quercetin payload nanosized emulsion: in vitro and in vivo activity against B16-F10 melanoma. J Nanosci Nanotechnol 2016;16(2):1275–81.

[119] Li QC, et al. Enhanced therapeutic efficacy and amelioration of cisplatin-induced nephrotoxicity by quercetin in 1,2-dimethyl hydrazine-induced colon cancer in rats. Indian J Pharmacol 2016;48(2):168–71.

[120] Demir MG, et al. Effect of transtympanic injection of melatonin on cisplatin-induced ototoxicity. J Int Adv Otol 2015;11(3):202–6.

[121] Jang H, et al. Melatonin prevents cisplatin-induced primordial follicle loss via suppression of PTEN/AKT/FOXO3a pathway activation in the mouse ovary. J Pineal Res 2016;60(3):336–47.

[122] Guo Y, et al. Oral alpha-lipoic acid to prevent chemotherapy-induced peripheral neuropathy: a randomized, double-blind, placebo-controlled trial. Support Care Cancer 2014;22(5):1223–31.

[123] Gedlicka C, et al. Amelioration of docetaxel/cisplatin induced polyneuropathy by alpha-lipoic acid. Ann Oncol 2003;14(2):339–40.

[124] Pachman DR, et al. The search for treatments to reduce chemotherapy-induced peripheral neuropathy. J Clin Invest 2014;124(1):72–4.

[125] Tomizawa K, et al. A retrospective study of UFT and oral leucovorin plus PSK combination adjuvant chemotherapy in patients with stage III colon cancer. Gan to Kagaku Ryoho 2012;39(4):571–5.

[126] Ohwada S, et al. Beneficial effects of protein-bound polysaccharide K plus tegafur/uracil in patients with stage II or III colorectal cancer: analysis of immunological parameters. Oncol Rep 2006;15(4):861–8.

[127] Ghoreishi Z, et al. Omega-3 fatty acids are protective against paclitaxel-induced peripheral neuropathy: a randomized double-blind placebo controlled trial. BMC Cancer 2012;12:355.

[128] Schloss JM, et al. A randomised, placebo-controlled trial assessing the efficacy of an oral B group vitamin in preventing the development of chemotherapy-induced peripheral neuropathy (CIPN). Support Care Cancer 2017;25(1):195–204.

[129] Schloss JM, et al. Chemotherapy-induced peripheral neuropathy (CIPN) and vitamin B12 deficiency. Support Care Cancer 2015;23(7):1843–50.

[130] Kidd PM. The use of mushroom glucans and proteoglycans in cancer treatment. Altern Med Rev 2000;5(1):4–27.

[131] Badr El-Din NK, et al. Enhancing the apoptotic effect of a low dose of paclitaxel on tumor cells in mice by arabinoxylan rice bran (MGN-3/biobran). Nutr Cancer 2016;68(6):1010–20.

[132] Biswal BM, et al. Effect of Withania somnifera (Ashwagandha) on the development of chemotherapy-induced fatigue and quality of life in breast cancer patients. Integr Cancer Ther 2013;12(4):312–22.

[133] Guven C, Taskin E, Akcakaya H. Melatonin prevents mitochondrial damage induced by doxorubicin in mouse fibroblasts through AMPK-PPAR gamma-dependent mechanisms. Med Sci Monit 2016;22:438–46.

[134] de Morree ES, et al. Association of survival benefit with docetaxel in prostate cancer and total number of cycles administered: a post hoc analysis of the Mainsail study. JAMA Oncol 2017;3(1):68–75.

[135] Cortes EP, et al. Adriamycin cardiotoxicity: early detection by systolic time interval and possible prevention by coenzyme Q10. Cancer Treat Rep 1978;62(6):887–91.

[136] Mythili Y, et al. Effect of DL-alpha-lipoic acid on cyclophosphamide induced lysosomal changes in oxidative cardiotoxicity. Life Sci 2007;80(21):1993–8.

[137] Chua S, et al. The cardioprotective effect of melatonin and exendin-4 treatment in a rat model of cardiorenal syndrome. J Pineal Res 2016;61(4):438–56.

[138] Cvetkovic Z, et al. Distribution of plasma fatty acids is associated with response to chemotherapy in non-Hodgkin's lymphoma patients. Med Oncol 2013;30(4):741.

[139] Fahrmann JF, Hardman WE. Omega 3 fatty acids increase the chemo-sensitivity of B-CLL-derived cell lines EHEB and MEC-2 and of B-PLL-derived cell line JVM-2 to anti-cancer drugs doxorubicin, vincristine and fludarabine. Lipids Health Dis 2013;12:36.

[140] Davis L, Kuttan G. Effect of Withania somnifera on cyclophosphamide-induced urotoxicity. Cancer Lett 2000;148(1):9–17.

[141] Fritz H, et al. Polysaccharide K and Coriolus versicolor extracts for lung cancer: a systematic review. Integr Cancer Ther 2015;14(3):201–11.

[142] Sookprasert A, et al. Melatonin in patients with cancer receiving chemotherapy: a randomized, double-blind, placebo-controlled trial. Anticancer Res 2014;34(12):7327–37.

[143] Marinac CR, et al. Prolonged nightly fasting and breast cancer prognosis. JAMA Oncol 2016;2(8):1049–55.

22

Cancer – Advanced II

Part A: Manuela Boyle
Part B: Teresa Mitchell-Paterson

RECOVERY AND RESTORATION POST CANCER

Survivorship

Worldwide, the number of cancer survivors continues to increase due to both advances in early detection and treatment, and the ageing and growth of the population. It has been estimated that more than 15.5 million Americans with a history of cancer were alive on 1 January 2016, with this number projected to reach more than 20 million by 1 January 2026 (see Fig. 22.1).[1] Similar to the US, current data (2016) from the Australian population shows that the three most prevalent cancers among males are prostate, colorectal and melanoma. Among females, breast, uterine and colorectal cancers have been recorded to be the most prominent.

In clinical practice, it is widely recognised that cancer survivors have unique medical and psychosocial needs, requiring proactive assessment and management by primary care providers. In a longitudinal study conducted by Verdecchia et al.,[2] incidence and survival were modelled by cancer type, sex and age group from 1975 to 2012. Data found that more than half (56%) of all survivors were diagnosed within the past 10 years.[3,4] Nearly half of all cancer survivors (47%) are aged 70 years or older, although age distribution varies by cancer type. For example, most of the prostate cancer survivors (64%) are aged 70 years or older, compared with only one-third of melanoma survivors (see Fig. 22.2).[1]

BREAST CANCER (FEMALE)

Recent data collection shows that there are an estimated 3.5 million women living in the US with a history of invasive breast cancer. Of these, 75 per cent of breast cancer survivors (more than 2.6 million women) are aged 60 years or older, while 7% are younger than 50 years (see Fig. 22.2).[1] Most of the surveyed cancer survivors had undergone surgical treatment for breast cancer either in the form of a breast-conserving surgery also known as

lumpectomy, or in the form of mastectomy. Interestingly, survivorship has shown to be the same regardless of the choice of surgery – lumpectomy or mastectomy.[5,6] It is common for some breast cancer patients to undergo both a lumpectomy and a mastectomy, due to either tumour characteristics (i.e. locally advanced stage, large or multiple tumours) or to a pre-existing medical condition.[7] Furthermore, recent data have reported an increase in the proportion of women with non-metastatic disease undergoing contralateral preventive mastectomy.[8]

Statistics show that most women diagnosed with stage I or II breast cancer generally prefer to undergo a breast-conserving surgery, with only 36% choosing to receive a mastectomy to improve chances of survival[1] (see Fig. 22.3). This proportion has been shown to change for patients at stage III and stage IV, with a much smaller percentage opting for a lumpectomy and a clear majority preferring a mastectomy, followed by radiation and/or chemotherapy. Among women with hormone-receptor-positive breast cancer regardless of the stage, 79% receive hormonal therapy.[9] For survivors of breast cancer, reconstruction may involve the use of a saline or silicone implant, a tissue flap or a combination of both.[10,11]

PAEDIATRIC CANCERS

It is estimated that currently in the US alone, there are 65 190 children cancer survivors aged from birth to 14 years, and 47 180 adolescent survivors aged 15–19 years. The three most commonly diagnosed cancers are leukaemia (30%), brain and central nervous system tumours (26%) and soft tissue sarcomas (7%). Among adolescents, the most common cancers are brain and central nervous system tumours (20%), followed by leukaemia (14%) and Hodgkin lymphoma (HL) (13%).[12]

Childhood cancer survivors may experience chronic long-term effects of chemotherapy, with some symptoms expected to occur months or years after diagnosis or treatment. It is noticeable that for those paediatric patients who received aggressive chemotherapy and radiation therapy treatment in the 1970s and 1980s, there is a demonstrated increased risk of secondary cancers and cardiomyopathies.[13] A study by Armstrong et al. reported that 50% of childhood cancer survivors are estimated to develop a significant chronic health condition by the time they reach the age of 50 years.[14] Furthermore, another

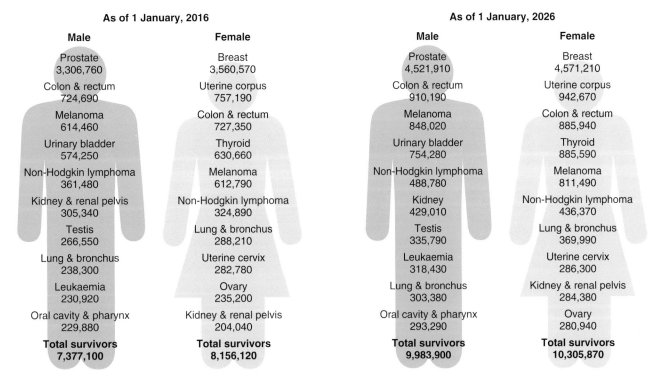

FIGURE 22.1 The estimated number of US cancer survivors

Miller KD, Siegel RH, Lin CC et al. Cancer treatment and survivorship statistics, 2016. *CA: A Cancer Journal for Clinicians* 2016;66(4):271–89.

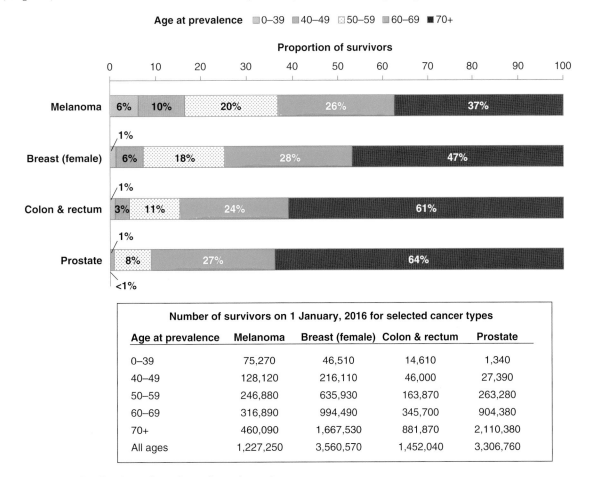

FIGURE 22.2 Age distribution of survivors for selected cancer types

Miller KD, Siegel RH, Lin CC et al. Cancer treatment and survivorship statistics, 2016. *CA: A Cancer Journal for Clinicians* 2016;66(4):271–89.

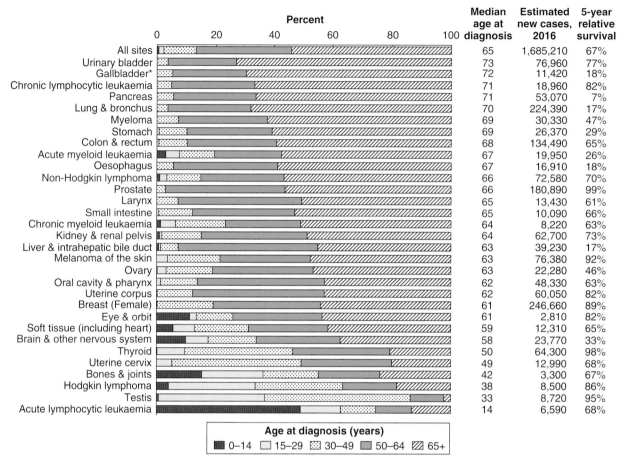

FIGURE 22.3 Age distribution of new cases (%), median age at diagnosis, estimated number of new cases, and 5-year relative survival by cancer type

Miller KD, Siegel RH, Lin CC et al. Cancer treatment and survivorship statistics, 2016. *CA: A Cancer Journal for Clinicians* 2016;66(4):271–89.

investigation has demonstrated that the majority of childhood cancer survivors who were diagnosed and treated with common chemotherapy drugs between 1962 and 2001 experienced ongoing pulmonary dysfunction.[15] In the past two decades, the decline of side effects and cancer recurrence in children has been attributed to the reduced use of cranial and abdominal radiation.[14] However, it is well established that cognitive impairment secondary to chemotherapy still affects up to one-third of childhood cancer survivors.[16] Furthermore, childhood cancer survivors who were treated with surgery, radiation and some chemotherapies affecting the reproductive organs have been found to be infertile.[17]

COLON AND RECTAL CANCERS

Current statistics estimate that in the US there are 1.4 million men and women with a previous diagnosis of colon and/or rectal cancers. Most colon cancer sufferers are aged 60 years and older, with a small minority aged 50 years and younger[1] (see Fig. 22.2). On the other hand, patients affected by rectal cancer tend to be younger at diagnosis compared with those individuals diagnosed

with colon cancer (median age, 63 vs 70 years, respectively).[10]

Many survivors with a previous diagnosis of stage I and II colon cancer are given the choice to have either a partial or a total colectomy, depending on the position of the tumour mass. Approximately two-thirds of individuals diagnosed with stage III disease generally are scheduled to receive chemotherapy following a colectomy (see Fig. 22.4). For patients with rectal cancer, proctectomy or proctocolectomy is the most common treatment (61%) for stage I disease.[1] Chemotherapy is the general treatment for all stage IV rectal cancers.

Survivors of colon and/or rectal cancer who have been treated with chemotherapy often experience both chronic neuropathies[18] and chronic diarrhoea,[19] as well as chronic bowel dysfunction (including increased stool frequency, incontinence, radiation proctitis and perianal irritation), particularly among those treated with pelvic radiation.[20] Survivors may also suffer from bladder dysfunction, sexual dysfunction and negative body image following a colostomy.[21] However, research findings have shown that colorectal cancer survivors are often at risk of contracting

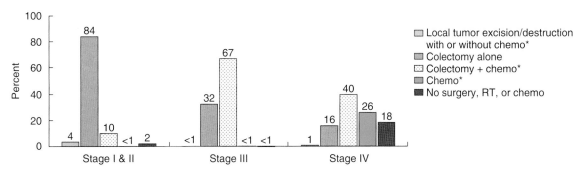

FIGURE 22.4 Colon cancer treatment patterns (%) by stage, 2013

Miller KD, Siegel RH, Lin CC et al. Cancer treatment and survivorship statistics, 2016. *CA: A Cancer Journal for Clinicians* 2016;66(4):271–89.

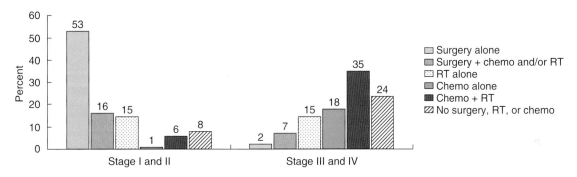

FIGURE 22.5 Non-small cell lung cancer treatment patterns (%) by stage, 2013

Miller KD, Siegel RH, Lin CC et al. Cancer treatment and survivorship statistics, 2016. *CA: A Cancer Journal for Clinicians* 2016;66(4):271–89.

secondary cancers arising from other organs of the gastrointestinal tract.[22]

LEUKAEMIAS AND LYMPHOMAS

Although acute myeloid leukaemia (AML) is the most common type of cancer among children aged from birth to 14 years, the clear majority (92%) of patients with a blood-borne cancer are diagnosed at age 20 years and older with acute lymphocytic leukaemia. Adults diagnosed with leukaemia are affected by either acute myeloid leukaemia (AML) or chronic lymphocytic leukaemia.[23] The 5-year relative survival rate for children and adolescents is estimated to be 65%, rapidly declining to 50%, 32% and 6% for patients aged 20–49 years, 50–64 years and 65 years and older, respectively.

Subdivision exists also among lymphomas, with HL and non-Hodgkin's lymphoma (NHL) identified as the two main types. NHLs can be further divided into indolent and aggressive categories, each of which includes many subtypes that progress and respond to treatment differently. Prognosis and treatment depends on the stage and type of lymphoma. Although both HL and NHL occur in children and adults, most HL cases (64%) are diagnosed before age 50 years, whereas most NHL cases (85%) occur in those aged 50 years and older. Chemotherapy is the standard treatment for the most common types of leukaemia and lymphoma, with most patients undergoing stem cell transplantation, often in combination with chemotherapy.[24]

Survivors of leukaemia and lymphoma have been shown to experience several long-term and late effects. For example, documented health issues affecting those individuals who receive stem cell transplantation have been identified as being recurrent infections, infertility, serious anaemia requiring routine blood transfusions and chronic graft-versus-host disease, which can cause skin changes, dry mucous membranes (eyes, mouth, vagina), joint pain, weight loss, shortness of breath and fatigue. Furthermore, cancer survivors who were treated with anthracyclines commonly report cardiovascular problems.[25]

LUNG CANCER

Generally, the median age for a diagnosis of lung cancer is 70 years. Lung cancer is classified as small cell lung cancer (SCLC) (13% of cases) or non-small cell (NSCLC) (83%). SCLC survivors receive chemotherapy and thoracic radiation therapy. The treatment protocol for those individuals diagnosed with stage I and II NSCLC is surgery, with a minority of these cases also receiving chemotherapy and/or radiation therapy after the main intervention[1] (see Fig. 22.5). Recently, targeted therapy drugs, such as monoclonal antibodies, angiogenesis inhibitors, epidermal growth factor receptor (EGFR) inhibitors and anaplastic lymphoma kinase inhibitors have become part of the treatment for NSCLC due to some recorded and consistent positive results. These types of drugs are growing to be a preferred option after research has demonstrated that many survivors of lung cancers who had received conventional oncological treatment showed impaired pulmonary function.[26] The recorded side effects of most targeted drugs, when administered in maximum doses, are: immune mediated toxicities, colitis, nephritis and endocrinopathy. Lung cancer survivors who are typically smokers and have chosen not to quit smoking after treatment have been found to be at an increased risk for subsequent smoking-related cancers, especially lung, head and neck, and oesophageal, as well as other smoking-related health problems. It is interesting to note that, differently from other cancer survivors, these individuals commonly feel blame and low self-esteem due to the social perception that lung cancer is a self-inflicted disease.[27]

MELANOMA

Melanoma is a cancer that has been linked to occupational and recreational exposure to ultraviolet radiation. As such, it is often detected in younger individuals who may have spent time in the outdoors.[10] Surgery is regarded as the primary conventional oncological treatment for most melanoma sufferers, and until a few years ago, these individuals were also treated with adjuvant immunotherapy such as ipilimumab, an anticytotoxic T-lymphocyte-associated protein. Following the mapping of the Human Genomic Project (2003), the identification of BRAF mutations has led to the creation of chemotherapeutic inhibitors, which have been shown to improve survival for melanoma patients.[28] Research data confirm that melanoma survivors treated with BRAF inhibitors have an increased risk of developing squamous cell skin carcinomas.[29]

Although the 5-year and 10-year relative survival rates for people with melanoma are high, it is critical that these cancers are identified and diagnosed at a localised stage with regular medical check-ups, and that behavioural risk factors are correctly addressed.[30]

PROSTATE CANCER

Typically, survivors of prostate cancer are over the age of 70 years, with a small minority identified under the age of 50 years[1] (see Fig. 22.2). Most men diagnosed with prostate cancers following a prostate-specific antigen (PSA) testing receive different types of treatment, depending on the extent of disease, age and pre-existing conditions. Most younger patients (<65 years) are generally likely to be treated with radical prostatectomy followed by radiation therapy, whereas about half of men aged 75 years or older often are spared from surgery or radiation. For men who were diagnosed with a less aggressive prostate cancer, active surveillance is the commonly recommended approach.[31] Survivors of prostate cancer who display a rising of PSA and who are not responding to hormonal therapy are generally prescribed specific drugs such as abiraterone and enzalutamide.[32]

Data show that the 5-year relative survival rate approaches 100% for patients with localised disease who have chosen and adhered to active vigilance and declined surgery and/or radiotherapy to minimise risk of chronic

urinary incontinence, erectile dysfunction and inflammatory bowel conditions.[33,34] It is common for prostate cancer survivors who are receiving hormonal treatment to experience long-term loss of libido, hot flushes, night sweats, irritability, breast development, osteoporosis, obesity and type 2 diabetes.[35,36] Some of the literature has reported a higher risk for prostate cancer survivors placed on hormonal therapy to experience cardiovascular risk factors compared to the healthy population.[37]

Limitations of self-management skills in recovery

Cancer survivors may struggle to self-manage following primary treatment where either confidence is low or support is lacking. Supporting physical recovery and improving self-confidence are important aspects of the healing path for most survivors.[38] It has been recognised that people face challenges when primary cancer treatment comes to an end. Individuals may face a range of problems including fatigue, concerns about recurrence, dealing with others' expectations that life should be 'back to normal', having to adjust expectations about physical ability, concerns about leaving the hospital system,[39] concerns about the impact on family and friends and unmet supportive care needs.[40]

The time of transition from active treatment to follow-up has been associated with distress due to the loss of frequent medical monitoring and support. Most of all, cancer survivors who have completed treatment are typically overwhelmed by feelings of abandonment, vulnerability and the loss of a 'safety net'.[41] Thus, the problems of cancer survivorship are broader than the physical consequences and psychological distress of cancer diagnosis and treatment, and, like people with other chronic illnesses, cancer survivors need to work on rebuilding and integrating their disrupted identities into new and changed identities.[42] Many cancer patients are reported to become 'lost' in this transition from patient to survivor.[43] Karnilowicz[44] argues that chronic illness identity is mediated through psychological ownership of illness, and that the experience of owning an illness is fixed in the idea of control. The greater the level of control, the more likely control is experienced psychologically as part of self, with a close and ongoing interaction between an individual's psychological state and their social environment. Creating the conditions to enable people to self-manage this transition and restore order in their disrupted lives is a necessary step that needs to be taken to empower cancer survivors.

CLINICIAN CONSIDERATIONS

Clinicians can create programs for self-management and allow for a fundamental shift in the way that healthcare is delivered. Survivorship may involve engaging the patients in seeking personal resources and encouraging them in being proactive in seeking out information and support; managing symptoms, thoughts and expectations; carefully planning activities; and making connections with others with similar experiences. Examples include helping cancer survivors in maintaining a positive outlook on life and organising activities to allow for physical challenges, such as fatigue or mobility problems following primary treatment.[45] Thus, it is recommended that clinicians maintain contact with cancer survivors even after their treatment is completed. A model of restorative emotional wellbeing for cancer survivors by Lent suggests that two key facets for restoration of emotional wellbeing are the individual's characteristics and the environmental supports and resources available to them.[46] Failing to provide appropriate long-term support across the spectrum of problems faced following primary treatment may have negative consequences for a successful recovery[47] and may prevent patients from returning to productive lives, both socially and economically.[48]

Stress, depression and cancer survivorship

Recent research studies have identified extreme suppression of anger as the most common psychological trait among 160 elderly breast cancer patients.[49] Other studies have confirmed that further to extreme anger, suppression, repression or restraint of anger are emotions generally exhibited by breast cancer patients.[50] Epidemiological studies have reported that participation in psychological support groups is typically associated with better health outcomes for these patients, calling for an integration of such a modality in cancer management and treatment.[51] With such a consistent evidence pointing to a link between emotional distress and chronic disease, the question is whether suppressed anger could also be identified as an indicative factor in the progression of the disease after diagnosis.

A complete eradication of a malignant tumour is not always achieved even after the completion of a conventional aggressive treatment. In many instances, interventions of complementary and alternative medicine have been shown to achieve excellent results and to work well in conjunction with conventional approaches, as tumours increasingly meet the definition of chronic diseases.[52] Treatment protocols of some cancers such as breast, prostate and colon cancer can last for months; individuals on certain oral chemotherapeutic regimens, particularly for breast cancer and some forms of leukaemia, often require chemotherapeutic interventions for 5–10 years. Even after the completion of a treatment protocol, cancer survivors generally need to receive ongoing physical care from multiple specialists in order to manage the long-term residue of the illness and its treatment.[53]

In addition to dealing with severe concerns brought about by their diagnosis, cancer patients and their families must cope with the stresses caused by physically demanding chemotherapy and radiation therapy treatments, which often result in physical impairment, disability, fatigue and pain.[54] Physical debilitation further contributes to emotional distress, depression and anxiety, inevitably leading to substantial social problems, such as the inability to work and sudden loss of income. Furthermore, the presence of preexisting psychological and social stressors often caused by weak or absent social supports and/or lack of health insurance has been shown to contribute to cancer patients' emotional distress, with physical, psychological and social stressors resulting from and contributing to each other.[55]

Pre-existing conditions

Compared to healthy people, at the time of diagnosis, adults with or without a history of cancer more frequently report a fair or poor state of health (30%), other existing chronic medical conditions (42%), one or more physical limitations in performing activities of daily living (11%), other functional disabilities (58%) and, among those under the age of 65, a chronic inability to work because of an existing health condition is commonly recorded (17%).[56] Data collected between 1998 and 2005 by the National Health Interview Survey in the US indicate that there is a strong link between a history of cancer and the onset of permanent poor health and disability.[57] Further research studies have demonstrated the connection between cancer survivors and the development of cardiovascular disease. These studies have also shown that when a history of cancer and chronic disease coexist, there is a 10-fold higher risk for disability to occur. Survivors of childhood cancers have been found to suffer with a higher incidence of chronic diseases in their early or middle adult years. A large retrospective study conducted on over 10 000 adult cancer survivors has produced some alarming statistics: 62% of individuals between the ages of 18 and 48 who had been diagnosed with cancer before the age of 21 had developed at least one chronic disease, with 27% of them being affected by severe or life-threatening conditions such as kidney failure and congestive heart failure. Although on average chronic health conditions have been estimated to appear about 17 years after the cancer diagnosis, even after 30 years from a previous cancer diagnosis, three-quarters of individuals with a previous history of cancer have been shown to suffer with significant chronic illnesses.[58]

The incidence of psychological distress varies considerably depending on type of cancer, time since diagnosis, amount of pain, degree of physical impairment and prognosis. A comprehensive study conducted on 4500 older adult cancer patients indicated that the rate of significant psychological distress expressed by individuals varied from 29% to 43% depending on the type of cancer being diagnosed[58] and the degree of depression and anxiety displayed.[59] Those individuals diagnosed with cancer who do not develop a mental health condition have been found to experience various forms of psychological distress, including guilt, anger, confusion, fear and sadness.[60] Furthermore, anxiety, concerns about body image, lack of communication with family members, changes in sexual function and a general heightened sense of vulnerability are commonly felt by cancer patients. Moreover, cancer patients often face spiritual and existential issues involving their faith and the meaning of end of life. In response to these and other stresses, cancer patients often report feelings of isolation, anger and diminished self-esteem.[61]

The role of caregivers and supporters for cancer recovery

A diagnosis of cancer has been shown to profoundly affect the patient's family members. A meta-analysis conducted on the psychological distress recorded by both patients and their primary caregivers has shown the psychological distress experienced by these individuals to be as severe as that demonstrated by the individual diagnosed with cancer.[62] Moreover, research studies on husbands/partners/daughters and friends of women diagnosed with breast cancer have documented that the degree of depression and anxiety expressed by the patient was reflected in these individuals in a bidirectional way.[63] Likewise, family members expressing a positive attitude have been shown to beneficially improve the mental health status of cancer patients. Predominantly family members, but also friends, often provide substantial amounts of emotional and logistical support to cancer patients. The estimated value of their non-reimbursed care and support has been shown to exceed US$1 billion annually.[64] Furthermore, when cancer patients experience acute or long-term inability to care for themselves or to carry out their roles in the family, family members often step in to take up these roles. Taking on these responsibilities requires considerable adaptation and re-adaptation as the course of the disease changes.

CLINICIAN CONSIDERATIONS

Counselling/psychotherapy

Psychotherapy is efficacious in ameliorating cancer-related distress, anxiety and depression, with newer models focusing on meaning and adaptive coping. Although there is not a strong evidence base for the impact of psycho-oncology on survival, psychological factors clearly impact on adherence to cancer treatment. Most survivors do well overall, but concerns relate to the long-term impact of specific treatments or special populations including children.[65] Studies have shown that the psychological response to breast cancer, such as a fighting spirit or an attitude of helplessness and hopelessness towards the disease, are a prognostic factor with an influence on survival and recovery. Watson et al. demonstrated there was a significantly increased risk of relapse or death at 5 years in women with high scores on the helplessness and hopelessness category of the mental adjustment to cancer scale compared with those with a low score in this category.[66]

Nutritional medicine – dietary support

IMPACT OF NUTRITIONAL AND DIETARY CHOICES ON CANCER SURVIVORSHIP

Healthcare practitioners can significantly improve survivorship by facilitating preventive health behaviours. A study conducted on 450 breast cancer survivors showed that following the clinician's recommendation to engage in exercise resulted in a noticeable increase in physical activity.[67] This study illustrates the importance of supporting lifestyle changes and applying a holistic approach in clinical settings for the benefit of survivorship. For example, a growing number of individuals have been made aware of the link between obesity and the onset of cancer due to the widespread use of early detection,[68] with the additional weight gain being a frequent complication of treatment.[69]

It is well known that cancer can cause profound metabolic and physiological alterations, affecting the nutrient requirements for macro- and micronutrients.[70] Symptoms such as anorexia, early satiety, changes in taste and smell and disturbances of the bowel are common side effects of cancer and cancer treatment, leading to malnutrition. Poor nutritional status and cancer cachexia can occur early in the course of some cancers[71]; therefore, consuming enough kilojoules to prevent additional weight loss is vital for survivors.[72] Providing individualised nutritional advice can improve dietary intake and potentially decrease some of the toxicities associated with cancer treatments.

DIETARY RECOMMENDATIONS POST TREATMENT

The Mediterranean diet follows the traditional dietary pattern of the inhabitants of the Mediterranean countries. It is characterised by a varied menu based on local and seasonal vegetables and fruits, fish, legumes, whole grains, olive oil, herbs and spices. It typically includes many bioactive components such as carotenoids, antioxidant vitamins (vitamins C, E and A), lycopene, resveratrol, flavonoids, polyphenols and dietary fibre, with a beneficial ratio of polyunsaturated fatty acids of omega-6 family to omega-3.[73]

Epidemiological studies were launched in 1993 under the auspices of the International Agency for Research on Cancer and World Health Organization to assess the impact of diet on the development and progression of cancer in terms of practical aspects and the promotion of healthy dietary habits.[74] The study involved 521 468 people, including 366 521 women aged from 39 to 69 years. The study was performed in 10 countries and it included 24 195 people – 7272 men and 16 923 women – with diagnosed cancer. The diet was rich in polyphenols, resveratrol, pomegranate, lycopene, olive oil, herbs and spices.

Polyphenols are natural antioxidants, protecting the body against reactive oxygen species (ROS) and reactive nitrogen species (RNS). They also have demonstrated ability to chelate iron and copper ions with vasodilatory ability. They also show antibacterial, antiviral, anti-inflammatory and anti-thrombotic properties.[75]

Resveratrol is a natural phytoalexin, present in skins of red fruits, including grapes. It has a demonstrated and wide range of cytotoxic, anti-fungal, anti-microbial, anti-viral and cytoprotective ability. Resveratrol is found in the two forms of cis and trans isomers. Trans-resveratrol is a stilbenoid present in the common grape vine *Vitis vinifera*.[76] The second form of resveratrol, cis-resveratrol, is formed because of isomerisation of trans-resveratrol and after the dissolution of the polymer molecule of resveratrol of grape skins during fermentation, by the action of UV rays and high pH. Furthermore, resveratrol affects the regulation and the balance of a healthy metabolism due to the activation of protein SIRT1.[77] Resveratrol plays an important role in the prevention of cancer by blocking the process of initiation, promotion and progression. As a phyto-oestrogen, it regulates the expression of numerous genes associated with the development of breast cancer, including a tumour suppressor BRCA1 gene.[78]

Urolithin B is a metabolite of ellagic acid in pomegranate and is formed under the influence of the bacterial flora in the gastrointestinal tract. Urolithin B has a demonstrated ability to inhibit aromatase activity (the enzyme responsible for the conversion of androgens into oestrogen) as well as the process of proliferation of tumour cells in the mammary gland, as demonstrated in several in vitro studies.[79]

One of the best known natural antioxidants is lycopene, the bright red carotenoid pigment found in tomatoes. Lycopene has been shown to hold anti-tumour activity, due to its antioxidant, anti-inflammatory and immunomodulatory properties as well as its ability to express the protective antioxidant response element (ARE) gene. Furthermore, lycopene competes with oestrogen for oestrogen receptors ERα and ERβ. The Mediterranean diet, rich in fresh and cooked tomatoes, may be a preventive measure in reducing the risk of cancer.[80]

The Mediterranean diet is also rich in olive oil. The effects of vitamin E, which is found in large quantities in olive oil, are primarily due to its ability to protect against lipid peroxides and free radicals. Lower concentrations of vitamin E have been correlated with an increase in the incidence of some cancers.[81] Further studies have shown that alpha-tocopherol inhibits premalignant stages of breast cancer in women.[82] The effect of olive oil in the prevention of the recurrence of breast cancer was observed in a study carried out in Spain in 2003–2009. The study involved 4282 women aged 60–80 years, randomly assigned to three groups: 1) the Mediterranean diet with the addition of extra virgin olive oil; 2) Mediterranean diet supplemented with a variety of nuts; or 3) control diet with a reduced fat content. After the average follow-up of 4.8 years, 35 confirmed cases of cancer of the breast were identified. Based on the finding of this research study, the following observations were made: for every 1000 women using the Mediterranean diet with an increased amount of extra virgin olive oil, only 1.1 had a recurrence of breast cancer compared to 1.8 and 2.9 in the control group.[83]

For the preparation of dishes, the Mediterranean diet proposes a variety of herbs and spices which contain bioactive components with anti-cancer properties. Some of these agents are apigenin and quercetin (basil, oregano), rosmarinic acid (rosemary), curcumin (turmeric), gingerol (ginger), allicin (garlic) and apigenin (basil, marjoram). The beneficial effects of herbs and spices is likely to be due to their antioxidant, anti-inflammatory and anti-microbial properties as well as to their ability to inhibit the bioactivation of carcinogens in the body.[84] Of special interest is rosemary extract, with its documented anti-cancer activity against the onset of breast cancer by decreasing the expression of ER-α receptor HER2.

Clinician considerations

- For individuals experiencing anorexia or early satiety, and who are at risk of becoming underweight, consuming smaller, more frequent meals with minimal liquids consumed during meals can help to increase food intake. Liquids can and should be consumed in between meals to avoid dehydration.
- For individuals who cannot meet their nutritional needs through foods alone, wholesome, homemade, nutrient-dense beverages or foods can improve the intake of energy and nutrients.
- For individuals who are unable to meet their nutritional needs through these measures and who are at risk of becoming malnourished, targeted nutritional and botanical support may be needed to improve gut function and absorption, and energy.

NUTRITIONAL ASSESSMENT

Gastrointestinal malabsorption and dysfunction are determinants of the overall nutritional status of an individual. The best possible diet will be of little value unless it is digested and assimilated. Recognised causes of malabsorption are: achlorhydria, pancreatic and bile insufficiency, inflammation of the small bowel, bacterial infection of the bowel and diarrhoea. Symptoms associated with malabsorption are: bloating, wind, burping, nausea, abdominal pain and spasm.[85]

The role of a healthy diet and sufficient physical activity in cancer prevention have been well documented,[86] and it is widely accepted that a poor diet, lack of exercise, smoking and excessive alcohol consumption can increase an individual's risk of developing cancer. There is a growing body of evidence for the need to implement lifestyle interventions that aim to enhance healthy eating and weight management, as well as to promote physical activity. These are demonstrated strategies for the reduction of some of the adverse effects of cancer treatments, disease progression and other health outcomes.[68] Besides the potential beneficial effect on recurrence, a healthy diet and regular physical activity may contribute to a reduced risk of comorbid conditions, such as other cancers, cardiovascular disease and diabetes.[87]

In 2007, a comprehensive report by the World Cancer Research Fund (WCRF) – *Food, Nutrition, Physical Activity, and the Prevention of Cancer: A Global Perspective* – set out some recommendations based on the systematic review of randomised control trials on the effects of nutritional and physical activity interventions on cancer survival. It concluded that there is emerging evidence that some aspects of food, nutrition or physical activity may help prevent recurrence of cancer[88] (see Table 22.1). More recent specific guidance on diet and physical activity for cancer survivors has been made available by the British Association of Sport and Exercise Sciences, with recommendations on exercise and cancer survivorship, and by the American College of Sports Medicine, with its detailed booklet on diet/physical activity for cancer survivors.[89]

Nutritional oncology, as an integrated approach, was initially defined in the mid 1990s as the field of science and medicine that researches the interaction of nutrients and

TABLE 22.1 Summary of potential catabolic and anabolic forces in the cancer patient

Note: Check with interaction databases for current information on supplements and herbs or discuss with medical team before use. The statement 'no known contraindications' is for general use during cancer supportive therapy.

Nutrient	Dosage range	Comments (references[90,91] unless otherwise stated)
Alpha-lipoic acid	General dose 600 mg/day[92] 600 mg IV once a week for 3–5 weeks then 600 mg t.d.s. during chemotherapy[93]	May interfere with radiation treatment – caution with chemotherapy, apply safe dosing May be contraindicated with blood thinning medication[92]
Calcium	1000–1300 mg/day[92]	No known contraindications
CoQ10	150–300 mg per day[92]	May interfere with some chemotherapy, protects against doxorubicin cardiotoxicity[92]
Flaxseed	25 g/day[94]	Generally deemed safe during therapy
Fruits and vegetables	191–500 g/day[95,96] Fisetin content of foods[97] Apigenin content of foods[98]	Beneficial effects
Glutamine	15 g twice daily[93,99]	Conflicting research. It is imperative the clinician review the specific patient's history presentation and health history prior to prescribing to make an informed and judicious decision
Indole-3-carbinols	Diet containing[100] 300–800 mg/d[91]	Food grade appears safe, supplement not to be taken with tamoxifen or similar oestrogen blocking agents
Intravenous vitamin C	30–100 mg[101]	Discuss with oncologist and healthcare providers – not without GDP6 testing
Lycopene	2 serves of tomato paste/sauce per week as minimum[102,103] 15–45 mg/day[91]	No known side effects
Mediterranean diet	[104–106]	No suggested negative effects
Melatonin	3–20 mg daily[91]	No known side effects
Olive oil	To be administered as per daily guidelines for fat intake for height and weight – 5% of daily intake[83]	No known adverse effects
Omega-3	Doses vary EPA 180 mg/DHA 120 mg[107] 2 g EPA during chemotherapy[108] 4.9 g/day EPA and 3.2 g/day DHA[109]	No known side effects
Pyridoxal-5-phosphate (PLP) B6	25–300 mg/day[91]	Conflicting evidence
Proanthocyanidins	200–500 mg/day[91]	No known side effects[110]
Probiotics	Healthy microbiome, to be chosen according to patient needs[111]	No known side effects
Quercetin	500–4000 mg/day[91]	Not to be utilised with taxanes
Resveratrol	15–200 mg/day[91]	No known adverse effects
Selenium	50 micrograms[112]	Caution with kidney or liver damage
Shark cartilage	200 mL/day[91]	No known side effects[113]
Vitamin A	350 000–500 000 IU/day[109]	Not with active liver disease and radiotherapy
Vitamin D	To attain a blood level of 89–90 nmol/mL to 200 nmol/mL[114,115]	Monitor blood levels with general practitioner or oncologist
Vitamin E	400–800 IU/day[91]	May increase risk of bleeding
Zinc	Zinc:copper ratio[116] 15–45 mg/day[91]	No known side effects[90,117,118]

TABLE 22.1 Summary of potential catabolic and anabolic forces in the cancer patient—cont'd

Nutrient	Dosage range	Comments (references[90,91] unless otherwise stated)
Phytotherapy		
Astragalus membranaceus	1–2 g/day or as standardised dose suggests[91]	Generally deemed safe during therapy
Common herbs and spices	Ad lib in food[119]	No known side effects
Fermented wheat	9 g/day[91]	No known side effects
Essiac formula tea	4–8 g/day[91]	Unknown[120]
Ginkgo biloba	120 mg twice daily[93]	May increase risk of bleeding, caution with ER+ cancers, not during chemotherapy
Green tea	6–9 Japanese-sized cups, approximately 180 mL, equivalent to 1–2 g of EGCG in humans[121]	No known adverse effects
Genistein	Mixed doses recommended including 39–47 mg per day[122] and 6–11 g/day[123]	Caution with ER+ cancers, conflicting reports – NOT during chemotherapy[124]
Glycyrrhiza glabra	Herbalist advice required and blood pressure monitoring, 3–10 mL/day standardised extract[91]	Adjunctive with cisplatin[125]
Moringa oleifera folia	No dose evidence in humans[126]	Unknown
Curcuma longa	Powdered 1–3 g/day[123] 12 g/day curcumin[123]	May increase bleeding, not with letrozole, erlotinib, exemestane, cyclophosphamide, anastrozole May enhance FOLFOX[127]
Withania somnifera	3–6 g/day[91]	Caution with chemotherapy
Zingiber officinalis	As decoction[128]	May increase risk of bleeding
Mushrooms	Polysaccharides 1 mg per kg body weight[91]	No known side effects[129]
Rosmarinus officinalis	1–4 mL t.d.s.[128]	Not to be taken with tamoxifen or similar oestrogen blocking agents
Sanguinaria canadensis	Not for safe use	[130]

Source: https://accc-cancer.org/oncology_issues/supplements/Integrating-Nutrition-nto-Your-Cancer-Program-MA02.pdf.

nutritional factors with cancer, including cancer prevention, adjunctive therapy and supportive nutritional intervention.[131] In the past decade, this field of medicine has gained a broader scope with the creation of a system aimed at assessing nutritional risks and deficits and how they may affect clinical outcomes. Extensive progress has also been made in understanding catabolic stresses (both cytokine mediated and not cytokine mediated) that contribute to progressive weight loss and malnutrition. Finally, researchers have been able to publish data and to develop integrated algorithmic approaches incorporating medical, nutritional, physical and psychological interventions that work synergistically with the unique individuality of each patient. This approach is illustrated in Table 22.1 and demonstrates the importance of addressing all three primary components of intervention: the nutrition of the host, the hormonal milieu of the host (including both classic hormones and cytokines) and exercise.

CARCINOGENS AND ANTI-CARCINOGENS: INTEGRATIVE MEDICINE STRATEGIES FOR PREVENTION AND PREVENTION OF RECURRENCE

A multitude of epidemiological and preclinical studies point to the connection between dietary habits and cancer risk, with the former showing strong evidence of impacting on incidence and biological behaviour of the latter. Although the risk of breast, prostate, colon, lung and liver cancers is frequently associated with dietary patterns, some inconsistencies have been noticed due to the intrinsic multi-factorial nature of cancer cells. The recognition of genes and pathways regulating cell growth and development, and determining a response to hormones and other chemicals synthesised by the body, has paved the way for the identification of molecular targets by which dietary components may influence cancer prevention. It is certainly plausible that bridging knowledge about these unique cancer cellular characteristics with the molecular targets for nutrients can be used to assist in minimising cancer risk.[132]

Chemoprevention strategies represent therapeutic interventions at early stages of carcinogenesis, before the onset of invasive cancer. Effective chemoprevention aims at treating early neoplastic lesions before the onset of clinical signs or symptoms. Preclinical, clinical and epidemiological research data provide considerable support for cancer chemoprevention as an attractive therapeutic preventive strategy.[133] Interestingly, although retinoids have shown positive documented effects in treating specific premalignant lesions and reducing incidence of secondary tumours, a carotenoid (beta-carotene) was shown as inactive in prevention of lung cancers in high-risk individuals.[134]

Along with nutritional supplementation, lifestyle risk-reducing strategies and stress management have been shown to be viable interventions for those considered to be at high risk of developing cancer.[135] While the cause and nature of certain human cancers are known, definitive preventive guidelines are still lacking, possibly partly due to inherent biostatistical limitations in the identification and interpretation of complex carcinogenic risk factors. Recently, two divergent control strategies have emerged: 1) regulatory programs aimed at eliminating specific quantities of pollutants following a quantitative risk analysis; and 2) a biological research effort aimed at understanding the biological mechanisms of carcinogens and their matching anti-carcinogens. Current research indicates that the eliminatory approach will have little impact on the cancer burden and that the biological approach represents the better alternative, regardless of the need for major investments in fundamental research and manpower.[136] Despite the accumulating evidence supporting a direct correlation between environmental pollution and tumorigenesis, there is still a lack of intervention at both public and private levels, possibly due to a lack of formal input to appropriate national bodies by experts in chemical carcinogenesis.

Physical activity and exercise in cancer survivorship

Epidemiological studies have linked low levels of physical activity and obesity and with an increased risk of breast cancer.[137] Other clinical and epidemiological studies have identified obesity and weight gain as an equally important negative prognostic factor for breast cancer survivors.[69] Physical activity has been associated with lean body mass[138] and optimal body composition of breast cancer survivors.[139] It is therefore remarkable that despite the evidence suggesting that regular physical activity can protect against weight gain, decrease breast cancer risk and potentially improve breast cancer prognosis, efforts to encourage physical activity are not a routine part of the cancer treatment or rehabilitation process.[138]

A review of the literature has pointed out that a clear majority of the breast cancer studies report that physical activity is associated with a reduction in breast cancer and all-cause mortality. Other research has found strong evidence of an association between physical activity and disease outcomes for colorectal cancer survivors.[140] This evidence was sufficiently compelling to justify the first ever randomised controlled exercise intervention trial among colon cancer survivors.[141]

Other compelling evidence has shown that obesity and a sedentary lifestyle are highly prevalent among cancer survivors, with a growing number of publications demonstrating a significant association between obesity, low levels of physical activity and cancer recurrence.[142] With most cancer survivors not currently engaged in recommended physical activities, targeted exercise therapy has the potential to benefit many cancer survivors by improving quality of life and preventing recurrence.

CLINICIAN CONSIDERATIONS

It is recommended that cancer survivors keep themselves physically active. At the same time, it is desirable that primary healthcare practitioners are aware of the benefits of exercise by endorsing validated physical activity guidelines. The positive therapeutic outcome of exercise in cancer patients was published for the first time by Winningham in 1983.[143] In her study, a 10-week bicycle ergometer training program of 30 minutes, three times per week was shown to produce a substantial increase in physical performance of breast cancer survivors post chemotherapy compared with control patients who did not train. In further studies, Winningham et al. showed that individualised exercise programs can reduce mood disturbance, relieve somatic complaints, reduce total body weight and increase physical performance of breast cancer survivors.[144] In recent studies, exercise has also been shown to improve outcome of patients who had undergone prior myeloablative therapies. The exercise program consisted of walking on a treadmill for 30 minutes daily for the duration of 6 weeks. The results were consistent with a general improvement of physical performance and a reduction of lactate.[145]

In a randomised controlled study, cancer survivors who could sustain a 6-week endurance training program after high-dose chemotherapy and peripheral blood stem cell transplantation showed significantly lower fatigue scores and higher haemoglobin compared to others who did not train.[146] Another study has shown that exercise dramatically improves haemoglobin levels in cancer survivors suffering with severe anaemia due to chronic renal failure caused by the activation, production and release of haematopoietic growth factors.[147]

The improvement of physical performance has broader ramifications, including an increased feeling of control, independence and self-esteem, and related social interaction, with a tangible reduction of anxiety and fear.

PART B

TREATMENTS TO SUPPORT CANCER CARE AND PREVENTION

Prostate cancer

PREVENTION

Oxidative stress and diet have been the main oncogenic factors realised in prostate cancer. There is a demonstrated higher level of oxidation in prostate cancer tissue than in non-cancerous prostate tissue.[148] Oxidation and, therefore, reactive oxygen species initiate inflammatory prostaglandins, leukotrienes and eicosanoids, ameliorating anti-inflammatory enzymes such as COX-2 and LOX, a key aim in therapy.[149,150] A diet linked to high fat intake may increase the risk of prostate cancer. High fat may increase testosterone levels, which may increase the rate of development of prostate cancer cells, coupled with a low intake of vitamin E, D, selenium and lycopene.[90,151]

EXERCISE

Moore et al.[152] studied pooled data from 1.44 million participants from 12 prospective European and US self-reported physical activity surveys (95% confidence) over 26 types of prostate cancers. Although physical activity did not lower the risk of incidence, it demonstrated a high confidence level in the attenuation of malignancies in prostate cancer patients (95% CI).[152] An Australian study utilising exercise in medically induced androgen-deprived prostate cancer demonstrated benefits in patients combining both cardiovascular intensity of 70–85% (estimated maximum heart rate for 20–30 minutes and resistance training for 20–30 minutes) and resistance training.[153] Major upper and lower muscle groups were targeted, with 6–12 repetitions lifting 60–85% of one repetition with a maximum of 1–4 sets. Duration was set at 150 minutes of exercise per week over 3 months. It was concluded that exercise minimised severe hypogonadism and morbidity.[153]

DURING ACTIVE CANCER

Herbal medicine

ROSMARINUS OFFICINALIS

In a mini review, the phenolic properties of rosemary diterpenes canosinic acid and carnosol exhibited potent antioxidant activity via inhibition of lipid peroxidation.[154,155] In DU-145 and prostate cancer antigen 3, and prostate cancer cell lines in vitro, carnosic acid verified anti-proliferative, apoptotic and cytotoxic properties. Carnosol has also revealed anti-proliferative, cell-cycle-arresting regulatory properties, while modulating multiple signalling pathways, including mTOR and PI3K. Surprisingly, it has an additional benefit to prostate cancer patients in that carnosol can attenuate both androgen receptors and oestrogen receptor alpha in vitro (cancer cell lines) and in vivo in mice studies.[154,155]

GREEN TEA EGCG

Metastatic disease progresses via many mechanisms where the family of proteolytic enzymes (matrix metalloproteinases or MMPs) remodel the extracellular matrix. High levels of MMP-2/9 are found to be elevated in metastatic disease.[156] Tissue inhibitors of matrix metalloproteinases inhibit MMPs. Green tea polyphenols and epigallocatechin-3-gallate (EGCG) significantly reduce MMP-2/9's invasive ability via TIMP-3 induction, and may delay prostate cancer progression.[156]

URTICA DIOICA (NETTLE)

In prostate cancer antigen 3 cell lines, nettle induces apoptosis via an increase in caspase-3 and -9 mRNA expression, and concurrently decreases Bcl-2.[157]

PYGEUM AFRICANUM (PYGEUM)

Pygeum demonstrates its effect by mediating the androgen receptor site via transcriptional activity. The active principle is atraric acid, an inhibitor of amino/carboxy (N/C) terminal interaction with androgen receptors.[158]

CURCUMA LONGA (TURMERIC)

Curcumin demonstrates its effect by mediating the androgen receptor pathways via transcriptional activity. However, curcumin compounds demonstrate multiple anti-cancerous potential in the attenuation of both testosterone and dihydrogen testosterone, and is a valuable addition to active therapy.[159]

ESSIAC FORMULA

Low dose Essiac formulations demonstrate inhibition of tumour cells grown in vitro via T-lymphocyte proliferation. Some, but not all, of the components of the formula suggest anti-tumour effects; specifically, slippery elm (*Ulmus fulva*) and burdock root (*Arctium lappa*) contain quercetin as well as several other antioxidants which may be of benefit.[160] Indian rhubarb root (*Rheum officinale*) and sheep sorrel (*Rumex acetosella*) have few human or animal studies.[160] More studies are required.[120]

Nutritional medicine

DIETARY SUPPORT

It is recommended that a reduction of pro-inflammatory omega-6 fats, found in vegetable oils, hydrogenated foods, meat and dairy, and a reduction of sugars and refined flours will drive inflammation down, coupled with the increase of anti-inflammatory omega-3 fats and beneficial nutrients.[161] A large ($n = 1294$) study conducted on Italian men suggests that an inflammatory diet is a predictor for prostate cancer risk and progression. Men with higher inflammatory diets as measured via a dietary inflammatory index categorically suggest elevated risk factors (95% CI).[162,163]

ZINC

Zinc citrate is an ionophore and has the ability to exhibit anti-proliferative effects via mitochondrial apoptogenesis through increasing malignant cell zinc levels.[164] Prostate zinc levels present with deficiency; therefore, increasing zinc may attenuate the disease. However, there are limited human trials, but compelling evidence. Zinc is additionally stated to inhibit the migration activity of malignant cells.[90,164,165]

OMEGA-3 FATTY ACIDS

A low intake of omega-6 and rich omega-3 diets correlates with lower incidences of cancer generally. There has been controversy about the use of omega-3 in prostate cancer therapy; however, the media have exploited the issue.[166] It has conversely been established that the ratio of dietary omega-6 to omega-3 is the most important factor rather than a bombardment of omega-3 supplementation. If the intake of supplements matches that of an omega-3-rich diet, there should not be an issue. The findings are consistent in both animal and human trials. Omega-3, when coupled with Taxotere, was found to be more effective in inhibiting growth in metastatic prostate cancer than when using Taxotere alone.[161]

LYCOPENE

Lycopene is a potent carotenoid, which has been demonstrated to slow the growth of tumours and lower PSA levels in prostate cancer.[102] In the Health Professionals Follow-up Study, there was a relational association between higher intakes of tomatoes and tomato products and a lowered risk of prostate cancer.[103] In some ways, even a modest two serves a week of tomato sauce may have a protective effect in ERG-positive prostate cancer, but not in ERG-negative disease. However, by increasing the intake of all forms of lycopene, there was a decreased risk in both subtypes. Lycopene in the form of simply adding tomato sauce to a diet may be enough to reduce transmembrane protease serine 2 in ERG-positive disease.[103]

SELENIUM

As previously discussed, the oxidation of fats plays an important role in prostate cancer. Selenium reduces lipopolysaccharide TLR4-NF-κB signalling, which may reduce inflammation via inhibition of vascular endothelial growth factor (VEGF) and inflammatory cytokines in prostate cancer. It is also a cofactor in glutathione peroxidase, which theoretically reduces radical oxygen-induced fat rancidity.[167]

QUERCETIN

Previous studies have found that quercetin attenuates the reduction of cancer growth.[168] Mechanistic factors are obtained through reduction of androgen receptor expression, suppression of proliferation and induction of apoptosis.[168] A review of the material indicates that daily intake of red wine, tea, onions and apples provides approximately 10–100 mg of quercetin. Quercetin is a hydrophilic glycoside and is difficult to absorb. It relies on effective glucuronidation, sulfation and methylation to reach its active potency 3-O-methyl-quercetin, quercetin-3-O-glucuronide and isorhamnetin 3-O-glucuronide.[168] The small and large intestine, colon and kidney also play a metabolic role. Yang et al.[168] presented a very impressive table of the multiple molecular mechanisms cascading the anti-prostate cancer effect of quercetin. An intraperitoneal dose of 150 mg/kg suppressed tumour growth.[169] Similarly, Sharmila et al.[170] suggested that a 200 mg/kg dose, which induced superoxide dismutase, catalase and apoptotic proteins, decreased protein kinase B (PKB), also known as Akt, androgen-induced AR target gene expressions and insulin growth factors. Large doses are needed to achieve effect.

SOY ISOFLAVONES

Soy isoflavones have a complex multi-functional effect on the metabolism of prostate cancer, not restricted to chemoprotection, antioxidant, DNA repair, potentiation of chemo- and radio-therapeutic therapy, inhibition of angiogenesis, metastasis, antagonism of oestrogen and androgen-mediated signalling pathways.[171] They are also protective of the milieu surrounding the cells enhancing immunity, endothelial strength and in the growth factors of fibroblastic stromal cells.[171] In a review of the data on

soy flavonols, the level of intake to achieve a reduced or stabilised PSA in 50% of the treated-food-based group was 450 mg genistein, 300 mg daidzein and other isoflavones daily.[172] Additionally, soy consumption as a food may reduce the risk of progression to advanced prostate cancer due to its effect on endogenous oestrogen metabolism. The markers for proliferation, free testosterone and PSA levels were also reduced in the isoflavone-treated group, identifying that soy proteins may potentially slow progression rate.[172]

VITAMIN D

There is still significant conflict regarding vitamin D supplementation during active cancer. In a review of five studies, three studies suggested an inverse relationship between higher circulating 25(OH) D and risk of fatal prostate cancer, with one cohort representing a statistically significant result.[173] Unfortunately, there was little heterogeneity between the studies. Previous studies support higher levels of vitamin D.[174]

SUPPORT DURING RADIOTHERAPY

Herbal medicine

SERENOA REPENS (SAW PALMETTO)

A small clinical trial proved inconclusive on the lower urinary tract symptom benefits of saw palmetto during active radiation treatment. However, as no toxicity was reported, the research on this herb warrants further investigation.[175]

Nutritional medicine

LYCOPENE

In a small study, lycopene supported quality of life (QOL) when used in conjunction with radiotherapy treatment.[176]

MELATONIN

A meta-analysis of randomised controlled trials regarding efficacy and safety of adjuvant melatonin therapy in radiotherapy and chemotherapy in solid tumours suggested improvements of remission, side effects and remission, and 1-year survival rates.[177]

SUPPORT DURING CHEMOTHERAPY

Herbal medicine

GREEN TEA EPIGALLOCATECHIN GALLATE (EGCG) AND QUERCETIN

In castration-resistant metastatic cancer, EGCG combined with quercetin (found in onions and apples) may enhance the efficacy of docetaxel, specifically in two cell lines LAPC-4-AI (three fold) and prostate cancer antigen 3 (eight fold). The therapy was more effective than docetaxel itself via the inhibition of PI3K/Akt and signal inducers and transcription activators. EGCG and quercetin were shown to downregulate chemoresistance.[178]

CURCUMA LONGA (TURMERIC)

There is promising evidence for the use of curcuminoids in dual therapy (animal studies). The delivery method is via nanoparticles.[179] However, it may be seen that turmeric may safely be used to enhance the effect of chemotherapy.[179]

Nutritional medicine

MELATONIN

A meta-analysis of randomised controlled trials regarding efficacy and safety of adjuvant melatonin therapy in radiotherapy and chemotherapy in solid tumours suggested improvements of remission, side effects and remission, and 1-year survival rates.[177]

Bowel – colorectal cancer (CRC)

PREVENTION

Exercise

The continuous update program of the WCRF[180] suggests that physical activity shows positive benefits for the reduction of risk for CRC. The evidence is considered convincing, with the greater frequency and intensity of exercise producing greater benefits (meta-analysis 11% decreased risk of colorectal and 12% decreased risk of colon cancer). The recommendations are to exercise at least 30 minutes per day as there are links to a dose–response effect. Exercise may protect against colon cancer by reducing insulin levels and resistance and decreasing inflammation.[181]

Nutritional medicine – dietary

A meta-analysis of fibre intake suggested a 21% decreased risk with the consumption of wholegrain fibre, including both soluble and insoluble fibres, in the diet assisting short-chain fatty acid production and gut flora fermentation, which increases butyrate-causing cell arrest, apoptosis and a reduction of cell differentiation.[180,181]

Preclinical evidence and animal studies suggested garlic inhibits colon tumour formation and growth inhibition in laboratory studies, largely due to the allyl sulfur component of the food. In a meta-analysis and mini review of case control studies, garlic was associated with probably a 37% reduction in the risk of CRC.[182]

Calcium foods restrain cell proliferation and encourage apoptosis. The findings from the Nurses' Health Study and the Health Professionals Follow Up Study suggested higher calcium intakes from various sources are associated with a lower risk of colon cancer. The analysis also stated that there appears to be a lower risk when calcium foods are consumed for up to 10 years prior to diagnosis.[183]

High red meat and processed meat consumption has long been surmised to be a risk factor for CRC.[181] It appears that the way meat is cooked and the amount of meat are of importance. Red meat includes kangaroo, beef, lamb and pork; processed meat is any meat that has been manufactured and processed with added chemicals.[184,185] Guidelines are to limit the intake of the aforementioned meat and meat products to less than 500 g per week, where there is an increased risk with red meat of 17% per 100 g/day and processed meat of 18% per 50 g/day. Fibre intake with red meat such as beans, legumes and wholegrains, and the intake of resistant starches are

thought to lower the risk.[186] This is partially due to the reduced contact time in the colon of carcinogenic byproducts – heterocyclical amines, polycyclical aromatic hydrocarbons and N-nitroso compounds, plus cytotoxic alkenals from fat peroxidation.[181,186]

Alcoholic beverage consumption shows a 10% increased risk per 10 g ethanol/day for bowel cancer. Therefore, limiting consumption to no more than two drinks a day for men and one drink a day for women is prudent.[181]

Other suggestions[181]:
- Be as lean as possible without being underweight.
- Avoid sweet energy-dense foods.
- Eat the minimum five serves of vegetables and two serves of fruit per day.
- Limit sodium intake.
- Do not smoke.

DURING ACTIVE CANCER

Herbal medicine

GREEN TEA EGCG

Du et al.[187] stated that EGCG polyphenol is among the most effective CRC cell preventive, demonstrating a high anti-proliferative effect, inducing cell death in the G1 phase of cell cycle growth (human cell culture).

GENISTEIN

In one of the first studies, Xiao et al.[122] demonstrated that genistein from soy food at a non-toxic, dietary dose inhibits human CRC metastasis. Adopting a Chinese or Japanese diet where the intake of genistein is between 39 and 47 mg, respectively, proves a historically lower incidence of CRC than Western diets. Genistein modulates epigenetic histone action in DNA, although multiple pathways are also alluded to.[122]

CURCUMA LONGA (TURMERIC)

There are many proposed biochemical signalling pathways suggested to be stunted by the use of turmeric as an anti-cancerous agent. The studies are largely in human tissue, with many difficulties faced raising the intake of turmeric to a chemopreventive level. Liposomal treatment is now being adopted. However, this is not backed by clinical trials at this time.[188] The herb exhibits many anti-inflammatory properties where curcumin alone does not work as effectively as the entire herb. In its entire state, it contains structural gradients which assist it to function effectively in the suppression of nuclear factor-κB. It is still deemed useful as an adjunct therapy for CRCs.[188]

Nutritional medicine

OVERALL DIET

The WCRF and Perera[95,181] suggest the same dietary recommendations for prevention are also recommended for survivors and active cancers.

CALCIUM

The calcium-sensing receptor (CaSR) is downregulated in malignant CRCs, leading to a reduction in tumour apoptosis and poor tumour differentiation. In an in vivo animal study, a lack of CaSR led to a statistically noticeable increase in markers for proliferation.[189] How this translates to humans is unknown. However, the WCRF[180] suggests a calcium-rich diet, and where this is not possible, calcium and vitamin D supplements may be of assistance.

OMEGA-3 FATTY ACIDS

Osiecki[90] suggests omega-3 acts as an inflammation modulator, differentiation preventer, tumour necrosing factor and stabiliser of membrane fluidity.

SELENIUM

Selenium is perhaps the most studied chemotherapeutic agent. In doses of 50 micrograms (above the RDI) or more (toxic level 350–700 micrograms), it has been suggested to be both preventive and therapeutic.[112] In vivo selenium may regulate cell cycles, stimulate apoptosis and inhibit tumour cell migration. Selenium is also suggested to sensitise cancer cells to cell death via tumour necrosis apoptosis-inducing ligand and to increase efficacy of doxorubicin.[112]

QUERCETIN AND RESVERATROL

Human in vitro studies support the use of quercetin as a regulatory factor increasing colon cancer cell apoptosis via various mechanisms. In combination with resveratrol, the impact is more potent. Tandem use creates inhibition of reactive oxygen species. The combination may also induce caspase-3 cleavage and increase poly(ADP-ribose) polymerase separation.[190,191]

VITAMIN D

Low levels of vitamin D 25-hydroxyvitamin D are associated with increased risk of both colorectal risk and morbidity, with higher levels of vitamin D correlating to a better prognosis. A suggested level is 30 ng/mL for risk reduction, equating to 89–90 nmol/mL.[192,193]

SUPPORT DURING RADIOTHERAPY

Herbal medicine

CURCUMA LONGA (TURMERIC)

Curcumin may sensitise CRC cells via multiple molecular pathways, enhancing the effects of radiotherapy. Modulation of apoptosis, reactive oxidation scavenging, anti-inflammatory adaptations and inhibition of survival signals are among the known pathways.[194]

SUPPORT DURING CHEMOTHERAPY

Herbal medicine

GREEN TEA EGCG

EGCG is capable of targeting colorectal stem cells in chemoresistant CRC. EGCG enhances the effect of FOLFOX (5FU/leucovorin/oxaliplatin) in vitro (animal studies) as seen in the reduction and inhibition of Notch- and polycomb-repressive complexes (among multiple pathways), leading to cell death.[195,196]

CURCUMA LONGA (TURMERIC)

Curcumin may inhibit chemoresistance to FOLFOX response by 50%, occurring via its effect on endothelial growth factor receptor (EGFR) and insulin-like growth factors 1 receptor (IGF-1R). In vitro curcumin reduced oxaliplatin resistance and increased efficacy.[127,197]

Nutritional medicine

VITAMIN D

Low levels of vitamin D 25-hydroxyvitamin D are associated with increased risk of both colorectal risk and morbidity, with higher levels of vitamin D correlating to a better prognosis. A suggested level is 30 ng/mL for risk reduction, equating to 89–90 nmol/mL.[192,193]

INTRAVENOUS VITAMIN C (IVC)

With a noted approximate 50% rate of human CRCs expressing KRAS or BRAF gene aberrations, vitamin C (dehydroascorbate) was utilised in cultured human CRC cells, a promising study whereby vitamin C increased oxidative-stress-depleting glutathione, inactivating glyceraldehyde 3-phosphate dehydrogenase, impairing tumour growth.[198]

MELATONIN

A meta-analysis of randomised controlled trials regarding efficacy and safety of adjuvant melatonin therapy in radiotherapy and chemotherapy in solid tumours suggested improvements of remission, side effects and remission, and 1-year survival rates.[177] Melatonin markedly reduces cell to cell contact and reduces the spread and formation of colon cancer cells.[199]

Breast cancer

PREVENTION

The WCRF[200] findings from the continuous update project reviewed 85 studies with over 164 416 participants from early diagnosis to those living with breast cancer. Lifestyle factors suggested that women who exercise both prior to and post diagnosis have a greater chance of survival; the findings were coupled with healthy weight management. Family history is strongly correlated and early detection provides a more advantageous outcome.

Nutritional medicine – dietary

Dietary aspects for lowering the risk of dying from breast cancer relate to diets containing fibre. Both pre- and post-diagnosis fibre intake may lower the risk of the disease being fatal.

Consuming soy products after diagnosis may confer lower risk – without enough compelling evidence for or against ingestion pre diagnosis.[200] This is confirmed by a recent epidemiological meta-analysis, which highlighted that soy consumption reduces the risk in Asian demographics but not Western countries.[201] A theoretical assumption may be that this is due to the different fermentation and production of soy in other countries, among other factors. High-fat diets – predominantly saturated fat – provide an increased risk of fatality.[200] Lignans, zeaxanthine, lutein, beta-carotene and vitamin A show possible inverse trends. However, in meta-analysis, broad spectrum antioxidants rather than a focus on individual antioxidants are more likely to provide better outcomes.[202]

A Mediterranean-style diet is also recommended from a randomised, single-blind, controlled field trial in Spain spanning 6 years. Many factors of the diet promote good health; notably, the diet contained a higher level of extra virgin olive oil than other diets, at an estimated 5% of total calorie intake.[83]

Other suggestions

The Rotterdam Study suggested family history, reproductive history, weight gain, moderate alcohol consumption, postmenopausal hormone therapy and the absence of breastfeeding as risk factors.[202]

DURING ACTIVE CANCER

Herbal medicine

ASTRAGALUS MEMBRANACEUS (ASTRAGALUS)

Isolated principle astragloside III from *Astragalus membranaceus* has demonstrated potential therapeutic use via an induction of apoptotic cell signalling pathways, inducing a decreased cancer cell survival in vitro, coupled with inhibition of tumour growth in vivo.[203] The flavonoidal compounds from *A. complanatus* also demonstrate anti-cancer effects on human breast cell apoptosis, proliferation and metastasis in vitro. Identified mechanisms for suppression of BRACA1 gene expression was downregulation of BCL-2 and FAK proteins and caspase-9/BCL-2 increase, inducing cancer cell death and metastasis regulation.[204]

WITHANIA SOMNIFERA (ASHWAGANDHA)

Cell culture and animal studies suggest the alkaloids of ashwagandha possess anti-tumorigenic properties. Withanaloids are reported to induce apoptotic pathways, reducing tumour weight in breast cancer cells.[205] A further study suggested that the internal pH of the cells can affect the efficacy of treatment with ashwagandha in human breast cancer cells. Clinically, this equates to the inclusion of bicarbonate soda ingestion prior to taking the herb.[206] Other components of the herb such as the steroidal lactone withaferin A have been suggested to have possible immunomodulatory actions. *Withania* may modulate mitochondrial viability, regulate apoptosis, decrease reactive oxygen species, improve endothelial function and reduce inflammation.[207]

GREEN TEA

EGCG has been shown to be beneficial in numerous cancers, including breast cancer lines MDA-MB-231, HS578T and MCF-7. The proposed dose is 6–9 Japanese-sized cups – approximately 180 mL, equivalent to 1–2 g of EGCG in humans.[121]

Nutritional medicine

OVERALL DIET

Definitive trials for preventive dietary factors for treatment during active breast cancer have yet to be conducted. However, the WCRF[95] states that people who have active cancer should follow preventive dietary suggestions.

FLAXSEED

The exact mechanism whereby dietary addition of flaxseed modifies oestrogen-dependent (ER+) microenvironment is largely unknown. A proposed pathway is that flaxseed has an effect on leptin, which decreases extracellular VEGF, enhancing an anti-tumorigenic environment, suppressing cancer growth. A suggested dose is 25 g per day.[94]

OMEGA-3 FATTY ACIDS

A consumption of a diet rich in omega-3 proves a significant relationship between its effect on microRNA-21, reducing carcinogenesis and modulating cell growth in breast cancer MCF-7 cell lines. Alpha-linolenic acid with docosahexaenoic acid (DHA) and eicosapentaenoic acid (EPA) reduces ER+ growth in breast cancer cells, demonstrating once more that protection of the microenvironment in reducing growth of cancer cells is an important consideration.[208]

VITAMIN D

A proposal for an Italian study in women with histologically confirmed active breast cancer ($n = 506$) stage II and III without metastasis requires the cohorts to follow a low GI diet with exercise and vitamin D.[114] The theoretical basis for the trial is to reduce factors that may increase recurrence risk by influencing blood glucose regulation, high oestrogen and insulin-like growth factors, based on previous findings. This intervention will review inflammation, impaired cellular apoptosis and differentiation.[114] Higher serum levels of vitamin D have been seen to increase the survival rate and reduce breast cancer recurrence when seen in a Mediterranean-style lifestyle and dietary pattern.[114] The intervention suggests a theoretically significant outcome by reducing recurrence by 12%. Suggestions for vitamin D serum levels for the trial are 80 ng/mL, which converts to Australian levels of almost 200 nmol/L, which is significantly higher than current guidelines.[114] In a meta-analysis on the mortality of breast cancer patients after diagnosis and vitamin D levels, the serum level of 25-hydroxyvitamin D 30–80 ng/mL, equivalent to 74.88 to 199.68 nmol/L, is confirmed to demonstrate longer survival times in breast cancer patients.[115]

INTRAVENOUS VITAMIN C (IVC)

IVC was first utilised by Linus Pauling suggesting the selective toxicity of high-dose vitamin C to some forms of cancer. A small Singaporean trial ($n = 9$) administered titrated doses of 15 mg to 100 g with the appropriate carrier magnesium chloride in various cancers.[101] In a single case ER and PR positive invasive, cerbB2 negative ductal carcinoma with dietary modification, exercise and cessation of smoking, there was a noted tumour reduction; surgery was still suggested.[101] In a patient with stage 11 ductal carcinoma grade 3, of the same nature as patient one, after lumpectomy there were no further masses or lesions seen after 6 months of IVC treatment, with cancer markers reduced to the normal range. More trials are needed.[101]

INDOLE-3-CARBINOLS

A significant modifiable risk factor is the ingestion of fruit and a diet containing vegetables with indole-3-carbinols. This was demonstrated for the treatment of ER but not ER+ breast cancers.[100] The study-specific multi-variable relative risks were a 95% confidence interval. The results furthermore showed significance in the ingestion of indole-3 vegetables alone, with no statistical benefit with fruit ingestion alone.[100]

IODINE

While iodine intake is required for thyroid health, approximately 60–80% of iodine is found in extra thyroid tissue. Dietary deficiency is associated with the pathology of breast diseases including cancer. Both thyroid and breast tissue share common iodide gathering abilities, forming protective factors in cells and averting peroxidative damage.[209] Iodine may also positively bind oestrogen at receptor binding sites in MCF-7 cells.[210] The study was based on a proprietary brand 5–10% iodide solution, reporting affectation of 43 genes involved in proliferation, differentiation and cell cycle growth. This implies that iodide may act in an anti-oestrogenic fashion and may be a useful adjunct in therapy.[211]

CURCUMA LONGA (TURMERIC)

Curcumin demonstrates suggestive evidence exerting anti-cancer effects through multiple molecular signalling networks including human epidermal growth factor receptor 2 (HER2), proliferation and oestrogen receptor pathways. Other potential attributes are the regulation of apoptotic activity and microRNA in breast cancer cells.[212] In the aggressive triple-negative breast cancer (TNBC) where there is no expression of epidermal growth factor receptor 2, progesterone receptor or oestrogen receptor, MDA-MB-231 TNBC cells treated with curcumin demonstrate apoptosis. The mechanism of downregulation of extracellular regulated protein kinase and phosphorylated epidermal growth factor in the treated group had a 26.34% apoptosis where the control was 2.76%. There was a significant benefit found in the treated group.[213]

RESVERATROL

Sinha et al.[214] suggested phytochemicals as a means of chemoprevention and for treatment options in active cancer. Resveratrol is a non-flavonoid polyphenol found in berries, grapes, pomegranate and lesser known foods such as peanuts and soybeans. Resveratrol may play a role in epigenetic alterations, apoptosis, reduction of tumour cell proliferation and metastasis, and sensitising tissue to chemotherapeutic medications in vitro and in vivo.

MELATONIN

In vitro studies support the hypothesis that longer elevated maintenance of melatonin levels during sleep cycles plays a vital role in regressing metastatic breast cancer progression. The mechanism to date is seen as inhibition of RSK2, which reduces mechanisms that promote tumour growth and metastasis. Treatment with melatonin has been shown to be valuable in HER2 positive and negative breast cancer cells.[215]

SUPPORT DURING RADIOTHERAPY

Nutritional medicine

MELATONIN

Pre-treatment melatonin may decrease expression of oestrogen-synthesising proteins, allowing radiotherapy to be more therapeutically beneficial. Melatonin doubles the efficacy of radiotherapy via the regulation of p53, demonstrating greater efficacy than radiotherapy alone.[216]

VITAMINS C AND E

See chemotherapy treatment.

SUPPORT DURING CHEMOTHERAPY

Herbal medicine

ASTRAGALUS MEMBRANACEUS (ASTRAGALUS)

A study on injections of astragalus as dual therapy with chemotherapy are promising, with no known detrimental effect on oestrogen treatment. A systematic review of treatments suggests that astragalus can reduce the haematopoietic consequences and death of normal cells. It may promote T cell subsets, therefore improving cell immunity, improve nutritional status, maintain or increase weight during treatment, reduce fatigue and protect bone marrow suppression.[217]

Nutritional medicine

RESVERATROL

Resveratrol may play a role in epigenetic alterations, apoptosis, reduction of breast tumour cell proliferation and metastasis and sensitising tissue to chemotherapeutic medications in vitro and in vivo.[218]

COENZYME Q10 (COQ10)

A study suggested breast cancer tissue has lower levels of CoQ10 during treatment with doxorubicin. Doxorubicin induces cardiotoxicity due to an increase in reactive oxygen species and damage to the cardiac tissue.[219] In conjunction with chemotherapy, CoQ10 did not interfere with the anti-neoplastic ability or the induction of apoptosis in breast cancer cell lines.[219] Breast cancer patients undergoing treatment in a small multi-institutional, randomised trial ($n = 57$) were given CoQ10 with L-carnitine to reduce the fatigue side effects subjectively experienced during chemotherapy. Global fatigue scores were significantly different in the treatment group.[220]

MELATONIN

Anti-metastatic actions are seen in ERa-, HER2+, SKBR-3 breast tumour cell line and ERa-positive MCF-7 cells with melatonin treatment. HER2 drives transcription factors that increase drug resistance and metastasis in breast cancer. Both endogenous and exogenous melatonin has a significant effect on downregulating mechanistic stimulators of metastasis and reduces the progression of breast cancer.[215]

OMEGA-3 FATTY ACIDS

Dietary omega-3 benefits breast cancer patients by increasing the efficacy or reducing the side effects of treatment. In cross-sectional studies, higher intakes of omega-3 are associated with lower risk of cancer-related mortality by raising global health status. In a very small case trial, fish oil supplementation (EPA 180 mg/DHA 120 mg) improved breast cancer patients' quality of life.[107]

VITAMINS C AND E

Supplementation before and after diagnosis of breast cancer, radiation and hormonal therapy demonstrates protective features against chemotherapy toxicity via increased super oxidase dismutase (SOD), glutathione, catalase and glutathione peroxidase, with notable decline in DNA and malondialdehyde damage.[107,214] The Shanghai Breast Cancer Survival study related a decrease in mortality and recurrence of the disease with multivitamin, or vitamin E or C, 6 months prior to treatment.[107,221]

QUERCETIN

In vitro quercetin demonstrates an ability to reduce resistance of breast cancer cells to chemotherapy and re-sensitise cells during both tamoxifen and chemotherapy.[222] Studies suggest it may potentiate cisplatin, ribavirin, topotecan, doxorubicin (Adriamycin), genistein and carboxyamidotriazole.[222–224]

Note: genistein should not be supplemented during chemotherapy as it suggests potential drug interactions with efficacy of treatment.[124]

GLUTAMINE

In a systematic review, 11 of 15 studies reported the effectiveness of oral glutamine in reducing mucositis, with a weight-loss dosing range of 30 g per day in a divided dose.[99]

Melanoma of the skin

PREVENTION

There is little data from the WCRF's Continuous Upgrade Project regarding prevention of melanoma. However, worldwide melanoma incidence rates are rising annually. Prevention is primarily based on limiting exposure to ultraviolet radiation.[225] Indoor sun beds do not decrease risk. Melanoma is the most common cancer in adolescence and young adults in Australia.[225]

Nutritional medicine – dietary

A systematic review of 18 studies suggested that there is a demonstrated protective factor with the ingestion of fish, fruit and vegetables. The risk reduction is reported as 35–37%, 40–57% and 34–46%, respectively. This trend suggests that dietary intakes of vitamin A, D, C and E plus beta-carotene may be a risk reduction factor.[104,105] Dietary suggestions are not unlike the parameters of the Mediterranean diet, where a similar ingestion of nutrients is purported to engage an approximate 40% decreased risk for melanoma.[106]

Other recommendations

SUN PROTECTION

Avoid the sun where possible; protecting the skin from direct contact and using protective filters are currently suggested. However, there is some controversy over the potential toxicity of zinc oxide, para-aminobenzoic acid (PABA) and other filtration chemicals. Currently, there is a lack of substantial research to support cessation of use of sun filters.[106] PABA and its derivatives may cause allergy and have the potential to penetrate the skin due to a low molecular weight. Vitamin D deficiency is also deemed to pose a supplementary risk for development of the disease. It is accepted that there are some positive effects of UV (and UVB) radiation in moderation such as stress reduction, mental wellbeing and vitamin D_3 synthesis.[104] The generation of melanoma is caused by suppressed skin immune response, with increased risk of photocarcinogenesis due to a loss of protective factors. To reduce skin damage, the minimal erythmal dose is suggested – this may vary from person to person and is based upon the amount of radiation that is needed to cause redness and therefore inflammation in the cutaneous layers.[106]

WEIGHT LOSS

Adipose tissue is a known pro-inflammatory which may possibly pose some risk in the initiation of melanoma.[111]

HEALTHY MICROBIOME

Current research in animals is demonstrating the impact of the microbiome on melanoma. The results appear to be relevant in that in mouse studies, the gut immune response may antagonise tumour development. More studies are needed.[111]

DURING ACTIVE CANCER

Herbal medicine

SANGUINARIA CANADENSIS ('BLACK SALVE')

Caution is raised by Mazzio et al.[130] for the use of black salve (also known as bloodroot) topically as there are no studies to suggest benefits. Sanguinarine (toxic benzophenanthridine alkaloid) causes skin corrosion and scar tissue, which may induce a potentially innocuous basal cell to form an aggressive malignant cancer. The herb does possess some suggestive therapeutic value. However, the small therapeutic dose range of this herb prevents it from safe use.[130]

ROSMARINUS OFFICINALIS FOLIA (ROSEMARY)

The anti-melanogenic effects of rosemary are currently under investigation. The components thought to demonstrate promise are the bioactive principles ursolic acid, 12-O-methyl carnosic acid and oleanic acid, with the latter demonstrating the highest cytotoxicity. Ursolic acid and its various isomers, including betulinic acid, demonstrate a milder inhibitory effect on tyrosinase, an enzyme critical to the precipitation of melanogenesis. Rosemary demonstrates a positive downregulation of tyrosinase expression in human cell animal studies.[226]

ATRACTYLODES MACROCEPHALAE RHIZOME (ATRACTYLODES)

Early studies suggest the herb may have a use in the treatment of melanoma cells.[227] Atractylodis is a herb widely used in traditional Chinese formulations. The herb exhibits a cytotoxic action in melanoma cells via multiple mechanisms, including ERK/GSK38 AT-I-induced G1 phase arrest, leading to apoptosis. Further studies are needed.[227]

GREEN TEA EGCG

The polyphenol EGCG significantly inhibit a variety of human melanoma cell lines in vitro. The mechanism is downregulation of histone deactylase, which is known to induce DNA damage. EGCG decreases histone deactylase proteins via a proteasomal degradation, leading to cell death.[228] Epigenic alterations are driven by acetylation and deacetylation. Thereby, the polyphenols are a valuable adjunct to therapy. Other mechanisms demonstrated were a decrease in the cell cycle via cyclins and cyclin-dependent kinases of the G1 phase, and positive influence on tumour suppressor proteins.[228]

CURCUMA LONGA (TURMERIC)

Curcumin has the ability to suppress melanoma cells via multiple signalling pathways exerting a powerful anti-tumorigenic effect. Possible pathways include reduction of invasion, cell cycle arrest and autophagy.[229]

Nutritional medicine

OVERALL DIET

Definitive trials for preventive dietary factors in dietary treatment during active melanoma have yet to be conducted. However, the WCRF[95] states that people who have active cancer should follow preventive dietary suggestions. The inclusion of cold-water fish, fruit and dark green leafy vegetables to increase dietary intakes of vitamins A, D, C and E and carotenoids may be a risk reduction factor.[91,104,105] Epidemiological studies between Western and Japanese diets suggest the possibility of ingestion of brown seaweed. Brown seaweed contains active principles of ascophyllan, fucoidan, fucoxanthin, galactolipids and prebiotics properties, which may be of benefit.[230] In both single isolated fractions and as a food, brown seaweed demonstrates a decrease in melanoma cell growth, suppressed skin mRNA expression, an increase in cell arrest and slower tumour adhesion, invasion and migration in animal studies.[230]

BIOACTIVE GRAPE SEED PROANTHOCYANIDINS

In a single study of in vivo human cell xenograft melanoma cells, the trial suggested that beta-catenin, which is associated with the rapid growth of melanoma cells, can be inhibited with the use of grape seed extract.[110]

RESVERATROL

Resveratrol manifests the induction of autophagy with an associated inhibition of ceramide formation via the Akt/mTOR pathway.[231]

OMEGA-3 FATTY ACIDS

Omega-3 long-chain DHA provides an anti-neoplastic inhibitory effect on the growth of human melanoma cells. DHA decreases MMP-2, MMP-13 and MT1-MMP expression while potently increasing the activity of beta-catenin. The action of beta-catenin promotes melanocyte-inducing transcription factor, which prevents the invasive action of melanoma cells in vitro.[232]

QUERCETIN

The plant form of quercetin found in a methanolic extract of *Lawsonia inermis*, or Henna as it is commonly known, inhibits melanoma tyrosinase activity, therefore reducing the production of melanin. Quercetin is found to inhibit proliferation by decreasing matrix metalloproteinase-9, tyrosinase-related protein (TRP)-1 and TRP-2 mRNA expression, leading to spontaneous apoptosis. Other constituents of the plant include luteolin and several other flavonoids.[90,233]

SUPPORT DURING RADIOTHERAPY

Resveratrol

Resveratrol may enhance the efficacy of radiotherapy in radio-resistant melanoma cell lines. Resveratrol reduces colonisation, proliferation and density of melanoma cells, supporting increased apoptosis via decreasing the expression of cyclin B, D, cdk2 and cdk4.[234]

SUPPORT DURING CHEMOTHERAPY

Herbal medicine

GLYCYRRHIZA GLABRA (LIQUORICE)

A flavone extraction of liquorice, liquiritigenin demonstrates synergistic properties in enhancing the action of cisplatin in autophagy of melanoma cells via multiple mechanistic actions. Dual therapy upregulated PTEN protein level and downregulated protein expression of MMP-2/9, PI3K, p-AKT. Both of these actions inhibit tumour metastasis progression.[125]

Nutritional medicine

CoQ10

CoQ10 acts as a protector of mitochondrial function during chemotherapy and serves as an intercellular antioxidant. During chemotherapy, CoQ10 levels are altered. Recent studies suggest that CoQ10 may impact on the expression of transcription, cell signalling, cellular transport and metabolism associating CoQ10 as a gene regulator. Administering CoQ10 during chemotherapy has not been shown to interfere with treatment and serves to provide multiple benefit to the patients' wellbeing.[235]

MELATONIN AND VITAMIN D

Melatonin and vitamin D have demonstrated protective factors and can be utilised as an adjuvant during any stage of the disease and during therapy for metastatic melanoma.[236] Melatonin is non-toxic, and vitamin D levels do not rise to pose toxicity without heavy supplementation, which is easily monitored via blood levels. It is suggested that both agents be used prophylactically and as deterrents to progressive disease.[236]

OMEGA-3 FATTY ACIDS

Chemotherapy promotes an inflammatory cytokine response by macrophages within tumour microenvironments. Omega-3 acts as an endogenous regulator of inflammation and protects the lipid membrane of the surrounding tumour site from invasion. Omega-3 upregulates maresin 1, which can be enhanced via the ingestion of DHA. Moreover, maresin 1 decreases the pro-inflammatory cytokines produced during cisplatin therapy and is therefore a positive adjunct to treatment.[237]

FERMENTED WHEAT EXTRACT

This is a patented product and as such research may have bias. Patel[238] discusses the benefits of wheatgerm extract fermented with *Saccharomyces cerevisiae* as having potential benefit as a complementary adjunct in melanoma treatment. Challem[239] supports its use, stating that there are over 100 studies including clinical trials to demonstrate efficacy. The nutrient contains benzoquinones, which are suggested to inhibit glucose uptake by cancer cells.

QUERCETIN

Quercetin may sensitise melanoma cells to decarbazine therapy via regulation of reactive oxygen species.[90]

Lung cancer

PREVENTION

Worldwide, lung cancer is the most common cause of deaths attributed to cancer. Systematic review of the evidence suggests that eliminating tobacco smoking is the best strategy for prevention.[240]

Nutritional medicine – dietary

ANTIOXIDANTS AND CAROTENOIDS

A recent systematic review and meta-analysis of 18 studies suggested that antioxidants and carotenoids in fruit and vegetables reduce the risk of lung cancer.[240] The relative risk estimates were higher for the combination of fruit and vegetables, rather than either fruit or vegetable intake alone. The results yield ingestion was marginally significant for current smokers and significantly inverse for former or non-smokers. Findings also suggested that for each 100 g/day increase of combined fruit and vegetables, the inverse relationship became more significant. This amplifies the notion that there is a dose-responsive association to the benefits. The consumption of 400 g/day of plant food or more did not provide greater benefit.[240] The Mediterranean diet is a proposed protective diet to reduce the risk of most cancers, including lung cancer.[240]

Although carotenoids, the precursor to vitamin A also known as retinal, from plant foods prove beneficial, the ingestion of large doses of retinol vitamin A from animal foods may increase free radical production.[241] However, this is suggested to be dose dependent. As the safe oral supplemental dose of vitamin A retinol in lung cancer is largely unknown, it would be prudent not to supplement with retinol.[242] Foods containing high levels of retinol are beef liver, fatty fish, cheese and milk, although no studies have suggested lowering the intake of food-based retinol.

HIGHER VITAMIN AND FIBRE DIETS

In a 5–7-year study of participants ($n = 4336$) where 178 of the participants were diagnosed with lung cancer, vegetable fat combined with fruit and vegetables consumption provided a significant risk reduction. It is assumed that respondents consuming higher vitamin and fibre diets present a reduced incidence of the disease.[243]

Herbal medicine

GREEN TEA EGCG

Green tea is suggested as both a preventive and a chemotherapeutic for the delay of cancer onset, and as a primary preventive.[121] In an early prospective Japanese study, Nakachi et al.[244] found that drinking 10 cups (150 mL) of green tea per day significantly delayed the onset of cancer in the general population, where a large proportion of the population (males) are heavy smokers.

SUPPORT DURING ACTIVE CANCER

Herbal medicine

ASTRAGALUS MEMBRANACEUS (ASTRAGALUS)

Astragalus root has been utilised in traditional Chinese herbal medicine for many years. Li et al.[245] support previous findings of over 65 clinical trials that the use of astragalus in combination with herbal therapeutic formulae has benefit in the treatment of NSCLC.[246] The herb provides immune-modulating, restorative and anti-tumour effects in vivo and in vitro by improving natural killer cell activity, inhibiting cytokines and stimulating macrophage activity.[245]

GREEN TEA EGCG

The polyphenol EGCG significantly inhibits tumour cell mass and human lung cell lines in vitro. A proprietary anti-inflammatory drug Sulindac in combination with EGCG has a noted effect on reducing the number of tumours in animal studies, via upregulation of genes that arrest growth and damage to DNA in PC-9 cells.[247]

CURCUMA LONGA (TURMERIC)

The lipophilic polyphenol curcumin, found in turmeric, acquired from the rhizome is well known for its anti-cancer properties. However, the effects of curcumin are enhanced by components in the oil of turmeric – primarily the chemical elemene. In China, this is the focus of the anti-cancerous properties of the herb along with turmerin, turmerone, furanodiene, curdione, bisacurone, cyclocurcumin, calebin A and germacrone.[248] Most studies focus on curcumin as the phenolic with the most diverse anti-tumour activity in NSCLC.[249,250]

Nutritional medicine

OVERALL DIET

Definitive trials for preventive dietary factors in the treatment during active lung cancer have yet to be conducted. However, the WCRF[95] states that people who have active cancer should follow preventive dietary strategies. Giacosa et al.[251] suggest the target for dietary parameters is a combination of a healthy lifestyle and the avoidance of smoking as a priority, combined with the Mediterranean dietary protocol.

MELATONIN

Melatonin exerts an induction of cellular apoptosis in cultured human lung adenocarcinoma, via multiple pathways. The nutrient expresses an inhibitory effect on cell adhesion, migration and intracellular glutathione levels increasing caspase-3 activities and reactive oxygen species. Additionally, melatonin downregulates proliferation and cell signalling.[252]

SHARK CARTILAGE

Once thought to be pure folklore, purified matrilin-1 from the cartilage of sharks has been able to demonstrate an inhibitory effect on neovascularisation both in vivo and in vitro in human lung cancer cell lines. The mechanism is thought to be that of capillary endothelial cell proliferation and elevated expression of PECAM1, VEGFR and VE-cadherin.[253] Physicians Data Query Cancer Information Summaries[113] suggest in a very small ($n = 22$) study that shark cartilage propriety brand AE-941 (Neovastat) may lengthen the survival of patients with NSCLC. There is potential for bias in the study.

OMEGA-3 FATTY ACIDS

Based on statistically significant follow-up studies (over a 20-year period), the principle that low-dose aspirin may decrease the risk of some cancers due to its effects on cyclooxygenase-2, EPA and DHA was examined in respect of similar actions. Higher omega-3 to omega-6 intakes lessen the risk and progression of lung adenocarcinomas via their anti-inflammatory (reduction of PGE_2) tissue membrane support roles. Both autocrine and paracrine complementary effects are noted via downregulation of the isotypes EP1–4, which oppose apoptosis and enhance proliferation, and increase both the risk of lung cancer and the risk of spread.[254]

VITAMIN D

High vitamin D_3 intake may result in the inhibition of tumour growth in NSCLC via its effect on EGFR. Vitamin D is proposed to induce E-cadherin in directly opposing action on the EGFR.[255] It is known that low levels of vitamin D may increase the growth of EGFR lung cancers, as stated in early studies by White.[256]

SUPPORT DURING RADIOTHERAPY

Herbal medicine

ASTRAGALUS MEMBRANACEUS (ASTRAGALUS)

In China, astragalus-containing herbal therapy is often prescribed in combination with other herbs during active cancers. The saponins from the herb exert an anti-carcinogenic activity in some cancers, and are suggested to be of benefit to patients undergoing radiotherapy for NSCLC. He et al.,[257] in a meta-analysis of 29 studies ($n = 2547$ patients) with NSCLC, demonstrated increased tumour response, survival and performance and reduced side effects when the herb was co-administered.[257]

SUPPORT DURING CHEMOTHERAPY

Herbal medicine

GREEN TEA EGCG

In human graft cells, EGCG in combination with anti-inflammatories provides a synergistic effect by inhibiting tumour growth in human lung cancer cells and provides viable co-administration during chemotherapy.[247]

ASTRAGALUS MEMBRANACEUS (ASTRAGALUS)

Astragalus improves the QOL in patients undergoing chemotherapy with vinorelbine and cisplatin. The herb assists in enhancing immune response and reducing immunosuppression, which may allow for treatment to continue.[257,258]

Nutritional medicine

CoQ10

CoQ10 acts as a protector of mitochondrial function during chemotherapy and serves as an intercellular antioxidant. During chemotherapy, CoQ10 levels are altered. Recent studies suggest that CoQ10 may impact on the expression of transcription, cell signalling, cellular transport and metabolism associating CoQ10 as a gene regulator. Administering CoQ10 during chemotherapy has not been shown to interfere with treatment and serves to provide multiple benefits to the patient's wellbeing.[235]

MELATONIN

In NSCLC, patients with specific epidermal growth factor mutations become resistant to drug therapy. Melatonin was utilised with gefitinib to target TKI-resistant H1975 cells. The combination therapy demonstrated an effective decrease in cellular activity and downregulated the growth of epidermal growth factor activity inducing apoptosis.[259]

SHARK CARTILAGE

In vivo studies suggest a proprietary brand of shark cartilage AE-941 (Neovastat) enhanced the effects of cisplatin in Lewis lung cancer.[113]

Mudge et al.[237] suggest that omega-3 upregulates maresin 1 that may decrease the pro-inflammatory cytokines produced during cisplatin therapy in NSCLC and is therefore a positive adjunct to treatment. To that end, as shark cartilage demonstrates similar properties, it may pose as a novel adjunctive therapy.

OMEGA-3 FATTY ACIDS

Chemotherapy promotes an inflammatory cytokine response by macrophages within tumour microenvironments. Omega-3 acts as an endogenous regulator of inflammation and protects the lipid membrane of the surrounding tumour site from invasion. Omega-3 upregulates maresin 1, which can be enhanced via the ingestion of DHA. Moreover, maresin 1 decreased the pro-inflammatory cytokines produced during cisplatin therapy and is therefore a positive adjunct to treatment.[237]

FISETIN

Fisetin is a dietary flavonoid (3,3′,4′,7-tetrahydroxyflavone) found in strawberries, blueberries, kiwi fruit, apples, persimmon, onions, grapes and cucumbers. The skin of fruit is particularly high in the flavonoid, which in preclinical studies suggests cancer inhibition via apoptosis, angiogenesis, invasion, alterations in cell cycle and metastasis, demonstrating a non-toxic benefit.[97] Cisplatin in combination with fisetin demonstrates enhanced apoptosis via inactivation of MAPK pathways and suppression of survivin in NSCLC. The flavonoid additionally impacts on caspase-3 activation, reduces lipid peroxidation and inhibits PI3K/Akt/mTOR. Dose is reported (in animals) as 25 mg/kg/BW.[97]

Non-Hodgkin lymphoma (NHL)

PREVENTION

NHL accounts for approximately 70% of B cell lymphoma.[260] The Memorial Sloan Kettering Cancer Center[261] states there are no particular preventive measures for decreasing lymphoma occurrence. However, suggested risk factors include having a human T cell leukaemia/lymphotropic virus, *Helicobacter pylori* bacteria and exposure to various pesticides – specifically for NHL, prolonged use of herbicides. Diffuse large B cell lymphoma subtype is the most common NHL in Western countries. There is a strong correlation between higher BMI in certain subtypes of NHL, as evidenced by Breitenstein et al.[262] A healthy lifestyle, with lowered BMI, is also advocated in a review of the evidence.[263] A multi-ethnic cohort study ($n = 2339$) suggested higher mortality rates with the consumption of dairy and a better outlook for those who consumed legumes on a regular basis.[264] A systematic review and meta-analysis conducted in the US, Europe and Asia suggested a favourable risk reduction with light alcohol consumption in 10% of respondents.[265]

SUPPORT DURING ACTIVE CANCER

There are many forms of NHL – not all have been widely researched with herbal or nutrient intervention.

Herbal medicine

CURCUMA LONGA (TURMERIC)

Turmeric diferuloylmethane component may have a role to play in inhibiting histone deacetylase and reducing the proliferation, and increasing apoptosis in B-NHL Raji cell lines.[266] Additionally, turmeric may induce tumour cell

differentiation, apoptosis and cell arrest in T cell lymphoma lines. However, evidence is from animal studies and relatively scarce.[267]

GREEN TEA EGCG

In an MCL Jeko-1 and BL Raji cell line study, green tea EGCG demonstrated growth inhibition via caspase activation and anti-oncogenic proteins that induce apoptosis, which may suggest green tea may be useful in active B cell lymphoma treatment.[268]

Nutritional medicine

OVERALL DIET

Survivors of NHL demonstrate a higher antioxidant and phytochemicals intake from fruit and vegetables. The increased nutrients may lead to tumour inhibition via their influence on immune function and antioxidant detoxification.[264] Earlier studies state an association with meat, high sugar intake, fat, dairy and milk with increased risk, and possibly decreased survival.[269–271] Leo et al.[264] state the evidence is conflicting. Legume consumption is possibly protective. Fish and meat at a low level predict a better survival. However, high meat consumption was inversely correlated.[264]

OMEGA-3 FATTY ACIDS

A literature review (1998–2012) on the use of EPA and DHA from omega-3 fatty acids renders promising results.[272] The essential fatty acids prohibit inflammatory markers (IL-1, IL-6 and tumour necrosis factor-alpha [TNF-α]) secreted by malignant cells, which are identified as prompting their own growth. Fish oils are lipid mediators and decrease arachidonic acid metabolism in haematological neoplasm. This suggests omega-3's action is a possible immunomodulatory, eliciting a protective response in malignant cells.[272]

ZINC

Higher levels of serum copper with a disturbed copper to zinc ratio are found in early stage NHL. In advanced NHL cases, low zinc levels are noted. High copper levels can be utilised to stimulate angiogenic activity, particularly where low protective micronutrient zinc is seen.[116] VEGF and zinc regulate tumour progression, and increased levels of VEGF are linked with poor outcomes for patients with solid tumours. The ratio of copper to zinc is both diagnostic and prognostic in haematological tumours. Zinc levels need to be within range to predict a favourable prognosis.[116]

VITAMIN D

A prospective study of newly diagnosed patients with NHL ($n = 983$) suggested associations between insufficient (<62.5 nmol/L) serum levels of vitamin D 25(OH)D to be predictive of lower survival rates.[273] As the reference range is 50–140 nmol/L in Australian pathology results, this study suggested that 50 nmol/L would be considered insufficient. Higher vitamin D levels, both serum and converted metabolically active 1,25(OH)$_2$D, are associated with lower event-free survival and overall survival. This is likely to be due to vitamin-D-modulated induction of cellular differentiation, apoptotic promotion and inhibitory actions on proliferation of lymphoma cell lines.[273]

RESVERATROL

Studies have been conducted on the use of resveratrol on NHL since 2000.[274,275] Resveratrol, despite its very low oral absorption and expression in the blood stream, demonstrates the capacity in vivo to create active metabolites via resveratrol sulfates and glucoronides and piceatannol (stilbene) possessing anti-cancerous actions.[276] The dose range orally is in dispute as it ranges from 0.03 g to 5 g daily. However, there is a confirmed sensitivity of leukaemia and lymphoma cells where resveratrol is found to be cytotoxic, triggering apoptosis and autophagy.[276]

SUPPORT DURING RADIOTHERAPY

Nutritional medicine

MELATONIN

Melatonin use is strongly recommended to reduce the side effects of radiotherapy, demonstrating low toxicity over a wide range of doses, with uses in both initial and advanced metastatic cancers.[277]

SELENIUM

Short-term selenium supplementation during radiation therapy is generally deemed safe and improves QOL by reducing radiotherapy-induced side effects. Selenium provides anti-cancer effects via selenoproteins, which limit DNA and oxidative damage. It may also assist in the conjugation and detoxification of carcinogens.[278]

SUPPORT DURING CHEMOTHERAPY

Herbal medicine

GREEN TEA EGCG

As previously stated, EGCG is known to act in tumour regulation in Jeko-1 and Raji cells. Although yet to be thoroughly studied with all chemotherapeutic agents, the addition of EGCG to first-line therapy seems noteworthy. EGCG protects mitochondrial function, concurrently inducing apoptosis in imatinib-resistant chronic myelogenous leukaemia. The authors suggest it is a potential therapy in B cell lymphomas.[268]

CURCUMA LONGA (TURMERIC)

There is promising evidence for the use of curcuminoids in dual therapy in advanced cancer treatment. It appears that turmeric may safely be used to enhance the effect of chemotherapy and may sensitise cancer cells to medication. However, this has not been specifically studied in NHL.[279]

Nutritional medicine

MELATONIN

Melatonin has a demonstrated role to play in antiproliferative, angiogenetic and differentiation in solid and liquid tumours including NHL.[280] In a small case

study, patients treated with chemotherapy, retinoids and melatonin demonstrated a percentage of cure rate and increased prognosis. Todisco[280] and Di Bella et al.[277] suggest its use in all oncological diseases.

QUERCETIN

Quercetin may re-sensitise non-Hodgkin's follicular lymphoma to first-line therapy. Many patients experience recurrent relapses of the disease when resistance to medication occurs, which may shorten prognosis. Bcl-2 overexpression favourably leads to apoptosis; quercetin may release the blocked pathway of Bcl-2 (via multiple pathways) in the mitochondria and increase the efficacy of Apo2L/TRAIL medication.[260]

ACETYL-L-CARNITINE

As a critical component of mitochondrial function, acetyl-L-carnitine was investigated to mitigate peripheral neuropathy where chemotherapeutic agents bortezomib and doxorubicin were utilised. Acetyl-L-carnitine demonstrated a reduction of peripheral neuropathy without reducing the response rate, with high tolerability by the patients.[281]

General cancer support (unknown primary site)

PREVENTION

The WCRF[95] suggests the following for general cancer prevention:
- Avoid energy-dense foods, fast food (large portions, higher fat content), high-kilojoule sugar drinks.
- Increase non-starchy vegetables and fruit to at least 600 g per day: five portions of vegetables of varying colour, two of fruit.
- Eat unprocessed grains and legumes/pulses.
- Reduce starch roots and tubers to ensure adequate non-starchy vegetables.
- Avoid sodium in excess (2 g sodium per day is suggested).
- Avoid grains, legumes and cereals that are mouldy.
- Limit red meat to under 500 g, very little if any to be processed deli meats (population averages are 300 g per week).
- Do not drink alcohol, or if it is consumed, drink within national guidelines.
- Supplements must be discussed with the primary healthcare team.

Nutritional medicine – dietary

The overwhelming suggestion for the prevention of cancers in general from numerous studies is the Mediterranean diet.[96] The principles of the diet are high vegetable oil/extra virgin olive oil; low saturated fats; fruit and vegetables (191–500 g/day); wholegrain cereal; legumes; limited amounts of fish, chicken and meat, dairy; with occasional reserved consumption of egg, alcohol and sweets. Additionally, there is a distinct absence of additives where the inclusion of fresh herbs is documented.[96] The potential success of the Mediterranean diet is the high nutritive bioactive polyphenolic and phytosterol content of the foods.[282] The vast variance of the intakes of food groups across the Mediterranean is noted and dose references are limited due to such wide parameters. However, the dietary patterning compared to a Western diet is the likely key to its success.[96]

Other suggestions[95]

- Avoid central adiposity.
- Stay within the BMI reference range for your population, preferably in Western ethnicity, 21–23.
- Ensure throughout childhood and adolescence the range is at the lower end of normal of 21.
- Start with 30 minutes of exercise per day and increase to 60 minutes of vigorous physical activity every day, with limited sedentary habits.
- Encourage breastfeeding exclusively for a 6-month period. This is beneficial for both mother and child.
- Cancer survivors and those living with the disease should follow preventive measures.

SUPPORT DURING ACTIVE CANCER

Herbal medicine

TUMOURICIDAL HERBS

In a study, 347 herbal remedies were evaluated for a dose-dependent tumouricidal effect.[128] The herbal family classifications with the most potent demonstration of apoptotic events were (from most potent to least): Arecaceae, Verbenaceae, Clusiaceae, Dryopteridaceae, Berberidaceae, Umbelliferae, Solanaceae, Chenopodiaceae, Boraginaceae, Hydrangeaceae, Zygophyllaceae, Rhamnaceae, Fabaceae, Burseraceae, Salicaceae, Dipsacaceae, Papaveraceae and Dioscoreaceae. The greatest response (LD_{50} <0.1 mg/mL) was from the extracts of wild yam *Dioscorea villosa* root, a popular Western herb, and the lesser known teasel root, balm of Gilead bud and frankincense. This is a surprising result as dioscorea is not a well-studied or utilised herbal therapy for cancer therapy. Diosgenin has been studied and is known to produce pro-apoptotic effects, reduce proliferation via downregulation of NF-κB, Akt, cyclin D, G2/M arrest, c-Myc and induction of pro-PARP cleavage/DNA fragmentation.[130]

ASTRAGALUS MEMBRANACEUS (ASTRAGALUS)

Isolated principles astragaloside I, II, III and IV from *Astragalus membranaceus* have demonstrated potential therapeutic use in multiple cancers, via an induction of apoptotic cell signalling pathways. Astragalus induces decreased cancer cell survival in vitro coupled with inhibition of tumour growth via downregulation of endothelial growth factors in vivo.[203]

ASTRAGALUS MEMBRANACEUS (ASTRAGALUS) AND CODONOPSIS PILOSULA (CODONOPSIS)

Randomised control trials on traditional Chinese medicine utilise injected forms of *Astragalus membranaceus* and *Codonopsis pilosula* to improve Qi energy, erythropoiesis, immune function and QOL.[283]

WITHANIA SOMNIFERA (ASHWAGANDHA)

Cell culture and animal studies suggest the alkaloids of ashwagandha possess anti-tumourigenic properties and possibly can be utilised as preventive therapy. Interestingly, the root has been the most studied part of the herb, whereas the leaf also demonstrates anti-cancerous therapeutic potential.[205] Withania is also hepatoprotective. The alkaloids and withanolides are possibly enhanced by the other elements of the plant's constituents. The herb demonstrates an unusual approach to autophagy via multiple cellular signalling pathways, via binding to cysteine in B-tubulin, inhibitor of NF-κB kinase subunit beta, glial fibrillary acidic protein and vimentin, additionally modulating heat shock response and proteasomal degradation.[205]

GREEN TEA (EGCG)

EGCG has been shown to be beneficial in numerous cancers. The proposed dose is 6–9 Japanese-sized cups – approximately 180 mL, equivalent to 1–2 g of EGCG in humans.[121] A large Japanese study ($n = 8552$) spanning 10 years followed green tea consumers (419 developed a demonstrated cancer). The onset of cancer in females who consumed 10 cups of green tea per day was 7.3 years later than those who drank three cups. In males, it was 3.2 years, but the male group may have been confounded by cigarette smoking. The study states that EGCG and various other catechins from the plant target and suppress cancer stem cells from various human cancer tissues.[121]

CURCUMA LONGA (TURMERIC)

Curcumin demonstrates suggestive evidence exerting anti-cancer effects through multiple molecular signalling networks.[284]

Nutritional medicine

OVERALL DIET

The WCRF[95] states that people who have active cancer should follow preventive dietary suggestions.

COMMON HERBS AND SPICES

Kitchen spices contain bioactive components, anthocyanins, phenylpropanoids, alkaloids, terpenes and flavonoids. These chemicals scavenge free radicals and support tissue at a cellular level.[119] Some have been studied for chemoprotective purposes, several demonstrating arrest of cytochrome P450, cyclooxygenase-2 and isozyme CYP 1A1, the action of which demonstrates reduction of signal transducers and activators. They also downregulate cell cycle proteins decreasing stimulation of caspases and suppress κB initiation. Spices pose anti-inflammatory and immune regulatory actions, pointing to their use in cancer therapy.[119]

Herbs and spices discussed by Bhagat et al. are[119]: *Pimpinella anisum L., Ocimum sanctum, Nigella sativa, Cinnamomum tamala/cassia, Elettaria cardamomum, Eugenia caryophyllata, Coriandrum sativum, Trigonella foenum-graecum, Allium sativa, Foeniculum vulgare,*

Zingiber officinalis, Stigmata croci, Papaver somniferum and *Curcuma longa*.

MUSHROOMS (*LENTINUS EDODES* AND *GANODERMA LUCIDUM*)

A review of *Lentinus edodes* and *Ganoderma lucidum* suggested the action of therapy is the regulation of NK cells providing desirable survival outcomes in advanced cancer patients. QOL was improved via a decrease in adverse effects of treatment (chemotherapy and radiotherapy) and of the cancer itself in terms of reduced fatigue, anxiety and depression.[129]

MELATONIN

There is support for the hypothesis that elevated melatonin levels are useful in a range of different cancer tumours. Melatonin demonstrates amplification of cytotoxicity and cytostatic events, even where the direct effect of melatonin on tumours seems unresponsive. Melatonin has been found to complement conventional drug therapy via reduced Sirt1 and elevated p53/MDM2p ratios.[285]

OMEGA-3 FATTY ACIDS

Several types of cancers demonstrate an intracellular deficit of omega-3 and omega-6. This is thought to reduce the effects of chemotherapy and increase generation of lipid peroxides. Fish oils may reduce overexpression of integrin-linked kinase, which increases neoplastic risk. This is achieved via an increase in anchorage-dependent cell growth, tumour angiogenesis, invasion and migration of cancer cells.[284]

VITAMIN D

Higher pre-diagnostic vitamin D levels are associated with superior overall cancer survival.[286] A recent study suggests the gene regulatory factors that permit the action of 1,25D involve vitamin D receptor and retinoic X receptor interaction. The complex initiation affects a governing effect on DNA sequencing.[287]

Vitamin D cofactors

The binding receptor for vitamin D (VDR) is activated by 1,25-dihydroxyvitamin D_3 (1,25D). The action of 1,25D regulates genes that influence mood, calcium and phosphate metabolism and feedback of mineral ions, and assists xenobiotic detoxification, immune regulation, oxidative stress reduction, inflammation. Furthermore, it exerts anti-cancer and cardiovascular protective properties.[288] Nutrients that encourage VDR ligand receptor complex include polyunsaturated fatty acids, anthocyanidins and curcumin via an initiation of signalling. It is suggested that resveratrol potentiates VDR signalling via SIRT1's deacetylation of protein enzymatic reaction contributing to healthy cellular regulation.[288,289]

INTRAVENOUS VITAMIN C (IVC)

IVC was first utilised by Linus Pauling suggesting the selective toxicity of high dose vitamin C to some forms of cancer.[101] A recent review of the evidence stated there is no clear evidence to suggest the benefits.[290] However, this is largely a lack or inconsistency of evidence. In vitro and in vivo studies are promising.[291]

RESVERATROL

Mahabir et al.[284] suggest selective phytochemicals as a means of chemoprevention and for treatment options in active cancer. Resveratrol is a non-flavonoid polyphenol found in berries, grapes, pomegranate and lesser known foods such as peanuts and soybeans. Leischner et al.[292] state that resveratrol powerfully modulates immune function of NK cells. Resveratrol may play a role in epigenetic alterations, apoptosis, reduction of tumour cell proliferation and metastasis, sensitising tissue to chemotherapeutic medications in vitro and in vivo.[284]

QUERCETIN

Broccoli, onions, apples, berries and tea contain quercetin. We may consume as much as 25 mg/day from food. Quercetin binds with free radicals to form less reactive phenoxy radicals. The anti-kinase activity of the nutrient promotes anti-inflammatory, anti-proliferative effects and initiates apoptosis.[284]

SUPPORT DURING RADIOTHERAPY

Nutritional medicine

MELATONIN

Melatonin use is strongly recommended to reduce the side effects of radiotherapy, demonstrating low toxicity over a wide range of doses, with uses in both initial and advanced metastatic cancers.[277]

SELENIUM

Short-term selenium supplementation during radiation therapy is generally deemed safe and improves QOL by reducing radiotherapy-induced side effects. Selenium provides anti-cancer effects via selenoproteins, which limit DNA and oxidative damage. It may also assist in the conjugation and detoxification of carcinogens.[278]

SUPPORT DURING CHEMOTHERAPY

Herbal medicine

ASTRAGALUS MEMBRANACEUS (ASTRAGALUS)

A study on injections of astragalus as dual therapy with chemotherapy is promising, with no known detrimental effect on oestrogen treatment. A systematic review of treatments suggested that astragalus can reduce the haematopoietic consequences and death of normal cells. It may promote T cell subsets, therefore improving cell immunity, improve nutritional status, maintain or increase weight during treatment, reduce fatigue and protect bone marrow suppression.[217] In combination therapy with 5-FU, the polysaccharides of astragalus ameliorated cardiotoxicity via decreased and partial reversal of SOD and caspase-3 activation of 5-FU.[293]

Nutritional medicine

RESVERATROL

Mahabir et al.[284] suggest selective phytochemicals as a means of chemoprevention and for treatment options in active cancer.

CoQ10

CoQ10 functions as an oxidative phosphorylatory promoter in mitochondrial cells. Decreased levels are seen with the cytotoxicity associated with chemotherapy treatment. CoQ10 has been confirmed as a safe supplement, although sufficient human randomised controlled clinical trials have not been demonstrated.[294]

MELATONIN

Melatonin has demonstrated suppressive effects on neoplastic growth in various tumours.[295] Much research has been conducted around its ability to induce apoptosis in cancer cells, anti-metastatic effects and reduced telemerase activity but melatonin also modulates sleep response of cancer patients, which is a known comorbidity.[296] The nutrient also demonstrated antidepressive and anxiolytic actions where cancer patients demonstrate higher levels of mental angst for obvious reasons.[297] It is suggested as an adjuvant therapy despite, in some cases, not having a direct anti-tumouristatic effect.[295]

OMEGA-3 FATTY ACIDS

Omega-3 at a dose of 2 g EPA per day is suggested during chemotherapy. The suggestions are based on limited evidence but a well-validated safety profile in recent clinical trials. It is suggested that omega-3 supplements be given during chemotherapy as they improve tolerability of treatment and improve patient outcomes.[108]

QUERCETIN

Quercetin has a well-documented ability to enhance chemotherapy and radiotherapy sensitisation as well as act as a chemoprotective and radioprotective, posing advantages in dual use during active treatment.[298]

GENISTEIN

Genistein should not be supplemented during chemotherapy as it suggests potential drug interactions with efficacy of treatment.[124]

GLUTAMINE

In a systematic review, 11 of 15 studies reported the effectiveness of oral glutamine in reducing mucositis, with a weight-loss dosing range of 30 g per day in a divided dose.[99]

Renal cancer

PREVENTION

Epidemiological evidence is shifting away from previous limited risk factor parameters for renal cancer such as obesity, cigarette smoking and hypertension. New studies are suggesting genetics play the largest part, influenced by levels of physical activity, exposure to trichloroethylene, alcohol and a demonstrated higher prevalence in women than men. Risk genome typing is being employed to provide scanning ability for potential genetic implications in renal carcinogenesis.[299] The Mayo Clinic[300] suggests older age as an additional risk factor.

SUPPORT DURING ACTIVE CANCER

Herbal medicine

GREEN TEA (EGCG)

Gu et al.[301] suggest that the major catechins EGCG can reduce DNA methyltransferase. DNA methyltransferase is linked to a renal tissue overexpression of factor pathway inhibitor-2, a carcinogenesis-promoter. EGCG can downregulate factor pathway inhibitor-2, which inhibits growth and upregulates apoptosis in renal cell carcinoma cell line 786-0.

CURCUMA LONGA (TURMERIC)

There is a lack of substantial evidence for the use of turmeric in renal cell cancer. General research is suggestive that curcumin may inhibit endothelial growth factor C lymphangiogenesis in animal studies in vivo and in vitro. This may suppress proliferation, migration and cell cycle progression, demonstrating an anti-metastatic effect.[302]

MUSHROOMS – *GANODERMA LUCIDUM* AND *LENTINUS EDODES*

Generally, mushrooms have been utilised in traditional Chinese medicine for centuries. Constituents of mushrooms have demonstrated apoptotic, anti-angiogenic and anti-growth expression in a multitude of cancers.[303,304] Although evidence is still scarce, the following have been noted for urological cancers, but not for renal cancer: *Ganoderma lucidum* may inhibit human urethral and bladder cancer[305]; *Lentinus edodes* co-administration demonstrated a reduction of tumour progression in bladder cancer patients during active treatment with gemcitabine and demonstrates in vitro inhibition of tumour cell proliferation.[306,307]

Nutritional medicine – dietary

OVERALL DIET

The WCRF[95] suggests the same dietary recommendations for prevention are also useful in active cancer treatment.

ALCOHOL

The strongest dietary evidence for renal cancer states moderate ingestion of alcohol may decrease the risk of renal cancer where 30 g or two drinks are consumed per day. Conversely, the ingestion of higher levels, although not directly related to renal cancer (insufficient evidence), is related to several other cancer risks.[308]

WATER

There is also limited evidence that arsenic-containing water may present a risk.[308]

MEAT CONSUMPTION

In a meta-analysis of premenopausal women, there was a reported association between meat and processed meat intake and renal cancer, particularly clear cell adenocarcinomas.[309,310]

WHOLEGRAINS AND CRUCIFEROUS VEGETABLES

Protective dietary factors are suggested with wholegrains and the ingestion of cruciferous vegetables at least once a week, rather than none or occasional consumption.[311,312]

Nutritional medicine

VITAMIN D

Higher levels of circulating vitamin D are associated with a lower risk of renal cell carcinoma.[313]

In the largest study of its kind a meta-analysis (n = 130 609 participants and n = 1815 active renal cancer patients), higher levels of circulating vitamin D suggested an inverse relationship with renal cancer risk by approximately 21%.[314] Muller et al.[315] provide evidence that vitamin D is associated with longer survival rates if vitamin D is higher at time of diagnosis.

GENISTEIN

MicroRNA has become a topic of conversation in modulation of Wnt signalling. Wnt signalling passes messages into a cell through receptors on the cell surface determining the fate of cell migration, patterning and organogenesis.[316] Genistein has a potent effect on the Wnt signalling pathways in renal cell carcinoma by decreasing microRNA's effect, promoting apoptosis and concomitantly inhibiting proliferation and invasion.[316]

SHARK CARTILAGE

Alschuler et al.[91] suggest, from earlier studies, the potential for a proprietary shark cartilage to inhibit angiogenesis and increase survival rate in advanced renal cell cancer with a daily dose of 240 mL per day. Simard et al.[317] discuss the potential for inhibition of VEGFR2 and MMPs by the extract expressing a mechanistic action on the tissue plasminogen activator gene. However, the cells were pretreated with N-acetylcysteine (NAC), and therefore it is not known if shark cartilage alone or the synergy of NAC and shark cartilage is responsible for the action.

SUPPORT DURING CHEMOTHERAPY

Herbal medicine

MUSHROOMS – GANODERMA LUCIDUM AND LENTINUS EDODES

As previously discussed.

ASTRAGALUS MEMBRANACEUS (ASTRAGALUS)

The addition of astragalus-based herbal therapy has a long history of benefiting renal tissue. However, no human trials for renal cancer have been elucidated, and murine trials are old in terms of research currency. Astragalus demonstrates increases in circulating cytokines interferon-γ, IL-2R, IL-13, IL-6 and TNF-α. It therefore may be a positive adjuvant to drug therapy for immune function, wound healing ability and blood flow stability.[318]

Nutritional medicine

OMEGA-3 FATTY ACIDS

Kinase inhibitors such as regorafenib are associated with cancer cell resistance to responsive treatment after 1–2 years. Regorafenib is involved in the downregulation of soluble epoxide hydrolase (sEH).[219] sEH results in increases in DHA-derived epoxydocosapentaenoic acid, which proves anti-carginogenic. In vivo tests confirm that the combination of regorafenib and DHA reduces tumour invasion as well as p-VEGFR in animal studies of human renal cell carcinoma. Similar data reveals this action in vitro. There are no known current clinical trials for omega-3 alone. However, evidence is promising.[319]

VITAMIN D

A cross-sectional study suggested that vitamin D deficiency is seen in 90% of advanced cancer patients in palliative care. The authors concluded that there is a positive correlation between improved physical and mental function, wellbeing and reduced fatigue in patients with higher levels of serum vitamin D.[320]

Pancreatic cancer

PREVENTION

A meta-analysis of pooled summarised results of 117 studies reported that an estimated two-thirds of the major risk factors for pancreatic cancer are modifiable.[321] This gives great hope for those with hereditary predisposition to the disease.

The most well-established risk factor for pancreatic cancer is tobacco smoking; other considerations are alcohol consumption, chlorinated hydrocarbon solvents (occupational), diet and certain nutrients (discussed below), anthropometric measures and physical activity levels, past medical history such as impaired fasting blood glucose, cholecystectomy, *helicobacter pylori*, atopic allergy or hay fever, hepatitis C, certain medications, heredity and genetic factors, and population.[321]

DURING ACTIVE CANCER

Herbal medicine

The research is promising. In a recent article, 12 herbal compounds were found to be of benefit in human in vivo and in vitro pancreatic cancer cell lines via four or more mechanisms. Curcumin will be discussed, as the compound has the highest level of evidence above other therapy. Others include sulforaphane, quercetin, resveratrol, genistein, EGCG, benzyl isothiocyanate, thymoquinone, dihydroartemisinin, curcubitacin B, perillyl alcohol and apigenin.[322]

CURCUMA LONGA (TURMERIC)

In human and animal in vitro studies of pancreatic cancer cell lines such as AsPC1, MiaPaCa-2 and BxPC-3, potent cytotoxic effects were seen. In vivo curcumin reduced proliferation and angiogenesis and induced apoptosis.[323] The herb has poor bioavailability; therefore, large doses are needed for effect. No dose-limiting toxicity is reported at

12 g/day; however, some patients did report nausea and diarrhoea. Generally, dosing is set at 8 g/day. A small (*n* = 16) phase 1 clinical trial stated that oral Theracurmin® may allay the side effects of high dosing. Utilised alongside chemotherapy, the supplement did not increase adverse effects. The dose of Theracurmin® is suggested at approximately 400 mg/day.[323] Further trials are required to find no-observed-adverse-effect level.

Nutritional medicine – dietary

OVERALL DIET

Evidence is modest to poor due to research variabilities.

INCREASED RISK

High consumption of red and processed meat and soft drinks, and increases of 25 g of fructose/day increase risk.[321]

PROTECTIVE

There is supportive evidence for the consumption of fruit and vegetables, particularly citrus, and dietary folate (green leafy vegetables) being protective, with possible inverse relationships with consumption of tea (green and black), more so than coffee.[91,321,324] As there are no exact measures of the quantity of fruit and vegetables required, it is prudent to utilise the National Health and Medical Research Council's recommendations of five serves of vegetables and two of fruit per day as a standard approach.

PROTEIN

There is a possible need to increase protein levels 60–80 g/day to maintain muscle mass and body weight, with pancreatic enzyme support.[91] Metabolic increases in protein catabolism are found to negatively impact on survival and QOL in pancreatic cancer patients. In animal pancreatic cancer studies, higher protein intake and lower carbohydrate intake have proven to be advantageous by slowing tumour growth and preventing initiation.[325] There is a paucity of human studies. However, in a small human trial (*n* = 8), cachectic pancreatic cancer patients demonstrated protein anabolism when oral amino acid feeding was administered.[326] There may be a need to include digestive enzyme support to assist with protein digestion due to the inability of normal pancreatic function. However, cachexia is complicated and not solely due to protein digestion inability.[91,327]

Nutritional medicine

VITAMIN D

The evidence for concrete therapeutic ingestion is poor. One pooled analysis suggested no association of increased risk with low 25(OH)D status.[328] A single meta-analysis suggested higher risk with higher concentration (>100 nmol/L), whereas another single meta-analysis suggested 30% risk reduction with high vitamin D levels.[329,330] Dosage of 1000–5000 IU daily to reach vitamin D serum requirements is recommended. Lorenc et al.[331] suggest a vitamin D target range of >75 nmol/L.

GENISTEIN

Genistein has been shown to increase in vitro pro-apoptosis in pancreatic cancer cell lines through the caspase-9 and MMP-9 pathway. The nutrient may prohibit adhesion by binding to and inhibiting MEK4, which reduces the production of MMP-2 and decreases cellular invasion.[332–334] Pavese et al.[123] suggest low in vitro concentration levels are effective. Considering soy ingestion of Western (1 g/day) versus Asian populations (6–11 g/day) and the inverse relationship between intake and pancreatic cancer, Asian dosing would be prudent. A 10 g intake of tempeh will provide 2.4 mg of genistein, whereas the suggested dose in clinical trials is 2–8 mg per kg of body weight per day, which is 27 times higher than the average daily consumption. Therefore, a person weighing 60 kg would have to consume 600 g of various soy foods per day to reach a therapeutic dose. Although effective in animal studies, supplemental intake in human trials has yet to be confirmed to provide the same protective effect. The suggested dose range is approximately 3500 mg per day in a divided dose.[335] (Further information on the genistein content of foods can be found on the USDA nutrient database.)

MELATONIN

In pancreatic cancer cell lines, high-dose melatonin has been demonstrated to stimulate caspase-9 and caspase-3 activating apoptotic pathways. It may also decrease angiogenesis and reduce proliferation of pancreatic cancer through VEGF. In a small clinical study, there was a demonstrated higher 1-year survival rate in the melatonin-treated group.[336,337] Additional benefits of melatonin are immune modulation. In animal studies, it has been shown to increase the efficacy of oncostatic medications.[338] Dosage range is suggested between 3 and 20 mg daily, to be avoided in bipolar disorders.[91]

OMEGA-3 FATTY ACIDS

Fish oils have been seen to be supportive, reducing cachexia in pancreatic cancer patients.[109] In in vitro animal studies, EPA and DHA were found to suppress MIA-PaCa-2 human pancreatic cancer xenografts, the action of which induces oxidative stress and cancer cell death.[339] A recent systematic evaluation of 11 randomised controlled trials of EPA and DHA intervention versus traditional diet (95% CI) suggested EPA/DHA is safe and may confer a positive effect on survival and clinical outcomes for pancreatic cancer patients.[340] The recommended dose in humans for weight stabilisation would relate to a high dose of 4.9 g/day of EPA and 3.2 g/day of DHA.[109] Contraindications with other medications must be considered.

SELENIUM

It is established that low levels of selenium are associated with an increased risk and that survivors of pancreatic surgery have low serum blood levels.[341] A meta-analysis of five studies found an association between selenium supplementation and the reduction of pancreatic and other gastrointestinal cancers (RR 0.76).[342] An early trial of selenium coupled with beta-carotene suggested reduced rate of pancreatic cancer growth.[343] Dose range is based on approximately 100 micrograms taken in from food and 200 micrograms as supplement, with no adverse effect seen at doses triple this amount.[92,344,345]

SUPPORT DURING CHEMOTHERAPY

Herbal and supplemental assistance is generally considered safe and efficacious to date.

Herbal medicine

Most herbal therapy is not advised with taxane chemotherapy as it may interfere with the action of the drugs.

ADJUVANTS

- Green tea as an adjuvant to treatment[126]
- *Moringa oleifera* folia as an adjuvant
- In Panc-1, p34 and COLO 357 cultured human pancreatic cancer cells, *Moringa* leaf extract both alone and in conjunction with a taxane chemotherapeutic agent enhanced the cytotoxic effect of the drug by inhibiting NF-κB signalling.[346]

Nutritional medicine

- Probiotics for the reduction of chemotherapy-induced diarrhoea and gut health[347]
- L-glutamine to reduce gastric side effects of medications, increase energy and reduce inflammation[348]
- Ginger to reduce nausea and adjuvant[128]
- Melatonin increases QOL survival rate and reduces cachexia[349]
- Fish oil increases drug uptake and suppresses survival pathways for cancer cell growth[109]

Bladder cancer

PREVENTION

The WCRF[350] suggests that prevention is based on limiting smoking as smokers have a six-fold increased risk for bladder cancer compared to those who have never smoked. Although not likely in Australia, the infestation of the bladder by parasites is a risk factor for squamous cell carcinomas. The most significant finding is that of occupational and environmental toxins such as arsenic in water, and exposure to polyaromatic hydrocarbons and aromatic amines, inducing a significantly elevated risk. Other risk factors include long-term catheter use, other cancer treatment, chronic infections, being male, older age, family history and treatment for diabetes.[241]

Nutritional medicine – dietary

Findings of contaminated drinking water (arsenic) associated with bladder cancer are very strong. Contamination can occur from natural deposits and from run off from industrial and agricultural wastes. This may not be prevalent in Australia, but countries such as Chile, Mexico, India, Cambodia and Bangladesh are implicated.

In terms of foods, there is some evidence that a higher intake of protective factors of polyphenols and bioflavonoids in a diet rich in fruit and vegetables decreases the risk, as does the consumption of tea.[351]

Other suggestions

Adoption of the Mediterranean diet and lifestyle pyramid suggests protective factors for most cancers. The requisites for the diet are the limitation of sweets, alcohol and red and processed meat, favouring white meat and seafood, eggs, legumes and moderate dairy (low fat), with high consumption of olives, nuts, seeds, spices, herbs and water, as well as liberal physical activity and traditional living with non-toxic cleaning practices.[241]

DURING ACTIVE CANCER

Herbal medicine

GREEN TEA (EGCG)

Guohua et al.[352] suggest green tea polyphenol EGCG is both preventive and beneficial in treatment (animal studies). In vitro studies demonstrate a potent induction of apoptosis, suppression of metastasis and cell cycle arrest. Chen et al.[353] state that EGCG inhibits transitional cell carcinoma of bladder cell lines. In novel technically advanced models of cancer therapy, catechin nanoparticle drug delivery systems have a high cellular uptake both in vivo and in vitro, demonstrating an enhanced anti-tumour activity.[354]

CURCUMA LONGA (TURMERIC)

A recent in vitro study on a branded registered turmeric extract showed decreased cell viability, induction of apoptosis, cell cycle dysregulation and reduced clonogenicity.[355] The theory regarding autophagy is strongly supported by various other studies on the use of turmeric in bladder cancer treatment in active cancer.[355–357]

Nutritional medicine – dietary

OVERALL DIET

Definitive trials for the prevention of dietary factors in the treatment of bladder cancer during active cancer have yet to be conducted. However, preliminary findings are as detailed in the Prevention section.[95] Increased fruit and vegetable intakes and potentially the reduction of meat and fat intakes are recommended.[358] Michaud et al.[359] suggest that cruciferous vegetables have the most potent anti-bladder cancer risk reduction.

ALLYL ISOTHIOCYANATE

The chemical component allyl isothiocyanate is found abundantly in cruciferous vegetables, horseradish, wasabi and mustard. A low oral dose has been suggestive of inhibiting the proliferation of human bladder carcinoma cell lines in vitro at a dose of 1 mg/kg. As discussed, previous studies suggested a human diet high in cruciferous vegetables concurs with the animal findings.[359] The exact mechanism is unknown; however, the actions are postulated to act via MMP-2 and MMP-9 inhibition.[360]

APIGENIN

Apigenin occurs naturally in the hydroxylated form in onions, parsley, oranges, onions and tea. The nutrient demonstrates in human bladder cancer T-24 cell line the ability to inhibit cell proliferation and tumour cell proliferation as well as the induction of angiogenesis, purportedly via sub-G1 and G2/M phase reduction.[98]

Nutritional medicine

VITAMIN B₆ – PYRIDOXAL-5-PHOSPHATE (PLP)

PLP is needed to regulate homocysteine. A gene mutation that renders antiquitin inactive can inactivate the metabolic reactions of B_6 (and therefore conversion of B_6 to PLP) and lead to increases in homocysteinaemia.[361] There is an assumed link between high-circulating B_6 and low homocysteine being preventive. Certainly, low homocysteinaemia and high B_6 reflect improved disease outcomes in solid tumour neoplastic bladder cancer patients. B_6/PLP may modulate the adaptive response of tumour cells.[361]

OMEGA-3 FATTY ACIDS

A diet consisting of low omega-3 demonstrated a predictive factor for bladder cancer in Italian subjects. The dietary inflammatory index was studied in $n > 12000$ subjects over a period of 11 years. In cases with histologically confirmed bladder cancer and cancer-free subjects, higher dietary pro-inflammatory foods increased risk and negative outcomes, linking a suggestive reasoning to increase anti-inflammatory dietary omega-3.[362]

SELENIUM

As discussed in the CRC section, selenium is perhaps the most studied chemotherapeutic agent. In doses of 50 micrograms (above the RDI) or more (toxic level 350–700 micrograms), it has been suggested to be both preventive and therapeutic. In vivo, selenium may regulate cell cycles, stimulate apoptosis and inhibit tumour cell migration. Selenium is also suggested to sensitise cancer cells to spontaneous cell death via TNF-related apoptosis-inducing ligand and to increase efficacy of doxorubicin.[112]

QUERCETIN

The natural polyphenol quercetin has demonstrated potential in human cancer cell lines as an anti-cancer treatment. The suggestive mechanism is via induction of apoptosis and inhibition of migratory cell activity through activation of AMPK pathways. Quercetin preserves cellular energy homeostasis and regulates cellular metabolism.[363]

VITAMIN D

Low levels of vitamin D 25-hydroxyvitamin D are associated with increased risk of urothelial bladder cancer, patient risk and morbidity. Higher levels of vitamin D and an effective vitamin D receptor cell correlate with a more promising prognosis. This suggests that vitamin D therapy may be necessary, particularly in patients with ineffective vitamin D receptor cells.[364]

SUPPORT DURING RADIOTHERAPY

Nutritional medicine – dietary

There is a potential role for a dietary strategy to include anti-inflammatory foods such as the Mediterranean diet. Radiotherapy creates an acute inflammatory response cycling the fibrotic process in radical pelvic radiotherapy.[365] Diets high in long-chain fatty acids and total fat are pro-inflammatory, with an associated low bile production. Medium-chain triglycerides such as olive oil do not stimulate pancreatic lipase, which may be a factor in protecting gut mucosa from proteolysis. Additionally, it is implied that a low lactose intake would benefit recovery due to acute lactose intolerance during treatment.[365]

SUPPORT DURING CHEMOTHERAPY

Herbal medicine

GREEN TEA (EGCG)

EGCG is potentially an adjuvant treatment in bladder cancer. However, studies are animal and cell based. EGCG may regulate angiogenesis and arrest growth in selective known bladder tumour cell lines.[366]

Nutritional medicine

OMEGA-3 FATTY ACIDS

DHA presents anti-inflammatory, anti-angiogenic, anti-invasive and anti-metastatic properties via multiple biochemical pathways. Recently, the nutrient has demonstrated the ability to enhance the uptake of anti-cancer drugs while still performing regulation of oxidation and inhibiting cell invasion. Another potential benefit is the action of anti-cachexic properties exerted by DHA in bladder and other cancers.[367]

RESVERATROL

Resveratrol may protect in situ bladder cancer cells and induce apoptosis via Bcl-2 family of pro-apoptotic proteins. Oral bioavailability is poor and therefore large amounts of the nutrient are needed.[90,366]

QUERCETIN

Quercetin may inhibit cell proliferation, reduce inflammation and induce DNA damage in human bladder cancer cells, with possible chemotherapeutic sensitising effects.[90,368]

MELATONIN

A meta-analysis of randomised controlled trials regarding efficacy and safety of adjuvant melatonin therapy in radiotherapy and chemotherapy in solid tumours suggested improvements of remission, side effects and remission, and 1-year survival rates.[177] Many tumours do not respond to chemotherapy treatment. Melatonin influences apoptosis in most tumour cells. It is a considered adjuvant to therapy, possibly via its action on caspase activation and intrinsic apoptotic pathways.[369]

REFERENCES

[1] Miller KD, Siegel RH, Lin CC, et al. Cancer treatment and survivorship statistics, 2016. CA Cancer J Clin 2016;66(4):271–89.

[2] Verdecchia A, De Angelis G, Capocaccia R. Estimation and projections of cancer prevalence from cancer registry data. Stat Med 2002;21:3511–26.

[3] DeSantis CE, Lin CC, Mariotto AB, et al. Cancer treatment and survivorship statistics, 2014. CA Cancer J Clin 2014;64:252–71.

[4] Siegel R, DeSantis C, Virgo K, et al. Cancer treatment and survivorship statistics, 2012. CA Cancer J Clin 2012;62:220–41.

[5] Jatoi I, Proschan MA. Randomized trials of breast-conserving therapy versus mastectomy for primary breast cancer: a pooled analysis of updated results. Am J Clin Oncol 2005;28:289–94.

[6] Litiere S, Werutsky G, Fentiman IS, et al. Breast conserving therapy versus mastectomy for stage I-II breast cancer: 20 year follow-up of the EORTC 10801 phase 3 randomised trial. Lancet Oncol 2012;13:412–19.

[7] McGuire KP, Santillan AA, Kaur P, et al. Are mastectomies on the rise? A 13-year trend analysis of the selection of mastectomy versus breast conservation therapy in 5865 patients. Ann Surg Oncol 2009;16:2682–90.

[8] Kummerow KL, Du L, Penson DF, et al. Nationwide trends in mastectomy for early-stage breast cancer. JAMA Surg 2015;150:9–16.

[9] American College of Surgeons, Commission on Cancer. National Cancer Database, 2013 Data Submission. Chicago, IL: American College of Surgeons; 2015.

[10] Howlader N, Noone AM, Krapcho M, et al. SEER cancer statistics review, 1975–2012. Bethesda, MD: National Cancer Institute; 2015. seer.cancer.gov/csr/1975_2012/. (based on November 2014 SEER data submission).

[11] Vona-Davis L, Rose DP. The influence of socioeconomic disparities on breast cancer tumor biology and prognosis: a review. J Womens Health (Larchmt) 2009;18:883–93.

[12] Siegel RL, Miller KD, Jemal A. Cancer statistics, 2016. CA Cancer J Clin 2016;66:7–30.

[13] Thompson CA, Mauck K, Havyer R, et al. Care of the adult Hodgkin lymphoma survivor. Am J Med 2011;124(12):1106–12.

[14] Armstrong GT, Oeffinger KC, Chen Y, et al. Modifiable risk factors and major cardiac events among adult survivors of childhood cancer. J Clin Oncol 2013;31:3673–80.

[15] Hudson MM, Ness KK, Gurney JG, et al. Clinical ascertainment of health outcomes among adults treated for childhood cancer. JAMA 2013;309:2371–81.

[16] Castellino SM, Ullrich NJ, Whelen MJ, et al. Developing interventions for cancer-related cognitive dysfunction in childhood cancer survivors [serial online]. J Natl Cancer Inst 2014;106(8):dju186.

[17] Barton SE, Najita JS, Ginsburg ES, et al. Infertility, infertility treatment, and achievement of pregnancy in female survivors of childhood cancer: a report from the Childhood Cancer Survivor Study cohort. Lancet Oncol 2013;14(9):873–81.

[18] Gamelin E, Bossi L, Quasthoff S. Clinical aspects and molecular basis of oxaliplatin neurotoxicity: current management and development of preventive measures. Semin Oncol 2002;29:21–33.

[19] Ramsey SD, Berry K, Moinpour C, et al. Quality of life in long term survivors of colorectal cancer. Am J Gastroenterol 2002;97:1228–34.

[20] Emmertsen KJ, Laurberg S, Rectal Cancer Function Study Group. Impact of bowel dysfunction on quality of life after sphincter-preserving resection for rectal cancer. Br J Surg 2013;100:1377–87.

[21] Schover LR, van der Kaaij M, van Dorst E, et al. Sexual dysfunction and infertility as late effects of cancer treatment. EJC Suppl 2014;12:41–53.

[22] Primrose JN, Perera R, Gray A, et al. Effect of 3 to 5 years of scheduled CEA and CT follow-up to detect recurrence of colorectal cancer: the FACS randomized clinical trial. JAMA 2014;311:263–70.

[23] Dohner H, Weisdorf DJ, Bloomfield CD. Acute myeloid leukemia. N Engl J Med 2015;373:1136–52.

[24] Dohner H, Estey EH, Amadori S, et al. Diagnosis and management of acute myeloid leukemia in adults: recommendations from an international expert panel, on behalf of the European LeukemiaNet. Blood 2010;115:453–74.

[25] Pui CH, Robison LL, Look AT. Acute lymphoblastic leukaemia. Lancet 2008;371:1030–43.

[26] Poghosyan H, Sheldon LK, Leveille SG, et al. Health-related quality of life after surgical treatment in patients with non-small cell lung cancer: a systematic review. Lung Cancer 2013;81:11–16.

[27] Chambers SK, Dunn J, Occhipinti S, et al. A systematic review of the impact of stigma and nihilism on lung cancer outcomes [serial online]. BMC Cancer 2012;12:184.

[28] Davies H, Bignell GR, Cox C, et al. Mutations of the BRAF gene in human cancer. Nature 2002;417:949–54.

[29] Hodi FS, O'Day SJ, McDermott DF, et al. Improved survival with ipilimumab in patients with metastatic melanoma. N Engl J Med 2010;363:711–23.

[30] Balamurugan A, Rees JR, Kosary C, et al. Subsequent primary cancers among men and women with in situ and invasive melanoma of the skin. J Am Acad Dermatol 2011;65:S69–77.

[31] Albertsen PC, Hanley JA, Fine J. 20-year outcomes following conservative management of clinically localized prostate cancer. JAMA 2005;293:2095–101.

[32] Ryan CJ, Smith MR, de Bono JS, et al. Abiraterone in metastatic prostate cancer without previous chemotherapy. N Engl J Med 2013;368:13–48.

[33] Birkhahn M, Penson DF, Cai J, et al. Long-term outcome in patients with a Gleason score ≤ 6 prostate cancer treated by radical prostatectomy. BJU Int 2011;108:660–4.

[34] Taylor KL, Luta G, Miller AB, et al. Long-term disease-specific functioning among prostate cancer survivors and noncancer controls in the prostate, lung, colorectal, and ovarian cancer screening trial. J Clin Oncol 2012;30:2768–75.

[35] Alibhai SM, Duong-Hua M, Sutradhar R, et al. Impact of androgen deprivation therapy on cardiovascular disease and diabetes. J Clin Oncol 2009;27:3452–8.

[36] Saylor PJ, Smith MR. Metabolic complications of androgen deprivation therapy for prostate cancer. J Urol 2013;189:S34–42.

[37] Levine GN, D'Amico AV, Berger P, et al. Androgen-deprivation therapy in prostate cancer and cardiovascular risk: a science advisory from the American Heart Association, American Cancer Society, and American Urological Association: endorsed by the American Society for Radiation Oncology. CA Cancer J Clin 2010;60:194–201.

[38] Foster C, Fenlon D. Recovery and self-management support following primary cancer treatment. Br J Cancer 2011;105(Suppl. 1):S21–8.

[39] Jefford M, Karahalios E, Pollard A, et al. Survivorship issues following treatment completion – results from focus groups with Australian cancer survivors and health professionals. J Cancer Surviv 2008;2(1):20–32.

[40] Armes J, Crowe M, Colbourne L, et al. Patients' supportive care needs beyond the end of cancer treatment: a prospective, longitudinal survey. J Clin Oncol 2009;27(36):6172–9.

[41] Ward S, Viergutz G, Tormey D, et al. Patients' reactions to completion of adjuvant breast cancer therapy. Nurs Res 1992;42(6):362–6.

[42] Bury M. Chronic illness as biographical disruption. Sociol Health Illn 1982;4(2):167–82.

[43] Hewitt M, Rowland JH, Yancik R. Cancer survivors in the United States: age, health and disability. J Gerontol A Biol Sci Med Sci 2003;58(1):82–91.

[44] Karnilowicz W. Identity and psychological ownership in chronic illness and disease state. Eur J Cancer Care (Engl) 2011;20(2):276–82.

[45] Foster C, Roffe L, Scott I, et al. Self-management of problems experienced following primary cancer treatment: an exploratory study. London: Macmillan Cancer Support; 2010.

[46] Lent RW. Restoring emotional well-being: a theoretical model. In: Feuerstein M, editor. Handbook of cancer survivorship. New York: Springer; 2007. p. 231–48.

[47] Maher EJ, Makin W. Life after cancer treatment – a spectrum of chronic survivorship conditions. Clin Oncol 2007;19:743–5.

[48] Corner J. Addressing the needs of cancer survivors: issues and challenges. Expert Rev Pharmacoecon Outcomes Res 2008;8(5):443–51.

[49] Singh U, Verma N. Psychopathology among female breast cancer patients. Journal of the Indian Academy of Applied Psychology 2007;33(1):61–71.

[50] Schlatter MC, Cameron LD. Emotional suppression tendencies as predictors of symptoms, mood, and coping appraisals during AC chemotherapy for breast cancer treatment. Ann Behav Med 2010;40(1):15–29.

[51] Monti DA, Kash KM, Kunkel EJ. Psychosocial benefits of a novel mindfulness intervention versus standard support in distressed women with breast cancer. Psychooncology 2013;22(11):2565–75.

[52] Coussens L, Werb Z. Inflammation and cancer. Nature 2002;420:860–7.

[53] Foà C, Copelli P, Cornelli MC. Meeting the needs of cancer patients: identifying patients', relatives' and professionals' representations. Acta Biomed 2014;85(3):41–51.

[54] Byar KL, Berger AM. Impact of adjuvant breast cancer chemotherapy on fatigue, Other symptoms, and quality of life. Oncol Nurs Forum 2006;33(1):21–30.

[55] Carver CS, Scheier MF, Weintraub JK. Assessing coping strategies: a theoretically based approach. J Pers Soc Psychol 1999;56:267–83.

[56] Parry C, Kent E, Mariotto A, et al. Cancer Survivors: a booming population. Cancer Epidemiol Biomarkers Prev 2011;20:1996–8.

[57] Centers for Disease Control and Prevention. National Health Interview Survey. Available from: https://www.cdc.gov/nchs/nhis/nhis_2005_data_release.htm.

[58] Oeffinger KC, Mertens AC, Sklar CA. Chronic health conditions in adult survivors of childhood cancer. N Engl J Med 2006;355(15):1572–82.

[59] Spiegel D, Giese-Davis J. Depression and cancer: mechanisms and disease progression. Biol Psychiatry 2003;54(3):269–82.

[60] Giacobbi PR Jr, Stancil M, Hardin B. Physical activity and quality of life experienced by highly active individuals with physical disabilities. Adapt Phys Activ Q 2008;25(3):189–207.

[61] Roland KB, Rodriguez JL, Patterson JR. A literature review of the social and psychological needs of ovarian cancer survivors. Psychooncology 2013;22(11):2408–18.

[62] Hodges LJ, Humphris GM, Macfarlane G. A meta-analytic investigation of the relationship between the psychological distress of cancer patients and their carers. Soc Sci Med 2005;60(1):1–12.

[63] Badger T, Segrin C, Dorros SM. Depression and anxiety in women with breast cancer and their partners. Nurs Res 2007;56(1):44–53.

[64] Hayman JA, Langa KM, Kabeto MU. Estimating the cost of informal caregiving for elderly patients with cancer. J Clin Oncol 2001;19(13):3219–25.

[65] Levin T, Kissane D. Psychooncology – the state of its development in 2006. Eur J Psychiatry 2006;20.

[66] Watson M, Haviland JS, Greer S. Influence of psychological response on survival in breast cancer: a population-based cohort study. Lancet 1999;354(9187):1331–6.

[67] Rock CL, Doyle C, Demark-Wahnefried W, et al. Nutrition and physical activity guidelines for cancer survivors. CA Cancer J Clin 2012;62:242–74.

[68] Pekmezi DW, Demark-Wahnefried W. Updated evidence in support of diet and exercise interventions in cancer survivors. Acta Oncol 2011;50:167–78.

[69] Chlebowski RT, Aiello E, McTiernan A. Weight loss in breast cancer patient management. J Clin Oncol 2002;20:1128–43.

[70] Schattner M, Shike M. Nutrition support of the patient with cancer. In: Shils ME, Shike M, Ross AC, et al, editors. Modern nutrition in health and disease. 10th ed. Philadelphia, PA: Lippincott Williams & Wilkins; 2006. p. 1290–313.

[71] Fearon K, Strasser F, Anker SD. Definition and classification of cancer cachexia: an international consensus. Lancet Oncol 2011;12:489–95.

[72] Blum D, Omlin A, Baracos VE, et al; European Palliative Care Research Collaborative. Cancer cachexia: a systematic literature review of items and domains associated with involuntary weight loss in cancer. Crit Rev Oncol Hematol 2011;80:114–44.

[73] Itsiopoulos C, Hodge A, Kaimakamis M. Collaborative Group on Hormonal Factors in Breast Cancer: breast cancer and hormone replacement therapy: collaborative reanalysis of data from 51 epidemiological studies of 52,705 women with breast cancer and 108,411 women without breast cancer. Mol Nutr Food Res 2009;53:227–39.

[74] Gonzalez CA. The European prospective investigation into cancer and nutrition (EPIC). Public Health Nutr 2006;9(1A):124–6.

[75] Ullah MF, Khan MW. Food as medicine: potential therapeutic tendencies of plant derived polyphenolic compounds. Asian Pac J Cancer Prev 2008;9:187–95.

[76] Todaro A, Palmeri R, Barbagallo RN, et al. Increase of trans-resveratrol in typical Sicilian wine using β-glucosidase from various sources. Food Chem 2008;4:1570–5.

[77] Lagouge M, Argmann C, Gerhart-Hines Z, et al. Resveratrol improves mitochondrial function and protects against metabolic disease by activating SIRT1 and PGC-1α. Cell 2006;6:1–14.

[78] Le Corre L, Fustier P, Chalabi N, et al. Effects of resveratrol on the expression of a panel of genes interacting with the BRCA1 oncosuppressor in human breast cell lines. Clin Chim Acta 2004;344:115–21.

[79] Adams LS, Zhang Y, Seeram NP, et al. Pomegranate ellagitannin-derived compounds exhibit antiproliferative and antiaromatase activity in breast cancer cell in vitro. Cancer Prev Res (Phila) 2010;3:108–13.

[80] Divisi D, Di Tommaso S, Salvemini S, et al. Diet and cancer. Acta Biomed 2006;77:118–23.

[81] Cardenas E, Ghosh R. Vitamin E: a dark horse at the crossroad of cancer management. Biochem Pharmacol 2013;86(7):845–52. doi:10.1016/j.bcp.2013.07.018.

[82] Jiang Q. Natural forms of vitamin E as effective agents for cancer prevention and therapy. Adv Nutr 2017;8(6):850–67. doi:10.3945/an.117.016329.

[83] Toledo E, Salas-Salvadó J, Donat-Vargas C, et al. Mediterranean diet and invasive breast cancer risk among women at high cardiovascular risk in the PREDIMED trial: a randomized clinical trial. JAMA Intern Med 2015;175:1752–60.

[84] Kaefer CM, Milner JA. The role of herbs and Spice in cancer prevention. J Nutr Biochem 2008;19:347–61.

[85] Bauer J, Jurgens H, Fruhwald MC. Important aspects of nutrition in children with cancer. Adv Nutr 2011;2(2):67–77.

[86] Chan JM, Gann PH, Giovannucci EL. Role of diet in prostate cancer development and progression. J Clin Oncol 2005;23:8152–60.

[87] Jones LW, Demark-Wahnefried W. Diet, physical activity, and complementary therapies after primary treatment for cancer. Lancet Oncol 2006;7:1017–26.

[88] Bekkering T, Beynon R, Davey Smith G, et al. A systematic review of RCTs investigating the effect of dietal and physical activity interventions on cancer survival, updated report World Cancer Research Fund; 2006. Available from: http://www.dietandcancerreport.org/.

[89] Schmitz KH, Courneya KS, Matthews C, et al. American College of Sports Medicine roundtable on exercise guidelines for cancer survivors. Med Sci Sports Exerc 2010;42(7):1409–26. Erratum in: Med Sci Sports Exerc 2011;43(1):195.

[90] Osiecki H. Cancer: the importance of clinical nutrition in prevention and treatment. Eagle Farm, Qld: Bioconcepts Publishing; 2012.

[91] Alschuler LN, Gazella KA. The definitive guide to cancer: an integrative approach to prevention, treatment and healing. 3rd ed. Berkeley: Celestial Arts; 2012.

[92] Braun L, Cohen M. Herbs and natural supplements: an evidence-based guide. Chatswood, NSW: Elsevier Health Services; 2010.

[93] Badreldin HA. Amelioration of oxaliplatin neurotoxicity by drugs in humans and experimental animals: a minireview of recent literature. Basic Clin Pharmacol Toxicol 2009;106(4):272–9.

[94] Morad V, Abrahamsson A, Kjölhede P, et al. Adipokines and vascular endothelial growth factor in normal human breast tissue in vivo – correlations and attenuation by dietary flaxseed. J Mammary Gland Biol Neoplasia 2016;21(1):69–76.

[95] World Cancer Research Fund International Cancer prevention recommendations; 2016. Available from: http://www.wcrf.org/int/research-we-fund/our-cancer-prevention-recommendations.

[96] Davis C, Bryan J, Hodgeson J, et al. Definition of the Mediterranean diet: a literature review. Nutrients 2015;7(11):9139–53.

[97] Lall RK, Adhami VM, Mukhtar H. Dietary flavonoid fisetin for cancer prevention and treatment. Nutr Cancer 2016;60(6):1396–405.

[98] Shi MD, Shiao CK, Lee YC, et al. Apigenin, a dietary flavonoid, inhibits proliferation of human bladder cancer T-24 cells via

blocking cell cycle progression and inducing apoptosis. Cancer Cell Int 2015;15:33.

[99]   Sayles C, Hickerson SC, Bhat RR, et al. Oral glutamine in preventing treatment-related mucositis in adult patients with cancer: a systematic review. Nutr Clin Pract 2016;31(2):171–9.

[100]   Jung S, Spiegelman D, Baglietto L, et al. Fruit and vegetable intake and risk of breast cancer by hormone receptor status. J Natl Cancer Inst 2013;105(3):219–36.

[101]   Yuen CFR, Chong SLG, Lim KM. Effects of high doses of vitamin C on cancer patients in Singapore: nine cases. Integr Cancer Ther 2016;15(2):197–204.

[102]   Clinton SK. Tomatoes, lycopene, and prostate cancer. Cancer Prev Res (Phila) 2014;8(10).

[103]   Graff RE, Pettersson A, Lis RT, et al. Dietary lycopene intake and risk of prostate cancer defined by ERG protein expression. Am J Clin Nutr 2016;103(3):851–60.

[104]   deWaure C, Quaranta G, Guilano MR, et al. Systematic review of studies investigating the association between dietary habits and cutaneous malignant melanoma. Public Health 2015;129(8): 1099–113.

[105]   Skotarczak K, Osmola-Mankowsa A, Lodyga M, et al. Photoprotection: facts and controversies. Eur Rev Med Phamacol Sci 2015;19:98–112.

[106]   Erdmann F, Lortet-Tieulent J, Schuz J, et al. International trends in the incidence of malignant melanoma 1953–2008 – are recent generations at higher or lower risk? Int J Cancer 2013;132: 385–400.

[107]   Mansara P, Kerkar M, Deshpande R, et al. Improved antioxidant status by omega-3 fatty acid supplementation in breast cancer patients undergoing chemotherapy: a case series. J Med Case Rep 2015;9:148.

[108]   Morland SL, Martins KJB, Masurak VC. n-3 polyunsaturated fatty acid supplementation during cancer chemotherapy. J Nutr Intermed Metab 2016;5:107–16.

[109]   Persson C, Glimelius B, Ronnelid J, et al. Impact of fish oil and melatonin on cachexia in patients with advanced gastrointestinal cancer: a randomized pilot study. Nutrition 2005;21(2):170–8.

[110]   Vaid M, Singh T, Prasad R, et al. Bioactive proanthocyanidins inhibit growth and induce apoptosis in human melanoma cells by decreasing the accumulation of β-catenin. Int J Oncol 2015; 48(2):624–34.

[111]   Merlino G, Herlyn M, Risher DE, et al. The state of melanoma: challenges and opportunities. Pigment Cell Melanoma Res 2016;29(4):404–16.

[112]   Sanmartin C, Plano D, Sharma AK, et al. Selenium compounds, apoptosis and other types of cell death: an overview for cancer therapy. Int J Mol Sci 2012;13(8):9649–72.

[113]   PDQ Integrative, Alternative, and Complementary Therapies Editorial Board. Cartilage (bovine and shark) (PDQ®): health professional version 2018. In: PDQ cancer information summaries. Bethesda (MD): National Cancer Institute (US); 2018. [Internet].

[114]   Augustin LS, Libra M, Crispo A, et al. Low glycemic index diet, exercise and vitamin D to reduce breast cancer recurrence: rationale for the design of a clinical trial. FASEB J 2016; 30(1(Suppl. 1168)):2.

[115]   Mohr SB, Gorham ED, Kim J, et al. Meta-analysis of vitamin D sufficiency for improving survival of patients with breast cancer. Anticancer Res 2014;34:31163–6.

[116]   Elgezawy E, Elgizawy S, Zaineldeen M, et al. Overview of angiogenesis in Upper Egypt non-Hodgkins lymphoma patients. Quality in Primary Care 2016;24(3):125–32.

[117]   Costello LC, Franklin RB, Zou J, et al. Evidence that human prostate cancer is a ZIP1-deficient malignancy that could be effectively treat with a zinc ionophore (clioquinol) approach. Chemotherapy 2015;4(2):152.

[118]   Franklin RB, Costello LC. Zinc as an anti-tumour agent in prostate cancer and in other cancers. Arch Biochem Biophys 2007;463(2):211–17.

[119]   Bhagat N, Chaturvedi A. Spices as an alternative therapy for cancer treatment. Systematic Reviews in Pharmacy 2016;7(1):46–56.

[120]   Leggett S, Koczwara B, Miller M. The impact of complementary and alternative medicines on cancer symptoms, treatment side effects, quality of life, and survival in women with breast cancer – a systematic review. Nutr Cancer 2014;67(3):373–91.

[121]   Fujiki H, Sueoka E, Watanabe T, et al. Primary cancer prevention by green tea, and tertiary cancer prevention by the combination of green tea catechins and anticancer compounds. J Cancer Prev 2015;20(1):1–4.

[122]   Xiao X, Liu Z, Wang R, et al. Genistein suppresses FLT4 and inhibits human colorectal cancer metastasis. Oncotarget 2014;6(5):3225–39.

[123]   Pavese JM, Farmer RL, Bergan RC. Inhibition of cancer cell invasion and metastisis by genistein. Cancer Metastasis Rev 2010;29(3):465–82.

[124]   Rigalli JP, Tocchetti GN, Arana MR, et al. The phytoestrogen genistein enhances multidrug resistance in breast cancer cell lines by translational regulation of ABC transporters. Cancer Lett 2016;376(1):165–72.

[125]   Shi H, Wu Y, Wang Y, et al. Liquiritigenin potentiates the inhibitory effects of cisplatin on invasion and metastasis via downregulation MMP-2/9 and PI3 K/AKT signaling pathway in B16F10 melanoma cells and mice model. Nutr Cancer 2015;67(5):761–70.

[126]   Lucumberri E, Dupertuis YM, Miralbell R, et al. Green tea polyphenol epigallocatechin-3-gallate (EGCG) as adjuvant in cancer therapy. Clin Nutr 2013;32(6):894–903.

[127]   Irving GRB. A novel approach to enhancing the effectiveness of chemotherapy: combining curcumin with FOLFOX chemotherapy for metastatic colorectal cancer. Leicester: University of Leicester, College of Medicine; 2014. Available from: https://lra.le.ac.uk/ handle/2381/35981.

[128]   Saxena R, Rida PCG, Kucuk O, et al. Ginger augmented chemotherapy: a novel multitarget nontoxic approach for cancer management. Mol Nutr Food Res 2016;60(6):1364–73.

[129]   Patel S, Goyal A. Recent developments in mushrooms as anti-cancer therapeutics: a review. 3 Biotech 2012;2(1):1–15.

[130]   Mazzio EA, Soliman KFA. In vitro screening for the tumoricidal properties of international medicinal herbs. Phytother Res 2009;23(3):385–98.

[131]   Block G, Patterson B, Subar A. Fruits, vegetables, and cancer prevention: a review of epidemiological evidence. Nutr Cancer 1992;18:1–29.

[132]   Milner JA. 2007 Strategies for cancer prevention: the role of diet. Br J Nutr 2007;87(S2):S265–72.

[133]   Fisher B, Costantino JP, Wickerham DL, et al. Tamoxifen for prevention of breast cancer: report of the national surgical adjuvant breast and bowel project P-1 study. J Natl Cancer Inst 1998;90:1371–88.

[134]   Dragnev KH, Rigas JR, Dmitrovsky E. The retinoids and cancer prevention mechanisms. Oncologist 2000;5(5):361–8.

[135]   Lamson DW, Brignall MS. Natural agents in the prevention of cancer, part two: preclinical data and chemoprevention for common cancers. Altern Med Rev 2001;6(2):167–87.

[136]   Gadd GM. New horizons in geomycology. Environ Microbiol Rep 2017;9(1):4–7.

[137]   Brown J, Byers T, Doyle C. Nutrition and physical activity during and after cancer treatment: an American Cancer Society guide for informed choices. CA Cancer J Clin 2003;53(5):268–91.

[138]   Irwin ML, Yasui Y, Ulrich C. Effect of exercise on total and intra-abdominal body fat in postmenopausal women: a randomized controlled trial. JAMA 2003;289(3):323–30.

[139]   Rock CL, Demark-Wahnefried W. Can lifestyle modification increase survival in women diagnosed with breast cancer? J Nutr 2002;132(Suppl. 11):3504S–7S.

[140]   Haydon AM, Macinnis RJ, English DR, et al. Effect of physical activity and body size on survival after diagnosis with colorectal cancer. Gut 2006;55(1):62–7.

[141]   Courneya KS, Booth CM, Gill S. The colon health and life-long exercise change trial: a randomized trial of the national cancer institute of Canada clinical trials group. Curr Oncol 2008;15(6):279–85.

[142]   Irwin ML. Physical activity interventions for cancer survivors. Br J Sports Med 2009;43:32–8.

[143]   Winningham ML. Effects of a bicycle ergometry program on functional capacity and feelings of control of patients with breast cancer [dissertation]. Columbus, OH: Ohio State University; 1983.

[144]   Winningham ML, MacVicar MG, Bondoc M, et al. Effect of aerobic exercise on body weight and composition in patients with breast

cancer on adjuvant chemotherapy. Oncol Nurs Forum 1989;16: 683–9.

[145] Dimeo F, Bertz H, Finke J, et al. An aerobic exercise program for patients with haematological malignancies after bone marrow transplantation. Bone Marrow Transplant 1996;18:1157–60.

[146] Dimeo F, Tilmann MH, Bertz H, et al. Aerobic exercise in the rehabilitation of cancer patients after high dose chemotherapy and autologous peripheral stem cell transplantation. Cancer 1997;79:1717–22.

[147] Clyne N, Ekholm J, Jogestrand T, et al. Effects of exercise training in predialytic uremic patients. Nephron 1991;59:84–9.

[148] Wu X, Daniels G, Lee P, et al. Lipid metabolism in prostate cancer. Am J Clin Exp Urol 2014;2(2):111–20.

[149] Nelson WG, De Marzo AM, Isaacs WB. Prostate cancer. N Engl J Med 2003;349:366–81.

[150] Coussens LM, Werb Z. Inflammation and cancer. Nature 2002;420: 860–7.

[151] Udensi KU, Tchounwou PB. Oxidative stress in prostate hyperplasia and carcinogenesis. J Exp Clin Cancer Res 2016;35:139.

[152] Moore SC, Lee MI, Weiderpass E, et al. Association of leisure-time physical activity with risk of 26 types of cancer in 1.44 million adults. JAMA Intern Med 2016;176(6):816–25. doi:10.1001/jamainternmed.2016.1548.

[153] Cormie P, Galvao DA, Spry N, et al. Can supervised exercise prevent treatment toxicity in patients with prostate cancer initiating androgen deprivation therapy: a randomized controlled trial. Urological Oncology 2014;115(2):256–66.

[154] Petiwala SM, Puthenveetil AG, Johnson JJ. Polyphenols from the Mediterranean herb rosemary (Rosmariunus officinalis) for prostate cancer. Front Pharmacol 2013;4:29.

[155] Petiwala SM, Berhe S, Li G, et al. Rosemary (Rosmarinus officinalis) extract modulates CHOP/GADD153 to promote androgen receptor degradation and decreases xenograft tumour growth. PLoS ONE 2014;9(3):e89772.

[156] Deb G, Thakur VS, Shankar E, et al. Abstract 2609: epigenetic reactivation of TIMP-3 in human prostate cancer cells by green tea polyphenols. Cancer Res 2016;76(14):2609.

[157] Mohammadi A, Mansoori B, Aghapour M, et al. Urtica dioica dichloromethane extract induce apoptosis from intrinsic pathway on human prostate cancer cells (PCa3). Cell Mol Biol (Noisy-le-grand) 2016;62(3):78–83.

[158] Hessenkemper W, Roediger J, Bartsch S, et al. A natural androgen receptor antagonist induces cellular senescence in prostate cancer cells. Mol Endocrinol 2014;28(11):1831–40.

[159] Zhou DY, Ding N, Du ZY, et al. Curcumin analogues with high activity for inhibiting human prostate cancer cell growth and androgen receptor activation. Mol Med Rep 2014;10(3):1315–22.

[160] Ottenweller J, Putt K, Blumentahl EJ, et al. Inhibition of prostate cancer-cell proliferation by Essiac®. The Journal of Alternative and Complementary Medicine 2004;10(4):687–91.

[161] Ma IV, Mouradian M, Sorreta AG, et al. Abstract 906: decreasing omega-6 to omega-3 polyunsaturated fatty acid dietary ratios inhibit tumorigenesis in prostate cancer cells in vitro and in vivo. Prevention Research 2015;75(Suppl. 15).

[162] Shivappa N, Bosetti C, Zucchetto A, et al. Association between dietary inflammatory index and prostate cancer among Italian men. Br J Nutr 2015;113(2):278–83.

[163] Graffouillere L, Deschasaux M, Mariotti F, et al. The dietary inflammatory index is associated with prostate cancer risk in French middle aged adults in a prospective study. J Nutr 2016;146(4):785–91.

[164] Costello LC, Franklin RB, Zou J, et al. Evidence that human prostate cancer is a ZIP1-deficient malignancy that could be effectively treat with a zinc ionophore (clioquinol) approach. Chemotherapy 2015;4(2):152.

[165] Franklin RB, Costello LC. Zinc as an anti-tumour agent in prostate cancer and in other cancers. Arch Biochem Biophys 2007;463(2):211–17.

[166] Alexander W. Prostate cancer risk and omega-3 fatty acid intake from fish oil. P T 2013;38(9):561–4.

[167] Pei Z, Li H, Guo Y, et al. Sodium selenite inhibits the expression of VEGF, TGFβ1 and IL-6 induced by LPS in human PC3 cells via TLR4-NF-κB signaling blockage. Int Immunopharmacol 2010;10(1):50–6.

[168] Yang F, Song L, Wang H, et al. Quercetin in prostate cancer: chemotherapeutic and chemopreventive effects, mechanisms and clinical application potential (review). Oncol Rep 2015;33(6):2659–68.

[169] Asea A, Ara G, Teicher BA, et al. Effects of the flavonoid drug quercetin on the response of human prostate tumors to hyperthermia in vitro and in vivo. Int J Hyperthermia 2001;17:347–56.

[170] Sharmila G, Bhat FA, Arunkumar R, et al. Chemopreventive effect of quercetin, a natural dietary flavonol on prostate cancer in in vivo model. Clin Nutr 2014;33:718–26.

[171] Mahmoud AM, Yang W, Bosland MC. Soy isoflavones and prostate cancer: a review of molecular mechanisms. J Steroid Biochem Mol Biol 2014;140:116–32.

[172] van Die MD, Bone KM, Williams SG, et al. Soy and soy isoflavones in prostate cancer: a systematic review and meta-analysis of randomized controlled trials. BJU Int 2014;113(5b):E119–30.

[173] Shui IM, Mondul AM, Lindstrom S, et al. Circulating vitamin D, vitamin D-related genetic variation, and risk of fatal prostate cancer in the National Cancer Institute Breast and Prostate Cancer Cohort Consortium. Cancer 2015;121(12):1949–56.

[174] Areti A, Yerra VG, Naidu VGM, et al. Oxidative stress and nerve damage: role in chemotherapy induced peripheral neuropathy. Redox Biol 2014;2:289–95.

[175] Wyatt GK, Sikorskii A, Safikhani A, et al. Saw palmetto for symptom management during radiation therapy for prostate cancer. J Pain Symptom Manage 2016;51(6):1046–54.

[176] Datta M, Taylor ML, Firzzell B. Dietary serum lycopene levels in prostate cancer patients undergoing intensity-modulated radiation therapy. J Med Food 2013;16(12):1131–7. [Abstract].

[177] Wang YM, Jun BZ, Ai F, et al. The efficacy and safety of melatonin in concurrent chemotherapy or radiotherapy for solid tumors: a meta-analysis of randomized controlled trials. Cancer Chemother Pharmacol 2012;69(5):1213–20.

[178] Wang P, Henning SM, Heber D, et al. Sensitization to docetaxel in prostate cancer cells by green tea and quercetin. J Nutr Biochem 2015;26(4):408–15.

[179] Lakshmanan VK. Therapeutic efficacy of nanomedicines for prostate cancer: an update. Investig Clin Urol 2016;57(1): 21–9.

[180] World Cancer Research Fund. Continuous update project: colorectal cancer; 2011. Available from: http://wcrf.org/int/research-we-fund/continuous-update-project-findings-reports/colorectal-bowel-cancer.

[181] Perera PS, Thompson RL, Wiseman MJ. Recent evidence for colorectal cancer prevention through healthy food, nutrition, and physical activity: implications for recommendations. Curr Nutr Rep 2012;1(1):44–54.

[182] Chiavarini M, Minellie L, Faiani R. Garlic consumption and colorectal cancer risk in man: a systematic review and meta-analysis. Public Health Nutr 2015;19(2):308–17.

[183] Zhang X, Keum NN, Wu K, et al. Calcium intake and colorectal cancer risk: results from the nurses' health study and health professionals follow-up study. Int J Cancer 2016;139(10):2232–42.

[184] Larsson SC, Wolk A. Meat consumption and risk of colorectal cancer: a meta-analysis of prospective studies. Int J Cancer 2006;119(11):2657–64.

[185] Alexander DD, Miller AJ, Cushing CA, et al. Processed meat and colorectal cancer: a quantitative review of prospective epidemiologic studies. Eur J Cancer Prev 2010;19(5):328–41.

[186] Ward HA, Norat T, Overvad K, et al. Pre-diagnostic meat and fibre intakes in relation to colorectal cancer survival in European prospective investigation into cancer and nutrition. Br J Nutr 2016;116(2):316–25.

[187] Du JG, Zhang Z, Wen XD, et al. Epigallocatechin gallate (EGCG) is the most effective cancer chemopreventive polyphenol in green tea. Nutrients 2012;4(11):1679–91.

[188] Durak Z, Em Buber SM, Devrim E, et al. Aqueous extract from turmeric (Curcuma longa) inhibits adenosine deaminase activity significantly in cancerous and non-cancerous human gastric and colon tissues. Food and Nutrition Report 2015;1(1):24–6.

[189] Aggarwal A, Prinz-Wohlgenannt M, Tennakoon S, et al. The calcium-sensing receptor: a promising target for the prevention of colorectal cancer. Biochim Biophys Acta 2015;1853(9):2158–67.

[190] Kim GT, Lee SE, Kim YM. Quercetin regulates sestrin 2-AMPK-mTOR signaling pathway and induces apoptosis via increased intracellular ROS in HCT116 colon cancer cells. J Cancer Prev 2013;18(3):264–70.

[191] Follo-Martinez AD, Banerjee N, Li X, et al. Resveratrol and quercetin in combination have anticancer activity in colon cancer cells and repress oncogenic microRNA-27a. Nutr Cancer 2012;65(3):494–504.

[192] Mezawa H, Sugiura T, Watanabe M, et al. Serum vitamin D levels and survival of patients with colorectal cancer: post-hoc analysis of a prospective cohort study. BMC Cancer 2010;10:347.

[193] Gandini S, Boniol M, Haukka J, et al. Meta-analysis of observational studies of serum 25-hydroxyvitamin D levels and colorectal, breast and prostate cancer and colorectal adenoma. Int J Cancer 2011;128:1414–24.

[194] Park W, Ruhul Amin ARM, Chen ZG, et al. New perspectives of curcumin in cancer prevention. Cancer Prev Res (Phila) 2013;6(5):387–400.

[195] Tran HMT, Oscar A, Carmago T, et al. Sa1953 elipallocatechinb-3-gallate (EGCG) targets cancer stem-like cells and enhances 5-flouracil chemosensitivity in chemoresistant colorectal cancer. Gastroenterology 2015;148(4(Suppl. 1)):S365–6.

[196] Toden S, Tran HM, Tovar-Camargo OA, et al. Epigallocatechin-3-gallate targets cancer stem-like cells and enhances 5-fluorouracil chemosensitivity in colorectal cancer. Oncotarget 2016;7(13):16158–71.

[197] Zhou E, You T, Wang WM, et al. Curcumin combined FOLFOX induced cell apoptosis of gastric cancer and its mechanism research. Europe PMC 2013;33(6):810–13. [Abstract].

[198] Yun J, Mullarky E, Lu C, et al. Vitamin C selectively kills KRAS and BRAF mutant colorectal cancer cells by targeting GAPDH. Science 2015;350(6266):1391–6.

[199] Srinivasan V, Gobbi G, Shillcutt SD, et al; Taylor & Francis Group. Melatonin: therapeutic value and neuroprotection. Boca Raton: CRC Press; 2015.

[200] World Cancer Research Fund International/American Institute for Cancer Research. Continuous Update Project Report: diet, nutrition, physical activity, and breast cancer survivors; 2014. Available from: www.wcrf.org/sites/default/files/Breast-Cancer-Survivors-2014-Report.pdf.

[201] Bahrom S, Idris NRN. Soy intake and breast cancer risk: a meta-analysis of epidemiological studies. AIP Conf Proc 2016;1739(2016):020075. http://dx.doi.org/10.1063/1.4952555.

[202] Pantavos A, Ruiter R, Feskens EF, et al. Total dietary antioxidant capacity, individual antioxidant intake and breast cancer risk: the Rotterdam Study. Int J Cancer 2015;136(9):2178–86.

[203] Wang S, Tang L, Feiyu C. Astragaloside III from Astragalus membranaceus antagonizes breast cancer growth. Afr J Tradit Complement Altern Med 2015;12(3):183–6.

[204] Zhu J, Zhang H, Zhu Z, et al. Effects and mechanism of flavonoids from Astragalus complanatus on breast cancer growth. Naunyn Schmiedebergs Arch Pharmacol 2015;388(9):965–72.

[205] Palliyaguru D, Singh SV, Kensler TW. Withania somnifera: from prevention to treatment of cancer. Mol Nutr Food Res 2016;60(6):1342–53.

[206] Khan MA, Ahmad R, Trivedi A, et al. Determination of combined effect of pH and Withania somnifera on human breast cancer cell line MDA MB-231. Austin J Cancer Clin Res 2015;2(6):1–5.

[207] Dar NJ, Hamid A, Ahmad M. Pharmacologic overview of Withania somnifera, the Indian Ginseng. Cell Mol Life Sci 2015;72:4445.

[208] LeMay-Nedjelski L, Mason J, Taibi A, et al. Omega-3 polyunsaturated fatty acids (n-3 PUFAs) decrease growth and microRNA-21 expression of estrogen receptor-positive (ER+) MCF-7 breast cancer cells. FASEB J 2016;29(Suppl. 1).

[209] Amadi EN, Njoku OO, Ufele NA. Iodine deficiency and its proliferation in cancer increase. American Journal of Life Science Researches 2016;4(2):46–9.

[210] Stoddard FR, Brooks AD, Eskin BA, et al. Iodine alters gene expression in the MCF7 breast cancer cell line: evidence for an anti-estrogen effect of iodine. Int J Med Sci 2008;5(4):189–96.

[211] Soriano O, Delgado G, Anguiano B, et al. Antineoplastic effect of iodine and iodide in dimethylbenz[a]anthracene-induced mammary tumors: association between lactoperoxidase and estrogen-adduct production. Endocr Relat Cancer 2011;18:529–39.

[212] Wang Y, Yu J, Cui R, et al. Curcumin in treating breast cancer: a review. J Lab Autom 2016;21(6):723–31.

[213] Sun XD, Liu XE, Huang DS. Curcumin induces apoptosis of triple-negative breast cancer cells by inhibition of EGFR expression. Mol Med Rep 2012;6(6):1267–70.

[214] Suhail N, Bilal N, Khan HY, et al. Effect of vitamins C and E on antioxidant status of breast-cancer patients undergoing chemotherapy. J Clin Pharm Ther 2012;37(1):22–6.

[215] Mao L, Summers W, Xiang S, et al. Melatonin represses metastasis in HER2-positive human breast cancer cells by suppressing RSK2 expression. Mol Cancer Res 2016;14(11):1159–69.

[216] Alonso- Gonzalez C, Gonsalez A, Martinez-Campa C, et al. Melatonin enhancement of the radiosensitivity of human breast cancer cells is associated with the modulation of proteins involved in estrogen biosynthesis. Cancer Lett 2016;370(1):145–52.

[217] Li Y, Han N, Chen Z, et al. Systematic review and meta-analysis of shenqi furzheng and chemotherapy combination in the treatment of breast cancer. Bangladesh J Pharmacol 2016;11:793–801. Available from: http://www.banglajol.info/index.php/BJP/article/view/27200/19858.

[218] Sinha D, Sarkar N, Biswas J, et al. Resveratrol for breast cancer prevention and therapy: preclinical evidence and molecular mechanisms. Semin Cancer Biol 2016;40(41):209–32.

[219] Greenlee H, Shaw J, Lau YKI, et al. Lack of effect of coenzyme Q10 on doxorubicin cytotoxicity in breast cancer cell cultures. Integr Cancer Ther 2012;11(3):242–50.

[220] Iwase S, Kawaguchi R, Yotsumoto D, et al. Efficacy and safety of an amino acid jelly containing coenzyme Q10 and l-carnitine in controlling fatigue in breast cancer patients receiving chemotherapy: a multi-institutional, randomized, exploratory trial (JORTC-CAM01). Support Care Cancer 2016;24(2):637–46.

[221] Nechuta S, Lu W, Chen Z, et al. Vitamin supplement use during breast cancer treatment and survival: a prospective cohort study. Cancer Epidemiol Biomarkers Prev 2011;20(2):262–71.

[222] Smith AJ, Oertle J, Warren D, et al. Quercetin: a promising flavonoid with a dynamic ability to treat various diseases, infections, and cancers. Journal of Cancer Therapy 2016;7:83–95.

[223] Oh SJ, Kim O, Lee JS, et al. Inhibition of angiogenesis by quercetin in tamoxifen-resistant breast cancer cells. Food Chem Toxicol 2010;48:3227–34.

[224] Du G, Lin H, Yang Y, et al. Dietary quercetin combining intratumoural doxorubicin injection synergistically induces rejection of established breast cancer in mice. Int Immunopharmacol 2010;10819–26.

[225] Innacone MR, Youlden DR, Baade PD, et al. Melanoma incidence trends and survival in adolescents and young adults in Queensland, Australia. Int J Cancer 2015;136(3):603–9.

[226] Kai H, Maeda A, Nagatomo A, et al. Ursolic acid and 12-O-methylcarnosic acid from the leaves of Rosmarinus officinalis L. suppressed melanin production with downregulation of tyrosinase expression in HMV-II melanoma cells. Planta Med 2015;81.

[227] Mori H, Xu Q, Sakamoto O, et al. Mechanisms of antitumor activity of aqueous extracts from Chinese herbs: their immunopharmacological properties. Jpn J Pharmacol 1989;49:423–31.

[228] Prasad R, Katiyar SK. Polyphenols from green tea inhibit the growth of melanoma cells through inhibition of class I histone deacetylases and induction of DNA damage. Genes Cancer 2015;6(1–2):49–61.

[229] Zhao G, Han X, Zheng S, et al. Curcumin induces autophagy, inhibits proliferation and invasion by downregulating AKT/mTOR signaling pathway in human melanoma cells. Oncol Rep 2015;35(2):1065–74.

[230] Teas J, Irhimeh MR. Melanoma and brown seaweed: an integrative hypothesis. J Appl Psychol 2016;29(2):941–8.

[231] Wang M, Yu T, Zhu C, et al. Resveratrol triggers protective autophagy through the ceramide/Akt?mTOR pathway in melanoma B16 cells. Nutr Cancer 2014;66(3):435–40. Available from: https://www.tandfonline.com/doi/abs/10.1080/01635581.2013.878738#.

[232] Serini S, Zinzi A, Vasconcelos RO, et al. Role of β-catenin signaling in the anti-invasive effect of the omega-3 fatty acid DHA in human

melanoma cells. J Dermatol Sci 2016;84(2):149–59. Available from: http://www.sciencedirect.com/science/article/pii/S092318111630127X. [Abstract].

[233] Nakashima S, Oda Y, Nakamura S, et al. Inhibitors of melanogenesis in B16 melanoma 4A5 cells from flower buds of Lawsonia inermis (Henna). Bioorg Med Chem Lett 2015;25(13):2702–6.

[234] Fang Y, Bradley MJ, Cook KM, et al. A potential role for resveratrol as a radiation sensitizer for melanoma treatment. J Surg Res 2013;183(2):645–53.

[235] Soni A, Monica V, Vivek K, et al. Coenzyme Q10 therapy in current clinical practice. Int J Mol Sci 2015;3(4):817–25.

[236] Slominski AT, Carlson JA. Melanoma resistance: a bright future for academicians and a challenge for patient advocates. Mayo Clin Proc 2014;89(4):429–33.

[237] Mudge D, Kieran MW, Bielenberg D, et al. Abstract 1170: Maresin 1: a potent endogenous anti-inflammatory and pro-resolving inhibitor of primary tumor growth and metastasis. Cancer Res 2014;74(19). Available from: http://cancerres.aacrjournals.org/content/74/19_Supplement/1170.short.

[238] Patel S. Fermented wheat germ extract: a dietary supplement with anticancer efficacy. Nutritional Therapy and Metabolism 2014;32(2):61–7.

[239] Challem J. Fermented wheat germ extract – an adjunct treatment for cancer? Current Controversies in Nutrition. Alternative and Complementary Therapies 2012;18(4):199–201. doi:10.1089/act.2012.18401.

[240] Vieira AR, Abar L, Vingeliene S, et al. Fruit, vegetables and lung cancer risk: a systematic review and meta-analysis. Ann Oncol 2016;27(1):81–96. doi:10.1093/annonc/mdv381.

[241] Giacosa A, Bareale R, Bavaresco L, et al. Cancer prevention in Europe: the Mediterranean diet as a protective choice. Eur J Cancer Prev 2013;22:90–5.

[242] de Bittencourt Pasquali MA, Gelain DP, Zeidan-Chulia F, et al. Vitamin A (retinol) downregulates the receptor for advanced glycation endproducts (RAGE) by oxidant-dependent activation of p38 MAPK and NF-kB in human lung cancer A549 cells. Cell Signal 2013;25(4):939–54.

[243] Gnagnarella P, Maisonneuve P, Bellomi M, et al. Nutrient intake and nutrient patterns and risk of lung cancer among heavy smokers: results from the COSMOS screening study with annual low-dose CT. Eur J Epidemiol 2013;28(6):503–11.

[244] Nakachi K, Matsuyama S, Miyake S, et al. Preventive effects of drinking green tea on cancer and cardiovascular disease: epidemiological evidence for multiple targeting prevention. Biofactors 2000;13:49–54. doi:10.1002/biof.5520130109.

[245] Li SG, Chen HY, Ou-Yang CS, et al. The efficacy of Chinese herbal medicine as an adjunctive therapy for advanced non-small cell lung cancer: a systematic review and meta-analysis. PLoS ONE 2013;8(2):e57604.

[246] Dugoua JJ, Wu P, Seely D, et al. Astragalus-containing Chinese herbal combinations for advanced non-small-cell lung cancer: a meta-analysis of 65 clinical trials enrolling 4751 patients. Lung Cancer 2010;1:85–100. doi:10.2147/lctt.s7780.

[247] Fujiki H, Imai K, Nakachi K, et al. Innovative strategy of cancer treatment with the combination of green tea catechins and anticancer compounds. Cancer Cell Microenviron 2015;2(4):e886. Available from: http://smartscitech.com/index.php/CCM/article/view/886/pdf_114. Review.

[248] Aggarwal BB, Yuan W, Li S, et al. Curcumin-free turmeric exhibits anti-inflammatory and anticancer activities: identification of novel components of turmeric. Mol Nutr Food Res 2013;57(9):1529–42. Review.

[249] Lu Y, Wei C, Xi Z. Curcumin suppresses proliferation and invasion in non-small cell lung cancer by modulation of MTA1-mediated Wnt/β-catenin pathway. In Vitro Cell Dev Biol Anim 2014;50(9):840–50.

[250] Gupta SC, Kismali G, Aggarwal BB. Curcumin, a component of turmeric: from farm to pharmacy. Biofactors 2013;39(1):2–13.

[251] Giacosa A, Barale R, Bavaresco L, et al. Cancer prevention in Europe: the Mediterranean diet as a protective choice. Eur J Cancer Prev 2013;22(1):90–5.

[252] Fan C, Pan Y, Yang Y, et al. HDAC1 inhibition by melatonin leads to suppression of lung adenocarcinoma cells via induction of

[253] Foradori MJ, Chen Q, Fernandez CA, et al. Matrilin-1 is an inhibitor of neovascularization. J Biol Chem 2014;289:14301–9. Available from: http://www.jbc.org/content/289/20/14301.full.

[254] DiNicolantonio JJ, McCarty MF, Chatterjee S, et al. A higher dietary ratio of long-chain omega-3 to total omega-6 fatty acids for prevention of COX-2-dependent adenocarcinomas. Nutr Cancer 2014;66(8):1279–84.

[255] Verone-Boyle AR, Shoemaker S, Attwood K, et al. Diet-derived 25-hydroxyvitamin D3 activates vitamin D receptor target gene expression and suppresses EGFR mutant non-small cell lung cancer growth in vitro and in vivo. Oncotarget 2016;7(1):995–1013.

[256] White JH. Profiling 1,25-dihydroxyvitamin D3-regulated gene expression by microarray analysis. J Steroid Biochem Mol Biol 2004;89–90(1–5):239–44.

[257] He H, Zhou X, Wang Q, et al. Does the course of Astragalus-containing Chinese herbal prescriptions and radiotherapy benefit to non-small-cell lung cancer treatment: a meta-analysis of randomized trials. Evid Based Complement Alternat Med 2013;2013:426207. Available from: http://dx.doi.org/10.1155/2013/426207. Review.

[258] Lee G, Kim SK. Therapeutic effects of phytochemicals and medicinal herbs on chemotherapy-induced peripheral neuropathy. Molecules 2016;21(9):1252. doi:10.3390/molecules21091252.

[259] Yun M, Kim EO, Lee D, et al. Melatonin sensitizes H1975 non-small-cell lung cancer cells harboring a T790M-targeted epidermal growth factor receptor mutation to the tyrosine kinase inhibitor gefitinib. Cell Physiol Biochem 2014;34:865–72. doi:10.1159/000366305.

[260] Jacquemin G, Ganci V, Gallouet AS, et al. Quercetin-mediated Mcl-1 and survivin downregulation restores TRAIL-induced apoptosis in non-Hodgkin's lymphoma B cells. Haematologica 2012;97(1):38–46.

[261] Memorial Sloan Kettering Cancer Center. Prevention & risk factors for lymphoma; 2016. Available from: https://www.mskcc.org/cancer-care/types/lymphoma/prevention-risk-factors.

[262] Breitenstein MK, O'Byrne MM, Feldman AL, et al. Body mass index shows etiologic heterogeneity for risk of diffuse large B cell lymphoma (DLBCL) subtype defined by cell-of-origin [Abstract]. Cancer Res 2016;76(Suppl. 14). In: Proceedings of the 107th Annual Meeting of the American Association for Cancer Research; 2016 Apr 16–20; New Orleans, LA. Philadelphia (PA): AACR, Abstract nr 1762.

[263] DePergola G, Silvestris F. Obesity as a major risk factor for cancer. J Obes 2013;2013:291546.

[264] Leo QJN, Ollberding NJ, Wilkens LR, et al. Nutritional factors and non-Hodgkin lymphoma survival in an ethnically diverse population: the Multiethnic Cohort. Eur J Clin Nutr 2015;70:41–6. doi:10.1038/ejcn.2015.139.

[265] Rota M, Porta L, Pelucchi C, et al. Alcohol drinking and risk of leukemia – a systematic review and meta-analysis of the dose–risk relation. Cancer Epidemiol 2014;38(4):330–45.

[266] Liu HL, Chen Y, Cui GH, et al. Curcumin, a potent anti-tumor reagent, is a novel histone deacetylase inhibitor regulating B-NHL cell line Raji proliferation. Acta Pharmacol Sin 2005;26(5):603–9.

[267] Piekarz RL, Frye R, Turner M, et al. Phase II multi-institutional trial of the histone deacetylase inhibitor romidepsin as monotherapy for patients with cutaneous T cell lymphoma. J Clin Oncol 2009;27:5410–17.

[268] Wang J, Xie Y, Feng Y, et al. Epigallocatechingallate induces apoptosis in B lymphoma cells via caspase-dependent pathway and Bcl-2 family protein modulation. Int J Oncol 2015;46:1507–15.

[269] Franceschi S, Serraino D, Carbone A, et al. Dietary factors and non-Hodgkin's lymphoma: a case-control study in the northeastern part of Italy. Nutr Cancer 1989;12:333–41.

[270] Talamini R, Polesel J, Montella M, et al. Food groups and risk of non-Hodgkin lymphoma: a multicenter, case-control study in Italy. Int J Cancer 2006;118:2871–6.

[271] Zheng T, Holford TR, Leaderer B, et al. Diet and nutrient intakes and risk of non-Hodgkin's lymphoma in Connecticut women. Am J Epidemiol 2004;159:454–66.

[272] da Silva Borges Betiati D, de Oliveira PF, de Quadros Camargo C, et al. Effects of omega-3 fatty acids on regulatory T cells in

hematologic neoplasms. Rev Bras Hematol Hemoter 2013;35(2): 119–25.

[273] Drake MT, Maurer MJ, Link BK, et al. Vitamin D insufficiency and prognosis in non-Hodgkin's lymphoma. J Clin Oncol 2010;2(27):4191–8.

[274] Bernhard D, Tinhofer I, Tonko M, et al. Resveratrol causes arrest in the S-phase prior to Fas-independent apoptosis in CEM-C7H2 acute leukemia cells. Cell Death Differ 2000;7:834–42.

[275] Dorrie J, Gerauer H, Wachter Y, et al. Resveratrol induces extensive apoptosis by depolarizing mitochondrial membranes and activating caspase-9 in acute lymphoblastic leukemia cells. Cancer Res 2001;61:4731–9.

[276] Frazzi R, Tigano M. The multiple mechanism of cell death triggered by resveratrol in lymphoma and leukemia. Int J Mol Sci 2014;15(3):4977–93. doi:10.3390/ijms15034977.

[277] Di Bella G, Mascia F, Gualano L, et al. Melatonin anticancer effects. Int J Mol Sci 2013;14(2):2410–30. Review.

[278] Puspitasari IM, Abdulah R, Yamazaki C, et al. Updates on clinical studies of selenium supplementation in radiotherapy. Radiat Oncol 2014;9:124. Available from: https://ro-journal.biomedcentral.com/articles/10.1186/1748-717X-9-125.

[279] Chakraborty C, Doss CGP, Sarin R, et al. Can the chemotherapeutic agents perform anticancer activity though miRNA expression regulation? Proposing a new hypothesis. Protoplasma 2015;252(6):1603–10.

[280] Todisco M. Chronic lymphocytic leukemia: long-lasting remission with combination of cyclophosphamide, somatostatin, bromocriptine, retinoids, melatonin, and ACTH. Cancer Biother Radiopharm 2009;24:353–5.

[281] Callander N, Markovina S, Eickhoff J, et al. Acetyl-l-carnitine (ALCAR) for the prevention of chemotherapy-induced peripheral neuropathy in patients with relapsed or refractory multiple myeloma treated with bortezomib, doxorubicin and low-dose dexamethasone: a study from the Wisconsin Oncology Network. Cancer Chemother Pharmacol 2014;74(4):875–82.

[282] Zamora-Ros R, Andres-Lacueva C, Lameula-Raventós RM, et al. Estimation of dietary sources and flavonoid intake in a Spanish adult population (Epic-Spain). J Am Diet Assoc 2010;110:390–8.

[283] Ramzan I. Phytotherapies: efficacy, safety and regulation. Hoboken. New Jersey: John Wiley & Sons, Inc.; 2015.

[284] Mahabir S, Pathak Y, Taylor & Francis Group. Nutraceuticals and health: review of human evidence. Boca Raton: CRC Press; 2014.

[285] Bizzari M, Proietti S, Cucina A, et al. Molecular mechanisms of the pro-apoptotic actions of melatonin in cancer: a review. Expert Opin Ther Targets 2013;17(12):1483–96.

[286] Weinstein SJ, Mondul A, Albanes D. Association between pre-diagnostic circulating 25-hydroxyvitamin D and cancer survival [Abstract]. Cancer Res 2016;76(Suppl. 14). In: Proceedings of the 107th Annual Meeting of the American Association for Cancer Research; 2016 Apr 16–20; New Orleans, LA. Philadelphia (PA): AACR, Abstract nr 3416.

[287] Christakos S, Dhawan P, Verstuyf A, et al. Vitamin D, metabolism, molecular mechanism of action, and pleiotropic effects. Physiol Rev 2016;96(1):365–408.

[288] Haussler MR, Saini RK, Sabir MS, et al. Vitamin D nutrient-gene interactions and healthful aging, molecular basis of nutrition and aging. A volume in the molecular nutrition series. US: Elsevier Inc; 2016. p. 449–71. doi:10.1016/B978-0-12-801816-3.00033-9.

[289] Kaeberlein M, McDonagh T, Heltweg B, et al. Substrate-specific activation of sirtuins by resveratrol. J Biol Chem 2005;280(17):17038–45.

[290] Goodman A. Vitamin C and cancer. AIMS Medical Science 2016;3(1):41–51. Review.

[291] Chen Q, Polireddy K, Chen P, et al. The unpaved journey of vitamin C in cancer. Can J Physiol Pharmacol 2015;10(27):1–9.

[292] Leischner C, Burkard M, Pfeiffer MM, et al. Nutritional immunology: function of natural killer cells and their modulation by resveratrol for cancer prevention and treatment. Nutr J 2016;15(47). doi:10.1186/s12937-016-0167-8.

[293] Wu D, Jiang Z, Gong B. Astragalus polysaccharide protects cardiomyocytes from 5-fluorouracil-induced injury via decreasing ROS production. Int J Clin Exp Med 2016;9(6):11058–64.

[294] Saha SP, Whayne TF Jr. Coenzyme Q-10 in human health: supporting evidence? South Med J 2016;109(1):1–21.

[295] Cardinali D, Escames G, Acuna-Castroviejo D, et al. Melatonin-induced oncostasis, mechanisms and clinical relevance. J Integr Oncol 2016;S1. Available from: http://www.omicsgroup.org/journals/melatonininduced-oncostasis-mechanisms-and-clinical-relevance-2329-6771-S1-006.pdf.

[296] Otte JL, Carpenter JS, Manchanda S, et al. Systematic review of sleep disorders in cancer patients: can the prevalence of sleep disorders be ascertained? Cancer Med 2015;4:183–200.

[297] Irwin MR, Olmstead R, Carroll JE. Sleep disturbance, sleep duration, and inflammation: a systematic review and meta-analysis of cohort studies and experimental sleep deprivation. Biol Psychiatry 2016;80(1):40–52.

[298] Brito AF, Riberio M, Abrantes AM, et al. Quercetin in cancer treatment, alone or in combination with conventional therapeutics? Curr Med Chem 2015;22(26):3025–39.

[299] Chow WH, Dong LM, Devesa SS. Epidemiology and risk factors for kidney cancer. Nat Rev Urol 2010;7:245–57. doi:10.1038/nrurol.2010.46.

[300] Mayo Clinic Staff. Kidney cancer: risk factors. Mayo Clinic; 2016. Available from: http://www.mayoclinic.org/diseases-conditions/kidney-cancer/basics/risk-factors/con-20024753.

[301] Gu B, Ding Q, Xia G, et al. EGCG inhibits growth and induces apoptosis in renal cell carcinoma through TFPI-2 overexpression. Oncol Rep 2009;21(3):635–40.

[302] Wang W, Sukamtoh E, Xiao H, et al. Curcumin inhibits lymphaniogenesis in vitro and in vivo. Molecular Nutrition 2015;59(12):2345–54.

[303] Kaur G, Verma N. Nature curing cancer – review on structural modification studies with natural active compounds having anti-tumor efficiency. Biotechnol Rep (Amst) 2015;6:64–78.

[304] Roupas P, Keogh J, Noakes M, et al. The role of edible mushrooms in health: evaluation of the evidence. J Funct Foods 2012;4:687–709.

[305] Sadava D, Still DW, Mudry RR, et al. Effect of Ganoderma on drug-sensitive and multidrug-resistant small-cell lung carcinoma cells. Cancer Lett 2009;277:182–9.

[306] Sun M, Zhao W, Xie Q, et al. Lentinan reduces tumor progression by enhancing gemcitabine chemotherapy in urothelial bladder cancer. Surg Oncol 2015;24:28–34.

[307] Jeff IB, Yuan X, Sun L, et al. Purification and in vitro anti-proliferative effect of novel neutral polysaccharides from Lentinus edodes. Int J Biol Macromol 2013;52:99–106.

[308] World Cancer Research Fund International/American Institute for Cancer Research Continuous Update Project Report: Diet, nutrition, physical activity and kidney cancer; 2015. Available from: http://www.wcrf.org/int/research-we-fund/continuous-update-project-findings-reports/kidney-cancer.

[309] Alexander DD, Cushing CA. Quantitative assessment of red meat or processed meat consumption and kidney cancer. Cancer Detect Prev 2009;32(56):340–51.

[310] DellaValle CT, Daniel CR, Aschebrook-Kilfoy B, et al. Dietary intake of nitrate and risk of renal cell carcinoma in the NIH-AARP Diet and Health Study. Br J Cancer 2013;108:205–12. doi:10.1038/bjc.2012.522. www.bjcancer.com.

[311] Chatenoud L, Tavani A, La Vecchia C, et al. Whole grain food intake and cancer risk. Int J Cancer 1998;77(1):24–8.

[312] Bosetti C, Filomeno M, Riso P, et al. Cruciferous vegetables and cancer risk in a network of case-control studies. Ann Oncol 2012;23(8):2198–203. Available from: http://annonc.oxfordjournals.org/content/early/2012/02/10/annonc.mdr604.short.

[313] Mondul AM, Weinstein SJ, Moy KA, et al. Vitamin D binding protein, circulating vitamin D and risk of renal cell carcinoma. Int J Cancer 2014;134(110):2699–706.

[314] Lin G, Ning L, Gu D, et al. Examining the association of circulating 25-hydroxyvitamin D with kidney cancer risk: a meta-analysis. Int J Clin Exp Med 2015;8(11):20499–507.

[315] Muller DC, Scelo G, Saridze D, et al. Circulating 25-Hyrdoxyvitamin D3 and survival after diagnosis with kidney cancer. Cancer Epidemiol Biomarkers Prev 2015;24(8):1277–81.

[316] Hirata H, Ueno K, Tanaka Y, et al. Abstract 4394: Genistein downregulates onco-miR-1260b and inhibits Wnt-signaling in renal cancer cells. Cancer Res 2014;74(19). doi:10.1158/1538-7445.AM2014-4394.

[317] Simard B, Ratel D, Dupre I, et al. Shark cartilage extract induces cytokines expression and release in endothelial cells and induces E-selectin, plasminogen and t-PA genes expression through an antioxidant-sensitive mechanism. Cytokine 2013;61(1):104–11.

[318] Denzler K, Moore J, Harrington H, et al. Characterisation of the physiological response following in vivo administration of Astragalus membranaceus. Evid Based Complement Alternat Med 2016;2016:6861078. doi:10.1155/2016/6861078.

[319] Kin J, Ulu A, Wan D, et al. Addition of DHA synergistically enhances the efficacy of regorafenib for kidney cancer. Mol Cancer Ther 2016;15(5):890–8.

[320] Martinez-Alonso M, Dusso A, Ariza G, et al. Vitamin D deficiency and its association with fatigue and quality of life in advanced cancer patients under palliative care: a cross-sectional study. Palliat Med 2016;30(1):89–96.

[321] Maisonneuve R, Lowenfels AB. Risk factors for pancreatic cancer: a summary review of meta-analytical studies. Int J Epidemiol 2014;44(1):186–98. Available from: http://ije.oxfordjournals.org/content/44/1/186.full.

[322] Azimi H, Khakshur AA, Abdollohi M, et al. Potential new pharmacological agents derived from medicinal plants for the treatment of pancreatic cancer [Abstract]. Pancreas 2015;44(1):11–15. Available from: http://www.ncbi.nlm.nih.gov/pubmed/25493374.

[323] Bimonte S, Barbieri A, Leongito M, et al. Curcumin anticancer studies in pancreatic cancer. Nutrients 2016;8(7):433. doi:10.3390/nu8070433.

[324] Genkinger JM, Li R, Spiegelman D, et al. Coffee, tea, and sugar-sweetened carbonated soft drink intake and pancreatic cancer risk: a pooled analysis of 14 cohort studies. Cancer Epidemiol Biomarkers Prev 2012;21:305–18.

[325] Ho VW, Leung K, Hsu A, et al. A low carbohydrate, high protein diet slows tumor growth and prevents cancer initiation. Cancer Res 2011;71(13). Available from: http://cancerres.aacrjournals.org/content/71/13/4484.

[326] Van Dijk DPJ, Marcel CG, van de Poll AGW, et al. Effects of oral meal feeding on whole body protein breakdown and protein synthesis in cachectic pancreatic cancer patients. J Cachexia Sarcopenia Muscle 2015;6(3):212–21. Available from: http://onlinelibrary.wiley.com/doi/10.1002/jcsm.12029/full.

[327] Nicolini A, Ferrari P, Masoni MC, et al. Malnutrition, anorexia and cachexia in cancer patients: a mini-review on pathogenesis and treatment. Biomed Pharmacother 2013;67(8):807–17.

[328] Stolzenberg-Solomon RZ, Jacobs EJ, Arslan AA, et al. Circulating 25-hydroxyvitamin D and risk of pancreatic cancer: cohort consortium Vitamin D pooling project of rarer cancers. Am J Epidemiol 2010;172:81–93.

[329] Wolpin BM, Ng K, Bao Y, et al. Plasma 25-hydroxyvitamin D and risk of pancreatic cancer. Cancer Epidemiol Biomarkers Prev 2012;21:82–91.

[330] Liu SL, Zhao YP, Dai MH, et al. Vitamin D status and the risk of pancreatic cancer: a meta-analysis. Chin Med J 2013;126:3356–9.

[331] Lorenc R, Karczmarewicz E, Kryskiewicz E, et al. Vitamin D provision and supplementation standards. Standardy Medyczne/Pediatria 2012;9:595–604.

[332] Buchler P, Gukovskaya AS, Mouria M, et al. Prevention of metastatic pancreatic cancer growth in vivo by induction of apoptosis with genistein, a naturally occurring isoflavonoid. Pancreas 2003;26(3):264–73.

[333] Gu Y, Zhu CF, Dai Y, et al. Inhibitory effects of genistein on metastasis of human hepatocellular carcinoma. World J Gastroenterol 2009;15(39):4952–7.

[334] Xu L, Ding Y, Catalona WJ, et al. Mek4 function, genistein treatment, and invasion of human prostate cancer cells. J Natl Cancer Inst 2009;101(16):1141–55.

[335] Takimoto CH, Glover K, Huang X, et al. Phase I pharmacokinetic and pharmacodynamic analysis of unconjugated soy isoflavones administered to individuals with cancer. Cancer Epidemiol Biomarkers Prev 2003;12(11 Pt 1):1213–21.

[336] Lissoni P, Ardizzoia A, Meregalli S, et al. A clinical-study of immunotherapy versus endocrine therapy versus chemotherapy in the treatment of advanced pancreatic adenocarcinoma. Oncol Rep 1994;1(6):1277–80.

[337] Lissoni P, Paolorossi F, Tancini G, et al. A phase II study of tamoxifen plus melatonin in metastatic solid tumour patients. Br J Cancer 1996;74(9):1466–8.

[338] Jaworek J, Leja-Szpak A. Melatonin influences pancreatic cancerogenesis. Histol Histopathol 2014;29(4):423–31.

[339] Fukui M, Sung Kang K, Okada K, et al. EPA, an omega-3 fatty acid, induces apoptosis in human pancreatic cancer cells: role of ROS accumulation, caspase-8 activation, and autophagy induction. J Cell Biochem 2012;114:192–203.

[340] Morland SL, Martins SJB, Mazurak VC. n-3 polyunsaturated fatty acid supplementation during cancer chemotherapy. J Nutr Intermed Metab 2016;2016(5):107–16.

[341] Armstrong T, Strommer L, Ruiz-Jasbon F, et al. Pancreaticoduodenectomy for peri-ampullary neoplasia leads to specific micronutrient deficiencies. Pancreatology 2007;7(1):37–44.

[342] Bjelakovic G, Nikolova D, Simonetti RG, et al. Antioxidant supplements for preventing gastrointestinal cancers. Cochrane Database Syst Rev 2008;16(3):CD004183.

[343] Appel MJ, Woutersen RA. Effects of dietary beta-carotene and selenium on initiation and promotion of pancreatic carcinogenesis in azaserine-treated rats. Carcinogenesis 1996;17(7):1411–16.

[344] Council for Responsible Nutrition. Vitamin and mineral safety. 3rd ed. 2013. Available from: http://www.crnusa.org/safety/updatedpdfs/31-CRNVMS3-SELENIUM.pdf.

[345] Reid ME, Stratton MS, Lillico AJ, et al. A report of high-dose selenium supplementation: response and toxicities. J Trace Elem Med Biol 2004;18(1):69–74.

[346] Berkovich L, Earon G, Ron I, et al. Moringa oliefera aqueous leaf extract down-regulates nuclear factor-KappaB and increases cytotoxic effect of chemotherapy in pancreatic cancer cells. BMC Complement Altern Med 2013;13:212. doi:10.1186/1472-6882-13-212.

[347] Wang YH, Yao N, Wei KK, et al. The efficacy and safety of probiotics for prevention of chemoradiotherapy-induced diarrhea in people with abdominal and pelvic cancer: a systematic review and meta-analysis. Eur J Clin Nutr 2016;70(11):1246–53.

[348] Schlemmer M, Suchner U, Schapers B, et al. Is glutamine deficiency the link between inflammation, malnutrition and fatigue in cancer patients? Clin Nutr 2015;34(6):1258–65.

[349] Von Haehling S, Anker SD. Treatment of cachexia: an overview of recent developments. Int J Cardiol 2015;184:736–42.

[350] World Cancer Research Fund International/American Institute for Cancer Research. Continuous Update Project Report: Diet, nutrition, physical activity and bladder cancer; 2015. Available from: www.wcrf.org/bladder-cancer-2015.

[351] Cancer Council Australia. Understanding bladder cancer; 2016. Available from: http://www.cancer.org.au/about-cancer/types-of-cancer/bladder-cancer.html.

[352] Guohua H, Lei Z, Yefei R, et al. Downstream carcinogenesis signaling pathways by green tea polyphenols: a translational perspective of chemoprevention and treatment for cancers. Curr Drug Metab 2014;15(1):14–22.

[353] Chen D, Wan SH, Yang H, et al. EGCG, green tea polyphenols and their synthetic analogs and prodrugs for human cancer prevention and treatment. Adv Clin Chem 2011;53:155–77.

[354] Chen Z, Yu T, Zhou B, et al. Mg(II)-Catechin nanoparticles delivering siRNA targeting EIF5A2 inhibit bladder cancer cell growth in vitro and in vivo. Biomaterials 2016;81:125–34.

[355] Kang K, Ho JN, Kook HR, et al. Theracurmin® efficiently inhibits the growth of human prostate and bladder cancer cells via induction of apoptotic cell death and cell cycle arrest. Oncol Rep 2015;35(3):1463–72.

[356] Su CL, Fan YW. Induction of autophagy and inhibition of oncoprotein aurora-A activity in curcumin-enhanced chemosensitivity of Grade III human bladder cancer T24 cells to FDA-approved anticancer drugs. FASEB J 2015;29(1):S752.1.

[357] Sun X, Deng QF, Liang ZF, et al. Curcumin reverses benzidine-induced cell proliferation by suppressing ERK1/2 pathway in human bladder cancer T24 cells. Exp Toxicol Pathol 2016;68(4):215–22.

[358] Silberstein J, Parsons JK. Evidence-based principles of bladder cancer and diet. Urology 2010;75(2):340–6.

[359] Michaud DS, et al. Fruit and vegetable intake and incidence of bladder cancer in a male prospective cohort. J Natl Cancer Inst 1999;91:605–13.

[360] Battacharya A, Tang L, Li Y, et al. Inhibition of bladder cancer development by allyl isothiocyanate. Carcinogenesis 2010;31(2):281–6. doi:10.1093/carcin/bgp303.

[361] Galluzzi L, Vacchelli E, Michels J, et al. Effects of vitamin B6 metabolism on oncogenesis, tumour progression and therapeutic responses. Oncogene 2013;32:4995–5004.

[362] Shivappa N, Hebert JR, Rosato V, et al. Dietary inflammatory index and risk of bladder cancer in a large Italian case-control study. Urology 2017;100:84–9.

[363] Su Q, Peng M, Zhang Y, et al. Quercetin induces bladder cancer cells apoptosis by activation of AMPK signaling pathway. Am J Cancer Res 2016;6(2):498–508.

[364] Bunch CL, Johnson CS, Trump DL. Abstract 1190: Pretreatment with 1,25 dihydroxyvitamin D3 modulates p73 levels and activity to increase pro-apoptotic effects of cisplatin in bladder cancer. Cancer Res 2016;76(Suppl. 14). In: Proceedings of the 107th Annual Meeting of the American Association for Cancer Research; 2016 Apr 16–20; New Orleans, LA. Philadelphia (PA): AACR, Abstract nr 1190.

[365] Wedlake LJ, Shaw C, Whelan K, et al. Systematic review: the efficacy of nutritional interventions to counteract acute gastrointestinal toxicity during therapeutic pelvic radiotherapy. Aliment Pharmacol Ther 2013;37(11):1046–56.

[366] Philippou Y, Hadjipavlou M, Khan S, et al. Complementary and alternative medicine (CAM) in prostate and bladder cancer. BJU Int 2013;112(8):1073–9.

[367] Merendino N, Costantini L, Manzi L, et al. Dietary ω-3 polyunsaturated fatty acid DHA: a potential adjuvant in the treatment of cancer. Biomed Res Int 2013;2013. doi:10.1155/2013/310186. Article ID 310186.

[368] Orsolic N, Karac I, Sirovina D, et al. Chemotherapeutic potential of quercetin on human bladder cancer cells. J Environ Sci Health A Tox Hazard Subst Environ Eng 2015;51(9):776–81. Part A.

[369] Sanchez-Hidalgo MM, Guerrero J, Villegas I, et al. Melatonin, a natural programmed cell death inducer in cancer. Curr Med Chem 2012;19(22):3805–21.

23

HIV (human immunodeficiency virus)

Leah Hechtman, Dr Janet Schloss

HIV STATISTICS (WORLD HEALTH ORGANIZATION [WHO] HIV/AIDS STATISTICS AND DATA)[1]

- In 2015, 36.7 million people in the world were living with HIV.
- In 2015, 2.1 million people worldwide were newly infected with HIV.
- Over 90% of these people are in developing countries; 150 000 were under the age of 15.
- Every day, approximately 5753 people contract HIV, which is about 240 people every hour.
- In 2015, 1.1 million people died from AIDS-related illnesses.
- Since the disease was recognised, 78 million people have contracted HIV and 35 million have died of AIDS-related causes.
- By December 2015, 17 million people living with HIV (46% of the total) had access to anti-retroviral therapy. (See Table 23.1, Fig. 23.1 and Table 23.2.)

AIDS STATISTICS[1,2]

East and southern Africa (46% of the global new HIV infections)

In 2015, 19 million people (more than half of whom were women) were living with HIV in eastern and southern Africa. In 2015, approximately 960 000 people became newly infected with HIV, while 470 000 people died of AIDS-related causes.

Western and central Africa

In 2015, 6.5 million people (nearly 60% women) were living with HIV in western and central Africa. Approximately 410 000 people became newly infected in 2015, and 330 000 people died of AIDS-related causes.

Asia and the Pacific

Approximately 300 000 people became newly infected in 2015 in the Asia/Pacific region, bringing the total number of people living with HIV there to 5.1 million. AIDS had claimed around 180 000 lives within the Asian region by 2015.

Latin America and the Caribbean

Around 100 000 new HIV infections and 50 000 AIDS-related deaths were seen in the Latin America and Caribbean area in 2015. Currently, 2 million people live with HIV.

North Africa and the Middle East

It is estimated that 230 000 people are living with HIV in this region, with 21 000 people becoming newly infected in 2015. Approximately 12 000 adults and children died of AIDS in North Africa and the Middle East in 2015.

Eastern Europe and central Asia

In 2015, 190 000 people were newly infected with HIV, 1.5 million people lived with HIV, and AIDS claimed 47 000 lives.

Western and central Europe and North America

In 2015, approximately 91 000 new cases of HIV were diagnosed, bringing the number of people living with HIV in this region to 2.4 million. In 2015, 22 000 people died of AIDS.

CLASSIFICATION

Classification of HIV status is primarily determined by a patient's CD4+ levels.

Early HIV infection – CD4+ >500 (cells/mL)

No unusual conditions likely. Emphasise good health habits and healthcare maintenance.

Intermediate stages – CD4+ 200–500 (cells/mL)

Increased risk for shingles (zoster), thrush (*Candida*), skin infections, bacterial sinus and lung infections, and TB.

TABLE 23.1 HIV prevalence in selected countries[2]

Regional data—2015

| Region | People living with HIV (total) | New HIV infections | | | AIDS-related deaths (total) | Total number accesing anti-retrovial therapy |
		Total	Aged 15+	Aged 0–14		
Eastern and southern Africa	19.0 million (17.7 million–20.5 million)	960 000 (830 000–1.1 million)	910 000 [790 000– 1.1 million)	56 000 (40 000–76 000)	470 000 (390 000–560 000)	10 million
Latin America and the Caribbean	2.0 million (1.7 million–2.3 million)	100 000 (86 000–120 000)	100 000 (84 000–120 000)	2100 (1600–2900)	50 000 (41 000–59 000)	1.1 million
Western and central Africa	6.5 million (5.3 million–7.8 million)	410 000 (310 000–530 000)	350 000 (270 000–450 000)	66 000 (47 000–87 000)	330 000 (250 000–430 000)	1.8 million
Asia and the Pacific	5.1 million (4.4 million–5.9 million)	300 000 (240 000–380 000)	280 000 (220 000–350 000(	19 000 (16 000–21 000)	180 000 (150 000–220 000)	2.1 million
Eastern Europe and central Asia	1.5 million (1.4 million–1.7 million)	190 000 (170 000–200 000)	190 000 (170 000–200 000)	—	47 000 (39 000–55 000)	320 000
Middle East and North Africa	230 000 (160 000–330 000)	21 000 (12 000–37 000)	19 000 (11 000–34 000)	2100 (1400–3200)	12 000 (8700–16 000)	38 000
Western and central Europe and North America	2.4 million (2.2 million–2.7 million)	91 000 (89 000–97 000)	91 000 (88 000–96 000)	—	22 000 (20 000–24 000)	1.4 million

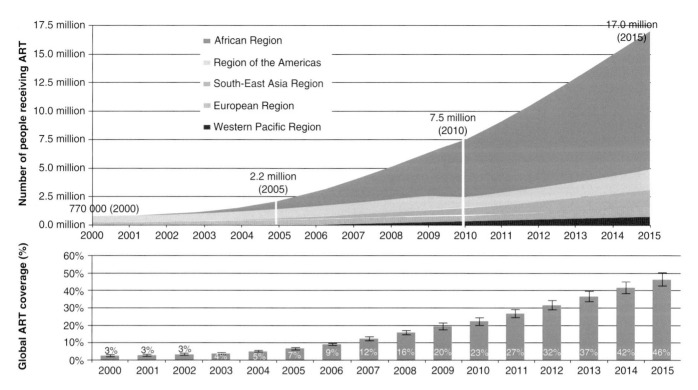

FIGURE 23.1 Estimated number of people receiving anti-retroviral therapy globally and by WHO region and percentage coverage globally, 2000–2015

Opportunistic infections, such as *Pneumocystis carinii* pneumonia (PCP), *Mycobacterium avium intracellulare* complex (MAC) and cytomegalovirus (CMV), are rare.

ADVANCED HIV INFECTION – CD4+ 50–200 (CELLS/ML)

Increased risk for PCP and other opportunistic infections. Preventive treatment for PCP is indicated. If counts are fewer than 100, consider preventive treatment for MAC, CMV and invasive fungal infections.

CD4+ <50 (cells/mL)

Increased risk for opportunistic infections, including MAC and CMV. Continue preventive medication.

AIDS DEFINITION

AIDS is currently defined as the presence of one of 25 conditions indicative of severe immunosuppression or HIV infection in an individual with a CD4+ cell count of <200 cells per cubic mm of blood. AIDS is therefore the end point of an infection that is continuous, progressive and pathogenic. With the prevalence of HIV in the developing world, HIV and its complications will be with us for generations. Table 23.3 outlines a person's risk of developing AIDS in 6 years based on their viral load and CD4 count.

AETIOLOGY

Transmission

Transmission of HIV requires contact with body fluids containing infected cells (lymphocytes), free virions or plasma. This includes the following:
- blood
- semen
- cervical and vaginal secretions
- breast milk
- cerebrospinal fluid (CSF)
- synovial fluid
- wound exudates
- saliva or droplet nuclei produced by coughing or sneezing (theoretically possible but extremely rare)
- not transmitted by casual contact or close non-sexual contact.

MOST COMMON MEANS OF TRANSMISSION

- Sharing a contaminated needle.
- Transmission of HIV by needle-stick injury (1/300) is less frequent than transmission of hepatitis B (lower number of HIV virions in the blood of most infected patients)
- Sexual relations.

TABLE 23.2 WHO worldwide HIV data[1]								
	2000	**2005**	**2010**	**2011**	**2012**	**2013**	**2014**	**2015**
People living with HIV	28.9 million (26.5 million–31.7 million)	31.8 million (29.4 million–34.5 million)	33.3 million (30.8 million–36.1 million)	33.9 million (31.4 million–36.7 million)	34.5 million (31.9 million–37.4 million)	35.2 million (32.6 million–36.1 million)	35.9 million (33.3 million–38.9 million)	36.7 million (34.0 million–39.8 million)
New HIV infections (total)	3.2 million (2.9 million–3.5 million)	2.5 million (2.3 million–2.8 million)	2.2 million (2.0 million–2.5 million)	2.2 million (1.9 million–2.5 million)	2.2 million (1.9 million–2.4 million)	2.1 million (1.9 million–2.4 million)	2.1 million (1.9 million–2.4 million)	2.1 million (1.8 million–2.4 million)
New HIV infections (aged 15+)	2.7 million (2.5 million–3.0 million)	2.1 million (1.9 million–2.3 million)	1.9 million (1.7 million–2.1 million)	1.9 million (1.7 million–2.2 million)	1.9 million (1.7 million–2.2 million)	1.9 million (1.7 million–2.2 million)	1.9 million (1.7 million–2.2 million)	1.9 million (1.7 million–2.2 million)
New Infections (aged 0–14)	490 000 (430 000–560 000)	450 000 (390 000–510 000)	290 000 (250 000–350 000)	270 000 (220 000–330 000)	230 000 (190 000–290 000)	200 000 (160 000–250 000)	160 000 (130 000–220 000)	150 000 (110 000–190 000)
AIDS- related deaths	1.5 million (1.3 million–1.8 million)	2.0 million (1.7 million–2.3 million)	1.5 million (1.3 million–1.7 million)	1.4 million (1.2 million–1.7 million)	1.4 million (1.2 million–1.6 million)	1.3 million (1.1 million–1.5 million)	1.2 million (990 000–1.4 million)	1.1 million (940 000–1.3 million)
People accessing treatment	770 000	2.2 million	7.5 million	9.1 million	11 million	13 million	15 million	17 million
Resources available for HIV (low- and middle-income countries)	4.8 billion	9.4 billion	15.9 billion	18.3 billion	19.5 billion	19.6 billion	19.2 billion	19 billion

TABLE 23.3 Risk of AIDS in 6 years			
	CD4 count		
Viral load	<350	350–500	>500
>55 000	93%	79%	67%
20 000–55 000	73%	57%	50%
7000–20 000	42%	40%	26%
<7000	19%	22%	15%

- Sexual practices involving no exposure to bodily fluids are safe.
- Fellatio and cunnilingus appear to be relatively, but not absolutely, safe.
- Greatest risk is through genital intercourse, especially anal-receptive intercourse.
- Sexual practices producing mucosal trauma before or during intercourse increase the risk – latex condoms or dams decrease risk but do not eliminate risk; oil-based lubricants decrease the protection provided.
- HIV transmission may be more likely in the presence of herpes, syphilis, trichomoniasis and possibly other sexually transmitted infections.

Most common individuals at risk

Those at high risk for contracting HIV include:
- Recipients of blood products from blood transfusion prior to 1985 (especially between 1980 and 1985).
- Men engaging in male-to-male sex – especially the recipient of anal sex.
- IV drug users.
- Those having sex with an individual at high risk.
- Those who are promiscuous, having multiple partners, especially since 1980 and without protection (condoms).
- Heterosexual people with greater than one sex partner in the past 12 months.
- Non-condom users in the past 6 months.
- Females are at higher risk than males.
- Child born to an HIV-positive mother.
- Those with lowered immunity.
- Minority groups.
- Regular sexual partners of people in the aforementioned groups.
    It is important to remember that HIV is not only in the homosexual community.

HIV OVERVIEW

HIV is caused by one of two related retroviruses: HIV-1 and HIV-2. HIV-1 is found throughout the world. Multiple subtypes (or clades) exist, including clades A to N. The majority of infections in the Western world are caused by HIV-1 clade B. HIV-2 was first identified in West Africa in 1986 and has been found to have a genetic sequence approximately 50% similar to HIV-1. HIV-2 is considered less virulent than HIV-1 and shows lower rates of sexual and perinatal transmission. It has also been found to have

a lower viral load with a slower rate of CD4 cell decline. This results in a slower rate of disease progression in infected people. Research shows that the virus is mutating, and multiple subtypes are spreading throughout the world.[3] The existence of multiple clades raises the theoretical possibility that a single individual could become infected with multiple subtypes of the virus.[4]

    HIV results in a wide range of clinical manifestations, varying from asymptomatic carrier states to severely debilitating and fatal disorders related to defective cell-mediated immunity. It was identified in 1984 as the cause of an epidemic of severe immunosuppression – acquired immune deficiency syndrome (AIDS). AIDS diagnosis was typically achieved from opportunistic infection or malignancy.

Pathogenesis
HIV LIFE CYCLE
Binding and fusion

HIV begins its life cycle when it binds to a CD4 receptor on the target cell through the interaction of the viral gp120 and gp41 transmembrane proteins with CD4 and chemokine receptors on the cell's membrane. The virus then fuses with the host cell. After fusion, the virus releases ribonucleic acid (RNA) into the host cell.

MEDICATION INTERACTION

Fusion inhibitors are designed to inhibit this process by altering the cellular receptor sites.

    Newer medications, CCR5 inhibitors, are designed to prevent the virus from entering uninfected CD4-T cells – the target for HIV.

REVERSE TRANSCRIPTION

Reverse transcriptase converts the single-stranded HIV RNA to double-stranded HIV DNA.

MEDICATION INTERACTION

Nucleoside/tide reverse transcriptase inhibitors (NRTIs) and non-nucleoside reverse transcriptase inhibitors (NNRTIs) are designed to affect this process.

Integration

The newly formed HIV DNA enters the host cell's nucleus, where integrase 'hides' the HIV DNA (provirus) within the host cell's own DNA. The provirus is then permanently integrated into the host DNA and may remain inactive (dormant) for several years, producing few or no new copies of HIV, or can become activated and initiate the production of large chains of new viral RNA subunits, independent of the host cell's replication process.

MEDICATION INTERACTION

Newly developed integrase inhibitors inhibit this part of the process.

TRANSCRIPTION

When the host cell receives a signal to become active, the provirus uses a host enzyme called RNA polymerase to create copies of the HIV genomic material, as messenger RNA (mRNA). The mRNA is used as a blueprint to make long chains of HIV proteins (i.e. is translated in the cytoplasm to viral polypeptides).

Cleavage or assembly

Protease cuts the long chains of HIV proteins into smaller individual proteins. As the smaller HIV proteins come together with copies of HIV's RNA genetic material, a new virus particle is assembled.

MEDICATION INTERACTION

Protease inhibitors block the action of the protease enzyme and thereby prevent the reassembly of new viral polypeptides.

Packaging

New RNA viruses are wound up tightly and encapsulated into new viral particles. Zinc atoms in the shape of a finger are used to wrap up the viral RNA.

MEDICATION INTERACTION

Zinc finger inhibitors are being developed to interfere with this part of the process. The inner core of HIV is called the nucleocapsid. It is held together by structures called 'zinc fingers'. Zinc finger inhibitors (or zinc ejectors) are drugs that can break apart these structures and prevent the virus from functioning.

Budding

The newly assembled virus pushes out ('buds') from the host cell. During budding, the new virus steals part of the cell's outer envelope. This envelope, which acts as a covering, is studded with protein/sugar combinations called HIV glycoproteins. These HIV glycoproteins are necessary for the virus to bind CD4 and co-receptors. The new copies of HIV can now move on to infect other cells.

MEDICATION INTERACTION

As mentioned earlier, newer medications, CCR5 inhibitors, are designed to prevent the virus from entering uninfected CD4-T cells – the target for HIV.

The cellular picture

There is a loss of one cell type throughout the course of the disease: *CD4+ T4 helper cells* (see Box 23.1). As such, a fall in the CD4+ cells always precedes disease. In advanced disease, there is a loss of another cell type: *CD8+ cytotoxic killer cells* (see Box 23.1). This loss suggests an infectious agent (i.e. a virus).

HIV/CD4 interaction

HIV primarily infects CD4+ T-lymphocytes. Continuous viral replication occurs throughout the course of HIV disease. Up to 10 billion virions are produced and cleared daily, and the half-life of an HIV-infected CD4 cell is 1.3 days. Most CD4 cells turn over rapidly and some belong to a latent pool with a long half-life.

BOX 23.1 CD4 and CD8 cells

CD4 – helper T cells

These cells display CD4 on the surface, so are also known as T4 cells or TH cells. They recognise antigen fragments associated with major histocompatibility complex (MHC)-II molecules. Their function is to co-stimulate all other lymphocytes, secrete cytokines (interleukin-2) and have an autocrine function in that they co-stimulate themselves to proliferate and secrete more interleukin (positive feedback effect causes formation of many more helper T cells).

CD8 – cytotoxic T cells

These cells display CD8 on the surface, so are known as T8 or Tc or killer T cells. They recognise antigen fragments associated with MHC-I molecules (e.g. cells infected with virus, tumour cells, tissue transplants). Co-stimulation is required by cytokine from helper T cells.

SIGNS AND SYMPTOMS: STAGES OF INFECTION

Acute onset

Acute onset (acute anti-retroviral syndrome) resembles common influenza. Most people experience this syndrome 2–6 weeks after initial infection, and it often goes undiagnosed as HIV due to its similarity to the flu. Signs and symptoms might include fever; fatigue; lymphadenopathy; pharyngitis; maculopapular rash on the face, head and trunk; mucocutaneous ulceration of mouth/oesophagus/genitals; myalgia; night sweats; diarrhoea; headache; nausea and vomiting; hepatosplenomegaly; weight loss; thrush; neurological symptoms (aseptic meningitis, encephalitis, peripheral neuropathy, facial palsy, Guillain–Barré syndrome, brachial neuritis, cognitive impairment or psychosis); thrombocytopenia; leucopenia; and transaminase elevation.

Insidious onset

Insidious onset may present as an AIDS-associated opportunistic infection or as unexplained progressive fatigue, weight loss, fever, diarrhoea or generalised lymphadenopathy.[5]

Stage 1: primary infection

When people first become infected with HIV, they may in many cases experience a flu-like illness, sometimes accompanied by a rash, which is referred to as seroconversion illness. Not all people who have been exposed to HIV will experience seroconversion illness – some people do not have any symptoms at all. They present with a high virus titre (up to 10 million viruses per mL blood) and mild symptoms (if at all), and there is a fall in CD4+ cells (but recovers) and a rise in CD8+ cells (but recovers).

Macrophages are infected. HIV is now not replicating in resting T4 cells and most are resting in the peripheral circulation. At this time, most replication is in lymph nodes in macrophages and dendritic cells. Symptoms are flu-like or mononucleosis-like as the cellular immune response is within weeks. Anti-viral antibodies and cytotoxic T cells rise to high levels and persist for years as they are very effective at keeping the virus in the circulation at low levels.

The CD8 cells rise transiently while CD4 cells fall, but almost recover again. The loss of these CD4 cells may result from direct infection of T cells in the circulation. Although antibodies lower HIV in blood, infection persists in the lymph nodes and in macrophages. Macrophages bring HIV into the body if sexually transmitted.

Stage 2: asymptomatic infection

For a number of years following infection, many people with HIV remain well and symptom-free. The virus almost disappears from circulation as there is good cytoxic T cell response. Soluble antibodies appear later against both surface and internal proteins, and most of the virus comes from recently activated (dividing) and infected CD4+ cells. CD4+ cell production compensates for loss due to lysis of cells by virus production and destruction of infected cells by cytotoxic T lymphocytes.

Stage 3A: symptomatic illness

The symptoms people might experience at this stage include diarrhoea, minor skin conditions, minor oral (mouth) conditions, lack of energy, night sweats, and/or persistently swollen glands lasting longer than 2 months. It is described as a latency of virus and of symptoms. The virus persists in extravascular tissues, specifically in the lymph node dendritic cells. Resting CD4+ memory cells (which last a very long time as it is a very stable population of cells) carry the provirus, and the patient presents with persistent infection with no or minor symptoms – night sweats, generalised lymphadenopathy, diarrhoea.

The virus persists as a provirus in resting memory T cells. Reactivation of cells occurs, contributing to overall viral load, but this does not at this stage significantly affect CD4 cell numbers. Nevertheless, CD4 cells drop in number throughout infection.

Stage 3B: the beginning of disease

During this stage there is a massive loss of CD4+ cells as the CD4+ cells are the targets of the virus. Cells that proliferate to respond to the virus are killed by it – this is called clonal deletion. Dendritic cells present antigen and virus to CD4 cells just as they are activated. Epitope variation allows more and more HIV to escape from the immune response just as the response wanes. There is apoptosis of CD4+ cells. It is important to remember that HIV patients with high T4 cell counts do not develop AIDS.

Stage 4: advanced disease (AIDS)

At this stage, HIV will have done great damage to a body's ability to cope with illness and infection. People with AIDS experience severe symptoms, and are at risk of opportunistic illnesses.

CD8+ cells destroy more CD4+ cells. CD4 cell loss means virus and infected cells are no longer controlled. As CD4+ cells fall below 200 per cubic mm, virus titre rises rapidly and the remaining immune response collapses. The CD8+ cell number collapses. Opportunistic infections develop. Death occurs in ≈ 2 years without intervention.

Complications

Obviously, the main complication is the progression of AIDS. It is essential to watch patients' CD4+, CD8+ and CD4 to CD8 ratio to monitor their health and disease progression.

WHO clinical staging of HIV/AIDS for adults and adolescents[6]

The clinical staging and case definitions of HIV for resource-constrained settings were developed by the WHO in 1990 and revised in 2007. Staging is based on clinical findings that guide the diagnosis, evaluation and management of HIV/AIDS, and does not require a CD4 cell count. This staging system is used in many countries to determine eligibility for anti-retroviral therapy, particularly in settings in which CD4 testing is not available. Clinical stages are categorised as 1 to 4, progressing from primary HIV infection to advanced HIV/AIDS. These stages are defined by specific clinical conditions or symptoms. For the purpose of the WHO staging system, adolescents and adults are defined as individuals aged ≥15 years.

PRIMARY HIV INFECTION

- Asymptomatic
- Acute retroviral syndrome.

CLINICAL STAGE 1

- Asymptomatic
- Persistent generalised lymphadenopathy.

CLINICAL STAGE 2

- Moderate unexplained weight loss (<10% of presumed or measured body weight)
- Recurrent respiratory infections (sinusitis, tonsillitis, otitis media and pharyngitis)
- Herpes zoster
- Angular cheilitis
- Recurrent oral ulceration
- Papular pruritic eruptions
- Seborrhoeic dermatitis
- Fungal nail infections.

CLINICAL STAGE 3

- Unexplained severe weight loss (>10% of presumed or measured body weight)
- Unexplained chronic diarrhoea for >1 month
- Unexplained persistent fever for >1 month (>37.6°C, intermittent or constant)
- Persistent oral candidiasis (thrush)
- Oral hairy leukoplakia
- Pulmonary tuberculosis (current)
- Severe presumed bacterial infections (e.g. pneumonia, empyema, pyomyositis, bone or joint infection, meningitis, bacteraemia)

- Acute necrotising ulcerative stomatitis, gingivitis or periodontitis
- Unexplained anaemia (haemoglobin <8 g/dL)
- Neutropenia (neutrophils <500 cells/μL)
- Chronic thrombocytopenia (platelets <50 000 cells/μL).

CLINICAL STAGE 4

- HIV wasting syndrome
- *Pneumocystis* pneumonia
- Recurrent severe bacterial pneumonia
- Chronic herpes simplex infection (orolabial, genital or anorectal site for >1 month or visceral herpes at any site)
- Oesophageal candidiasis (or candidiasis of trachea, bronchi or lungs)
- Extrapulmonary tuberculosis
- Kaposi sarcoma
- Cytomegalovirus infection (retinitis or infection of other organs)
- Central nervous system toxoplasmosis
- HIV encephalopathy
- Cryptococcosis, extrapulmonary (including meningitis)
- Disseminated nontuberculosis *Mycobacterium* infection
- Progressive multifocal leukoencephalopathy
- *Candida* of the trachea, bronchi or lungs
- Chronic cryptosporidiosis (with diarrhoea)
- Chronic isosporiasis
- Disseminated mycosis (e.g. histoplasmosis, coccidioidomycosis, penicilliosis)
- Recurrent nontyphoidal *Salmonella* bacteraemia
- Lymphoma (cerebral or B cell non-Hodgkin)
- Invasive cervical carcinoma
- Atypical disseminated leishmaniasis
- Symptomatic HIV-associated nephropathy
- Symptomatic HIV-associated cardiomyopathy
- Reactivation of American trypanosomiasis (meningoencephalitis or myocarditis).

CONDITIONS ASSOCIATED WITH HIV/AIDS

As the immune system plummets, the incidence of immune deviations and increased susceptibility to infection rises. AIDS has been directly linked to an increased incidence of malignancies. Kaposi sarcoma, non-Hodgkin lymphoma and cervical cancer are AIDS-defining illnesses in HIV-infected patients. Other neoplastic diseases associated with AIDS include Hodgkin's disease, anal cancer, testicular cancer, melanoma, non-melanomatous skin cancers, lung cancer and primary central nervous system (CNS) lymphoma. Leiomyosarcoma has been reported as a rare complication of HIV infection in children.

Progressive cytopenias (anaemia, thrombocytopenia, leucopenia) commonly occur in HIV-infected patients. The pathophysiological mechanisms are multifactorial and include direct effects of HIV on haematopoietic precursor cells, alterations in the microenvironment of the bone marrow and immunological destruction of peripheral blood cells. The severity of these changes relates to the infections or malignancies superimposed on AIDS and the myelosuppressive effects of anti-retroviral, anti-infective and anti-neoplastic therapies.

Wasting syndrome

Wasting syndrome is categorised as an involuntary weight loss of greater than 10% of baseline body weight and accompanied by greater than 30 days of chronic fever, weakness or diarrhoea. It is linked to disease progression and death. Losing just 5% of body weight can have the same negative effects. Wasting is still a problem for people with AIDS, even people whose HIV is controlled by medications.

AIDS WASTING SYNDROME CRITERIA

AIDS wasting syndrome must meet one of the following criteria:
- unintentional weight loss of >10% over 12 months
- unintentional weight loss of >7.5% over 6 months
- body cell mass (BCM) loss of >5% over 6 months
- men: BCM <35% of total body weight (TBW) and body mass index (BMI) <27 kg/m²
- women: BCM <23% of TBW and BMI <27 kg/m²
- BMI <20 kg/m².
  Research shows that BCM is a better predictor of survival than CD4 counts.

Lipodystrophy/lipoatrophy

Lipodystrophy/lipoatrophy refers to metabolic and morphological alterations among HIV patients receiving highly active anti-retroviral treatment (HAART). It comprises insulin resistance, lipidaemia, abdominal and torsocervical fat accumulation, fat depletion in the extremities and the face, and increased risk for diabetes, heart disease and stroke.[7]

MANAGEMENT OF LIPODYSTROPHY

- Monitor cholesterol and triglyceride levels.
- The first biochemical signal of lipodystrophy is raised triglyceride levels.

Peripheral neuropathy

It is estimated that 42% of people with HIV/AIDS experience some peripheral nerve damage. It can be caused by the virus itself, by NRTIs, other medication or complications, or as a result of opportunistic infections (e.g. cytomegalovirus, candidiasis [thrush], herpes, tuberculosis).[8] Neuropathy can also result from other associated causes such as heavy alcohol consumption, diabetes and vitamin deficiency (B vitamins).

Diarrhoea

This is a common complaint and an issue that can greatly affect quality of life. An HIV+ person might develop diarrhoea for numerous reasons, and the specific aetiology guides the choice of treatment. Causes might include HIV-associated enteropathy, HAART side effects (see specific medications; particularly an issue with protease inhibitors [PIs]), antibiotic side effects, gastrointestinal infections and food allergies or intolerances. An osmotic-type diarrhoea can also result from the consumption of too many indigestible gel caps (from medications and supplements) building up in the lumen of the intestines.

Psychological conditions

- Depression
- Anxiety
- Post-traumatic stress disorder
- Sexual dysfunction
- Substance abuse
- Suicidal ideations and suicide attempt/s.

Blood deficiencies

- Macrocytic anaemia
- Microcytic (iron-deficient) anaemia
- Thrombocytopenia
- Neutropenia
- Lymphocytopenia.

Cancers

- Non-Hodgkin lymphomas
- Primary central nervous system lymphoma
- Hodgkin's disease
- Cervical cancer
- Anal cancer.

DIFFERENTIAL DIAGNOSIS

Due to the confirmation of disease diagnosis, differential diagnosis is not essential. It is important to consider and reflect on the various opportunistic infections possible for a thorough overview of the patient.

Opportunistic infections

As the HIV epidemic evolved in the early 1980s, its diverse manifestations were described and categorised. Patients with opportunistic infections or malignancies were defined as having AIDS. Opportunistic infections and malignancies occur with increasing frequency in patients with declining immune function. See Table 23.4.

NATUROPATHIC DIAGNOSIS

Due to the nature of this condition, naturopathic diagnosis relies on allopathic assessment and confirmation of the presence of disease. Furthermore, it follows traditional assessment and diagnostic strategies for management of patients, remembering that everyone is individual.

Investigations

INITIAL ASSESSMENT: HIV ANTIBODIES

Assessment is conducted via an enzyme-linked immunosorbent assay (ELISA) test and/or Western blot method. It typically takes at least 6 weeks following infection with the virus for antibodies to be detected; however, antibodies generally appear within 3 months after infection with HIV, but may take up to 6 months in some people. The Western blot test is the most sensitive laboratory test for HIV antibodies; ELISAs are used more often, however, as they are less costly and require less time. Table 23.5 compares the various methods used.

VIRAL LOAD

The viral load test measures the amount of HIV virus in a person's blood. A CD4+ cell count helps measure the strength of a person's immune system, whereas a viral load test indicates how active HIV is in their body. Together, these two tests are used to monitor how a person is responding to HIV infection and to HIV treatment.

Viral load is assessed through three different techniques. It is imperative that the same technique is used throughout patient care for more accurate comparison as each can produce different readings.

Quantitative polymerase chain reaction (Q-PCR)

- Commercially known as the Amplicor HIV-1 Monitor Test.
- Most sensitive and can detect very low levels of virus in blood.
- Requires less blood (100–200 µL).
- Gives a viral load value twice as high as b-DNA. As such, it is prudent to use the same method of testing for subsequent assessments.

Branched-chain DNA, or quantiplex (b-DNA)

- Most accurate in quantifying high levels of the virus.
- Requires most blood (2 mL).

Nucleic acid sequence-based amplification (NASBA)

- Requires less blood (100–200 µL).

VIRAL LOAD QUANTITY

The range of viral load can be from <50/mL (undetectable) to millions/mL. A viral load below 10 000 copies/mL is considered 'low', whereas a viral load above 100 000 copies/mL is considered 'high'. Viral load is affected by external stimuli, including another infection or recent vaccination. It is also important to note that approximately 2% of the viral load is in the blood. This assessment does not measure how much HIV is in other body tissues, including lymph nodes, spleen or brain. HIV levels in lymph tissue and semen go down when blood levels go down, but not at the same time or the same rate.

Some research suggests women have lower loads than men (especially in the first few years of infection); however, they have the same viral load at AIDS diagnosis.

T/B/NK CELL SUBSETS: CD3, CD4, CD8, CD19, CD56

CD4+ (found on T helper cells)

CD4+ is a glycoprotein predominantly found on the surface of helper T cells. In humans, it is a receptor for HIV, enabling the virus to gain entry into its host. When HIV infects humans, it infects CD4 cells more frequently than other cells as the HIV mRNA is integrated within the cell. As such, when CD4 cells multiply to fight an infection, they also make more copies of HIV. Regular measurement of CD4+ T lymphocyte count is therefore essential to

	TABLE 23.4 Potential opportunistic infections as the disease progresses		
Body system	**CD4+ >500 early**	**CD4+ 200–500 intermediate**	**CD4+ <200 severe**
Respiratory	Interstitial lung disease	TB, sinusitis	PCP CMV Non-Hodgkin lymphoma Other opportunistic infections
Digestive	Sjögren's syndrome Anorexia	Bacterial gastroenteritis Rotavirus gastroenteritis Oral candidiasis Cryptosporidiosis Hairy leukoplakia GIT Karposi sarcoma and lymphoma	Herpes simplex infections Microsporidiosis Enteritis, colitis, cholangitis Oesophageal *Candida* and ulceration
Nervous	Demyelinating diseases Polymyositis Bell's palsy Guillain–Barré syndrome	Bell's palsy AIDS dementia TIAs Herpes zoster CNS lymphoma	TIAs Nephropathies – sensory, autonomic Hypomania Toxoplasmosis, Cryptococcus, CMV, CNS lymphoma
Haematopoietic	Idiopathic thrombocytopenia Lymphadenopathy Malaise	Kaposi sarcoma Lymphoma (non-Hodgkin)	
Eye	Vasculopathies/vasculitis Ocular inflammation Reiter's syndrome Sicca syndrome	Blepharitis Herpes zoster Molluscum contagiosum Herpes simplex Optic neuritis	Karposi sarcoma Toxoplasmosis CMV retinitis Herpes simplex keratitis
Oral cavity		Gingivitis Candidiasis Hairy leukoplakia Lymphoma Herpes simplex	Non-Hodgkin lymphoma Herpes simplex
Integumentary	Tinea Seborrhoeic dermatitis Impetigo	Tinea Seborrhoeic dermatitis Warts Molloscum contagiosum Herpes zoster Herpes simplex Pityriasis versicolor	Papular/follicular eruptions Kaposi sarcoma Opportunistic infections
Musculoskeletal	Arthralgias Arthritis Vasculitis Lupus-like syndrome	Arthralgias Arthritis Vasculitis Lupus-like syndrome	Arthralgias Arthritis Vasculitis Lupus-like syndrome

AIDS = acquired immune deficiency syndrome; CNS = central nervous system; CMV = cytomegalovirus; GIT = gastrointestinal tract; PCP = *Pneumocystis carinii* pneumonia; TB = tuberculosis; TIA = transient ischaemic attack

assess the progress of the disease and the health of the patient. Percentage of CD4+ cells within total lymphocyte count is also essential.

Normal levels: 600–1500/mm³. Classification of the progression of HIV is determined by a patient's CD4 count.

CD4+ percentage

Alternatively, a CD4 percentage can be ordered.
Normal levels: 28–58%.

CD8+ (found on the surface of killer T cells)

CD8+ is a glycoprotein on the surface of killer T cells that enhances binding with MHC molecules. CD8 binds to human leukocyte antigen (HLA) class I on some other cell, which allows the T cell receptor protein to dock to HLA-I and check the antigen ('Ag'), which HLA is presenting.

Normal levels: 300–800/mm³.

CD4:CD8

Normal = 2:0. In HIV, the ratio is inverted. CD8+ cell level rises, CD4+ cells decrease.

RESISTANCE TESTING

Therapeutic drug monitoring (TDM)

TDM is used to help individualise anti-HIV therapy by measuring the amount of drug in an individual's plasma or

TABLE 23.5 Comparison of assessment methods	
ELISA (EIA)	First screening tool. Inexpensive, sensitive. Performed on blood (typically), but can use saliva or urine. Takes 3.5–4 hours for results
Rapid test	Takes 20–40 minutes by taking a sample from the buccal mucosa to assess for HIV antibodies. Small margin of error, so must be confirmed by a WB
Western blot (WB) assay or indirect immunofluorescence assay (IFA)	Performed if ELISA or rapid test is positive. Used as a confirmatory test
Detuned ELISA	Used in research settings after HIV antibodies are confirmed by a WB. Can determine if an HIV infection is recent (within the past 6 months), so can be useful to determine treatment options

TABLE 23.6 Monitoring the patient	
Assessment	**Justification**
Fasting glucose, insulin, HBA1c	Assess blood sugar level (BSL), query medication side effects
Cholesterol profile including triglycerides	Assess cholesterol levels, query medication side effects
Liver function tests (LFT)	Assess liver function, query medication side effects
Urea and electrolytes (U and E)	Assess kidney function, query medication side effects. Assess blood levels of protein to protect against wasting
Full blood count and erythrocyte sedimentation rate (FBC + ESR)	Assess for presence of anaemia, query medication side effects, assess level of infection from opportunistic infections
Urinalysis	Especially important if taking protease inhibitors
Pap smear	Assess for koilocytotic changes and bacterial dysbiosis
Hepatitis, sexually transmitted infections (STIs)	Holistic assessment of the patient
Other assessments specific to presentation	Such as chest X-ray, skin swabs, etc.

CSF. This enables an individualised assessment of drug metabolism and can enable accurate assessment to calculate the lowest plasma drug concentration to be effective to still inhibit HIV. Some, but not all, studies have shown that using TDM to guide treatment decisions increases the chance of successful viral suppression and can assist in minimising side effects. However, drug level monitoring is not appropriate for all anti-HIV drugs. A study published in 2016 identified that the CD4 to CD8 ratio is inversely associated with carotid intima-media thickness and can be a predictor of heart disease in HIV-infected patients. This now allows clinicians to identify HIV-infected patients who are at risk of developing atherosclerosis and coronary heart disease and offer appropriate interventions.[9]

Genotypic resistance assay

The purpose of this test is to detect the presence of known virus mutations associated with drug resistance. It is used to compare the genetic code of the sample of HIV virus being tested against a 'wildtype' (the most common form of HIV virus). This test can only be performed if the patient has a viral load over about 2000 copies/mL of blood.

Phenotypic assay

Measures the virus's ability to grow in the presence of different combinations of anti-retroviral treatments. This test provides a direct and quantitative measure of the likelihood of resistance developing for individual treatments, and can also be used to determine the optimal dosing of treatments.

Virtual phenotype

Genotype test that is interpreted with the aid of a large database of samples of known genotype and phenotype data. Results are dependent on the number of known matches, and are a simpler method of determining the likelihood of developing resistance.

Abacavir hypersensitivity

Genetic test used to determine the likelihood of a possibly fatal side effect of abacavir (anti-viral medication), known as abacavir hypersensitivity reaction. Wherever possible, it should be performed prior to commencing abacavir.

MONITORING THE PATIENT

See Table 23.6.

SPECIFIC NATUROPATHIC INVESTIGATIONS

See Table 23.7.

Therapeutic considerations

CLINICAL DECISION MAKING AND RATIONALE

Complementary and allopathic medicine (CAM) – a combined approach to treatment

A review published in 2013 reported that a lifetime use of CAM by HIV-positive people ranged from 30 to 90%, with national studies suggesting CAM is used by around 55%. The most common CAM utilised included vitamins, herbs and supplements, followed by prayer, meditation and spiritual approaches. People with HIV using CAM rarely rejected conventional medicine, rather choosing to combine the both for best life expectancy.[10]

TABLE 23.7 Specific naturopathic investigations	
Assessment	**Justification**
Vitamin D	Assess nutrient status and immune- potential
DHEA	Assess impact of DHEA on immune function and hormone cascades
Serum *Candida* Abs	Assess impact of *Candida* spp. on health progression
GI profile	Assess for presence of parasites and query digestive absorption of dietary (and supplemental) intake of nutrients
Co-factor viruses (serum and antibody) e.g. Epstein–Barr virus (EBV), cytomegalovirus (CMV), mycoplasma, toxoplasmosis	Assess for underlying infection and modify treatment accordingly
Homocysteine and MTHFR	Strong links with development and progression of disease. Monitor patient and treat accordingly
IgG and IgE food allergy profile	Assess to ensure no dietary impact on absorption of nutrients
Coeliac profile	Assess to ensure no dietary impact on absorption of nutrients or proinflammatory condition that would compromise health
Thyroid panels	Ensure no thyroid effects are noted and contribute to poor immune response
Iron studies	Ensure iron status is replete for optimal immune function
B$_{12}$ and folate	Assess nutrient status and modify treatment accordingly
Zinc and copper	Assess nutrient status and modify treatment accordingly
Amino acid studies	Due to wasting potential, assessment can indicate protein deficiency and associated amino acid deficiencies
General nutrient and toxic element profile or hair mineral analysis	Assess nutrient and toxic element status

DHEA = dehydroepiandrosterone; GI = gastrointestinal; MTHFR = methylenetetrahydrofolate reductase.

Other considerations

Naturopathy considers a holistic assessment of the patient paramount to accurately determining potential triggers and aggravators for optimal health. These include underlying herpes infection, undiagnosed or underlying intestinal parasites, poor digestive environment, low protein status, nutrient deficiencies, hormonal imbalances, substance abuse or emotional distress.

HOMOCYSTEINE

Elevations in homocysteine have been implicated in HIV-infected patients, particularly in HIV-infected men with lipodystrophy characteristics, including elevated plasma insulin and low levels of adiponectin.[11] Elevated total plasma homocysteine has been established as an independent risk factor for thrombosis and cardiovascular disease,[12] and has been associated with the development and progression of HIV/AIDS.[13] Investigations and supportive treatment are thus essential for successful outcome.

INTESTINAL PARASITES AND VIRAL LOAD

HIV-infected patients are at high risk of gastrointestinal infections that cause diarrhoea, especially when the infections are associated with parasites. Data on parasitic infestations in HIV-infected patients has mostly been conducted in developing countries, particularly poverty-stricken areas. However, parasitic infection can also be found in HIV patients in developed countries.[14] Hence, an interesting correlation has been shown in a number of studies. When HIV patients have been treated with anti-worming medications, it has been associated with a decreased HIV viral load. Albendazole prescribed daily for 3 days at baseline, 3 and 6 months or a dose of 40 mg/kg of praziquantel if schistosomiasis detected showed marked reduction in HIV viral load in 56 HIV-positive adults (p = 0.04).[15] Similarly to homocysteine, this is an important consideration for treatment for both assessment and prescriptions.

Therapeutic application
ALLOPATHIC PERSPECTIVE

Over the past 25 years, there have been a number of changes in the ways HIV infection is understood and managed. These changes have led to great improvements in treatment and management of HIV infection and have greatly increased the range of options available. Since the advent of HAART involving combinations of anti-viral drugs, deaths from AIDS have dramatically declined, and people with HIV on treatments have a much longer life expectancy. There are a number of changes that have led to these improvements[16]:

1 We have a clearer understanding of how HIV works inside the body.

2   The use of the viral load test measuring the amount of HIV circulating in blood is now standard practice in Australia, Europe and North America. The results of this test can help in making treatment decisions. They can also show how well the treatments are working against HIV.

3   Genotyping and phenotyping assays (resistance testing) are used to measure the likelihood of resistance to anti-viral drugs and can provide an indication of which drugs and combinations of drugs are working.

4   We have a clearer idea of the short- and long-term side effects sometimes experienced by people using these drugs and how to manage most of them.

Current recommendations

See Table 23.8.

Classes of HIV medications

1   Nucleoside analogues and NRTIs (also known as 'nukes')
2   NNRTIs ('non-nukes')
3   Protease inhibitors
4   Fusion inhibitors
5   Integrase inhibitors
6   CCR5 entry inhibitors.

Combination therapy

In line with the current international treatment guidelines, widely supported by existing research, it is now standard practice to commence and maintain people on a combination of at least three drugs from two of these classes, or more. The most common combinations include two NRTIs, in combination with either an NNRTI or a PI. Newer multi-combination medications have been produced, and the product Atripla (efavirenz + emtricitabine + tenofovir) is considered the first-line treatment for all new infections.

Medications used in HIV are listed in Table 23.9.

Medication timing

There are no concrete guidelines as to when to start treatment; however, a few guidelines have been developed based on current research. These include:

1   *Recent infection.* A number of smaller studies have suggested that a short course (3 months) of treatment for people with recent HIV infection could help the body's immune system make a more effective response against HIV infection, stabilising the CD4 count to delay CD4 cell decline and the need to take treatments in the future. Unfortunately, there are no studies that strongly suggest any long-term benefit to early treatment. There is also evidence that people with recent HIV infection have higher levels of the HIV virus in their semen, thereby increasing the likelihood of sexual transmission of HIV. Treating people in the first few weeks of HIV infection could help reduce the risk of HIV transmission to sexual partners.[16]

2   *Chronic infection but remain well.* The current treatment guidelines (as of 2008) recommend treatment be offered whenever the CD4 cell count falls below 350. The pendulum is now swinging back towards earlier treatment of people who are well, and some experts would now recommend commencing treatment at CD4 counts about 350. The viral load is less important in determining when to start medication, but if the viral

TABLE 23.8 Current recommendations for medication		
CD4 count	**Viral load**	**Medication indication**
<200	Any	Recommended
200–350	Any	Offered
350+	>100 000	Considered
350+	<100 000	Deferred
Any	Any	Recommended with presence of AIDS-defining illness or with severe symptoms of HIV infection

TABLE 23.9 HIV medications[17]		
Single-table regimens		
Drug	Abbreviation	Generic names
Atripla	N/A	Efavirenz + tenofovir disoproxil fumarate + emtricitabine
Complera	N/A	Rilpivirine + tenofovir disoproxil fumerate + emtricitabine
Genvoya	N/A	Elvitegravir + tenofovir alafenamide + emtricitabine + cobicistat
Odefsey	R + FTC + TAF	Rilpivirine + emtricitabine + tenofovir alafenamide
Stribild	Quad	Elvitegravir + cobicistat + tenofovir disoproxil fumarate + emtricitabine
Triumeq	Triumeq	Dolutegravir + abacavir + lamivudine
Doultegravir + rilpivirine	DTG + RPV	Dolutegravir + rilpivirine
Doravirine + tenofovir disoproxil fumarate + lavivudine	N/A	Doravirine + tenofovir disoproxil fumarate + lamivudine

Continued

TABLE 23.9 HIV medications[17]—cont'd

Nucleoside/nucleotide reverse transcriptase inhibitors (NRTIs)

Drug	Abbreviation	Generic names
Combir*	AZT + 3TC	Zidovudine + lamivudine
Descovy	FTC + TAF	Emtricitabine + tenofovir alafenamide
Emtriva	FTC	Emtricitabine
Epivir	3TC	Lamivudine
Epzicom	ABC + 3TC	Abacavir + lamivudine
Retrovir	AZT	Zidovudine
Trizivir	ABC + AZT + 3TC	Abacavir + zidovudine + lamivudine
Truvada	TDF + FTC	Tenofovir disoproxil fumarate + emtricitabine
Videx EC	DdI	Didanosine
Viread	TDF	Tenofovir disoproxil fumarate
Zerit	D4T	Stavudine
Ziagen	ABC	Abacavir

Non-nucleoside reverse transcriptase inhibitors (NNRTIs)

Drug	Abbreviation	Generic names
Edurant	RPV	Rilpivirine
Intelence	ETR	Etravirine
Rescriptor	DLV	Delavirdine
Sustiva	EFV	Efavirenz
Viramune and Viramune XR	NVP	Nevirapine
Doravirine	N/A	Doravirine

Protease inhibitors (PIs)

Drug	Abbreviation	Generic names
Aptivus	TPV	Tipranavir
Crixivan	IDV	Indinavir
Evotaz	ATV/c	Atazanavir + cabicistat
Invirase	SQV	Saquinavir
Kaletra	LPV/r	Lopinavir + ritonavir
Lexiva	FPV	Fosamprenavir
Norvir	RTV	Ritonavir
Prezcobix	DRV/c	Darunavir + cabicistat
Prezista	DRV	Darunavir
Reyataz	ATV	Atazanavir
Viracept	NFV	Nelfinavir

Integrase inhibitors

Drug	Abbreviation	Generic names
Isentress	RAL	Raltegravir
Tivicay	DTG	Dolutegravir
Vitelta	EVG	Elvitegravir

Entry inhibitors

Drug	Abbreviation	Generic names
Fuzeon	ENF	Enfuvirtide
Selzentry	MVC	Maraviroc

Pharmacokenetic enhancers

Drug	Abbreviation	Generic names
Tybost	N/A	Cobicistat

load is greater than 100 000 per mL, this might be another factor in starting treatment earlier rather than later. The goal of treatment is to prevent progression of HIV disease and the development of symptoms. Currently, no clear long-term benefits have been established for the commencement of HIV treatment for people who are well (i.e. do not have symptoms of HIV infection) and have CD4 counts above 350, although a number of studies do suggest that there may be some benefit in starting with a CD4 count between 350 and 500.[16]

3 *People with a history of AIDS-defining illness, a CD4 count below 200 or severe symptoms of HIV regardless of CD4 count.* Treatment is recommended for any person with symptoms of HIV disease – including neurological HIV disease – or who has experienced an AIDS-defining illness (opportunistic infection) in the past. The goal of treatment is both improvement in health and the prevention of further damage to the immune system or reoccurrence of an AIDS-defining illness.[16]

4 *Pregnant women.* The recommended goal of HIV anti-viral treatment is to reduce HIV viral load, and therefore decrease the chances of vertical transmission from mother to baby.

Medication breaks

The concept of 'drug holidays' was historically recommended as it was believed to help the body adjust to the high toxic burden from the medication. In 2008, a large international trial was used to compare the people who continuously took their drugs and people who took treatment breaks.

The Strategies for Management of Anti-Retroviral Therapy (SMART) trial[18] was a large international trial designed to determine which of two distinct HIV treatment strategies yielded a better clinical outcome over the long term. The trial enrolled HIV-positive participants with CD4+ cell counts of more than 350 cells/mm³ of blood. (CD4+ cells are a type of infection-fighting white blood cell and are a primary target of HIV.) Volunteers were randomised to receive one of two anti-retroviral treatment (ART) strategies: continuous drug therapy, designed to suppress viral load as much as possible (the viral suppression, or VS, arm); or episodic ART (the drug conservation, or DC, arm). The use of ART in the DC arm was determined by the participant's CD4+ cell count: trial participants in the DC arm began ART when CD4+ cell counts fell below 250 cells/mm³, with the aim of suppressing viral load and increasing the CD4+ cell count, and discontinued ART when counts were above 350 cells/mm³. The study, initially designed to last 9 years, was stopped after only 2 years due to the high number of people who took regular treatment breaks who developed AIDS-defining illnesses. The results of this study clearly show that treatment breaks are associated with a rapid fall in CD4 counts and an increase in viral load and illness, as well as the development of multi-drug resistance. As such, it is recommended to continue HAART treatment for greatest clinical outcome.

A study published in 2016 addressed single (STR)- versus multiple (MTR)-tablet HIV regimens. Data was drawn from the Veterans Healthcare Administration with a total of 15 602 (6191 STR and 9411 MTR) patients meeting study criteria. After controlling for baseline covariates, it was found that single treatment regimens had twice the odds of being adherent, 31% significantly lower risk of hospitalisation and 21% higher odds of having an undetectable viral load during follow-up.[19]

HISTORICAL PERSPECTIVE

HIV was first officially recognised in 1981 when five cases of pneumonia as a result of infection with *Pneumocystis jirovecii* were reported in homosexual men. Because of the affected population group, initially the US Centers for Disease Control and Prevention believed that the disease was confined to homosexual males. However, by the end of the year, the infection was observed in heterosexual male injection drug users as well as in countries outside the US.[20] Just short of 2 years later, a retrovirus known as human immunodeficiency virus (or HIV) was isolated from a French homosexual male with AIDS.[21] Two years later, testing procedures were put in place, and by 1985, only 5 years after the initial discovery of HIV, over 17 000 cases of AIDS had been reported from 71 countries to the WHO.

Despite its official recognition in 1981, there is evidence to suggest that HIV existed long before this, with HIV found in a plasma sample taken in 1959 from a male living in the Democratic Republic of Congo.[22] A 2008 study suggested the origin of HIV to be between 1884 and 1924, much earlier than previous estimates.[23]

NATUROPATHIC PERSPECTIVE

The prime objective when treating HIV-positive patients is to integrate our treatment and services within a comprehensive healthcare team. It is expected that most patients will be taking HAART, and as such, treatment will need to complement and enhance the positive effects of HAART and minimise (or treat) side effects.

At all times, it is imperative to focus on encouraging and supporting optimal health in every aspect of a person's life. This may include nutritional, environmental, emotional, mental, sexual and social aspects. Improvements in quality of life and wellbeing should be paramount for all treatment objectives.

Dietary and supplemental recommendations should be encouraged to support optimal nutritional levels. Any deficiency can and will increase the potential for HIV to replicate. Specifically, it is beneficial to provide nutrients that support optimal function and address known triggering deficiencies.

Specifically, naturopathic treatments aim to address the following:
- reduce HIV viral load
- strengthen the immune system
- increase the CD4 count
- reduce oxidative stress and free radical damage

- reduce inflammation
- 'hit it hard and hit it early' to 'delay HAART for as long as possible'.

STAGES OF TREATMENT

When considering treating HIV-positive patients, it is beneficial to consider structuring treatment in a three-stage approach.

Stage 1. CAM only treatment

- Blood parameters are within normal limits – CD4/CD8, neutrophils, white blood cells, platelets, HIV viral load
- Monitor parameters while on herbal treatment
- Recently seroconverted, and those still well, even if already long infected
- Energy levels, sleep and digestion are good
- Patients are well and stable. Immune function is good (the patient is not getting sick regularly).

NATUROPATHIC OBJECTIVE

- Be proactive in treatments.
- Aim to maintain good health.
- Primarily focus on natural treatments and monitor progress closely.
- Avoid the Western medical approach of 'wait and see' for illness to present itself. Conventional strategy is to wait for sickness to start and then prescribe anti-viral medications.

Stage 2. CAM and HAART – as an adjunct

- Patients are already developing some health issues from their HIV, or those who have been stable for a long time but are now declining
- They are not ill enough for medical intervention so are usually able to utilise natural therapies alone for 3–4 months
- Feeling ill regularly and parameters are declining
- Alternative strategies are able to often halt, if not reverse, the immune system's decline.

NATUROPATHIC OBJECTIVE

- Naturopathic regime for 2–4 months without HAART while monitoring the above parameters monthly
- Introduce HAART if the natural therapies fail to stop the decline in parameters
- CAM especially beneficial for HAART side effects (lipodystrophy syndrome)
- Needs constant vigilant monitoring
- Initial symptoms are greatly relieved and controlled through using various alternative strategies – diarrhoea, fatigue, urticaria, bloating and so on.

Stage 3. HAART only or HAART and minimal CAM

- Very unwell
- Many AIDS-defining conditions and symptoms have emerged

- CD4 count is consistently dropping
- Natural killer (NK) cells are unable to perform their tasks as a back-up system for the failure of the CD4s.

NATUROPATHIC OBJECTIVE

- Drug approach is best implemented at this stage in conjunction with alternative medicines
- Introduce HAART and natural therapies concurrently
- Be aware of HAART only times/restrictions
- Consider herb/drug interactions
- Utilise alternative strategies
- Treatment of side effects from medications
- Optimum GIT health
- Enhance immune system functioning
- Assist in optimum nutrient and drug absorption and utilisation
- Complement medication's anti-viral actions
- Utilise herbal anti-viral medications in conjunction as they appear to further decrease the possibilities of drug resistance
- Medication usage is very important and therapeutic benefits far outweigh the toxic side effects at this stage.

NUTRITIONAL MEDICINE (DIETARY)

Limited research has been conducted on the dietary intake, body weight changes or activity levels influencing metabolic dysfunction in HIV-infected individuals and ART use. It has been found that HIV-infected individuals with or without ART are at greater risk of developing insulin resistance compared to HIV-uninfected individuals. This has been associated with altered levels of adipokines such as adiponectin, soluble tumour necrosis factor (TNF) receptor 1 and decreased leptin. In addition, HIV impairs glycolysis, which adversely impacts on glucose metabolism. Therefore, they are at higher risk of developing diabetes, cardiovascular disease and other metabolic disorders, which can be managed through dietary assistance and exercise.[24]

Dietary therapeutic objectives

- Implement a low-glycaemic-index (GI) diet utilising wholefoods (e.g. Mediterranean diet) has been suggested and trialled with benefit.
- Prevent wasting, lipid imbalance or other major side effects associated with medications.
- Provide wholesome, organic and nourishing foods to support the body and repair the immune system.
- A higher than normal intake of nutrients is required due to malabsorption and medication side effects, as well as disease manifestations.
- It is very important to maintain a healthy, highly nutritious, wholefood diet – food should provide nutrition and sustenance and should not cause any extra pressure on the body.
- Increase vegetable juices to cleanse the body.
- Reduce animal products as much as possible, particularly the fat and skin on meats.
- Encourage liver-stimulating foods such as bitter greens.

- Encourage high-fibre foods to support healthy bowel transit time.
- Avoid saturated, rancid and trans fats to reduce cardiovascular risk.
- Avoid refined carbohydrates and sugars to prevent lipodystrophy aggravation.
- Ensure protein needs are met and calculate based on patient's weight to prevent wasting.
- Ensure hydration needs are met and calculate based on patient's weight to prevent dehydration.
- Avoid alcohol, non-organic foods and other liver stressors.
- Only drink filtered/purified water to further reduce the burden on the body.
- Identify food allergies/intolerances as they will compromise nutritional absorption and immunity.

Specific dietary treatments
DIETARY INCLUSIONS
Whole lemon drink

The whole lemon drink is a strongly advocated dietary modification for HIV patients. Patients and clinicians report improvements in biochemicals, weight stabilisation (helps to gain or lose weight depending on the patient), decreases TNF and inflammation, improves digestion and bloating, assists those on HAART and increases oxygenation levels.

One interesting paper[25] assessed the treatment of oral thrush with lemon juice (*Citrus limon*) and lemongrass (*Cymbopogon citratus*). Oral thrush is a frequent complication of HIV infection. In the Moretele Hospice in South Africa, due to financial constraints, the treatment routinely given to patients with oral thrush is either lemon juice directly into the mouth or a lemongrass infusion made from lemongrass grown and dried at the hospice. These two remedies have been found to be very efficacious and, therefore, are used extensively. Gentian violet, the first-line medication for oral thrush in South Africa, is not preferred by primary health clinic patients because of its visible purple stain, which leads to them being stigmatised as HIV positive. *Cymbopogon citratus* and *Citrus limon* have known antifungal properties and results of the randomised controlled trial showed positive outcomes. This is especially useful for financially challenged patients.

> ### Whole lemon drink: recipe
>
> Whole organic lemon – cut into quarters and place in a blender
> Add 1.5 cups of water
> Add 1–2 dessertspoons of organic flaxseed oil
> Add 1–3 capsules lecithin (1.2 g)
> Add 500 IU capsule of vitamin E (broken)
> Add knob of ginger
> Blend for 40–45 seconds
> Strain and press pulp
> Divide liquid into two serves
> Drink whole lemon drink before and during breakfast and dinner.

Wholefood diet

Nutrient status is recognised as an important determinant of HIV outcomes[26]; thus, a diet that is rich in wholefoods that contain an array of nutrients is going to be most beneficial for HIV-positive patients. Studies demonstrate that HIV-positive subjects consuming a diet based upon fruit, vegetables and low-fat dairy show consistently better CD4 counts and higher BMIs than those subjects whose diet is based on fast food.[26]

This type of diet is similar to the Mediterranean diet, which has been recommended for HIV-infected individuals.[24]

Protein

Protein is essential for immune function, growth and repair, so adequate protein intake is critical in patients with HIV/AIDS. In spite of this, protein malnutrition and wasting are commonly observed in this patient population. Supplementation with whey protein (40 g/twice daily) has been found to increase CD4 cell counts over a 3-month period, but failed to increase weight or lean body mass in patients with HIV.[23,27] Whey protein may not be tolerated by all patients. Therefore, it is imperative that, first, the correct protein is chosen (e.g. whey, rice, soy, etc.), and second, that it is of good quality (i.e. without sugars and colours, has minimal preservatives, etc.).

Momordica charantia (bitter melon)

Momordica charantia has been used medicinally in Indian and Thai cultures due to its anti-viral and immune-boosting properties.[28] Researchers have discovered a number of ribosome-inactivating proteins from within *M. charantia* that act against multiple stages of the HIV viral life cycle, on acute infection as well as replication in chronically infected cells.[29] One of these proteins, MAP30, when used together with anti-retroviral drugs, was found to improve anti-HIV therapy. The action of MAP30 is additionally exciting as it displays itself to be active against infection and replication of HIV cells, but is non-toxic to normal cells.[30] Furthermore *M. charantia* is known to exert beneficial effects on healthy blood sugar. Therefore, in patients with HIV who present with insulin resistance, dietary intake of *M. charantia* is likely to be beneficial.

HOW TO USE BITTER MELON

Somewhat misleadingly, the taste and appearance of bitter melon are actually nothing like a melon; however, bitter melon is extremely bitter. Therefore, some patients may view the suggestion of its addition to their diet with some resistance.

Bitter melon can be prepared by extracting juices from fresh leaves and fruits and adding purified water to the extract to control the potency.[28] Another preparation involves bringing 1 kg of leaves and fruits in 3.8 L of purified water to a boil, allowing it to simmer for 5 minutes, filtering the decoction in a sterile strainer and storing it in the refrigerator.

This therapy can be administered either orally or via the rectum via an enema if taste is an issue, but should be consumed on a daily basis. Rebultan[28] describes a client partaking in bitter melon therapy whose energy level increased rapidly and whose physical stamina and appetite improved. One year after therapy began, his CD4 count increased greatly. Later, his CD4 to CD8 ratios had returned to normal.

Spirulina platensis (blue-green algae)

Spirulina platensis is a filamentous cyanobacterium that provides rich concentrations of beneficial nutrients in a natural form. Spirulina has been referred to as the 'poor man's HAART'[31] and has been observed to inhibit the HIV virus both in vitro and in vivo. Spirulina has a beneficial effect on the immune system, with it being shown to increase the phagocytic activity of macrophages, increase accumulation of NK cells into tissue and activation and mobilisation of T and B cells.[32] Spirulina contains phycocyanin, a rare blue pigment unique to spirulina. Phycocyanin is a powerful antioxidant and immune system stimulant.

Spirulina is a complete protein and contains all 22 essential amino acids; this further adds to its therapeutic benefits for patients with HIV, as many tend to be protein malnourished. Interestingly, it has been noted that the Kanembu tribe of Chad, in Africa, who consume high quantities of blue-green algae, have a lower incidence of HIV/AIDS (2–3%) compared to other African countries (40%) where blue-green algae is not consumed.[31] Thus, it would appear that regular consumption of dietary algae may help prevent HIV infection and suppress viral load among those infected.

Macrobiotic foods

Umeboshi are pickled plums (although they are actually a species of apricot) from the macrobiotic tradition. Umeboshi are used medicinally for their alkalising properties and their ability to stimulate digestion and relieve fatigue.[33] Sea vegetables such as wakame, kombu, arame, nori and hijiki may also be useful; these are high in minerals and other nutrients that may not be found in land foods as a result of soil depletion. Many sea vegetables also display anti-viral properties that may help to inhibit replication of the HIV virus. For example, fucoidan, a constituent within the brown seaweed Adenocystis utricularis, displays potent anti-HIV activity in vivo and has been shown to interfere with all stages of viral replication.[34]

DIETARY EXCLUSIONS

Caffeine

Caffeine is a diuretic that encourages the loss of much needed nutrients from the body. Excessive intake of caffeine is also associated with a negative effect on bone health in patients with HIV, who have an increased risk of osteoarthritis (see section on calcium), and in whom caffeine intake is likely to further promote bone loss. Furthermore, caffeine places stress on the adrenals; in this patient population, it is recognised that stress and depression are substantial, and therefore implementing strategies that nurture the adrenals rather than deplete them is preferential. Currently, no studies have been conducted on caffeine and HIV-infected individuals.

Alcohol

As with caffeine, alcohol depletes the body of much needed nutrients, increases reactive oxygen species and impairs immune status in patients with HIV.[35] Intake of alcohol is high in many patients with HIV; however, it is important to counsel patients on the link between intake of alcohol and increased progression of disease. Among patients who have a history of alcohol problems and are receiving ART, alcohol consumption has been associated with higher HIV RNA levels and lower CD4 counts.[36] Lower CD4 cell counts have also been observed in individuals not on ART with heavy intake of alcohol.[37] Additionally, alcohol may also increase the risk of developing HIV-related symptoms such as lipodystrophy.[38]

Another factor that needs to be discussed with patients regarding binge drinking is that alcohol intake may encourage risk-taking behaviour such as unprotected sexual intercourse (increasing risk of transmission of the HIV virus to others), as well as less adherence with medications.[39] Furthermore, in patients who already have coexisting liver disease such as hepatitis infection, the removal of alcohol from the diet is even more important. It must also be acknowledged that alcohol may be used as a coping mechanism. Therefore, before removing it completely, this issue needs to be addressed.

Sugar

Many Western diets contain high quantities of sugar, but in the patient with HIV infection, this must be reduced or omitted. A high-refined diet including large amounts of processed sugar foods increases the risk of metabolic disorders, diabetes, cardiovascular disease and immune suppression, all of which are adverse events for HIV-infected people. In one paper, it was shown that 2–4 teaspoons of sugar suppressed neutrophil function by 92%.[37] It is important to remember that one can of soft drink can contain up to 10 teaspoons of sugar. Avoiding all sources is essential.

Many high-sugar foods (e.g. lollies) are devoid of nutrients and will thus create a nutrient-deficit diet where nutritious foods could have been consumed instead. Minimising sugar from the diet will also reduce oral candidiasis in HIV-positive patients.[40] Similar benefits would result for systemic candidiasis as blood glucose levels have been linked with increased Candida status in the body. Moreover, high glucose intake from processed foods increases the development of insulin resistance, which as mentioned, is common among HIV-infected individuals.

Carbohydrate-rich foods

Refined carbohydrate foods are highly processed and tend to be stripped of beneficial nutrients. In a similar manner to the recommendations made above with regards to sugar, refined carbohydrates are likely to increase insulin resistance and provide a feeding ground for microbial pathogens in patients with oral Candida. Starchy carbohydrates are also likely to be too heavy on the digestion of patients with HIV who have poor appetite and feel overly full before the meal is consumed. For these reasons, refined carbohydrates should not make up the majority of the meal.

Preservatives, colourings, additives

Preservatives, colourings and additives are foreign substances to the body and their ingestion places extra stress on the body to aid in their breakdown and removal. Furthermore, the very presence of these substances in a food implies the food is not fresh and thus is unlikely to provide the same health benefits as fresh foods.

Trans fatty acids

Increased intake of saturated fat has been demonstrated to contribute to hypertriglyceridaemia among HIV-infected patients, many of whom display metabolic abnormalities.[41] Trans fatty acids have been shown to increase the risk of cardiovascular disease. Therefore, increased saturated fat

intake should be targeted for dietary modification in this population.

OTHER DIETARY CONSIDERATIONS

Vegetarian diet

A vegetarian diet may be of use in patients with HIV if implemented correctly. A vegetarian diet that is based upon an array of fresh wholefoods with optimal fruit, vegetables and protein is likely to be medicinally therapeutic. However, a vegetarian diet based on tinned and processed foods such as cereals for breakfast, banana bread for morning tea and a cheese sandwich for lunch is unlikely to bring about the same benefits, as it is not producing the nutrients required for a healthy body.

A well-designed vegetarian diet that encompasses a wide variety of plant foods has been shown to provide a number of therapeutic benefits.[42] Thus, if implementing a vegetarian diet, it is important for patients to receive adequate education on how to plan their diets to ensure both adequate nutrient intake and maximum benefit.

SAMPLE DAILY DIET

On waking		
Water with slippery elm powder		Assists with healthy digestive function, which is known to be compromised in patients with HIV (see the slippery elm section for more information).
Breakfast	Smoothie made from soaked oats, flaxseed, seasonal fruit, greens, cinnamon and kefir.	A smoothie provides an easy-to-assimilate nutrient breakfast. Oats, flaxseed, fruit and greens are rich in fibre. Increased fibre improves insulin resistance and decreases hyperlipidaemia associated with HAART in HIV-infected adults.[43,44] The addition of cinnamon further helps to improve insulin resistance, while the fruit and greens provide a source of immune-boosting nutrients. Kefir provides a source of beneficial bacteria. Supplementing combined ART with probiotics in individuals infected with HIV may improve GI tract immunity and reduce microbial translocation, reducing inflammation and improving prognosis.[45]
	Steamed salmon with lemon and dill served with brown rice, beetroot, feta, corn and pickles.	Reduced serum level of micronutrients is common in HIV disease[46];thus, a nutrient-rich diet is advocated. Adequate protein is required for immune function, which is imperative since protein intakes have been found to be below RDIs in some populations. Omega-3 fatty acids have been shown to decrease depressive symptoms in individuals with HIV[47] as well as reduce elevated triglycerides; thus, oily fish should be consumed regularly in the diet. Increased saturated fats assists with the development of lipodystrophy[48] and should be replaced with monounsaturated fatty acids coming from avocado, nuts and seeds. Probiotic support is required for immune health if consumed regularly.
	Miso broth with tamari, gai lan, nori, ginger, pumpkin and noodles.	Leafy green vegetables such as gai lan are a source of folate and magnesium. Lower intakes of both folate and magnesium are associated with higher incidences of depression in individuals living with HIV.[49] Miso is a source of both prebiotics and probiotics for immune and gut health.
Snacks	Basil and garlic pesto with crackers Fresh fruit and vegetables Green tea Bitter melon juice	Basil is antimicrobial to help prevent opportunistic infections. Garlic is a potent anti-viral and immune stimulant. Fresh fruit and vegetables support healthy immune function Constituents within green tea display anti-HIV-1 activity Bitter melon/gourd displays anti-HIV activity and may also be used as a dietary strategy to decrease HIV associated hyperlipidaemia. It can be found at the greengrocers or Asian shops.

NUTRITIONAL MEDICINE (SUPPLEMENTAL)

Therapeutic objectives

- Address constitutional symptoms if present and address any underlying genetic weakness that may aggravate or potentiate the disease.
- Prevent and support medication side effects (both minor and major).
- Prevent and support symptoms of immunosuppression.
- Provide antioxidants to protect against and treat the medication's toll on the body.
- Provide specific anti-viral therapy and immunomodulation using other non-drug treatments.

Specific nutrients required

VITAMIN B COMPLEX

Regular intake of B vitamins has been suggested by Zha et al.[50] to slow down the development of AIDS in asymptomatic HIV-infected patients by preventing immune compromisation due to vitamin B deficiencies and compensating for nutrient deficiencies induced by the retrovirus infection.

Requirements for vitamin B1 appear to be increased in patients with HIV/AIDS due to moderate to severe thiamine deficiencies being observed in patients,[51] which may correlate to HIV-related symptoms of fatigue and lethargy. Most importantly, patients with adequate intakes of vitamins B and C have been shown to have a decreased progression from HIV to AIDS.[52] Vitamin B_1 and vitamin B_2 have also been suggested to reduce lactic acidosis, a rare but life-threatening condition fairly common in HIV-infected individuals which is thought to result from the use of HAART. A deficiency of vitamin B_1 and vitamin B_2 are thought to contribute to hyperlactic acidaemia; thus, supplementation may reduce high levels of lactic acid.[53] Niacin has been suggested to help manage dyslipidaemia in patients with HIV[54,55] in addition to providing other benefits such as assisting protein, carbohydrate and fat metabolism.

Vitamin B_6 is one of the key B vitamins for patients with HIV due to its assistance with immune function. However, a deficiency of vitamin B_6 is common in patients with HIV, and has been shown to be related to the disease state. For example, overtly deficient subjects display much lower lymphocyte responsiveness to the mitogens phytohaemagglutinin and pokeweed and reduced natural killer cell cytotoxicity when compared to individuals with adequate vitamin B_6.[56] Vitamin B_6 has also been suggested to be helpful in reducing psychological stress in patients with HIV infection, possibly through its biochemical involvement with neurotransmitters.[57]

A deficiency of vitamin B_{12} is commonly observed in patients with HIV and may occur due to a number of factors, including chronic diarrhoea and malabsorption.[58,59] A deficiency in vitamin B_{12} leads to pernicious anaemia and can alter immune function. Therefore, testing for all patients is highly recommended.

NIACIN AND LIPODYSTROPHY

Sixteen patients with intra-abdominal fat (IAF) area >70 cm were given niacin therapy at median dose of 3000 mg/day ≥6 months. Results indicated that IAF was decreased by 26.9% in 81% of patients (13/16) who took niacin for 1 year. The same participants' high-density lipoprotein (HDL) cholesterol also increased from 35.4 to 43.1 mg/dL, leading the authors to make an association between niacin, reduced IAF and increased HDL.[60]

VITAMIN A

Vitamin A is an important nutrient for T immune function in patients with HIV infection; however, deficiency is common.[61] A vitamin A deficiency increases cytotoxicity to natural killer cells[62] as well as T cell counts, including the CD4 cells. Observational studies suggest that advanced HIV disease may suppress the release of vitamin A from the liver.[63] However, other contributing factors for a deficiency of vitamin A may also include poor dietary intake or malabsorption issues.

BETA-CAROTENE

Beta-carotene is a carotenoid and is an essential nutrient for normal growth, development, immune function and vision. Supplementation with beta-carotene (180 mg/day) in HIV-positive patients resulted in an increase in total white blood cell count (p = 0.01), a percentage change in CD4 count (p = 0.02) and a percentage hange in CD4 to CD8 ratios (p = 0.02) compared to placebo, revealing beta-carotene to have an immune-stimulating effect in patients positive for HIV.[64]

VITAMIN C

Vitamin C is required for the growth and repair of tissues, is an important cofactor for collagen production, aids in wound healing and assists the immune system. Low plasma levels of vitamin C have been found in individuals with HIV, suggesting that requirements for vitamin C for people who are HIV positive are increased.[65] However, there are limited good-quality studies examing vitamin C status or vitamin C supplementation in HIV-infected individuals.

VITAMIN D

Vitamin D is a potent immune modulator, with numerous studies highlighting its function within the immune system. There is considerable evidence to support its prescription in a number of autoimmune conditions and cancer. A number of studies have now been conducted on vitamin D status in HIV-infected individuals as well as medication-induced vitamin D deficiencies. García-Álvarez et al.[66] examined vitamin D status in a cross-sectional study evaluating bacterial DNA translocation. The authors found that optimal (no less than 75 nmol/L) vitamin D plasma levels were associated with lower bacterial translocation and inflammation in HIV and hepatitis C co-infected patients.

It has also been found that the introduction of the efavirenz-based combination anti-retroviral therapy (cART) has been associated with a vitamin D deficiency. A study published in August 2016[67] found that low plasma cholesterol levels, high CYP3A activity and high plasma efavirenz concentrations were significant predictors of an early vitamin D-induced deficiency. It is suggested that supplementation with vitamin D occur in all patients being administered cART.

VITAMIN E

High serum levels of vitamin E have been linked with slower HIV-1 disease progression.[68] Vitamin E deficiencies have been identified in patients with HIV, in particular patients on new anti-retroviral medication. There was a significant association between low cholesterol levels and very low vitamin E status, mainly due to the relationship between liposoluble vitamins and lipid profiles.[69] Vitamin E supplementation (800 IU/day) has shown association with reduced viral load.[70]

SELENIUM

Selenium levels are highly significant in relation to predicting AIDS-related mortality. In addition, the HIV virus has been found to manufacture selenoproteins that are involved in the regulation of viral replication, which may lead to lower selenium levels in HIV-infected individuals.[71] Selenium displays significant immune and antioxidant defence mechanisms likely to be beneficial in patients with HIV infection. Selenium is indicated to slow HIV proliferation, decrease HIV-associated mortality, decrease anxiety in HIV+ recreational drug users and decrease hospitalisation and cost of caring for HIV+ patients. It is considered to be a prime deficiency of long duration in most patients and is found with or without diarrhoea and malabsorption. Levels of selenium reduce as the disease progresses and correlate with albumin levels, lean body mass and total lymphocyte count – all markers of immune function. Deficiency is associated with heart disease, anaemia, thrush (especially oral) and a reduction in CD4+ count.

A number of clinical trials have assessed the role of selenium on various health parameters, with promising results. A randomised clinical trial published in 2015 examined the effect of selenium supplementation on CD4-T cell counts, viral suppression and time to anti-retroviral therapy (ART) in ART-naïve HIV-infected patients in Rwanda. Of the 300 patients, 149 received 200 micrograms of selenium daily for 24 months. The rate of CD4 depletion was reduced by 43.8%, with no other statistically significant results found.[72]

Burbano et al. evaluated the impact of selenium chemoprevention (200 micrograms/day) on hospitalisations in 186 HIV-positive individuals with a history of illegal drug use over a 2-year period.[73] At 2 years, total hospital admission rates as a result of opportunist infections and HIV-related infections were reduced in the selenium group compared to the placebo. As a result, the cost for hospitalisation decreased 58% in the selenium group, compared to a 30% decrease in the placebo group. In the final analyses, selenium therapy continued to be a significant independent factor associated with lower risk of hospitalisation, leading the authors to conclude that

selenium supplementation appears to be a beneficial adjuvant treatment to decrease hospitalisations as well as the cost of caring for HIV-1-infected patients. This study was not without its methodological errors (e.g. limited external validity); however, it provides an insight into the action of selenium's use in patients with HIV infection.

ESSENTIAL FATTY ACIDS

HIV is characterised by gradual destruction of the immune system. Thus, the omega-3 fatty acids that are known for their immune-modulating action have been suggested to be useful for patients with HIV infection. Omega-3 fatty acids may also be well utilised to help manage coexisting symptoms such as hyperlipidaemia and metabolic syndrome, which may be caused by anti-retroviral therapy. A number of studies have demonstrated the efficacy of supplementation with omega-3 fatty acids in HIV, with beneficial results seen with regards to a reduction of serum triglycerides[74,75] and decreased arachidonic acid.[75]

Omega-3 fatty acid supplementation has also been found to improve depressive symptoms in HIV-infected individuals within 8 weeks of supplementation without any significant adverse reactions.[47]

ZINC

Zinc plays a key role in maintaining a healthy immune system as well as functioning as an antioxidant in patients with HIV infection. Deficiency is common in individuals with HIV and is said to be the most prevalent micronutrient abnormality observed in HIV infection.[76] Zinc can be shuttled from blood to tissue in times of stress or illness; thus, plasma levels may not reflect its true concentration in the body. A study assessing breast milk composition in HIV-infected and HIV-uninfected mothers found that zinc levels were significantly lower in HIV-infected women compared to those not infected.[77]

Deficiency of zinc is associated with impaired immunity and increased risk of infection. In illegal drug users, low plasma levels of zinc are estimated to account for a three-fold increase in HIV-related mortality.[78] Baum et al. note that the correct quantity of zinc administered is crucial as deficiency, as well as excessive dietary intake of zinc, has been linked with declining CD4 cell counts and reduced survival.[76]

In one paper,[79] oral zinc sulfate (0.45 mg/kg/day elemental zinc) for 10 weeks showed a significant increase in mean CD4+ cells (from 280 to 390/mm^3) (p <0.05). In addition, oral zinc (12 mg daily for 30 days) + AZT caused a decreased risk of opportunistic infections.

IRON

Iron deficiency is a common manifestation in HIV and occurs due to various reasons. These include alterations in the metabolism of iron and the direct inhibitory effect of HIV on red cell precursors, as well as such factors as dietary deficiency, anaemia of chronic disease and medication use.[80] A study conducted in Ghana assessed the prevalence of anaemia and markers of iron homeostasis in HIV patients. In this cohort, the authors found that anaemia was common and related to HAART status and disease progression. The authors' conclusion was that HIV itself was the most important cause of anaemia and treatment of HIV should be a priority, rather than iron supplementation.[81] Although this was the authors' conclusion, if a person is iron deficient, iron supplementation should be initiated.

COPPER

Copper is an antioxidant and has been found to inhibit viral replication.[82] Deficiencies of copper are associated with AZT therapy and AIDS. It is necessary as part of some of the enzymes that help inactivate free radicals. Supplementation is not recommended unless found deficient, but it is an important mineral to test.

COENZYME Q10 (COQ10)

CoQ10 is found in every cell of the body and is required for ATP production in the cell mitochondria, and thus may be useful for managing symptoms of fatigue in patients with HIV infection. A randomised clinical trial addressing the effect of rosuvastatin on plasma CoQ10 in HIV-infected individuals on anti-retroviral therapy found that 10 mg of rosuvastatin daily decreases CoQ10 concentrations in this cohort. This study assessed 147 patients, 78% which were male and 68% African American.[83]

In a small study involving seven patients, patients with AIDS and HIV were observed to have lower concentrations than controls of CoQ10.[84] Deficiency of CoQ10 was noted to increase with severity of the disease; for example, patients with AIDS were more deficient in CoQ10 than patients with HIV. Supplementation with CoQ10 (despite poor compliance) produced encouraging results in those patients who finished the study.

CoQ10 also functions as an antioxidant and has been shown to contribute to healthy oxidant defence mechanisms in male patients with HIV when used with other antioxidants.[85] Coenzyme supplementation has also been suggested for HIV-infected patients looking to counteract mitochondrial damage as a side effect from certain medications, such as the anti-retroviral drug zidovudine. Drug-related side effects such as skeletal myopathy have been shown to respond well to supplementation with 300 mg/day CoQ10 without cessation of drug therapy.[86] The dose of CoQ10 may be lowered as symptoms abate and then held at a maintenance dose.

PROBIOTICS

A majority of research has recently focused on probiotics and the microbiome in many different disease states. For HIV-infected patients, a systematic review published in 2016 assessed the effect of probiotics on CD4 counts. The overall conclusion collectively suggested that daily consumption of probiotics over a prolonged period of time may improve CD4 counts in HIV-infected people.[87] Other studies have assessed the microbiome alterations in HIV-infected people, concluding that the microbiome plays an important role in the pathogenesis of HIV disease, and also that the modulation of the microbiome could be an important therapeutic target to improve HIV-infected

patients' health.[88] A report from the 8th International Yakult Symposium put forward recommendations in gastroenterology guidelines regarding the proactive approach and benefit of probiotic supplementation in HIV-infected patients.[89]

In addition, the use of anti-retroviral medication for HIV is associated with a high prevalence of diarrhoea and gastrointestinal upset. Given the discomfort symptoms such as these can cause, and the known benefits of probiotics in reducing these uncomfortable symptoms, supplementation with probiotics is highly recommended. A combination of probiotics, soluble fibre and glutamine has been found to significantly reduce diarrhoea in HIV-positive males with diarrhoea (2+ liquid stools/day) as a result of medication.[90] The men were administered a combination of probiotics (1.2 g/day) and soluble fibre (11 g/day) over a 12-week period. At 4 weeks, patients with persistent diarrhoea were also given 30 g/day L-glutamine. Diarrhoea completely resolved in 10 of 28 subjects, with the mean number of stools per day declining. Fifteen subjects did not obtain full relief with probiotics and fibre, but the number of stools passed each day decreased substantially after administration of glutamine. In their study, Wolf et al. found faecal levels of lactobacilli in HIV-positive males to be lower than those of the general population.[91] They examined safety and tolerance with administration of *Lactobacillus rueteri* in HIV-positive males, finding it to be tolerated well. While no differences were noted in bowel function, faecal odour and consistency were improved. A specific strain of lactobacillus isolated from the human mouth is under development. This probiotic has been found to block HIV transmission via breastfeeding by capturing the HIV and binding to its envelope.[92]

ALPHA-LIPOIC ACID

Alpha-lipoic acid is a powerful antioxidant with many therapeutic benefits in managing HIV infection. Early in vitro studies demonstrated alpha-lipoic acid's ability to inhibit the replication of the HIV-1 virus.[93] Other studies have demonstrated the ability of alpha-lipoic acid to inhibit NF-κB activation in human T cells by scavenging reactive oxygen species, thus blocking the activation of NF-κB, and subsequently, HIV transcription.[94] Decreased glutathione levels are common in patients with HIV or AIDS; however, alpha-lipoic acid improved functional reactivity of lymphocytes to T cell mitogens in HIV patients with history of unresponsiveness to HAART.[95]

In one small clinical trial, 11 AIDS-diagnosed patients were prescribed 450 mg lipoic acid daily for 14 days. Results were impressive and showed increased plasma ascorbate, increased total glutathione, increased total plasma thiols and increased CD4 and CD4 to CD8 ratios. What was most impressive was the significant increase in CD4+ count (6 out of 10 cases) and decrease in lipid peroxide levels in all participants.[96]

ACETYL-L-CARNITINE

It is recognised that many patients with HIV/AIDS are likely to be deficient in carnitine due to such factors as increased risk of malabsorption or medication use. Supplementation with acetyl-L-carnitine has demonstrated positive results in patients on high-dose NRTI medications, as many of these medications inhibit mitochondrial function[97] and promote oxidation. A mouse study found that acetyl-L-carnitine may prove to be preventive for neurological side effects of anti-retroviral therapy in mothers on fetus/newborns. The authors noticed that supplementation of acetyl-L-carnitine throughout the entire pregnancy was effective in preventing/ameliorating the neurochemical, neuroendocrine and behavioural adverse effects induced by AZT in the offspring.[98]

N-ACETYLCYSTEINE (NAC)

Higher risk of cardiovascular disease has been found in HIV-infected individuals compared to the general population, particularly in older persons.[99] A randomised, double-blind, three-arm, parallel-group, placebo-controlled, 8-week pilot trial in HIV-infected people aged 50 years old or older receiving virologically suppressive ART was conducted. It assessed the safety and efficacy of a registered NAC supplement. The three arms consisted of NAC 900 mg twice daily, NAC 1800 mg twice daily or matching placebo. The supplements were generally well tolerated in this study. The results found that the levels of glutathione in red blood cells increased substantially and flow-mediated dilation also increased, suggesting an improvement in endothelial function. No changes in malondialdehydra were noted; therefore, benefit may not be due to antioxidant activity.[100]

CALCIUM

Skeletal modifications including reduced bone density and bone insufficiency fractures have been observed in a number of studies in patients with long-term HIV infection, with a meta-analysis of 11 cross-sectional studies published over approximately a 40-year period observing that 15% out of a group of 884 HIV patients had osteoporosis and 52% had osteopenia.[101] A number of reasons have been proposed for the bone loss observed in HIV-infected individuals, including medication use, malabsorption and dietary insufficiency, as well as the possibility that bone loss may occur as a direct result of the HIV virus itself affecting osteoclast function[102] – all theories are likely to be influential.

A randomised trial assessing vitamin D and calcium for bone loss in anti-retroviral therapy assessed 165 HIV-infected patients over 48 weeks. The study found that supplementation with vitamin D (800 IU daily) and calcium (500 mg daily) for 48 weeks was statistically significant in mitigating the loss of bone mineral density seen with intiation of efavirenz/emtricitabine/tenofovir, particularly in the hip.[103] Therefore, from both a medical and naturopathic perspective, it is imperative to supplement with calcium and vitamin D_3 to prevent long-term fracture complications in HIV-infected patients.

MAGNESIUM

Given its multiple roles in the body, adequate intake of magnesium is essential in patients with HIV infection.

Intake of magnesium may help with complaints of fatigue due to magnesium's role in the mitochondria, as well deviations in mood due to magnesium's role in healthy neurotransmitter function. Magnesium has been used successfully in HIV-negative individuals for managing symptoms of insulin resistance and cardiovascular disease.[104] Thus, it is also likely to provide similar benefits in patients who are HIV positive. Low magnesium levels have been found in individuals positive for HIV, and have been found to occur early in the disease. Bogden et al.[105] found that the lowest erythrocyte magnesium concentrations occurred in HIV-infected subjects who consumed alcoholic beverages. Thus, this is something that must be acknowledged when assisting patients who regularly consume alcohol.

CHROMIUM

Many patients with HIV are on multiple medications; one side effect of these multi-drug regimens is insulin resistance. In fact, these drug regimens are estimated to increase insulin resistance by up to 50%.[106] As with the general population, insulin resistance predisposes patients with HIV infection to increased risk of diabetes, cardiovascular disease and metabolic syndrome.

A randomised, double-blind, placebo-controlled trial of participants receiving 500 micrograms of chromium picolinate or placebo twice daily for 2 months was conducted in HIV-infected patients on anti-retroviral therapy. Of the 43 participants enrolled, 39 completed the study. However, chromium supplementation was found not to be effective for reducing insulin resistance in these HIV-infected patients. These findings were based on the glucose tolerance test and insulin level tests.[107]

Nevertheless, supplementation with chromium has been shown to have beneficial effects in some individuals with HIV; these improvements are seen in insulin resistance[106] and other metabolic abnormalities such as triglycerides, body fat mass and trunk mass.[105]

Dosage requirements

The dosage requirements listed below are based on adult doses and what is reported in the literature.

- B complex: 1–2 high-potency B complex with added B vitamins as below, depending on presentation:
- B_1: 100 mg/day
- B_6: 50 mg/day
- B_9: 400–1000 micrograms/day
- B_{12}: 1000 micrograms cyanocobalamin sublingual or activated form
- Vitamin A: 25 000–100 000 IU/day for a few weeks[108]
- Beta-carotene: 180 mg/day
- Vitamin C: 2000 mg/t.i.d[108]
- Vitamin D: investigation results dependent. Minimum of 1000 IU/day
- Vitamin E: 400 IU b.i.d. (mixed tocopherols)[108]
- Essential fatty acids. For reducing hyperlipidaemia associated with HAART, omega-3 fatty acids 300 mg containing EPA: 180 mg/day and DHA: 120 mg/day (× 9 capsules).[74] For healthy cell membranes: 5 g/day

- Calcium: 400–1000 mg/day (depending on severity of lipodystrophy; higher doses should be split so no more than 500 mg are ingested in a dose)
- Chromium: 200–400 micrograms/day (depending on severity of lipodystrophy)
- Copper: 2 mg/day
- Iron: assess blood levels first. Highest dose should not be higher than 25–50 mg/day
- Magnesium: 300–500 mg/day
- Selenium: 400 micrograms/day
- Zinc: 25–50 mg/day
- CoQ10: 30–100 mg t.d.s. (between meals)[108]
- Probiotics – dependent upon condition; for example, strain and dose will be dependent upon symptom (e.g. diarrhoea versus *Candida*)
- Alpha-lipoic acid: 200 mg/day t.d.s.[108]
- Acetyl-L-carnitine: 2–6 g/day (away from food)
- NAC: 1000–4000 mg/b.i.d.[108]
- Protein: calculate based on patient's weight and general health. Range may be between 0.8 and 1.4 g/kg.

HERBAL MEDICINE

Therapeutic objectives

- Support patients taking allopathic medications and associated side effects.
- Provide antioxidant herbal medicine to reduce oxidative stress.
- Improve nutritional status, GIT absorption, heal and seal the GIT, improve lymphatic function in GIT. It is important to remember that HIV is a lymphatic disease as well, and the GALT – gut-associated lymphoid tissue – is strongly associated. The more dysfunctional the gut, the more HIV disease seems to progress.
- Address constitutional symptoms if present and address any underlying genetic weakness that may aggravate or potentiate the disease.
- Prevent and support medication side effects (both minor and major).
- Prevent and support symptoms of immunosuppression.
- Provide antioxidant herbal medicines to protect and address medication's toll on the body.
- Provide specific anti-viral therapy and immunomodulation using other non-drug treatments.

HAART and herbal medicine – potential side effects

The combination of HAART and herbal medicine opens many questions for both patient and practitioner. HAART can initiate a toxic overload to the body. The human body is constantly bombarded with exposure to environmental toxins including xenoestrogens from plastics, pesticides, heavy metals in fertilisers, and others. It is believed that this overload is compounded by the toxicity caused by HAART. When herbal medicines are added into the equation, it may occasionally cause a detoxification reaction.

QUESTIONS FOR THE PRACTITIONER

When presented with a potential reaction, practitioners should ask themselves the following questions:
- Are the side effects caused by drug–drug or herb–drug interactions? If there is any doubt, discontinue the herbal medicine for at least 3 days to see if the symptoms resolve.
- If the symptoms resolve, was:
  1 the dose of the herbal medicine too high?
  2 the herbal medicine introduced too fast?
- If the symptoms do not resolve, the reaction is most likely connected to the medication.

CLINICAL SITUATION

We are presented with a number of queries regarding the interaction of herbal medicines and HAART. For safety, it is prudent to avoid concurrent application; however, it is beneficial to review the evidence of published papers and assess whether a study mirrors a clinical situation. In a clinical scenario, it is likely that some patients will be on both herbal treatment and HAART concurrently. Does science mirror this clinical situation or are the two treatments given separately or intermittently, as appears the case with the cited drug–herb interactions in the literature? Look at the following example and acknowledge that questions are required when considering the clinical efficacy of the study design and delivery.

Example of herb–drug interaction

The best known negative herb–drug interaction in herbal medicine is that between *Hypericum perforatum* (St John's wort) and indinavir. In one study, *H. perforatum* was shown to decrease indinavir levels. As such, it is absolutely contraindicated while a patient is taking medications, especially NNRTIs and PIs. St John's wort has been noted to increase the action of the hepatic cytochrome P450 enzyme system, which may decrease the efficacy of these medications.

When reviewing the results of one study,[109] published in *The Lancet*, we can see that the study design was poor.

STUDY RESULTS

Day 1: 3 × 800 mg indinavir at 8-hourly intervals
Day 3: 300 mg of St John's wort (0.3% hypericin) t.d.s. for 14/7
Day 16: (day 14 of St John's wort) 3 × 800 mg indinavir at 8-hourly intervals
Results: St John's wort ↓ indinavir in the blood between 57% and 81%. A reduction in indinavir exposure → the development of drug resistance and treatment failure.

A study addressing clinically relevant pharmacokinetic herb–drug interactions for anti-retroviral therapy was published in 2015.[110] From this study, the recommendations in Table 23.10 were made.

Herbal medicine classes

See Table 23.11.

TABLE 23.10 Herb–drug interations with anti-retroviral medication[110]

Recommendation	Botanical	Reason
AVOID	St John's wort (*Hypericum perforatum*)	Increases drug clearance and decreases drug exposure
	Black pepper (*Piper species*)	Is a potent inhibitor of several CYP450 enzymes. Increased clearance of nevirapine by almost 170%
	Grapefruit juice	Increased the oral bioavailability of saquivavir by 200% and the clearance by 50%.
Use with caution	African potato (*Hypoxis hemerocallidea*)	Inhibits CYP3A4 – further studies required to ascertain increased clearance of ARTs
	Ginkgo (*Ginkgo biloba*)	May be used with ritonavir. As anti-retroviral drugs are primarily metabolised by CYP3A4, ginkgo is recommended to not be used with them
	Ginseng (*Panax* spp.)	Case studies have reported interactions. Ginseng has also been found to alter CYP3A4 substrates
	Garlic (*Allium sativum*)	Fresh garlic and an odourless garlic supplement produced a dose-related inhibitory response on human CYP3A4. However, garlic is popular among HIV-infected people; although side effects are noted, minor clearance of medication has also been found
	Goldenseal (*Hydrastic Canadensis*)	Inclusive data on clearance. One study showed it was safe with minimal clearance, but another study showed 70% increased clearance.
	Kava kava (*Piper methysticum*)	Clincial studies on drug metabolism are mixed.

TABLE 23.11 Herbal medicine classes

Class	Indication
Adaptogen, adrenal restorative, nervine tonic, tonic	To rebuild and restore the body from stressors, to support sleep and energy restoration
Depurative, alterative	To support the body's eliminatory channels
Lymphatic	To support the lymphatic system for the clearance of toxic material
Anthelmintic, anti-parasitic	To eradicate GIT parasites
Anti-microbial, anti-bacterial, anti-fungal, anti-viral	To address infection specific to subtype
Immune enhancing	To support the immune response
Anti-emetic	To reduce nausea and vomiting associated with medications
Bitter	To stimulate appetite and support protein digestion
Astringent	To restore and balance bowel transit time and improve nutrient absorption
Antioxidant	To reduce oxidative damage and associated disease progression
Hepatoprotective	To protect and restore hepatobiliary function
Hypoglycaemic	To reduce blood sugar levels associated with medication side effects
Pancreatic trophorestorative	To reduce blood sugar levels and restore pancreatic function associated with medication side effects
Hypolipidaemic	To reduce blood lipid levels associated with medication side effects
Hypocholesterolaemic	To reduce blood lipid levels associated with medication side effects

Specific herbal medicines

ALLIUM SATIVUM (GARLIC)

Allium sativum is an immune stimulant that has been shown to stimulate the proliferation of lymphocytes, interleukin-2, TNF-α and interferon-gamma, as well as enhancing the natural killer cells. *A. sativum* exhibits specific anti-fungal, anti-bacterial,[111] anti-parasitic and anti-viral[112] properties against a wide range of bacteria, viruses and fungi. Thus, it may be useful for enhancing the immune system in HIV-infected patients, as well as managing microbial conditions associated with HIV such as *Candida*, which commonly presents in patients with HIV.

Attention has also focused on ajoene, a constituent within *A. sativum* that appears to protect CD+ cells from attack by HIV early in the viral life cycle.[113] Ajoene has demonstrated anti-HIV activity that is said to be 45 times more powerful than the drug dextran sulfate; however, ajoene is only found in fresh *A. sativum*. This may be the reason why garlic is popular with HIV-infected patients, in addition to its cholesterol-lowering properties. However, due to its possible affect on CYP3A4, it does need to be used with caution in combination with ART. A study assessing short-term garlic supplementation and highly active ART found that using garlic as needed, rather than daily, did not impact on HAART adherence level, HIV viral load or CD4+ cell counts.[114] Therfore, using garlic when needed is recommended for HIV-infected patients, but daily for long periods.

ALOE VERA (ALOE VERA)

Aloe vera demonstrates anti-viral and immune properties. Traditionally, it is used in South Africa for the treatment of HIV-infected individuals.[115] Aloe vera contains over 75 potentially active constituents[116]; of these, acemannan, a complex sugar, is used for its immune-enhancing and retroviral action,[117] and has been suggested for use in HIV. In vitro studies[118] have confirmed the efficacy of acemannan in vitro, as did a small pilot study undertaken by Pulse in 1990,[119] which observed that patients administered 1200 mg/day of acemannan (in combination with other supplements) resulted in improved symptoms including better energy levels, decreased shortness of breath and cough, a reduction in lymph node size and weight gain. Patients' T4 helper lymphocytes also increased, and Karnofsky scores (a tool to assess wellbeing) showed significant improvement at 6 months of treatment. However, a subsequent study utilising a higher dose of acemannan (1600 mg/day) failed to replicate these positive results.

A preliminary trial of aloe vera was conducted on 10 young HIV-infected women in Nigeria. A blend of 30–40 mL of aloe vera gruel was given daily instead of ART, as the women did not meet the criteria for commencing HAART. The results found that the women gained weight steadily and increased their CD4+ count, which was similar to those on HAART. Although only preliminary data, the results suggest that aloe ingestion in HIV-infected patients prior to commencing HAART may be beneficial.[120]

ANDROGRAPHIS PANNICULATA (ANDROGRAPHIS)

Andrographis displays anti-viral and immune-modulating properties that have been shown to be beneficial to patients with HIV. Experimental studies reveal that andrographolide inhibits viral replication in HIV-infected cells.[121]

A phase I dose-escalating clinical trial was conducted in 13 HIV-positive patients and five HIV-uninfected, healthy volunteers.[122] Patients were administered andrographolide, of which the planned regimen was 5 mg/kg bodyweight for the first 3 weeks, escalating to 10 mg/kg bodyweight for weeks 4–6. From week 6 onwards, no more andrographolide was administered due to numerous adverse reactions (deemed to be mild to moderate, e.g. loose stools, metallic taste) in all but one patient; of note is the fact that these reactions had all dissipated by week 9. A decline in CD4+ count in HIV is associated with a declined ability to mount an immune response. However, in these patients, a significant rise in the mean CD4+ lymphocyte level of HIV subjects occurred after administration of 10 mg/kg andrographolide (from a baseline of 405 cells/mm(3) to 501 cells/mm(3); p = 0.002), revealing the therapeutic action of andrographis in HIV. While there were no statistically significant changes in mean plasma HIV-1 RNA levels throughout the trial, the authors proposed that andrographolide may inhibit HIV-induced cell cycle dysregulation, leading to a rise in CD4+ lymphocyte levels in HIV-1-infected individuals.

ARCTOSTAPHYLOS UVA-URSI (UVA URSI)

Ursolic acid, a constituent of *Arctostaphylos uva-ursi*, has demonstrated anti-HIV activity.[123]

ASTRAGALUS MEMBRANACEUS (ASTRAGALUS)

Astragalus membranaceus has traditionally been used to enhance the body's natural defence systems. In vivo and in vitro studies[124] reveal *A. membranaceus* to exhibit immune-modulating and immune-restorative properties that may be well utilised in patients with HIV. Furthermore, astragalus, via its function as an adaptogen, may also help to rejuvenate the immune system of HIV-infected persons.

A. membranaceus in combination with other botanicals is widely used in traditional Chinese medicine for management of HIV-related symptoms.[125,126] As yet, no studies could be found assessing the efficacy of *A. membranaceus* in isolation for management in HIV.

BAPTISIA TINCTORIA (WILD INDIGO)

Baptisia tinctoria displays immune-modulating and immune-stimulating properties, suggested to occur as a result of increased macrophage activity within the body.[127] As yet, no studies have been undertaken assessing its effects in HIV-infected individuals; however, it may be useful for its immune-enhancing properties.

A study assessing the botanicals used in Zambia for HIV/AIDS-infected patients found that 94 medicinal plant species were used to manage skin infections, diarrhoea, sexually transmitted infections, tuberculosis, coughs, malaria and oral infections associated with HIV/AIDs. Eighteen of the most commonly used plants included: *Achyranthes aspera L., Lannea discolor (Sond.) Engl., Hyphaene petersiana Klotzsch ex Mart., Asparagus racemosus Willd., Capparis tomentosa Lam., Cleome hirta Oliv., Garcinia livingstonei T. Anderson, Euclea divinorum Hiern, Bridelia cathartica G. Bertol., Acacia nilotica Delile, Piliostigma thonningii (Schumach.) Milne-Redh., Dichrostachys cinerea (L.) Wight and Arn., Abrus precatorius L., Hoslundia opposita Vahl., Clerodendrum capitatum (Willd.) Schumach., Ficus sycomorus L., Ximenia americana*

L. and *Ziziphus mucronata* Willd. Considering medical treatment in Zambia for HIV/AIDs is difficult due to staff shortages and patients face long queues and the stigma of having HIV/AIDs, it is not surprising that they would use tradional herbal remedies instead of medical assistance.[128]

BUPLEURUM FALCATUM (BUPLEURUM)

Bupleurum falcatum is a traditional Chinese medicine well known for its effects on the liver, where it exerts anti-inflammatory and hepatoprotective[129] actions, suggesting it may be useful in hepatitis associated with HIV. In vitro studies demonstrate that *B. falcatum* in combination with other botanicals can exert anti-HIV effects.[130,131] Currently, there are no published studies of patients with HIV infection and bupleurum.

CAMELLIA SINENSIS (GREEN TEA)

Camellia sinensis is well known for its powerful antioxidant actions. However, a specific anti-viral constituent within *C. sinensis* also shows great promise in the management of HIV. This constituent, epigallocatechin gallate (EGCG), has been shown to exert its effects via a number of mechanisms. EGCG prevents replication of HIV strains.[132] It has also been shown to prevent the binding of the HIV virus to human T lymphocytes,[133] including inhibiting the activity of HIV-1 reverse transcriptase[134] (which leads to a decrease in HIV p24 antigen concentration), as well as interfering with HIV-1 viral infection by virion destruction.[132] In a recent study, EGCG was found to inhibit HIV-1 infectivity on human CD4+ T cells and macrophages in a dose-dependent manner by preventing the attachment of HIV-1-glycoprotein 120 to the CD4 molecule.[133] This inhibition was achieved using physiological concentrations. Thus, experts are now suggesting EGCG to be a 'natural anti-HIV agent' and a possible candidate for alternative therapy in HIV-1 therapy.[135] Clinical trials in patients with HIV are warranted to further assess the efficacy of *C. sinensis* and its constituents.

CANNABIS SATIVA (MARIJUANA)

Neuropathic pain has been suggested to affect up to 30% of patients with HIV, significantly affecting quality of life and day-to-day functioning.[136] *Cannabis sativa* contains tetrahydrocannabinol, which displays analgesic properties likely to assist in the relief of pain associated with HIV. In a small randomised clinical trial, patients with HIV smoking cannabis at maximum tolerable dose (1–8% tetrahydrocannabinol [THC]), in combination with allopathic analgesics they were already taking, experienced a reduction in neuropathic pain (from strong to mild–moderate) compared to placebo.[136] Furthermore, improvements were experienced in mood disturbance and quality of life.

While the results from this study are heartening, it must be acknowledged that production and sale of *C. sativa* or medicinal cannabis is still illegal in a number of countries. Another aspect that needs to be recognsied is that its use (particularly long term) is also associated with

a number of potentially negative side effects. While smoking was used as a vehicle for *C. sativa*, it has been observed that this may not be the best means of administration due to increased risk of cough and lung complications. Ellis et al. note that vaporisation and mucosal sprays are currently approved in the UK and Canada, and therefore may be better transmission routes than smoking.[136] Now medicinal cannabis is available in oil form, with the US, Canada and the UK standarising production for cannabinoids and THC concentrations.

CURCUMA LONGA (TURMERIC)

Curcumin, the main active ingredient within *Curcuma longa*, has been shown to reduce viral infectivity.[137] In vitro studies have found that cucumin inhibits Tat transactivation of the HIV-1-LTR genome, inflammatory moleucles (interleukins, TNF-α, NF-κB, COX-2) and HIV-associated various kinases such as tyrosine kinase, PAK1, MAPK, PKC, cdk and others. As well as these actions, curcumin has been found to enhance the effect of HAART and minimises their side effects.[138]

In addition, it is effective as a hypocholesterolaemic/hypolipidaemic herbal medicine. Aside from these properties, curcumin shows promising results in the management of HIV-related symptoms such as diarrhoea. Eight patients with HIV-associated diarrhoea were administered 1862 mg/day of curcumin for approximately 10 months.[139] Resolution of diarrhoea and normalisation of stool quality occurred within 13 +/− 9.3 days. Mean number of bowel movements per day dropped from 7 +/− 3.6 to 1.7 +/− 0.5. All patients bar one also gained weight while taking curcumin (10.8 +/− 8.9 lb). A number of patients also experienced an end to bloating and abdominal pain.

ECHINACEA SPP. (ECHINACEA)

Echinacea is well known for its immunological effects and is commonly used for infections. Its use is controversial in HIV. Some have suggested that echinacea weakens the immune system's ability to control HIV,[140] while others suggest that echinacea may increase immune-mediated HIV-killing activity.[141] In vivo and in vitro studies are promising, revealing that L-chicoric acid, a constituent of the *Echinacea* spp., inhibits HIV-1 integration in vivo and is a non-competitive but reversible inhibitor of HIV-1 integrase in vitro.[142,143]

An open-label trial investigating the potential use of *E. purpurea* (500 mg every 8 hours for 14 days) in 15 HIV-infected patients receiving ART with etravirone was conducted. Echinacea was well tolerated and all participants finished the study. No interaction was found with etravirone, and the authors stated that the use of echinacea with etravirone was safe, with no dose adjustment necessary on the medication.[144] This study was a follow on from the researchers' previous study of another 15 HIV-infected patients on darunavir-ritonavir ART. They were given 500 mg of echinacea every 6 hours for 14 days. Similar to the other trial, echinacea was found to be safe and well tolerated, with no interactions noted.[145]

ELEUTHEROCOCCUS SENTICOSUS (SIBERIAN GINSENG)

While some individuals infected with HIV view it as a challenge to be met, others may view it as a major obstacle they are unable to cross. As a clinician, it is important to acknowledge the wide range of acute as well as ongoing challenges/stressors that individuals with HIV encounter on a daily basis; these include such things as the social stigma associated with having HIV, side effects as a result of medications and physical symptoms such as fatigue.[146] As yet, there are no studies assessing the effects of *Eleutherococcus senticosus* in patients with HIV. However, administration is likely to be well utilised in the majority of patients due to the adaptogenic property of *E. senticosus*. Adaptogens such as *E. senticosus* help patients adapt to the stresses of everyday living,[147] as well as helping to manage concomitant symptoms such as stress and fatigue. Furthermore, *E. senticosus* demonstrates immune-modulating effects,[147] which may also be useful for patients with HIV infection.

GANODERMA LUCIDUM (REISHI)

Ganoderma lucidum is a medicinal mushroom used therapeutically in Asia for over 2000 years. It has been reported to have a number of pharmacological effects; those relevant to HIV include immune-modulating, antioxidant and anti-viral (including anti-HIV) properties.[148] A number of constituents have been identified within *G. lucidum* for this anti-HIV activity; they include ganoderiol F and ganodermanontriol, found to be active as anti-HIV-1 agents,[149] as well as other triterpenoids such as ganodermanondiol and ganolucidic acid A, which show significant anti-HIV-1 protease activity.[150] As yet, no published controlled studies have been undertaken assessing the effects of *G. lucidum* in patients with HIV.

GLYCYRRHIZA GLABRA (LIQUORICE)

Glycyrrhizin, the active constituent in *Glycyrrhiza glabra* radix, exhibits potent immune-stimulating properties as well as anti-viral[151] and anti-HIV activity. Glycyrrhizin has been shown to enhance NK cell effects as well as induce interferon.[152] Although clinical human research examining glycyrrhizin's effects in HIV is minimal, one early human study demonstrated good results when glycyrrhizin was administered by drop infusion to patients with AIDS, with clinical improvement seen in almost half the individuals observed via improvement in CD4 to CD8 ratio and inhibition of HIV replication.[153] Further clinical studies utilising liquid extracts would be interesting to see if these same effects may be achieved.

HYDRASTIS CANADENSIS (GOLDENSEAL)

Hydrastis canadensis contains berberine, the active constituent within it deemed responsible for its actions. Berberine is said to kill a wide range of microbes and may also activate white blood cells, making them more effective at fighting infection and strengthening the immune system. Recent studies in animals suggest that berberine may be a complementary therapeutic agent for HIV infection due to its ability to inhibit HIV-protease-inhibitor-induced inflammatory response by modulating endoplasmic reticulum stress signalling pathways.[50] *H. canadensis* has traditionally been used as a bitter stomachic herb to aid digestion and relieve symptoms of mild digestive disorders through enhancement of bile flow and liver function. Estimates suggest that 50–93% of patients with HIV experience significant GI complaints during the course of the illness.[154] Abdominal pain and diarrhoea are both reported; however, diarrhoea is most prevalent, with up to 14% of patients said to be affected. *H. canadensis* may be useful to kill pathogens implicated as an infective cause of diarrhoea as well as infections of the gut, such as *Candida*.

HYPERICUM PERFORATUM (ST JOHN'S WORT)

Hypericum perforatum has been identified as having anti-viral properties thought to be useful in infectious conditions.[155] Experimental studies reveal *H. perforatum* to contain a protein, p27(SJ), that in laboratory studies has been found to suppress transcription of the HIV-1 genome in several human cell types.[156,157] Aside from its action on the HIV virus, *H. perforatum* may also be used to help manage coexisting symptoms such as depression due to its antidepressant action. Depression is prevalent in subjects with HIV, with some studies observing up to 58%[158] of individuals feeling depressed; this is a substantial percentage considering rates of depression in the general population are thought to be less than one-third of this. Because *H. perforatum* induces the cytochrome P450 enzyme system, caution should be exercised in patients taking medications, particularly anti-retrovirals.

LENTINUS EDODES (SHIITAKE)

Lentinus edodes may be used to provide general support to the immune system for the individual with HIV due to its immune-stimulating,[159] antioxidant and anti-microbial[160] properties. One such constituent is lentin, a potent anti-fungal protein from shiitake mushrooms which demonstrates inhibitory effects on the activity of HIV-1 reverse transcriptase.[161] Another constituent, lentinan, a beta-1,3 glucan isolated from *L. edodes*, demonstrates immune-modulating properties, which may also be useful in patients with HIV infection.

OLEA EUROPAEA (OLIVE LEAF)

Olea europaea displays anti-viral properties and has been shown to inhibit acute infection as well as cell-to-cell transmission of HIV-1, blocking the HIV virus entry into the host cell.[162] Further studies are required in humans to confirm these results.

PANAX GINSENG (KOREAN GINSENG)

Korean red ginseng is one of the most widely clinically researched botanicals for the management of HIV in humans. In Korea, Korean red ginseng has been utilised since 1991 as a medicine to be used in isolation or in combination with allopathic drugs for patients with HIV infection due to its ability to maintain or even increase CD4 T cell counts for long periods[163] by preventing depletion of CD4 cells,[163] even when used in isolation. Long-term intake of Korean red ginseng has been found to delay disease progression in HIV-1-infected patients.[164]

An open-label, single-centre trial investigating *Panax ginseng* in 12 healthy HIV-infected patients on lopinavir-ritonavir was conducted. It found that 500 mg twice daily of *P. ginseng* for 2 weeks in conjunction with ART lopinavir-ritonavir was safe, with no interaction noted.[165] Therefore, supplementation with Korean ginseng is recommended for HIV-infected patients.

PHYLLANTHUS AMARUS (PHYLLANTHUS)

Phyllanthus spp. have been used traditionally in Ayurvedic, Chinese and Indonesian herbal medicine for a wide range of conditions, including those of viral origin.[166] *P. amarus* displays antioxidant, anti-inflammatory[167] and anti-viral properties.[168] Its anti-viral properties have been particularly well received in patients with viral hepatitis.[166] This suggests that it may also be well utilised in other viral conditions such as HIV. In vitro and in vivo studies reveal the ability of *P. amarus* to inhibit HIV replication by cleverly targeting different steps of the HIV life cycle, thereby presenting multiple anti-viral activities.[168] Acknowledging these results and those seen in patients with viral hepatitis virus, *P. amarus* appears to be a promising botanical for the management of HIV, and clinical studies undertaken in humans are likely to be well received.

PHYTOLACCA DECADRA (POKE ROOT)

The pokeweed anti-viral protein, a ribosome-inhibitory protein isolated from the leaves or seeds of *Phytolacca americana*, is a potent inhibitor of HIV-1 replication.[169]

SCUTELLARIA BAICALENSIS (BAICAL SKULLCAP)

Baicalin is a flavonoid present in the Chinese botanical *Scutellaria baicalensis*, which has been found to inhibit HIV-1 infection and replication in vitro.[170] Baicalin appears to block HIV infection at the level of viral infection, a process that involves interaction between HIV-1 envelope proteins and the cellular CD4 and chemokine receptors.[171] In animal studies, baicalin has been observed to reduce gastrointestinal side effects induced by ritonavir (a protease inhibitor drug, commonly used in AIDS), thus reducing drug-induced side effects.[172] *S. baicalensis* also demonstrates anti-allergic and anti-inflammatory properties, and may therefore also be useful in the management of symptoms that manifest concurrently with HIV where there is inflammation (e.g. hepatitis) or allergy (e.g. hayfever).

SILYBUM MARIANUM (ST MARY'S THISTLE)

The liver is responsible for numerous biochemical functions in the body, including metabolism of alcohol and other drugs, detoxification, conjugation and secretion of bilirubin, synthesis of bile salts and cholesterol and fatty acid metabolism. Optimal liver function is therefore paramount. People with HIV may present with liver impairment and inflammation due to damage from medications, concomitant hepatitis, alcohol or drug abuse.[173]

In vitro studies have shown that silymarin blocks hepatitis C virus infection and T cell proliferation. It has also been found to inhibit the replication of HIV-1 in TZM-bl cells, PBMCx and CEM cells, therefore displaying cytoprotection by suppressing virus infection, immune activation and inflammation, which is relevant for HIV and HIV/HCV co-infected patients.[174] Administration of *Silybum marianum*, a hepatoprotective and restorative, is highly suggested.

TABEBUIA SPP. (PAU D'ARCO)

Tabebuia spp. display potent anti-fungal properties,[175] and are thus highly regarded in naturopathic medicine for the management of fungal infections which are common in immune-compromised HIV patients. *Cryptococcus neoformans* is a fungal infection that has been identified as the fourth most common cause of life-threatening infection in AIDS patients.[175] Other common fungal infections in HIV include *Candida* (thrush, as it is sometimes called), which may present orally (visible when you examine the tongue) or systemically in the gut. Although most naturopaths are familiar with the *Candida albicans* strain, it is important to note that other strains exist; for example, *C. dubliniensis* is an opportunistic yeast implicated in oropharyngeal candidiasis in patients with HIV.[176] For oral thrush, *Tabebuia* spp. may be gargled and then swallowed; for systemic fungal infections; *Tabebuia* spp. may be consumed internally; while for fungal infections on the skin surface, *Tabebuia* spp. may be applied topically in a cream as well as consumed internally. Horopito (*Psuedowintera*) is a New Zealand herb that also has strong anti-fungal activity which can also be used.

ULMUS SPP. (SLIPPERY ELM)

Ulmus spp. have been traditionally used to maintain healthy digestive function and to relieve symptoms of gastrointestinal disturbances. Both Grieve[177] and Felter et al.[178] advocate its use as a demulcent for irritated mucous membranes of the stomach and bowel, suggesting its administration in the form of a mucilaginous drink to be consumed frequently throughout the day. Modern science confirms traditional use of *U. rubra*, revealing it to have anti-inflammatory and antioxidant properties.[179] *U. rubra* contains mucilage, which functions to coat the mucous membranes, acting as a barrier to the lining of the digestive system and soothing irritation or inflammation.[180] As yet, there is a scarcity of human clinical trials assessing the effects of *U. rubra* in patients with HIV infection; however, it is logical to assume that *U. rubra* may be well utilised due to the actions detailed above.

U. rubra may be particularly useful in patients with HIV who exhibit poor gut function as a result of drug degradation, and may help ameliorate concomitant symptoms of HIV such as diarrhoea and gastritis. The *British Herbal Compendium* indicates *U. rubra* for inflammation and ulceration of the gastrointestinal tract, such as oesophagitis, gastritis, colitis and gastric or duodenal ulcers.[180] Acknowledging traditional methods, it would appear that *U. rubra* is best consumed frequently in the form of a drink.

UNCARIA TOMENTOSA (CAT'S CLAW)

Uncaria tomentosa is a botanical traditionally found in the highlands of the Peruvian Amazon. It is revered for its effects on the immune system. Modern studies confirm the immune-enhancing effects, revealing it to contain anti-viral constituents.[181] Few studies have assessed the effects of *U. tomentosa* in HIV. However, in their review, Mukhtar et al. detail beneficial effects in a small study in which individuals with HIV taking *U. tomentosa* showed an increase in CD4+ counts.[182]

LIFESTYLE RECOMMENDATIONS

General recommendations

1   Exercise and breathing exercises to increase oxidation, circulation and general wellbeing are important for all patients.
2   Psychological support and counselling are crucial for long-term survival and to assist in maintaining a positive outlook.
3   ALWAYS use a condom or dams for any sexual contact.
4   Avoid sharing toothbrushes, razors, tweezers and any other instruments that may come into contact with blood.
5   Reduce the burden on the liver by encouraging natural cleaning products and natural hair, body and skin care.
6   Eliminate and avoid tobacco, alcohol and recreational drugs.
7   Ensure sleep requirements are met, with at least 8 hours per night (minimum).
8   Sleep should be encouraged before 10 pm and patients should support waking close to sunrise to regulate circadian rhythm.

Party with care

Hard partying with heavy recreational drugs drives the adrenals into exhaustion – our bodies are not invincible. Dehydration can set in quickly and the adrenals are no longer able to produce enough cortisol to regulate stress and inflammation in the body. When our bodies become tired and depleted, people often forget about eating fresh fruit, vegetables and protein. This leads to not getting the right fuel to keep fit and healthy, which can increase the susceptibility to infections.

Interactions with HAART and ecstasy

Patients who use PIs or NNRTIs can develop life-threatening complications when taking concurrent ecstasy (3,4-methylenedioxymethamphetamine, also known as MDMA, 'E' or 'X'). Both PIs and NNRTIs increase the levels of ecstasy in the blood. A case in the UK highlighted that haemolytic anaemia developed while taking HAART and MDMA.[183]

Social contact and support

Social contact and support is essential for all patients. In one study, the importance of social support and social network factors as modifiers of the rate of decline of CD4 lymphocyte level was highly evident, as seen in Table 23.12.[183]

TABLE 23.12 Social network factors as modifiers of the rate of decline of CD4 lymphocyte level

Results	Half-life of T4 count
Males with highest family contact	20.3 years
Males with lowest family contact	7.4 years (p = 0.03)
Males with highest social participation	14.7 years
Males with lowest social participation	6.3 years (p = 0.10)

CASE STUDY

OVERVIEW

JC was a 47-year-old man who had contracted HIV 25 years prior from unprotected sexual intercourse with a male. He had previously been treated with anti-retroviral drugs, but felt sick on them and had stopped taking them. He had remained in reasonable health until 2 months ago when he began having night sweats, was sick constantly with diarrohea, had severe stomach pain and had lost 12 kg of weight within a week. On presentation to the hospital, they noted that the patient had a fever, hepatospenomegaly (enlarged spleen), weight loss and diarrhoea. He also had a skin lesion which was caused by leishmania, identified by a biopsy. He was initially treated with N-methyl-glucamine-antimony and amphotericin B deoxycholate. However, due to the toxicity, this was later changed to tenofovir, lamivudine and lopinavir/ritonavir. JC's diet was poor due to work and consisted of fast food and frequent meal skipping. He consumed high quantities of sugar, caffeine, alcohol and refined products.

CLINICAL EXAMINATION

Weight 92 kg, Height 194 cm
Temperature: 35.4°C
Sores on his arms
Mild bruising on legs and upper arms
Abdominal pains and distention

INVESTIGATIONS

Blood testing that precipitated medication prescription included:

Test	Result
CD4	154 cells/mm³
Viral load	208 000 copies/mL
Haemoglobin	102 g/L

Test	Result
RCC	4.1×10^{12}/L
MCV	123 fL
WCC	10.4×10^9/L
Vitamin D$_3$	29 ng/mL
Gamma-glutamyl transpeptidase (GGT) (liver function test otherwise normal)	210 U/L
Glucose (fasting)	6.9 nmol/L
Pancreatic enzyme test:	
Amylase	460 U/L
Lipase	530 U/L

TREATMENT PROTOCOL

Treatment was multifactorial due to the number of presenting variables. Dietary modifications were paramount to the success of long-term treatment and longevity. Lengthy discussion regarding the importance of caring for the body through food was made and JC was cautious but open to making changes. The main issue at present was the pancreatitis, fatty liver, high white cell count (as there was still an infection) and anaemia. JC was also presenting with pre-diabetes. He was still experiencing diarrhoea and severe pain abdominally.

HERBAL MEDICINE

Herbal medicines were not chosen in the initial appointment, as treatment focused on nutritional and lifestyle modifications.

NUTRITIONAL MEDICINE

Dietary

Marked dietary improvements were suggested with menu ideas, modifications to existing dietary intake and explanation regarding importance of inclusion of key foods and exclusion of negative contributing foods. Specific recommendations were as follows:

- A major decrease in processed foods, processed sugar, and caffeine
- NO alcohol was to be consumed
- Reduction of carbohydrate consumption due to increased blood glucose level (BGL)
- Protein choices were discussed looking at approximately 1.4 g of protein/kg of body weight a day. This was particulary due to the loss of weight and increased diarrhoea he was experiencing.
- Optimal hydration calculated based on JC's weight to improve glomerular filtration rate (eGFR)
- Encouraged increased intake of fresh fruits and vegetables and wholefoods with a focus on organic sources
- Avoidance of saturated, rancid and trans fats
- Whole lemon drink to be drunk daily to stimulate liver function and assist in weight management
- New menu ideas, new foods to try such as bitter melon.

Supplemental

Nutrient	Dose	Justification
High potency B complex (activated)	1 capsule b.i.d.	To normalise red blood cell parameters and support optimal blood sugar levels
Zinc	50 mg/day	To support the immune system, assist healing of connective tissue
Vitamin D	5000 IU/day	To address deficiency
Selenium	100 micrograms/day	To support immune function and increase CD4 count
Alpha-lipoic acid	400 mg b.i.d.	To reduce oxidation and inhibit HIV replication

LIFESTYLE/EDUCATION

Strong emphasis to sustain supportive social network and reduce drinking by himself each night (avoidance of all alcohol was emphasised due to pancreatitis). New habits needed to be formed, so a focus was placed on changing his daily routine. Sleep at a minimum of 8–10 hours per night was encouraged. Exercise was encouraged, with walking to start with about 15–20 minutes a day.

FOLLOW-UP

Treatment was modified periodically to support progressive changes in JC's health. At each appointment, different nutritional and lifestyle education was conducted to ensure patient motivation and compliance. It also enabled significant changes to eventuate in JC's life that were able to be maintained.

Referral was organised for a number of key naturopathic investigations to further direct treatment, and JC was encouraged to organise resistant testing for his medication regimen to ensure greatest outcome.

At the second appointment, a herbal formula was prescribed and consisted of:

Herbal medicine	Ratio	Quantity	Rationale
Silybum marianum	STD Ext	60 mL	Hepatoprotective and hepatotrophorestorative
Astragulus membranaceus	1:2	60 mL	Immune stimulant for chronic low immune function
Panax ginseng	1:2	40 mL	Adaptogen, adrenal restorative, immune support
Withania somnifera	1:1	40 mL	Adaptogen, nervine tonic, blood tonic

REFERENCES

[1] World Health Organisation. HIV/AIDS data and statistics. Geneva: WHO; 2016.

[2] UNAIDS. 2030 – ending the AIDS epidemic. 2015 global statistics; 2016. Available from https://www.who.int/hiv/pub/arv/global-AIDS -update-2016_en.pdf?ua=1.

[3] Takebe Y, Kusagawa S, Motomura K. Molecular epidemiology of HIV: tracking AIDS pandemic. Pediatr Int 2004;46:236–44.

[4] Rahman I, Biswas S, Kirkham PA. Regulation of inflammation and redox signaling by dietary polyphenols. Biochem Pharmacol 2006;72:1439–52.

[5] Pizzorno J, Murray M. Textbook of natural medicine. US: Elsevier; 2007.

[6] World Health Organization. WHO case definitions of HIV for surveillance and revised clinical staging and immunological classification of HIV-related disease in adults and children. Geneva: World Health Organization; 2007.

[7] Wanke CA, Falutz J, Shevitz A, et al. Clinical evaluation and management of metabolic and morphologic abnormalities associated with human immunodeficiency virus. Clin Infect Dis 2002;34:248–59.

[8] Smyth K, Affandi J, McArthur JC, et al. Prevalence of and risk factors for HIV – associated neuropathy in Melbourne, Australia 1993–2006. HIV Med 2007;8(6):367–73.

[9] Bernal Morell E, Serrano Cabeza J, Muñoz Á, et al. The CD4/CD8 ratio is inversely associated with carotid intima-media thickness progression in human immunodeficiency virus-infected patients on antiretroviral treatment. AIDS Res Hum Retroviruses 2016;32(7): 648–53.

[10] Lorenc A, Robinson N. A review of the use of complementary and alternative medicine and HIV: issues for patient care. AIDS Patient Care STDS 2013;27(9):503–10.

[11] Deminice R, Vassimon H, Machado AA, et al. Plasma homocysteine levels in HIV-infected men with and without lipodystrophy. Nutrition 2013;29(11–12):1326–30.

[12] Desouza C, Keebler M, McNamara OB, et al. Drugs affecting homocysteine metabolism: impact on cardiovascular risk. Drugs 2002;62(4):605–16.

[13] Müller F, Svardal A, Aukrust P, et al. Elevated plasma concentration of reduced homocysteine in patients with human immunodeficiency virus infection. Am J Clin Nutr 1996; 63(2):242–6.

[14] Del Pilar-Morales EA, Cardon-Rodríguez Z, Bertrain-Pasarell J, et al. Multiple simultaneous gastrointestinal parasitic infections in a patient with human immunodeficiency virus. P R Health Sci J 2016;35(2):97–9.

[15] Wolday D, Mayaan S, Mariam ZG, et al. Treatment of intestinal worms is associated with decreased HIV plasma viral load. JAIDS 2002;31:58–62.

[16] National Association of People with HIV Australia. HIV tests and treatments; 2019. Available from https://www.afao.org.au/ wp-content/uploads/2018/12/HIV-in-Australia-2019_No-Bleed.pdf.

[17] HIV & AIDS Medications; 2016. Available from https://www .healthline.com/health/hiv-aids/medications-list#hiv-drug-classes.

[18] The Strategies for Management of Antiretroviral Therapy (SMART) Study Group. Inferior clinical outcome of the CD4+ cell count – guided antiretroviral treatment interruption strategy in the SMART study: role of CD4+ cell counts and HIV RNA levels during follow-up. J Infect Dis 2008;197(8):1145–55. https://doi.org/ 10.1086/529523.

[19] Sutton SS, Hardin J, Bramley TJ, et al. Single- versus multiple-tablet HIV regimens: adherence and hospitalisation risks. Am J Manag Care 2016;22(4):242–8.

[20] Merson MH, O'Malley J, Serwadda D, et al. The history and challenge of HIV prevention. Lancet 2008;372(9637):475–88.

[21] Barré-Sinoussi F, Chermann J, Rey F, et al. Isolation of a T-lymphotropic retrovirus from a patient at risk for acquired immune deficiency syndrome (AIDS). Science 1983;220: 868–71.

[22] Zhu T, Korber B, Nahmias AJ, et al. An African HIV-1 sequence from 1959 and implications for the origin of the epidemic. Nature 1998;39:1594–7.

[23] Worobey M, Gemmel M, Teuwen DE, et al. Direct evidence of extensive diversity of HIV-1 in Kinshasa by 1960. Nature 2008; 455:661–4.

[24] Willig AL, Overton E. Metabolic complications and glucose metabolism in HIV infection: a review of the evidence. Curr HIV/ AIDS Rep 2016;13(5):289–96.

[25] Wright SC, Maree J, Sibanyoni M. Treatment of oral thrush in HIV/ AIDS patients with lemon juice and lemon grass (Cymbopogon citratus) and gentian violet. Phytomedicine 2009;16(2–3):118–24.

[26] Hendricks KM, Mwamburi D, Newby PK, et al. Dietary patterns and health and nutrition outcomes in men living with HIV infection. Am J Clin Nutr 2008;88(6):1584–92.

[27] Sattler FR, Rajicic N, Mulligan K, et al. ACTG 392 Study Team. Evaluation of high-protein supplementation in weight-stable HIV-positive subjects with a history of weight loss: a randomized, double-blind, multicenter trial. Am J Clin Nutr 2008;88(5):1313–21.

[28] Rebultan SP. Bitter melon therapy: an experimental treatment of HIV infection. AIDS Asia 1995;2(4):6–7.

[29] Lee-Huang S, Huang P, Chen HC, et al. Anti-HIV and anti-tumor activities of recombinant MAP30 from bitter melon. Gene 1995;161(2):151–6.

[30] Puri M, Kaur I, Kanwar RK, et al. Ribosome inactivating proteins (RIPs) from Momordica charantia for anti viral therapy. Curr Mol Med 2009;9(9):1080–94.

[31] Teas J, Hebert J, Fitton JH, et al. Algae – a poor man's HAART? Med Hypotheses 2004;62(4):507–10.

[32] Khan Z, Bhadiouria P, Bisen PS. Nutritional and therapeutic potential of Spirulina. Curr Pharm Biotechnol 2005;6(5):373–9.

[33] Belleme J, Belleme J. Japanese foods that heal. Hong Kong (China): Tuttle Publishing; 2007.

[34] Trinchero J, Ponce N, Córdoba OL, et al. Antiretroviral activity of fucoidans extracted from the brown seaweed Adenocystis utricularis. Phytother Res 2009;23(5):707–12.

[35] Haorah J, Heilman D, Diekmann C, et al. Alcohol and HIV decrease proteasome and immunoproteasome function in macrophages: implications for impaired immune function during disease. Cell Immunol 2004;229(2):139–48.

[36] Samet JH, Horton N, Traphagen ET, et al. Alcohol consumption and HIV disease progression: are they related? Alcohol Clin Exp Res 2003;27(5):862–7.

[37] Sanchez A, Reeser J, Lau HS, et al. Role of sugars in human neutrophilic phagocytosis. Am J Clin Nut 1973;26(11):1180–4.

[38] Cheng DM, Libman H, Bridden C, et al. Alcohol consumption and lipodystrophy in HIV-infected adults with alcohol problems. Alcohol Clin Exp Res 2009;43(1):65–71.

[39] Wilcox RD. Alcohol and HIV: a serious cocktail for transmission and medication adherence. HIV Clin 2009;21(1):1–4.

[40] Hilton JF, MacPhail L, Pascasio L, et al. Self-care intervention to reduce oral candidiasis recurrences in HIV-seropositive persons: a pilot study. Community Dent Oral Epidemiol 2004;32(3):190–200.

[41] Joy T, Keogh H, Hadigan C, et al. Dietary fat intake and relationship to serum lipid levels in HIV-infected patients with metabolic abnormalities in the HAART era. AIDS 2007;21(12): 1591–600.

[42] Mann JI. Optimizing the plant-based diet. Asia Pac J Clin Nutr 2000;9(Suppl. 1):S60–4.

[43] Lazzaretti RK, Kuhmmer R, Sprinz E, et al. Dietary intervention prevents dyslipidemia associated with highly active antiretroviral therapy in human immunodeficiency virus type 1–infected individuals – a randomized trial. J Am Coll Cardiol 2012;59:979–88.

[44] Stradling C, Chen YF, Russell T, et al. The effects of dietary intervention on HIV dyslipidaemia: a systematic review and meta-analysis. PLoS ONE 2012;7:e38121.

[45] d'Ettorre G, Ceccarelli G, Giustini N, et al. Probiotics reduce inflammation in antiretroviral treated, HIV-infected individuals: results of the 'Probio-HIV' Clinical Trial. PLoS ONE 2015;10(9):doi:10.1371/journal.pone.0137200. e0137200.

[46] Carter GM, Indyk D, Johnson M, et al. Micronutrients in HIV: a Bayesian meta-analysis. PLoS ONE 2015;10(4):doi:10.1371/journal. pone.0120113. e0120113.

[47] Ravi S, Khalili H, Abbasian L, et al. Effect of omega-3 fatty acids on depressive symptoms in HIV-positive individuals: a randomized, placebo-controlled clinical trial. Ann Pharmacother 2016; 50(10):797–807. doi:10.1177/1060028016656017.

[48] Samaras K, Wand H, Law M, et al. Dietary intake in HIV-infected men with lipodystrophy: relationships with body composition, visceral fat, lipid, glucose and adipokine metabolism. Curr HIV Res 2009;7(4):454–61.

[49] Purnomo J, Jeganathan S, Begley K, et al. Depression and dietary intake in a cohort of HIV-positive clients in Sydney. Int J STD AIDS 2012;23(12):882–6. doi:10.1258/ijsa.2012.012017.

[50] Zha W, Liang G, Xiao J, et al. Berberine inhibits HIV protease inhibitor-induced inflammatory response by modulating ER stress signaling pathways in murine macrophages. PLoS ONE 2010; 5(2):e9069.

[51] Butterworth RF, Gaudreau C, Vincelette J, et al. Thiamine deficiency and Wernicke's encephalopathy in AIDS. Metab Brain Dis 1991;6:207–12.

[52] Tang AM, Graham N, Kirby AJ, et al. Dietary micronutrient intake and risk of progression to acquired immunodeficiency syndrome (AIDS) in human immunodeficiency virus type-1 (HIV-1)-infected homosexual men. Am J Epidemiol 1993;138:937–51.

[53] Bowers JM, Bert-Moreno A. Treatment of HAART-induced lactic acidosis with B vitamin supplements. Nutr Clin Pract 2004;19(4): 375–8.

[54] Oh J, Hegele R. HIV-associated dyslipidaemia: pathogenesis and treatment. Lancet Infect Dis 2007;7(12):787–96.

[55] Chow DC, Tasaki A, Ono J, et al. Effect of extended-release niacin on hormone-sensitive lipase and lipoprotein lipase in patients with HIV-associated lipodystrophy syndrome. Biologics 2008;2(4): 917–21.

[56] Baum MK, Mantero-Atienza E, Shor-Posner G. F et al. Association of vitamin B6 status with parameters of immune function in early HIV-1 infection. J Acquir Immune Defic Syndr 1991;4(11): 1122–32.

[57] Shor-Posner G, Feaster D, Blaney NT, et al. Impact of vitamin B6 status on psychological distress in a longitudinal study of HIV-1 infection. Int J Psychiatry Med 1994;23(3):209–22.

[58] Rule SA, Hooker M, Costello C, et al. Serum vitamin B12 and transcobalamin levels in early HIV disease. Am J Hematol 1994; 47(3):167–71.

[59] Ehrenpreis ED, Carlson S, Boorstein HL, et al. Malabsorption and deficiency of vitamin B12 in HIV-infected patients with chronic diarrhea. Dig Dis Sci 1994;39(10):2159–62.

[60] Fessel WJ, Follansbee S, Rego J. High density lipoprotein cholesterol is low in HIV-infected patients with lipodystrophic fat expansions: implications for pathogenesis of fat redistribution. AIDS 2002;16(13):1785–9.

[61] Visser ME, Maartens G, Kossew G, et al. Plasma vitamin A and zinc levels in HIV-infected adults in Cape Town. South Africa. Br J Nutr 2003;89(4):475–82.

[62] Semba RD, Lyles C, Margolick JB, et al. Vitamin A supplementation and human immunodeficiency virus load in injection drug users. J Infect Dis 1998;177(3):611–61.

[63] Mehta S, Fawzi W. Effects of vitamins, including vitamin A, on HIV/AIDS patients. Vitam Horm 2007;75:355–83.

[64] Coodley GO, Nelson H, Loveless MO, et al. Beta-carotene in HIV infection. J Acquir Immune Defic Syndr 1993;6(3):272–6.

[65] Stephensen CB, Marquis G, Jacob RA, et al. Vitamins C and E in adolescents and young adults with HIV infection. Am J Clin Nutr 2006;83(4):870–9.

[66] García-Alvarez M, Berenguer J, Jiménez-Sousa MÁ, et al. Optimal vitamin D plasma levels are associated with lower bacterial DNA translocation in HIV/hepatitis C virus coinfected patients. AIDS 2016;30(7):1069–74.

[67] Nylén H, Habtewold A, Makonnen E, et al. Prevalence and risk factors for efavirenz-based antiretroviral treatment-associated severe vitamin D deficiency: a prospective cohort study. Medicine (Baltimore) 2016;95(34):e4631.

[68] Tang AM, Graham N, Semba RD, et al. Association between serum vitamin A and E levels and HIV-1 disease progression. AIDS 1997;11(5):613–20.

[69] Itinoseki Kaio DJ, Rondó P, Luzia LA, et al. Vitamin E concentrations in adults with HIV/AIDS on highly active antiretroviral therapy. Nutrients 2014;6(9):3641–52.

[70] Allard JP, Aghdassi E, Chau J, et al. Effects of vitamin E and C supplementation on oxidative stress and viral load in HIV-infected subjects. AIDS 1998;12(13):1653–9.

[71] Patrick L. Nutri and HIV-part one-bete carotene and selenium. Altern Med Rev 1999;4(6):403–13.

[72] Kamwesiga J, Mutabazi V, Kayumba J, et al. Effect of selenium supplementation on CD4+ T-cell recovery, viral suppression and morbidity of HIV-infectged patients in Rwanda: a randomized controlled trial. AIDS 2015;29(9):1045–52.

[73] Burbano X, Miguez-Burbano M, McCollister K, et al. Impact of a selenium chemoprevention clinical trial on hospital admissions of HIV-infected participants. HIV Clin Trials 2002;3(6):483–91.

[74] Carter VM, Woolley I, Jolley D, et al. A randomised controlled trial of omega-3 fatty acid supplementation for the treatment of hypertriglyceridemia in HIV-infected males on highly active antiretroviral therapy. Sex Health 2006;3(4):287–90.

[75] Woods MN, Wanke C, Ling PR, et al. Effect of a dietary intervention and n-3 fatty acid supplementation on measures of serum lipid and insulin sensitivity in persons with HIV. Am J Clin Nutr 2009;90(6):1566–78.

[76] Baum MK, Campa A, Lai S, et al. Zinc status in human immunodeficiency virus type 1 infection and illicit drug use. Clin Infect Dis 2003;37(Suppl. 2):S117–23.

[77] Fouché C, van Niekerk E, du Plessis LM. Differences in breast milk composition of HIV-infected and HIV uninfected mothers of premature infants: effects of antiretroviral therapy. Breastfeed Med 2016;11(9):doi:10.1089/bfm.2016.0087.

[78] Baum MK, Shor-Posner G, Lai S, et al. High risk of HIV-related mortality is associated with selenium deficiency. J Acquir Immune Defic Syndr Hum Retroviral 1997;15:370–430.

[79] Patrick L. Nutrients and HIV: part two – vitamins A and E, zinc, B-vitamins, and magnesium. Altern Med Rev 2000;5(1):39–51.

[80] Adetifa I, Okomo U. Iron supplementation for reducing morbidity and mortality in children with HIV. Cochrane Database Syst Rev 2009;(1):CD006736.

[81] Obirikorang C, Issahaku R, Osakunor DN, et al. Anaemia and iron homeostasis in a cohort of HIV-infected patients: a cross-sectional study in Ghana. AIDS Res Treat 2016;2016:1623094.

[82] Davis DA, Branca A, Pallenberg AJ, et al. Inhibition of the human immunodeficiency virus-1 protease and human immuno-deficiency virus-1 replication by bathocuproine disulfonic acid Cu1+. Arch Biochem Biophys 1995;322:127.

[83] Morrison JT, Longenecker C, Mittelsteadt A, et al. Effect of rosuvastatin on plasma coenzyme Q10 in HIV-infected individuals on antiretroviral therapy. HIV Clin Trials 2016;17(4):140–6.

[84] Folkers K, Langsjoen P, Nara Y, et al. Biochemical deficiencies of coenzyme Q10 in HIV-infection and exploratory treatment. Biochem Biophys Res Commun 1988;153(2):888–96.

[85] Batterham M, Gold J, Naidoo D, et al. A preliminary open label dose comparison using an antioxidant regimen to determine the effect on viral load and oxidative stress in men with HIV/AIDS. Eur J Clin Nutr 2001;55(2):107–14.

[86] Rosenfeldt FL, Mijch A, McCrystal G, et al. Skeletal myopathy associated with nucleoside reverse transcriptase inhibitor therapy: potential benefit of coenzyme Q10 therapy. Int J STD AIDS 2005;16(12):827–9.

[87] Miller H, Ferris R, Phelps BR. The effect of probiotics on CD4 counts among people living with HIV: a systematic review. Benef Microbes 2016;7(3):345–51.

[88] Williams B, Landay A, Presti RM. Microbiome alterations in HIV infection a review. Cell Microbiol 2016;18(5):645–51.

[89] Thomas LV, Suzuki K, Zhao J. Probiotics: a proactive approach to health. A symposium report. Br J Nutr 2015;114(Suppl. 1): S1–15.

[90] Heiser CR, Ernst J, Barrett JT, et al. Probiotics, soluble fiber, and L-glutamine (GLN) reduce nelfinavir (NFV)- or lopinavir/ritonavir (LPV/r)-related diarrhea. J Int Assoc Physicians AIDS Care (Chic Ill) 2004;3(4):121–9.

[91] Wolf BW, Wheeler K, Ataya DG, et al. Safety and tolerance of Lactobacillus reuteri supplementation to a population infected with the human immunodeficiency virus. Food Chem Toxicol 1998;36(12):1085–94.

[92] No authors listed. Probiotic blocks HIV transmission via breastfeeding. AIDS Patient Care STDS 2008;22(8):687.

[93] Baur A, Harrer T, Peukert M, et al. Alpha-lipoic acid is an effective inhibitor of human immuno-deficiency virus (HIV-1) replication. Klin Wochenschr 1991;69(15):722–4.

[94] Suzuki YJ, Aggarwal B, Packer L. Alpha-lipoic acid is a potent inhibitor of NF-kappa B activation in human T cells. Biochem Biophys Res Commun 1992;189(3):1709–15.

[95] Jariwalla RJ, Lalezari J, Cenko D, et al. Restoration of blood total glutathione status and lymphocyte function following alpha-lipoic acid supplementation in patients with HIV infection. J Altern Complement Med 2008;14(2):139–46.

[96] Fuchs J, Schöfer H, Milbradt R, et al. Studies on lipoate effects on blood redox state in human immunodeficiency virus infected patients. Arzneimittelforschung 1993;43:1359–62.

[97] Aukrust P, Müller F, Svardal AM, et al. Disturbed glutathione metabolism and decreased antioxidant levels in human immunodeficiency virus-infected patients during highly active antiretroviral therapy. J Infect Dis 2003;188:232–8.

[98] Zuena AR, Giuli C, Venerosi Pesciolini A, et al. Transplacental exposure to AZT induces adverse neurochemical and behavioural effects in a mouse model: protection by L-acetylcarnitine. PLoS ONE 2013;8(2):e55753.

[99] Triant VA, Lee H, Hadigan C, et al. Increased acute myocardial infarction rates and cardiovascular risk factors among patients with human immunodeficiency virus disease. J Clin Endocrinol Metab 2007;92:2506–12.

[100] Gupta SK, Kamendulis LM, Clauss MA, et al. A randomized, placebo-controlled pilot trial of N-acetylcysteine on oxidative stress and endothelial function in HIV-infected older adults receiving antiretroviral treatment. AIDS 2016;30(15):2389–91. doi:10.1097/QAD.0000000000001222.

[101] Brown TT, Qaqish R. Antiretroviral therapy and the prevalence of osteopenia and osteoporosis: a meta-analytic review. AIDS 2006;20:2165–74.

[102] Paccou J, Viget N, Legrout-Gérot I, et al. Bone loss in patients with HIV infection. Joint Bone Spine 2009;76(6):637–41.

[103] Overton ET, Chan E, Brown TT, et al. Vitamin D and calcium attenuate bone loss with antiretroviral therapy initiation: a randomized trial. Ann Intern Med 2015;162(12):815–24.

[104] Volpe SL. Magnesium, the metabolic syndrome, insulin resistance, and type 2 diabetes mellitus. Crit Rev Food Sci Nutr 2008;48(3):293–300.

[105] Bogden JD, Kemp F, Han S, et al. Status of selected nutrients and progression of human immunodeficiency virus type 1 infection. Am J Clin Nutr 2000;72(3):809–15.

[106] Feiner JJ, McNurlan M, Ferris RE, et al. Chromium picolinate for insulin resistance in subjects with HIV disease: a pilot study. Diabetes Obes Metab 2008;10(2):151–8.

[107] Stein SA, McNurlan M, Phillips BT, et al. Chromium therapy for insulin resistance associated with HIV-disease. J AIDS Clin Res 2013;4(9):239.

[108] Standish LJ, Ruhland J, DiDomenico B, et al. HIV/AIDS: naturopathic medical principles and practice. In: Pizzorno J, Murray P, editors. Textbook of natural medicine. US: Elsevier; 2007.

[109] Piscitelli SC, Burstein A, Chaitt D, et al. Indinavir concentrations and St John's wort. Lancet 2000;355:547–8.

[110] Fasinu PS, Gurley B, Walker LA. Clinically relevant pharmacokinetic herb-drug interactions in antiretroviral therapy. Curr Drug Metab 2015;17(1):52–64.

[111] Gomaa NF, Hashish M. The inhibitory effect of garlic (Allium sativum) on growth of some microorganisms. J Egypt Public Health Assoc 2003;78(5–6):361–72.

[112] Goncagul G, Ayaz E. Antimicrobial effect of garlic (Allium sativum). Recent Pat Antiinfect Drug Discov 2010;5(1):91–3.

[113] No authors listed. Garlic extract for HIV? Treatmentupdate 1998;10(3):1–2.

[114] Liu C, Wang C, Robison E, et al. Short-term garlic supplementation and highly active antiretroviral treatment adherence, CD4+ cell counts, and human immunodeficiency virus viral load. Althern Ther Health Med 2012;18(1):18–22.

[115] Babb DA, Pemba L, Seatlanyane P, et al. Use of traditional medicine by HIV-infected individuals in South Africa in the era of antiretroviral therapy. Psychol Health Med 2007;12(3):314–20.

[116] Surjushe A, Vasani R, Saple DG. Aloe vera: a short review. Indian J Dermatol 2008;53(4):163–6.

[117] Womble D, Helderman J. The impact of acemannan on the generation and function of cytotoxic T-lymphocytes. Immunopharmacol Immunotoxicol 1992;14(1–2):63–77.

[118] Kahlon JB, Kemp M, Carpenter RH, et al. Inhibition of AIDS virus replication by acemannan in vitro. Mol Biother 1991;3(3):127–35.

[119] Pulse TL, Elizabeth U. A significant improvement in a clinical pilot study utilizing nutritional supplements, essential fatty acids and stabilized aloe vera juice in 29 HIV seropositive, ARC and AIDS patients. Journal of Advancement in Medicine 1990;3(4).

[120] Olatunya OS, Olatunya A, Anyabolu HC, et al. Preliminary trial of aloe vera gruel on HIV infection. J Altern Complement Med 2012;18(9):850–3.

[121] Chang RS, Yeung H. Inhibition of growth of human immunodeficiency virus in vitro by crude extracts of Chinese medicinal herbs. Antiviral Res 1988;9(3):163–75.

[122] Calabrese C, Berman S, Babish JG, et al. A phase I trial of andrographolide in HIV positive patients and normal volunteers. Phytother Res 2000;14(5):333–8.

[123] Kashiwada Y, Nagao T, Hashimoto A, et al. Anti-AIDS agents 38. Anti-HIV activity of 3-O-acyl ursolic acid derivatives. J Nat Prod 2000;63(12):1619–22.

[124] Cho WCS, Leung KN. In vitro and in vivo immunomodulating and immunorestorative effects of Astragalus membranaceus. J Ethnopharmacol 2007;113(1):132–41.

[125] Wei JA, Sun L, Chen YX. Effects of ailing granule on immuno-reconstruction in HIV/AIDS patients. Zhongguo Zhong Xi Yi Jie He Za Zhi 2006;26(4):319–21.

[126] Kusum M, Klinbuayaem V, Bunjob M, et al. Preliminary efficacy and safety of oral suspension SH, combination of five Chinese medicinal herbs, in people living with HIV/AIDS: the phase I/II study. J Med Assoc Thai 2004;87(9):1065–70.

[127] Monograph NS. Wild Indigo; 2009. Available from https://www.scu.edu.au/southern-cross-plant-science/facilities/medicinal-plant-garden/monographs/baptisia-tinctoria/#d.en.196646.

[128] Cinsembu KC. Ethnobotanical study on plants used in the management of HIV/AIDs-related Diseases in Livingstone, Southern Province, Zambia. Evid Based Complement Alternat Med 2016;2016:4238625.

[129] Moga M. Alternative treatment of gallbladder disease. Med Hypotheses 2003;60(1):143–7.

[130] Inada Y, Watanabe K, Kamiyama M, et al. In vitro immunomodulatory effects of traditional Kampo medicine (Sho-saiko-to: SST) on peripheral mononuclear cells in patients with AIDS. Biomed Pharmacother 1990;44(1):17–19.

[131] Buimovici-Klein E, Mohan V, Lange M, et al. Inhibition of HIV replication in lymphocyte cultures of virus-positive subjects in the presence of Sho-saiko-to, an oriental plant extract. Antiviral Res 1990;14(4–5):279–86.

[132] Fassina G, Buffa A, Benelli R, et al. Polyphenolic antioxidant (-)-epigallocatechin-3-gallate from green tea as a candidate anti-HIV agent. AIDS 2002;16(6):939–41.

[133] Nance CL, Shearer W. Is green tea good for HIV-1 infection? J Allergy Clin Immunol 2003;112:851–3.

[134] Nakane H, Ono K. Differential inhibition of HIV-reverse transcriptase and various DNA and RNA polymerases by some catechin derivatives. Nucleic Acids Res 1989;21:115–16.

[135] Nance CL, Siwak E, Shearer WT. Preclinical development of the green tea catechin, epigallocatechin gallate, as an HIV-1 therapy. J Allergy Clin Immunol 2009;123(2):459–65.

[136] Ellis RJ, Toperoff W, Vaida F, et al. Smoked medicinal cannabis for neuropathic pain in HIV: a randomized, crossover clinical trial. Neuropsychopharmacology 2009;34(3):672–80.

[137] Riva DA, Fernández-Larrosa P, Dolcini GL, et al. Two immunomodulators, curcumin and sulfasalazine, enhance IDV antiretroviral activity in HIV-1 persistently infected cells. Arch Virol 2008;153(3):561–5.

[138] Prasad S, Tyagi A. Curcumin and its analogues: a potential natural compound against HIV infection and AIDS. Food Funct 2015;6(11):3412–19.

[139] Conteas CN, Panossian A, Tran TT, et al. Treatment of HIV-associated diarrhea with curcumin. Dig Dis Sci 2009;54(10):2188–91.

[140] No authors listed. Are echinacea and HIV not a good mix? Treatmentupdate 1999;11(1):3.

[141] Berman S, Justis J, Tilles JG, et al. Dramatic increase in immune mediated HIV killing activity induced by Echinacea angustifolia. Int Conf AIDS 1998;12:582.

[142] Reinke RA, Lee D, McDougall BR, et al. L-chicoric acid inhibits human immunodeficiency virus type 1 integration in vivo and is a noncompetitive but reversible inhibitor of HIV-1 integrase in vitro. Virology 2004;326(2):203–19.

[143] Robinson WE Jr. L-chicoric acid, an inhibitor of human immunodeficiency virus type 1 (HIV-1) integrase, improves on the in vitro anti-HIV-1 effect of zidovudine plus a protease inhibitor (AG1350). Antiviral Res 1998;39:101–11.

[144] Moltó J, Valle M, Miranda C, et al. Herb-drug interaction between Echinacea purpurea and etravirine in HIV-infected patients. Antimicrob Agents Chemother 2012;56(10):5328–31.

[145] Moltó J, Valle M, Miranda C, et al. Herb-drug interaction between Echinacea purpurea and darunavir-ritonavir in HIV-infected patients. Antimicrob Agents Chemother 2011;55(1):326–30.

[146] Farber EW, Bhaju J, Campos PE, et al. Psychological well-being in persons receiving HIV-related mental health services: the role of personal meaning in a stress and coping model. Gen Hosp Psychiatry 2010;32(1):73–9.

[147] No authors listed. Eleutherococcus senticosus. Altern Med Rev Monograph 2006;11(2):151–5.

[148] Sanodiya BS, Thakur G, Baghel RK, et al. Ganoderma lucidum: a potent pharmacological macrofungus. Curr Pharm Biotechnol 2009;10(8):717–42.

[149] el-Mekkawy S, Meselhy M, Nakamura N, et al. Anti-HIV-1 and anti-HIV-1-protease substances from Ganoderma lucidum. Phytochemistry 1998;49(6):1651–7.

[150] Min BS, Nakamura N, Miyashiro H, et al. Triterpenes from the spores of Ganoderma lucidum and their inhibitory activity against HIV-1 protease. Chem Pharm Bull (Tokyo) 1998;46(10):1607–12.

[151] Fiore C, Eisenhut M, Krausse R, et al. Antiviral effects of Glycyrrhiza species. Phytother Res 2008;22(2):141–8.

[152] Mori K, Sakai H, Suzuki S, et al. Effects of glycyrrhizin (SNMC: stronger neo-minophagen C) in hemophilia patients with HIV infection. Tohoku J Exp Med 1989;158:25–35.

[153] Gotoh Y, Tada K, Yamada M, et al. Administration of glycyrrhizin to patients with human immunodeficiency virus infection. Igaku no Ayumi 1987;140:619–20.

[154] Al Anazi AR. Gastrointestinal opportunistic infections in human immunodeficiency virus disease. Saudi J Gastroenterol 2009;15(2):95–9.

[155] Birt DF, Widrlechner M, Hammer KD, et al. Hypericum in infection: identification of anti-viral and anti-inflammatory constituents. Pharm Biol 2009;47(8):774–82.

[156] No author listed. Protein in St John's wort may suppress HIV-1 gene expression. Research suggests interesting possibilities. AIDS Alert 2005;20(15):138–9.

[157] Darbinian-Sarkissian N, Darbinyan A, Otte J, et al. p27(SJ), a novel protein in St John's wort, that suppresses expression of HIV-1 genome. Gene Ther 2006;13(4):288–95.

[158] Mayne TJ, Vittinghoff E, Chesney MA, et al. Depressive affect and survival among gay and bisexual men infected with HIV. Arch Intern Med 1996;156:2233–8.

[159] Dattner A. Herbal and complementary medicine in dermatology. Dermatol Clin 2004;22(3):325–32.

[160] Kitzberger C, Rozangela P, Junior A, et al. Antioxidant and antimicrobial activities of shiitake (Lentinula edodes) extracts obtained by organic solvents and supercritical fluids. J Food Eng 2007;80(2):631–8.

[161] Ngai PH, Ng T. Lentin, a novel and potent antifungal protein from shitake mushroom with inhibitory effects on activity of human immunodeficiency virus-1 reverse transcriptase and proliferation of leukemia cells. Life Sci 2003;73(26):3363–74.

[162] Lee-Huang S, Zhang L, Huang PL, et al. Anti-HIV activity of olive leaf extract (OLE) and modulation of host cell gene expression by HIV-1 infection and OLE treatment. Biochem Biophys Res Commun 2003;307(4):1029–37.

[163] Sung H, Kang S, Lee MS, et al. Korean red ginseng slows depletion of CD4 T cells in human immunodeficiency virus type 1-infected patients. Clin Diagn Lab Immunol 2005;12(4):497–501.

[164] Cho YK, Kim Y, Lee I, et al. The effect of Korean red ginseng (KRG), zidovudine (ZDV), and the combination of KRG and ZDV on HIV-infected patients. J Korean Soc Microbiol 1996;31:353–60.

[165] Calderón MM, Chairez CL, Gordon LA, et al. Influence of Panax ginseng on the steady state pharmacokinetic profile of lopinavir-ritonavir in healthy volunteers. Pharmacotherapy 2014;34(11):1151–8.

[166] Thyagarajan SP, Subramanian S, Thirunalasundari T, et al. Effect of Phyllanthus amarus on chronic carriers of hepatitis B virus. Lancet 1988;2:764–6.

[167] Kiemer AK, Hartung T, Huber C, et al. Phyllanthus amarus has anti-inflammatory potential by inhibition of iNOS, COX-2, and cytokines via the NF-kappaB pathway. J Hepatol 2003;38:289–97.

[168] Notka F, Meier G, Wagner R. Concerted inhibitory activities of Phyllanthus amarus on HIV replication in vitro and ex vivo. Antiviral Res 2004;64(2):93–102.

[169] Uckun FM, Chelstrom L, Tuel-Ahlgren L, et al. TXU (anti-CD7)-pokeweed antiviral protein as a potent inhibitor of human immunodeficiency virus. Antimicrob Agents Chemother 1998;42:383–8.

[170] Li BQ, Fu T, Yan YD, et al. Inhibition of HIV infection by baicalin – a flavonoid compound purified from Chinese herbal medicine. Cell Mol Biol Res 1993;39(2):119–24.

[171] Li BQ, Fu T, Dongyan Y, et al. Flavonoid baicalin inhibits HIV-1 infection at the level of viral entry. Biochem Biophys Res Commun 2000;276(2):534–8.

[172] Mehendale S, Aung H, Wang CZ, et al. Scutellaria baicalensis and a constituent flavonoid, baicalein, attenuate ritonavir-induced gastrointestinal side-effects. J Pharm Pharmacol 2007;59(11):1567–72.

[173] Hernandez V. Liver function and HIV-1 infection. STEP Perspect 1995;7(2):13–15.

[174] McClure J, Lovelace E, Elahi S, et al. Silibinin inhibits HIV-1 infection by reducing cellular activation and proliferation. PLoS ONE 2012;7(7):e41832.

[175] Portillo A, Vila R, Freixa B, et al. Antifungal activity of Paraguayan plants used in traditional medicine. J Ethnopharmacol 2001;76(1):93–8.

[176] Chunchanur SK, Nadgir S, Halesh LH, et al. Detection and antifungal susceptibility testing of oral Candida dubliniensis from human immunodeficiency virus-infected patients. Indian J Pathol Microbiol 2009;52(4):501–4.

[177] Grieve M. A modern herbal. New York: Dover Publications; 1971.

[178] Felter H, Lloyd J. King's American dispensatory. 18th ed. Portland, OR: Eclectic Medical Publications; Reprinted 1983, originally 1905.

[179] Leonard SS, Keil D, Mehlman T, et al. Essiac tea: scavenging of reactive oxygen species and effects on DNA damage. J Ethnopharmacol 2006;103(2):288–96.

[180] Bradley PR. British herbal compendium. Bournemouth, UK: British Herbal Medicine Association; 1992.

[181] Keplinger K, Laus G, Wurm M, et al. Uncaria tomentosa (Willd.) DC. – Ethnomedicinal use and new pharmacological, toxicological and botanical results. J Ethnopharmacol 1998;64(1):23–34.

[182] Mukhtar M, Arshad M, Ahmad M, et al. Antiviral potentials of medicinal plants. Virus Res 2008;131:111–20.

[183] Persson L, Ostergren P, Hanson BS, et al. Social network, social support and the rate of decline of CD4 lymphocytes in asymptomatic HIV-positive homosexual men. Canadian AIDS Treatment Information Exchange (CATIE) News September 2002;12.

24

Lyme disease and co-infections

Dr Nicola McFadzean Ducharme

INTRODUCTION

Lyme disease is an infectious disease caused by the bacteria *Borrelia burgdorferi*, along with other strains of *Borrelia* such as *garinii*, *afzelii* and *andersonii*. Collectively, they are known as *Borrelia burgdorferi sensu lato*. Worldwide, the *Borrelia burgdorferi sense lato* complex consists of at least 23 genospecies or genomospecies.[1]

Borrelia are spiral-shaped bacteria called spirochaetes, similar to *Treponema palladium*, the bacteria that causes syphilis. Their long, spiral shape facilitates their burrowing into body tissues and gives them certain attributes that are vital to their virility. *B. burgdorferi* is officially not classified Gram positive or Gram negative, but does stain Gram negative by default, and acts in a manner closer to the behaviour of Gram-negative bacteria.[2]

As well as existing in spirochaete form, *Borrelia* bacteria have the ability to morph into other forms – notably, a cell-wall-deficient, or L-form, and a round-body, or cyst form. These three morphologically different presentations of the same bacteria can help to explain the ability of the bacteria to produce persistent infection and chronic disease.[3,4]

Research shows that these forms can morph back and forth, forming cell-wall-deficient or cyst formation colonies, and then revert back to their original spirochaete form, depending on environmental conditions.[5]

This phenomenon is not unique to *Borrelia* bacteria; however, it does add to the complexity of the disease and, as evidenced in the section on treatment, influences the way treatment protocols must be designed.

Another factor adding to the complexity of *Borrelia* is the existence of biofilm colonies. A biofilm occurs when a group of bacteria adhere to one another and to other surfaces within the body and produce an extracellular polymeric substance (EPS) that is made up of extracellular DNA, proteins and polysaccharides. This slimy, sticky matrix provides an environment where the bacteria are sheltered from the immune system and, in the case of Lyme disease, from antimicrobial agents such as antibiotics too. It provides an environment where the bacteria can hide and evade host defences, and allows them to survive in diverse environmental conditions.[6]

It has been stated that the virulence and persistence of *Borrelia* spp. and their apparent resistance to treatment is due both to their ability to morph into cell-wall-deficient and cystic states, and their ability to create biofilm.[3]

BROADENING THE DEFINITION OF LYME DISEASE

While the textbook definition of Lyme disease is infection with *B. burgdorferi*, in clinical practice, this definition becomes too limited. In reality, Lyme disease includes borreliosis as well as a range of co-infections that are commonly transmitted along with it. These co-infections include *Babesia*, *Bartonella* and *Ehrlichia* and *Rickettsia* spp.

Babesia is a malaria-like illness caused by a parasite called a piroplasm, rather than a bacterium. This is significant, as many antibiotic therapies will not be effective against *Babesia*. Common species include *Babesia microti* and *B. duncani*. *Babesia* inhabits the red blood cells and can cause haemolysis and haemoglobinuria with resultant anaemia.

Bartonella is also known as cat scratch fever (*B. henselae*), Carrion's disease (*B. bacilliformins*) and trench fever (*B. quintana*), depending on the strain. *B. henselae* often creates scratches on the skin that come and go. Striae ranging from white to red to purple that flare and remit are also common. In the bacterial family, *Bartonella* can produce symptoms that overlap closely with those of borreliosis, but tends to have stronger neurological and psychiatric manifestations than musculoskeletal.

Human ehrlichiosis, first recognised in the US in 1986, is caused by several species of bacteria of the subfamily *Rickettsiaceae*. Human granulocytic ehrlichia and human monocyctic ehrlichia are two variants of this co-infection, infecting the granulocytes and monocytes respectively. Both strains cause the same clinical presentation, so are jointly referred to as ehrlichiosis.

Rickettsiae, other than those causing ehrlichiosis, belonging to either the spotted or typhus fever group, are also tick borne and can co-exist with *Borrelia*. They are small, Gram-negative bacteria and are highly prevalent in Australia.

The signs and symptoms of these co-infections will be examined in the following sections, along with their respective treatment protocols. Dr Richard Horowitz, one of the leading American Lyme-literate physicians, in a presentation at the International Lyme and Associated Disease Society conference in 2014, stated that while 20 years ago he would see patients that were infected simply with *B. burgdorferi*, he now estimates that over 80% of his patients are infected with at least one co-infection, many of them multiply co-infected.

Dr Horowitz is also a proponent of looking at a broad definition of Lyme disease, beyond that of a simple infectious process. He coined the term multiple systemic infectious diseases syndrome (MSIDS), which states that Lyme disease should be looked at within the context of the broad systemic impact on the body, but also in the context of co-factors that contribute to its severity and chronicity, such as other opportunistic infections (including candida, mycoplasma and viruses), methylation issues, mould toxicity, heavy metal toxicity, adrenal and hormonal dysfunction and chronic inflammatory states. In reality, in a chronic Lyme patient, many of these factors will indeed be at play and must be addressed holistically.

STAGES OF LYME DISEASE

There are three main stages of Lyme disease. Borreliosis can be categorised into early localised, early disseminated and chronic infection. Certainly, a previously healthy person with an acute case of Lyme disease will have a much better prognosis and easier treatment path than the chronically ill patient if the infection is identified, accurately diagnosed and accurately treated. The problem lies in the fact that fewer than 50% of patients with Lyme disease recall a tick bite, and fewer than 50% of patients recall a rash.[7]

Early localised Lyme

In early localised Lyme, the classic sign is the erythema migrans, or bull's eye rash (see Fig. 24.1). This may occur at the bite site within a few days up to a month, and appears as a target shape with a red circular rash and central clearing. Many erythema migrans rashes are misdiagnosed as ringworm, which is also non-itchy and has a rounded shape, or a spider bite. Some rashes do not

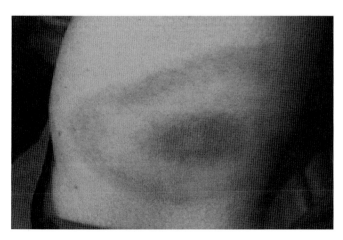

FIGURE 24.1 Erythema migrans rash[8]

have the signature target presentation and may be more diffuse, lack the central clearing, cover larger areas of the body and be patchier. This leads to yet further confusion over an accurate diagnosis.

In early localised Lyme, we can see flu-like illness, headaches, myalgia and malaise.

Early disseminated Lyme

Here the bacteria are spreading throughout the body and causing a wider array of systemic symptoms. Neurological symptoms, such as burning and shooting pains, cognitive changes and psychological symptoms, are common. Migratory arthralgias and myalgias are common, and cardiac involvement, such as palpitations and chest pain, can result. This is in addition to the symptoms in early localised Lyme listed above.

Early disseminated Lyme, while still being acute, is a more severe presentation and may need more aggressive antimicrobial therapy to overcome it.

Chronic Lyme disease

Chronic Lyme disease is defined as illness that exists beyond 1 year. Symptoms are typically multi-systemic and can become severe, including arthralgias, myalgias, cognitive deficits, headaches and migraines, debilitating fatigue, sleep disturbance and many more (see symptom list). Symptoms tend to wax and wane, sometimes on a random schedule, but often flare every month following the reproductive cycle of the *Borrelia* bacteria.

Joseph Burrascano, MD, author of *Advanced Topics in Lyme Disease: Diagnostic Hints and Treatment Guidelines for Lyme and Other Tick-borne Illnesses*, suggests that to be categorised as chronic Lyme disease, three criteria must be present[9]:

1   Duration greater than 1 year.
2   Major neurological involvement or active arthritic symptoms.
3   Active *Borrelia* infection despite prior antibiotic therapy.

Chronic Lyme disease has become quite a political issue. To give a brief synopsis, the Infectious Diseases Society of America (IDSA) contends that chronic Lyme disease does not even exist, and that all cases of Lyme can be cured with 14–28 days of antibiotic therapy. Its position is that symptoms that persist beyond antibiotic therapy are classified as 'post-Lyme syndrome' and are the result of factors such as ongoing inflammation, tissue damage, depression and even psychosomatic illness.

There are many studies that demonstrate the persistence of *Borrelia*, even after the IDSA-recommended courses of antibiotics. However, its position stands and has influenced positions of other governments and health agencies, including those in Australia. Once its treatment guidelines are adopted, any consideration of Lyme as a chronic illness is refuted and often denied. This has contributed to widespread misdiagnosis, under-diagnosis and the inability of patients to find adequate and informed medical care.

At the time of writing, there is little recognition of the existence of chronic Lyme disease in Australia, despite studies showing the presence of *Borrelia* in ticks and patients who tested positive through polymerase chain reaction (PCR) testing but had never left the country.[10]

The political climate of Lyme and co-infections makes it challenging for practitioners and patients alike.

The existence of Lyme as a chronic illness is supported by the International Lyme and Associated Diseases Society (ILADS) (www.ilads.org). It has a bank of research to substantiate its position on the chronicity of Lyme disease as well as a published set of treatment guidelines.

Much of this chapter refers to the treatment of patients with chronic Lyme disease. In a previously healthy patient, with sufficient antimicrobial treatment, an acute case of Lyme can be overcome. It is the chronically ill patients who are most challenged in their health and need a holistic and multi-systemic approach to their care.

EPIDEMIOLOGY OF LYME DISEASE

Lyme disease is currently the most prevalent vector-borne disease in the US, with more than 100 000 cases reported by the US Centers for Disease Control and Prevention (CDC) since its discovery in 1982.[11]

Newer reports show that the CDC is aware of the gross underestimation of cases; its new estimates are that 300 000 people are infected with Lyme disease each year, 10 times more than previously reported.[12] Another reason for the under-reporting of Lyme disease cases is that, as mentioned earlier, fewer than 50% of patients with Lyme disease recall a tick bite, and less than 50% of cases recall any rash.[13]

Boys aged 5–9 are the most affected group in the US,[14] followed by both males and females aged 60–64 years.[15]

Occupations such as forest workers, hunters, rangers, gamekeepers, farmers and military field personnel have a higher incidence of infection, which has been documented by both antibody prevalence in the blood and disease incidence.[16]

Lyme disease is also the fastest growing vector-borne disease in Europe[17] and has been found in over 80 nations worldwide.[18]

While accurate numbers of cases in Australia are impossible to predict due to lack of health agency tracking, a study investigating the incidence of Lyme disease, *Babesia*, *Bartonella* and *Rickettsia* identified a much greater incidence than previously reported. Further, endemic cases of human *Babesia* and *Bartonella* disease in Australia with coexisting *Borrelia* infection have been documented, demonstrating local acquisition in patients who have never been abroad.[10]

Even as far back as 1998, a study was published in the *Medical Journal of Australia* describing the results of testing from 1024 patients who presented with erythema migrans rash, arthritis and radiculopathy.[19] It found that of these patients, 20% tested positive on a Western blot against *B. burgdorferi*, *garinii* or *afzelii*. Of these positive results, 56% were due to *B. garinii*, 34% to *B. afzelii* and only 10% to *B. burgdorferi*.

This reflects what is still considered relevant today: Australian Lyme disease is caused more by European strains of *Borrelia* (*garinii* and *afzelii*) than American strains (*burgdorferi*).

HOW IS LYME TRANSMITTED?

Lyme disease is considered to be a tick-borne pathogen; that is, it is transmitted through the bite of a tick. Nymph ticks are the most common ticks to harbour and transmit Lyme disease. They are the size of a poppy seed and are, therefore, very difficult to spot on the body.

Australia is home to between 750 and 900 species of ticks. The paralysis tick, *Ixodes holocyclus*, appears to be responsible for most bites to humans on the east coast of Australia; however, the brown dog tick *Rhipicephalus sanguineus* and the bush tick *Haemaphysalis longicornis* have both been found to harbour *Borrelia* spirochaetes. Given the disease-carrying potential of ticks in general, it is wise to consider any tick a possible vector for *Borrelia* and co-infections.

Animals that have been found to carry *Borrelia* include bandicoots, grey and red kangaroos, rats, other rodents and cattle.

Thus, factors that influence transmission of Lyme are those that influence the patterns of vectors: climate factors include rainfall, humidity and temperature; human behaviour patterns include building expansions and locations of homes that enter into high-prevalence areas; patterns of recreation and leisure include hiking, camping and other outdoor activities; and patterns of travel into forested, rural areas, as well as across countries and nations.

It is important to consider that other vectors may be able to transmit *Borrelia* bacteria. Several global studies support this.

Dr Steven Luger reported in the *New England Journal of Medicine* a case in which a patient was bitten by a fly and presented with Lyme symptoms 13 days later[20] and a German study reported a patient who developed arthritis and was seropositive for *Borrelia* following a fly bite.[21]

Several studies have reported *Borrelia* spirochaetes being identified in mosquitoes and fleas, and also in mites. These tests actually found the spirochaetes in the insects themselves.[22–25]

Other important routes of transmission include sexual transmission and transmission from mother to baby in utero.

There are several studies demonstrating sexual transmission of Lyme disease. Given that *Borrelia* is a spirochaete not unlike *Treponema* – the cause of syphilis – which is considered a sexually transmitted disease, it seems logical that *Borrelia* could also be transmitted that way.

Dr Gregory Bach, DO, a physician in Pennsylvania, observed that many partners and spouses of his patients were also presenting with Lyme disease, despite no known personal experience of a tick bite. He also noted that sexually active couples had more antibiotic treatment failures, which indicated that one partner might be reinfecting the other.

He conducted blood tests on those partners, as well as their semen and vaginal secretions. Semen samples of his male patients (who had tested positive for Lyme via PCR and/or Western blot tests) and of male partners of female patients were positive 40% of the time. In the semen itself, spirochaetes were detected in 14 of 32 Lyme patients. Further, he found that all positive semen and vaginal secretions resulted in positive Lyme titres and/or PCR tests in their sexual partners.

Another study also demonstrated the presence of *Borrelia* spirochaetes in semen and vaginal fluids. This study also noted a distinct *Borrelia* strain in a sexually active couple that was different from other strains found in other couples, supporting the premise of *Borrelia* transmission via shared genital secretions.

This study divided patients into three groups – a control group of subjects without evidence of Lyme disease, random subjects who tested positive for Lyme disease, and married heterosexual subjects engaging in unprotected sex who had tested positive for Lyme disease.

Results showed that the control subjects tested negative for *Borrelia* bacteria in semen and vaginal secretions. Of the positive Lyme patients, all of the women had *Borrelia* spirochaetes in their vaginal secretions, while half the men had *Borrelia* spirochaetes in their semen. The sexually active couples showed identical strains of *Borrelia* in their semen and vaginal secretions, indicating that those strains had been shared.[26]

This study supports the probability of sexual transmission of Lyme disease. Case reports also support the idea of sexual transmission; people engage in sexual relations with symptomatic individuals and quickly become symptomatic with the exact same symptoms themselves.

Another mode of transmission is congenital – mother to baby in utero. Studies have demonstrated that transplacental transmission of *Borrelia* is possible, and that gestational Lyme is associated with problems including fetal death, hydrocephalus, cardiovascular anomalies, neonatal respiratory distress, hyperbilirubinaemia, intrauterine growth retardation, cortical blindness, sudden infant death syndrome and maternal toxaemia of pregnancy.[27]

There are 46 cases of congenital Lyme disease documented in peer-reviewed research studies. These cases mostly reflect babies that have been stillborn or died shortly after birth, as autopsy examination gives information that is not possible to gather from live children (such as biopsies of brain tissue). Many other children have been born with congenital Lyme but do not have life-threatening presentations.

Several studies have demonstrated the link between *Borrelia* spirochaetes in fetal tissue and in babies and adverse outcomes. One study reported a woman who developed Lyme disease in her first trimester of pregnancy but was not treated with antibiotics. The infant was born at 35 weeks gestation and died of congenital heart disease during the first week of life. Histological examination showed the *Borrelia* spirochaete in the spleen, kidneys and bone marrow of the infant.[28]

Another case reported a baby born at term weighing only 2.5 kg and stillborn.[29] *Borrelia* was cultured from the liver, and spirochaetes were found in the heart, adrenal glands, liver, brain and placenta.

Outcomes in congenital Lyme are related to whether or not the mother was treated with antibiotics. In a presentation at the ILADS annual conference in Toronto, Canada, in 2011, paediatric Lyme expert Charles Ray Jones, MD, stated his opinion that mothers with Lyme disease had a 50% chance of passing Lyme onto their children, mothers who were treated with one antibiotic had a 25% chance and women who were treated with two antibiotics had a 5% chance.

In a published review of 95 cases of pregnant women with Lyme disease who were treated with antibiotics (66 of them parenterally – intravenously [IV] or intramuscular [IM] injection, 19 of them with oral antibiotics and 10 women with no treatment). Adverse outcomes were seen in 8 of 66 parenterally treated women, 6 of 19 orally treated women and 6 of 10 untreated women. In other words, 60% of untreated women had adverse outcomes compared with 12% and 31% of treated mothers (parenteral and oral, respectively). Loss of the pregnancy and cavernous haemangioma were the most common adverse outcomes.[30]

There is also evidence of *Borrelia* spirochaetes in breast milk; however, the possibility and incidence of transmission this way is less clear. *Borrelia* has been detected in breast milk based on PCR testing.[31] No studies of maternal–infant transmission have been published; however, most doctors who are experts in the treatment of chronic Lyme disease still recommend that women either do not breastfeed or remain on antibiotic therapy throughout.

SIGNS AND SYMPTOMS OF LYME DISEASE

Lyme disease is often called 'the great imitator' because it mimics so many other illnesses. Many patients have received diagnoses over the course of their illness that may match their symptoms, while Lyme disease may have always been the underlying trigger, or at least a contributor. Following is a list of diagnoses that are common in Lyme patients:

- chronic fatigue syndrome
- fibromyalgia
- multiple sclerosis
- ALS/motor neurone disease
- Parkinson's disease
- Alzheimer's disease
- autism spectrum disorders
- rheumatoid arthritis
- Hashimoto's thyroiditis and other thyroid disorders
- autoimmune diseases including lupus and Sjogren's syndrome
- juvenile arthritis
- encephalitis.

These are just a few examples. There are many more that could be mistakenly given, even though the problem may have been Lyme disease all along. There are also times, of course, when both diagnoses are accurate and relevant, but Lyme may have triggered the comorbidity.

Signs and symptoms of Lyme disease are many and varied. Each person presents somewhat differently, and symptom pictures will change over time. In fact, one hallmark of Lyme disease is that symptoms wax and wane, sometimes in a regular/cyclical fashion, but sometimes erratically and without a predictable pattern.

The list below represents signs and symptoms of Lyme disease.[32] The list is extensive. However, patients will typically present with many if not most of these. Having 30–40 symptoms on their list is not uncommon.

Skin

- Rash at the site of the bite
- Rash on other parts of the body
- Raised rash, disappearing and recurring
- Striae (stretch marks) that may be red or purple
- Scratches on the skin (like cat scratches)
- Lumps (nodules) under the skin

Head, face, neck

- Unexplained hair loss
- Headaches, mild or severe
- Seizures
- Pressure in head, white matter lesions in brain (MRI)
- Twitching of facial or other muscles
- Facial paralysis (Bell's palsy)
- Tingling of the nose, tongue or cheek
- Facial flushing
- Stiff or painful neck
- Jaw pain or stiffness
- Dental problems (unexplained), tooth pain
- Sore throat, clearing throat a lot, phlegm, hoarseness, runny nose
- Difficulty swallowing, feeling as if something is stuck in the throat

Eyes/vision

- Double or blurry vision
- Increased floaters
- Pain in the eyes or swelling around the eyes
- Hypersensitivity to light
- Flashing lights
- Phantom images in the periphery of vision

Ears/hearing

- Decreased hearing in one or both ears, plugged ears
- Buzzing in the ears
- Pain in the ears, oversensitivity to sounds
- Ringing in one or both ears

Digestive and excretory systems

- Diarrhoea
- Constipation
- Irritable bladder (trouble starting, stopping)
- Interstitial cystitis
- Upset stomach (nausea or pain)
- GORD (gastro-oesophageal reflux disease)

Musculoskeletal system

- Bone pain, joint pain or swelling, carpal tunnel syndrome
- Stiffness of joints, back, neck, tennis elbow
- Muscle pain or cramps
- Fibromyalgia
- Tendonitis

Respiratory and circulatory systems

- Shortness of breath
- Air hunger – cannot get full/satisfying breath
- Chronic cough
- Chest pain or rib soreness
- Night sweats or unexplained chills
- Heart palpitations or extra beats
- Endocarditis
- Heart blockage

Neurological system

- Tremors or unexplained shaking
- Burning or stabbing sensations in the body
- Weakness, peripheral neuropathy or partial paralysis
- Pressure in the head
- Numbness in the body, tingling, pinpricks
- Poor balance, dizziness, difficulty walking
- Increased motion sickness
- Light-headedness, wooziness

Psychological/psychiatric

- Mood swings, irritability, bipolar disorder
- Unusual depression
- Disorientation (getting or feeling lost)
- Feeling as if you are losing your mind
- Over-emotional reactions, crying easily
- Too much sleep, or insomnia
- Difficulty falling or staying asleep
- Narcolepsy, sleep apnoea
- Panic attacks, anxiety
- Obsessive–compulsive disorder (OCD) traits

Cognitive

- Memory loss (short or long term)
- Confusion, difficulty in thinking
- Difficulty with concentration or reading
- Speech difficulty (slurred or slow)
- Word finding difficulty
- Stammering speech
- Forgetting how to perform simple tasks

Reproduction and sexuality

- Loss of sex drive
- Sexual dysfunction
- Unexplained menstrual pain, irregularity
- Unexplained breast pain, discharge
- Testicular or pelvic pain
- Vulvodynia

General wellbeing

- Phantom smells
- Unexplained weight gain or loss
- Extreme fatigue
- Swollen glands/lymph nodes
- Unexplained fevers (high or low grade)
- Continual infections (sinus, kidney, eye, etc.)
- Symptoms seem to change, come and go
- Pain migrates (moves) to different body parts
- Early on, experienced a 'flu-like' illness from which the patient has not recovered completely
- Low body temperature
- Allergies/ chemical sensitivities
- Alcohol sensitivity

In the allopathic medical model, body systems are divided up into specialties. This contributes to the difficulty that chronic Lyme disease patients have with finding the right treatment. Lyme patients see neurologists, rheumatologists, cardiologists, endocrinologists, gastroenterologists, and so on, but all these specialists examine and treat their particular area/system of expertise, often at the expense of seeing the whole person and the totality of their symptoms. Subsequently, Lyme disease patients often experience a fragmentation of their care that might bring them symptom relief in certain areas, but does not address the underlying cause.

Symptoms of co-infections

We discussed that the definition of Lyme disease generally includes co-infections because they are such a common component in the infectious process, and the symptom list above reflects the totality of Lyme and co-infection symptoms.

Having said that, it is important to recognise the more specific symptoms of co-infections in order to identify them accurately and treat them effectively. There is much overlap with symptoms of strict borreliosis, but there are a few key hallmark symptoms that stand out to help identify each one.[33]

BORRELIA

- Gradual onset of symptoms
- Multi-system – for example, joint pain along with cardiac involvement; cognitive deficits with fatigue and muscle/joint pain
- Migratory pain from joint to joint
- Fatigue and lethargy, worse in the afternoon
- Four-week cycles
- Stiff, crackly joints
- Headaches originating in the neck
- Slow response to treatment with initial flare (Herxheimer reaction), improvement over weeks with monthly symptom flare
- Erythema migrans rash in 25–50%

BARTONELLA

- Gradual onset of initial illness
- Central nervous system symptoms out of proportion to musculoskeletal

- Central nervous system irritability including muscle twitches, tremors, insomnia, seizures, agitation, anxiety, severe mood swings, outbursts and antisocial behaviour; OCD traits
- Headaches – feel like ice picks in the head
- Gastritis or abdominal pain, bowel problems (irritable bowel syndrome)
- Tender subcutaneous nodules along the extremities, especially the outer thigh, shins and triceps
- Occasional lymphadenopathy (swollen, enlarged lymph nodes)
- Striae or stretch marks that are new or out of place; can be white or red/purple in colour
- Pain in the sides and back of the ribs
- Pain in soles of the feet, painful to walk in the morning
- Tachycardia (rapid heartbeat)
- Photophobia (light sensitivity)
- Rapid response to treatment but a rapid return of symptoms if treatment is stopped too early

BABESIA

- Night sweats and sometimes day sweats as well
- Shortness of breath, air hunger, sighing
- Dry, chronic cough
- Fullness in the throat, difficulty swallowing
- Severe headaches – dull, all over head, feel like head is in a vice
- Dizziness, light-headedness
- Capillary angiomas, especially on breasts
- Vasculitis (red skin with white splotches)
- Hormone imbalance
- Easy bruising
- Burning symptoms
- Head/tooth/sinus/jaw symptoms
- Bell's palsy
- Nausea
- Ear ringing
- Blurry vision
- Vivid/violent dreams, nightmares
- Flushing
- Flare-ups every 4–6 days
- Failure to respond to Lyme treatment
- Feeling of spaciness, wooziness and impending doom

EHRLICHIA/ANAPLASMA

- Rapid onset of initial illness
- Headaches – sharp, knife-like, and often behind the eyes
- Muscle pain, not joint pain, can be mild or severe
- Neurological symptoms – seizure disorders, shooting pains
- Tendon pain
- Pain in the right upper quadrant of the abdomen
- Low white blood cell count, elevated liver enzymes
- Rapid response to treatment

RICKETTSIA

- Fever/chills
- Headaches
- Confusion
- Aching muscles

- Gastrointestinal symptoms – nausea, loss of appetite
- Swelling of lymph nodes
- Malaise

TESTING FOR LYME DISEASE

Testing for Lyme disease is notoriously difficult and somewhat controversial. The lack of reliability and sensitivity in testing, combined with the immune-suppressive effects of the illness itself, have contributed to the misdiagnosis and under-diagnosis of patients.

It should be stressed that Lyme disease is a clinical diagnosis that is based on history, signs, symptoms and clinical presentation, and backed up with lab testing. It is possible to have a negative test result but have all the symptoms of Lyme disease, and potentially a history of a tick bite, and respond to antimicrobial therapy.

Types of tests

Lab tests for Lyme disease can be classified in two categories – direct and indirect tests. Direct tests look for the pathogens or parts of the pathogens themselves, while indirect tests measure an antibody/immune response to the pathogens. It is optimal to combine several different methods of testing to enhance the likelihood of getting useful and accurate diagnostic information. Sensitivity and specificity of these tests varies.

PCR TEST

Polymerase chain reaction (PCR) tests evaluate bodily fluids such as whole blood, serum, urine and cerebrospinal fluid for DNA fragments of the bacteria. The PCR test has good specificity; that is, if a DNA sequence is found that matches the *Borrelia* bacteria, it is a clear diagnosis. It is not highly sensitive, however, especially in chronically ill patients, because *Borrelia* is known to use its corkscrew shape to burrow into tissues, rather than staying in the blood stream. PCR inhibitors in host blood may also play a role.[34]

For this reason, PCR tests may be more sensitive in acute cases of Lyme. PCR testing can also be run on breast milk, semen and tissues from biopsy. It is advantageous to run PCR tests on more than one sample type to maximise the chances of an accurate result. Also, it is important that PCR tests be sensitive to multiple strains of *Borrelia*, not only *B. burgdorferi*.

FISH TEST

Fluorescence in situ hybridisation (FISH) tests also looks for genetic information – in this case, the ribosomal RNA of particular pathogens in the blood. This ribosomal RNA indicates active infection with the pathogen. At the time of writing, FISH tests are available in the US but not Australia for *Babesia* and *Bartonella* (not *Borrelia*). PCR tests are also available for these co-infections, along with antibody tests. FISH tests reportedly have high sensitivity and specificity – 100% and >98%, respectively.[35]

CULTURE

A culture test is when a small amount of blood is taken from a patient and placed in a medium that promotes the growth of that specific bacteria. Bacterial growth and cell characteristics will be assessed over a period of time, assessing short-term growth over a few days to longer-term growth over several weeks. A culture test can be more sensitive and more specific than other direct and indirect tests, and also be validated further by PCR testing. At the time that the culture test was released in the US (by Advanced Labs), the lab was predicting a sensitivity of 94% and specificity of 100%, which surpasses that of the ELISA or Western blot tests.[36]

At the time of writing, a *Borrelia* culture test is not available in Australia.

ELISA TEST

An enzyme-linked immunosorbent assay (ELISA) test is probably the most widely run test as a preliminary screen for Lyme disease. It is not a highly sensitive test and should not be considered reliable. The College of American Pathologists states that a screening test should have 95% sensitivity to be considered an adequate screening test, and the ELISA does not meet that criterion.[37]

The IDSA has required a two-tiered approach to testing, whereby an ELISA test is the first test run, reflexing to Western blot only if the ELISA is positive. This two-tiered approach has been adopted by other countries, including Australia, and contributes to the under-diagnosis and under-reporting of Lyme disease cases.

Studies show that 56% of Lyme patients test negative using the two-tiered approach recommended by the CDC.[38] In fact, 52% of patients with chronic disease are negative by ELISA but positive by Western blot.[39]

The other issue with the sensitivity of the ELISA test is that Lyme disease is inherently immune suppressive. Low white blood cell count is the norm, indicating lowered immune response. Indirect tests, by definition, are measuring an immune response to *Borrelia* – and yet the *Borrelia* is suppressing the immune response. This further reduces sensitivity and underpins the frequent seronegativity of Lyme patients – especially the most chronically ill and the most severe cases.

This is true of any indirect test – they all measure immune response – and is one of the main reasons why Lyme disease should be primarily a clinical diagnosis based on history, symptoms and clinical presentation, and secondarily, a diagnosis based on lab work.

WESTERN BLOT TEST

The Western blot test is one of the most common tests used in the diagnosis of Lyme disease. Lyme-literate practitioners will order Western blot tests and PCR tests most commonly, and will rarely, if at all, order ELISA tests.

The Western blot is prone to the same limitations of indirect tests. When there is an infection suppressing the immune response, measuring the immune response to that infection may not bring the most accurate information. However, by virtue of its methodology, it has greater sensitivity than the ELISA test.[40,41]

Western blots are run on IgG and IgM antibodies. The test reports specific 'bands' that represent different parts of the *Borrelia* antigen. A positive antibody response to that part of the *Borrelia* bacteria will show up as band activity on the test result.

Once again, politics influences which bands are considered clinically significant. In the US, the IDSA restricts the number of bands reported to three – the 23–24 kDa, 39 kDa and 41 kDa. Other labs consider a wider array of bands to be clinically significant, adding 31 kDa, 34 kDa and 83–93 kDa to the above. Band 41 is not a highly specific band because there may be cross-reactivity with other bacteria and viruses. However, the other bands are more Lyme specific and, therefore, more indicative of infection. The CDC requires 5 of 10 bands for IgG surveillance purposes, while other labs will recognise 2 of 5 bands.

Bands are typically reported as negative, indeterminate or positive, with the positive being graded on a scale of one to four. The benefit of this is that even if the test reports negative, seeing the specific bands that are showing some activity can be clinically useful. If a test report shows three Lyme-specific bands showing indeterminate, it will report as negative, whereas a knowledgeable clinician would recognise those bands as clinically relevant information.

T CELL TEST

Western blot, ELISA and other antibody tests measure the humoral immune response to *Borrelia* and co-infections, which does not always bring reliable information and results. The T cell test measures the cellular immune response – it measures T cells that are reactive to specific infections. A lab in Germany that offers this test (called elispot) claims that its test will detect just one reactive cell in 100 000, and that it is between 20 and 200 times more sensitive than the ELISA test.[42]

Another benefit of the T cell test is that the T cells should become non-reactive 4–8 weeks after successful completion of therapy, while antibodies can persist and lead to confusion as to whether the infection has been eradicated. Therefore, the T cell test may be a better choice for monitoring therapy outcome.

Elispot testing is currently available for *B. burgdorferi* and *B. miyamotoi*, and anaplasma/*Ehrlichia*.

Testing for co-infections

Co-infections can also be evaluated by laboratory testing, and should be done so alongside the *Borrelia* testing. While false negatives can occur, it is important to gather as much information as possible relating to co-infections, given that co-infections are such a significant part of the Lyme disease puzzle.

Just as there are many strains of *Borrelia*, there are many strains of the common co-infections too, and testing is not available for all of them. The predominant tests are listed below:

* *Babesia duncani*
* *Babesia microti*
* *Bartonella henselae*
* *Bartonella quintana*
* Human monocytic *Ehrlichia* (HME)
* Human granulocytic *Ehrlichia* (HGE)
* *Rickettsia typhi*
* *Rickettsia rickettsia*

The type of testing done for co-infections varies between different labs and different regions.

The direct tests run for these co-infections are PCR tests and FISH tests. Indirect tests including antibody tests are also commonly run. Both IgG and IgM antibodies should be tested. Elispot tests are offered for some of the co-infections, more frequently by European laboratories.

Similar challenges occur in testing for co-infections due to the immune-suppressing effects of the illness, and so ideally, at last one direct and one indirect test would be combined for maximum results.

Other tests to order

Because Lyme disease is complex and multisystem, comprehensive testing can help identify areas that have been impacted on and need restorative treatment. The following list is a sample of other tests that may be helpful and warranted in Lyme patients:

* CD-57 – an immune marker that can reflect the degree of immunosuppression due to Lyme disease, and hence the severity of the Lyme infection.
* Adrenal testing – preferably salivary cortisol testing to give measurements morning, noon, afternoon and evening to check the circadian rhythm of production. Also dehydroepiandrosterone (DHEA) and pregnenolone.
* Thyroid testing – TSH, free T3, free T4, reverse T3, thyroid antibodies.
* Reproductive hormones – testosterone (free and total), oestradiol, progesterone.
* Iron studies – iron, ferritin, iron-binding capacity – important especially in babesiosis, which can cause haemolysis of red blood cells and therefore impact on iron levels.
* Autoimmune markers – rheumatoid arthritis (RA) factor and antinuclear antibody (ANA).
* Neurotoxin markers such as C4a and C3a.
* Heavy metal testing – hair or urine, provoked with chelator optimal.
* Mould/mycotoxin levels.

TREATMENT OF LYME DISEASE

Before we get into more detailed discussions of both allopathic and naturopathic approaches to Lyme disease, it is helpful to examine some of the complicating factors of treatment in general:

1 Treatment will vary depending on the phase of infection – whether it is in the acute phase or chronic phase. Acute Lyme is much easier to treat successfully, but due to the lack of an accurate diagnosis in the early phases, many cases are not caught and persist into chronicity.

2 There is no one treatment plan or protocol that will fit everyone. Especially in chronic disseminated Lyme, there can be a multitude of factors at play, including

comorbidity with mould and heavy metal toxicity, methylation defects, chronic inflammatory states and opportunistic infections such as mycoplasma and *Candida*. This complicates the treatment process exponentially. Treatment protocols must be tailored to the individual, and some trial and error is inherently part of the process.

3 Co-infections must be given due consideration early in treatment planning, as untreated co-infections can hinder recovery from Lyme disease. As discussed, laboratory testing is not 100% reliable for any of these infections, and especially for co-infections. Thus, a good understanding of symptomatology is necessary to have good discernment about co-infections and be able to treat appropriately based on clinical presentation. Treat the dominant co-infection first; that is, the one that seems to be creating the most symptomatology.

4 Patients can get worse in the early phases of treatment before they get better. This is due to a phenomenon called the Jarisch–Herxheimer reaction (for more information, see below). Integrative approaches to treatment can help offset this response, especially through detoxification therapies to promote the removal of the endotoxins released and therapies to manage inflammatory responses in the body.

5 Treatment must be multisystem and holistic. Chronic infections such as these can cause damage to, and symptoms within, each and every system of the body. Hormone balance is important, with special attention paid to the hypothalamic–pituitary–adrenal axis. Adequately addressing each area can lead to complicated treatment regimens, which can be overwhelming to the patient and lead to treatment fatigue and compliance issues.

Herxheimer reactions

The Jarisch–Herxheimer reaction, also called a Herxheimer reaction or Herx reaction, results from the release of endotoxin-like products when bacteria are killed, leading to a worsening of a patient's symptoms. Common symptoms of Herxheimer reactions are fevers, chills, headaches, tachycardia, myalgia and anxiety.

The Herxheimer reaction is a situation of both toxicity and inflammation. There is an increase in inflammatory cytokines during this time, including tumour necrosis factor-alpha (TNF-α), interleukin-6 and interleukin-8.[43,44]

Typical symptoms of toxicity and inflammation can be present, but most people report that a Herxheimer reaction feels like all their typical symptoms but exacerbated. This can help to distinguish between a Herxheimer reaction and a side effect of a new medication or therapy. If it is typical symptoms for them but worse, it points more to a Herxheimer reaction. New symptoms such as gastrointestinal distress, rashes or headaches can be more indicative of a side effect or adverse treatment reaction. Also, Herxeimer reactions tend to take a few days to build, while adverse reactions and side effects tend to be more immediate.

Many patients welcome Herxheimer reactions to some extent as it shows them that their treatment is indeed

having an effect. The important thing is adequate education and warning as to what may occur, coaching as to when to persist with treatment and when to back off, and modalities that they can use to help them with detoxification and reducing the inflammatory state that has been produced.

Allopathic treatment of Lyme disease

The basis of allopathic treatment of Lyme disease is antibiotic therapy. The way antibiotics are prescribed will depend on whether the case is acute or chronic.

If treated promptly in the acute phase, Lyme disease can be successfully treated and eradicated with a relatively short course of antibiotics. Once it becomes chronic, treatment is significantly more complex and can require long-term courses of multiple antibiotics. One of the factors that attract criticism from some practitioners in chronic Lyme is the number of antibiotics that are prescribed, the duration of prescription and the fact that, in Lyme treatment, doses required are often higher than typical. A good example is doxycycline, which has been found to be bacteriostatic at doses of 100 mg twice daily, which means that, at that dose, it will halt the progression of the *Borrelia* spirochaetes; whereas it is bacteriocidal at 200 mg twice daily, which means that at that dose it is sufficiently powerful to eradicate *Borrelia*. Kill kinetics indicate that a large spike in blood and tissue levels is more effective than sustained levels, which is why with doxycycline, oral doses of 200 mg twice daily are more effective than 100 mg four times daily.[45] The dose of 200 mg twice daily is double the typical dosing used in other conditions, and physicians and chemists without this knowledge specific to *Borrelia* may find the dose startling.

As discussed, acute Lyme disease may not appear on testing for several weeks, by which time the opportunity for prompt treatment has been lost. Thus, there is a valid argument for treating prophylactically after a known tick bite, whether or not an erythema migrans rash and/or flu-like symptoms have appeared.

According to the IDSA, the standard treatment regimen for acute Lyme disease is[46]:

- No prophylactic treatment necessary for known tick bite, although a single dose of doxycycline (maximum 200 mg) may be offered to adults and children older than age 8, providing that the medication is given within 72 hours of the bite.
- For symptomatic acute Lyme:
  - Erythema migrans/Lyme arthritis:
    - > doxycycline 100 mg twice daily; or
    - > amoxicillin 500 mg three times daily; or
    - > cefuroxime 500 mg twice daily
    - > for 14 days (14–21 days)
  - Early neurological Lyme/Lyme carditis:
    - > ceftriaxone 2 g daily for 14 days (range 10–28 days).

The conflict between the IDSA and the ILADS is reflected even in the acute antibiotic protocols each recommends. The ILADS has its own evidence-based treatment guidelines and ILADS the following position statements[12]:

- It is impossible to state a meaningful success rate for the prevention of Lyme disease by a single 200 mg dose of doxycycline because the sole trial of that regimen utilised an inadequate observation period and unvalidated surrogate end point.
- Success rates for treatment of an erythema migrans rash were unacceptably low, ranging from 52.2% to 84.4% for regimens that used 20 or fewer days of azithromycin, cefuroxime, doxycycline or amoxicillin/phenoxymethylpenicillin (rates were based on patient-centred outcome definitions and conservative longitudinal data methodology).
- In a well-designed trial of antibiotic retreatment in patients with severe fatigue, 64% in the treatment arm obtained a clinically significant and sustained benefit from additional antibiotic therapy.

The philosophy behind ILADS' statements and in its guidelines includes the following[13]:

- The optimal treatment regimen for the management of known tick bites, erythema migrans rashes and persistent disease has not yet been determined. Accordingly, it is too early to standardise restrictive protocols.
- Given the number of clinical variables that must be managed and the heterogeneity within the patient population, clinical judgment is crucial to the provision of patient-centred care.
- Based on the Grading of Recommendations Assessment, Development and Evaluation model, ILADS recommends that patient goals and values regarding treatment options be identified and strongly considered during a shared decision-making process.

In a nutshell, ILADS argues that the IDSA protocols may be too short, too restrictive, not have enough individualisation and not take into account the clinical judgment of the practitioner. It states that there is not enough evidence of the efficacy of the IDSA guidelines to make them universally accepted without any question or challenge.

ILADS' treatment guidelines suggest the following:

- Amoxicillin, cefuroxime or doxycycline as first-line agents for the treatment of erythema migrans.
- Azithromycin is cited as an acceptable agent, particularly in Europe, based on trials showing it to either outperform or be as effective as other first-line agents.[47–50]
- Initial antibiotic therapy should employ 4–6 weeks of:
  - amoxicillin 1500–2000 mg daily in divided doses
  - cefuroxime 500 mg twice daily
  - doxycycline 100 mg twice daily or a minimum of 21 days of azithromycin 250–500 mg daily.
- Paediatric dosing for the individual agents is as follows:
  - amoxicillin 50 mg/kg/day in three divided doses, with a maximum daily dose of 1500 mg
  - cefuroxime 20–30 mg/kg/day in two divided doses, with a maximum daily dose of 1000 mg
  - azithromycin 10 mg/kg on day 1 then 5–10 mg/kg daily, with a maximum daily dose of 500 mg. For children 8 years and older, doxycycline is an additional option. Doxycycline is dosed at 4 mg/kg/day in two divided doses, with a maximum daily

dose of 200 mg. Higher daily doses of the individual agents may be appropriate in adolescents.[12]

Dr Richard Horowitz treats acute Lyme disease with a 2-month regimen of the following[51]:

- First month:
  - doxycycline 200 mg – twice daily
  - hydroxychloroquine 200 mg – twice daily or
  - tinidazole 500 mg – twice daily.
- Second month:
  - cefuroxime 500 mg – twice daily
  - azithromycin 500 mg – once daily or clarithromycin 500 mg – twice daily
  - hydroxychloroquine 200 mg – twice daily or tinidazole 500 mg – twice daily.

Antibiotic therapy for chronic Lyme disease

Antibiotic therapy for chronic Lyme disease is influenced by the morphology of the bacteria, which can morph back and forth between spirochaete, cell-wall-deficient form and cyst form. To adequately address chronic infection, medications must be given for all three forms. *Borrelia* tries to evade immune defences and antimicrobial therapy by morphing into the cyst form, where it is better protected. If medications are not included that address those cyst forms, the infection can be pushed into that state, which can bring symptom relief to the patient, as it is a more dormant state. Yet, when antibiotic therapy is ceased, the microbes can morph back to the spirochaetes and cell-wall-deficient forms, which are more active, pushing the patient into a relapsing state.

According to Lyme-literate physician Joseph Burrascano, MD:

> It has been recognised that B. burgdorferi *can exist in at least two, and possibly three different morphologic forms: spirochete, spheroplast (or l-form), and the recently discovered cystic form (presently, there is controversy whether the cyst is different from the l-form). L-forms and cystic forms do not contain cell walls, and thus beta lactam antibiotics will not affect them. Spheroplasts seem to be susceptible to tetracyclines and the advanced erythromycin derivatives. Apparently, Bb can shift among the three forms during the course of the infection. Because of this, it may be necessary to cycle different classes of antibiotics and/or prescribe a combination of dissimilar agents.*[45]

A further note on cystic forms:

> When present in a hostile environment, such as growth medium lacking some nutrients, spinal fluid, or serum with certain antibiotics added, Bb can change into a cyst form. This cyst seems to be able to remain dormant, but when placed into an environment more favorable to its growth, the cyst can revert into the spirochete form. The conventional antibiotics used for Lyme, such as the penicillins, cephalosporins, etc do not kill the cystic form of Bb, yet there is laboratory evidence that metronidazole will kill it. Therefore, the trend now is to treat the chronically infected patient who has resistant disease by combining metronidazole with one or two other antibiotics to target all forms of Bb.[45]

TABLE 24.1 Medication summary		
Form of *borrelia*	Medication class	Commonly used examples
Spirochaetes	Penicillins	Amoxicillin, bicillin LA
	Cephalosporins	Cefuroxime, ceftriaxone, cefdinir
Cell wall deficient	Macrolides	Azithromycin, clarithromycin
	Tetracyclines	Doxycycline, minocycline
Cyst forms		Tinidazole, metronidazole
		Hydroxychloroquine (Plaquenil)
		Nitazoxanide (Alinia)

TABLE 24.2 Common dosages		
Penicillins		
Amoxicillin	1000 mg	3–6 daily
Augmentin XR	2000 mg	2 × daily
Bicillin LA	0.9 million units	2 vials injected IM 3 × weekly
Cephalosporins		
Cefuroxime	500 mg	3 × daily
Ceftriaxone	2 g	2 g twice daily IV 4 days/week
Cefdinir	600 mg	2 × daily
Macrolides		
Azithromycin	500 mg	1 × daily
Clarithromycin	500 mg	2 × daily
Telithromycin	800 mg	1 × daily
Tetracyclines		
Minocycline	100 mg	3–4 × daily
Doxycycline	100 mg	2 twice daily
Tetracycline	500 mg	3–4 × daily
Cyst-form medications		
Metronidazole	500 mg	2 × daily; 2 weeks on/2 weeks off
Tinidazole	500 mg	2 × daily; 2 weeks on/2 weeks off
Plaquenil	200 mg	2 × daily
***Babesia* medications**		
Mepron	750 mg/5 mL	1–2 tsp twice daily
Malarone	250/100 mg	2 twice daily
Lariam	250 mg	1 every five days
Alinia	500 mg	2 × daily
***Bartonella, ehrlichia, anaplasma* and *rickettsia* medications**		
Rifampicin	300 mg	2 × daily
Levaquin	500 mg	1 × daily
Bactrim DS	800/160 mg	2 × daily

Because antibiotic therapy for chronic Lyme can be long term and involve multiple medications, care must be taken to minimise side effects and offset any negative impact of antibiotics where possible. Liver and kidney function must be checked monthly to screen for any abnormalities. White blood cell counts, often low in chronic Lyme disease anyway, frequently drop further. *Candida* overgrowth is fairly common and is possibly the most problematic sequelae of long-term antibiotics. These three considerations will be discussed further in the section on naturopathic approaches to Lyme disease, but suffice it to say that naturopaths and integrative health practitioners are uniquely placed and well qualified to offer optimal support in these areas.

Tables 24.1 and 24.2 are summaries of the medication classes used for different forms of *Borrelia*. The ultimate goal of therapy is to combine medications for spirochaete forms, cell-wall-deficient forms and cyst forms. Medication choices depend largely on the sensitivity of the patient, any medication allergies and prior therapy. Medications to address co-infections must be added also.

ANTIBIOTIC THERAPY DURING PREGNANCY AND BREASTFEEDING

Starting in the early 1980s, the Lyme Disease Foundation in Hartford, Connecticut, kept a pregnancy registry over an 11-year period. It found that women who took adequate amounts of antibiotics during pregnancy showed a very low, in fact almost zero, transmission rate to their baby.

Medications utilised in pregnancy include:
- amoxicillin – 1 g four times daily
- bicillin LA – 1 injection three times weekly
- cefuroxime – 1 g every 12 hours
- azithromycin – 500 mg daily.

At the ILADS annual conference in 2011, paediatric Lyme specialist Charles Ray Jones cited the following figures:
- Pregnant women with active Lyme disease who do not take antibiotics have a 50% chance of passing the infection to their child.
- Women who take one antibiotic during pregnancy have a 25% chance of passing Lyme disease to their child.
- Women who take two antibiotics during pregnancy have less than a 5% chance of passing Lyme disease on to their child.

Obviously, many women are reluctant to take antibiotics during pregnancy for fear of harming their baby. Certainly, there are specific medications that are *not* appropriate, such as the tetracycline class of antibiotics, metronidazole and tinidazole. The medications listed above are deemed safe in pregnancy. Although taking antibiotics during pregnancy is not ideal, it is a far better choice than risking the transmission of Lyme disease to a baby, which could then impact on their entire life. Since *Borrelia* spirochaetes have been detected in breast milk by PCR testing, the antibiotic regimens above should be continued if breastfeeding.

ANTIBIOTIC THERAPY FOR CHILDREN

Children can be treated with antibiotic therapy, but the medication choices and dosages will be adjusted for them. Tetracyclines are not used in children 8 years and younger because of their ability to cause a permanent discolouration of the teeth.

Antibiotics considered safe and effective for children include:
- amoxicillin – 50 mg/kg/day divided into doses every 8 hours
- cefuroxime axetil – 125–500 mg every 12 hours based on weight
- azithromycin – 250–500 mg daily depending on their weight
- tinidazole – 125–250 mg daily depending on weight. May be pulsed 2 days per week.

ANTIBIOTIC THERAPY FOR CO-INFECTIONS

Co-infections must be addressed concurrently with *Borrelia* for the best chance of recovery for the patient. Untreated co-infections are one of the biggest hindrances to recovery.

The co-infection *Babesia* is a malaria-like protozoan parasite; therefore, the medications that treat Lyme are unlikely to help *Babesia*. *Babesia* requires malarial medications. *Bartonella*, *Ehrlichia* and *Rickettsia* are bacteria, like *Borrelia*, so there is more crossover between medications for these co-infections (see Table 24.3).

Allopathic supportive therapy

Another aspect in allopathic treatment of Lyme disease involves medications to provide symptomatic relief and supportive medications. These may be pain medications, sleep medications, cognitive enhancers, antidepressant medications and anxiety medications, to name just a few. Individuals suffering from chronic Lyme disease experience severe and unrelenting symptoms, so providing symptomatic relief can be necessary. Issues arise when those medications produce side effects of their own or when stopping them can provoke withdrawal reactions, such as with benzodiazepine withdrawal. Supportive medications can be life saving, but should not replace addressing the underlying cause of the symptoms.

NATUROPATHIC APPROACHES TO LYME DISEASE AND CO-INFECTIONS

The following section discusses naturopathic approaches to Lyme disease treatment.

There are several different treatment priorities in treating Lyme disease and co-infections, only part of which is eradicating the pathogens themselves. As previously stated, treatment must be holistic and address many of the secondary impacts of the illness.

TABLE 24.3 Commonly used medications for co-infections		
Babesia		
Atovaquone + proguanil (Malarone)	250/100 mg	2 twice daily
Atovaquone (Wellvone)	750 mg/5 mL	5 mL twice daily
Nitazoxanide (Alinia)	500 mg	1 twice daily
Artemether/ lumefantrine (Riamet)	20/120 mg	4 tablets twice daily for 3 consecutive days per month
Sulfamethoxazole/ trimethoprim (Bactrim DS)	800/160 mg	1 twice daily
Bartonella		
Rifampicin	300 mg b.i.d.	
Doxycycline	200 mg b.i.d.	
Azithromycin	500 mg q.d.	
SMX/TMP	800/160 mg b.i.d.	
Levofloxacin	750 mg b.i.d.	
Ciprofloxacin	500 mg b.i.d.	
Ehrlichia/ rickettsia		
Doxycycline	200 mg b.i.d.	
Rifampicin	300 mg b.i.d.	

The following section is divided into the following modality classifications:
- Nutrition (dietary)
- Nutrition (supplements)
- Nutrition (micronutrients)
- Herbal medicine
- Amino acids
- Lifestyle factors.

Within each modality, you will find the information organised by treatment priority.

Primary treatment priorities for Lyme patients include:
- antimicrobial therapy to kill pathogens
- inflammation reduction
- immune system support
- detoxification support.

Secondary considerations and symptomatic support include:
- brain chemistry and mood balance
- sleep support
- energy/adrenal support
- digestive support.

Nutritional therapy (dietary)

Nutrition makes a profound difference in the outcomes of Lyme disease patients and should not be underestimated.

For many patients, however, the dietary recommendations can be a whole new concept, and quite overwhelming and challenging. Encouraging gradual, step-by-step changes and providing consistent support and practical guidance, such as shopping lists and easy recipe ideas, will help with compliance. It is also useful to remind patients that in an illness in which they can feel so helpless and powerless, nutrition is one area that they have complete control over; they can feel empowered about that.

REDUCING INFLAMMATION

This is one of the key goals in nutritional therapy. Inflammation is a logical secondary effect of chronic infection and can produce a wide array of symptoms of its own. Lyme disease is primarily an infectious illness, and secondarily an inflammatory disorder. The key approach nutritionally is to avoid pro-inflammatory foods and eat anti-inflammatory foods.

Pro-inflammatory foods

GLUTEN

Gluten is one of the most inflammatory foods. It is found in oats, rye, barley and wheat, and is pervasive in processed foods today. It is thought that in the Australian population, 1 in 100 is gluten intolerant, 1 in 70 has coeliac disease and 56% carry the gene for gluten intolerance.[52]

Gluten can create inflammation in a number of different ways. It can trigger an IgE food allergy, which is an immediate and usually obvious immune reaction – what we consider a food allergy. It can also cause an IgG immune response, also known as a type IV delayed hypersensitivity response. This reaction can take up to 72 hours to manifest, and the symptoms may be subtle and not always directly related to the immune system. Fatigue, brain fog and mood changes are common manifestations, especially in Lyme patients who are prone to those things anyway. The third way gluten can cause inflammation is by triggering an autoimmune response. Coeliac disease is the most extreme form of this; however, there are grades of gluten intolerance, which do not always fit the diagnostic criteria for coeliac. Testing may involve anti-gliadin and transglutaminase antibodies as well as genetic markers for gluten intolerance. Some patients who could tolerate gluten well in their past may find themselves becoming intolerant to it over the course of their Lyme illness, and even those who do not show laboratory markers in line with gluten intolerance may still feel better avoiding it, simply from an inflammatory standpoint.

In one study, researchers assessed the likelihood of developing coeliac disease by observing gluten presentation on CD4 T cells. It states:

> In the presence of gluten, this could become a self-amplifying loop that could cause limited tissue damage locally. This tissue damage would lead to the release of TG2 that will modify native gluten peptides into high affinity ligands for human leukocyte antigen (HLA)-DQ2 and/or HLA-DQ8, thereby expanding the gluten-specific CD4+ T cell

> responses and leading to additional tissue damage: the initiation of a second self-amplifying loop. Alternatively, infections occurring in the gastrointestinal tract would generate a proinflammatory milieu that might lead to loss of tolerance to native gluten peptides and generate tissue damage simultaneously and thus, initiate deamidation by TG2.[53]

Infections such as *Borrelia* and *Bartonella* can infect the gut; therefore, we see here the connection between Lyme disease and the onset of gluten intolerance.

Any of these mechanisms (IgE, IgG and autoimmune) will create immune activation in the gut. Immune activation by nature leads to an inflammatory process that can impact on not only gut function, but systemic symptoms too.

One of the things gluten can do is promote leaky gut, where the cell junctions of the intestinal wall open up and allow the passage of larger than normal food molecules to pass through, thus leading to even more immune activation and inflammation. Gluten does this by stimulating zonulin, a substance that regulates the permeability of the gut wall. Eating gluten triggers more zonulin, which makes the intestinal wall more permeable, which leads to food particle passage across the intestinal lining, which triggers an immune response (the immune system is trained that single amino acids, sugars and fatty acids are 'normal', whereas molecules containing groups of these are treated as 'invaders'), which creates cytokines, chemokines and other chemical mediators of inflammation. These can then travel throughout the body and lead to inflammatory symptoms such as headache/migraine, joint pain, fatigue, myalgia and cognitive deficits, to name just a few.[54,55]

Gluten has one other key negative impact. Zonulin regulates gut permeability, but it also regulates the permeability of the blood–brain barrier. So along with 'leaky gut', it promotes 'leaky brain'. When the blood–brain barrier is compromised and rendered more permeable, it is more open to the influx of cytokines and chemokines, toxins including heavy metals and ammonia, and other harmful substances. This leads to a worsening of 'Lyme brain' – cognitive deficits such as brain fog, memory loss, word-finding difficulties, problems with focus and concentration, depression and anxiety. These are some of the symptoms that Lyme patients struggle with the most, so avoiding the gluten-containing foods that can make it worse is key.

In one study, researchers observed how cereal grains affected human behaviour and mental health:

> In vitro, antibodies against gluten removed from human blood attack cerebellar proteins and components of the myelin sheath that insulate nerves. They also attack an enzyme involved in the production of GABA – our prime inhibitory neurotransmitter, whose dysregulation is implicated in both anxiety and depression.[54]

DAIRY

Dairy is the second food category that can be pro-inflammatory. Studies show that a diet containing A1 beta-casein had pro-inflammatory effects in the gut, with increased levels of inflammatory markers and immunoglobulins, leukocyte infiltration and Toll-like receptor expression.[56]

Cow dairy is the most inflammatory, followed by sheep dairy, and then goat dairy. Goat dairy is the closest in molecular structure to human dairy, has the smallest fat molecules and the lowest ratio of casein. Pasteurised dairy products are hard to digest because they are treated in a way that kills off naturally occurring enzymes and cultures. Raw dairy contains more of these beneficial ingredients, but can also contain bacteria that would normally be killed off in the pasteurisation process. In an immunosuppressed Lyme disease patient, this may present a further risk to their health.

Dairy does not trigger autoimmune reactions in the same way that gluten does, but many patients have IgG sensitivities to dairy. IgG food sensitivity tests are so helpful in discerning the degree of sensitivity in patients, but they also give more of a detailed breakdown of dairy. Most tests will differentiate between casein, whey, different types of cheese, yoghurt, milk and goat's milk.

Casein and whey are the two key proteins in dairy. Of the two, casein is the more problematic: it comprises 80% of the proteins in dairy and the majority of proteins in cheese, and takes several hours to break down and digest as it coagulates and forms a gel in the stomach. Whey protein digests quickly and more easily, and has some helpful roles such as promoting glutathione production and providing a ready source of amino acids. For these reasons, there may be some patients who avoid dairy products in general but still tolerate a pure whey protein isolate. Still others cannot tolerate dairy, but fare well on kefir, which is fermented. Kefir has the added benefit of containing cultures and probiotics that can assist in maintaining healthy gut flora. Again, IgG food sensitivity testing can provide information that helps to guide these choices in different individuals. Food and symptom diaries can also help patients see correlations between certain food groups and flare-ups or improvements in their symptoms.

SATURATED FATS

Saturated fats can be a source of inflammation in the body as they promote prostaglandins that fuel inflammation. Saturated fats are naturally occurring fats found in nature such as in red meat and dairy. Another source of inflammatory fats is trans fatty acids, which are found in processed foods. These fats may have originated as vegetable oils but have been treated with heat and pressure to make them more solid and give them a longer shelf life. They are often labelled as hydrogenated or partially hydrogenated oils and are found in chips, biscuits, lollies, cakes and crackers. Lyme patients are encouraged to eat a wholefoods diet low in processed foods of any kind. High-sugar, high-fat foods, such as fast foods and pastries, should be avoided, not only because of their unhealthy fat content, but many are made from gluten-containing grains, dairy and sugar, all of which are detrimental. Unhealthy fats such as these promote PG2 production – the prostaglandins that increase inflammation, constrict blood vessels and encourage blood clotting.

On the other hand, anti-inflammatory fats can help to reduce inflammation in the body and help with symptom control. Healthy fats promote PG1 and PG3 production. PG1 prostaglandins reduce inflammation and inhibit blood clotting. PG3 prostaglandins have mixed function within the body, but are generally considered anti-inflammatory as they help to reduce the rate at which PG2 are formed.

Anti-inflammatory fats are unsaturated fats – classified as omega-3, omega-6 and omega-9. Omega-3s have the greatest effect in reducing inflammation as they produce the lowest number of prostaglandins: they produce PG1 and PG3, which act to counter PG2 production, and they compete with omega-6 fatty acids on the binding sites of the COX1 enzyme, thus reducing omega-6's conversion to PG2.

A review in the *British Journal of Clinical Pharmacology* looked at omega-3's anti-inflammatory properties.[57] It found substantial evidence that omega-3 fatty acids are able to inhibit a number of aspects of inflammation, including leukocyte chemotaxis, adhesion molecule expression and leukocyte–endothelial adhesive interactions, production of eicosanoids such as prostaglandins and leukotrienes from the omega-6 fatty acid arachidonic acid, production of inflammatory cytokines and T cell reactivity.

Most people also get omega-6 and omega-9 fatty acids through their diet (prevalent in vegetable oils, nuts and seeds), whereas omega-3 fatty acids are less common. Fish and flax are the richest sources of omega-3, with fish oil having a much stronger effect. One study found flaxseed oil to inhibit the production of cytokines by 30% in 4 weeks, whereas 9 g of fish oil for another 4 weeks inhibited IL-1 by 80% and TNF-α by 74%.[58]

Eating seafood and incorporating flax oil into a smoothie or as a salad dressing or food topping can be good ways to get more omega-3. Supplementation can be an important consideration in those with high levels of inflammation, as is frequently the case in Lyme disease.

Cruciferous vegetables and carotenoids both exhibit anti-inflammatory activity in the body. One study of 1005 middle-aged Chinese women found that a higher intake of cruciferous vegetables was associated with significantly lower circulating concentrations of the pro-inflammatory markers TNF-α, IL-1β and IL-6, after accounting for a wide range of potential confounding variables, including socioeconomic status, dietary and non-dietary lifestyle factors, BMI, health conditions and medication use.[59]

The carotenoids, particularly lycopene and beta-carotene, concentrated in deeply coloured items such as carrots, tomatoes and dark green vegetables, are other dietary antioxidants that function to reduce oxidative stress in vivo and blood markers of inflammation.[60]

OTHER INFLAMMATORY FOODS

Other foods that should be avoided are any foods that create immune activation for that person, regardless of what they are. Again, food sensitivity testing is a quick, easy way to assess these, but elimination diets can be a good tool to use too. One limitation of the elimination diet in Lyme patients is the time required to do the restriction phase and reintroduction phase. Since Lyme symptoms typically wax and wane, acting in a cyclical fashion, it can be hard for patients to differentiate what is a reaction to a reintroduced food versus what is a natural flare of their symptoms, which may happen every few days or every month regardless of dietary or treatment changes.

Any food can cause inflammation in certain individuals. Garlic, bananas or blueberries may show high IgG reactions. These foods are generally regarded as healthy foods and not problematic for most. Some people may react to almond, which can be important because many people change their milk to almond milk, thinking that they are doing the right thing in avoiding dairy. This is where individuation of diet is important.

SUPPORTING IMMUNE FUNCTION

A large part of dietary modification to support immune function means eradicating foods that cause immune activation, as discussed in the prior section on inflammation.

The diet can also be tailored to promote healthy immune function. This mostly entails a diet that is high in fresh fruit and vegetables in order to provide the vitamins, minerals and enzymes needed to assist in the composition of cells, enhance cell-to-cell communication and provide catalysts for the thousands of biochemical reactions in our bodies, including those reactions necessary for our immune systems to function well. Deficiencies of particular nutrients can compromise the body's ability to create antibodies and elements of cell-mediated immunity.

Malnutrition will decrease antibody production, so ensuring adequate kilojoule intake is important. Some Lyme patients have such compromised digestive function and such profound nausea that getting adequate kilojoules can be challenging. Loss of appetite is also a common symptom of Lyme disease. Strategies must be employed to encourage small, frequent meals and utilise protein smoothies, broths and soups, which can be easier to digest, and light but nutrient-rich foods. Protein intake is important. Amino acids are the building blocks of cells and tissues, and are needed to create the antibodies that are needed to overcome infection. Lean, organic, high-quality proteins should be eaten with each meal to provide these amino acids. If not well tolerated, protein powders can be utilised once or twice daily.

Another major element in dietary modification for Lyme disease is reducing overall sugar intake and eradicating any refined sugars. Naturally occurring sugars, such as in honey, maple syrup and fruit, do not have the immunosuppressive effects of refined sugars, but may still need to be restricted for reasons relating to digestive health and *Candida*. However, from an immune-support standpoint, the key is omitting any refined sugars as they have a profoundly suppressive effect on the immune system.

Eating or drinking 100 g of sugar, the equivalent of one medium bottle of soft drink, can reduce immune function by up to 40%. The immune-suppressing effects of sugar, including a reduction in the ability of neutrophils to engulf bacteria, start less than 30 minutes after ingestion and can last for up to 10 hours.[61]

Secondarily, sugar causes the pancreas to secrete insulin, which can stay in the bloodstream long after the sugar has been metabolised. One of the things insulin does is suppress growth hormone production from the pituitary, and growth hormone is one of the key regulators of the immune system.

Since refined sugar contains virtually no vitamins, minerals or other micronutrients, sugar consumption decreases overall micronutrient intake by an average of almost 20%.[61,62]

Finally, glucose competes with vitamin C for absorption into white blood cells. Vitamin C acts as an antioxidant and promotes healthy immune function. Reducing sugar ingestion to allow vitamin C uptake is going to have a more beneficial impact on overall immune function.

Many patients with Lyme disease resort to sugar because of their profound fatigue. They try to get energy however they can, even if the boost is short term and followed by energy crashes. Others resort to high-sugar foods for emotional reasons, to try to cheer themselves up during very trying times. Withdrawing from sugar can be very difficult for them but is crucial to their recovery.

ENCOURAGING DETOXIFICATION AND ELIMINATION

This is another significant consideration for Lyme patients – second only perhaps to reducing inflammation. As patients move through antimicrobial therapy, the toxins produced in the killing off of the bacteria (the Herx reaction), as well as the pre-existing toxic load that patients may be predisposed to due to HLA/methylation factors, such as heavy metals and ammonia, must be cleared from the body. Modalities such as nutrient supplementation, herbal medicine and homeopathy are crucial, but dietary choices can assist greatly in the process too.

The first thing to think about in assisting the body in detoxification is to stop the influx of toxins. This means shifting the diet towards organic to reduce pesticides, fertilisers and other chemicals coming into the body. Meats and poultry should be grass fed, organic and hormone/antibiotic free. Seafood should be low-mercury types. Water should be filtered and free of pollutants such as heavy metals. Two litres of water should be drunk each day to help flush toxins out of the body. Caffeine and alcohol should be avoided, as they can place additional stress on the liver.

Given that the liver is the key organ of detoxification in the body, foods to support liver function are useful. These include onions, garlic, broccoli, beetroot, spinach, asparagus, artichokes, Brazil nuts and walnuts. Cayenne pepper is both anti-inflammatory and supports detoxification. Lemon is a good cleansing agent.

Green juices and smoothies are a good way to get concentrated nutrients to the cells in a way that does not stress the digestive system. Juices may be better for those who have highly inflamed GI systems, as sometimes the fibre content of blended smoothies can be irritating and hard to digest. For those who tend towards constipation, the fibre content of smoothies may be helpful. Juices are ideal, as the nutrients are easy to digest and assimilate, additional elements such as ginger, garlic and cayenne can be added, and they assist the liver and kidney in the detoxification process.

Elimination is another consideration in supporting detoxification. Toxins have to be able to find their way out of the body. There are other ways to assist this, such as infra-red sauna and coffee enemas, but from a dietary standpoint, make sure that the kidneys are flushing well by drinking plenty of water and herbal teas made from ingredients such as dandelion, juniper berry, cranberry and tart cherry.

Elimination through the bowel is especially important and can be challenging given that many Lyme patients experience either constipation or diarrhoea. Adequate dietary fibre intake to ensure at least once daily bowel movements can be helpful. High water intake is also important. As per the information on gluten and dairy as inflammatory foods, eliminating those often leads to healthier bowel function.

SUPPORTING HEALTHY DIGESTION

There are many different stressors on the digestive systems of Lyme patients. Overall, immune activation and inflammation can render them more reactive to various foods such as gluten and dairy (as discussed in the section on nutrition and inflammation). Those on antibiotic therapy can experience gastritis, oesophagitis and intestinal distress from the irritating effects of those medications. *Borrelia* and co-infections can inhabit the gut lining and cause symptoms of their own. Opportunistic infections, such as *Blastocystis hominis*, *Cryptosporidium parvum*, *Giardia lamblia* and *Entamoeba histolytica*, are not uncommon and should be screened for. *Candida* overgrowth and other changes in the gut microbiome can produce symptoms too.

Much of the naturopathic approach to these stressors rests on antimicrobial therapy and supplementation to reduce inflammation.

Dietary modifications are largely geared around reducing any additional stress through inflammatory foods such as gluten, dairy and IgG food intolerances. Soothing, healing foods should be used: bone broth can help to heal leaky gut and provide high-level nutrition to those with compromised gut function; slippery elm powder can be added to smoothies and drinks; aloe vera juice can soothe and heal the gut mucosa; and deglycyrrhizinated liquorice can help with oesophagitis. Yeast also tend to grow in more inflamed and compromised environments, so identifying sources of inflammation and eradicating them also helps prevent yeast overgrowth.

The second nutritional consideration in helping digestive function is the microbial balance, especially vis-à-vis *Candida* overgrowth, and maintaining healthy gut flora. This is especially important for those on antibiotics. Avoiding sugar and highly processed foods will reduce the overgrowth of yeast and unwanted bacteria. This is the most important thing patients can do in this area, and its importance must be stressed to them. For people with existing *Candida* issues, even restriction in fruit intake may be necessary for a period of time. For some, eating a grain-free diet is required and helps them to feel better.

This can be hard to adhere to, but for those with severe digestive irritation, it might be necessary.

Fermented foods can play a big role in promoting healthy gut flora. These include fermented vegetables such as kimchi, kefir and kombucha. It is important to caution patients about store-bought varieties, as they are often pasteurised, which takes away much of their benefit, and frequently have added sugars to make them more palatable. Suggest specific brands that are known to have the best health-giving benefits.

SUPPORTING ADRENAL AND THYROID FUNCTION

Lyme disease patients often have major hormonal irregularities impacting on adrenal and thyroid hormones. This is largely due to the impact of infections on the hypothalamic–pituitary axis, which then filter down the pathway to the endpoint hormones. Imbalances in these hormones can worsen typical Lyme symptoms such as fatigue, insomnia, brain fog, anxiety and depression. Diet can be used to support hormone balance.

Adrenals

Adrenal stress is profound in Lyme disease. With a chronic stressor on the body such as systemic infection, the adrenals will overcompensate by producing an excess of cortisol for a period of time, but ultimately, cortisol levels will fall and adrenal exhaustion will ensue.

Poor nutrition is a stressor on the adrenals too, so people who are not conscious of their diet may be adding to the stress on their adrenals.

Eating for adrenal health involves a few different principles. The first is to eat small amounts of food frequently. This helps to keep cortisol levels regulated, as cortisol will not be called in to help regulate fluctuating levels of blood sugar and insulin. It also tends to help people maintain sustained levels of energy, rather than have to endure the spikes and crashes involved with eating less frequently.

The second principle is to eat a high-quality protein with every meal. Eating protein promotes glucagon, the opposing hormone to insulin. Since insulin can promote inflammation, weight gain through energy storage, high cholesterol and heart disease, it is important to produce glucagon to balance it. High-carbohydrate, low-protein meals will produce mostly insulin in the body; high-protein and high-fat meals will produce a balance of insulin and glucagon. This is important for the regulation of blood sugar and management of inflammation in Lyme patients.

Thyroid

Thyroid function is frequently impacted on in Lyme patients and may need to be regulated through the use of herbs, nutrients or supplemental hormone therapy. Hypothyroidism is the prevalent condition seen. Hashimoto's thyroiditis, involving a period of hyperthyroidism followed by a longer-term hypothyroidism, is also common. This is an autoimmune thyroid condition which has been associated with gluten intolerance (also autoimmune).[63]

One study showed that 10 of 14 patients with Hashimoto's thyroiditis had genotypes compatible with coeliac disease (three patients had DQ heterodimer A1*0501, B1*0201, four had DRB1*04 and one had A1*0101, B1*0501). Six of these 14 patients showed an increased density of γδ+ T-cell-receptor-bearing intraepithelial lymphocytes and signs of mucosal T cell activation, both typical of coeliac disease.[64]

Therefore, in thyroid dysfunction, gluten should be avoided, especially where autoimmune markers such as anti-thyroid peroxidase (TPO) and anti-thyroglobulin levels are elevated on blood work.

One of the contributing factors to low thyroid function is low iodine levels, which is fairly common in Lyme patients. Eating iodine-rich foods, including asparagus, kelp, seafood, sesame seeds, Swiss chard, sea salt, spinach, turnip greens and seaweed, can help.

Another factor can be a deficiency in tyrosine, an amino acid necessary for the production of T3 and T4. A high-protein diet will ensure that amino acids are available to the body for hormone production.

There are some foods that block thyroid hormone production and thyroid function (termed goitrogens), and these should be avoided in people with low thyroid function. These include cabbage, broccoli, swede, cauliflower, kale, Brussels sprouts and peanuts. Cooking these foods can help limit the goitrogens associated with them; however, some need total avoidance.

SAMPLE DAILY DIET

BREAKFAST	Chocolate chai smoothie: almond milk, cacao, chia, ginger, cardamom, cloves, cinnamon, banana and gluten-free oats.	Fatigue is a common complaint in Lyme disease; thus, foods rich in B vitamins such as oats, and foods rich in magnesium such as bananas, cacao and almonds are required for energy production as well as to help manage psychological symptoms such as depression. Notably, magnesium deficiency has been found in individuals with Lyme disease, and supporting healthy levels may function to stimulate impaired immunity.[65] Oats are high in fibre, which assists in maintaining stable blood sugar levels. In vivo studies reveal hyperglycaemia is associated with reduced ability of neutrophils to uptake and kill *B. burgdorferi* as well as impaired clearance of bacterial DNA in multiple tissues, including the brain, heart, liver, lung and knee joint.[66]
LUNCH	Baked sweet potato filled with basil, rocket and garlic pesto. Marinated tofu. Sauerkraut and side salad.	Supporting the immune system is crucial in Lyme disease to assist in countering the immune evasion mechanisms exhibited by Lyme disease spirochaetes and minimise effects of co-infections such as *Candida*. Foods with immune-boosting properties, including ample fruit, vegetables, herbs and spices, are advocated. To support antimicrobial properties to eradicate infection and resolve symptoms,[67] a diet that emphasises foods with anti-bacterial properties such as garlic, ginger, onion and basil would also be useful. Probiotic foods may be useful to enhance immunity and gut microbiome balance.
DINNER	Slow-cooked organic chicken, ginger, turmeric, spring onions, shiitake mushroom and basmati rice congee with tamari.	Centring the diet on potent anti-inflammatory agents and immune regulators is imperative. Systemic autoimmune joint diseases (i.e. RA, PsA, SpA) may follow Lyme disease,[68] with 45–60% of individuals with Lyme disease manifesting some form of arthritis[69]; thus, consumption of anti-inflammatory herbs and spices such as ginger and turmeric to downregulate inflammation and modulate the immune system is suggested. Due to Lyme disease sharing many similar properties to autoimmune diseases, a gluten-free, dairy-free, anti-inflammatory diet should be followed.
SNACK	Blueberries and walnuts Salsa and guacamole with gluten-free crackers	Foods chosen as snacks are reflective of their affinity for the neurological and cardiovascular system since both these systems are attacked by *B. burgdorferi*. Antioxidant constituents that are known to be able to cross the blood–brain barrier, such as anthocyanins in blueberries and omega-3 fatty acids in walnuts, are recommended for their neuroprotective abilities where they counteract neuro-inflammation that drives depression. Salsa is a source of lycopene. Although no studies exist examining its role as food as medicine in Lyme disease, lycopene displays cardioprotective properties. Thus, hypothetically, it may be useful counteract inflammation associated with Lyme carditis.

Nutritional therapy (supplements)

ANTIMICROBIAL

Colloidal silver

Colloidal silver has a long history of use as an antimicrobial, including the World Health Organization's use of it to purify water in developing countries. True colloidal silver is nanoparticles of silver suspended in a liquid suspension. It works by binding to the cell wall, moving through the cell membrane and disabling essential metabolic functions of the cell.

While human studies directly involving Lyme disease are limited, it appears that colloidal silver also impacts on the biofilm development of certain other bacteria, including *Staphylococcus aureus*, which also may have important implications for biofilm eradication in Lyme.[70]

There are in vitro studies that demonstrate that colloidal silver does have potent antimicrobial activity against *Borrelia*, and many case reports back that up. Dr M. Paul Farber, author of *The Micro-Silver Bullet: A Scientifically Documented Answer to the Three Largest Epidemics in the World: Lyme Disease, Aids Virus, Yeast Infection, and the Common Cold*, cites[71]:

> *Two studies have been conducted with colloidal silver and its effectiveness against* Borrelia burgdorferi. *The first study conducted at Fox Chase Cancer Center, Philadelphia, Pennsylvania, showed growth inhibition in low concentrations (2–10 ppm) and much faster action in higher concentrations (15–75 ppm).*
>
> *The Department of Health and Human Services, Rocky Mountain Laboratories, tested cultured spirochetes of the* Borrelia burgdorferi … *using 150 ppm and 15 ppm colloidal silver … none of the treated cultures contained live spirochetes after 24 hours.*

Safety of colloidal silver is an obvious consideration, as some colloidal silver products are simply specks of silver in suspension, which the body could have trouble clearing. High-quality silver used for medicinal purposes should be nanoparticles of silver, between 1 nanometer and 100 nanometers in size.

Dose: up to 10 mL b.i.d. at 5–10 ppm.

INFLAMMATION REDUCTION

Reducing inflammation is another high priority in the naturopathic treatment of Lyme disease. Inflammation is a byproduct of chronic inflammation and contributes significantly to many Lyme symptoms, ranging from joint pain to cognitive dysfunction.

Proteolyic enzymes

Proteolytic enzymes such as bromelain are significant regulators of the inflammatory response. They increase the activity of macrophages and increase the potency of natural killer cells. Most importantly, they have the ability to break down antigen–antibody complexes and even

prevent their formation in the first place. These antigen–antibody complexes are an inherent part of the chronic infectious process, but if prolonged can contribute to a chronic inflammatory state. They also break down plasma proteins and inflammatory debris. One study demonstrated that bromelain has the ability to inhibit the expression of INF-γ and TNF-α, two distinctly inflammatory markers.[72]

The other benefit of proteolytic enzymes is reducing fibrin, a fibrous mesh that forms in areas of tissue damage. Excessive fibrin can impede the flow of blood and can contribute to hypercoagulation, which is a common finding in Lyme patients. Hypercoagulation can lead to a reduction in oxygenation to the tissues and can impede the tissues' ability to shuttle wastes and toxins out of the cells.

Further, excess fibrin can contribute to the formation of biofilm which, as discussed, provides a polysaccharide matrix structure within which the bacteria themselves can hide and evade antimicrobial therapy. Therefore, proteolytic enzymes not only play a role in inflammation itself, but in the breaking down of biofilm.

Dose: 100–300 mg b.i.d.–t.d.s.

Lumbrokinase

Lumbrokinase is an enzyme sourced from *Lumbricus rubellus*, a species of earthworm. It has been shown to contain six proteolytic enzymes that act to reduce blood clots, decrease fibrinogen levels, regulate hypercoagulation and dissolve biofilm.[73,74]

Lumbrokinase is utilised in Lyme treatment to break down biofilm, which is the polysaccharide matrix created by the bacteria in the body and which houses and protects the bacteria. Breaking down biofilm to expose the bacteria to the antimicrobial effects of herbs and antibiotics is a vital part of the treatment process.

Nattokinase is another biofilm agent, sourced from soybeans instead of earthworms. Consequently, it would be a better choice for vegans. However, lumbrokinase has demonstrated greater efficacy in clinical studies for *Borrelia*. Nattokinase has been shown to destroy biofilms of *S. aureus* and *Bacillus subtilis*.[75,76]

Serrapeptase, which is from the digestive systems of silkworms, is yet another option.

Dose: lumbrokinase 20 mg b.i.d. between meals.
Dose: serrapeptase 100 000–200 000 units q.d.

IMMUNE SYSTEM SUPPORT

Immune support is crucial in Lyme treatment because Lyme disease is immune suppressive. White blood cell counts are frequently low or on the low end of normal in this population, providing even more of a challenge for overcoming infection. Antibiotic therapy can also cause leukopenia, which is another reason why it is important for the patient to have monthly blood testing done that includes a full blood count with differential.

Transfer factors

Transfer factors are molecules that support and modulate immune function. They contain antigen-related information, helping the host immune system recognise, and better respond to, external threats. They help to train and sensitise the immune system. They also transfer recognition signals between immune cells, alerting naïve immune cells about a potential threat.[77]

Transfer factors also boost natural killer cell activity, a vital part of immune defence. They work on the Th1 cellular immunity and help to balance Th1/Th2 balance. They can be general or antigen specific, and are available for *Borrelia*, mycoplasma, viruses and so on. They are generally derived from cow colostrum or chicken egg yolk.

Dose: 500–1000 mg q.d.

Beta-glucans

Beta-glucans are polysaccharides that are naturally occurring in the cell walls of yeasts, bacteria, fungi and cereals. While beta-glucans can have diverse effects including helping with cardiovascular function, reducing blood levels of saturated fats and balancing blood sugar regulation, in Lyme treatment, they are chosen for their immune-balancing properties. Most of the ones used are sourced from medicinal mushrooms such as shiitake, maitake and reishi, or the yeast *Saccromyces cerevisiae* (although the final product is not yeast containing).

Beta-glucans are immunomodulating, meaning they can strengthen immune function and also dampen detrimental immune hyperactivation. Beta-glucans can activate macrophages, neutrophils and T cells, setting off a cascade of heightened cellular immune response.[78]

Their ability to strengthen and activate macrophages is one of their key benefits in Lyme treatment, as it is postulated that *Borrelia* can actually invade macrophages and weaken their activity.[79]

They also can assist in the phagocytosis of the *Borrelia* bacteria, through their influence on the complement receptor 3. Phagocytosis of *Borrelia* is dependent on complement receptor 3, which in turn requires an immune element called CD-14. In cases of deficient CD-14, beta-glucans were found to compensate and allow for greater phagocytosis.[80]

Dose: 50–200 mg q.d.

Colostrum

Colostrum is a high-protein substance found in the milk of mammals. While naturally produced to protect offspring early in their lives as their immune system develops, bovine colostrum has been used in human supplements to confer similar immune-boosting properties.

It is rich in antibodies, lactoferrin and other immune agents that provide bacteriostatic, bacteriocidal, anti-viral, anti-inflammatory and immunomodulatory protection against infection.[81]

It also modulates inflammation by binding and, hence, interfering with the bioactivity of TNF-α.[82]

Studies also show that, along with IgG antibody protection, colostrum also contains IgA (albeit in lesser amounts), an anti-inflammatory antibody that plays a large role in immune protection in the mucosal membranes.[83] Given that *Borrelia* and related infections can invade gastrointestinal tissues, and given the prevalence of

intestinal bacterial and fungal imbalances, this provides significant benefit to Lyme patients.

Dose: 500–1000 mg q.d.

DETOXIFICATION SUPPORT

Detoxification will make a tremendous difference to the outcomes of Lyme treatment. More sensitive patients may experience Herxheimer reactions at even low doses of antimicrobial therapy, but even those who are not highly sensitive can experience Herxes and will need additional detox support to help clear the toxins that were released from the killing off of the bacteria. Additionally, patients on antibiotic therapy will benefit from extra liver and kidney support as their systems are additionally taxed from the medications.

It is helpful to look at a patient's methylation status as that can play such a pivotal role in immune health and detoxification capability. See Chapter 7 for detailed information.

Glutathione

Glutathione is a substance made up of three amino acids – glutamine, cysteine and glycine – and is produced in the liver. Glutathione is considered the 'master antioxidant' in the body; it plays a vital role in countering reactive oxidant species, especially in the brain, which consumes the greatest amount of oxygen and, therefore, creates the most oxidative stress. It is known to be neuroprotective, as it prevents neuronal death associated with amyloid plaque deposits. Glutathione production depletes with age, indicating a potential for supplementation especially in older populations.[84]

Glutathione is also a major detoxification agent. It neutralises and clears heavy metals and other toxins from the body. While the body does produce its own supply of glutathione, excess toxic stress will deplete it, thus creating a higher need. If the body's production does not keep up with need, toxins will accumulate in the body.

Glutathione supply can be boosted by moderate exercise, but many Lyme patients are not able to do even that. Supplementation with N-acetylcysteine or S-adenosyl methionine (SAMe) may provide precursors, and undenatured whey protein can also stimulate endogenous production. Glutathione is often given intravenously, which optimises absorption but can also produce significant detoxification responses in Lyme patients, especially when given at higher doses. Liposomal glutathione is the optimal form for oral supplementation as reduced glutathione is rapidly degraded in the gastrointestinal tract.

Dose: 400–1000 mg q.d. PO (liposomal preferred); 500–2000 mg IV.

ENERGY/ADRENAL SUPPORT

Lyme disease can cause significant disturbances in hormone regulation, in particular, the hypothalamic–pituitary–adrenal axis. The chronic stressors of Lyme disease tax the adrenal glands, often resulting in imbalances in cortisol and DHEA levels. The first stage of the chronic stress response is elevated cortisol as the body tries to compensate for the additional need. This is more likely in the earlier stages of disease. In later stages of the chronic stress response, cortisol is likely to be depleted, and DHEA is often low too. This is a major contributor to the chronic fatigue in Lyme disease, and so adrenal support is a priority.

Phosphatidylserine is a naturally occurring phospholipid that is produced in the body, and occurs in highest concentrations in the brain, lungs, liver, heart and skeletal muscle. It has been shown to lower excess cortisol levels by blunting the cortisol response – specifically, by altering the interactions with receptors to reduce the release of corticotropin releasing factor, which in turn would increase adrenocorticotropic hormone (ACTH), which would then reduce cortisol. Studies have shown this effect to occur using exercise as a short-term stressor on the body, but have also validated a similar response with mental and emotional stressors.[85]

Low cortisol levels can also be balanced with adaptogenic herbs. DHEA supplementation may be indicated with patients with low levels of DHEA and also can act as a precursor to cortisol. Liquorice root is a herb known to have cortisol-boosting properties, but care must be taken because of its oestrogen-promoting effects and also possible hypertensive side effects. Some patients with critically low cortisol benefit from hydrocortisone supplementation for a period of time; however, natural/herbal remedies may be safer and more effective long term.

Another aspect of energy support for Lyme disease patients is mitochondrial support. The mitochondria are the powerhouses of the cell where adenosine triphosphate (ATP) is produced. Nutrients such as NADH, co-enzyme Q10 (CoQ10) and acetyl-L-carnitine can enhance metabolic processes and energy production.

Agents that help to repair the membranes of the mitochondrial wall have also been used to assist energy production in Lyme patients. Mitochondrial cell walls can become damaged over the course of chronic illness through prolonged inflammatory response and increase in free radical production and oxidative stress. Thus, repairing cell membranes and increasing membrane fluidity by providing phospholipid support can lead to increased nutrients entering the cells and greater mitochondrial output.

NT factor is one variant of glycophospholipids that can be used for lipid replacement therapy. Another is phosphotidylcholine (PC). PC can be given orally or intravenously.

Dose: phosphatidylserine 100–200 mg q.d.
Dose: DHEA 5–25 mg q.d.
Dose: NADH 5–10 mg q.d.
Dose: CoQ10 100–400 mg q.d.
Dose: acetyl-L-carnitine 500–2000 mg q.d.
Dose: phosphatidylcholine 500–2000 mg q.d.

DIGESTIVE SUPPORT

Supporting the digestive systems of Lyme patients is important. First, because many of them suffer from digestive issues as part of their illness, but also because for those on antibiotic therapy, gastritis and overgrowth of *Candida* are two of the most common side effects they must overcome.

Probiotics

Top priority in all patients is a high-quality, high-potency probiotic to replenish any good flora that might be killed by antibiotics or other antimicrobials. Probiotics must be separated by any antimicrobials (pharmaceutical or herbal) by at least 2 hours to prevent it being adversely impacted itself. Probiotics will be the most important step in supporting digestive function and the top priority for those on antibiotics to prevent the overgrowth of *Candida albicans*. Strains that have been found to be most helpful include *Lactobacillus acidophilus*, *L. casei*, *L. plantarum*, *Bifidobacterium lactis*, *B. longum*, and *B. bifidum*. They are beneficial to the host by balancing the gastrointestinal microflora.[86]

Key benefits of probiotics in Lyme treatment include that they:
* resist enteric pathogens
* aid in lactose digestion
* modulate the immune system
* enhance nutrient value
* reduce inflammation of the intestinal tract.

Supplementation with kefir and kombucha can also help maintain healthy microbial balance in the gut. The main polysaccharide in kefir grains is kefiran. Kefiran is known to possess anti-inflammatory, anti-fungal and anti-bacterial properties.[87,88]

Kombucha is a drink that is fermented from black tea by a symbiotic colony of bacteria and yeast, which results in a liquid that contains several species of beneficial flora, including lactic acid, acetic acid, bacteria and *Saccharomyces boulardii* (a yeast that has health-promoting properties and functions like a probiotic in the body).

Reducing irritation and inflammation of the gastrointestinal system can help patients to tolerate their antimicrobial treatments. Dietary modifications are obviously important here too to reduce any source of further inflammation.

Dose: 50–200 billion CFUs q.d. at least 2 hours away from antimicrobials.

SLEEP SUPPORT

Melatonin

The pineal gland produces the hormone melatonin to regulate the body's internal time-keeping system, pubertal development and seasonal adaptation. When there are changes in melatonin production and melatonin receptor expression, circadian rhythm sleep disorders may arise.[89,90]

Many Lyme patients have sleep disturbances, including sleep pattern reversal, where they cannot sleep at night but then sleep most of the day.

Melatonin can help them to fall asleep at an appropriate hour. Sustained-release melatonin is more appropriate for people who wake during the night as melatonin has a short half-life and wears off quickly.

Dose: 1–3 mg h.s.

Nutritional therapy (micronutrients)

Lyme disease can cause nutrient depletion, and evaluations of vitamin and mineral status are important to identify specific ones in patients.

VITAMIN C

Because of its significance in immune function, vitamin C should be considered an important supplement. Liposomal vitamin C offers superior absorption without the risk of digestive distress caused by some forms of vitamin C. Some patients do very well with intravenous vitamin C as larger amounts can be given than oral forms – between 5 and 100 g, given by slow drip.

Dose: 500–2000 mg PO; 5–100 g IV.

B VITAMINS

B vitamins are important for energy production and to help the body manage the stress response associated with chronic disease. They can help neurological symptoms significantly too. Beyond the scope of this chapter, but worth stressing, is the importance of evaluating Lyme patients for methylation defects and treating them accordingly with methylated (or non-methylated) B vitamins. Methylfolate and methyl-B_{12} are perhaps the most significant, but should be given with other B vitamins to prevent imbalance. Also of significance is the evaluation of pyroluria, a metabolic illness where abnormal porphyrins carry out zinc and B_6 from the body. Supplementation with activated B_6 (pyridoxal-5-phosphate) in combination with zinc and magnesium can help to restore healthy levels.

Dose: methyl-folate 500–1000 micrograms; methyl-B_{12} 1000–5000 micrograms daily, sublingual or IM preferred; pyridoxal-5-phosphate 50–100 mg.

VITAMIN D

Traditionally thought of as being most important for bone health, vitamin D is an important vitamin for immune modulation; it also functions as a hormone in the body. Deficiency of vitamin D is associated with increased autoimmunity as well as increased susceptibility to infection.[91] Vitamin D receptors and vitamin D metabolising enzymes are found in many immune cell types including antigen-presenting cells, T cells, B cells and monocytes. Research shows that vitamin D leads to a shift from a pro-inflammatory to a more anti-inflammatory immune status. It inhibits the secretion of pro-inflammatory Th1 (IL-2, interferon-γ, TNF-α), Th9 (IL-9) and Th22 (IL-22) cytokines while promoting the production of more anti-inflammatory Th2 cytokines (such as IL-3, IL-4, IL-5, IL-10).[92]

Vitamin D is often depleted in chronic Lyme patients, so testing and possible supplementation should be considered.

Dose: 1000–5000 IU q.d.

ZINC

Zinc is a vital mineral, because of both its connection with pyroluria (which appears to be common in Lyme patients) and its general immune-enhancing properties. Zinc is crucial for the normal development and function of immune cells including neutrophils, macrophages and natural killer cells. Antibody production is also compromised in zinc deficiency.[93]

Dose: 25–50 mg q.d.

MAGNESIUM

Perhaps the most depleted mineral in Lyme patients is magnesium. *Borrelia* and *Bartonella* both require magnesium to duplicate thus depleting the body's stores rapidly. While some practitioners argue that magnesium should not be supplemented so as not to 'feed' the pathogens, in reality, many patients benefit significantly from magnesium supplementation. This is particularly for its effects on muscle relaxation and relief from spasms, bowel function (offsetting constipation) and assistance with balancing mood and promoting better sleep.

Dose: 300–1000 mg q.d. in divided doses. Can be taken h.s. to promote sleep.

MOLYBDENUM

Molybdenum is a trace mineral that can assist with detoxification in Lyme treatment. Molybdenum boosts the production of certain enzymes in the body known as molybdoenzymes. Sulfite oxidase helps to break down sulfites into sulfates, which can then be eliminated from the body. A subset of Lyme patients is sensitive to sulfites, so this can be a helpful mineral in those circumstances.

Perhaps most importantly, molybdenum stimulates the production of aldehyde oxidase and aldehyde dehydrogenase – enzymes that are necessary to break down aldehydes such as formaldehyde and acetylaldehyde. Alcohol metabolism is one source of acetylaldehydes, but another important potential source for Lyme patients is *Candida albicans*. *C. albicans* produces aldehydes in the gastrointestinal tract by sugar fermentation. These aldehydes can have neurotoxic effects. Aldehydes can bind with the neurotransmitters serotonin and dopamine, creating secondary metabolites that can cause neuronal cell death.[94,95]

Aldehydes also damage cell membranes of red blood cells, compromising their function and impacting on haemoglobin levels and oxygenation to the brain.[96]

Finally, aldehydes disable the formation of tubulin in the brain, which then undermines the structural support of dendrites, leading to dendritic atrophy and death.[97]

Individuals with an overgrowth of *Candida* may benefit from supplementation of molybdenum to help metabolise those detrimental compounds.[98,99]

Dose: 30–200 micrograms q.d.

Herbal medicine
ANTIMICROBIAL THERAPY

Herbal regimens for Lyme disease and co-infections can be very effective in eradicating the pathogens underlying the illness without the toxicity and side effects of antibiotics.

The following herbs are just a sampling of what can be used in each category, but represent options that are commonly used and have shown efficacy in the treatment of Lyme disease.

HERBAL THERAPY FOR BORRELIA

Uncaria tomentosa (cat's claw)

Uncaria tomentosa (cat's claw) is a medicinal herb from the Amazon rainforest that has anti-inflammatory, anti-bacterial, anti-viral, immune-modulating and antioxidant properties. It is one of the more popular herbs for treating chronic Lyme disease. Cat's claw contains quinovic acid glycosides, which are natural precursors to quinolones, a class of pharmaceutical antibiotics (that includes Cipro and Levaquin). These compounds give it strong antimicrobial properties; however, the same side effect of tendon pain and damage that can come with the quinolone antibiotics can occur with cat's claw, so care must be taken.

Cat's claw also has anti-inflammatory properties. An Austrian study published in the April 2002 *Journal of Rheumatology* showed that rheumatoid arthritis patients treated with 60 mg a day of a standardised extract of cat's claw for 1 year experienced a reduction in the number of painful and swollen joints.[100]

The mechanisms for its anti-inflammatory properties are the inhibition of TNF-α production, as well as its ability to scavenge free radicals.[101]

Dose: tincture 10–30 drops b.i.d.

Dipsacus sylvestris (teasel root)

Teasel root is considered a valuable antimicrobial herb in the treatment of Lyme disease. Some sources believe that it helps to bring spirochaetes into the bloodstream from the tissues, making them more vulnerable to antimicrobials.[102]

One study looked at the expression of genes associated with the immune system in fibroblasts infected with Lyme disease after treatment with teasel root. The results suggested that the herb did indeed have anti-bacterial and anti-inflammatory effects in human cells infected with Lyme.[103]

Dose: tincture 5–10 drops b.i.d.

Olea europaea (olive leaf)

Olive leaf extract has a wide variety of uses in Lyme treatment, but it is one of the stronger and more effective antimicrobials. Olive leaf contains high amounts of phenolics, in particular oleuropein. Its benefits include being anti-bacterial, anti-viral, anti-fungal and anti-protozoal. Olive leaf extract also has protective effects on the cardiovascular system, and has anti-inflammatory and antioxidant properties.[104]

Of high priority for Lyme patients, olive leaf is neuroprotective and can help mitigate the cognitive impairment commonly experienced in Lyme. One of the ways it does that is by improving the permeability of the blood–brain barrier and reducing brain oedema.[105]

Dose: capsules 500 mg t.d.s.

Origanum vulgare (oil of oregano)

Oil of oregano contains high concentrations of two substances called carvacrol and thymol, which are largely responsible for its strong anti-bacterial qualities.[106]

The impact of oil of oregano appears to be dose and concentration dependent, and is equal between Gram-positive and Gram-negative bacteria.

It is also a powerful anti-fungal. A study of several essential oils, including oregano, and three major anti-fungal medications (fluconazole, itraconazole and triclomazole) showed that yeast had higher sensitivity levels overall to the essential oils than the medications. The essential oils affected mainly the cell wall and membranes of the yeast.[107]

Oil of oregano also has been shown to act in a synergistic fashion with certain other antimicrobials, notably the antibiotic doxycycline and biological silver nanoparticles, both of which are used in Lyme treatment.[108,109] Georgetown University researchers found that oil of oregano appeared to be as effective as traditional antibiotics in reducing infection. Oil of oregano at relatively low doses was found to be efficacious against *Staphylococcus* bacteria and was comparable in its germ-killing properties to antibiotic drugs such as streptomycin, penicillin and vancomycin.[110]

Oil of oregano is also a potent antimicrobial against *Borrelia*, *Bartonella* and *Candida*, and therefore is an important natural agent in Lyme treatment.

Dose: capsules 50 mg b.i.d.–t.d.s.

Citrus paradisi (grapefruit seed)

Grapefruit seed extract is a good option for patients with Lyme disease, as it is a natural agent that has been shown to be effective against cystic forms of *Borrelia*. Grapefruit seed extract works by disrupting the bacterial membrane and liberating cytoplasmic contents.[111]

One study showed that at low concentrations, grapefruit seed extract caused herniation and disruption of the cell membranes, with a leaking out of the contents of the cell, even just 15 minutes after contact. Then, at higher concentrations, grapefruit seed extract eradicated the bacteria and cysts completely.[112]

The fact that grapefruit seed extract reduced the conversion of spirochaetes to cyst forms makes it a highly valuable part of Lyme treatment.

Dose: capsules 250 mg b.i.d.

HERBAL THERAPY FOR CO-INFECTIONS

Artemisia annua (wormwood)

Artemisia annua has been used in the treatment of malaria, mostly because of the anti-malarial compound it contains, known as artemisinin. Because *Babesia* is a malaria-like illness, artemisinin also has a place in its treatment.

A. annua is the only known source of the sesquiterpene artemisinin (qinghaosu). Its biological activities relate to the presence of secondary metabolites such as sesquiterpenoids, aliphatic hydrocarbons, aromatic hydrocarbons, aromatic ketones, flavonoids, terpenoids and steroids.[113]

Pharmaceutial companies have created synthetic versions of artemisinin, in the forms of artesunate and artemether. They are typically used in combination with other anti-parasitic agents to prevent resistance. Naturally occurring artemisinin has good blood–brain barrier penetration, lower toxicity levels and a moderate half-life in the body, so it is a credible choice for babesiosis. Unlike other antiprotozoal agents, artemisinin also appears to be effective against all stages of the life cycle, not just the mature parasites.[114]

In a study by Kim et al., researchers evaluated the anti-inflammatory, antioxidant and antimicrobial effects of *A. annua* using the DPPH radical scavenging assay. The results demonstrated that artemisinin has anti-inflammatory, antioxidant and antimicrobial activities.[115]

Dose: 200–400 mg q.d.; can pulse at higher doses up to 500 mg t.d.s. 4 days on/3 days off. Higher doses can be hard to tolerate.

Cryptolepis sanguinolenta (cryptolepis root)

The aqueous root extract of *Cryptolepis sanguinolenta* has been used as an anti-malarial agent for decades, and for this reason, it has benefit for patients with the *Babesia* co-infection. The major indoloquinoline alkaloid isolated from *C. sanguinolenta* is cryptolepine. Cryptolepine has been reported to have various biological activities such as anti-fungal and anti-bacterial activity against both Gram-positive and Gram-negative organisms.[116,117]

Of further benefit to Lyme patients, cryptolepis has anti-inflammatory and analgesic effects on patients suffering from osteoarthritis.[118]

Dose: tincture 60–120 drops b.i.d.

Houttuynia cordata (chameleon)

Houttuynia cordata is commonly used as a herbal tea in Japan to promote health. In one study, researchers demonstrated the anti-bacterial, bacteriostatic and antibiofilm effect of *H. cordata* poultice ethanol extract (eHCP) against *S. aureus* and MRSA. The findings support that eHCP has the ability to inhibit IL-8 and CCL20 productions from *S. aureus* without any cytotoxic effect.[119]

The mechanisms of its action are not fully known, but preliminary studies demonstrate that houttuynia extracts can increase levels of hydrogen peroxide, which in turn, leads to bacterial cell death.[119]

H. cordata is a herb that has been used in Lyme treatment, most specifically against the co-infection *Bartonella*. Clinical reports validate its use against *Bartonella*, although specific research is lacking for this use. Houttuynia has also been shown to help inhibit biofilm formation of *C. albicans* in the oral cavity, which further gives it relevance for Lyme patients.[120]

Dose: capsules 250 mg t.d.s.

IMMUNE SUPPORT

Astragalus membranaceus (astragalus)

Astragalus has a long history of use as a tonic and immune strengthener, boosting the number and activity of immune cells. Astragalus works by stimulating several factors of the immune system, including enhancing phagocytic activity of monocytes and macrophages, increasing interferon production and natural killer cell activity, enhancing T cell activity and potentiating other anti-viral mechanisms. Astragalus has also been demonstrated to have anti-inflammatory activity. It is often used with other adaptogenic/tonic herbs such as liquorice and ginseng.

There is some controversy as to whether astragalus should be avoided in late-stage Lyme because of its tendency to boost Th1 immune response; chronic, late-stage Lyme tends to be Th1 dominant. Herbalist Stephen Buhner cautions against its use and suggests that astragalus is a better herb for acute Lyme and early in infection. (See his website www.buhnerhealinglyme.com.)[121]

Dose: 1000 mg q.d.

INFLAMMATION REDUCTION

Curcuma longa (turmeric)

Curcumin, a component of turmeric, is one of the most useful anti-inflammatory agents, and is widely used in Lyme treatment. It also has very strong antioxidant capabilities, and is immune supportive and immune balancing in autoimmune processes.

Curcumin's anti-inflammatory actions come from its ability to reduce pro-inflammatory cytokines such as IL-1, IL-6, COX-2, MMP-9, NF-κB, CRP, TNF and others. Studies have shown multiple pathways and mechanisms by which curcumin reduces inflammation.

Curcumin also has antioxidant properties. It increases levels of vitamins C and E in the body, and prevents lipid peroxidation and oxidative damage.[122]

Curcumin can improve mitochondrial enzymes and boost glutathione levels, adding to its antioxidant, detoxification and ATP-producing benefits.

Curcumin has been shown to be neuroprotective by reducing oxidative damage caused by D-galactose, a reducing sugar that can lead to mitochondrial dysfunction and death of neurons. It is also neuroregenerative – meaning it can promote the development of new, healthy neurons by increasing neuron stem cell growth in the brain by up to 80%.[123] Studies showed that it increased both the numbers of stem cells produced as well as the number of fully differentiated mature cells.

It also helps reduce neuropathic pain by inhibiting TNF-α and nitric oxide release.[124]

There are many human studies showing the efficacy of curcumin in reducing inflammation, while having an excellent safety profile.

Dose: capsules 500 mg t.d.s.

Boswellia serrata (boswellia, frankincense)

Boswellia is a herb that has long been used as an anti-inflammatory, with wide usage in arthritis and arthritic conditions. The main active constituents of boswellia are the boswellic acids, most importantly acetyl-11-keto-beta-boswellic acid (AKBA). AKBA has demonstrated many significant immunomodulatory and inflammation-modulating effects in preclinical research.[125]

Boswellia works in a couple of different ways. It inhibits 5-lipoxygenase, an agent that promotes inflammatory leukotrienes. It can also reduce inflammation through the inhibition of the proinflammatory enzyme human leukocyte esterase. To date, boswellia is the only compound that has been found that works on both 5-lipoxygenase and human leukocyte esterase.[126]

Because it works on the 5-lipoxygenase and not the COX-2 inhibition as non-steroidal anti-inflammatory drugs (NSAIDs) do, it can provide relief from pain and inflammation without the gastrointestinal side effects of the medications. NSAIDs, by default, block COX-1 enzymes too, which are necessary for a healthy gastrointestinal mucosal lining.

In an animal study comparing the efficacy of 5-LOXIN™, a standardised extract from boswellia, to that of the anti-inflammatory drug ibuprofen, 5-LOXIN™ produced a 27% reduction in inflammation, compared to 35% for ibuprofen.[127]

Another study comparing 5-LOXIN™ to the anti-inflammatory steroid drug prednisone found that 5-LOXIN™ produced a 55% reduction in inflammation, similar to the effects of prednisone.[128]

Thus, boswellia has a comparable benefit to anti-inflammatory medications, but with a much better side effect and safety profile. It is considered safe and well tolerated.

Another way to utilise boswellia is the essential oil frankincense. The essential oil is a highly concentrated source of boswellic acids and can have profound anti-inflammatory benefits. The essential oil can be used topically on areas of pain and inflammation, often diluted in a carrier oil such as fractionated coconut oil.

Dose: capsules 500 mg t.d.s.

Polygonum cuspidatum (Japanese knotweed)

The dried root of Japanese knotweed is a traditional Chinese medicinal herb, which has been widely distributed in the world. It can now be found in Asia and North America. Pharmacological and clinical studies have indicated that this herb has anti-viral, antimicrobial, anti-inflammatory, neuroprotective, anti-tumour, chemoprotective and cardioprotective functions. Main active compounds include anthraquinones, resveratrol and stilbenes.[129]

Antimicrobial effects have seen in prevention of oral disease in relation to biofilms, as demonstrated by a study showing the inhibitory effects against ATP-ase and production of *Streptococcus mutans* in biofilms.[130]

Anti-inflammatory properties have also been attributed to Japanese knotweed as a potent agent for rheumatoid arthritis treatment. Research has shown ethyl acetate extract suppressed serotonin-induced swelling, as well as inhibiting positive responses of C-reactive protein and rheumatoid factor, when compared to untreated controls.[131]

One of the most important aspects of Lyme treatment is to interrupt the pro-inflammatory cytokine cascade. Japanese knotweed is known to be a very strong inhibitor of cytokine cascades initiated by bacteria. In Lyme disease, there is a spirochaete-stimulated release of a number of

matrix metalloproteinases (MMPs). Currently, this is the only herb that is known to specifically block MMP-1 and MMP-3 induction.

Emodin, an anthraquinone, has been shown to inhibit the expression of inflammatory-associated genes including iNOS, TNF-α, interleukin-1, IκB kinase (IKK)-alpha, and IKK-gamma and to inhibit the nuclear translocation of NF-κB on LPS-induced inflammatory responses in RAW 264.7 macrophages.[132]

There are many additional mechanisms responsible for the therapeutic properties of this herb. Its role as a capillary stimulant is important in increasing blood flow to areas where Lyme spirochaetes reside, such as eyes, skin, heart and joints. According to Stephen Buhner,[121] this herb is an anti-spirochaetal, indicated for prevention and acute onset Lyme, as well as *Bartonella* co-infections. In addition, it has immune modulatory and protective properties against Lyme neurotoxins, Lyme arthritis, Lyme carditis, dermatoborreliosis, memory and cognitive decline, as well as reduction in Herxheimer reactions and headaches.

Dose: capsules 500 mg up to 10 capsules q.d. in divided doses.

Andrographis paniculata (andrographis)

Andrographis is an important constituent of at least 26 Ayurvedic formulas in Indian pharmacopoeia. In traditional Chinese medicine, it is seen as a herb used to rid the body of heat and fever and to dispel toxins from the body.[133] Diterpenes, flavonoids, xanthones, noriridoides and other miscellaneous compounds have been isolated from this plant. Extract and pure compounds of the plant have been reported for their anti-microbial, cytotoxic, anti-protozoan, anti-inflammatory, antioxidant, immunostimulant, anti-diabetic, anti-infective, anti-angiogenic, hepato-renal protective, sex hormone/sexual function modulation and liver enzymes modulation.[134,135]

The phytochemistry of this plant is quite complex, spanning many different body systems and mechanisms of action. Research has shown an alleviation in lipopolysaccharide-induced release of pro-inflammatory mediators, such as NO, IL-1β and IL-6, inflammatory mediators, such as PGE$_2$ and TXB$_2$, and allergic mediators. Additional anti-inflammatory effects can be attributed to its interference with COX-enzyme activity and downexpression of genes involved in the inflammatory cascade.[136]

One of the reasons it may be helpful in treatment of Lyme is due to its ability to activate adenylate cyclase, increasing cAMP, which is important for preventing damage to cell membranes. In this way, symptoms of nerve cell irritation, such as headaches, tingling, burning, numbness, stabbing sensations, tremors and unexplained lactation, can be reduced.[137]

Dose: capsules 400 mg b.i.d.

DETOXIFICATION SUPPORT

Smilax glabra (sarsaparilla)

Smilax glabra is a herb that has detoxifying and anti-inflammatory properties. The polysaccharides contained in the rhizomes have been shown to reduce nitric oxide, TNF-α and IL-6, thus modulating inflammatory response.[138]

Another study showed a reduction in COX-2 activity and COX expression.[139]

The major benefit of *S. glabra* in terms of detoxification is its ability to cross the blood–brain barrier. Other species of smilax do not have that capability. *S. glabra* is able to neutralise neurotoxins and can play a significant role in mitigating Herxheimer reactions, particularly where they include the worsening of neurological symptoms.

Research also shows that *S. glabra* can protect the brain against lead-induced oxidative stress. Administration of an extract from *S. glabra* reduced blood and tissue levels of lead significantly, while also increasing protective antioxidants such as superoxide dismutase and glutathione.[140]

Given that many Lyme patients have methylation defects that may impair detoxification pathways and predispose them to accumulation of toxic metals, and given that metals such as lead and mercury have been found in biofilm, substances that support detoxification of these toxins play a significant role in treatment approaches.

Dose: tincture 30–60 drops b.i.d.

Liver support herbs

Other than the specific detoxification agents discussed, there are many possibilities for liver support herbs, including *Taraxacum officinale* (dandelion root), *Cynara scolymus* (artichoke), *Glycyrrhiza* spp. (liquorice root), *Silybum marianum* (milk thistle), *Mahonia aquifolium* (oregon grape root) and *Schisandra chinensis* (magnolia).

Supporting liver function is one of the highest priorities in Lyme treatment for those who are on antibiotic therapy. Elevations in liver enzymes are always a possibility, especially in chronic cases where multiple antibiotics are being used on a long-term basis. Patients on antibiotics should have routine blood testing done on a monthly basis to monitor liver enzyme levels.

Dose: tinctures 40–60 drops b.i.d. in combination.

BRAIN CHEMISTRY AND MOOD BALANCE

Hypericum perforatum (St John's wort)

St John's wort has been used successfully in mild to moderate depression. It works by inhibiting the reuptake of serotonin, dopamine and noradrenaline (norepinephrine) as well as the enzymes monoamine oxidase and catechol-O-methyltransferase, which allows more conversion of dopamine to noradrenaline. It also binds to GABA receptors.[141] St John's wort may also enhance memory properties due to the constituent hyperforin.[142]

Dose: capsule 300 mg t.d.s.

SLEEP SUPPORT

Valeriana officinalis (valerian)

Numerous studies have demonstrated that valerian improves both the ability to fall asleep quickly and the quality and depth of sleep throughout the night. Valerian contains over 150 constituents that are calming to the nervous system, with valerenic acid as its main constituent.

One review of data on valerian showed that 80% of patients experienced some improvement in sleep compared to placebo. Of six studies that measured 'hangover effect', valerian measured equally with placebo.[143]

Other herbs that have been demonstrated to help with sleep include *Humulus lupulus* (hops), *Passiflora incarnata* (passionflower), *Matricaria recutita* and *Chamomilla recutita* (chamomile), and *Scutellaria lateriflora* (skullcap). Amino acids already discussed may also assist in sleep promotion, including 5-HTP, GABA and L-theanine.

Assisting patients in getting adequate sleep is a high priority as many experience significant insomnia and resort to prescription sleep medications and strong medications, such as benzodiazepines, both of which have significant side effect profiles and the potential for dependence.

Dose: tincture 2–5 mL t.d.s.

NEUROPROTECTIVES

Hericium erinaceus (lion's mane)

Lion's mane is a traditional Chinese medicinal mushroom that was commonly prescribed for stomach ailments and cancer prevention, with additional medicinal properties emerging. Indications for lion's mane include aiding in digestion, stimulating nerve growth factor (NGF) in the central and peripheral nervous system, repairing neurological degradation from senility, improving cognitive function and memory loss, and improving reflexes.

Memory and cognitive dysfunction from chronic Lyme disease and Lyme disease co-infections can be severe. Once the infections have invaded the brain and central nervous system, they are capable of causing numerous cognitive deficits, including short- and long-term memory loss, difficulty retaining new information, compromised ability to read and write, and an inability to make new memories.[144]

Neurotrophic factors are important in promoting the growth and differentiation of neurons. NGF is essential for the maintenance of the basal forebrain cholinergic system. Hericenones and erinacines isolated from the medicinal mushroom *Hericium erinaceus* can induce NGF synthesis in nerve cells.[145]

The cognitive benefits of lion's mane stem from the potent neuroprotective properties of the mushroom and its ability to restore myelin along the axons in the brain – a process that is highly beneficial for those with Lyme disease and Lyme disease co-infections, as many of the cognitive deficits from these diseases result from the bacteria's affinity for breaking down myelin sheath in the brain. To date, lion's mane is the only mushroom that displays promising potential for nerve regeneration due to its ability to stimulate synthesis of NGF.[145,146]

Dose: 2–3 mL b.i.d.

Amino acids

BRAIN CHEMISTRY AND MOOD BALANCE

Many patients with Lyme disease experience depression and anxiety, and many take pharmaceutical medications to try to relieve them. Amino acid therapy can provide significant relief, and could be considered as an alternative, providing the raw materials the body can use to produce more neurotransmitters, thus supporting neurotransmitter pathways without the side effects of medications.

5-HTP

Used as a precursor to serotonin, the amino acid 5-HTP can bring significant relief from depression. In larger doses taken before bed, it can also be used as a sleep aid. 5-HTP crosses the blood–brain barrier and is freely converted to serotonin without biochemical feedback inhibition.[147]

Studies have also shown 5-HTP to be beneficial for patients with migraines and symptoms of fibromyalgia, including tender points, pain intensity, sleep quality, morning stiffness, anxiety and fatigue.[148,149]

Dose: 50–100 mg q.d.; up to 200 mg h.s. for sleep promotion.

GABA

GABA is an inhibitory neurotransmitter, just as serotonin is an inhibitory neurotransmitter. Low GABA levels can lead to anxiety, noise sensitivity and aggressive behaviour; therefore, GABA supplementation can also calm the brain and balance mood. Interestingly, GABA can also promote gastric motility – low levels can lead to decreased bowel function – and can help reduce gastro-oesophageal reflux. This may be significant in the subset of Lyme patients who experience GORD and gastroparesis. GABA has shown profound benefit for those patients who struggle with anxiety.[150–152]

Dose: 200–500 mg b.i.d.

L-theanine

L-theanine is another amino acid that has proven efficacy in states of anxiety and also insomnia. L-theanine comes from green tea leaves and blocks the binding of L-glutamic acid to glutamate receptors in the brain. It promotes GABA as well as the production of alpha brain waves, further inducing a relaxed state.

Being a GABA agonist, it can also have benefits in promoting restful sleep and reducing the stress response.[153]

Dose: 200–400 mg b.i.d.

Tyrosine

Tyrosine is the precursor to the catecholamine neurotransmitters dopamine, noradrenaline (norepinephrine) and adrenaline (epinephrine), which make up more of the stimulatory, excitatory neurotransmitters. Tyrosine can benefit depression and can also promote mental alertness.[154]

Dose: 500–1000 mg b.i.d.

Lifestyle factors

Patients benefit from undertaking additional measures at home that support detoxification.

DRY SKIN BRUSHING

Dry skin brushing can assist with lymphatic clearing by aiding in the manual return of toxins into the central blood stream from the periphery. This is especially important in patients who are mostly bedbound as they are not getting the muscular contractions necessary to stimulate lymph flow.

EPSOM SALTS BATHS

Bathing in magnesium sulfate salts stimulates detoxification and can bring significant relief from Herxheimer reactions. Some patients are heat sensitive, so care must be taken to not overheat the bath water. The magnesium component of the Epsom salts can help ease muscle aches and spasms, while the sulfur component provides the detoxification effect.

COFFEE ENEMAS

Coffee enemas can provide a rapid elimination of toxins via two key mechanisms. First, the palmitates of coffee stimulate glutathione-S-transferase, which helps to remove toxins from the blood. Second, the enema stimulates peristalsis within the intestines, which helps to move toxins through the intestines and out through the rectum. Many patients find that coffee enemas bring immediate and profound relief from Herxheimer reactions and general symptoms of pain, fatigue, depression, anxiety, headaches and migraines.

CONCLUSION

Lyme is complex, multifactorial, multisystemic and challenging to treat. Simply addressing infection is clearly not enough; a truly holistic approach is necessary, with consideration of the many areas that are impacting on each individual. This can be very overwhelming for patient and practitioner alike, so sensitivity to that and a step-by-step, manageable approach will set up the patient for success.

There are yet other areas that frequently impact on Lyme patients that were not covered in depth in this chapter, but are worth mentioning. Mould toxicity, methylation defects, pyroluria and heavy metal toxicity are co-stressors that are frequently present and can be closely related but hard to delineate, due to overlap of symptoms.

Another consideration in treating Lyme patients is to be understanding of their illness experience to date. Lyme is frequently misdiagnosed and under-diagnosed; therefore, many patients have seen multiple doctors, often over many years, and failed to receive an accurate diagnosis or effective treatment. Many have been told that their illness is in their heads (because of the lack of medical findings to support any other diagnosis). Some have post-traumatic stress disorder in response to their experience. Many are angry, resentful and feel that the medical community has let them down. Friends and family often do not fully understand their illness, and patients are often told how well they look, when in reality they may be struggling to get out of bed each morning and in significant pain. The human side of the Lyme disease experience cannot be overlooked. Counselling can help patients to work through this, and addressing the emotional elements can in fact accelerate their physical healing. Children need modifications to their school and social schedules to help them adapt, and it is recommended that the family unit participate in support of some kind (therapy, counselling etc.) to be able to understand and support one another.

There is a huge need for recognition of Lyme disease and practitioners who can recognise it and treat it. These patients are complex but also highly self-educated and motivated. An integrative approach is the usually the best approach, and a team of practitioners may need to be involved. Naturopathic and allied health practitioners are in a unique position to help patients manage this multisystem illness that frequently is missed in allopathic medical communities, and have the tools required to effect significant change in patients. There is a clear need for more research into the mechanisms and therapeutics, especially with regards to chronic Lyme disease. Until more research is carried out, there will continue to be a lot of misunderstanding, misdiagnosis and mistreatment of this population.

CASE STUDY

A 43-year old female presented with a diagnosis of Lyme disease, *Babesia* and *Bartonella* based on clinical presentation from a previous practitioner. Her Western blot had reported as indeterminate, so other doctors she had seen had been hesitant to treat her for Lyme based on the ambiguity of the lab work.

Prior to seeing me, she had done some homeopathic treatments with a local practitioner with no positive response.

HPI

Patient was working as a photographer and spent time in woodsy areas in a Lyme-endemic area doing photo shoots. She was also working in a colour photo lab, which was exposing her to chemicals daily, and she was studying full time. Her stress level was high, and gradually, health issues arose. Initial symptoms included a sore throat, sinus issues and feeling run down.

She had been diagnosed with pernicious anaemia as a child and had some ongoing GI issues, but otherwise had enjoyed good health prior to the onset of these symptoms.

After a couple of months, she experienced what she described as a 'health crash'. She rested a lot, with moderate improvements. She saw another practitioner who started her on low doses of herbal medicines for Lyme, which triggered major anxiety, depression and panic attacks. She started taking houttuynia in response (a herb for *Bartonella*), which alleviated those symptoms immediately.

She added some essential oils, based on a lecture she had attended, and was cycling oregano, thyme, clove and

---

cassia in 2-week pulses. She felt more well on the 2 weeks on than the 2 weeks off.

The patient presented to me after this with major symptoms of fatigue, always feeling like she was on the verge of the flu, cognitive issues such as short-term memory loss, and problems with focus and concentration. She was experiencing night sweats, air hunger and tightness in her chest. She had experienced pain in the soles of her feet, but that had resolved with the houttuynia. She also felt some dizziness and some mild anxiety and suffered from a low libido. She did not have severe joint or muscle pain, but did have more general aches with the flu-like episodes.

She was supplementing with ozonated oils, allicin, houttuynia, essential oils, curcumin, B_{12}, D, probiotic, CLO, NT factor, trace minerals, CoQ10, zinc and iron.

FIRST TREATMENT PLAN

Patient was on a lot of good supportive supplements already. I wanted to support her detoxification further so I added the following:
- Liposomal glutathione – start with ¼ teaspoon in water first thing in the morning on an empty stomach (can eat/drink 10 minutes later). Work up to 1 teaspoon daily.
- Smilax – 30 drops twice daily in water.
- Detox Support Formula – 30 drops twice daily in water.
I also wanted to help her cognitive function and her energy levels, so I prescribed:
- Frankincense – 2 drops twice daily under the tongue.
- Energy Multiplex – 3 capsules in the morning.

This patient clearly had co-infections: *Bartonella*, based on severe anxiety, panic attacks, pain in the soles of the feet (a hallmark symptom) and a positive response to houttuynia; and *Babesia*, based on night sweats, air hunger, low-grade fevers, chills and tightness in the chest.

To try to get better discernment on these, I undertook a co-infection provocation in which I gave a herb that targets *Borrelia* for the first week, then added a herb that targets *Babesia* in the second week and a herb that targets *Bartonella* in the third week. This helped me to decipher what co-infection is playing what role based on symptom improvements and/or Herxheimer responses.

Provocation:
- Teasel root – 10 drops twice daily in water. Herb for *Borrelia*.
  Wait 1 week, then add:
- Artemisinin SOD – 2 twice daily. Herb for *Babesia*.
  Wait 1 week, then add:
- HH2 – 1 capsule three times daily. Herb for *Bartonella*.
  All other supplements were to remain the same so as not to create too many variables. Patient was to take notes on reactions and follow up with me in 6 weeks.

VISIT TWO, 3 MONTHS LATER

Patient reported results of the co-infection provocation:
- Teasel had given her a sore throat, headaches, fevers and night sweats, from which she would wake up feeling more well than the day before.
- Artemisinin gave her quite significant Herxing – severe anxiety, splitting headache, head pressure and dizziness,

but no sweats or fevers. That Herx was worse than any other she had experienced in treatment to date.

- HH2 gave some head pressure, anxiety and tightness in the chest.

Based on this provocation, it was clear that *Babesia* was playing a major role (provoked with the artemisinin). We added activated charcoal to help bind the toxins that had been released, and her Herxheimer reactions subsided.

Patient was also doing infrared sauna and Epsom salts baths to help with detoxification.

Concurrently, her primary care doctor gave her Nature Throid, based on blood work showing hypothyroidism, but the thyroid hormone made her sweat profusely, even at low doses, so she discontinued it.

Patient was instructed to continue on current herbal protocol and supplements, increase her detox modalities and return in 2 months. Coffee enemas were suggested, but patient was not sure if she was going to do them.

VISIT THREE, 2 MONTHS LATER

Patient was feeling much better and more stable, with fewer ups and downs of symptoms. Herxheimer reactions had subsided, she was tolerating treatment well and feeling improvement. She wanted to get more aggressive with herbal antimicrobials.

Herbal supplement plan:

- A-BAB – ½ drop twice daily. This is a combination formula from Byron White Herbs for *Babesia*.
- Artemisinin – 2 twice daily. For *Babesia*.
- Teasel root – had been at 5 drops twice daily. Advised that she could go up to 10 drops twice daily.
- Lyme Support Formula – 10 drops twice daily. Blend of samento, guaiacum, andrographis, olive leaf extract and Japanese knotweed.
- A-BART or houttuynia – 5 drops of each twice daily.
- Grapefruit seed extract – 2 capsules twice daily; for cyst forms of Lyme and anti-fungal.
- Anti-viral tincture – 40 drops twice daily (melissa and larrea). Patient had high titres of EBV and CMV on labwork.

For immune boosting:

- Transfer Factor Multi-immune – 2 at night.
- Lauricidin – 1 scoop daily.
- Low-dose naltrexone – 1.5 mg, working up to 4.5 mg. This is an immune modulator that also helps to boost endogenous endorphin production. It can help with mood, energy, sleep and pain.

VISIT FOUR, 2 MONTHS AFTER VISIT THREE

Low-dose naltrexone was helping her sleep, but she was still struggling a bit. She wakes feeling tired and often needs a nap mid-afternoon. She has added acupuncture to her plan and feels that is helping.

She also started coffee enemas, which help dramatically calm her anxiety and relieve cognitive issues.

Overall, patient is improving substantially – more good days now than bad, flu-like episodes resolved, body aches resolved and dizziness resolved.

Biggest issues now are sleep quality and daytime fatigue. Patient feels fatigue is secondary to insomnia, more than a Lyme symptom of its own, as her energy is much better following nights of good sleep.

Treatment plan focused on sleep:

- PheniTropic (Biotics) – 2 before bed. This is a GABA derivative that crosses the blood–brain barrier better than regular GABA and assists sleep.
- Serenity Restful Complex (doTERRA) – 2 before bed. This is a blend of lavender essential oil, L-theanine, passionflower, chamomile and lemon balm.

The only new thing added to her Lyme protocol was an enzyme to help break down biofilm to ensure that her antimicrobials were able to reach the pathogens:

- Boluoke (lumbrokinase) – 1 twice daily on an empty stomach (at least 1 hour apart from foods, meds and supplements).

Patient is feeling 80% improved by this stage. The focus is still on *Babesia* primarily, and *Borrelia/Bartonella* secondarily. Detoxification herbs and modalities were crucial in allowing her to tolerate quite an aggressive herbal antimicrobial protocol. Patient was highly self-motivated and was compliant with a gluten-free, sugar-free and dairy-free diet.

Treatment will continue for 2 months beyond resolution of her symptoms, at which time antimicrobials will be gradually discontinued and a maintenance plan will be designed to support immune function and detoxification long term. I also anticipate more adrenal support being included at our next visit.

REFERENCES

[1] Scott JD, Anderson JF, Durden LA, et al. Prevalence of the Lyme disease Spirochete, Borrelia burgdorferi, in blacklegged ticks, ixodes scapularis at Hamilton-Wentworth, Ontario. Int J Med Sci 2016;13(5):316–24. doi:10.7150/ijms.14552.

[2] Tawadros M. Borrelia burgdorferi. n.d. Available from http://web.uconn.edu/mcbstaff/graf/Student%20presentations/Bburgdorferi/bburgdorferi.html.

[3] Stricker R, Johnson L. Lyme disease: the next decade. Infect Drug Resist 2011;4:1–9. doi:10.2147/idr.s15653.

[4] Domingue G, Woody H. Bacterial persistence and expression of disease. Clin Microbiol Rev 1997;10:320–44.

[5] Dienes L, Weinberger H. The L forms of bacteria. Bacteriol Rev 1951;15:245–88.

[6] Sapi E, Bastian SL, Mpoy CM, et al. Characterization of Biofilm formation by Borrelia burgdorferi in vitro. PLoS ONE 2012;7(10):doi:10.1371/journal.pone.0048277. e48277.

[7] Stricker RB, Lautin A. The Lyme wars: time to listen. Expert Opin Investig Drugs 2003;12(10):1609–14. doi:10.1517/eoid.12.10.1609.21835.

[8] Gathany J. Erythema migrans – erythematous rash in Lyme disease. 2006. Available from https://en.wikipedia.org/wiki/Lyme_disease#/media/File:Erythema_migrans_-_erythematous_rash_in_Lyme_disease_-_PHIL_9875.jpg.

[9] Burrascano J. Advanced topics in Lyme disease: diagnostic hints and treatment guidelines for Lyme and other tick-borne illness. 2005. Available from International Lyme and Associated Diseases, http://www.ilads.org/files/burrascano_0905.pdf.

[10] Mayne P. Emerging incidence of Lyme borreliosis, babesiosis, bartonellosis, and granulocytic ehrlichiosis in Australia. Int J Gen Med 2011;4:845–52. doi:10.2147/ijgm.s27336.

[11] Brownstein JS, Holford TR, Fish D. A climate-based model predicts the spatial distribution of the Lyme disease vector Ixodes

scapularis in the United States. Environ Health Perspect 2003;111(9):1152–7. doi:10.1289/ehp.6052.

[12] International Lyme and Associated Diseases Society. Basic information about Lyme disease from ILADS. 2016. Available from http://www.ilads.org/lyme/about-lyme.php.

[13] International Lyme and Associated Diseases Society. Treatment guidelines for Lyme disease from ILADS. Evidence assessments and guideline recommendations in Lyme disease: the clinical management of known tick bites, erythema migrans rashes and persistent disease. 2016. Available from http://www.ilads.org/lyme/treatment-guideline.php#sthash.3BzAOGUa.dpuf.

[14] Centers for Disease Control and Prevention. Data and statistics. 2015. Available from http://www.cdc.gov/lyme/stats.

[15] Nelson CA, Saha S, Kugeler KJ, et al. Incidence of clinician-diagnosed Lyme disease, United States, 2005–2010. Emerg Infect Dis 2015;21(9):1625–31. doi:10.3201/eid2109.150417.

[16] Lindgren E, Jaenson T. Lyme borreliosis in Europe: influences of climate and climate change, epidemiology, ecology and adaptation measures. 2006. Available from WHO Regional Office for Europe, http://www.euro.who.int/__data/assets/pdf_file/0006/96819/e89522.pdf.

[17] European Centre for Disease Prevention and Control. Lyme Borreliosis in Europe. 2014. Available from http://ecdc.europa.eu/en/healthtopics/vectors/world-health-day-2014/documents/factsheet-lyme-borreliosis.pdf.

[18] Lyme Disease Association. Lyme in 80+ countries worldwide. 2013. Available from https://www.lymediseaseassociation.org/about-lyme/cases-stats-maps-a-graphs/940-lyme-in-more-than-80-countries-worldwide.

[19] Hudson B, Barry R, Shafren D, et al. Does Lyme borreliosis exist in Australia? Journal of Spirochetal and Tick Borne Diseases 1994;1(2):46–51.

[20] Luger S. Lyme disease transmitted by a biting fly. N Engl J Med 1990;322:1752.

[21] Herzer P, Wilske B, Preac-Mursic V, et al. Lyme arthritis: clinical features, serological, and radiographic findings of cases in Germany. Klin Wochenschr 1986;64(5):206–15. doi:10.1007/bf01711648.

[22] Pokorný P. Incidence of the spirochete Borrelia burgdorferi in arthropods (Arthropoda) and antibodies in vertebrates (Vertebrata). Cesk Epidemiol Mikrobiol Imunol 1989;38(1):52–60.

[23] Hubálek Z, Halouzka J. Juřicová Z. Investigation of haematophagus arthropods for borreliae – summarized data, 1988–1996. Folia Parasitol (Praha) 1998;45:67–72.

[24] Magnarelli L, Anderson J. Tick and biting insects infected with the etiologic agent of Lyme disease, Borrelia burgdorferi. J Clin Microbiol 1988;26(8):1482.

[25] Zákovská A, Capková L, Sery O, et al. Isolation of Borrelia afzelii from overwintering Culex piniens biotype molestus mosquitoes. Ann Agric Environ Med 2006;13(2):345–8.

[26] Middelveen MJ, Burke J, Sapi E, et al. Culture and identification of Borrelia spirochetes in human vaginal and seminal secretions. F1000Res 2014;3:309. doi:10.12688/f1000research.5778.2.

[27] MacDonald A. Gestational Lyme Borreliosis: implications for the fetus. Rheum Dis Clin North Am 1989;15(4):657–77.

[28] Schlesinger P, Duray P, Burke B, et al. Maternal-fetal transmission of the Lyme disease spirochete, Borrelia burgdorferi. Ann Intern Med 1985;103(1):67–8.

[29] MacDonald A, Benach J, Burgdorfer W. Stillbirth following maternal Lyme disease. N Y State J Med 1987;87:615–16.

[30] Lakos A, Solymosi N. Maternal Lyme borreliosis and pregnancy outcome. Int J Infect Dis 2010;14(6):e494–8. doi:10.1016/j.ijid.2009.07.019.

[31] Schmidt B, Aberer E, Stockenhuber C, et al. Detection of Borrelia burgdorferi DNA by polymerase chain reaction in the urine and breast milk of patients with Lyme borreliosis. Diagn Microbiol Infect Dis 1995;21(3):121–8.

[32] CanLyme. Symptoms. n.d. Available from https://canlyme.com/lyme-basics/symptoms/.

[33] McFadzean N, Burrascano JJ. The beginner's guide to Lyme disease: diagnosis and treatment made simple. San Diego, CA: BioMed Publishing Group; 2012. p. 76–8.

[34] Aguero-Rosenfeld ME, Wang G, Schwartz I, et al. Diagnosis of Lyme borreliosis. Clin Microbiol Rev 2005;18(3):484–509. doi:10.1128/CMR.18.3.484-509.2005.

[35] Igenex.Com. Welcome to IGeneX, Inc. n.d. Available from http://search-id.com/d/igenex.com.

[36] Sapi E, Pabbati N, Datar A, et al. Improved culture conditions for the growth and detection of Borrelia from human serum. Int J Med Sci 2013;10(4):362–76. doi:10.7150/ijms.5698.

[37] Bakken L, Callister S, Wand P, et al. Interlaboratory comparison of test results for detection of Lyme disease by 516 participants in the Wisconsin State Laboratory of Hygiene/College of American Pathologist proficiency testing program. J Clin Microbiol 1997;35(3):537–43.

[38] Stricker RB, Johnson L. Let's tackle the testing. BMJ 2007;335(7628):1008. doi:10.1136/bmj.39394.676227.be.

[39] Donta ST. Late and chronic Lyme disease. Med Clin North Am 2002;86(2):341–9. doi:10.1016/s0025-7125(03)00090-7.

[40] Steere A. Lyme disease. N Engl J Med 2001;345:115–25.

[41] Rossler D, Eiffert H, Jauris-Heipke S, et al. Molecular and immunological characterization of the p83/100 protein of various Borrelia burgdorferi sensu lato strains. Med Microbiol Immunol 1995;184(1):23–32. doi:10.1007/bf00216786.

[42] ArminLabs GmbH. Elispot. 2014. Available from http://www.arminlabs.com/en/tests/elispot.

[43] Vidal V, Scragg IG, Cutler SJ, et al. Variable major lipoprotein is a principal TNF-inducing factor of louse-borne relapsing fever. Nat Med 1998;4(12):1416–20. doi:10.1038/4007.

[44] Kaplanski G, Granel B, Vaz T, et al. Jarisch-Herxheimer reaction complicating the treatment of chronic Q fever endocarditis: elevated TNFα and IL-6 serum levels. J Infect 1998;37(1):83–4. doi:10.1016/s0163-4453(98)91120-3.

[45] Burrascano J. Advanced topic in Lyme disease. Diagnostic hints and treatment guidelines for Lyme and other tick borne illnesses. 16th ed. 2008. Available from https://www.researchednutritionals.com/wp-content/uploads/2016/04/Burrascanos-Advanced-Topics-in-Lyme-Disease-_12_17_08.pdf.

[46] Wormser GP, Dattwyler RJ, Shapiro ED, et al. The clinical assessment, treatment, and prevention of Lyme disease, human granulocytic anaplasmosis, and Babesiosis: clinical practice guidelines by the infectious diseases society of America. Clin Infect Dis 2006;43(9):1089–134. doi:10.1086/508667.

[47] Strle F, Ružič E, Cimperman J. Erythema migrans: comparison of treatment with azithromycin, doxycycline and phenoxymethylpenicillin. J Antimicrob Chemother 1992;30(4):543–50. doi:10.1093/jac/30.4.543.

[48] Strle F, Cimperman J, Maraspin V, et al. Azithromycin versus doxycycline for treatment of erythema migrans: clinical and microbiological findings. Infection 1993;21(2):83–8. doi:10.1007/bf01710737.

[49] Weber K, Wilske B, Preac-Mursic V, et al. Azithromycin versus penicillin V for the treatment of early lyme borreliosis. Infection 1993;21(6):367–72. doi:10.1007/bf01728915.

[50] Barsic B, Maretic T, Majerus L, et al. Comparison of Azithromycin and Doxycycline in the treatment of Erythema migrans. Infection 2000;28(3):153–6. doi:10.1007/s150100050069.

[51] Horowitz R. Lyme disease & babesiosis: updates on diagnosis and treatment 2011. 2011. Available from http://www.ilads.org/media/videos/videos_horowitz.php.

[52] Tye-Din J. The problem of coeliac disease in Australia. Australian Coeliac 2013. Dec 2013. Available from http://search.informit.com.au/documentSummary;dn=792500089102977;res=IELHEA.

[53] Tjon JM-L, van Bergen J, Koning F. Celiac disease: how complicated can it get? Immunogenetics 2010;62(10):641–51. doi:10.1007/s00251-010-0465-9.

[54] Bressan P, Kramer P. Bread and other edible agents of mental disease. Front Hum Neurosci 2016;10:doi:10.3389/fnhum.2016.00130.

[55] Asmar RE, Panigrahi P, Bamford P, et al. Host-dependent zonulin secretion causes the impairment of the small intestine barrier function after bacterial exposure. Gastroenterology 2002;123(5):1607–15. doi:10.1053/gast.2002.36578.

[56] Pal S, Woodford K, Kukuljan S, et al. Milk intolerance, beta-casein and lactose. Nutrients 2015;7(9):7285–97. doi:10.3390/nu7095339.

[57] Calder PC. Omega-3 polyunsaturated fatty acids and inflammatory processes: nutrition or pharmacology? Br J Clin Pharmacol 2013;75(3):645–62. doi:10.1111/j.1365-2125.2012.04374.x.

[58] Caughey G, Mantzioris E, Gibson R, et al. The effect on human tumor necrosis factor alpha and interleukin 1 beta production of diets enriched in n-3 fatty acids from vegetable oil or fish oil. Am J Clin Nutr 1996;63:116–22.

[59] Jiang Y, Wu S-H, Shu X-O, et al. Cruciferous vegetable intake is inversely correlated with circulating levels of proinflammatory markers in women. J Acad Nutr Diet 2014;114(5):700–8.e2. doi:10.1016/j.jand.2013.12.019.

[60] Johnston C. Functional foods as modifiers of cardiovascular disease. Am J Lifestyle Med 2009;3(1 Suppl.):39S–43S. doi:10.1177/1559827609332320.

[61] Sanchez A, Reeser J, Lau H, et al. Role of sugars in human neutrophilic phagocytosis. Am J Clin Nutr 1973;26:1180–4.

[62] Ringsdorf WJ, Cheraskin E, Ramsay RJ. Sucrose, neutrophilic phagocytosis and resistance to disease. Dent Surv 1976;52(12): 46–8.

[63] Collin P, Salmi J, Hällström O, et al. Autoimmune thyroid disorders and coeliac disease. Eur J Endocrinol 1994;130:137–40.

[64] Valentino R, Savastano S, Maglio M, et al. Markers of potential coeliac disease in patients with Hashimoto's thyroiditis. Eur J Endocrinol 2002;146(4):479–83. doi:10.1530/eje.0.1460479.

[65] Cristea V, Crişan M. Lyme disease with magnesium deficiency. Magnes Res 2003;16(4):287–9.

[66] Javid A, Zlotnikov N, Pětrošová H, et al. Hyperglycemia impairs neutrophil-mediated bacterial clearance in mice infected with the Lyme disease pathogen. PLoS ONE 2016;11(6):e0158019.

[67] Halperin JJ. Chronic Lyme disease: misconceptions and challenges for patient management. Infect Drug Resist 2015;8:119–28.

[68] Arvikar SL, Crowley JT, Sulka KB, et al. Autoimmune arthritides, rheumatoid arthritis, psoriatic arthritis, or peripheral spondyloarthritis following Lyme disease. Arthritis Rheumatol 2017;69(1):194–202.

[69] Borchers AT, Keen CL, Huntley AC, et al. Lyme disease: a rigorous review of diagnostic criteria and treatment. J Autoimmun 2015;57:82–115.

[70] Goggin R, Jardeleza C, Wormald P-J, et al. Colloidal silver: a novel treatment for staphylococcus aureus biofilms? Int Forum Allergy Rhinol 2014;4(3):171–5. doi:10.1002/alr.21259.

[71] Borwick S. Colloidal silver and Lyme disease. 2016. Available from The Silver Edge, http://thesilveredge.com/colloidal-silver-and-lyme-disease.shtml#.WBjbS3eZNm8.

[72] Stopper H, Schinzel R, Sebekova K, et al. Genotoxicity of advanced glycation end products in mammalian cells. Cancer Lett 2003;190(2):151–6. doi:10.1016/s0304-3835(02)00626-2.

[73] Cooper E. New enzyme complex isolated from earthworms is potent fibrinolytic. ACAM Integrative Medicine Blog. 2009. Available from https://www.acam.org/blogpost/1092863/185721/New-Enzyme-Complex-Isolated-from-Earthworms-is-Potent-Fibrinolytic.

[74] Cooper EL, Hirabayashi K. Origin of innate immune responses: revelation of food and medicinal applications. J Tradit Complement Med 2013;3(4):204–12. doi:10.4103/2225-4110.119708.

[75] Zapotoczna M, McCarthy H, Rudkin JK, et al. An essential role for coagulase in Staphylococcus aureus biofilm development reveals new therapeutic possibilities for device-related infections. J Infect Dis 2015;212(12):1883–93. doi:10.1093/infdis/jiv319.

[76] Hsu R, Lee K, Wang J, et al. Amyloid-degrading ability of nattokinase from Bacillus subtilis natto. J Agric Food Chem 2009;57(2):503–8.

[77] Lawrence HS, Borkowsky W. Transfer factor – current status and future prospects. Biotherapy 1996;9(1–3):1–5. doi:10.1007/bf02628649.

[78] Akramiene D, Kondrotas A, Didziapetriene J, et al. Effects of beta-glucans on the immune system. Medicina (Kaunas) 2007;43(8):597–606.

[79] Chronic Lyme Disease. Beta glucan for treating Lyme disease. n.d. Available from http://www.chroniclymedisease.com.

[80] Hawley KL, Martín-Ruiz I, Iglesias-Pedraz JM, et al. CD14 targets complement receptor 3 to lipid rafts during phagocytosis of Borrelia burgdorferi. Int J Biol Sci 2013;9(8):803–10. doi:10.7150/ijbs.7136.

[81] Rodriguez NA, Miracle DJ, Meier PP. Sharing the science on human milk feedings with mothers of very-low-birth-weight infants. J Obstet Gynecol Neonatal Nurs 2005;34(1):109–19. doi:10.1177/0884217504272807.

[82] Buescher ES, McWilliams-Koeppen P. Soluble tumor necrosis factor-α (TNF-α) receptors in human colostrum and milk bind to TNF-α and neutralize TNF-α bioactivity. Pediatr Res 1998;44(1):37–42. doi:10.1203/00006450-199807000-00006.

[83] Cakebread JA, Humphrey R, Hodgkinson AJ. Immunoglobulin A in bovine milk: a potential functional food? J Agric Food Chem 2015;63(33):7311–16. doi:10.1021/acs.jafc.5b01836.

[84] Kowalska K, Milnerowicz H. The influence of age and gender on the pro/antioxidant status in young healthy people. Ann Clin Lab Sci 2016;46(5):480–8.

[85] Starks MA, Starks SL, Kingsley M, et al. The effects of phosphatidylserine on endocrine response to moderate intensity exercise. J Int Soc Sports Nutr 2008;5(1):11. doi:10.1186/1550-2783-5-11.

[86] Kailasapathy K, Chin J. Survival and therapeutic potential of probiotic organisms with reference to Lactobacillus acidophilus and Bifidobacterium spp. Immunol Cell Biol 2000;78(1):80–8. doi:10.1046/j.1440-1711.2000.00886.x.

[87] Cevikbas A, Yemni E, Ezzedenn FW, et al. Antitumoural antibacterial and antifungal activities of kefir and kefir grain. Phytother Res 1994;8(2):78–82. doi:10.1002/ptr.2650080205.

[88] Rodrigues KL, Carvalho JC, Schneedorf JM. Anti-inflammatory properties of kefir and its polysaccharide extract. Inflammopharmacology 2005;13(5–6):485–92. doi:10.1163/156856005774649395.

[89] Claustrat B, et al. The basic physiology and pathophysiology of melatonin. Sleep Med Rev 2005;9:11–24.

[90] Pandi-Perumal S, Trakht I, Srinivasan V, et al. Physiological effects of melatonin: role of melatonin receptors and signal transduction pathways. Prog Neurobiol 2008;85(3):335–53.

[91] Aranow C. Vitamin D and the immune system. J Investig Med 2011;59(6):881–6.

[92] Prietl B, Treiber G, Pieber TR, et al. Vitamin D and immune function. Nutrients 2013;5(7):2502–21. doi:10.3390/nu5072502.

[93] Shankar A, Prasad A. Zinc and immune function: the biological basis of altered resistance to infection. Am J Clin Nutr 1998;68(2):447S–63S.

[94] Epp L, Mravec B. Chronic polysystemic candidiasis as a possible contributor to onset of idiopathic Parkinson's disease. Bratisl Lek Listy 2006;107(6–7):227–30.

[95] Maruyama W, Naoi M. Cell death in Parkinson's disease. J Neurol 2002;249:183–9.

[96] Tsuboi KK, Thompson DJ, Rush EM, et al. Acetaldehyde-dependent changes in hemoglobin and oxygen affinity of human erythrocytes. Hemoglobin 1981;5(3):241–50. doi:10.3109/03630268108997548.

[97] Tuma DJ, Jennett RB, Sorrell MF. The interaction of acetaldehyde with tubulin. Ann N Y Acad Sci 1987;492(1):277–86. doi:10.1111/j.1749-6632.1987.tb48681.x.

[98] Truss C. Metabolic abnormalities in patients with chronic candidiasis: the acetaldehyde hypothesis. J Orthomolecular Psychiatry 1984;13(2):66–93.

[99] Schmitt W, et al. Molybdenum for Candida albicans patients and other problems. The Digest of Chiropractic Economics 1991;31(4):56–63.

[100] Mur E, Hartig F, Eibl G, et al. Randomized double blind trial of an extract from the pentacyclic alkaloid-chemotype of Uncaria tomentosa for the treatment of rheumatoid arthritis. J Rheumatol 2002;29(4):678–81.

[101] Sandoval M, Charbonnet RM, Okuhama NN, et al. Cat's claw inhibits TNF-α production and scavenges free radicals: role in cytoprotection. Free Radic Biol Med 2000;29(1):71–8. doi:10.1016/s0891-5849(00)00327-0.

[102] Lyme. Teasel root and Lyme disease treatment. 2011. Available from http://www.tiredoflyme.com/teasel-root.html/.

[103] Stawonogi W. Zależności w układzie żywiciel-ektopasożyt-patogen. Poland: Koliber; 2016. p. 207–15.

[104] Stevenson L, et al. Oxygen radical absorbance capacity (ORAC) report on olive leaf. Australia's olive leaf extracts. Lismore, NSW: Southern Cross University. 2005.

[105] Mohagheghi F, Bigdeli MR, Rasoulian B, et al. The neuroprotective effect of olive leaf extract is related to improved blood–brain barrier permeability and brain edema in rat with experimental focal cerebral ischemia. Phytomedicine 2011;18(2–3):170–5. doi:10.1016/j.phymed.2010.06.007.

[106] Lambert RJW, Skandamis PN, Coote PJ, et al. A study of the minimum inhibitory concentration and mode of action of oregano essential oil, thymol and carvacrol. J Appl Microbiol 2001;91(3):453–62. doi:10.1046/j.1365-2672.2001.01428.x.

[107] Bona E, Cantamessa S, Pavan M, et al. Sensitivity of Candida albicans to essential oils: are they an alternative to antifungal agents? J Appl Microbiol 2016;121(6):1530–45. doi:10.1111/jam.13282.

[108] Valcourt C, Saulnier P, Umerska A, et al. Synergistic interactions between doxycycline and terpenic components of essential oils encapsulated within lipid nanocapsules against gram negative bacteria. Int J Pharm 2016;498(1–2):23–31. doi:10.1016/j.ijpharm.2015.11.042.

[109] Scandorieiro S, de Camargo LC, Lancheros CAC, et al. Synergistic and additive effect of oregano essential oil and biological silver nanoparticles against multidrug-resistant bacterial strains. Front Microbiol 2016;7:doi:10.3389/fmicb.2016.00760.

[110] Georgetown University Medical Center. Oregano oil may protect against drug-resistant bacteria, Georgetown researcher finds. 2001. Available from Science Daily, https://www.sciencedaily.com/releases/2001/10/011011065609.htm.

[111] Heggers JP, Cottingham J, Gusman J, et al. The effectiveness of processed grapefruit-seed extract as an antibacterial agent: II. Mechanism of action and in vitro toxicity. J Altern Complement Med 2002;8(3):333–40. doi:10.1089/10755530260128023.

[112] Brorson Ø, Brorson S. Grapefruit seed extract is a powerful in vitro agent against motile and cystic forms of Borrelia burgdorferi sensu lato. Infection 2007;35(3):206–8. doi:10.1007/s15010-007-6105-0.

[113] Brown GD. The biosynthesis of artemisinin (Qinghaosu) and the phytochemistry of artemisia annua L. (Qinghao). Molecules 2010;15(11):7603–98. doi:10.3390/molecules15117603.

[114] Li J, Zhou B. Biological actions of Artemisinin: insights from medicinal chemistry studies. Molecules 2010;15(3):1378–97. doi:10.3390/molecules15031378.

[115] Kim W-S, Choi WJ, Lee S, et al. Anti-inflammatory, antioxidant and antimicrobial effects of artemisinin extracts from Artemisia annua L. Korean J Physiol Pharmacol 2014;19(1):21. doi:10.4196/kjpp.2015.19.1.21.

[116] Sawer IK, Berry MI, Ford JL. The killing effect of cryptolepine on Staphylococcus aureus. Lett Appl Microbiol 2005;40(1):24–9. doi:10.1111/j.1472-765x.2004.01625.x.

[117] Mills-Robertson FC, Tay SCK, Duker-Eshun G, et al. In vitro antimicrobial activity of ethanolic fractions of Cryptolepis sanguinolenta. Ann Clin Microbiol Antimicrob 2012;11(1):16. doi:10.1186/1476-0711-11-16.

[118] Hanprasertpong N, Teekachunhatean S, Chaiwongsa R, et al. Analgesic, anti-inflammatory, and chondroprotective activities of Cryptolepis buchanani extract: in vitro and in vivo studies. Biomed Res Int 2014;2014:1–8. doi:10.1155/2014/978582.

[119] Sekita Y, Murakami K, Yumoto H, et al. Anti-bacterial and anti-inflammatory effects of ethanol extract from Houttuynia cordata poultice. Biosci Biotechnol Biochem 2016;80(6):1205–13. doi:10.1080/09168451.2016.1151339.

[120] Sekita Y, Murakami K, Yumoto H, et al. Preventive effects of Houttuynia cordata extract for oral infectious diseases. Biomed Res Int 2016;2016:doi:10.1155/2016/2581876.

[121] Buhner S. Healing Lyme – natural healing of Lyme borelliosis and the coinfections Chlamydia and spotted fever rickettsioses. 2nd ed. US: Raven Press; 2016.

[122] Rai B, Jasdeep K, Reinhilde J, et al. Curcumin exhibits anti-pre-cancer activity by increasing levels of vitamin C and E, and preventing lipid peroxidation and oxidative damage. J Oral Sci 2010;52(2).

[123] Hucklenbroich J, Klein R, Neumaier B, et al. Aromatic-turmerone induces neural stem cell proliferation in vitro and in vivo. Stem Cell Res Ther 2014;5(4):100. doi:10.1186/scrt500.

[124] Sharma S, Kulkarni SK, Agrewala JN, et al. Curcumin attenuates thermal hyperalgesia in a diabetic mouse model of neuropathic pain. Eur J Pharmacol 2006;536(3):256–61. doi:10.1016/j.ejphar.2006.03.006.

[125] Appleton J. Turmeric and frankincense in inflammation: an update. Natural Medicine Journal 2013;3(9).

[126] Safayhi H, Rall B, Sailer E, et al. Inhibition by boswellic acids of human leukocyte elastase. J Pharmacol Exp Ther 1997;281(1):460–3.

[127] Roy S, Khanna S, Shah H, et al. Human genome screen to identify the genetic basis of the anti-inflammatory effects of Boswellia in microvascular endothelial cells. DNA Cell Biol 2005;24(4):244–55. doi:10.1089/dna.2005.24.244.

[128] Roy S, Khanna S, Krishnaraju AV, et al. Regulation of vascular responses to inflammation: inducible matrix metalloproteinase-3 expression in human microvascular endothelial cells is sensitive to antiinflammatory boswellia. Antioxid Redox Signal 2006;8(3–4):653–60. doi:10.1089/ars.2006.8.653.

[129] Zhang H, Li C, Kwok S-T, et al. A review of the pharmacological effects of the dried root of Polygonum cuspidatum (Hu Zhang) and its constituents. Evid Based Complement Alternat Med 2013;2013.

[130] Pandit S, Kim HJ, Park SH, et al. Enhancement of fluoride activity against Streptococcus mutans biofilms by a substance separated from Polygonum cuspidatum. Biofouling 2012;28(3):279–87.

[131] Han JH, Koh W, Lee HJ, et al. Analgesic and anti-inflammatory effects of ethyl acetate fraction of Polygonum cuspidatum in experimental animals. Immunopharmacol Immunotoxicol 2012;34(2):191–5.

[132] Li HL, Chen HL, Li H, et al. Regulatory effects of emodin on NF-κB activation and inflammatory cytokine expression in RAW 264.7 macrophages. Int J Mol Med 2005;16(1):41–7.

[133] Deng WL. Preliminary studies on the pharmacology of the Andrographis product dihydroandrographolide sodium succinate. Newslett Clin Herb Med 1978;8:26–8.

[134] Singh PK, Roy S, Dey S. Antimicrobial activity of andrographis paniculata. Fitoterapia 2003;74:692–4.

[135] Chandrasekaran CV, Gupta A, Agarwal A. Effect of an extract of Andrographis paniculata leaves on inflammatory and allergic mediators in vitro. J Ethnopharmacol 2010;129:203–7.

[136] Parichatikanond W, Suthisisang C, Dhepakson P, et al. Study of anti-inflammatory activities of the pure compounds from Andrographis paniculata (Burm.f.) Nees and their effects on gene expression. Int Immunopharmacol 2010;10:1361–73.

[137] Yang A-J, Li C-C, Lu C-Y, et al. Activation of the cAMP/CREB/inducible cAMP early repressor pathway suppresses andrographolide-induced gene expression of the π class of glutathione S-transferase in rat primary hepatocytes. J Agric Food Chem 2010;58(93):1993–2000.

[138] Chuan-li L, Wei Z, Min W, et al. Polysaccharides from Smilax glabra inhibit the pro-inflammatory mediators via ERK1/2 and JNK pathways in LPS-induced RAW264.7 cells. Carbohydr Polym 2015;122:428–36. doi:10.1016/j.carbpol.2014.11.035.

[139] Shu X-S, Gao Z-H, Yang X-L. Anti-inflammatory and anti-nociceptive activities of Smilax china L. Aqueous extract. J Ethnopharmacol 2006;103(3):327–32. doi:10.1016/j.jep.2005.08.004.

[140] Xia D, Yu X, Liao S, et al. Protective effect of Smilax glabra extract against lead-induced oxidative stress in rats. J Ethnopharmacol 2010;130(2):414–20. doi:10.1016/j.jep.2010.05.025.

[141] Butterweck V. Mechanism of action of St John's wort in depression: what is known? CNS Drugs 2003;17(8):539–62.

[142] Klusa V, Germane S, Nöldner M, et al. Hypericum extract and hyperforin: memory-enhancing properties in rodents. Pharmacopsychiatry 2001;34(Suppl. 1):61–9. doi:10.1055/s-2001-15451.

[143] Bent S, Padula A, Moore D, et al. Valerian for sleep: a systematic review and meta-analysis. Am J Med 2006;119(12):1005–12. doi:10.1016/j.amjmed.2006.02.026.

[144] White SM. Herbs and supplements for memory and cognitive support during lyme treatment. ProHealth. 2016. Available from https://www.prohealth.com/library/herbs-and-supplements-for-memory-and-cognitive-support-during-lyme-treatment-7197.

[145] Lai P-L, et al. Neurotrophic properties of the Lion's mane medicinal mushroom, Hericium erinaceus (higher basidiomycetes) from Malaysia. Int J Med Mushrooms 2013;15(6).

[146] Burke V. Lion's mane mushroom – unparalleled benefits for your brain and nervous system. GreenMedInfo. 2016. Available from

https://rcf.fr/sites/default/static.rcf.fr/le_champignon_qui_protege_le_cerveau.pdf.

[147] Hinz M, Stein A. 5-HTP efficacy and contraindications. Neuropsychiatr Dis Treat 2012;8:323–8. doi:10.2147/ndt .s33259.

[148] De Giorgis G, Miletto R, Iannuccelli M, et al. Headache in association with sleep disorders in children: a psychodiagnostic evaluation and controlled clinical study–L-5-HTP versus placebo. Drugs Exp Clin Res 1987;13:425–33.

[149] Puttini P, Caruso I. Primary fibromyalgia syndrome and 5-hydroxy-L-tryptophan: a 90-day open study. J Int Med Res 1992;20:182–9.

[150] Yasko DA. Autism: pathways to recovery. 2004. Bethel, ME: Neurological Research Institute, LLC.

[151] Yasko DA. Autism: pathways to recovery. 2007. Bethel, ME: Neurological Research Institute, LLC.

[152] Yasko DA. Autism: pathways to recovery. 2009. Bethel, ME: Neurological Research Institute, LLC.

[153] Juneja LR, Chu D-C, Okubo T, et al. L-theanine – a unique amino acid of green tea and its relaxation effect in humans. Trends Food Sci Technol 1999;10(s 6–7):199–204. doi:10.1016/S0924-2244(99)00044-8.

[154] Fernstrom J. Can nutrient supplements modify brain function? Am J Clin Nutr 2000;71(6 Suppl.):1669S–75S.

Index

Interactions table

HERB/NUTRIENT–DRUG INTERACTIONS TABLES

Compiled by Liesl Blott

Potential herb–drug and nutrient–drug interactions are described in the following tables. These tables have been formulated to include information on interactions between herbal medicines, nutrients/nutritional medicines and drugs. They include a summary of the potential outcome, a graded recommendation and a comments section that explains the nature of each interaction in more detail.

The recommendations are broadly divided into four categories: avoid, caution, monitor and beneficial. Factors that were taken into account when determining these interaction categories include currently available evidence and safety data; potential severity and clinical consequences; the likelihood of an interaction; whether the interaction is based on clinical studies or extrapolated from case studies, laboratory or animal studies; and commonly applied integrative prescribing principles. However, new safety data and evidence are constantly emerging, and best practice regarding some of these interactions may change with time.

The tables do not include information on possible contraindications, for example use in pregnancy, nor do they include herb–herb, herb–nutrient or nutrient–nutrient interactions.

Practitioners are encouraged to use the interactions tables as a guide, but to apply professional judgment on the appropriateness of use of a combination of herb–drug or nutrient–drug for each individual patient. It is imperative that health practitioners investigate whether there are any known safety concerns or interactions when prescribing herbal or nutritional medicines for patients already taking pharmaceutical medicines.

Health practitioners of all disciplines are encouraged to make use of available resources to allow for informed decisions, so as to optimise patient wellbeing without compromising patient safety. When recommending complementary medicines in combination with pharmaceutical medicines, both anticipated benefits and potential risks should be taken into consideration.

ACNM herbal interactions table				
Herbal medicine	**Drug/drug class**	**Potential outcome**	**Recommendations**	**Comments**
Achillea millefolium	Acid-reducing drugs (antacids, H_2 antagonists, proton pump inhibitors)	Theoretical decreased drug effect	Monitor – may not be clinically significant	Yarrow may increase gastric acidity. Use may theoretically antagonise drug action, resulting in decreased drug effect.
	Anticoagulant/ antiplatelet drugs	Theoretical increased risk of bleeding	Caution with use of this combination	Yarrow may have antiplatelet properties. Combined use with anticoagulant and antiplatelet drugs will theoretically increase the risk of bleeding and bruising.
	Barbiturates e.g. phenobarbital	Theoretical increased sedation	Caution with use of this combination	Yarrow may theoretically prolong barbiturate-induced sleep time.
	Lithium	Theoretical increased risk of drug toxicity	Caution with use of this combination	Yarrow may have diuretic properties. Combined use may theoretically precipitate lithium toxicity.

LEGEND

■ Combination okay to use
■ Use of combination should be monitored
■ Use combination with caution
■ Avoid combination

Continued

ACNM herbal interactions table—cont'd				
Herbal medicine	**Drug/drug class**	**Potential outcome**	**Recommendations**	**Comments**
Actaea racemosa	Androgen blockade chemotherapies	Theoretical decreased drug adverse effects	May be beneficial – medical supervision recommended	Androgen deprivation in prostate cancer patients can result in hot flushes and decreased libido. Black cohosh may theoretically reduce vasomotor symptoms in patients taking drugs that reduce androgen levels. Benefits are speculative and more data is required.
	Cisplatin	Possible reduced drug effects	Avoid combination	Preliminary evidence suggests that black cohosh may decrease the cytotoxic effects of cisplatin on breast cells. Avoid combination until further data becomes available.
	Chemotherapy drugs	Variable effects possible	Avoid combination	Variable effects have been reported with concomitant use of black cohosh and chemotherapeutic agents. Some studies have shown a decreased effect and others an increased drug action and risk of toxicity, depending on the agent. Concomitant use should be avoided unless under strict medical supervision.
	CYP2D6 substrates	Theoretical increased drug levels	Caution with use of this combination	Limited evidence suggests black cohosh may modestly inhibit CYP2D6. Theoretically, this can result in increased drug levels and risk of toxicity of drugs metabolised by this enzyme.
	Hepatotoxic drugs	Possible increased risk of liver toxicity	Caution with use of this combination	The risk of liver damage may be increased with concomitant use of black cohosh and hepatotoxic drugs.
	HMGCoA reductase inhibitors (statins)	Possible increased risk of liver toxicity	Caution with use of this combination	One case report describes a patient who was taking atorvastatin who developed significantly raised liver enzymes after commencement of black cohosh. It is unclear if this was due to the drug, the herb or the combination.
	Hormone replacement therapy (HRT)	Possible additive effects	Combination may be beneficial	Black cohosh may theoretically provide additive benefits for the reduction of menopause symptoms such as hot flushes and night sweats when used with HRT. Theoretically, concomitant use may allow for lower HRT doses. Direct research investigating the safety and efficacy of combined use is lacking.
	Tamoxifen	Possible reduction of hot flushes	Caution with use of this combination	Some studies suggest that black cohosh may help to treat hot flushes in women with a history of breast cancer and taking tamoxifen. Appropriateness of use is, however, the subject of debate as the oestrogenic effects of black cohosh may also potentially have negative consequences. Medical supervision is recommended.

ACNM herbal interactions table—cont'd				
Herbal medicine	**Drug/drug class**	**Potential outcome**	**Recommendations**	**Comments**
Aesculus hippocastanum	Anticoagulant/ antiplatelet drugs	Theoretical increased risk of bleeding	Caution with use of this combination	Horse chestnut may have antiplatelet properties. Concomitant use with anticoagulant or antiplatelet drugs will theoretically increase the risk of bleeding.
	Antidiabetic drugs	Possible additive effects possible	Caution with use of this combination	Horse chestnut may lower blood glucose levels. Additive effects are theoretically possible, increasing the risk of hypoglycaemia. Caution is advised until more data becomes available.
	Lithium	Increased risk of drug toxicity	Caution with use of this combination	Horse chestnut may have diuretic properties. Combined use may theoretically precipitate lithium toxicity. The combination should be used with caution or avoided.
Agaricus blazei	Antidiabetic drugs	Possible additive effects	Caution with use of this combination	Clinical research suggests agaricus mushrooms may lower blood glucose levels by decreasing insulin resistance in type 2 diabetics. Additive effects are theoretically possible, which increases the risk of hypoglycaemia.
Agrimonia eupatoria	Antidiabetic drugs	Theoretical additive effects	Caution with use of this combination	Agrimony may theoretically lower blood glucose levels, based on one animal study. Findings are inconclusive.
Albizia lebbeck	Antidepressant drugs (SSRIs, SNRIs)	Theoretical risk of serotonin syndrome	Monitor – may not be clinically significant	Albizia may theoretically increase serotonin levels based on animal studies. Patients should be monitored but this effect has not yet been demonstrated in humans.
	Antihistamines	Theoretical additive effects	Combination may be beneficial – monitor	Additive, beneficial effects are theoretically possible as albizia inhibits early processes of allergy sensitisation and may reduce allergic response.
	CNS depressant drugs including barbiturates	Theoretical increased risk of sedatin	Monitor – may not be clinically significant	Albizia may theoretically enhance drug sedative adverse effects. Animal studies suggest that albizia may potentiate phenobarbital-induced sleep time.
Alchemilla vulgaris	Oral drugs	Theoretical decreased drug absorption	Monitor – may not be clinically significant	The high tannin content of Lady's mantle may theoretically impair absorption of some drugs due to precipitation interactions. Significance is unknown, but dosage separation is advised.
Aletris farinosa	Acid-reducing drugs (antacids, H_2 antagonists, proton pump inhibitors)	Theoretical decreased drug effect	Monitor – may not be clinically significant	True unicorn root may increase gastric acidity. Use may theoretically counteract drug action, resulting in decreased drug effect.
	Oestrogens	Theoretical altered drug effect	Monitor – may not be clinically significant	True unicorn root may have oestrogenic activity and so may theoretically interfere with the effects of hormone replacement therapy (HRT) or oral contraceptives due to competition for oestrogen receptors. Evidence of this interaction is lacking. Women with hormone sensitive conditions should avoid this herb.

Continued

ACNM herbal interactions table—cont'd				
Herbal medicine	Drug/drug class	Potential outcome	Recommendations	Comments
Allium cepa	Anticoagulant/ antiplatelet drugs	Theoretical increased risk of bleeding	Caution with use of this combination	Limited data suggests onion may have antiplatelet activity at high doses. There is a theoretical interaction with anticoagulant and antiplatelet drugs, increasing the risk of bleeding.
	Antidiabetic drugs	Possible additive effects possible	Caution with use of this combination	Onion may lower blood glucose levels. Additive effects are theoretically possible, increasing the risk of hypoglycaemia. Caution is advised until more data becomes available.
	CYP450 substrates (CYP2E1)	Theoretical risk of increased drug levels	Monitor – may not be clinically significant	Animal research suggests that onion powder may inhibit CYP2E1. This may theoretically increase drug levels of agents metabolised by this enzyme; however, this has not yet been demonstrated in humans.
	Lithium	Increased risk of drug toxicity	Caution with use of this combination	Onion may have diuretic properties. Combined use may theoretically precipitate lithium toxicity. The combination should be used with caution.
Allium sativum	Anticoagulant/ antiplatelet drugs	Theoretical increased risk of bleeding	Caution with use of this combination	Garlic has antiplatelet activity and may theoretically interact with anticoagulant and antiplatelet drugs. Clinical studies have not reported changes to the pharmacokinetics or pharmacodynamics of warfarin, nor an increased incidence of adverse effects. Caution is advised, however, with doses >7g/day of garlic. Normal therapeutic doses appear safe.
	Antihypertensive drugs	Theoretical additive effects	Combination may be beneficial – monitor	Garlic may have a small effect in lowering blood pressure, so additive effects are theoretically possible. The interaction may be beneficial but patients should be monitored for hypotension.
	Anti-retroviral drugs – protease inhibitors (e.g. saquinavir)	Possible decreased drug effect	Avoid combination	Garlic extract has been shown to significantly reduce blood concentrations of saquinavir, potentially reducing drug effectiveness in the management of HIV. High-dose garlic supplements should be avoided with saquinavir. A study with ritonavir showed only a small non-statistically significant change in drug concentration, but caution is advised with use of supplemental garlic and all drugs in this class until more data becomes available. The effect of dietary garlic is unknown.
	CYP450 substrates (CYP2E1)	Theoretical increased risk of drug toxicity	Caution with use of this combination	Preliminary evidence suggests garlic oil may inhibit the activity of CYP2E1 by 39%. Theoretically, this may increase the risk of toxicity of drugs metabolised by this enzyme.

ACNM herbal interactions table—cont'd				
Herbal medicine	**Drug/drug class**	**Potential outcome**	**Recommendations**	**Comments**
Allium sativum cont'd	CYP450 substrates (CYP3A4)	Theoretical decreased drug effectiveness	Caution with use of this combination	Preliminary evidence suggests garlic may induce the activity of CYP3A4, although results from different studies have been mixed. Caution is advised due to a theoretical risk of decreased drug effectiveness with concurrent use of garlic and drugs metabolised by this enzyme.
	Isoniazid	Theoretical decreased drug effect	Avoid combination	Animal studies report that garlic can significantly reduce isoniazid plasma concentrations. The combination should be avoided until further data becomes available.
	Lipid-lowering agents e.g. statins	Theoretical additive effects	Combination may be beneficial – monitor	Garlic is reported to lower cholesterol and a study suggests it may potentiate the effects of lipid-lowering drugs. The combination appears well tolerated and may be beneficial.
Aloe barbadencis	Antidiabetic drugs	Theoretically additive effects	Caution with use of this combination	Some clinical research has reported that oral aloe vera may lower blood glucose levels in patients with type 2 diabetes, although other studies have reported no effect. Concomitant use may theoretically be additive and beneficial, but caution is advised due to a risk of hypoglycaemia.
	Cancer therapy (chemotherapy or radiotherapy)	Possible improved response; possible reduced drug adverse effects	May be beneficial – medical supervision recommended	Results of a clinical study suggest that the addition of aloe vera to chemotherapy in patients with advanced cancer may lead to improved survival and reduced tumour progression, compared to placebo. More research is needed, but the combination may be beneficial under medical supervision. Topical aloe vera may also reduce inflammation of the oral mucosa caused by chemotherapeutic agents or radiation therapy.
	Corticosteroids – topical	Theoretical improved drug effect	Combination may be beneficial	An animal study conducted on rodent paws reported that the addition of topical aloe vera to topical hydrocortisone was more effective in reducing inflammation and oedema than topical hydrocortisone alone. Theoretically, combined use may be beneficial; however, the effect has not been demonstrated in clinical trials.
	Digoxin	Theoretical increased risk of adverse effects	Avoid combination	Long-term excessive use of oral aloe vera may theoretically lead to loss of potassium, which potentially increases the risk of drug toxicity.
	Diuretics	Theoretical increased risk of adverse effects	Caution with use of this combination	Oral aloe vera has a laxative effect. Excessive use may lead to loss of potassium, which increases the risk of hypokalaemia when used with potassium-depleting diuretics such as thiazide and loop diuretics.

Continued

ACNM herbal interactions table—cont'd				
Herbal medicine	**Drug/drug class**	**Potential outcome**	**Recommendations**	**Comments**
Aloe barbadencis cont'd	Laxatives	Additive effects with increased risk of adverse effects	Caution with use of this combination	The combination of oral aloe vera and stimulant laxatives may increase the risk of fluid and electrolyte loss.
	Sevoflurane	Theoretical increased risk of bleeding	Caution with use of this combination	A case report describes excessive intraoperative blood loss in a patient who was administered sevoflurane for anaesthesia and had taken high-dose oral aloe vera prior to surgery. While it was proposed that aloe vera may have enhanced drug antiplatelet effects, evidence is inconclusive.
Althaea officinalis	Antidiabetic drugs	Theoretical additive effects	Caution with use of this combination	Marshmallow may theoretically have hypoglycaemic effects. Concomitant use may theoretically be additive and beneficial, but caution is advised due to a risk of hypoglycaemia.
	Lithium	Theoretical increased risk of drug toxicity	Caution with use of this combination	Marshmallow may have diuretic properties. Theoretically, combined use may reduce lithium excretion and increase the risk of lithium toxicity.
	Oral drugs	Theoretical impaired drug absorption	Caution with use of this combination	The mucilage in marshmallow may theoretically impair absorption of some drugs.
Ammi visnaga	Digoxin	Theoretical decreased drug effect	Caution with use of this combination	In vitro and in vivo evidence suggests that a constituent of this herb, Visnadine (visnadin) may have negative inotropic effects. This may theoretically oppose drug action. Significance is unknown, but caution is advised.
	Hepatotoxic drugs	Theoretical additive effects	Monitor – may not be clinically significant	A constituent of this herb may increase liver transaminases. Theoretically, concomitant use with hepatotoxic drugs will increase the risk of liver damage.
	Photosensitising drugs	Theoretical increased risk of photosensitivity	Monitor – may not be clinically significant	This herb may cause photosensitivity. Additive adverse effects are theoretically possible.
Andrographis paniculata	5-aminosalicylates (e.g. mesalazine, sulphasalzine)	Possible additive effects possible	Combination may be beneficial – medical supervision recommended	The combination may lead to improved clinical response and mucosal healing, based on limited research in patients with ulcerative colitis. Caution is advised until more long-term safety data becomes available.
	Anticoagulant/ antiplatelet drugs	Theoretical increased risk of bleeding	Caution with use of this combination	Andrographis has antiplatelet activity. Concomitant use with anticoagulant or antiplatelet drugs will theoretically increase the risk of bleeding and bruising.
	Anti-rheumatoid arthritis agents (e.g. prednisone, methotrexate)	Possible additive effects possible	May be beneficial – medical supervision recommended	Andrographis has been shown to reduce pain, swelling and inflammation associated with rheumatoid arthritis in a small study. The combination may be additive and beneficial, but caution is advised until more safety data becomes available.
	Immunosuppressant drugs	Theoretical risk of decreased drug effect	Caution with use of this combination	Andrographis has immunomodulatory activity which may theoretically counteract drug immunosuppressant effects.

ACNM herbal interactions table—cont'd				
Herbal medicine	Drug/drug class	Potential outcome	Recommendations	Comments
Anethum graveolens	Antidiabetic drugs	Possible additive effects	Caution with use of this combination	Dill may theoretically lower blood glucose levels, based on animal studies. Concomitant use may theoretically be additive and beneficial, but caution is advised due to a risk of hypoglycaemia.
	Lithium	Increased risk of drug toxicity	Caution with use of this combination	Dill may have diuretic properties. Theoretically, combined use may reduce lithium excretion and increase the risk of lithium toxicity.
Angelica sinensis/ polymorpha	Anticoagulant/ antiplatelet drugs	Theoretical increased risk of bleeding	Caution with use of this combination	Dong quai may have antiplatelet activity based on limited data. Concomitant use with anticoagulant and antiplatelet drugs will theoretically increase the risk of bleeding and bruising. A case report describes a woman who was taking warfarin and experienced fluctuations in INR when she started taking dong quai.
	Oestrogens	Theoretical altered drug effect	Caution with use of this combination	Dong quai may have oestrogenic activity. Theoretically, this herb may interfere with the effects of hormone replacement therapy (HRT) due to competition for oestrogen receptors. Evidence of this interaction is lacking.
Apium graveolens	Antidepressant drugs e.g. venlafaxine	Theoretical increased risk of adverse effects	Avoid combination	A case report describes an interaction between celery root extract, St John's wort and venlafaxine, which led to mania and hallucinations.
	Anticoagulant/ antiplatelet drugs	Theoretical increased risk of bleeding	Caution with use of this combination	In vitro research has reported that two of the constituents found in celery have antiplatelet activity. Concomitant use with anticoagulant and antiplatelet drugs theoretically increases the risk of bleeding and bruising.
	Antihypertensive drugs	Additive effects theoretically possible	Caution with use of this combination	Anecdotal evidence suggests that celery may lower blood pressure. Concomitant use may be additive, with a theoretical risk of hypotension. Clinical significance is unclear.
	CYP450 substrates (CYP1A2)	Theoretical increased drug effect	Caution with use of this combination	In vitro and animal research suggest celery may inhibit CYP1A2. Theoretically, concomitant use with drugs that are CYP1A2 substrates may result in increased drug effects and risk of adverse effect.
	L-Thyroxine (Levothyroxine)	Theoretical decrease in drug effect	Caution with use of this combination	Case reports suggest that celery seed tablets may interact with thyroxine, leading to reduced drug effect. Caution is advised until more data becomes available.
	Lithium	Increased risk of drug toxicity	Caution with use of this combination	Celery may have diuretic properties. Theoretically, combined use may reduce lithium excretion and increase the risk of lithium toxicity.

Continued

ACNM herbal interactions table—cont'd				
Herbal medicine	**Drug/drug class**	**Potential outcome**	**Recommendations**	**Comments**
Apium graveolens cont'd	Paracetamol	Theoretical increased drug effect	Monitor – may not be clinically significant	Animal research suggests celery juice may prolong the effects of paracetamol. It has been proposed that this is due to the inhibition of CYP450 enzyme activity.
	PUVA therapy	Increased risk of phototoxicity	Caution with use of this combination	Celery may increase the risk of phototoxicity when used with PUVA therapy according to limited data.
Armoracia rustica	L-thyroxine (Levothyroxine)	Theoretical decreased drug effect	Monitor – may not be clinically significant	Theoretically, horseradish may exacerbate hypothyroidism or interfere with drug action. Clinical significance is unknown, but patients should be monitored.
Arctium lappa	Anticoagulant/ antiplatelet drugs	Theoretical increased risk of bleeding	Caution with use of this combination	Burdock may have antiplatelet properties. Concomitant use with anticoagulant and antiplatelet drugs will theoretically increase the risk of bleeding and bruising.
	Antidiabetic drugs	Theoretical additive effects	Caution with use of this combination	Burdock may theoretically lower blood glucose levels, based on animal studies. Findings are inconclusive, but caution is advised due to a risk of hypoglycaemia.
Arctostaphylos uva-ursi	Lithium	Increased risk of drug toxicity	Caution with use of this combination	This herb may have diuretic properties. Theoretically, combined use may reduce lithium excretion and increase the risk of lithium toxicity. A case report describes an interaction between lithium and a herbal combination that included bearberry, that led to drug toxicity.
Artemesia annua	CYP450 substrates (CYP2B6, CYP3A4)	Theoretical decreased drug effects	Monitor – clinical significance unknown	In vitro evidence suggests this herb may induce CYP2B6 and CYP3A4 activity. Theoretically, this may result in increased metabolism and decreased therapeutic effects of drugs that are CYP2B6 or CYP3A4 substrates.
Artemisia herba-alba	Antidiabetic drugs	Theoretical additive effects	Caution with use of this combination	Artemisia may theoretically lower blood glucose levels, based on animal studies. Findings are inconclusive, but caution is advised due to a theoretical risk of hypoglycaemia.
Asparagus racemosus	Lithium	Increased risk of drug toxicity	Caution with use of this combination	Shatavari may have diuretic properties. Theoretically, combined use may reduce lithium excretion and increase the risk of lithium toxicity.
	Metoclopramide	Possible additive effects	Caution with use of this combination	Limited evidence suggests that shatavari may help to promote lactation. Additive effects are theoretically possible when used concomitantly with metoclopramide, a drug sometimes prescribed to promote lactation. There is currently insufficient clear data on the effectiveness or safety of this combination and caution is advised.

ACNM herbal interactions table—cont'd				
Herbal medicine	**Drug/drug class**	**Potential outcome**	**Recommendations**	**Comments**
Astragalus membranaceus	Chemotherapeutic agents (e.g. cyclophosphamide, cisplatin)	Interaction may be beneficial – herb may improve patient QoL measures	May be beneficial – medical supervision recommended	Limited research suggests that astragalus may improve quality of life and patient wellbeing while reducing drug-related adverse effects such as fatigue, nausea and vomiting, pain and loss of appetite. Further study is needed to confirm results, but adjunctive use of astragalus may be beneficial.
	Immunosuppressant drugs	Theoretical decreased drug effect	Caution with use of this combination	Astragalus has immuno-stimulant activity which may theoretically counteract drug immunosuppressant effects. Clinical significance is unclear, but caution is advised.
	Interferon alpha (IFN-α)	Theoretical additive or synergistic effect	May be beneficial – medical supervision recommended	Astragalus may increase endogenous interferon production by leukocytes, based on limited data. Theoretically, concomitant use with therapeutic interferon-alpha may have additive beneficial effects. Data is limited and medical supervision is strongly recommended.
	Lithium	Increased risk of drug toxicity	Caution with use of this combination	Astragalus may have diuretic properties. Theoretically, combined use may reduce lithium excretion and increase the risk of lithium toxicity.
Avena sativa	Antihypertensive drugs	Additive effects possible	Combination may be beneficial	Beta-glucan, found in oats, has been shown to reduce blood pressure, particularly in obese individuals with hypertension. Concurrent use may be additive and potentially beneficial, but monitor for hypotension.
	Immunosuppressant drugs	Theoretical risk of decreased drug effect	Caution with use of this combination	Beta-glucan, found in oats, may have immune-stimulant effects. Theoretically, this may counteract drug immunosuppressant action; however, clinical significance is unclear.
	Lipid-lowering drugs	Additive effects possible	Combination may be beneficial	Beta-glucan, found in oats, has been shown to significantly reduce cholesterol. Additive beneficial effects may be seen with concurrent use.
Azadirachta indica	Antidiabetic drugs	Theoretical additive effects	Caution with use of this combination	Neem may theoretically lower blood glucose levels, based on limited data. Concomitant use may theoretically be additive and beneficial, but caution is advised due to a risk of hypoglycaemia.
	Immunosuppressant drugs	Theoretical decreased drug effect	Caution with use of this combination	Neem may have immune-stimulant activity according to animal studies. Theoretically, this may counteract drug immunosuppressant effects. Clinical significance is unclear, but caution is advised.
	Lithium	Increased risk of drug toxicity	Caution with use of this combination	Neem may have diuretic properties. Theoretically, combined use may reduce lithium excretion and increase the risk of lithium toxicity.

Continued

ACNM herbal interactions table—cont'd				
Herbal medicine	**Drug/drug class**	**Potential outcome**	**Recommendations**	**Comments**
Bacopa monniera	Acetylcholinesterase inhibitors	Possible increased drug effects and adverse effects	Caution with use of this combination	Bacopa appears to inhibit acetylcholinesterase, which can increase acetylcholine levels. Concomitant use of bacopa and acetylcholinesterase (AChE) inhibitors, such as donepezil, used for Alzheimer's disease, may theoretically have additive beneficial effects. Caution is advised as there is an increased risk of cholinergic side effects.
	Anticholinergic drugs	Theoretical decreased drug effect	Caution with use of this combination	Bacopa appears to increase acetylcholine levels and may theoretically oppose the action of drugs with an anticholinergic action. Significance is unclear, but caution is advised.
	Cholinergic drugs	Theoretical additive drug effect	Caution with use of this combination	Bacopa appears to increase acetylcholine levels and may theoretically have additive effects when used in combination with drugs with cholinergic actions. Significance is unclear.
Barosma betulina	Anticoagulant/ antiplatelet drugs	Theoretical increased risk of bleeding	Caution with use of this combination	Buchu may have antiplatelet properties. Concomitant use with anticoagulant and antiplatelet drugs will theoretically increase the risk of bleeding and bruising.
	Lithium	Increased risk of drug toxicity	Caution with use of this combination	Buchu may have diuretic properties. Theoretically, combined use may reduce lithium excretion and increase the risk of lithium toxicity.
Berberis aquifolium	Cyclosporin	Theoretical increased risk of drug toxicity	Caution with use of this combination	A clinical study reported that berberine, which is a constituent of Oregon grape, significantly increased drug serum levels in renal-transplant patients. This may have been due to inhibition of CYP3A4. Theoretically, concomitant use will increase the risk of drug toxicity.
	CYP3A4 substrates	Theoretical increased drug levels	Caution with use of this combination	Oregon grape may inhibit CYP3A4 activity based on limited data. Theoretically, this may lead to increased drug levels and risk of toxicity of drugs metabolised by this enzyme. More data is needed to determine significance of this interaction.
Berberis vulgaris	Anticholinergic drugs	Theoretical increased risk of adverse effects	Monitor – clinical significance unknown	Barberry may have anticholinergic properties based on in vitro evidence. Theoretically, concomitant use with anticholinergic drugs, such as antihistamines and tricyclic antidepressants, may result in additive effects and adverse effects.
	Anticoagulant/ antiplatelet drugs	Theoretical increased risk of bleeding	Caution with use of this combination	In vitro and animal studies suggest that berberine, a constituent of barberry, may inhibit platelet aggregation. There is a theoretical increased risk of bleeding, although this has not been demonstrated in human studies.
	Antidiabetic drugs	Theoretical additive effects	Caution with use of this combination	Berberine, a constituent of barberry, may lower blood glucose levels and have additive effects. Caution is advised due to an increased risk of hypoglycaemia.

		ACNM herbal interactions table—cont'd		
Herbal medicine	**Drug/drug class**	**Potential outcome**	**Recommendations**	**Comments**
Berberis vulgaris cont'd	Antihypertensive drugs	Theoretical additive effects	Monitor – may not be clinically significant	Berberine, a constituent of barberry, may have hypotensive effects. Additive effects are theoretically possible if used in combination with antihypertensive drugs. Monitor for hypotension.
	Cholinergic drugs	Theoretical decreased drug effect	Monitor – clinical significance unknown	Barberry may have anticholinergic properties based on in vitro evidence. Theoretically, concurrent use may decrease the effects of cholinergic drugs e.g. donepezil, tacrine.
	CNS depressant drugs	Increased risk of sedative effects	Caution with use of this combination	Animal research suggests that berberine, a constituent of barberry, may have sedative effects. There is a theoretical risk of excessive drowsiness when used with CNS depressant drugs.
	Cyclosporin	Increased risk of drug toxicity	Avoid this combination	A clinical study reported that berberine, which is a constituent of barberry, significantly increased drug serum levels in renal-transplant patients. This may have been due to inhibition of CYP3A4. Theoretically, concomitant use will increase the risk of drug toxicity.
	CYP450 substrates (CYP3A4)	Theoretical increased risk of drug toxicity	Caution with use of this combination	Preliminary evidence suggests berberine may inhibit activity of CYP3A4. Theoretically, this may lead to increased drug levels and risk of toxicity of drugs metabolised by this enzyme. More data is needed to determine significance of this interaction.
Berberine extract/ Berberine-containing herbs	Anticoagulant/ antiplatelet drugs	Theoretical increased risk of bleeding	Caution with use of this combination	In vitro and animal studies suggest that berberine may inhibit platelet aggregation. There is a theoretical increased risk of bleeding, although this has not been demonstrated in human studies. Caution is advised.
	Antidiabetic drugs	Theoretical additive effects	Caution with use of this combination	Berberine may lower blood glucose levels and have additive effects when used concomitantly with antidiabetic drugs. Caution is advised due to an increased risk of hypoglycaemia.
	Antihypertensive drugs	Theoretical additive effects	Monitor – may not be clinically significant	Berberine may have hypotensive effects. Additive effects are theoretically possible if used in combination with antihypertensive drugs. Monitor for hypotension.
	CNS depressant drugs	Increased risk of sedative effects	Caution with use of this combination	Animal research suggests that berberine may have sedative effects. There is a theoretical risk of excessive drowsiness when used with CNS depressant drugs.
	Cyclosporin	Increased risk of drug toxicity	Avoid this combination	A clinical study reported that berberine significantly increased drug serum levels in renal-transplant patients. This may have been due to inhibition of CYP3A4. Theoretically, concomitant use will increase the risk of drug toxicity.

Continued

ACNM herbal interactions table—cont'd				
Herbal medicine	**Drug/drug class**	**Potential outcome**	**Recommendations**	**Comments**
Berberine extract/ Berberine-containing herbs cont'd	CYP450 substrates (CYP2C9, CYP2D6, CYP3A4)	Theoretical increased risk of drug toxicity	Caution with use of this combination	Preliminary evidence suggests berberine may inhibit activity of CYP2C9, CYP2D6 and CYP3A4. Theoretically, herbal medicines containing berberine may increase drug levels and increase the risk of toxicity if used concomitantly with substrates of these enzymes.
Boswellia serrata	Antidiabetic drugs	Theoretical additive effects	May be beneficial – medical supervision recommended	One study reported that boswellia extract improved glucose levels and cholesterol levels compared to placebo when used in combination with conventional anti-diabetic medication. More study is needed to confirm findings.
	Anti-inflammatory drugs	Theoretical additive effects	Combination may be beneficial	Boswellia has anti-inflammatory properties and may provide an additive effect when used with anti-inflammatory drugs for conditions such as arthritis.
	CYP450 substrates (CYP1A2, CYP2C9, CYP2C19, CYP2D6, CYP3A4)	Theoretical increased risk of drug toxicity	Caution with use of this combination	In vitro studies suggest boswellia may inhibit activity of CYP1A2, CYP2C19, CYP2C9, CYP2D6 and CYP3A4. Concurrent use of boswellia may theoretically increase drugs levels of drugs metabolised by these enzymes, and increase the risk of toxicity.
	Immunosuppressant drugs	Theoretical decreased drug effectiveness	Caution with use of this combination	Boswellia may have immuno-stimulant activity according to in vitro studies. This may theoretically counteract drug immunosuppressant effects, although evidence is limited.
	Sulphasalazine	Additive effects possible	May be beneficial – medical supervision recommended	Clinical research suggests boswellia may improve symptoms of ulcerative colitis. Additive effects are theoretically possible with concomitant use, but medical supervision is recommended.
Brassica oleracea	CYP450 substrates (CYP1A2, CYP2A6)	Theoretical decreased drug effects	Monitor – clinical significance unknown	In vitro evidence suggests broccoli may induce CYP1A2 and CYP2A6 activity. Theoretically, this may result in increased metabolism and decreased therapeutic effects of drugs that substrate for these enzymes.
Bupleurum falcatum	Anticoagulant/ antiplatelet drugs	Theoretical increased risk of bleeding	Caution with use of this combination	Bupleurum may have antiplatelet properties. Concomitant use with anticoagulant and antiplatelet drugs will theoretically increase the risk of bleeding and bruising.
	Antidiabetic drugs	Theoretical compromised disease management	Caution with use of this combination	Animal research suggests that saikosaponins, constituents of bupleurum, can increase blood glucose. Concomitant use with antidiabetic drugs may theoretically interfere with blood glucose control and management of diabetes.
	Immunosuppressant drugs	Theoretical decrease in drug effectiveness	Caution with use of this combination	Bupleurum may have immuno-stimulant activity according to animal studies. This may theoretically counteract drug immunosuppressant effects, although evidence is limited.

| **ACNM herbal interactions table—cont'd** | | | | |
Herbal medicine	Drug/drug class	Potential outcome	Recommendations	Comments
Calendula officinalis	CNS depressant drugs	Theoretical increased risk of sedative effects	Monitor – unlikely to be clinically significant	Animal studies suggest oral calendula may have sedative effects. Concomitant use with CNS depressant drugs may theoretically increase sedation.
	Radiation therapy	Possible decreased adverse effects	May be beneficial – medical supervision recommended	Preliminary evidence suggests that topical application of calendula may help to ameliorate dermatitis in patients receiving radiation therapy for breast cancer.
Camellia sinensis	Alcohol	Theoretical increased risk of adverse effects	Monitor – unlikely to be clinically significant	Alcohol reduces caffeine metabolism. Theoretically, concomitant intake will increase the risk of caffeine-related adverse effects.
	Amphetamines	Theoretical increased risk of CNS effects	Caution with use of this combination	Caffeine in green tea may have additive CNS stimulat effects if taken concomitantly with amphetamines.
	Anticoagulant/ antiplatelet drugs	Theoretical increased risk of bleeding	Caution with use of this combination	Catechins in green tea are reported to have antiplatelet activity. The interaction has not been reported in human studies; however, people taking warfarin should avoid excessive consumption of green tea.
	Antidiabetic drugs	Theoretical altered drug effects	Monitor – unlikely to be clinically significant	Caffeine in green tea may affect blood glucose levels according to some sources, but data is conflicting. Patients should be monitored, but it seems unlikely that the interactions will be clinically relevant based on current data.
	Antifungal agents	Theoretical increased caffeine effects	Monitor – unlikely to be clinically significant	Preliminary evidence suggests that caffeine metabolism may be decreased by some antifungal agents such as e.g. fluconazole and terbinafine. Theoretically, this may result in increased caffeine-related adverse effects. Evidence is inconclusive.
	Bortezomib	Theoretical decreased drug effect	Avoid combination	Green tea polyphenols such as EGCG were reported to block this drug's antineoplastic effects in animal studies. Avoid use of green tea in patients taking boronic acid-based proteasome inhibitors such as bortezomib until further data becomes available.
	Cimetidine	Theoretical increased caffeine effects	Monitor – unlikely to be clinically significant	Cimetidine may reduce clearance of caffeine in green tea, which theoretically increases the risk of caffeine-related adverse effects.
	Clozapine	Theoretical decreased drug effects	Caution with use of this combination	Animal studies suggest green tea may reduce drug concentrations, although the clinical significance of these findings is unclear. Caffeine has also been shown to exacerbate psychotic symptoms. Caution is advised as this drug has a narrow therapeutic index.

Continued

ACNM herbal interactions table—cont'd				
Herbal medicine	**Drug/drug class**	**Potential outcome**	**Recommendations**	**Comments**
Camellia sinensis cont'd	CNS depressants	Theoretical decreased CNS effects	Monitor – may not be clinically significant	Caffeine in green tea may theoretically oppose the action of CNS depressant drugs and reduce drug effects.
	CNS stimulants	Theoretical increased CNS effects	Monitor – may not be clinically significant	Caffeine in green tea may have additive CNS stimulant effects if taken concomitantly with CNS stimulant drugs.
	Disulfiram	Theoretical increased caffeine effects	Monitor – may not be clinically significant	Disulfiram may reduce clearance of caffeine in green tea, which theoretically increases the risk of caffeine-related adverse effects.
	Doxorubicin	Theoretical decreased adverse effects and increased drug effect	May theoretically be beneficial – medical supervision recommended	Preliminary evidence suggests green tea polyphenols may reduce doxorubicin-induced cardiotoxicity. In addition, experimental in vitro data suggests that EGCG and theanine may enhance drug activity. While human studies are required to confirm these effects, there is a theoretical beneficial interaction.
	Ephedrine	Increased risk of stimulatory effects	Avoid combination	Use of ephedrine with caffeine-containing products may increase the risk of excessive stimulatory effects.
	Fluvoxamine	Theoretical increased caffeine levels	Monitor – may not be clinically significant	Fluvoxamine may reduce caffeine metabolism, theoretically increasing the risk of caffeine-related adverse effects.
	Hepatotoxic drugs	Increased risk of hepatotoxicity	Caution with use of this combination	Green tea extract supplements have been linked to several cases of hepatoxicity. Concurrent use with hepatotoxic drugs will have additive effects.
	Iron	Theoretical decreased mineral absorption	Monitor – may not be clinically significant	Tea polyphenols may form chelates with non-heme iron and reduce absorption. This interaction may not be significant, but dose administration should be separated.
	Lithium	Increased risk of drug toxicity	Caution with use of this combination	Abrupt withdrawal of caffeine can increase serum lithium levels and increase risk of adverse effects and drug toxicity.
	Monoamine oxidase inhibitors (MAOIs)	Theoretical risk of hypertensive crisis	Caution with use of this combination	Theoretically, high intake of caffeine, which is found in green tea, may precipitate a hypertensive crisis in patients taking MAOIs.
	Nadolol	Possible decreased drug effect	Avoid combination	Clinical trial evidence suggests that green tea catechins may inhibit organic anion-transporting polypeptides (OATP), resulting in decreased drug levels and antihypertensive effect.
	Oral contraceptives	Theoretical increased caffeine effects	Monitor – may not be clinically significant	Oral contraceptives may reduce clearance of caffeine in green tea, which theoretically increases the risk of caffeine-related adverse effects.
	Phenylpropanolamine	Theoretical increased risk of hypertension	Caution with use of this combination	Phenylpropanolamine and caffeine in green tea may have additive effects on raising blood pressure. Caution is advised with this combination.

ACNM herbal interactions table—cont'd				
Herbal medicine	**Drug/drug class**	**Potential outcome**	**Recommendations**	**Comments**
Camellia sinensis cont'd	Quinolone antibiotics	Theoretical increased caffeine effects	Monitor – may not be clinically significant	Quinolone antibiotics may reduce clearance of caffeine in green tea, which theoretically increases the risk of caffeine-related adverse effects.
	Theophylline	Theoretical increased risk of adverse effects	Caution with use of this combination	Caffeine in green tea may theoretically increase drug effects and adverse effects. Caution is advised but the interaction may not be clinically significant.
	Verapamil	Theoretical increased caffeine effects	Caution with use of this combination	Verapamil may increase plasma caffeine concentration by 25% according to some research. Concomitant use may theoretically increase the risk of caffeine-related adverse effects.
Cannabis spp	CNS depressant drugs	Additive effects and adverse effects	Caution with use of this combination	Preliminary evidence suggests cannabidiol has sedative and hypnotic effects. Excessive sedation is theoretically possible when used in combination with CNS depressant drugs.
	CYP450 substrates (CYP1A1, CYP1A2, CYP1B1, CYP2B6, CYP2C9, CYP2C19, CYP2D6, CYP3A4, CYP3A5)	Theoretical increased risk of drug toxicity	Caution with use of this combination	In vitro and animal research shows that cannabidiol, in cannabis, may inhibit CYP1A1, CYP1A2, CYP1B1, CYP2B6, CYP2C9, CYP2C19, CYP2D6, CYP3A4 and CYP3A5. Theoretically, concomitant use may increase the risk of drug toxicity of drugs metabolised by these enzymes. Caution is advised until more data becomes available.
Cantharanthus rosea	Antidiabetic drugs	Theoretical additive effects	Caution with use of this combination	Madagascar periwinkle may lower blood glucose levels. Additive effects are theoretically possible, increasing the risk of hypoglycaemia.
	Lithium	Increased risk of drug toxicity	Caution with use of this combination	Madagascar periwinkle may have diuretic properties. Theoretically, combined use may reduce lithium excretion and increase the risk of lithium toxicity.
Capsella bursa-pastoris	CNS depressant drugs	Theoretical additive effects	Monitor – may not be clinically significant	Shepard's purse may theoretically have additive sedative effects, based on limited data.
	Thyroid hormone	Theoretical altered drug effect	Monitor – may not be clinically significant	Concomitant use may theoretically interfere with drug therapy, based on limited data. Significance is unknown.
Capsicum spp	ACE-Inhibitors (ACE-I)	Theoretical increased risk of drug-induced cough	Monitor – may not be clinically significant	A case report describes a woman, who was previously stabilised on an ACE-I, experiencing a cough when she applied topical capsaicin cream. This may be due to an increase in bradykinin levels. The interaction is unlikely to be of significance in most individuals.

Continued

ACNM herbal interactions table—cont'd				
Herbal medicine	**Drug/drug class**	**Potential outcome**	**Recommendations**	**Comments**
Capsicum spp cont'd	Acid-reducing medication	Worsening or improved outcomes –conflicting data	Monitor – unlikely to be beneficial	Data is conflicting. Preliminary observational evidence suggested that regular intake of dietary chili may be associated with a lower incidence of peptic ulcers. Some sources have suggested that cayenne may have gastroprotective effects. Other sources have, however, stated that cayenne is gastro-irritant and may worsen gastric conditions. A small preliminary clinical study reported that 2.5g/day of red pepper may improve symptoms of dyspepsia, possibly by desensitising gastric nociceptive C-fibres. Results of a clinical trial, however, showed no improvement in duodenal ulcers compared to placebo when patients consumed chili peppers. No benefits were reported in a study investigating the use of capsicum or cayenne in IBS.
	Analgesics and NSAIDs	Additive effects possible	Combination may be beneficial	Topical use of capsaicin may have additive effects for reduction of pain.
	Anticoagulant/ antiplatelet drugs	Theoretical increased risk of bleeding	Caution with use of this combination	Capsicum (capsaicin) may have antiplatelet properties. Combined oral use with anticoagulant and antiplatelet drugs will theoretically increase the risk of bleeding and bruising. An observational study suggested that capsicum may increase the risk of bleeding when used with warfarin.
	Antidiabetic drugs	Theoretical additive effects	Caution with use of this combination	Oral use of high-dose capsicum may increase the risk of hypoglycaemia, according to limited data.
	Theophylline	Theoretical increased drug absorption and risk of adverse effects	Caution with use of this combination	Oral capsaicin may enhance theophylline absorption, based on animal research.
Carica papaya	Anticoagulant/ antiplatelet drugs	Theoretical increased risk of bleeding	Caution with use of this combination	Papaya may have antiplatelet properties. Concomitant use with anticoagulant and antiplatelet drugs may theoretically increase the risk of bleeding and bruising. Significance is unknown.
	Antidiabetic drugs	Additive effects possible	Caution with use of this combination	Fermented papaya may lower blood glucose levels, based on limited study. Additive, potentially beneficial effects are possible. Caution is advised until more data becomes available.
Carum carvi	Antidiabetic drugs	Theoretical additive effects	Monitor – may not be clinically significant	Caraway may theoretically lower blood glucose levels, based on animal data. Additive effects are theoretically possible, increasing the risk of hypoglycaemia.
	CNS depressant drugs	Theoretical additive effects	Monitor – may not be clinically significant	Caraway may theoretically have sedative effects, due to the constituent carvone, according to animal studies. Significance in humans is unknown.

ACNM herbal interactions table—cont'd				
Herbal medicine	**Drug/drug class**	**Potential outcome**	**Recommendations**	**Comments**
Carum carvi cont'd	L-Thyroxine (Levothyroxine)	Theoretical increased risk of hypothyroidism	Avoid combination	A case report describes a significant increase in thyroid stimulating hormone (TSH) in a patient who took caraway with thyroxine. TSH returned to normal once caraway was stopped. Caution is advised until further safety data becomes available.
	Lithium	Increased risk of drug toxicity	Caution with use of this combination	Caraway may have diuretic properties, which could theoretically precipitate lithium toxicity. The combination should be used with caution or avoided.
Centella asiatica	CNS depressant drugs	Theoretical additive effects	Caution with use of this combination	Gotu kola may have sedative effects, leading to a theoretical increased risk of sedation if used concomitantly with CNS depressant drugs.
	Hepatotoxic drugs	Theoretical increased risk of hepatotoxicity	Caution with use of this combination	Based on case reports, some concerns have been raised that concomitant use of gotu kola with hepatoxic drugs may theoretically increase the risk of liver damage.
Cetraria islandica	Oral drugs	Theoretical impaired drug absorption	Monitor – may not be clinically significant	The mucilage content of Iceland moss may theoretically interfere with drug absorption, although clinical significance has not been established.
Chamaelirium luteum	Lithium	Increased risk of drug toxicity	Caution with use of this combination	False unicorn may have diuretic properties, which could theoretically precipitate lithium toxicity. The combination should be used with caution.
Chelidonium majus	Hepatotoxic drugs	Theoretical increased risk of hepatotoxicity	Caution with use of this combination	Greater celandine has been linked to several cases of hepatotoxicity. Concerns have been raised that concomitant use of this herb with hepatotoxic drugs may increase the risk of liver damage.
	Immunosuppressant drugs	Theoretical decreased drug effect	Caution with use of this combination	A semi-synthetic derivative of chelidonine, a constituent of greater celandine, may stimulate the immune response in cancer patients, according to preliminary evidence. Theoretically, this may decrease the effects of immunosuppressant drugs. Caution is advised until more data becomes available.
Cinnamomum zeylanicum	Antidiabetic drugs	Theoretical additive effects	Caution with use of this combination	Cinnamon may lower blood glucose levels and additive effects are theoretically possible. The combination may be beneficial, but caution is advised due to a risk of hypoglycaemia.
Citrus paradisi	Aliskiren	Decreased drug concentration	Caution with use of this combination	Studies have reported a significant decrease in drug concentration with this combination, which may lead to reduced drug effect. The proposed mechanism for this interaction is due to inhibition of the organic anion-transporting protein polypeptide 2B1 (OATP2B1). Separate dose administration by at least 4 hours if concurrent use is deemed necessary.

Continued

ACNM herbal interactions table—cont'd				
Herbal medicine	**Drug/drug class**	**Potential outcome**	**Recommendations**	**Comments**
Citrus paradisi cont'd	Amiodarone	Increased drug plasma concentration and risk of adverse effects	Avoid combination	Grapefruit juice has been shown to significantly inhibit CYP3A4 enzyme activity. Studies have reported a significant increase in drug concentration with this combination, which increases the risk of adverse effects and drug toxicity.
	Artemether	Increased drug plasma concentration and risk of adverse effects	Avoid combination	Grapefruit juice has been shown to significantly inhibit CYP450 enzyme activity. Studies have reported a significant increase in drug concentration with this combination, which increases the risk of adverse effects and drug toxicity.
	Benzodiazepines e.g. midazolam, diazepam	Increased drug plasma concentration and risk of adverse effects	Avoid combination	Grapefruit juice has been shown to significantly inhibit CYP3A4 enzyme activity. Studies have reported a significant increase in drug concentration with this combination, which increases the risk of adverse effects and drug toxicity. This interaction has been reported especially with diazepam and midazolam. It does not appear to occur with alprazolam.
	Budesonide	Increased drug plasma concentration and risk of adverse effects	Caution with use of this combination	Grapefruit juice has been shown to significantly inhibit CYP3A4 enzyme activity. Studies have reported an increase in drug concentration with this combination, which increases the risk of adverse effects and drug toxicity.
	Buspirone	Increased drug plasma concentration and risk of adverse effects	Avoid combination	Studies have reported a significant increase in drug concentration with this combination, which increases the risk of adverse effects and drug toxicity.
	Caffeine	Increased risk of caffeine-related adverse effects	Caution with use of this combination	Studies have reported an increase in caffeine concentration with this combination, which increases the risk of adverse effects.
	Calcium channel blockers e.g. verapamil, amlodipine, nifedipine	Increased drug plasma concentration and risk of adverse effects	Avoid combination	Studies have reported a significant increase in drug concentration with this combination, which increases the risk of adverse effects and drug toxicity. It has been proposed that this is due to inhibition of CYP3A4 activity, but some sources suggest other mechanisms may also be involved.
	Carbamazepine	Increased drug plasma concentration	Avoid combination	Increased drug absorption and plasma concentrations have been reported.
	Carvedilol	Increased drug plasma concentration	Avoid combination	Grapefruit juice is reported to increase drug bioavailability.
	Celiprolol	Decreased drug concentration	Avoid combination	Grapefruit juice is reported to decrease drug bioavailability. The proposed mechanism for this interaction is due to inhibition of the organic anion-transporting protein polypeptide (OATP).
	Cisapride	Increased drug plasma concentration and risk of adverse effects	Avoid combination	Increased plasma concentrations have been reported.

ACNM herbal interactions table—cont'd				
Herbal medicine	**Drug/drug class**	**Potential outcome**	**Recommendations**	**Comments**
Citrus paradisi cont'd	Clomipramine	Increased drug plasma concentration and risk of adverse effects	Caution with use of this combination	Increased plasma concentrations have been described in two case reports.
	Clopidogrel	Decreased drug concentration	Avoid combination	Grapefruit juice has been reported to significantly decrease drug concentrations, which could reduce effectiveness as an antiplatelet drug.
	Colchicine	Increased drug plasma concentration and risk of adverse effects	Caution with use of this combination	In vitro evidence has reported that grapefruit juice increases drug absorption by inhibiting P-gp.
	Cyclosporin	Increased drug bioavailability	Avoid combination	Evidence suggest an increase in drug bioavailability with use of this combination.
	CYP450 substrates (CYP1A2, CYP2C19, CYP2C9)	Risk of increased drug plasma concentration and adverse effects	Caution with use of this combination	Preliminary evidence suggests grapefruit juice may inhibit CYP1A2, CYP2C19 and CYP2C9. Interactions have not been reported in human studies to date and significance is unclear.
	CYP450 substrates (CYP3A4)	Risk of increased drug plasma concentration and adverse effects	Avoid combination	Grapefruit juice has been shown to significantly inhibit CYP34A enzyme activity. When taken orally, effects of grapefruit juice on CYP3A4 appear to last at least 48 hours.
	Dextromethorphan	Increased drug concentration and risk of adverse effects	Caution with use of this combination	A pharmacokinetic study reported increased concentration of dextromethorphan when taken in combination with grapefruit juice. It has been proposed that the interaction is due to inhibition of CYP3A4.
	Docetaxel	Increased drug plasma concentration and risk of adverse effects	Avoid combination	A case report describes an interaction with use of this combination, leading to increased drug concentrations and a reduction in white blood cell count.
	Erythromycin	Increased drug plasma concentration and risk of adverse effects	Caution with use of this combination	A study reported increased absorption of erythromycin when taken in combination with grapefruit juice.
	Etoposide	Decreased drug concentration and effect	Avoid combination	Studies have reported a significant decrease in drug concentration with this combination, which may lead to reduced drug effect. The proposed mechanism for this interaction is inhibition of the organic anion-transporting protein polypeptide (OATP).
	Fexofenadine	Decreased drug concentration and effect	Caution with use of this combination	Studies have reported a significant decrease in drug concentration with this combination, which may lead to reduced drug effect. The proposed mechanism for this interaction is inhibition of the organic anion-transporting protein polypeptide (OATP).
	Fluvoxamine	Increased drug plasma concentration	Caution with use of this combination	Increased drug plasma concentrations have been reported.
	Halofantrine	Increased drug plasma concentration and risk of adverse effects	Avoid combination	Increased drug plasma concentrations have been reported in a small clinical study. This may lead to an increased risk of prolonged QT interval.

Continued

ACNM herbal interactions table—cont'd				
Herbal medicine	**Drug/drug class**	**Potential outcome**	**Recommendations**	**Comments**
Citrus paradisi cont'd	HMGCoA reductase inhibitors (statins) e.g. atorvastatin, simvastatin	Increased drug plasma concentration and risk of adverse effects	Avoid combination	Grapefruit juice has been shown to significantly inhibit CYP3A4 enzyme activity. Studies have reported a significant increase in drug concentration with this combination, which increases the risk of adverse effects and drug toxicity.
	Itraconazole	Altered drug levels possible	Caution with use of this combination	Data on effect of grapefruit juice on this drug is conflicting and significance is unclear. Caution with use until further data becomes available.
	L-Thyroxine (levothyroxine)	Possible decreased drug effect	Caution with use of this combination	A modest decrease in drug effect has been reported. The proposed mechanism for this interaction is due to inhibition of the organic anion-transporting protein polypeptide (OATP).
	Losartan	Possible decreased drug concentration	Caution with use of this combination	A study in healthy volunteers reported decreased drug concentrations with use of this combination. Clinical significance is unclear.
	Methadone	Increased drug plasma concentration	Caution with use of this combination	An increased drug concentration has been reported with this combination. Clinical significance is unclear.
	Methylprednisolone	Increased drug plasma concentration	Avoid combination	Studies have reported an increase in drug concentration with this combination, which increases the risk of adverse effects and drug toxicity.
	Nadolol	Theoretical decreased drug effect	Caution with use of this combination	Grapefruit juice may theoretically decrease drug bioavailability due to inhibition of the organic anion-transporting polypeptide (OATP1A2). It is not known if this interaction is clinically significant.
	Nilotinib	Increased drug plasma concentration	Caution with use of this combination	Increased drug concentration and drug absorption have been reported with this combination.
	Oestrogens	Increased drug plasma concentration	Caution with use of this combination	Increased plasma concentrations have been reported. It has been proposed that this is due to inhibition of CYP3A4.
	Organic anion-transporting polypeptide substrates (OATP)	Possible decreased drug absorption and drug effect	Avoid combination	In vitro and clinical evidence show that grapefruit juice inhibits organic anion-transporting polypeptides (OATP). This reduces bioavailability of oral drugs that are OATP substrates. Separation of dose administration by at least 4 hours may help to avoid this interaction as the effect appears to only last for a short time.
	Oxycodone	Increased drug concentration and risk of adverse effects	Avoid combination	An increase in drug concentration has been reported with this combination. Oxycodone is metabolised by CYP3A4.
	Praziquantel	Increased drug concentration and risk of adverse effects	Avoid combination	Studies have reported a significant increase in drug concentration with this combination, which increases the risk of adverse effects and drug toxicity.

ACNM herbal interactions table—cont'd				
Herbal medicine	**Drug/drug class**	**Potential outcome**	**Recommendations**	**Comments**
Citrus paradisi cont'd	Primaquine	Possible increased drug bioavailability	Caution with use of this combination	An increase in drug bioavailability has been reported. Clinical significance is unclear.
	Quinidine	Altered drug effect	Caution with use of this combination	Grapefruit juice has been reported to decrease drug absorption, clearance and metabolism, and to prolong drug half-life. Clinical significance is unclear.
	Regorafenib	Theoretical increased drug concentrations and risk of toxicity	Avoid combination	Grapefruit juice has been shown to significantly inhibit CYP3A4 enzyme activity. While no direct interaction has been reported, this drug is a CYP3A4 substrate.
	Repaglinide	Small increase in serum drug concentration	Caution with use of this combination	A small but significant increase in drug concentration has been reported with use of this combination.
	Saquinavir	Increased drug absorption	Caution with use of this combination	Increased drug absorption has been reported with use of this combination. This interaction does not appear to occur with indinavir, another protease inhibitor.
	Scopolamine	Increased drug concentration and risk of adverse effects	Avoid combination	An increased drug concentration has been reported with this combination. Scopolamine is metabolised by CYP3A4.
	Sertraline	Increased drug plasma concentration and risk of adverse effects	Caution with use of this combination	Two studies have reported a significant increase in drug concentration with this combination, which increases the risk of adverse effects and drug toxicity.
	Sildenafil	Increased drug concentration and risk of adverse effects	Caution with use of this combination	An increased drug concentration has been reported with this combination. Sildenafil is metabolised by CYP3A4.
	Sunitinib	Possible increase in drug plasma concentration	Caution with use of this combination	A modest increase in drug levels has been reported with use of this combination. This interaction may not be clinically significant, but caution is advised.
	Tacrolimus	Increased drug bioavailability and risk of adverse effects	Avoid combination unless under strict medical supervision	Studies have reported a significant increase in drug bioavailability with this combination. It has been proposed that this may enhance drug action, but strict medical supervision is required due to a lack of reliable safety and efficacy data.
	Talinolol	Possible increased drug bioavailability	Caution with use of this combination	An increase in drug bioavailability may occur with this combination. The clinical significance is unclear.
	Terfenadine	Possible increased drug concentrations	Avoid combination	An increase in drug absorption and plasma concentration have been reported with this combination. Clinical significance is unclear.
	Theophylline	Possible decreased drug concentrations	Caution with use of this combination	A modest decrease in drug levels has been reported. The mechanism of this interaction is unknown.

Continued

ACNM herbal interactions table—cont'd				
Herbal medicine	**Drug/drug class**	**Potential outcome**	**Recommendations**	**Comments**
Citrus paradisi cont'd	Ticagrelor	Increased drug plasma concentration and risk of bleeding	Avoid combination	Grapefruit juice has been shown to significantly inhibit CYP3A4 enzyme activity. Studies have reported a significant increase in drug concentration with this combination, which increases the risk of adverse effects and drug toxicity.
	Tolvaptan	Increased drug plasma concentration and risk of adverse effects	Caution with use of this combination	Studies have reported an increase in drug concentration with this combination. This may lead to an increased extent and duration of diuretic effect, and an increased risk of adverse effects and drug toxicity.
	Toremifene	Theoretical increased drug plasma concentration and risk of adverse effects	Avoid combination	Grapefruit juice has been shown to significantly inhibit CYP3A4 enzyme activity. While an interaction between grapefruit juice and this drug has not been demonstrated directly, the drug is a CYP3A4 substrate. There is a theoretical risk of prolonged QT interval.
	Warfarin	Theoretical increased risk of bleeding	Caution with use of this combination	A case report describes an increase in INR in a patient taking large doses of grapefruit juice while on warfarin. A small clinical study, however, reported that daily consumption of grapefruit juice did not affect INR in a group of men taking warfarin. Caution is recommended until more safety data becomes available.
Cnicus benedictus	Acid-reducing drugs e.g. antacids, H_2 antagonists, proton pump inhibitors	Theoretical decreased drug effect	Monitor – may not be clinically significant	Blessed thistle may increase gastric acidity. Use may theoretically counteract drug acid-reducing action, resulting in decreased drug effect.
Codonopsis pilosula	Anticoagulant/ antiplatelet drugs	Theoretical increased risk of bleeding	Caution with use of this combination	Preliminary clinical research suggests codonopsis has antiplatelet activity. Concomitant use with anticoagulant and antiplatelet drugs may theoretically increase the risk of bleeding and bruising.
Coffea arabica	Alcohol	Theoretical increased caffeine effects	Monitor – may not be clinically significant	Alcohol reduces caffeine metabolism. Theoretically, concomitant intake will increase the risk of caffeine-related adverse effects.
	Alendronate	Reduced drug bioavailability	Caution with use of this combination – separate doses	Coffee significantly reduces drug bioavailability. Doses should be separated by at least 2 hours.
	Anticoagulant/ antiplatelet drugs	Theoretical increased risk of bleeding	Monitor – may not be clinically significant	Caffeine is reported to have antiplatelet activity; however, an interaction between coffee and anticoagulant/antiplatelet drugs has not been reported in humans.
	Clozapine	Theoretical disease exacerbation	Caution with use of this combination	The caffeine content of coffee may exacerbate psychotic symptoms and increase drug effects and toxicity at high doses (400–1000 mg daily of caffeine).
	CNS stimulant drugs	Enhanced stimulatory effects	Caution with use of this combination	Concomitant use of caffeine in coffee and CNS stimulant drugs will increase the risk of adverse effects due to additive stimulatory actions.

ACNM herbal interactions table—cont'd				
Herbal medicine	Drug/drug class	Potential outcome	Recommendations	Comments
Coffea arabica cont'd	Disulfiram	Theoretical increased caffeine effects	Monitor – may not be clinically significant	Disulfiram may reduce clearance of caffeine, which theoretically increases the risk of caffeine-related adverse effects.
	Ephedrine	Enhanced stimulatory effects	Avoid combination	Ephedrine may enhance the stimulatory effects of caffeine. The combination has been associated with an increased risk of life-threatening or debilitating adverse effects such as hypertension, myocardial infarction, stroke, seizures and death.
	L-Thyroxine (Levothyroxine)	Possible decreased drug absorption	Caution with use of this combination	It has been proposed that coffee may form insoluble complexes with L-thyroxine in some patients. Dose administration should be separated.
	Monoamine oxidase inhibitors	Theoretical risk of hypertensive crisis	Caution with use of this combination	Theoretically, high intake of caffeine in coffee may precipitate a hypertensive crisis in patients taking MAOIs.
	Phenylpropanolamine	Theoretical increased risk of hypertension	Caution with use of this combination	Phenylpropanolamine and caffeine may have additive effects on raising blood pressure. Caution is advised with this combination.
	Quinolone antibiotics	Theoretical increased caffeine effects	Monitor – may not be clinically significant	Quinolones reduce caffeine metabolism. Theoretically, there is an increased risk of caffeine-related adverse effects.
	Theophylline	Theoretical increased risk of drug toxicity	Caution with use of this combination	Caffeine in coffee may inhibit drug metabolism and increase the risk of adverse effects.
Coleus forskohlii	Anticoagulant/ antiplatelet drugs	Unpredictable effect	Caution with use of this combination	Coleus may increase the rate of warfarin metabolism, leading to a reduced anticoagulant action, according to animal studies. There is, however, evidence that forskolin, a constituent of coleus, may inhibit platelet aggregation and adhesion, which potentially increases the risk of bleeding and bruising.
	Antihypertensive drugs	Theoretical additive effects	Caution with use of this combination	Coleus may lower blood pressure, based on limited studies. Additive effects are possible, increasing the risk of hypotension.
	CYP450 substrates (CYP2C9, CYP3A4)	Theoretical decrease in drug effects	Caution with use of this combination	Laboratory and animal studies suggest that coleus may induce CYP2C9 and CYP3A4. Theoretically, this may result in an increased rate of drug metabolism and decreased drug effect. Clinical significance is unclear, but caution is advised.
	Nitrates	Additive coronary vasodilatory effect	Avoid combination	Limited research suggests that additive vasodilatory effects are possible, due to the constituent forskolin. The combination should be avoided unless under medical supervision.
	Vasodilatory drugs including calcium channel blockers	Additive vasodilatory effects	Caution with use of this combination	Limited research suggests that additive vasodilatory effects are possible, due to the constituent forskolin. Caution is advised.

Continued

ACNM herbal interactions table—cont'd				
Herbal medicine	**Drug/drug class**	**Potential outcome**	**Recommendations**	**Comments**
Commiphora myrrha/molmol	Anticoagulant/ antiplatelet drugs	Theoretical decreased drug effect	Caution with use of this combination	One case report and in vitro studies suggest myrrh may decrease effectiveness of warfarin. Caution is advised, but clinical significance is unclear based on current data.
	Antidiabetic drugs	Theoretical additive effects	Caution with use of this combination	Myrrh may have hypoglycaemic effects. Additive effects are theoretically possible, increasing the risk of hypoglycaemia.
Commiphora mukul	Anticoagulant/ antiplatelet drugs	Theoretical increased risk of bleeding	Caution with use of this combination	Guggul may have antiplatelet activity. Concomitant use may theoretically increase the risk of bleeding and bruising. Clinical significance is unclear.
	CYP450 substrates (CYP3A4)	Theoretical decreased drug effects	Monitor – clinical significance is unclear	In vivo evidence suggests that guggul may induce CYP3A4 enzyme activity. Theoretically, this may result in increased rate of drug metabolism and decreased drug effects.
	Diltiazem	Possible decreased drug effects	Monitor – clinical significance is unclear	One small study reported that guggul may reduce drug bioavailability. Significance is unknown.
	L-Thyroxine Levothyroxine	Theoretical altered drug effects	Monitor – clinical significance is unclear	High-dose intake of guggul may theoretically interfere with drug action.
	Propranolol	Possible decreased drug effects	Monitor – clinical significance is unclear	One small study reported that guggul may reduce drug bioavailability. Significance is unknown.
	Tamoxifen	Theoretical altered drug effects	Caution with use of this combination	High-dose intake of guggul may theoretically interfere with drug action through oestrogen-alpha receptor agonist activity.
Coptic chinensis	Cyclosporin	Theoretical increased risk of drug toxicity	Caution with use of this combination	Berberine, a constituent of this herb, may reduce rate of metabolism of cyclosporin and increase risk of drug toxicity.
	CYP3A4 substrates	Theoretical increased drug levels	Caution with use of this combination	This herb may inhibit CYP3A4 activity based on limited data. Theoretically, this may result in increased drug levels and risk of toxicity of drugs metabolised by this enzyme. More data is needed to determine significance of this interaction.
Cordyceps spp	Anticoagulant/ antiplatelet drugs	Theoretical increased risk of bleeding	Caution with use of this combination	Animal research suggests cordyceps may have antiplatelet effects. There is a theoretical increased risk of bleeding with concomitant use, but this has not been reported in humans.
	Chemotherapy	Theoretical improved outcomes	Caution with use of this combination	Preliminary evidence suggests cordyceps may improve quality of life and cellular immunity in patients undergoing cancer chemotherapy. Concomitant use may be beneficial, but caution is advised until more data becomes available.

ACNM herbal interactions table—cont'd				
Herbal medicine	**Drug/drug class**	**Potential outcome**	**Recommendations**	**Comments**
Cordyceps spp cont'd	Cyclosporin	Theoretical decreased drug effects	Avoid combination	A small clinical study reported that cordyceps reduced the immunosuppressive effects of cyclosporin in patients who had undergone renal transplantation. Other research has reported that cordyceps may help to ameliorate cyclosporin-induced nephrotoxicity. Avoid combination unless under strict medical supervision.
	Immunosuppressant drugs	Theoretical decreased drug effects; possible improved outcomes	Caution with use of this combination	Theoretically, cordyceps may reduce drug immunosuppressive effects by stimulating the immune system. Preliminary evidence has, however, suggested that use of cordyceps in renal-transplant patients may have beneficial effects. Research has suggested that adjunctive use of cordyceps with immunosuppressive therapy may result in reduced hepatotoxicity and nephrotoxicity, reduced number of infections and reduced drug requirements. Concomitant use may potentially be beneficial under strict medical supervision.
	Testosterone	Theoretical additive effects	Monitor – clinical significance is unclear	Animal research suggests cordyceps may increase testosterone levels. Clinical significance is unknown based on current data.
Crataegus spp	Antihypertensive drugs	Possible additive effects	Caution with use of this combination	Hawthorn has been shown to lower blood pressure and may reduce heart rate. Additive beneficial effects are possible with antihypertensive drugs, but caution is advised due to a risk of hypotension.
	Digoxin and cardiac glycosides	Theoretical additive effects	May be beneficial – medical supervision recommended	Hawthorn appears to improve cardiac output and combined use may theoretically potentiate drug effects. This interaction may be beneficial, but medical supervision is advised as there is currently insufficient data to determine risks and benefits of concomitant use.
	Diuretics	Theoretical additive effects in heart failure	May be beneficial – medical supervision recommended	Hawthorn may provide additional cardiovascular benefits in patients with congestive heart failure which could theoretically lead to improved outcomes. Limited data suggests a potential benefit with concurrent use. Caution is advised until more data becomes available.
	Doxorubicin	Theoretical decreased drug cardiotoxicity	May be beneficial – medical supervision recommended	It has been speculated that hawthorn may provide cardioprotective effects and help to reduce risk of cardiotoxicity in patients taking doxorubicin. Further research is needed to investigate the risks and benefits of this interaction.

Continued

ACNM herbal interactions table—cont'd				
Herbal medicine	**Drug/drug class**	**Potential outcome**	**Recommendations**	**Comments**
Crataegus spp cont'd	Lipid-lowering drugs	Theoretical additive effects	Combination may be beneficial	Hawthorn may theoretically reduce serum cholesterol and potentiate drug lipid-lowering effects.
	Nitrates	Theoretical additive effects	Avoid combination	Hawthorn may have additive vasodilatory effects when used with nitrates. The combination should be avoided unless under medical supervision.
	Phosphodiesterase-5 inhibitors	Theoretical additive effects	Avoid combination	Hawthorn may have additive vasodilatory effects when used with phosphodiesterase-5 inhibitors, such as sildenafil. The combination should be avoided unless under medical supervision.
Crocus sativus	Antihypertensive drugs	Theoretical additive effects	Monitor – clinical significance is unclear	Animal studies suggest saffron may have hypotensive properties. Additive effects are theoretically possible, with an increased risk of hypotension.
	Calcium channel blockers	Theoretical additive effects	Caution with use of this combination	Additive coronary vasodilatory effects are possible, based on animal research, which suggests saffron may have negative inotropic and chronotropic activity.
Curcuma longa	Alcohol	Possible reduced organ damage	May be beneficial – medical supervision recommended	Animal models suggest that curcumin may provide some protective effects against alcoholic liver and pancreatic disease. This may theoretically be a useful adjunct therapy in those with high alcohol ingestion.
	Anticoagulant/antiplatelet drugs	Theoretical increased risk of bleeding	Caution with use of this combination	Turmeric is reported to have antiplatelet activity in vitro. Theoretically, concurrent use with anticoagulant or antiplatelet drugs increases the risk of bleeding. Caution is advised until more data becomes available.
	Antidiabetic drugs	Theoretical additive effects	Caution with use of this combination	Turmeric may have hypoglycaemic effects. Clinical significance of this interaction is unclear, but additive effects are theoretically possible.
	CYP450 substrates (CYP1A1, CYP1A2, CYP3A4)	Theoretical increased drug effect	Monitor – may not be clinically significant	In vitro and animal research suggests that curcumin may inhibit liver metabolising activity of CYP1A1, CYP1A2 and CYP3A4. This has not been demonstrated in humans, although a case report describes a possible interaction with tacrolimus, a CYP3A4 substrate.
	Dexamethasone	Theoretical increase in drug levels	Caution with use of this combination	Turmeric may increase drug blood levels, based on preliminary data. There is a theoretical increase in drug effects and adverse effects, although data is limited.
	Non-steroidal anti-inflammatory drugs (NSAIDs)	Theoretical additive effects	Combination may be beneficial	Additive effects are possible with concomitant use which may be beneficial for the management of conditions such as arthritis. No negative drug-herb interactions have been reported, but monitoring is suggested.

ACNM herbal interactions table—cont'd				
Herbal medicine	**Drug/drug class**	**Potential outcome**	**Recommendations**	**Comments**
Curcuma longa cont'd	Sulphasalazine	Theoretical increased drug levels	Caution with use of this combination	Preliminary evidence suggests turmeric may increase blood levels of drug. Combined use may theoretically increase drug effects and adverse effects.
	Tacrolimus	Theoretical increased drug levels	Caution with use of this combination	Animal studies and a case report suggest that turmeric may increase drug levels. Combined use may theoretically increase drug effects and adverse effects. Caution is advised until more safety data becomes available.
	Talinolol	Possible reduced drug bioavailability	Caution with use of this combination	Preliminary clinical evidence suggests curcumin may decrease drug bioavailability. Caution is advised until more data becomes available.
Cynara scolymus	Lipid-lowering drugs	Theoretical additive effects	Combination may be beneficial	Additive, beneficial effects are theoretically possible. No negative drug-herb interactions have been reported.
Dioscorea villosa	Oestrogens e.g. HRT and oral contraceptives	Theoretical additive effects	Monitor – may not be clinically significant	In vitro evidence suggests wild yam may have oestrogenic and anti-oestrogenic effects. Clinical evidence of an interaction is lacking, but monitoring is advised with concomitant use.
Echinacea purpurea/ angustifolia	Antineoplastic drugs e.g. etoposide	Theoretical increased risk of drug toxicity	Avoid combination	A case report suggests that use of echinacea with etoposide resulted in increased drug toxicity. Avoid this combination until further data becomes available.
	Asthma or atopic medication	Herb may trigger allergic reactions and asthma	Avoid combination	There are several case reports that echinacea caused allergic reactions and exacerbated asthma in predisposed individuals, leading to effects including anaphylaxis, urticaria and bronchospasm. Although the incidence of reported interactions is rare, caution or avoidance of echinacea is recommended in patients requiring regular asthma or atopic medication.
	Cyclophosphamide	Theoretical decreased drug effect	Caution with use of this combination	Echinacea has immuno-stimulant activity which may theoretically counteract drug effect. The clinical significance is unknown, but caution is advised.
	CYP450 substrates (CYP1A2)	Theoretical increased drug levels	Caution with use of this combination	Echinacea may inhibit CYP1A2 based on limited study. There is a theoretical risk of increased drug levels and toxicity.
	CYP450 substrates (CYP3A4)	Theoretical altered drug effect	Caution with use of this combination	Some literature suggests that echinacea may induce CYP3A4, while other sources suggest it may inhibit CYP3A4. It has been proposed that this herb may induce hepatic CYP3A4 and inhibit intestinal CYP3A4. The effects may theoretically balance each other out. The interaction may not be clinically relevant, but caution is advised until more data becomes available.

Continued

ACNM herbal interactions table—cont'd				
Herbal medicine	**Drug/drug class**	**Potential outcome**	**Recommendations**	**Comments**
Echinacea purpurea/ angustifolia cont'd	Immunosuppressant drugs	Theoretical decreased drug effect	Caution with use of this combination	Echinacea has immuno-stimulant activity which may theoretically counteract drug immunosuppressant effects. Evidence of an interaction is limited, but caution is advised.
	Warfarin	Theoretical decreased drug	Monitor – may not be clinically significant	A study conducted in healthy male volunteers suggests that echinacea may increase drug clearance. This did not appear to have a clinically relevant effect on INR.
Echium amoenum	Antidepressant drugs (SSRIs)	Possible improved outcomes	Caution with use of this combination	Results of two small clinical trials suggest an additive beneficial effect with concomitant use of SSRIs and Iranian borage in the management of anxiety or depression. No differences in frequency of adverse effects have been reported so far. Patients should be monitored and caution is advised until more data becomes available.
	Benzodiazepines	Theoretical additive effects	Caution with use of this combination	Iranian borage may have anxiolytic properties according to animal studies and preliminary clinical research. Additive effects and an increased risk of adverse effects are theoretically possible. Patients should be monitored and caution is advised until more data becomes available.
Eleutherococcus senticosus	Alcohol	Increased risk of sedation	Caution with use of this combination	Siberian ginseng may have additive sedative effects when used in combination with alcohol.
	Anticoagulant/ antiplatelet drugs	Theoretical increased risk of bleeding	Monitor – clinical significance is unclear	A constituent of Siberian ginseng is reported to have antiplatelet activity in vitro. There is a theoretical risk of increased bleeding, but significance is unclear.
	Antidiabetic drugs	Theoretical additive effects	Monitor – clinical significance is unclear	Siberian ginseng may have hypoglycaemic effects. Additive effects are theoretically possible, increasing the risk of hypoglycaemia. Caution is advised until more data becomes available.
	Chemotherapy	Possible reduced drug adverse effects	Combination may be beneficial – medical supervision recommended	Limited evidence suggests Siberian ginseng may reduce adverse effects associated with chemotherapy and enhance general stress resistance. Data is limited and medical supervision is recommended.
	CNS depressant drugs	Increased risk of sedation	Caution with use of this combination	Siberian ginseng may have additive sedative effects when used in combination with CNS depressant drugs.
	CYP450 substrates (CYP1A2, 2C9, 2D6, 3A4)	Theoretical increased risk of drugs effects and adverse effects	Caution with use of this combination	In vitro and animal studies suggest that Siberian ginseng may inhibit activity of CYP 1A2 and CYP2C9. Caution is advised until more data becomes available. Siberian ginseng has also been shown to inhibit CYP2D6 and 3A4 in vitro and in animal models, but this effect does not appear to be relevant in human studies.

ACNM herbal interactions table—cont'd				
Herbal medicine	**Drug/drug class**	**Potential outcome**	**Recommendations**	**Comments**
Eleutherococcus senticosus cont'd	Digoxin	Theoretical risk of increased drug levels	Caution with use of this combination	One case report associated Siberian ginseng with an elevation in serum digoxin levels. Drug toxicity was not reported, but caution is advised until further safety data becomes available.
	Immunosuppressant drugs	Theoretical decrease in drug effectiveness	Caution with use of this combination	Siberian ginseng may theoretically counteract drug immunosuppressant effects due to herb immunostimulating activity. Evidence of an interaction is limited, but caution is advised.
	Lithium	Theoretical increased risk of drug toxicity	Caution with use of this combination	Siberian ginseng may have diuretic properties. Theoretically, combined use may reduce lithium excretion and increase the risk of lithium toxicity.
	P-gp substrates		Caution with use of this combination	Preliminary in vitro evidence suggests that Siberian ginseng may inhibit P-gp. This could theoretically increase drug effects, although there is currently insufficient data to determine if the interactions would be clinically important.
Ephedra sineca	Anticonvulsants	Increased risk of seizures	Caution with use of this combination	Ephedra is associated with triggering seizure activity and may therefore interfere with drug effectiveness. Use would be inappropriate in people with epilepsy or a history of seizures.
	Antidiabetic drugs	Possible decreased drug effects	Caution with use of this combination	Limited research suggests ephedra may raise blood glucose and potentially interfere with drug effectiveness and impair disease management.
	B-agonists e.g. salbutamol (Ventolin®)	Increased risk of adverse effects	Caution with use of this combination	Additive effects are possible, with an increased risk of adverse effects.
	Caffeine	Additive stimulant effects	Avoid combination	Evidence suggests that use of ephedra in combination with caffeine may increase the risk of potentially serious life-threatening or debilitating adverse effects.
	Cardiovascular drugs	Increased risk of cardiovascular events	Avoid combination	Ephedra has been reported to cause severe life-threatening or disabling adverse effects and there are case reports linking ephedra to hypertension, myocardial infarction and stroke. Those with pre-existing cardiovascular conditions appear to be at greater risk.
	Dexamethasone	Theoretical decreased drug effects	Caution with use of this combination	The ephedrine in ephedra may theoretically increase the rate of dexamethasone clearance and reduce drug effectiveness.
	Ergot derivatives	Theoretical risk of hypertension	Caution with use of this combination	There is a theoretical risk of hypertension due to the ephedrine in ephedra.
	Monoamine oxidase inhibitors (MAOIs)	Theoretical increased risk of adverse effects	Avoid combination	There is a theoretical increased risk of drug adverse effects based on drug and herb mechanisms of action and limited case reports.

Continued

ACNM herbal interactions table—cont'd				
Herbal medicine	**Drug/drug class**	**Potential outcome**	**Recommendations**	**Comments**
Ephedra sineca cont'd	Pseudoephedrine	Theoretical risk of hypertension	Caution with use of this combination	There is a theoretical risk of hypertension due to the ephedrine in ephedra.
	QT-interval prolonging drugs e.g. amiodarone	Increased risk of arrhythmias	Avoid combination	A small study reported that use of a combination product containing ephedra and caffeine increased the QT interval in healthy volunteers. Additive effects are theoretically possible with a combination of ephedra and drugs that prolong the QT interval, and may increase the risk of arrhythmias.
	Stimulant drugs	Increased risk of adverse effects	Avoid combination	There is a theoretical increased risk of hypertension and adverse cardiovascular effects with use of ephedra and drugs with CNS stimulant properties including phenylpropanolamine and pseudoephedrine.
	Theophylline	Increased risk of adverse effects	Avoid combination	The combination of ephedra with methylxanthine drugs such as theophylline will have additive stimulant actions and risk of adverse effects.
Equisetum arvense	Antidiabetic drugs	Theoretical additive effects	Monitor – clinical significance is unclear	Horsetail may lower blood glucose levels, based on limited data. Additive effects are theoretically possible, increasing the risk of hypoglycaemia. Caution is advised until more data becomes available.
	Diuretic drugs	Increased risk of potassium depletion	Caution with use of this combination	Horsetail may have diuretic properties. Concurrent use with potassium-depleting diuretics will increase the risk of hypokalaemia.
	Lithium	Theoretical increased risk of drug toxicity	Caution with use of this combination	Horsetail may have diuretic properties. Theoretically, combined use may reduce lithium excretion and increase the risk of lithium toxicity.
Eriodictyon crassifolium	Lithium	Theoretical increased risk of drug toxicity	Caution with use of this combination	This herb may have diuretic properties. Theoretically, combined use may reduce lithium excretion and increase the risk of lithium toxicity.
Eschscholzia californica	Benzodiazepines	Theoretical additive effects and adverse effects	Caution with use of this combination	Concurrent use of Californian poppy with benzodiazepines may theoretically lead to additive effects and an increased risk of adverse effects such as excessive drowsiness.
	CNS depressants	Theoretical additive effects and adverse effects	Caution with use of this combination	Concurrent use of Californian poppy with CNS depressant drugs may theoretically lead to additive effects and risk of adverse effects such as excessive drowsiness.
Eucalyptus globus	Antidiabetic drugs	Theoretical additive effects	Monitor – clinical significance is unclear	Eucalyptus may have hypoglycaemic effects, based on animal research. Significance is unknown, but additive effects are theoretically possible, increasing the risk of hypoglycaemia.
	CYP450 substrates (CYP1A2, CYP2C19, CYP2C9, CYP3A4)	Theoretical increased drug levels	Monitor – clinical significance is unclear	In vitro evidence suggests eucalyptus oil may inhibit CYP450 enzyme activity. This has not been demonstrated in humans to date.

ACNM herbal interactions table—cont'd				
Herbal medicine	**Drug/drug class**	**Potential outcome**	**Recommendations**	**Comments**
Eucalyptus globus cont'd	Phenobarbital	Theoretical decreased drug effect	Monitor – clinical significance is unclear	Preliminary animal research suggests that inhaling eucalyptus may reduce the amount of drug that reaches the brain. Clinical significance is not known.
Eugenia caryophyllata	Anticoagulant/ antiplatelet drugs	Theoretical increased risk of bleeding	Monitor – clinical significance is unclear	Laboratory studies suggest that eugenol, a constituent of clove, may have antiplatelet activity. This has not been demonstrated in humans, but monitoring is recommended.
Eupatorium perfoliatum	CYP450 substrates (CYP3A4)	Theoretical risk of decreased drug effect	Monitor – interaction is speculative	It has been proposed that boneset may theoretically induce CYP3A4, based on the fact that this herb belongs to the genus Eupatorium, and other plants of this genus have been shown to induce CYP3A4. There is no specific research investigating this effect with boneset.
Euphrasia spp.	Antidiabetic drugs	Theoretical additive effects	Monitor – clinical significance is unclear	It has been proposed that eyebright may have hypoglycaemic effects, based on animal studies. Clinical significance has not been established, but additive effects are theoretically possible, increasing the risk of hypoglycaemia.
Eurycoma longifolia	Propranolol	Risk of decreased drug effects	Caution with use of this combination	Results of a small clinical trial found that concomitant use of this herb and propranolol led to reduced drug bioavailability. This appears to be due to decreased drug absorption.
Filipendula ulmaria	Anticoagulant/ antiplatelet drugs including aspirin	Theoretical additive effects	Caution with use of this combination	Meadowsweet contains plant salicylates which have been shown to have anticoagulant properties in vitro and in animal studies. There is a theoretical increased risk of bleeding, but this is speculative and clinical significance is unknown.
Foeniculum vulgare	Anticoagulant/ antiplatelet drugs	Theoretical increased risk of bleeding	Monitor – clinical significance is unclear	Animal research suggests fennel may have some antithrombotic and antiplatelet effects.
	Ciprofloxacin	Theoretical decreased drug effect	Caution with use of this combination	Preliminary evidence suggests fennel may reduce drug bioavailability by nearly 50%. Caution with combination and separate dose administration.
	CYP450 substrates (CYP3A4)	Theoretical increased risk of drugs effects and adverse effects	Caution with use of this combination	In vitro evidence suggests fennel may inhibit activity of CYP3A4, which may theoretically increase the risk of drug effects and adverse effects.
	Oestrogens (e.g. oral contraceptives and HRT)	Theoretical additive effects	Caution with use of this combination	Some constituents of fennel have oestrogenic activity. Theoretically, large doses of fennel may affect drug action by competing for oestrogen receptor binding sites. Clinical significance is unclear.
	Tamoxifen	Theoretical decrease in drug effect	Caution with use of this combination	Some constituents of fennel have oestrogenic activity. Theoretically, large doses of fennel may decrease drug effectiveness. Clinical significance is unclear, but caution is advised.

Continued

ACNM herbal interactions table—cont'd				
Herbal medicine	Drug/drug class	Potential outcome	Recommendations	Comments
Fucus versiculosis	Anticoagulant/ antiplatelet drugs	Theoretical increased risk of bleeding	Monitor – may not be clinically significant	In vitro evidence suggests a constituent of kelp may have anticoagulant properties. Clinical research, however, suggests that a clinically relevant interaction is unlikely due to poor absorption. Patients should be monitored.
	Lithium	Case report of hyperthyroidism	Caution with use of this combination	A case reports describes hyperthyroidism with concomitant use of lithium and kelp.
	Thyroid medication	Additive effects	Caution with use of this combination	Kelp contains a significant amount of iodine. Evidence suggests concomitant use with thyroid medication may have additive effects and result in hypothyroidism. A case report describes iodine-induced thyrotoxicosis in a patient with an enlarged thyroid gland after ingestion of a kelp-containing tea.
Galega officinalis	Anticoagulant/ antiplatelet drugs	Theoretical increased risk of bleeding	Monitor – clinical significance is unclear	In vitro studies suggest goat's rue may have antiplatelet properties. There is a theoretical increased risk of bleeding and bruising when used with anticoagulant or antiplatelet drugs.
	Antidiabetic drugs	Theoretical additive effects	Monitor – clinical significance is unclear	Goat's rue may theoretically potentiate the hypoglycaemic effects of antidiabetic drugs. Clinical significance has not been established, but caution is advised. Dosage adjustments may be required.
Ganoderma lucidum	Anti-cancer therapy	Theoretical improved outcomes	Combination may be beneficial – medical supervision recommended	Animal studies suggest reishi extracts may provide protective benefits against the adverse effects associated with some antineoplastic drugs, including myelosuppression, and may improve therapeutic outcomes.Several mechanisms have been proposed. Further clinical trial evidence is needed to establish the benefits and risks associated with concomitant use.
	Anticoagulant/ antiplatelet drugs	Theoretical increased risk of bleeding	Monitor – clinical significance is unclear	Limited evidence suggests that high-dose use (···> 3g daily) of reishi mushrooms may have antiplatelet properties. This effect has not been shown at doses of <··· 1.5g daily.
	Antidiabetic drugs	Theoretical additive effects	Monitor – clinical significance is unclear	It has been proposed that reishi mushrooms may have hypoglycaemic effects based on animal studies. Additive effects are theoretically possible, with an increased risk of hypoglycaemia.
	Antihypertensive drugs	Theoretical additive effects	Monitor – clinical significance is unclear	Animal studies suggest reishi mushrooms may have hypotensive properties. Additive effects are theoretically possible, with an increased risk of hypotension.
	Antimicrobial therapy	Theoretical improved outcomes	Combination may be beneficial – medical supervision recommended	In vitro research has demonstrated synergy between reishi mushroom and several antibiotics. Reishi may have antibacterial properties and may enhance immune response.

ACNM herbal interactions table—cont'd				
Herbal medicine	**Drug/drug class**	**Potential outcome**	**Recommendations**	**Comments**
Ganoderma lucidum cont'd	Antiviral therapy	Theoretical improved outcomes	Combination may be beneficial – medical supervision recommended	In vitro research has demonstrated synergy between reishi mushroom and acyclovir. Reishi may have antiviral effects against HSV1 and HSV2 and may enhance immune response. More research is needed to establish safety and efficacy of concomitant use.
Garcinia mangostana	Anticoagulant/ antiplatelet drugs	Theoretical increased risk of bleeding	Caution with use of this combination	In vitro and animal research suggests mangosteen may have antiplatelet activity. There is a theoretical increased risk of bleeding, although data is limited.
Gentiana lutea	Antihypertensive drugs	Theoretical additive effects	Monitor – speculative	Traditional use suggests gentian may have hypotensive properties. Theoretically, the combination may have additive effects, but the interaction is speculative.
Ginkgo biloba	Antibiotics – aminoglycosides e.g. gentamycin	Theoretical decreased drug adverse effects	Monitor – unlikely to be of benefit	Animal research has reported that ginkgo may have protective effects against the ototoxicity and nephrotoxicity associated with use of gentamycin. Another study, however, reported that concomitant use of ginkgo increased the incidence of ototoxicity. Benefits in humans are considered unlikely. The doses used in animal studies were very high and do not translate to normal therapeutic doses of gingko. Theoretical benefits can also not be extrapolated to other antibiotics.
	Anticoagulants/ antiplatelet drugs	Possible increased risk of bleeding	Caution with use of this combination	Several studies suggest that ginkgo inhibits platelet aggregation, which appears to be due to the action of the constituent ginkgolide B. A number of case studies have described serious bleeding events in patients taking ginkgo. However, population-based studies and clinical trials have produced mixed results, with evidence suggesting that gingko may not exhibit significant effects on platelet aggregation with short-term use. Analysis of the records of a large medical database suggests that when warfarin and ginkgo are taken concurrently, there is a 38% increased risk of bleeding. This interaction has not been shown in studies with other anticoagulant or antiplatelet drugs. Caution is advised until further safety data becomes available, especially with longer-term use.
	Anticonvulsant drugs	Theoretical increased risk of seizures	Caution with use of this combination	Large amounts of ginkgotoxin, which is found in ginkgo seeds, has been shown to cause neurotoxicity and seizures. Only trace amounts of ginkgotoxin are found in ginkgo leaf and it has been proposed that toxicity and seizures are unlikely with use of ginkgo leaf extract. There are, however, anecdotal reports of seizures occurring in epileptic patients following use of ginkgo. Evidence is inconclusive, but caution is recommended.

Continued

ACNM herbal interactions table—cont'd				
Herbal medicine	**Drug/drug class**	**Potential outcome**	**Recommendations**	**Comments**
Ginkgo biloba cont'd	Antidepressant drugs	Theoretical decreased drug effects	Caution with use of this combination	Animal and in vitro studies suggest that ginkgo may increase serotonin reuptake, which could theoretically decrease drug efficacy. Significance is unclear.
	Antidiabetic drugs	Possible altered drug effects	Caution with use of this combination	Ginkgo may influence insulin secretion and metabolism in type 2 diabetics. Theoretically, gingko may alter response to antidiabetic drugs, with variable effects reported in different patients. The effect ginkgo has on insulin secretion may be patient-specific, and also relate to which antidiabetic medications are being taken.
	Buspirone	Theoretical risk of adverse effects	Caution with use of this combination	A case report describes the development of hypomania in a patient after adding ginkgo and St John's wort to her existing regimen of fluoxetine and buspirone.
	CYP450 substrates (CYP1A2, CYP2C9, CYP2D6, CYP3A4)	Theoretical increased risk of toxicity	Caution with use of this combination	Preliminary evidence suggests that ginkgo may modestly inhibit CYP1A2, CYP2C9 and CYP2D6. There is conflicting evidence as to whether ginkgo inhibits or induces CYP3A4. Theoretically, inhibition of these enzymes can reduce the rate of drug metabolism and increase risk of toxicity. Caution is advised until further data becomes available.
	CYP450 substrates (CYP2C19, CYP3A4)	Theoretical decreased drug effect	Caution with use of this combination	Preliminary evidence suggests that ginkgo may modestly induce CYP2C19 and CYP3A4. There is conflicting evidence as to whether ginkgo inhibits or induces CYP3A4. Enzyme induction may theoretically increase the rate of drug metabolism and decrease drug effectiveness. Caution is advised until further data becomes available.
	Donepezil	Possible additive effects	May be beneficial – medical supervision recommended	Co-administration of ginkgo and donepezil in a group of patients with Alzheimer's disease did not have a major effect on drug pharmacokinetics and pharmacodynamics. Effects may therefore be additive and beneficial, but monitoring is recommended.
	Fluoxetine	Theoretical risk of adverse effects	Caution with use of this combination	A case report describes the development of hypomania in a patient after adding ginkgo and St John's wort to her existing regimen of fluoxetine and buspirone.
	Haloperidol	Possible enhanced drug effect	May be beneficial – medical supervision recommended	Research suggests that gingko may enhance drug effects and reduce drug adverse effects in schizophrenic patients. A small but well-designed study reported that ginkgo enhanced the effectiveness of haloperidol in schizophrenic patients.

ACNM herbal interactions table—cont'd				
Herbal medicine	**Drug/drug class**	**Potential outcome**	**Recommendations**	**Comments**
Ginkgo biloba cont'd	HIV-drugs – non-nucleoside reverse transcriptase inhibitors (NNRTIs) e.g. efavirenz, raltegravir	Possible altered drug effect	Caution with use of this combination	Ginkgo may influence activity of drugs in this class, but results have been conflicting. Two case reports describe a reduction in concentration of efavirenz with use of gingko. A pharmacokinetic study showed a small effect on raltegravir, but clinical significance was unclear. It is possible that variations in response may relate to the different drugs in this class being metabolised by different CYP450 enzymes.
	HMGCoA reductase inhibitors (statins) e.g. atorvastatin and simvastatin	Theoretical decreased drug effects	Caution with use of this combination	Ginkgo has been shown to significantly increase the clearance of atorvastatin and simvastatin, which may theoretically reduce drug efficacy.
	Omeprazole	Possible decreased drug levels	Caution with use of this combination	Ginkgo has been shown to decrease plasma concentrations of omeprazole in a study conducted in healthy volunteers. It has been proposed that this was due to induction of CYP2C19.
	Selective serotonin-reuptake inhibitors (SSRIs)	Possible decreased drug-induced sexual dysfunction	May be beneficial – medical supervision recommended	Ginkgo may theoretically help to ameliorate symptoms of sexual dysfunction associated with use of SSRIs, based on limited and conflicting data. Preliminary data suggested a benefit, but subsequent data has not been as positive. Response may vary significantly between individuals.
Glycine max	Antibiotics	Theoretical decreased herbal action	Monitor – clinical significance is unclear	Theoretically, antibiotics may decrease the action of soy isoflavones by disturbing gastrointestinal bacteria. This may theoretically impair conversion of isoflavones to the active form. The interaction is speculative and only likely to be relevant with long-term antibiotic use.
	Antidiabetic drugs	Additive effects theoretically possible	Caution with use of this combination	Clinical research suggests that soy-based diets may reduce fasting blood glucose levels. Theoretically, concomitant use may have additive effects, which could be beneficial for the management of diabetes. Caution is advised due to the theoretical risk of hypoglycaemia.
	Antihypertensive drugs	Additive effects theoretically possible	Monitor – clinical significance is unclear	Clinical evidence suggests that soy protein may modestly lower blood pressure in individuals with hypertension. Effects may be additive, but patients should be monitored for hypotension.
	Chemotherapeutic drugs e.g. vincristine, vinblastine, cisplatin, daunorubicin	Theoretical beneficial interaction	Caution with use of this combination	In vitro evidence suggests soy isoflavones may potentially enhance drug anti-tumour effects with certain chemotherapeutic agents. Clinical significance is unknown and safety of this combination has not been established. Medical supervision is warranted.

Continued

ACNM herbal interactions table—cont'd				
Herbal medicine	**Drug/drug class**	**Potential outcome**	**Recommendations**	**Comments**
Glycine max cont'd	L-Thyroxine (Levothyroxine)	Possible decreased drug effects	Caution with use of this combination	Preliminary evidence suggests that soy-based formulas may decrease thyroxine levels in infants with congenital hypothyroidism. It is unclear if this interaction occurs in other patient populations. Soy may theoretically affect thyroid function, although this effect does not appear to be clinically significant based on current evidence.
	Monoamine oxidase inhibitors (MAOIs)	Theoretical increased risk of drug adverse effects	Avoid combination	Fermented soy products such as tofu and soy sauce contain tyramine, which may theoretically interact with MAOIs and increase the risk of a hypertensive crisis. The amount of tyramine in fermented soy products is usually relatively small, but concentrations can vary.
	Oestrogens e.g. HRT	Theoretical altered drug action	May be beneficial – medical supervision recommended	Data is conflicting on the interaction between soy and oestrogenic drugs. Some sources suggest that soy isoflavones theoretically inhibit the effects of HRT due to competition for oestrogen-binding receptors, while others suggest soy may have additive beneficial effects. Caution is advised until more data becomes available.
	Progesterone	Possible increased bone loss	Monitor – clinical significance is unclear	Results of a small clinical study suggest that while both soy milk and progesterone patches had bone-sparing effects when used alone, when used in combination it resulted in bone loss. Further data is required to establish clinical significance.
	Tamoxifen	May antagonise drug effect	Avoid combination	Soy may interfere with drug action due to the oestrogenic effects of soy isoflavones. Preliminary evidence suggests that the soy isoflavones genistein and diadzen may antagonise drug anti-tumour effect. Results from studies have been conflicting, which may be due to dose variations. Caution is advised until more data becomes available.
	Warfarin	Theoretical decreased drug effect	Caution with use of this combination	A case report describes a possible interaction between soy milk and warfarin. The data is inconclusive.
Glycyrrhiza glabra	Antihypertensive drugs	Theoretical decreased drug effect and increased hypertension	Caution with use of this combination	Licorice can significantly raise blood pressure with regular high-dose intake. This adverse effect appears to occur to a greater extent in patients with high blood pressure than in those with normal blood pressure.
	Cisplatin	Theoretical decreased drug effects	Caution with use of this combination	Licorice has been reported to reduce drug therapeutic effect in animal models. Clinical significance is unclear.

ACNM herbal interactions table—cont'd				
Herbal medicine	**Drug/drug class**	**Potential outcome**	**Recommendations**	**Comments**
Glycyrrhiza glabra cont'd	Corticosteroids	Theoretical increased drug adverse effects	Caution with use of this combination	High-dose intake of licorice may potentiate drug duration and activity and decrease drug excretion. This could theoretically lead to an increased risk of drug adverse effects. The combination may also increase the risk of potassium loss and potassium depletion.
	Cyclosporin	Theoretical decreased drug effects	Caution with use of this combination	Licorice has been reported to reduce drug therapeutic effects in animal models. Clinical significance is unclear, but caution is advised due to the risk of serious consequences.
	CYP450 substrates (CYP2B6)	Theoretical increased risk of adverse effects	Monitor – clinical significance is unclear	Licorice may inhibit activity of CYP2B6 based on in vitro studies. These interactions have not been demonstrated in humans.
	CYP450 substrates (CYP2C9)	Theoretical altered drug effects	Monitor – clinical significance is unclear	Evidence about the effect of licorice on CYP2C9 activity is conflicting. Some studies suggest licorice induces enzyme activity, while others suggest enzyme inhibition. Caution is advised until more data becomes available.
	CYP450 substrates (CYP3A4)	Theoretical decreased drug effects	Caution with use of this combination	Licorice appears to induce CYP3A4 metabolism, which may theoretically reduce drug effectiveness. Caution is advised until further data becomes available.
	Digoxin	Increased risk of drug adverse effects	Caution with use of this combination	There is an increased risk of potassium loss and drug adverse effects with regular consumption of large quantities of licorice. Small occasional consumption is not expected to affect digoxin efficacy or toxicity. Caution is advised.
	Diuretic drugs (thiazide and loop)	Increased risk of potassium loss	Caution with use of this combination	There is an increased risk of hypokalaemia with overuse of licorice in combination with potassium-depleting diuretics such as thiazides and loop diuretics.
	Non-steroidal anti-inflammatory drugs (NSAIDs)	Decreased drug gastric adverse effects	Combination may be beneficial	Licorice and DGL confer gastroprotective effects which may help to reduce the incidence of gastric irritation associated with NSAIDs and aspirin.
	Laxatives including herbal laxatives	Increased risk of potassium loss	Caution with use of this combination	The overuse or misuse of licorice in combination with stimulant laxatives increases the risk of potassium depletion, which may have health consequences.
	Oestrogens e.g. oral contraceptives and HRT	Theoretical increased drug adverse effects	Caution with use of this combination	Case reports suggest that licorice may increase the risk of drug adverse effects. Use with caution at high doses for > 2 weeks.
	Warfarin	Theoretical decreased drug effects	Caution with use of this combination	An animal study suggested that licorice may increase drug metabolism and decrease drug effects. The interaction is, however, speculative and there is currently no evidence that constituents of licorice have anticoagulant effects.

Continued

ACNM herbal interactions table—cont'd				
Herbal medicine	**Drug/drug class**	**Potential outcome**	**Recommendations**	**Comments**
Grifolia frondosa	Antidiabetic drugs	Possible additive effects	Caution with use of this combination	Preliminary clinical research suggests maitake mushrooms may lower blood glucose levels in type 2 diabetic patients. Concomitant use with antidiabetic drugs may result in additive effects and an increased risk of hypoglycaemia.
	Antihypertensive drugs	Theoretical additive effects	Caution with use of this combination	Animal research suggests maitake mushrooms may lower blood pressure. Theoretically, concomitant use with antihypertensive drugs may result in additive effects and an increased risk of hypotension.
	Warfarin	Theoretical increased risk of bleeding	Caution with use of this combination	A case report describes an increase in INR when a patient who was previously stabilised on warfarin commenced taking maitake mushrooms. It has been proposed that this may have been due to protein displacement of warfarin, resulting in increased anticoagulant effect. Caution is advised until more data becomes available.
Guaiacum officinale	Lithium	Increased risk of drug toxicity	Caution with use of this combination	This herb may have diuretic properties. Theoretically, combined use may reduce lithium excretion and increase the risk of lithium toxicity.
Gymnena sylvestre	Antidiabetic drugs	Possible additive effects	Caution with use of this combination	Gymnema has clinically relevant hypoglycaemic effects in type 2 diabetics according to a number of clinical studies. The combination will be additive and potentially be beneficial. Caution is recommended as dosage adjustments may be needed to avoid hypoglycaemia.
	Insulin	Additive effects possible	Caution with use of this combination	Gymnema has clinically relevant hypoglycaemic effects in type 1 diabetics. The combination will be additive and potentially beneficial. Caution is recommended as dosage adjustment may be needed to avoid hypoglycaemia.
Harpagophytum procumbens	Acid-reducing drugs e.g. H$_2$ antagonists and proton pump inhibitors	Theoretical decreased drug effect	Monitor – clinical significance is unclear	Devil's claw may increase gastric acidity. Use may theoretically counteract drug acid-reducing action, resulting in decreased drug effect. More data is needed to establish relevance.
	CYP450 substrates (CYP2C19, CYP2C9, CYP3A4)	Theoretical increased risk of drug toxicity	Monitor – clinical significance is unclear	Limited in vitro studies suggest that devil's claw may inhibit CYP2C19, CYP2C9 and CYP3A4. This may theoretically lead to increased drug serum levels and risk of toxicity with drugs metabolised by these enzymes. These interactions are speculative and have not been demonstrated in humans.
	Non-steroidal anti-inflammatory drugs (NSAIDs)	Possible additive effects possible	Combination may be beneficial	Additive anti-inflammatory effects may allow for a decrease in NSAID dose and this will reduce the risk of drug adverse effects. This beneficial interaction is supported by evidence.

ACNM herbal interactions table—cont'd				
Herbal medicine	**Drug/drug class**	**Potential outcome**	**Recommendations**	**Comments**
Harpagophytum procumbens cont'd	Warfarin	Theoretical increased risk of bleeding	Caution with use of this combination	A case report describes symptoms of purpurea in a patient that took devil's claw with warfarin. Findings were inconclusive, but caution is recommended.
Hericium erinaceus	Anticoagulant/ antiplatelet drugs	Theoretical increased risk of bleeding	Caution with use of this combination	In vitro evidence suggests this herb has antiplatelet activity. Combined use with anticoagulant and antiplatelet drugs will theoretically increase the risk of bleeding and bruising.
	Antidiabetic drugs	Theoretical additive effects	Caution with use of this combination	Animal studies suggest this herb may lower blood glucose levels. Additive effects are theoretically possible, increasing the risk of hypoglycaemia. Caution is advised until more data becomes available.
Hibiscus sabdariffa	Antidiabetic drugs	Theoretical additive effects	Caution with use of this combination	Preliminary evidence suggests roselle may lower blood glucose levels. Effects may be additive, with a theoretical risk of hypoglycaemia.
	Antihypertensive drugs	Theoretical increased risk of hypotension	Monitor – clinical significance is unclear	Limited studies suggest that roselle may lower blood pressure. The interaction may be beneficial but patients should be monitored for hypotension.
	Chloroquine	Reduced drug effect	Avoid combination	Roselle has been shown to significantly reduce the bioavailability of chloroquine. Concomitant use may reduce drug efficacy and should be avoided.
Hippophea rhamnoides	Anticoagulant/ antiplatelet drugs	Theoretical increased risk of bleeding	Caution with use of this combination	Limited research suggests sea buckthorn has antiplatelet properties. Concomitant use with anticoagulant and antiplatelet drugs will theoretically increase the risk of bleeding and bruising.
	Antihypertensive drugs	Theoretical increased risk of hypotension	Monitor – clinical significance is unclear	Limited studies suggest that sea buckthorn may have hypotensive properties. Additive beneficial effects are theoretically possible, but monitor for hypotension.
Humulus lupulus	Alcohol	Increased risk of sedation	Caution with use of this combination	Hops may potentiate the sedative effects of alcohol.
	CNS depressant drugs	Increased risk of sedation	Caution with use of this combination	Hops may potentiate the sedative effects of CNS depressant drugs.
	CYP450 substrates (CYP1A1, CYP1A2, CYP1B1)	Theoretical increased risk of adverse effects	Monitor – may not be clinically significant	Hops may inhibit CYP1A1, CYP1A2 and CYP1B1 enzymes according to in vitro studies. This may theoretically increase the risk of drug adverse effects, although this interaction has not been reported in humans.
	CYP450 substrates (CYP3A4)	Theoretical decreased drug effects	Monitor – may not be clinically significant	Hops may induce CYP3A4 enzyme based on in vitro studies. Theoretically, combined use may decrease drug effect. Caution is advised although this interaction has not been demonstrated in humans.

Continued

ACNM herbal interactions table—cont'd				
Herbal medicine	**Drug/drug class**	**Potential outcome**	**Recommendations**	**Comments**
Humulus lupulus cont'd	Oestrogen e.g. oral contraceptives & HRT or anti-oestrogenic drugs	Theoretical altered drug effect	Monitor – may not be clinically significant	In vitro studies suggest that certain hops constituents can bind to oestrogen receptors and potentially alter drug efficacy. The interaction may not be clinically relevant, but patients can be monitored.
Hydrastis canadensis	Anticoagulant/ antiplatelet drugs	Theoretical increased risk of bleeding	Caution with use of this combination	In vitro and animal studies suggest that berberine, a constituent of goldenseal, may inhibit platelet aggregation. There is a theoretical increased risk of bleeding, although this has not been demonstrated in human studies. Caution is advised.
	Antidiabetic drugs	Theoretical additive effects	Caution with use of this combination	Berberine in goldenseal may lower blood glucose levels, theoretically increasing the risk of hypoglycaemia.
	Antihypertensive drugs	Theoretical additive effects	Caution with use of this combination	Berberine in goldenseal may have hypotensive effects, theoretically having additive effects. The interaction may not be clinically significant, but monitor for hypotension.
	Antimicrobial agents	Theoretical additive effects	Combination may be beneficial	Constituents of goldenseal have antimicrobial effects against several organisms. Due to poor absorption of the alkaloids, it is unclear if the serum concentrations will be sufficiently high to make a clinical difference. There is, however, a theoretical additive effect.
	CNS depressant drugs	Theoretical additive effects	Caution with use of this combination	Berberine in goldenseal may have sedative effects. Theoretically, this may result in additive effects and a risk of excessive sedation, although clinical significance of this interaction is unclear.
	Cyclosporin	Risk of increased drug effects	Caution with use of this combination	A clinical study reported that berberine, which is a constituent of goldenseal, significantly increased drug serum levels in renal-transplant patients. Theoretically, concomitant use may increase the risk of drug toxicity.
	CYP2D6 substrates	Theoretical risk of increased drug effects	Caution with use of this combination	Goldenseal has been shown to significantly inhibit CYP2D6 enzyme activity, theoretically leading to an increased risk of drug toxicity and adverse effects.
	CYP450 substrates (CYP2D9, CYP2E1, 3A4)	Theoretical risk of increased drug effects	Caution with use of this combination	Goldenseal may inhibit CYP2C9, CYP2E1 and CYP3A4 enzyme activity based on in vitro studies. This may theoretically lead to an increased risk of drug toxicity and adverse effects, although clinical significance is unclear.
	Digoxin	Risk of increased drug effects	Caution with use of this combination	A small increase in drug peak levels has been reported with use of this combination. Caution is advised until more data becomes available.
	Laxatives	Risk of decreased drug effect	Monitor – may not be clinically significant	Goldenseal may have an anti-diarrhoeal effect. This may theoretically reduce effectiveness of laxatives.

ACNM herbal interactions table—cont'd				
Herbal medicine	**Drug/drug class**	**Potential outcome**	**Recommendations**	**Comments**
Hydrastis canadensis cont'd	Midazolam	Risk of increased drug effects	Caution with use of this combination	Goldenseal has been shown to increase midazolam blood concentrations in two clinical studies.
	P-gp substrates	Possible altered drug effects	Caution with use of this combination	There is conflicting data as to whether goldenseal affects P-gp or not, and if so, whether it inhibits or induces P-gp. Caution is advised until more data becomes available.
	Tacrolimus	Risk of increased drug effects	Caution with use of this combination	An increased incidence of drug adverse effects was reported in a case study where goldenseal and tacrolimus were used concurrently.
Hypericum perforatum	Antidepressant drugs (SSRIs e.g. paroxetine or SNRIs e.g. venlafaxine)	Increased risk of serotonin-related adverse effects	Avoid combination	Concomitant use of St John's wort and selective serotonin antagonists (SSRI antidepressants) may increase the risk of adverse effects and serotonin syndrome. The combination should be avoided.
	Antidepressants (tricyclics e.g. amitriptyline, nortriptyline)	Decreased drug effect	Caution with use of this combination	St John's wort may reduce drug effect due to induction of the CYP3A4 enzyme and P-gp drug transporter.
	Antiepileptic drugs (barbiturates e.g. phenytoin, phenobarbital)	Decreased drug effect	Avoid combination	St John's wort may increase the rate of drug metabolism, which can potentially result in decreased drug effect. The interaction is considered likely to be clinically significant, and may lead to an increased risk of seizures.
	Antineoplastic drugs	Decreased drug effect	Avoid combination	St John's wort may increase the rate of drug metabolism, which can potentially result in decreased drug effect. The interaction is considered likely to be clinically significant.
	Benzodiazepines (e.g. alprazolam, midazolam)	Decreased drug effect	Avoid combination	St John's wort may increase the rate of drug metabolism, which can potentially result in decreased drug effect. The interaction is considered likely to be clinically significant.
	Buproprion	Decreased drug effect	Caution with use of this combination	St John's wort may increase the rate of drug metabolism, which can potentially result in decreased drug effect. The interaction is considered likely to be clinically significant.
	Clopidogrel	Theoretical increased risk of bleeding	Caution with use of this combination	Preliminary evidence suggest St John's wort may increase antiplatelet activity of clopidogrel, which could potentially increase the risk of bleeding. Evidence is inconclusive.
	Contraceptive drugs	Decreased drug effect	Avoid combination	St John's wort may increase the rate of drug metabolism, which can potentially result in decreased drug effect. The interaction is considered likely to be clinically significant and may increase the risk of break-through bleeding and unplanned pregnancy.

Continued

ACNM herbal interactions table—cont'd				
Herbal medicine	Drug/drug class	Potential outcome	Recommendations	Comments
Hypericum perforatum cont'd	Cyclosporin	Decreased drug effect	Avoid combination	St John's wort may increase the rate of drug metabolism, which can potentially result in decreased drug effect. The interaction is considered likely to be clinically significant.
	CYP450 substrates (CYP3A4 & CYP2C19)	Decreased drug effects	Avoid combination	St John's wort significantly induces cytochrome P450 enzymes CYP2C19 and CYP3A4. This has been shown to increase the rate of clearance of drugs metabolised via these pathways, potentially leading to reduced drug concentration and drug effectiveness. A significant number of medicinal drugs are metabolised via these two pathways, especially CYP3A4.
	CYP450 substrates (CYP1A2, CYP2B6, CYP2C9)	Decreased drug effects	Caution with use of this combination	St John's wort may moderately induce activity of CYP1A2, CYP2B6 and CYP2C9. This may increase the rate of drug metabolism, leading to reduced drug effect. The extent of enzyme induction appears to be less pronounced than the effect on CYP3A4 and CYP2C19.
	Dextromethorphan	Increased risk of serotonin-related adverse effects	Caution with use of this combination	Concomitant use of St John's wort and dextromethorphan may increase the risk of adverse effects and serotonin syndrome.
	Digoxin	Decreased drug effect	Avoid combination	St John's wort may increase the rate of drug metabolism, which can potentially result in decreased drug effect. The interaction is considered likely to be clinically significant.
	Docetaxel	Decreased drug effect	Avoid combination	St John's wort may increase the rate of drug metabolism, which can potentially result in decreased drug effect. The interaction is considered likely to be clinically significant and may compromise cancer treatment.
	Fenfluramine	Increased risk of serotonin-related adverse effects	Avoid combination	Concomitant use of St John's wort and fenfluramine may increase the risk of adverse effects and serotonin syndrome.
	Gliclazide	Decreased drug effect	Caution with use of this combination	St John's wort may increase the rate of drug metabolism, which can potentially result in decreased drug effect.
	HMGCoA reductase inhibitors (statins) e.g. simvastatin	Decreased drug effect	Caution with use of this combination	St John's wort may increase the rate of drug metabolism, which can potentially result in decreased drug effect. A study describes a 28% reduction in plasma concentrations of simvastatin.
	Imatinib	Decreased drug effect	Avoid combination	St John's wort may increase the rate of drug metabolism, which can potentially result in decreased drug effect. The interaction is likely to be clinically significant.

ACNM herbal interactions table—cont'd				
Herbal medicine	**Drug/drug class**	**Potential outcome**	**Recommendations**	**Comments**
Hypericum perforatum cont'd	Irinotecan	Decreased drug effect	Avoid combination	St John's wort may increase the rate of drug metabolism, which can potentially result in decreased drug effect. The interaction is likely to be clinically significant.
	Methadone	Decreased drug effect	Avoid combination	St John's wort may increase the rate of drug metabolism, which can potentially result in decreased drug effect. The interaction is likely to be clinically significant.
	Methylphenidate	Decreased drug effect	Monitor – may not be clinically significant	A case report describes a decrease in drug effectiveness in a man who had been stabilised on methylphenidate and commenced use of St John's wort.
	Monoamine oxidase inhibitors	Increased risk of adverse effects	Caution with use of this combination	Concomitant use of St John's wort and drugs in this class may increase the risk of adverse effects and serotonin syndrome.
	Non-nucleoside reverse transcriptase inhibitors (NNRTIs)	Decreased drug effect	Avoid combination	St John's wort may increase the rate of drug metabolism, which can potentially result in decreased drug effect. The interaction is likely to be clinically significant and may result in treatment failure of HIV.
	Omeprazole	Decreased drug effect	Caution with use of this combination	St John's wort may increase the rate of drug metabolism, which can potentially result in decreased drug effect.
	Photosensitising drugs	Increased risk of photosensitivity	Caution with use of this combination	St John's wort may increase the risk of photosensitivity due to the hypericin content. Clinical significance is unclear, but caution is recommended.
	P-glycoprotein (P-gp) substrates	Decreased efficacy with drugs that areP-gp substrates	Avoid combination	St John's wort induces P-glycoprotein (P-gp), which may lead to decreased drug effect. P-gp is a transport protein that can actively pump drugs out of cells.
	Psoralen plus UVA therapy	Increased risk of photosensitivity	Caution with use of this combination	St John's wort may increase the risk of photosensitivity reactions due to the hypericin content.
	Protease inhibitors (e.g. indinavir)	Decreased drug effect	Avoid combination	St John's wort may increase the rate of drug metabolism, which can potentially result in decreased drug effect. The interaction is likely to be clinically significant and may result in treatment failure of HIV.
	Proton-pump inhibitors (e.g. omeprazole)	Decreased drug effect	Caution with use of this combination	St John's wort may increase the rate of drug metabolism, which can potentially result in decreased drug effect.
	Tacrolimus	Decreased drug effect	Avoid combination	St John's wort may increase the rate of drug metabolism, which can potentially result in decreased drug effect. The interaction is likely to be clinically significant.
	Tramadol	Increased risk of serotonin-related adverse effects	Avoid combination	Concomitant use of St John's wort and tramadol may theoretically increase the risk of adverse effects and serotonin syndrome.

Continued

ACNM herbal interactions table—cont'd				
Herbal medicine	**Drug/drug class**	**Potential outcome**	**Recommendations**	**Comments**
Hypericum perforatum cont'd	Triptans (e.g. sumatriptan, zolmitriptan) for migraines	Increased risk of serotonin-related adverse effects	Avoid combination	Concomitant use of St John's wort and selective serotonin agonists (triptans) may theoretically increase the risk of adverse effects and serotonin syndrome. Case reports describe interactions between St John's wort and 'triptan' drugs, used for migraines.
	Tyrosine kinase inhibitors (e.g. imatinib)	Decreased drug effect	Avoid combination	St John's wort may increase the rate of drug metabolism, which can potentially result in decreased drug effect. The interaction is likely to be clinically significant.
	Warfarin	Decreased drug effect – risk of clotting	Avoid combination	St John's wort may increase the rate of drug metabolism, which can potentially result in decreased drug effect. This may increase the risk of clotting. The interaction is likely to be clinically significant.
	Zolpidem	Decreased drug effect	Avoid combination	A small study reported a reduction in zolpidem serum levels with concurrent use of St John's wort.
Inula helenium	CYP450 substrates (CYP2C19, CYP3A4)	Theoretical decreased drug effects	Caution with use of this combination	In vitro and animal studies suggest that a constituent of elecampane, alantolactone, may induce CYP3A4 and CYP2C19 enzyme activity. This may theoretically result in increased rate of drug metabolism and decreased efficacy. Clinical significance is unknown.
	CNS depressant drugs	Theoretical additive sedative effects	Caution with use of this combination	Sedative effects have been observed with use of elecampane in animal models. There is a risk of additive sedation with concomitant use. Clinical significance is unclear.
Iris versicolor	Digoxin	Theoretical increased risk of drug adverse effects	Avoid this combination	Theoretically, the combination of blue flag with digoxin increases the risk of drug adverse effects. Clinical evidence of this interaction is lacking, but caution is advised due to potentially serious consequences.
	Diuretics	Theoretical increased risk of potassium loss	Caution with use of this combination	There is an increased risk of hypokalaemia with overuse of blue flag in combination with potassium-depleting diuretics such as thiazides and loop diuretics.
	Warfarin	Theoretical increased risk of bleeding	Caution with use of this combination	Blue flag has stimulant laxative effects and may cause diarrhoea. This may theoretically elevate INR and increase the risk of bleeding with excessive intake of herb.
Juglans cinerea	Corticosteroids	Increased risk of potassium loss	Caution with use of this combination	Overuse of this herb may compound drug-induced potassium loss.
	Digoxin	Increased risk of drug adverse effects	Caution with use of this combination	Overuse of this herb may compound drug-induced potassium loss, leading to an increased risk of drug adverse effects and toxicity.

ACNM herbal interactions table—cont'd				
Herbal medicine	**Drug/drug class**	**Potential outcome**	**Recommendations**	**Comments**
Juglans cinerea cont'd	Diuretics	Increased risk of potassium loss	Caution with use of this combination	Overuse of this herb in combination with potassium-depleting diuretics, such as thiazides and loop diuretics, increases the risk of potassium loss.
	Stimulant laxatives	Increased risk of diarrhoea and loss of electrolytes	Caution with use of this combination	Both herb and drug have laxative effects, and may lead to loss of electrolytes.
Juniperus communis	Antidiabetic drugs	Theoretical additive effects	Monitor – clinical significance is unclear	Juniper may have hypoglycaemic properties based on animal studies. Additive effects are theoretically possible, increasing the risk of hypoglycaemia. Caution is advised until more data becomes available.
	Diuretics	Possible additive effects	Monitor – clinical significance is unclear	Juniper has been shown to have diuretic properties. Additive effects are theoretically possible, but the clinical significance has not been established.
Lavendula officinalis	Antidepressant drugs, including imipramine	Potentially beneficial additive effects	May be beneficial – medical supervision recommended	Oral lavender may improve management of mild to moderate depression. Concomitant use may be beneficial, but caution is recommended until more data becomes available.
	Antihypertensive drugs	Theoretical additive effects	Monitor – may not be clinically significant	Lavender oil in combination with other essential oils as aromatherapy may slightly lower blood pressure. Additive effects are theoretically possible. The interaction may be beneficial, but patients should be monitored for hypotension.
	Barbiturates	Theoretical increased effects and sedation	Caution with use of this combination	Lavender may theoretically potentiate the effects of barbiturates and increase the risk of sedation.
	Benzodiazepines	Possible additive effects and increased risk of sedation	Caution with use of this combination	Lavender may theoretically potentiate the effects of benzodiazepines and increase the risk of sedation. Clinical studies have reported that oral lavender has beneficial anxiolytic effects.
	CNS depressant drugs	Theoretical increased effects and sedation	Caution with use of this combination	Lavender may theoretically potentiate the effects of CNS depressant drugs and increase the risk of sedation.
Lentinus edodes	Immunosuppressant drugs	Theoretical decreased drug effect	Caution with use of this combination	Shiitake mushrooms may have immuno-stimulant activity based on laboratory studies. Theoretically this could counteract drug immunosuppressant effects. Clinical significance is unclear, but caution is advised.
Leonurus cardiaca	CNS depressant drugs including benzodiazepines	Possible additive effects and adverse effects	Caution with use of this combination	Evidence suggests motherwort has additive effects when used with CNS depressant drugs such as benzodiazepines. The combination may lead to excessive drowsiness.
Lepidium meyenii	Antidepressant drugs (SSRIs, SNRIs)	Possible decreased drug adverse effects	Combination may be beneficial	Maca may help to alleviate sexual dysfunction caused by SSRIs/SNRIs. This is according to the findings of a small clinical trial conducted in postmenopausal women who were taking these drugs for depression.

Continued

ACNM herbal interactions table—cont'd				
Herbal medicine	**Drug/drug class**	**Potential outcome**	**Recommendations**	**Comments**
Leptandra virginica	Digoxin	Altered drug effects	Caution with use of this combination	Theoretically, overuse or abuse of black root may increase the risk of adverse effects of cardiac glycosides such as digoxin. Some other sources suggest black root may reduce drug effectiveness by binding to the drug in the GI tract. Evidence is inconclusive, but caution is advised.
	Diuretics	Theoretical risk of hypokalaemia	Caution with use of this combination	Black root may lead to diuretic-induced potassium loss. There is a theoretical increased risk of hypokalaemia when used with potassium-depleting diuretics.
Leptospermum scoparium	Antibiotics for wound healing	Theoretical additive effect	Combination may be beneficial	Topical use of manuka honey may improve wound healing and have antimicrobial properties. Theoretically, honey dressings may provide an additive beneficial effect when used with antibiotics.
Linum usitatissimum	Anticoagulant/antiplatelet drugs	Theoretical increased risk of bleeding	Monitor – may not be clinically significant	Flaxseed may have antiplatelet properties. Concomitant use with anticoagulant and antiplatelet drugs will theoretically increase the risk of bleeding and bruising. The interaction is unlikely to be clinically significant at normal therapeutic doses.
	Antidiabetic drugs	Theoretical additive effects	Monitor – may not be clinically significant	Flaxseed may lower blood glucose levels. Additive effects are theoretically possible, increasing the risk of hypoglycaemia. Clinical significance at normal therapeutic doses is unclear.
	Antihypertensive drugs	Theoretical additive effects	Monitor – may not be clinically significant	Flaxseed may slightly lower diastolic pressure, leading to a theoretical additive effect. Clinical significance at normal therapeutic doses is unclear.
	Furosemide	Theoretical decreased drug absorption	Monitor – may not be clinically significant	Preliminary in vitro research suggests flaxseed may decrease drug absorption. The clinical significance is unknown.
	Ketoprofen	Theoretical decreased drug absorption	Monitor – may not be clinically significant	Preliminary in vitro research suggests flaxseed may decrease drug absorption. The clinical significance is unknown.
	Oestrogens e.g. HRT and oral contraceptives	Theoretical decreased drug effect	Monitor – may not be clinically significant	Flaxseed may theoretically have mild oestrogenic effects. Theoretically, the lignans in flaxseed may compete with oestrogens for binding sites and reduce drug effect. The interaction is speculative.
	Paracetamol	Theoretical decreased drug absorption	Monitor – may not be clinically significant	Preliminary in vitro research suggests flaxseed may decrease drug absorption. The clinical significance is unknown.
Lobelia inflata	Lithium	Theoretical increased risk of drug toxicity	Caution with use of this combination	Lobelia may have diuretic properties. Theoretically, this might decrease drug excretion and potentiate the risk of drug toxicity.

ACNM herbal interactions table—cont'd				
Herbal medicine	**Drug/drug class**	**Potential outcome**	**Recommendations**	**Comments**
Lobelia inflata cont'd	Nicotine replacement therapy	Theoretical additive effects	May be beneficial – medical supervision recommended	Some studies suggest a possible benefit for lobelia as an aid to smoking cessation, although results have been conflicting. Theoretically, combined use may be beneficial, under appropriate medical supervision.
Lycopus virginicus	L-Thyroxine (levothyroxine)	Possible reduced drug effect	Avoid combination	Bugleweed may reduce drug effect by blocking peripheral conversion of thyroxine to T3.
Magnolia spp	Alcohol	Theoretical additive sedative effects	Caution with use of this combination	Magnolia may have sedative properties. Theoretically, concomitant use with alcohol may lead to excessive drowsiness and decreased motor function.
	Anticoagulant/ antiplatelet drugs	Additive effects theoretically possible	Monitor – may not be clinically significant	Magnolia may have some antiplatelet properties. The combination may theoretically increase the risk of bleeding, although this has not been demonstrated in humans.
	Barbiturates	Theoretical additive sedative effects	Caution with use of this combination	Magnolia may have sedative properties. Theoretically, concomitant use with barbiturates may lead to excessive drowsiness and decreased motor function.
	Benzodiazepines	Theoretical additive sedative effects	Caution with use of this combination	Magnolia may have sedative properties. Theoretically, concomitant use with benzodiazepines may lead to excessive drowsiness and decreased motor function.
	CNS depressant drugs	Theoretical additive sedative effects	Caution with use of this combination	Magnolia may have sedative properties. Theoretically, concomitant use with CNS depressant drugs may lead to excessive drowsiness and decreased motor function.
Marrubium vulgare	Antidiabetic drugs	Theoretical additive effects	Monitor – may not be clinically significant	White horehound may slightly lower blood glucose. Preliminary clinical research suggests this effect may not be clinically significant when used in combination with antidiabetic drugs.
	Antihypertensive drugs	Theoretical additive effects	Monitor – may not be clinically significant	White horehound may lower blood pressure according to animal research. Theoretically, this may increase the risk of hypotension when used with antihypertensive drugs.
Matricaria recutita	Anticoagulant/ antiplatelet drugs	Case report of increased bleeding	Monitor – may not be clinically significant	One case report describes internal bleeding and raised INR following ingestion of 4–5 cups of chamomile tea and use of a chamomile-based skin lotion in an elderly woman taking warfarin. Caution is recommended until more data becomes available.
	Antidiabetic drugs	Theoretical additive effects	Combination may be beneficial	Chamomile may have hypoglycaemic effects. The interaction may be beneficial and improve outcomes based on limited research, but patients should be monitored for hypoglycaemia.

Continued

ACNM herbal interactions table—cont'd				
Herbal medicine	Drug/drug class	Potential outcome	Recommendations	Comments
Matricaria recutita cont'd	CNS depressant drugs including benzodiazepines	Theoretical additive sedative effects	Caution with use of this combination	Chamomile has sedative effects and may theoretically interact with CNS depressants drugs, including benzodiazepines, leading to additive effects and adverse effects.
	CYP450 substrates (CYP2C9, CYP2D6, CYP3A4)	Theoretical risk of increased adverse effects	Monitor – may not be clinically significant	Chamomile may inhibit activity of CYP2D6, CYP2C9 and CYP3A4 according to in vitro studies. This may theoretically increase the risk of drug-related adverse effects, although this interaction has not been reported in humans.
	Oestrogen e.g. HRT and oral contraceptives	Theoretical altered drug effects	Monitor – may not be clinically significant	Chamomile may have oestrogenic effects and may theoretically interact with oestrogenic drugs. The interaction may not be clinically significant, but patients should be monitored.
	Tamoxifen	Theoretical altered drug effects	Caution with use of this combination	Chamomile may have oestrogenic effects and theoretically interact with anti-oestrogen drugs (e.g. tamoxifen). Oral chamomile should be avoided in hormone-sensitive tumours until more safety data becomes available.
Medicargo sativa	Antidiabetic drugs	Theoretical additive effects	Monitor – may not be clinically significant	Alfalfa may have hypoglycaemic properties based on animal research and one case report. Additive effects are theoretically possible, increasing the risk of hypoglycaemia. Caution is advised until more data becomes available.
	Immunosuppressant drugs	Theoretical decreased drug effects	Caution with use of this combination	Alfalfa may theoretically counteract drug immunosuppressant effects due to herb immune-stimulating activity. Evidence of an interaction is limited, but caution is advised. Alfalfa has been shown to exacerbate symptoms of SLE and should be avoided in these patients.
	Oestrogen (e.g. HRT and oral contraceptives)	Theoretical altered drug effects	Caution with use of this combination	Alfalfa contains isoflavonoids with oestrogenic properties. Theoretically, this may interfere with drug effects at high dose, although data is limited.
	Photosensitising drugs	Increased risk of photosensitivity	Caution with use of this combination	Excessive intake of alfalfa may potentiate drug-induced photosensitivity reactions.
	Warfarin	Decreased drug effect	Avoid combination	Alfalfa contains high amounts of vitamin K. Concurrent use can oppose drug action and increase the risk of clotting.
Melissa officinalis	Alcohol	Increased risk of sedation	Caution with use of this combination	Lemon balm may potentiate the sedative effects of alcohol.
	Antidiabetic drugs	Theoretical additive effects	Monitor – may not be clinically significant	Lemon balm may have hypoglycaemic properties based on one animal study. Additive effects are theoretically possible, increasing the risk of hypoglycaemia. More study is needed to assess the clinical significance of this effect.
	Barbiturates	Increased risk of sedation	Caution with use of this combination	Lemon balm may potentiate the sedative effects of barbiturates.

ACNM herbal interactions table—cont'd				
Herbal medicine	**Drug/drug class**	**Potential outcome**	**Recommendations**	**Comments**
Melissa officinalis cont'd	CNS depressant drugs	Increased risk of sedation	Caution with use of this combination	Lemon balm may potentiate the sedative effects of CNS depressant drugs
	Thyroid hormones	Theoretical altered thyroid function	Monitor – may not be clinically significant	Theoretically, lemon balm may alter thyroid function and reduce thyroid hormone levels based on animal and in vitro studies. Evidence is weak.
Mentha x piperita	Acid-reducing drugs (antacids, H_2-antagonsist and proton pump inhibitors)	Increased herbal adverse effects; decreased management of condition	Caution with use of this combination	Drugs that decrease stomach acid and raise gastric pH may cause premature dissolution of enteric-coated peppermint oil. In addition, peppermint oil may relax the lower oesophageal sphincter in some individuals, leading to increased risk of heartburn, reflux and GORD and potentially counteracting drug effects.
	CYP450 substrates (CYP1A2, CYP2C19, CYP2C9, CYP3A4)	Decreased drug metabolism with theoretical increased risk of adverse effects	Caution with use of this combination	Peppermint oil may inhibit activity of CYP1A2, CYP2C19, CYP2C9 and CYP3A4. This may theoretically increase blood levels of drugs metabolised via these enzyme pathways. The interactions appear to only occur at very high doses of peppermint oil, but caution is advised.
	Cyclosporin	Increased risk of drug effects and adverse effects	Caution with use of this combination	Peppermint oil may inhibit drug metabolism by inhibition of CYP3A4. This may theoretically increase drug bioavailability and the risk of adverse effects. An interaction between cyclosporin and peppermint oil has not been reported in human studies, but caution is advised.
	Felodipine	Increased risk of drug effects and adverse effects	Caution with use of this combination	A small clinical study reported that peppermint oil increased drug bioavailability and theoretically increased the risk of adverse effect. Peppermint has been shown to inhibit CYP3A4 enzyme activity in animal and in vitro studies. Patients taking felodipine with peppermint oil should be monitored for hypotension and other drug adverse effects.
	Simvastatin	Increased risk of drug effects and adverse effects	Monitor – may not be clinically significant	Preliminary animal research suggests peppermint oil may increase drug bioavailability and theoretically increase the risk of adverse effects. Clinical significance is unclear.
	Iron	Decreased iron absorption	Monitor – may not be clinically significant	High intake of peppermint tea has been shown to inhibit iron absorption. Dose separation is advised.
Mentha spicata	CNS depressant drugs	Increased risk of sedation	Monitor – may not be clinically significant	Spearmint may have sedative effects, based on animal studies. Theoretically, this may potentiate the sedative effects of CNS depressant drugs, although clinical significance is unknown.
	Hepatotoxic drugs	Theoretical increased risk of liver damage	Monitor – may not be clinically significant	Animal research suggests that high-dose spearmint tea may increase markers of liver damage (AST and ALT). Theoretically, excessive intake may have additive detrimental effects on the liver when used with hepatotoxic drugs.

Continued

ACNM herbal interactions table—cont'd				
Herbal medicine	Drug/drug class	Potential outcome	Recommendations	Comments
Menyanthes trifoliata	Anticoagulant / antiplatelet drugs	Theoretical additive effects	Monitor – may not be clinically significant	Bogbean may theoretically have some antiplatelet properties although data is limited. Concomitant use with anticoagulant and antiplatelet drugs will theoretically increase the risk of bleeding and bruising.
Momordica charantia	Antidiabetic drugs	Possible additive effects possible	Caution with use of this combination	Bitter melon has hypoglycaemic properties and may have additive effects when used with antidiabetic drugs. This interaction may be beneficial, but supervision is required due to the risk of hypoglycaemia.
Moringa oleifera folia	Antidiabetic drugs	Theoretical additive effects	Caution with use of this combination	Animal research suggests moringa may lower blood glucose levels. Concomitant use with antidiabetic drugs may result in additive effects and an increased risk of hypoglycaemia.
	Antihypertensive drugs	Theoretical additive effects	Monitor – may not be clinically significant	Animal research suggests moringa pod may lower blood pressure. Theoretically, concomitant use with antihypertensive drugs may result in additive effects and an increased risk of hypotension. This effect may not apply to other plant parts.
	CYP450 substrates (CYP3A4)	Theoretical increased drug levels	Monitor – may not be clinically significant	In vitro evidence suggests moringa may inhibit CYP3A4 activity. Theoretically, this may result in raised drug plasma levels and an increased risk of adverse effects and toxicity if taken with drugs that are CYP3A4 substrates.
	L-thyroxine (Levothyroxine)	Theoretical decreased drug effects	Monitor – may not be clinically significant	Theoretically, moringa may reduce effectiveness of L-thyroxine. Preliminary animal research suggests moringa may inhibit peripheral conversion of T4 to T3.
Morus alba	Antidiabetic drugs	Possible additive effects	Caution with use of this combination	White mulberry has hypoglycaemic properties according to limited studies. Additive effects are theoretically possible, increasing the risk of hypoglycaemia. Caution is advised until more data becomes available.
Mucuna pruriens	Anaesthesia	Possible increased risk of cardiac arrhythmias	Caution with use of this combination	Theoretically, this herb may increase the risk of cardiac arrhythmias with certain anaesthetics (cyclopropane and halogenated hydrocarbons), due to the L-dopa constituent. Patients should be advised to withdraw herbal therapy 2 weeks prior to surgery.
	Antidiabetic drugs	Theoretical risk of hypoglycaemia	Caution with use of this combination	Limited data suggests this herb may have hypoglycaemic effects. Additive effects are theoretically possible, increasing the risk of hypoglycaemia. Caution is advised until more data becomes available.
	Anti-Parkinson's disease drugs	Possible additive effects	May be beneficial – medical supervision recommended	This herb contains L-dopa. Preliminary evidence suggests this herb may help to improve symptoms of Parkinson's disease when used in combination with conventional drugs for Parkinson's disease.

ACNM herbal interactions table—cont'd				
Herbal medicine	**Drug/drug class**	**Potential outcome**	**Recommendations**	**Comments**
Mucuna pruriens cont'd	Antipsychotic drugs	Possible decreased drug effects	Caution with use of this combination	This herb appears to have dopaminergic effects and so may theoretically decrease the antidopaminergic effects of some antipsychotic medications. Caution is advised.
	Levodopa	Possible additive effects	May be beneficial – medical supervision recommended	This herb contains L-dopa. Preliminary evidence suggests this herb may lead to quicker onset of action, duration of action and higher drug levels when used with levodopa. While theoretically this may be beneficial, medical supervision is required due to a risk of toxicity.
	Methyldopa	Increased risk of adverse effects	Avoid combination	Additive hypotensive effects are possible when used with methyldopa. Methyldopa may also inhibit peripheral decarboxylation of the herb constituent, L-dopa, which increases the risk of L-dopa toxicity.
	Monoamine oxidase inhibitors (MAOIs)	Increased risk of adverse effects	Avoid combination	An increased risk of hypertensive crisis has been proposed with this combination, due to the L-dopa constituent. The risk appears greatest with non-selective MAOIs.
	Tricyclic antidepressants	Increased risk of adverse effects	Caution with use of this combination	Rare reports suggest concomitant use may lead to hypertension and dyskinesia. Caution is advised until further data becomes available.
Myrtilli fructus	Anticoagulant / antiplatelet drugs	Additive effects theoretically possible	Caution with use of this combination	Preliminary evidence suggests that bilberry may inhibit platelet aggregation at high dose, due to the anthocyanidin content. Combined use may increase the risk of bleeding and bruising.
	Antidiabetic drugs	Additive effects theoretically possible	Caution with use of this combination	Bilberry may have hypoglycaemic properties according to limited animal and human research findings. Additive effects are theoretically possible, increasing the risk of hypoglycaemia.
Nepeta cataria	CNS depressant drugs	Increased risk of sedation	Monitor – may not be clinically significant	Catnip may have sedative effects, based on limited research. Theoretically, this may potentiate the sedative effects of CNS depressant drugs, although clinical significance is unknown.
	Lithium	Increased risk of drug toxicity	Caution with use of this combination	Catnip may have diuretic properties. Theoretically, combined use may reduce lithium excretion and increase the risk of lithium toxicity.
Nigella sativa	Analgesics	Theoretical additive effects	Monitor – may not be clinically significant	Animal studies suggest that nigella may have analgesic effects at high doses.
	Anticoagulant/ antiplatelet drugs	Theoretical additive effects	Caution with use of this combination	Preliminary evidence suggests that nigella may inhibit platelet aggregation. Combined use with anticoagulants may theoretically may increase the risk of bleeding.
	Anticonvulsants	Theoretical additive effects	Monitor – may not be clinically significant	A small clinical study reported that nigella had anticonvulsant effects. Clinical significance is unknown, but caution is advised.

Continued

ACNM herbal interactions table—cont'd				
Herbal medicine	**Drug/drug class**	**Potential outcome**	**Recommendations**	**Comments**
Nigella sativa cont'd	Antidiabetic drugs	Theoretical additive effects	Monitor – may not be clinically significant	Nigella may have hypoglycaemic properties according to limited animal and human research findings. Additive effects are theoretically possible, increasing the risk of hypoglycaemia. Caution is advised until more data becomes available.
	Antihypertensive drugs	Possible additive effects	Monitor – may not be clinically significant	Nigella may have mild hypotensive effects, and so theoretically enhance the effects of drugs that lower blood pressure. Significance is unclear.
	Antineoplastic drugs	Possible additive beneficial effects theoretically possible	Combination may be beneficial – medical supervision recommended	Preliminary evidence suggests that constituents of nigella may have antineoplastic activity. Nigella may potentiate the drug effects of some antineoplastic drugs, according to some animal studies. There may theoretically be potential for beneficial interactions, but further research is required to determine significance.
	Cisplatin	Theoretical decreased drug adverse effects	Combination may be beneficial	The constituent thymoquinone may be protective against cisplatin-induced nephrotoxicity based on animal models. More data is required.
	CNS depressant drugs	Theoretical increased risk of sedation	Monitor – may not be clinically significant	Nigella may have sedative effects, based on animal studies. Theoretically, this may potentiate the sedative effects of CNS depressant drugs.
	Doxorubicin	Theoretical decreased drug adverse effects	Combination may be beneficial	The constituent thymoquinone may be protective against doxorubicin-induced cardiotoxicity based on animal models. More data is required.
	Immunosuppressant drugs	Theoretical decreased drug effect	Caution with use of this combination	Nigella may have immuno-stimulant properties based on animal and in vitro research which could theoretically antagonise the effects of immunosuppressant drugs. Some animal studies have, however, suggested nigella may suppress immune function. Caution is advised until more data becomes available.
Nigra alba	Antidiabetic drugs	Additive effects theoretically possible	Monitor – may not be clinically significant	Black mulberry may have hypoglycaemic properties according to limited studies. Additive effects are theoretically possible when used with antidiabetic drugs, but significance is unclear. Monitor for hypoglycaemia.
Ocimum tenuiflorum	Anticoagulant/ antiplatelet drugs	Theoretical additive effects	Monitor – may not be clinically significant	Holy basil may have antiplatelet properties according to animal research. Concomitant use with anticoagulant and antiplatelet drugs will theoretically increase the risk of bleeding and bruising.
	Phenobarbital	Theoretical increased risk of sedation	Monitor – may not be clinically significant	Results of an animal study suggest that holy basil may increase phenobarbital-induced sleeping time. Clinical significance is unclear. It is unknown whether this interaction would apply to other barbiturates or CNS depressant drugs, but patients should be monitored.

ACNM herbal interactions table—cont'd				
Herbal medicine	**Drug/drug class**	**Potential outcome**	**Recommendations**	**Comments**
Olea europea	Anticoagulant/ antiplatelet drugs	Theoretical additive effects	Monitor – may not be clinically significant	Olive leaf extract may have antiplatelet properties according to limited research. Concomitant use with anticoagulant and antiplatelet drugs will theoretically increase the risk of bleeding and bruising.
	Antidiabetic drugs	Theoretical additive effects	Monitor – may not be clinically significant	Olive leaf extract was found to lower blood glucose concentrations and improve glucose regulation in a small study. Additive effects are therefore theoretically possible. Patients should be monitored for hypoglycaemia with concomitant use.
	Antihypertensive drugs	Theoretical additive effects	Monitor – may not be clinically significant	Olive leaf extract may have hypotensive properties and additive effects are theoretically possible. The interaction may be beneficial but patients should be monitored for hypotension.
Origanum vulgare	Anticoagulant/ antiplatelet drugs	Theoretical additive effects	Monitor – may not be clinically significant	Oregano may have antiplatelet / anticoagulant properties according to limited research. Concomitant use with anticoagulant and antiplatelet drugs will theoretically increase the risk of bleeding and bruising.
	Antidiabetic drugs	Theoretical additive effects	Monitor – may not be clinically significant	Oregano may lower blood glucose concentrations according to animal and in vitro studies. Additive effects are theoretically possible, increasing the risk of hypoglycaemia.
Paeonia lactiflora	Anticoagulant/ antiplatelet drugs	Theoretical additive effects	Monitor – may not be clinically significant	White peony may have antiplatelet / anticoagulant properties according to limited research. Concomitant use with anticoagulant and antiplatelet drugs will theoretically increase the risk of bleeding and bruising.
	Phenytoin	Theoretical decreased drug effect	Caution with use of this combination	Limited research suggest white peony root may reduce phenytoin plasma levels, which could theoretically decrease drug effectiveness.
Panax ginseng	Anticoagulant/ antiplatelet drugs	Theoretical increased risk of bleeding	Caution with use of this combination	In vitro studies suggest that panax ginseng may inhibit platelet aggregation; however, research conducted in humans has not shown a clinically relevant effect. Caution is advised until more data becomes available.
	Antidiabetic drugs	Possible additive effects	Caution with use of this combination	Evidence suggests that panax ginseng may have hypoglycaemic properties. Additive effects are possible, with an increased risk of hypoglycaemia.
	Caffeine	Additive stimulant effects	Caution with use of this combination	Theoretically, caffeine may exacerbate the stimulant effects of panax ginseng.
	Cancer therapy (chemotherapy and radiotherapy)	Possible improved quality of life and outcomes	May be beneficial – medical supervision recommended	Preliminary research suggests panax ginseng may improve quality of life, psychological and social wellbeing and reduce mortality in breast cancer patients. Medical supervision is recommended.

Continued

ACNM herbal interactions table—cont'd				
Herbal medicine	**Drug/drug class**	**Potential outcome**	**Recommendations**	**Comments**
Panax ginseng cont'd	CYP450 substrates (CYP2D6, CYP3A4)	Theoretical increased risk of drug toxicity	Caution with use of this combination	Limited evidence suggests that panax ginseng may inhibit CYP2D6 and CYP3A4. However, findings of one study with midazolam suggested that panax ginseng may induce CYP3A4. Caution is advised until further data becomes available about the nature and extent of effect on CYP450 enzymes.
	Digoxin	Theoretical increased risk of drug toxicity	Caution with use of this combination	Panax ginseng may lead to an increase in serum digoxin levels according to limited data. This would theoretically increase the risk of drug adverse effects and toxicity.
	Imatinib	Theoretical increased risk of hepatotoxicity	Caution with use of this combination	A case report describes drug-induced hepatoxicity when panax ginseng was added to an established regimen of imatinib.
	Immunosuppressant drugs	Theoretical decreased drug effectiveness	Caution with use of this combination	The immune-stimulant properties of panax ginseng may theoretically counteract the action of immunosuppressant drugs.
	Insulin	Possible additive effects	Caution with use of this combination	Evidence suggests that panax ginseng may have hypoglycaemic properties. Additive effects are possible, with an increased risk of hypoglycaemia.
	Midazolam	Possible decreased drugs effect	Caution with use of this combination	Clinical research suggests that panax ginseng may reduce drug plasma concentration, theoretically decreasing drug effect. It has been proposed that this interaction was due to CYP3A4 induction.
	Monoamine oxidase inhibitors (MAOIs)	Possible increased risk of adverse effects	Caution with use of this combination	Concomitant use of panax ginseng and phenelzine may result in symptoms of mania, insomnia, headache and tremors according to some case reports. Caution is advised until more data becomes available.
	Nifedipine	Theoretical altered drug effects	Caution with use of this combination	One study reported that panax ginseng may inhibit drug metabolism, which would theoretically increase the risk of adverse effects. This interaction has not been reported in other studies.
	Oestrogens	Theoretical altered drug effects	Caution with use of this combination	Panax ginseng appears to have oestrogenic effects due to ginsenosides. Theoretically, large doses may compete with hormone replacement therapy for oestrogen receptors and alter drug activity. Clinical significance is unclear.
	Raltegravir	Increased risk of liver toxicity	Caution with use of this combination	A case report suggests that concomitant use of panax ginseng with raltegravir resulted in elevated liver enzymes.
	Stimulant drugs	Additive stimulant effects	Caution with use of this combination	Theoretically, panax ginseng may exacerbate the effects of stimulant drugs. Caution is advised.

ACNM herbal interactions table—cont'd				
Herbal medicine	**Drug/drug class**	**Potential outcome**	**Recommendations**	**Comments**
Panax notoginseng	Oestrogenic and anti-oestrogenic drugs	Speculative effects	Monitor – speculative interaction	Panax notoginseng may have oestrogenic effects based on in vitro studies. Theoretically, this herb may interact with oestrogens and anti-oestrogenic drugs; however, this interaction is speculative.
Panax quinquefolius	Antidiabetic drugs	Possible additive effects	Caution with use of this combination	Clinical evidence suggests that American ginseng has hypoglycaemic properties. Additive effects are theoretically possible, increasing the risk of hypoglycaemia. Caution is advised until more data becomes available.
	Antineoplastic drugs (breast cancer)	Improved quality of life	May be beneficial – medical supervision recommended	Clinical evidence suggests that use of American ginseng may improve quality of life in patients with breast cancer whilst undergoing treatment.
	Immunosuppressant drugs	Theoretical decrease in drug effectiveness	Caution with use of this combination	The immune-stimulant properties of American ginseng may theoretically counteract the action of immunosuppressant drugs. Caution is advised.
	Monoamine oxidase inhibitors (MAOIs)	Increased risk of adverse effects	Caution with use of this combination	One case report describes how concomitant use of phenelzine and an unspecified ginseng resulted in insomnia, headache and tremors. Another case report suggests this combination may result in hypomania. Caution is advised.
	Warfarin	Decreased drug effectiveness	Avoid combination	Evidence from a randomised control trial (RCT) reported that America ginseng significantly reduced INR, warfarin plasma concentrations and drug effectiveness. Concomitant use should be avoided.
Passiflora incarnate	Barbiturates	Increased risk of sedation	Caution with use of this combination	Passionflower may potentiate the sedative effects of barbiturates.
	Benzodiazepines	Increased risk of sedation	Caution with use of this combination	A case report describes a suspected interaction between lorazepam and a combination of passionflower and valerian. Concomitant use led to symptoms including excessive drowsiness, dizziness, shaking and palpitations.
	CNS depressant drugs	Increased risk of sedation	Caution with use of this combination	Passionflower may potentiate the sedative effects of CNS depressant drugs.
Pelargonium sidoides	Anticoagulant/ antiplatelet drugs	Additive effects theoretically possible	Monitor – may not be clinically significant	Pelargonium (Umckaloabo) may have antiplatelet properties according to limited research. The combination may theoretically increase the risk of bleeding and bruising, although this has not been shown in studies.
	Immunosuppressant drugs	Theoretical decrease in drug effect	Caution with use of this combination	Pelargonium may have immuno-stimulant properties which could theoretically antagonise the effects of immunosuppressant drugs.

Continued

ACNM herbal interactions table—cont'd				
Herbal medicine	**Drug/drug class**	**Potential outcome**	**Recommendations**	**Comments**
Peumus boldo	Anticoagulant/ antiplatelet drugs	Theoretical increased risk of bleeding	Caution with use of this combination	Boldo may have antiplatelet properties according to limited evidence and an isolated case report. Concomitant use may theoretically increase the risk of bleeding and bruising.
	Hepatotoxic drugs	Theoretical increased risk of liver damage	Caution with use of this combination	Boldo may cause hepatotoxicity. Theoretically, the risk of liver damage is increased if boldo is used concomitantly with hepatotoxic drugs.
	Lithium	Increased risk of drug toxicity	Caution with use of this combination	Boldo may have diuretic properties. Theoretically, combined use may reduce lithium excretion and increase the risk of lithium toxicity.
	Tacrolimus	Possible decreased drug effectiveness	Avoid combination	A case report describes sub-therapeutic drug levels of tacrolimus following co-administration of boldo. Avoid this combination until further data becomes available.
Picrorhiza kurroa	Antidiabetic drugs	Possible additive effects	Monitor – may not be clinically significant	Picrorhiza may have hypoglycaemic properties according to limited animal studies. Additive effects are theoretically possible, increasing the risk of hypoglycaemia. Caution is advised until more data becomes available.
	Immunosuppressant drugs	Theoretical decreased drug effects	Caution with use of this combination	Picrorhiza appears to have immune-stimulant properties. This could theoretically antagonise the effects of immunosuppressant drugs. Caution is advised until further data becomes available.
Pimpinella anisum	Oestrogens e.g. oral contraceptives & HRT	Theoretical altered drug effects	Monitor – may not be clinically significant	In vitro studies have reported both oestrogenic and anti-oestrogenic effects with anise. This appears to be due to mechanisms relating to oestrogen-receptors modulation. The significance in humans is not known, but caution is advised.
	Tamoxifen	Theoretical altered drug effects	Caution with use of this combination	In vitro studies have reported both oestrogenic and anti-oestrogenic effects with anise. This appears to be due to mechanisms relating to oestrogen-receptors modulation. The significance in humans is not known, but caution is advised.
Pinus pinaster	Anticoagulant/ antiplatelet drugs	Theoretical increased risk of bleeding	Caution with use of this combination	Pycnogenol may have antiplatelet properties according to clinical research. Concomitant use may theoretically increase the risk of bleeding and bruising.
	Antidiabetic drugs	Possible additive effects	Caution with use of this combination	Pycnogenol appears to have hypoglycaemic properties according to human studies. Additive effects are theoretically possible, increasing the risk of hypoglycaemia. Caution is advised until more data becomes available.

	ACNM herbal interactions table—cont'd			
Herbal medicine	**Drug/drug class**	**Potential outcome**	**Recommendations**	**Comments**
Pinus pinaster cont'd	Antihypertensive drugs (e.g. Ramipril)	Possible protective effects on renal function in patients at risk	May be beneficial – medical supervision recommended	A small study reported that pycnogenol conferred protective effects on renal function in a group of patients taking ramipril, who had advanced hypertension and a history of cardiovascular events.
	Cardiovascular drugs	Possible improved disease management	May be beneficial – medical supervision recommended	Pycnogenol appears to have antioxidant, antiplatelet and anti-inflammatory effects. A small study reported that pycnogenol was effective in improving endothelial function and reducing oxidative stress in patients with stable coronary artery disease.
	Immunosuppressant drugs	Theoretical decreased drug effects	Caution with use of this combination	Pycnogenol may have immuno-stimulant properties which could theoretically antagonise the effects of immunosuppressant drugs. Significance is unclear, but caution is advised until further data becomes available.
Piper longum	Propranolol	Theoretical increased drug bioavailability	Monitor – may not be clinically significant	Piperine, a constituent of Indian long pepper, may increase drug bioavailability based on a small preliminary study.
	Theophylline	Theoretical increased drug bioavailability	Monitor – may not be clinically significant	Piperine, a constituent of Indian long pepper, may increase drug bioavailability based on a small preliminary study.
Piper methysticum	Alcohol	Increased risk of sedation and liver damage	Avoid combination	Kava may potentiate the sedative effects of alcohol. There is also concern that concomitant use may increase the risk of hepatotoxicity.
	Benzodiazepines	Increased risk of sedation; may help with drug withdrawal	Avoid combination unless under medical supervision	Kava may potentiate the sedative effects of benzodiazepines. Kava may, however, also assist in benzodiazepine withdrawal. The combination should be avoided unless under close medical supervision.
	CNS depressant drugs	Increased risk of sedation	Avoid combination	Kava may potentiate the sedative effects of CNS depressant drugs.
	CYP450 substrates (CYP1A2, CYP2C19, CYP2C9, CYP2E1)	Increased risk of drug effects and adverse effects	Caution with use of this combination	Preliminary evidence suggests kava may significantly inhibit CYP2E1. This would theoretically decrease the rate of drug metabolism, which may result in an increased risk of adverse effects. It appears unlikely that kava will affect drugs metabolised by CYP1A2, CYP2D6, CYP2C19 or CYP3A4 based on current research, but caution is advised.
	Haloperidol	Theoretical increased risk of adverse effects	Caution with use of this combination	A case report describes symptoms of atrial flutter and hypoxia following co-administration of oral kava and intramuscular haloperidol and lorazepam.
	Hepatotoxic drugs	Increased risk of hepatotoxicity	Caution with use of this combination	Concomitant use of kava with hepatotoxic drugs may increase the risk of liver damage. This may include high-dose paracetamol.

Continued

ACNM herbal interactions table—cont'd				
Herbal medicine	**Drug/drug class**	**Potential outcome**	**Recommendations**	**Comments**
Piper methysticum cont'd	Levodopa	Symptoms of Parkinson's disease may worsen based oncase reports	Avoid combination	Several case reports describe how the combination of kava with levodopa has led to a significant increase in the number and duration of severe Parkinson's symptoms.
	Paracetamol	Increased risk of hepatoxicity at high drug dose	Caution with use of this combination	Kava may theoretically increase the risk of paracetamol-induced liver damage. This is unlikely to be a concern with normal therapeutic doses, but caution is advised.
	P-glycoprotein substrates	Theoretical increased drug effect	Caution with use of this combination	Kava may inhibit P-gp, based on limited data. Theoretically, this may increase drug effects of P-gp substrates, although this has not been demonstrated in human studies.
Piscidia erythrina/ piscipula	CNS depressant drugs	Theoretical increased risk of sedation	Caution with use of this combination	Jamaican dogwood may theoretically potentiate sedative adverse effects when used concomitantly with CNS depressant drugs.
Plantago ovata	Anticoagulants	Possible reduced drug absorption	Caution with use of this combination	Ispaghula may reduce drug absorption and theoretically reduce drug effect. No clinically significant interactions with warfarin have been reported.
	Antidiabetic drugs	Theoretical additive effects	May be beneficial – medical supervision recommended	Ispaghula may reduce blood glucose levels in patients with type 2 diabetes and potentially have additive effects. Close monitoring is recommended.
	Antihypertensive drugs	Theoretical additive effects	May be beneficial – medical supervision recommended	Ispaghula may reduce blood pressure. Additive beneficial effects are theoretically possible when used concomitantly with antihypertensive drugs. Monitor for hypotension.
	Carbamazepine	Reduced drug absorption possible	Caution with use of this combination	Ispaghula may reduce drug absorption and may theoretically interfere with drug effect.
	Lithium	Reduced drug absorption possible	Caution with use of this combination	Ispaghula may reduce drug absorption and theoretically reduce drug effect. An interaction between ispaghula and lithium salts has been described in one case report.
Polygonum multiflorum	Antidiabetic drugs	Theoretical additive effects	Caution with use of this combination	This herb may have hypoglycaemic properties. Additive effects are theoretically possible when used with antidiabetic drugs. Significance is unclear based on current evidence, but caution is advised due to a risk of hypoglycaemia.
	CYP450 substrates (CYP1A2, CYP2C19, CYP2C9, CYP3A4)	Theoretical risk of increased drug levels	Caution with use of this combination	In vitro evidence suggests this herb may inhibit activity of CYP1A2, CYP2C19, CYP2C9 and CYP3A4. There is a theoretical risk of increased drug levels and adverse effects with drugs metabolised by these enzymes. Clinical significance in humans is unknown based on current evidence.

ACNM herbal interactions table—cont'd

Herbal medicine	Drug/drug class	Potential outcome	Recommendations	Comments
Polygonum multiflorum cont'd	Digoxin	Theoretical increased risk of drug toxicity	Caution with use of this combination	Overuse of anthraquinone laxative herbs may theoretically increase the risk of hypokalaemia, which increases the risk of digoxin cardiotoxicity.
	Diuretics	Theoretical increased risk of hypokalaemia	Caution with use of this combination	This herb may result in potassium loss. Theoretically, there is an increased risk of hypokalaemia when used in combination with potassium-depleting diuretic drugs such as loop and thiazide diuretics.
	Hepatotoxic drugs	Increased risk of liver damage	Caution with use of this combination	Case reports suggest this herb may be hepatotoxic. There is a theoretical increased risk of liver damage when used concomitantly with hepatotoxic drugs.
	Oestrogens	Theoretical altered drug effect	Monitor – may not be clinically significant	This herb may have oestrogenic activity based on in vitro studies. Theoretically, high-dose use may interfere with HRT and oral contraceptive drugs due to competitive binding at oestrogen receptors.
	Stimulant laxatives	Theoretical additive effects	Caution with use of this combination	This herb has stimulant laxatives properties. Theoretically, concomitant use with stimulant laxatives drugs will increase the risk of fluid and electrolyte depletion.
	Warfarin		Caution with use of this combination	A case report describes acute hepatitis and an elevated INR when a patient, previously stabilised on warfarin, commenced intake of this herb. It has been proposed that this may have been due to diarrhoea caused by the herb's laxative effect.
Punica grantum	ACE-Inhibitors (ACE-I)	Theoretical additive effects	Caution with use of this combination	Pomegranate may have an action similar to ACE-inhibitors, leading to additive effects and an increased risk of hypotension. Monitor for hypotension and for signs of potassium depletion.
	Antihypertensive drugs	Theoretical additive effects	Caution with use of this combination	Pomegranate may modestly lower blood pressure. Additive effects are theoretically possible, with an increased risk of hypotension.
	Carbamazepine	Theoretical increased drug levels	Caution with use of this combination	Animal models suggest pomegranate juice may decrease the rate of carbamazepine metabolism and increase the serum levels.
	CYP450 substrates (CYP2C9, CYP2D6)	Theoretical increased drug levels	Caution with use of this combination	Animal models suggest pomegranate may inhibit activity of CYP2C9 and CYP2D6, which may theoretically lead to increased drug levels and adverse effects. Clinical significance in humans is currently unknown.
	CYP450 substrates (CYP3A4)	Theoretical altered drug levels	Caution with use of this combination	Evidence about the effect of pomegranate on CYP3A4 is contradictory. Some research has reported enzyme inhibition, while other studies have reported enzyme induction, and some have reported no effect. Caution is advised at high doses until more data becomes available.

Continued

ACNM herbal interactions table—cont'd				
Herbal medicine	**Drug/drug class**	**Potential outcome**	**Recommendations**	**Comments**
Punica grantum cont'd	Rosuvastatin	Theoretical increased drug adverse effects	Caution with use of this combination	A case report describes a patient on rosuvastatin that developed rhabdomyolysis 3 weeks after commencing pomegranate juice, 200 ml taken twice weekly. It is possible the patient was predisposed to this adverse effect as there was a history of elevated levels of creatine kinase.
	Tacrolimus	Theoretical increased drug levels	Avoid combination	A case report describes elevated drug levels while consuming concentrated pomegranate popsicles. More data is required to determine significance.
	Warfarin	Theoretical increased risk of bleeding	Caution with use of this combination	High intake of pomegranate juice may increase bleeding time in patients taking warfarin, based on two case reports. Warfarin is a CYP2C9 substrate and animal models have reported that pomegranate juice may inhibit this metabolising enzyme, potentially leading to increased drug levels.
Rehmannia glutinosa	Antidiabetic drugs	Theoretical additive effects	Caution with use of this combination	Rehmannia may have hypoglycaemic properties. Additive effects are theoretically possible, increasing the risk of hypoglycaemia. Caution is advised until more data becomes available.
	Irbesartan	Improved disease management in chronic renal disease	May be beneficial – medical supervision recommended	The results of one study of 480 patients with chronic renal disease suggest that the combination of rehmannia with irbesartan is more effective in reducing proteinuria than irbesartan alone.
Rhamnus purshiana	Corticosteroids	Theoretical increased risk of potassium loss	Caution with use of this combination	Overuse of cascara may compound drug-induced potassium loss. The interaction is speculative, but caution is advised.
	Digoxin	Theoretical risk of increased drug adverse effects	Caution with use of this combination	Overuse of cascara may compound drug-induced potassium loss, which may theoretically increase the risk of drug toxicity. The interaction is speculative, but caution is advised.
	Diuretics	Increased risk of potassium loss	Caution with use of this combination	Overuse of cascara in combination with potassium-depleting diuretics, such as thiazide and loop diuretics, may increase the risk of hypokalaemia.
	Stimulant laxatives	Increased risk of diarrhoea and electrolyte loss	Caution with use of this combination	Additive stimulant laxative effects may occur with concomitant use of this drug class and cascara. This may result in diarrhoea and loss of electrolytes.
Rheum palmatum	Corticosteroids	Increased risk of potassium loss	Caution with use of this combination.	Overuse of rhubarb may compound drug-induced potassium loss. The interaction is speculative, but caution is advised.
	Digoxin	Increased risk of drug toxicity	Caution with use of this combination	Overuse of rhubarb may compound drug-induced potassium loss, which theoretically increases the risk of drug toxicity. The interaction is speculative, but caution is advised.

ACNM herbal interactions table—cont'd				
Herbal medicine	**Drug/drug class**	**Potential outcome**	**Recommendations**	**Comments**
Rheum palmatum cont'd	Diuretics	Increased risk of potassium loss	Caution with use of this combination	Overuse of rhubarb in combination with potassium-depleting diuretics, such as thiazide and loop diuretics, may increase the risk of hypokalaemia. The interaction is speculative, but caution is advised.
	Nephrotoxic drugs	Increased risk of renal failure	Caution with use of this combination	A case report described renal failure linked to a rhubarb-containing supplement, possibly due to the anthraquinone constituent. The patient was also taking diclofenac (NSAID). It is unclear how much effect was due to rhubarb alone.
	Stimulant laxatives	Increased risk of diarrhoea and loss of electrolytes	Caution with use of this combination	Additive stimulant laxative effects may occur with concomitant use of this drug class and rhubarb. This may result in diarrhoea and loss of electrolytes.
Rhodiola rosea	Adriamycin	Theoretical decreased drug adverse effects	Combination may be beneficial	Preliminary evidence suggest rhodiola may reduce severity of drug-induced liver dysfunction. More data is needed to determine significance and likelihood of benefit.
	Antidepressant drugs e.g. paroxetine, escitalopram	Theoretical increased risk of adverse effects	Caution with use of this combination	A case report describes an interaction which appears to have been due to the addition of rhodiola to paroxetine in patient with depression. The patient experienced restlessness, trembling and a disordered state of consciousness. Another case report describes significant tachycardia occurring in a patient who took rhodiola in combination with escitalopram. Caution is advised.
	Antidiabetic drugs	Theoretical additive effects	Caution with use of this combination	Animal and in vitro studies suggest rhodiola may have hypoglycaemic properties due to alpha-glucosidase activity. Additive effects are theoretically possible, increasing the risk of hypoglycaemia. Caution is advised until more data becomes available.
	Antihypertensive drugs especially ACE-inhibitors	Possible additive effects	Monitor – may not be clinically significant	Animal and in vitro studies suggest rhodiola may lower blood pressure due to inhibition of angiotensin-converting enzyme (ACE). Additive effects are theoretically possible, with an increased risk of hypotension.
	CYP3A4 substrates	Theoretical increased risk of adverse effects	Monitor – may not be clinically significant	In vitro research suggests that rhodiola may inhibit CYP3A4. Theoretically, this may increase drug levels and the risk of adverse effects, although significance in humans has not been established.
	Immunosuppressant drugs	Theoretical decreased drug effects	Caution with use of this combination	Rhodiola may have immuno-stimulant properties which could theoretically antagonise the effects of immunosuppressant drugs. Significance is unclear, but caution is advised until further data becomes available.

Continued

ACNM herbal interactions table—cont'd				
Herbal medicine	**Drug/drug class**	**Potential outcome**	**Recommendations**	**Comments**
Rhodiola rosea cont'd	Monoamine oxidase inhibitors (MAOIs)	Theoretical altered drug effects	Caution with use of this combination	In vitro studies suggest that rhodiola may inhibit MAO-A receptors. There is a theoretical interaction with MAOI antidepressants, although effect and significance are unknown.
	P-glyocoprotein (P-gp) substrates	Theoretical increased drug effects	Caution with use of this combination	Rhodiola may inhibit P-gp, based on limited data. This may theoretically increase drug effects, although this has not been demonstrated in human studies.
Ricinus communis	Diuretics	Increased risk of hypokalaemia	Caution with use of this combination	Overuse of castor oil may exacerbate potassium loss due to diuretics.
Rosmarinus officinalis	Anticoagulant/ antiplatelet drugs	Theoretical increased risk of bleeding	Caution with use of this combination	In vitro and animal research suggests that rosemary may have antithrombotic and antiplatelet effects. Concomitant use with anticoagulant and antiplatelet drugs will theoretically increase the risk of bleeding and bruising.
	Iron supplements	Reduced iron absorption	Caution with use of this combination	Rosemary has been shown to reduce absorption of dietary iron and may theoretically decrease absorption of iron supplements. Dosage separation is recommended.
	P-glyocoprotein (P-gp) substrates	Theoretical increased drug effect	Caution with use of this combination	Rhodiola may inhibit P-gp, based on limited data. This may theoretically increase drug effects, although this has not been demonstrated in human studies.
Rumex acetosa	Mineral supplements (calcium, iron and zinc)	Possible reduced mineral absorption	Monitor – may not be clinically significant	Sorrel contains oxalates which may theoretically bind to minerals and reduce absorption. Clinical significance is unclear, but dosage separation is advised.
Rumex crispus	Digoxin	Theoretical increased risk of drug toxicity	Avoid this combination	Chronic use of yellow dock may result in potassium loss, which increases the risk of drug toxicity.
	Diuretics	Theoretical increased risk of potassium loss	Caution with use of this combination	Overuse of yellow dock in combination with potassium-depleting diuretics, such as thiazide and loop diuretics, will increase the risk of hypokalaemia.
Salix alba	Anticoagulant/ antiplatelet drugs	Theoretical increased risk of bleeding	Avoid this combination	Willow bark has been shown to have antithrombotic and antiplatelet activity. Concomitant use with anticoagulant and antiplatelet drugs will theoretically increase the risk of bleeding and bruising. Caution is also recommended with use of willow bark in combination with other salicylate-containing herbs, or herbs with anticoagulant properties.
	NSAIDs and opioid analgesics	Theoretical additive effects	Combination may be beneficial – monitor	Willow bark extract has been shown to provide additive pain-relieving effects when used in combination with NSAIDs or opioid drugs for rheumatic pain. There was no direct evidence of an interaction in this study, but patients should be monitored.

	ACNM herbal interactions table—cont'd			
Herbal medicine	**Drug/drug class**	**Potential outcome**	**Recommendations**	**Comments**
Salvia miltiorrhiza	Anticoagulant/ antiplatelet drugs	Possible increased risk of bleeding	Avoid this combination	Dan shen appears to have anticoagulant effects. A series of case reports suggest that dan shen may affect the pharmacokinetics of warfarin, leading to an increased INR and risk of bleeding. Avoid use with warfarin.
	Antihypertensive drugs	Possible additive effects	Caution with use of this combination	Dan shen may lower blood pressure; therefore there is a theoretical increased risk of hypotension when used with antihypertensive drugs. An in vitro study reported that dan shen may potentiate effects of captopril.
	CYP450 substrates (CYP3A4)	Theoretical decreased drug effects	Caution with use of this combination	Preliminary evidence suggests dan shen may induce CYP3A4 enzyme activity. This could theoretically lead to an increased rate of metabolism and decreased drug effect in drugs that are CYP3A4 substrates.
	Digoxin	Theoretical increased risk of drug toxicity	Avoid this combination	Dan shen has structural and pharmacological similarities to cardiac glycosides. Concomitant use could theoretically have additive effects and increase the risk of arrhythmias and drug toxicity.
	Midazolam	Theoretical decreased drug effect	Caution with use of this combination	A small study reported that dan shen significantly increased the rate of drug clearance, leading to decreased drug effect.
Salvia officinalis	Acetylcholinesterase inhibitors	Theoretical increase in drug effects and adverse effects	Caution with use of this combination	In vitro research suggests sage may inhibit acetylcholinesterase. Additive effects are theoretically possible with concomitant use of sage and acetylcholinesterase (AChE) inhibitors, such as donepezil, used for Alzheimer's disease. The interaction may potentially be beneficial, but there is an increased risk of cholinergic adverse effects.
	Anticholinergic drugs	Theoretical decreased drug effect	Monitor – may not be clinically significant	In vitro research suggests sage may increase acetylcholine levels. This may theoretically oppose the action of drugs with an anticholinergic action. Significance has not been established.
	Antidiabetic drugs	Theoretical additive effects	Caution with use of this combination	Preliminary research suggests that sage may have hypoglycaemic properties. Additive effects are theoretically possible, increasing the risk of hypoglycaemia. Caution is advised until more data becomes available.
	Cholinergic drugs	Theoretical additive drug effect	Monitor – may not be clinically significant	In vitro research suggests sage may increase acetylcholine levels. Theoretically, there may be additive effects when used in combination with drugs with cholinergic actions. Significance is unclear.
	CNS depressant drugs	Theoretical increased sedative effects	Monitor – may not be clinically significant	Some constituents of sage may have sedative effects. There is a theoretical risk of additive effects and adverse effects.

Continued

ACNM herbal interactions table—cont'd				
Herbal medicine	**Drug/drug class**	**Potential outcome**	**Recommendations**	**Comments**
Salvia officinalis cont'd	CYP450 substrates (CYP2C19, CYP2C9, CYP2D6, CYP3A4)	Theoretical increased risk of adverse effects.	Monitor – may not be clinically significant	Preliminary evidence suggests that sage may inhibit activity of CYP2C19, CYP2C9, CYP2D6 and CYP3A4 enzymes. This may theoretically increase drug concentrations and the risk of adverse effects. These interactions have not been demonstrated in human studies.
Sambucus nigra	Antidiabetic drugs	Theoretical additive effects	Caution with use of this combination	Elderflower may have hypoglycaemic properties according to in vitro studies. Additive effects are theoretically possible, increasing the risk of hypoglycaemia. Caution is advised until more data becomes available.
	Immunosuppressant drugs	Theoretical decreased drug effect	Caution with use of this combination	Elderberry may have immune-stimulant properties which could theoretically antagonise the effects of immunosuppressant drugs. Caution is advised.
Sceletium tortuosum	CNS depressant drugs	Theoretical increased risk of sedation	Monitor – may not be clinically significant	Sceletium may have sedative effects, based on in vitro studies. Theoretically, this may potentiate the sedative effects of CNS depressant drugs.
Schisandra chinensis	Benzodiazepines e.g. midazolam	Risk of increased drug levels and adverse effects.	Caution with use of this combination	A small study reported an interaction between schisandra and midazolam, leading to an increased drug concentration and theoretical increased risk of adverse effects. It is unclear if this is a drug class effect, but caution is advised with all benzodiazepines.
	CYP2C9 substrates	Theoretical decreased drug effects	Monitor – may not be clinically significant	Schisandra may induce activity of CYP2C9 based on animal models. This may theoretically lead to reduced drug effect of drugs metabolised by this enzyme pathway.
	CYP3A4 substrates	Theoretical altered drug effects	Monitor – may not be clinically significant	Schisandra has been shown to inhibit CYP3A4 enzyme activity in some animal studies, with other animal studies reporting that this herb induced CYP3A4 activity. Caution is advised until more data becomes available.
	Phenobarbital	Increased risk of sedation	Caution with use of this combination	Schisandra may potentiate the sedative effects of phenobarbital based on animal studies.
	Sirolimus and tacrolimus	Risk of increased drug levels and adverse effects	Avoid this combination	Schisandra has been shown to significantly increase concentration of both sirolimus and tacrolimus (immunosuppressants) in separate small studies conducted in healthy volunteers. Avoid this combination until further safety data becomes available.
	Warfarin	Theoretical decreased drug effects	Caution with use of this combination	Animal models suggest that schisandra may decrease warfarin levels, theoretically leading to decreased drug effect.

ACNM herbal interactions table—cont'd				
Herbal medicine	**Drug/drug class**	**Potential outcome**	**Recommendations**	**Comments**
Scutellaria baicalensis	Alcohol	Increased risk of sedation	Caution with use of this combination	Baical skullcap may theoretically potentiate the sedative effects of alcohol. Clinical significance is unclear, but caution is advised.
	Anticoagulant/ antiplatelet drugs	Theoretical increased risk of bleeding	Caution with use of this combination	Baical skullcap may have antiplatelet activity. Concomitant use with anticoagulant and antiplatelet drugs will theoretically increase the risk of bleeding and bruising.
	Antidiabetic drugs	Theoretical additive effects	Caution with use of this combination	Baical skullcap may enhance the antidiabetic effect of metformin, based on animal research. Additive effects are theoretically possible, increasing the risk of hypoglycaemia. Caution is advised until more data becomes available.
	Antihypertensive drugs	Theoretical additive effects	Monitor – may not be clinically significant	Baical skullcap may lower blood pressure. Additive effects are theoretically possible, with an increased risk of hypotension.
	Benzodiazepines	Theoretical additive effects	Caution with use of this combination	Baical skullcap may potentiate the therapeutic and sedative effects of benzodiazepines.
	CNS depressant drugs	Theoretical additive effects	Caution with use of this combination	Baical skullcap may potentiate the therapeutic and sedative effects of CNS depressant drugs.
	Cyclosporin	Theoretical decreased drug effects	Avoid this combination	An animal study reported a significant decrease in drug plasma levels with use of this combination. Avoid until further data becomes available.
	CYP450 substrates (CYP1A2, CYP2C19)	Theoretical increased risk of adverse effects	Monitor – may not be clinically significant	In vitro evidence suggests that baical skullcap may inhibit CYP1A2 and CYP2C19 enzyme activity. Theoretically, this may increase drug concentrations and risk of adverse effects.
	Oestrogens	Theoretical altered drug effects	Monitor – may not be clinically significant	In vitro evidence suggest baical skullcap may have oestrogenic activity. Concomitant use of high doses may theoretically interfere with the action of oral contraceptives and HRT.
	Lithium	Theoretical increased risk of drug toxicity	Caution with use of this combination	Baical skullcap may have diuretic properties. Theoretically, combined use may reduce lithium excretion and increase the risk of lithium toxicity.
	Rosuvastatin	Possible reduced drug effects	Avoid this combination	Baicalin, a constituent of baical skullcap, was reported to reduce the serum concentration of rosuvastatin in one small study. It has been proposed that this may relate only to specific genotypes, but caution is advised until more data becomes available.
Scutellaria lateriflora	CNS depressant drugs	Theoretical additive effects	Caution with use of this combination	Skullcap may potentiate the therapeutic and sedative effects of CNS depressant drugs.

Continued

ACNM herbal interactions table—cont'd				
Herbal medicine	**Drug/drug class**	**Potential outcome**	**Recommendations**	**Comments**
Serenoa repens	Androgenic drugs e.g. testosterone	Theoretical decreased drug effects	Monitor – clinical significance is unclear	Saw palmetto may reduce the effectiveness of androgenic drugs such as testosterone. Monitor for signs of decreased drug effect.
	Anticoagulant/ antiplatelet drugs	Theoretical increased risk of bleeding	Caution with use of this combination	Saw palmetto may have antiplatelet activity. Concomitant use with anticoagulant and antiplatelet drugs will theoretically increase the risk of bleeding and bruising.
	Finasteride and other drugs used for BPH	Possible additive effects	Combination may be beneficial	Additive effects are theoretically possible, which may improve disease management. There does not appear to be any evidence of negative interactions, but patients should be monitored.
	Oestrogen (HRT and oral contraceptives)	Theoretical altered drug effects	Caution with use of this combination	Saw palmetto may have anti-oestrogenic effects. Concomitant use with oestrogenic drugs such as HRT and oral contraceptives may theoretically interfere with drug action.
Silybum marianum	Antidiabetic drugs	Possible additive effects	May be beneficial – medical supervision recommended	St Mary's thistle may lower blood glucose levels, HBA1c and insulin resistance in type 2 diabetics, according to clinical research. Additive, potentially beneficial effects are possible, but caution is advised due to an increased risk of hypoglycaemia.
	CYP450 substrates (CYP2C9, CYP2D6)	Theoretical increased drug concentrations and risk of adverse effects	Monitor – may not be clinically significant	Preliminary evidence suggests that St Mary's thistle may inhibit CYP2C9 and CYP2D6 enzymes, theoretically increasing drug concentrations and risk of adverse effects.
	CYP450 substrates (CYP2C9, CYP2D6, CYP3A4)	Theoretical altered drug effects	Monitor – may not be clinically significant	There is contradictory evidence as to whether St Mary's thistle has an effect on CYP3A4 and if so whether it inhibits or induces enzyme activity. Patients should be monitored.
	Doxorubicin and cisplatin	May increase drug effect	Combination may be beneficial – medical supervision recommended	Limited evidence suggests St Mary's thistle may increase tumour sensitivity to the chemotherapeutic action of these drugs, while also reducing drug toxicity. Clinical significance is unclear and medical supervision is recommended.
	Hepatotoxic substances	Theoretical protect effects	Combination may be beneficial – medical supervision recommended	Milk thistle is reported to have hepatoprotective effects and may be beneficial in combination with hepatotoxic drugs.
	Metronidazole	Risk of decreased drug concentrations	Monitor – may not be clinically significant	A constituent of St Mary's thistle, silymarin, was reported to reduce drug concentrations in a small study. The interaction may not be clinically significant, but patients should be monitored.
	Risperidone	Theoretical increased drug bioavailability	Caution with use of this combination	A pharmacokinetic study in rats reported that regular use of St Mary's thistle increased drug bioavailability, possibly due to inhibition of P-gp. Clinical significance has not been established.

	ACNM herbal interactions table—cont'd			
Herbal medicine	**Drug/drug class**	**Potential outcome**	**Recommendations**	**Comments**
Silybum marianum cont'd	Sirolimus	Theoretical increase in drug concentration	Caution with use of this combination	Pharmacokinetic research suggests the constituent silymarin may decrease the clearance of sirolimus in hepatically impaired renal-transplant patients. Caution is advised.
	Tamoxifen	Theoretical increase in drug concentration	Caution with use of this combination	Preliminary animal research suggests the constituent silibinin may increase drug plasma concentration. Clinical significance in humans is unknown, but caution is advised.
Smilax ornata	Digoxin	Theoretical increased drug effect and adverse effect	Caution with use of this combination	Sarsaparilla may theoretically increase drug absorption, which could theoretically lead to increased drug levels and risk of toxicity.
	Lithium	Theoretical increased risk of drug toxicity	Caution with use of this combination	Sarsaparilla may have diuretic properties. Theoretically, concomitant use may reduce lithium excretion and increase the risk of lithium toxicity.
Solidago spp.	Diuretics	Theoretical additive effects	Monitor – may not be clinically significant	Goldenrod may have diuretic properties. Additive effects are theoretically possible. Monitor for hypotension and loss of fluid and electrolytes.
Tabebuia avellanedae	Anticoagulant/ antiplatelet drugs	Theoretical increased risk of bleeding	Caution with use of this combination	Pau d'arco may have anticoagulant properties at high doses based on limited evidence. Concomitant use with anticoagulant and antiplatelet drugs will theoretically increase the risk of bleeding and bruising.
Tanacetum parthenium	Anticoagulant/ antiplatelet drugs	Theoretical increased risk of bleeding	Caution with use of this combination	Feverfew may inhibit platelet aggregation, based on in vitro studies. Concomitant use with anticoagulant and antiplatelet drugs will theoretically increase the risk of bleeding and bruising. This interaction has not been demonstrated in human studies.
	CYP450 substrates (CYP1A2, CYP2C19, CYP2C8, CYP2C9, CYP2D6, CYP3A4)	Theoretical increased risk of drug toxicity	Monitor – may not be clinically significant	Preliminary evidence suggests feverfew may inhibit several CYP450 enzymes (CYP1A2, CYP2C19, CYP2C8, CYP2C9, CYP2D6, CYP3A4). Theoretically, this may reduce the rate of drug metabolism and increase the risk of toxicity. Interactions have not been demonstrated in human studies.
Taraxacum officinale	Anticoagulant/ antiplatelet drugs	Theoretical increased risk of bleeding	Caution with use of this combination	Dandelion root may inhibit platelet aggregation. Concomitant use with anticoagulant and antiplatelet drugs will theoretically increase the risk of bleeding and bruising. Significance is unclear, but caution is advised.
	Antidiabetic drugs	Theoretical additive effects	Caution with use of this combination	Dandelion extract may have hypoglycaemic properties. Additive effects are theoretically possible, increasing the risk of hypoglycaemia. Caution is advised until more data becomes available.

Continued

ACNM herbal interactions table—cont'd				
Herbal medicine	Drug/drug class	Potential outcome	Recommendations	Comments
Taraxacum officinale cont'd	CYP450 substrates (CYP1A2)	Theoretical increased risk of drug toxicity	Monitor – may not be clinically significant	Preliminary evidence suggests dandelion may inhibit CYP1A2. This interaction has not been demonstrated in human studies.
	Lithium	Theoretical increased risk of drug toxicity	Caution with use of this combination	Dandelion may have diuretic properties. Theoretically, concomitant use may reduce lithium excretion and increase the risk of lithium toxicity.
	Potassium-sparing diuretics e.g. spironolactone	Increased risk of hyperkalaemia; possible additive diuretic actions	Monitor – may not be clinically significant	Dandelion leaf contains significant amounts of potassium. Theoretically, concomitant use of dandelion and potassium-sparing diuretics will have additive effects and an increased risk of hyperkalaemia. Additive diuretic actions are also possible with use of dandelion leaf in combination with diuretic drugs.
	Quinolone antibiotics	Theoretical decreased drug bioavailability	Monitor and separate doses	The high mineral content of dandelion may theoretically form insoluble complexes with drugs in this class and reduce absorption and bioavailability. Doses should be separated.
Terminalia arjuna	Antidiabetic drugs	Theoretical additive effects	Caution with use of this combination	This herb may have hypoglycaemic properties, based on animal research. Theoretically, concomitant use with antidiabetic drugs may result in additive effects and a risk of hypoglycaemia.
Thuja occidentalis	Anticonvulsant drugs	Increased risk of seizures	Caution with use of this combination	Thuja may lower seizure threshold due to the constituent thujone, which has neurotoxic properties. This may theoretically increase the risk of seizures and reduce drug effectiveness.
	Immunosuppressant drugs	Theoretical decrease in drug effect	Caution with use of this combination	Thuja may have immuno-stimulant properties which could theoretically antagonise the effects of immunosuppressant drugs.
Thymus vulgaris	Anticoagulant/ antiplatelet drugs	Theoretical increased risk of bleeding	Caution with use of this combination	Thyme may have antiplatelet properties. Concomitant use with anticoagulant and antiplatelet drugs will theoretically increase the risk of bleeding and bruising.
Tilia spp	Lithium	Theoretical increased risk of drug toxicity	Caution with use of this combination	Linden may have diuretic properties. Theoretically, concomitant use may reduce lithium excretion and increase the risk of lithium toxicity.
Tinospora cordifolia	Antidiabetic drugs	Theoretical additive effects	Caution with use of this combination	This herb may have hypoglycaemic properties, leading to theoretical additive effects. Clinical significance is unclear.
	Immunosuppressant drugs	Theoretical decrease in drug effect	Caution with use of this combination	This herb may have immune-stimulant properties which could theoretically antagonise the effects of immunosuppressant drugs.
Tribulus terrestris	Antidiabetic drugs	Theoretical additive effects	Caution with use of this combination	Tribulus may have hypoglycaemic properties. Additive effects are theoretically possible, increasing the risk of hypoglycaemia. Caution is advised until more data becomes available.

ACNM herbal interactions table—cont'd				
Herbal medicine	**Drug/drug class**	**Potential outcome**	**Recommendations**	**Comments**
Tribulus terrestris cont'd	Antihypertensive drugs e.g. ACE-inhibitors	Theoretical additive effects	Monitor – may not be clinically significant	Animal studies suggest that tribulus may lower blood pressure due to inhibition of angiotensin-converting enzyme (ACE). Additive effects are theoretically possible, with an increased risk of hypotension.
	Androgenic drugs	Theoretical additive effects	Caution with use of this combination	Theoretically, the combination may have additive effects. There does not appear to be evidence of a negative interaction, but caution is advised.
	Erectile dysfunction drugs	Theoretical additive effects	Caution with use of this combination	Theoretically, concomitant use may have additive beneficial effects. There does not appear to be evidence of a negative interaction, but caution is advised.
	Lithium	Theoretical increased risk of drug toxicity	Caution with use of this combination	Tribulus may have diuretic properties. Theoretically, concomitant use may reduce lithium excretion and increase the risk of lithium toxicity.
	Testosterone	Theoretical additive effects	Caution with use of this combination	Concomitant use may have additive effects. There does not appear to be evidence of a negative interaction, but caution is advised.
Trifolium pratense	Anticoagulant/ antiplatelet drugs	Theoretical increased risk of bleeding	Caution with use of this combination	Red clover may inhibit platelet aggregation. Concomitant use with anticoagulant and antiplatelet drugs will theoretically increase the risk of bleeding and bruising. No effects on coagulation or prothrombin time were seen in a 12-month study using red clover 378 mg daily. Clinical significance is thus unclear, but caution is advised.
	Contraceptive drugs	Possible altered drug effect	Caution with use of this combination	Theoretically, high-dose red clover may compete with contraceptive drugs for oestrogen receptor binding sites. Significance is unclear.
	CYP450 substrates (CYP1A2, CYP2C19, CYP2C9, CYP3A4)	Theoretical risk of increased drug adverse effects	Monitor – may not be clinically significant	Preliminary evidence suggests red clover may inhibit the activity of CYP1A2, CYP2C19, CYP2C9 and CYP3A4 enzymes. This may theoretically increase drug levels and risk of adverse effects when used concomitantly with drugs that are substrates for these enzymes. So far, interactions have not been reported in humans.
	Hormone replacement therapy (HRT)	Possible altered drug effects	Caution with use of this combination	Theoretically, high-dose red clover may compete with HRT for oestrogen receptor binding sites. Significance is unclear.
	Lipid-lowering drugs	Possible additive effects	Combination may be beneficial – monitor	Red clover may have favourable effects on serum lipids, especially in postmenopausal women. It does not appear to have negative interactions with lipid-lowering drugs based on current evidence.

Continued

ACNM herbal interactions table—cont'd				
Herbal medicine	Drug/drug class	Potential outcome	Recommendations	Comments
Trifolium pratense cont'd	Methotrexate	Theoretical increased risk of drug toxicity	Caution with use of this combination	A case study describes adverse effects consistent with drug toxicity including severe vomiting and epigastric pain when red clover was added to an existing regimen of methotrexate in a woman with psoriasis.
	Tamoxifen	Theoretical antagonistic action	Caution with use of this combination	It has been proposed that red clover may antagonise drug effects due to the herb's oestrogenic actions. Caution is advised until more data becomes available.
Trigonella-foenum graecum	Anticoagulant/ antiplatelet drugs	Theoretical increased risk of bleeding	Caution with use of this combination	Fenugreek may inhibit platelet aggregation. Concomitant use with anticoagulant and antiplatelet drugs will theoretically increase the risk of bleeding and bruising.
	Antidiabetic drugs	Possible additive effects	Caution with use of this combination	Fenugreek has been shown to reduce blood glucose concentrations in patients with type 2 diabetes. Additive, beneficial effects are possible. Caution is advised as there is a risk of hypoglycaemia.
	Theophylline	Theoretical decreased drug effects	Monitor – may not be clinically significant	Limited animal research suggests fenugreek may reduce drug effects. Clinical significance is unknown, but patients should be monitored.
Turnera diffusa	Antidiabetic drugs	Theoretical additive effects	Caution with use of this combination	Damiana may have hypoglycaemic properties based on animal research. Additive effects are theoretically possible, increasing the risk of hypoglycaemia. Caution is advised until more data becomes available.
Ulmus fulva	Oral drugs	Possible decreased drug absorption	Monitor and separate dose. May not be clinically significant	The mucilage content of slippery elm may theoretically slow the absorption and reduce serum levels of some oral drugs. Clinical significance is unclear, but separation of dose administration is recommended. Caution is advised in particular with drugs with a narrow therapeutic index.
Uncaria tomentosa	Anticoagulants/ antiplatelet dugs	Theoretical increased risk of bleeding	Caution with use of this combination	Constituents in cat's claw may inhibit platelet aggregation. The combination will theoretically increase the risk of bleeding, although clinical significance is unclear.
	Antihypertensive drugs	Additive effects theoretically possible	Monitor – may not be clinically significant	Cat's claw may lower blood pressure. Additive effects are theoretically possible if used concomitantly with antihypertensive drugs. Monitor for hypotension.
	CYP3A4 substrates	Theoretical increased risk of drug adverse effects	Monitor – may not be clinically significant	Preliminary evidence suggests cat's claw may inhibit the activity of CYP3A4. This may theoretically increase drug levels and risk of adverse effects when used concomitantly with drugs that are CYP3A4 substrates.
	Immunosuppressant drugs	Theoretical decrease in drug effect	Caution with use of this combination	Cat's claw may have immuno-stimulant properties which could theoretically antagonise the effects of immunosuppressant drugs.

ACNM herbal interactions table—cont'd				
Herbal medicine	**Drug/drug class**	**Potential outcome**	**Recommendations**	**Comments**
Uncaria tomentosa cont'd	Protease inhibitors e.g. atazanavir, ritonavir, saquinavir	Theoretical increased risk of drug adverse effects	Caution with use of this combination	A case study describes a possible interaction between atazanavir and cat's claw leading to increased drug levels and risk of toxicity.
Urtica dioica	Antidiabetic drugs	Theoretical additive effects	Monitor – a clinically significant interaction appears unlikely	Stinging nettle may have hypoglycaemic properties according to animal studies, and limited clinical research. Additive effects are theoretically possible, increasing the risk of hypoglycaemia.
	Antihypertensive drugs	Theoretically additive effects	Monitor – a clinically significant interaction appears unlikely	Stinging nettle may lower blood pressure according to animal studies. Additive effects are theoretically possible if used concomitantly with antihypertensive drugs. Monitor for hypotension.
	Lithium	Theoretical increased risk of drug toxicity	Caution with use of this combination	Stinging nettle may have diuretic properties. Theoretically, concomitant use may reduce lithium excretion and increase the risk of lithium toxicity.
	Warfarin	Theoretical decreased drug effect	Caution with use of this combination	Stinging nettle contains significant amounts of vitamin K. Concomitant use of stinging nettle with warfarin may antagonise drug effects.
Vaccinium macrocarpon	Atorvastatin	Theoretical increased risk of drug adverse effects	Caution with use of this combination	A case report describes upper backpain, rhabdomyolysis and abnormal liver function after high intake of cranberry juice in a patient taking atorvastatin. It has been proposed that this was due to inhibition of CYP3A4 activity, leading to increased drug concentration.
	CYP450 substrates (CYP2CP, CYP3A4)	Theoretical increased risk of drug adverse effects	Caution with use of this combination	Cranberry may inhibit activity of CYP2C9 and CYP3A4, although data has been conflicting. Current evidence suggests the effect on CYP2C9 may not be clinically relevant, but that some cranberry products may affect CYP3A4 activity. Variations in effect may relate to differences in the concentration of triterpenes in various cranberry products. Patients should be monitored and cranberry should be used with caution with drugs with a narrow therapeutic index.
	Non-steroidal anti-inflammatory drugs (NSAIDs)	Theoretical increased drug effect	Monitor – may not be clinically significant	In vitro evidence suggest cranberry may inhibit metabolism of some NSAIDs due to an effect on CYP2C9. This has not been shown in human studies. Clinical research reported no significant changes to drug plasma levels when cranberry was used in combination with diclofenac, nor when used in combination with flurbiprofen.

Continued

ACNM herbal interactions table—cont'd				
Herbal medicine	**Drug/drug class**	**Potential outcome**	**Recommendations**	**Comments**
Vaccinium macrocarpon cont'd	Warfarin	Possible increased INR, but data is conflicting	Caution with use of this combination	Evidence is conflicting. A small number of case reports have suggested that cranberry may interact with warfarin leading to increased INR. A possible interaction was also reported in two small studies. However, no clinically relevant interactions have been found between cranberry and warfarin in clinical pharmacokinetic studies. Other studies investigating this interaction have also failed to report changes to warfarin plasma levels or INR.
Vaccinium myrtillus	Anticoagulants/antiplatelet dugs	Theoretical increased risk of bleeding	Caution with use of this combination	Anthocyanidin extracts from bilberry can inhibit platelet aggregation. Concomitant use with anticoagulant and antiplatelet drugs will theoretically increase the risk of bleeding and bruising. Clinical significance is unclear.
	Antidiabetic drugs	Possible additive effects	Caution with use of this combination	Bilberry may have hypoglycaemic properties. The combination could be additive and beneficial, but monitor for hypoglycaemia.
Valeriana officinalis	Alcohol	Increased risk of sedation	Caution with use of this combination	Valerian may potentiate the sedative effects of alcohol. Caution is advised.
	Benzodiazepines	Increased effects and risk of sedation	Caution with use of this combination	Valerian may have additive effects and potentiate the sedative effects of benzodiazepines.
	CNS depressant drugs including barbiturates	Increased effects and risk of sedation	Caution with use of this combination	Valerian may have additive effects and potentiate the sedative effects of CNS depressant drugs.
	CYP450 substrates (CYP3A4)	Theoretical altered drug effect	Monitor – interaction may not be clinically significant	Results from in vitro studies have been conflicting. Some findings suggest valerian may inhibit CYP3A4 and other findings suggest it may induce CYP3A4. It has been proposed that a modest interaction may occur at doses of 1000 mg daily of valerian, but is unlikely at low doses. Caution is advised until further data becomes available.
Viscum album	Antihypertensive drugs	Theoretical additive effects	Monitor – interaction may not be clinically significant	Preliminary research suggests European mistletoe may have hypotensive properties. Theoretically, this may result in additive effects and a risk of hypotension. Clinical significance is unknown.
	Hepatotoxic drugs	Theoretical increased risk of liver damage	Monitor – may not be clinically significant	Case studies suggest European mistletoe may adversely affect liver function in some individuals. There is a theoretical increased risk of liver damage when used concomitantly with hepatotoxic drugs, but significance is unknown.
	Immunosuppressant drugs	Theoretical decrease in drug effect	Caution with use of this combination	European mistletoe may have immuno-stimulant properties which could theoretically antagonise the effects of immunosuppressant drugs.

ACNM herbal interactions table—cont'd				
Herbal medicine	**Drug/drug class**	**Potential outcome**	**Recommendations**	**Comments**
Verbena officinalis	CYP450 substrates (CYP2B1)	Theoretical risk of increased adverse effects	Monitor – may not be clinically significant	In vitro research suggests verbena can significantly inhibit CYP2B1 enzyme activity. Theoretically, this may increase levels of drugs metabolised by this enzyme; however, this interaction has not been reported in humans.
Vitex agnus-castus	Dopamine receptor antagonists – including antipsychotic drugs	Theoretical decreased drug effects	Monitor – may not be clinically significant	Chaste tree may have dopaminergic activity. Concurrent use with dopamine antagonists may theoretically result in decreased drug effects. Caution is advised, although there are no clinical studies in humans to confirm this interaction.
	Dopamine agonists	Theoretical additive effects	Monitor – may not be clinically significant	Chaste tree may have dopaminergic effects and so may theoretically potentiate drug effects.
	Metoclopramide	Theoretical decreased drug effects	Monitor – may not be clinically significant	Chaste tree may interfere with drug action due to the dopaminergic effects of this drug.
	Oestrogenic drugs (e.g. contraceptive drugs and HRT)	Theoretical decreased drug effects	Monitor – may not be clinically significant	Chaste tree appears to have weak hormone-modulating activity and may theoretically interfere with drug action. This interaction is hypothetical and has not been supported by evidence.
Vitis vinifera	Anticoagulants/ antiplatelet dugs	Theoretical increased risk of bleeding	Caution with use of this combination	Grape may inhibit platelet aggregation. Concomitant use with anticoagulant and antiplatelet drugs will theoretically increase the risk of bleeding and bruising. Clinical significance is unclear.
	CYP450 substrates (CYP2C9, CYP3A4)	Theoretical increased risk of adverse effects	Monitor – may not be clinically significant	Preliminary in vitro evidence suggests that grape may inhibit activity of CYP2C9 and CYP3A4. This interaction has not been reported in humans and significance is unknown.
Withania somnifera	Antidiabetic drugs	Additive effects theoretically possible	Caution with use of this combination	Preliminary evidence suggests that withania may have hypoglycaemic properties. Additive effects are theoretically possible, increasing the risk of hypoglycaemia. Caution is advised until more data becomes available.
	Antihypertensive drugs	Additive effects theoretically possible	Monitor – may not be clinically significant	Withania may lower blood pressure according to animal studies. Additive effects are theoretically possible, with an increased risk of hypotension.
	Antipsychotic drugs e.g. haloperidol	Theoretical decreased drug effects	May be beneficial – medical supervision recommended	Animal studies suggest withania may reduce drug-induced adverse effects such as dyskinesia. Clinical relevance is unclear, but may theoretically be beneficial.
	Benzodiazepines	Increased risk of sedation	Caution with use of this combination	Preliminary evidence suggests that withania may potentiate the effects of benzodiazepines. Caution is advised.
	Clomipramine	Improved management of OCD	May be beneficial – medical supervision recommended	A small study describes improved outcomes in patients with obsessive compulsive disorder when withania was added to existing drug therapy.

Continued

ACNM herbal interactions table—cont'd				
Herbal medicine	**Drug/drug class**	**Potential outcome**	**Recommendations**	**Comments**
Withania somnifera cont'd	CNS depressant drugs	Increased risk of sedation	Caution with use of this combination	Theoretically, concomitant use may have additive effects and an increased risk of excessive sedation.
	Chemotherapeutic agents	Improved patient wellbeing	May be beneficial – medical supervision recommended	Withania has been found to significantly improve quality of life and reduce fatigue in breast cancer patients undergoing chemotherapy. Medical supervision is recommended.
	Immunosuppressant drugs	Theoretical decrease in drug effect	Caution with use of this combination	Withania may have immuno-stimulant properties which could theoretically antagonise the effects of immunosuppressant drugs.
Zanthoxylum spp	Acid-reducing drugs (antacids, H_2 antagonists, proton pump inhibitors)	Theoretical decreased drug effect	Monitor – may not be clinically significant	Prickly ash may increase gastric acidity. Use may theoretically antagonise drug action, resulting in decreased drug effect.
Zanthoxylum simulans	Anticoagulants/ antiplatelet dugs	Theoretical increased risk of bleeding	Caution with use of this combination	Chinese prickly ash may inhibit platelet aggregation based on in vitro research. Concomitant use with anticoagulant or antiplatelet drugs may theoretically increase the risk of bleeding.
Zea mays	Antidiabetic drugs	Theoretical additive effects	Caution with use of this combination	Corn silk may have hypoglycaemic properties according to animal research. Additive effects are theoretically possible, increasing the risk of hypoglycaemia. Caution is advised until more data becomes available.
	Antihypertensive drugs	Theoretical additive effects	Monitor – may not be clinically significant	Corn silk may theoretically lower blood pressure due to the herb's diuretic properties. Additive effects are theoretically possible, with an increased risk of hypotension. Clinical significance is unclear.
	Diuretics – potassium depleting e.g. loop and thiazides	Theoretical increased risk of hypokalaemia	Monitor – may not be clinically significant	Diuretic effects with increased potassium loss have been reported in animal studies. Theoretically, concomitant use of corn silk with potassium depleting diuretics increases the risk of hypokalaemia. Monitor for signs of potassium depletion.
	Warfarin	Theoretical decreased drug anticoagulant effect	Caution with use of this combination	Corn silk contains vitamin K. Theoretically, high-dose intake of corn silk will increase vitamin K levels and could antagonise the activity of anticoagulants such as warfarin and reduce drug anticoagulant effect.
Zingiber officinale	Anaesthetics	Possible decreased drug-induced nausea	May be beneficial – medical supervision recommended	Limited research suggests ginger may reduce severity of anaesthetic-induced post-operative nausea and vomiting if taken pre-treatment.
	Anticoagulant/ antiplatelet dugs	Theoretical increased risk of bleeding	Caution with use of this combination	Ginger appears to inhibit thromboxane synthetase and decrease platelet aggregation. Excessive intake of ginger may theoretically increase the risk of bleeding when used with anticoagulant/ antiplatelet drugs.

ACNM herbal interactions table—cont'd

Herbal medicine	Drug/drug class	Potential outcome	Recommendations	Comments
Zingiber officinale cont'd	Antidiabetic drugs	Additive effects theoretically possible	Monitor – may not be clinically significant	Preliminary evidence suggests that ginger may have hypoglycaemic properties, although data has been inconclusive. Additive effects are theoretically possible, increasing the risk of hypoglycaemia.
	Anti-emetic drugs	Additive effects theoretically possible	Combination may be beneficial	Ginger has anti-emetic properties and may have additive beneficial effects when used concomitantly with anti-emetic drugs. Theoretically, this may allow for a lower drug dose.
	Chemotherapy (e.g. cisplatin)	Possible decreased drug-induced nausea	May be beneficial – medical supervision recommended	Limited research suggests ginger may reduce severity of nausea associated with certain chemotherapeutic agents.
	Nifedipine	Additive effects theoretically possible	Avoid combination	A synergistic effect on platelet aggregation was observed between ginger 1g and nifedipine 10 mg in a small study of hypertensive patients. The combination should be avoided.
	Tacrolimus	Theoretical increased risk of drug toxicity	Avoid combination	An animal study reported increased drug levels when ginger was given concomitantly with tacrolimus. The combination should be avoided due to an increased risk of drug toxicity.
Zizyphus jujube / spinosa	Antidiabetic drugs	Theoretical additive effects	Caution with use of this combination	Animal research suggests that zizyphus may have hypoglycaemic properties. Additive effects are theoretically possible, increasing the risk of hypoglycaemia. Clinical significance is unclear, but caution is advised until more data becomes available.
	CNS depressant drugs	Theoretical increased risk of sedation	Caution with use of this combination	Zizyphus may theoretically potentiate sedative adverse effects when used with CNS depressant drugs, based on animal studies.

ACNM NUTRIENT AND NUTRITIONAL SUPPLEMENTS INTERACTIONS TABLE

Nutrient/ supplement	Drug/drug class	Potential outcome	Recommendations	Comments
3-diindolylmethane (DIM)	CYP450 substrates (CYP1A2)	Theoretical decreased drug effect	Monitor – may not be clinically significant	In vitro evidence suggests that diindolylmethane may induce CYP1A2, which could theoretically increase the rate of drug metabolism and reduce drug efficacy. This has not been demonstrated in humans.
	Diuretics	Theoretical increased risk of hyponatraemia	Monitor – may not be clinically significant	A small study conducted in men with prostate cancer reported that high dose intake of diindolylmethane resulted in asymptomatic hyponatraemia. Theoretically, the risk of hyponatraemia is increased when used with diuretics.
	Oestrogens (e.g. HRT and oral contraceptives)	Theoretical altered drug effect	Monitor – may not be clinically significant	Diindolylmethane may have mild oestrogenic and anti-oestrogenic effects. Theoretically, high-dose intake may interfere with drug action.

Continued

ACNM NUTRIENT AND NUTRITIONAL SUPPLEMENTS INTERACTIONS TABLE—cont'd				
Nutrient/ supplement	Drug/drug class	Potential outcome	Recommendations	Comments
5-Hydroxytryptophan (5-HTP)	Antidepressant drugs (SSRIs and SNRIs)	Increased risk of serotonin-related adverse effects	Avoid combination	Concomitant use of 5-HTP and SSRIs or SNRIs may increase the risk of adverse effects and serotonin syndrome. The combination should be avoided as the consequences are potentially serious.
	Carbidopa	Increased risk of serotonin-related adverse effects	Caution with use of this combination	Concomitant use of 5-HTP and carbidopa may increase the risk of serotonergic adverse effects. Limited research suggests the combination may enhance drug therapy, but there is insufficient data to be clear on the benefits vs the risks.
	CNS depressants	Increased risk of drowsiness	Caution with use of this combination	Additive sedative effects are possible and may lead to excessive drowsiness.
	Dextromethorphan	Increased risk of serotonin-related adverse effects	Caution with use of this combination	Concomitant use of 5-HTP and dextromethorphan may increase the risk of adverse effects and serotonin syndrome.
	Monoamine oxidase inhibitors (MAOIs)	Increased risk of serotonin-related adverse effects	Avoid combination	Concomitant use of 5-HTP and MAOIs may increase the risk of adverse effects and serotonin syndrome.
	Tramadol	Increased risk of serotonin-related adverse effects	Caution with use of this combination	Concomitant use of 5-HTP and tramadol may increase the risk of adverse effects and serotonin syndrome.
Acetyl L-carnitine	Anticoagulants/ antiplatelet dugs	Theoretical increased risk of bleeding	Caution with use of this combination	Acetyl L-carnitine may theoretically potentiate drug effects and increase the risk of bleeding.
Activated charcoal	Oral medications	Theoretical decreased drug absorption	Caution with use of this combination	Activated charcoal may theoretically bind to, and reduce, absorption of several drugs and supplements. Dosages should be separated by a minimum of 2 hours.
Adenosine	Antigout drugs	Theoretical decreased drug effectiveness	Monitor – may not be clinically significant	Adenosine triphosphate can cause hyperuricaemia and uricosuria. This may theoretically reduce drug effectiveness.
	Dipyridamole	Risk on nutrient toxicity	Avoid combination	Dipyridamole decreases metabolism of adenosine and may increase risk of toxicity.
	Methylxanthines	Theoretical decreased nutrient effect	Monitor – may not be clinically significant	Aminophylline, caffeine and theophylline may theoretically block adenosine effects due to a competitive antagonist action.
Agaricus mushrooms	Antidiabetic drugs	Theoretical additive effects	Caution with use of this combination	Some evidence suggests that agaricus mushrooms may lower blood glucose levels by decreasing insulin resistance in type 2 diabetics. Additive effects are possible, with an increased risk of hypoglycaemia.

ACNM NUTRIENT AND NUTRITIONAL SUPPLEMENTS INTERACTIONS TABLE—cont'd

Nutrient/ supplement	Drug/drug class	Potential outcome	Recommendations	Comments
Alpha-casozepine milk protein (casein peptides)	Antihypertensive drugs	Theoretical additive effects	Monitor – may not be clinically significant	Alpha-casozepine may lower blood pressure slightly according to limited research. Concomitant use will theoretically have additive effects. This may potentially be beneficial, but monitor for hypotension.
	Anxiolytic drugs e.g. benzodiazepines	Theoretical additive effects	Monitor – may not be clinically significant	Alpha-casozepine may have anxiolytic properties. Concomitant use will theoretically have additive effects, which may be beneficial. Patients should be monitored due to insufficient research data on the effects of combined use.
Alpha-lipoic acid	Antidiabetic drugs	Theoretical additive effects	Caution with use of this combination	Alpha-lipoic acid may have hypoglycaemic effects. The combination could be additive and beneficial, but drug dosage adjustments may be required.
	Cisplatin	Possible decreased drug-induced adverse effects	May be beneficial – medical supervision recommended	Preliminary research suggests alpha-lipoic acid may have some protective effects against drug-induced ototoxicity, peripheral sensory neuropathy and oxidative stress.
	L-Thryroxine (Levothyroxine)	Theoretical decreased drug effects	Caution with use of this combination	Animal research suggests that alpha-lipoic acid may reduce conversion of thyroxine to the active T3 form. Significance is unclear.
Aniseed	Oestrogens e.g. oral contraceptives & HRT	Theoretical altered drug effects	Monitor – may not be clinically significant	In vitro studies have reported both oestrogenic and anti-oestrogenic effects with anise. This appears to be due to mechanisms relating to oestrogen-receptors modulation. The significance in humans is not known, but caution is advised.
	Tamoxifen	Theoretical altered drug effects	Caution with use of this combination	In vitro studies have reported both oestrogenic and anti-oestrogenic effects with anise. This appears to be due to mechanisms relating to oestrogen-receptors modulation. The significance in humans is not known, but caution is advised.
Apple cider vinegar	Antidiabetic drugs	Theoretical additive effects	Caution with use of this combination	Apple cider vinegar may have additive effects when used with antidiabetic drugs. It has been shown to reduce postprandial blood glucose levels and decrease gastric emptying time in people with diabetes. While this could potentially be beneficial, caution is recommended.
	Digoxin	Theoretical increased risk of drug toxicity	Caution with use of this combination	Overuse of apple cider vinegar may theoretically decrease potassium levels and increase the risk of drug toxicity.
	Diuretics	Theoretical increased risk of hypokalaemia	Caution with use of this combination	Overuse of apple cider vinegar may theoretically decrease potassium levels and increase the risk of hypokalaemia.

Continued

ACNM NUTRIENT AND NUTRITIONAL SUPPLEMENTS INTERACTIONS TABLE—cont'd				
Nutrient/ supplement	Drug/drug class	Potential outcome	Recommendations	Comments
Arginine (L-Arginine)	ACE-Inhibitors (ACE-I)	Risk of hypotension and hyperkalaemia	Caution with use of this combination	Additive vasodilatory and blood pressure-lowering effects have been reported, which increases the risk of hypotension. Theoretically, combined use may also increase the risk of hyperkalaemia as both drug and nutrient can raise potassium levels. The combination may theoretically be beneficial, but careful monitoring is recommended.
	Angiotensin receptor blockers (ARBs)	Risk of hypotension and hyperkalaemia	Caution with use of this combination	Additive vasodilatory and blood pressure-lowering effects have been reported, which increases the risk of hypotension. Theoretically, combined use may also increase the risk of hyperkalaemia as both drug and nutrient can raise potassium levels. The combination may theoretically be beneficial, but careful monitoring is recommended.
	Anticoagulant/ antiplatelet drugs	Theoretical increased risk of bleeding	Caution with use of this combination	Preliminary evidence suggests arginine may decrease platelet aggregation. Concurrent use may theoretically increase the risk of bleeding.
	Antidiabetic drugs	Theoretical increased risk of hypoglycaemia	Caution with use of this combination	Preliminary evidence suggests arginine may decrease blood glucose levels in patients with type 2 diabetes. Concurrent use may theoretically be beneficial; however, there is an increased risk of hypoglycaemia.
	Antihypertensive drugs	Additive effect possible	Caution with use of this combination	Arginine increases nitric oxide levels which results in vasodilation. Additive blood pressure-lowering effects have been reported when used in combination with antihypertensive drugs. Concurrent use may theoretically be beneficial; however, there is an increased risk of hypotension.
	Diuretics	Increased risk of hyperkalaemia	Caution with use of this combination	Arginine intake may result in raised potassium levels. There is a theoretical increased risk of hyperkalaemia when used with potassium-sparing diuretics.
	Herpes treatments including antiviral drugs and lysine	Possible decreased disease management	Caution with use of this combination	Arginine may oppose the therapeutic action of agents used for the management of herpes simplex. High levels of arginine may stimulate viral replication of HSV.
	Nitrates	Additive vasodilatory effects possible	Caution with use of this combination	Caution is advised due to a risk of additive vasodilatory and hypotensive effects.
	Sildenafil and other phosphodiesterase-5 inhibitors	Additive effects possible	May be beneficial – medical supervision recommended	Arginine can lead to increased nitric oxide production, which may theoretically enhance drug effect in the management of erectile dysfunction. The combination may theoretically be beneficial; however, caution is advised due to an increased risk of vasodilation and hypotension.

ACNM NUTRIENT AND NUTRITIONAL SUPPLEMENTS INTERACTIONS TABLE—cont'd				
Nutrient/ supplement	**Drug/drug class**	**Potential outcome**	**Recommendations**	**Comments**
Ascorbic acid - See Vitamin C				
B-sitosterol	Ezetimibe	Decreased β-sitosterol absorption	Caution with use of this combination	Ezetimibe has been shown to inhibit absorption of β-sitosterol and may reduce levels by up to 41%.
	Pravastatin	Theoretical decreased β-sitosterol levels	Monitor – may not be clinically significant	Limited data suggests that pravastatin may lower β-sitosterol levels.
Beta-carotene	Anthelmintic drugs	Possible improved response	Combination may be beneficial	Vitamin A deficiency is associated with an increased risk of parasitic worm infections. In addition, worm infections, especially roundworm, can interfere with vitamin A absorption. Concurrent use of beta-carotene or vitamin A may assist with management of this condition, as well as supporting immunity and epithelial integrity.
	Cholestyramine	Reduced nutrient absorption	May be beneficial to address nutrient depletion	Cholestyramine may reduce nutrient absorption. Supplements may be required in some individuals. Separate dose administration.
	Colchicine	Reduced nutrient absorption	May be beneficial to address nutrient depletion	Colchicine reduces absorption of fat-soluble vitamins including beta-carotene. Supplements may be required to address nutrient depletion.
	Mineral oil	Risk of vitamin depletion	May be beneficial to address nutrient depletion	A moderate risk of nutrient depletion has been reported and supplements may be required in some individuals.
	Neomycin	Risk of nutrient depletion	May be beneficial to address nutrient depletion	Neomycin may damage the structure and affect function of the digestive tract lining. Long-term use may reduce absorption and increase excretion of beta-carotene.
	Orlistat	Reduced nutrient absorption	May be beneficial to address nutrient depletion	Orlistat reduces absorption of fat-soluble vitamins including beta-carotene. Supplements may be required to address nutrient depletion.
	Proton pump inhibitors	Risk of nutrient depletion	Combination may be beneficial to address nutrient depletion	Proton pump inhibitors may theoretically reduce absorption of beta-carotene. Increased intake of dietary carotenoid-rich foods may be beneficial. Individuals taking proton pump inhibitors should be monitored for signs of nutrient deficiencies.
Beta-glucan	Antihypertensive drugs	Additive effects possible	Combination may be beneficial	Beta-glucan has been shown to reduce blood pressure, particularly in obese individuals with hypertension. Concurrent use may be additive and potentially beneficial, but monitor for hypotension.
	Immunosuppressant drugs	Theoretical risk of decreased drug effect	Caution with use of this combination	Beta-glucans may have immune-stimulant effects. Theoretically, this may counteract drug immunosuppressant action; however, clinical significance is unclear.
	Lipid-lowering drugs	Additive effects possible	Combination may be beneficial	Beta-glucans have been shown to significantly reduce cholesterol. Additive beneficial effects may be seen with concurrent use.

Continued

	ACNM NUTRIENT AND NUTRITIONAL SUPPLEMENTS INTERACTIONS TABLE—cont'd			
Nutrient/ supplement	**Drug/drug class**	**Potential outcome**	**Recommendations**	**Comments**
Betaine HCl	Acid-reducing drugs (antacids, H$_2$-antagonists, proton pump inhibitors)	Theoretical decreased drug effect	Monitor – may not be clinically significant	Betaine may increase gastric acidity and concurrent use may theoretically counteract drug action.
Biotin	Anticonvulsant drugs	Nutrient depletion possible	May be beneficial to address nutrient depletion	Reduced plasma biotin levels have been observed in patients taking carbamazepine, phenobarbital and phenytoin. Clinical significance is unclear.
Blackcurrant oil	Anticoagulant/ antiplatelet drugs	Theoretical increased risk of bleeding	Caution with use of this combination	Gamma-linolenic acid (GLA), which is found in blackcurrant oil, may have antiplatelet properties. Concurrent use may theoretically increase the risk of bleeding.
	Anticonvulsant drugs	Theoretical increased risk of seizures	Caution with use of this combination	Theoretically, products containing gamma-linolenic acid (GLA), including blackcurrant oil, may lower seizure threshold and increase the risk of seizures. This interaction is based on anecdotal evidence and significance is unclear.
	Antihypertensive drugs	Theoretical risk of hypotension	Monitor – may not be clinically significant	Blackcurrant oil may decrease systolic blood pressure, based on limited data. There is a theoretical increased risked of hypotension when used concurrently with antihypertensive drugs.
	Phenothiazines	Theoretical increased risk of seizures	Caution with use of this combination	Theoretically, products containing gamma-linolenic acid (GLA), including blackcurrant oil, may increase the risk of seizures in people taking phenothiazines. This interaction is based on anecdotal evidence and significance is unclear.
Blueberry	Antidiabetic drugs	Possible additive effects	May be beneficial – monitor	Evidence suggests that blueberries and blueberry extract may lower blood glucose and improve glycaemic status. Additive beneficial effects are theoretically possible, but monitor for hypoglycaemia.
Bromelain	Anticoagulant/ antiplatelet drugs	Theoretical increased risk of bleeding	Caution with use of this combination	Bromelain may have antiplatelet properties, leading to a theoretical increased risk of bleeding.
Branched chain amino acids (BCAAs)	Antidiabetic drugs	Possible additive hypoglycaemic effects	Caution with use of this combination	Some evidence suggests that BCAA may stimulate release of insulin. Additive effects are theoretically possible, but may increase the risk of hypoglycaemia.
	Levodopa	Theoretical decreased drug effects	Caution with use of this combination	Theoretically, BCAA may compete with levodopa for transport systems. This may result in decreased drug effectiveness, although clinical significance is unclear.

ACNM NUTRIENT AND NUTRITIONAL SUPPLEMENTS INTERACTIONS TABLE—cont'd				
Nutrient/ supplement	Drug/drug class	Potential outcome	Recommendations	Comments
Caffeine	Alcohol	Theoretical increased caffeine levels	Monitor – may not be clinically significant	Alcohol reduces caffeine metabolism; therefore there is a theoretical increased risk of caffeine-related adverse effects.
	Alendronate	Reduced drug bioavailability	Caution with use of this combination – separate doses	Caffeine significantly reduces drug bioavailability. Doses should be separated by at least 2 hours.
	Anticoagulant/ antiplatelet drugs	Theoretical increased risk of bleeding	Monitor – may not be clinically significant	Caffeine is reported to have antiplatelet activity; however, an interaction between coffee and drugs in this class has not been reported in humans.
	Anticonvulsant drugs (e.g. carbamazepine, phenytoin, ethosuximide, valproate)	Theoretical decreased drugs effects	Caution with use of this combination	Animal models suggest that high-dose intake of caffeine may reduce drug anticonvulsant effects. The mechanism of this interaction and clinical significance is unclear.
	Cimetidine	Theoretical increased caffeine levels	Caution with use of this combination	Cimetidine may reduce caffeine metabolism, theoretically increasing the risk of caffeine-related adverse effects.
	Clozapine	Theoretical disease exacerbation	Caution with use of this combination	Caffeine may exacerbate psychotic symptoms and increase drug effects and toxicity at high doses (400–1000 mg daily of caffeine).
	CNS stimulant drugs	Enhanced stimulatory effects	Caution with use of this combination	Concomitant use of caffeine and CNS stimulant drugs will increase the risk of adverse effects due to additive stimulatory actions.
	Disulfiram	Theoretical increased caffeine levels	Monitor – may not be clinically significant	Disulfiram may reduce caffeine metabolism, theoretically increasing the risk of caffeine-related adverse effects.
	Diuretics	Theoretical increased risk of hypokalaemia	Caution with use of this combination	Excessive intake of caffeine may reduce potassium levels due to stimulation of the sodium-potassium pump. There is a theoretical increased risk of hypokalaemia when taken with potassium-depleting diuretics.
	Ephedrine	Enhanced stimulatory effects	Avoid combination	Ephedrine may enhance the stimulatory effects of caffeine. The combination has been associated with an increased risk of life-threatening or debilitating adverse effects such as hypertension, myocardial infarction, stroke, seizures and death.
	Fluvoxamine	Theoretical increased caffeine levels	Monitor – may not be clinically significant	Fluvoxamine may reduce caffeine metabolism, theoretically increasing the risk of caffeine-related adverse effects.
	L-Thyroxine (Levothyroxine)	Possible reduced drug absorption	Caution with use of this combination	It has been proposed that coffee may form insoluble complexes with thyroxine in some patients. Dosage separation is advised.

Continued

ACNM NUTRIENT AND NUTRITIONAL SUPPLEMENTS INTERACTIONS TABLE—cont'd				
Nutrient/ supplement	Drug/drug class	Potential outcome	Recommendations	Comments
Caffeine cont'd	Lithium	Theoretical increased risk of drug toxicity	Caution with use of this combination	Case reports suggest that abrupt withdrawal from caffeine may increase serum lithium levels.
	Monoamine oxidase inhibitors (MAOIs)	Theoretical risk of hypertensive crisis	Caution with use of this combination	Theoretically, high intake of caffeine may precipitate a hypertensive crisis in patients taking MAOIs.
	Phenylpropanolamine	Theoretical increased risk of hypertension	Caution with use of this combination	Concomitant use may have additive effects in raising blood pressure. Phenylpropanolamine may also raise serum caffeine levels according to limited data.
	Quinolone antibiotics	Theoretical increased caffeine levels	Monitor – may not be clinically significant	Quinolones reduce caffeine metabolism; therefore there is a theoretical increased risk of caffeine-related adverse effects.
	Theophylline	Theoretical increased risk of drug toxicity	Caution with use of this combination	Caffeine may inhibit drug metabolism and increase the risk of adverse effects.
	Verapamil	Theoretical increased caffeine levels	Caution with use of this combination	Verapamil may increase plasma caffeine concentration by 25% according to some research. Concomitant use may theoretically increase the risk of caffeine-related adverse effects.
Calcium	Acid-reducing drugs (H_2-antagonists and proton pump inhibitors (PPIs))	Risk of nutrient depletion	May be beneficial to address nutrient depletion	Some calcium salts, especially calcium carbonate, require adequate stomach acid to dissolve and allow for absorption. Drugs that raise gastric pH may theoretically reduce calcium absorption. Monitor for calcium depletion with long-term use of acid-reducing drugs.
	Aluminium salts (e.g. antacids)	Increased risk of aluminium absorption	Caution with use of this combination	Calcium citrate may increase the absorption of aluminium as aluminium hydroxide. Aluminium may be toxic, especially in those with renal disease. This interaction appears to be specific to the citrate salt.
	Antibiotics (tetracyclines and quinolones)	Reduced drug effect	Monitor – separate doses	Calcium supplements form complexes with these drugs and may reduce drug effectiveness. Separate doses by at least 2 hours.
	Anticonvulsant drugs (carbamazepine, phenobarbital, phenytoin, fosphenytoin)	Risk of nutrient depletion with long-term use	May be beneficial to address nutrient depletion	Use of some anticonvulsant drugs may result in a major calcium depletion. This is due to increased vitamin D metabolism resulting in decreased calcium absorption. Hypocalcaemia and osteomalacia have occurred, especially with prolonged therapy or concurrent use of more than one anticonvulsant drug. Most patients will need calcium and vitamin D supplements.

			ACNM NUTRIENT AND NUTRITIONAL SUPPLEMENTS INTERACTIONS TABLE—cont'd	
Nutrient/ supplement	**Drug/drug class**	**Potential outcome**	**Recommendations**	**Comments**
Calcium cont'd	Bisphosphonates (e.g. alendronate, risedronate, ibrandronic acid)	Reduced drug absorption	Beneficial interaction, but dosage separation is essential	Calcium significantly reduces absorption of oral bisphosphonates and may reduce drug effectiveness. Bisphosphonates should be taken at least 30 minutes before calcium supplements. It should be noted that use of bisphosphonates is contraindicated in individuals with hypocalcaemia; therefore adequate intake of calcium and vitamin D is important for both drug safety and efficacy, and to enhance disease management.
	Caffeine	Risk of nutrient depletion with long-term use	May be beneficial to address nutrient depletion	High caffeine intake may increase urinary excretion of calcium and has been associated with increased bone loss and risk of fractures in the elderly. Calcium supplements may be required with regular high intake.
	Calcipotriene	Increased risk of hypercalcaemia	Caution with use of this combination	Rare cases of hypercalcaemia have been reported with use of calcipotriene. Calcium supplements should be used with caution or avoided due to an increased risk of hypercalcaemia.
	Calcium channel blockers	Theoretical antagonistic effect	Monitor – may not be clinically significant	Calcium supplements may antagonise the effects of intravenous calcium channel blockers. There is no evidence that dietary or supplemental calcium interacts with oral calcium channel blockers.
	Ceftriaxone	Risk of deposition of a drug-nutrient complex	Avoid combination	Case reports describe an interaction in neonates where the combination of IV calcium with IV ceftriaxone has led to the precipitation of a drug-nutrient salt in the lungs and kidneys, which has led to death. While this interaction has not been reported in adults, caution and dosage separation are advised, especially with IV forms of calcium and ceftriaxone.
	Cholestyramine	Risk of nutrient depletion with long-term use	May be beneficial to address nutrient depletion	Cholestyramine may reduce vitamin D absorption which can then affect calcium absorption. Current evidence suggests this depletion is not significant in most patients, but monitoring is advised.
	Corticosteroids	Risk of mineral depletion with long-term use	May be beneficial to address nutrient depletion	Long-term intake of oral corticosteroids (equivalent to ⋯⟩ 7.5 mg prednisone daily) causes significant bone loss and increases the risk of osteoporosis and fractures. A major depletion is possible and supplements may be required.

Continued

ACNM NUTRIENT AND NUTRITIONAL SUPPLEMENTS INTERACTIONS TABLE—cont'd				
Nutrient/ supplement	Drug/drug class	Potential outcome	Recommendations	Comments
Calcium cont'd	Digoxin	Increased risk of drug toxicity	Caution with use of this combination	Hypercalcaemia may potentiate digoxin toxicity. Caution is recommended with high-dose intake of supplemental calcium.
	Diuretics – loop	Risk of nutrient depletion	May be beneficial to address nutrient depletion	Loop diuretics increase urinary excretion of calcium. Moderate risk of depletion.
	Diuretics – thiazides	Increased risk of hypercalcaemia	Caution with use of this combination	Thiazide diuretics decrease urinary excretion of calcium, theoretically increasing the risk of hypercalcaemia with high calcium intake.
	Integrase inhibitors (e.g. dolutegravir, elvitegravir, raltegravir)	Theoretical decreased drug effect	Avoid combination	Pharmacokinetic studies suggest calcium supplements decrease drug serum levels of integrase inhibitors, possibly due to a chelation interaction. These combinations should be avoided until more data becomes available as it may theoretically compromise HIV therapy.
	L-Thyroxine (Levothyroxine)	Possible decreased drug absorption	Caution with use of this combination – separate doses	Calcium may theoretically reduce drug absorption by forming insoluble complexes. Separate doses by at least 4 hours.
	Lithium	Theoretical increased risk of hypercalcaemia	Caution with use of this combination	Evidence suggest that long-term use of lithium may result in hypercalcaemia. Combined use of calcium supplements with lithium will theoretically increase this risk.
	Minerals (iron, magnesium)	Reduced mineral absorption	Monitor – separate doses	Calcium supplements may interfere with absorption of dietary and supplemental iron and magnesium. The interaction may not be clinically relevant unless there is a deficiency, but separation of dose administration is generally advised.
	Mineral oil	Risk of nutrient depletion with long-term use	May be beneficial to address nutrient depletion	Mineral oil may interfere with absorption of vitamin D and calcium. Some patients will need supplements with long-term use.
	Sotalol	Possible decreased drug absorption	Caution with use of this combination – separate doses	Calcium appears to reduce drug absorption, possibly by forming insoluble complexes. Dose administration should be separated.
	Stimulant laxatives	Risk of nutrient depletion with long-term use	May be beneficial to address nutrient depletion	Stimulant laxatives can moderately reduce calcium and vitamin D absorption. Advise patients not to use stimulant laxatives long term, and monitor for signs of nutrient depletion.

ACNM NUTRIENT AND NUTRITIONAL SUPPLEMENTS INTERACTIONS TABLE—cont'd

Nutrient/ supplement	Drug/drug class	Potential outcome	Recommendations	Comments
Calcium D-glucarate	Alcohol	Theoretical decreased calcium D-glucarate activity	Caution with use of this combination	Clinical research suggests alcohol may increase urinary excretion of calcium D-glucarate and decrease nutrient activity.
	Glucuronidated drugs	Theoretical increased drug clearance	Monitor – clinical significance is unknown	Theoretically, calcium D-glucarate may increase clearance of drugs that undergo Phase II glucuronidation metabolism. Examples of drugs metabolised via this pathway include atorvastatin, diazepam, digoxin, lamotrigine, lorazepam, paracetamol, morphine, oxazepam.
Carnitine (L-Carnitine)	Anticoagulants/ antiplatelet dugs	Theoretical increased risk of bleeding	Caution with use of this combination	L-carnitine may theoretically potentiate drug effects and increase the risk of bleeding.
	L-Thyroxine (levothyroxine)	Theoretical decreased drug effect	Caution with use of this combination	Theoretically L-carnitine may decrease effectiveness of L-thyroxine. L-carnitine appears to act as a peripheral thyroid hormone antagonist.
Celery	Antidepressant drugs e.g. venlafaxine	Theoretical increased risk of adverse effects	Avoid combination	A case report describes an interaction between celery root extract, St John's wort and venlafaxine, which led to mania and hallucinations.
	Anticoagulant/ antiplatelet drugs	Theoretical increased risk of bleeding	Caution with use of this combination	In vitro research has reported that two of the constituents found in celery have antiplatelet activity. Concomitant use with anticoagulant and antiplatelet drugs theoretically increases the risk of bleeding and bruising.
	Antihypertensive drugs	Additive effects theoretically possible	Caution with use of this combination	Anecdotal evidence suggests that celery may lower blood pressure. Concomitant use may be additive, with a theoretical risk of hypotension. Clinical significance is unclear.
	CYP450 substrates (CYP1A2)	Theoretical increased drug effect	Caution with use of this combination	In vitro and animal research suggest celery may inhibit CYP1A2. Theoretically, concomitant use with drugs that are CYP1A2 substrates may result in increased drug effects and risk of adverse effect.
	L-Thyroxine (Levothyroxine)	Theoretical decrease in drug effect	Caution with use of this combination	Case reports suggest that celery seed tablets may interact with thyroxine, leading to reduced drug effect. Caution is advised until more data becomes available.
	Lithium	Increased risk of drug toxicity	Caution with use of this combination	Celery may have diuretic properties. Theoretically, combined use may reduce lithium excretion and increase the risk of lithium toxicity.
	Paracetamol	Theoretical increased drug effect	Monitor – may not be clinically significant	Animal research suggests celery juice may prolong the effects of paracetamol. It has been proposed that this is due to inhibition of CYP450 enzyme activity.
	PUVA therapy	Increased risk of phototoxicity	Caution with use of this combination	Celery may increase the risk of phototoxicity when use with PUVA therapy according to limited data.

Continued

ACNM NUTRIENT AND NUTRITIONAL SUPPLEMENTS INTERACTIONS TABLE—cont'd

Nutrient/ supplement	Drug/drug class	Potential outcome	Recommendations	Comments
Chondroitin sulphate	Anticoagulant/ antiplatelet drugs	Theoretical increased risk of bleeding	Caution with use of this combination	Evidence suggests that a combination of chondroitin with glucosamine may potentiate the effects of warfarin, leading to an increased risk of bleeding. It is unclear whether the interaction is due to chondroitin, glucosamine or both.
	Non-steroidal anti-inflammatory drugs (NSAIDs)	Increased disease management in OA	Combination may be beneficial	The combination may lead to improved outcomes in patients with osteoarthritis and may result in reduced NSAID requirements.
Choline	Atropine	Theoretical decreased drug effects	Monitor – may not be clinically significant	Animal research suggests that concomitant administration of choline and atropine may result in decreased effects of atropine.
Chromium	Antidiabetic drugs	Possible additive effects	Caution with use of this combination	Chromium may lower blood glucose levels. Additive effects are possible when used with antidiabetic drugs, which may be beneficial, but caution is advised due to a risk of hypoglycaemia.
	Corticosteroids	Risk of nutrient depletion	May be beneficial to address nutrient depletion	Corticosteroids may increase urinary excretion of chromium. A moderate risk of chromium deficiency has been reported with long-term use.
	Insulin	Possible additive effects	Caution with use of this combination	Chromium has been shown to increase insulin sensitivity. Additive effects are possible and may be beneficial, but caution is advised due to a risk of hypoglycaemia.
	L-Thyroxine (Levothyroxine)	Possible decreased drug bioavailability	Caution with use of this combination	Clinical research suggests that chromium may bind to thyroxine and decrease drug absorption. Intake should be separated.
	Lipid-lowering drugs	May improve disease management	Combination may be beneficial	Chromium may have lipid-lowering properties and could have additive benefits in disease management.
Clove	Anticoagulant/ antiplatelet drugs	Theoretical increased risk of bleeding	Monitor – may not be clinically significant	In vitro studies have reported that a constituent of clove, eugenol, appears to have antiplatelet activity. No interactions have been reported in humans, but patients should be monitored.
Coenzyme Q10 (ubiquinol, ubidecarenone)	Antidiabetic drugs	Possible improved disease management; possible nutrient depletion	Combination may be beneficial	Research reports that people with type 2 diabetes tend to have lower CoQ10 levels and that CoQ10 supplements may help to improve glycaemic control. CoQ10 has also been shown to improve nerve conduction and reduce neuropathic pain in diabetic patients. Observational studies have proposed that some oral antidiabetic drugs may deplete CoQ10 levels, although further research is needed to investigate significance. The combination may be beneficial, but monitoring is advised.

ACNM NUTRIENT AND NUTRITIONAL SUPPLEMENTS INTERACTIONS TABLE—cont'd

Nutrient/ supplement	Drug/drug class	Potential outcome	Recommendations	Comments
Coenzyme Q10 (ubiquinol, ubidecarenone) cont'd	Antihypertensive drugs	Possible additive effects	Combination may be beneficial	CoQ10 can lower blood pressure according to research, with this effect being clinically relevant. Additive beneficial effects are theoretically possible, but monitor for hypotension.
	B-blockers	Possible nutrient depletion	May be beneficial to address nutrient depletion	In vitro studies suggest that B-blockers may lead to a reduction in CoQ10 levels, with secondary sources proposing that this may contribute to drug adverse effects such as fatigue. Concurrent use may theoretically be beneficial and could potentially support cardiovascular health in general.
	Doxorubicin	Possible decreased risk of drug toxicity	May be beneficial – medical supervision recommended	Preliminary evidence suggests that doxorubicin may decrease CoQ10 synthesis and that this may contribute to drug cardiotoxicity. CoQ10 has not been shown to affect drug pharmacokinetics; therefore may be useful as an adjunct therapy, under medical supervision.
	HMGCoA reductase inhibitors (statins)	Possible decreased risk of drug adverse effects	May be beneficial to address nutrient depletion	Statins block endogenous synthesis of CoQ10, which may lead to reduced serum levels. This dose-dependent interaction is considered a contributing factor for statin-induced adverse effects such as myalgia, fatigue and headache. Concerns have also been raised about the potential negative impact of reduced CoQ10 levels on cardiovascular function, particularly in those at risk. While there is a lack of consensus as to whether CoQ10 should be recommended routinely with statins, there are no known risks to use of this combination and it is potentially beneficial.
	Warfarin	Theoretical decreased drug effect	Caution with use of this combination	Data on this interaction is conflicting. CoQ10 is structurally similar to menaquinone and may theoretically have a vitamin K-like effect. Case reports suggest use of CoQ10 may reduce drug anticoagulant effect. Results of a small RCT trial, however, reported no significant change to warfarin pharmacokinetics with concurrent use of warfarin and CoQ10. Caution is advised until more data becomes available.

Continued

ACNM NUTRIENT AND NUTRITIONAL SUPPLEMENTS INTERACTIONS TABLE—cont'd				
Nutrient/ supplement	Drug/drug class	Potential outcome	Recommendations	Comments
Cocoa (also refer to interactions listed under Caffeine)	ACE-Inhibitors (ACE-I)	Additive effects possible	May be beneficial – medical supervision recommended	Cocoa may inhibit angiotensin converting enzyme activity according to limited research. Additive blood pressure-lowering effects are theoretically possible, but monitor for hypotension.
	Anticoagulant/ antiplatelet drugs	Theoretical increased risk of bleeding	Caution with use of this combination	Cocoa may have antiplatelet properties according to limited research. There is a theoretical increased risk of bleeding with this combination.
	Antidiabetic drugs	Theoretical altered drug affects	Caution with use of this combination	Cocoa may affect blood glucose regulation, with some reports suggesting an increased level of blood sugar and other reports suggesting a decreased level. Clinical significance of this interaction is unclear and caution is advised.
	Antihypertensive drugs	Additive effects possible	May be beneficial – medical supervision recommended	Cocoa may lower blood pressure. The combination may theoretically be beneficial, but caution is advised due to a risk of hypotension.
	Cardiovascular drugs	Possible improved disease management	May be beneficial – medical supervision recommended	A preliminary study reported that increased intake of high-flavonol cocoa helped to improve endothelial function and blood pressure in patients with coronary artery disease who were taking a combination of statins, aspirin, beta-blockers and ACE-I/ARB.
	Clozapine	Theoretical disease exacerbation	Caution with use of this combination	Caffeine, found in cocoa, may exacerbate psychotic symptoms and increase drug effects and toxicity at high doses.
	Lipid lowering drugs (statins)	Possible improved disease management	May be beneficial –medical supervision recommended	A preliminary study reported that increased intake of high-flavonol cocoa helped to improve endothelial function and blood pressure in patients with coronary artery disease who were taking a combination of statin, aspirin, beta-blocker and ACE-I/ARB.
Cod liver oil	Anticoagulant/ antiplatelet drugs	Theoretical increased risk of bleeding	Caution with use of this combination	Cod liver oil may have antiplatelet properties at high doses, leading to a theoretical increased risk of bleeding.
	Antihypertensive drugs	Possible additive effects	Caution with use of this combination	Cod liver oil may lower blood pressure. This may lead to additive beneficial effects, but monitor for hypotension.

ACNM NUTRIENT AND NUTRITIONAL SUPPLEMENTS INTERACTIONS TABLE—cont'd				
Nutrient/ supplement	Drug/drug class	Potential outcome	Recommendations	Comments
Colloidal silver	Antibiotics (quinolones and tetracyclines)	Theoretical decreased drug absorption	Caution with use of this combination	Colloidal silver may theoretically reduce drug absorption.
	Hepatotoxic drugs	Increased risk of liver damage	Caution with use of this combination	Colloidal silver may be hepatotoxic according to preliminary animal studies. Concurrent use with hepatotoxic drugs theoretically increases the risk of liver damage.
	L-Thyroxine (Levothyroxine)	Theoretical decreased drug absorption	Caution with use of this combination	Colloidal silver may theoretically reduce drug absorption.
	Penicillamine	Theoretical decreased drug absorption	Caution with use of this combination	Colloidal silver may theoretically reduce drug absorption.
Conjugated linoleic acid (CLA)	Anticoagulant/ antiplatelet drugs	Theoretical increased risk of bleeding	Caution with use of this combination	CLA may have antiplatelet properties. There is a theoretical increased risk of bleeding with concurrent use.
	Antihypertensive drugs (e.g. Ramipril)	Additive effects	Caution with use of this combination	CLA may reduce blood pressure and enhance drug effects. One study reported that CLA enhanced ramipril's blood pressure-lowering effects in obese hypertensive patients. The combination of CLA with antihypertensive drugs may be beneficial, but monitor for hypotension.
Copper	Contraceptive drugs	Increased copper levels	Monitor – may not be clinically significant	Contraceptive drugs may increase copper levels above reference levels according to some studies. Intake of supplemental copper while taking the contraceptive pill may theoretically lead to excessive copper levels.
	Penicillamine	Decreased drug effects	Caution with use of this combination	Copper chelates penicillamine and decreases drug absorption. Separate dose administration by at least 2 hours.
Cordyceps mushrooms	Anticoagulant/ antiplatelet drugs	Theoretical increased risk of bleeding	Monitor – may not be clinically significant	Animal research suggests cordyceps may have antiplatelet effects. There is a theoretical increased risk of bleeding with concomitant use, but this has not been reported in humans.
	Chemotherapy	Theoretical improved outcomes	Caution with use of this combination	Preliminary evidence suggests cordyceps may improve quality of life and cellular immunity in patients undergoing cancer chemotherapy. Concomitant use may be beneficial, but caution is advised until more data becomes available.
	Cyclosporin	Theoretical decreased drug effects	Avoid combination	A small clinical study reported that cordyceps reduced the immunosuppressive effects of cyclosporin in patients who had undergone renal transplantation. Other research has reported that cordyceps may help to ameliorate cyclosporin-induced nephrotoxicity. Avoid combination unless under strict medical supervision.

Continued

ACNM NUTRIENT AND NUTRITIONAL SUPPLEMENTS INTERACTIONS TABLE—cont'd				
Nutrient/ supplement	Drug/drug class	Potential outcome	Recommendations	Comments
Cordyceps mushrooms cont'd	Immunosuppressant drugs	Theoretical decreased drug effects	Caution with use of this combination	Cordyceps may theoretically reduce drug immunosuppressive effects by stimulating the immune system. Preliminary evidence has, however, suggested that use of cordyceps in renal-transplant patients may have beneficial effects. Research has suggested that adjunctive use of cordyceps with immunosuppressive therapy may result in reduced hepatotoxicity and nephrotoxicity, reduced number of infections and reduced drug requirements. Concomitant use may potentially be beneficial under strict medical supervision.
	Testosterone	Theoretical additive effects	Monitor – clinical significance is unclear	Animal research suggests cordyceps may increase testosterone levels. Clinical significance is unknown based on current data.
Creatine	Nephrotoxic drugs	Theoretical increased risk of kidney damage	Caution with use of this combination	Some cases of renal impairment after intake of creatine supplements have been reported, although most research suggests no adverse effect on kidney function. Theoretically, creatine may increase the risk of kidney damage when used with nephrotoxic drugs, although this effect has not been reported in humans.
Curcumin	Alcohol	Possible reduced organ damage	May be beneficial – medical supervision recommended	Animal models suggest that curcumin provides some protective effects against alcoholic liver and pancreatic disease. Curcumin may theoretically be a useful adjunct therapy in those with high alcohol ingestion.
	Anticoagulant/ antiplatelet drugs	Theoretical increased risk of bleeding	Caution with use of this combination	Curcumin is reported to have antiplatelet activity in vitro. Theoretically, concurrent use with anticoagulant or antiplatelet drugs increases the risk of bleeding. Caution is advised until more data becomes available.
	Antidiabetic drugs	Theoretical additive effects	Caution with use of this combination	Curcumin may have hypoglycaemic effects. Clinical significance of this interaction is unclear, but caution is advised.
	CYP450 substrates (CYP1A1, CYP1A2, CYP3A4)	Theoretical increased drug effect	Monitor – may not be clinically significant	In vitro and animal research suggest that curcumin may inhibit liver metabolising activity of CYP1A1, CYP1A2 and CYP3A4. This has not been demonstrated in humans, although a case report describes a possible interaction with tacrolimus, a CYP3A4 substrate.

ACNM NUTRIENT AND NUTRITIONAL SUPPLEMENTS INTERACTIONS TABLE—cont'd

Nutrient/ supplement	Drug/drug class	Potential outcome	Recommendations	Comments
Curcumin cont'd	Dexamethasone	Theoretical increase in drug levels	Caution with use of this combination	Curcumin may increase drug blood levels, based on preliminary data. Based on limited data, there is a theoretical risk of increased drug effects and adverse effects.
	Non-steroidal anti-inflammatory drugs (NSAIDs)	Theoretical additive effects	Combination may be beneficial	Additive effects are possible with concurrent use which may be beneficial for the management of conditions such as arthritis. No negative drug-herb interactions have been reported, but monitoring is suggested.
	Sulphasalazine	Theoretical increase in drug levels	Caution with use of this combination	Preliminary evidence suggests curcumin may increase blood levels of drug. Combined use may theoretically increase drug effects and adverse effects.
	Tacrolimus	Theoretical increase in drug levels	Caution with use of this combination	Animal studies and a case report suggest that curcumin may increase drug levels. Combined use may theoretically increase drug effects and adverse effects. Caution is advised until more safety data becomes available.
	Talinolol	Possible reduced drug bioavailability	Caution with use of this combination	Preliminary clinical evidence suggests curcumin may decrease drug bioavailability. Caution is advised until more data becomes available.

Ellagic acid – See Pomegranate

Epigallocatechin-3-gallate - See Green tea

Nutrient/ supplement	Drug/drug class	Potential outcome	Recommendations	Comments
Evening primrose oil	Anticoagulant/ antiplatelet drugs	Theoretical increased risk of bleeding	Caution with use of this combination	Gamma-linolenic acid (GLA), found in evening primrose oil, may have antiplatelet properties, leading to a theoretical increased risk of bleeding.
	Anticonvulsant drugs	Theoretical increased risk of seizures	Caution with use of this combination	Theoretically, products containing gamma-linolenic acid (GLA), including evening primrose oil, may lower seizure threshold and increase the risk of seizures. This interaction is based on anecdotal evidence and significance is unclear.
	Phenothiazines	Theoretical increased risk of seizures	Caution with use of this combination	Theoretically, products containing gamma-linolenic acid (GLA), including evening primrose oil, may increase the risk of seizures in people taking phenothiazines. This interaction is based on anecdotal evidence and significance is unclear.
	Protease inhibitors (e.g. lopinavir)	Possible increased drug levels	Caution with use of this combination	A case report describes a possible interaction between evening primrose oil and lopinavir in an HIV patient, which led to increased drug concentration.

Continued

ACNM NUTRIENT AND NUTRITIONAL SUPPLEMENTS INTERACTIONS TABLE—cont'd				
Nutrient/ supplement	Drug/drug class	Potential outcome	Recommendations	Comments
Evening primrose oil cont'd	Tamoxifen	Possible improved outcomes	May be beneficial – medical supervision recommended	Preliminary evidence suggests that gamma-linolenic acid (GLA), found in evening primrose oil, may improve outcomes in patients with breast cancer who are taking tamoxifen. Data is limited and medical supervision recommended.
Fermented wheat germ extract	Immunosuppressant drugs	Theoretical risk of decreased drug effect	Caution with use of this combination	Fermented wheat germ extract appears to stimulate immune function. This may theoretically oppose drug immunosuppressant effects.
Fibre	Oral medications	Theoretical decrease in drug effect possible	Monitor – separate doses	High fibre intake may theoretically affect absorption of some drugs. Clinical significance is unclear and will be variable. Dosage separation is suggested.

Fish oil - See Omega-3 essential fatty acids

Nutrient/ supplement	Drug/drug class	Potential outcome	Recommendations	Comments
Flaxseed	Anticoagulant/ antiplatelet drugs	Theoretical increased risk of bleeding	Monitor – may not be clinically significant	Flaxseed may have antiplatelet properties. There is a theoretical risk of additive effects, with an increased risk of bleeding. The interaction is unlikely to be clinically significant at normal therapeutic doses.
	Antidiabetic drugs	Theoretical additive effects	Monitor – may not be clinically significant	Flaxseed may have hypoglycaemic properties and additive effects are theoretically possible. Clinical significance at normal therapeutic doses is unclear.
	Antihypertensive drugs	Theoretical additive effects	Monitor – may not be clinically significant	Flaxseed may slightly lower diastolic pressure and additive effects are theoretically possible. Clinical significance at normal therapeutic doses is unclear.
	Furosemide	Theoretical decreased drug absorption	Monitor – may not be clinically significant	Preliminary in vitro research suggests flaxseed may decrease drug absorption. Clinical significance is unknown.
	Ketoprofen	Theoretical decreased drug absorption	Monitor – may not be clinically significant	Preliminary in vitro research suggests flaxseed may decrease drug absorption. Clinical significance is unknown.
	Oestrogens (e.g. HRT and oral contraceptives)	Theoretical decreased drug effect	Monitor – may not be clinically significant	Flaxseed may theoretically have mild oestrogenic effects. Theoretically, the lignans in flaxseed may compete with oestrogens for binding sites and may theoretically reduce drug effect. The interaction is speculative.
	Paracetamol	Theoretical decreased drug absorption	Monitor – may not be clinically significant	Preliminary in vitro research suggests flaxseed may decrease drug absorption. Clinical significance is unknown.

ACNM NUTRIENT AND NUTRITIONAL SUPPLEMENTS INTERACTIONS TABLE—cont'd				
Nutrient/ supplement	Drug/drug class	Potential outcome	Recommendations	Comments
Folic acid (Folate, folinic acid, 5-methyltetrahydrofolate (L-5MTHF), vitamin B9)	5-Fluorouracil	Theoretical increased risk of drug toxicity	Caution with use of this combination	Theoretically, high-dose folic acid may increase drug toxicity. Increased gastrointestinal adverse effects including stomatitis and diarrhoea have been described in clinical studies.
	Anticonvulsants (e.g. phenytoin)	Risk of vitamin depletion; risk of decreased seizure control	Combination may be beneficial to address nutrient depletion, but medical supervision is recommended	Anticonvulsants such as phenytoin may lead to a moderate nutrient depletion, especially with low dietary intake. Patients should be monitored and supplements may be required in some individuals. Conversely, some studies have reported that high-dose folic acid may cause a reduction in phenytoin blood levels and lead to an increased risk of seizures. High-dose intake of folic acid should be avoided unless under medical supervision.
	Carbamazepine	Risk of vitamin depletion; risk of decreased seizure control	Combination may be beneficial to address nutrient depletion, but medical supervision is recommended	Carbamazepine may reduce serum folate levels, which may theoretically contribute to drug-induced mild reductions in nerve conduction and mental changes. Megaloblastic anaemia has not been reported. Caution is advised, however, as folic acid supplements have been shown to reduce seizure control in some patients with epilepsy.
	Capecitabine	Theoretical increased risk of drug toxicity	Caution with use of this combination	Theoretically, high-dose folic acid may increase drug toxicity. A case report suggests that folic acid 15 mg daily contributed to drug toxicity symptoms including severe diarrhoea, vomiting, oedema, hand-foot syndrome and eventual death in a patient taking capecitabine. It is unclear if this interaction would occur at normal therapeutic doses.
	Cholestyramine	Risk of vitamin depletion	May be beneficial to address nutrient depletion	This drug is associated with a moderate risk of folic acid depletion. Patients should be monitored and doses should be separated. Supplements may be required in some individuals.
	Metformin	Risk of vitamin depletion	May be beneficial to address nutrient depletion	Metformin may reduce folic acid absorption according to some sources. Symptomatic folic acid deficiency seems unlikely, based on current evidence, but patients should be monitored. Long-term use of metformin is associated with an increased risk of raised homocysteine levels, although data on severity and clinical significance is conflicting.

Continued

	ACNM NUTRIENT AND NUTRITIONAL SUPPLEMENTS INTERACTIONS TABLE—cont'd			
Nutrient/ supplement	Drug/drug class	Potential outcome	Recommendations	Comments
Folic acid (Folate, folinic acid, 5-methyltetrahydrofolate (L-5MTHF), vitamin B9) cont'd	Methotrexate	Risk of vitamin depletion; risk of decreased drug efficacy in cancer	Caution with use of this combination	Methotrexate is a folic acid antagonist and can lead to a major folic acid depletion. Supplementation with folic acid is usually required in patients prescribed methotrexate for conditions such as rheumatoid arthritis or psoriasis. Use may help to reduce drug toxicity and side effects. Folic acid supplements may, however, oppose drug mechanism of action if methotrexate is prescribed for the management of cancer and could reduce drug efficacy. Medical supervision is required.
	Oral contraceptives	Risk of vitamin depletion	May be beneficial to address nutrient depletion	Folate levels may be reduced with long-term use of oral contraceptives. Supplements may be required in some individuals.
	Pyrimethamine	Risk of vitamin depletion; risk of decreased drug efficacy	Caution with use of this combination	This drug is a folic acid antagonist and can reduce serum folate levels. Folic acid supplements may antagonise drug action and reduce drug efficacy, depending on indication. Medical supervision is recommended.
	Retinoids	Risk of vitamin depletion	May be beneficial to address nutrient depletion	Isotretinoin has been shown to reduce serum folic acid in patients with acne. Good dietary intake should be maintained. Supplements may be required in some individuals, due to a moderate risk of depletion.
	Sulphasalazine	Risk of vitamin depletion	May be beneficial to address nutrient depletion	Moderate risk of depletion as drug reduces folic acid absorption. Patients should be monitored –supplements may be required in some individuals.
GABA	Antihypertensive drugs	Theoretical additive effects	Caution with use of this combination	Some evidence suggests that GABA may lower blood pressure. Additive beneficial effects are theoretically possible, but caution is advised due to a risk of hypotension.
Gamma-linolenic acid (GLA)	Anticoagulant/ antiplatelet drugs	Theoretical increased risk of bleeding	Caution with use of this combination	Gamma-linolenic acid (GLA) may have antiplatelet properties, leading to a theoretical increased risk of bleeding.
	Anticonvulsant drugs	Theoretical increased risk of seizures	Caution with use of this combination	Theoretically, gamma-linolenic acid (GLA) may lower seizure threshold and increase the risk of seizures. This interaction is based on anecdotal evidence and significance is unclear.
	Phenothiazines	Theoretical increased risk of seizures	Caution with use of this combination	Theoretically, gamma-linolenic acid (GLA) may increase the risk of seizures in people taking phenothiazines. This interaction is based on anecdotal evidence and significance is unclear.

ACNM NUTRIENT AND NUTRITIONAL SUPPLEMENTS INTERACTIONS TABLE—cont'd				
Nutrient/ supplement	Drug/drug class	Potential outcome	Recommendations	Comments
Garlic	Anticoagulant/ antiplatelet drugs	Theoretical increased risk of bleeding	Caution with use of this combination	Garlic has antiplatelet activity and may theoretically interact with anticoagulant and antiplatelet drugs. Clinical studies have not reported changes to the pharmacokinetics or pharmacodynamics of warfarin, nor an increased incidence of adverse effects. Caution is advised, however, with doses >7g/day of garlic. Normal therapeutic doses appear safe.
	Antihypertensive drugs	Theoretical additive effects	Combination may be beneficial – monitor	Garlic may have a small effect in lowering blood pressure, so additive effects are theoretically possible. The interaction may be beneficial but patients should be monitored for hypotension.
	Anti-retroviral drugs – protease inhibitors (e.g. saquinavir)	Possible decreased drug effect	Avoid combination	Garlic extract has been shown to significantly reduce blood concentrations of saquinavir, potentially reducing drug effectiveness in the management of HIV. High-dose garlic supplements should be avoided with saquinavir. A study with ritonavir showed only a small non-statistically significant change in drug concentration, but caution is advised with use of supplemental garlic and all drugs in this class until more data becomes available. The effect of dietary garlic is unknown.
	CYP450 substrates (CYP2E1)	Theoretical increased risk of drug toxicity	Caution with use of this combination	Preliminary evidence suggests garlic oil may inhibit the activity of CYP2E1 by 39%. Theoretically, this may increase the risk of toxicity of drugs metabolised by this enzyme.
	CYP450 substrates (CYP3A4)	Theoretical decreased drug effectiveness	Caution with use of this combination	Preliminary evidence suggests garlic may induce the activity of CYP3A4, although results from different studies have been mixed. Caution is advised due to a theoretical risk of decreased drug effectiveness with concurrent use of garlic and drugs metabolised by this enzyme.
	Isoniazid	Theoretical decreased drug effect	Avoid combination	Animal studies report that garlic can significantly reduce isoniazid plasma concentrations. The combination should be avoided until further data becomes available.
	Lipid-lowering agents e.g. statins	Theoretical additive effects	Combination may be beneficial – monitor	Garlic is reported to lower cholesterol and a study suggests it may potentiate the effects of lipid-lowering drugs. The combination appears well tolerated and may be beneficial.

Continued

ACNM NUTRIENT AND NUTRITIONAL SUPPLEMENTS INTERACTIONS TABLE—cont'd

Nutrient/ supplement	Drug/drug class	Potential outcome	Recommendations	Comments
Genistein – see Soy and soy isoflavones				
Germinated barley foodstuff	Antidiabetic drugs	Additive effects possible	Monitor – may not be clinically significant	Barley may theoretically enhance drug blood glucose lowering effects. Clinical significance is not clear.
Glucosamine sulphate	Anticoagulant/ antiplatelet drugs	Increased risk of bleeding	Avoid combination	Case reports suggest that the combination of warfarin and glucosamine, both with and without chondroitin, may increase INR and risk of bleeding and bruising. The combination should be avoided until more safety data becomes available.
	Antidiabetic drugs	Theoretical decreased disease management, although interaction appears unlikely	Monitor – may not be clinically significant	Preliminary research suggested that glucosamine may increase insulin resistance or decrease insulin production. Concerns were raised that use of glucosamine may decrease drug effectiveness and worsen disease management. Based on current clinical research, however, glucosamine does not appear to adversely affect blood glucose control or HbA1C. Patients should still be monitored.
	Non-steroidal anti-inflammatory drugs (NSAIDs)	Possible improved disease management; reduced need for drug therapy	Combination may be beneficial	Glucosamine sulphate can help to improve cartilage synthesis and repair, reduce disease progression and reduce symptoms of osteoarthritis. Glucosamine sulphate may reduce requirements for NSAID therapy in patients with knee OA, according to clinical research.
	Paracetamol	Theoretical decreased pain management	Monitor – unlikely to be clinically relevant	Two case reports in a survey suggested that concomitant use of glucosamine sulphate and paracetamol may lead to decreased pain control in patients with osteoarthritis. This interaction is considered speculative and unlikely to be clinically relevant. The combination is frequently used in practice.
Glutamine (L-glutamine)	Anticonvulsant drugs	Theoretical antagonistic effect	Caution with use of this combination	Glutamine may be metabolised to the excitatory neurotransmitter glutamate which could theoretically antagonise the anticonvulsant's effects. Clinical significance is unclear, but caution is advised.
	Antidiabetic drugs	Reduced cardiovascular risk	Combination may be beneficial	One study reported that glutamine supplementation was effective in improving cardiovascular risk factors in patients with type 2 diabetes.
	Anti-retroviral therapy	Possible decreased drug adverse effect	May be beneficial – medical supervision recommended	Preliminary clinical research reported that glutamine reduced severity of diarrhoea in HIV patients taking nelfinavir. More research is needed to investigate this possible beneficial interaction.

ACNM NUTRIENT AND NUTRITIONAL SUPPLEMENTS INTERACTIONS TABLE—cont'd

Nutrient/ supplement	Drug/drug class	Potential outcome	Recommendations	Comments
Glutamine (L-glutamine) cont'd	Chemotherapy	Possible improved disease management	May be beneficial – medical supervision recommended	Data is inconclusive, but glutamine may potentially have some benefits as an adjunct therapy in patients undergoing chemotherapy. Research suggests oral glutamine may decrease the incidence, severity and duration of mouth pain and oral mucositis in some patients undergoing cancer chemotherapy or bone marrow transplant. Research has suggested that glutamine may also help reduce drug-induced myalgia and arthralgia in patients taking paclitaxel. Other studies have suggested that glutamine may help to reduce chemotherapy-induced diarrhoea and chemotherapy-induced lymphocytopaenia. More research is needed but current evidence is promising.
	Human growth hormone	Possible improved disease management	May be beneficial – medical supervision recommended	Glutamine in combination with human growth hormone may decrease dependence on parenteral nutrition in some patients with short-bowel syndrome. Research findings have, however, been inconsistent.
	Lactulose	Theoretical decreased drug effects	Monitor – may not be clinically significant	Glutamine may theoretically reduce the drug effects due to an antagonistic action.
Glutathione	Alcohol	Risk of nutrient depletion	May be beneficial to address nutrient depletion	Alcohol may deplete glutathione levels and may theoretically reduce efficacy of glutathione supplements. Supplementation may be beneficial with regular excessive intake of alcohol.
	Chemotherapeutic agents	Reduced risk of drug toxicity	May be beneficial – medical supervision recommended	Evidence suggest that IV glutathione may help to prevent against toxicity induced by several chemotherapeutic agents. It is unclear if oral glutathione will have the same effect. More data is required to investigate clinical significance.
	Paracetamol	Risk of nutrient depletion	May be beneficial to address nutrient depletion	Paracetamol may deplete glutathione levels and may theoretically reduce efficacy of glutathione supplements. Supplementation may be beneficial with chronic or high-dose intake of paracetamol.
Glycine	Clozapine	Theoretical decrease in disease management	Caution with use of this combination	High-dose glycine was shown to interfere with drug antipsychotic activity in a small study of patients with schizophrenia.

Continued

ACNM NUTRIENT AND NUTRITIONAL SUPPLEMENTS INTERACTIONS TABLE—cont'd

Nutrient/ supplement	Drug/drug class	Potential outcome	Recommendations	Comments
Grapefruit	Aliskiren	Decreased drug concentration	Caution with use of this combination	Studies have reported a significant decrease in drug concentration with this combination, which may lead to reduced drug effect. The proposed mechanism for this interaction is due to inhibition of the organic anion-transporting protein polypeptide 2B1 (OATP2B1). Separate dose administration by at least 4 hours if concurrent use is deemed necessary.
	Amiodarone	Increased drug plasma concentration and risk of adverse effects	Avoid combination	Grapefruit juice has been shown to significantly inhibit CYP3A4 enzyme activity. Studies have reported a significant increase in drug concentration with this combination, which increases the risk of adverse effects and drug toxicity.
	Artemether	Increased drug plasma concentration and risk of adverse effects	Avoid combination	Grapefruit juice has been shown to significantly inhibit CYP450 enzyme activity. Studies have reported a significant increase in drug concentration with this combination, which increases the risk of adverse effects and drug toxicity.
	Benzodiazepines e.g. midazolam, diazepam	Increased drug plasma concentration and risk of adverse effects	Avoid combination	Grapefruit juice has been shown to significantly inhibit CYP3A4 enzyme activity. Studies have reported a significant increase in drug concentration with this combination, which increases the risk of adverse effects and drug toxicity. This interaction has been reported especially with diazepam and midazolam. It does not appear to occur with alprazolam.
	Budesonide	Increased drug plasma concentration and risk of adverse effects	Caution with use of this combination	Grapefruit juice has been shown to significantly inhibit CYP3A4 enzyme activity. Studies have reported an increase in drug concentration with this combination, which increases the risk of adverse effects and drug toxicity.
	Buspirone	Increased drug plasma concentration and risk of adverse effects	Avoid combination	Studies have reported a significant increase in drug concentration with this combination, which increases the risk of adverse effects and drug toxicity.
	Caffeine	Increased risk of caffeine-related adverse effects	Caution with use of this combination	Studies have reported an increase in caffeine concentration with this combination, which increases the risk of adverse effects.
	Calcium channel blockers e.g. verapamil, amlodipine, nifedipine	Increased drug plasma concentration and risk of adverse effects	Avoid combination	Studies have reported a significant increase in drug concentration with this combination, which increases the risk of adverse effects and drug toxicity. It has been proposed that this is due to inhibition of CYP3A4 activity, but some sources suggest other mechanisms may also be involved.

ACNM NUTRIENT AND NUTRITIONAL SUPPLEMENTS INTERACTIONS TABLE—cont'd

Nutrient/ supplement	Drug/drug class	Potential outcome	Recommendations	Comments
Grapefruit cont'd	Carbamazepine	Increased drug plasma concentration and risk of adverse effects	Avoid combination	Increased drug absorption and plasma concentrations have been reported.
	Carvedilol	Increased drug plasma concentration and risk of adverse effects	Avoid combination	Grapefruit juice is reported to increase drug bioavailability.
	Celiprolol	Decreased drug concentration	Avoid combination	Grapefruit juice is reported to decrease drug bioavailability. The proposed mechanism for this interaction is due to inhibition of the organic anion-transporting protein polypeptide (OATP).
	Cisapride	Increased drug plasma concentration and risk of adverse effects	Avoid combination	Increased plasma concentrations have been reported.
	Clomipramine	Increased drug plasma concentration and risk of adverse effects	Caution with use of this combination	Increased plasma concentrations have been described in two case reports.
	Clopidogrel	Decreased drug concentration	Avoid combination	Grapefruit juice has been reported to significantly decrease drug concentrations, which could reduce effectiveness as an antiplatelet drug.
	Colchicine	Increased drug plasma concentration and risk of adverse effects	Caution with use of this combination	In vitro evidence has reported that grapefruit juice increases drug absorption by inhibiting P-gp.
	Cyclosporin	Increased drug bioavailability	Avoid combination	Evidence suggest an increase in drug bioavailability with use of this combination.
	CYP450 substrates (CYP1A2, CYP2C19, CYP2C9)	Risk of increased drug plasma concentration and adverse effects	Caution with use of this combination	Preliminary evidence suggest grapefruit juice may inhibit CYP1A2, CYP2C19 and CYP2C9. Interactions have not been reported in human studies to date and significance is unclear.
	CYP450 substrates (CYP3A4)	Risk of increased drug plasma concentration and adverse effects	Avoid combination	Grapefruit juice has been shown to significantly inhibit CYP34A enzyme activity. When taken orally, effects of grapefruit juice on CYP3A4 appear to last at least 48 hours.
	Dextromethorphan	Increased drug concentration and risk of adverse effects	Caution with use of this combination	A pharmacokinetic study reported increased concentration of dextromethorphan when taken in combination with grapefruit juice. It has been proposed that the interaction is due to inhibition of CYP3A4.
	Docetaxel	Increased drug plasma concentration and risk of adverse effects	Avoid combination	A case report describes an interaction with use of this combination, leading to increased drug concentrations and a reduction in white blood cell count.
	Erythromycin	Increased drug plasma concentration and risk of adverse effects	Caution with use of this combination	A study reported increased absorption of erythromycin when taken in combination with grapefruit juice.

Continued

ACNM NUTRIENT AND NUTRITIONAL SUPPLEMENTS INTERACTIONS TABLE—cont'd

Nutrient/ supplement	Drug/drug class	Potential outcome	Recommendations	Comments
Grapefruit cont'd	Etoposide	Decreased drug concentration and effect	Avoid combination	Studies have reported a significant decrease in drug concentration with this combination, which may lead to reduced drug effect. The proposed mechanism for this interaction is inhibition of the organic anion-transporting protein polypeptide (OATP).
	Fexofenadine	Decreased drug concentration and effect	Caution with use of this combination	Studies have reported a significant decrease in drug concentration with this combination, which may lead to reduced drug effect. The proposed mechanism for this interaction is inhibition of the organic anion-transporting protein polypeptide (OATP).
	Fluvoxamine	Increased drug plasma concentration and risk of adverse effects	Caution with use of this combination	Increased drug plasma concentrations have been reported.
	Halofantrine	Increased drug plasma concentration and risk of adverse effects	Avoid combination	Increased drug plasma concentrations have been reported in a small clinical study. This may lead to an increased risk of prolonged QT interval.
	HMGCoA reductase inhibitors (statins) e.g. atorvastatin, simvastatin	Increased drug plasma concentration and risk of adverse effects	Avoid combination	Grapefruit juice has been shown to significantly inhibit CYP3A4 enzyme activity. Studies have reported a significant increase in drug concentration with this combination, which increases the risk of adverse effects and drug toxicity.
	Itraconazole	Altered drug levels possible	Caution with use of this combination	Data on effect of grapefruit juice on this drug is conflicting and significance is unclear. Caution with use until further data becomes available.
	L-Thyroxine (levothyroxine)	Possible decreased drug effect	Caution with use of this combination	A modest decrease in drug effect has been reported. The proposed mechanism for this interaction is due to inhibition of the organic anion-transporting protein polypeptide (OATP).
	Losartan	Possible decreased drug concentration	Caution with use of this combination	A study in healthy volunteers reported decreased drug concentrations with use of this combination. Clinical significance is unclear.
	Methadone	Increased drug plasma concentration and risk of adverse effects	Caution with use of this combination	An increased drug concentration has been reported with this combination. Clinical significance is unclear.
	Methylprednisolone	Increased drug plasma concentration and risk of adverse effects	Avoid combination	Studies have reported an increase in drug concentration with this combination, which increases the risk of adverse effects and drug toxicity.

ACNM NUTRIENT AND NUTRITIONAL SUPPLEMENTS INTERACTIONS TABLE—cont'd				
Nutrient/ supplement	Drug/drug class	Potential outcome	Recommendations	Comments
Grapefruit cont'd	Nadolol	Theoretical decreased drug effect	Caution with use of this combination	Grapefruit juice may theoretically decrease drug bioavailability due to inhibition of the organic anion-transporting polypeptide (OATP1A2). It is not known if this interaction is clinically significant.
	Nilotinib	Increased drug plasma concentration and increased absorption	Caution with use of this combination	Increased drug concentration and drug absorption have been reported with this combination.
	Oestrogens	Increased drug plasma concentration and risk of adverse effects	Caution with use of this combination	Increased plasma concentrations have been reported. It has been proposed that this is due to inhibition of CYP3A4.
	Organic anion-transporting polypeptide substrates (OATP)	Possible decreased drug absorption and drug effect	Avoid combination	In vitro and clinical evidence show that grapefruit juice inhibits organic anion-transporting polypeptides (OATP). This reduces bioavailability of oral drugs that are OATP substrates. Separation of dose administration by at least 4 hours may help to avoid this interaction as the effect appears to only last for a short time.
	Oxycodone	Increased drug concentration and risk of adverse effects	Avoid combination	An increase in drug concentration has been reported with this combination. Oxycodone is metabolised by CYP3A4.
	Praziquantel	Increased drug concentration and risk of adverse effects	Avoid combination	Studies have reported a significant increase in drug concentration with this combination, which increases the risk of adverse effects and drug toxicity.
	Primaquine	Possible increased drug bioavailability	Caution with use of this combination	An increase in drug bioavailability has been reported. Clinical significance is unclear.
	Quinidine	Altered drug effect	Caution with use of this combination	Grapefruit juice has been reported to decrease drug absorption, clearance and metabolism, and to prolong drug half-life. Clinical significance is unclear.
	Regorafenib	Theoretical increased drug concentrations and risk of toxicity	Avoid combination	Grapefruit juice has been shown to significantly inhibit CYP3A4 enzyme activity. While no direct interaction has been reported, this drug is a CYP3A4 substrate.
	Repaglinide	Small increase in serum drug concentration	Caution with use of this combination	A small but significant increase in drug concentration has been reported with use of this combination.
	Saquinavir	Increased drug absorption	Caution with use of this combination	Increased drug absorption has been reported with use of this combination. This interaction does not appear to occur with indinavir, another protease-inhibitor.

Continued

ACNM NUTRIENT AND NUTRITIONAL SUPPLEMENTS INTERACTIONS TABLE—cont'd

Nutrient/ supplement	Drug/drug class	Potential outcome	Recommendations	Comments
Grapefruit cont'd	Scopolamine	Increased drug concentration and risk of adverse effects	Avoid combination	An increased drug concentration has been reported with this combination. Scopolamine is metabolised by CYP3A4.
	Sertraline	Increased drug plasma concentration and risk of adverse effects	Caution with use of this combination	Two studies have reported a significant increase in drug concentration with this combination, which increases the risk of adverse effects and drug toxicity.
	Sildenafil	Increased drug concentration and risk of adverse effects	Caution with use of this combination	An increased drug concentration has been reported with this combination. Sildenafil is metabolised by CYP3A4.
	Sunitinib	Possible increase in drug plasma concentration	Caution with use of this combination	A modest increase in drug levels has been reported with use of this combination. This interaction may not be clinically significant, but caution is advised.
	Tacrolimus	Increased drug bioavailability and risk of adverse effects	Avoid combination unless under strict medical supervision	Studies have reported a significant increase in drug bioavailability with this combination. It has been proposed that this may enhance drug action, but strict medical supervision is required due to a lack of reliable safety and efficacy data.
	Talinolol	Possible increased drug bioavailability	Caution with use of this combination	An increase in drug bioavailability may occur with this combination. The clinical significance is unclear.
	Terfenadine	Possible increased drug concentrations	Avoid combination	An increase in drug absorption and plasma concentration have been reported with this combination. Clinical significance is unclear.
	Theophylline	Possible decreased drug concentrations	Caution with use of this combination	A modest decrease in drug levels has been reported. The mechanism of this interaction is unknown.
	Ticagrelor	Increased drug plasma concentration and risk of bleeding	Avoid combination	Grapefruit juice has been shown to significantly inhibit CYP3A4 enzyme activity. Studies have reported a significant increase in drug concentration with this combination, which increases the risk of adverse effects and drug toxicity.
	Tolvaptan	Increased drug plasma concentration and risk of adverse effects	Caution with use of this combination	Studies have reported an increase in drug concentration with this combination. This may lead to an increased extent and duration of diuretic effect, and an increased risk of adverse effects and drug toxicity.
	Toremifene	Theoretical increased drug plasma concentration and risk of adverse effects	Avoid combination	Grapefruit juice has been shown to significantly inhibit CYP3A4 enzyme activity. While an interaction between grapefruit juice and this drug has not been demonstrated directly, the drug is a CYP3A4 substrate. There is a theoretical risk of prolonged QT interval.

ACNM NUTRIENT AND NUTRITIONAL SUPPLEMENTS INTERACTIONS TABLE—cont'd

Nutrient/ supplement	Drug/drug class	Potential outcome	Recommendations	Comments
Grapefruit cont'd	Warfarin	Theoretical increased risk of bleeding	Caution with use of this combination	A case report describes an increase in INR in a patient taking large doses of grapefruit juice while on warfarin. A small clinical study, however, reported that daily consumption of grapefruit juice did not affect INR in a group of men taking warfarin. Caution is recommended until more safety data becomes available.
Green tea (epigallocatechin-3-gallate)	Alcohol	Theoretical increased risk of adverse effects	Monitor – unlikely to be clinically significant	Alcohol reduces caffeine metabolism. There is a theoretical increased risk of adverse effects with this combination.
	Amphetamines	Theoretical increased risk of CNS effects	Caution with use of this combination	Caffeine in green tea may theoretically have additive CNS effects.
	Anticoagulant/ antiplatelet drugs	Theoretical increased risk of bleeding	Caution with use of this combination	Catechins in green tea are reported to have antiplatelet activity. The interaction has not been reported in human studies; however, people taking warfarin should avoid excessive consumption of green tea.
	Antidiabetic drugs	Theoretical altered drugs effects	Monitor – unlikely to be clinically significant	Conflicting data suggests that that green tea may either increase or decrease blood sugar levels. Caution is advised until more data about this interaction becomes available.
	Antifungal agents	Theoretical decrease in metabolism of caffeine	Monitor – unlikely to be clinically significant	Some antifungal agents (e.g. fluconazole, terbinafine) may decrease caffeine metabolism, and will theoretically increase the risk of adverse effects at high doses. Evidence is inconclusive.
	Bortezomib	Theoretical decrease in drug effect	Avoid combination	Green tea polyphenols were reported to block drug anti-cancer effects in animal studies. Avoid until further data becomes available.
	Cimetidine	Increased effects of caffeine theoretically possible	Monitor – unlikely to be clinically significant	Cimetidine may reduce clearance of caffeine in green tea and theoretically increase the risk of caffeine-related adverse effects.
	Clozapine	Theoretical decrease in drug effect	Caution with use of this combination	Animal studies suggest green tea may reduce drug concentrations, although the clinical significance of these findings is unclear. Caffeine in green tea may potentially also exacerbate psychotic symptoms.
	Doxorubicin	Theoretical decreased drug adverse effects and enhanced drug action	May be beneficial – medical supervision recommended	Limited evidence suggests green tea polyphenols may reduce doxorubicin-induced cardiotoxicity. In addition, in vitro data suggests that EGCG and theanine may enhance drug activity. While human studies are required to confirm these effects, there is a theoretical beneficial interaction.
	Ephedrine	Increased risk of stimulatory effects	Avoid combination	Use of ephedrine with caffeine-containing products may increase the risk of excessive stimulatory effects.

Continued

		ACNM NUTRIENT AND NUTRITIONAL SUPPLEMENTS INTERACTIONS TABLE—cont'd		
Nutrient/ supplement	**Drug/drug class**	**Potential outcome**	**Recommendations**	**Comments**
Green tea (epigallocatechin-3-gallate) cont'd	Hepatotoxic drugs	Increased risk of hepatotoxicity	Caution with use of this combination	Green tea extract supplements have been linked to several cases of hepatoxicity. Concurrent use with hepatotoxic drugs will have additive effects.
	Iron	Theoretical decreased mineral absorption	Monitor – may not be clinically significant	Tea polyphenols may form chelates with non-heme iron and reduce absorption. This interaction does not appear to be clinically significant, based on current evidence, but separation of dose administration is recommended.
	Lithium	Increased risk of drug adverse effects if stopped suddenly	Caution with use of this combination	Abrupt withdrawal of caffeine can increase serum lithium levels and so increase the risk of adverse effects and drug toxicity.
	Monoamine oxidase inhibitors (MAOIs)	Increased risk of adverse effects	Caution with use of this combination	Theoretically, high intake of green tea or green tea extract may precipitate a hypertensive crisis when taken concurrently with MAOIs. This concern is based on the caffeine content of green tea.
	Theophylline	Theoretical increased risk of drug adverse effects	Caution with use of this combination	Caffeine in green tea may theoretically increase drug effects and adverse effects. The interaction may not be clinically relevant based on current data, but caution is advised.
Guar gum	Antidiabetic drugs	Theoretical additive effects	Monitor – may not be clinically significant	Guar gum may decrease blood glucose levels. Additive effects are possible, which may be beneficial, but caution is advised to reduce risk of hypoglycaemia.
	Antihypertensive drugs	Theoretical additive effects	Monitor – may not be clinically significant	Some evidence suggests that guar gum may lower blood pressure. Additive effects are theoretically possible, but caution is advised to reduce risk of hypotension.
	Digoxin	Theoretical decreased drug absorption	Caution with use of this combination	Guar gum may reduce drug absorption and theoretically decrease drug effect. Significance has not been established, but caution is advised.
	Metformin	Theoretical decreased drug absorption	Monitor – may not be clinically significant	Guar gum may reduce drug absorption and theoretically decrease drug effect. Significance has not been established.
	Oestrogens	Theoretical decreased drug absorption	Monitor – may not be clinically significant	Guar gum may reduce drug absorption and theoretically decrease drug effect. Significance has not been established.
	Penicillin	Theoretical decreased drug absorption	Monitor – may not be clinically significant	Guar gum may reduce drug absorption and theoretically decrease drug effect. Significance has not been established.

ACNM NUTRIENT AND NUTRITIONAL SUPPLEMENTS INTERACTIONS TABLE—cont'd				
Nutrient/ supplement	Drug/drug class	Potential outcome	Recommendations	Comments
Hesperidin	Anticoagulant/ antiplatelet drugs	Theoretical increased risk of bleeding	Monitor – may not be clinically significant	Hesperidin may have antiplatelet activity. There is a theoretical increased risk of bleeding, but clinical significance has not been established.
	Antihypertensive drugs	Theoretical additive effects	Monitor – may not be clinically significant	Some evidence suggests that hesperidin may lower blood pressure. Additive beneficial effects are theoretically possible, but caution is advised to reduce the risk of hypotension.
	CNS depressant drugs including benzodiazepines	Theoretical increased risk of sedation	Monitor – may not be clinically significant	Animal studies suggest hesperidin may have sedative effects due to opioid receptor activity. There is a theoretical increased risk of sedation when use with CNS depressant drugs.
	P-glycoprotein substrates	Theoretical increased drug effect	Monitor – may not be clinically significant	In vitro studies suggest hesperidin may inhibit p-glycoprotein. Theoretically, this could increase drug levels of p-glycoprotein substrates.
Indole-3-carbinol	CYP450 substrates (CYP1A2)	Theoretical increased drug levels	Monitor – clinical significance unclear	In vitro and in vivo evidence suggest indole-3-carbinol may inhibit CYP1A2. This could theoretically result in increased drug concentration and risk of drug toxicity, although clinical significance is not known.
Inositol	Anticonvulsant drugs carbamazepine, valproic acid	Theoretical decrease in inositol levels in the brain.	Monitor – may not be clinically significant	Carbamazepine and valproic acid have been shown to reduce inositol levels in the brain. This is possibly due to these drugs inhibiting an enzyme involved in inositol synthesis. The clinical significance of this is unknown, but caution is advised with use of inositol supplements in patients taking these drugs
	Lithium	Possible reduced drug effect	Caution with use of this combination	Lithium reduces inositol levels in the brain by inhibition of an enzyme involved in synthesis of inositol. Preliminary data also suggest that inositol supplements may reduce the therapeutic effects of lithium, and that dietary restriction of inositol may enhance effects of lithium. Caution is advised until more data becomes available.
Iodine	Amiodarone	Risk of excessive iodine	Caution with use of this combination	Amiodarone contains nearly 40% iodine and can increase iodine levels. Concomitant use with iodine supplements may result in excessive iodine levels and may adversely affect thyroid function.
	Anti-thyroid medication (e.g. carbimazole, propylthiouracil)	Increased risk of hypothyroidism	Avoid combination	Concomitant use may result in additive hypothyroid activity and may lead to hypothyroidism. The combination should be avoided.

Continued

ACNM NUTRIENT AND NUTRITIONAL SUPPLEMENTS INTERACTIONS TABLE—cont'd				
Nutrient/ supplement	Drug/drug class	Potential outcome	Recommendations	Comments
Iodine cont'd	Lithium	Theoretical increased risk of hypothyroidism	Caution with use of this combination	Lithium may inhibit thyroid function. Combined use may have additive hypothyroid effects.
	Metronidazole	Risk of mineral depletion	May be beneficial to address nutrient depletion	There is a moderate risk of iodine depletion. Patients should be monitored as supplements may be required in some individuals.
Iron	ACE-Inhibitors	Possible improvement of drug-induced cough	Combination may be beneficial	Oral iron supplementation may inhibit coughs induced by ACE-I, according to a study used ferrous sulphate 200 mg. This appears to be due to an effect on nitric oxide generation.
	Acid-reducing agents (e.g. antacids, H$_2$-antagonists, proton pump inhibitors)	Decreased iron absorption	Monitor – separate doses	Adequate gastric acid is important for iron absorption. Drugs that raise gastric pH may theoretically reduce iron absorption. Doses should be separated.
	Antibiotics (tetracyclines and quinolones)	Reduced drug effect	Caution with use of this combination	Iron supplements form complexes with these drugs and may reduce drug effectiveness. Separate doses by at least 2 hours.
	Bisphosphonates	Reduced drug absorption	Caution with use of this combination	Iron can reduce absorption of oral bisphosphonates and reduce drug efficacy. Separate doses by at least 2 hours.
	Chloramphenicol	Theoretical decreased response to mineral	Monitor – may not be clinically significant	Chloramphenicol interferes with maturation of erythrocytes and may reduce response to iron supplements in iron deficiency anaemia. The interaction is unlikely to be clinically significant as the antibiotic is generally only used short term.
	Integrase inhibitors (e.g. dolutegravir)	Reduced drug effect	Caution with use of this combination	Iron supplements may form complexes with drugs in this class and reduce drug effectiveness. Separate doses by at least 2 hours.
	L-Thyroxine (Levothyroxine)	Reduced drug effect	Caution with use of this combination	Iron supplements may form complexes with L-thyroxine and reduce drug effectiveness. Separate doses by at least 2 hours.
	Levodopa	Reduced drug effect	Caution with use of this combination	Iron supplements may form complexes with levodopa and reduce drug effectiveness. Separate doses by at least 2 hours.
	Methyldopa	Reduced drug effect	Caution with use of this combination	Iron supplements are known to form complexes with methyldopa and reduce drug effectiveness. Separate doses by at least 2 hours or avoid combination.

		ACNM NUTRIENT AND NUTRITIONAL SUPPLEMENTS INTERACTIONS TABLE—cont'd		
Nutrient/ supplement	**Drug/drug class**	**Potential outcome**	**Recommendations**	**Comments**
Iron cont'd	Minerals (calcium, zinc)	Reduced mineral absorption	Monitor – separate doses	Calcium may inhibit the absorption of haem and non-haem iron. This may not be clinically significant unless there is iron deficiency. Doses should be separated. Iron and zinc supplements can interfere with each other's absorption, especially if taken on an empty stomach due to competition for non-specific carriers. The interaction does not appear to be significant if the supplements are taken with food as the ions complex with food components. Take supplements with food or separate intake.
	Mycophenolate mofetil	Theoretical decreased drug absorption	Caution with use of this combination	It has been proposed that iron may form an insoluble chelate with this drug and decrease absorption. This has not been demonstrated in clinical studies, but caution is advised and dose administration should be separated.
	Penicillamine	Reduced drug effect	Caution with use of this combination	Iron supplements may form complexes with penicillamine and reduce drug effectiveness. Separate doses by at least 2 hours.
	Vitamin C	Increased vitamin absorption	Combination may be beneficial	Vitamin C (dietary and supplemental) improves absorption of iron if ingested at the same time.
Krill oil – see Omega-3 essential fatty acids				
L-Arginine – see Arginine				
L-Carnitine – see Carnitine				
L-Glutamine – see Glutamine				
L-Tryptophan – see Tryptophan				
Lactobacilli and Bifidobacteria – see Probiotics				
Lutein	Orlistat	Theoretical risk of nutrient depletion	May be beneficial to address nutrient depletion	Theoretically, long-term use of orlistat may result in lutein depletion due to reduced gastrointestinal absorption. Patients should be monitored. Supplements may be required in some individuals.
Lycopene	Anticoagulant/ antiplatelet drugs	Theoretical increased risk of bleeding	Caution with use of this combination	Lycopene may have antiplatelet effects based on in vitro studies. There is a theoretical increased risk of bleeding.
Lysine	Antiviral therapy (e.g. acyclovir, famciclovir)	Improved disease management	Combination may be beneficial	Lysine has been shown to be beneficial in reducing the recurrence of herpes simplex infections, and may reduce severity and healing times of herpes simplex infections. No negative interactions have been reported in the literature with use of lysine concurrently with antiviral therapy for herpes infection.

Continued

ACNM NUTRIENT AND NUTRITIONAL SUPPLEMENTS INTERACTIONS TABLE—cont'd				
Nutrient/ supplement	**Drug/drug class**	**Potential outcome**	**Recommendations**	**Comments**
Maca	Antidepressant drugs (SSRIs, SNRIs)	Possible decreased drug adverse effects	Combination may be beneficial	Maca may help to alleviate sexual dysfunction caused by SSRIs/SNRIs, according to the findings of a small clinical trial conducted in postmenopausal women who were taking these drugs for depression.
Magnesium	Alcohol	Risk of mineral depletion	May be beneficial to address nutrient depletion	High ingestion of alcohol may result in magnesium depletion. Alcohol impairs the kidneys' ability to conserve magnesium and so may result in increased urinary excretion. Supplements may be indicated in some individuals.
	Anticoagulant/ antiplatelet drugs	Theoretical increased risk of bleeding	Monitor – clinical significance unclear	In vitro evidence suggests magnesium sulphate may inhibit platelet aggregation. Some preliminary clinical research suggests that IV magnesium may increase bleeding time and reduce platelet activity, but results from research have been inconsistent and conflicting.
	Antibiotics (aminogylcosides)	Theoretical increased risk of neuromuscular adverse effects; theoretical risk of mineral depletion	Caution with use of this combination	An animal study reported that concurrent use of IV magnesium and aminoglycoside antibiotics led to neuromuscular weakness and possible paralysis. A case report describes respiratory failure in an infant with high blood magnesium levels after administration of gentamycin. Magnesium and aminoglycoside antibiotics both reduce presynaptic release of acetylcholine, which can affect neuromuscular function. Aminoglycosides have also been associated with nephrotoxicity which may increase urinary loss of magnesium.
	Antibiotics (tetracyclines and quinolones)	Reduced drug effect possible	Caution with use of this combination	Magnesium supplements form complexes with these drugs and may reduce drug effectiveness. Use with caution and separate doses by at least 2 hours.
	Antidiabetic drugs (sulphonylureas) e.g. glibenclamide, glipizide)	Theoretical increased drug absorption	Monitor – clinical significance unclear	Antacids containing magnesium hydroxide raise gastric pH, which is reported to increase absorption of glibenclamide and glipizide. This may theoretically increase the risk of hypoglycaemia.
	Amphotericin-B	Major risk of mineral depletion	May be beneficial to address nutrient depletion	There is a major risk of magnesium depletion associated with use of this antifungal agent (not marketed in Australia). Supplements may be required with long-term use.
	Bisphosphonates	Risk of decreased drug absorption	Caution with use of this combination – separate doses	Magnesium may reduce drug absorption and bioavailability by forming drug-mineral complexes. Separate dose administration by 2 hours.

ACNM NUTRIENT AND NUTRITIONAL SUPPLEMENTS INTERACTIONS TABLE—cont'd

Nutrient/supplement	Drug/drug class	Potential outcome	Recommendations	Comments
Magnesium cont'd	Calcium channel blockers	Additive effect possible	Combination may be beneficial – monitor	Magnesium may theoretically have an additive effect when used with calcium channel blockers at high doses. The interaction is likely to be beneficial at normal therapeutic doses, although there is a theoretical risk of hypotension. Caution is advised as some research has reported severe hypotension and neuromuscular blockade with concurrent use of IV magnesium and nifedipine.
	Corticosteroids (chronic use)	Risk of mineral depletion	May be beneficial to address nutrient depletion	Moderate risk of depletion. Patients should be monitored and supplements may be required in some individuals.
	Cyclosporin	Risk of mineral depletion	May be beneficial to address nutrient depletion	Moderate risk of depletion. Patients should be monitored and supplements may be required in some individuals.
	Digoxin	Risk of decreased drug effect; risk of mineral depletion	Caution with use of this combination	Clinical evidence suggests that oral magnesium hydroxide or magnesium trisilicate may reduce digoxin absorption, which could lead to decreased therapeutic effects. Digoxin may also result in increased urinary excretion of magnesium, resulting in a moderate risk of depletion. Patients should be monitored and supplements may be required in some individuals. Depletion increases the risk of arrhythmias and may have serious consequences. The likelihood of depletion is increased if the patient is also taking diuretics, e.g. in heart failure.
	Diuretics (loop and thiazide)	Risk of mineral depletion	May be beneficial to address nutrient depletion	Moderate risk of depletion. Patients should be monitored and supplements may be required in some individuals.
	Diuretics (potassium-sparing)	Possible risk of excessive magnesium	Monitor – may not be clinically significant	Potassium-sparing diuretics may also spare magnesium. Theoretically, concomitant use of magnesium supplements with potassium-sparing diuretics may result in raised magnesium levels; however, significance is not clear.
	Foscarnet	Risk of mineral depletion	May be beneficial to address nutrient depletion	Foscarnet may result in symptomatic hypomagnesaemia, possibly due to magnesium chelation and increased elimination. Magnesium levels should be monitored and supplements may be required in some patients.

Continued

ACNM NUTRIENT AND NUTRITIONAL SUPPLEMENTS INTERACTIONS TABLE—cont'd				
Nutrient/ supplement	Drug/drug class	Potential outcome	Recommendations	Comments
Magnesium cont'd	Minerals (calcium, zinc)	Reduced mineral absorption	Monitor – separate doses	Calcium may decrease absorption of magnesium. Magnesium does not appear to affect calcium absorption. High-dose zinc supplements may decrease magnesium absorption and increase magnesium excretion. These interactions may not be clinically relevant unless there is a deficiency, but dosage separation is generally advised.
	Oestrogens (e.g. oral contraceptives, HRT)	Risk of mineral depletion	May be beneficial to address nutrient depletion	There is a moderate risk of depletion with long-term use of oestrogens. Oestrogens enhance uptake of magnesium into soft tissue and bones which may lower serum levels. Patients should be monitored and supplements may be required in some individuals.
	Panitumumab	Risk of mineral depletion	May be beneficial to address nutrient depletion	Hypomagnesaemia has occurred with use of this drug, with decreased magnesium levels being reported in almost 40% of patients according to secondary sources. Monitor for signs of magnesium depletion.
	Penicillamine	Possible decreased drug absorption	Caution with use of this combination	Magnesium may reduce drug bioavailability by forming insoluble drug-mineral complexes. Dose administration should be separated and patients should be monitored for magnesium depletion with long-term drug use.
	Pentamidine	Major risk of mineral depletion	May be beneficial to address nutrient depletion	Symptomatic hypomagnesaemia has occurred with use of this drug, especially when given intravenously. Patients should be monitored and supplements will be needed in most patients with long-term use.
	Proguanil	Possible decreased drug absorption	Caution with use of this combination	A small study reported that concomitant use of magnesium trisilicate and the antimalarial drug proguanil resulted in a significant decrease in drug absorption. Separate dose administration by at least 3 hours.
	Proton pump inhibitors (PPIs)	Major risk of mineral depletion	May be beneficial to address nutrient depletion	PPIs inhibit the active transport of magnesium and long-term use may lead to severe hypomagnesemia with side effects including muscle spasm, tetany, hypokalaemia, hypoparathyroidism, hypocalcaemia, and seizures. A magnesium supplement will be required by most individuals who take PPIs long term.
	Tacrolimus	Major risk of mineral depletion	May be beneficial to address nutrient depletion	Tacrolimus reduces renal tubular reabsorption of magnesium. Hypomagnesaemia is reported in a significant proportion of people treated with tacrolimus. Supplements will be required in most individuals.

ACNM NUTRIENT AND NUTRITIONAL SUPPLEMENTS INTERACTIONS TABLE—cont'd				
Nutrient/ supplement	Drug/drug class	Potential outcome	Recommendations	Comments
Maitake mushrooms	Antidiabetic drugs	Possible additive effects	Caution with use of this combination	Preliminary clinical research suggests maitake mushrooms may lower blood glucose levels in type 2 diabetic patients. Concomitant use with antidiabetic drugs may result in additive effects and an increased risk of hypoglycaemia.
	Antihypertensive drugs	Theoretical additive effects	Caution with use of this combination	Animal research suggests maitake mushrooms may lower blood pressure. Theoretically, concomitant use with antihypertensive drugs may result in additive effects and an increased risk of hypotension.
	Warfarin	Theoretical increased risk of bleeding	Caution with use of this combination	A case report describes an increase in INR when a patient who was previously stabilised on warfarin commenced taking maitake mushrooms. It has been proposed that this may have been due to protein displacement of warfarin, resulting in increased anticoagulant effect. Caution is advised until more data becomes available.
Manganese	Antibiotics (e.g. tetracyclines and quinolones)	Reduced drug effect possible	Monitor – separate doses	Manganese supplements form complexes with these drugs, which may theoretically reduce drug effectiveness. Separate doses by at least 2 hours.
Mangosteen	Anticoagulant/ antiplatelet drugs	Theoretical increased risk of bleeding	Caution with use of this combination	In vitro and animal research suggests mangosteen may have antiplatelet activity. There is a theoretical increased risk of bleeding, although data is limited.
Medicinal mushrooms	*Refer to Agaricus mushroom, Cordyceps mushroom, Maitake mushroom, Reishi mushroom, Shiitake mushroom*			
Melatonin	Anticoagulant/ antiplatelet drugs	Possible increased risk of bleeding	Caution with use of this combination	Isolated case reports describe bleeding with use of warfarin and melatonin which suggests a possible interaction. More data is needed to confirm interaction.
	Anticonvulsant drugs	Possible increased risk of seizures	Caution with use of this combination	Some clinical evidence suggests that melatonin may increase the risk of seizures in certain patients, especially in neurologically disabled children. Melatonin may inhibit drug effects in these patients.
	Antidiabetic drugs	Possible altered disease management	Caution with use of this combination	Some evidence suggests that melatonin may impair glucose utilisation and increase insulin resistance. Other studies have reported improved glycaemic control, while still others have reported that melatonin has no effect on glucose levels. Caution is advised until more data becomes available.

Continued

ACNM NUTRIENT AND NUTRITIONAL SUPPLEMENTS INTERACTIONS TABLE—cont'd				
Nutrient/ supplement	**Drug/drug class**	**Potential outcome**	**Recommendations**	**Comments**
Melatonin cont'd	Antihypertensive drugs e.g. verapamil, nifedipine	Possible altered disease management	Caution with use of this combination	Melatonin may decrease blood pressure according to some studies. Other studies, however, report that melatonin may worsen blood pressure in patients taking antihypertensive drugs. Caution is advised until more data becomes available.
	Benzodiazepines	Possible reduced endogenous melatonin. Risk of excessive sedative effects with combined use	Caution with use of this combination	Theoretically, chronic intake of benzodiazepines may decrease endogenous melatonin levels. Additive effects are possible with combined use which may lead to excessive drowsiness and sedation.
	CNS depressant drugs	Risk of excessive sedative effects	Caution with use of this combination	Additive effects are possible which may lead to excessive drowsiness and sedation.
	Fluvoxamine	Risk of increased melatonin levels	Caution with use of this combination	Fluvoxamine can significantly increase melatonin levels and may lead to excessive drowsiness.
	Hypnotic drugs including zolpidem	Risk of excessive sedative effects	Caution with use of this combination	Additive effects are possible which may lead to excessive drowsiness and sedation.
	Immunosuppressant drugs	Possible decreased drug effect	Caution with use of this combination	Melatonin may have immuno-stimulant activity. This may theoretically interfere with immunosuppressive drug action.
	Methamphetamine	Theoretical increased drug adverse effects	Caution with use of this combination	Animal research suggests melatonin may exacerbate adverse effects of methamphetamine.
	Nifedipine	Possible decreased drug effect	Caution with use of this combination	Preliminary evidence suggests that melatonin may impair antihypertensive activity of nifedipine. Caution is advised until further data becomes available.
	Oestrogens	Risk of excessive sedative effects	Caution with use of this combination	Oestrogens may inhibit metabolism of melatonin, which may result in increased drowsiness and sedation.
	Propofol	Possible decreased drug requirement for anaesthesia	Caution with use of this combination	A study reported that the combination resulted in a decreased dose requirement of Propofol to induce anaesthesia.
	Psoralen medication e.g. 5-methoxypsoralen	Risk of excessive sedative effects	Caution with use of this combination	Drugs in this class may inhibit metabolism of melatonin, which may result in increased drowsiness and sedation.
	Seizure threshold lowering drugs	Possible increased risk of seizures	Caution with use of this combination	Some clinical evidence suggests a risk of increased frequency of seizures with this combination, especially in neurologically disabled children.

	ACNM NUTRIENT AND NUTRITIONAL SUPPLEMENTS INTERACTIONS TABLE—cont'd			
Nutrient/ supplement	**Drug/drug class**	**Potential outcome**	**Recommendations**	**Comments**
N-acetyl cysteine (NAC)	ACE-Inhibitors (ACE-I)	Theoretical additive effects	Caution with use of this combination	NAC may potentiate the blood pressure-lowering effects of ACE-I according to animal research. The interaction may potentially be beneficial, but caution is advised due to a risk of hypotension.
	Activated charcoal	Possible decreased effect of activated charcoal	Caution with use of this combination	NAC may possibly reduce the ability of activated charcoal to adsorb paracetamol and aspirin according to some studies. Activated charcoal does not appear to affect effectiveness of NAC.
	Anticoagulant/ antiplatelet drugs	Increased risk of bleeding	Caution with use of this combination	NAC may decrease platelet aggregation and prothrombin time, prolong coagulation time and increase blood loss in surgical patients.
	Antihypertensive drugs	Theoretical additive effects	Caution with use of this combination	NAC may potentiate the blood pressure-lowering effects of ACE-I according to animal research. This effect may theoretically also be seen with other antihypertensive drugs. The interaction may potentially be beneficial, but caution is advised due to a risk of hypotension.
	Chloroquine	Theoretical decreased drug effect	Caution with use of this combination	Animal research suggest NAC may reduce drug antimalarial effect by increasing cellular levels of glutathione.
	Clomiphene	Possible improved outcomes	May be beneficial – medical supervision recommended	NAC was shown to be a safe and effective adjuvant to clomiphene in improving induction of ovulation in patients with PCOS.
	Nitroglycerine (glyceryl trinitrate)	Increased risk of hypotension and severe headache	Avoid combination	Concurrent use of NAC and IV nitroglycerine may cause severe hypotension and intolerable headaches according to limited clinical research.
Nattokinase	Anticoagulant/ antiplatelet drugs	Theoretical increased risk of bleeding	Caution with use of this combination	Nattokinase may have antiplatelet effects based on in vitro and animal studies. There is a theoretical increased risk of bleeding.
	Antihypertensive drugs	Possible additive effects	Combination may be beneficial	Nattokinase has been shown to reduce blood pressure in clinical trials. Concurrent use may be additive and potentially beneficial, but monitor for hypotension.
New Zealand green-lipped mussel	NSAIDs	Possible additive effects	Combination may be beneficial	Additive beneficial effects are theoretically possible due to the anti-inflammatory effects of NZ green lipped mussel. No negative interaction has been reported with this combination.

Continued

ACNM NUTRIENT AND NUTRITIONAL SUPPLEMENTS INTERACTIONS TABLE—cont'd

Nutrient/ supplement	Drug/drug class	Potential outcome	Recommendations	Comments
Niacin (vitamin B3)	Alcohol	Increased risk of adverse effects	Caution with use of this combination	Alcohol may exacerbate flushing and pruritic associated with high-dose niacin supplementation.
	Anticoagulant/ antiplatelet drugs	Theoretical increased risk of bleeding	Caution with use of this combination	High-dose sustained release niacin may theoretically increase the risk of bleeding in patients taking anticoagulants and antiplatelet drugs.
	Antidiabetic drugs	Risk that condition may be exacerbated	Caution with use of this combination	High-dose niacin may impair glycaemic control, possibly aggravating insulin intolerance and increasing glucose production by the liver. About 10–35% of diabetic patients may need drug dose adjustments with high-dose niacin therapy.
	Antiepileptic drugs	Risk of vitamin depletion	May be beneficial to address nutrient depletion	A moderate risk of nutrient depletion has been reported with use of phenytoin and valproic acid.
	Antihypertensive drugs	Possible additive effects	Caution with use of this combination	Some evidence suggests that high-dose niacin may lower blood pressure in hypertensive individuals. This may potentially be beneficial, but monitor as there is an increased risk of hypotension.
	Antigout drugs	Possible decreased disease management	Caution with use of this combination	High-dose niacin may reduce urinary excretion of uric acid, potentially leading to hyperuricaemia. Drug dosage adjustment may be required if patients who commence treatment with high-dose niacin.
	Azathioprine	Risk of vitamin depletion	May be beneficial to address nutrient depletion	A moderate depletion of niacin has been reported with use of this drug. Supplements may be required in some individuals.
	Bile acid sequestrants	Possible decreased nutrient absorption and increased risk of myopathy	Caution with use of this combination	Bile acid sequestrants can bind niacin and decrease absorption. Doses should be separated. Some evidence suggests an increased risk of myopathy associated with concomitant use of high-dose niacin and bile acid sequestrants.
	Cycloserine	Risk of vitamin depletion	May be beneficial to address nutrient depletion	A moderate depletion of niacin has been reported with use of this drug. Supplements may be required in some individuals.
	Fluorouracil	Risk of vitamin depletion	May be beneficial to address nutrient depletion	A moderate depletion of niacin has been reported with use of this drug. Supplements may be required in some individuals.

	ACNM NUTRIENT AND NUTRITIONAL SUPPLEMENTS INTERACTIONS TABLE—cont'd			
Nutrient/ supplement	Drug/drug class	Potential outcome	Recommendations	Comments
Niacin (vitamin B3) cont'd	HMGCoA reductase inhibitors (Statins)	Possible additive lipid lowering effects	Combination may be beneficial	High-dose niacin may enhance drug lipid-lowering effects and the combination may be beneficial and result in improved outcomes. Case reports have, however, suggested an increased risk of muscle myopathy with this combination. Evidence of this interaction is limited and significance unclear.
	Isoniazid	Risk of vitamin depletion	May be beneficial to address nutrient depletion	A moderate depletion of niacin has been reported with use of this drug. Supplements may be required in some individuals.
	Levodopa/ carbidopa	Risk of vitamin depletion	May be beneficial to address nutrient depletion	A moderate depletion of niacin has been reported with use of this drug. Supplements may be required in some individuals.
Nicotinamide (Vitamin B3)	Anticoagulant/ antiplatelet drugs	Theoretical increased risk of bleeding	Caution with use of this combination	Concomitant use of high-dose nicotinamide with anticoagulant/ antiplatelet drugs may increase the risk of bleeding, based on case reports. Caution is advised until further safety data becomes available.
	Carbamazepine	Theoretical increased drug levels	Caution with use of this combination	Two case reports suggest that high-dose nicotinamide may increase drug levels. There is currently insufficient data to determine significance.
	Ethionamide	Risk of nutrient depletion	May be beneficial to address nutrient depletion	This drug has structural similarities to nicotinamide and may interfere with nutrient activity. There is a moderate risk of nutrient depletion. Supplements may be required in some individuals.
	Hepatoxic drugs	Theoretical increased risk of hepatoxicity	Caution with use of this combination	Nicotinamide has been associated with increased liver enzymes and liver damage at high doses. Theoretically, concomitant use may result in an increased risk of liver damage.
	Primidone	Theoretical increased drug levels	Caution with use of this combination	Limited case reports suggest that high-dose nicotinamide may reduce drug metabolism and increase drug levels. There is currently insufficient data to determine significance.
	Pyrazinamide	Risk of nutrient depletion	May be beneficial to address nutrient depletion	This drug has structural similarities to nicotinamide and may interfere with nutrient activity. There is a moderate risk of nutrient depletion. Supplements may be required in some individuals.

Continued

ACNM NUTRIENT AND NUTRITIONAL SUPPLEMENTS INTERACTIONS TABLE—cont'd

Nutrient/ supplement	Drug/drug class	Potential outcome	Recommendations	Comments
Omega-3 fatty acids (EPA and DHA)	Anticoagulant/ antiplatelet drugs	Possible additive effects, with theoretical increased risk of bleeding	Monitor, but unlikely to be clinically significant	There has long been concern that use of fish or krill oil supplements may increase the risk of bleeding with anticoagulant/antiplatelet drugs, due to the antiplatelet activity of EPA. A recent, large, retrospective analysis, however, found no reports of an interaction between warfarin and fish or krill oil. This supports findings of other studies that found no evidence of an interaction between warfarin and fish oil. Monitoring is advised at very high dose intake (equivalent to ⋯$\rightarrow$12g fish oil daily).
	Antihypertensive drugs	Possible additive effects	Combination may be beneficial	Omega-3 fatty acids as fish oils have been shown to have a small, but consistent blood pressure-lowering effect. Additive beneficial effects may be seen when used concomitantly with antihypertensive drugs.
	Chemotherapy	Possible improved outcomes	Combination may be beneficial	Omega-3 fatty acids may provide nutritional, anti-inflammatory and cardiovascular support and enhance overall patient management. There does not appear to be evidence of a negative interaction.
	Corticosteroids	Possible improved outcomes	Combination may be beneficial	Omega-3 supplements may improve management of inflammatory conditions, including RA and IBD. Theoretically, the combination may allow for lower dose requirements of corticosteroids. There does not appear to be evidence of a negative interaction.
	Cyclosporin	Possible reduced drug adverse effects	Combination may be beneficial	Some research evidence suggests omega-3 fatty acids may help to reduce blood pressure and preserve renal function in patients following organ transplantation. Results have been inconsistent.
	Lipid-lowering drugs – hypertriglyceridaemia	Possible additive effects	Combination may be beneficial	Omega-3 essential fatty acids as fish oils have been shown to significantly reduce triglyceride levels and may be beneficial as an adjunct therapy with drugs used to treat hypertriglyceridaemia.
	Non-steroidal anti-inflammatory drugs (NSAIDs)	Possible additive effects	Combination may be beneficial	Fish or krill oil can reduce inflammation, pain and swelling due to the EPA content. The combination will have an additive beneficial effect especially in the management of conditions such as arthritis.
	Sulphasalazine	Possible improved outcomes	Combination may be beneficial	Omega-3 fatty acid supplements may improve management of inflammatory conditions, including RA and IBD. Theoretically, the combination may allow for lower drug dose requirements. There does not appear to be evidence of a negative interaction.

	ACNM NUTRIENT AND NUTRITIONAL SUPPLEMENTS INTERACTIONS TABLE—cont'd			
Nutrient/ supplement	**Drug/drug class**	**Potential outcome**	**Recommendations**	**Comments**
Papain	Anticoagulants/ antiplatelet drugs	Theoretical increased risk of bleeding	Caution with use of this combination	Combined use may theoretically potentiate the erects of warfarin. Clinical significance is unclear.
Phosphatidylcholine	Acetylcholinesterase (AChE) inhibitors (e.g. donepezil, rivastigmine)	Theoretical increased risk of cholinergic adverse effects	Caution with use of this combination	Phosphatidylcholine may theoretically increase acetylcholine levels. The combination could theoretically increase the risk of cholinergic adverse effects.
	Anticholinergic drugs	Theoretical decreased drug effect	Caution with use of this combination	Phosphatidylcholine may theoretically increase acetylcholine levels. The combination could theoretically decrease effectiveness of anticholinergic drugs.
	Cholinergic drugs	Theoretical increased risk of cholinergic adverse effects	Caution with use of this combination	Phosphatidylcholine may theoretically increase acetylcholine levels. The combination could theoretically increase the risk of cholinergic adverse effects.
Phosphatidylserine	Acetylcholinesterase (AChE) inhibitors (e.g. donepezil, rivastigmine)	Theoretical increased risk of cholinergic adverse effects	Caution with use of this combination	Phosphatidylserine may theoretically increase acetylcholine levels. The combination could theoretically increase the risk of cholinergic adverse effects.
	Anticholinergic drugs	Theoretical decreased drug effect	Caution with use of this combination	Phosphatidylcholine may theoretically increase acetylcholine levels. The combination could theoretically decrease effectiveness of anticholinergic drugs.
	Cholinergic drugs	Theoretical increased risk of cholinergic adverse effects	Caution with use of this combination	Phosphatidylcholine may theoretically increase acetylcholine levels. The combination could theoretically increase the risk of cholinergic adverse effects.
Pomegranate	ACE-Inhibitors (ACE-I)	Theoretical additive effects	Caution with use of this combination	Pomegranate may have an action similar to ACE-Inhibitors, leading to a theoretical increased risk of hypotension and potassium depletion.
	Antihypertensive drugs	Theoretical additive effects	Caution with use of this combination	Pomegranate may moderately lower blood pressure, leading to a theoretical increased risk of hypotension.
	Carbamazepine	Theoretical risk of increased drug levels	Caution with use of this combination	Animal models suggest pomegranate juice may decrease the rate of drug metabolism and increase drug serum levels. Limited clinical research suggests this effect may not occur in humans. Caution is advised until more data becomes available.

Continued

ACNM NUTRIENT AND NUTRITIONAL SUPPLEMENTS INTERACTIONS TABLE—cont'd				
Nutrient/ supplement	Drug/drug class	Potential outcome	Recommendations	Comments
Pomegranate cont'd	CYP450 substrates (CYP2C9, CYP2D6, CYP3A4)	Theoretical risk of increased drug levels	Caution with use of this combination	Animal models suggest pomegranate may inhibit activity of CYP2C9 and CYP2D6. There is a theoretical risk of increased drug levels and adverse effects, but clinical significance in humans is currently unknown. There is contradictory evidence as to the effect of pomegranate on CYP3A4, with some reports suggesting enzyme inhibition, others suggesting enzyme induction and still others showing no effect.
	Rosuvastatin	Theoretical increased risk of drug adverse effects	Caution with use of this combination	A case report describes a patient on rosuvastatin that developed rhabdomyolysis 3 weeks after commencing pomegranate juice, 200 ml taken twice weekly. It is possible the patient was predisposed to this adverse effect as there was a history of elevated creatine kinase levels.
	Tacrolimus	Theoretical increased drug levels	Avoid combination	A case report describes elevated drug levels while consuming concentrated pomegranate popsicles. More data is required to determine significance.
	Warfarin	Theoretical increased risk of bleeding	Caution with use of this combination	High intake of pomegranate juice may increase bleeding time in patients taking warfarin, based on a two case reports. Until more safety data becomes available, patients taking warfarin should neither significantly increase, nor decrease, intake of pomegranate juice without medical supervision.
Potassium	ACE-Inhibitors (ACE-I)	Increased risk of hyperkalaemia	Caution with use of this combination	ACE-I have a potassium-sparing action. Concomitant use may theoretically increase the risk of hyperkalaemia. In practice, ACE-I are often prescribed with potassium-depleting diuretics, so this interaction may not be clinically relevant.
	Aminoglycosides	Risk of mineral depletion	Combination may be beneficial	Aminoglycosides may cause nephrotoxicity, which can lead to increased urinary loss of potassium. Patients should be monitored.
	Amphotericin-B	Major risk of mineral depletion	May be beneficial to address nutrient depletion	There is a major risk of potassium depletion associated with use of this antifungal agent (not marketed in Australia). Supplements may be required with long-term use.
	Angiotensin receptor blockers (ARBs)	Increased risk of hyperkalaemia	Caution with use of this combination	ARBs have a potassium-sparing action. Concomitant use may theoretically increase the risk of hyperkalaemia. In practice, ARBs are often prescribed with potassium-depleting diuretics, so this interaction may not be clinically relevant.

ACNM NUTRIENT AND NUTRITIONAL SUPPLEMENTS INTERACTIONS TABLE—cont'd				
Nutrient/ supplement	Drug/drug class	Potential outcome	Recommendations	Comments
Potassium cont'd	Cisplatin	Risk of mineral depletion	May be beneficial to address nutrient depletion	Cisplatin can cause renal tubular damage which may result in increased loss of electrolytes, including potassium.
	Corticosteroids	Risk of mineral depletion	May be beneficial to address nutrient depletion	Corticosteroids can cause sodium retention, resulting in a compensatory renal loss of potassium. Risk of hypokalaemia has been associated with drugs such as hydrocortisone, cortisone, fludrocortisone, prednisone and prednisolone.
	Diuretics – potassium depleting e.g. loop and thiazides	Major risk of mineral depletion	May be beneficial to address nutrient depletion	There is a major risk of potassium depletion associated with use of potassium depleting diuretics. Supplements may be required with long-term use.
	Diuretics – potassium sparing	Increased risk of hyperkalaemia	Caution with use of this combination	Concomitant use of potassium supplements with potassium-sparing diuretics may increase the risk of hyperkalaemia.
	Methylxanthines	Possible risk of mineral depletion	May be beneficial to address nutrient depletion	Theophylline and related drugs have been shown to reduce serum potassium levels. Patients should be monitored for signs of hypokalaemia.
	Penicillins	Possible risk of mineral depletion	May be beneficial to address nutrient depletion	Penicillins may theoretically promote potassium excretion. This is unlikely to be a concern with short-term antibiotic use, but monitor for signs of hypokalaemia with long-term use. Supplements may be required in some individuals.
	Stimulant laxatives	Possible risk of mineral depletion	May be beneficial to address nutrient depletion	Hypokalaemia has been reported with long-term use of stimulant laxatives, or acute use of high doses. Monitor for signs of depletion.
	Succinylcholine	Theoretical increased risk of hyperkalaemia	Caution with use of this combination	A case report describes the occurrence of hyperkalaemia following administration of succinylcholine. Theoretically, concurrent use of this drug and potassium supplements may increase the risk of hyperkalaemia; however, clinical significance is unclear.
Probiotics	Antibiotics	Reduced drugs adverse effects	Combination may be beneficial	Probiotics can reduce the risk of adverse effects of antibiotics such as gastrointestinal disturbances including diarrhoea, and urogenital disturbances such as thrush/candida. Dosage separation is recommended.
Propolis	Anticoagulant/ antiplatelet drugs	Theoretical increased risk of bleeding	Monitor – may not be clinically significant	In vitro evidence suggests that a constituent of propolis may inhibit platelet aggregation. The interaction is speculative.

Continued

ACNM NUTRIENT AND NUTRITIONAL SUPPLEMENTS INTERACTIONS TABLE—cont'd				
Nutrient/ supplement	**Drug/drug class**	**Potential outcome**	**Recommendations**	**Comments**
Proteolytic enzymes	See Bromelain, Papain			
Pumpkin seeds	Lithium	Theoretical increased risk of drug toxicity	Caution with use of this combination	Pumpkin may have diuretic properties. This may theoretically reduce drug excretion and increase the risk of drug toxicity. Significance is unclear.
Pycnogenol	Anticoagulant/ antiplatelet drugs	Theoretical increased risk of bleeding	Caution with use of this combination	Pycnogenol may have antiplatelet properties according to clinical research. Concomitant use may theoretically increase the risk of bleeding and bruising.
	Antidiabetic drugs	Possible additive effects	Caution with use of this combination	Pycnogenol appears to have hypoglycaemic properties according to human studies. Additive effects are theoretically possible, increasing the risk of hypoglycaemia. Caution is advised until more data becomes available.
	Antihypertensive drugs (e.g. Ramipril)	Possible protective effects on renal function in patients at risk	May be beneficial – medical supervision recommended	A small study reported that pycnogenol conferred protective effects on renal function in a group of patients taking ramipril, who had advanced hypertension and a history of cardiovascular events.
	Cardiovascular drugs	Possible improved disease management	May be beneficial – medical supervision recommended	Pycnogenol appears to have antioxidant, antiplatelet and anti-inflammatory effects. A small study reported that pycnogenol was effective in improving endothelial function and reducing oxidative stress in patients with stable coronary artery disease.
	Immunosuppressant drugs	Theoretical decreased drug effects	Caution with use of this combination	Pycnogenol may have immuno-stimulant properties which could theoretically antagonise the effects of immunosuppressant drugs. Significance is unclear, but caution is advised until further data becomes available.
Resveratrol	Anticoagulant/ antiplatelet drugs	Theoretical increased risk of bleeding	Monitor – may not be clinically significant	Resveratrol may have antiplatelet effects. There is a theoretical increased risk of bleeding. Monitor patients taking this combination, but clinical significance is unclear.
	CYP450 substrates (CYP1A1, CYP1A2, CYP1B1, CYP2C19, CYP2E1, CYP3A4)	Theoretical increased drug levels	Monitor – may not be clinically significant	In vitro evidence suggests resveratrol may inhibit activity of CYP1A1, CYP1A2, CYP1B1, CYP2C19, CYP2E1 and CYP3A4. Theoretically, this may lead to increased drug levels; however, these interactions have not been reported in humans.
Quercetin	Adriamycin	Theoretical decreased risk of drug-induced cardiotoxicity	May be beneficial – medical supervision recommended	Animal studies suggest quercetin may have a protective effect against drug-induced cardiotoxicity.
	Antihypertensive drugs	Possible additive effects	May be beneficial – medical supervision recommended	Quercetin can modestly lower blood pressure in people with mild hypertension. The combination may be beneficial, but monitor for signs of hypotension.

ACNM NUTRIENT AND NUTRITIONAL SUPPLEMENTS INTERACTIONS TABLE—cont'd				
Nutrient/ supplement	Drug/drug class	Potential outcome	Recommendations	Comments
Quercetin cont'd	Cisplatin	Theoretical increased drug effect	May be beneficial – medical supervision recommended	In vitro evidence suggests pre-treatment with quercetin may sensitise cervical cancer cells to drug-induced apoptosis. Clinical significance is not known.
	Cyclosporin	Possible increased drug effects	Caution with use of this combination	A small study in healthy volunteers found that pre-treatment with quercetin led to increased drug plasma levels and prolonged half-life. Caution is advised until more data becomes available.
	CYP450 substrates (CYP2C8, CYP2C9, CYP2D6, CYP3A4)	Theoretical increased drug levels	Monitor – may not be clinically significant	Preliminary evidence suggests quercetin may inhibit activity of CYP2C8, CYP2C9, CYP2D6 and CYP3A4. Theoretically, this may lead to increased drug levels and risk of adverse effects.
	Digoxin	Theoretical increased drug bioavailability	Caution with use of this combination	Quercetin may result in increased drug bioavailability according to the findings of an in vivo study. Caution is advised until more data becomes available, especially as this drug has a narrow therapeutic index.
	Diltiazem	Theoretical increased drug bioavailability	Caution with use of this combination	Quercetin may result in increased drug bioavailability according to the findings of an animal study. The interaction may not be clinically significant, but caution is advised until more data becomes available.
	Doxorubicin	Theoretical increased drug effect	May be beneficial – medical supervision recommended	In vitro studies suggest quercetin may potentiate drug anti-tumour effect. Further research is needed to investigate the relevance of this interaction.
	Haloperidol	Possible increased drug effects	May be beneficial – medical supervision recommended	Quercetin may reduce haloperidol-induced tardive dyskinesia, according to results from animal studies. A positive interaction is theoretically possible, although this effect has not yet been described in human studies.
	Iron	Possible decreased iron absorption	Monitor and separate dose administration	Quercetin chelates iron and may reduce bioavailability. Intake of quercetin and iron supplements should be separated by 2 hours.
	Paclitaxel	Theoretical increased drug effects	Caution with use of this combination	Quercetin may result in increased drug bioavailability according to the findings of an animal study. This drug is used in the treatment of cancer and the interaction could theoretically be beneficial under medical supervision, but drug dose adjustments may be required. Caution is advised until more data becomes available.

Continued

ACNM NUTRIENT AND NUTRITIONAL SUPPLEMENTS INTERACTIONS TABLE—cont'd				
Nutrient/ supplement	**Drug/drug class**	**Potential outcome**	**Recommendations**	**Comments**
Quercetin cont'd	P-glycoprotein substrates	Theoretical increased drug bioavailability	Caution with use of this combination	Preliminary evidence suggests quercetin may inhibit the gastrointestinal p-glycoprotein (P-gp) efflux pump. This may theoretically increase drug bioavailability of P-gp substrates. Significance is unclear based on current evidence, but caution is advised with use of high-dose quercetin in combination with P-gp substrates.
	Pioglitazone	Theoretical increased drug bioavailability	Caution with use of this combination	In vitro evidence suggest quercetin may increase drug bioavailability. While human data is not yet available, there is a theoretical increased the risk of adverse effects and drug toxicity. The antidiabetic drug has been associated with rare incidences of hepatic damage, heart failure and pulmonary oedema.
	Quinolone antibiotics	Theoretical decreased drug effect	Caution with use of this combination	Limited evidence suggests that quercetin may theoretically reduce drug action by competitive inhibition at the DNA gyrase binding site.
	Warfarin	Theoretical increased risk of bleeding	Caution with use of this combination	In vitro evidence suggest quercetin may increase warfarin levels by displacement at the human serum albumin (HSA) binding site. Significance is unknown.
Reishi mushrooms	Anti-cancer therapy	Theoretical improved outcomes	May be beneficial – medical supervision recommended	Animal studies suggest reishi extracts may provide protective benefits against the adverse effects associated with some antineoplastic drugs, including myelosuppression, and may improve therapeutic outcomes. Several mechanisms have been proposed.Further clinical trial evidence is needed to establish the benefits and risks associated with this combination.
	Anticoagulant/ antiplatelet drugs	Theoretical increased risk of bleeding	Monitor – clinical significance is unclear	Limited evidence suggests that high-dose use (⋯≥ 3g daily) of reishi mushrooms may have antiplatelet properties. This effect has not been shown at doses of 1.5g daily.
	Antidiabetic drugs	Theoretical additive effects	Monitor – clinical significance is unclear	It has been proposed that reishi mushrooms may have hypoglycaemic effects based on animal studies. Additive effects are theoretically possible, with an increased risk of hypoglycaemia.
	Antihypertensive drugs	Theoretical additive effects	Monitor – clinical significance is unclear	Animal studies suggest reishi mushrooms may have hypotensive properties. Additive effects are theoretically possible, with an increased risk of hypotension.

ACNM NUTRIENT AND NUTRITIONAL SUPPLEMENTS INTERACTIONS TABLE—cont'd				
Nutrient/ supplement	Drug/drug class	Potential outcome	Recommendations	Comments
Reishi mushrooms cont'd	Antimicrobial therapy	Theoretical improved outcomes	May be beneficial – medical supervision recommended	In vitro research has demonstrated synergy between reishi mushroom and several antibiotics. Reishi may have antibacterial properties and may enhance immune response.
	Antiviral therapy	Theoretical improved outcomes	May be beneficial – medical supervision recommended	In vitro research has demonstrated synergy between reishi mushroom and acyclovir. Reishi may have antiviral effects against HSV1 and HSV2 and may enhance immune response. More research is needed to establish safety and efficacy of this combination.
Saccaromyces boulardii	Antifungal drugs	Theoretical decreased drug effectiveness	Monitor – clinical significance is unclear	Theoretically, Saccharomyces boulardii may reduce antifungal action as it is a yeast; however, this interaction is speculative.
SAMe (S-adenosyl-L-methionine)	Antidepressant drugs (SSRIs, SNRIs, TCAs)	Possible improved disease management; increased risk of serotonin syndrome	Avoid combination unless under medical supervision	Some evidence suggests that concomitant use may be beneficial in patients who are not responding adequately to conventional antidepressant drugs. Strict medical supervision would be required with use of this combination as there an increased risk of serotonergic effects and serotonin syndrome.
	Dextromethorphan	Theoretical increased risk of serotonin syndrome	Caution with use of this combination	Theoretically, concurrent use may have additive serotonergic effects at high doses, which increases the risk of serotonin syndrome.
	Levodopa	Theoretical decreased drug effects	Caution with use of this combination	SAMe methylates levodopa, which may reduce drug effectiveness and theoretically worsen symptoms of Parkinson's disease.
	Monoamine oxidase inhibitors (MAOIs)	Increased risk of serotonin syndrome	Avoid combination	Concurrent use may have additive serotonergic effects, which increases the risk of serotonin syndrome. SAMe should be avoided in patients taking MAOI and for 2 weeks after discontinuation of MAOIs.
	Oral contraceptives	May be beneficial in women at risk of hepatobiliary dysfunction	Combination may be beneficial	Co-administration may be beneficial in patients at risk of hepatobiliary dysfunction, according to secondary sources. SAMe supports liver detoxification process, including production of glutathione.
	Tramadol	Theoretical increased risk of serotonin syndrome	Caution with use of this combination	Theoretically, concurrent use may have additive serotonergic effects at high doses, which increases the risk of serotonin syndrome.

Continued

		ACNM NUTRIENT AND NUTRITIONAL SUPPLEMENTS INTERACTIONS TABLE—cont'd		
Nutrient/ supplement	**Drug/drug class**	**Potential outcome**	**Recommendations**	**Comments**
Selenium	Antiplatelet/ anticoagulant drugs	Theoretical increased risk of bleeding	Caution with use of this combination	There is a theoretical increased risk of bleeding with this combination. Preliminary evidence suggest that selenium may reduce platelet aggregation. Animal studies suggest selenium may increase warfarin activity.
	Barbiturates	Theoretical prolonged sedative effects	Caution with use of this combination	Preliminary evidence suggests selenium may inhibit hepatic metabolism of barbiturates and prolong the sedative effects. This has not been demonstrated in humans but caution is advised.
	Corticosteroids	Possible nutrient depletion	Combination may be beneficial	Some evidence suggest that high-dose corticosteroids may increase urinary excretion of selenium and reduce plasma levels. Data is, however, conflicting. Some inflammatory conditions have also been associated with low selenium status. Selenium supplementation may theoretically be beneficial and could also support immunity.
	Cisplatin	Theoretical decrease in drug adverse effects	May be beneficial – more data is required	Preliminary evidence suggests cisplatin may lower selenium levels in humans. Furthermore, in vitro and animal studies suggest that selenium may help to reduce drug-induced nephrotoxicity, myeloid suppression and weight loss. There is insufficient evidence to know if selenium supplements would be beneficial.
	Clozapine	Theoretical nutrient depletion	May be beneficial – more data is required	Low plasma selenium levels have been observed in some patients taking clozapine. It has been speculated that this may contribute to drug-induced adverse effects; however, there is insufficient data to routinely recommend selenium supplements for patients taking clozapine.
	Doxorubicin	Theoretical decrease in drug adverse effects	May be beneficial – medical supervision recommended	Animal research suggests selenium may help to reduce risk of drug-induced cardiotoxicity without affecting drug efficacy.
	Heavy metals e.g. mercury, lead, arsenic, silver, cadmium	Theoretical decreased risk of heavy metal toxicity	Combination may be beneficial	Selenium may theoretically reduce risk of heavy metal toxicity by forming inert complexes with these metals.
	HMGCoA reductase inhibitors (statins)	Theoretical risk of decreased drug effect	Monitor – clinical significance is unclear	Reduced drug effectiveness was reported in a clinical study investigating the concomitant use of statins plus niacin, with an antioxidant combination of selenium, beta-carotene, vitamin C and vitamin E. It is not possible to determine how much of this can be attributed to selenium, or the clinical relevance of this interaction.

	ACNM NUTRIENT AND NUTRITIONAL SUPPLEMENTS INTERACTIONS TABLE—cont'd			
Nutrient/ supplement	**Drug/drug class**	**Potential outcome**	**Recommendations**	**Comments**
Selenium cont'd	Immunosuppressants	Theoretical risk of decreased drug effect	Monitor – clinical significance is unclear	Selenium may stimulate the immune system. There is a theoretical risk that this may interfere with immunosuppressant therapy, but appears unlikely at normal therapeutic doses.
Serrapeptase	Anticoagulant/ antiplatelet drugs	Theoretical increased risk of bleeding	Caution with use of this combination	Serrapeptase may have fibrinolytic activity. Combined use may theoretically increase the risk of bleeding.
Shark cartilage	Immunosuppressant drugs	Theoretical decreased drug effectiveness	Caution with use of this combination	Shark cartilage may stimulate immune response based on in vitro evidence. Theoretically, this could interfere with immunosuppressive therapy.
Shiitake mushrooms	Immunosuppressant drugs	Theoretical decreased drug effectiveness	Caution with use of this combination	Shiitake mushrooms may stimulate immune response based on in vitro evidence. Theoretically, this could interfere with immunosuppressive therapy. Clinical significance is unclear, but caution is advised until more research data becomes available.
Slippery elm powder	Oral drugs	Possible decreased drug absorption	Monitor and separate dose. May not be clinically significant	The mucilage content of slippery elm may theoretically slow the absorption and reduce serum levels of some oral drugs. Clinical significance is unclear, but doses should be separated.
Sodium	Antihypertensive drugs	Reduced drug effect/ increased drug requirements	Caution with use of this combination	High dietary intake of sodium can raise blood pressure and may lead to increased drug requirements. Patients on antihypertensive medication should avoid high sodium intake.
	Didanosine (NRTI)	Possible excessive sodium intake	Caution with use of this combination	Didanosine formulations contain a significant amount of sodium. The combination may lead to excessive sodium levels.
	Glucocorticoids e.g. hydrocortisone	Theoretical increased risk of hypernatraemia	Caution with use of this combination	Glucocorticoids may cause sodium retention. The magnitude of effect relates to drug dose and specific drug characteristics. Not all glucocorticoids result in clinically relevant sodium retention, but caution is advised with intake of sodium-containing foods and supplements.
	Lithium	Altered drug effect	Caution with use of this combination	High sodium intake can decrease drug concentrations by increasing lithium excretion. Conversely, a significant decrease in sodium intake can result in drug toxicity. Patients taking lithium should avoid significant alterations to sodium intake without medical supervision.
	Mineralocorticoids	Theoretical increased risk of hypernatraemia	Caution with use of this combination	Mineralocorticoids may cause sodium retention. The magnitude of effect relates to drug dose and drug mineralocorticoid potency.
	Tolvaptan	Theoretical increased risk of hypernatraemia	Caution with use of this combination	Concomitant use may increase the risk of sodium retention and hypernatraemia.

Continued

		ACNM NUTRIENT AND NUTRITIONAL SUPPLEMENTS INTERACTIONS TABLE—cont'd		
Nutrient/ supplement	**Drug/drug class**	**Potential outcome**	**Recommendations**	**Comments**
Sodium bicarbonate	Aminoglycosides	Theoretical increased risk of hypokalaemia	Caution with use of this combination	The combination theoretically increases the risk of hypokalaemia. Excessive intake of sodium bicarbonate has been associated with hypokalaemia. Aminoglycosides may cause nephrotoxicity, resulting in further loss of potassium.
	Amphotericin-B	Theoretical increased risk of hypokalaemia	Caution with use of this combination	The combination increases the risk of hypokalaemia, and potassium supplements may be required. Excessive intake of sodium bicarbonate has been associated with hypokalaemia. This drug increases urinary loss of potassium.
	Aspirin	Possible reduced drug effects	Caution with use of this combination	Sodium bicarbonate may increase elimination of salicylates such as aspirin. It is proposed that this is due to increased urinary pH.
	B2-agonists e.g. salbutamol	Theoretical increased risk of hypokalaemia	Caution with use of this combination	Excessive intake of sodium bicarbonate has been associated with hypokalaemia. The combination theoretically increases the risk of hypokalaemia.
	Cefpodoxime proxetil	Decreased drug concentrations	Caution with use of this combination	High-dose sodium bicarbonate may increase gastric pH and inhibit conversion of drug to the active form. A clinical study reported a significant decrease in drug plasma concentration when taken concomitantly with 12.6g oral sodium bicarbonate.
	Chlorpropamide	Possible reduced drug effect	Caution with use of this combination	High-dose sodium bicarbonate may alter urinary pH. A preliminary clinical study reported a significant increase in drug urinary excretion with this combination.
	Cisplatin	Theoretical increased risk of hypokalaemia	Caution with use of this combination	The combination theoretically increases the risk of hypokalaemia. Excessive intake of sodium bicarbonate has been associated with hypokalaemia. Cisplatin may affect renal function, resulting in further loss of potassium.
	Corticosteroids	Theoretical increased risk of hypokalaemia	Caution with use of this combination	The combination theoretically increases the risk of hypokalaemia. Excessive intake of sodium bicarbonate has been associated with hypokalaemia. Corticosteroids may cause hypokalaemia as a consequence of sodium retention and resulting compensatory renal excretion of potassium.
	Diuretics – loop and thiazide	Theoretical increased risk of hypokalaemia	Caution with use of this combination	Excessive intake of sodium bicarbonate has been associated with hypokalaemia. The combination theoretically increases the risk of hypokalaemia.

ACNM NUTRIENT AND NUTRITIONAL SUPPLEMENTS INTERACTIONS TABLE—cont'd

Nutrient/ supplement	Drug/drug class	Potential outcome	Recommendations	Comments
Sodium bicarbonate cont'd	Methylxanthines	Theoretical increased risk of hypokalaemia	Caution with use of this combination	Excessive intake of sodium bicarbonate has been associated with hypokalaemia. The combination theoretically increases the risk of hypokalaemia as theophylline and related compounds may reduce serum potassium levels.
	Penicillins	Theoretical increased risk of hypokalaemia	Caution with use of this combination	Excessive intake of sodium bicarbonate has been associated with hypokalaemia. Some penicillins are formulated as sodium salts, which may theoretically promote urinary excretion of potassium. The combination may theoretically increase the risk of hypokalaemia.
	Pseudoephedrine	Theoretical increased risk of drug toxicity	Caution with use of this combination	High intake of sodium bicarbonate may increase urinary pH. A case study describes a patient with persistent alkaline urinary who experienced hallucinations and personality changes while taking pseudoephedrine. Theoretically, the combination may reduce drug clearance and increase the risk of drug toxicity.
	Stimulant laxatives	Theoretical increased risk of hypokalaemia	Caution with use of this combination	Excessive use of stimulant laxatives may increase urinary excretion of potassium. Excessive intake of sodium bicarbonate has also been associated with hypokalaemia. The combination theoretically increases this risk.
Soy protein and soy isoflavones (e.g. genistein and daidzein)	Antibiotics	Theoretical decreased effect of soy isoflavones	Monitor – clinical significance is unclear	Theoretically, antibiotics may decrease the action of soy isoflavones by disturbing gastrointestinal bacteria, which may then impair conversion of isoflavones to the active form. The interaction is speculative and only likely to be relevant with long-term antibiotic use.
	Antidiabetic drugs	Possible additive effects	Caution with use of this combination	Clinical research suggest that soy-based diets may reduce fasting blood glucose levels. Theoretically, concurrent use may have additive effects, which could be beneficial for the management of diabetes. Caution is advised due to the risk of hypoglycaemia.
	Antihypertensive drugs	Possible additive effects	Monitor – clinical significance is unclear	Clinical evidence suggests that soy protein may modestly lower blood pressure in individuals with hypertension. Effects may be additive, but there is a theoretical risk of hypotension.
	Chemotherapeutic drugs (e.g. vincristine, vinblastine, cisplatin, daunorubicin)	Theoretical beneficial interaction	Caution with use of this combination	In vitro evidence suggests soy isoflavones may potentially enhance drug anti-tumour effects with certain chemotherapeutic agents. Clinical significance is unknown and safety of this combination has not been established. Medical supervision is warranted.

Continued

ACNM NUTRIENT AND NUTRITIONAL SUPPLEMENTS INTERACTIONS TABLE—cont'd

Nutrient/ supplement	Drug/drug class	Potential outcome	Recommendations	Comments
Soy protein and soy isoflavones (e.g. genistein and daidzein) cont'd	L-Thyroxine (Levothyroxine)	Possible decreased drug effects	Caution with use of this combination	Preliminary evidence suggests that soy-based formulas may decrease thyroxine levels in infants with congenital hypothyroidism. It is unclear if this interaction occurs in other patient populations. Soy may theoretically affect thyroid function, although this effect does not appear to be clinically significant based on current evidence.
	Monoamine oxidase inhibitors (MAOIs)	Theoretical increased risk of drug adverse effects	Avoid combination	Fermented soy products such as tofu and soy sauce contain tyramine, which may theoretically interact with MAOIs and increase the risk of a hypertensive crisis. The amount of tyramine in fermented soy products is usually relatively small, but concentrations can vary.
	Oestrogens (e.g. HRT)	Theoretical altered drug action	May be beneficial – medical supervision recommended	Data is conflicting on the interaction between soy and oestrogenic drugs. Some sources suggest that soy isoflavones may have additive beneficial effects when used with HRT, while others suggest soy theoretically inhibits the effects of HRT due to competition for oestrogen bind receptors. Caution is advised until more data becomes available.
	Progesterone	Possible increased bone loss	Monitor – clinical significance is unclear	Both soy milk and progesterone patches have bone-sparing effects when used alone; however, results of a small clinical study suggest that use of this combination resulted in bone loss. Further data is required to establish clinical significance of this interaction.
	Tamoxifen	May antagonise drug effect	Avoid combination	Preliminary evidence suggests that the soy isoflavones genistein and diadzen may antagonise drug anti-tumour effect. Soy may interfere with drug action due to the oestrogenic effects of soy isoflavones. Results from studies have, however, been conflicting, which may be due to dose variations. Caution is advised until more data becomes available.
	Warfarin	Theoretical decreased drug effect	Caution with use of this combination	A case report describes a possible interaction between soy milk and warfarin. The data is inconclusive but caution is advised.
Spirulina (Blue-green algae)	Anticoagulant/ antiplatelet drugs	Theoretical increased risk of bleeding	Caution with use of this combination	Spirulina may have antiplatelet properties. Concomitant use with anticoagulant and antiplatelet drugs will theoretically increase the risk of bleeding and bruising.
	Immunosuppressant drugs	Theoretical risk of decreased drug effect	Caution with use of this combination	Spirulina may have immunomodulatory activity which could theoretically oppose drug immunosuppressant effects.

ACNM NUTRIENT AND NUTRITIONAL SUPPLEMENTS INTERACTIONS TABLE—cont'd

Nutrient/ supplement	Drug/drug class	Potential outcome	Recommendations	Comments
Taurine	Antihypertensive drugs	Possible additive effects	Combination may be beneficial – monitor	Clinical evidence suggests taurine may lower blood pressure. Additive beneficial effects may be seen with use of this combination, but monitor to reduce the risk of hypotension.
	Lithium	Theoretical increased risk of drug toxicity	Caution with use of this combination	Taurine may have diuretic properties, which can theoretically reduce drug excretion and increase the risk of toxicity.
Theanine (L-Theanine)	Antihypertensive drugs	Theoretical additive effects	Combination may be beneficial – monitor	Animal studies suggest theanine may lower blood pressure. Additive beneficial effects may theoretically be seen with use of this combination, but monitor to reduce the risk of hypotension.
	Stimulant drugs	Theoretical decreased drug effects	Caution with use of this combination	Animal studies suggest that theanine may decrease drug effects. Significance is unclear.

Tocopherols and Tocotrienols – see Vitamin E

Nutrient/ supplement	Drug/drug class	Potential outcome	Recommendations	Comments
Tryptophan (L-Tryptophan)	Antidepressant drugs (SSRIs and SNRIs)	Theoretical risk of serotonin syndrome	Caution with use of this combination	Tryptophan is an endogenous precursor for the production of serotonin. Theoretically, the combination may increase the risk of serotonin syndrome.
	Antidepressant drugs (tricyclic antidepressants)	Possible synergistic effects	Caution with use of this combination	Synergistic beneficial effects are theoretically possible, but medical supervision is required.
	Benzodiazepines	Theoretical increased risk of adverse effects	Caution with use of this combination	Secondary sources suggest that concomitant use may increase the risk of adverse effects such as sexual disinhibition, reversible dyskinesia and reversible Parkinson's-like rigidity. There is insufficient data to comment on clinical relevance of this interaction.
	CNS depressant drugs	Increased risk of sedation	Avoid combination	Concomitant use may have additive effects and increase the risk of excessive sedation.
	Dextromethorphan	Theoretical risk of serotonin syndrome	Caution with use of this combination	Tryptophan is an endogenous precursor for the production of serotonin. Theoretically, the combination may increase the risk of serotonin syndrome.
	Monoamine oxidase inhibitors (MAOIs)	Theoretical risk of serotonin syndrome	Avoid combination	Tryptophan is an endogenous precursor for the production of serotonin. Theoretically, the combination may increase the risk of serotonin syndrome. Case reports describe adverse reactions with this combination including myoclonus, hyperreflexia, diaphoresis, confusion, hypomania, ocular oscillation and ataxia.

Continued

ACNM NUTRIENT AND NUTRITIONAL SUPPLEMENTS INTERACTIONS TABLE—cont'd				
Nutrient/ supplement	Drug/drug class	Potential outcome	Recommendations	Comments
Tryptophan (L-Tryptophan) cont'd	Phenothiazines	Theoretical increased risk of adverse effects	Caution with use of this combination	Secondary sources suggest that concomitant use may increase the risk of adverse effects such as sexual disinhibition, reversible dyskinesia and reversible Parkinson's-like rigidity. There is insufficient available data to comment on clinical relevance of this interaction.
	Tramadol	Theoretical risk of serotonin syndrome	Caution with use of this combination	Tryptophan is an endogenous precursor for the production of serotonin. Theoretically, the combination may increase the risk of serotonin syndrome.
Tyrosine	L-Thyroxine (Levothyroxine)	Theoretical additive effects	Caution with use of this combination	Tyrosine is a precursor to thyroid hormone. There is some concern that concomitant use may have additive effects. Dose adjustments may be required.
	Levodopa	Theoretical decreased drug effect	Caution with use of this combination	Tyrosine and levodopa compete for absorption by the same transport system. Theoretically, concomitant use may lead to decreased drug effectiveness.
Turmeric – see Curcumin				
Ubiquinol/Ubidecarenone– see Coenzyme Q10				
Vitamin A	Anthelmintic drugs	Possible improved response	Combination may be beneficial	Vitamin A deficiency is associated with an increased risk of parasitic worm infections. Concurrent use of beta-carotene or vitamin A may assist with management of condition, as well as supporting immunity and epithelial integrity.
	Bile acid sequestrants	Risk of vitamin depletion	May be beneficial to address nutrient depletion	Nutrient depletion has been reported, but may not be clinically significant unless there is long-term use of cholestyramine.
	Chemotherapeutic agents	Possible improved drug response	Caution with use of this combination	Epidemiological evidence suggests an association between higher dietary intake of vitamin A and a reduced risk of breast cancer and possibly some other forms of cancer although data is inconclusive. Adjunctive use of vitamin A with chemotherapeutic agents may improve outcomes based on some preliminary data although evidence is conflicting and inconclusive.
	Hepatotoxic drugs	Increased risk of hepatotoxicity	Caution with use of this combination	Theoretically, high-dose vitamin A may increase the risk of liver damage when used in combination with hepatotoxic drugs.
	HMGCoA reductase inhibitors (statins)	Possible increased vitamin A levels	Caution with use of this combination	Preliminary research suggests statins may increase serum retinol levels. The clinical significance is not known. Caution is advised with high-dose vitamin A supplements, especially in those with compromised liver function, until more data becomes available.

ACNM NUTRIENT AND NUTRITIONAL SUPPLEMENTS INTERACTIONS TABLE—cont'd				
Nutrient/ supplement	Drug/drug class	Potential outcome	Recommendations	Comments
Vitamin A cont'd	Retinoids e.g. isotretinoin	Risk of drug toxicity	Avoid combination	There is a major risk of additive toxic effects with concomitant use of vitamin A and retinoid drugs such as isotretinoin. The interaction is well established and the combination should be avoided.
	Mineral oil	Risk of vitamin depletion	May be beneficial to address nutrient depletion	A moderate risk of vitamin A depletion has been reported with long-term or regular use of mineral oil. Supplements may be required in some individuals.
	Neomycin	Risk of vitamin depletion	May be beneficial to address nutrient depletion	Neomycin may damage the structure and affect the function of the digestive tract lining. Long-term use may reduce absorption of vitamin A.
	Orlistat	Risk of vitamin depletion	May be beneficial to address nutrient depletion	A moderate risk of vitamin A depletion has been reported with long-term use of orlistat. Supplements may be required in some individuals.
	Tetracycline antibiotics	Increased risk of adverse effects	Caution with use of this combination	Long-term tetracyclines in combination with vitamin A increases the risk of benign intercranial hypertension. This interaction has been described in case reports.
	Warfarin	Theoretical increased risk of bleeding	Caution with use of this combination	Theoretically, high-dose vitamin A may increase the risk of bleeding if taken with warfarin. Vitamin A toxicity is associated with haemorrhage, possibly due to vitamin K antagonism.
Vitamin B1 (Thiamine)	Alcohol	Risk of vitamin depletion	May be beneficial to address nutrient depletion	It has been reported that 30–80% of alcoholics have clinical or biochemical signs of vitamin B1 deficiency. Vitamin B1 deficiency may lead to the development of Wernicke-Korsakoff syndrome and alcoholic neuropathy.
	Diuretic drugs	Risk of vitamin depletion	May be beneficial to address nutrient depletion	A moderate depletion of vitamin B1 has been reported with long-term use of diuretics due to increased excretion. The risk of depletion appears greatest in those taking loop diuretics and if over 60 years, especially where dietary intake is inadequate. There is a concern that vitamin B1 deficiency may worsen heart failure.
	Oestrogens e.g. oral contraceptives	Risk of vitamin depletion	May be beneficial to address nutrient depletion	A small reduction in vitamin B1 levels has been noted in women taking oral contraceptives long term. The depletion may not be clinically significant, but monitor for signs of deficiency.

Continued

ACNM NUTRIENT AND NUTRITIONAL SUPPLEMENTS INTERACTIONS TABLE—cont'd				
Nutrient/ supplement	Drug/drug class	Potential outcome	Recommendations	Comments
Vitamin B2 (Riboflavin, Riboflavin -5-phosphate)	Antibiotics	Risk of vitamin depletion	May be beneficial to address nutrient depletion	Long-term use of antibiotics may interfere with bacterial synthesis of vitamin B2. This interaction may not be clinically relevant, but monitor for signs of depletion with long-term antibiotic use.
	Oestrogens e.g. oral contraceptives	Risk of vitamin depletion	May be beneficial to address nutrient depletion	A small reduction in vitamin B2 activity has been noted in women taking oral contraceptives long term. The depletion may not be clinically significant, but monitor for signs of deficiency.
	Tricyclic antidepressants (TCAs)	Risk of vitamin depletion	May be beneficial to address nutrient depletion	Tricyclic antidepressants may interfere with conversion of vitamin B2 to the active form FAD. The interaction does not appear to be important clinically, but monitor for signs of deficiency.

Vitamin B3 – see Niacin and Nicotinamide

Vitamin B6 (Pyridoxine, pyridoxyl-5-phosphate (PLP))	Amiodarone	Possible increased risk of photosensitivity	Caution with use of this combination	Preliminary evidence suggests that vitamin B6 may exacerbate drug-induced photosensitivity. Data is conflicting and inconclusive, with some sources suggesting vitamin B6 provides a protective effect.
	Anticonvulsant drugs e.g. phenobarbital, phenytoin	Risk of decreased drug levels with high vitamin intake	Caution with use of this combination	Preliminary evidence suggests that high-dose vitamin B6 (200 mg daily) can reduce plasma levels of phenobarbital and phenytoin, possibly due to increased drug metabolism. Concerns have also been raised about the potential for interactions between high-dose vitamin B6 and other anticonvulsant drugs.
	Antihypertensive drugs	Additive effects possible	Combination may be beneficial	Vitamin B6 may lower blood pressure in hypertensive patients. Additive beneficial effects are possible, but monitor for hypotension.
	Cycloserine	Major risk of vitamin depletion	May be beneficial to address nutrient depletion	A major risk depletion of vitamin B6 has been reported with use of cycloserine. It has been proposed that this depletion contributes to drug-induced neurotoxicity and seizures. Most patients will require supplementation with long-term use.
	Diuretics (loop)	Risk of vitamin depletion	May be beneficial to address nutrient depletion	Loop diuretics may theoretically increase urinary excretion of vitamin B6. Monitor for signs of deficiency; however, this depletion does not appear to be clinically significant based on current data.
	Hydralazine	Risk of vitamin depletion	May be beneficial to address nutrient depletion	This drug may lead to a moderate depletion of vitamin B6 with long-term use. Patients should be monitored for depletion and supplements may be required in some individuals, especially in those presenting with paraesthesia, numbness and tingling.

ACNM NUTRIENT AND NUTRITIONAL SUPPLEMENTS INTERACTIONS TABLE—cont'd				
Nutrient/ supplement	Drug/drug class	Potential outcome	Recommendations	Comments
Vitamin B6 (Pyridoxine, pyridoxyl-5-phosphate (PLP)) cont'd	Isoniazid	Risk of vitamin depletion	May be beneficial to address nutrient depletion	This drug may lead to a moderate depletion of vitamin B6 with long-term use, which could lead to a peripheral neuritis. Patients should be monitored for depletion and supplements may be required in some individuals.
	Levodopa (without carbidopa)	Theoretical decreased drug effect	Combination may be beneficial	Vitamin B6 enhances levodopa peripheral metabolism and may reduce anti-Parkinson's disease effect. In practice, this interaction is unlikely as levodopa is usually co-prescribed with carbidopa, and this negates this effect.
	Methotrexate	Possible reduced vitamin levels	May be beneficial – medical supervision recommended	Some sources suggest that chronic inflammatory diseases such as rheumatoid arthritis may be associated with a lower vitamin B6 status. Use of methotrexate has also been associated with raised homocysteine levels due to an interference in vitamin B6 and folic acid-dependent reactions. Monitor for signs of deficiency, although significance is unclear based on current data.
	Penicillamine	Major risk of vitamin depletion	May be beneficial to address nutrient depletion	A major risk of vitamin B6 depletion has been associated with this drug. Penicillamine inhibits the activity of vitamin B6 by forming an inactive complex with pyridoxal phosphate. Most patients will require supplementation with long-term use.
	Oestrogens (oral contraceptives and HRT)	Risk of vitamin depletion	May be beneficial to address nutrient depletion	Oestrogens can interfere with vitamin B6 metabolism and may theoretically reduce levels, or increase nutrient requirements. Evidence from one recent study suggests that vitamin B6 supplementation may help to reduce the incidence of drug-related adverse effects such as nausea, headache and depression. Monitor for signs of deficiency, but the risk of depletion is not considered to be clinically significant in most individuals.
	Theophylline	Risk of vitamin depletion	May be beneficial to address nutrient depletion	Theophylline intake may theoretically result in a moderate vitamin B6 deficiency and it has been proposed that this may contribute to drug adverse effects. Theophylline inhibits pyridoxal kinase, which catalyses phosphorylation of vitamin B6 to the active form pyridoxal-5-phosphate. Monitor for signs of deficiency. Supplements may be required in some individuals.

Continued

ACNM NUTRIENT AND NUTRITIONAL SUPPLEMENTS INTERACTIONS TABLE—cont'd				
Nutrient/ supplement	Drug/drug class	Potential outcome	Recommendations	Comments
Vitamin B9 – see Folic acid				
Vitamin B12 (Cyanocobalamin, methylcobalamin, hydroxycobalamin)	Acid-reducing drugs e.g. H$_2$-antagonists and proton pump inhibitors (PPIs)	Risk of vitamin depletion	May be beneficial to address nutrient depletion	Absorption of dietary vitamin B12 may be compromised with regular intake of acid-reducing drugs. Stomach acid is required to release vitamin B12 from protein so that it can be absorbed. Monitor for vitamin B12 depletion with long-term use (>2 years) of acid-reducing drugs.
	Aminosalicylic acid	Risk of vitamin depletion	May be beneficial to address nutrient depletion	Aminosalicylic acid may significantly reduce absorption of vitamin B12. Megaloblastic anaemia has been reported with long-term use of this drug. Monitor for signs of deficiency.
	Anticonvulsant drugs e.g. phenytoin	Risk of vitamin depletion	May be beneficial to address nutrient depletion	A moderate vitamin B12 depletion has been reported with use of anticonvulsant drugs, especially phenytoin, phenobarbital and primidone. Patients should be monitored and supplements may be required in some individuals.
	Aspirin	Risk of vitamin depletion	May be beneficial to address nutrient depletion	There is a moderate risk of depletion with long-term use of aspirin. Patients should be monitored and supplements may be required in some individuals.
	Chloramphenicol	Risk of delayed response to vitamin supplementation	Monitor – may not be clinically significant	Limited case reports suggest that chloramphenicol can delay response to vitamin B12 supplementation. Monitor if the combination is required.
	Colchicine	Risk of vitamin depletion	May be beneficial to address nutrient depletion	There is a moderate risk of vitamin B12 depletion with use of colchicine. Colchicine disrupts normal intestinal mucosal function, which may lead to malabsorption of some nutrients. Patients should be monitored and supplements may be required in some individuals.
	Metformin	Risk of vitamin depletion	May be beneficial to address nutrient depletion	Metformin can deplete vitamin B12 and folic acid with long-term use. This can lead to raised homocysteine levels and an increased risk of cardiovascular disease and other conditions related to hyperhomocysteainaemia. Megaloblastic anaemia has also been reported with long-term use of metformin. Patients should be monitored and supplements may be required in some individuals.
	Zidovudine	Possible increased risk of drug related adverse effects	May be beneficial – medical supervision recommended	Some research suggests that low vitamin B12 levels may increase the risk of drug-related adverse effects. A higher incidence of comprised vitamin B12 status has also been reported in individuals with HIV infection. While data is inconclusive, vitamin B12 status should be monitored in HIV positive patients.

ACNM NUTRIENT AND NUTRITIONAL SUPPLEMENTS INTERACTIONS TABLE—cont'd				
Nutrient/ supplement	**Drug/drug class**	**Potential outcome**	**Recommendations**	**Comments**
Vitamin C (Ascorbic acid)	Aluminium (e.g. in antacids)	Risk of increased aluminium absorption and toxicity	Monitor and separate doses	Vitamin C may increase aluminium absorption which is potentially toxic. The interaction may not be clinically significant, unless renally impaired, but dosage separation is recommended.
	Chemotherapy	Possible enhanced disease management	May be beneficial with medical supervision	Use of high-dose IV vitamin C in the management of cancer is controversial. Vitamin C may enhance therapeutic effects of some drugs. There is, however, concern that the antioxidant action may also interfere with drug efficacy for certain chemotherapeutic agents. Medical supervision is required to determine appropriateness of use for the individual.
	Corticosteroids	Theoretical vitamin depletion	May be beneficial to address nutrient depletion	Vitamin C requirements may be increased in patients taking corticosteroids based on in vitro and animal studies.
	Indinavir	Possible decreased drug absorption	Caution with use of this combination	Concomitant use of 1g vitamin C with indinavir resulted in a small reduction in drug absorption in a preliminary pharmacokinetic study. Clinical significance is unclear but caution is advised.
	Iron	Enhanced iron absorption	Combination may be beneficial	Vitamin C enhances the absorption of iron. The combination is often used to manage iron deficiency.
	Oestrogens	Theoretical increase in plasma oestrogen levels	Monitor – interaction may not be clinically significant	Limited evidence suggests that vitamin C supplements may increase plasma oestrogen levels in women who are vitamin C deficient. Vitamin C supplements do not appear to have an effect on oestrogen in the absence of deficiency and a clinically relevant interaction appears unlikely.
	Propranolol	Theoretical decreased drug absorption	Monitor – interaction may not be clinically significant	Preliminary data suggests that pre-treatment with vitamin C 2g may reduce propranolol absorption and metabolism. Patients should be monitored with use of this combination, but the interaction may not be clinically relevant.
	Warfarin	Theoretical decreased drug effect – conflicting data	Caution with use of this combination	Data on the interaction between warfarin and vitamin C is conflicting. A small study concluded that vitamin C does not affect warfarin's anticoagulant effects. However, several case reports describe a possible interaction between warfarin and high-dose vitamin C, leading to reduced drug effect. Caution is advised until more data becomes available.

Continued

ACNM NUTRIENT AND NUTRITIONAL SUPPLEMENTS INTERACTIONS TABLE—cont'd

Nutrient/ supplement	Drug/drug class	Potential outcome	Recommendations	Comments
Vitamin D	Aluminium (e.g. in antacids)	Risk of increased aluminium absorption and toxicity	Monitor – separate doses	Vitamin D increases aluminium absorption which is potentially toxic. The interaction may not be clinically significant, but dosage separation is recommended.
	Anticonvulsant drugs e.g. carbamazepine, phenobarbital, phenytoin	Risk of nutrient depletion	May be beneficial to address nutrient depletion	Anticonvulsant drugs may lead to a moderate vitamin D depletion by increasing liver metabolism of vitamin D to inactive compounds. Hypocalcaemia and osteomalacia have been reported with long-term use, especially where other risk factors for vitamin D deficiency are present. Patients taking anticonvulsant drugs should be monitored. Supplements may be required in some individuals.
	Atorvastatin	Possible decreased drug bioavailability	Caution with use of this combination	Limited evidence suggests that vitamin D supplements may decrease atorvastatin bioavailability. Caution is advised until more data becomes available.
	Calcipotriene	Theoretical increased risk of hypocalcaemia	Caution with use of this combination	Calcipotriene is a vitamin D analogue used in the management of psoriasis. Theoretically, concomitant use of vitamin D supplements with this drug may increase the risk of hypercalcaemia.
	Calcium channel blockers e.g. diltiazem, verapamil	Theoretical risk of reduced drug effect	Caution with use of this combination	High-dose intake of vitamin D (in the absence of deficiency) may increase the risk of hypercalcaemia and theoretically reduce drug effectiveness. Clinical significance is unclear.
	Cholestyramine	Risk of nutrient depletion	May be beneficial to address nutrient depletion	There is a risk of a moderate risk of vitamin D depletion with use of cholestyramine. Patients should be monitored and supplements may be required in some individuals.
	Corticosteroids (chronic use)	Risk of nutrient depletion	May be beneficial to address nutrient depletion	Long-term intake of oral corticosteroids (equivalent to ⋯⋙ 7.5 mg prednisone daily) causes significant bone loss and increases the risk of osteoporosis and fractures. This is mainly due to disturbances in calcium metabolism; however, vitamin D supplements may be required to improve calcium absorption.
	Digoxin	Increased risk of hypercalcaemia	Caution with use of this combination	High-dose intake of vitamin D, in the absence of a deficiency, can increase the risk of hypercalcaemia and risk of fatal cardiac arrhythmias in patient taking digoxin.
	Orlistat	Risk of major nutrient depletion	May be beneficial to address nutrient depletion	There is a significant risk of vitamin D deletion with use of orlistat. Patients should be monitored for vitamin D depletion and a supplement will be needed in most individuals. Doses should be separated by at least 2 hours.

ACNM NUTRIENT AND NUTRITIONAL SUPPLEMENTS INTERACTIONS TABLE—cont'd

Nutrient/ supplement	Drug/drug class	Potential outcome	Recommendations	Comments
Vitamin D cont'd	Rifampicin/Rifampin	Risk of nutrient depletion	May be beneficial to address nutrient depletion	Rifampicin may increase vitamin D metabolism and may result in an increased risk of osteomalacia with long-term use. Patients should be monitored and supplements may be required in some individuals.
	Stimulant laxatives (chronic use)	Risk of nutrient depletion	May be beneficial to address nutrient depletion	Moderate risk of depletion. Patients should be monitored and supplements may be required in some individuals.
Vitamin E (Tocopherols & tocotrienols)	Anticoagulant/ antiplatelet drugs	Theoretical increased risk of bleeding	Caution with use of this combination	There is an increased risk of bleeding with the combined use of warfarin and vitamin E, especially at higher doses. Vitamin E inhibits platelet aggregation and reduces vitamin K-dependent clotting factors. People with low levels of vitamin K appear to be at a greater risk of an interaction.
	Anticonvulsant drugs (e.g. phenytoin, phenobarbital)	Risk of nutrient depletion	May be beneficial to address nutrient depletion	A moderate risk of nutrient depletion has been reported with use of anticonvulsant drugs. Supplements may be required in some individuals.
	Beta-carotene	Reduced nutrient absorption	Monitor – may not be clinically significant	High-dose vitamin E (⋯>800iu) may reduce absorption of beta-carotene. Clinical significance is unclear.
	Chemotherapeutic agents	Possible reduced drug effects – controversial	Caution with use of this combination	The use of antioxidants including vitamin E in patients on chemotherapy is controversial. It has been proposed that vitamin E may protect tumour cells from chemotherapeutic drugs that work by inducing oxidative stress and so theoretically reduce drug effectiveness. Avoid high-dose supplements unless under medical supervision.
	Cholestyramine	Risk of nutrient depletion	May be beneficial to address nutrient depletion	Vitamin E depletion has been reported with use of cholestyramine. This interaction may not be clinically significant unless there is long-term use. Patients on this drug should be monitored for signs of depletion.
	Cyclosporin	Theoretical increased risk of drug toxicity	Caution with use of this combination	Some evidence suggests that certain forms of vitamin E may increase cyclosporin absorption, which could theoretically lead to drug toxicity. The combination should be used with caution until further data becomes available.
	HMGCoA reductase inhibitors (statins)	Risk of nutrient depletion	May be beneficial to address nutrient depletion	Some reports suggest that statins may lower vitamin E levels; however, clinical significance is unclear based on current data.
	Nitrates	Decreased risk of drug adverse effects	May be beneficial to address nutrient depletion	Oral vitamin E (300–600 mg/day) may help to prevent development of nitrate tolerance to transdermal patches.
	Orlistat	Risk of nutrient depletion	May be beneficial to address nutrient depletion	Orlistat may result in a moderate vitamin E depletion. Supplements may be required in some individuals, but dose administration should be separated.

Continued

ACNM NUTRIENT AND NUTRITIONAL SUPPLEMENTS INTERACTIONS TABLE—cont'd				
Nutrient/ supplement	Drug/drug class	Potential outcome	Recommendations	Comments
Vitamin K	Antibiotics (long term)	Risk of nutrient depletion	Monitor – may not be clinically significant	Long-term antibiotics use may alter synthesis of vitamin K2 by disturbing normal gut flora. The clinical significance of this interaction is unclear.
	Anticoagulant/ antiplatelet drugs	Risk of decreased drug effect and clotting	Avoid combination	High intake of vitamin K antagonises the activity of anticoagulants such as warfarin and will reduce drug anticoagulant effect, leading to an increased risk of clotting. Anticoagulants will also affect the activity of vitamin K. Significant dietary changes that alter vitamin K intake may also potentially lead to an interaction. The combination should be avoided, or only used under medical supervision.
	Antidiabetic drugs	Theoretical risk of hypoglycaemia	Caution with use of this combination	High intake of vitamin K1 has been reported to increase insulin sensitivity and reduce postprandial glucose levels. Clinical significance is unclear.
	Cholestyramine	Risk of nutrient depletion	May be beneficial to address nutrient depletion	Vitamin K depletion has been reported with use of cholestyramine. This interaction may not be clinically significant unless there is long-term use. Patients on this drug should be monitored for signs of depletion.
	Orlistat	Risk of nutrient depletion	May be beneficial to address nutrient depletion	Orlistat may result in a moderate vitamin K depletion. Supplements may be required in some individuals, but dose administration should be separated.
	Rifampicin	Risk of nutrient depletion	May be beneficial to address nutrient depletion	A moderate risk of nutrient depletion has been reported with long-term use of rifampicin. Supplements may be required in some individuals.
Whey protein	Albendazole	Theoretical risk of decreased drug effect	Monitor – separate doses	Animal research suggests high intake of whey protein prior to intake of oral albendazole may delay or hinder drug effects. Significance is unknown, but separation of dose administration is recommended.
	Antibiotics (quinolones and tetracyclines)	Possible decreased drug absorption	Monitor – separate doses	Secondary sources suggest intake of whey protein may decrease drug absorption. Significance is unknown, but separation of dose administration is recommended.
	Levodopa	Possible decreased drug absorption	Caution with use of this combination	Secondary sources suggest intake of whey protein may decreased drug absorption. Significance is unknown, but separation of dose administration is recommended.

ACNM NUTRIENT AND NUTRITIONAL SUPPLEMENTS INTERACTIONS TABLE—cont'd

Nutrient/ supplement	Drug/drug class	Potential outcome	Recommendations	Comments
Zinc	ACE-Inhibitors	Risk of nutrient depletion	May be beneficial to address nutrient depletion	There is a moderate risk of zinc depletion with this class of antihypertensive drugs. Patients should be monitored and supplements may be required in some individuals.
	Androgens	Possible synergistic effects.	Combination may be beneficial	Zinc helps to support male sexual function and to maintain male sexual health. Concurrent use may provide a synergistic benefit.
	Antibiotics (tetracyclines and quinolones)	Reduced drug effect	Monitor – separate doses	Zinc supplements form complexes with these drugs and may reduce drug effectiveness. Separate doses by at least 2 hours.
	Antibiotic – cephalexin	Reduced drug effect	Monitor – separate doses	Zinc supplements may reduce drug concentration and effectiveness. Separate doses by at least 3 hours.
	Antidepressant drugs	Possible improved outcomes	Combination may be beneficial	Zinc supplements may improve drug efficacy and the management of depression.
	Antiretroviral therapy e.g. zidovudine	Possible improved outcomes	May be beneficial – medical supervision recommended	Preliminary evidence suggests that use of zinc supplements in combination with zidovudine (AZT) may reduce the risk of opportunistic infections in patients with HIV. Zinc supports immune function, but a higher incidence of zinc deficiency has been reported in patients with HIV. Drugs used for the management of HIV such as zidovudine and other NRTIs may theoretically deplete zinc due to their mechanism of action. Some concerns have been raised, however, that elevating zinc levels may not be appropriate, especially in later stages of disease. Supplements may be beneficial but medical supervision is recommended as data is inconsistent.
	Corticosteroids	Theoretical risk of nutrient depletion	May be beneficial to address nutrient depletion	Ongoing use of corticosteroids may theoretically lead to a reduction in zinc levels. Based on current evidence, the risk of depletion appears to be low and supplementation will not be needed in most patients.
	Diuretics	Risk of nutrient depletion	May be beneficial to address nutrient depletion	Diuretics may increase urinary extraction of zinc. Long-term use of diuretics will increase the risk of depletion. Many patients take diuretics in combination with ACE-I, which further increases the risk of zinc depletion.
	Methylphenidate	Increased drug effect possible	Combination may be beneficial	Drug efficacy has been shown to improve with supplementation of 15 mg elemental zinc/day for ⋯⋗ 6 weeks. Assess appropriateness of high-dose zinc for younger patients.

Continued

ACNM NUTRIENT AND NUTRITIONAL SUPPLEMENTS INTERACTIONS TABLE—cont'd

Nutrient/supplement	Drug/drug class	Potential outcome	Recommendations	Comments
Zinc cont'd	Minerals (calcium, iron, magnesium)	Reduced nutrient absorption	Monitor – separate doses	Calcium supplements may decrease dietary zinc absorption. High-dose zinc supplements may decrease magnesium absorption and increase magnesium excretion. These interactions may not be clinically relevant unless there is a deficiency, but dosage separation is generally advised. Iron and zinc supplements can interfere with each other's absorption, especially if taken on an empty stomach due to competition for non-specific carriers. The interaction does not appear to be significant if the supplements are taken with food as the ions complex with food components.
	Oestrogens (HRT and oral contraceptives)	Theoretical risk of nutrient depletion	May be beneficial to address nutrient depletion	Ongoing use of intake of oestrogens may lead to a reduction in zinc levels; however, data is conflicting. Based on current evidence, the risk of depletion appears to be low and supplementation will not be needed in most patients. Monitor.

REFERENCES

Al-Jenoobi FI, Al-Thukair AA, Alam MA, et al. Effect of Curcuma longa on CYP2D6- and CYP3A4-mediated metabolism of dextromethorphan in human liver microsomes and healthy human subjects. Eur J Drug Metab Pharmacokinet 2014;online ahead of print.

Azadmehr A, Ziaee A, Ghanei L, et al. A Randomized Clinical Trial Study: anti-oxidant, anti-hyperglycemic and anti-hyperlipidemic effects of olibanum gum in Type 2 Diabetic Patients. Iran J Pharm Res 2014;13(3):1003–9.

Baskaran K, Ahamath BK, Shanmugasundaram KR, et al. Antidiabetic effect of a leaf extract from Gymnema sylvestre in non-insulin dependent diabetes mellitus patients. J Ethnopharmacol 1990;30:295–305.

Biswal BM, Sulaiman SA, Ismail HC, et al. Effect of Withania somnifera (Ashwagandha) on the development of chemotherapy-induced fatigue and quality of life in breast cancer patients. Integr Cancer Ther 2013;12(4):312–22.

Blonk M, Colbers A, Poirters A, et al. Effect of ginkgo biloba on the pharmacokinetics of raltegravir in healthy volunteers. Antimicrob Agents Chemother 2012;56(10):5070–5.

Bodinet C, Freundenstein J. Influence of Cimicifuga racemosa on the proliferation of estrogen receptor-positive human breast cancer cells. Breast Cancer Res 2002;76:1–10.

Bonetto N, Santelli L, Battistin L, et al. Serotonin syndrome and rhabdomyolysis induced by concomitant use of triptans, fluoxetine and hypericum. Cephalalgia 2007;27(12):1421–3. [Epub 2007 Sep 14].

Bossaer JB, Odle BL. Probable etoposide interaction with Echinacea. J Diet Suppl 2012;9(2):90–5. doi:10.3109/19390211.2012.682643.

Braun L, Cohen M. Herbs and natural supplements: an evidence-based guide. 4th ed. Elsevier Churchill Livingston; 2015.

Brown BG, Zhao XQ, Chait A, et al. Simvastatin and niacin, antioxidant vitamins, or the combination for the prevention of coronary disease. N Engl J Med 2001;345:1583–93.

Burgos RA, Hancke JL, Bertoglio JC, et al. Efficacy of an Andrographis paniculata composition for the relief of rheumatoid arthritis symptoms: a prospective randomized placebo-controlled trial. Clin Rheumatol 2009;28(8):931–46.

Campbell NR, Kara M, Hasinoff BB, et al. Norfloxacin interaction with antacids and minerals. Br J Clin Pharmacol 1992;33(1):115–16.

Campbell N, Paddock V, Sundaram R. Alteration of methyldopa absorption, metabolism, and blood pressure control caused by ferrous sulfate and ferrous gluconate. Clin Pharmacol Ther 1988;43(4):381–6.

Chan TY. Drug interactions as a cause of overanticoagulation and bleedings in Chinese patients receiving warfarin. Int J Clin Pharmacol Ther 1998;36(7):403–5.

Chedraui P, et al. Effect of Trifolium pratense-derived isoflavones on the lipid profile of postmenopausal women with increased body mass index. Gynecol Endocrinol 2008;24(11):620–4.

Chen HW, Lin IH, Chen YJ, et al. A novel infusible botanically-derived drug, PG2, for cancer-related fatigue: a phase II double-blind, randomized placebo-controlled study. Clin Invest Med 2012;35(1):E1–11.

Chen MF, Shimada F, Kato H, et al. Effect of oral administration of glycyrrhizin on the pharmacokinetics of prednisolone. Endocrinol Jpn 1991;38(2):167–74.

Chen M-F, Shimanda F, Kato H, et al. Effect of oral administration of glycyrrhizin on the pharmacokinetics of prednisolone. Endocrinol Jpn 1991;38:167–75.

Cui Y, Shu X-O, Gao Y-T, et al. Association of ginseng use with survival and quality of life among breast cancer patients. Am J Epidemiol 2006;163:64553.

Day E, Bentham P, Callaghan R, et al. Thiamine for prevention and treatment of Wernicke-Korsakoff Syndrome in people who abuse alcohol. Cochrane Database Syst Rev 2013;(7):CD004033.

de Maat MMR, Hoetelmans RMW, Mathot RAA, et al. Drug interaction between St John's wort and nevirapine. AIDS 2001;15(3):420–1.

Dhamija P, Malhotra S, Pandhi P. Effect of oral administration of crude aqueous extract of garlic on pharmacokinetic parameters of isoniazid and rifampicin in rabbits. Pharmacology 2006;77:100–4.

Ding Y, Jia Y, Li F, et al. The effect of staggered administration of zinc sulfate on the pharmacokinetics of oral cephalexin. Br J Clin Pharmacol 2011;doi:10.1111/j.1365-2125.2011.04098.x.

Enseleit F, Sudano I, Périat D, et al. Effects of Pycnogenol on endothelial function in patients with stable coronary artery disease: a double-blind, randomized, placebo-controlled, cross-over study. Eur Heart J 2012;33(13):1589–97.

Fan L, Zhang W, Guo D, et al. The effect of herbal medicine baicalin on pharmacokinetics of rosuvastatin, substrate of organic anion-transporting polypeptide 1B1. Clin Pharmacol Ther 2008;83(3):471–6. [Epub 2007 Sep 12].

Golden EB, Lam PY, Kardosh A, et al. Green tea polyphenols block the anticancer effects of bortezomib and other boronic acid-based proteasome inhibitors. Blood 2009;113(23):5927–37.

Guo L, Bai SP, Zhao L, et al. Astragalus polysaccharide injection integrated with vinorelbine and cisplatin for patients with advanced non-small cell lung cancer: effects on quality of life and survival. Med Oncol 2012;29(3):1656–62.

Gupta I, et al. Effects of gum resin of Boswellia serrata in patients with chronic colitis. Planta Med 2001;67(95):391–5.

Gupta A, Gupta R, Lal B. Effect of Trigonella foenum-graecum (Fenugreek) seeds on glycaemic control and insulin resistance in Type 2 Diabetes Mellitus: a double blind placebo controlled study. J Assoc Physicians India 2001;49:1057–61.

Harada T, Ohtaki E, Misu K, et al. Congestive heart failure caused by digitalis toxicity in an elderly man taking a licorice-containing chinese herbal laxative. Cardiology 2002;98(4):218.

Heiss C, Jahn S, Taylor M, et al. Improvement of endothelial function with dietary flavanols is associated with mobilization of circulating angiogenic cells in patients with coronary artery disease. J Am Coll Cardiol 2010;56(3):218–24.

Hernandez-Munoz G, Pluchino S. Cimicifuga racemosa for the treatment of hot flushes in women surviving breast cancer. Maturitas 2003;44(Suppl. 1):S59–65.

Hurrel RF, Reddy M, Cook JD. Inhibition of non-haem iron absorption in man by polyphenolic-containing beverages. Br J Nutr 1999;81(4):289–95.

Jacobson JS, Troxel AB, Evans J, et al. Randomized trial of black cohosh for the treatment of hot flashes among women with a history of breast cancer. J Clin Oncol 2001;19(10):2739–45.

JAMA 2004;291(2):216–21.

Jiang X, Williams K, Liauw WS, et al. Effect of ginkgo and ginger on the pharmacokinetics and pharmacodynamics of warfarin in healthy subjects. Br J Clin Pharmacol 2005.

Isso AA, Ernst E. Interactions between herbal medicines and prescribed drugs: an updated systematic review. Drugs 2009;69(13):1777–98.

Khalid Z, Osuagwu FC, Shah B, et al. Celery root extract as an inducer of mania induction in a patient on venlafaxine and St John's Wort. Postgrad Med 2016;128(7):682–3.

Kassi E, et al. Greek plant extracts exhibit selective estrogen receptor modulator (SERM)-like properties. J Agric Food Chem 2004;52(23):6956–61.

Kenny FS, Pinder SE, Ellis IO, et al. Gamma linolenic acid with tamoxifen as primary therapy in breast cancer. Int J Cancer 2000;85:643–8.

Krivoy N, Pavlotzky E, Chrubasik S, et al. Effect of salicis cortex extract on human platelet aggregation. Planta Med 2001;67:209–12.

Kurnik D, Loebstein R, Rabinovitz H, et al. Over-the-counter vitamin K1-containing multivitamin supplements disrupt warfarin anticoagulation in vitamin K1-depleted patients. A prospective, controlled trial. Thromb Haemost 2004;92(5):1018–24.

Lau WC, Carville DG, Guyer KE, et al. St John's Wort enhances the platelet inhibitory effect of clopidogrel in clopidogrel 'resistant' healthy volunteers. J Am Coll Cardiol 2005;45:382A.

Lau WC, Welch TD, Shields T, et al. The effect of St John's Wort on the pharmacodynamic response of clopidogrel in hyporesponsive volunteers and patients: increased platelet inhibition by enhancement of CYP3A4 metabolic activity. J Cardiovasc Pharmacol 2011;57(1):86–93.

Li R, Guo W, Fu Z, et al. A study about drug combination therapy of Schisandra sphenanthera extract and Rapamycin in healthy subjects. Can J Physiol Pharmacol 2012;90(7):941–5. [Epub 2012 Jun 12].

Li Y, Xue WJ, Tian PX, et al. Clinical application of Cordyceps sinensis on immunosuppressive therapy in renal transplantation. Transplant Proc 2009;41(5):1565–9.

Lissoni P, Rovelli F, Brivio F, et al. A randomized study of chemotherapy versus biochemotherapy with chemotherapy plus Aloe arborescens in patients with metastatic cancer. In Vivo 2009;23(1):171–5.

Lydeking-Olsen E, Beck-Jensen JE, Setchell KD, et al. Soymilk or progesterone for prevention of bone loss–a 2 year randomized, placebo-controlled trial. Eur J Nutr 2004;43(4):246–57.

Maged AM, Elsawah H, Abdelhafez A, et al. The adjuvant effect of metformin and N-acetylcysteine to clomiphene citrate in induction of ovulation in patients with Polycystic Ovary Syndrome. Gynecol Endocrinol 2015;31(8):635–8.

Malsch U, Kieser M. Efficacy of kava-kava in the treatment of non-psychotic anxiety, following pretreatment with benzodiazepines. Psychopharmacology (Berl) 2001;157:277–83.

Mansour A, Mohajeri-Tehrani MR, Qorbani M, et al. Effect of glutamine supplementation on cardiovascular risk factors in patients with type 2 diabetes. Nutrition 2015;31(1):119–26.

Mathijssen RHJ, Loos WJ, Sparreboom A, et al. Effects of St. John's wort on irinotecan metabolism. J Natl Cancer Inst 2002;94(16):1247–9.

McBride BF, et al. Electrocardiographic and hemodynamic effects of a multicomponent dietary supplement containing ephedra and caffeine: a randomized controlled trial.

Mills S, Bone K. The essential guide to herbal safety. Churchill Livingstone: Elsevier; 2005.

Moltó J, Valle M, Miranda C, et al. Effect of milk thistle on the pharmacokinetics of Darunavir-Ritonavir in HIV-infected patients. Antimicrob Agents Chemother 2012;56(6):2837–41.

Mosby's Handbook of drug-herb and drug-supplement interactions. Mosby; 2003.

Natural Medicines databases. Therapeutic Research Center; 2017.

Neuvonen PJ. Interactions with the absorption of tetracyclines. Drugs 1976;11(1):45–54.

Persky VW, Turky ME, Wang L, et al. Effect of soy protein on endogenous hormones in postmenopausal women. Am J Clin Nutr 2002;75:145–53.

Piscitelli SC, Burstein AH, Welden N, et al. The effect of garlic supplements on the pharmacokinetics of saquinavir. Clin Infect Dis 2002;34:234–8.

Pryce R, Bernaitis N, Davey AK, et al. The use of fish oil with warfarin does not significantly affect either the international normalised ratio or incidence of adverse events in patients with atrial fibrillation and deep vein thrombosis: a retrospective study. Nutrients 2016;8(9).

Pyevich D, Bogenschutz MP. Herbal diuretics and lithium toxicity. Am J Psychiatry 2001;158(8):1329.

Qiu H, Fu P, Fan W, et al. Treatment of primary chronic glomerulonephritis with Rehmannia glutinosa acteosides in combination with the angiotensin receptor blocker irbesartan: a randomized controlled trial. Phytother Res 2014;28(1):132–6.

Rahimi R, et al. Induction of clinical response and remission of inflammatory bowel disease by use of herbal medicines: a meta-analysis. World J Gastroenterol 2013;19(34):5738–49.

Rajnarayana K, Reddy MS, Vidyasagar J, et al. Study on the influence of silymarin pretreatment on metabolism and disposition of metronidazole. Arzneimittelforschung 2004;54(2):109–13.

Raskin HN, Fishman RA. Pyridoxine-deficiency neuropathy due to hydralazine. N Engl J Med 1965;273:1182–5.

Rockwell S, Liu Y, Higgins SA. Alteration of the effects of cancer therapy agents on breast cancer cells by the herbal medicine black cohosh. Breast Cancer Res Treat 2005;90:233–9.

Samman S, Sandström B, Toft MB, et al. Green tea or rosemary extract added to foods reduces nonheme-iron absorption. Am J Clin Nutr 2001;73(3):607–12.

Sandborn WJ, Targan SR, Byers VS, et al. Andrographis paniculata extract (HMPL-004) for active ulcerative colitis. Am J Gastroenterol 2013;108(1):90–8.

Scambia G, De Vincenzo R, Ranelletti FO, et al. Antiproliferative effect of silybin on gynaelogical malignancies: synergism with cisplatin and doxorubicin. Eur J Cancer 1996;32:877–82.

Schelosky L, Raffauf C, Jendroska K, et al. Kava and dopamine antagonism. J Neurol Neurosurg Psychiatry 1995;58(5):639–40.

Segal R, Pilote L. Warfarin interaction with Matricaria chamomilla. CMAJ 2006;174(9):1281–2.

Sharma RD, Sarkar A, Hazra DK, et al. Use of fenugreek seed powder in the management of non-insulin dependent diabetes mellitus. Nutr Res 1996;16(8):1331–9.

Shi S, Klotz U. Drug interactions with herbal medicines. Clin Pharmacokinet 2012;51(2):77–104.

Sigurjónsdóttir HA, Franzson L, Manhem K, et al. Liquorice-induced rise in blood pressure: a linear dose-response relationship. J Hum Hypertens 2003;17(2):125–31.

Sigurjonsdottir HA, Manhem K, Axelson M, et al. Subjects with essential hypertension are more sensitive to the inhibition of 11 beta-HSD by liquorice. J Hum Hypertens 2003;17(2):125–31.

Shanmugasundaram ERB, Rafeswari G, Baskaran K, et al. Use of Gymnema sylvestre leaf extract in the control of blood glucose in insulin-dependent diabetes mellitus. J Ethnopharmacol 1990;30:281–94.

Stargrove MB, Treasure J, McKee DL. Herb, nutrient and drug interactions. Clinical implications and therapeutic strategies. Mosby: Elsevier; 2008.

Stoddard GJ, Archer M, Shane-McWhorter L, et al. Ginkgo and warfarin interaction in a large veterans administration population. AMIA Annu Symp Proc 2015;2015:1174–83.

Terzic MM, Dotlic J, Maricic S, et al. Influence of red clover-derived isoflavones on serum lipid profile in postmenopausal women. J Obstet Gynaecol Res 2009;35(6):1091–5.

Turkistani A, Abdullah KM, Al-Shaer AA, et al. Alkatheri K. Melatonin premedication and the induction dose of propofol. Eur J Anaesthesiol 2007;24(5):399–402. [Epub 2006 Nov 10].

Uehleke B, Müller J, Stange R, et al. Willow bark extract STW 33-I in the long-term treatment of outpatients with rheumatic pain mainly osteoarthritis or back pain. Phytomedicine 2013;20(11):980–4.

Ulbricht CE, Basch EM. Natural standard. Herb and supplement reference. Evidence-based clinical reviews. Mosby: Elsevier; 2005.

Var C, Keller S, Tung R, et al. Supplementation with vitamin B6 reduces side effects in Cambodian women using oral contraception. Nutrients 2014;6(9):3353–62. doi:10.3390/nu6093353.

Wainstein J, Ganz T, Boaz M, et al. Olive leaf extract as a hypoglycemic agent in both human diabetic subjects and in rats. J Med Food 2012;15(7):605–10.

Walker AF, Marakis G, Morris AP, et al. Promising hypotensive effect of hawthorn extract: a randomized double-blind pilot study of mild, essential hypertension. Phytother Res 2002;16(1):48–54.

Xin HW, Wu XC, Li Q, et al. Effects of Schisandra sphenanthera extract on the pharmacokinetics of midazolam in healthy volunteers. Br J Clin Pharmacol 2009;67(5):541–6.

Xin HW, Wu XC, Li Q, et al. Effects of Schisandra sphenanthera extract on the pharmacokinetics of tacrolimus in healthy volunteers. Br J Clin Pharmacol 2007;64:469–75.

Yamamoto T, Hatanaka M, Matsuda J, et al. Clinical characteristics of five elderly patients with severe hypokalemia induced by glycyrrhizin derivatives. Nippon Jinzo Gakkai Shi 2010;52(1):80–5.

Yuan CS, Wei G, Dey L. American ginseng reduces warfarin's effect in healthy patients. A randomized, controlled trial. Ann Intern Med 2004;141(1):123–6.

Zemestani M, Rafraf M, Asghari-Jafarabadi M. Chamomile tea improves glycemic indices and antioxidants status in patients with type 2 diabetes mellitus. Nutrition 2016;32(1):66–72.